Contents

Alexander's
CARE
OF THE PATIENT
IN SURGERY

15th Edition

Jane Rothrock, PhD, RN, CNOR, FAAN
Adjunct Professor, Perioperative Programs
Delaware County Community College
Media, Pennsylvania

Associate Editor
Donna McEwen, RN, BSN, CNOR(E)
Clinical Training Instructional Designer
Optum—Shared Services
San Antonio, Texas

ELSEVIER
MOSBY

3251 Riverport Lane
St. Louis, Missouri 63043

ALEXANDER'S CARE OF THE PATIENT IN SURGERY, 15th EDITION ISBN: 978-0-323-08942-5

Notices

Knowledge and best practice in this field are constantly changing. As new research and experience broaden our understanding, changes in research methods, professional practices, or medical treatment may become necessary.

Practitioners and researchers must always rely on their own experience and knowledge in evaluating and using any information, methods, compounds, or experiments described herein. In using such information or methods they should be mindful of their own safety and the safety of others, including parties for whom they have a professional responsibility.

With respect to any drug or pharmaceutical products identified, readers are advised to check the most current information provided (i) on procedures featured or (ii) by the manufacturer of each product to be administered, to verify the recommended dose or formula, the method and duration of administration, and contraindications. It is the responsibility of practitioners, relying on their own experience and knowledge of their patients, to make diagnoses, to determine dosages and the best treatment for each individual patient, and to take all appropriate safety precautions.

To the fullest extent of the law, neither the Publisher nor the authors, contributors, or editors, assume any liability for any injury and/or damage to persons or property as a matter of products liability, negligence or otherwise, or from any use or operation of any methods, products, instructions, or ideas contained in the material herein.

Library of Congress Cataloging-in-Publication Data

Alexander's care of the patient in surgery.—15th edition / [edited by] Jane Rothrock ; associate editor, Donna McEwen.
  p. ; cm.
  Care of the patient in surgery
  Includes index.
  ISBN 978-0-323-08942-5 (pbk. : alk. paper)
  I. Rothrock, Jane C., 1948- editor of compilation. II. McEwen, Donna R., editor of compilation. III. Title: Care of the patient in surgery.
  [DNLM: 1. Perioperative Nursing. 2. Nursing Care. 3. Operating Room Nursing. 4. Surgical Procedures, Operative—nursing. WY 161]
  RD99.24
  617′.0231—dc23

                                                                                2014000316

Acquisitions Editor: Terry Hines Burnham
Developmental Editor: Laura Selkirk
Publishing Services Manager: Jeff Patterson
Project Manager: Jeanne Genz
Design Direction: Jessica Williams

Printed in Canada

Last digit is the print number: 9 8 7 6 5 4 3 2

Working together
to grow libraries in
developing countries

www.elsevier.com • www.bookaid.org

Contributors

Jacqueline R. Bak, RN, MSN, CNOR, RNFA, CST
Director of Perioperative Programs
Delaware County Community College
Media, Pennsylvania
Chapter 9: Wound Healing, Dressings, and Drains

Kay A. Ball, RN, PhD, CNOR, FAAN
Associate Professor, Nursing Department
Otterbein University
Westerville, Ohio;
Consultant
K & D Medical Inc.
Lewis Center, Ohio
Chapter 8: Surgical Modalities

Robert M. Blumm, BS, MS, PA-C, DFAAPA
Senior Surgical PA, Department of Plastic Surgery
St. Joseph Hospital
Bethpage, New York;
Chairman, PA Advisory Board
New York City, New York
Chapter 22: Reconstructive and Aesthetic Plastic Surgery

Barbara A. Bowen, RN, MSN, CRNP, CRNFA
President
Perioperative Consulting & Surgical Services, LLC
Collegeville, Pennsylvania;
Consultant
Stryker Performance Solutions
Chicago, Illinois
Chapter 20: Orthopedic Surgery

Brian D. Campbell, BS, BSN, CRNA, COL (USAR Ret.)
Staff Anesthetist
Winchester Anesthesia Associates
Winchester, Massachusetts
Chapter 5: Anesthesia

Susan A. Carzo, RN, BSN, CNOR
RNFA/Staff Nurse, Operating Room
Winchester Hospital
Winchester, Massachusetts
Chapter 14: Gynecologic and Obstetric Surgery

Maya Nicole Clark-Cutaia, RN, BSN, MSN, PhD, ACNP-BC
Ruth L. Kirschstein T32 Postdoctoral Fellow
Center for Global Women's Health and Center for Health Equity
    Research
University of Pennsylvania, School of Nursing
Philadelphia, Pennsylvania
Chapter 13: Hernia Repair

Troy J. DeRose, RN, MSN, CRNP, ANCC-C, RNFA, CORLN
Certified Registered Nurse Practitioner
Department of Otolaryngology—Head and
    Neck Surgery
Thomas Jefferson University Hospital
Philadelphia, Pennsylvania
Chapter 19: Otorhinolaryngologic Surgery

Leigh Ann DiFusco, RN, MSN, CNOR, PCNS-BC
Clinical Nurse Specialist, Cardiac Care Unit
The Children's Hospital of Philadelphia
Philadelphia, Pennsylvania
Chapter 26: Pediatric Surgery

Terri Fink, RN, BSN, CNOR
Registered Nurse First Assistant
University Medical Center at Princeton
Plainsboro, New Jersey
Chapter 22: Reconstructive and Aesthetic Plastic Surgery

Allison Lindsey Flanagan, RN, MSN, CNOR
Staff Nurse, Operating Room
Paoli Hospital
Paoli, Pennsylvania;
Adjunct Faculty, Perioperative Nursing Program
Delaware County Community College
Media, Pennsylvania
Chapter 27: Geriatric Surgery

Maria Arlene Gapac LeMin, RN, BSN, CNOR, RNFA
Clinical Coordinator, Cardiac Surgery
Penn Presbyterian Medical Center
Philadelphia, Pennsylvania
Chapter 23: Thoracic Surgery

David P. Gawronski, RN, MSN, CNOR
Perioperative Educator/Manager
Mercy Hospital of Buffalo
Buffalo, New York
Chapter 28: Trauma Surgery

Sarah Krizman Germanovich, BSN, MSN, CNOR
Staff Nurse, Operating Room
Thomas Jefferson University Hospital;
Adjunct Faculty, Nursing
Thomas Jefferson University Hospital School
    of Nursing
Philadelphia, Pennsylvania
Chapter 21: Neurosurgery

Pauline A. Heizenroth, RN, MSN, CNOR
Perioperative Nurse/Clinical Nurse Educator
Bryn Mawr Hospital Surgicenter
Bryn Mawr, Pennsylvania;
Perioperative Nurse
Paoli Surgery Center
Paoli, Pennsylvania
Chapter 6: Positioning the Patient for Surgery

Denise Jackson, BSN, MSN
Clinical Nurse Specialist, Certified RN First Assistant
Shannon Health System and The Better Weigh Center;
Clinical Supervisor, APRN, RNFA Program
Angelo State University
San Angelo, Texas
Chapter 11: Gastrointestinal Surgery

Helene P. Korey Marley, RN, BSN, CNOR, CRNFA
Clinical Service Coordinator, Operating Room
Pennsylvania Hospital
Philadelphia, Pennsylvania
Chapter 15: Genitourinary Surgery

Rachael Larner, RN, BSN, MSN
Senior Professional Nurse, Post Anesthesia
    Care Unit
UPMC Hamot
Erie, Pennsylvania
*Chapter 30: Integrative Health Practices: Complementary and
    Alternative Therapies*

Maria C. Marinelli, BSN, MSN, RNFA, CNOR
BSN Nursing Faculty
Thomas Jefferson University School of Nursing
Philadelphia, Pennsylvania
Chapter 16: Thyroid and Parathyroid Surgery

James R. McCarthy, RN, AS
Certified Registered Nurse, First Assistant
Perioperative Nursing Services
Temple University Hospital
Philadelphia, Pennsylvania
Chapter 7: Sutures, Needles, and Instruments

Eileen Mielcarek, BSN, RNFA, COE
Practice Administrator
Mielcarek Eye Lifetime Vision Center
RNFA, Perioperative, Operating Room
Main Line Health Care (MLHC) Riddle Hospital
Media, Pennsylvania
Chapter 18: Ophthalmic Surgery

Ellen Murphy, RN, MS, JD, FAAN
Professor Emerita, College of Nursing
University of Wisconsin-Milwaukee
Milwaukee, Wisconsin
Chapter 2: Patient Safety and Risk Management

Janice A. Neil, RN, PhD, CNE
Associate Professor and Chair
Undergraduate Nursing Science Junior Division
East Carolina University
Greenville, North Carolina
*Chapter 12: Surgery of the Liver, Biliary Tract, Pancreas,
    and Spleen*

Jan Odom-Forren, RN, PhD, CPAN, FAAN
Assistant Professor, College of Nursing
University of Kentucky
Lexington, Kentucky
Chapter 10: Postoperative Patient Care and Pain Management

Rebecca M. Patton, RN, MSN, CNOR, FAAN
Atkinson Scholar in Perioperative Nursing
Case Western Reserve University
Cleveland, Ohio;
Immediate Past President
American Nurses Association
Washington, DC
Chapter 3: Workplace Issues and Staff Safety

Elizabeth Pearsall, RN, BSN, CNOR
Staff Nurse, Perioperative Services
Taylor Hospital
Ridley Park, Pennsylvania;
Adjunct Faculty, Nursing and Allied Health
Delaware County Community College
Media, Pennsylvania
Chapter 17: Breast Surgery

Jennifer Schaadt, MS, MBA
Principal Consultant
Integrated Services Management
Siemens Medical
Cary, North Carolina
Chapter 29: Interventional and Image-Guided Procedures

Patricia C. Seifert, RN, MSN, CNOR, CRNFA, FAAN, RNFA
Cardiovascular Operating Room
Inova Heart and Vascular Institute
Falls Church, Virginia;
Former Editor-in-Chief, *AORN Journal*
Denver, Colorado
Chapter 25: Cardiac Surgery

Cynthia Spry, RN, MA, MS, CNOR, CBSPDT
Independent Consultant
New York City, New York
Chapter 4: Infection Prevention and Control

Victoria Steelman, RN, PhD, CNOR, FAAN
Assistant Professor, College of Nursing
The University of Iowa
Iowa City, Iowa
Chapter 1: Concepts Basic to Perioperative Nursing

Joseph H. Viveiros, RN, CNOR
RNFA/Staff Nurse
Winchester Hospital
Winchester, Massachusetts
Chapter 14: Gynecologic and Obstetric Surgery

Maryann Papanier Wells, RN, PhD, FAAN
Nurse Manager, Perioperative Nursing
Hospital of the University of Pennsylvania
Philadelphia, Pennsylvania
Chapter 27: Geriatric Surgery

Patricia Wieczorek, RN, MSN, CNOR
Nurse Manager, Perioperative Services
The Johns Hopkins Hospital
Baltimore, Maryland
Chapter 24: Vascular Surgery

Clinical Consultants

Gerald A. Acker, MD
Director of Cosmetic Surgery
Catholic Health Services of Long Island
Roslyn, New York

Gregory Artz, MD
Assistant Professor, Co-Director for Jefferson Center for Balance
   and Hearing
Department of Otolaryngology, Head and Neck Surgery
Thomas Jefferson University Hospital
Philadelphia, Pennsylvania

James Black, MD
Associate Professor Vascular Surgery
The Johns Hopkins Hospital
Baltimore, Maryland

David Cognetti, MD
Assistant Professor, Co-Director for Jefferson Center for Head
   and Neck Surgery
Department of Otolaryngology, Head and Neck Surgery
Thomas Jefferson University Hospital
Philadelphia, Pennsylvania

Alan S. Crandall, MD
Professor of Ophthalmology
Senior Vice Chair and Director of Glaucoma and
   Cataracts
Co-Director of Moran International Division
Moran Eye Center, University of Utah
Salt Lake City, Utah

Glen A. Dixon, Jr., MD
Obstetrics and Gynecology
Winchester Hospital
Winchester, Massachusetts

Marc A. Drimmer, MD
Princeton Plastic Surgery Associates;
Chief of the Department of Plastic Surgery
University Medical Center at Princeton
Princeton, New Jersey

Ginger D. Elmore, RN, BSN, ASLCN Certified
Registered Nurse Clinician III
James Madison University and Legal Nurse Consulting
   Center
Charlotte, North Carolina

Arlan F. Fuller, Jr., MD
Clinical Vice President for Oncology Services
Winchester Hospital
Winchester, Massachusetts

Allen S. Gabroy, MD, FACS
Chief of Surgery
Taylor Hospital
Ridley Park, Pennsylvania

Maureen W. Hemingway, RN
Clinical Nurse Specialist
Massachusetts General Hospital
Boston, Massachusetts

Lori J. Howell, MS, RN
Executive Director, Center for Fetal Diagnosis and Treatment
The Children's Hospital of Philadelphia
Philadelphia, Pennsylvania

David Kaczorowski, MD
Attending Cardiac Surgeon
York Hospital
York, Pennsylvania

Sean P. Larner, DO
ENT Resident
Department of Otolaryngology and Facial Plastic Surgery
Millcreek Community Hospital
Erie, Pennsylvania

Maureen Lewis, BSN, CNOR, CRNFA
RN First Assistant
Riddle Hospital, Main Line Health
   System
Media, Pennsylvania

Frederic Ramsey, MD
Staff Anesthesiologist
Winchester Anesthesia Associates
Winchester, Massachusetts

Angela N. Reeves, BS, RT(R)
Product Manager, Interventional Radiology
Siemens Healthcare
Malvern, Pennsylvania

Marc Rosen, MD
Vice Chairman for Clinical Affairs
Jefferson Medical College;
Associate Professor, Department of Otolaryngology, Head and
   Neck Surgery
Thomas Jefferson University Hospital
Philadelphia, Pennsylvania

Heather Rozencwaig, RN, MSN, CRNP
Inpatient Care Coordinator
Department of Otolaryngology, Head and
  Neck Surgery
Thomas Jefferson University Hospital
Philadelphia, Pennsylvania

Eric Sarin, MD
Cardiac Surgeon
Inova Fairfax Hospital;
Inova Heart and Vascular Institute
Falls Church, Virginia

Katie Schrack, MD
Ophthalmologist
Mielcarek Eye Lifetime Vision Center
Media, Pennsylvania

Peter F. Sharkey, MS, MD
Professor of Orthopedic Surgery
Thomas Jefferson University Hospital, Rothman
  Institute
Philadelphia, Pennsylvania

Brittany Shumway, PA-C
Inpatient Care Coordinator
Department of Otolaryngology, Head and Neck Surgery
Thomas Jefferson University Hospital
Philadelphia, Pennsylvania

Ariana L. Smith, MD
Assistant Professor of Surgery/Urology
Pelvic Medicine and Reconstructive Surgery
Hospital of the University of Pennsylvania, Division of Urology
Philadelphia, Pennsylvania

Kevin Smith, BS, RN, MHA
Staff Nurse
Temple University and St. Joseph's University
Philadelphia, Pennsylvania

Dorothy M. Urschel, MS, ACNP-BC, FNP-BC, CCRN, MBA, NEA-BC
Director of Cardiovascular Surgery and Critical Care Services
Daemen College
Amherst, New York

Reviewers

Patricia C. Albaugh, RN, CNOR, CRNFA
Certified RNFA
UPMC Hamot
Erie, Pennsylvania

Robert M. Blumm, PA-C, BS, MS, DFAAPA
Senior Surgical PA
Department of Plastic Surgery
St. Joseph Hospital
Bethpage, New York;
Chairman, PA Advisory Board
New York City, New York

Jay Bowers, BSN, RN, CNOR, TNCC
Clinical Nurse Educator
WVU Healthcare
Morgantown, West Virginia

Amy Broadhurst, RN, BS, BSN, CNOR
Perioperative Staff
Christiana Care Health System
Newark, Delaware

Susan L. Bugajsky, BS, PA, RN
Professor/Coordinator of Surgical Technology
Prairie State College
Chicago Heights, Illinois

Susan A. Carzo, BSN, RN, CNOR
RNFA/Staff Nurse
Operating Room
Winchester Hospital
Winchester, Massachusetts

Monica Cisneros, RN, MSN, ANP-BC, CRNFA
Independent Board Certified RN First Assistant
Hackensack University and Medical Center
Hackensack, New Jersey

Jessikah Clark, BSN, RN
Robotic Surgery Resource Nurse and Coordinator
Barnes-Jewish Hospital
St. Louis, Missouri

Thomas M. Connor, ADN
Resource Nurse Urology
Barnes-Jewish Hospital
St. Louis, Missouri

Mary Ellen Cook, BSN, RN, CNOR
Senior Professional Nurse
UPMC Hamot
Erie, Pennsylvania

Theresa M. Criscitelli, EdD, RN, CNOR
Assistant Director of Professional Nursing Practice and Education
Winthrop University Hospital
Mineola, New York

Richard G. Cuming, RN, MSN, EdD, CNOR, NEA-BC
Nurse-Executive
Operations Management
Performance Management & Innovation Group
Tenet Healthcare Corporation
Dallas, Texas

Lynda Custer, CST, MA in Education
Surgical Technology Program Director
Baker College of Clinton Township
Clinton Township, Michigan

Nan DeStefano, RN, BSN, CNOR, RNFA
Urology Specialty Coordinator
Phoenixville Hospital
Phoenixville, Pennsylvania

Mary Dillard, MSN, MA, RN, CNOR
Clinical Educator, Perioperative Services
Barnes-Jewish Hospital
St. Louis, Missouri

Beth Fitzgerald, MSN, RN, CNOR
Perioperative Nurse Residency Manager
Perioperative Simulation Coordinator
VEST Center
Christiana Care Health System
Newark, Delaware

Denise Gautsch, MAED, BS, CST
Program Director, Surgical Technology
Cape Fear Community College
Wilmington, North Carolina

David P. Gawronski, RN, MSN, CNOR
Perioperative Educator/Manager
Mercy Hospital of Buffalo
Buffalo, New York

Elizabeth Genazzio, RN, BSN, MA, CNOR, RNFA
Perioperative Nurse, First Assistant
Lankenau Medical Center
Wynnewood, Pennsylvania

Carol A. Hager, RN, BSN, MSN, CRNP, CRNFA
Nurse Practitioner, Bayview Breast Care
UPMC Hamot
Erie, Pennsylvania

Lynne B. Hendricks, RN, BSN, CNOR
Clinical Educator
Jackson Memorial Hospital
Miami, Florida

Julia Hinkle, RN, MHS, CNOR
Professor/Program Chair, Surgical Technology
Ivy Tech Community College
Evansville, Indiana

Jennifer L. Hogan, RN, BSN
OR Staff Nurse
Bryn Mawr Hospital
Bryn Mawr, Pennsylvania

Jan Holbrook, MSN, RN, CCRN, FBN/FPN
Affiliate Assistant Professor
Goldfarb School of Nursing
Barnes-Jewish Hospital
St. Louis, Missouri

Captain John J. Kane, Sr., NC, USN, RN, MS, MSN, CNOR
Deputy Program Director
Air Force and Navy Surgical Technologist Program
Director of Navy Hospital Corps School
Fort Sam Houston, Texas

Maureen Lewis, MSN, CRNP, CRNFA, CNOR
RN First Assistant for Orthopedics
Riddle Hospital
Media, Pennsylvania

Brenda K. Mandic, RN, ADN, CNOR
Cardiothoracic Clinical Specialist
UPMC Hamot
Erie, Pennsylvania

Tanya M. Marandola, MSN, RN, CNOR
Staff RN, Ophthalmology Coordinator
Roxanna Cannan Arsht Surgicenter
Christiana Care Health Services
Wilmington, Delaware

Eileen Mielcarek, BSN, RNFA, COE
Practice Administrator
Mielcarek Eye Lifetime Vision;
RNFA, Perioperative
Operating Room
Main Line Health Care (MLHC) Riddle Hospital
Media, Pennsylvania

Deborah D. Moore, BSN, RN, CNOR
Staff Nurse
Crozer Chester Medical Center
Upland, Pennsylvania

Rosemary A. Nagler, RN, BS, MSNed, SBL, CNOR
Chairperson Health Careers
Clinical Education Coordinator
School of Surgical Technology
Western Suffolk BOCES
Northport, New York

Mary Fran Palmatier, RN, BSN, CNOR, CRNFA
Clinical Nurse Educator, Surgical Services
St. Vincent Hospital, Allegheny Health Network
Erie, Pennsylvania

Carol R. Ritchie, RN, MSN, CNOR, TNCC
Clinical Educator
Scottsdale Healthcare, Osborn Campus
Scottsdale, Arizona

Tamara R. Rosov, BSN, RN, CNOR
Main or Control Desk Manager
MedStar Washington Hospital Center
Washington, District of Columbia

Laura L. Ross, RN, BSN, CNOR, RNFA
Senior Professional Nurse
UPMC Hamot
Erie, Pennsylvania

Meranda D. Scherer, BSN, RNFA, CNOR
Transplant Surgical Assistant
Resource Nurse for Transplant and Hepatobiliary
Barnes-Jewish Hospital
St. Louis, Missouri

Linda M. Schultz, PhD, CRRN
Assistant Professor
Maryville University
St. Louis, Missouri

Shelley D. Schwartz, RN, BSN, CNOR, RNFA
RNFA and Process Improvement Coordinator for Surgical
     Services
Aria Health
Philadelphia, Pennsylvania

Karen Siverd, RN, CNOR
Senior Professional Staff Nurse
UPMC Hamot
Erie, Pennsylvania

Cynthia L. Thomas, RN, BA, CNOR
Clinical Educator, Perioperative Services
Scottsdale Healthcare
Scottsdale, Arizona

Margaret Mary Thomas, RN, BS, CNOR
Registered Nurse
Bryn Mawr Hospital
Bryn Mawr, Pennsylvania

Cynthia Ann Toale, RN, BSN, CNOR
Associate Unit Nurse Manager, Operating Room
UPMC Hamot
Erie, Pennsylvania

Anne Van Landingham, RN, BSN, MSN
Medical Careers Magnet Program
Apopka High School
Apopka, Florida

Joseph Viveiros, RN, CNOR
RNFA/Staff Nurse
Winchester Hospital
Winchester, Massachusetts

Theresa M. Wadas, PhD-c, DNP, MSN, ACNP-BC, FNP-BC
Clinical Faculty and Coordinator, Adult Acute Care Nurse
Practitioner and RNFA Program, School of Nursing
University of Alabama at Birmingham
Birmingham, Alabama

Marion Knapp Wardle, RN, MSM, CNOR
Director of Perioperative Education/Quality and Patient Safety
Bascom Palmer Eye Institute/Anne Bates Leach Eye Hospital
Miami, Florida

Kathleen A. Wernicki, RN, BSN, CPAN
Senior Professional Nurse
UPMC Hamot
Erie, Pennsylvania

Deborah E. Wisinski, RN, BSN, CNOR
ENT Specialty Resource Nurse/Staff Nurse
St. Vincent Hospital, Allegheny Health Network
Erie, Pennsylvania

Abigail A. Wolfe, BSN, RN
Registered Nurse, Operating Room
Christiana Care Health System
Newark, Delaware

About the Author

JANE C. ROTHROCK, PhD, RN, CNOR, FAAN

To Rick Lynch and Harold Hutt—
two incredible, loving and generous men
who have taught me
about resilience,
being open-minded about change,
and the importance of balance,
and done it with grace,
tact, and diplomacy.
I love you, my brothers.

Dr. Jane Rothrock has practiced and taught perioperative nursing since 1969. In 1979 she joined the faculty of Delaware County Community College, where she is an Adjunct Professor in the college's Perioperative Programs. Her responsibilities include entry-level, postbasic RN education for perioperative nursing and advanced skill preparation for RN first assistants. During her 35-year tenure at the college, Jane has helped to educate more than 4000 registered nurses in the professional practice of perioperative patient care.

Jane's decades of experience include not only as a faculty member but also as an author and speaker. She has taught at the University of Pennsylvania, been an OR director, and served as the preceptor for many graduate students. She has authored five perioperative nursing textbooks, published more than 50 articles, and presented a host of topics to nursing audiences across the United States and internationally. Jane is an AORN past president and has chaired the AORN Project Team on Professional Practice Issues, the AORN Project Team on a Professional Practice Model for Perioperative Nursing, and the Perioperative Academic Curriculum Task Force. She is an evidence reviewer for AORN's Evidence-based Recommended Practices for Perioperative Patient Care. She has received a number of distinguished awards, and is very active in both nursing and community organizations. Jane is a past vice chair of NOLF, a past member of the ANCC Magnet Commission, a past president of the ASPAN Foundation, and a past president of the AORN Foundation Board of Trustees. She served on ASPAN's first National Clinical Guideline Panel to develop a Guideline on Prevention of Unplanned Hypothermia in Adult Surgical Patients. In 2000, Jane became a Fellow of the American Academy of Nursing (FAAN).

Jane began her nursing education with a diploma from Bryn Mawr School of Nursing. She received her BSN and MSN from the University of Pennsylvania and was the first recipient of a doctoral degree from Widener University in suburban Philadelphia, earning her PhD in nursing in 1987.

Preface

The fifteenth edition of *Alexander's Care of the Patient in Surgery* has been updated to reflect both new and essential key concepts in perioperative nursing practice and increased sophistication and complexity of surgical procedures. The multimedia resource, first introduced in the thirteenth edition, strongly enhances the elemental goal of this textbook: to provide a comprehensive basic reference that will assist perioperative practitioners to meet the needs of the patients they care for safely, cost-effectively, and efficiently during surgical interventions.

As the standard in perioperative nursing for more than 50 years, *Alexander's Care of the Patient in Surgery* is written primarily for professional perioperative nurses, but it is also useful for nursing students, surgical technologists, healthcare industry representatives, medical students, interns, residents, and government officials concerned with healthcare issues. Perioperative nurses, RN first assistants, clinical nurse specialists, nurse practitioners, surgeons, surgical technologists, and educators from many geographic areas of the United States have served as contributors and reviewers for this text, providing a vast range of perioperative patient care knowledge and procedural information.

This thoroughly revised edition highlights current techniques and innovations in surgery. More than a thousand illustrations, including many new photographs and drawings, help familiarize the reader with contemporary procedures, methods, and equipment. Classic illustrations, particularly of surgical anatomy, have been preserved to enhance the text. New to this edition are features highlighting patient-centered care and patient-centered communication, a chapter summary of Key Points and a Critical Thinking question. There is a thorough laboratory values appendix in which readers can review normal lab values and ranges. As in the previous edition, readers will find Ambulatory Surgery Considerations, Evidence for Practice, Patient and Family Education, Patient Safety, Research Highlights, Sample Plans of Care, and Surgical Pharmacology features.

Enhanced in the fifteenth edition is the Evolve website. With its learner resources, readers are able to access animations, AHRQ case studies, answers to the critical thinking questions, flashcards, interactive study questions, OR Live links, and scenario packets.

Also enhanced in the fifteenth edition are resources for instructors and clinical educators. In addition to the learner resources listed previously, instructor resources contain a lesson plan for each chapter with the following elements: case studies, answers to critical thinking questions, learning objectives, suggested content for lectures and class activities, clinical learning scenarios for each covered surgical procedure, PowerPoint lecture slides with speaker notes, and an image collection of more than 1000 images to use in teaching. Instructors and clinical educators will also find a test bank with more than 750 questions as well as more than 50 customizable competency assessments for use in clinical settings or simulation laboratories as learners practice new perioperative nursing skills and techniques. Overall, this textbook imparts state-of-the-art information and resources that reflect contemporary practice and promote the delivery of comprehensive perioperative patient care.

Unit I, Foundations for Practice, provides information on basic principles and patient care requisites deemed essential to the care of all recipients of perioperative patient care. The nursing process, a model for developing therapeutic nursing interventional knowledge, reflects a six-step process that includes the identification of desired patient outcomes. Interest in patient outcomes and their improvement continues to be an essential element of nursing. The collection of health data requires clear identification of contributions to patient outcomes and quantification of these contributions. Perioperative nurses must continue to link their interventions to outcomes. This relationship is presented in Chapter 1 and explicated in each Sample Plan of Care throughout the text. Research Highlights continue to be included in every chapter, reflecting the steady increase in the amount and quality of research relevant to perioperative patient care. As current findings of new research are important to use in clinical practice, the editors and authors of *Alexander's Care of the Patient in Surgery* are committed to supporting this research-practice relationship. The Research Highlights will help perioperative nurses implement research findings in their practice and patient care activities. Chapter 1 also sets the stage for an emphasis on patient and family education and discharge planning throughout the text. Chapters in Units II and III address specific patient and family education and discharge planning relevant for patients undergoing one or more of the respective specialty surgical procedures. As the responsibilities of perioperative nurses become greater with regard to those important care components, it is imperative that we effectively educate patients and families. With the length of stay in healthcare facilities continuing to decrease, patients and families must be informed and prepared to deal appropriately with postoperative needs after discharge. Pain management, addressed in Chapter 10, is also reflected in many of the chapters on surgical specialties, because all perioperative nurses recognize its importance in patient discharge planning.

Chapter 2 focuses on patient safety and risk management along with a review of the use of social media and patient privacy issues. As perioperative nurses and surgical technologists face increasing workloads and workplace stress, this fifteenth edition emphasizes the need for workplace safety in Chapter 3. When pressure in the surgical suite mounts, nurses and surgical technologists may feel the need to work faster, even if it means taking shortcuts. The chapter on workplace safety stresses the need for personal safety at work and explores such issues as noise in the OR, and workplace violence and bullying. The remaining chapters in Unit I focus on perioperative precepts guiding infection prevention; anesthesia; patient positioning; sutures, needles, and instruments; surgical modalities; wound healing; and caring for the postoperative patient in the PACU and on the transfer unit.

The chapters within *Unit II, Surgical Interventions,* include more than 400 contemporary and traditional specialty surgical interventions, with descriptions of open, minimally invasive surgical procedures and robotic-assisted surgery. Each chapter provides a helpful review of pertinent anatomy and details the steps of surgical procedures. Perioperative nursing considerations are again presented within the nursing process framework. Current NANDA International–approved nursing diagnoses and Sample Plans of Care for each surgical specialty aim to help perioperative nurses plan, implement, and evaluate individualized perioperative patient care. Each of these chapters also provides an example of Evidence for Practice related to the surgical specialty. In 2014 and beyond, perioperative nurses can expect to find a continuing emphasis on evidence-based nursing as a means to provide care that is effective and yields improved outcomes. The integration of evidence-based practice with the perioperative nurse's individual clinical expertise leads to optimal care provision, the foundation of perioperative patient care. Improving the quality of patient care and effecting safe outcomes are at the heart of all of our efforts to achieve excellence in whatever setting we encounter the patient undergoing an operative or other invasive procedure.

Incorporation of Surgical Pharmacology in the fifteenth edition reflects the ongoing emphasis on medication safety in the United States. Medication errors can occur anywhere in the medication-use system, from prescribing to administering a drug. *Alexander's Care of the Patient in Surgery* joins the nationwide health professional education campaign aimed at reducing the number of common but preventable sources of medication errors. Providing information about select medications and dosages used in surgical specialties, the Surgical Pharmacology feature is intended to promote safe medication practices among perioperative practitioners to help avoid serious, even potentially fatal, consequences of medication errors.

To further facilitate the perioperative nurse's focus on safe patient care, Patient Safety features in each chapter succinctly review a practice to assist perioperative practitioners in developing a core body of knowledge about safe patient care. We intend this feature not only to raise awareness about patient safety applications but also simultaneously foster communication and ongoing dialogue in perioperative practice settings regarding application of recommended patient safety strategies and use of robust process improvement initiatives, all to improve quality and safety.

The unique needs of pediatric, geriatric, and trauma surgery patients are presented in *Unit III, Special Considerations*. The chapter Interventional and Image-Guided Procedures reflects processes of care in sophisticated hybrid OR suites, where enhanced capabilities merge open and interventional surgery in a multidisciplinary environment. The chapter Integrative Health Practices: Complementary and Alternative Therapies was introduced in the twelfth edition. Perioperative nurses frequently encounter patients who use such therapies, some of which are nonpharmacologic and some of which involve medications. This chapter explores alternative medical systems, mind-body interventions, biologically based therapies, manipulative and body-based methods, and energy therapies. Numerous treatments and systems within each category are discussed.

Many expert perioperative practitioners, RN first assistants, clinical nurse specialists, and educators have contributed to this fifteenth edition, and I owe a debt of gratitude to all of them for sharing their expertise in the development of this text. I give ongoing thanks to my partner, Alan Zulick, for his help during copyedits and page proofs. I also acknowledge the valuable assistance of editors, reviewers, photographers, and illustrators who have contributed their time and expertise to the revision of this text. The team I had the privilege of working with at Elsevier is talented and eager to support perioperative practitioners in their commitment to excellence in patient care. Laura Selkirk, I would clone you and give you as a gift to all of my nurse editor colleagues if I could—you walk the entire journey with each edition of this book with supreme aplomb! Donna McEwen, my Associate Editor, is not only a masterful editor but also an instructional design expert. The Evolve website is the elegant and robust feature that it is due to her acumen and talent. Christine Smith is a clinical nurse specialist who develops the test bank and competencies. Clearly, I work with a team to be admired and esteemed for their contributions to this edition.

Alexander's Care of the Patient in Surgery is written by and for perioperative nurses. Its premise is underscored by the clear understanding that perioperative nursing is a caring and intellectual endeavor, requiring critical thinking, technical acumen, and clinical reasoning and decision-making to improving patient outcomes. With the multimedia package accompanying this fifteenth edition, *Alexander's Care of the Patient in Surgery* invites you to journey with us as we meet the challenges and opportunities of perioperative nursing in the twenty-first century.

Jane C. Rothrock

Contents

CHAPTER 1

Concepts Basic to Perioperative Nursing

VICTORIA M. STEELMAN

Overview of Perioperative Nursing Practice

Perioperative nursing is the nursing care provided to patients before, during, and after surgical and invasive procedures. Nurses practice this specialty in surgical suites, ambulatory surgery centers, endoscopy suites, laser centers, interventional radiology departments, mobile surgical units, and physicians' offices across the United States and the world. Perioperative nursing includes a broad array of cutting-edge innovations, such as remote surgery, virtual endoscopy, robotics, computerized navigation systems for neurosurgery, transplanted tissue and organs, biologic materials that are absorbed to replace worn-out body parts, radiofrequency identification (RFID), transoral approaches (natural orifice surgery), and electronic health records (EHRs). In this high-tech era, perioperative patient care is very different than it was in the past.

In the past, the term *operating room (OR)* nursing was used to describe the care of patients in the immediate preoperative, intraoperative, and postoperative phases of the surgical experience (Figure 1-1). This term implied that nursing care activities were limited to the physical confines of the surgical suite. The term may have contributed to stereotypic images of the OR nurse who took care of the OR and its equipment, but who had little if any interaction or nursing responsibility for medicated and anesthetized patients in the surgical suite. With such an image, nurses practicing outside the OR had difficulty crediting important elements of the nursing process and patient care accountability to the nurse who practiced "behind the double doors" of the surgical suite.

Today, *perioperative nursing* implies the delivery of comprehensive patient care within the preoperative, intraoperative, and postoperative periods of the patient's experience during operative and other invasive procedures, using the framework of the nursing process. In doing so, the perioperative nurse assesses the patient—collects, organizes, and prioritizes patient data; establishes nursing diagnoses; identifies desired patient outcomes; develops and implements a plan of nursing care; and evaluates that care in terms of outcomes achieved by and for the patient. Throughout, the perioperative nurse functions both independently and interdependently. As with nurses in other specialties, the perioperative nurse collaborates with other healthcare professionals, makes appropriate nursing referrals, and delegates and supervises other personnel in providing safe and efficient patient care.

When nurses practice perioperative nursing in its broadest sense, care may begin in the patient's home, a clinic, a physician's office, the patient care unit, the presurgical care unit, or the holding area. After the surgical or invasive procedure, care may continue in the postanesthesia care unit (PACU) and evaluation of patient outcomes may extend onto the patient care unit, in the physician's office, in the patient's home, in a clinic, or through written or telephone patient surveys.

When nurses practice perioperative nursing in its more limited sense, patient care activities may be confined to the common areas of the surgical suite. Assessment and data collection may take place in the holding area, whereas evaluation may take place on discharge from the OR. Regardless of the way nurses practice perioperative nursing in a healthcare setting, it remains based on the nursing process and professional nursing practice.

The perioperative nurse also functions as a patient advocate during times of vulnerability. This specialty requires a broad knowledge base, instant recall of nursing science, an intuitive ability to be guided by nursing experience, and diversity of thought and action, as well as great stamina and flexibility. Whether a generalist or a specialist, the perioperative nurse depends on knowledge of surgical anatomy, physiologic alterations and their consequences for the patient, intraoperative risk factors, potentials for and prevention of patient injury, and psychosocial implications of surgery for the patient and family. This knowledge enables the perioperative nurse to anticipate needs of the patient and surgical team and to rapidly initiate safe and appropriate nursing interventions. This too is part of patient advocacy—that is, doing for the patient what needs to be done to provide a safe and caring environment. The Association of periOperative Registered Nurses (AORN) has asserted the significance of such safety by reaffirming that staffing of healthcare personnel must ensure that patients undergoing surgical and invasive procedures have a perioperative nurse as circulator in the OR, and also that the core activities of perioperative nursing care (assessment, diagnosis, outcome identification, planning, and evaluation) be completed by a perioperative nurse (AORN, 2012a).

A significant part of perioperative nursing is the delivery of scientifically based care. Such care implies understanding the rationale for certain activities and interventions, knowledge of how and when to implement them, and the skills to evaluate safety, cost-effectiveness, and outcomes of the care delivered. This knowledge empowers the perioperative nurse to anticipate and prepare for the next steps of the surgical procedure and understand their concomitant implications for the patient and for the surgical team. Scientific nursing interventions, critical thinking and clinical reasoning, and caring, comforting behaviors are at the heart of perioperative nursing. Unit II focuses on surgical procedures common to inpatient and ambulatory settings. Each chapter in Unit II contains a Sample Plan of Care with suggested nursing interventions. A fundamental assumption throughout this textbook is that perioperative nursing is a blend of technical and behavioral care and that critical thinking is the underpinning for caring for patients professionally. Good clinical judgment derives from critical thinking (Sullivan, 2012). Critical thinking requires purposeful, outcomes-directed thought and is driven by patient need. It is based on the nursing process and nursing science. Further, critical thinking requires knowledge, skills, and experience guided by professional standards and ethics and grounded in constant reevaluation, self-correction, and continual striving to improve.

Perioperative Patient Focused Model

AORN has developed a model to describe the important relationship between the patient and the perioperative nursing care provided. The Perioperative Patient Focused Model (AORN, 2012b) consists of domains or areas of nursing concern: nursing diagnoses, nursing interventions, and patient outcomes. These domains are in continuous interaction with the health system that encircles the focus of perioperative nursing practice—the patient (AORN, 2011a).

Three of these domains—behavioral responses, patient safety, and physiologic responses—reflect phenomena of concern to perioperative nurses and comprise the nursing diagnoses, interventions, and outcomes that surgical patients or their families experience. The fourth domain, the health system, comprises the structural data elements and focuses on clinical processes and outcomes.

The model illustrates the dynamic nature of the perioperative patient experience and the nursing presence throughout that process. Working in a collaborative relationship with other members of the healthcare team and the patient, the nurse establishes outcomes, identifies nursing diagnoses, and provides nursing care. The nurse intervenes within the context of the healthcare system to help the patient achieve the highest attainable health outcomes (physiologic, behavioral, and safety) throughout the perioperative experience.

The Perioperative Patient Focused Model (AORN, 2011b) emphasizes the outcomes-driven nature of perioperative patient care. Perioperative nurses possess a unique understanding of desired outcomes that apply to all patients. In contrast to some nursing specialties in which nursing diagnoses are derived from signs and symptoms of a condition, much of perioperative nursing care is preventive in nature, based on knowledge of risks inherent to patients undergoing surgical and invasive procedures. Perioperative nurses identify these risks and potential problems in advance, and direct nursing interventions toward prevention of undesirable outcomes, such as injury and infection. Based on an individual patient assessment, the perioperative nurse identifies relevant nursing diagnoses. This information guides the nursing interventions for each patient. From admission through discharge and home follow-up, the perioperative nurse plays a major role in managing the patient's care. Research based on the Perioperative Patient Focused Model (AORN, 2011b) continues to test and validate the contributions of perioperative nurses to patient outcomes in the variety of settings in which this nursing specialty is practiced.

Standards of Perioperative Nursing Practice

Perioperative nursing is a systematic, planned process—a series of integrated steps. For professional nursing, national standards establish the full expectations of the professional role within which the nurse practices. In the 1960s, the American Nurses Association (ANA) engaged in standards development. First published in 1973, these standards helped to shape nursing practice. Specialty nursing organizations, including AORN, have worked with the ANA to develop their own standards and guidelines using the ANA framework. This collaboration has resulted in the use of common language and a consistent format for the profession.

Perioperative Nursing Practice Standards

AORN (2013a) has developed a set of standards for perioperative nursing care (Box 1-1). These standards are authoritative statements that define and enumerate the responsibilities for which perioperative nurses are accountable. The standards represent a comprehensive approach to meeting the healthcare needs of surgical patients.

AORN's nursing standards are categorized as either structure or process. AORN (2013a) *Standards of Perioperative Administrative Practice* are *structure* standards that describe organizational characteristics, administrative and fiscal accountabilities, personnel qualifications, and facilities and environmental requirements. These standards provide authoritative guidance for professionals in administrative roles and provide the structure within which perioperative patient care should be provided.

Process standards relate to nursing activities, interventions, and interactions. They are used to explicate clinical, professional, and quality objectives in perioperative nursing. The three AORN (2013a,b) process standards are the *Standards of Perioperative Nursing, Standards of Perioperative Professional Practice,* and *Quality and Performance Improvement Standards for Perioperative Nursing.*

FIGURE 1-1 Thomas Eakins, *The Agnew Clinic,* 1889. In this painting, reforms and advancements in surgical techniques and procedures are apparent. Surgeons wear gowns, instruments are sterilized, ether is used, and the patient is covered. An OR nurse is a prominent member of the team.

BOX 1-1

Standards of Perioperative Nursing Practice

- *Standards of Perioperative Administrative Practice*
- *Standards of Perioperative Nursing*
- *Standards of Perioperative Professional Practice*
- *Quality and Performance Improvement Standards for Perioperative Nursing*

From the Association of periOperative Registered Nurses: *Perioperative standards and recommended practices,* Denver, 2013, The Association.

Standards of Perioperative Nursing constitute standards of care and professional performance (AORN, 2013a). Standards of care are based on and describe the application of the nursing process in perioperative nursing. They include the collection and analysis of health data, identification of expected outcomes, planning and implementation of patient care, and evaluation of the effects of this care on patient outcomes.

AORN (2013a) *Standards of Perioperative Professional Practice* require, in part, that the perioperative nurse evaluate the effectiveness of nursing practice and the quality of that practice. These professional practice standards also require perioperative nurses to evaluate their own practice. Achieving certification (certified nurse, operating room [CNOR]), pursuing lifelong learning, and maintaining competency and current knowledge in perioperative nursing are hallmarks of the professional. One of the standards focuses on the importance of evidence-based practice (EBP) and participation in the generation of new knowledge through research. The pace and complexity of advances in surgical procedures, minimally invasive surgery, new technologies, professional nursing issues, ongoing healthcare reform measures, continuing changes in recommended practices, and the burgeoning body of nursing research and best practice guidelines demand constant professional education and development. Perioperative professionals must continue to research patient outcomes, to link nursing interventions to outcomes, and to develop methods that conserve resources when implementing interventions. Other standards of professional practice address ethics, collaboration, and collegiality.

The third set of *process* standards, AORN (2013b) *Quality and Performance Improvement Standards for Perioperative Nursing,* delineate perioperative nurses' responsibilities to evaluate the patient care provided and to optimize patient outcomes. This set of standards underscores the importance of analyzing and using data to improve patient care.

Nursing Process

Looking at nursing as a process brings it into perspective as a system of critical thinking that provides the foundation for nursing actions (Figure 1-2). The focus of the nursing process is the patient, and prescribed nursing interventions are those that meet patient needs. Given the setting and the nature of the work, perioperative nursing is particularly susceptible to being seen as only an accumulation of mechanical techniques and the execution of surgeon orders. By using the nursing process, however, perioperative nurses can focus on the patient and, at the same time, use skills and knowledge to care for patients and to make independent judgments and clinical decisions. Use of the nursing process, nursing plans of care, clinical pathways, and best practices (discussed later in this chapter) has become an integral part of patient care.

In its simplest form, the nursing process defined by the ANA consists of the following six steps: assessment, nursing diagnosis, outcome identification, planning, implementation, and evaluation. The process is dynamic and continual. Also, in all areas of nursing practice, certain responsibilities are inherent in the nursing process: (1) providing culturally and ethnically sensitive, age-appropriate care; (2) maintaining a safe environment; (3) educating patients and their families; (4) ensuring continuity and coordination of care through discharge planning and referrals; and (5) communicating information.

Assessment. *Assessment* is the collection and analysis of relevant health data about the patient. Sources of data may be a preoperative

Assessment...	Review medical record, validate important findings, corroborate with patient. Analyze, interpret, and prioritize information.
Nursing Diagnosis...	Synthesize data collected; then label clinical judgment about the patient as a nursing diagnosis. Can be actual or risk for. Based on patient assessment and perioperative nurse's clinical reasoning and critical thinking.
Outcome Identification...	Because perioperative nursing is largely preventive, generic outcomes have been identified that apply to all patients undergoing an operative or other invasive procedure. Additional outcomes are identified based on individual patient assessment and nursing diagnosis. Some outcomes are mutually formulated by the nurse and patient. Guide implementation of nursing interventions. Should be specific, realistic, and measurable.
Planning...	Incorporate information into a plan for the patient's care. Identify nursing interventions to achieve identified outcomes.
Implementation...	Carry out nursing plan of care. Gather equipment and supplies; participate in/guide/supervise patient preparation, transfer to OR bed, anesthesia induction, antimicrobial skin preparation, draping, patient positioning, time-out, monitoring of physiologic alterations during surgery, and patient discharge (transfer from OR bed, hand-off to PACU or other postoperative unit).
Evaluation...	Determine whether outcomes were met; use outcome statements. Incorporate outcomes that have been met and those that are pending in hand-off report to nurse in PACU discharge area.

FIGURE 1-2 The steps of the nursing process are interrelated, forming a continuous cycle of thought and action. *PACU,* Postanesthesia care unit.

interview with the patient and the patient's family; review of the planned surgical or invasive procedure; review of the patient's medical record; examination of the results of diagnostic tests; and consultation with the surgeon and anesthesia provider, unit nurses, or other personnel. Data collection focuses on these major elements: (1) the patient's current diagnosis, physical status, and psychosocial status (including literacy, language skills, and spiritual, ethnic, cultural, and lifestyle information relevant to the delivery of patient-specific care); (2) previous hospitalizations or surgical interventions, and serious illnesses; and (3) the planned surgical

PATIENT-CENTERED CARE

One aspect of patient-centered care is communication. The perioperative nurse communicates with the patient with courtesy and respect, listens to the patient, and explains things the way the patient can understand them. The nurse might verify a patient procedure during the preoperative verification process thus:

"My name is Victoria Steelman. Today I will be the nurse taking care of you during your operation. I see on your consent form that Dr. Maxwell has said he is going to do a right total hip replacement. Can you point to where your operation will be? Tell me in your words what the name of this operation is. Is there information I can give you or note that you still need? I want you to know that it is okay to ask questions and expect answers that you understand. That is our job and we want to do it right for you."

PATIENT SAFETY

Involving Patients in Marking the Surgical Site

Perioperative nurses collectively value the goal of patient safety. One way to facilitate this goal is to improve involvement of patients in their care through information and education. The Joint Commission (TJC) Speak Up campaigns are safety initiatives that encourage patients to take an active role in their healthcare. *Help Avoid Mistakes in Your Surgery* offers a patient the following information about marking the surgical site and the time-out:

- A healthcare professional will mark the spot on your body where the surgeon will operate. Make sure that only the correct part and nowhere else is marked. This helps avoid mistakes.
- Marking usually happens when you are awake. Sometimes you cannot be awake for the marking. If this happens, a family member or friend or another healthcare worker can watch the marking. They can make sure that your correct body part is marked.
- Your neck, upper back, or lower back will be marked if you are having spine surgery. The surgeon will check the exact place on your spine in the OR after you are asleep.
- Ask your surgeon if he or she will take a "time-out" just before your surgery. This is done to make sure the surgeon does the right surgery on the right body part on the right person.

TJC also offers surgery patients these tips to further encourage active involvement:

- You and your surgeon should agree on exactly what will be done during the operation.
- Ask to have the surgical site marked with a permanent marker and to be involved in marking the site. This means that the site cannot be easily overlooked or confused (for example, surgery on the right knee instead of the left knee).
- Ask questions. You should speak up if you have concerns. It is okay to ask questions and expect answers that you understand.
- Think of yourself as an active participant in the safety and quality of your healthcare. Studies show that patients who are actively involved in making decisions about their care are more likely to have good outcomes.

Modified from The Joint Commission: *Speak up: help avoid mistakes in your surgery*, available at www.jointcommission.org/Speak_Up_Help_Avoid_Mistakes_in_Your_Surgery/, 2009. Accessed January 16, 2013.

or invasive procedure and the patient's understanding of this plan. Implementing patient-centered care (Patient-Centered Care) requires the perioperative nurse to encourage the patient's active involvement in his or her care as part of patient safety. Of primary importance are the patient's and family's understanding of the scheduled procedure and the patient's participation in activities such as marking the surgical site (Patient Safety) (the Universal Protocol for correct site surgery, along with other National Patient Safety Goals, is discussed in Chapter 2) (TJC, 2013). The perioperative nurse also assesses risk factors that may contribute to negative outcomes.

The perioperative nurse proactively reports any concerns (e.g., abnormal laboratory values, or issues related to the patient's lack of understanding of the planned procedure) to the surgeon, documents all data collected, and notes any referrals that he or she makes.

The assessment format varies from institution to institution but always includes the physiologic and psychosocial aspects of the patient. In some settings the assessment is done in stages by one or more perioperative nurses. A perioperative nurse may perform an assessment in the presurgical care unit or by telephone before the day of surgical admission. In such cases the nurse in the OR verifies parts of the assessment previously done and completes the remainder. For a perioperative nurse caring for a healthy patient, assessment may mean only a thoughtful, brief review of the assessments previously done, a short patient interview, review of the medical record and surgical procedure, and a mental rehearsal of the resources and knowledge necessary to guide the patient successfully through an operative course. At other times, the perioperative nurse assesses all aspects of the patient and the patient's condition thoroughly, along with preoperative and postoperative reviews.

When developing guidelines for preoperative assessment, patient and family education, and discharge planning, the perioperative nurse considers the following:
- What is the best EBP?
- Is relevant, concise patient information already available to the perioperative nursing staff?
- Is enough information available for perioperative nurses to consider patient care needs when preparing the room (e.g., special equipment, accessory items, instruments, sutures)?
- Is sufficient time available to initiate a meaningful perioperative nurse-patient interaction?
- Are surgical patients satisfied with their perioperative nursing care (do they express feelings of comfort and satisfaction

regarding their care in the surgical setting) and do they have knowledge of the perioperative nurse's role?
- Is there continuity of care between the perioperative unit and other nursing care units?

Being able to exchange information about patients in face-to-face meetings, by telephone, or by written messages is helpful for unit and perioperative nurses. A thorough assessment made and recorded by the preoperative nurse can accompany patients to the OR and serve as a guide for the perioperative nurse, who then completes a more focused preoperative patient assessment. With the burgeoning number of ambulatory surgery procedures, preoperative assessment is often integrated with preadmission testing. Some institutions hold group preoperative sessions. These not only help nurses get to know the patients, but also permit nurses to impart information on common routines, reactions, sensations, and nursing procedures that will take place preoperatively, intraoperatively, and postoperatively. The perioperative setting determines the type of interaction that may occur. The use of preoperative phone calls and on-line questionnaires has also gained wide acceptance. The important point is that some form of assessment, patient and family education, and discharge planning must be done. The particular facility and nursing staff determine how to accomplish it.

Assessment requires that the nurse know and understand the patient as a feeling, thinking, and responsible individual who is a candidate for a surgical or invasive procedure. Data identified through assessment help the perioperative nurse meet unique patient needs throughout the surgical intervention. Based on the data collected, recorded, and interpreted during patient assessment, the perioperative nurse then formulates a nursing diagnosis.

Nursing Diagnosis. *Nursing diagnosis* is the process of identifying and classifying data collected in the assessment in a way that provides a focus to plan nursing care. Nursing diagnoses have evolved since they were first introduced in the 1950s. Today they are identified, named, and classified according to human response patterns and functional health patterns. The authoritative organization responsible for delineating the accepted list of nursing diagnoses is the North American Nursing Diagnosis Association International (NANDA-I) (Box 1-2). Each NANDA-I–approved nursing diagnosis has a set of components, as follows: a definition of the diagnostic term; its defining characteristics (i.e., the requisite pattern of signs and symptoms or cues that make the meaning of the diagnosis clear); and its related or risk factors (i.e., causative or contributing factors that are useful in determining whether the diagnosis applies to a particular patient). For perioperative patients, many nursing diagnoses are "risk" diagnoses, meaning that they are not evidenced by signs or symptoms because the problem has yet to occur and nursing interventions are directed at prevention.

Not all patient problems encountered in the perioperative setting can be described by the list of accepted NANDA-I nursing diagnoses. Perioperative nurses must participate in describing and naming new nursing diagnoses that characterize unique perioperative patient problems. NANDA-I has established a "to be developed" category to designate nursing diagnoses that are partially developed and deemed useful to the nursing profession; perioperative nurses may develop unique diagnostic labels and definitions, and work to develop and validate them further through this process. This constructive process becomes even more important as healthcare moves toward the use of information systems to document nursing practice.

Outcome Identification. *Outcome identification* describes the desired or favorable patient condition that can be achieved through nursing interventions (Box 1-3). The study of patient outcomes is not new. To be useful for assessing the effectiveness of nursing care, patient outcomes should be "nursing-sensitive"; they should be influenced by nursing and describe a patient state that can be measured and quantified. Nursing-sensitive patient outcomes derive from nursing diagnoses and direct the interventions that resolve the

---

BOX 1-2

Selected Perioperative Nursing Diagnoses

- Ineffective **A**irway clearance
- **A**nxiety
- Risk for **A**spiration
- Risk for imbalanced **B**ody temperature
- Readiness for enhanced **C**omfort
- Ineffective **C**oping
- Risk for imbalanced **F**luid volume
- Impaired **G**as exchange
- **H**yperthermia
- **H**ypothermia
- Risk for **I**nfection
- Risk for **I**njury
- Deficient **K**nowledge
- Acute **P**ain
- Risk for **P**erioperative positioning injury
- Risk for impaired **S**kin integrity
- Delayed **S**urgical recovery
- Ineffective **T**hermoregulation
- Ineffective peripheral **T**issue perfusion
- Impaired **U**rinary elimination

From NANDA-International: *NANDA nursing diagnoses: definition and classification 2012-2014,* Philadelphia, 2012, Author.

BOX 1-3

Selected PNDS Desired Patient Outcomes

- O.30 The patient's procedure is performed on the correct site, side, and level.
- O.10 Patient is free from signs and symptoms of injury related to thermal sources.
- O.20 The patient is free from signs and symptoms of unintended retained objects.
- O.40 Patient's specimen(s) is managed in the appropriate manner.
- O.50 Patient's current status is communicated throughout the continuum of care.
- O.60 Patient is free from signs and symptoms of injury caused by extraneous objects.
- O.80 Patient is free from signs and symptoms of injury related to positioning.
- O.130 Patient receives appropriately administered medication(s).
- O.280 Patient is free from signs and symptoms of infection.
- O.290 Patient is at or returning to normothermia at the conclusion of the immediate postoperative period.
- O.300 Patient's fluids, electrolyte, and acid-base balances are maintained at or improved from baseline levels.
- O.310 Patient's respiratory status is consistent with or improved from baseline levels established preoperatively.
- O.320 Patient's cardiovascular status is maintained at or improved from baseline levels.
- O.500 Patient or designated support person demonstrates knowledge of the expected psychosocial responses to the procedure.
- O.550 Patient or designated support person demonstrates knowledge of the expected responses to the operative or invasive procedure.
- O.700 Patient or designated support person participates in decisions affecting his or her perioperative plan of care.
- O.720 Patient's value system, lifestyle, ethnicity, and culture are considered, respected, and incorporated in the perioperative plan of care.
- O.740 Patient's right to privacy is maintained.

PNDS, Perioperative Nursing Data Set.
From the Association of periOperative Registered Nurses: PNDS—*perioperative nursing data set,* ed 3, Denver, 2011, The Association.

nursing diagnoses. They are the standards or criteria by which the effectiveness of interventions is measured. Outcomes are stated in terms of expected or desired patient behavior and must be specific and measurable. The appropriate time to measure perioperative nursing-sensitive outcomes varies.

Some outcomes from intraoperative nursing interventions can be measured or evaluated immediately. Others occur over a longer period. In this textbook, the use of the phrase "the patient will" indicates an outcome that is expected to occur over time. Identification of expected and desired outcomes unique to the surgical patient provides the opportunity to prioritize care, becomes a basis for continuity of care, and directs evaluation (outcomes research). In this type of research, the relationship between patient characteristics, the processes of care (i.e., what the perioperative nurse does, described under Implementation), and the outcomes of that care are studied, enhancing the perioperative nurse's ability to improve care. In many instances outcomes research results in the identification of a "best practice" to improve patient care (Whittemore, 2009).

Planning. After collecting and interpreting patient data, identifying appropriate nursing diagnoses, and establishing desired outcomes, the perioperative nurse begins *planning* the nursing care for the patient. Planning requires use of nursing knowledge and information about the patient and the intended surgical or invasive procedure in order to prepare the surgical environment and to plan patient care. Perioperative nurses check equipment for proper functioning, ensure that requisite supplies and positioning devices are available, and use their knowledge of anatomy to have proper instruments and sutures on hand for the procedure to be performed. They also modify routines based on unique patient information, such as allergies, transmissible infections, and risk of hypothermia, deep vein thrombosis, infection, or pressure injury. They know the sequence of steps in the operative or other invasive procedure and use surgeons' preference cards, nursing care guides, and other resources such as computerized data sheets to prepare the room and equipment for the patient and surgical team.

Planning is preparing in advance for what will or may happen and determining the priorities for care. Planning based on patient assessment results in knowing the patient and the patient's unique needs so that alterations in events such as positioning requirements or the surgical process are anticipated and readily accommodated. Planning also requires knowledge of the patient's psychosocial state and feelings about the proposed operation so that the perioperative nurse can provide explanation, comfort, and emotional support.

Effective communication with other members of the healthcare team is essential, and miscommunication in the OR easily can occur (Gillespie et al, 2012). Briefings before the procedure allow for opportunities to improve safety and efficiency of care by ensuring that team members understand the plan of care, are prepared for potential changes, and discuss any safety concerns (Figure 1-3). Debriefings at the end of the procedure provide an opportunity to discuss changes that should be made based on lessons learned (Research Highlight).

Implementation. *Implementation* is performing nursing care activities and interventions that were planned as well as responding with critical thinking and orderly action to changes in the surgical procedure, patient's condition, or emergencies (Box 1-4). Implementation uses established standards of nursing care, recommended practices, clinical practice guidelines, and best practices. During this phase of the nursing process the perioperative nurse continues to

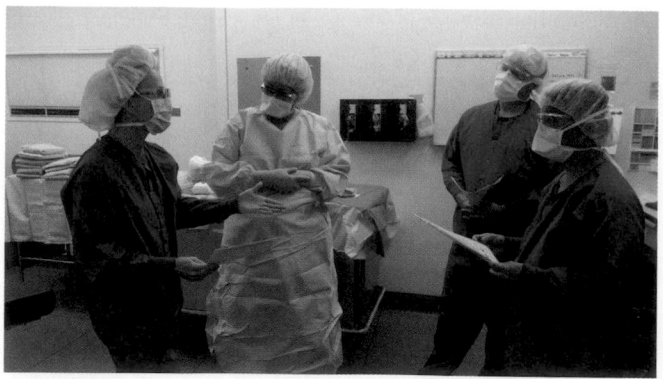

FIGURE 1-3 The surgical team at the Portland VA Medical Center conducts a briefing before surgery. This briefing allows team members to finalize the plan for the patient's care, anticipate potential changes in the patient's needs, and discuss potential safety concerns effectively.

assess the patient to determine the appropriateness of selected interventions and to alter interventions as necessary to achieve desired outcomes of care. Interventions are the "work of nursing." Many interventions used in perioperative nursing address patient safety issues (Patient Safety). The study of nursing interventions links nursing diagnoses with interventions and outcomes, and leads to validation of selected interventions or the development of new ones. Likewise, clinical practice, decision making, and EBP are enhanced by their study. The study of nursing interventions also helps to deliver cost-effective care by quantifying resource allocation.

Finally, implementation also means being the patient's advocate by recognition of patient concerns and unmet needs. Advocacy, a part of nurse-caring, encompasses caring behaviors that promote emotional and physical comfort. Caring behaviors include establishing a "connection" with the patient, responding to each patient's individuality, and meeting patient and family expectations. The role of patient advocate is especially important in surgical settings when patients are sedated or unconscious and unable to speak for themselves. As caring patient advocates, perioperative nurses advance the best interests of their patients.

Delegation. A team delivers perioperative patient care and different categories of team personnel assist in a host of direct and indirect patient care activities. The surgical team usually consists of a surgeon and assistants at surgery (e.g., resident, interns, physician assistant [PA], registered nurse first assistant [RNFA], certified nurse practitioner [CNP], or certified first assistant [CFA]), an anesthesia provider, a circulating nurse, and a scrub person, who may be either a surgical technologist or an RN. Other members of the healthcare team, such as nursing assistants, orderlies, environmental services personnel, and patient care technicians, support the surgical team. During implementation of patient care, the perioperative nurse may delegate certain nursing activities to these personnel, often called *unlicensed assistive personnel (UAP)*. These healthcare workers emerged during the nursing shortages of World War I and World War II and became part of a team model of delivering patient care. In the 1980s, delivery models shifted the skill mix away from assistive personnel, and RNs were the principal caregivers in primary nursing models. During the fiscally constrained 1990s, however, healthcare facilities began to reintroduce assistive personnel, who have less training and receive lower salaries than nurses. Instead of using UAP in narrowly defined job

RESEARCH HIGHLIGHT

Surgery Briefings and Debriefings

Teamwork and effective communication are essential to safe perioperative patient care. Failures of communication and teamwork are common root causes in serious adverse events in the OR. To improve communication, the practice of team briefings before and debriefing after surgery have been modeled on the aviation industry. The goal of briefing is to ensure that all team members are prepared for the surgical plan and any changes to the plan. During debriefings, team members discuss any opportunities for future improvement.

Researchers in a large midwestern hospital studied use of briefing and debriefing tools to identify clinical and operational "defects" in an OR. Bandari and colleagues (2012) found a total of 6202 reported defects over 3½ years—an average of 141 defects per month. During the first 6 months, 2760 defects were identified, of which 46% surfaced during briefings; the remaining 54% arose during debriefings. The most common issues were related to equipment (48%) and communication (31%). Of the 3442 defects identified during subsequent months of the study, the most common issues were central processing department (CPD) instrumentation (22%) and communication/safety (15%). Overall, 87% of 80 respondents agreed that briefings were effective for revealing defects, and 76% agreed that debriefings were likewise effective. The researchers concluded that briefings and debriefings are practical and effective strategies to identify potential surgical defects in the OR.

In a prospective cohort study in a large teaching hospital on the East Coast, Berenholtz and colleagues (2009) evaluated use of a standardized one-page briefing and debriefing tool to improve interdisciplinary communication and teamwork in the OR. The briefing portion was completed after the patient's final positioning, but before the incision. The debriefing portion was completed by the circulating nurse after the first closing counts. A survey of 40 perioperative caregivers elicited perceptions of interdisciplinary communication and teamwork in the OR and the average time taken to complete the briefing and debriefing tool. Over 18 months, surgical teams conducted 37,133 briefings and debriefings. The majority of caregivers perceived that the briefing and debriefing tool improved interdisciplinary communication and teamwork. On average, briefings took 2.9 minutes (range, 1-5 minutes) to complete, and debriefings took 2.5 minutes (range, 1-5 minutes) to complete. Researchers concluded that using a standardized briefing and debriefing tool is a practical and feasible way to improve perceptions of interdisciplinary communication and teamwork in the OR.

Modified from Bandari J et al: Surfacing safety hazards using standardized operating room briefings and debriefings at a large regional medical center, *Jt Comm J Qual Patient Saf* 38(4):154–160, 2012; Berenholtz SM et al: Implementing standardized operating room briefings and debriefings at a large regional medical center, *Jt Comm J Qual Patient Saf* 35(8): 391–397, 2009.

BOX 1-4

Selected PNDS Perioperative Nursing Interventions

- A.10 Confirms patient identity.
- A.20 Verifies operative procedure, surgical site, and laterality.
- Im.60 Uses supplies and equipment within safe parameters.
- E.10 Evaluates for signs and symptoms of physical injury to skin and tissue.
- Im.20 Performs required counts.
- E.50 Evaluates results of the surgical count.
- Im.330 Manages specimen handling and disposition.
- E.40 Evaluates correct processes have been performed for specimen handling and disposition.
- Im.500 Provides status reports to designated support person.
- E.800 Ensures continuity of care.
- Im.10 Implements protective measures prior to operative or invasive procedure.
- Im.80 Applies safety devices.
- Im.160 Maintains continuous surveillance.
- A.280.1 Identifies physical alterations that require additional precautions for procedure-specific positioning.
- Im.120 Implements protective measures to prevent skin/tissue injury due to mechanical sources.
- Im.210 Administers prescribed solutions.
- Im.220 Administers prescribed medications.
- Im.300 Implements aseptic technique.
- Im.300.1 Protects from cross-contamination.
- Im.270 Performs skin preparations.
- Im.280 Implements thermoregulation measures.
- Im.370 Monitors physiologic parameters.
- E.260 Evaluates response to thermoregulation measures.
- A.520.1 Preserves and protects the patient's autonomy, dignity, and human rights.

PNDS, Perioperative Nursing Data Set.
From the Association of periOperative Registered Nurses: *PNDS—perioperative nursing data set*, ed 3, Denver, 2011, The Association.

categories (e.g., clerical, housekeeping, orderly, patient transport), the trend in the late 1990s was to create a set of multiskilled assistive personnel who could assist nurses in multiple activities rather than in just a single area.

As the use of UAP quickly grew in the 1990s, questions and concerns arose about the proper scope of delegated activities that nurses formerly performed. Each state's board of nursing defines the scope of practice for registered nurses, based on the nursing process. Further, each state's nurse practice act—a state law that protects the health and safety of the public—establishes legal qualifications for

who can practice nursing. Implementation of the plan of care and the interventions to accomplish it are part of the nursing process. Therefore, guidelines for proper delegation of some of these interventions became necessary. Delegation transfers to a competent person the authority to perform a selected nursing task in a selected situation according to the "five rights" of delegation (Box 1-5). The perioperative nurse who delegates a task retains accountability for that delegation. Nursing functions of performing assessments, determining nursing diagnoses, establishing patient outcomes, developing the plan of care, and evaluating patient outcomes, as well as nursing interventions that require independent nursing knowledge, skills, or judgment, cannot be delegated (ANA and NCSBN, 2012). Perioperative nurses need to understand that institutional policy cannot contradict the nurse practice act of their state. Although tasks and procedures may be delegated to unlicensed members of the surgical team, the perioperative nurse remains responsible for supervising care because supervision cannot be delegated. Accordingly, the perioperative nurse must assess the patient and the competency level of personnel to determine which team member has the skill to provide the necessary care. Using UAP appropriately assists the profession of perioperative nursing to be better prepared for the challenge of maintaining high-quality patient care services even when nurse shortages occur.

PATIENT SAFETY

Perioperative Patient Safety Issues

Much of the work of perioperative nursing involves patient safety, protecting patients from risks related to the procedure, positioning, equipment, and the environment. It is essential that nurses assess risks to their patients and implement interventions to minimize these risks proactively. Steelman and colleagues (2013) surveyed perioperative nurses to identify what safety issues they consider to be the highest priority. They obtained 3137 usable responses. The majority of nurses considered preventing wrong site, procedure, or patient surgery (69%) and preventing retained surgical items (61%) to be high-priority safety issues in need of heightened attention. More than one third of respondents identified preventing medication errors, failures in instrument reprocessing, pressure injuries, and surgical fires to be high-priority issues as well.

The top rated issues are:

1. Preventing wrong site/procedure/patient surgery
2. Preventing retained surgical items
3. Preventing medication errors
4. Preventing failures in instrument reprocessing
5. Preventing pressure injuries
6. Preventing specimen management errors
7. Preventing surgical fires
8. Preventing perioperative hypothermia
9. Preventing burns from energy devices
10. Responding to difficult intubation/airway emergencies

Steelman VM et al: Priority patient safety issues identified by perioperative nurses, *AORN J* 97(4):402–418, 2013.

Documenting Interventions. Accurate documentation of nursing care is integral to all phases of the nursing process, especially implementation of the plan of care. A description of the patient, nursing diagnoses and desired patient outcomes, nursing care given, and the patient's response to care (outcomes) should be included in the patient record. Documentation of the nursing care given should include more than technical aspects of care, such as counts or application of the electrosurgical (ESU) dispersive pad. Nursing care documentation should be associated with assessment and nursing diagnoses, with preestablished outcomes against which appropriateness and effectiveness of care may be judged. The form for this documentation may include standardized protocols and interventions; space should be provided to add interventions that are unique to individual patients or to describe variances in care. Documentation should require little time to complete, be specific to the perioperative setting, and provide continuity across the various areas in surgery, from presurgical holding areas to the PACU. Most facilities incorporate computerized documentation systems to enhance retrievability of data for evaluation of care and patient outcomes.

Syntegrity. In 1993 AORN recognized the need to describe and define the unique contributions of perioperative nurses to patient outcomes. After 6 years of research and validation, the Perioperative Nursing Data Set (PNDS) was recognized as a specialty nursing language, providing a uniform and systematic method to document the basic elements of perioperative nursing care (AORN, 2011b). The third edition of the PNDS has since been incorporated into an electronic framework called Syntegrity. Similar to the *Perioperative Patient Focused Model*, the PNDS begins with desired patient

BOX 1-5

The Five Rights of Delegation

- **The Right task.** The perioperative nurse determines that this task is delegable for a specific patient, taking into consideration such factors as potential for harm, complexity of the task, necessary problem solving, and predictability of the outcome. Routine tasks performed according to a standardized procedure and which have predictable outcomes are safest to delegate.
- **The Right circumstances.** The perioperative nurse considers the patient care setting, resources available, and other relevant factors. Tasks delegated must not require independent nursing judgment.
- **The Right person.** The perioperative nurse is the right person to delegate the right task to the right person to be performed on the right patient. The perioperative nurse must be familiar with the job description of the unlicensed assistive personnel (UAP) along with the person's capabilities, knowledge and skill level, and learning needs to ensure that safe, quality patient care is provided. In this way the nurse matches tasks to the UAP's skills, qualifications, and competence.
- **The Right communication and direction.** The perioperative nurse provides a clear, specific, and concise description of the task, with key information relating to its objectives, rationale, limits, and expectations. There should be an opportunity for questions and clarifying instructions. Information which the perioperative nurse needs to know from the person performing the task must be identified. Communication should be direct and not provided through others.
- **The Right supervision and evaluation.** The perioperative nurse appropriately monitors the task or person performing it, evaluates results or patient outcomes or both, intervenes if necessary, and provides feedback. Providing immediate feedback or identifying a problem with performance as it occurs is essential to upholding standards of care and performance expectations.

Perioperative nurses must be involved actively in providing the assessment, evaluation, and judgment needed to coordinate and supervise perioperative patient care. When delegating care activities, perioperative nurses retain accountability for analyzing and evaluating the outcomes of delegated tasks. Activities that rely on the nursing process, such as performing assessments, making nursing diagnoses, establishing plans of care, providing extensive patient and family education, and planning for patient discharge, cannot be delegated.

Modified from the *National Council of State Boards of Nursing response to the PEW taskforce principles and vision for health care workforce regulation*, Chicago, 1996, The Council; Cherry B, Jacob SR: *Contemporary nursing: issues, trends and management*, ed 5, St Louis, 2010, Mosby; Hauden N, Galura C: *Ulrich and Canale's nursing care planning guides: prioritization, delegation and critical thinking*, ed 7, St Louis, 2011, Saunders.

outcomes. Each outcome is defined and interpreted and presents criteria by which to measure outcome achievement. Subsequently, nursing interventions to achieve the desired patient outcomes are noted, along with suggested nursing activities to support the interventions. Of special import is the opportunity for perioperative nurses to use Syntegrity to document assessments, interventions, and outcomes electronically, enabling Syntegrity to compare clinical outcomes from large patient populations within an institution and even across institutions. Syntegrity can be used to guide research, develop best practices, and support EBP.

Evaluation. *Evaluation* is checking, observing, and appraising the results of what was done. Although evaluation is traditionally listed as the last phase of the nursing process, it is an integral, systematic, and ongoing component of providing safe, effective—and good—perioperative patient care. Evaluation focuses on the patient's progress in attaining identified outcomes. When feasible and appropriate, the patient and family should participate in the evaluation process. The attainment of outcomes, any revisions to nursing diagnoses or desired outcomes, and the plan of care are documented. Because perioperative patient care processes and interventions often are interdisciplinary, healthcare facilities may need to use additional evaluation methods.

Evaluation of the patient's progress toward desired outcomes extends throughout the postoperative period and beyond. It is essential that critical information be shared with nurses responsible for care postoperatively. Communication during this transition of care, referred to as a hand-off or handover, is critical to patient safety and continuity of care (Research Highlight).

Performance improvement activities, notably by monitoring important aspects of care, problem identification, problem solving, and peer review, may be part of overall system evaluation. Often referred to as *quality improvement (QI) programs,* overall system evaluations by interdisciplinary teams address areas for improvement in patient care, identify problems, propose solutions, and monitor and evaluate the effectiveness of improvements. This topic is discussed in more detail later.

Institutional Standards of Care

Healthcare facilities have developed additional standards to communicate expectations of performance. Perioperative departments have responsibility, delegated through administrative governance of the institution, to develop policies and procedures, often called *surgical services standards of care.* Policies are written statements that outline responsibilities and appropriate actions in specific circumstances. To be effective, a policy should be consistent with national and state practice standards, be realistic and achievable, be consistently followed except where prior approval of deviation has been obtained, and be based on evidence and reasoned and rational thinking.

Procedures are written guides to implementing policies. They describe detailed chronologic sequences of activities as they relate to particular policies. Policies and procedures are usually combined into a manual that is kept readily available as a perioperative care resource in departments where operative or other invasive procedures occur. Many facilities have moved to an on-line manual as well, to provide easy access in multiple patient care locations. Participation of staff members in policy and procedure development increases their knowledge of the subject matter and generates a sense of ownership. This results in meaningful and authoritative interpretation of approved policy and procedure to peers and furthers successful implementation.

Evidence-Based Practice

Perioperative nursing relies on a strong foundation of traditions designed to provide excellent patient care. These traditions include many aspects of direct patient care as well as control of the environment in which care is provided. Perioperative nurses have an ethical responsibility to review practices and to modify them, based on the best available scientific evidence. Using research to guide practice is called EBP. This process can be used proactively to evaluate alternative ways of providing care, such as using different patient positioning surfaces or developing patient education materials. EBP can also be used to problem solve, as when investigating a serious

RESEARCH HIGHLIGHT

Postoperative Handovers

When the care of a patient is transferred from one caregiver to another (patient "handovers" or "hand-offs"), it is essential to provide a set of comprehensive data to ensure continuity of care and to allow the next caregiver to anticipate potential changes in the patient's condition. Since 2003, studies on handover failures revealed that they lead to delays in treatment and serious adverse events (Mazzocco et al, 2009). The postoperative handover between the surgical and anesthesia team and the perianesthesia care unit (PACU) nurse provides critical information that the PACU nurse needs to prioritize patient assessments, develop a plan of care, and respond effectively to emergencies. Some essential data include airway management, vital signs, fluid and electrolyte management, risk factors for complications, and pain management.

Segall and colleagues (2012) systematically reviewed the research on postoperative handovers to the PACU or intensive care unit (ICU) nurse. Some 31 studies met the inclusion criteria and 18 cross-sectional studies characterized current postoperative handover practices. Fourteen of the studies proposed recommendations supported by evidence; four tested the effectiveness of structured interventions; and five described educational programs and development of electronic or printed transfer reports. Recommendations supported by evidence from the studies include the following actions:

- Prepare monitors, equipment, and fluids prior to patient arrival.
- Complete urgent tasks before the verbal handover report.
- Set aside time for the handover; avoid multitasking and limit conversations.
- Permit only patient-specific conversation and urgent interruptions.
- Require the presence of all relevant members of the OR and postop teams.
- Permit only one team member to speak/report at a time.
- Provide an opportunity to ask questions and voice concerns.
- Document the handover.
- Use supporting documentation when relevant/possible (e.g., lab results).
- Use a checklist or protocol with standardized processes.
- Provide formal team training.

The authors conclude that following these recommendations has potential for improving postoperative handovers and the safety of patient care.

Modified from Mazzocco K et al: Surgical team behaviors and patient outcomes, *Am J Surg* 197(5):678–285, 2009; Segall N et al: Can we make postoperative patient handovers safer? A systematic review of the literature, *Anesth Analg* 115(1):102–115, 2012.

adverse event or other clinical problem, such as hypothermia, a pressure injury, or a retained surgical sponge. EBP is the hallmark of excellence in perioperative patient care because it promotes decisions based on scientific evidence rather than opinions (Steelman, et al, 2011).

EBP is a systematic, thorough process by which to identify a clinical issue, collect and evaluate the best evidence, design and implement a practice change, and evaluate the process (Carey et al, 2009). The change may be how patients are assessed for risk, an intervention, patient or staff education, or a change in supplies or equipment. Some changes that have been implemented through this process based on early work of nurses are double-gloving to reduce sharps injuries (Stebral and Steelman, 2006); asking patients to shower preoperatively twice with chlorhexidine gluconate (Pottinger et al, 2006); administering antibiotics within 60 minutes before the surgical incision (Spalter and Wyatt, 2006); using forced-air warming devices to prevent perioperative hypothermia (Evidence for Practice)(Paulikas, 2009); and administering a combination of blood products (massive transfusion protocol) for control of hemorrhage (Enticott et al, 2012).

When there is not enough evidence to guide practice, perioperative nurses should collaborate with a nurse researcher in a research study to address the practice issue or to identify, review, and evaluate evidence about it. One model used in many healthcare facilities is the Iowa Model of Evidence-Based Practice to Promote Quality Patient Care (Figure 1-4).

EBP has become an integral part of many national quality initiatives. One such initiative, the Surgical Care Improvement Project (SCIP), is a national quality partnership endorsed by many organizations and focused on improving care of surgical patients by using EBP to significantly reduce surgical complications. Endorsing organizations include the American College of Surgeons (ACS), American Society of Anesthesiologists (ASA), AORN, Centers for Disease Control and Prevention (CDC), and The Joint Commission (TJC, 2012). Some core measures of SCIP address prophylactic antibiotics, normothermia, prevention of deep vein thrombosis (DVT), and blood glucose control (TJC, 2012). The Centers for Medicare & Medicaid Services (CMS) require that healthcare facilities receiving reimbursement by Medicare report their level of compliance with these core measures; noncompliance can result in reduced payment for services (USDHHS and CMS, 2011).

Performance Improvement

Continuing trends in healthcare have seen increased control of costs, more efficient use of resources and supplies, decreased length of stay for surgical patients, and a shift of many surgical procedures from inpatient to ambulatory care settings (Ambulatory Surgery Considerations). Concomitantly, there is a keener awareness of the need for continued improvement in delivery of perioperative patient care. TJC has taken a strong position on the need to monitor and evaluate the quality and appropriateness of care delivery continually to resolve any identified problems, while striving constantly to improve delivery systems and processes. In 1994, TJC instituted performance assessment, measurement, and improvement as the core of its standards. This represented an evolution from quality assurance to continuous quality improvement, and finally to performance improvement (PI). Such a transition underscored the belief that measuring outcomes and improving care are essential elements of effective healthcare delivery. PI efforts encompass improvements in quality and effectiveness, based on ethical and economic perspectives.

A surgical services PI program should be based on established standards of care and the intent of each standard reflected in realistic and measurable outcomes. A plan to measure and improve care, including the scope of care and important aspects of that care, should be in place. Specific quality indicators must be identified that reflect all important aspects of care. Thresholds that identify the level of acceptable variance for each indicator are then established. Measurement methods include retrospective or concurrent review of medical records, review of adverse event reports, utilization review, patient surveys and interviews, and peer review. Emphasis has evolved from process auditing to the current emphasis on structure, process, and outcome indicators. Some facilities have

▌ EVIDENCE FOR PRACTICE

Perioperative Hypothermia

Unplanned hypothermia (core temperature less than 96.8°F (36°C) is among the most common complications of surgery. It results from impaired thermoregulation caused by anesthesia and heat lost into the surgical environment. Shortly after induction of anesthesia, body heat rapidly shifts from the body's core to its periphery. This heat redistribution results in a core temperature drop of about 2.7°F (1.6°C) during the first hour after induction of anesthesia. All anesthetized surgical patients are at risk of hypothermia.

Overwhelming evidence demonstrates that even mild hypothermia may:

- Significantly increase the risk of morbid cardiac events, including ventricular tachycardia
- Cause coagulopathy and increase blood loss, resulting in potential increased requirements for volume expansion/transfusion
- Impair antibody- and cell-mediated immune defenses and diminish oxygen availability in the peripheral wound tissues, resulting in an increased risk of surgical site infection (SSI)
- Impair drug metabolism, increase plasma concentration of intravenous anesthetic agents, and increase duration of action of neuromuscular blocking agents as well as duration of postanesthesia recovery

Blankets reduce heat loss in only about a third of nonanesthetized individuals. Applying heated cotton blankets is slightly more effective, but the benefit is brief. Active warming is required to prevent perioperative hypothermia. The most common method of active warming is forced air warming (FAW), which involves a blanket with small holes distributing warm air over the skin surface, heating peripheral tissues, and minimizing the core-to-periphery temperature gradient. Numerous clinical trials have demonstrated that intraoperative FAW is an effective intervention for preventing perioperative hypothermia.

To be most effective, FAW should be initiated preoperatively (Cobbe et al, 2012) as well as intraoperatively. Prewarming patients with FAW before induction of anesthesia minimizes heat loss more effectively than warmed cotton blankets. The application of FAW preoperatively is more effective in maintaining normothermia than using FAW intraoperatively alone. Cobbe and colleagues (2012) note that starting FAW on maximum fan speed and temperature settings and titrating down as necessary for patient comfort, appears preferable to starting at a low fan speed and temperature setting and titrating up as tolerated. Titration of settings during warming should be informed by assessments of thermal comfort and signs of adverse effects, such as sweating and thermal discomfort, rather than body temperature readings alone. Based on similar studies, warming patients using active methods (e.g., FAW) preoperatively and intraoperatively has become a standard, evidence-based practice (AORN, 2013).

Modified from Association of periOperative Registered Nurses (AORN): Recommended practices for prevention of unplanned perioperative hypothermia. In *Perioperative standards and recommended practices,* Denver, 2013, The Association; Cobbe K et al: Preventing inadvertent hypothermia: comparing two protocols for preoperative forced-air warming, *J Perianesth Nurs* 27(1):18–24, 2012; Hooper VD et al: ASPAN's evidence-based clinical practice guideline for the promotion of perioperative normothermia: second edition, *J Perianesth Nurs* 25:346–365, 2010; Lynch S: Reducing the risk of unplanned perioperative hypothermia, *AORN J* 92(5):553–565, 2010; Winslow EH: Are postoperative adult patients' thermal comfort ratings and temporal artery thermometer readings accurate indices for identifying hypothermia? *J Perianesth Nurs* 27(3):e42–e43, 2012.

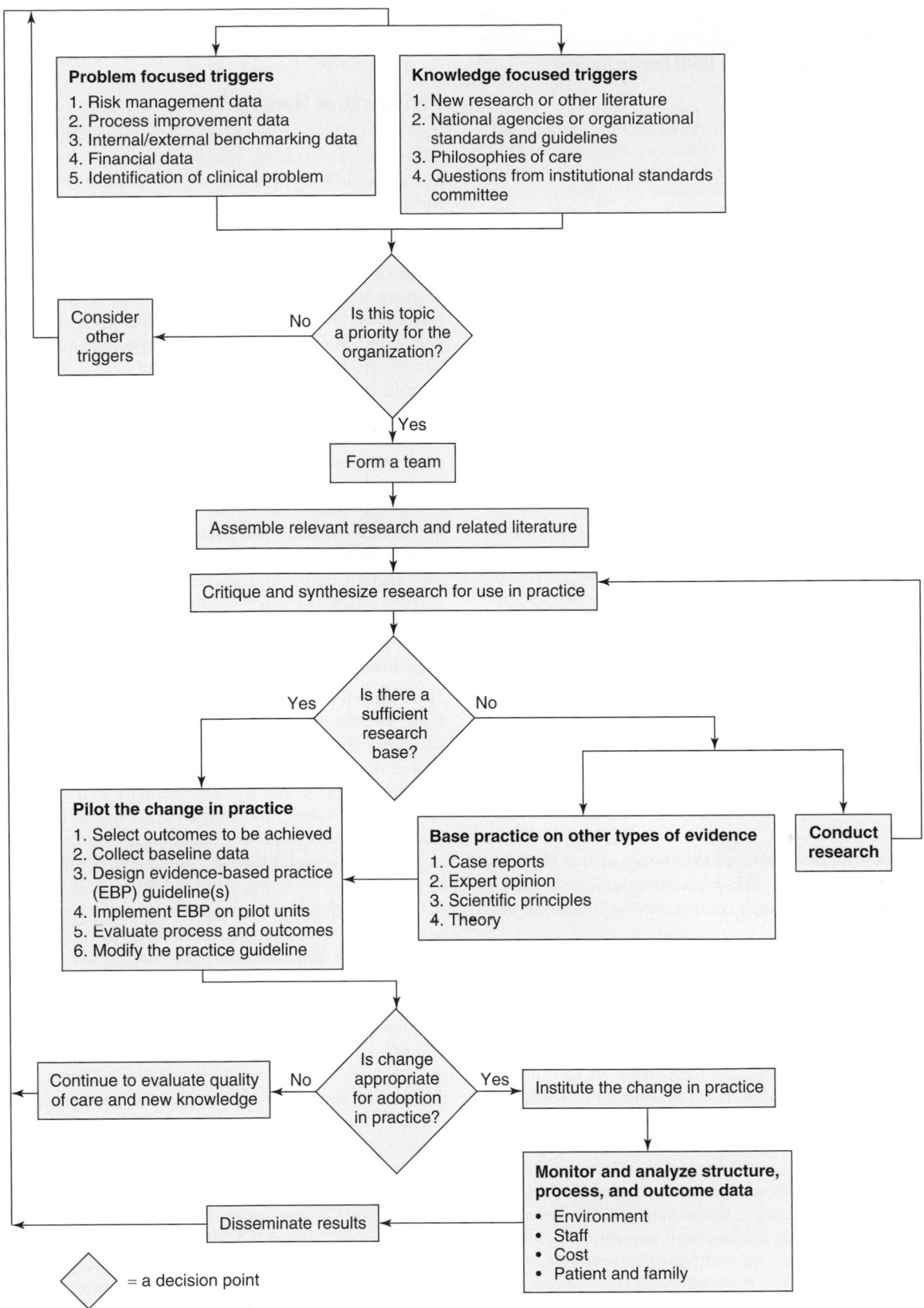

Problem focused triggers
1. Risk management data
2. Process improvement data
3. Internal/external benchmarking data
4. Financial data
5. Identification of clinical problem

Knowledge focused triggers
1. New research or other literature
2. National agencies or organizational standards and guidelines
3. Philosophies of care
4. Questions from institutional standards committee

Is this topic a priority for the organization?

No → Consider other triggers

Yes

Form a team

Assemble relevant research and related literature

Critique and synthesize research for use in practice

Is there a sufficient research base?

Yes

No

Pilot the change in practice
1. Select outcomes to be achieved
2. Collect baseline data
3. Design evidence-based practice (EBP) guideline(s)
4. Implement EBP on pilot units
5. Evaluate process and outcomes
6. Modify the practice guideline

Base practice on other types of evidence
1. Case reports
2. Expert opinion
3. Scientific principles
4. Theory

Conduct research

Is change appropriate for adoption in practice?

No → Continue to evaluate quality of care and new knowledge

Yes → Institute the change in practice

Monitor and analyze structure, process, and outcome data
• Environment
• Staff
• Cost
• Patient and family

Disseminate results

◇ = a decision point

FIGURE 1-4 The Iowa Model of Evidence-Based Practice to Promote Quality Patient Care is one model used in some healthcare settings to identify opportunities to improve care; evaluate evidence; and design, implement, and evaluate evidence-based practice changes.

AMBULATORY SURGERY CONSIDERATIONS

The Functional Recovery Index (FRI) for Ambulatory Surgery Patients

Ambulatory surgery centers regularly perform complex procedures on higher risk patients. Therefore, it becomes important not only to determine patients' readiness for discharge from the ambulatory surgery center but also how well patients fare in their recovery and rehabilitation after discharge. Researchers in Toronto developed a research tool to evaluate recovery after ambulatory surgery, focusing on functional abilities after discharge. The research instrument, called the Functional Recovery Index (FRI), takes about 4 to 5 minutes to complete. There are 14 queries that patients answer on a scale of 0 (no difficulty with activity) to 10 (extreme difficulty with activity). The items are grouped according to important recovery activities such as pain, social activity, lower limb activity, and general physical activity. Responses are summed; the lower the score, the more superior the patient's recovery. The sum of the answer scores can be adjusted for a query that is not applicable or that the patient did not answer. As is usual during development of a research tool, tests were undertaken for validity and reliability. In the FRI, internal consistency for three factors was Cronbach α = 0.90, 0.89, and 0.86, respectively. Interrater reliability as assessed in 264 patients was 0.99, indicating high reliability. Convergent validity testing for FRI compared to a verbal rating scale pain score was 0.76. Discriminant validity testing showed that the type of surgery was significant and that both intermediate surgery and major surgery were associated with higher FRI scores than minor surgery, not an unusual finding. The tool developers concluded that the FRI has excellent reliability, good validity, adequate responsiveness, and general acceptability.

Modified from Wong J et al: Development of the functional recovery index for ambulatory surgery and anesthesia, *Anesthesiology* 110(3):596–602, 2009.

implemented multiple programs used in industry, such as Six Sigma and Lean Sigma, to assess and refine processes to improve efficiency. These efforts underscore nursing's commitment to improving processes and outcomes of care.

Performance measurement and improvement approaches facilitate the delivery of safe, high-quality perioperative patient care. When processes are understood, they can be improved through a systematic plan of action. Involvement on teams that perform surgical services performance assessments and create improvement plans strengthens the staff's commitment to meet standards and enhance program effectiveness. TJC supports the evolution to an information technology infrastructure (i.e., EHR) in which performance measurement becomes an integral part of the care delivery process. As current uses of data expand and improve, objectives will still include the use of data for research activities directed at improving quality of care and identifying and disseminating EBPs. Perioperative nurses can anticipate that measurement requirements and performance expectations will change over time with new technologies and care practices as they affect the quality and safety of care. TJC and insurance companies also expect healthcare organizations to evaluate patients' perception of care and to use this information to improve the system of care delivery. The objectives of future TJC activities are likely to focus on the following:

- Continued expansion and coordination of nationally standardized core measurement capabilities

- Increased use of measurement data for quality improvement, benchmarking, accountability, decision making, accreditation, and research

Perioperative Nursing Roles

The nursing profession and the healthcare culture in the United States continue to change rapidly in response to many elements. An aging population, with the over-65 population already topping some 40 million, continues to create significant increases in demands for health services. As baby boomers turn 65, the over-85 segment of the population is projected to triple by 2050. Referred to as the "longevity revolution," in 2030 it is anticipated that one in five residents in the United States will be older than 85. New ambulatory settings for the delivery of health services, including operative and other invasive procedures, will continue to develop, as will community-based clinics, school-linked clinics, mobile clinics, and drive-in health centers. Healthcare organizations that are able to respond quickly to change will have an edge in the healthcare industry of the future. Likewise, perioperative nurses who understand the need for clinical and service quality, cost-effectiveness, information management, coordinated patient-centered care, efficiency, the special needs of an aging surgical population, and the importance of patient satisfaction will be able to anticipate and position themselves for this future. Roles in case management, care coordination, informatics, the healthcare industry, consulting, management, advanced practice nursing, and research are all very real possibilities for future-oriented perioperative nurses.

Traditional Perioperative Roles

There are two traditional perioperative nursing roles: the circulating nurse and the scrub person. The circulating nurse remains "nonscrubbed" and uses the nursing process to assess the patient, identify desired outcomes, formulate nursing diagnoses, choose a plan of care, implement or delegate interventions, and evaluate outcomes of the care provided. Among many other responsibilities, the circulating nurse manages patient positioning, antimicrobial skin preparation, medications, implants, specimens, warming devices, and surgical counts. As noted, AORN (2012a) reaffirmed its position statement advocating the requirement that there be a registered nurse circulator for every patient undergoing surgery or other invasive procedure and that this nurse manage the care of only one patient at a time.

The scrub person assembles needed instruments and supplies in a manner to maximize safety and efficiency. This role requires an in-depth knowledge of each step of the surgical procedure and the certain ability to anticipate each and every instrument and supply that will be needed. Many instruments are complex and require assembly. Instruments are positioned on the sterile table so that the scrub person can prepare each instrument as it will be used and quickly transfer it to the surgeon, often without being asked. This role is highly technical and either a registered nurse or a surgical technologist (ST) may assume it. The ST who functions as the scrub person may be certified (CST). The certifying agency for STs is the National Board of Surgical Technology and Surgical Assisting (the NBSTSA). Surgical technology students who graduate from an accredited surgical technology program are eligible for and must sit for the certification exam. Many of these programs result in an associate degree.

The scrub person and circulating nurse form an important partnership in ensuring patient safety. They work closely and effectively together throughout the procedure. Close teamwork keeps communication open, minimizes the risk of errors, and promotes the cost-effective use of supplies. Based on mutual respect, teamwork enhances quality in the workplace.

The CNOR is available to perioperative nurses who function in traditional or nontraditional roles. This credential represents demonstrated knowledge of clinical practices and standards as well as a marked level of professional achievement. It also demonstrates proficiency in support of quality patient care and sets a standard of commitment to the profession of perioperative nursing (Competency and Credentialing Institute, 2013a).

Registered Nurse First Assistant

The role of the perioperative registered nurse first assistant (RNFA) in surgery is an expanded perioperative nursing role that requires formal academic education (AORN, 2012). In 1984, AORN approved an official statement on the RNFA and has revised the statement regularly to reflect changes in the RNFA's role. The RNFA works collaboratively with the surgeon (and the patient and surgical team) by handling and cutting tissue, using instruments and medical devices, providing exposure and hemostasis, and suturing, all as components of assisting-at-surgery behaviors. AORN has developed standards for RNFA educational programs (AORN, 2011a), and certification is available for this role (CRNFA) (Competency and Credentialing Institute, 2013b). Many experienced perioperative nurses obtained this education. Effective January 1, 2020, the education level for entry into an RNFA program and subsequent RNFA practice will be the baccalaureate degree. AORN recommends RNs who were practicing as RNFAs prior to 2020 and do not have a baccalaureate degree be permitted to continue to practice as RNFAs. Performing as an RNFA allows an experienced perioperative nurse to expand clinical knowledge and skills and to assume additional responsibility for preoperative and postoperative patient management while still remaining directly involved with intraoperative patient care. The RNFA has gained wide professional acceptance as a highly skilled member of the surgical team. Functioning in this role is another way perioperative nurses can develop professionally to meet the changing needs of healthcare delivery.

Advanced Practice Registered Nurse

Advanced practice registered nurses (APRNs) include certified nurse practitioners (CNPs), certified registered nurse anesthetists (CRNAs), certified nurse midwives (CNMs), and clinical nurse specialists (CNSs). Acute-care CNPs fill gaps in providing care for patients who are more acutely ill and whose medical-surgical problems are more complex. Opportunities within this role are expanding rapidly (Aleshire et al, 2012). CNPs are employed in acute care hospitals and ambulatory surgery centers across the country. Some CNPs focus primarily on the preoperative phase of patient care, using their advanced knowledge to assess patients and order preoperative medications and treatment. Other CNPs combine this role with that of the first assistant, allowing them to use their advanced practice skills throughout the perioperative care continuum. Some CNSs also provide licensed independent care to individual patients. However, the traditional role of the CNS involves primarily indirect care within the perioperative leadership team. As part of the management team, the CNS provides support for the care of groups of patients through leadership, education, consultation, management, and research. CNSs have assumed a significant leadership role in the implementation of EBP changes in healthcare settings (Steelman, 2009).

APRNs must have graduate nursing education (at least a master's degree). In 2004, the American Association of Colleges of Nursing (AACN) published a position statement advocating for the doctor of nursing practice degree as the minimum educational preparation for APRNs. These educational programs are available across the country and have a standardized core curriculum (Raines, 2010).

Emerging Roles

As patient needs change and technology advances, new perioperative nursing roles develop to meet these needs. Some of these roles include care coordinator, family liaison, robotics coordinator, and informatics specialist. Some healthcare organizations have established the role of care coordinator in specific programs such as trauma, bariatrics, cardiac care, and organ transplant to meet the unique challenges and complexities of these specific patient populations. The role of care coordinator provides an opportunity for the perioperative nurse to develop more in-depth skills to meet the needs of a specific population of surgical patients.

As early as the late 1990s the perioperative nursing role of family or surgical liaison evolved to serve as a communication link between the OR and the family during surgery. The liaison translates information from the surgical team to the family, often serving to clarify and answer questions that require an understanding of events in the OR. Hospitals and ambulatory surgery centers have implemented this perioperative nursing role to enhance patient and family satisfaction.

Another emerging role in perioperative nursing is that of robotics coordinator. Both the number and the types of procedures performed with surgical robots have increased dramatically. Robots are now commonly used for general, cardiovascular, pediatric, and urologic surgery. The complexity of the equipment and requisite troubleshooting demand additional specialized skills. The evolution of robotic technology and rapid expansion of its use have created many challenges for the perioperative team. Some healthcare facilities have developed a new role, the robotics coordinator, to coordinate this technology, provide complex troubleshooting, and train personnel (Zender and Thell, 2010). The robotics coordinator may also serve as a public liaison by providing marketing and public educational opportunities about the robotics surgery program.

Informatics is another specialty in which some perioperative nurses are focusing. Nursing informatic systems have applications for practice, administration, education, and research (Baker, 2012). Pressure for more efficient management of fiscal, material, and human resources has stimulated the development of electronic information systems for diverse functions in perioperative patient care settings. A well-designed information system can synthesize large volumes of data efficiently into meaningful reports to support decision making. Newer nursing applications include point-of-care clinical systems, electronic health and medical records, Internet-based patient education, research, and telemedicine and telenursing. The growing field of nursing informatics is an interaction of cognitive science, computer science, and informatics, all of which are based on a foundation of nursing science (Figure 1-5) (Baker, 2012; Ozbolt and Saba, 2008). Perioperative nurse informatics specialists have the opportunity to develop clinical nursing systems that incorporate nursing care protocols, critical paths, best practices, the PNDS, and patient education materials that track patients over time. Such systems allow sharing information across wide networks as patients access healthcare at different points and times over a continuum of care. Future technology systems may include interactive computer/television by which perioperative nurses will remotely

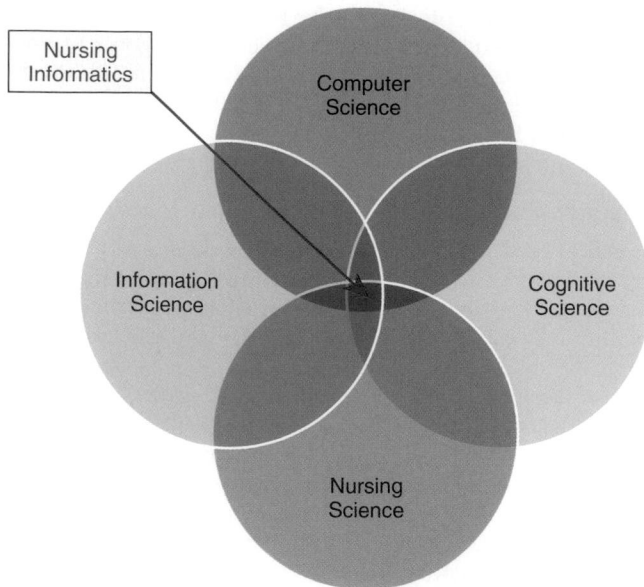

FIGURE 1-5 Nursing informatics Venn diagram.

communicate with their patients over phone or cable lines, allowing the perioperative nurse to view the patient's wound or discuss recovery and rehabilitation from surgery.

Perioperative nursing is an exciting, ever-changing specialty. The opportunities for continual learning and challenges are endless. As we move into the future, these opportunities will continue to grow and evolve. Perioperative nurses need to identify their professional goals and develop strategic plans to accomplish these goals, including enhancing their skill sets and education. This strategy will position the perioperative nurse well for exciting roles in the future.

KEY POINTS

- Perioperative nursing is a complex specialty that uses the nursing process to provide high-quality patient care.
- The Perioperative Patient Focused Model provides a framework for perioperative nursing standards.
- The Perioperative Nursing Data Set (PNDS) is a standardized language to document patient care in order to enhance retrievability of data for evaluation of patient care.
- Evidence-based practice is a systematic process by which to identify an issue, collect and evaluate the best evidence, and make the best clinical decisions.
- Perioperative nurses work with a team of professionals and unlicensed assistive personnel to provide patient care; effective, extensive, and ongoing communication within the team is essential to accomplish safe patient care.
- There are a variety of perioperative nursing roles, including circulating nurse, scrub nurse, registered nurse first assistant (RNFA), advanced practice registered nurse (APRN), and emerging roles such as robotics coordinator and informatics specialist.

CRITICAL THINKING QUESTION

When reviewing your assignment for the day, you note that you are caring for a 45-year-old male patient undergoing a left nephrectomy. When you interview him in the preoperative area, what questions will you ask him in order to protect his rights? What questions will you ask him to achieve other important desired outcomes?

⊖volve *The answers to the Critical Thinking Question can be found at http://evolve.elsevier.com/Rothrock/Alexander.*

REFERENCES

Aleshire ME et al: The future of nurse practitioner practice: a world of opportunity, *Nurs Clin North Am* 47(2):181–191, 2012.

American Nurses Association, National Council of State Boards of Nursing: Joint statement on nursing delegation, ANA/NCSBN, available at www.ncsbn.org/Joint_statement.pdf. Accessed June 1, 2012.

Association of periOperative Registered Nurses (AORN): AORN standards for RN first assistant education programs, *AORN J* 94(1):49–52, 2011a.

Association of periOperative Registered Nurses (AORN): *PNDS—perioperative nursing data set*, ed 3, Denver, 2011b, The Association.

Association of periOperative Registered Nurses (AORN): *Position statement: registered nurse first assistants*, Denver, 2012, The Association.

Association of periOperative Registered Nurses: *Position statement: one perioperative registered nurse circulator dedicated to every patient undergoing a surgical or other invasive procedure*, Denver, 2012a, The Association, available at www.aorn.org/Clinical_Practice/Position_Statements/Position_Statements.aspx. Accessed January 16, 2013.

Association of periOperative Registered Nurses (AORN): *Position statement: APRN in the perioperative setting*, Denver, 2013, The Association, available at www.aorn.org/Clinical_Practice/Position_Statements/Position_Statements.aspx. Accessed January 16, 2013.

Association of periOperative Registered Nurses (AORN): Standards of perioperative nursing. In *Perioperative standards and recommended practices*, Denver, 2013a, The Association.

Association of periOperative Registered Nurses (AORN): Quality and performance improvement standards for perioperative nursing. In *Perioperative standards and recommended practices*, Denver, 2013b, The Association.

Baker JD: Nursing informatics, *Periop Nurs Clin* 7(2):151–160, 2012.

Carey M et al: The cycle of change: implementing best-evidence clinical practice, *Int J Qual Health Care* 21(1):37–43, 2009.

Competency and Credentialing Institute: *CNOR certification and recertification candidate handbook*, available at www.cc-institute.org/docs/default-document-library/2011/07/27/CNOR_candidate_handbook.pdf, 2013a. Accessed January 16, 2013.

Competency and Credentialing Institute: *CRNFA certification and recertification candidate handbook*, available at www.cc-institute.org/docs/default-document-library/2011/07/27/CRNFA_candidate_handbook.pdf?Status=Master, 2013b. Accessed January 16, 2013.

Enticott JC et al: A review on decision support for massive transfusion: understanding human factors to support the implementation of complex interventions in trauma, *Transfusion* Apr 15, 2012.

Gillespie BM et al: Interruptions and miscommunications in surgery: an observational study, *AORN J* 95(5):576–590, 2012.

Ozbolt JG, Saba VK: A brief history of nursing informatics in the United States of America, *Nurs Outlook* 56:199–205, 2008.

Paulikas CA: Prevention of unplanned hypothermia, *AORN J* 89(4):701–713, 2009.

Pottinger J et al: Skin preparation, *Periop Nurs Clin* 1:203–210, 2006.

Raines CF: The doctor of nursing practice: a report on progress, March 21, 2010, available at www.aacn.nche.edu/leading-initiatives/dnp/DNP Forum3-10.pdf. Accessed June 1, 2012.

Spalter AW, Wyatt DA: Antibiotic prophylaxis and surgical site infection: are we doing enough to ensure quality? *Periop Nurs Clin* 1:211–222, 2006.

Stebral LL, Steelman VM: Double gloving for surgical procedures: an evidence-based practice project, *Periop Nurs Clin* 1:251–260, 2006.

Steelman VM: The advanced practice nurse: an essential part of the perioperative leadership team, *Periop Nurs Clin* 4:51–56, 2009.

Steelman VM et al: Selection of a method to rate the strength of scientific evidence for AORN recommendations, *AORN J* 93(4):433–444, 2011.

Sullivan AE: Critical thinking in clinical nurse education: application of Paul's model of critical thinking, *Nurse Educ Pract* Apr 12, 2012.

The Joint Commission: Surgical care improvement project, 2012 (August), available at www.jointcommission.org//surgical_care_improvement_project. Accessed January 16, 2013.

The Joint Commission: Universal protocol, 2013, available at www.joint commission.org/assets/1/18/NPSG_Chapter_Jan2013_HAP.pdf. Accessed January 16, 2013.

U.S. Department of Health and Human Services, Centers for Medicare & Medicaid Services: Medicare program: proposed changes to the hospital inpatient prospective payment systems for acute care hospitals (CMS-1518-P), *Fed Regist* 76:25788–26084, May 5, 2011.

Whittemore R: How can nursing intervention research reduce the research-practice gap? *Can J Res* 41:7–15, 2009.

Zender J, Thell C: Developing a successful robotic surgery program in a rural hospital, *AORN J* 92:72–86, 2010.

CHAPTER 2

Patient Safety and Risk Management

ELLEN K. MURPHY

Think about what happens in the perioperative setting. Patients' natural pain, communication, and reflex and infection defenses are purposefully diminished or obliterated. Their bodies are positioned on very firm flat surfaces and in unnatural positions. Then their bodies are further traumatized with instruments, fibers, drugs, and other foreign materials. It is no wonder that more than one quarter of the reported sentinel events from 2006 through 2012 occurred in the perioperative setting (Table 2-1).

Although patient safety should be, and is, a paramount concern to nurses in all settings, nowhere is it more imperative than in the immediate perioperative period. Additionally, many elements of perioperative patient safety are coextensive with those of workplace safety (see Chapter 3).

This chapter describes the evolution of perioperative patient safety and the management of injury risks as a collective responsibility of the entire healthcare team.

History

Patient safety remains a primary concern for members of the surgical team. *Primum non nocere* or "First, do no harm," is a longstanding imperative for physicians and nurses. Early operating room (OR) nursing textbooks written by OR nurses included counting sponges among nursing duties (e.g., Smith, 1924). Perioperative nursing textbooks and curricula continued to include substantial content on infection control, positioning, safe medication practices, and counts through World War II. The first edition of this very textbook by Edythe Alexander (1943) included content on asepsis, the importance of correct side surgery, proper blood handling, and proper tourniquet application. Alexander did not use the word "safety," but she described the purpose of "perfecting every detail . . . to insure that patients . . . have every chance to overcome the disease or injury with which they are afflicted" (1943, p. 7).

After World War II, safety activities increased and became more formalized. The Joint Commission for the Accreditation of Hospitals (JCAH), now The Joint Commission, emerged. Nursing groups and publications increasingly emphasized their patient safety content. The American Nurses Association (ANA) published its *Code for Nurses,* which included provisions on patient safety and privacy, and the Association of Operating Room Nurses (now, the Association of periOperative Registered Nurses [AORN]) organized in the early 1950s. From the beginning, AORN's conferences and publications were replete with patient safety information. Its first conference in 1954 included programs on methods improvement, explosion prevention, bacteria destruction, the surgeon-nurse relationship, and positioning (Glass and Murphy, 2002). AORN published its first *Standards of Operating Room Practice* in 1974. Its *Technical Standards* soon followed, and by the 1980s it published

and regularly updated its *Recommended Practices* (RPs). AORN soon became and remains the primary resource and a fundamental authority for evidence-based perioperative safety practices (e.g., the RP on sterile technique [AORN, 2013]).

Safety as an Individual Responsibility

Throughout the 1980s, healthcare authorities viewed professionals' errors and their effects on patient safety primarily as the individual practitioner's responsibility. The legal and professional licensure systems tended to reinforce this approach. Any finding of negligence required that at least one individual had failed to do what a similarly situated, reasonable, and prudent professional would have done under similar circumstances. Likewise, professional licensure related to the abilities and behavior of the individual licensee.

In 1991, Brennan, Leape, and others proposed that despite individual best efforts by professionals, mistakes continued and were, in fact, more common than previously thought (Brennan et al, 1991). Their findings, combined with James Reason's influential book *Human Error* (1990), spawned a plethora of new safety-related groups (Box 2-1), as well as fresh research and literature based on the role of systems, human factors, and their relationship to human error in healthcare. Researchers and authorities began to recognize human errors leading to patient injuries not so much as an individual's shortcoming, deserving of blame or punishment, but more as a result of *system failures* in patient care areas such as the perioperative setting. Similarly, Leape (1994), Cook and Woods (1994), and others urged that the legal and professional licensure systems' continued focus on individual error was misplaced if adverse patient events were to be effectively prevented. They urged an emphasis on transparent systems that required open reporting, investigation, innovation, and dissemination. The aviation and nuclear systems' parallel examination of human factors served as models for ideas that led to relative success in preventing injury attributable to human error. Communication and teamwork have been identified as key factors to promote patient safety.

In the first edition of this textbook, Alexander noted that "to get the best result from a surgical operation, the surgeon and his assistants, the operating room nurse and the entire staff must work as a team" (1943, p. 8). Despite AORN and its partner professional associations' emphasis on safety and teamwork, however, patient injuries caused by human error in perioperative settings continue (Pronovost and Colantuoni, 2009; TJC, 2012b).

Concentrated Emphasis on Systems

This earlier work took on urgency in 1999. The Institute of Medicine (IOM) landmark work, *To Err Is Human,* spurred major additional safety initiatives when it reported that at least 44,000, and

TABLE 2-1

Summary Data of Perioperative Sentinel Events Reviewed by The Joint Commission

Type of Sentinel Event	Number of Events from 2004 to 2012
Anesthesia-related event	94
Fall	538
Fire	98
Infection-related event	153
Med equipment-related	193
Medication error	378
Op/postop complication	719
Transfusion error	114
Unintended retention of a foreign body*	773
Wrong-patient, wrong-site, wrong-procedure	928
All others[†]	3006
Total Incidents Reviewed	**6994**

*Category added in 2005.
[†]Examples include criminal event, infant abduction, suicide, and perinatal death/injury.
Modified from www.jointcommission.org/assets/1/18/2004_4Q_2012_SE_Stats_Summary.pdf. Accessed February 11, 2013.

perhaps as many as 98,000, patients died in U.S. hospitals every year as a result of preventable adverse events (IOM, 1999). Even the lower figure exceeded the number of deaths resulting from motor vehicle accidents, breast cancer, or acquired immunodeficiency syndrome (AIDS). The IOM report did not focus solely on perioperative errors. However, it did refer to Reason's (1990) theory that complex, tightly coupled systems are most prone to accidents, and specified the surgical suite, along with emergency departments and intensive care units, as examples of complex, tightly coupled systems. Moreover, when one considers the incredibly complex highly invasive surgical procedures and number of team members and disciplines involved, juxtaposed with anesthetized patients who are unable to detect pain or otherwise defend themselves, patient vulnerability and the consequent need for protection by all team members are strikingly apparent. More than 4000 surgical "never events" occurred each year between 1990 and 2010 in the United States, according to the findings of a retrospective study of national malpractice data (Johns Hopkins Malpractice Study, 2012).

Brennan and colleagues (1991) studied 30,121 randomly selected hospital records, found adverse events occurred in 3.7% of hospitalizations, and concluded that substandard care had caused substantial numbers of patient injuries. In part 2 of that study, Leape and colleagues (1991) found that nearly half (48%) of adverse events were associated with surgery. Their results were consistent with those of earlier investigators, who had found half of all hospital-based, potentially compensable events (i.e., injuries from substandard care) arose from treatment in the OR. The Joint Commission (TJC) findings from 2006 to 2012 (TJC, 2012b) are

BOX 2-1

Select Perioperative Safety-Related Entities

CAPS (Consumers Advancing Patient Safety) is a consumer-led nonprofit organized as a voice for individuals, families, and healthcare professionals. CAPS is committed to contributing the consumer perspective to research, educating both consumers and providers, and developing solutions to help create healthcare systems that are safe, compassionate, and just. patientsafety.org.

ECRI Institute is a nonprofit organization dedicated to using the discipline of applied scientific research to discover which medical procedures, devices, drugs, and processes, including fire safety, best improve patient care. www.ecri.org.

IHI (Institute for Healthcare Improvement) works with healthcare providers and leaders throughout the world to enhance delivery of safe and effective healthcare. An independent not-for-profit organization based in Cambridge, Massachusetts, IHI focuses on motivating and building the will for change; identifying and testing new models of care in partnership with patients and healthcare professionals; and ensuring the broadest possible adoption of best practices and effective innovations. www.ihi.org.

IOM (Institute of Medicine) was chartered in 1970 as a component of the National Academy of Sciences. The Institute works outside the framework of government to ensure scientifically informed analysis and independent guidance. The IOM's mission is to serve as adviser to the nation to improve health by providing unbiased, evidence-based, and authoritative information and advice on health and science policy. www.iom.edu.

ISMP (Institute for Safe Medication Practices) is the nation's only nonprofit organization devoted entirely to medication error prevention and safe medication use. ISMP focuses on helping healthcare practitioners keep patients safe and leading efforts to improve the medication use process. www.ismp.org.

NQF (National Quality Forum) is a public-private partnership created to develop and implement a national strategy for healthcare quality measurement and reporting by building consensus on goals, endorsing standards, and monitoring their attainment through education and outreach. This group's 27 Safe Practices are widely accepted. Nurses are expressly included in its membership. www.qualityforum.org.

SCIP (Surgical Care Improvement Project) is a national quality partnership interested in improving surgical care by significantly reducing surgical complications. It was established by CMS to provide healthcare quality improvement news, resources, and data reporting tools and applications. SCIP created an original goal of reducing by 25% the national incidence of three types of surgical complications by 2010 (surgical site infections, perioperative myocardial infarction, and deep vein thrombosis/pulmonary embolism [DVT/PE]). New SCIP measures have been added and are among measures that acute care hospitals must disclose to receive full annual payment updates from Medicare (Patterson, 2011). Seven of the SCIP measures are included in the measures determining how much hospitals will be paid in fiscal year (FY) 2013. www.cms.gov/qualityimprovementorgs.

The Leapfrog Group is a voluntary program aimed at mobilizing employer purchasing power to alert America's health industry that "big leaps" in healthcare safety, quality, and customer value will be recognized and rewarded. It reports comparison data on providers. www.leapfroggroup.org.

In addition, many states have state-based coalitions that encourage cost-effective, safe, quality healthcare.

similarly consistent with those findings: Individual efforts of the best nurses, surgeons, and anesthesia providers, combined with a recognized need for teamwork, are not sufficient to prevent injury—and are especially insufficient in the perioperative setting.

This shift away from emphasis on individual responsibility to a broader systems approach that began in the 1990s has accelerated since 2000. Advances in surgical instrumentation and health information systems, as well as in social media and consumerism, have combined to alter the context of perioperative care dramatically. This change in context requires a new and more inclusive, global approach to safety.

New terms and phrases have joined the patient safety lexicon, such as "e-iatrogenesis," "better systems for patient safety," "shared decision making," and *C. diff.* Checklists and tools for measuring safety practices have multiplied (e.g., the Institute for Healthcare Improvement (IHI) Global Trigger Tool for Measuring Adverse Events, Partnerships for Patients and IHI Improvement Blogs; the National Quality Forum's (NQF) Safe Practices Quality Positioning System; and National Priorities Partnerships to the Leapfrog Group's Health User Group Dashboards). Safety scholars have published influential treatises for the professions and the public that have raised everyone's awareness of checklist initiatives (e.g., Conley, 2011; Gawande, 2009).

Despite the impressive initial effectiveness of checklists (Haynes et al, 2009), barriers to their adoption (Fourcade et al, 2012) and a parallel need for flexibility, leadership, and teamwork different from current practice (Walker, 2012) have been identified. Various voluntary and governmental standards have so proliferated that matrices are published by still other groups to compare or provide crosswalks between them.

Major Association Safety Activities

TJC and TJC International, especially their National Patient Safety Goals (NPSGs), are excellent sources for safety information applicable to systems and facilities wherein invasive procedures take place. The AORN *Perioperative Standards and Recommended Practices* is the best source for information specific to perioperative nursing practices. Major government agencies that provide financial incentives and research resources for patient safety are also useful sources for safety information for facilities and individual professionals.

The Joint Commission

TJC has long been involved with quality and safety. It sharpened its systems-based safety focus in the mid-1990s when it established its Sentinel Event Policy. That policy first encouraged and then required self-reporting of medical errors and root cause analyses of them. Based on cumulative data, TJC published its first NPSGs in 2003. It then recognized the need for standardized methods of patient identification and established the Universal Protocol (discussed later in this chapter) in 2004. By 2005, the World Health Organization (WHO) formed the Collaborative Centre for Patient Safety Solutions, comprised of TJC and TJC International. TJC also is a founding member of the National Patient Safety Foundation (NPSF), collaborates with the National Quality Forum (NQF), and is an affiliate of Consumers Advancing Patient Safety (CAPS).

Sentinel Events. TJC designated unexpected occurrences involving death or risk of serious physical or psychologic injuries as sentinel events. It chose the word "sentinel" to indicate that these events signal the need for immediate investigation and response through root cause analysis, a systematized process to identify variations in performance that cause or could cause a sentinel event. Suggested steps in such an analysis are briefly summarized in the Patient Safety box on page 19. Whereas TJC data collection focuses on sentinel events, it also recognizes the value of analyzing "close calls" to improve patient safety (Wu, 2011).

TJC categorizes errors reported to it and publishes their frequencies. Examples of perioperative care errors are those that are (1) related to anesthesia; (2) caused by medical equipment; (3) caused by medication error; (4) result in infection, fires, and transfusion reactions; (5) are operative or postoperative; or (6) give rise to unintended retained surgical items (RSIs) or wrong site/patient/procedure surgery. The summary of sentinel events published in 2013 reveals that of 6994 total incidents reviewed from 2004 through 2012, nearly 25% of all incidents reviewed most likely occurred in an operative setting (RSI, referred to by TJC as retained foreign object [RFO], and wrong site procedures). Add in the number of events that could have occurred in the perioperative setting (falls, transfusion and medication errors) and the percentage might reach closer to the 50% figure that Leape and Brennan found in the early 1990s.

National Patient Safety Goals. Another TJC initiative relates to NPSGs for hospitals and office-based surgery, derived from reported sentinel events. NPSGs are reviewed, updated, or retired each year. See the Patient Safety box on page 19 for an overview of the 2013 NPSGs for hospitals and the Patient Safety box on page 20 for elements of performance for the NPSG related to labeling medications.

TJC also publishes NPSGs for office-based surgery. These are not excerpted here because the goals for patients in both settings are almost the same. Although initially surprising, this similarity is understandable. Even though patients in office-based surgery settings tend to be of healthier physical status classifications as set out by the American Society of Anesthesiologists (ASA) (see Chapter 5), one could argue that error prevention procedures in office-based surgery facilities nevertheless must be rigorous because these smaller facilities are less likely to have available the hospitals' wider array of emergency and corrective equipment and personnel. In addition, office-based and ambulatory perioperative staff provides most patient and family discharge education and preparation, unlike inpatient care settings (Ambulatory Surgery Considerations) (Patient and Family Education). Finally, causes of infection and patient defenses against infection do not differ based on the location of the surgical procedure.

Universal Protocol. TJC introduced its required safety practice under the nomenclature, Universal Protocol, now incorporated into the NPSGs. Key features of the Universal Protocol, as codified in the NPSGs, are performing a preoperative verification process; marking the operative site; and conducting a time-out immediately before starting the procedure. A properly performed time-out includes information about the patient and procedure, as discussed in more detail later in this chapter.

U.S. Government Agencies

Centers for Medicare & Medicaid Services. As part of the U.S. Department of Health and Human Services (DHHS), the Centers for Medicare & Medicaid Services (CMS) is the federal agency charged with administration (including regulations for payment) of

PATIENT SAFETY

Root Cause Analysis

The Joint Commission (TJC) Root Cause Analysis and Action Plan tool has 24 analysis questions. TJC framework is intended to provide a template for organizing and answering analysis questions. Not all questions are listed here:

1. What happened?
2. Why did that happen?
   - What was the intended process flow? List pertinent steps in the process—use those identified in policy, procedure, protocols, or guidelines in effect at time of event. In the OR these might be, for example, the site verification protocol, procedures for soft good, sharps counts, patient identification protocols, or fall risk/fall prevention guidelines for perioperative patient positioning.
   - Were there steps in the policy, procedure, protocol, or guideline that did not occur as intended?
   - What human factors are relevant? Consider staff-related factors such as fatigue, inattention, lack of clinical reasoning/critical thinking skills, and rushing to completed task. Disruptions in the flow of a surgical procedure, such as teamwork and communication failures, may contribute significantly to the event.
   - Were there problems with equipment that affected the outcome?

- What factors in the environment were controllable? These factors should be specific to the event.
- What external factors in the environment were uncontrollable (these are factors that cannot be changed)?

3. What other factors are involved?
   - Was the staff properly qualified and competent for their responsibilities at the time of the event? Address staffing levels, staff performance in this part of the analysis.
   - To what degree was all necessary information available when needed?
   - Was communication among participants adequate for this situation?
   - How does the organization's culture support risk reduction? Are there barriers to communicating potential risk factors?
   - How is the prevention of adverse outcomes communicated as a high priority?

Root cause analysis involves an action plan addressing "what can be done to prevent this?" Root cause analysis concentrates on systems and processes, not individuals. It is characterized by a structured "sense-making conversation."

Modified from Cassin BR, Barach PE: Making sense of root cause analysis investigations of surgery-related adverse events, *Surg Clin North Am* 92(1):101–115, 2012; *Framework for conducting a root cause analysis and action plan*, revised February 28, 2013, available at www.jointcommission.org/Framework_for_Conducting_a_Root_Cause_Analysis_and_Action_Plan. Accessed March 18, 2013.

PATIENT SAFETY

Select Hospital-Based Surgery National Patient Safety Goals That Apply to Perioperative Patient Care

Identify patients correctly.
- Use at least two ways to identify patients, such as both the patient's name and date of birth.
- Conduct a preprocedure verification process.
- Preoperatively, mark the procedure site; if possible, do so with the patient involved.
- Label container used for blood and other specimens in the presence of the patient.

Make sure that the correct patient gets the correct blood type when receiving a transfusion.
- Read back spoken (verbal) or phone orders to the person who gave the order.
- Refer to and use a list of abbreviations and symbols that are not to be used.
- Use a two-person verification process (or one person plus bar coding) to match the blood or blood component to order and to the patient. One of these two people must be the person involved in blood/blood component administration.
- Report critical test results on an institutionally determined basis.

Use medications safely (see Patient Safety: Elements of Performance for Medication Safety on page 20 for recommendations for medication safety).
- Prior to the procedure start, label all medicines in syringes, basins, and medication cups, or other medical devices that are not already labeled. This must be done for all medications both on and off the sterile field.
- Label when transferring any medication from the original packaging to another container. This is done in the location where the

procedure will take place (such as the OR or other procedure room).
- Labels, both on and off the sterile field, include medication name, strength, quantity; diluent and volume; expiration date or expiration time.
- Take extra care when anticoagulants are administered.
- Review medication labels during any relief of personnel during the procedure. Immediately discard any medication or solution found unlabeled.
- Record all medications administered on the patient's record.
- Discard any unused medication or solution at the end of the procedure

Prevent surgical site infections.
- Use hand hygiene guidelines from the WHO or CDC.
- Use evidence-based practices to prevent infections (e.g., antimicrobial prophylaxis, hair removal).
- Use evidence-based practices to prevent central line–associated bloodstream infections (CLABSI) and catheter-associated urinary tract infections (CAUTIs).
- Use policies and procedures based on evidence to prevent surgical site infection.

Perform a time-out immediately before the procedure to prevent surgical errors.
- Use a facility-defined standardized procedure to ensure correct person, procedure, and site.
- Involve all immediate members of the surgical/procedure team in the time-out. They must agree that this is the correct patient, the correct site, and the correct procedure to be performed.
- Document the completion of the time-out.

Modified from The Joint Commission: *2013 hospital national patient safety goals,* available at jointcommission.org/assets/1/18/NPSG_Chapter_Jan2013_HAP.pdf. Accessed February 10, 2013.

PATIENT SAFETY

Elements of Performance for Medication Safety

1. In perioperative and other procedural settings, label medications and solutions that are not immediately administered both on and off the sterile field. Label them as soon as they are prepared. This applies even if only one medication is used.

   Note: An immediately administered medication is one that an authorized staff member prepares or obtains, takes directly to a patient, and administers to that patient without any break in the process.

2. In perioperative and other procedural settings, labeling occurs when any medication or solution, either on or off the sterile field, is transferred from its original packaging to another container.

3. In perioperative and other procedural settings both on and off the sterile field, medication or solution labels include the following:
   • Medication name
   • Strength
   • Quantity
   • Diluent and volume (if not apparent from the container)
   • Expiration time, when expiration occurs in less than 24 hours

   Note: The date and time are not necessary for short procedures, as defined by the hospital.

4. Verify all medication or solution labels both verbally and visually. Verification is done by two individuals qualified to participate in the procedure whenever the person preparing the medication or solution is not the person who will be administering it.

5. Immediately discard any medication or solution found unlabeled.

6. Remove all labeled containers on the sterile field and discard their contents at the conclusion of the procedure.

   Note: This does not apply to multiuse vials that are handled according to the institution's infection control practices.

7. All medications and solutions both on and off the sterile field and their labels are reviewed by entering and exiting staff responsible for the management of medications.

Modified from The Joint Commission: *2013 Hospital national patient safety goals,* available at jointcommission.org/assets/1/18/NPSG_Chapter_Jan2013_HAP.pdf. Accessed March 24, 2013.

AMBULATORY SURGERY CONSIDERATIONS

Postoperative Telephone Calls

Office-based and ambulatory perioperative staff provides most patient and family discharge education and preparation, unlike inpatient care settings. Commonly they also contact patients postoperatively to determine whether there are any problems or concerns. In reviewing the timing for such postoperative phone calls, Flanagan's research explored themes of postoperative patient calls at different time periods and discovered the following:

• At 12 hours postoperatively, patients expressed relief that their procedure was completed. Their primary symptom was nausea (Odom-Forren [2011] reports that approximately one third of ambulatory surgery patients experience postdischarge nausea and vomiting [PDNV]).

• At 24 hours postoperatively, patients expressed feelings of being unprepared and unable to manage by themselves. They needed resources to help with their care; they had symptoms of pain, nausea, and fatigue and reported decreased mobility.

• By 72 hours postoperatively, patients were more able to function on their own and continued to experience fatigue, but felt "abandoned." They did not yet feel "back to normal" and had concerns about missing work and their inability to manage other role functions and activities. However, they were now able to ask more questions and felt more comfortable expressing their concerns over the phone.

Patient and family education and preparation for discharge are critical to the well-being of surgery patients. Each of the chapters in this book that reviews a surgical specialty has a discussion of this critical aspect of perioperative nursing care in order to assist both the nurse and the patient in discussing and anticipating what will be needed during the postoperative recovery and convalescence period.

Modified from Flanagan J: Postoperative telephone calls: timing is everything, *AORN J* 90(1):41–51, 2009; Odom-Forren J: Measurement of postdischarge nausea and vomiting for ambulatory surgery patients: a critical review and analysis, *J PeriAnesth Nurs* 26(6):372–383, 2011.

PATIENT AND FAMILY EDUCATION

Ambulatory Surgery

The continued success of ambulatory surgery has been achieved in part through patient education and satisfaction with this environment of care. Below is an example of educational information for patients and their families when ambulatory surgery is scheduled:

Ambulatory surgery means you can go home the same day as your surgery, or with a hospital stay of less than 24 hours. Ambulatory procedures are just as safe as those in a hospital. Usually, ambulatory surgery patients are quite satisfied with the care they receive. Once you and your surgeon decide on an ambulatory procedure, someone will discuss some of the following topics with you and a member of your family (it is a good idea to have a family member with you to help you remember things, but it is not required):

• Why is ambulatory surgery a good choice for me?
• What type of ambulatory surgery facility will I go to?
• What happens during my preoperative visit?
• What important things will I have to do to prepare for the procedure?
• What happens during the surgery?
• Will I go to a recovery room?
• Are there special things I need to do to take care of myself at home?
• When should I call my doctor after the surgery?

Modified from *Outpatient surgery*, available at www.nursingconsult.com/nursing/patient-education/full-text?handout_id=45020&docId=10087&filter_id=0&filter_by=&sort_by=title&sort_order=asc&page=&otherid=48616&english=true&tab=cond&specId=1398823441&specName=&sortOrd=&parentpage=search&story_title=Outpatient Surgery-SportsMed (subscription required). Document revised 8/29/12. Accessed January 17, 2013.

the Medicare, Medicaid, and multiple state Children's Health Insurance Programs (CHIP), part of Medicaid. It also administers the Health Insurance Portability and Accountability Act (HIPAA) (discussed later) and several other health-related federal programs. Significant to patient safety is the decision by CMS to impose financial *disincentives* for selected unsafe patient care outcomes by refusing to pay for the extra cost of treatment to correct those outcomes. Conversely stated, the agency responsible for paying Medicare claims now provides a financial *incentive* for safe patient care.

Nonreimbursable claims most relevant to perioperative patient care include the following (CMS, 2012):
- Pressure ulcers, stages III and IV
- Falls and trauma
- Surgical site infections (SSIs) after bariatric surgery, certain orthopedic procedures, and coronary artery bypass surgery (mediastinitis)
- Vascular catheter-associated infections
- Catheter-associated urinary tract infections (CAUTIs)
- Administration of incompatible blood
- Air embolism
- Foreign objects unintentionally retained after surgery
- Wrong patient, wrong procedure, or wrong site surgeries
- Deep vein thrombosis (DVT)
- Pulmonary emboli associated with knee and hip replacements
- High readmission rates to facility within 30 days of discharge

CMS regularly reviews and adds conditions pursuant to its federal rule-making process (e.g., it added specific types of readmissions within 30 days of discharge, effective 2013).

CMS notes that it does not consider these listed patient safety concerns more important than others. Rather, it has chosen the selected concerns to emphasize that the facilities deemed responsible now must bear directly otherwise avoidable financial costs of insufficient patient safety controls. Furthermore, CMS regulations prohibit passing these costs on to patients. Most private insurance companies have adopted similar provisions. Thus from a purely risk management standpoint, in addition to potential indirect costs arising from negligence awards and settlements (which can be insured against), facilities now bear the risk of direct, uninsurable, and potentially severe cost disincentives if they fail to avoid the listed conditions though the institution of safe practices.

Agency for Healthcare Research and Quality (AHRQ). As one of the 12 agencies within DHHS, the AHRQ's mission is to improve the quality, safety, efficiency, and effectiveness of healthcare for all Americans. This agency is committed to improving care safety and quality by developing successful partnerships and generating the knowledge and tools required for long-term improvement. The central goal of its research is measurable improvements in healthcare in America. These measurable goals include improved quality of life and patient outcomes, lives saved, and value gained.

The overall focus of AHRQ activities is threefold:
- *Safety and quality:* reduce the risk of harm
- *Effectiveness:* improve healthcare outcomes by encouraging the use of evidence
- *Efficiency:* transform research into practice

This agency serves healthcare clinicians, facilities and systems, consumers, policymakers, purchasers and payers, and academic healthcare. AHRQ offers nurses and other providers extensive evidence-based resources related to patient safety on its website (ahrq.gov).

The World Health Organization

The United Nations (UN) created WHO to function as its health oversight and coordination authority for all UN member nations who in turn have joined WHO. In 2004, WHO launched the World Alliance on Patient Safety, by which it began to examine patient safety in acute as well as in primary care settings relevant to all WHO member nations. Its action initiatives include Clean Care is Safer Care and Safe Surgery Saves Lives. The focus of the Clean Care campaign is hand hygiene (also referenced in TJC's NPSGs); it resulted in release of a 2009 WHO guideline for surgical hand preparation (Evidence for Practice). Salient points in the guideline section titled Surgical Hand Preparation: State of the Art include discussion of the time required for preoperative hand antisepsis, encouragement of brushless hand scrubs, and review of antimicrobial hand scrub preparations.

WHO's Safe Surgery Saves Lives initiative led to publication of its Surgical Safety Checklist. Similar in content to TJC's Universal Protocol, the WHO checklist adds a third phase, the Sign Out that

---

▌EVIDENCE FOR PRACTICE

WHO Guidelines on Surgical Hand Hygiene

Steps before starting surgical hand antisepsis (scrub):

Key Steps
- Keep nails short and pay attention to them when washing your hands—most microbes on hands come from beneath the fingernails.
- Do not wear artificial nails or nail polish.
- Remove all jewelry (rings, watches, bracelets) before entering the OR.
- Wash hands and arms with a nonmedicated soap before entering the OR and/or if hands are visibly soiled.
- Clean under the nails with a nail file. Nail brushes should not be used because they may damage the skin and encourage shedding of cells. If used, nail brushes must be sterile and used once only (single use). Reusable nail brushes may be resterilized for each use.

Procedural Steps
- Start timing. Scrub each side of each finger, between the fingers, and the back and front of the hand for 2 minutes.
- Proceed to scrub the arms, keeping the hand higher than the arm at all times. This helps to avoid recontamination of the hands by water from the elbows and prevents bacteria-laden soap and water from contaminating the hands.
- Wash each side of the arm from wrist to elbow for 1 minute.
- Repeat the process on the other hand and arm, keeping hands above elbows at all times. If the hand touches anything at any time, the scrub must be lengthened by 1 minute for the area that has been contaminated.
- Rinse hands and arms by passing them through the water in one direction only, from fingertips to elbow. Do not move the arm back and forth through the water.
- Proceed to the OR holding hands above elbows.
- At all times during the scrub procedure, care should be taken not to splash water onto surgical attire.
- Once in the OR, hands and arms should be dried using a sterile towel and aseptic technique before donning gown and gloves.

WHO, World Health Organization.
Modified from *WHO guidelines on hand hygiene in health care,* available at http://whqlibdoc.who.int/publications/2009/9789241597906_eng.pdf. Accessed January 8, 2013.

includes team reviews of outcomes and concerns to be included in the handover (the international term for "hand-off") to postanesthesia recovery caregivers (Evidence for Practice). Haynes and colleagues (2009) hypothesized that implementation of the *WHO Surgical Safety Checklist* would reduce complications and deaths associated with surgery. They compared outcomes of surgical patients in eight countries representing widely diverse economic circumstances and patient populations, and found that a 1.5% prechecklist rate of death declined to 0.8% (p = 0.003) with use of the checklist. They also found inpatient complications occurred in 11% of patients before the checklist was implemented and in 7% after introduction of the checklist. They also confirmed tangible improvements in safety outcomes after implementation of the checklist (Haynes et al, 2009; 2011). Notable about WHO's entry into surgical patient safety is recognition that perioperative adverse events causing complications before, during, and after surgery is a *public health* problem worldwide.

The Association of periOperative Registered Nurses

For nearly 60 years AORN has addressed perioperative patient safety issues. It represents perioperative patients and perioperative nurses in multiple policy settings, collaborates with TJC, WHO, other nursing associations and surgical alliances, and many safety coalitions to formulate safety statements that directly affect perioperative patient care. AORN provides an array of standards, RPs, guidelines, publications, videos, and tool kits that specifically address patient safety from the perioperative team's point of view. Tool kits include subjects such as fire safety, correct site surgery, sharps safety, hand-off communications, safe patient handling, and cultural and human factors. RPs and tool kits are evidence based to the extent possible. These AORN undertakings aim to develop real-world strategies to implement perioperative patient care practices. Along with TJC and WHO recommendations, AORN recommendations should be reflected and adopted, to the extent possible, within institutional policies and procedures, and educational curricula.

Other Patient Safety Groups/Coalitions/Companies

Major professional associations representing other perioperative team members (e.g., American College of Surgeons [ACS], American Society of Anesthesiologists [ASA], American Association of Nurse Anesthetists [AANA], Association of Surgical Technologists [AST]) have also issued multiple position statements and clinical recommendations related to patient safety. Many of these are co-issued or mutually endorsed with AORN. This reflects the increasing systems approach to perioperative safety. Additionally, many coalitions with similar patient safety interests have emerged as not-for-profit entities to gather and disseminate data, guidelines, protocols, and goals. For-profit groups are also included in what now may fairly be called a "patient safety industry." (A partial listing of additional patient safety groups is noted in Box 2-1.)

Perioperative Nursing Safety Issues

Communication and Teamwork

Communication underpins many patient safety issues. Implementation of both the Universal Protocol and the WHO checklist requires enhanced communication within a culture of teamwork (discussed later) (Research Highlight). Hand-off/handover protocols have joined traditional clinical written documentation records to improve communication further in perioperative settings.

Research continues in the use of perioperative patient care checklists in a variety of settings and situations (Research Highlight).

Checklists and protocols alone, however, cannot enhance meaningful communication without an equal commitment to teamwork, trust, and respect. Ultimately, improved communication is imbedded in human factors, culture, and social systems, all of which are more complex than checklists, mnemonics, and acronyms (Bliss et al, 2012; de Vries et al, 2011).

Clinical Documentation

The written clinical record is the historical anchor of communicating perioperative patient information. Evidence suggests, however, that a written (or digital) record is inadequate as the sole perioperative communication tool. More enhanced communication initiatives such as safer surgery briefings and hand-offs now augment the written record. Nonetheless, whether documented on paper or digitally, the clinical record remains foundational in assuring a safer patient experience and provision of information to future care areas.

Facilities where operative and other invasive procedures occur maintain records of each operation that must comply with state and federal regulations as well as with accreditation requirements. Those operative records include preoperative diagnosis, surgery performed, a description of findings, specimens removed, postoperative diagnosis, and names of all individuals participating in intraoperative care. Additional key components include positioning and stabilizing devices, electrosurgical unit number and settings, medications, and evidence of ongoing assessment and additional actions taken (a sample intraoperative record is shown in Figure 2-1). The operative record is a permanent part of the patient's medical record. Note that nearly all components of perioperative clinical documentation relate directly or indirectly to patient safety and injury prevention.

RESEARCH HIGHLIGHT

Outcomes of Checklist with Team Training Use

The use of surgical safety checklists to reduce perioperative adverse events has steadily increased. Although results are very encouraging, to be effective the checklist fosters, but also requires improved teamwork and communication.

This study used the AORN comprehensive surgical checklist; training sessions based on the book *Crucial Conversations* and other communication theories; data from the American College of Surgeons (ACS) National Surgical Quality Improvement Program (NSCIP); and trained observers to assess checklist completion and team communication.

The study was a prospective cohort design. Three 60-minute team training sessions were held for surgical services staff. The sample consisted of high-risk adult general surgery procedures that required general, spinal, or epidural anesthesia, excluding trauma and transplant surgeries. The trained observers remained in the room for the entire surgical procedure. Control group data were from in the ACS NSCIP database.

This study demonstrated that the use of a comprehensive surgical safety checklist with implementation of structured team training sessions produced statistically significant reductions in 30-day morbidity among high-risk general surgery patients. The authors noted that team training allows the checklist to facilitate communication and prevents checklist completion from becoming a perceived administrative task.

Modified from Bliss LA et al: Thirty-day outcomes support implementation of a surgical safety checklist, J Am Coll Surg 215(6):766–776, 2012.

EVIDENCE FOR PRACTICE
Surgical Safety Checklist

Surgical Safety Checklist

World Health Organization | **Patient Safety**
A World Alliance for Safer Health Care

Before induction of anaesthesia

(with at least nurse and anaesthetist)

Has the patient confirmed his/her identity, site, procedure, and consent?
☐ Yes

Is the site marked?
☐ Yes
☐ Not applicable

Is the anaesthesia machine and medication check complete?
☐ Yes

Is the pulse oximeter on the patient and functioning?
☐ Yes

Does the patient have a:

Known allergy?
☐ No
☐ Yes

Difficult airway or aspiration risk?
☐ No
☐ Yes, and equipment/assistance available

Risk of >500ml blood loss (7ml/kg in children)?
☐ No
☐ Yes, and two IVs/central access and fluids planned

Before skin incision

(with nurse, anaesthetist and surgeon)

Confirm all team members have introduced themselves by name and role.

Confirm the patient's name, procedure, and where the incision will be made.

Has antibiotic prophylaxis been given within the last 60 minutes?
☐ Yes
☐ Not applicable

Anticipated Critical Events

To Surgeon:
☐ What are the critical or non-routine steps?
☐ How long will the case take?
☐ What is the anticipated blood loss?

To Anaesthetist:
☐ Are there any patient-specific concerns?

To Nursing Team:
☐ Has sterility (including indicator results) been confirmed?
☐ Are there equipment issues or any concerns?

Is essential imaging displayed?
☐ Yes
☐ Not applicable

Before patient leaves operating room

(with nurse, anaesthetist and surgeon)

Nurse Verbally Confirms:
☐ The name of the procedure
☐ Completion of instrument, sponge and needle counts
☐ Specimen labeling (read specimen labels aloud, including patient name)
☐ Whether there are any equipment problems to be addressed

To Surgeon, Anaesthetist and Nurse:
☐ What are the key concerns for recovery and management of this patient?

Revised 1 / 2009   © WHO, 2009

This checklist is not intended to be comprehensive. Additions and modifications to fit local practice are encouraged.

RESEARCH HIGHLIGHT

Checklists for Surgical Crisis Events

Efficacy of using surgical safety checklists has been well established. Data from this study suggest that checklist use may also improve adherence to lifesaving processes during OR patient crises such as cardiac arrest and massive hemorrhage. Although these do not occur frequently, estimated incidence of such events in a facility that does 10,000 procedures per year is 146 OR-related crises annually.

Arriaga and colleagues used a simulated OR to investigate using checklists to improve crisis event management. Seventeen OR teams were exposed to106 simulated intraoperative crises (e.g., air embolism, cardiac arrest, anaphylaxis). They measured whether the teams adhered to 47 key lifesaving processes with and without checklist use.

Each crisis was taped via multiscreen, synchronized videography. Interrater reliability was established and all videos were then reviewed.

Teams using checklists had nearly a 75% reduction in failure to adhere to critical steps in management of the simulated surgical crisis (6% missed with checklists; 23% without checklist use). The authors conclude that hospitals and ambulatory surgery centers should consider checklist implementation for common OR patient crises.

Modified from Arriaga AF et al: Simulation based trial of surgical-crisis checklists, *N Engl J Med* 368:246–253, 2013.

Proper perioperative nursing documentation describes assessment, planning, and implementation of perioperative patient care reflecting individualization of care and evaluation of patient outcomes. Any and every unusual or significant incident pertinent to patient outcomes must be documented as well as all remediation efforts related to the patient's care. The facility's risk manager may require additional documentation. Only objective information directly related to the specific patient is included in the patient's record (e.g., it is inappropriate to record personal opinions or to describe circumstances surrounding an event except as they appear to affect the patient directly).

Thoughtfully designed perioperative nursing documentation tools include defined elements in a format to minimize time needed for the documentation process (e.g., checklists). Ideally, collaboration with preoperative, postanesthesia care unit (PACU), and postoperative nursing units will produce one documentation tool used across all areas, avoiding duplication of patient data by different nursing staff. Increasingly, settings where operative and other invasive procedures are performed use electronic records to enter and track patient care information. Coordination of the content included in the intraoperative record with that in the surgeon's and anesthesia provider's intraoperative content can reduce documentation time and provide a more integrated record that streamlines workflow and reduces documentation errors.

Documentation of perioperative patient care in the clinical record simultaneously serves risk management functions. Documentation requirements serve as reminders of actions needed to provide safe care, thus prompting risk reduction strategies and preventing injury. Information in the clinical record also enhances continuity of care, thus reducing future injury. If a patient injury does occur, documentation that preventive measures or other actions to mitigate risks were taken may lessen the likelihood of a successful lawsuit.

Hand-offs/Handovers

As noted, written documentation alone, however crucial, is insufficient to ensure patient safety as care responsibility passes from one team or individual caregiver to another. As they reviewed the evidence related to hand-offs, Friesen and colleagues (2008) defined the transfer of information and responsibility for care of the patient from one provider to another as a hand-off or (internationally) handover. Standardized approaches to hand-off communication further reduce risk for error.

TJC, AORN, and WHO uniformly recommend that time-outs (or "safer surgery briefings"), as well as pre- and postoperative hand-offs, be formalized. In healthcare settings, occasions for transfer-of-care processes, such as hand-offs, include nursing shift changes, temporary relief or coverage, nursing and physician hand-offs from one department to another, various other transfers of information in inpatient settings, and interhospital transfers. The purpose of hand-off communication and reports is to provide essential, up-to-date, and specific information about the patient. Standardized hand-off communication must include an opportunity to ask and respond to questions. For examples of strategies to assist in effective and efficient hand-off communication and reports, see the Patient Safety box on page 28.

Amato-Vealey and colleagues (2008) identified and further developed elements of effective hand-off communication for use at each perioperative hand-off stage, using the SBAR mnemonic (Situation, Background, Assessment, Recommendation). For identification of critical elements for hand-offs from preoperative to intraoperative, see Box 2-2; for hand-offs intraoperatively between scrub persons, see Box 2-3; and for hand-offs from intraoperative to PACU or another postanesthesia recovery area, see Box 2-4.

Like advancements in other segments of perioperative safety, communication, although improved, remains developmentally in process. Healy and associates (2012) argue that a new view of communication is needed to improve perioperative safety. They describe reengineering the system of communication for safety that includes not only immediate informational needs, but also an account of the broader ergonomic and human factors that shape improved communication (Shouhed et al, 2012).

Wrong Site, Person, or Procedure Surgery

Surgery that is the wrong procedure or surgery performed on the wrong site or person includes any operative or other invasive procedure performed on the wrong patient, wrong body part, wrong side of the body, or at the wrong level of the otherwise correctly identified anatomic structure, such as in spinal surgery. Evidence shows that wrong site surgery can not only devastate the patient and family but also negatively affect the entire perioperative team including the facility itself (Mulloy and Hughes, 2008). All institutions accredited by TJC must comply with the Universal Protocol found at TJC's NPSG at UP.01.01.01 Conduct a preprocedure verification process; UP.01.02.01 Mark the procedure site; and UP.01.03.01 A time-out is performed before the procedure begins.

- *Preoperative verification process* ensures that all relevant documents (e.g., the history and physical examination, surgical consent, required laboratory studies) and imaging studies (properly labeled and displayed) are available before the start of the procedure. Preprocedure verification is best conducted when the patient can be involved and should be complete before the patient leaves the preprocedure area. The surgical team must

Text continued on p. 29

Instruction:
To be completed by RN.   Page 1 of 3

CASE PARTICIPANTS	
Attending surgeon:	Resident:
Attending surgeon:	Resident:
Attending surgeon:	Resident:
Assistant:	Assistant:
Anesthesiologist:	Anesthetist:
Perfusionist:	Autotransfusionist:
X-Ray tech:	Laser operator:
Circulating nurse:	Scrub person:
Circ relief: Time in: Out:	Scrub relief: Time in: Out:
Circ relief: Time in: Out:	Scrub relief: Time in: Out:
Circ relief: Time in: Out:	Scrub relief: Time in: Out:
Other/observer:	Other/observer:

CASE TIMES

Patient in O.R.: _____ Anesthesia induction: _____ Incision/start: _____ Closure/end: _____ Patient out: _____

Recovery in O.R. Start: _____   Recovery in O.R. Stop: _____

ARRIVAL TO O.R.

Via: ☐ Ambulatory ☐ Stretcher ☐ Patient bed ☐ Other: _____ ☐ Personal items to O.R.: _____

Pre-op skin condition: ☐ Dry and intact ☐ Other: _____

Safety strap applied ☐ Abdomen ☐ Thighs ☐ Other: _____

PLAN OF CARE

☐ Allergies verified ☐ Perioperative history and assessment reviewed ☐ Standard plan of care implemented

Plan of care exceptions: ☐ Latex precautions ☐ Contact precautions ☐ Airborne precautions ☐ Droplet precautions

☐ Other: _____

PATIENT POSITIONING

Body position: ☐ Supine ☐ Prone ☐ Lithotomy ☐ Sitting ☐ Lateral right side up ☐ Lateral left side up

            ☐ Other: _____

LEFT arm: ☐ Board ☐ Side ☐ Chest ☐ Arm holder   RIGHT arm: ☐ Board ☐ Side ☐ Chest ☐ Arm holder

Traction weight_____lbs. ☐ Positioned by self ☐ Positioned by (initial):_____

Positioning device/site:

☐ Andrews bed ☐ Axillary roll ☐ Donut ☐ Fracture table ☐ Gel pads ☐ Hall Relton frame ☐ Jackson table

☐ Mayfield headrest ☐ McGuire positioner ☐ LamiRolls ☐ Stirrups ☐ Stryker frame ☐ VacPac

☐ Other/Comments: _____

INTERMITTENT COMPRESSION DEVICES	☐ N/A

Serial #:_____   Setting:_____mmHg   ☐ To O.R. with compression device on

Device type: ☐ Calf ☐ Thigh ☐ Bilateral ☐ Left ☐ Right   Applied by (initial):_____

SKIN PREP	☐ N/A

Hair removal method: ☐ None ☐ Dry clip ☐ Dry shave ☐ Wet clip ☐ Wet shave   Hair removed by (initial):_____

In O.R. Pre-op scrub: ☐ Betadine scrub ☐ Chlorhexidine ☐ Other: _____

Prep agent: ☐ Betadine ☐ Chloraprep ☐ Other: _____

22280 S(15730)(0808)C

FIGURE 2-1 Sample intraoperative report.

Continued

CATHETERS, DRAINS, TUBES	☐ N/A

Catheter/drain description: _____ ☐ Straight catheter

Location: _____ Collection device: _____

Balloon fill amount: _____ Inserted by (initial): _____ Date: _____ Time: _____

Drainage description: _____

☐ Present on arrival ☐ Removed at end of case

ESU/OTHER EQUIPMENT	☐ N/A

Type: ☐ Monopolar ☐ Other: _____ Serial #: _____ Settings: _____ Cut _____ Coag

    Grounding pad site: _____ Applied by (initial): _____

    ☐ Bipolar ☐ Tripolar   Serial #: _____ Setting: _____ Coag

    ☐ Argon beam coagulator   Serial #: _____ Beam Setting: _____

TOURNIQUET #1	☐ N/A

Tourniquet side: ☐ Left ☐ Right   Site: ☐ Thigh ☐ Calf ☐ Upper arm ☐ Forearm ☐ Ankle

Pressure _____ mmHg Time inflated: _____ Deflated: _____ Time inflated: _____ Deflated: _____

Pressure _____ mmHg Time inflated: _____ Deflated: _____ Time inflated: _____ Deflated: _____

Applied by (initial): _____ Serial #: _____ ☐ Tourniquet applied but not inflated

TOURNIQUET #2	☐ N/A

Tourniquet side: ☐ Left ☐ Right   Site: ☐ Thigh ☐ Calf ☐ Upper arm ☐ Forearm ☐ Ankle

Pressure _____ mmHg Time inflated: _____ Deflated: _____ Time inflated: _____ Deflated: _____

Pressure _____ mmHg Time inflated: _____ Deflated: _____ Time inflated: _____ Deflated: _____

Applied by (initial): _____ Serial #: _____ ☐ Tourniquet applied but not inflated

EXPLANTS	☐ N/A

Explant description: _____

LASER DATA	☐ N/A

Laser type/model/serial #: _____ Laser time: _____ ☐ Standby

X-RAYS and IMAGES	☐ N/A

Type: ☐ Angiography ☐ Flat plate ☐ Fluoroscan/self image ☐ Fluoroscopy

CELLSAVER	☐ N/A

☐ Used

GENERAL CASE DATA

O.R.: _____ ☐ ASA class: _____ ☐ Return to O.R. ☐ See implant record

Pre-op diagnosis: _____

Post-op diagnosis: _____ ☐ Same as Pre-op

SURGICAL PROCEDURE

Procedure performed: _____

_____

_____

_____

Anesthesia type: ☐ General ☐ M.A.C. ☐ Spinal ☐ Block (type) _____ ☐ Epidural ☐ Local

Wound class: ☐ 1 ☐ 2 ☐ 3 ☐ 4

FIGURE 2-1, cont'd Sample intraoperative report.

Continued

MEDICATIONS					☐ N/A
Medication	Dose	Route	Given by (Initial)	Date	Time

Hemostatic agents: _____

IRRIGATION			☐ N/A
Irrigation	Additives	Estimated In	Estimated Out

FAMILY COMMUNICATION   ☐ N/A

☐ By Phone ☐ In person Communicated to: _____

Communicated by (initial): _____ Date: _____ Time: _____

SPECIMENS/CULTURES

Number of specimen: Tissue:_____ Frozen section:_____ Culture:_____ Fluid:_____ Foreign body:_____ ☐ None

Examined and disposed per Dr. (Print Name):_____

Skin/bone freezer: Description:_____

PACKING   ☐ N/A

Packing type:_____ Packing site: _____

DEPARTURE FROM O.R.

Post-op skin condition excluding operative site: ☐ Dry and intact ☐ Unchanged ☐ Other, description:_____

Via: ☐ Ambulatory ☐ Bed ☐ Crib ☐ ICU bed ☐ Post-op chair ☐ Stretcher ☐ Surgilifter ☐ Other:_____

Destination: ☐ PACU☐ PACU Phase I ☐ PACU Phase II ☐ Home ☐ Other:_____

Dressings:_____

COMMENTS

Abbreviations:
ASA–American Society of Anesthesiology   Coag–Coagulation   M.A.C.–Monitored Anesthesia Care   O.R.–Operating Room
Circ–Circulator   ESU–Electrosurgical Unit   Op–Operative   PACU–Post Anesthesia Care Unit

Initial	Signature/Title	Print Name	Initial	Signature/Title	Print Name

FIGURE 2-1, cont'd Sample intraoperative report.

PATIENT SAFETY

Strategies to Assist in Effective Hand-off Communication

1. *Use clear language.* Avoid unclear or potentially confusing terms. When appropriate, define the terms you are using. Use only approved abbreviations and avoid jargon that could be misinterpreted.
2. *Incorporate effective communication techniques* such as the SBAR technique (situation, background, assessment, and recommendations), MAPS (medications, allergies, procedure/pertinent information, special needs), or other mnemonic or acronym to facilitate sequence and type of information. Limit interruptions and distractions (consider a "no interruption zone" or "protected hour"), focus on information being exchanged, and allocate sufficient time to this important task. Keep the report patient-centered, and avoid irrelevant details. Use read-back, report-back, or check-back techniques to ensure common understanding about information exchanged. There must be an opportunity for each caregiver to ask and respond to questions.
3. *Standardize shift-to-shift and caregiver-to-caregiver (relief) reporting.* A consistent format increases the information staff members accurately record and improves their ability to plan patient care. Keep reports concise and accurate.
4. *Standardize perioperative nursing reports to the perianesthesia care unit (PACU) or postoperative ambulatory surgery units.* Consider essential information such as reporting the procedure done, duration (and whether longer or shorter than expected), complexity of the procedure (greater than, less than, or as expected), whether there were events or deviations from the expected course, implants, medications administered, current status of vital signs (including temperature and warming methods used), pulses, incision/dressings/drains, estimated blood loss, blood/blood products/fluids administered, and urinary output.
5. *Use technology.* Communication systems that transmit information across settings and providers improve consistency and coordination. Automated electronic perioperative records can facilitate transitions by providing consistent, accessible information about surgical patients and their care in the OR. Staff members should be able to access readily essential components of care, such as whether a newly ordered medication was administered, whether laboratory studies were done, or if a do not resuscitate (DNR) order is in place.

Modified from DeJohn P: ASCs take steps to improve handoffs, *OR Manager* 25(1):26–27, 29, 2009; Lewis TP et al: Tips to reduce dangerous interruptions by healthcare staff, *Nursing 2012* 42(11):65–67, 2012; Ortega L, Parsh B: Improving change-of-shift report, *Nursing* 43(2):68, 2013.

BOX 2-2

Elements of the Preoperative to Intraoperative Hand-off Communication Using SBAR

Situation
- Name of patient and date of birth
- Name of operative or invasive procedure to be performed, including modifiers and site
- Pertinent documents present and consistent

Background
- Elements of patient history pertinent to surgery
- Medical clearance
- Patient allergies and nothing per mouth (NPO) status
- Patient's vital signs and pain level
- Medication profile and medications taken today
- Specific laboratory results
- Code status of patient

Assessment
- Patient's current level of understanding of the surgery
- Special patient needs or precautions
- Pertinent aspects of the patient's emotional and spiritual status
- Pertinent cultural implications
- Anesthesia requests

Recommendations
- State whether the patient has been seen preoperatively by the surgeon and anesthesia care provider.
- Determine whether the patient is ready for surgery.
- Allow an opportunity for preoperative and intraoperative staff members to ask questions or voice concerns.

From Amato-Vealey EJ et al: Hand-off communication: a requisite for patient safety, *AORN J* 88(5):766, 2008.

BOX 2-3

Elements of the Intraoperative Hand-off Communication Between Scrub Persons Using SBAR

Situation
- Name of patient
- Name of procedure being performed
- Pertinent information about the procedure (what is the progress of the surgery, have any additional/different surgical procedures been discussed?)

Background
- Elements of patient history pertinent to surgery (e.g., allergies)
- Who are the members of the surgical team (names, roles)?
- Special instruments, suture, other items being used
- What is the blood loss and will hemostatic adjuncts be needed?
- What medications and fluids are on the sterile field (review each label together quietly)?
- Specifics about any equipment issues/special needs/back table and Mayo setup

Assessment
- What is the status of specimens?
- Have any counts been done? Which ones? Do a transfer of care count together quietly.
- What is the anticipated amount of time remaining in the procedure?
- Have any complications been discussed/anticipated?
- Have there been any problems with anesthesia?

Recommendations
- Note any special requests for closure/dressings/drains noted by the surgical team or special requests noted by the anesthesia provider.
- Prepare to introduce the relief scrub person.
- Allow an opportunity for relief scrub person to ask questions or voice concerns prior to "breaking scrub" by person being relieved.

BOX 2-4

Elements of the Intraoperative to PACU Hand-off Communication Using SBAR

Situation
- Name of patient and date of birth
- Full name of operative or invasive procedure performed, including modifiers and site

Background
- Type of anesthesia administered and name of anesthesia care provider
- Intraoperative medications administered, including dose and time
- IV fluids administered
- Estimated blood and urine loss
- Pertinent information related to the surgical site such as dressings, tubes, drains, or packing
- Any significant OR events

Assessment
- Hemodynamic stability
- Airway and oxygenation status
- Thermal status (e.g., presence of hypothermia or hyperthermia)
- Urine output
- Presence or absence of surgical complications
- Level of pain
- Method of pain management

Recommendations
- Assist with transfer of lines and equipment.
- Ensure that immediate postoperative orders have been completed.
- Discharge from the PACU when stable.
- Allow opportunity for intraoperative and PACU staff members to ask questions or voice concerns, especially when equipment and information hand-off occur simultaneously.

PACU, Perianesthesia care unit.
From Amato-Vealey EJ et al: Hand-off communication: a requisite for patient safety, *AORN J* 88(5):766, 2008; van Rensen et al: Multitasking during patient handover in the recovery room, *Anesth Analg* 15(6):1183–1187, 2012.

---

agree that this is the correct patient and the planned procedure on the specified side and site. The preprocedure verification process also includes confirming availability of necessary equipment, which is reconfirmed during the time-out.

- *Marking the surgical site* must occur so that the intended site of incision or insertion is clear and unambiguous. Procedures that involve left/right distinction, multiple structures, or multiple levels (spinal surgery) require specific marking. The marking also must be unambiguous; initials, a "yes," or a line at or near the incision site are all acceptable. The marking methodology should be consistently used throughout the facility. The person performing the procedure, who is accountable for it, and who will be present when the procedure is performed, must personally mark the site, and the patient should be involved in the marking if possible. The markings must remain visible after the patient has been prepped and draped. Facilities should have a provision in place for patients who refuse site marking.
- *Taking the time-out.* Facilities must have a procedure to implement the time-out before starting the procedure or making the surgical incision. The surgeon or other physician who is conducting the procedure must be present for the time-out. If separate teams are to perform distinct segments of a multiple

procedure surgery, there must be a time-out *before each procedure.* This does not apply to patients in whom the same surgical team is performing multiple aspects of a single procedure. Specific situations requiring two time-outs are those in which hospital policy or law/regulation requires two separate consents (e.g., for a cesarean section followed by a tubal ligation). During the time-out, active involvement and communication among all surgical team members is expected while all participants confirm and agree that they have the correct patient, correct side and site, and the correct procedure to be performed. Many facility procedures include verification that the patient is in the correct position and that any needed equipment, supplies, or implants are correct and available, and sterile if indicated; the presence and review of relevant imaging studies; and that all prep solutions have dried to minimize surgical fire risks.

Since establishment of the Universal Protocol and WHO's Safe Surgery Saves Lives Checklist, the professional literature has asserted wide acceptance and general success in reducing errors (Haynes et al, 2011). Reducing errors does serve to reduce 30-day mortality (van Klei et al, 2012), but the authors caution that "the effect depended crucially on checklist compliance" (p. 49). Other articles have also identified barriers to implementation acceptance and a need for a broader systems approach if the checklist is to achieve its desired potential (e.g., Fourcade et al, 2012; McNamara, 2012; Walker et al, 2012). Increasingly comprehensive safety systems depend on compliance for effectiveness (Brooke et al, 2012). Unanticipated positive consequences have emerged from the implementation of checklists during surgery, such as reduction in conversion rates from laparoscopic cholecystectomy to open procedures (Robb et al, 2012) and the potential for reduced malpractice claims (de Vries et al, 2011) (Research Highlight).

Retained Surgical Items

RSIs are a concern of AORN, TJC, WHO, and all facilities where surgery is performed. Although clinically different, wrong-site surgery and RSIs are similar from safety and risk management perspectives. They both also share top positions in TJC's top 10 annual sentinel events. The physiologic, financial, and public relations consequences from both wrong-site surgery and RSIs are potentially severe. In ORs, conducting count processes according to evidence-based policies (audible, visual, and concurrent) are considered a key risk reduction and patient safety strategy (Grant-Orser, 2012).

Soft goods such as surgical sponges are one of the most frequent inadvertently retained items (Martindell, 2012). Moreover, in about 80% of retained sponge cases, counts were reported as "correct" at the conclusion of the procedure (Gibbs, 2011). Physiologic consequences of an RSI include possible infection, obstruction, fistula formation, perforation or consequent pain, suffering and possible death, and the likely need for additional surgery.

A voluntary national surgical patient safety initiative, NoThing Left Behind, investigated why RSIs continue and attempted to develop practices to reduce their persistence. Participating facilities aggregated data related to RSIs. Analysis revealed that the attribution of increased retention risk to patient or procedure characteristics such as those described by Rowlands (2012) (e.g., obesity, complexity of procedure, increased number of personnel emergencies) only partially explained incorrect surgical counts. Gibbs (2011) concludes that the OR culture and environment in which the patient has the procedure is also a major risk determinant. Thus prevention of RSIs, once thought of as a straightforward matter of counting to 10, has joined the human factors/systems analysis research cadre that focuses on perioperative patient safety issues. Gibbs also urges a greater effort at a common nomenclature that includes replacing the word "count" with "account" to more accurately reflect the complexity of the process.

RESEARCH HIGHLIGHT ▐▐

The Malpractice Claim Cost of "Never Events" That Do Occur

Despite emphases on controlling costs and avoiding never events, little is known about costs of never events and their nonfinancial effects on patients and families or the characteristics of providers involved. Researchers used the National Practitioner Data Bank to identify malpractice settlements and judgments against surgery and anesthesia providers of surgical never events that occurred from 1999 to 2010 (dentists, nurses, pharmacists, and social workers were excluded). They identified 9744 paid malpractice reports with a mean payment of $133,055 and the highest payment of $7,082,528. The highest median payment was associated with wrong procedure events and the lowest was for retained surgical items. The total costs were estimated at $1.3 billion, without including legal fees, additional inpatient costs (not paid by CMS or many insurance providers), disability care, lost workdays, or harm to provider reputation.

Data revealed that 6.6% of the events resulted in patient mortality. Data also suggested there may be individual provider factors involved because 12.4% of the physicians involved had claims for more than one never event.

The authors recognize that several national and local programs have been initiated to reduce frequency of surgical never events including TJC, CMS, and the NQF as well as those initiated in individual facilities and systems. Yet surgical never events still occur, emphasizing the need to monitor patterns of these errors better and identify effective approaches to eliminating them.

CMS, Centers for Medicare & Medicaid Services; *NQF,* National Quality Forum; *TJC,* The Joint Commission.

Modified from Mehtsen W et al: Surgical never events in the United States, *Surgery* 153(4):465–472, 2013.

As noted, CMS and many private insurers now refuse payment for remedial treatment such as otherwise unnecessary surgery to remove a sponge or to treat the physiologic consequences of its inadvertent retention. The healthcare facility must absorb the costs of extended hospitalization and required corrective treatment; it also may be deemed responsible for the entire cost of care for patients whose condition requires readmission within 30 days of discharge. Additional financial losses may arise from defending any resultant malpractice litigation, impaired public reputation, and the need to respond to licensing and regulatory body inquiries.

Prevention of RSIs. Facilities should have an established system to prevent RSIs that reflects AORN's *RP for Prevention of Retained Surgical Items* (AORN, 2013). Key components of that RP appear in the Patient Safety box below, as does the sample count record in Figure 2-2. The policy should also incorporate human factors and keep interruptions, distractions, and repetition-induced attention deficits to their minimum (Coiera, 2012).

Two persons counting aloud, combined with the surgeon's manual exploration and the scrub person's mental tracking of sponges and other counted objects in the wound (situational awareness), have long been mainstay approaches to prevent RSIs. Situational awareness may be defined as the perioperative nurse's and scrub person's perception of relevant clinical cues in the count environment, their comprehension of the importance of those cues, and their identification of required interventions based on those cues (Sitterding et al, 2012). New sponge-tracking technologies have emerged to enhance risk reduction strategies to prevent inadvertent retention of RSIs. These include sequentially numbered sponges, bar coding, and radiofrequency identification (RFID) products (Goldberg and Feldman, 2012).

Typically, sequentially numbered sponge products are prepackaged, presterilized sponges in groups of 5 or 10 in sequentially numbered packages. When using such numbered systems, surgical teams are more likely to detect a missing/retained sponge because they must account for each numbered, individual sponge rather than account simply for an aggregate number. The usual tenets of

---

PATIENT SAFETY

Key Components of Counts to Prevent Retained Surgical Items (RSIs)

Research indicates that a discrepancy of a count at any time during a surgical procedure is a safety variance associated with elevated RSI risk. Counts of soft goods such as radiopaque sponges, sharps, and instruments should be performed, reported to the surgical team at each count in step 4, below, and recorded:

1. Before the procedure to establish the baseline number of soft goods, sharps, and instruments
2. When new items are added to the field
3. At time of permanent relief of either the scrub person or the circulator (although items within the body cavity may not be directly visible)
4. When cavity (e.g., heart, uterus, peritoneum) closure begins; when final closure begins; and at end of procedure when counted items no longer used. As the first layer of closure begins, the scrub person and circulating nurse count all items consecutively in a standardized routine such as proceeding from sterile field to Mayo stand to back table and then off the field, or vice versa. The count is done audibly, visibly, and concurrently. This is referred to as the "second" count.
5. At time of instrument assembly for sterilization

Methods
- Items should be counted audibly and viewed concurrently by two people, one of whom is the circulating nurse for each count.
- The circulating nurse informs the surgeon of the results of the closing counts.
- Individual pieces of assembled units should be accounted for separately; account for all pieces of a broken item.
- Preprinted sheets/preformatted screens should be used to record the counts.
- To the extent possible, procedure setup should be standardized with the minimum number of counted items needed.

Modified from AORN: Recommended practices for prevention of retained surgical items. In *Perioperative standards and recommended practices,* 2013, Denver, The Association; Stawicki SPA et al: Retained surgical items: a problem yet to be solved, *J Am Coll Surg* 216(1):15–22, 2013.

Purpose: To document sponge, sharps and instrument counts for invasive procedures.

Date: _____

COUNTS	BASELINE	CAVITY IN CAVITY	BEFORE WOUND CLOSURE	FINAL - SKIN CLOSURE	PERMANENT RELIEF	TEMPORARY RELIEF
Time:						
Sponges						
Sharps						
Miscellaneous items						
Instruments						
Circulator initials:						
Scrub initials:						

FINAL COUNT

Sponges	☐ Correct	☐ Correct with packed sponges		☐ Unresolved
Sharps	☐ Correct	☐ N/A		☐ Unresolved
Miscellaneous items	☐ Correct			☐ Unresolved
Instruments	☐ Correct	☐ Correct with packed instruments		☐ Unresolved

CORRECT WITH INTENTIONALLY PACKED SPONGES/INSTRUMENTS

Wound was packet with: _____   _____
                    (number)   (name of item)

Packing communication log initiated: ☐ Yes   **Purple arm band applied:** ☐ Yes   _____ (RN initials)

UNRESOLVED COUNT

Name of unresolved item: _____

☐ Physician notified: _____
                                 (name of physician)

X-ray taken: ☐ Yes ☐ No, reason: _____   _____ (RN initials)

Initial	Signature/Title	Print Name	Initial	Signature/Title	Print Name

Instructions:
1. To be completed by RN assigned to the procedure.
2. Record sponge, sharps, and miscellaneous items on dry erase board per policy.
3. Instruments are counted and recorded on the inventory list. If baseline instrument count is not indicated per the policy, document N/A (not applicable).
4. Record the time each count is performed in the appropriate column.
5. Initials and signatures are required for the RN and scrub person that performed each count.
6. Permanent relief is an RN and/or scrub person that provides relief for the circulating RN or scrub person for the remainder of the procedure or until the next shift. A complete sponge, sharps, miscellaneous item, and instrument count is required for permanent relief.
7. Temporary relief is an RN and/or scrub person that provides relief for the circulating RN or scrub person for lunch relief/break. A sponge, sharps, and miscellaneous item count is required.
8. RN performing final count will check appropriate boxes:
   - Correct
   - Unresolved
   - N/A when applicable

FIGURE 2-2 Count record.

counting remain: counts are performed *audibly, concurrently, and visibly.* Count policies and practices in the institution should be standardized with little variability among staff members (Edel, 2012). Distractions are minimized; some institutions take a "pause for the cause" while counts are in progress.

RFID and bar-code technologies are also incorporated into equipment to prevent RSIs. RFID systems tag instruments, soft goods such as sponges, and other items likely to enter the body during a procedure and use a scanning wand through tissues to ascertain the location of these items before the procedure ends. Bar-code scanning systems require the scanning of items as a procedure begins and/or as they are put into the body and again as they are removed from the body and/or as a procedure ends.

Other technologic approaches will continue to emerge. No matter which RSI prevention system a facility adopts, none is a cure-all or infallible. All technologies require precise use, as designed and in accordance with the manufacturer's instructions. As with any new technology or approach, all team members must be alert to possible unintended consequences of its use (e.g., electrical interference with other equipment or overreliance on the additional margin of safety provided by an approach, which may lead to less vigilance).

Incorrect Counts. An "incorrect" or unreconciled count occurs when the number of items on the count record or worksheet fails to match the number of items recovered during a closing count. All incorrect closure counts must be reported immediately, and attempts made to resolve every discrepancy. If a count remains unresolved, the circulating nurse must again notify the surgeon of the unresolved count, and a search must be made for the missing item, including the surgical wound, field, floor, linen, and trash (this is the rationale that linen and trash must not leave the OR until the end of the procedure). All personnel must direct their immediate attention to locating the missing item. If it is not found, an x-ray film may be taken and read by the radiologist or surgeon as specified in institutional policy. If the x-ray is negative, the count is recorded as incorrect or unreconciled and the x-ray results noted on the patient's intraoperative record. An incident/occurrence/event report should be initiated according to institution policy. Accurate counting and recording of soft goods, sharps, and instruments are essential for the protection of the patient, personnel, and the institution, and are integral to effective risk management.

Care and Handling of Specimens

During the many years perioperative patient care has included safe handling of surgical specimens, laboratory medicine's safety practices focused on the analysis of the surgical specimen. The WHO World Alliance on Patient Safety now recognizes that to improve patient safety further in laboratory medicine, the pre- and postanalytic stages are equally important. As with checklists and communication, this WHO initiative urges adoption of requirements for multidisciplinary, multistage, and multisystem approaches (McCoy et al, 2009). Like other areas of patient safety, laboratory errors occur more frequently than commonly believed (Zarbo, 2009). Bixenstine and colleagues (2013) found specimen errors in 2.9% of cases they reviewed. The errors included problems with specimen containers (1.2% of containers with errors) and specimen requisitions (2.3% of requisitions with errors). Their analysis of errors only included specimens before they reached the pathology laboratory (from the OR to pathology). There is a wide potential for errors in surgical specimens, including unlabeled specimens, empty

containers, incorrect side designation (called wrong "laterality"), incorrect or no identified tissue site, or incorrect or no patient names. As with preventing RSIs, technologies such as bar coding and RFID chips methods may reduce the frequency of specimen labeling errors (Layfield and Anderson, 2010).

TJC addresses specimen handling in the *2013 National Patient Safety Goals,* requiring use of at least two patient identifiers when collecting specimens for clinical testing. It also requires action to improve timeliness of reporting critical laboratory results. Accurate and timely communication and delivery of specimens are presumptively necessary in timely reporting of results. The care and handling of specimens raise considerations unique to perioperative settings, and again AORN's *RPs for Care and Handling of Specimens in the Perioperative Environment* provides the best guidance. (The Patient Safety box on page 33 summarizes key points in safe specimen care and handling.)

Proper management of specimens is critical to the outcome of a patient's surgery. It is the responsibility of the surgical team to identify, document, and care properly for specimens. Common specimens include blood, soft tissue, bone, body fluids, and removed foreign bodies. Complete and accurate identification and labeling of specimens and timely delivery to the proper laboratory for analysis are imperative. A mislabeled specimen may result in misdiagnosis and consequently inappropriate treatment of the patient. At a minimum, each specimen must bear a label with the correct patient name and identification number, specific origin of the specimen, and laterality (e.g., Jane Doe, 100001, right breast biopsy). The surgeon should provide descriptive information about the specimen (e.g., "suture tag at 6 o'clock"). The nurse should "repeat back" to the surgeon information being sent to the laboratory (e.g., patient name, type of specimen, source/location, required tests, special handling needs). All specimens and their disposition must be documented in the patient's intraoperative record.

Handling of each specimen occurs according to specific protocols established by the receiving laboratory. Generally the surgical team handles all tissue in order to preserve its integrity, keeping specimens moist and transporting them to the laboratory as soon as possible. Standard transmission-based precautions govern specimen transport to protect individuals who must handle the specimen (see Chapter 4). Labels should identify the need for precautions and the presence of biohazardous material. Formalin is frequently used to preserve specimens if they are not taken to the laboratory immediately. It is a hazardous substance that can cause watery eyes and respiratory irritation. Direct contact will injure human tissue. Gloves must be worn and adequate ventilation provided in areas where formalin is handled. Institutional policy should describe procedures to follow in case of spills.

Specimens for Frozen Section. When immediate tissue identification or identification of malignancy is needed, specimens are quick-frozen, sliced, stained, and examined in the laboratory under a microscope. This method of tissue examination is called *frozen section.* Specimens for frozen section usually are placed on moistened Telfa or into a dry covered specimen container to prevent drying. They are *never* placed in saline solution or formalin *nor are they ever* transported on a counted sponge. The results of frozen-section analysis are communicated to the surgeon intraoperatively. If the hospital has no system for direct pathologist-surgeon communication, the perioperative nurse receives the telephone report of a frozen section. Because this is considered an especially critical test result, the nurse "reads back" the test result to the pathologist

PATIENT SAFETY

Key Points in Handling Specimens in the Perioperative Environment

1. Assessment of specimen collecting and handling needs begins when the procedure is scheduled. The perioperative nurse and surgeon should discuss specimen information such as anticipated specimens, particular needs, specific information that needs to be communicated to pathology, and specimen identifiers (improve the communication loop).
2. Procedures for correct patient and specimen identification should include consistent and accurate information on labels and forms. Specimen labels should include at least two identifiers.
3. Communication begins with the surgeon and follows this pathway:
   - The surgeon hands a specimen to the scrub person and tells him/her what the specimen is, what process is needed in the lab, and whether there are any special labeling needs or information to include on the requisition slip for the pathology lab.
   - The scrub person hands off the specimen to the circulating nurse, repeating what the surgeon said.
   - The circulating nurse receives the specimen, places it in the container, and labels the specimen container according to information provided by the surgeon and scrub person, repeating back the label information.
   - The circulating nurse completes the necessary lab requisition and follows institution-prescribed steps for sending the specimen to the lab.
   - During the debriefing at procedure end, the circulating nurse announces all specimens obtained; if no specimens were obtained, that is also announced.
4. Institute methods to prevent transmissible infection/contamination of personnel and specimens including the proper use of preservatives/solutions as well as use of tight, appropriate sized lids for specimen containers.
5. Forensic specimens may require unique handling to preserve the chain of evidence.

Modified from Minato H: Rinsho byori, *Jpn J Clin Pathol* 59(3):299–304, 2011; Raising the bar for safety in the handling of surgical specimens, *OR Manager* 28(8), 2012, available at www.ormanager.com/2012/08/01/raising-the-bar-for-safety-in-the-handling-of-surgical-specimens/ (subscription required). Accessed February 11, 2013; Steelman VM: *Three top emerging patient safety issues*, 2012, available at aorn.org/News.aspx?id=22778&terms=surgical%20specimens. Accessed January 7, 2013.

and surgeon and receives a repeat-back from the pathologist and surgeon to verify accurate communication of the results.

Risks for Burns: Electrical and Light

Electrical hazards in the OR include electric shock, fire, burns, and explosions. Electrical burns result from current flowing through the body and emerging in a concentrated area to ground and can occur from touching an uninsulated wire, a damaged plug, or an ungrounded piece of metal equipment. Electrosurgical units (ESUs; sometimes called the "Bovie") send a specified current from the ESU through the active electrode (often referred to as a "pencil") or other ESU electrode to create sufficient heat to cut or coagulate the vessel touched by the pencil or other instrument. The current then exits the body through a dispersive electrode (sometimes called the "ground pad") and returns to the ESU. Chapter 8 contains a thorough discussion of electrical safety.

Fires and Explosions

Surgical fires are one of the top 10 technology hazards identified by the ECRI Institute (ECRI, 2013). Fires and explosions in all settings require three components: (1) ignition source/heat, (2) fuel, and (3) oxygen (or another source of oxygenation [e.g., H_2O_2]). Nurses in perioperative settings can decrease risks of burns from fires by considering these "fire triangle" requirements during procedures and working with the perioperative team to reduce each to no more than necessary. Elimination of any single component of the triangle will prevent fire. If elimination of at least one component is not possible, the perioperative team's goal is to keep each component as distant from each other in either time and/or space as possible.

Ignition/heat sources serve to provide the energy to initiate the oxidation chemical reaction, that is, ignition. In the OR, concentrated sources of energy such as sparks from static electricity, ESUs, and lasers are key sources of heat and ignition. Oxygen or an oxygen-nitrogen composition such as nitrous oxide (N_2O), administered via

prong or mask, is the usual oxygenation source. Room air (21% O_2) can serve as the oxygenation source but only if there is a sufficiently fine fuel (e.g., powders). A common fuel source is disposable drapes (which can also trap oxygenation sources in its folds). Fuels can literally be anything that burns, even mascara (Raqqad, 2010).

Fire and explosion prevention strategies involve separation of ignition/heat sources, fuel, and oxygen in time and/or space. Speed of the ignition reaction depends on temperature, particle size, and the concentration of the reactant fuel. Space separation strategies involve keeping (or eliminating) possible sources of igniting sparks (e.g., ESUs and lasers) as far from anesthesia and the patient's head and throat as possible and using room air rather than more concentrated oxygen or N_2O as much as possible. Nitrous oxide, like free oxygen, is an oxidizing agent but only in the presence of a fire or explosion, which then breaks down its chemical bonds; an explosion, however, can be even more violent when N_2O is present than with O_2 alone because when a fuel burns in N_2O, it produces more heat than burning in O_2 alone.

Not surprisingly, procedures using ESUs and lasers around the face and neck (i.e., near O_2 or O_2/N_2O) provide the greatest risk (Haith et al, 2012). Even so, as with all surgeries, ESU-active electrodes should be kept in holsters and not allowed to rest on drapes; lasers and ESU-active electrodes should not be allowed to touch fine gauze or sponges, especially alcohol-soaked sponges (Herman et al, 2009). See the Patient Safety box on page 34 for additional safe practice specifics.

Risk for Chemical Burns

Chemical burns most commonly occur during or after surgical site skin preparation (prep). Skin prep solutions should be applied with care to prevent pooling, which can lead to chemical burns to the skin. Towels should be tucked under the patient along the area to be prepped to catch any dripping solution and removed upon completion of skin prep (these towels are sometimes called "drip" towels). In addition to being a chemical irritant, prep solution can

PATIENT SAFETY

Surgical Fire Prevention

At the Start of Each Surgery:
- Enriched O_2 and N_2O atmospheres can vastly increase flammability of drapes, plastics, and hair. Be aware of possible O_2 enrichment under drapes.
- Do not apply drapes until all flammable preps have fully dried; remove spilled or pooled prep agent.
- Fiberoptic light sources can start fires; complete all cable connections before activating the source, and place the source in standby mode when disconnecting cables.
- Moisten sponges to make them ignition resistant in oropharyngeal and pulmonary surgery.
- Include fire risk and prevention status in briefing/time-out.

During Head, Face, Neck, and Upper Chest Surgery:
- Use medical-grade air for open delivery to the face if the patient can maintain a safe blood O_2 saturation without supplemental O_2.
- If the patient cannot maintain a safe blood O_2 saturation without extra O_2, secure the airway with a laryngeal mask airway or tracheal tube.

Exceptions: When patient verbal responses may be required during surgery (e.g., carotid artery surgery, neurosurgery, pacemaker insertion) and when open O_2 delivery is required to keep the patient safe:
- At all times, deliver the minimum O_2 concentration necessary (titrate O_2 to patient's needs) for adequate oxygenation and increase as necessary.
- Stop supplemental O_2 at least 1 minute before and during use of electrosurgery, electrocautery, or laser, if possible.

Surgical team communication is essential for this recommendation.
- Keep fenestration towel edges as far from the incision as possible.
- Arrange drapes to minimize O_2 buildup underneath.
- Coat head hair and facial hair (e.g., eyebrows, beard, mustache) within the fenestration with water-soluble surgical lubricating jelly to make them nonflammable.
- For coagulation, use bipolar electrosurgery, not monopolar electrosurgery.

During Oropharyngeal Surgery (e.g., Tonsillectomy):
- Scavenge deep within the oropharynx with a metal suction cannula to catch leaking O_2 and N_2O.
- Moisten gauze or sponges and keep them moist, including those used with uncuffed tracheal tubes.

When Using Electrosurgery Units (ESU), Electrocautery, or Laser:
- The surgeon should be made aware of open O_2 use.
- Activate the unit only when the active tip is in view (especially if looking through a microscope or endoscope).
- Deactivate the unit before the tip leaves the surgical site.
- Place electrosurgical electrodes in a holster or another location off the patient.
- Place lasers in standby mode when not in active use.
- Do not place rubber catheter sleeves over electrosurgical electrodes.

Modified from Bruley ME: *New recommendations for surgical fire prevention and management,* AORN Congress, March 5, 2013, San Diego, CA; Silverstein KL, Joseph S: *Prevention of surgical fires,* 2011, available at www.medscape.org/viewarticle/753330?src=cmemp. Accessed March 18, 2013.

serve as the fuel component of the fire triangle that may be ignited by a spark from an active electrode of the ESU or even from a discharge of static electricity. Thus inappropriate use of prep solution can also cause thermal burns. Ignition of prep vapors can also occur as solution evaporates. Solutions used for skin prep must dry before application of surgical drapes.

Pressure Injuries

Pressure injuries include nerve compression (peroneal and ulnar nerves are particularly susceptible); nerve stretching (e.g., brachial plexus extension); and pressure ulcers (especially on the coccyx, heels, or back of head in supine position). Pressure or the lack thereof also may cause vessel stasis and DVT. Each surgical position has its own predictable pressure risks and methods of prevention. As a rule, however, the surgical team should remember that increasing the area of contact or reducing the force pushing on that area will decrease pressure. An easy to remember formula is pressure equals force divided by area ($P = F/A$). Thus both increasing area and decreasing force lessen pressure. This formula explains why both thin and obese patients are at risk for pressure injuries during surgery. Thin patients tend to have a smaller area (e.g., the coccyx) directly in contact with the OR bed or a positioning device. Obese patients, on the other hand, have more force from their increased weight and body mass. Padding typically reduces pressure by increasing the area over which a force is applied. Reminding

scrubbed personnel not to lean on the patient reduces force applied to an area, thus also avoiding pressure increases.

Medication Administration

Like all perioperative safety concerns, medication administration safety must be examined within the context of its multidisciplinary system. That system includes medication prescribing, transcribing, procurement and dispensing, as well as administering (AORN, 2013). Medication administration in the OR/invasive procedure room is complicated, compared with that found in other nursing care areas, in that the OR often requires that the circulating nurse and scrub person jointly prepare a medication that will be administered by a third person, usually the surgeon. Moreover, two potentially lethal medications are frequently used on the field, for example epinephrine and heparin, and both are clear and come in widely disparate dosages. Additionally, aseptic technique requires the medication be administered by someone other than the person removing the medication from its original container. Checking for allergies, important in all areas, takes on new dimensions as well because anesthetics may disguise allergic reactions.

Vigilance in following established safe medication practices is crucial. Consider a "No interruption zone" or "Do not disturb" time during important activities in medication preparation (ISMP, 2012). Perioperative personnel must pay particular attention to acknowledging medication name, and concentrations, labeling

PATIENT SAFETY

Potential Risks Associated with Medication Errors in the Perioperative Setting

- Inconsistent communication
- Confusion in medication order due to muffled verbal orders through surgical masks
- Incomplete, ambiguous, or incorrectly spoken or illegible written orders
- Necessary removal of medication from the manufacturer's packaging for use on sterile field
- Inconsistent labeling of medication on and off sterile field
- Medication dispensed to the sterile field usually handled by multiple licensed and unlicensed individuals before reaching the licensed person actually administering the medication
- Patient condition may require rapid interventions
- Sensory distractions inherent in environment (noise such as talking, music, alarms)
- Interruptions by other healthcare staff

Modified from AORN: Recommended practice for medication safety. In *Perioperative standards and recommended practices*, 2013, Denver, The Association; Lewis TP et al: Tips to reduce dangerous interruptions by healthcare staff, *Nursing 2012* 42(11):65–67, 2012; Treiber LA, Jones JH: Medication errors, routines, and differences between perioperative nurses and non-perioperative nurses, *AORN J* 96(3):285–294, 2012.

TABLE 2-2

Do Not Use Abbreviations

Use	Do Not Use	Reason
units	U or u	Mistaken as "0", "4," or "cc"
0.1 mg	.1 mg	No leading zero results in easily missed decimal point (i.e., 10 times the dose)
0.1 mg or 1 mg	.10 mg or 1.0 mg	Trailing zero results in easily missed decimal point (i.e., 10-100 times the intended dose)
mcg or micrograms	μg	Mistaken for mg
morphine sulfate	MS	Mistaken for MSO_4 and $MgSO_4$
morphine sulfate	MSO_4	Mistaken for MS and $MgSO_4$
magnesium sulfate	$MgSO_4$	Mistaken for MS and MSO_4
International unit	IU	Mistaken for IV and 10
daily	Q.D.	Mistaken for Q.O.D.; the period after the Q can be mistaken for an "I"
every other day	Q.O.D.	Mistaken for Q.O.D.; the period after the Q can be mistaken for an "I" and the "O" can be mistaken for "I"
left ear	as	Confused with left eye (os)
right ear	ad	Confused with right eye (od)

solutions in syringes and containers on and off the sterile field, and performing read-backs/repeat-backs. Tedious as it may seem, the complete name and concentration of the drug should appear on the administration device; thus "lidocaine 2% with epinephrine 1 : 100,000" and not "epi." The Patient Safety box above lists some potential risks of medication errors in the perioperative setting.

Team members also must follow policies and procedures strictly to double check the medication or solution before it is dispensed to the sterile field. Medications and medication containers (e.g., syringes, cups, basins), both on and off the sterile field, must be labeled fully and accurately with medication names and concentrations (see Patient Safety: Elements of Performance for Medication Safety, p. 20); furthermore, processes must be established and used to verify labels. Scrub persons should identify medications by announcing the name of the medication being passed to the surgeon, along with its concentration. A repeat-back confirmation from the surgeon ensures the correct dose of medication or solution. The institution's "Do not use" list of abbreviations must be observed and applied to all medication orders and medication-related documentation that are handwritten or on preprinted forms (Table 2-2).

TJC's list of look-alike/sound-alike drugs, based on findings from the Institute for Safe Medication Practices (ISMP), should be readily available to all perioperative personnel (see Table 2-2 for potentially problematic drug names, potential errors and consequences, and specific safety strategies).

Federal agencies, TJC, and individual institutions increasingly look to bar-code medication administration (BCMA) systems to reduce medication errors. Adoption of BCMA systems is likely to accelerate because BCMA has become a criterion of the "meaningful use" of health information technology (CMS, 2012). Empiric studies have found a reduction in errors after BCMA implementation. Unfortunately, precursors to errors, such as workarounds, interruptions, and patient and technology characteristics, continue (IOM, 2011). As with adoption of any new system, perioperative

nurses must recognize unique factors arising from the use of BCMA in perioperative settings and remain vigilant for possibly unintended consequences.

Risk for Fluid or Electrolyte Imbalance

Blood Loss. Measuring blood loss is a vital procedure in the surgical management of critically ill or elderly patients, patients undergoing complex procedures, trauma and organ transplant patients, patients with abnormal bleeding or clotting time or with extensive renal/liver disease, and infants. Some anesthesia providers prefer to estimate blood loss via visual inspection of drapes, suction canisters, and used soft goods such as sponges. When blood loss estimates must be more accurate, weighing sponges provides a reliable means of judging the amount of blood lost and of gauging the need for transfusion. The weight of dry, unused sponges and the weight of the plastic bag for soiled sponges must first be determined and then excluded from the weight tally. Grams (g) measured are converted to milliliters (mL) on a 1 : 1 basis, and blood loss estimates are reported to the anesthesia provider. The setup to weigh sponges requires a gram scale and plastic bags to hold soiled sponges. (Box 2-5 details the procedure.) The estimated blood loss may be part of the hand-off report in ORs that use a surgical Apgar score.

Blood and Blood Products. Maintenance of circulating blood volume is crucial during surgical procedures; this is accomplished with administration of whole blood or blood components. Blood

---

BOX 2-5

Procedure to Measure Blood Loss by Weighing Sponges

1. Weigh a dry, radiopaque sponge in a plastic bag, then adjust the scale to register zero.
2. Place used, bagged sponges on the scale.
3. Record the scale reading: 1 g equals 1 mL of blood loss.
4. Note the blood loss on the record.
5. Add subsequent weight to the preceding weight each time sponges are weighed so that a running total blood loss, calculated from sponges, is available.
6. Measure blood in the suction canister(s) at regular intervals, subtracting the amount of any irrigating solution used.
7. Add the amount of blood loss calculated from suction canisters to the total recorded from sponges to obtain accurate blood loss estimates.
8. Report blood loss totals to anesthesia provider/surgical team at regular intervals if blood/blood product replacement therapy is being considered for the patient.

PATIENT-CENTERED CARE

When Adams and Tolich (2011) sought to identify how well patients understand the role of blood transfusion in their treatment and whether it caused them discomfort, they discovered that relying on consent forms or other written materials wasn't adequate to explain risks and benefits of the procedure and that patients had concerns about the safety of the blood supply. Also, patients valued their nurse's information. When a patient is receiving blood or a blood component, consider including the following as part of your patient-centered communication:

- Provide information and clarification (as appropriate to patient condition).
- Do not hesitate to address safety.
- Discuss how blood is administered.
- Assure the patient that it won't "hurt."
- Review signs/symptoms you want the patient (or patient's family) to watch for.
- Invite the patient to express concerns or fears.

Modified from Adams KW, Tolich D: Blood transfusion: the patient's experience, AJN 111(9):24–30, 2011.

---

products are literally life savers but can be fatal if improperly stored or administered. American Association of Blood Banks' (AABB, 2011) standards and technical manuals should be incorporated into facility policy and must be followed exactly. Whole blood is rarely administered unless the patient has an acute, massive loss (often empirically determined as a loss that exceeds one third of the circulating volume, or approximately 1500 mL for an adult). Instead, packed red blood cells (PRBCs) that improve oxygen-carrying capacity and oxygen transport to tissues, with or without crystalloid or colloid solutions, are administered to maintain intravascular blood volume. Crystalloid solutions include normal saline and lactated Ringer's solution; colloid solutions include albumin, purified protein factors, dextran, and hydroxyethyl starch (hetastarch). If coagulopathy is an issue, fresh frozen plasma (FFP) platelets and cryoprecipitate should be considered. When blood or any blood products must be given, appropriate precautions are necessary to reduce the hazards of its administration. Despite which product is administered, blood management is a patient-centered care measure provided by nurses (Tolich et al, 2013) (Patient-Centered Care).

Elective surgery patients who may need blood products during surgery have a pretransfusion sample taken 1 to 7 days (facility policy and patient history dependent) before surgery to ensure compatibility and to avoid antibodies that may emerge in response to exposure through blood transfusions, pregnancy, or environmental factors or as a consequence of the patient's disease process. *Type* refers to the test to determine the ABO and Rh blood type. *Screen* refers to the test for unexpected antibodies. *Crossmatching* refers to the test for the compatibility of the recipient's serum and the donor's red blood cells. It is crucial to identify the patient correctly before the pretransfusion blood sample is drawn and then to ensure that the sample is properly labeled. Improperly identified pretransfusion blood samples can result in acute hemolytic transfusion reactions at the time of transfusion, and death.

A patient having an elective surgical procedure for which blood has been requested should not be anesthetized without verification that the requested blood products are typed, crossmatched, and available, and that informed consent to receive blood products has been documented (Figure 2-3). This should be part of the preoperative verification process and then reverified during the time-out. An institutional blood requisition form, with complete and accurate patient identification information, should be sent to the blood bank when blood or blood products are being requested. Included on or with this requisition should be the number of units desired. Many institutions have computerized ordering and the same information is required.

If the patient is sent to the OR directly from the emergency department or trauma admitting area without a chart, all patient identification information must be printed plainly on a piece of paper. The perioperative nurse should contact the blood bank to explain the emergency situation and facilitate release of the needed blood products.

Precise and accurate blood product storage conditions are important to ensure patient safety and to avoid wasting improperly stored products. Whole blood and blood products must be stored under continuously monitored conditions in accordance with AABB rules and U.S. Food and Drug Administration (FDA) regulations. Storage temperatures must be documented and all storage equipment for blood products must be properly maintained and tested, including function checks on alarms. The return of unused blood products must comply with facility policy; further, each component presents specific requirements for proper maintenance and return (e.g., thawed cryoprecipitate and platelets must be maintained at room temperature [22° C]; and red cells and thawed plasma must be kept refrigerated at 4° C).

Before administration of any blood product, the circulating nurse and anesthesia provider (or a second licensed individual) must confirm that a signed consent is on the medical record, and then proceed with the following:

- The unit number on the blood product corresponds with the unit number on the blood requisition. Facilities using electronic records will return a "transfusion card" or "crossmatch card" as verification that this unit can be given to this patient in lieu of the requisition.
- The name, birth date, and number on the patient's identification band agree with the name, birth date, and number on the slip with the blood product.

BLOOD/BLOOD PRODUCTS CONSENT

My doctor _____, has advised that I may require a blood transfusion.
(Type or print doctor or practitioner names[s])

The amount of blood products I receive is a choice my doctor will make based on my needs. I understand that all blood is screened for hepatitis, HIV (AIDS virus), and other contagious conditions.

I consent to receive blood or blood products now and during my hospital stay.

The risks, benefits, and alternatives to receiving blood products have been explained to me.

I certify that I have had the above information regarding treatments and alternative procedures explained to me. In addition, I have been offered the opportunity to ask questions and they have been answered to my satisfaction.

_____ ___/___/___ _____   _____ ___/___/___ _____
Signature of Patient or Decision Maker   Date   Time   Doctor or Practitioner Signature/Title   Date   Time

_____   _____
Relationship to Patient   Doctor or Practitioner Print Name or ID#

_____ ___/___/___ _____
Witness Signature   Date   Time

_____
Witness Print Name

Telephone Consent:

_____   _____
Name of person providing consent   Relationship to Patient if Decision Maker

_____ ___/___/___ _____   _____ ___/___/___ _____
Witness Signature   Date   Time   Witness Signature   Date   Time

_____   _____
Witness Print Name   Witness Print Name

If revoked: Write "REVOKED" on form
My signature below acknowledges my decision to revoke my consent for blood/blood products documented above on this form.

_____   _____ ___/___/___ _____
Signature of Patient or Decision Maker   Relationship to Patient   Date   Time

_____   _____ ___/___/___ _____
Witness Signature   Witness Print Name   Date   Time

Interpretation: The information presented orally to the O patient   O representative   O decision maker was interpreted into (language):
_____ . The person for whom the information was interpreted stated s/he understood the interpretation.

_____   _____
Interpreter Name   Agency and ID# (if applicable)

_____   _____ ___/___/___ _____
Signature/Title   Print Name or ID#   Date   Time

FIGURE 2-3 Consent for blood/blood products.

- The patient's name on the slip with the blood product corresponds with the name on the requisition.
- The blood group indicated on the blood product corresponds with that of the patient.
- The date and time of expiration have not been reached.
- The blood product bag is free of leaks, damage, or signs of possible bacterial contamination (e.g., presence of fine gas bubbles, discoloration, clots, or excessive air in the bag).

Both individuals who verify this information must sign the slip that comes with the blood product. If a discrepancy arises with any of these checks, the blood product must not be infused until and unless resolution of the discrepancy occurs.

When it becomes apparent that more blood products will be needed than originally anticipated, the perioperative nurse should request the blood bank prepare a specified number of units in advance of the actual need to transfuse. This procedure allows the blood bank time to crossmatch the units carefully, without rushing and jeopardizing patient safety. Crossmatch requisitions should be sent for any additional units requested. If a significant amount of blood product has been required, a new, properly labeled sample with a blood grouping requisition may be needed to have an adequate sample for crossmatching although blood banks prefer using the original undiluted sample when possible.

Rapid blood transfusion requires warming of blood products to prevent hypothermia, which may induce cardiac arrest. Blood products should be warmed during passage through the transfusion set. The warming device must incorporate a temperature sensing device and a warning system to detect malfunction to prevent hemolysis or other damage to blood components (AABB, 2011). Blood must *never* be warmed in a microwave because its uneven, rapid heating can cause hemolysis. The probability of a transfusion reaction increases in direct proportion to the number of units transfused. The circulating nurse should remain alert for any signs of reaction, including the following:

- Hyperthermia
- Increased intraoperative bleeding
- Weak pulse
- Hypotension
- Visible hemoglobinuria
- Vasomotor instability
- Greatly decreased or no urinary output

If any such suspicious signs of reaction occur, the circulating nurse should assist the anesthesia provider to do the following:

1. Stop the transfusion. The tubing is disconnected and a new infusion of fluid such as 0.9% sodium chloride is begun to maintain venous access.
2. Report the reaction to the surgeon and blood bank immediately.
3. Anticipate possible order for stat antihistamines.
4. Return the unused portion of the blood product, the IV tubing used during the transfusion, and a properly labeled sample of the patient's blood to the blood bank.
5. Send a urine sample to the laboratory if requested.
6. Monitor the patient's reaction carefully.
7. Complete an incident/occurrence/event report covering the suspected reaction. The report might include time and date of reaction, type and amount of blood/blood product infused, and times transfusion started and stopped. Signs and symptoms, in the order of occurrence, along with the patient's vital signs, any urine or blood samples sent to the laboratory for analysis, any treatment given, and the patient's response should all be noted.

A suspected transfusion reaction report must be sent to the blood bank.

Any unused blood product should be returned to the blood bank as soon as the patient leaves the OR. Returned blood can be reissued if it has not been allowed to warm to a temperature greater than 10° C. External blood bag thermometers (e.g., HemoTemp II), similar to a skin contact tape thermometer, are used on blood product bags by many blood banks to quickly identify blood that has exceeded safe storage temperatures.

Autotransfusion—the reinfusion of a patient's own blood intraoperatively—is used with increasing frequency in surgery. Predated autologous blood donation is in decreasing use. During intraoperative autotransfusion (cell salvage), blood is collected as it is lost during the surgical procedure and reinfused to the patient after it is filtered or washed. This technique can be lifesaving in emergency situations, as with major trauma, or in procedures with major blood loss, as in liver transplantation. It is also used for patients who refuse blood based on religious beliefs.

Maintaining Fluid and Electrolyte Balance

The body's fluids and electrolytes play a key role in maintaining homeostasis, transporting necessary oxygen and nourishment to the cells, removing waste products of cellular metabolism, and helping to maintain body temperature. Electrolytes are also essential to transmission of nerve impulses, regulation of water distribution, contraction of muscles, generation of adenosine triphosphate (ATP, needed for cellular energy), regulation of acid-base balance, and hemostasis (clotting blood). The intake, distribution, and output of water and electrolytes, regulated by the renal and pulmonary systems, normally maintain fluid and electrolyte balance.

Fluid and electrolyte imbalances may occur rapidly in the surgical patient, and can be caused by numerous factors, including preoperative fluid and food restrictions, intraoperative fluid loss, or the stress of surgery. The surgical patient is unable to regulate body fluid and electrolyte requirements by normal activities of drinking, eating, excreting, and breathing unaided. It is therefore imperative that the perioperative nurse collaborate in monitoring the fluid and electrolyte status of the patient intraoperatively.

Body Fluids. The adult human body is approximately 60% water, although water content varies by age, gender, and body mass. In the elderly, body water content averages 45% to 55% of body weight, whereas it ranges from 70% to 80% in infants. Older adults are at higher risk for fluid imbalance because they have less fluid reserve, whereas the very young are at risk for fluid problems because a greater percentage of their body weight is water. Both age groups have a decreased ability to compensate for fluid loss. Muscular tissue contains more water than the same amount of adipose tissue; men generally have higher water content because they usually have more lean muscle mass than women.

Body fluids are distributed in two main functional compartments—intracellular and extracellular. *Intracellular fluids (ICFs)* are liquids within cell membranes that contain dissolved substances essential to fluid and electrolyte balance and metabolism. ICFs constitute approximately 70% of the body's fluid. Consequently, anything that affects water loss at the intracellular level has significant implications for the entire body. *Extracellular fluids (ECFs)* (30% of the body's fluid) are fluids in compartments outside the cells of the body, including plasma, intravascular fluids, fluids in the gastrointestinal (GI) tract, and cerebrospinal fluid (CSF).

Fluid spacing is a term used to classify distribution of body water. *First spacing* is the normal distribution of fluid in extracellular and intracellular compartments. *Second spacing* refers to excess accumulation of interstitial fluid (edema), and *third spacing* occurs when fluid accumulates in areas that normally have no fluid or only a minimal amount of fluid. This fluid accumulation occurs with burns, ascites, peritonitis, or small-bowel obstruction. Third spacing traps fluid away from normal fluid compartments and results in a deficit in useful fluid volume.

Electrolytes. Electrolytes (Table 2-3) are found in both ICFs and ECFs. When dissolved in water, electrolytes dissociate into ions and are able to carry an electric charge. Positively charged ions are called cations, and negatively charged ions are anions.

The electrolytes found in ICFs and ECFs are essentially the same, but concentrations in each compartment differ. The primary ICF cation is potassium, and the primary ECF cation is sodium. The primary ICF anion is phosphate, and the primary ECF anion is chloride. Fluids and electrolytes move between the ICF and ECF spaces to facilitate body processes, such as acid-base balance, tissue oxygenation, response to drug therapies, and response to illness. Diffusion, active transport, and osmosis control these movements.

Diffusion, Active Transport, and Osmosis. *Diffusion* is the movement of molecules from an area of high concentration to one of low concentration and can take place with or without a membrane separating the concentration gradient. When diffusion occurs, movement continues until there is an equal concentration of molecules. Diffusion across membranes is particularly important in regulating fluid transport and balance in the body.

Active transport is a process by which molecules move across a cell membrane against a concentration gradient (i.e., from an area of low concentration to an area of high concentration) with the impetus of external energy. A so-called "sodium-potassium pump" moves sodium out of the cell and potassium into the cell to maintain the intracellular and extracellular concentration differences of sodium and potassium. ATP is the energy source for this sodium-potassium pump.

Osmosis is the movement of a fluid through a semipermeable membrane from a solution that has a lower solute concentration to one that has a higher solute concentration (Figure 2-4). The

semipermeable membrane prevents movement of solute particles. The concentration of these particles is measured in a unit called the osmole (osm). *Osmolality* is the term used to express the concentration of a solution in milliosmoles per kilogram (mOsm/kg) of water. A solution with the same osmolality as blood plasma is called *isotonic*. Isotonic solutions, such as 0.9% normal saline or lactated Ringer's solution administered intravenously, prevent the shift of fluid and electrolytes from intracellular compartments. A *hypotonic* IV solution (0.45% saline or 2.5% dextrose) has a lower concentration of solutes than that found in plasma and moves water into the cells. Administration of a *hypertonic* IV solution (5% dextrose in normal saline or 5% dextrose in lactated Ringer's solution) with a greater concentration of solutes than that of plasma moves water out of the cells.

Preoperative Considerations. Preoperative laboratory analysis of electrolyte levels should be checked and abnormalities corrected to within normal limits before any surgical procedure, unless the surgery is needed to correct a life-threatening problem. Preexisting conditions, such as diabetes mellitus, liver disease, or renal insufficiency, may worsen with surgical stress, increasing a patient's risk of fluid and electrolyte imbalances. Diagnostic procedures that require the administration of IV dyes may produce osmotic diuresis, with resulting urinary excretion of water and electrolytes. Preoperative steroids or diuretics affect the excretion of water and electrolytes; diuretics, used in the management of hypertension, cause the loss of potassium. Preoperative surgical regimens, such as bowel-cleansing routines, may increase fluid loss from the GI tract. Medical management, such as gastric suction, can also affect fluid and electrolyte balance in the surgical patient, as can preoperative fluid restriction.

Preoperative fluid restrictions are used to reduce nausea, vomiting, and aspiration risks in the surgical patient. Many healthcare facilities and providers are changing this practice because newer anesthetic agents tend to cause less nausea and vomiting than in the past. Prolonged fluid restrictions may not be necessary in healthy patients before surgery; thus black coffee or pulp-free juice may be ingested safely 2 to 3 hours before surgery, without an increase in gastric volume (see Chapter 5).

Deficient Fluid Volume. The most common patient problems associated with fluid and electrolyte imbalances during surgery include deficient fluid volume (DFV), water imbalance, and potassium imbalance. DFV is an imbalance in isotonic body fluids related to decreased intravascular, interstitial, or intracellular fluid. Very young and very old surgical patients are affected most rapidly by fluid losses from bleeding; inadequate intake because of previous nothing per os (mouth) (NPO) status; inadequate IV fluid replacement; excessive cutaneous losses from fever and sweating; third-space fluid losses attributable to bowel obstructions, ascites, or peritonitis; excessive GI losses resulting from diarrhea, vomiting, GI suctioning, or fistulas; evaporation of fluid from the exposed peritoneum during open abdominal surgery; shifting of intravascular fluid into the surgical site (third-space edema); and inhalation of dry gases. Third-space fluid losses cannot be measured directly, but can be considerable after extensive dissection of tissue. Intraoperative use of an electrolyte solution, such as lactated Ringer's solution, for fluid replacement can help to correct intraoperative third-space fluid losses.

The effect of fluid loss on the surgical patient depends on the amount of fluid lost and the speed at which the fluid is lost. A

Before osmosis   After osmosis

Selectively permeable membrane

Concentrated salt solution

Dilute salt solution

FIGURE 2-4 Osmosis is the movement of solvent molecules across a membrane to an area of higher solute concentration. The solvent moves because the solute cannot pass through the membrane. The result of osmosis is two solutions, separated by a selectively permeable membrane, that are equal in concentration.

TABLE 2-3

Electrolyte Functions and Regulators

Electrolyte	Reference Range	Functions	Regulation
Sodium (Na^+)	135-145 mmol/L	Maintains blood volume Controls water shifting between compartments Major cation involved in sodium-potassium pump necessary for nerve impulse conduction Interacts with calcium to maintain muscle contraction Major cation in bicarbonate and phosphate acid-base buffer system	Renin-angiotensin-aldosterone system • Retains sodium and water is passively absorbed
Potassium (K^+)	3.5-5 mmol/L	Affects osmolality Major cation involved in sodium-potassium pump necessary for nerve impulse conduction Promotes nerve impulse conduction, especially in heart and skeletal muscles Assists in conversion of carbohydrates to energy and of amino acids to protein Promotes glycogen storage in liver Assists maintenance of acid-base balance through cellular exchange with hydrogen	Renin-angiotensin-aldosterone system • Kidneys excrete potassium in exchange for sodium
Calcium (Ca^{2+})	2.2-2.7 mmol/L or 9-11 mg/dL	Nonionized form promotes strong teeth and bones Promotes blood coagulation Promotes nerve impulse conduction; decreases neuromuscular irritability Strengthens and thickens cell membrane Assists in absorption and utilization of vitamin B_{12} Activates enzymes for many chemical reactions Inhibits cell membrane permeability to sodium Activates actin-myosin muscle contraction	Parathyroid hormone, calcitonin, and vitamin D • Increases calcium reabsorption from bone • Increases calcium reabsorption by inhibiting phosphate reabsorption from kidney tubules • Increases calcium absorption from gastrointestinal tract
Chloride (Cl^-)	98-108 mmol/L	Inhibits smooth muscle contraction Regulates extracellular fluid volume Promotes acid-base balance through exchange with bicarbonate in red blood cells (chloride shift) Promotes protein digestion through hydrochloric acid; acid pH required for activation of protease	Renin-angiotensin-aldosterone system • Kidneys excrete chloride if body fluids are acidic and reabsorb it if body fluids are alkalotic
Magnesium (Mg^{2+})	0.7-1.2 mmol/L 1.5-2.5 mEq/L or 1.8-3 mg/dL	Promotes metabolism of carbohydrates, fats, and proteins Activates many enzymes (B_{12} metabolism) Promotes regulation of Ca^{2+}, PO_4^{2-}, K^+ Promotes nerve impulse conduction, muscle contraction, and heart function Powers sodium-potassium pump Promotes conversion of adenosine triphosphate to adenosine diphosphate for energy release	Kidneys • Increases or decreases magnesium reabsorption in kidney tubules according to need
Phosphate (HPO_4^-)	0.8-1.5 mmol/L or 2.5-4.5 mg/dL	Nonionized form promotes bone and teeth rigidity Promotes acid-base balance through phosphate buffer system Necessary for adenosine triphosphate production	Parathyroid hormone, calcitonin, and vitamin D • Increases phosphate resorption from bone • Inhibits phosphate reabsorption in kidney tubules • Increases phosphate absorption in gastrointestinal tract as needed

Modified from Harkreader H et al: *Fundamentals of nursing: caring and clinical judgment*, ed 3, St Louis, 2007, Saunders.

patient who loses a large amount of fluid (>500 mL) or loses fluid rapidly exhibits symptoms of shock; immediate fluid replacement therapy is required. A slow loss of fluid may be compensated through albumin synthesis and erythropoiesis.

Sodium and Water Imbalances. Sodium is a cation in ECF; sodium plays a major role in maintaining the osmolality and water balance of ECF. Because cell membranes are permeable to water, sodium also affects ICF volume, as well as helps to maintain acid-base balance in the body. The sodium-potassium pump plays a vital role in neuromuscular activity.

Hyponatremia (serum sodium level <135 mEq/L) can be caused by increased excretion of sodium with diuretic therapy and the abnormal loss of sodium through nasogastric (NG) suctioning and third spacing. Patients undergoing procedures such as transurethral resection of the prostate (TURP) or similar procedures are at risk for dilutional hyponatremia and volume overload, caused by absorption of the irrigation solution used. Given that saline is a good conductor of electrical current, fluids that contain no electrolytes (e.g., glycine, sorbitol, and mannitol) must be used to irrigate when using electrical current in tissue dissection during these procedures.

Potassium Imbalances. Potassium is the major ICF cation and is necessary for contraction of skeletal, smooth, and cardiac muscle. It is also necessary for cardiac contractions and for peristaltic movements of the GI tract. Potassium plays a major role as well in the transmission of nerve impulses by regulating neuromuscular excitability and in the formation of muscle protein by transporting glucose into the cells with insulin. It is also elemental in maintaining acid-base balance and ICF osmotic pressures.

Hypokalemia (serum potassium concentration <3.5 mEq/L) can occur intraoperatively as a result of the suctioning of large amounts of body fluids or using diuretic therapy and other drugs (e.g., mannitol) that increase renal flow. Signs and symptoms of hypokalemia include cardiac effects, such as ectopy, dysrhythmias, conduction abnormalities, and altered sensitivity to digitalis. The neuromuscular effects of hypokalemia include muscle weakness; its smooth muscle effects include gastric distention, paralytic ileus, and urinary retention.

Treatment of hypokalemia includes IV replacement when the deficit is severe, as in the development of cardiovascular or other serious symptoms. Potassium irritates veins on infusion; the infusion site therefore requires monitoring for redness, heat, swelling, and site pain—all signs of chemical phlebitis. Overcorrection and subsequent hyperkalemia must be avoided by monitoring serum potassium levels at frequent intervals (often every 2 to 4 hours).

Hyperkalemia (serum potassium level of more than 5 mEq/L) can arise during surgery via massive transfusions of stored blood; decreased excretion of potassium caused by hypovolemia or renal failure; and shifting of potassium from the cells into the ECF caused by acidosis, tissue breakdown from surgery, crush injuries, or burns. Drugs infused during surgery can also induce hyperkalemia; such drugs include antiinflammatory agents, β-adrenergic receptor blockers, digitalis, succinylcholine, heparin, and the penicillins.

Signs and symptoms of hyperkalemia include neuromuscular symptoms such as weakness and paresthesias in the arms and legs. Smooth muscle symptoms include diarrhea and abdominal distention. Excess potassium can cause serious cardiac symptoms

such as ventricular dysrhythmias, heart block, and asystole. Cardiac side effects of hyperkalemia are treated by calcium gluconate infusion. Sodium bicarbonate or insulin-glucose infusions can shift ECF potassium into the cells, reducing the plasma's potassium level.

Patient Rights

Protection of patients' personal, ethical, and legal rights underlies patient safety and risk management. Many nurses equate patients' legal rights with negligence, malpractice, and informed consent. As described in the following text, these are only some of the many legal and ethical concerns in myriad perioperative settings, although legal and ethical issues interrelate as do all components in healthcare.

Freedom from Negligent Treatment

Malpractice is negligence by a professional in the performance of a professional act. Provision of safe care to the patient is the best protection for the nurse and facility from malpractice claims. This is because it is impossible to sue healthcare providers for malpractice without an injury; almost always this must be a physical injury. To be successful in a malpractice case, the injured patient must prove that the member(s) of the surgical team departed from the standard(s) of care applicable to their profession and that this breach of applicable standard(s) caused the injury.

If an injury occurs, both the professional licensure and civil legal systems require the team to act to prevent it from worsening. Risk management should be notified and become involved immediately after injury occurs in order to minimize the likelihood of the patient or his or her representative bringing suit and if that fails, to prepare a defense.

Many injuries that do occur in the immediate perioperative period are extremely difficult to defend successfully. Injuries resulting from RSIs, wrong site surgery, wrong patient surgery, wrong side surgery, fires and other burns, and intraoperative pressure ulcers are all subject to a legal doctrine, in Latin called *res ipsa loquitur* ("the thing speaks for itself"), because these injuries ordinarily do not occur in the absence of some form of negligence. This means that unless the defense can prove there was no negligence (proving a negative is always difficult, if not impossible), the injured party will prevail. Even in potential *res ipsa loquitur* cases, patients who feel they have been treated with respect and dignity may be likely to accept sometimes less than perfect results, may be less inclined to litigate, and may be more likely to cooperate with postinjury treatment, regardless of fault.

Privacy

A patchwork of state statutes attempts to protect confidentiality, to ensure patients' access to their healthcare records, and to preserve healthcare data privacy. Simultaneously, federal law provides that patients must consent for their health information to be used for treatment, payment, or business purposes. The federal Health Insurance Portability and Accountability Act (HIPAA) imposes privacy and security rules that limit use or disclosure of protected health information in order to ensure patient privacy rights with respect to this information. Healthcare facilities accordingly must have administrative procedures to protect the privacy and confidentiality of all patient information. Facility policies should include protocols specific to perioperative settings, such as those governing or limiting the presence of healthcare industry representatives or other visitors in the OR.

Another federal statute, the Patient Safety and Quality Improvement Act (PSQIA) established a voluntary medical error reporting system to enhance the data available to assess and resolve patient safety and quality issues. To encourage reporting and analysis of medical errors, PSQIA created federal confidentiality protections for patient safety information. That law also sets forth an exception to HIPAA rules requiring patients' consent to disclose information about an error that occurred in the course of their treatment. Many states also have mandatory medical error reporting systems that likewise make exceptions to their confidentiality rules. Additional information on PSQIA is available at www.hhs.gov/ocr/privacy/psa/understanding.

Perioperative nurses ethically must protect patient privacy even if HIPAA, state laws, or facility protocols do not specifically address a privacy issue. Team members exercise care to protect patients' bodies from any more exposure than is required by a procedure. Likewise, comments made in or out of patient care areas about patient appearance, lifestyle, or social status, for example, are never appropriate unless required for safe care of that patient.

Privacy and Social Media

Widespread use of social media has raised a new challenge for patient privacy protection. Adoption and even the definition of social media is rapidly evolving (von Muhlen and Ohno-Machado, 2012). Although social media provide many benefits, including patient access to their records and facilitating patient partnership in their care, confidentiality pitfalls are rife. Inappropriate discussions of patient information in elevators, in cafeterias, or in social settings after work can now wind up being "overheard" worldwide. In that light, all healthcare professionals, employees, and facilities themselves must recognize that they have a heightened obligation to protect patient privacy by avoiding such inappropriate discussions entirely and absolutely. A refinement of HIPAA was passed in 2009 called the HITECH Act. Students, unlicensed and licensed healthcare workers, and retired healthcare workers uniformly have a continuing duty to observe and protect patient privacy rights under HIPAA and HITECH (Terry, 2011-2012).

The consequences of violating patient privacy rights via inappropriate use of social media may result in both employer and licensure disciplinary actions, possibly including termination of employment, suspension and revocation of license, fines, and other serious penalties. A 2010 survey of state boards of nursing by the National Council of State Boards of Nursing (NCSBN) revealed that 33 of 46 responding state boards had received complaints of nurses violating patient privacy by posting patient information and/or photographs on social networking sites. Twenty six of those 33 state boards reported taking disciplinary action based on these complaints, ranging from reprimand to license suspension (NCSBN, 2011) (Box 2-6).

In addition to violating federal and state patient privacy laws, posting anonymous patient photographs on social media can also violate another federal statute, the Video Voyeurism Prevention Act of 2004, which provides that whoever photographs, films, or records (by any means), and disseminates an image of a private area of an individual who has a reasonable expectation of privacy without the individual's consent shall be fined or imprisoned up to 1 year or both. Every healthcare facility should have a social media use policy. Several professional associations have developed or are developing such a policy. In addition to legal and ethical considerations, inappropriate postings can harm the reputation of the student/

Social Media Myths and Recommendations for Use

Common myths about social media:
- A post or communication is accessible only by the intended recipient.
- Once a post is deleted it is no longer accessible.
- Posting private information is okay as long as the patient is otherwise unidentified.
- Setting privacy settings is sufficient to ensure privacy.

How to avoid problems:
- Remember that legal and ethical obligations to protect privacy and confidentiality apply at all times and places, not just to care settings and care hours.
- Do not post any patient image or any other information that might degrade or embarrass a patient, even if otherwise unidentified.
- Do not disclose any information gained within the nurse-patient relationship unless there is a patient related need to disclose.
- Do not take photos or videos of patients on personal devices. Follow facility policy for taking same on facility-provided devices.
- Follow facility policies precisely for work-related postings, and use of personal and facility computers, cameras, and other electronic devices in the workplace.

Modified from NCSBN: *White paper: a nurse's guide to the use of social media*, 2011, available at www.ncsbn.org/Social_Media.pdf. Accessed February 10, 2013.

---

professional posting them and jeopardize future graduate program admission and employment prospects.

Patient Autonomy

Courts in the United States have long recognized that every adult has the right to determine what happens to his or her body (e.g., *Schloendorff v. Society of New York Hospitals,* 105 N.E.92 [N.Y., 1914]). This legal right is also an ethical right recognized under the ethical principle of respect for persons as autonomous beings (Beauchamp and Childress, 2008). In perioperative settings, these rights enjoy protections via the informed consent process for the procedure itself and/or for any research interventions; and via patient wishes expressed in advance directives for healthcare.

Informed Consent

The current professional literature may seem to place less emphasis on informed consent as it focuses more on other aspects of patient safety. However, courts continue to affirm the patient's right to informed consent (e.g., *Singer v Rodriguez et al,* 2012). Usually, the informed consent case also involves a physical injury due to other lapses in the safety system, but both aspects of such cases are equally important in the respectful treatment of patients.

Except in emergencies, surgical procedures should not be performed without documentation of the patient's consent in the chart (Figure 2-5). How to document this "informed consent" should be described in facility policy, but documentation is typically accomplished by means of a signed consent form and/or the primary surgeon's entry into the progress notes, which may or may not also be signed by the patient. The surgeon or practitioner performing the procedure is legally responsible to inform the patient about the proposed operation or other invasive procedure and its inherent

Date of procedure: _____/_____/_____

CONSENT FOR PROCEDURE

I,_ _____ , request and give consent to _____
(Type or print patient name)   (Type or print doctor or practitioner name(s))

to perform the following procedure(s) _____
(Please list site and side if appropriate)

_____

The benefits, risks, complications, and alternatives to the above procedure(s) have been explained to me.

I understand that the procedure(s) will be performed at the facility by and under supervision of my doctor or practitioner. My doctor or practitioner may use the services of other doctors or practitioners, or members of the resident staff as he or she deems necessary or advisable.

I authorize my doctor or practitioner and his or her associates and assistants to perform such additional procedures, which in their judgment are necessary and appropriate to carry out my diagnosis or treatment.

I authorize the hospital to retain, photograph, preserve and use for scientific, teaching purposes, or to make other dispositions of, at their convenience, any specimens, tissues, or parts taken from my body during the course of this operation.

I consent to observers in the procedure area in accordance with hospital policy. I consent to a healthcare industry representative being present during the procedure, if necessary, to provide technical assistance or to perform calibration of equipment. I consent to photography or video taping of my surgical procedure for educational purposes, provided my identity remains anonymous and confidential.

I consent to the administration of sedation or analgesia during my procedure. The risks, benefits, and alternatives to receiving sedation or analgesia have been explained to me.

If anesthesia is required, I consent to the administration of anesthesia by members of the Department of Anesthesiology. I also consent to the use of non-invasive and invasive monitoring techniques as deemed necessary. I understand that anesthesia involves risks that are in addition to those resulting from the operation itself including, but not limited to, dental injury, hoarseness, vocal cord injury, infection, nerve injury, corneal abrasion, seizures, heart attack, stroke and even death.

If applicable, I consent to the use of fluoroscopy. I understand that prolonged exposure to fluoroscopy may result in skin reactions, such as redness, irritation or a burn.

Please initial one of the following statements (females 55 years and under):
————To the best of my knowledge I am not pregnant.   ————I believe I am pregnant.

I certify that I have read and understand the above consent statements. In addition, I have been offered the opportunity to ask my doctor or practitioner any questions I have regarding the procedure(s) to be performed and they have been answered to my satisfaction. I acknowledge that I have been given no guarantee or assurance as to the results that may be obtained from the procedure(s).

_____ ___/___/___ _____		_____ ___/___/___ _____
Signature of Patient or Decision Maker Date Time		Doctor or Practitioner Signature/Title Date Time
_____		_____
Relationship to Patient		Doctor or Practitioner Print Name or ID#
_____ ___/___/___ _____		
Witness Signature Date Time		
_____		
Witness Print Name		

Telephone Consent:

_____   _____
Name of person providing consent   Relationship to Patient if Decision Maker

_____ ___/___/___ _____   _____ ___/___/___ _____
Witness Signature   Date   Time   Witness Signature   Date   Time

_____   _____
Witness Print Name   Witness Print Name

Interpretation: The information presented orally to the O patient O representative O decision maker was interpreted into (language): _____ . The person for whom the information was interpreted stated s/he understood the interpretation.

_____   _____
Interpreter Name   Agency and ID# (if applicable)

_____   _____   ___/___/___ _____
Staff Signature/Title   Print Name or ID#   Date   Time

FIGURE 2-5 Consent for procedure.

risks, benefits, alternatives, and complications before obtaining the patient's oral and documented consent.

The patient must receive this information in terms that he or she can understand. TJC (2012a) also suggests, that to meet health literacy needs, consent materials be written at a fifth grade or lower reading level, subjected to readability tests, designed with bullet points to divide complex material, and translated into the patient's language whenever possible.

The patient also must be informed who will perform the procedure and when practitioners other than the primary surgeon will perform important parts of the procedure, even when under the primary surgeon's supervision. Nurses with concerns about the adequacy of the patient's understanding should report their concerns to the operating surgeon, or anesthesia provider if the concerns involve the anesthesia consent.

Consent documentation must be complete before administration of preoperative medications. On the patient's arrival in the OR, the circulating nurse and anesthesia provider are responsible to verify that consent documentation is in the chart and is correct, properly signed, and witnessed before administration of anesthesia. Typically, consent documentation encompasses the following:

- The patient's name (and legal guardian, if applicable)
- Name of facility where the procedure is being performed
- Specific name of the surgical procedure (or when multiple procedures are being done, the names of those procedures) in terms the patient understands
- Site/side of the planned procedure
- Name of the practitioner(s) performing the procedure or important aspects of it
- Risks of the procedure
- Alternative procedures, treatments, or therapies
- Signature of the patient (or legal guardian, if applicable)
- Date and time consent is obtained
- Statement that the procedure was explained to the patient (or legal guardian or both if applicable)
- Name and signature of the person who explained the procedure, usually the primary surgeon or physician performing the procedure
- Signature of person witnessing the consent, often a perioperative team member

Nurses who are involved as witnesses to the signing of the consent form attest only to the validity of the patient signature, time, and date, and not to the adequacy of the patient's understanding because that assurance remains the duty of the surgeon or physician performing the procedure.

Advance Directives and DNR Orders

Many of the 50 states had statutes to allow patients to make their wishes regarding their future known in a legally recognized fashion if they were unable to do so when a life-threatening situation arose. Then, in the wake of the first U.S. Supreme Court case to deal with the issue, *Cruzan v. Director, Missouri Department of Health,* 497 U.S. 261 (1990), Congress in 1991 passed the Patient Self-Determination Act (PSDA) to extend legal protection to all U.S. citizens and residents. Under PSDA, patients have the legal right to accept or refuse medical treatment, including resuscitation, even if refusal will likely result in death. That law also provides that all patients admitted to Medicare and Medicaid recipient providers must be asked whether they have executed, or wish to be given information about, such an advance healthcare directive,

and that information must be included in the patient's healthcare record. If a patient arrives in a preoperative area with such a directive, the perioperative nurse should immediately clarify with the surgeon and/or anesthesia provider if there has been a presedation discussion with the patient as to the effect the directive should have in the immediate perioperative period. The law does not address this issue, but an automatic suspension or continuation of advance directives or DNR orders is not justified under either legal or ethical analysis. Again, facility policy should describe a perioperative procedure that preserves the patient's right to legal and ethical self-determination.

Veracity and Fidelity

Veracity includes providing accurate information. Fidelity (or loyalty) carries with it an implicit promise of truth telling and promise keeping. Both principles relate to respect for patients and their autonomy—that patients are entitled to full and accurate information and disclosure; and both principles are likewise inherent in trust, which also is foundational for patient safety. These principles relate most directly to the patient's right to informed consent. Within the patient safety and risk management context, however, veracity and fidelity also demand transparency in disclosure of adverse events to the patient/family. Some states (e.g., Pennsylvania, Florida, and Utah) legally require patient notification when an error occurs (Griffin, 2008).

Griffin reviewed data that demonstrated transparency, and disclosure after an error has occurred can minimize the consequences of litigation. In fact, articles encouraging full disclosure often do so more as a risk management issue than as an issue concerning patient rights. In any event, one consequence of the renewed emphasis on patient safety and patient rights has been to merge the heretofore separate systems of perioperative care provision, risk management, and quality improvement under a patient safety rubric that has enhanced the effectiveness of each.

KEY POINTS

- Management of patient safety and prevention of injury risks is a collective responsibility of the entire perioperative care team.
- Major government, regulatory and accrediting agencies, and associations address key elements of patient safety.
- The AORN *Perioperative Standards and Recommended Practices* is the best source for information specific to perioperative nursing practices.
- Meaningful communication and a commitment to teamwork, trust, and respect are characteristic in workplace cultures that emphasize patient safety.
- Enhanced communication initiatives such as safer surgery briefings, clinical perioperative records (written or digital) and hand-offs are foundational in assuring a safer patient experience and care transitions between providers and units responsible for perioperative patient care.
- Communication for safety in perioperative settings includes a wide array of protocols and topics (such as the time-out, counts, surgical specimens, electrical and chemical safety, and proper positioning) to prevent patient harm.
- Maintaining fluid and electrolyte balance is a collaborative effort that prevents deficient volume in the surgical patient.
- Protection of a patient's personal, ethical, and legal rights underlies patient safety and risk management in perioperative care settings.

CRITICAL THINKING QUESTION

At 1600, Nurse Steve tweeted: awful day. fat guy fell off table. busted shoulder. MD blames me! Strap on!!!! pooled prep. 2d degree burns! allergic to I !!!!!! Camouflaged d/t drape fire.

Earlier that day:

Mike Jones, a 56-year-old construction worker enters the OR for removal of a suspicious mass left upper scapular areas under MAC. History and physical review reveals 40-year history for smoking and has COPD and hypertension. Ht = 70 inches and wt = 120 kg.

Mr. Jones was not yet sedated and able to move himself onto the table and lay supine attended by Carole, the anesthesia provider. When surgeon came in, Carole says, "I note you suggested prone; I'd rather do this right lateral—OK with you?" The surgeon responded, "Sure, whatever," and left to scrub.

Steve, the circulating nurse, gathers the pillows and axillary roll, then stands by Jones's side and loosens the safety strap. The anesthesia provider tells Mr. Jones to lie on his right side and bend his knees up until comfortable. Anesthesia positioned his right arm extended on an armboard. Steve places the axillary roll, a pillow between Jones's legs and under left elbow, and reattaches safety strap across Jones's upper thighs. He looks at Carole to say, "OK?" "Yup, thanks" was the response. Steve then proceeded with the prep; there was a little pooling of the iodine-based solution but since the case was so short and the surgeon was already gowning and gloving and said ready to drape, Steve just left it. After draping finished, Steve helped the scrub move the Mayo and back table to the left of the surgeon and the incision site as Carole adjusted the oxygen mask on the patient's face and announced she was now injecting the fentanyl and midazolam (Versed). Steve rolled the ESU unit next to the back table and reminded everyone to avoid ESU use when the patient was receiving enriched oxygen. He then called the time-out and read the checklist. All checked out, except his heart sank when Carole answered "Iodine" to allergies question. But everything was ready for the local injection and it was a short case.

Steve returned to his computer, facing the wall, to document. He glanced over to check for incision time and as he did so he heard a thump. He immediately checked the field and saw Mr. Jones's legs sliding down the other side of the table. He said, "What?" and ran to the patient's side. Carole had been turned from the patient documenting her sedatives and drawing up a sustaining dose. The surgeon and scrub tech were looking at each other at the Mayo stand discussing whether the deeper incision required a 10 blade or 15. Everyone's attention immediately turned to Jones. First they assessed breathing, then alignment, and an orthopedic surgeon came from the next room to assess Jones's shoulder, then the incision site and a second-degree skin burn was noted. A team was called to safely get the patient back on the table. His shoulder was x-rayed as positioned by the orthopedic surgeon; he was repositioned, reprepped, and the surgery proceeded.

Mr. Jones required extra sedative but was still hyperventilating. Carole began bagging with enriched O_2 under the drape so as not to interfere with the sterile field. The mass involved more bleeding than anticipated. The surgeon requested the ESU. In the confusion of the fall everyone forgot the time-out warning to avoid ESU use when the patient was receiving enriched oxygen. The surgeon activated the ESU tip and ignited a flame flashback from under the drape.

1. Could this fall have been prevented?
   * If not, why not?
   * If yes, by whom?
   * If yes, by doing what?

2. Could these burns have been prevented?
   * By whom?
   * Doing what?
3. What did the team do correctly immediately after the fall?
4. Was lateral really the indicated position for this patient?
5. What should Steve have done differently throughout Mr. Jones's perioperative care and why? Are there ethical and privacy issues that should be addressed with Steve?

evolve *The answers to the Critical Thinking Question can be found at http://evolve.elsevier.com/Rothrock/Alexander.*

REFERENCES

American Association of Blood Banks (AABB): *Standards*, ed 27, Bethesda, MD, 2011, AABB.

Alexander EL: *Operating room technique*, St Louis, 1943, CV Mosby.

Amato-Vealey EJ et al: Hand-off communication: a requisite for patient safety, *AORN J* 88(5):763–770, 2008.

Association of periOperative Registered Nurses (AORN): *Perioperative standards and recommended practices*, Denver, 2013, The Association.

Beauchamp T, Childress J: *Principles of biomedical ethics*, ed 6, New York, 2008, University Press.

Bixenstine PJ et al: Developing and pilot testing practical measures of preanalytic surgical specimen defects, *Am J Med Qual*, January 2013, available at ajm. sagepub.com/content/early/2013/01/15/1062860612469824 (subscription required). Accessed February 11, 2013.

Bliss LA et al: Thirty-day outcomes support implementation of a surgical safety checklist, *J Am Coll Surg* 215(6):766–776, 2012.

Brennan T et al: Incidence of adverse events and negligence in hospitalized patients: results of the Harvard Medical Practice Study I, *N Engl J Med* 324(6):370–376, 1991.

Brooke BS et al: Variations in surgical outcomes associated with hospital compliance with safety practices, *Surgery* 151(5):651–659, 2012.

CMS: EHR incentive program stage 2, 2012, available at www.cms.gov/Regulations-and-Guidance/Legislation/EHRIncentivePrograms/Downloads/Stage2Overview_Tipsheet.pdf. Accessed February 11, 2013.

Coiera E: The science of interruption, *BMJ Qual Saf* 21(5):357–360, 2012.

Conley DM et al: Effective surgical safety checklist implementation, *J Am Coll Surg* 212(5):873–879, 2011.

Cook R, Woods D: Operating at the sharp end: the complexity of human error. In Bogner MS, editor: *Human errors in medicine*, Hinsdale, NJ, 1994, Lawrence Erlbaum Associates.

de Vries EN et al: Prevention of surgical malpractice claims by use of a surgical safety checklist, *Ann Surg* 253(3):624–628, 2011.

ECRI top 10 health technology hazards for 2013, *Health Dev* 41(11), 2012, available at www.ecri.org/Forms/Pages/ECRI-Institute-2013-Top-10-Hazards.aspxs. Accessed May 4, 2013. (This is a free registration hyperlink request to download the report.)

Edel EM: Surgical count practice variability and the potential for retained surgical items, *AORN J* 95(2):228–238, 2012.

Fourcade A et al: Barriers to staff adoption of a surgical safety checklist, *BMJ Qual Saf* 21(3):191–197, 2012.

Friesen MA et al: Handoffs: implications for nurses. In Hughes RG, editor: *Patient safety and quality: an evidence based handbook for nurses*, Agency Healthc Res Qual (2):285–332, 2008.

Gawande AA: *The checklist manifesto: how to get things right*, New York, 2009, Henry Holt and Company, LLC.

Gibbs VC: Retained surgical items and minimally invasive surgery, *World J Surg* 35(7):1532–1539, 2011.

Goldberg JL, Feldman DL: Implementing AORN recommended practices for prevention of retained surgical items, *AORN J* 95(2):205–218, 2012.

Glass LK, Murphy EK: *AORN emergence and growth*, Denver, 2002, Association of periOperative Registered Nurses, Inc.

Grant-Orser A et al: The lost sponge: Patient safety in the operative room, *Can Med Assoc J* 184(1):1275–1278, 2012.

Griffen FD: The impact of transparency on patient safety and liability, *Am Coll Surg* (Bull) 3(93):19–23, 2008.

Haith LR et al: Burn center management of operating room fire injuries, *J Burn Care Res* 33(5):649–653, 2012.

Haynes AB et al: A surgical safety checklist to reduce morbidity and mortality in a global population, *N Engl J Med* 360(5):491–499, 2009.

Haynes AB et al: Changes in safety attitude and relationship to decreased postoperative morbidity and mortality following implementation of a checklist-based surgical safety intervention, *BMJ Qual Saf* 20(1):102–107, 2011.

Healey AN et al: Engineering the system of communication for safer surgery, *Surg Endosc* 26(2):350–356, 2012.

Herman MA et al: Surgical fire during organ procurement, *Internet J Anesthesiol* 19(1), 2009.

Institute for Safe Medication Practices (ISMP): Side tracks on the safety express. Interruptions lead to errors and unfinished … wait, what was I doing? 2012, available at http://search.ismp.org/cgi-bin/hits.pl?in=517791&fh=80&ph=1&tk=gE%3FF%20E%3FFmu&su=bzkkWZttuuu.nEIW.%26VStfHuE-HkkHVEtYmPkHmYVHtEz%26uYVknm-H.YEWqnO%3D37&qy=qtGA&pd=1. Accessed February 10, 2013.

Institute of Medicine: *To err is human: building a safer health system*, Washington, DC, 1999, National Academy Press.

Institute of Medicine: *Health IT and patient safety*, Washington, DC, 2011, National Academy Press.

Johns Hopkins Malpractice Study: Surgical 'Never Events' Occur At Least 4,000 Times per Year, 12/19/2012. Available at www.hopkinsmedicine.org/news/media/releases/johns_hopkins_malpractice_study_surgical_never_events_occur_at_least_4000_times_per_year. Accessed May 4, 2013.

Layfield LJ, Anderson GM: Specimen labeling errors in surgical pathology: an 18-month experience, *Am J Clin Pathol* 134(3):466–470, 2010.

Leape L: Error in medicine, *JAMA* 272(23):1951–1957, 1994.

Leape LL et al: The nature of adverse events in hospitalized patients: results of the Harvard Medical Practice Study II, *N Engl J Med* 324(6):377–384, 1991.

Martindell D: Update on the prevention of retained surgical items, *Pa Patient Saf Adv* 9(3):106–112, 2012.

McCay L et al: Laboratory safety and the WHO world alliance for patient safety, *Clin Chem Acta* 404(1):6–11, 2009.

McNamara SA: National time out day: more than "a pause and a checklist," *AORN J* 95(6):805–814, 2012.

Mulloy D, Hughes RG: Wrong site surgery: a preventable medical error. In Hughes RG, editor: *Patient safety and quality: an evidence based handbook for nurses*, Rockville MD, 2008, Agency for Healthcare Research and Quality.

NCSBN: White paper: a nurse's guide to use of social media, 2011, available at www.ncsbn.org/Social_Media.pdf. Accessed February 10, 2013.

Patterson P: SCIP measures to weigh in Medicare pay starting in 2013, *OR Manager* 27(3):1, 7–10, 2011.

Pronovost PJ, Colantuoni E: Measuring preventable harm—helping science keep pace with policy, *JAMA* 301(12):1273–1275, 2009.

Raqqad NA, Liu C: Mascara: a cause of thermal burn after cautery for eye lid lesion excision; a case report, *J Clin Exp Ophthalmol* 1:105, 2010, available at www.omicsonline.org/2155-9570/2155-9570-1-105.php?aid=830. Accessed May 1, 2013.

Reason J: *Human error*, Cambridge, United Kingdom, 1990, Cambridge Press.

Robb WB et al: A 10-step intraoperative surgical checklist (ISC) for laparoscopic cholecystectomy—can it really reduce conversion rates to open cholecystectomy? *J Gastrointest Surg* 16(7):1318–1323, 2012.

Rowlands A: Risk factors associated with incorrect surgical counts, *AORN J* 96(3):272–284, 2012.

Shouhed D et al: Integrating human factors research in surgery—a review, *Arch Surg* 147(12):1141–1146, 2012.

Singer v Rodriguez et al, 2012, NYSlipOp 32147(U).

Sitterding MC et al: Understanding situation awareness in nursing work, *Adv Nurs Sci* 35(1):77–92, 2012.

Smith AA: *The operating room: a primer for pupil nurses*, ed 2, Philadelphia, 1924, Saunders.

Terry NP: Fear of Facebook: private ordering of social media risks incurred by healthcare providers, *Neb L Rev* 90:703–751, 2011–2012.

The Joint Commission (TJC): Advancing effective communication, cultural competence, and patient-and family-centered care: a roadmap for hospitals, 2012a, available at www.jointcommission.org/Advancing_Effective_Communication. Accessed January 18, 2013.

The Joint Commission (TJC): Sentinel event data summary as of December 31, 2012, 2012b, available at www.jointcommission.org/sentinel_event_statistics_quarterly. Accessed February 11, 2013.

Tolich DJ et al: Blood management—best practice transfusion strategy, *Nursing 2013* 43(1):41–47, 2013.

van Klei WA et al: Effects of the introduction of the WHO surgical safety checklist on in-hospital mortality: a cohort study, *Ann Surg* 255(1):44–49, 2012.

von Muhlen M, Ohno-Machado L: Reviewing social media use by clinicians, *J Am Med Inform Assoc* 19(5):777–781, 2012.

Walker IA et al: Surgical safety checklists: do they improve outcomes? *Br J Anaesth* 109(1):47–54, 2012.

Wu AW: *The value of close calls in improving patient safety: learning how to avoid and mitigate patient harm*, Oakbrook Terrace, IL, 2011, Joint Commission Resources.

Zarbo RJ: The Henry Ford production system: reduction of surgical pathology in-process misidentification defects by bar code-specified work process standardization, *Am J Clin Pathol* 131(4):468–477, 2009.

CHAPTER 3

Workplace Issues and Staff Safety

REBECCA M. PATTON

Increasingly there is recognition that patient and employee safety programs should be considered together instead of as two separate programs. The Joint Commission (TJC) recognizes synergy between patient safety and worker safety as instrumental in helping organizations to keep both their patients and healthcare workers safe (TJC, 2012a). If the goals of healthcare are to reduce the burden of illness, injury, and disability and to improve the health and functioning of patients, then unsafe working environments must be corrected in order to achieve these goals. Perioperative nurses play a critical role in making the workplace environment safer (Spratt et al, 2012). They strive daily to keep the operating room (OR) safe for patients, other members of the perioperative staff, and themselves.

Employers create a climate of safety for their employees and patients by providing a framework of institutional support. Factors that affect the safety climate include management commitment to safety, healthcare worker involvement in safety decisions, implementation of measures to reduce safety hazards in the work environment, opportunity for feedback on safety improvements, and individual accountability.

Yet even with strong institutional support, OR nurses and surgical technologists face daily challenges to their health and safety and the effectiveness with which they can do their jobs. Routine occupational activities, such as lifting patients and equipment, can cause back injuries and musculoskeletal disorders, and unsafe working environments can lead to occupational injuries from slips, trips, and falls. In addition, OR nurses and surgical technologists regularly face low-level but repeated exposure to numerous hazardous materials, including residues from medications, anesthetic gases, sterilization chemicals, radiation, latex, cleaning chemicals, and disinfection agents. Surgical team members also risk injuries from sharps and exposure to bloodborne pathogens, hazardous chemicals, and workplace violence. Risks specific to the perioperative environment are biologic, ergonomic, chemical, physical, psychosocial, and cultural.

Ergonomics

Perioperative nurses and surgical technologists routinely face a wide array of occupational hazards that place them at risk for work-related musculoskeletal injuries, a frequent and costly occupational issue in nursing (AORN, 2013). More than any other work-related injury or illness, musculoskeletal disorders (MSDs) are responsible for lost work time (Waters, 2010), the need for protracted medical care, and permanent disability among healthcare workers (ANA, 2008). Nurses are known to be at risk for work-related injuries, and many nurses accept musculoskeletal pain as part of their job, with 52% reporting musculoskeletal pain such as back pain (Hunter et al, 2010; Pompeii et al, 2009). The

extent of musculoskeletal injuries among nurses should be no surprise, given that nurses lift and turn patients and move heavy equipment every day.

Studies of back-related workers' compensation claims reveal that nursing personnel have high claim rates compared with other occupations (King, 2011). Back injuries affect approximately 38% of all nurses (ANA, 2008), and an estimated 12% of nurses who leave the profession each year do so because of back injuries (ANA, 2009).

The high incidence of MSDs among nurses is the cumulative effect of repeated patient handling events, often involving unsafe loads. OR nurses and surgical technologists often lift, transfer, or reposition patients on OR beds and transport vehicles, and assist with prepping with arms outstretched or bodies bent forward in awkward postures and positions. Several factors influence the level of ergonomic risk, including patient weight, transfer distance, extent of the workspace, instrument temperature, unpredictable patient behavior, and awkward positions such as stooping, bending, and reaching (Nelson et al, 2009).

Work in the perioperative environment particularly requires an unavoidable constant—moving and lifting large quantities of patient equipment and instrumentation daily. OR nurses and surgical technologists also face risk of injury by standing on floor lifts and platforms while holding instruments and equipment. An ergonomically healthier workplace can decrease or prevent injury to its workforce.

Safe Patient Handling and Movement

Concerted efforts to address workplace safety for perioperative nurses have been under way for some time. As early as 2005, ANA partnered with AORN, the National Institute for Occupational Safety and Health (NIOSH), and the James A. Haley Veterans Administration Medical Center (VAMC) in Tampa, Florida, to form the Workplace Safety Task Force. Its aim was to prepare a safe patient handling "algorithm" guidance document to support ergonomically healthy workplaces. The task force began by identifying high-risk tasks specific to perioperative nurses that specific ergonomic tools could address. These tasks included transferring patients on and off OR beds, repositioning patients on the OR bed, lifting and holding patients' extremities, standing for long periods, holding retractors for long periods, lifting and moving equipment, and sustaining awkward positions. Using current ergonomic safety concepts, scientific evidence, and technology, such as safe patient handling equipment, the task force developed seven ergonomic tools, or *algorithms,* to guide workplace safety in the perioperative setting. These clinical tools are incorporated in AORN's Safe Patient Handling Tool Kit (AORN, 2012).

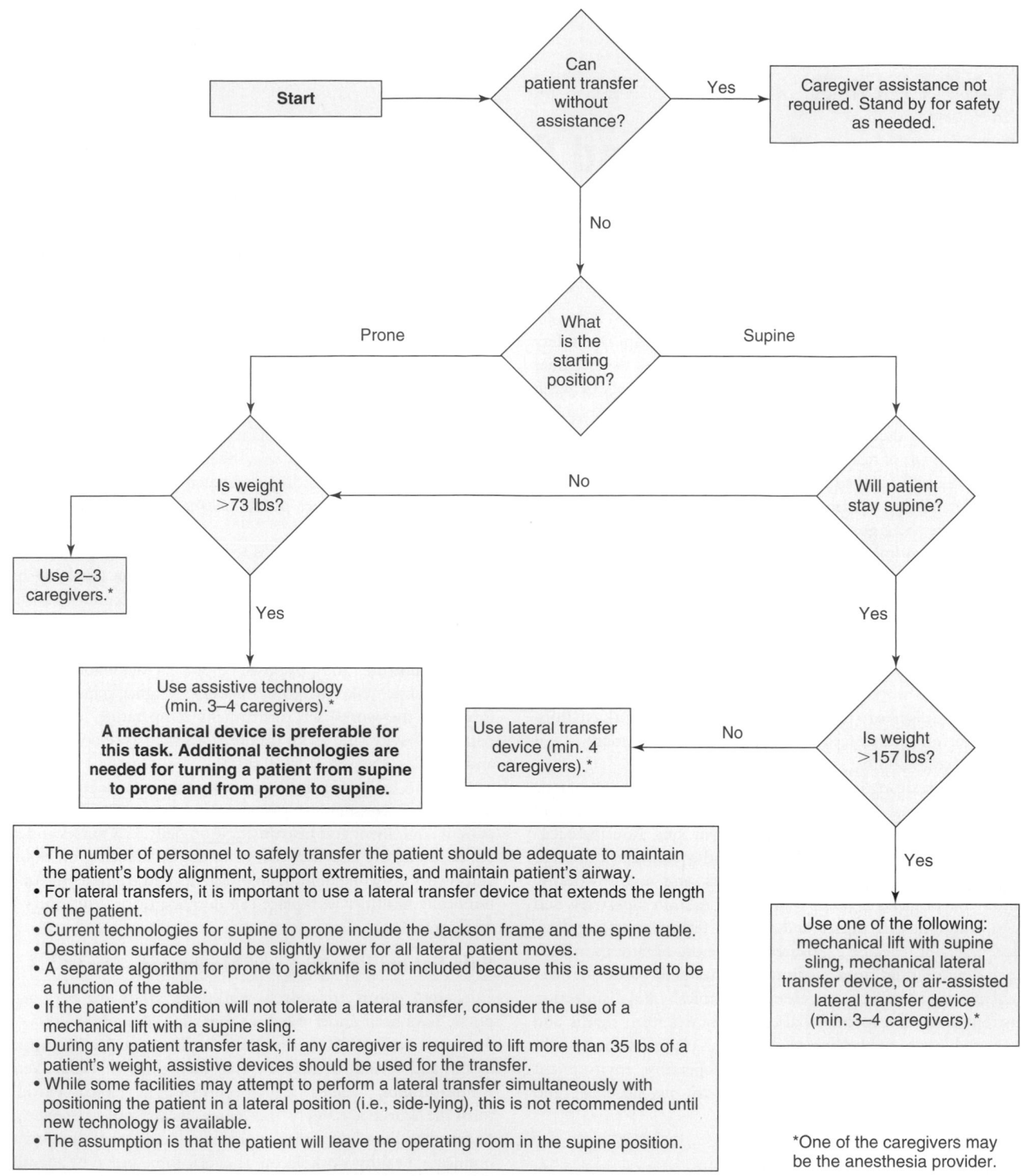

The flowchart contains the following elements:

Start → **Can patient transfer without assistance?**
- Yes → Caregiver assistance not required. Stand by for safety as needed.
- No → **What is the starting position?**

What is the starting position?
- Prone → **Is weight >73 lbs?**
- Supine → **Will patient stay supine?**

Is weight >73 lbs?
- (No) ← from "Will patient stay supine?" (No branch)
- Use 2–3 caregivers.*
- Yes → Use assistive technology (min. 3–4 caregivers).* **A mechanical device is preferable for this task. Additional technologies are needed for turning a patient from supine to prone and from prone to supine.**

Will patient stay supine?
- No → Is weight >73 lbs?
- Yes → **Is weight >157 lbs?**

Is weight >157 lbs?
- No → Use lateral transfer device (min. 4 caregivers).*
- Yes → Use one of the following: mechanical lift with supine sling, mechanical lateral transfer device, or air-assisted lateral transfer device (min. 3–4 caregivers).*

- The number of personnel to safely transfer the patient should be adequate to maintain the patient's body alignment, support extremities, and maintain patient's airway.
- For lateral transfers, it is important to use a lateral transfer device that extends the length of the patient.
- Current technologies for supine to prone include the Jackson frame and the spine table.
- Destination surface should be slightly lower for all lateral patient moves.
- A separate algorithm for prone to jackknife is not included because this is assumed to be a function of the table.
- If the patient's condition will not tolerate a lateral transfer, consider the use of a mechanical lift with a supine sling.
- During any patient transfer task, if any caregiver is required to lift more than 35 lbs of a patient's weight, assistive devices should be used for the transfer.
- While some facilities may attempt to perform a lateral transfer simultaneously with positioning the patient in a lateral position (i.e., side-lying), this is not recommended until new technology is available.
- The assumption is that the patient will leave the operating room in the supine position.

*One of the caregivers may be the anesthesia provider.

FIGURE 3-1 Lateral transfer from stretcher to and from the OR bed.

What is an algorithm? An algorithm is a set of rules for solving a problem in a finite number of discrete steps. In this case the algorithm is an ergonomic tool designed to help make decisions in performing various healthcare tasks. The tool directs the caregiver through a series of questions (diamond boxes in Figure 3-1) and provides optimal responses for action—specifically, whether assistive equipment should be used, what type of equipment would best support the task, and how many caregivers are needed to perform the task safely. The purpose of the algorithm is to standardize practice based on research and task analysis, rather than to allow each caregiver to rely solely on his or her own training and experience to make decisions.

The ergonomic tools should be used in the context of an assessment and plan of care for each patient. The plan of care is designed to communicate decisions about safe patient handling practices among all staff likely to participate in these tasks.

Seven Ergonomic Tools for Safe Patient Handling and Movement

This section explains the seven ergonomic tools for safe patient movement and handling.

Ergonomic Tool #1: Lateral transfer from stretcher to and from the OR bed is shown in Figure 3-1. Lifting and moving patients occurs frequently in perioperative settings, with patients transferring to and from transport carts and the OR bed. Many patients completely or partially depend on help with moving because of sedation and/or anesthesia. Lifting and moving patients is a hazardous patient care activity. Fully 38% of all nurses have suffered injuries related to moving, lifting, or repositioning patients, and about one half of all nurses have experienced chronic pain that they associate with these activities (Waters et al, 2011a).

Ergonomic Tool #2: Positioning and repositioning the patient on the OR bed into and from the supine position. The surgical team often repositions patients once they are on the OR bed to provide appropriate exposure of the surgical site. They frequently lift and maneuver the patient while simultaneously placing a positioning device. Ergonomic Tool #2 provides guidelines for repositioning the patient in a safe manner (Waters et al, 2011b).

Ergonomic Tool #3: Lifting and holding legs, arms, and head for prepping in a perioperative setting. OR nurses often lift or hold patients' limbs during skin prep. Ergonomic Tool #3 is a table that provides calculations to determine whether it is safe for only one caregiver to lift the weight of various limbs and the safe length of time the limbs can be lifted (Waters et al, 2011c).

Ergonomic Tool #4: Prolonged standing. This tool provides relief to OR nurses and surgical technologists who are often required to stand in one place for long periods during surgery. Prolonged standing can cause acute and chronic back, leg, and foot pain, as well as fatigue (Hughes et al, 2011).

Ergonomic Tool #5: Retraction. OR team members must sometimes hold retractors for long periods of time to expose the surgical site. This tool considers whether a self-retaining retractor can be used safely and, if not, how to determine an optimal working height and posture for the retracting team member (e.g., assistant in surgery, such as a physician's assistant [PA] or registered nurse first assistant [RNFA]) (Spera et al, 2011).

Ergonomic Tool #6: Lifting and carrying supplies and equipment. Members of the OR team lift and carry many types of supplies, instrument trays, and equipment. This tool uses the NIOSH lifting index (described following) to predict the risk of back pain from lifting specific objects in the OR (Waters et al, 2011d).

Ergonomic Tool #7: Pushing, pulling, and moving equipment on wheels. This tool makes recommendations on the number of people required to safely push or pull equipment on wheels; it is especially useful for prescribing safe movement of hospital and OR beds (Waters et al, 2011e).

The use of assistive devices is recommended for situations where manual lifting puts the caregiver at substantial risk of injury. According to ANA's Handle with Care campaign, the development of patient care ergonomics programs that include the use of assistive patient handling equipment and devices has essentially rendered "manual" patient handling unnecessary. A growing selection of equipment and devices is designed for the variety of patient handling tasks performed by nurses. Box 3-1 lists a number of such

---

BOX 3-1

Categories and Descriptions of Safe Patient Handling Equipment and Devices

Bed improvements to support transfer or repositioning: Beds that convert directly into chairs or are equipped with shearless pivot that minimizes slipping toward foot of bed when head is raised

Friction-reducing lateral-assist devices: Boards made with smooth, low-friction material used for patient transfer

Inflatable lateral-assist devices: Flexible mattress inflated with air to create a cushioned layer for patient transfer

Mechanical lateral-assist devices: Height-adjustable stretchers used for patient transfer

Powered full-body sling lifts: Portable or ceiling-mounted lift devices to lift and transfer highly dependent patients

Powered stand-assist and repositioning lifts: Lift with arm and/or back slings to assist patients with some weight-bearing ability

Sliding boards: Boards made of smooth, rigid, low-friction material for seated bed-to-chair or chair-to-toilet transfers that act as a supporting bridge

Stand-assist and repositioning aids: Secure devices, either freestanding or attached to beds, to help support patients to lift themselves

Transfer chairs: Chairs that convert into a stretcher, eliminating the transfer from a horizontal plane (bed or stretcher) to a seated position

Modified from de Castro AB: Handle with care: the American Nurses Association's campaign to address work-related musculoskeletal disorders, *Online J Issues Nurs* 9(3), 2004, available at www.nursingworld.org/MainMenuCategories/ANAMarketplace/ANAPeriodicals/OJIN/TableofContents?Volume92004/No3Sept04/HandlewithCare.aspx. Accessed July 6, 2013. Reprinted with permission.

---

patient handling devices. Figure 3-2 illustrates a ceiling lift device in use in the OR.

NIOSH Lifting Equation

The recommendation to use lifting devices for moving patients arises from a body of research that demonstrates that mechanical lifting equipment, as part of a program to promote safe patient handling, can significantly reduce musculoskeletal injuries among healthcare workers. In 1981 NIOSH developed a lifting equation to calculate recommended weight limits for specified two-handed, manual lifting tasks (Waters, 2007). Although NIOSH did not originally recommend the equation for the lifting of humans, it has revised the equation and now recommends it for many patient lifting activities under certain conditions (e.g., when the patient can follow directions or when an estimate of the weight the caregiver must handle is possible). The revised NIOSH lifting equation (RNLE), promulgated in 1991, provides a mathematical equation to determine the recommended weight limit (RWL) and lifting index (LI) for selected two-handed manual lifting tasks. RWL is defined for a specific set of task conditions and represents the weight of the load that nearly all healthy workers can perform over a substantial period (e.g., up to 8 hours) without an increased risk of developing lifting-related low back pain.

The concept behind the lifting equation is to start with a recommended weight that is considered safe for an ideal lift and then to reduce the weight as the task becomes more stressful (e.g., the distance of the load from the worker increases, the duration of the task increases, the type of handhold varies) (AORN, 2012). In

FIGURE 3-2 Ceiling lift.

general, the revised equation yields a recommended 35-pound maximum weight limit for use in patient handling tasks. When the weight to be lifted exceeds this limit, assistive devices should be used (Waters, 2007).

The formula produces a recommended weight limit that can be used to determine the lifting index. This lifting index may then be used to identify potentially hazardous lifting jobs or to compare the relative severity of two jobs for the purpose of selecting the better option. The equation has also been used to provide recommendations for lifting objects such as lead aprons, sterile packs, body positioning devices, and instrument pans or trays (AORN, 2012).

Slips, Trips, and Falls

Although slips, trips, and falls (STFs) may occur in many places throughout a hospital or ambulatory surgery center, the OR is of special focus here because it is where critical patient care occurs. An STF that disables a worker is expensive in terms of direct and indirect costs, but a disabling fall of an OR team member may adversely affect a patient as well. A fall in the OR can cause direct patient injury, disrupt the surgical procedure, contribute to surgical errors, and delay the current surgery as well as other scheduled surgeries while other staff attend to or replace the injured staff member (Brogmus et al, 2007).

STFs remain a leading cause of serious injury among hospital workers (Hughes, 2009), accounting for a large proportion of injuries to healthcare workers who lose time from work. Hospitals are responsible for STF incidence rates 67% higher than those in other U.S. private industries (Collins et al, 2008). STFs account for

nearly 14% of all workers' compensation costs (Brogmus et al, 2007). The average cost to an employer when a worker experiences a fall is $12,470 (Hughes, 2009).

STF Causes and Prevention

STFs arise from many factors, including wet floors, uneven floor surfaces, low-profile equipment and cords, cluttered or poorly lit walkways, and improper footwear. Historically, STF incidents largely appeared to be unpreventable, and blame has been laid more often than not on carelessness of the fall victim. Research has shown, however, that a comprehensive STF-prevention program can significantly reduce workers' compensation claims. To a large degree, STFs are preventable (Collins and Bell, 2012).

Wet Floors. In one 10-year study, STFs resulting from liquids (e.g., water; fluid; and slippery, greasy, and slick spots) were the most common cause (24%) of STF workers' compensation claims (Bell et al, 2008). Planning to avoid wet spots, however, can reduce the rate of falls. Providing lids for all cups or other open containers being transported, for example, helps to avoid spills. Likewise, installing paper-towel holders in high-spill areas, such as near scrub sinks, nursing stations, and elevators, helps employees clean up spills easily and promptly (Hughes, 2009).

Wet floors should be signaled by placing highly visible "Caution: Wet Floor" signs, preferably 4 feet tall and with flashing lights, in areas that have been recently mopped (Hughes, 2009). Housekeeping staff should be equipped with beepers so that they can be quickly alerted to spill areas. In a NIOSH study, employees were able to call a housekeeping hotline to report a spill and were encouraged to use pop-up caution signs placed throughout the hospital to cover spills until housekeeping arrived. The hospital also purchased highly visible yellow absorption towels that employees could toss onto a spill until it was cleaned (Bell et al, 2008).

In the OR, liquids on the floor can make an otherwise slip-resistant surface hazardous (Brogmus et al, 2007). Using a dripless, brush-free gel solution for surgical hand scrubs minimizes water splashes. In addition, when used at the surgical site, gel-based skin preps are less likely to run than liquid prep solutions. They are also less likely to pool under patients or to drip and pool on the floor or OR bed.

Pads can be used to temporarily cover a spill that occurs in an OR because fluids spilled during surgery are hazardous (Hughes, 2009). Fluid solidifiers usually are composed of a granulated substance that can be sprinkled onto a spill or poured into a container with fluid. Fluid solidifiers absorb liquid and solidify the fluid into gel. Adding a fluid solidifier in a liquid medical-waste container or on a fluid spill on the floor serves to control fluid and to reduce the risk of slips and falls (Brogmus et al, 2007). Effective containment also includes adequate waste containers for the planned procedure and readily available waste-control supplies, including absorptive products.

Uneven Floor Surfaces. Falls on the same level also occur at transition areas, such as from dry to wet, on uneven surfaces, or from one type of floor surface to another. Healthcare facilities should ensure that there are no uneven surfaces, including thresholds, on floors. In stairwells with potentially low visibility, the nosing on the top and bottom steps can be painted to provide visual cues.

Obstructed Pathways. Pathways must be kept clear, particularly of low-profile equipment and cords that can be overlooked easily in patients' rooms, hallways, ORs, or other care areas (Hughes, 2009). If possible, cords should not cross walkways; if this is impossible, cords should be covered or taped. Extension cords are also often found under desks and at nursing stations; where feasible, cord organizers, cord clamps, or retractable cord holders should be used to minimize these tripping hazards.

Keeping pathways clear is especially difficult in the OR, where multiple cables and cords are used in surgical procedures. Newer ORs are equipped with articulated ceiling-mounted booms that help keep cords off the floor and systems that integrate cables into the OR bed. Cords and cables in older ORs should be routed so that they do not stretch across walking paths, and they should be secured by bundling, taping, or braiding. Routing and securing cords makes it easier to check that all necessary cords are properly connected, and doing so makes it less likely that a patient will be injured or the procedure prolonged because someone trips on a cord (Brogmus et al, 2007).

Low-standing equipment and supplies are potential tripping hazards. These include buckets, rolling stools or stepstools, support structures for equipment, and supply containers. OR staff often has to navigate around intravenous (IV) tubing and poles. Consider marking mobile equipment such as stools with a bright color or a taped X to make them more visible and distinguishable from the floor. Also, even though protective and absorptive mats play a safety role, they too can pose a tripping hazard. Slip-resistant absorptive mats should be used, and soiled absorptive mats should be removed because a mat that is oversaturated can swell and become a slipping and tripping hazard.

Inadequate Lighting. Lighting throughout the healthcare facility must be adequate to visualize pathways, particularly stairways, when supplies or other items are being carried (Hughes, 2009). Adequate lighting is of specific and critical importance in the OR. Advancements in surgical technology, such as in minimally invasive surgery (MIS), have increased the use of light-emitting diode (LED) monitors in the OR. This increasingly requires dimming general room lighting while leaving the surgical site highly illuminated. Not only does this leave the rest of the OR dimly lit, but also the high illumination on the surgical site makes adapting one's vision to the dimmer room lighting more difficult. Dimmer lighting tends to heighten the risks of not seeing tripping hazards or fluids on the floor. High-quality monitors used during MIS have surface material that minimizes reflected light. Green filters on ambient lighting during MIS procedures minimize reflection of light off the monitors, provide some illumination for other perioperative team members, and reduce ocular fatigue.

Improper Footwear. Improper footwear increases the risk of STFs. Lessons can be learned from industries, such as food service and commercial fishing, in which antislip footwear is standard (Hughes, 2009). In its recommended practices for surgical attire, AORN suggests that shoes worn in the OR should have closed toes and backs, low heels, nonskid soles, and meet Occupational Safety and Health Administration (OSHA) standards as well as the healthcare facility's safety requirements (AORN, 2013).

Programmatic STF Prevention and Reduction

Given the diverse age, job duties, and experience of perioperative staff, an STF program is critical to create a safe work environment. During program development, each healthcare facility should conduct a hazard vulnerability analysis to study its unique hazards

so they can be appropriately addressed in a workplace safety program that includes targeted STFs (Collins and Bell, 2009; Hughes, 2009).

A comprehensive prevention program can significantly reduce injuries. NIOSH researchers in one study compared injury rates and workers' compensation costs for a 10-year period before, during, and after implementation of interventions; they found a 58% reduction in workers' compensation claims for STFs in the postintervention period (Bell et al, 2008). One key component of a successful STF prevention program is to educate workers about the importance of STF prevention and to encourage every employee to take personal responsibility for eliminating STF hazards. Whether this involves personally cleaning spills or cordoning off an area to alert fellow employees while waiting for housekeeping staff to arrive, a successful STF program requires that all hospital staff share responsibility for prevention (Collins and Bell, 2012).

Sharps Safety and Bloodborne Pathogens

Scope and Significance of Problem

In the high-risk perioperative environment, healthcare workers routinely face exposure to bloodborne pathogens (BBPs) and percutaneous injuries (PIs). Each year an estimated 385,000 needlesticks and other sharps-related injuries occur in the United States (Delisio, 2012)—an average of more than 1000 sharps injuries daily (CDC, 2010b). The OR, with 23% for needlesticks (Jagger et al, 2010) and 33% of PIs, has the highest proportion of needlesticks and overall PIs relative to those sustained in all other hospital settings (Research Highlight). In a 2007 study, nurses working in the OR and/or other perioperative settings had sharp device injury rates double those of nurses in other specialties in the United States and Canada—255 and 569 injuries per 1000 per year, respectively (Clarke et al, 2007). Despite passage of the 2007 Needlestick Safety and Prevention Act, while nonsurgical sharps injuries declined, surgical sharps injuries increased (DeJohn, 2012; Jagger et al, 2010).

Although the hepatitis B virus (HBV), the hepatitis C virus (HCV), and the human immunodeficiency virus (HIV) are the pathogens most commonly transmitted during patient care, injuries from needles and other sharp devices used in healthcare and laboratory settings are associated with the transmission of approximately 20 different pathogens (CDC, 2010b). In one study of the prevalence of BBPs in an urban, university-based general surgical practice, testing revealed that 38% of all operations involved patients infected with a BBP: 26% were infected with HIV, 4% with HBV, 35% with HCV, and 17% with both HIV and HCV (Davis, 2006). The risk of transmission after a needlestick or sharps injury is estimated to be 6 to 30 out of every 100 people for HBV, 3 to 10 out of every 1000 people for HCV, and 1 out of every 300 people for HIV.

Exposure to bloodborne pathogens occurs during all phases of the perioperative process, although cuts or needlestick injuries are more likely during the intraoperative phase of patient care. Risk of a sharps injury increases during more invasive, longer procedures that result in higher blood loss. Fatigue resulting from working extended hours coupled with the fast pace of the perioperative environment may also contribute to increased risk of PIs (AORN, 2013). Other factors that may contribute to surgical PIs include frequent handling of sharp instruments and items, prolonged contact with open surgical sites, presence of relatively large

RESEARCH HIGHLIGHT ‖

Scalpel Injuries and Sharps Safety

In surgical settings percutaneous injuries (PIs) from sharps are of grave concern. Scalpel blades are the second most frequent source of PIs in the OR and other procedural settings. Because of the seriousness of PIs, the researchers in this study conducted a literature review to determine levels of evidence for safety measures. Using a predetermined protocol, an independent assessment by two reviewers, and consensus decision, they identified 19 articles for inclusion in their review. Using the Hierarchy of Evidence model (see Evidence for Practice), they found little "high-level" evidence but were able to identify five strategies that had been studied:

1. *Use of cut-resistant gloves/liners:* This strategy decreased the number of glove perforations in comparison with double latex gloves alone but lessened the wearer's dexterity and tactile sensation; some wearers described double latex gloves as more comfortable.
2. *Benefit derived from the use of the hands-free passing technique:* The results supported this practice especially in procedures with more than 100 mL of blood loss.
3. *"Sharpless surgery":* Using the electrosurgical unit or other energy device to perform most of the surgical procedure was found to be feasible.
4. *Single-handed blade remover:* This prevented at least as many injuries as a safety scalpel.
5. *Various shoe materials:* This provided superior foot protection from a dropped sharp.

In the United States, sharps injury rates in the OR increased slightly from 2000 to 2010 and decreased by about 30% outside the OR. Using safety devices and work practices outside the OR is commonplace; implementing sharps safety measures in the OR continues to be lacking. While some known obstacles surrounding using sharps safety practices and devices in the OR include surgeon resistance, lack of awareness and training, and the unsatisfactory design of some safety devices, studies based on evidence assist in developing strategies to reduce PIs for members of the surgical team.

The focus on sharps safety is being championed by a number of individuals and associations, including AORN. Promotion of a culture of safety regarding PI prevention incorporates key sharps safety measures during perioperative patient care, including double-gloving, blunt suture needles for fascial closure, and a neutral/safe zone (the hands-free passing technique) when appropriate to avoid hand-to-hand passage of sharps.

Modified from Watt AM et al: Scalpel safety in the operative setting: a systematic review, *Surgery* 147(1):98–106, 2010.

quantities of blood, unsafe needle handling techniques (passing needles and using sharp rather than blunt needles), and failure to use a neutral zone for passing sharps between perioperative team members).

Although injuries from hollow-bore needles constitute the majority of percutaneous injuries in the healthcare field overall, the pattern of injuries inside the OR is somewhat different. Suture needle injuries (SNIs) are by far the predominant cause of PIs in the surgical setting. They account for as many as 77% of PIs (AORN, 2013) and are a primary cause of occupational exposure to BBPs among OR professionals.

Box 3-2 provides information on bloodborne pathogens and legislation.

Preventing Injuries During Surgery

Surgery involves precise, regimented actions that require planning, communication, and teamwork. Using these same elements can mitigate inherent hazards associated with sharp devices in the perioperative setting (AORN, 2013). AORN has developed a list of risk-reduction strategies that OR nurses can use to protect themselves from exposure injuries in surgery. Care in setting up the surgical work area includes placement of sharp items, constant awareness of the location of sharps and other sterile team members during surgery, and careful disposal of sharps after surgery. Such care contributes to ensuring a safe surgical environment for all participants. These risk-reduction strategies appear in the following sections.

Safe Handling Practices for Surgical Sharps. Observing safety precautions during all phases of surgery, from setup to cleanup, reduces the number of injuries and exposures for all OR personnel.

During preparation for surgery:
- Organize the work area (Mayo stand, back table) so that sharps are always pointed away from the person setting up.
- Establish a separate area, a neutral zone, to place a reusable sharp for safe handling during the procedure; include identification and agreement about this neutral zone in the preoperative briefing.
- Use standardized sterile field setups throughout the surgical services department.

During the procedure:
- Use neutral or hands-free techniques for passing sharp items, instead of passing hand to hand.
- Give verbal notification when passing a sharp device.
- Be aware of other sterile team members in and near the area when handling a sharp device.
- Keep track of, and account for, all sharp items throughout the procedure.
- Keep hands away from the surgical site when sharp items are in use (e.g., suturing, cutting).
- Use gloves and an instrument to pick up sharp items (e.g., suture needles, hypodermic needles, scalpel blades) that have fallen on the floor.

During postprocedure cleanup:
- Inspect the surgical setup used during the procedure for sharps.
- Transport reusable sharps in a closed, secure container to the designated cleanup area.
- Inspect the sharps container for overfilling before discarding disposable sharps in it.
- Do not place hands or fingers into a container to dispose of a device.
- Keep hands behind the sharp tip when disposing.

The Neutral Zone. The neutral zone has been defined as a location on the surgical field where sharps are placed in a predesignated sterile basin or tray or on a magnetic pad, from which the surgeon or assistant can retrieve them (AORN 2013; Burns, 2009). After use, the items are placed back in the neutral zone, and the scrub person retrieves them. This technique eliminates hand-to-hand passing of sharps between the surgeon and the scrub person, so that no two individuals touch the same sharp at the same time. Thus its name, the "hands-free technique" (HFT). Because it reduces the chance of accidental needle punctures and cuts, both the American College of Surgeons (ACS) and AORN recommend use

BOX 3-2

Bloodborne Pathogen Legislation

Protecting healthcare workers from bloodborne pathogens was largely neglected until the global AIDS epidemic of the 1980s. The CDC, the first federal agency to respond, in 1987 issued guidelines for Universal Precautions to protect workers at risk of exposure to patients' blood or body fluids.

In 1991 OSHA issued a rule for Occupational Exposure to Bloodborne Pathogens, based on the concept of Universal Precautions. The Needlestick Safety and Prevention Act, enacted in 2000, directed OSHA to revise its Bloodborne Pathogens Standard. OSHA subsequently revised its final rule to include a special focus on needlestick and other percutaneous exposures to bloodborne pathogens. OSHA's Bloodborne Pathogens Standard requires that engineering and work-practice controls be used to eliminate or minimize exposures to blood and other potentially infectious materials (OPIMs), including human body fluids, tissue, or organs; and HIV- or HBV-containing cell or tissue cultures.

In particular, the standard requires that sharps injuries in the surgical area be eliminated or minimized through the use of such measures as safe needles and other sharps devices, blunt-tip suture needles, needleless intravenous connectors, proper containers for sharps, a "no pass zone" for surgical instruments, and a method to pass equipment safely between surgeon and assistants. The standard also recommends use of scalpel blades with safety features; use of alternative cutting methods, when appropriate; and use of mechanical (self-retaining) retraction devices, when feasible. Other requirements include wearing appropriate personal protective equipment (PPE), such as gloves, gowns, face shields or masks, and shoe covers, if blood or OPIM exposure is anticipated, and adhering to the following practices regarding contaminated needles and sharps: contaminated needles and other sharps should not be bent, recapped, sheared, or broken; and they should be discarded immediately.

One unique feature of the Needlestick Safety and Prevention Act is the required participation of healthcare workers in evaluating and selecting safety-engineered needles and sharps; further, the act mandates employers to document evaluation and implementation of safety-engineered devices. Employers are also required to maintain a sharps injury log to document the types of devices causing injuries and an explanation of the circumstances of each incident.

Evidence shows that this legislation, particularly as it pertains to safety-engineered devices, has been successful. U.S. researchers identified more vigorous enforcement of safety guidelines. Within the United States, a study at Memorial Sloan-Kettering Cancer Center in New York explored the effects of adopting safety-engineered devices. After adoption there was an overall reduction in sharps injuries of 58%, with a 71% reduction in injuries from hollow-bore needles and a 75% reduction in injuries among nurses, the occupational group that typically sustains a high proportion of injuries. The same study found, however, that surgical settings are least likely to adopt safety-engineered devices, such as blunt suture needles and shielded scalpel blades. Professional associations like AORN have championed the focus on sharps safety. In 2012 AORN developed new resources for its Sharps Safety Tool Kit in collaboration with the American College of Surgeons to increase the awareness and implementation of sharps safety measures.

AIDS, Acquired immunodeficiency syndrome; *CDC,* Centers for Disease Control and Prevention; *HBV,* hepatitis B virus; *HIV,* human immunodeficiency virus; *OSHA,* Occupational Safety and Health Administration.

Modified from Jagger J et al: The impact of U.S. policies to protect healthcare workers from bloodborne pathogens: the critical role of safety-engineered devices, *J Infect Pub Health* 1:62–71, 2008; Occupational Safety and Health Administration (OSHA): *Bloodborne pathogens standard* 1910.1030, revised April 3, 2012, available at www.osha.gov/pls/oshaweb/owadisp.show_document?p_table=STANDARDS&p_id=10051. Accessed March 23, 2013; OSHA *Hospital eTool, surgical suite module, bloodborne pathogens (BBPs),* 2008, available at www.OSHA.gov/SLTC/etools/hospital/surgical/surgical.html#BloodbornePathogens. Accessed March 22, 2013; AORN: *Sharps safety tool kit,* available at www.aorn.org/Secondary.aspx?id=20948. Accessed March 21, 2013.

of the neutral zone to transfer sharps as a risk-mitigating strategy (IHWSC, 2010).

The following suggestions make valuable use of the neutral zone:

- A magnetic pad or basin may be used to create the neutral zone; if a basin is used, it should be placed on the field and not held by the scrub person.
- Dedicate the neutral zone to sharps only; these include suture and hypodermic needles, scalpels, and other sharp instruments.
- The scrub person and surgeon or assistants should confer on and agree about the best placement of sharps in the neutral zone.
- Place only one sharp at a time in the neutral zone.
- Announce the transfer of a sharp before placing it in the neutral zone (such as "knife down"); after the announcement, orient the sharp in the correct position in the neutral zone (i.e., place it such that the person picking it up does not have to alter its position in his or her hand).
- Include identification of the neutral zone during hand-off communications to relief scrub persons.

Personal Protective Equipment

The use of personal protective equipment (PPE) has proven effective against transmission of pathogens in the OR. For prevention of infection among OR nurses, two practices are particularly useful: double-gloving and the use of eye protection.

Double-Gloving

Glove barrier failure commonly occurs in the perioperative setting. The frequency of glove perforation during surgery has been studied extensively and found to range from 8% to 50% (Misteli et al, 2009). Glove failures can be caused by punctures, tears by sharp devices, or spontaneous failures; all these failures expose the wearer to BBPs. Studies have demonstrated that glove perforations often occur after an average of 40 minutes of glove use during surgical procedures. When two pairs of gloves are worn, in most instances only the outer glove perforates when punctured by a sharp device. In addition, research demonstrates that when two pairs of gloves are worn and a puncture occurs, the volume of blood transferred from a solid sharp device (e.g., suture needle) lessens by as much as 95%. AORN advises double-gloving during invasive procedures, noting that 18 clinical trials have demonstrated that double-gloving minimizes the risk of exposure to blood and that double-gloving reduces by as much as 87% the risk of exposure to blood and body fluids if the outer glove punctures (AORN, 2013). As part of double-gloving, use of a dark-colored glove against the skin can increase protection because it alerts the surgical team member when a glove defect occurs (Korniewicz and El-Masri, 2012). Another

RESEARCH HIGHLIGHT

Evaluation of an Antimicrobial Surgical Glove

Percutaneous injuries (PIs) expose the surgical team (and those downstream of handling the contaminated sharp items) to bloodborne pathogens. Standard Precautions, use of neutral passing zones (hands-free technique), and safety-engineered devices have helped decrease the incidence of such exposures. When they do occur, direct and indirect costs of managing exposure include time spent reporting, treating, and following up on the injuries; salaries and benefits for injured staff members; laboratory testing of exposure sources and exposed personnel; and postexposure prophylaxis. This study examined use of an antimicrobial glove to prevent transmission of HIV during simulated glove punctures.

Using an experimental design, the researchers evaluated passage of live human immunodeficiency virus (HIV-1) transferred via a contaminated blood-laden needle, using a standard double-layer glove (the control) and an antimicrobial benzalkonium chloride (BKC) surgical glove. Mean HIV viral loads were significantly reduced (P <0.01) following passage through the simulated puncture in the BKC surgical glove compared with passage through a simulated puncture in the nonantimicrobial glove. A pneumatically activated puncturing apparatus was used to ensure consistent and equal surgical glove perforation.

Cuts or needlesticks occur in many surgical procedures. Surgeons, assistants in surgery, and scrub persons are at highest risk for injury. Suture needles and scalpels are the most frequent sources of injury. The antimicrobial glove in this study was effective at reducing the risk for bloodborne virus transfer, which may be an innovation to add to the expanding field of occupational blood exposure prevention in the OR and other procedure settings.

Modified from Edmiston CE et al: Evaluation of an antimicrobial surgical glove to inactivate live human immunodeficiency virus following simulated glove puncture, *Surgery* 153(2):225–233, 2013.

potential for reducing transmission of bloodborne pathogens is an antimicrobial glove (Research Highlight).

Eye Protection

It is well documented that the conjunctivae serve as a transmission route for HIV and HCV. Therefore, it is required that all OR team members, regardless of proximity to the surgical site, wear protective eyewear as routinely as surgical masks.

Blunt Suture Needles

SNIs are the predominant cause of PIs in the surgical setting. Straight suture needles pose the highest risk of injury per needle use, but SNIs occur most often during suturing of fascia or muscles with curved sharp suture needles. According to the ACS, blunt suture needles permit suturing of fascia and other structures with minimal risk of injuring the surgeon, even when the surgeon's glove punctures. Published studies demonstrate that the use of blunt suture needles can reduce or eliminate SNIs (Sullivan, 2009). Blunt-tip suture needles can cut the risk of needlestick injuries by 69% (FDA et al, 2012). Along with use of a neutral zone, the ACS supports the adoption of blunt suture needles to minimize or eliminate needlestick injuries (Burns, 2009). The use of blunt suture needles has also been officially endorsed by AORN and the Council for Surgical and Perioperative Safety (Box 3-3).

Eliminating exposure to hazards is not a "once and done" effort. Often several diverse steps must occur simultaneously. These might

BOX 3-3

Blunt Suture Needles

The blunt suture needle does not have a sharp point; it dissects tissue as it is used, causing less tissue trauma than a conventional sharp-pointed needle. The risk of needlestick injury significantly lessens. The following organizations support the use of blunt suture needles in surgery:

- *The American College of Surgeons (ACS)* issued a statement on blunt suture needles, noting that the ACS supported "the universal adoption of blunt suture needles as the first choice for fascial suturing to minimize or eliminate needlestick injuries from surgical needles" and recommending that "blunt suture needles should be available in various sizes and with a range of suture adequate for different surgical applications."
- *The Council on Surgical and Perioperative Safety (CSPS)* endorses use of blunt suture needles as a recommended sharps safety measure.
- *NIOSH* strongly encourages the use of blunt-tip suture needles to decrease percutaneous injuries to surgical personnel.
- *U.S. Food and Drug Administration (FDA)* strongly encourages surgeons, OR supervisors, perioperative nurses, infection preventionists and other healthcare professionals to use and promote the use of blunt-tip suture needles instead of standard suture needles to suture fascia and muscle.
- *AORN* in its recommended practice for prevention of transmissible infections, notes that the use of blunt suture needles is a method for reducing injuries caused by needles.

Modified from American College of Surgeons: Statement on surgical patient safety, *Bull Am Coll Surg* 94(1):46–47, 2009; Association of periOperative Registered Nurses (AORN): Recommended practices for prevention of transmissible infections in the perioperative practice setting. In *Perioperative standards and recommended practices*, Denver, 2013, The Association; CSPS: *The CSPS endorses sharps safety measures to prevent injury during perioperative care. Sharps safety measures should include double-gloving, blunt suture needles for fascial closure, and the neutral zone when appropriate to avoid hand to hand passage of sharps,* modified February 5, 2009, available at www.cspsteam.org/information/information1.html. Accessed March 21, 2013; FDA, NIOSH and OSHA Joint Safety communication: *Blunt-tip surgical suture needles reduce needlestick injuries and the risk of subsequent bloodborne pathogen transmission to surgical personnel,* May 30, 2012, available at www.fda.gov/MedicalDevices/Safety/AlertsandNotices/ucm305757.htm. Accessed March 21, 2013; NIOSH: Use of blunt-tip suture needles to decrease percutaneous injuries to surgical personnel, *Safety Health Inform Bull,* publication no. 2008-101, 2008, available at www.cdc.gov/niosh/docs/2008-101/default.html. Accessed March 22, 2013.

be as different as hazard-proofing a room, changing the type of equipment used, and changing staff behavior by asking each team member to wear a particular type of protective garment. The Evidence for Practice box explains this approach as the Hierarchy of Controls model.

Responding to Exposure

OSHA regulations require healthcare organizations to protect their workers and to have a sharps injury and BBP exposure control plan (ECP) (Hart, 2011). By law, the plan must be written, communicated to all workers in the perioperative setting, regularly updated and uniformly supported and enforced by perioperative leadership (OSHA, 2012). At a minimum, the ECP must include the following:

- Determination of employee exposure
- Implementation of exposure control methods, including:
  - Standard Precautions
  - Engineering and work-practice controls

EVIDENCE FOR PRACTICE

Hierarchy of Controls

The Hierarchy of Controls model defines a method to control exposure to occupational hazards as a fundamental approach to protect workers. The hierarchy is used to determine a feasible and effective set of controls and can be summarized as follows:
- Elimination
- Substitution
- Engineering controls
- Administrative controls
- Personal protective equipment (PPE)

The concept of the hierarchy is that the control methods at the top of the list are potentially more effective and protective than those at the bottom. Elimination and substitution, although most effective at reducing hazards, also tend to be the most difficult to implement in an existing process. Administrative controls and PPE are frequently used with existing processes in which hazards are not particularly well controlled, but these methods for protecting workers have proven less effective than other measures and require significant effort by workers to achieve success.

Blood exposure prevention practices can be prioritized following the principles of the Hierarchy of Controls model. In the hierarchy for sharps injury prevention, for example, the first priority is to eliminate and reduce the use of needles and other sharps, when possible. The next step is to isolate the hazard, thereby protecting workers from an otherwise exposed sharp, through the use of an engineering control. When these strategies are not available or will not provide total protection, the focus shifts to work-practice controls, such as creating a neutral zone or using hands-free techniques, and PPE. Active involvement of the OR team and hospital management is essential because decisions about supplies, immunizations, and training, among other considerations, require continuous team efforts.

Modified from CDC, NIOSH: *NIOSH safety and health topic: engineering controls,* Cincinnati, 2010, last updated June 25, 2010, available at www.cdc.gov/niosh/topics/engcontrols. Accessed March 23, 2013.

- PPE, using a biohazard risk assessment to determine type of PPE for at-risk employees
- Written protocols for cleaning and decontamination
- Hepatitis B vaccination
- Postexposure evaluation and follow-up
- Communication of hazards to employees and training
- Recordkeeping
- Procedures to evaluate exposure incidents

If You Sustain an Injury

If a needlestick or other occupational contact (e.g., splashing or spraying) that could result in a bloodborne pathogen exposure does occur, the injured person should begin the following procedures *immediately.*

Immediate Response
- Wash with soap and water all wounds and skin sites that have been contacted by blood or body fluids. Flush mucous membranes with water.
- Alert your supervisor and initiate the injury reporting system used in your workplace.
- Identify the source patient; this patient should be tested for HIV, HBV, and HCV infections. Your workplace will begin the testing process by seeking patient consent.

- Immediately report to employee health, the emergency department (ED), or the designated facility.
- Get tested immediately and confidentially for HIV, HBV, and HCV infections.
- Get postexposure prophylaxis (PEP) using the Centers for Disease Control and Prevention (CDC) guidelines when the source patient is unknown or tests positive for HIV or HBV (there is no PEP for HCV). PEP medications for HIV should be started within 2 hours of exposure. PEP can be started after 2 hours from exposure; however, you should be evaluated as soon as possible after injury.
- Document the exposure in detail, for your own records as well as for the employer and for workers' compensation purposes. Employers must maintain a sharps injury log (described under EPINet below).
- Obtain an immediate evaluation and risk assessment.
- Initiate a postexposure treatment plan to include counseling, education, and follow-up testing.

Follow-up
- Obtain confidential postexposure testing at 6 weeks, 3 months, 6 months, and (depending on the risk), 1 year.
- Undergo monitoring and follow-up of PEP.
- Prevent exposing others until follow-up testing is complete.

EPINet

The Exposure Prevention Information Network (EPINet) is a voluntary surveillance system used to record and track PIs and blood and body fluid contacts. The EPINet system consists of a Needlestick and Sharp Object Injury Report (Figure 3-3), Blood and Body Fluid Exposure Report (Figure 3-4), and software to enter and analyze data from the forms (IHWSC, 2010). Since its introduction in 1992, hospitals throughout the United States and overseas have acquired EPINet.

The federal Needlestick Safety and Prevention Act of 2000 and the 2001 revised Bloodborne Pathogens Standards require healthcare facilities to maintain a sharps injuries log. The log must include, at a minimum, the type and brand of device involved in the exposure incident, the department where the exposure occurred, and an explanation of how it occurred. EPINet data can be used to help facilities target high-risk devices and products, identify injuries that may be prevented with safer medical devices, and evaluate new technology designed to prevent needlesticks. Data can also be used by institutions to share and compare information and successful prevention measures.

A Culture of Safety

A healthcare institution's culture of safety profoundly affects its success or failure in reducing employees' blood exposure risk. For sharps safety in particular, success factors include effective systematic review of exposure data, workers' perceptions of exposure risk, availability and use of safety devices, and comprehensive education on bloodborne pathogen exposure risk and safety device use (CDC, 2010b).

Protecting Yourself

You can take significant measures toward ensuring your safety and avoiding injuries from sharps if you do the following:
- Adopt and incorporate safe habits into daily work activities when preparing and using sharp devices.

Text continued on p. 61

Needlestick & Sharp Object Injury Report/OR

EPINet™
FOR MICROSOFT®ACCESS

Last Name: _____   First Name: _____

Injury ID: *(for office use only)* **S**_____   Facility ID: *(for office use only)* _____   **Completed By:** _____

EXPOSURE PREVENTION▶
INFORMATION NETWORK▶

EPINet is a trademark of the University of Virginia.
Windows is a registered trademark of
Microsoft Corporation in the United States and/or other countries.
Operates in Windows 95 and Windows 98 Environments.
© 2000 Becton, Dickinson and Company.
V1.2/US OR, L&D   1/2002

1)   **Date of Injury:** ☐☐ ☐☐ ☐☐☐☐   2)   **Time of Injury:** ☐☐ ☐☐

3)   **Surgical service:** _____
- ☐ 1   General
- ☐ 2   Cardiovascular
- ☐ 3   OB/C-Section
- ☐ 4   Gynecology
- ☐ 5   Orthopedic
- ☐ 6   ENT
- ☐ 7   Neurosurgery
- ☐ 8   Plastic
- ☐ 9   Urology
- ☐ 10 Oral/Dental
- ☐ 11 Transplants
- ☐ 12 Ophthalmology
- ☐ 13 Thoracic
- ☐ 99 Other service, describe: _____

4)   **Surgical procedure being performed:** _____

4a)   **Was it an endoscopic/laparoscopic procedure?**
☐ 1   Yes   ☐ 2 No   ☐ 3 Unknown   ☐ 4 Not Applicable

5)   **What is the job category of the injured worker:** (check one box only)
- ☐ 1   Surgeon *(attending)* specify specialty _____
- ☐ 2   Surgeon *(resident)* specify specialty _____
- ☐ 3   Ob/Gyn *(attending)*
- ☐ 4   Ob/Gyn *(resident)*
- ☐ 5   Anesthesiologist *(attending)*
- ☐ 6   Anesthesiologist *(resident)*
- ☐ 7   Nurse Anesthetist
- ☐ 8   Med Student, mark rotation→ ☐ surg ☐ anesth ☐ ob-gyn
- ☐ 9   Circulating nurse at time of incident → ☐ 1 RN ☐ 2 ORT ☐ 3 UAP
- ☐ 10 Scrub nurse at time of incident →   ☐ 1 RN ☐ 2 ORT ☐ 3 UAP
- ☐ 11 Other Nurse
- ☐ 12 Nursing Student
- ☐ 13 OR Attendant
- ☐ 14 Housekeeper
- ☐ 99 Other, describe: _____

6)   **Where did the injury occur?** (check one box only)
- ☐ 1   Pre-operative area
- ☐ 2   At the Mayo *(instrument)* stand
- ☐ 3   At the back table
- ☐ 4   In the operative site/wound
- ☐ 5   On the surgical field *(near operative site)*
- ☐ 6   On anesthesia machine
- ☐ 7   On anesthesia cart
- ☐ 8   At patient's puncture site *(intro of vascular cath/injection,etc)*
- ☐ 9   At site of injection into IV equipment
- ☐ 10 On OR floor
- ☐ 11 In the OR utility room
- ☐ 12 Post anesthesia care unit *(recovery room)*
- ☐ 99 Other, describe: _____

7)   **Was the source patient's identity known?** (check one box only)
☐ 1   Yes   ☐ 2 No   ☐ 3 Unknown   ☐ 4 Not Applicable

8)   **For what purpose was the sharp item originally used?** (check one box only)
- ☐ 1   Unknown/not applicable
- ☐ 2   Injection, intra-muscular/subcutaneous, or other injection through the skin *(syringe)*
- ☐ 3   To start IV or set up heparin lock *(IV catheter or winged set-type needle)*
- ☐ 4   To connect IV line *(intermittent IV/piggyback/IV infusion/other IV line connection)*
- ☐ 5   Injection into (or aspiration from) IV injection site or IV port
- ☐ 6   To place an arterial line/catheter
- ☐ 7   To place a central line/catheter
- ☐ 8   To place other non-vascular line/catheter
- ☐ 9   To draw venous blood sample
- ☐ 10 To draw arterial blood sample ▶ if used to draw blood was it?   ☐ 1 Direct stick?   ☐ 2 Draw from a Line?
- ☐ 11 To obtain a body fluid or tissue sample *(urine/CSF/amniotic fluid/other fluid, biopsy)*
- ☐ 12 Cutting *(surgery)*
- ☐ 13 Suturing muscle/fascia
- ☐ 14 Suturing skin
- ☐ 21 Suturing tissue not listed above, describe: _____
- ☐ 15 Electrocautery
- ☐ 16 Drilling/sawing
- ☐ 17 Retracting tissue/bone
- ☐ 18 Wiring/fixing
- ☐ 19 Using as a tool, not on patient
- ☐ 20 To contain a specimen or pharmaceutical *(glass items)*
- ☐ 99 Other; describe _____

9)   **Did the injury occur?** (check one box only)
- ☐ 1   Before use of item *(item broke/slipped, assembling device, etc.)*
- ☐ 2   During use of item *(item slipped, patient/colleague jarred item, etc)*
- ☐ 3   While manually retracting tissue in operative site
- ☐ 4   While retracting tissue using retractor or other instrument
- ☐ 5   Passing instruments, hand to hand
- ☐ 6   Passing instruments, hand-free transfer
- ☐ 7   Between incremental injections
- ☐ 8   In between uses of devices
- ☐ 9   Disassembling device or equipment
- ☐ 10 Sorting, disinfecting, and/or sterilizing instruments
- ☐ 11 While recapping a used needle
- ☐ 12 Withdrawing needle from rubber or resistant material
- ☐ 13 Other after use-before disposal *(in transit to trash, cleaning, left on bed, table, floor, or other inappropriate place, etc.)*
- ☐ 14 From item left on or near disposal container
- ☐ 15 While putting item into disposal container
- ☐ 16 After disposal, stuck by item protruding from opening of disposal container
- ☐ 17 Item pierced side of disposal container
- ☐ 18 After disposal, item protruded from **trash bag** or **inappropriate** waste container
- ☐ 99 Other, describe: _____

FIGURE 3-3 Needlestick and sharp object injury report for the OR.

10)   If the injury was sustained by an anesthesia team member, what anesthesia task was being performed at the time of injury?
Describe: _____

11)   At the time of the injury, was the sharp instrument/item? (check one box only)
☐ 1   Held by another person
☐ 2   Held by injured person
☐ 3   Not held by anyone

12)   The sharp item was: (check one box only)
☐ 1   Contaminated (known exposure to patient or contaminated equipment) ➡ **was there blood on the device?**   ☐ 1 Yes
☐ 2   Uncontaminated (no known exposure to patient or contaminated equipment)   ☐ 2 No
☐ 3   Unknown

13)   What type of device caused the injury? (check one box only)   ☐ Needle-*Hollow Bore*
☐ Surgical
☐ Glass

Which device caused the injury? (check one box from one of the three sections only)
Needles *(for suture needles see "**surgical instruments**")*

☐ 1   Disposable Syringe *(includes standard, insulin, tuberculin, etc)*
☐ 2   Pre-filled cartridge syringe *(includes Tubex™ *, Carpuject ™* - type syringes)*
☐ 3   Blood gas syringe *(ABG)*
☐ 4   Syringe, other type
☐ 5   Needle on IV line *(includes piggybacks & IV line connectors)*
☐ 6   Winged steel needle *(includes winged-set type devices)*
☐ 7   IV catheter stylet
☐ 8   Vacuum tube blood collection holder/needle *(includes Vacutainer™ *–type device)*

☐ 9   Spinal or epidural needle
☐ 10 Unattached hypodermic needle
☐ 11 Arterial catheter introducer needle
☐ 12 Central line catheter introducer needle
☐ 13 Drum catheter needle
☐ 14 Other vascular catheter needle *(cardiac etc.)*
☐ 15 Other non-vascular catheter needle *(ophthalmology, etc.)*
☐ 16 Huber-type needle
☐ 28 Needle, not sure what kind
☐ 29 Other needle, please describe: _____

Surgical instrument or other sharp items *(for glass items see "**glass**")*

☐ 30   Lancet (finger or heel sticks)
☐ 31   Suture needle
☐ 32   Scalpel blade, reusable handle
☐ 45   Scalpel blade, disposable scalpel
☐ 33   Razor
☐ 34   Pipette *(plastic)*
☐ 35   Scissors
☐ 360 Electro-cautery device, needle tip
☐ 361 Electro-cautery device, blade tip
☐ 362 Electro-cautery device, loop tip
☐ 37   Bone cutter
☐ 38   Bone chip
☐ 39   Perforating towel clip

☐ 40   Microtome blade
☐ 41   Trocar
☐ 42   Vacuum tube *(plastic)*
☐ 43   Specimen/Test tube *(plastic)*
☐ 44   Fingernails/Teeth
☐ 46   Retractors, skin/bone hooks
☐ 47   Staples/Steel sutures
☐ 48   Wire *(suture/fixation/guide wire)*
☐ 49   Pin *(fixation, guide pin)*
☐ 50   Drill bit/bur
☐ 51   Pickups/Forceps/Hemostats/Clamps
☐ 58   Sharp item, not sure what kind
☐ 59   Other sharp item: Describe: _____

Glass

☐ 60   Medication ampule
☐ 61   Medication vial *(small volume with rubber stopper)*
☐ 62   Medication/IV bottle *(large volume)*
☐ 63   Pipette *(glass)*
☐ 64   Vacuum tube *(glass)*
☐ 65   Specimen/Test tube *(glass)*

☐ 66   Capillary tube
☐ 67   Glass slide

☐ 78   Glass item, not sure what kind
☐ 79   Other glass item: Describe: _____

13a)   **Brand/Manufacturer of product:** (e.g., ABC Medical Company) _____

13b)   **Model:**
☐ 98 Known: Please specify: _____   ☐ 99 Unknown

14)   If the item causing the injury was a needle or sharp medical device, was it a" safety design" with a shielded, recessed, retractable, or blunted needle or blade?
☐ 1 Yes   ☐ 2 No   ☐ 3 Unknown

14a)   Was the protective mechanism activated?
☐ 1 Yes, fully   ☐ 2 Yes, partially   ☐ 3 No   ☐ 4 Unknown

14b)   Did incident happen?
☐ 1   Before activation
☐ 2   During activation
☐ 3   After activation
☐ 4   Unknown

FIGURE 3-3, cont'd   Needlestick and sharp object injury report for the OR.

Continued

Mark the location of the injury:

15)   Was the injury?
- ☐ 1   Superficial *(little or no bleeding)*
- ☐ 2   Moderate *(skin punctured, some bleeding)*
- ☐ 3   Severe *(deep stick/cut, or profuse bleeding)*

16)   If injury was to the hand, did the sharp item penetrate?
- ☐ 1   Single pair of gloves
- ☐ 2   Double pair of gloves
- ☐ 3   No gloves

17)   Dominant hand of the injured worker:
- ☐ 1   Right-handed
- ☐ 2   Left-handed

18)   Describe the circumstances leading to this injury *(please note if a device malfunction was involved)*:

_____
_____
_____
_____
_____
_____

Cost:

	Lab charges (Hb, HCV, HIV, other)
_____	Healthcare worker
_____	Source
	Treatment prophylaxis (HBIG, Hb vaccine, tetanus, other)
_____	Healthcare worker
_____	Source
_____	**Service charges** (Emergency Dept, Employee Health, other)
_____	**Other costs** (Workers' Comp, surgery, other)
_____	**TOTAL** (round to nearest dollar)

Is this incident OSHA reportable?
- ☐ 1   Yes   ☐ 2   No   ☐ 3   Unknown
  - **If yes**, days away from work? _____
  - Days of restricted work activity? _____

Does this incident meet the FDA medical device reporting criteria? (Yes, if a device defect caused serious injury necessitating medical or surgical intervention, or death occurred within 10 works days of incident.)
- ☐ 1   Yes *(If yes, follow FDA reporting protocol.)*   ☐ 2   No

* Tubex™ is a trademark of Wyeth Ayers; Carpuject™ is a trademark of Sanofi Winthrop; VACUTAINER™ is a trademark of Becton Dickinson. Identification of these products does not imply endorsement of these specific brands.

FIGURE 3-3, cont'd Needlestick and sharp object injury report for the OR.

Blood and Body Fluid Exposure Report/OR

EPINet™

FOR MICROSOFT®ACCESS

EXPOSURE PREVENTION►
INFORMATION NETWORK►

EPINet is a trademark of the University of Virginia.
Windows is a registered trademark of
Microsoft Corporation in the United States and/or other countries.
Operates in Windows 95 and Windows 98 Environments.
© 2000 Becton, Dickinson and Company.
V1.2/US OR, L&D   1/2002

Last Name: _____   First Name: _____

Exposure ID: *(for office use only)* **B**_____   Facility ID: *(for office use only)* _____

1) Date of exposure: ▢▢ ▢▢ ▢▢▢▢   2) Time of exposure: ▢▢ ▢▢

3) **Surgical service:** _____
- ▢ 1 General
- ▢ 2 Cardiovascular
- ▢ 3 OB/C-Section
- ▢ 4 Gynecology
- ▢ 5 Orthopedic
- ▢ 6 ENT
- ▢ 7 Neurosurgery
- ▢ 8 Plastic
- ▢ 9 Urology
- ▢ 10 Oral/Dental
- ▢ 11 Transplants
- ▢ 12 Ophthalmology
- ▢ 13 Thoracic
- ▢ 99 Other service, describe: _____

4) **Surgical procedure being performed:** _____

4a) **Was it an endoscopic/laparoscopic procedure?**
▢ 1 Yes   ▢ 2 No   ▢ 3 Unknown   ▢ 4 Not Applicable

5) **What is the job category of the injured worker:** (check one box only)
- ▢ 1 Surgeon *(attending)* specify specialty _____
- ▢ 2 Surgeon *(resident)* specify specialty _____
- ▢ 3 Ob/Gyn *(attending)*
- ▢ 4 Ob/Gyn *(resident)*
- ▢ 5 Anesthesiologist *(attending)*
- ▢ 6 Anesthesiologist *(resident)*
- ▢ 7 Nurse Anesthetist
- ▢ 8 Med Student, mark rotation→ ▢ surg ▢ anesth ▢ ob-gyn
- ▢ 9 Circulating nurse at time of incident → ▢ 1 RN ▢ 2 ORT ▢ 3 UAP
- ▢ 10 Scrub nurse at time of incident → ▢ 1 RN ▢ 2 ORT ▢ 3 UAP
- ▢ 11 Other Nurse
- ▢ 12 Nursing Student
- ▢ 13 OR Attendant
- ▢ 14 Housekeeper
- ▢ 99 Other, describe: _____

6) **If the injury was sustained by an anesthesia team member, what anesthesia task was being performed at the time of injury?**
Describe: _____

7) **Where Did the Exposure Occur?** (check one box only)
- ▢ 1 Pre-operative area
- ▢ 2 At the Mayo *(instrument)* stand
- ▢ 3 At the back table
- ▢ 4 In the operative site/wound
- ▢ 5 On the surgical field *(near operative site)*
- ▢ 6 On anesthesia machine
- ▢ 7 On anesthesia cart
- ▢ 8 At patient's puncture site *(intro of vascular cath/injection,etc)*
- ▢ 9 At site of injection into IV equipment
- ▢ 10 On OR floor
- ▢ 11 In the OR utility room
- ▢ 12 Post anesthesia care unit *(recovery room)*
- ▢ 99 Other, describe: _____

8) **Was the source patient's identity known?** (check one box only)
▢ 1 Yes   ▢ 2 No   ▢ 3 Unknown   ▢ 4 Not Applicable

9) **Which body fluids were involved in the exposure?** (check all that apply)
- ▢ Blood or blood products
- ▢ Vomit/gastric contents
- ▢ Sputum
- ▢ Saliva
- ▢ CSF
- ▢ Peritoneal fluid
- ▢ Pleural fluid
- ▢ Amniotic fuid
- ▢ Urine
- ▢ Other, describe: _____

Was the body fluid visibly contaminated with blood?   ▢ Yes   ▢ No   ▢ Unknown

10) **Was the exposed part:** (check all that apply)
- ▢ Intact skin
- ▢ Non-intact skin
- ▢ Eyes *(conjunctiva)*
- ▢ Nose *(mucosa)*
- ▢ Mouth *(mucosa)*
- ▢ Other, describe: _____

11) **Did the blood or body fluid:** (check all that apply)
- ▢ Touch unprotected skin
- ▢ Touch skin between gap in protective garments
- ▢ Touch skin through tear in glove
- ▢ Soak through barrier garment or protective garment
- ▢ Soak through clothing/undergarments

12) **Which barrier garments were worn at the time of exposure:** (check all that apply)
- ▢ Single pair latex/vinyl gloves
- ▢ Double pair latex/vinyl gloves
- ▢ Goggles
- ▢ Eyeglasses *(not a protective item)*
- ▢ Eyeglasses with side shields
- ▢ Face shield
- ▢ Surgical mask
- ▢ Surgical mask with attached eyeshield
- ▢ Surgical gown, disposable
- ▢ Surgical gown, reusable
- ▢ Other, describe: _____

12a) **If surgical gown, was it?**
- ▢ 1 Fabric, standard single layer
- ▢ 2 Fabric, reinforced
- ▢ 3 Plastic, reinforced/coated
- ▢ 4 Composite construction *(multi-layer laminate)*

FIGURE 3-4 Blood and body fluid exposure report for the OR.

Continued

13) Was the exposure the result of: (check one box only)

□ 1 Direct patient contact
□ 2 Touched contaminated equipment/surface
□ 3 Touched contaminated drapes/sheets/gowns, etc.
□ 4 Specimen container leaked/spilled/broke
□ 5 Tubing *(blood, suction, drain, etc.)* leaked/disconnected/broke
□ 6 Bag/pump leaked/spilled/broke

□ 7 Trach/NG tubing broke/sprayed
□ 8 Suction canister spilled/leaked/broke
□ 9 Other irrigation/fluid container spilled/leaked/broke
□ 10 Other equipment/operator failure
□ 11 Unknown
□ 99 Other, describe: _____

If equipment failure, please specify: **Equipment type:** _____

Manufacturer: _____

14) For how long was the blood or body fluid in contact with your skin or mucous membranes? (check one)

□ 1 Less than 5 minutes
□ 2 5-14 minutes
□ 3 15 minutes to 1 hour
□ 4 More than 1 hour

15) How much blood/body fluid came in contact with your skin or mucous membranes? (check one)

□ 1 Small amount (up to 5 cc, or up to 1 teaspoon)
□ 2 Moderate amount (up to 50 cc, or up to quarter cup)
□ 3 Large amount (more than 50 cc)

16) Location of the exposure:

Write the number of the location of up to three exposed body parts in the blanks below.

Largest area of exposure: _____

Middle area of exposure: _____

Smallest area of exposure: _____

17) Describe the circumstances leading to this exposure *(please note if a device malfunction was involved)*:

_____
_____
_____
_____
_____
_____
_____
_____

Cost:

_____ **Lab charges** *(Hb, HCV, HIV, other tests)*
            Healthcare worker
_____ Source
            Treatment prophylaxis *(HBIG, Hb vaccine, tetanus, other)*
_____ Healthcare worker
_____ Source
_____ **Service charges** *(Emergency Dept, Employee Health, other)*
_____ **Other costs** *(Worker's Comp, surgery, other)*
_____ **TOTAL** *(round to nearest dollar)*

Is this incident OSHA reportable?   □ 1 Yes   □ 2 No   □ 3 Unknown
   If yes, days away from work? _____
   Days of restricted work activity? _____

Does this incident meet the FDA medical device reporting criteria? (Yes, if a device defect caused serious injury necessitating medical or surgical intervention, or death occurred within 10 works days of incident.)

□ 1 Yes (If yes, follow FDA reporting protocol)   □ 2 No

FIGURE 3-4, cont'd Blood and body fluid exposure report for the OR.

- Observe local, state, and federal (OSHA) regulations.
- Comply with methods to protect yourself from disease transmission (e.g., get the hepatitis B vaccination).
- Participate in education about bloodborne pathogens, and follow recommended infection prevention practice.
- Know the location in your department of the exposure control plan.
- Finally, follow the exposure control policy if injured, including *immediately* reporting the incident and commencing exposure response procedures (AORN, 2013).

Waste Anesthetic Gases

Scope and Significance of Problem

The first use of surgical anesthesia in the United States occurred in 1842 when diethyl ether was administered to a patient. Since then many anesthetic agents have been administered to patients to provide freedom from pain during surgical procedures. Advances in anesthetic agents have eliminated the risk of explosion caused by formerly used anesthetic agents such as diethyl ether and cyclopropane. Developments in chlorofluorocarbon chemistry have resulted in halogenated, nonflammable, volatile agents; these have reduced the risk of explosion and flammability. OR workers at occupational risk include anesthesia care providers, perioperative nurses, surgical technologists, postanesthesia care unit (PACU) nurses, and others who work in settings where anesthetics are administered, such as office-based surgery.

Waste anesthetic gases (WAGs) are small amounts of gases that may leak either from the patient's anesthetic breathing circuit into the OR air while anesthesia is being administered or from exhalation of the patient during recovery (OSHA, 2008b). Both mechanisms of exposure create risks for OR personnel. Research on the effects of waste anesthetic gas exposure started appearing in the literature in 1967. Short-term exposure causes lethargy and fatigue, and long-term exposure may be linked to spontaneous abortion, congenital abnormalities, infertility, premature births, cancer, and renal and hepatic disease. Today, perioperative staff members are exposed to trace amounts of waste anesthetic gas, and although this exposure cannot be eliminated, it can be controlled.

OR personnel are more prone to being exposed to WAGs in facilities with no automatic scavenging systems or with no automated ventilation, in facilities with anesthesia systems in poor working order, or in recovery areas such as the PACU with inadequate systems. Where scavenging and ventilation systems are in place, OR personnel nevertheless can be exposed when leaks occur in the anesthetic breathing circuits because of poor maintenance of tubing, connectors, or valves, or because of circuits with loose connections. Gases can also escape during connection and disconnection of the system. In addition, poor-fitting patient masks or endotracheal tube connections can cause gases to escape into the air, making induction of anesthesia another occasion when gas leakage places OR staff at risk. Other mechanisms of potential exposure include defects in rubber and plastic tubing and hoses; selected anesthesia techniques; improper practices such as gas flow control valves being left open after use; liquid anesthetic spills; and improperly inflated tracheal tubes, which can allow WAGs to escape into the ambient OR air.

PACU personnel are exposed to WAGs from patients who have received anesthetics and then are admitted to the PACU or another postanesthesia recovery area. These postoperative patients eliminate anesthetics through their respiratory tracts by simply exhaling.

Given the close proximity of PACU nurses to their patients (i.e., within the nurses' breathing zone), they are exposed to varying concentrations of anesthetic agents. In contrast to the OR, ambient air in the PACU may contain multiple WAGs. Detection of the levels of WAGs without monitoring air samples in the breathing zone is deceiving because PACU nurses may be unable to detect the presence of agents until the concentrations are above the NIOSH-recommended exposure limit.

Exposure to high WAG concentrations can cause headaches, fatigue, irritability, nausea, drowsiness, liver and kidney disease, and difficulties with judgment and coordination. Some studies show that long-term exposure to low concentrations of WAGs appears to have no adverse health effects, whereas other studies show links to miscarriage, genetic damage, and cancer for perioperative personnel (and their spouses), with further links to birth defects in their children (CDC and NIOSH, 2007b). In light of these latter studies, healthcare facilities are required to develop, implement, measure, and control practices to reduce anesthetic gas exposure to the lowest practical level. Exposure levels must be measured every 6 months and maintained at less than 25 parts per million (ppm) for nitrous oxide and 2 ppm for halogenated agents to be compliant with OSHA standards (Smith, 2010).

Chemicals

Chemicals are used in OR settings for many purposes, including sterilization and disinfection of equipment, cleaning, specimen preservation, and anesthesia. Some commonly used chemicals include disinfectants and sterilants (e.g., glutaraldehyde, ortho-phthalaldehyde, ethylene oxide, hydrogen peroxide, peracetic acid), tissue preservatives (i.e., formalin), antiseptic agents (e.g., hand hygiene products, surgical prep solutions) (AORN, 2013), and methyl methacrylate (MMA) (used to cement orthopedic prostheses and in certain neurosurgical procedures to aid in reconstruction of cranial bone).

Exposure to chemicals occurs through several routes. Toxic exposure effects can be limited to the site of exposure or result in a systemic effect. The following are three main routes of exposure to toxic chemicals:

1. *Inhalation* is the introduction of toxic chemicals, radioisotopes, or pathogens via the respiratory tract. Gases or vapors of volatile liquids are the most commonly inhaled chemicals, although it is possible to inhale chemicals as aerosols or dusts. Inhaled chemical agents are generally quickly absorbed because of lung vascularity and large surface area, with exposure symptoms manifesting within 1 to 3 days after exposure.
2. *Skin contact or absorption through mucous membranes* is slower than inhalation. Mucous membranes include the mouth, eyes, and nose. Nonintact skin integrity (exposed skin that is chapped, abraded, or afflicted with dermatitis) can also lead to exposures.
3. *Ingestion* is the least common route of exposure. Ingestion may be the result of unintentional exposures from the hand (including cuticle tears and nail biting) or mouth, such as swallowing saliva containing trapped airborne particles.

The amount of chemical absorbed by the body varies, depending on duration of exposure, concentration of the chemical, and various environmental factors. Toxicity can be acute or chronic. Acute toxicity usually results from an accidental spill of a chemical. Exposure is sudden and results in an emergency. Chronic toxicity results from repeated exposure to low levels of a chemical over a prolonged period (CDC and NIOSH, 2007a).

Exposure limits for many chemicals used in healthcare help to provide a safer environment. Exposure limits published by OSHA are the only legally recognized regulatory limits. OSHA defines a permissible exposure limit (PEL) as the amount of exposure to a chemical permitted as a time-weighted average (TWA) (OSHA, 2006). Recommended exposure limits (RELs) are occupational exposure limits developed and recommended by NIOSH, providing protection over a working lifetime. NIOSH uses a TWA for up to a 10-hour workday during a 40-hour workweek (CDC and NIOSH, 2007a). A short-term exposure limit (STEL) is a designated value that should not be exceeded anytime during the workday, based on a 15-minute TWA (CDC and NIOSH, 2007). For example, for glutaraldehyde, the NIOSH REL is 0.2 ppm, with an OSHA PEL of zero (CDC and NIOSH, 2007a).

Responsibility to inform workers about chemical hazards and to use control measures, including providing PPE, rests with the employer. The OSHA Hazard Communication Standard (29 CFR 1910.1200, 1915.99, 1917.28, 1918.90, 1926.59, and 1928.21) requires all manufacturers and importers of hazardous chemicals to develop safety data sheets (SDSs) (formerly known as material safety data sheets [MSDSs]) for all chemicals and mixtures of chemicals (OSHA, 2012). Employers must make these data sheets readily available to all employees who could be exposed to hazardous products.

The purpose of the OSHA standards is to ensure evaluation of all hazardous chemicals produced or imported and transmission of information concerning such hazardous chemicals to employers and employees. This transmission occurs by comprehensive hazard communication programs that must include container labeling and other forms of warning, SDSs, and employee training (OSHA, 2012). SDSs initially arose as tools for workers with health and safety roles in the chemical industry. With the expansion of federal and state right-to-know laws and regulations, however, the need for information on SDSs expanded to the healthcare industry.

A typical SDS includes the following sections:
- Material identity, including chemical and common names
- Hazardous ingredients
- Cancer-causing ingredients
- List of physical and chemical hazards and characteristics
- List of health hazards, including acute and chronic effects
- Whether OSHA, the International Agency for Research on Cancer, or the National Toxicology Program lists the material as a carcinogen
- Limits to which a worker can be exposed
- Routes of entry
- Specific target organs likely to be damaged with exposure, and medical problems exacerbated by exposure
- Precautions and safety equipment
- Emergency and first aid procedures
- Firefighting information
- Procedures for cleanup of leaks and spills
- Safe handling precautions
- Identity of the organization responsible for the SDS, date of issue, and emergency phone number

The *NIOSH Pocket Guide to Chemical Hazards* offers useful information about several hundred chemicals (CDC and NIOSH, 2007a). It is important that healthcare workers are aware of chemicals they are exposed to in their work settings and take necessary precautions to use PPE and other means to eliminate or reduce their occupational risks. Measures may include attending training provided by the employer and being familiar with information about occupational exposures, such as the chemicals inventoried on their work unit. These inventories should be located on each unit and be easily accessible.

Another form of chemical exposure in perioperative settings is exposure to hazardous drugs. Exposure can result from handling hazardous drugs as well as working near sites where they are used. The drugs can be in the air, on surfaces in the work area, on medical equipment, or in the urine or feces of patients. Work practices and training are important to minimize occupational risks of hazardous drug exposure.

Related to hazardous drug exposure and chemical risk are reproductive hazards found in perioperative patient care settings, with implications for males as well as females. Occupational exposure to reproductive hazards can cause effects before or after conception, with different outcomes. Before conception, exposure effects include reduced fertility, unsuccessful fertilization, implantation problems, fetal abnormality, reduced libido, or menstrual dysfunction. Maternal exposure can result in low-birth-weight infants, birth defects, developmental difficulties, behavioral difficulties, cancer, or even fetal demise. Men who suffer workplace exposure can introduce harm to a woman's reproductive system and offspring (OSHA, 2010). Awareness of reproductive hazards, prevention strategies, and work practices to minimize risks is key to dealing with reproductive hazards in the workplace.

New bioengineered drugs target specific locations in the human body. These are evolving and potentially creating new hazardous risks to healthcare workers.

As healthcare facilities become more environmentally sensitive, they take more steps to reduce chemical exposures by eliminating or reducing the use of chemicals, seeking safer alternatives for substances such as cleaning agents, using engineering controls such as ventilation, and using chemical storage to isolate chemicals (Markkanen et al, 2009).

Standard Precautions

The CDC's Standard Precautions aim to reduce transmission of microorganisms from both recognized and unrecognized sources of infection. Standard Precautions apply to all patients receiving care, regardless of diagnosis or presumed infection status. They are considered the first and most important tier of precautions; as such, they are the primary strategy for successful infection prevention and control. Standard Precautions apply to (1) blood; (2) all body fluids, secretions, and excretions (except sweat), regardless of whether they contain visible blood; (3) mucous membranes; and (4) nonintact skin. Perioperative personnel historically have relied on numerous, differing sets of precautions to protect themselves and others from BBPs and other infectious diseases. Today, consistent application of these precautions and frequent handwashing by all members of the perioperative team serve to protect the healthcare provider and to minimize cross-infection of pathogens among patients (refer to Chapter 4 for further discussion of Standard- and Transmission-Based Precautions).

Immunizations and Infectious Disease Exposure

Contact with infected patients or infectious material puts healthcare workers at risk for occupational-acquired infection. Many diseases and infections are preventable through immunizations and vaccines. It is therefore essential for nurses and other healthcare workers to establish and maintain their immunity in cooperation with their employers. Healthcare organizations providing direct patient care should develop a comprehensive immunization program for workers.

HBV is a major infectious risk for healthcare workers as a result of percutaneous and permucosal exposure to blood or other potentially infectious material. Through a joint advisory notice in 1987, the Departments of Labor and Health and Human Services initiated rule making to regulate exposure to HBV. The resulting federal standard issued in December 1991 mandated that hepatitis B vaccine be made available at the employer's expense to all healthcare workers occupationally exposed to blood or other potentially infectious materials (Smith, 2010). It is important for healthcare workers to have a hepatitis B antibody titer to evaluate their immune response to a vaccine series. Once immunity is documented, there is no need for booster doses even if titer levels drop.

Seasonal influenza and its complications are responsible for more than 36,000 deaths and more than 200,000 hospitalizations each year (ANA, 2011; CDC, 2010a). Despite the well-documented seriousness of seasonal influenza cases, according to the CDC less than 50% of healthcare workers secure vaccination annually (ANA, 2011). Patients transmit influenza to healthcare workers and, in turn, healthcare workers who are clinically or subclinically infected with influenza can transmit seasonal influenza to patients or others. Studies demonstrate seasonal influenza antibodies in healthcare workers who did not recall ever having a respiratory tract infection. By receiving the seasonal influenza vaccination, healthcare workers protect themselves, their patients, and their families.

Inactivated influenza vaccine and live attenuated influenza vaccine (LAIV) are widely available for workers in the healthcare professions. LAIV is approved only for nonpregnant healthy persons, ages 5 to 49 years. Healthcare workers caring for severely immunocompromised patients should not receive LAIV. Instead, the inactivated influenza vaccine is the preferred vaccine for workers who come into direct contact with this group of patients. Workers can secure guidance on which vaccine to take from their occupational or employee health department.

TJC requires accredited organizations to offer influenza vaccinations to staff, including volunteers and licensed independent practitioners with close patient contact (TJC, 2012b). Accredited organizations are required to establish annual immunization programs to educate employees about influenza and to offer the vaccine onsite (ANA, 2011).

Healthcare-associated infections (HAIs) with measles, mumps, and rubella are all well documented. Previously, birth before 1957 was considered acceptable evidence of measles immunity. Serologic studies of healthcare workers, however, conclude that up to 10% of those born before 1957 are not immune to measles.

HAIs from varicella-zoster virus (VZV) are also well documented. Patients who are at increased risk for varicella infection are pregnant women; premature infants born to susceptible mothers; infants born at less than 28 weeks' gestation or who weigh less than 1000 g, regardless of maternal immune status; and immunocompromised people of all ages (including individuals undergoing immunosuppressive therapy, have malignant disease, or are immunodeficient). Sources of healthcare-associated varicella infection include patients, hospital employees, and hospital visitors who are infected with either varicella or zoster. Generally, a reliable history of chickenpox is a valid measure of VZV immunity.

Recent increases in rates of pertussis (an acute, infectious cough illness) among healthcare workers (Updated Recommendations, 2013) led to a recommendation that they receive one dose of tetanus toxoid, reduced diphtheria toxoid, and acellular pertussis vaccine (Tdap). Immunity to pertussis wanes 5 to 10 years after childhood immunization, leading to susceptibility to pertussis among adults.

Each year, recommendations for routine use of vaccines in children, adolescents, and adults in the United States are developed by the CDC's Advisory Committee on Immunization Practices (ACIP). Routine immunization of healthcare workers against tuberculosis, HAV, meningococcal disease, typhoid fever, or vaccinia (smallpox) (Lee et al, 2012) is not currently recommended by the ACIP.

Should an exposure to an infectious or communicable disease occur in the clinical area, chemoprophylaxis may be available. Healthcare workers should report the exposure to their occupational health department or other provider according to the facility's procedures and receive proper follow-up. Infectious exposures outside the workplace should also be reported for the protection of patients and coworkers. Postexposure work restrictions may range from restricting contact with high-risk patients to furlough for healthcare workers without immunity.

Exposure of healthcare workers to diphtheria, pneumococcal disease, or tetanus is not significantly more than that of the general population; healthcare professionals therefore should elect to receive these immunizations from their primary care providers. In addition to immunization records maintained by their employers, healthcare workers should also maintain accurate *personal* records of all their immunizations and exposures, including any prophylaxis or laboratory studies.

Immunizations are part of a comprehensive workplace infection control program. Guidance for development of a program is available from OSHA, CDC, and the department of health in the state in which the facility is located. The recommended and required vaccinations vary by state and depend on legislation at either the state or the federal level. To further evaluate compliance with recommended or required vaccinations, healthcare workers should consult with the occupational or employee health department at their workplace.

Radiation Safety

Radiologic imaging studies are invaluable diagnostic and treatment tools. At the same time, radiation presents environmental safety concerns for patients and staff. Many surgical procedures use radiologic studies performed immediately before, during, or after surgery, increasing the potential for radiation exposure. X-rays of all frequencies can damage tissues and may produce long-term effects. The effects of radiation are dose-dependent and cumulative: the larger the dose or the more frequent the exposure, the greater the risk of toxic effects of radiation.

Sources of radiation exposure in the OR include (1) ionizing sources—portable radiography (x-ray) machines and portable fluoroscopy units (C-arm)—and (2) nonionizing sources—lasers (laser safety discussion appears more extensively in Chapter 8). Ionizing radiation is used in diagnostic, interventional, and therapeutic procedures, but can damage living tissues and may produce long-term effects (AORN, 2013). Expanding use of x-ray imaging during interventional surgery has dramatically increased exposure of many OR personnel to ionizing radiation in recent years (Chapter 29 discusses interventional and image-guided radiology departments and procedures). Acute exposure to ionizing radiation can result in dermatitis and reddening of the skin (erythema) at the point of exposure, and large, full-body exposures can lead to radiation poisoning, symptoms of which may include nausea, vomiting, diarrhea, weakness, and death.

In radiation protection, the guiding philosophy is ALARA—as low as reasonably achievable (U.S. Nuclear Regulatory Commission, 2012). Typically, reducing the patient dose also reduces the dose to healthcare workers. Therefore, performing optimized procedures is an important aspect of radiation protection. Optimization includes performing only necessary studies and performing them sufficiently well that they do not need to be repeated.

In diagnostic radiology, the main source of occupational doses is radiation that scatters as the x-ray beam passes through the patient, particularly from fluoroscopically guided procedures. Healthcare workers who do not protect themselves from scatter radiation are especially at risk when performing interventional procedures, given significantly increased exposure time and proximity during the procedure (AORN, 2013). Personnel stand near patients for long times, and angulated geometries with C-arm equipment may result in high personnel doses from backscatter.

For all procedures, time, distance, and shielding affect dose levels sustained. Accordingly, guidelines for radiation safety are based on the principles of time, distance, and shielding. When exposed to radiation at a constant rate, the total dose equivalent received depends on the length of time exposed. If the distance from the point source of radiation doubles, exposure quarters. Passage through materials also reduces the amount of radiation (AORN, 2013).

Members of the surgical team should avoid unnecessary exposure to radiation sources and comply with practices that reduce potential exposure. Personnel in the OR maintain the greatest practical distance (at least 6 feet) from the radiation source or remain behind leaded shielding when ionizing radiation use occurs during surgery. Personnel assisting with radiologic procedures should not hold the patient manually during a study because the risk of exposure by the direct beam arises (AORN, 2013). Members of the sterile scrub team should wear protective devices and move as far from the radiation source as possible while still adhering to aseptic technique. Nonessential personnel should leave the room.

Protective equipment reduces the intensity of radiation exposure. Radiation safety devices include mobile rigid shields on wheels; ceiling-suspended transparent barriers; flexible leaded aprons (e.g., wraparound), vests, skirts, thyroid shields, and gloves; and leaded safety eyeglasses with side shields (AORN, 2013). AORN recommends that personnel who may have to stand with their back to the radiation beams wear wraparound aprons to decrease their risk of exposure, and that personnel nearest to the radiation beam shield their upper chest and neck and upper legs.

OSHA has established mandatory, health-based limits on occupational exposure to ionizing radiation and provides a series of guidelines that hospitals can use to protect staff from excess radiation exposure. OSHA requires that employees working with radiation sources be monitored for exposures and be informed of their levels of exposure at least once a year (ANA, 2007).

OSHA also recommends that film badges or an equivalent be used for long-term monitoring. A film badge is a passive dosimeter for personal exposure monitoring that should be worn whenever an employee works with x-ray equipment, radioactive patients, or radioactive materials. Depending on the work setting, dosimeters may be worn at collar, chest, or waist level. Personnel who work in high-dose fluoroscopy settings may be asked to wear two badges for additional monitoring. Ring badges (used to measure beta and gamma doses to the hand) should be worn on the hand closest to radiation sources (OSHA, 2008a).

Leaded garments should be handled carefully and examined regularly to ensure the integrity of shielding; they should not be folded during storage, and they should undergo regular radiologic testing to ensure effective shielding. Staff-development programs on radiation safety should occur periodically to reinforce radiation safety practices and to correct misconceptions or unrealistic practices relating to radiation exposure and monitoring.

The American College of Radiology (ACR) recommends that facilities adopt the following safety measures to protect personnel:
- Implement a radiation-exposure monitoring program, as required by the Nuclear Regulatory Commission or appropriate state agencies
- Perform systematic inspection of interlock systems
- Provide appropriate room shielding
- Perform routine leak testing of all sealed sources, as required by regulatory agencies
- Furnish appropriate safety equipment for use of sealed sources (ACR, 2009)

Latex Allergy

Natural rubber latex allergy is a serious medical problem for a growing number of patients and a disabling occupational disease among healthcare workers. Latex allergy develops from exposure to natural rubber latex and plant cytosol, used extensively to manufacture medical gloves and other devices, as well as numerous consumer products. Allergic reactions to latex range from skin disease to asthma and anaphylaxis that can result in chronic illness, disability, career loss, and death.

Historically, latex has been the material of choice for surgical gloves because it is flexible and maintains tactile sensitivity for the wearer. Although natural rubber latex has been a common component in thousands of medical and consumer products for many years, latex sensitivity is a relatively new problem for patients and healthcare personnel. Clinicians were aware of contact dermatitis from chemicals in rubber as early as the 1930s; they did not recognize, however, systemic allergic reactions to latex proteins until the 1970s. Latex allergy erupted in the United States shortly after the CDC introduced its Universal Precautions in 1985. Today, researchers hypothesize that the latex allergy outbreak is the result of multiple factors, including increased latex exposure and deficiencies in manufacturing, among others. Latex allergy affects between 8% and 12% of workers in all health disciplines, but it affects only about 1% of the general population.

Individuals can experience three reactions to latex. First, *irritant contact dermatitis* is the most common reaction, characterized by dry, reddened, itchy, or cracked hands. Irritant contact dermatitis is not a true allergic reaction. Second, *allergic contact dermatitis* (also called *chemical contact dermatitis*) is a delayed cell-mediated, type IV localized allergy caused by chemicals used to manufacture rubber products. The most common contact sensitizers are the accelerators: thiurams, mercaptobenzothiazoles (MBTs), and carbamates. Allergic contact dermatitis is a delayed reaction, usually appearing 6 to 48 hours after exposure. Symptoms are similar to those from irritant contact dermatitis (i.e., pruritus, edema, erythema, vesicles, drying papules, crusting and thickening of the skin), except that the reaction may extend beyond the actual point of contact.

Third and most serious is a true latex allergy, a type I, immunoglobulin E (IgE)–mediated hypersensitivity reaction that involves systemic antibody formation in reaction to proteins in products made from natural rubber latex. Natural rubber latex contains up to 240 potentially allergenic protein fragments, and different people may be sensitized to different combinations of latex allergens. Synthetic latexes are not involved in latex allergy. A true latex allergic response is immediate, IgE mediated, and anaphylactic. The onset of anaphylactic reaction usually occurs within minutes of contact with the proteins, with symptoms that may include generalized urticaria, wheezing, dyspnea, laryngeal edema, bronchospasm, tachycardia, angioedema, hypotension, and cardiac arrest. Many serious anaphylactic reactions have occurred when a latex product (e.g., surgical gloves) directly contacts mucous membranes during surgical procedures. This situation permits a rapid introduction of latex antigen directly into the vascular circulation.

Traditionally it was assumed that sensitization to latex resulted only from cutaneous absorption in healthcare workers or from direct mucosal contact during clinical treatment. Studies have confirmed that latex protein allergens effectively bind to glove powder and, when airborne, can remain suspended for prolonged periods. Inhalant exposure is an additional risk factor for sensitization to latex allergens.

Healthcare professionals should use the following strategies to reduce their risk of allergic reaction to latex:

- Use powder-free gloves that are low in protein and chemical allergens.
- Use nonlatex gloves for activities that are not likely to involve contact with infectious materials (OSHA, 2008b).
- Be aware that hypoallergenic gloves do not reduce the risk of latex allergy, although they may reduce reactions to chemical additives in the latex.
- When wearing latex gloves, do not use oil-based hand creams or lotions, which can cause glove deterioration.
- After removing latex gloves, wash hands with a mild soap and dry thoroughly.
- Learn to recognize the symptoms of latex allergy, which may include skin rashes; urticaria; flushing; pruritus; nasal, eye, or sinus symptoms; asthma; and shock.

Institutions need to develop strategies to limit the occupational exposure of healthcare workers to latex. If a latex-free environment cannot be created, the goal is to create a latex-safe environment, one in which the facility makes all reasonable efforts to remove high-allergen and airborne latex sources (Goodman and Spry, 2014). This includes switching to low-allergen, powder-free gloves. Cornstarch powder on powdered latex gloves is an efficient allergen carrier and contributes to airborne contamination, especially in ORs and invasive-procedure rooms where glove use is high. The use of low-allergen, powder-free gloves reduces airborne latex allergen sources to below detectable levels, reducing occupational exposure. In addition, appropriate latex-free gloves should be provided for healthcare workers with known latex sensitivity or for procedures in which patients have known sensitivity or allergy.

Box 3-4 provides valuable information on latex allergy.

Workplace Violence

Violence in the workplace affects patient care and healthcare workers and undermines a culture of safety. The Occupational Safety and Health Act of 1970 ensures every working person a safe and healthful workplace, free from recognized hazards that may cause death or serious physical harm. *Workplace violence* may be as any physical assault, threatening behavior, or verbal abuse occurring in the workplace. The healthcare sector leads other industries in workplace violence. OSHA has no federal standard on workplace violence.

Workplace violence can occur in various forms, from bullying and verbal abuse to physical abuse, assault and even homicide. Patients are the main perpetrators of physical violence, whereas staff are the main perpetrators of psychologic violence (also often referred to as lateral or horizontal violence, in which nurses inflict psychologic injury on one another) (ANA, 2013).

Prevention of workplace violence necessarily follows an analysis of workplace risk factors and incidence rates at the facility. Risk factors and solutions include environmental, work-practice, and training solutions. Environmental risk factors include the availability of guns or other weapons among patients and visitors; presence of mentally ill patients with little or no follow-up care; availability of medications or money; unrestricted movement of the general public throughout facilities; presence of gang members, drug or alcohol abusers, trauma patients, or distraught family members; and poorly lit parking areas. Work practices contributing to workplace violence include long waits in emergency or clinic areas, low staffing levels, isolated work with patients during examinations or treatment, and lack of staff training in recognizing and managing aggressive behavior. Victims are often untrained or newly hired staff nurses. Perpetrators often have a history of violent behavior and have been diagnosed with psychosis, substance abuse disorders, or dementia.

Workplace violence is preventable and is never acceptable (Strickler, 2013). Environmental solutions include controlled access doors, metal detectors, alarm systems, panic buttons, handheld noise devices, and cell phones; lockable staff areas, such as lounges and bathrooms; curved mirrors and adequate lighting; and well-lit parking areas. Work practices that help prevent workplace violence include identification of high-risk patients, including flagging charts, both hard copy and electronic; proper training of staff; avoidance of employees working alone, particularly in secluded areas; easy and effective processes to report suspicious behavior, harassment, threats, or violent assaults; careful supervision of the movement of psychiatric patients within the facility; and use of a team approach to prevent workplace violence. Training should include review of prevention policies, reporting procedures, support systems, and action plans; identification of risk factors that cause or contribute to violence; early identification of warning signs of escalating behavior; tools to diffuse violent situations; and review of system and policy failures.

Workplace bullying is another form of workplace violence. Bullying often involves vindictive, cruel, malicious, or humiliating attempts to undermine individuals or groups of employees. Colleagues, employers, management, patients, patients' families, or visitors can be responsible for bullying in the healthcare setting. Behaviors can be exhibited as sadistic or aggressive behavior over time, spreading rumors, exclusion from meetings, reduced opportunities for advancement, humiliation, ridicule, unwarranted private or public criticism, changing work responsibilities unreasonably or without justification, deliberately withholding information to affect work performance, punishing others for being competent, and overworking or overloading to punish (ICHRN, 2007).

Harmful effects of bullying include a decline in the quality of patient care delivery; poor staff relations; low morale; increase in stress and stress-related illness; feelings of shock, disbelief, shame, guilt, anger, fear, and powerlessness; depression; self-blame with decreased self-confidence that can endanger patients; sleeplessness and loss of appetite; increased cost to employers and the healthcare system; increased absenteeism and use of sick time; poor

---

BOX 3-4

Latex Allergy

Latex allergy is an immunoglobulin E (IgE)–mediated reaction to proteins retained in finished natural rubber latex products.

Etiology and Incidence

Latex is the milky sap of the rubber tree *Hevea brasiliensis*. This natural rubber product contains proteins. Latex allergy is the reaction to certain proteins in the latex rubber. These allergies emerged in the 1990s as one of the most pervasive problems in healthcare. It remains a serious and growing problem, and healthcare workers are at increasing risk to acquire latex allergies. Estimates are that an allergy caused by repeated exposure to latex protein allergens develops in about 1 in 10 healthcare professionals; indeed, more than half of healthcare workers report some reaction to latex gloves. Children with spina bifida and individuals with chronic illnesses who require frequent operations are especially susceptible to latex allergy.

Pathophysiology

The amount of latex exposure necessary to produce sensitization or an allergic reaction is unknown. Increasing exposure to latex proteins increases the risk of developing allergic symptoms. Although latex-containing products have only 2% to 3% protein, this protein is thought to be the allergen in type I hypersensitive individuals. The precise protein responsible for causing allergic contact dermatitis latex type I hypersensitivity remains unknown and may differ among individuals.

Risk Factors by Occupational Status

- Healthcare professionals: surgery personnel, emergency care workers, and obstetrics workers are at highest risk
- Children with spina bifida or others with conditions requiring frequent operations
- People with congenital urogenital abnormalities requiring indwelling catheters
- Employees in the rubber industry
- Individuals with history of other IgE-dependent allergies (e.g., rhinitis, asthma, or food allergies) with a positive skin test

Clinical Manifestations—Immediate Type I Hypersensitivity

Clinical signs include local skin redness, dryness, and itching after contact with latex. Inhalation of particles results in respiratory symptoms, such as rhinitis, sneezing, itchy eyes, scratchy throat, or asthma. More severe systemic manifestations include anaphylaxis with bronchospasm, laryngeal edema, respiratory distress, or respiratory failure.

Complications

Complications may include anaphylactic shock and respiratory and cardiac arrest, leading to death.

Diagnostic Tests
History

Diagnostic significance in an individual's history includes atopic history, hives under latex gloves, hand dermatitis related to gloves, allergic conjunctivitis after rubbing eyes following hand contact with latex, swelling around mouth after dental procedures or inflation of a balloon, and vaginal burning after pelvic examination or contact with latex condom.

Immunologic Evaluation

Immunologic evaluation comprises skin prick, intradermal, and patch contact skin tests and serologic testing (e.g., radioallergosorbent test [RAST] or enzyme-linked immunosorbent assay [ELISA]). The FDA has approved a standardized latex reagent for skin testing for research only, not for public use.

Therapeutic Management
Medications

Medications include epinephrine for reaction (may be autoinjector carried by allergic individual), β-agonist inhaler, prednisone, and other anaphylactic life-supporting medications.

General

Immediate assessment and interventions for acute reaction include cardiac monitoring and, if needed, respiratory support.

Prevention and Promotion
For latex-sensitive individuals:
- Avoid all items containing latex.
- Avoid environments with high levels of circulating aeroallergens (e.g., ORs, emergency departments, blood banks).
- Wear MedicAlert bracelet or tag.
- Carry autoinjector for use at first signs of anaphylaxis.

FDA, U.S. Food and Drug Administration.

---

performance; reduced productivity; loss of creative problem-solving capacity; and attrition (ICHRN, 2007).

Bullying risk factors in the workplace include stress, tension, and frustration; poor management skills; inadequate or nonexistent policies; lack of training to recognize or cope with bullying; shift work and demanding workloads; working alone (ICHRN, 2007); and lack of reporting systems or punishment of perpetrators (Hughes, 2008).

Most hospitals and ambulatory surgery centers have a code of conduct defining acceptable and disruptive or inappropriate behaviors that undermine a culture of safety. Leaders are expected to create and implement a process to manage behavior or behaviors that undermine this culture of safety. Perioperative nurses should be able to practice in an environment where they communicate, collaborate, and respect each other's role and skill set (AORN, 2013).

Workplace violence in any form negatively affects healthcare workers and patients. It harms workers professionally and personally, and it alters the quality of care provided to patients. The perioperative area is not excluded from the effect or incidence of workplace violence. Nurses and other healthcare workers in this setting need education and training to recognize workplace violence in all forms, including lateral violence (Koch, 2012) (violence between coworkers), in order to create a safe working environment that promotes teamwork and collaboration in the perioperative setting. Unit-level leadership and structural empowerment play key roles in creating healthy work environments and supporting cultures of safety (Laschinger et al, 2011).

KEY POINTS

- Patient and employee safety programs should be considered together instead of as two separate programs.
- Perioperative nurses and surgical technologists routinely face a wide array of occupational hazards that place them at risk for work-related musculoskeletal injuries.

- Concerted efforts to address workplace safety for perioperative nurses have been under way for some time.
- Ergonomic tools for safe patient movement and handling help the nurse determine whether assistive equipment should be used, what type of equipment would best support the task, and how many caregivers are needed to perform the task safely.
- Slips, trips and falls are caused by many factors, including wet floors, uneven floor surfaces, low-profile equipment and cords, cluttered or poorly lit walkways, and improper footwear.
- In perioperative patient care, healthcare workers routinely face exposure to bloodborne pathogens (BBPs) and percutaneous injuries (PIs).
- Observing safety precautions during all phases of surgery, from setup to cleanup, reduces the number of injuries and exposures for all OR personnel.
- OSHA regulations require healthcare organizations to protect their workers and to have a sharps injury and BBP exposure control plan.

CRITICAL THINKING QUESTION

You are a senior in your nursing program and have just finished your perioperative nursing rotation. You've been provided with a list of topics on safety and workplace issues and must select one to present to your class, with a focus on the OR. When you were working with the circulating nurse, she spoke about a culture of safety, and how the OR today was different from when she started working there 40 years ago. Then, she got a "needlestick" from a patient who was HBV positive. She uses her personal experience to share with you what the OR and what the circulating nurse do today to be sure this doesn't happen. What is the key information you will focus on to present to your class about exposure control plans and personal protective equipment in the OR?

evolve *The answer to the Critical Thinking Question can be found at http://evolve.elsevier.com/Rothrock/Alexander.*

REFERENCES

American College of Radiology (ACR): *ACR practice guideline for radiation oncology,* Reston, VA, Res. 8, 2009, available at www.acr.org/-/media/ACR/Documents/PGTS/guidelines/Radiation_Oncology.pdf. Accessed March 22, 2013.

American Nurses Association: *Environmental working group: nurses' health: a survey on health and chemical exposures,* 2007, available at www.ewg.org/research/nurses-health. Accessed March 23, 2013.

American Nurses Association: *Safe patient handling and movement* (pamphlet), Washington, DC, 2008.

American Nurses Association: *Handle with care backgrounder,* 2009, available at www.nursingworld.org/MainMenuCategories/Occupationaland Environmental/occupationalhealth/handlewithcare/Backgrounder. Accessed March 22, 2013.

American Nurses Association: *ANA backgrounders: influenza season,* 2011-2012, available at www.nursingworld.org/FunctionalMenuCategories/MediaResources/MediaBackgrounders/Seasonal-Influenza-Backgrounder.pdf. Accessed March 22, 2013.

American Nurses Association: *Workplace violence,* updated January 15, 2013, available at www.nursingworld.org/workplaceviolence. Accessed March 21, 2013.

Association of periOperative Registered Nurses (AORN): Guidance statement: sharps injury prevention in the perioperative setting, 2012. In *Perioperative standards and recommended practices,* Denver, CO, 2013, AORN.

Association of periOperative Registered Nurses (AORN): *Safe patient handling tool kit,* Denver, 2012, available at www.aorn.org/Secondary.aspx?id=20930. Accessed March 21, 2013.

Association of periOperative Registered Nurses (AORN): *Perioperative standards and recommended practices,* Denver, 2013, the Association.

Bell JL et al: Evaluation of a comprehensive slip, trip and fall prevention programme for hospital employees, *Ergonomics* 51(12):1906–1925, 2008.

Brogmus G et al: Best practices in OR suite layout and equipment choices to reduce slips, trips, and falls, *AORN J* 86(3):384–398, 2007.

Burns RP: *Governor's committee on surgical practice in hospitals and ambulatory settings: an update,* 2009, available at www.facs.org/fellows_info/bulletin/2009/burns0809.pdf. Accessed March 21, 2013.

CDC, NIOSH: *NIOSH pocket guide to chemical hazards, Publication No. 2005-149, Cincinnati,* 2007a, available at www.cdc.gov/niosh/docs/2005-149/pdfs/2005-149.pdf. Accessed March 22, 2013.

CDC, NIOSH: *Waste anesthetic gases: occupational hazards in hospitals, NIOSH Publication No. 2007-151, Cincinnati,* 2007b, available at www.cdc.gov/niosh/docs/2007-151/. Accessed March 22, 2013.

Centers for Disease Control and Prevention (CDC): Influenza vaccination of health-care personnel, *MMWR* 55:1–16, 2010a, available at www.hhs.gov/ash/initiatives/hai/hcpflu.html. Accessed March 22, 2013.

Centers for Disease Control and Prevention (CDC): *Workbook for designing, implementing, and evaluating a sharps injury prevention program,* 2010b, available at www.cdc.gov/sharpssafety/index.html. Accessed March 22, 2013.

Clarke SP et al: Sharp-device injuries to hospital staff nurses in 4 countries, *Infect Control Hosp Epidemiol* 28:473–478, 2007.

Collins JW, Bell JL: Prevention of slip, trip, and fall (STF) hazards for workers in hospital settings. In Charney W, editor: *Essentials of modern hospital safety,* ed 4, Los Angeles, 2009, Lewis.

Collins JW, Bell JL: *Slipping, tripping, and falling at work,* June 11, 2012, available at www.medscape.com/viewarticle/765348. Accessed March 23, 2013.

Collins JW et al: Multidisciplinary research to prevent slip, trip, and fall (STF) incidents among hospital workers. In *Contemporary ergonomics,* Nottingham, U.K., 2008, Taylor and Francis.

Davis MS: Sharps safety in the operating room, advances in engineered sharps injury prevention technology: suturing, 1–24, 2006. Adapted from Davis, MS: *Advanced precautions for today's OR: the operating room professional's handbook for the prevention of sharps injuries and blood borne exposures,* ed 2, Atlanta, 2001, Sweinbinderp.

DeJohn P: Is your ASC ready for closer scrutiny on sharps safety? *OR Manager* 28(2):26–28, 30, 2012.

Delisio N: Bloodborne infection from sharps and mucocutaneous exposure: a continuing problem, *Am Nurse Today* 7(5):33–38, 2012.

FDA, NIOSH and OSHA Joint Safety Communication: *Blunt-tip surgical suture needles reduce needlestick injuries and the risk of subsequent bloodborne pathogen transmission to surgical personnel,* 2012, available at www.fda.gov/MedicalDevices/Safety/AlertsandNotices/ucm305757.htm. Accessed March 21, 2013.

Goodman T, Spry C: *Essentials of perioperative nursing,* ed 5, Burlington, MA, 2014, Jones & Bartlett.

Hart PD: Complying with bloodborne pathogen standards: Protecting health care workers and patients, *AORN J* 94(4):393–399, 2011.

Hughes NL: Bullies in health care beware, *Am Nurs Today* 3(11):44–45, 2008.

Hughes NL: Slips, trips, and falls of healthcare workers, *Am Nurs Today* 4(3):38, 2009.

Hughes N et al: AORN ergonomic tool 4: solutions for prolonged standing in perioperative settings, *AORN J* 9(6):767–774, 2011.

Hunter B et al: Savings costs, saving health care providers' backs, and creating a safe patient environment, *Nurs Econ* 28(2):130–134, 2010.

International Centre for Human Resources in Nursing (ICHRN): *Workplace bullying in the health sector,* 2007, available at www.icn.ch/images/stories/documents/publications/fact_sheets/19l_FS-Bullying_Health_Sector.pdf. Accessed March 22, 2013.

International Healthcare Worker Safety Center (IHWSC): *Moving the sharps safety agenda forward in the United States: consensus statement and call to action,* 2010, available at http://c.ymcdn.com/sites/www.wocn.org/resource/resmgr/advocacy___policy/consensus_statement_sharps_i.pdf. Accessed March 21, 2013.

Jagger J et al: Increase in sharps injuries in surgical settings versus nonsurgical settings after passage of national needlestick legislation, *J Am Coll Surg* 210:496–502, 2010.

King C: Health care worker safety in surgery, *AORN J* 94(5):457–468, 2011.

Koch J: Lateral violence: Tools managers can use to help shift the culture, *OR Manager* 28(8):1, 6–8, 2012.

Korniewicz D, El-Masri M: Exploring the benefits of double gloving during surgery, *AORN J* 95(3):328–336, 2012.

Laschinger S et al: Situational and dispositional influences on nurses' workplace well-being: the role of empowering unit leadership, *Nurs Res* 60(2):124–131, 2011.

Lee JJ et al: *Vaccinia, Medscape reference*, updated January 12, 2012, available at http://emedicine.medscape.com/article/231773-overview. Accessed March 21, 2013.

Markkanen P et al: *Cleaning in healthcare facilities: reducing human health effects and environmental impacts*, 2009, available at www.sustainableproduction.org/downloads/CleaninginHealthcareFacilities.pdf. Accessed March 22, 2013.

Misteli H et al: Surgical glove perforation and the risk of surgical site infection, *Arch Surg* 144:553–558, 2009.

Nelson AL et al: *The illustrated guide to safe patient handling and movement*, New York, 2009, Springer.

Occupational Safety and Health Administration: *Permissible exposure limits (PELs)*, 2006, available at www.osha.gov/dsg/topics/pel/index.html. Accessed March 22, 2013.

Occupational Safety and Health Administration: *Hospital eTool, healthcare wide hazards module, latex allergy*, 2008a, available at www.OSHA.gov/SLTC/etools/hospital/hazards/latex/latex.html. Accessed March 22, 2013.

Occupational Safety and Health Administration (OSHA): *Waste anesthetic gases*, last reviewed May 2008b, available at www.osha.gov/SLTC/wasteanestheticgases/index.html. Accessed March 22, 2013.

Occupational Safety and Health Administration: *Reproductive hazards*, 2010, available at www.osha.gov/SLTC/reproductivehazards/index.html. Accessed March 22, 2013.

Occupational Safety and Health Administration: *Regulations (standards—29 CFR), hazard communication—1910.1200*, 2012, available at www.osha.gov/pls/oshaweb/owadisp.show_document?p_table=standards&p_id=10099. Accessed March 22, 2013.

Pompeii LA et al: Musculoskeletal injuries resulting from patient handling tasks among hospital workers, *Am J Indust Med* 52(7):571–578, 2009.

Smith FD: Management of exposure to waste anesthetic gases, *AORN J* 91(4):482–494, 2010.

Spera P et al: AORN ergonomic tool 5: tissue retraction in the perioperative setting, *AORN J* 94(1):54–58, 2011.

Spratt D et al: Workplace safety equals patient safety, *AORN J* 96(3):235–244, 2012.

Strickler J: When it hurts to care: workplace violence in healthcare, *Nursing* 43(4):58–62, 2013.

Sullivan S: Blunt needles for the reduction of needlestick injuries during cesarean delivery: a randomized controlled trial, *Obstet Gynecol* 114: 211–216, 2009.

The Joint Commission (TJC): *Improving patient and worker safety: opportunities for synergy, collaboration and innovation*, Oakbrook Terrace, IL, 2012a. The Joint Commission, available at www.jointcommission.org/joint_commission_publications_for_physicians.aspx. Accessed March 22, 2013.

The Joint Commission (TJC): *R3 report: requirement, rationale, reference—influenza vaccination for licensed independent practitioners and staff, Issue 3, May* 2012b, available at www.jointcommission.org/assets/1/18/R3_Report_Issue_3_5_18_12_final.pdf. Accessed March 22, 2013.

Updated recommendations for use of tetanus toxoid, reduced diphtheria toxoid, and acellular pertussis vaccine (Tdap) in pregnant women—advisory committee on immunization practices (ACIP), 2012, *MMWR* 62(7):131–138, 2013.

U.S. Nuclear Regulatory Commission: *ALARA*, updated December 10, 2012, available at www.nrc.gov/reading-rm/basic-ref/glossary/alara.html. Accessed March 21, 2013.

Waters T: Introduction to ergonomics for healthcare workers, *Rehabil Nurs* 35(5):185–191, 2010.

Waters T et al: AORN ergonomic tool 1: lateral transfer of a patient from a stretcher to an OR bed, *AORN J* 93(3):334–339, 2011a.

Waters T et al: AORN ergonomic tool 2: positioning and repositioning the supine patient on the OR bed, *AORN J* 93(4):445–449, 2011b.

Waters T et al: AORN ergonomic tool 3: lifting and holding the patient's legs, arms, and head while prepping, *AORN J* 93(5):589–592, 2011c.

Waters T et al: AORN ergonomic tool 6: lifting and carrying supplies and equipment in the perioperative setting, *AORN J* 94(2):173–179, 2011d.

Waters T et al: AORN ergonomic tool 7: pushing, pulling, and moving equipment on wheels, *AORN J* 94(3):254–260, 2011e.

Waters TR: When is it safe to manually lift a patient? *AJN* 107(8):53–58, 2007.

CHAPTER 4

Infection Prevention and Control

CYNTHIA SPRY

Advancements in surgical interventions and the science of infection prevention and control continue to evolve and have become increasingly complex. The complexity is derived from the changes in the healthcare environment, the advancements in minimally invasive and advanced surgical procedures, and the development of new, highly technical instrumentation and equipment. This chapter provides an overview of the etiology of infection, including emerging drug-resistant bacteria, and identifies various methods to control infection in the perioperative environment. Use of Standard Precautions along with engineering and work-practice controls assists perioperative practitioners in reducing the transmission of pathogenic organisms. Perioperative patient care is based on surgical aseptic principles. Careful adherence to these principles supports infection prevention and control, ultimately improving surgical patient safety and outcomes. Each member of the surgical team must demonstrate the highest integrity in the application of this knowledge. Finally, the potential for bioterrorism has forced the United States along with the rest of the world to strengthen security and emergency readiness. If a bioterrorist attack resulted in massive exposure or illness, perioperative personnel could and would be mobilized to serve in a variety of locations. Perioperative personnel need to be familiar with the most likely biologic weapons and the levels of precautions required for patient and personnel safety.

Causes of Infection

The human body has three lines of defense to combat infection. The first line of defense consists of *external barriers,* such as the skin and mucous membranes, which are usually impervious to most pathogenic organisms. The second line of defense is the *inflammatory response,* which prevents an invading pathogen from reproducing and possibly involving other tissue. The third line of defense, the *immune response,* is triggered after the inflammatory response. When a break in this defense mechanism occurs, the possibility for infection increases (Box 4-1 lists term definitions).

Microorganisms That Cause Infection

Microorganisms are living organisms that are too small to be seen with the naked eye. These organisms include bacteria, fungi, protozoa, algae, and viruses. Microorganisms are classified to determine appropriate treatment for an infection. Each organism is assigned two names; the genus is the first name, and the specific epithet (species) is the second. Bacteria are further described by shape, motility, growth in aerobic or anaerobic environments, and reaction to staining processes (Figure 4-1). Scientific names can be assigned to organisms in various ways. *Staphylococcus aureus* is a microorganism commonly found on the skin. *Staphylo* describes the clustered arrangement of the cells; *coccus* (Greek *kokkos,* "berry") indicates that they are shaped like spheres. The species *aureus* is Latin for

"golden," the color of the colonies of the bacterium. Bacteria cause most surgical site infections (SSIs). Gram-positive cocci, as a group, are the most common cause of SSIs. The organisms most commonly found in postoperative SSIs include staphylococcal, enterococcal, pseudomonal, and streptococcal species. *S. aureus* is the most frequently identified organism.

Staphylococci. Staphylococci are gram-positive cocci. They are facultative anaerobes but grow best under aerobic conditions. Staphylococci can be found in the indigenous flora of the skin and mucous membranes of the nasopharynx, urethra, and vagina. They are resistant to drying, heat, and high salt concentrations.

The two recognized species of staphylococci are *S. aureus* and *S. epidermidis.* Staphylococci are called *coagulase positive* when they are capable of clotting plasma and *coagulase negative* when the plasma clumps them. Coagulase-positive staphylococci are more virulent or pathogenic than coagulase-negative staphylococci. *S. aureus* is hemolytic, parasitic, pathogenic, and coagulase positive. *S. epidermidis* is parasitic, less pathogenic, and coagulase negative. *S. aureus* is a long-recognized cause of surgical site infections. More recently, *S. epidermidis* has been implicated in infections of prosthetic devices and indwelling medical devices (CDC, 2008a; Geipl 2009; Widerstrom et al, 2012). The skin surface is the most common site of *S. epidermidis.* Approximately 30% to 70% of individuals carry staphylococci on their skin. This can lead to contamination of clothing and dispersal of the microorganisms. For no known reason individuals who are skin carriers of staphylococci differ in the rate at which they shed the microorganisms. There is no obvious difference in hygiene and skin condition between light and heavy shedders, and no other contributing factor is apparent. Heavy shedders seem to be in normal good health.

S. aureus infections in hospitals can lead to prolonged hospital stays and may result in death. *S. aureus* is a medically important human pathogen that is found in the nares of approximately one third of the population (Pynnonen et al, 2011). Human nasal and throat cavities are the most important reservoirs that continually replenish the external environment. Among perioperative personnel, *S. aureus* has been found most commonly in the respiratory passages. The potential for patient infection increases greatly as the personnel carrier rate increases. Nasal carriers also may be skin carriers. Carriers usually harbor either coagulase-positive (pathogenic) or coagulase-negative (nonpathogenic) staphylococci; seldom are there both types, and rarely more than one strain is identified. Because an individual may be a carrier of staphylococci one day and a noncarrier the next, frequent swab testing of the nose as an infection control measure is impractical. Staphylococci survive for long periods in the air, dust, debris, bedding, and clothing. Pathogenic staphylococci grow in the sweat, urine, and tissue and on the human

---

BOX 4-1

Definition of Terms

Aeration: Method by which absorbed ethylene oxide (EO) is removed from EO-sterilized items.

Aerobes: Microorganisms unable to live and reproduce without access to free atmospheric oxygen, such as *Mycobacterium tuberculosis*.

Anaerobes: Bacteria able to survive only in the absence of molecular oxygen, such as *Clostridium perfringens*.

Bioburden: Amount of microbial load and organic debris on an item before sterilization.

Biofilm: A thin coating containing biologically active organisms that have the ability to grow in water, solutions, or in vivo and coat the surface of structures or devices. Biofilms may contain viable and nonviable microorganisms that may adhere to a surface and are trapped within organic matter.

Biologic indicator: A sterilization process–monitoring device commercially prepared with a known population of highly resistant spores to test the effectiveness of the sterilization process being used.

Carrier: Person who harbors one or more specific pathogens in the absence of discernible clinical disease.

Cohorting: The practice of grouping patients who are colonized or infected with the same pathogen.

Contamination: Presence of pathogenic microorganisms on or in animate or inanimate objects. This term generally is used in reference to a specific object, substance, or tissue that contains microorganisms, especially disease-producing microorganisms.

Deep incisional surgical site infection (SSI): Infection involving deep soft tissue, fascia, and muscle.

Dynamic air removal: Mechanically assisted air removal from a sterilizer's chamber. This includes prevacuum and steam flush, pressure pulsed steam sterilizers.

Facultative bacteria: Bacteria with enzyme systems that permit them to live and reproduce with or without free oxygen.

Flash sterilization: See Immediate-use steam sterilization (IUSS).

Gram stain: A procedure for staining bacteria that is the first step in classifying and differentiating them into two large groups (gram-positive and gram-negative) based on the chemical and physical properties of their cell walls.

Immediate-use steam sterilization (IUSS): Steam sterilization process of instruments intended to be used immediately. Items subject to IUSS may not be stored for use at a later time. Immediate use is the shortest time possible between the time the item(s) is removed from the sterilizer and aseptically transferred to the sterile field.

Immunity: Resistance to infection.

Infection: Invasion and multiplication of microorganisms in body tissues, causing cellular injury attributable to competitive metabolism, toxins, intracellular replication, or antigen-antibody response.

Infectious agent: Parasite (bacterium, spirochete, fungus, virus, or any other type of organism) that is capable of producing infection.

Healthcare-associated infections (HAIs): Infections acquired by patients during hospitalization, with confirmation of diagnosis by clinical or laboratory evidence. The infective agents may originate from endogenous sources, as from one tissue to another within the patient (self-infection), or from exogenous sources, as acquired from objects or other patients within the hospital (cross-infection). HAIs, which are often referred to as hospital-acquired or nosocomial infections, may not become apparent until after the patient has left the hospital.

Opportunists: Microorganisms of low virulence and requiring large numbers to produce infection.

Organ or space SSI: Infection involving any part of the anatomy other than the incision.

Parasites: Microorganisms that reside on or within the bodies of living organisms called hosts to find the environment and food they require for life and reproduction. Some microorganisms are obligatory parasites, meaning that they depend on their hosts for survival and reproduction. Other microorganisms are facultative parasites, meaning that they normally reside on dead matter, but may receive nourishment from living matter. All disease-producing microorganisms are parasites; however, not all parasites are disease-producing.

Pathogen: Any disease-producing agent or microorganism.

Primary pathogens: Highly virulent organisms that are capable of producing disease in low numbers.

Resident microorganisms: Organisms that habitually live in the epidermis, deep in the crevices and folds of the skin.

Reuse: The repeated or multiple uses of any medical device whether marketed as a reusable or single-use device. Repeated/multiple uses may be on the same patient or on a different patient with applicable reprocessing of the device between each use.

Source: Object, substance, or individual from which an infectious agent passes to a host. In some cases transfer is direct from the reservoir, or source, to the host.

Spore: Dormant stage of some bacteria that is reversible under favorable conditions. Common spore-forming bacteria include *Clostridium perfringens*, *Clostridium botulinum*, *Clostridium tetani*, and *Bacillus anthracis*.

Sterilization process–monitoring device: A device used to monitor specific sterilization processes. These devices can be biologic, physical, or chemical.

Superficial SSI: Infection involving skin and subcutaneous tissue as opposed to deep tissue.

Surgical site (incisional) infection: Infection involving body-wall layers that have been incised.

Toxins: Protein molecules released by bacteria to affect host cells at a distant site.

Transient microorganisms: Organisms with a very short life span, such as the normal flora present on the skin surface of humans. Gram-negative bacteria are transient on the hands of hospital personnel and account for 60% of infections.

Virulence: The potency of a pathogen measured in the numbers required to kill the host.

Virus: Ultramicroscopic infectious agent that replicates itself only within cells of living hosts.

---

skin. They are more difficult to destroy than many other non–spore-forming organisms. Cleanliness of the environment; proper handling; and, when appropriate, sterilization of linens and equipment; and adherence to adequate hand hygiene practices are important controls to prevent transmission of infection (AORN, 2013a).

Enterococci. Enterococci are gram-positive organisms that are found in the normal flora of the gastrointestinal and female genital tracts. These organisms are responsible for many serious healthcare-associated infections, including surgical site infections, bacterial endocarditis, septicemia, and urinary tract infections (UTIs).

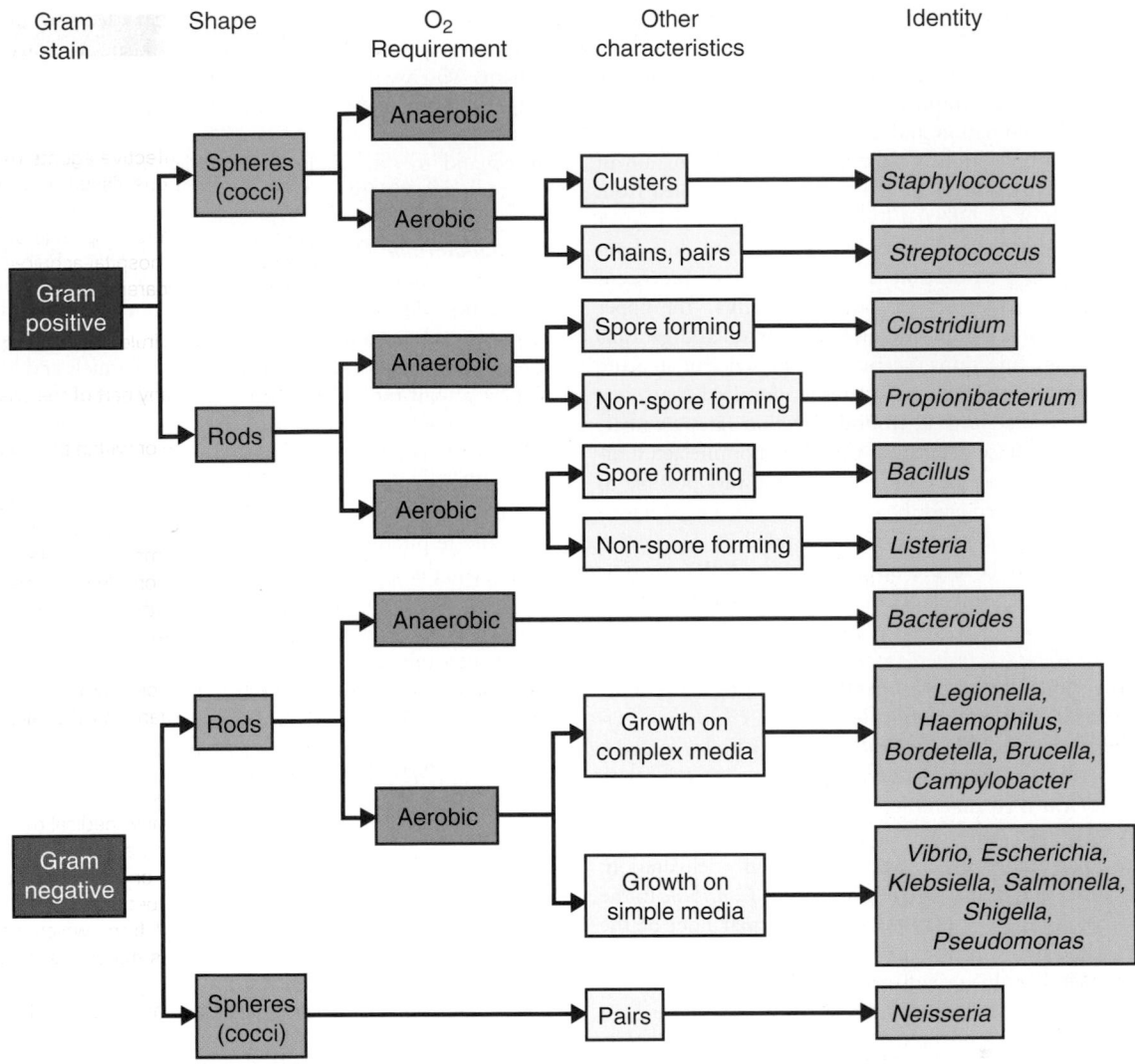

FIGURE 4-1 Types of gram-positive and gram-negative bacteria.

Enterococci also have been implicated in polymicrobial wound infections (CDC, 2007a; Scheithauer et al, 2012). Enterococcal infections are most often healthcare associated and seen in patients with comorbid conditions.

Pseudomonads. The most common aerobic species of pseudomonads pathogenic to humans is *Pseudomonas aeruginosa.* It thrives in moist environments and is found frequently in soil, water, sewage, debris, and air. It also can be found in the normal flora of the skin and intestines. *P. aeruginosa* was considered a microorganism of slight pathogenic power but is now known to be associated with many infections in humans, including surgical site infections. *P. aeruginosa* seems to be pathogenic only when it is introduced into areas where normal defenses are absent, when it is superimposed on staphylococcal infection, or when it is present in a mixed infection. It may attack a debilitated patient who has extensive burns or major trauma. The organism is often seen in critical care and burn units. *P. aeruginosa* is resistant to most antimicrobial agents. Other species of pseudomonads have been associated with infections caused by contaminated intravascular cannulae (as from the use of pressure transducers) or by the lumens of equipment (such as endoscopes

used in gastrointestinal [GI] studies). An important preventive measure is proper environmental sanitation and strict adherence to aseptic technique.

Streptococci. Most streptococci are gram-positive, non–spore-forming facultative microorganisms. They are normally found in the indigenous flora of the upper respiratory, genitourinary, and GI tracts. Streptococci are classified as alpha, beta, or gamma according to chemical factors, biochemical tests, and their action on red blood cells.

Group A streptococci account for most streptococcal infections in humans. Known as the *flesh-eating bacteria* because of their ability to cause necrotizing fasciitis, group A streptococci are of concern because of the sporadic and deadly outbreaks of community-acquired and healthcare-associated infection (CDC, 2006a; Ramirez et al, 2011). An example is *Streptococcus pyogenes,* which is responsible for most soft tissue infections, otitis media, pharyngitis, impetigo, septicemia, and surgical site infections. Virulent streptococci are more serious invaders than staphylococci. Streptococci tend to involve wide areas of tissue and cause necrosis without localization. Streptococci are usually sensitive to penicillin, whereas staphylococci may not be. Streptococci also occur in mixed infections with other pathogens.

In surgical wounds, streptococci can be introduced into the incision and spread via the lymph vessels and nodes. This distribution can result in inflammation and cellulitis. Streptococcal transmission occurs by droplet transmission and by contamination of the environment. Inhalation of infectious droplets expelled from the nose and mouth of an infected individual is considered direct contact. Indirect contact occurs when infected air and dust from the environment enter a susceptible host. Group A streptococcus can be carried in the nasal passages, anus, or vagina. The upper respiratory tract is not a significant reservoir for microorganisms that cause surgical site infections except in the presence of an acute upper respiratory tract infection. In several randomized controlled studies, it was found that surgical wound infection rates are unaffected by the use or nonuse of surgical masks by noninfected individuals during the operative procedure. It is not always possible to know who might be infected, and the use of masks during operative procedures continues to be strongly recommended in the prevention of SSIs. Most bacteria in the operating room (OR) environment are shed from the skin of perioperative personnel (AORN, 2013b).

Clostridia. The clostridia bacteria are spore-forming, anaerobic, gram-positive bacilli that produce virulent toxins. *Clostridium difficile* is a bacterium in the *Clostridium* genus, which also includes *C. perfringens* (gas gangrene), *C. tetani* (tetanus), and *C. botulinum* (botulism). *C. difficile* is an anaerobic, gram-positive, spore-forming bacillus. *C. difficile* is an overgrowth in the colon that can manifest symptoms of diarrhea, colitis, toxic megacolon, dehydration, colonic perforation, and death. The overgrowth of *C. difficile* in the colon usually results from alterations in the normal flora of the colon that are associated with the use of antibiotics (CDC, 2006a; Gould et al, 2008). For this organism to cause disease, *C. difficile* must already be in the GI system. Subsequently, there must be a change in the normal flora of the colon to allow the organism to grow and produce toxins. The two toxins produced are toxin A, which is an enterotoxin causing excretion of large amounts of fluid from the bowel, and toxin B, which is cytotoxic. Toxin B attacks and disintegrates cells of the intestines. Additionally, *C. difficile* produces tissue-degrading enzymes, which produce an inflammatory response within the colon that can result in a spectrum of disease entities.

In its spore form, *C. difficile* can withstand drying and heat and may be resistant to many disinfectants. The spores can survive up to 5 months in the environment. *C. difficile* can be transmitted between individuals and by touching objects contaminated with the organism. In the healthcare environment, *C. difficile* has been cultured in rooms of infected individuals 40 days after discharge. *C. difficile* also has been cultured from healthcare workers' shoes, fingernails, fingertips, and the underside of rings (Mitchum, 2009).

Several interventions can assist in the prevention of *C. difficile* transmission in the healthcare environment, including following Contact Precautions, handwashing with antimicrobial soap and water, using personal protective equipment (PPE), cleaning and disinfecting all surfaces and equipment, and cleaning and disinfecting reusable devices in the perioperative suite. The use of disposable equipment only is recommended for infected patients (CDC, 2010a). Additionally, clinical practice guidelines from the Society for Healthcare Epidemiology of America (SHEA) and the Infectious Diseases Society of America (IDSA) recommend that in a setting in which there is an outbreak or an increased rate of *C. difficile* infection to instruct visitors and healthcare workers caring for patients who are infected with *C. difficile* to wash their hands with soap, or antimicrobial soap and water. Further, they recommend that the frequency and duration of antimicrobial therapy be minimized and to implement an antimicrobial stewardship program (Cohen et al, 2010).

Mycobacterium Tuberculosis. *M. tuberculosis* is a non–spore-forming, nonmotile, aerobic bacillus. These bacilli can infect almost any tissue—skin, bones, kidney, lymph nodes, intestinal tract, and fallopian tubes—and cause tuberculosis (TB). Tubercle bacilli spread in the host through the lymphatic channels and bloodstream and by way of the alveoli and GI tract. Tuberculosis is responsible for more than 3 million deaths a year and is the most opportunistic infection associated with human immunodeficiency virus (HIV) (Neil, 2008).

Tubercle bacilli are transmitted directly by means of discharge from the respiratory tract (e.g., by inhalation of droplets expelled during coughing or kissing) and, less frequently, through the digestive tract. *M. tuberculosis* is carried via airborne droplet nuclei when infected people sneeze, cough, or speak. These nuclei particles are less than 5 micrometers in size and contain up to three bacteria, allowing them to be kept airborne for a prolonged period (CDC, 2006a). Infection occurs when individuals inhale these infected droplet nuclei. The droplet nuclei travel through the nasal passages, upper respiratory tract, and bronchi to reach the lung alveoli, where they are engulfed by macrophages and spread throughout the body. Symptoms of TB are dependent on the part of the body infected, but may be vague at the onset and include fever, fatigue, loss of appetite, cough, fever, and night sweats.

Generally 2 to 10 weeks after initial infection, an immune response limits additional multiplication and spread of the bacilli. Some of the bacilli can remain dormant for many years, however, a condition referred to as *latent tuberculosis infection*. Individuals with latent TB usually have positive purified protein derivative (PPD) results, but they exhibit none of the symptoms of active TB and are considered noninfectious. The probability that a person who is exposed to *M. tuberculosis* will become *infected* depends on the concentration of infectious droplet nuclei and the duration of exposure. When infected, an individual has approximately a 10% risk of developing active TB in his or her lifetime. The risk is greatest during the first 2 years after initial exposure. In individuals with compromised immune systems, there is a higher risk that latent TB will progress into active TB (CDC, 2006a). Latent TB is treated with isoniazid or rifampin. Active TB is treated with a combination of medications (e.g., isoniazid, rifampin, ethambutol, pyrazinamide) (Neil, 2008).

Viruses. Viruses are classified as small particles rather than living cells because viruses have no metabolic activity and must receive all sustenance for survival from a host cell. Viral pathogens are transmitted via the oral and respiratory tracts (e.g., poxvirus, rhinovirus), the intestinal and urinary tracts (e.g., poliovirus, hepatitis A virus, hepatitis E virus), and the genital tract (e.g., herpes simplex 2, HIV) and through blood and some blood products (e.g., HIV, hepatitis B virus, hepatitis C virus, hepatitis D virus, and others). Some viruses have multiple routes of transmission.

When a virus invades a host cell, it combines with the host cell's nucleic acid (deoxyribonucleic acid [DNA] or ribonucleic acid [RNA]) and reprograms the host cell metabolism to accommodate virus replication. Virus replication stimulates the antibody defense in the host. The presence of viruses may be detected by identifying the virus-specific antibodies that are produced by the infected individual's immune system, by detecting the antigens elaborated by the virus and present in the blood, or by growing a culture of the virus itself. Detection of virus-specific antibodies or antigens is termed *seropositivity,* or *seroconversion.* Viruses are susceptible to destruction by high-level disinfection—a process that destroys most disease-producing microorganisms.

Hepatitis. Hepatitis is defined as a widespread inflammation of the liver, often caused by a virus. It can be acute or chronic. Symptoms include hepatomegaly, right upper quadrant abdominal pain, and jaundice. Hepatitis is a frequently reported viral disease in the United States, with six identified strains (A through E and G).

Hepatitis A virus (HAV) is the causative agent of what is referred to as *infectious hepatitis.* HAV is spread through the fecal-oral route and can be prevented by proper hand hygiene. It is very common in underdeveloped countries with poor sanitation practices. HAV constitutes slightly less than half of all hepatitis cases reported in the United States and usually has an uneventful course and recovery. Immunization against HAV is available and has helped decrease the incidence of this strain of hepatitis.

Hepatitis B virus (HBV) is the causative agent for what is sometimes referred to as *serum hepatitis.* This worldwide virus has reached near-epidemic levels but is preventable via vaccination and the strict use of Universal Precautions. HBV can be transmitted by blood or body fluids, such as serum, saliva, semen, and vaginal fluids. It has an incubation period of 6 weeks to 4 months, depending on the type and amount of exposure. Almost 30% of infected individuals are asymptomatic; individuals with symptoms experience fatigue, abdominal pain, nausea, vomiting, and jaundice. Chronic hepatitis infection leads to progressive liver disease and possible death and is a leading cause of liver transplants. Most adults with HBV recover without incidence and develop immunity, but a small percentage may not develop immunity and will become carriers of the virus. HBV vaccine is recommended, by government regulation, for healthcare workers who may be exposed to blood and body fluids. Postexposure prophylaxis for percutaneous or permucosal exposure to HBV depends on the vaccination status of the healthcare worker. The risk of a susceptible person developing clinical HBV ranges from 1% to 31%, depending on the source person's HBV status (Davenport and Myers, 2009). The Occupational Safety and Health Administration (OSHA) mandates that all healthcare workers report blood and body fluid exposures, and perioperative personnel should follow the institutional protocol for exposure reporting.

Hepatitis C virus (HCV) transmission is most often associated with direct exposure to blood (e.g., via intravenous or subcutaneous routes) or other infectious materials. The average incubation period is 7 weeks. Currently there is no vaccine for the prevention of HCV. Individuals who contract HCV infection are prone to develop chronic infection. A high proportion of this population is asymptomatic and develops chronic liver disease, such as cirrhosis, hepatocellular carcinoma, and portal hypertension. As with HBV, a small proportion of individuals infected with HCV die. Prevention of HCV requires strict use of Universal Precautions, implementation of and adherence to sharps safety programs, compliance with exposure reporting protocols, and completion of a postexposure treatment plan. It is crucial that all perioperative personnel be educated regarding the risk for and prevention of all bloodborne infections, including HCV. These education programs should be conducted routinely and updated for accurate information inclusive of the Centers for Disease Control and Prevention (CDC) guidelines. The risk of HCV transmission after percutaneous exposure is about 1.8% (Davenport and Myers, 2009).

Hepatitis D virus (HDV) requires the coinfection of HBV. HDV is transmitted by blood and body fluids. The incubation period is generally 14 to 56 days. Individuals immunized against HBV have protection against contracting HDV. HDV is suspected when individuals present with HBV superinfection. Treatment is supportive for acute infections. With chronic HDV infections, antiviral therapies and liver transplants may be required.

Hepatitis E virus (HEV) is spread by the fecal-oral route. HEV is similar to HAV in the transmission and disease process. Most outbreaks have occurred in developing countries, where fecally contaminated water is found to be the source. The incubation period is 15 to 64 days. No vaccine is available for the prevention of HEV. Prevention is similar to that for HAV, with the use of proper hand hygiene. Treatment for HEV is supportive and the infection generally resolves on its own. The prevalence of HEV in the United States is low.

Hepatitis G virus is a bloodborne pathogen, with a comparable rate of infection as that of HCV in units of banked blood. It is spread in a manner similar to HBV and HCV dissemination, by percutaneous or permucosal exposure. There is no vaccine to prevent hepatitis G virus infection. Similar to HBV and HCV, prudent and consistent use of barrier protection (e.g., Standard Precautions) is recommended. There are no concrete data at present on the chronic nature of this viral disease (CDC, 2006a).

Human Immunodeficiency Virus. HIV is a retrovirus (e.g., a virus that carries genetic information in the RNA instead of the DNA) that attacks the immune system by destroying T-helper lymphocytes. Healthy individuals generally have 800 to 1000 T-helper cells/mm^3 in their blood. Infection with HIV reduces these numbers, and when a person is HIV positive and his or her T-cell count falls below 200 cells/mm^3 (or the person is HIV positive and is diagnosed with an atypical or opportunistic infection and/or cancer), a diagnosis of acquired immunodeficiency syndrome (AIDS) is made (Sampson and Workman, 2013). The period from HIV exposure to actual development of AIDS has been reported to be 12 years or longer. During this time the individual is a carrier of the virus. HIV has been isolated from all body fluids (e.g., blood, semen, vaginal secretions, saliva, tears, breast milk, cerebrospinal fluid, amniotic fluid, and urine) of infected individuals. Symptoms that result from HIV infection may be attributed to other causes and include fever, night sweats, chills, muscle aches, and headache.

Occupational exposure to HIV can occur by percutaneous injury (e.g., a needlestick or cut with a sharp instrument) or by mucous membrane or nonintact skin (e.g., exposed skin that is abraded) exposure to blood, tissue, or other body fluids that are potentially infectious. The CDC estimates that there is an average transmission rate of 0.3% per sharps injury (CDC, 2006b). Mucous membrane exposure is associated with a 0.09% transmission risk, and exposure through nonintact skin is probably lower (Davenport and Myers, 2009). If exposure occurs, appropriate postexposure management should take place as a part of the workplace safety program. The source patient should be informed of the incident. Serology testing should be done according to institutional policy and governmental requirements. Policies should be established for instances in which source patient consent cannot be obtained. The healthcare worker should be counseled about the risk of infection, and he or she should be evaluated clinically and serologically for evidence of HIV infection as soon as possible after exposure.

TABLE 4-1

Postexposure Prophylaxis (PEP) for Occupational HIV Exposure*

Basic PEP	Expanded PEP
Two drugs: zidovudine plus lamivudine or emtricitabine; or stavudine plus lamivudine or emtricitabine; or lopinavir/ritonavir	Three or more drugs: zidovudine plus lamivudine or emtricitabine plus lopinavir/ritonavir; or stavudine plus lamivudine or emtricitabine plus lopinavir/ritonavir; or tenofovir plus lamivudine or emtricitabine plus lopinavir/ritonavir
Small-volume (few drops) exposure to mucous membranes or nonintact skin Source patient is HIV positive, asymptomatic with known low viral load Source patient is HIV positive, symptomatic or AIDS with high viral load	Large-volume (major splash) exposure to mucous membranes or nonintact skin Source patient is HIV positive, symptomatic or AIDS with high viral load
Large-volume (major splash) exposure to mucous membranes or nonintact skin Source patient is HIV positive, asymptomatic with known low viral load Optional when source patient is unknown or known with HIV factors	Less severe percutaneous injury (solid needle or superficial injury) Source patient is HIV positive, symptomatic or AIDS with high viral load
Less severe percutaneous injury (solid needle or superficial injury) Source patient is HIV positive, asymptomatic with known low viral load Optional when source patient is unknown or known with HIV factors	More severe percutaneous injury (large-bore hollow needle, deep punctures, visible blood on device, needle was in patient's artery or vein) Source patient is HIV positive, asymptomatic with known low viral load Source patient is HIV positive, symptomatic or AIDS with high viral load

*PEP should be supported by policies and procedures that include sharps management, exposure documentation, and a procedure for staff members to follow if a percutaneous needlestick occurs. The key to any PEP plan is for the staff member to be able to undergo assessment as soon as possible after exposure so that if the administration of antiretroviral medication is recommended that the staff member is able to begin taking them before 72 hours to prevent the virus from rapidly replicating within the body. Medications need to be taken for 28 days.

AIDS, Acquired immunodeficiency syndrome; *HIV,* human immunodeficiency virus.

Modified from Sampson JG, Workman ML: Care of patients with HIV disease and other immune deficiencies. In Ignatavicius DD, Workman ML, editors: *Medical-surgical nursing: patient-centered collaborative care,* ed 7, St Louis, 2013, Saunders.

Postexposure prophylaxis (PEP) regimens (Table 4-1) should be supervised by an expert in the management of exposures; follow-up should be provided for adherence to PEP; and adverse events, including seroconversion, should be monitored. Timely postexposure management and administration is important, and an exposure incident should be treated as an urgent medical condition.

Multidrug-Resistant Organism Infections: Emerging and Resurging Organisms

Historical Perspective. The first antibiotics, sulfonamides, were introduced in 1935 to treat staphylococcal and streptococcal infections. Penicillin was introduced in the 1940s during World War II, followed by the discovery of streptomycin in the mid- to late 1940s. Although the introduction of these medications was viewed as miraculous and did save many lives, in the mid-1940s strains of previously susceptible microorganisms began showing resistance to some of these medications. During the 1960s, cephalosporin and semisynthetic penicillins were developed, and it was believed that the problem of healthcare-associated infections was solved. Many gram-negative bacteria were found to be susceptible to these new drugs. By the late 1970s, however, strains of *S. aureus* resistant to penicillin, methicillin, cephalosporins, aminoglycosides, clindamycin, erythromycin, and other antibiotics were isolated in hospital outbreaks of infection. This situation led to the development of new antibiotics, including carbapenems, cephamycins, and fluoroquinolones. These broad-spectrum antimicrobials were bactericidal at low concentrations and led to a false sense of euphoria during the 1980s, when it was believed that, at last, resistance to these antimicrobials would be impossible (Sandlin, 2008).

In the 1990s it became evident that the potential for resistance to any and all antimicrobials existed as healthcare-associated outbreaks of multidrug-resistant tuberculosis (MDR-TB) occurred. Significant outbreaks of methicillin-resistant *Staphylococcus aureus* (MRSA) (Surgical Pharmacology) and vancomycin-resistant *Enterococcus* (VRE) also occurred in the 1990s. More recently *Klebsiella,* a gram-negative bacteria associated with surgical site infection, has shown resistance to the carbapenems (CDC, 2010b). In some cases, organisms seemed to acquire resistance almost immediately on exposure to the particular antibiotic. As fewer new antimicrobial drugs are being developed by the pharmaceutical industry, many consider the 1990s to be the beginning of the postantibiotic era (Sandlin, 2008) (see Surgical Pharmacology).

Mechanisms of Resistance. Similar to their unwilling human hosts, pathogenic bacteria have an instinct to survive. When faced with an antimicrobial attack, they assemble their defensive resources. These microorganisms have the remarkable capability to incapacitate the threatening antibiotic and to mutate and outwit the most lethal clinical weapons. Although carrying only a single chromosome, bacteria by nature have extra minichromosomes called *plasmids.* These plasmids are hearty, and some may survive even the most aggressive antibiotic attack. Surviving plasmids are resistant and reproduce in kind, creating dominant organisms within the host. In addition, incompletely or ineffectively treated infections create the potential for reinfection with resistant organisms (CDC, 2006a).

Microbial resistance can be divided into three categories: (1) presence of a naturally resistant strain of an organism before any drugs are administered, (2) acquisition of a drug-resistant strain from an external source, and (3) drug resistance from treatment-related causes. Occurrence of naturally resistant strains of organisms without any exposure to drugs can occur by intrinsic resistance, genetic mutation, or transfer of genetic material. Some microorganisms possess genes that make them resistant to an antibiotic. These genes may always be present in the microorganism but remain in an inactive stage until challenged by an antibiotic. Genetic mutation can occur spontaneously in the course of rapid multiplication of the microbe. These antibiotic-resistant mutants reproduce within

SURGICAL PHARMACOLOGY

Treating Methicillin-Resistant *Staphylococcus aureus* (MRSA)

In the past, vancomycin was the only alternative for treating MRSA. With the increased use of vancomycin, however, strains of *S. aureus* with reduced susceptibility to vancomycin began to appear. Newer antibiotics include daptomycin, linezolid, teicoplanin, and quinupristin-dalfopristin.

Medication/Category	Dosage/Route	Purpose/Action	Adverse Reactions	Nursing Implications
Vancomycin	500-1000 mg IV q 12 hr	Indicated for the treatment of serious, life-threatening infections by Gram-positive bacteria that are unresponsive to other less-toxic antibiotics. Acts by inhibiting proper cell wall synthesis in Gram-positive bacteria.	• Anaphylaxis/anaphylactoid reaction • Hypotension, severe (rapid IV use) • Thrombophlebitis • Tissue necrosis (if extravasated) • Vasculitis • Exfoliative dermatitis • Stevens-Johnson syndrome • Toxic epidermal necrolysis • Rash w/eosinophilia and systemic symptoms • Interstitial nephritis • Nephrotoxicity • Ototoxicity • Neutropenia • Thrombocytopenia • *C. difficile*–associated diarrhea	Vancomycin may be confused with azithromycin, clindamycin, gentamicin, tobramycin, valacyclovir, vecuronium, vibramycin Monitor BUN/Cr and WBC at baseline, and periodically. Vancomycin can cause temporary or permanent hearing loss. Instruct patient to stop using this medication and call physician at once if he/she has any hearing problems or ringing in the ears.
Daptomycin (Cubicin)	4-6 mg/kg IV q 24 hr for 2-6 wk	Bacteremia, staphylococcal skin/skin structure infections, complicated bacterial infections caused by gram-positive organisms. Acts by disrupting multiple aspects of bacterial cell membrane function. Appears to bind to the membrane and cause rapid depolarization, resulting in a loss of membrane potential leading to inhibition of protein, DNA and RNA synthesis, which results in bacterial cell death.	• *C. difficile*–associated diarrhea • Superinfection • Pneumonia, eosinophilic • Hypersensitivity reaction • Anaphylaxis • Skin reaction, severe • Thrombocytopenia • Myopathy • Rhabdomyolysis • Peripheral neuropathy	Cubicin may be confused with Cleocin. Monitor BUN/Cr and WBC count at baseline, and periodically. Gently swirl but do not shake the medication bottle when mixing. After mixing daptomycin with a diluent, store in the refrigerator and use it within 48 hours. Do not freeze.
Linezolid (Zyvox)	600 mg IV/ PO q 12 hr for 14-28 days	Infections, VREF It is used for the treatment of serious infections caused by gram-positive bacteria that are resistant to several other antibiotics. Acts as a protein synthesis inhibitor, stopping the growth of bacteria by disrupting their production of proteins.	• Superinfection • *C. difficile*–associated diarrhea • Anemia • Leukopenia • Pancytopenia • Thrombocytopenia • Lactic acidosis • Peripheral neuropathy • Optic neuropathy • Vision loss • Serotonin syndrome • Anaphylaxis • Stevens-Johnson syndrome • Seizures	Zyvox may be confused with: Avelox, Vioxx, Ziox, Zithromax, Zosyn, Zovirax, or Zyflo. Monitor CBC weekly. Obtain ophthalmic exam if therapy extends beyond 3 months. Advise patient to avoid eating foods high in tyramine during treatment as this could lead to dangerously elevated blood pressure. Medication should be given slowly, over 2 hours.

Continued

SURGICAL PHARMACOLOGY

Treating Methicillin-Resistant *Staphylococcus aureus* (MRSA)—cont'd

Medication/Category	Dosage/Route	Purpose/Action	Adverse Reactions	Nursing Implications
Teicoplanin	IV/IM initially: 6 mg/kg on the first day, then 3 mg/kg/day. Severe infection: 6 mg/kg q 12 hr for the first three doses, then 6 mg/kg/day	An antibiotic used in the prophylaxis and treatment of serious infections caused by gram-positive bacteria, including MRSA and *Enterococcus faecalis*. Acts by inhibiting bacterial cell wall synthesis.	• Fever • Injection site problems such as abscess or pain • Itching • Redness of the skin • Skin rash or rashes	
Quinupristin-dalfopristin (Synercid)	7.5 mg/kg IV q 8 hr	A combination of two antibiotics used to treat infections by staphylococci and by VREF. Protein synthesis inhibitors in a synergistic manner. Whereas each of the two is only a bacteriostatic agent, the combination shows bactericidal activity.	• *C. difficile*–associated diarrhea • Superinfection • Anaphylactoid reaction • Angioedema	Most often given in a hospital setting. Medication must be given slowly through an IV infusion, and can take up to 1 hour or longer to complete. Usually given for at least 7 days, or longer for more severe infections.

BUN, Blood urea nitrogen; *CBC*, complete blood count; *Cr*, creatinine; *DNA*, deoxyribonucleic acid; *IV*, intravenous; *IM*, intramuscular; *PO*, by mouth; *RNA*, ribonucleic acid; *VREF*, vancomycin-resistant *Enterococcus faecium*; *WBC*, white blood cell.
Modified from http://online.epocrates.com. Accessed December 13, 2012; http://www.nhs.uk/medicine-guides/pages/MedicineSideEffects.aspx?condition=Bacterialinfections&medicine=Teicoplanin&preparation=. Accessed December 13, 2012.

the host. New genetic material also can be transferred into bacteria by means of free DNA that contains resistant genes (CDC, 2006a).

Introduction of drug-resistant microorganisms can occur through a person or an inanimate object. Bacteria become mobile and accessible to humans on the hands or clothing of care providers, through instruments and procedures, or through food. Resistant microorganisms may travel from distant parts of the world by means of infected travelers. Surgical instruments that have been ineffectively cleaned and processed can contribute to the spread of resistant organisms. Use of antibiotics in agriculture and in animal feed products also has contributed to the development of resistant organisms. When the food is ingested, resistant genes may be spread to humans (CDC, 2006a).

Drug resistance from treatment-related causes is often the result of misuse (e.g., incorrect use, overuse, or underuse) of antibiotics. It is believed that 50% of all antibiotic use in the United States can be characterized by misuse in one form or another, and efforts to reduce surgical site infections include appropriate prophylactic antibiotic use in surgical patients (Evidence for Practice). It is estimated that half of all antibiotic prescriptions written are not warranted. During antibiotic therapy, the patient may have had a few resistant organisms. By natural selection, as the susceptible organisms are killed, the resistant organisms multiply and become predominant. Inadequate drug therapy may contribute to the phenomenon and may be the fault of the patient, the provider, or both. Failure to perform sensitivity testing along with inappropriate dosing can contribute to resistance. If the patient is noncompliant with the prescribed regimen or discontinues the drug prematurely, he or she may also be contributing to drug resistance (CDC, 2012a).

Perioperative Considerations

Methicillin-Resistant *Staphylococcus aureus* (MRSA). MRSA infections, which occur in almost 130,000 cases in hospitals each year, lead to more than 5500 deaths annually (Ignatavicius, 2013). Common sites in which MRSA can be found include wounds (e.g., burns, surgical incisions, abrasions), chest tubes, intravenous catheter tips, intraabdominal abscesses, nasal passages, and the groin. *S. aureus* is one of the most frequently isolated organisms in postoperative surgical site infections. Surgical patients at risk for the development of MRSA infection include high-risk patients with underlying disease, patients who have a prolonged hospitalization, patients who have had previous antimicrobial therapy, patients who receive care in an intensive care unit, and patients who have been in proximity to another patient colonized with MRSA (Ignatavicius, 2013). Patients may present with unrecognized colonization or become infected by caregivers who carry MRSA in their nose or on their skin. The ambient environment is rarely a source of MRSA except for some reported cases in burn units.

The primary mode of transmission for MRSA is most likely direct contact transmission from the hands of healthcare personnel. The organism has been recovered from the hands of personnel after they touched contaminated material and before they washed their hands. It also has been shown that MRSA can be carried in the nares of personnel and transferred to patients by hand contact. The

▌EVIDENCE FOR PRACTICE

Prevention of Surgical Site Infections: Surgical Care Improvement Project

Many studies suggest that surgical site infections (SSIs) are among the most common complications of surgical patient care. SSIs increase morbidity and consume additional resources. The Centers for Medicare & Medicaid Services consider SSIs to be largely preventable and therefore do not reimburse healthcare facilities when SSIs occur after coronary artery bypass; bariatric surgery; and orthopedic surgery involving the spine, neck, shoulder, or elbow.

SSIs include superficial incisions, deep incisions, and organ/space infections. These have been defined in the Centers for Disease Control and Prevention (CDC) National Nosocomial Infections Surveillance (NNIS) system and are recognized worldwide. Surgical patients often receive some form of antibiotic prophylaxis. The Surgical Care Improvement Project (SCIP) is a national partnership of organizations committed to improving the safety of surgical care through the reduction of postoperative complications. In 2005 the SCIP launched a multiyear campaign to reduce surgical complications, and efforts are still underway. One of the targeted areas is SSIs.

Evidence for Practice Identified by Surgical Care Improvement Project to Reduce SSIs

Although some surgical complications are unavoidable, surgical care can be improved through decisions and subsequent care focusing on evidence-based practice recommendations. Research shows that delivering antibiotics to a patient within 1 hour of beginning surgery can dramatically decrease SSI rates, yet this practice is not followed in all situations.

Postoperative complications impose a substantial mortality-to-morbidity ratio on patients. The cost to the healthcare community is overwhelming. One approach to improving outcomes from surgery is to promote adherence to process of care measures such as administering prophylactic antibiotics. The purpose of antibiotic prophylaxis is to reduce intraoperative microbial contamination sufficiently to preclude microbial presence to reduce infection. The antimicrobial used should be safe, inexpensive, and bactericidal against a broad spectrum of the most probable contaminants for the intervention. Key measures identified in the SCIP to reduce surgical site infections and affect outcomes are the following:

- A prophylactic antibiotic should be administered within 1 hour before surgical intervention.
- The appropriate prophylactic antibiotic should be selected for surgical patients.
- Prophylactic antibiotics should be discontinued within 24 hours after surgery.
- Patients undergoing cardiac surgery should have their 6 AM postoperative glucose level controlled.
- Hair of surgical patients should be removed using the appropriate method.
- Patients undergoing colorectal surgery should reach immediate postoperative normothermia.
- Surgery patients should reach immediate postoperative normothermia.

Modified from The Commonwealth Fund: *Case study: the National Surgical Quality Improvement Program*, 2005, available at www.commonwealthfund.org/Innovations/Case-Studies/2005/May/Case-Study—The-National-Surgical-Quality-Improvement-Program.aspx. Accessed December 14, 2012; Centers for Disease Control and Prevention: *National nosocomial infections surveillance system*, available at www.cdc.gov/ncidod/hip/SURVEILL. Accessed December 14, 2012; Surgical Care Improvement Project—A National Quality Partnership, available at www.medqic.org/scip. Accessed December 14, 2012; Rosenberger L et al: The surgical care improvement project and prevention of post-operative infection, including surgical site infection, *Surg Infect* 12(3):163–168, 2011; Olson KM: Prevention of surgical site infections: improving compliance with the surgical care improvement project measures, July 2009, available at www.medscape.com/viewarticle/705366_1. Accessed December 14, 2012.

importance of hand hygiene cannot be overemphasized (AORN, 2013a; CDC, 2008a).

Because MRSA is transmitted by contact, perioperative protocols should be used when caring for these patients. They should include the following:

- Segregate the patient, using Contact Precaution guidelines.
- Wear a gown and gloves whenever there is potential for contact with contaminated fluids or materials.
- Implement strict hand hygiene practices.
- Limit patient transportation to essential movement only.
- Clean and disinfect patient care equipment as close as possible to the time of use (AORN, 2013c).

In healthcare facilities, MRSA causes serious and sometimes fatal infections, including necrotizing fasciitis. MRSA resists almost every antibiotic except intravenous vancomycin. One treatment for resistant MRSA is tigecycline (Tygacil). Tigecycline is an antibiotic related to the tetracycline family that was first used in 2005. This drug is formulated to retain activity against some bacteria that are resistant to tetracyclines and provides an expanded broad spectrum of activity for patients with complicated SSIs. Minocycline and doxycycline are also used in the treatment of MRSA.

Vancomycin-Resistant Enterococci. Enterococci are intrinsically resistant to cephalosporins, semisynthetic penicillins, and clindamycin. Some strains also have acquired resistance to erythromycin, chloramphenicol, tetracycline, fluoroquinolones, and vancomycin (CDC, 2006c). The incidence of VRE infections in the United States has increased rapidly in recent years and now is difficult or impossible to treat. Patients at the greatest risk of VRE infection are those with a prolonged stay in the critical care unit, intraabdominal or cardiothoracic surgical procedures, presence of indwelling central venous catheters, presence of urinary catheters, extended hospital stays, multiple antimicrobial therapies, and proximity to infected individuals. Because the enterococcal plasmid carrying the resistant gene can be transferred to organisms such as *S. aureus*, VRE infections are of serious concern (CDC, 2006c; Droboni et al, 2009).

The CDC has issued recommendations regarding the use of vancomycin, including identifying situations in which vancomycin should and should not be used; establishing education programs for practitioners, susceptibility testing, isolation procedures, and dedication of equipment and devices; verifying procedures for cleaning and disinfecting the environment; and minimizing movement of personnel between patients with and without VRE (CDC, 2006c; Droboni et al, 2009).

VRE can be transmitted directly from patient to patient, through the hands of healthcare providers, or through contact with contaminated environmental surfaces and equipment used for patient care. As with MRSA, Contact Precautions should be followed when caring for patients infected with VRE. Perioperative protocols are similar to protocols for MRSA patients and should include the following:

- Segregate patients, using Contact Precaution guidelines.
- Wear a gown and gloves when in contact with contaminated materials.
- Implement strict hand hygiene practices.
- Limit patient transportation to essential movement only.
- Clean and disinfect patient care equipment as close as possible to the time of use (AORN, 2013c; CDC, 2007a).

Germicides commonly used for cleaning and disinfecting in hospitals are effective against VRE. Isopropyl alcohol and sodium hypochlorite (bleach) are highly effective. With a 10-minute exposure time, some phenolic and some quaternary ammonium compounds also are effective. These are less effective at shorter exposure times. Hydrogen peroxide has been found to be ineffective. No relationship seems to exist between microbial resistance to antibiotics and increased resistance to germicides (CDC, 2008a). Perioperative personnel should routinely consult the manufacturer's written instructions and follow Environmental Protection Agency (EPA) recommendations when selecting germicides for surface cleaning (AORN, 2013d).

Vancomycin Intermediate–Resistant *Staphylococcus aureus.* In 1996 the first known incidence of vancomycin intermediate–resistant *S. aureus* (VISA) occurred in Japan when the organism was isolated from a surgical site infection and undrained abscess. The first occurrence of the organism in the United States was seen 1 year later. A patient that had been treated with vancomycin for multiple episodes of peritoneal MRSA developed bacterial strains moderately resistant to vancomycin, which was the treatment of choice for MRSA. Although the organism showed only intermediate levels of resistance, the CDC viewed this occurrence as an early warning that strains of *S. aureus* with full resistance to vancomycin may emerge (CDC, 2006c). Vancomycin is ineffective for the treatment of vancomycin-resistant *S. aureus* (VRSA) and VISA.

Multidrug-Resistant *Mycobacterium tuberculosis* (MDR-TB). Outbreaks of TB have heightened concern about healthcare-associated transmission of this disease. Transmission is most likely to occur from patients with unrecognized pulmonary or laryngeal tuberculosis and those who do not take their TB medication regularly. Populations at greatest risk of developing TB or MDR-TB are the elderly, indigent, minorities, immigrants from countries where TB and MDR-TB are prevalent, and HIV-infected individuals (CDC, 2006b). Transmission also occurs as a result of procedures such as bronchoscopy, endotracheal intubation, endotracheal suctioning, and open abscess irrigation, inclusive of inadequate equipment disinfection. Extensively drug-resistant TB (XDR-TB) is now a threat in many Asian countries and the former Soviet Union. This strain of TB is very difficult to treat because of its resistance to the primary medications used to treat TB (e.g., isoniazid and rifampin) as well as many of the secondary medications used (e.g., fluoroquinolone, amikacin, kanamycin, and capreomycin) (Neil, 2008).

The CDC's *Guidelines for Preventing the Transmission of* Mycobacterium tuberculosis *in Health-Care Settings* emphasize the following:

- Importance of control measures, including engineering controls and personal respiratory protection, including fit-tested, personal respirators when indicated
- Use of risk assessment to develop a tuberculosis-control plan
- Early detection and treatment of patients with tuberculosis
- Screening programs for healthcare workers

- Training and education for healthcare workers
- Evaluation of the tuberculosis-control program (CDC, 2005)

Prions: Creutzfeldt-Jakob Disease. Creutzfeldt-Jakob disease (CJD) is an infectious, human prion disease that is a fatal neurodegenerative disease of the central nervous system. CJD is one of a group of encephalopathies known as *transmissible spongiform encephalopathies (TSEs)*. Other human forms of TSE are Gerstmann-Sträussler-Scheinker syndrome and *new variant CJD (nvCJD)* or *variant CJD (vCJD)* (CDC, 2008b).

CJD is caused by a self-replicating prion. Prions are a unique class of organisms that have no detectable DNA or RNA. These small proteinaceous agents are abnormal isoforms of normal cellular proteins. The incubation period for CJD varies from months to years to decades. Symptoms include rapidly progressing dementia, memory loss, rapid physical and mental deterioration, and a distinctive electroencephalogram reading. Positive diagnosis can be made only by direct examination of affected brain tissue. Most cases occur randomly and for unknown reasons when the patient is between 50 and 75 years old. Death typically occurs within 1 year of symptom onset (CDC, 2012b). In contrast, vCJD has an earlier onset (between 18 and 41 years of age). Patients exhibit initial psychiatric symptoms and then neurologic symptoms differing from those of CJD, and the course of illness averages 14 months. The disease is always fatal (CDC, 2008b). According to the CDC, there is strong epidemiologic and laboratory evidence to support a causal association between vCJD and bovine spongiform encephalopathy (also known as *mad cow disease*).

CJD can be familial (i.e., inherited in the form of a mutant gene) or sporadic (no family history and no known source of transmission). Approximately 90% of cases are sporadic. Only about 1% of cases result from person-to-person transmission, and those are primarily the result of iatrogenic (medically related) exposure. Exposures have occurred via transplantation of contaminated central nervous system tissue, such as dura mater or corneas, from injections of pituitary hormone extracts, and by use of contaminated surgical instruments or stereotactic depth electrodes (CDC, 2008b).

CJD and other TSEs are unusually resistant to conventional chemical and physical decontamination methods. The causative prions are resistant to steam autoclaving, dry heat, ethylene oxide gas, and chemical disinfection with formaldehyde or glutaraldehyde as normally used in the healthcare environment (AORN, 2013e). Glutaraldehyde and formaldehyde act as fixatives, causing the prions to become more stable and less susceptible to normal sterilization/disinfection protocols. Special protocols for instrument care after exposure to prions should be followed (AAMI, 2012). Some institutions use disposable instrument sets for diagnostic brain biopsies to rule out CJD or TSE. Processes being investigated for cleaning and sterilizing devices contaminated with prions include the use of an alkaline cleaning agent and vaporized hydrogen peroxide (VHP) sterilization. Protocols for handling CJD are evolving as researchers learn more about prions and their destruction. Table 4-2 lists options from which an acceptable protocol for care of instruments and equipment exposed to the CJD prion can be developed.

Preventing Infection

Asepsis

The term *asepsis* means the absence of infectious organisms. Asepsis is directed at cleanliness and the elimination of all infectious agents. Surgical asepsis is designed to exclude all microbes, whereas medical

TABLE 4-2

Care of Items Exposed to the Creutzfeldt-Jakob Disease Prion

Tissue Infectivity	Item/Device (Using Spaulding Classification System)	Cleanable	Heat/Moisture Stable	Disposition
High infectivity	Critical/semicritical instruments/devices	If easily cleaned	If yes	1. Thoroughly clean with detergent germicide 2. Autoclave at 272°F (134°C) prevacuum sterilizer for 18 min (extended cycle) *or* 3. Autoclave instruments at 121°C (250°F) in gravity sterilizer for 1 hour *or* 4. Immerse in 1N NaOH (1 normal sodium hydroxide) for 60 min at room temperature. After 60 min, remove items from NaOH, rinse, and steam sterilize at 250°F (121°C) in gravity sterilizer or 273°F (134°C) for 1 hour 5. After processing according to one of above options, prepare instruments in usual fashion and sterilize for future use
			If no	Discard
	Critical/semicritical instruments/devices	If impossible to clean	NA	Discard
	Noncritical instruments/devices	If cleanable	NA	1. Clean according to routine procedures 2. Disinfect with a 1:5 to 1:10 dilution of sodium hypochlorite (bleach) or 1N NaOH, choosing solution that would be least damaging to items 3. Continue processing according to routine procedures
		Noncleanable	NA	Discard
	Environmental surfaces	NA	NA	1. Cover surface with plastic-backed sheet 2. Incinerate material after use 3. Clean with detergent then spot decontaminate with a surface with 1:5 to 1:10 dilution of sodium hypochlorite (bleach)—preferable 15-minute contact time 4. Wipe entire surface using routine facility decontamination procedures for surface decontamination
Medium/low/no infectivity	Critical/semicritical/noncritical instruments/devices	Cleanable	NA	1. Clean, disinfect, or sterilize according to routine procedures
		Noncleanable	NA	Discard
	Environmental surfaces	NA	NA	1. Cover surface with disposable, impermeable material 2. Dispose of material according to facility policy 3. Disinfect surface with OSHA-recommended agent for decontamination of blood-contaminated surfaces (e.g., 1:10 or 1:100 dilution of sodium hypochlorite [bleach])

Research into processing of medical devices contaminated with prions is ongoing, and institutional policies relating to processing of prion contaminated devices should periodically consult the World Health Organization and the Centers for Disease Control to determine if recommendations have changed.

NA, Not applicable; *OSHA*, Occupational Safety and Health Administration.

Modified from Rutala W, Weber D: Guideline for disinfection and sterilization of prion-contaminated medical instruments, *Infect Control Hosp Epidemiol* 31(2), 2010.

asepsis is designed to exclude microbes associated with communicable diseases. Practices that restrict microorganisms in the environment and on equipment and supplies and that prevent normal body flora from contaminating the surgical wound are termed *aseptic techniques.* The goal of each aseptic practice is to optimize primary wound healing, prevent surgical infection, and minimize the length of recovery from surgery. For perioperative practitioners, surgical aseptic principles and practices are the foundation for infection control efforts in the perioperative arena.

Infection control practices should primarily focus on prevention. Transmission of infection involves a chain of events, including the presence of a pathogenic agent, reservoir, portal of exit, transmission, portal of entry, and host susceptibility. Prevention occurs when there is a break in the chain of transmission. Infection control practices involve personal and administrative measures. Personal measures should include fitness for work and application of aseptic principles. Administrative measures should include provision of adequate physical facilities, appropriate surgical supplies, and

AMBULATORY SURGERY CONSIDERATIONS

Infection Prevention in Ambulatory Settings

The Centers for Disease Control and Prevention (CDC) note that more than three quarters of all operations in the United States are performed on an outpatient basis. Care provided in outpatient settings must minimize or eliminate the risks of healthcare-associated infections (HAIs). In response to outbreaks of the transmission of gram-negative and gram-positive bacteria, mycobacteria, viruses and parasites in ambulatory settings, the CDC published the *Guide to Infection Prevention in Outpatient Settings: Minimum Expectations for Safe Care*. The document represents the absolute minimum for safe care in ambulatory care settings. The fundamental elements needed to prevent the transmission of infectious agents in ambulatory care settings include the following:

- Administrative measures
  - Develop and maintain infection prevention and occupational health programs
  - Ensure sufficient and appropriate supplies necessary for adherence to Standard Precautions (e.g., hand hygiene products, personnel protective equipment [PPE], injection equipment)
  - Ensure at least one individual with training in infection prevention is employed by or regularly available to the facility
  - Develop written infection prevention policies and procedures appropriate for the services provided by the facility and based on evidence-based guidelines, regulations, or standards
- Education and training of healthcare personnel
  - Provision of job- or task-specific infection prevention education and training to all healthcare personnel (HCP)

- Training focusing on principles of both HCP safety and patient safety; presented at employee orientation and repeated regularly (e.g., annually)
- Initial and repeated documented competencies as appropriate for the specific HCP positions
- Monitoring and reporting of HAIs
  - Adherence to local, state, and federal requirements regarding HAI surveillance, reportable diseases, and outbreak reporting
  - Performance of regular audits and competency evaluations of HCP adherence to infection prevention practices
- Adherence to Standard Precautions
  - Observation of sound practices for hand hygiene
  - Utilization of PPE
  - Observation of safe injection practices
  - Provision for cleaning and disinfection of environmental surfaces
  - Provision for cleaning, disinfecting and/or sterilizing medical equipment
  - Observation of respiratory hygiene/cough etiquette

A wealth of information regarding infection prevention in ambulatory settings is available from a variety of sources, including a checklist published by the Centers for Medicare & Medicaid Services. The checklist captures all the elements of a sound infection prevention program and is a valuable resource for establishing and maintaining a program.

Modified from Centers for Disease Control and Prevention (CDC): *Guide to infection prevention in outpatient settings: minimum expectations for safe care,* 2011, available at www.cdc.gov/hai/pdfs/guidelines/ambulatory-care-04-2011.pdf. Accessed December 16, 2012; Centers for Medicare & Medicaid Services (CMS): *Ambulatory surgical center infection control surveyor worksheet,* 2010, available at www.cms.gov/Regulations-and-Guidance/Guidance/Manuals/downloads/som107_exhibit_351.pdf. Accessed December 18, 2012; Oregon Patient Safety Commission: *Infection prevention program development toolkit, 2012,* available at http://oregonpatientsafety.org/healthcare-professionals/infection-prevention-toolkit/section-1-infection-prevention-program-development/473/. Accessed December 18, 2012.

operational controls in the perioperative area. Standards for inpatient and outpatient settings should be established and followed (Ambulatory Surgery Considerations).

As new organisms emerge, and known organisms become more resistant, the importance of patient education as a risk reduction strategy cannot be minimized. In addition to practicing sound infection control practices, nurses partner with the patient through effective education about infection control measures to maximize the potential for perioperative safe care (Patient and Family Education).

Universal, Standard, and Transmission-Based Precautions

Universal Precautions. In 1985, in response to the growing number of individuals testing positive for HIV, the CDC published recommendations for the use of Universal Precautions (CDC, 2006b). Reports of hospital personnel becoming infected with HIV after a needlestick or skin exposure to a patient's blood created an urgent need for new and better measures to protect personnel from patient transmission of infection. With knowledge that many patients with bloodborne infections are undiagnosed, Universal Precautions, for the first time, placed emphasis on applying Blood and Body Fluid Precautions (previously a category in the 1993 *Guidelines for Isolation Precautions in Hospitals*) universally to all

individuals regardless of their presumed infection status. Universal Precautions expanded the Blood and Body Fluid Precautions by recommending masks and eye protection to prevent mucous membrane exposures in addition to the routine use of barrier protection, such as gowns and gloves. Universal Precautions also emphasized the prevention of needlestick injuries and the use of ventilation devices when resuscitation was performed. The CDC continued to recommend the use of Universal Precautions until 1987, when a new system of isolation called *Body Substance Isolation* (BSI) was proposed. BSI directed isolation of *all* moist and potentially infectious body substances (e.g., blood, feces, urine, sputum, saliva, wound drainage, other body fluids) for all individuals regardless of their infection status. This was accomplished primarily with the use of gowns and gloves. Because of the similarities yet differences between Universal Precautions and BSI, confusion reigned. In 2007 the CDC further expanded the *Guidelines for Isolation Precautions.*

OSHA issued a rule for *Occupational Exposure to Bloodborne Pathogens* to address workplace safety. This document was based on the concept of Universal Precautions. OSHA subsequently revised its final rule to include a special focus on needlestick and other percutaneous exposures to bloodborne pathogens (OSHA, 1991). The revised rule addressed "sharps with engineered sharps injury protections" (non-needle devices or needle devices with built-in

PATIENT AND FAMILY EDUCATION

Patient Education for Surgical Site Infection Prevention

The Joint Commission has established several National Safety Patient Goals (NPSGs) to provide organizational guidance for key patient safety issues. One of these goals, NPSG 7, focuses on how organizations reduce the patient's risk for developing a healthcare-associated infection (HAI). In addition to implementing hand hygiene measures and other evidence-based practices to prevent HAIs and surgical site infections (SSIs), organizations are also required to provide adequate education about SSI prevention to patients having surgical procedures as well as their families. Education can be provided by any means the organization chooses (e.g., printed materials, verbal teaching, classes), but there must be some documentation within the patient's record that the education occurred. Items that might be included in a patient handout are included below.

Millions of people have surgery each year. Every surgery has risks, but some can be prevented. One way for patients to help lower their risk for problems from surgery is to learn about some of the things that can cause infection and talk with a member of their surgical care team before surgery about the type of care they should receive. Here are some questions that patients often ask about SSIs.

What Is an SSI?

An SSI is an infection that occurs after surgery in the part of the body where the surgery took place. Most patients who have surgery do not develop an infection. However, infections develop in about 1 to 3 out of every 100 patients who have surgery.

The following are some of the common symptoms of a surgical site infection:

- Redness and pain around the area where you had surgery
- Drainage of cloudy foul-smelling fluid or pus from your surgical wound
- Fever

Can SSIs Be Treated?

Yes. Most surgical site infections can be treated with antibiotics. The antibiotic given to you depends on the bacteria (germs) causing the infection. Sometimes patients with SSIs also need another surgery to treat the infection.

What Are Some of the Practices Performed in Healthcare Facilities to Prevent SSIs?

To prevent SSIs, physicians, nurses, and other healthcare providers:

- Clean their hands and arms up to their elbows with an antiseptic agent just before the surgery.
- Clean their hands with soap and water or an alcohol-based hand rub before and after caring for each patient.
- If necessary may remove some of your hair immediately before surgery using electric clippers if the hair is in the same area where the procedure will occur. Personnel should not shave you with a razor. Using a razor to remove hair before surgery can lead to an infection because of the risk of leaving small cuts on the skin where bacteria can grow and possible gain access to the surgical wound.

- Wear special hair covers, masks, gowns, and gloves during surgery to keep the surgery area clean.
- Administer antibiotics before your surgery starts. In most cases, antibiotics are given within 60 minutes before the surgery starts and should be stopped within 24 hours after surgery. Given properly, antibiotics can greatly lower your chances of getting an infection after surgery.
- Clean the skin at the site of your surgery with a special soap that kills germs.

What Can I Do to Help Prevent SSIs?

Before your surgery:

- Tell your physician about other medical problems you may have. Health problems such as allergies, diabetes, and obesity could affect your surgery and your treatment.
- Quit smoking. Patients who smoke get more infections. Talk to your doctor about how you can quit before your surgery.
- Do not shave near where you will have surgery. Shaving with a razor can irritate your skin and make it easier for bacteria to proliferate and to develop an infection.

At the time of your surgery:

- Speak up if someone tries to shave you with a razor before surgery. Ask why you need to be shaved and talk with your surgeon if you have any concerns.
- Ask if you will get antibiotics before surgery.

After your surgery:

- Make sure that your healthcare providers clean their hands before examining you; either with soap and water or with an alcohol-based hand rub. *If you do not see your providers clean their hands, please ask them to do so.*
- Do not let family and friends who visit you touch the surgical wound or dressings.
- Ask family and friends to wash their hands with soap and water or an alcohol-based hand rub before and after visiting you. If you do not see them clean their hands, ask them to do so.

What Do I Need to Do When I Go Home from the Healthcare Facility?

- Before you go home, your physician or nurse should explain everything you need to know about taking care of your wound. Make sure you understand how to care for your wound before you leave the hospital.
- Always clean your hands before and after caring for your wound.
- Before you go home, make sure you know who to contact if you have questions or problems after you get home.
- If you have any symptoms of an infection, such as redness and pain at the surgery site, drainage, or fever, call your physician immediately.

If you have additional questions, please ask your physician or nurse.

Modified from The Joint Commission: Educating patients on SSI prevention, *OR Manager* 25(7):21–22, 2009; Surgical Care Improvement Project: *Tips for safer surgery*, available at www.fascrs.org/gedownload!/Content%20-%20Tips%20for%20Safer%20Surgery.pdf?item_id=488002&version_id=488003. Accessed December 9, 2012; The Society for Healthcare Epidemiology of America: *FAQs about surgical site infections*, available at www.shea-online.org/Assets/files/patient%20guides/NNL_SSI.pdf. Accessed December 9, 2012.

safety features to reduce the potential for injury) and "needleless systems" (alternative delivery devices using blunt cannulae, catheter ports or connectors, or other non-needle devices). Other revisions focused on the review and updating of exposure control plans, solicitation of employee input, and improved record keeping. The following is a summary of the requirements of the *Final Rule: Occupational Exposure to Bloodborne Pathogens* (OSHA, 2001):

1. Each facility must develop and implement an exposure control plan that defines exposure and implements the requirements of the final rule. This plan is to be reviewed and revised annually

with information provided to all employees. The plan must reflect changes in available technology to reduce exposure to bloodborne pathogens and implementation of appropriate technology to that end. Nonmanagerial employee input must be solicited in selecting technology to be implemented in the practice setting.

2. Engineering and work-practice controls must be used to eliminate or minimize employee exposure. Examples follow:

   a. The employer must provide everything necessary for proper hand hygiene.

   b. Contaminated needles must not be recapped or removed unless such action is required by a specific medical procedure. Such recapping or removal must be accomplished by the use of a mechanical device or one-handed technique.

   c. A clamp or other mechanical device should be used to disassemble a knife blade and handle.

   d. Sharps are to be placed in labeled or color-coded, puncture-resistant, leakproof containers for disposal.

   e. Specimens of blood or body fluids must be placed in containers that prevent leakage and are labeled or color-coded. Warning labels must be affixed to containers of regulated waste, refrigerators and freezers containing blood or potentially infectious materials, and other containers used to transport blood or potentially infectious materials (Figure 4-2). The labels must be fluorescent orange or orange-red.

   f. Food and drink are not to be kept in the same storage area where blood or other potentially infectious materials are present.

   g. PPE must be provided by the employer at no cost to the employee. Appropriate PPE shall include but is not limited to gloves, gowns, face shields or masks, and eye protection. Protective eyewear must have solid side shields. Gloves are to be worn when contact with blood or body fluids is anticipated. Disposable gloves are to be replaced as soon as possible after contamination occurs. Disposable gloves are not to be washed or decontaminated for reuse. Some facilities may have educational signs posted to assist employees in recognition of appropriate PPE (Figure 4-3).

   h. Signs must be posted at the entrance to work areas of potential contamination. These signs are to bear the biohazard legend with the following information: name of infectious agent, special requirements for entering the area, and name and telephone number of the responsible individual.

   i. Housekeeping provisions are to ensure that the workplace is clean and sanitary. A written schedule for cleaning and a method of decontamination must be established. All equipment and working surfaces must be cleaned and decontaminated after contact with blood or other potentially infectious materials.

   j. Contaminated laundry must be placed in a labeled or color-coded container that is recognized by all employees.

FIGURE 4-2 Biohazard label.

BODY SUBSTANCE ISOLATION IS FOR ALL PATIENT CARE | BODY SUBSTANCES INCLUDE ORAL SECRETIONS, BLOOD, URINE AND FECES, WOUND OR OTHER DRAINAGE.

Wash hands.

Wear gloves when likely to touch body substances, mucous membranes or nonintact skin.

Wear plastic apron when clothing is likely to be soiled.

Wear mask/eye protection when likely to be splashed.

DO NOT RECAP.

Place intact needle/syringe units and sharps in designated disposal container. **Do not** break or bend needles.

© 1987 San Diego Forms

FIGURE 4-3 Example of universal symbols for blood and body fluid protection.

k. All employees are to receive education and training about safe handling of hazardous substances and materials. Information must be provided to all occupationally exposed employees at no cost to them. Individuals must receive training at the time of employment and annually thereafter. Individual employee training records are to be maintained by the employer for the duration of employment plus 30 years. The healthcare worker is highly encouraged to receive the HBV vaccine after obtaining the required information about the risk of exposure and about the vaccine. If the employee chooses not to accept the vaccination, the employer must have the employee sign a letter of declination.

l. Employees should report all exposures to blood and body fluids for postexposure evaluation.

m. Employers who are required to maintain a log of occupational injuries and illnesses must maintain a sharps injury log that acts as a tool for identifying high-risk practice areas and for evaluating various devices in use. This log must protect the confidentiality of the injured employee. Log information should include the type and brand of the device, the practice area in which the injury occurred, and an explanation of how the incident occurred.

The bloodborne pathogen regulation is enforceable by OSHA at the federal and state levels. This regulation is based on the concept of Universal Precautions to serve and protect healthcare providers and to minimize the transfer of pathogens from one patient to another. Surveyors for OSHA may engage in onsite visits to healthcare facilities. Unannounced visits may occur at any site where an employee exposure occurs. The visit may be a result of a verbal or written employee concern, referral from another regulatory agency, or random inspection.

Standard Precautions. By the early 1990s the controversy regarding Universal Precautions and BSI had escalated. There was considerable confusion about which body fluids required special care under either Universal Precautions or BSI. There were also concerns about the need for additional precautions to prevent airborne, droplet, and contact transmission of other infectious agents. With this in mind, the CDC developed a single set of precautions incorporating the major features of Universal Precautions and BSI (CDC, 2007b). These precautions are called *Standard Precautions,* and they are designed to reduce the transmission risk of bloodborne and other pathogens. Additional precautions based on routes of transmission for patients known or suspected to be infected or colonized with highly transmissible or epidemiologically significant pathogens are included in the document.

Standard Precautions are intended to reduce the transmission of microorganisms from recognized and unrecognized sources of infection. Standard Precautions should be applied to all patients receiving care regardless of their diagnosis or presumed infection status. They are considered the first, and most important, tier of precautions and as such are a primary strategy for successful infection prevention and control. Standard Precautions apply to (1) blood, (2) all body fluids and secretions and excretions (except sweat) regardless of whether they contain visible blood, (3) mucous membranes, and (4) nonintact skin. Standard Precautions include the following:

1. *Hand hygiene.* Hand hygiene is the most important factor in preventing the spread of infection. Hands are to be washed whenever they are in contact with blood, body fluids, secretions, excretions, and contaminated items, whether or not gloves are worn. Hands are washed immediately after gloves are removed, between patient contacts, and when otherwise indicated to avoid transfer of microorganisms to other patients or environments. Sometimes it is necessary to wash hands between tasks and procedures on the same patient to prevent cross-contamination of different body sites. A plain (nonantimicrobial) soap should be used for routine handwashing. When special circumstances such as hyperendemic conditions occur, an antimicrobial soap or an antiseptic hand rub (waterless antiseptic agent) should be used. The hand rub antiseptic agent is most effective if the hands are clean before the antimicrobial agent is applied. For effectiveness, a sufficient amount of the agent must be used for the hand rub. Manufacturers' written instructions should be followed. An additional amount of hand rub agent may be necessary.

2. *Gloves.* Clean, nonsterile gloves should be worn when touching blood, body fluids, secretions, excretions, and contaminated items. Freshly donned gloves should be worn when touching mucous membranes and nonintact skin. Gloves should be changed between tasks and patient procedures and after contact with material that may contain high concentrations of organisms. Gloves should be removed immediately after use and hands washed before engaging in another task or giving care to another patient.

3. *Masks, eye protection, face shields.* A mask and eye protection or a face shield is to be worn at any time patient care activities are likely to generate sprays or splashes of blood or body fluids, secretions, and excretions. These protective devices help protect the mucous membranes of the nose, mouth, and eyes.

4. *Gowns.* Clean, nonsterile gowns are to be worn at any time patient care activities are likely to generate sprays or splashes of blood or body fluids, secretions, and excretions. Gowns help protect the skin and prevent soiling of clothing. The activity to be performed and the amount and type of fluid likely to be encountered dictate the degree of protective barrier necessary in the gown. Gowns should be removed immediately after use and hands washed before engaging in other activities or giving care to another patient.

5. *Sharps.* Needles, scalpels, and other sharps should be handled in a manner to avoid injury. Needles should never be recapped using any technique that directs the point of the needle toward any body part. If recapping is necessary, it should be done using a mechanical device or a one-handed scoop technique. Used needles should not be removed from disposable syringes, and they should not be bent, broken, or otherwise manipulated by hand. Used disposable sharps should be placed in puncture-resistant containers located as close as possible to the point-of-sharps use. Reusable sharps should be contained in a puncture-resistant container for transport to the point of decontamination.

6. *Patient care equipment.* Single-use items should be discarded after use. Reusable equipment must be cleaned and reprocessed to ensure safe use for another patient. Equipment soiled with blood, body fluids, secretions, and excretions should be handled carefully to prevent exposure of skin and mucous membranes, contamination of clothing, and transfer of organisms to patients, personnel, and the environment.

7. *Linens.* Linens soiled with blood, body fluids, secretions, or excretions should be handled in a manner to avoid skin and mucous membrane exposure, clothing contamination, and transfer of microorganisms to other patients, personnel, and the environment.

8. *Environmental control.* Adequate procedures for routine care and cleaning of environmental surfaces, beds, and associated

equipment are to be developed, and the use of these procedures is monitored on a regular basis.

9. *Patient placement.* Patients who contaminate the environment or who are unable to maintain appropriate hygiene or environmental control are to be housed in a private room with appropriate air handling and ventilation. If a private room is unavailable, the infection control professional may determine a method for cohorting patients with similar infectious organisms (CDC, 2007b).

Transmission-Based Precautions. Transmission-Based Precautions are the second tier of infection prevention, designed for patients known or suspected to be infected by epidemiologically important pathogens spread by airborne or droplet transmission or by contact with dry skin or contaminated surfaces. They may be used singly or in combination with one another if the patient has a disease that has multiple routes of transmission and are to be used in addition to Standard Precautions.

Airborne Precautions. Airborne transmission occurs by dissemination of droplet nuclei from evaporated droplets that can remain suspended in the air for long periods or by dissemination of dust particles that contain the infectious agent. Droplet nuclei are particles 5 μm or smaller in size. Airborne microorganisms can be dispersed widely depending on air currents and can be inhaled by or deposited on a susceptible host. In addition to Standard Precautions, Airborne Precautions include the following:

1. Patients are to be placed in private, negative-pressure rooms. The air exchange should be at a rate of 6 to 12 exchanges per hour with air discharged to the outdoors or circulated through high-efficiency particulate-arresting (HEPA) filters before being circulated to other areas of the facility.
2. Caregivers must wear OSHA-specified respiratory protection when caring for patients with known or suspected tuberculosis. If susceptible personnel care for patients with rubeola (measles) or varicella (chickenpox), respiratory protection should be worn. If the caregiver is immune to rubeola and varicella, respiratory protection is unnecessary.
3. All precautions for preventing transmission of tuberculosis should be implemented if the patient is known or suspected to have tuberculosis.
4. A surgical mask should be placed over the patient's nose and mouth for Airborne Infection Isolation Precautions when the patient must be transported from one location to another. Patient transport should be limited to essential purposes only.

Droplet Precautions. Droplet Precautions are used for patients known or suspected to be infected with microorganisms that are transmitted by large droplets (>5 μm). These droplets can be generated when the patient sneezes, coughs, or talks. Droplet Precautions are used in addition to Standard Precautions. Droplet Precautions include the following:

1. Patients are to be placed in private rooms when available. If this is not possible, the patient should be placed in a room with another patient who is infected with the same organism and with no other infection. If this is not possible, a 3-foot spatial separation should be maintained between the infected patient and other patients in the same room. For Droplet Precautions no special air handling is required.
2. Caregivers should wear a mask when working within 3 feet of the patient.
3. Patients should be transported only for essential purposes. When transport is necessary, a mask should be placed over the

patient's nose and mouth to minimize dispersal of droplets (CDC, 2007b).

Contact Precautions. In addition to Standard Precautions, Contact Precautions should be used for patients known or suspected to be infected or colonized with epidemiologically important organisms that can be transmitted by (1) direct contact, as occurs when the caregiver touches the patient's skin, or (2) indirect contact, as occurs when the caregiver touches patient care equipment or environmental surfaces in the patient's room. Contact Precautions include the following:

1. Patients should be placed in private rooms. If this is not possible, the patient should be placed in a room with another patient who is infected with the same organism and with no other infection. If this is not possible, patient placement must be determined on an individual basis, depending on the organism involved.
2. Gloves should be worn on entering the patient's room. Gloves should be changed after handling infective material that might contain a high concentration of microorganisms. When patient care activities have been completed, gloves should be removed before leaving the patient's room. Hands should be washed after glove removal. To avoid transferring microorganisms to others, no environmental surfaces in the patient's environment should be touched after the hands have been washed.
3. Gowns should be worn on entering the patient's room if there is a probability that the caregiver's clothing will be in contact with the patient or the environmental surfaces or if the patient is incontinent, has diarrhea, or has an ileostomy or colostomy. The gown should be removed before leaving the patient's room, and care should be exercised to avoid contact with environmental surfaces.
4. Patient transportation should be limited to essential transport only and Contact Precautions maintained to avoid contamination of personnel, visitors, or the environment.
5. Patient care equipment should be dedicated to a single patient and not be shared between patients. If this is impossible, equipment must be cleaned and disinfected thoroughly before being used for another patient (CDC, 2007b).

Perioperative staff members traditionally have relied on numerous types of precautions to protect themselves and others from bloodborne pathogens and other infectious diseases. Implementing these precautions within the surgical environment requires critical thinking skills and sound nursing judgment. Consistent application of these precautions by all members of the perioperative team serves to protect the healthcare provider and to minimize cross-infection of pathogens among patients (AORN, 2013f).

Infection Control and Bioterrorism. The potential for bioterrorism is a reality. The CDC has identified agents that may pose a risk to the national security because of their (1) easy dissemination or transmission from person to person, (2) potential to cause high mortality and have a major public health impact, (3) potential to cause public panic and social disruption, and (4) necessity for special action for public health preparedness (CDC, 2007) (Table 4-3). Perioperative personnel should have a basic knowledge and understanding of the agents most likely to be encountered and the levels of precautions required for patient and personnel safety. Communication, collaboration, and coordination are required in the face of any bioterrorist event or natural disaster. Communities need emergency plans for such matters, such as guarding patient data and protecting information systems, linking quickly and easily with

TABLE 4-3

Bioterrorism Agents*

Agent	Transmission	Incubation	Symptoms	Management
Anthrax (Bacillus anthracis)	Cutaneous: Direct contact Inhalation: Droplet, aerosolization	Cutaneous: 1-7 days Inhalation: 1-6 days on average, may be as late as 2 months	Cutaneous: Itching, progressing to papular and vesicular lesions, eschar, edema, ulceration, and sloughing. If untreated may spread to lymph nodes and bloodstream. Fatality: 5%-20%. Inhalation: Influenza-like with progression to high fever dyspnea, stridor, cyanosis, and shock. Chest wall edema and hemorrhagic meningitis may be present. Death is universal in untreated cases and may occur in 95% of cases not treated within 24-36 hours.	Standard Precautions. Special attention should be given to protection and containment of any draining wounds, inclusive of cutaneous lesions.
Smallpox (variola major/variola minor viruses)	Usually prolonged face-to-face contact is required. Also spread through direct contact with infected body fluids or contaminated objects. Rarely spread by virus carried in the air	Typically 12-14 days	High fever, malaise, head and body aches and sometimes vomiting. Rash develops over face and spreads to extremities. Rash soon becomes vesicular and then pustular. All lesions progress at same rate. Fever continues throughout course of disease, and growing and expanding pustules are very painful. Historical, variola major fatality rate is at 30%.	Standard, Droplet, Airborne, and Contact Precautions for patients with vesicular rash pending diagnosis. Avoid contact with organism while handling contaminated bedding. Wear protective attire to include gloves, gown, and N95 respirator. Vaccine does not give reliable lifelong immunity. Previously vaccinated persons are considered susceptible. After exposure, initiate Airborne Precautions and observe for unprotected contact (from days 10-17). Vaccinate within 2-3 days of exposure. One case is a public health emergency because of highly communicable nature of this disease. Consult CDC and local health agencies at earliest opportunity.
Plague (Yersinia pestis)	Pneumonic plague: Aerosolized bacteria carried on respiratory droplets from infected person Bubonic plague: Bites from fleas or infected rodent. Does not spread from person to person	Pneumonic plague: 1-3 days Bubonic plague: 2-8 days	Pneumonic: Fever, headache, and weakness, with rapid progression to pneumonia with dyspnea, chest pain, cough, and bloody or watery sputum. Respiratory failure and shock may follow within 2-4 days. Bubonic: Symptoms include swollen, tender lymph nodes (buboes), fever, headache, chills, and weakness.	Standard and Droplet Precautions. Patients should be placed in private rooms or cohorted with "like" patients. Transport should be limited to essential movement only, and patient should wear mask during transport. Contact Precautions until decontamination is complete.

Continued

TABLE 4-3

Bioterrorism Agents—cont'd

Agent	Transmission	Incubation	Symptoms	Management
Tularemia (*Francisella tularensis*)	Bites of ticks, deerflies, and other arthropods that have eaten infected animal tissue; by handling infected animal carcasses; by eating or drinking contaminated food or water; or by inhaling infected aerosols	1-14 days (average 3-5 days)	Depending on route of exposure, skin ulcers, inflamed eyes, sore throat, oral ulcers, swollen and painful lymph nodes, and pneumonia. When bacteria are inhaled, symptoms include sudden fever, chills, headache, muscle aches, joint pain, cough, and progressive weakness. Symptoms may progress to chest pain, dyspnea, bloody sputum, and respiratory failure.	Standard Precautions
Botulism (*Clostridium botulinum*)	Foodborne: Ingestion of preformed toxin Wound: When wounds are infected with *C. botulinum* that secretes toxin; injection drug users are at risk for wound botulism	Foodborne: Within hours of ingesting food, but can occur up to 8 days later	Early symptoms of botulism include gastrointestinal distress, nausea, and vomiting. Symptoms progress to diplopia, blurred vision, drooping eyelids, slurred speech, difficulty swallowing, dry mouth, and muscle weakness. If not treated, the disease progresses to respiratory paralysis and paralysis of arms and legs. Botulinum toxin is most poisonous substance known.	Standard Precautions

*The information about bioterrorism and the identified biologic weapons presented in this table represents current knowledge at the time of publication. The CDC updates its website with the most current information from throughout the world. Practitioners are encouraged to update their knowledge continually by consulting the CDC website (www.cdc.gov) and other experts in the field. The Health Alert Network (HAN) is the CDC's surveillance system. It connects local, state, and national public agencies with high-speed and satellite Internet access. The extent of precautions necessary can be quickly determined by using this system.
Modified from Centers for Disease Control and Prevention (CDC): *Anthrax information for health care providers,* available at www.bt.cdc.gov/agent/anthrax/anthrax-hcp-factsheet.asp. Accessed December 16, 2012; CDC: *Smallpox overview,* available at www.bt.cdc.gov/agent/smallpox. Accessed December 16, 2012; CDC: *Plague overview,* available at www.bt.cdc.gov/agent/plague. Accessed December 16, 2012; CDC: *Key facts about tularemia,* available at www.bt.cdc.gov/agent/tularemia. Accessed December 16, 2012; CDC: *Facts about botulism,* available at www.bt.cdc.gov/agent/botulism. Accessed December 16, 2012; Ignatavicius DD: *Care of patients with infection.* In Ignatavicius DD, Workman ML, editors: *Medical-surgical nursing: patient-centered collaborative care,* ed 7, St Louis, 2013, Saunders.

state and federal resources, ensuring culturally competent communication and care, accessing mental health resources, and identifying agencies that can partner with one another to provide services. Each institution must be compliant with The Joint Commission's (TJC) requirements for periodic testing of emergency management systems and their associated plans.

Engineering Practices to Prevent Infection

Environment of Care. The surgical suite should be designed in such a way as to minimize and control the spread of infectious organisms. Either a central-core, race track, or a single-corridor design may be used. With the central-core design, sterile equipment and supplies should be contained within the central-core area, which is surrounded by ORs and a peripheral corridor. The single-corridor design places the ORs on either side of a single corridor, with separate storage rooms, usually along the corridor, to house sterile equipment and supplies. If a single-corridor design is used, sterile and contaminated items must be separated by either space or time.

That is, sterile, wrapped, or containerized items can pass contaminated items in the corridor when the contaminated items are covered or otherwise contained.

Floors in the ORs should be hard, seamless, easily cleaned, and contiguous with the walls. This design eliminates the sharp angle where the floor and walls meet, where bacteria can become lodged and proliferate. Floors should be monolithic and joint free. Walls may be constructed of any hard surface that is easily cleaned and hard enough to withstand the impact of surgical equipment that may accidentally be pushed into the wall during transport. If ceramic tile is used, smooth-surface grouting mortar should be used. This grout provides a surface nearly as smooth as the tile itself; eliminating concerns that surface roughness may attract and retain bacteria. Painted walls are less desirable because the paint flakes and peels, particularly in areas of higher humidity. If a hard-finish epoxy paint is used, it is only as good as the surface beneath it. Equipment banged into a wall may cause damage and expose construction material to the environment. A soft-colored, matte-finished wall may be preferred to reduce reflectance and glare (AIA, 2010).

Doors in the ORs may swing or slide. If sliding doors are used, they should not recess into the wall but should slide over the adjoining wall to facilitate housekeeping. Cabinets should be recessed into the wall if possible. This configuration allows for maximum use of open floor space in ORs. Size and configuration of ORs are discussed in detail by the American Institute of Architects (AIA)/Academy of Architecture for Health. Stainless-steel cabinets are preferred because the surfaces remain smooth and are easily cleaned. Wooden cabinets quickly become damaged with cracks and crevices where bacteria can collect and proliferate. Wooden cabinets are difficult to clean and disinfect and should be avoided in ORs. Cabinet doors may be of either the swinging or the sliding type. A cleaning protocol should be established for the tracks if sliding doors are used. For noncabinet shelving, open wire shelves are preferred because dust and bacteria do not accumulate, and air can circulate freely around shelf contents (AIA, 2010).

Scrub sinks should be located adjacent to each OR, with a single area serving two ORs if possible. Ideally, scrub sinks are located in a room or alcove adjacent to the peripheral or single corridor of the OR. Scrub sinks should not be within the central-core area because aerosolization and splashing may occur where sterile items are stored, contaminating the environment.

Each surgical suite must contain an enclosed soiled workroom exclusive for its own use. The workroom should contain a flushing hopper, receptacles for waste and soiled linen, a handwashing sink, and a work counter. If the area is used as a holding area as part of a larger system for collection and disposal of soiled materials, the flushing hopper is not required (AIA, 2010).

Heating, Ventilation, Air Conditioning.
To control bioparticulate matter in the OR environment, ventilating air should be delivered to the room at the ceiling and exhausted near the floor and on walls opposite to those containing inlet vents. Airflow should be in a downward directional flow, moving down and through the location with a minimum of draft, to the floor and exhaust portals (AIA, 2010).

Air pressure in the OR should be greater than that in the surrounding corridor; this is called "positive pressure" in relation to corridors and adjacent areas. This positive pressure helps maintain the unidirectional airflow in the room and minimizes the amount of corridor air (less clean area) entering the OR (more clean area). Each OR should have a minimum of 15 total air exchanges per hour, with the equivalent of at least 3 replacements being of outside air to satisfy exhaust needs of the system. No recirculating devices, such as cooling fans or room humidifiers or dehumidifiers, are to be used. These units create a turbulent airflow and may recirculate settled bacteria. Doors to ORs should be kept closed to maintain correct ventilation, airflow, and air pressure. To minimize static electricity and to reduce the potential for bacterial growth, relative humidity in the OR should be maintained between 30% and 60%. A lower relative humidity may support accumulation of static electricity, whereas the presence of a higher humidity may cause condensation of ambient moisture, which may result in damp materials and supplies. This dampness supports bacterial growth. Temperatures in ORs should be maintained at 68° to 73° F (20° to 23° C) (AIA, 2010).

Practices to Prevent Infection

Preparing items for use in surgery and other invasive procedures requires thorough cleaning and drying of the items followed by either sterilization or high-level disinfection process. The efficacy of the sterilization or high-level disinfection process depends in part on cleaning to lower or limit the amount of bioburden present on the item to the lowest level possible.

Preparation of Items/Instruments for Sterilization and High-Level Disinfection

Cleaning. To prevent infection, all items that come into contact with the patient or sterile field should be systematically decontaminated after a surgical procedure. Handling, transport, and cleaning methods must be selected to prevent cross-contamination to other patients, exposure of personnel to bloodborne pathogens, and damage to instruments. The cleaning and decontamination methods chosen should be economic and of demonstrated effectiveness (Research Highlight). Items may be cleaned manually, by mechanical means, or by a combination of the two (AAMI, 2012). Increased productivity, greater cleaning effectiveness, and increased employee safety may result from use of mechanical cleaning methods. Some mechanical cleaning equipment is designed to remove microorganisms through a cleaning and rinsing action, whereas others clean

---

RESEARCH HIGHLIGHT ▐▐

Surgical Instrument Cleaning

The tenet that items that are not clean cannot be sterilized and debris that remains inside or outside of a surgical instrument after disinfection poses a threat to patient safety is basic to the core of infection control in the perioperative environment. In this study, authors undertook a project to investigate the efficacy of automated instrument reprocessing for cleaning suction tips. The multidisciplinary team focused on suction tips because they accumulate the maximum amount of debris after use compared with other instruments.

In the first round of the study the team verified that the existing cleaning procedures conformed to industry and manufacturers' standards. They then used fiberoptic digital photography to document debris not seen by the naked eye, but visible when magnified on a video screen. Of the previously cleaned and disinfected 144 suction tips selected for testing taken directly from the inventory shelf, 100% showed visible debris. The team then subjected the suction tips to a variety of different cleaning techniques in an attempt to reach 100% cleanliness. Despite successive use of manual rinsing and brushing, soaking in enzymatic solution, using an automatic reprocessor and an ultrasonic machine, a number of suction tips were still not visibly clean as seen through the camera system.

In a second round of testing, the team added chemical testing and expanded the number of instruments and variation in washing methods to include a total of 350 instruments. Again, using successive cleaning techniques, the team demonstrated that fewer than 5% of the suction tips were completely visibly cleaned at the end of the process.

At the end of their project the authors concluded that due to the increasing complexity and sophistication of medical instruments, some instruments may be impossible to clean, even with the use of rigorous methods and strict attention to detail. They note that as instruments become more complex, cleaning processes must also become more complex and that challenges presented by instrument cleaning warrant additional study to ensure patient safety.

Modified from Azizi J: Uphill grime: process improvement in surgical instrument cleaning, *AORN J* 96:152–162, 2012.

and destroy specific types of microorganisms by thermal or chemical means. The most commonly used mechanical cleaners are ultrasonic cleaners, washer disinfectors/decontaminators, and cart washers.

All workers handling soiled surgical instruments, whether in the OR, a substerile room, or a central decontamination area, must wear PPE sufficient to prevent contact with any blood or other body fluid. This generally means scrub attire covered with a liquid-resistant gown, coverall, or sleeved apron; hair covering; surgical face mask; eye protection; and gloves suitable to the task. In the event that fluids may pool on the floor, liquid-proof boots or shoe covers are recommended.

Instruments should be kept as free as possible from gross soil and other debris during the surgical procedure. Throughout the surgical procedure, the scrub person should wipe used instruments with sponges moistened with sterile water. When blood is allowed to dry on an instrument, it may cause pitting, rusting, or corrosion. Sterile water should be used rather than saline, which can cause pitting and damage to instrument surfaces. Initial decontamination should begin immediately on completion of the surgical procedure (AAMI, 2012; AORN, 2013e). All instruments that can be immersed are disassembled, and box locks are opened to allow solution to contact all soiled surfaces. These instruments should be placed in a basin, solid-bottom container system, or bin with a lid. Scissors and lightweight instruments should be placed on top. Heavy retractors should be placed in a separate tray.

Some instruments have sharp or pointed edges, such as scissors, forceps with teeth, perforating towel clamps, curettes, and rongeurs. These items can penetrate the gloves and skin, creating a portal of entry for infectious organisms. Sharp instruments must not be placed in a basin or tray in such a way that a worker would have to reach into the container to retrieve the instrument, risking injury. An enzyme solution, foam or spray, or a towel moistened with water can be added to the instruments to begin the process of breaking down any proteinaceous materials that may remain on the instruments and is useful in preventing debris from drying. Either should be used if there will be a delay in processing. Soiled instruments should be contained within leakproof containers, or trays inside plastic bags when they are transported from the OR for cleaning and decontamination. Soiled instruments should never be cleaned in a sink used for handwashing or a surgical scrub. Contaminated instruments should be transported to and cleaned only in a dedicated decontamination area. If sharps are being transported, the container should be puncture-resistant. Means of containing instruments include plastic, rubber, or metal bins with lids; solid-bottom sterilization container systems with the lids and filters in place; or simply placement of the instrument tray in a plastic bag. All soiled containment packages should be labeled with the biohazard symbol to warn handlers as to the nature of the contents. Transporting instruments while they are soaking is discouraged because of the possibility of a liquid spill and its associated clean-up problems as well as the difficulty of safely disposing the contaminated liquid (AAMI, 2012).

In the decontamination area, an initial cold water rinse with tap water or a soak in cool water with a protein-dissolving and blood-dissolving enzyme helps remove blood, tissue, and gross debris from device lumens, joints, and serrations. After completion of this pretreatment, the instruments should be processed in a mechanical washer or manually washed if a mechanical system is not available (AAMI, 2012) or if the device cannot tolerate mechanical washing.

Mechanical processing is usually accomplished with a washer disinfector/decontaminator and an ultrasonic cleaner. Washer disinfector/decontaminator cycles vary to some degree and may include an initial cool water rinse to remove protein debris, an enzymatic-solution soak, a detergent wash, ultrasonic cleaning, a hot water rinse, a liquid chemical germicide rinse, a lubrication cycle, and drying. Soiled utensils such as basins and trays should also pass through a mechanical washer. Some washers provide cycles specific to delicate or specialty instruments. When endoscopic devices or other items with a lumen are cleaned, a cleaning apparatus for these items can be attached to the many washer disinfectors/decontaminators (AAMI, 2012; CDC, 2008a).

The ultrasonic cleaning process is designed to remove fine soil from crevices and lumens of complex devices and from box-lock areas and serrations of instrumentation. It should be used only after gross debris has been removed. Ultrasonic energy occurs in waveforms and is generated by transducers on the sides or bottom of a specially constructed chamber that is filled with water or a water and detergent solution. The ultrasonic waves pass through the water, creating tiny bubbles that collapse or implode. This creates a negative pressure, which pulls debris away from surfaces. This process is known as *cavitation*. Ultrasonic cleaning is not biocidal, and after sonication the instruments should be rinsed to remove the loose debris.

Not all items tolerate the energy waves of the ultrasonic process. For example, lensed instruments should not be subject to ultrasonic cleaning because the energy can compromise the integrity of the lens seal. Dissimilar metals, such as stainless steel, titanium, copper, and lead, should not be ultrasonically processed at the same time. The energy waves, combined with the heat and detergent solution, can cause electrolysis to occur, plating one metal onto others, potentially ruining the instruments. Some manufacturers recommend that microsurgery instruments not be subjected to ultrasonic cleaning because of their delicate design and the fact that they may contain several types of metal. The detergent or enzyme cleaner used in the ultrasonic machine should be selected carefully and manufacturer's instructions should be consulted to determine compatibility with the ultrasonic cleaner machine and with the device. The corrosiveness and overall effectiveness of some solutions can be dramatically affected by the combination of heat and ultrasonic energy in such a machine. The water in the ultrasonic cleaner should be replaced when it is visibly soiled or at regularly scheduled intervals. Ultrasonic cleaners should be cleaned according to the manufacturer's written instructions for use.

Some instruments, such as air-powered and some microsurgical instruments, do not tolerate immersion in water or cannot tolerate the heat or pressures involved in mechanical processes. These items must be manually cleaned using an appropriate detergent for the type of material and the type of soil on the item. If protein or other organic soil is present, the detergent should have an alkaline pH (>7). If inorganic soil is present, the detergent should have an acid pH (<7). The degree of alkalinity or acidity should be selected so that the instrument or item itself is not damaged in the cleaning process. Using acidic or harshly alkaline solutions, however, can remove the protective passivation layer from the instrument, resulting in irreparable pitting and other corrosive activity. Although a neutral pH detergent is often selected for the foregoing reasons, written instructions from the instrument manufacturer should be consulted to determine appropriate cleaning products and procedures (AAMI, 2009b). If instruments are manually cleaned, they should be submerged in warm water with an appropriate detergent and then cleaned and rinsed while submerged. Cleaning in this fashion helps protect personnel from aerosolization or splashing of infectious material and from injury caused by sharp objects. Harsh abrasives should not be used for manual cleaning because they damage the protective surfaces of instruments, contribute to corrosion, and can impede sterilization (AORN, 2013e). The detergent manufacturer's instructions for concentration, water temperature, and contact time should be followed. Brushes used to clean lumens should be long enough to exit the distal end of the lumen. Brush diameter should be appropriate to lumen diameter. Brushing should be done under the surface of the water to prevent aerosolization and splashing of contaminants. Bristle diameter should be large enough to allow consistent contact with the inner walls of the lumen but small enough so as not to collapse when inserted. Brushes should be either single-use disposable or should be decontaminated at least daily.

Items that were soiled with blood or body fluids and that have been cleaned only may not have been sufficiently decontaminated to allow safe handling by workers not wearing protective attire and may require a microbicidal process, such as soaking in a liquid chemical germicide or liquid chemical sterilant. The device manufacturer's instructions should be consulted to determine if decontamination using a microbicidal process is required after cleaning and prior to packaging and sterilization. If there is no method suitable to further decontamination of the item, because of damage to the item, cost, or unavailability, workers in the preparation area should wear protective gloves when handling, inspecting, assembling, and packaging these items for sterilization.

The final step before sterilization for reuse includes instrument preparation and packaging. These activities should occur in a clean area, separate from the area where decontamination occurs. Instruments should be inspected for cleanliness and functionality. Soiled instruments should be returned to the decontamination area for further cleaning. Instruments with movable parts may be treated with a water-soluble lubricant solution that contains an antimicrobial agent to retard growth in the lubricant solution. Broken or worn instruments should be set aside for repair. Instruments are then assembled into sets according to set content lists prepared by perioperative nursing staff.

Packaging and Sterilizer Loading. Packaging of surgical supplies and their arrangement in loads in the sterilizer are factors that govern the effectiveness of sterilization. The prime function of a package containing a surgical item is to permit sterilization of the contents and to ensure the sterility of the contents up to the time the package is opened. Provision must be made for the contents to be removed without contamination. To be effective, packaging material should have the following characteristics:

- Allows for adequate air removal and sterilant penetration
- Provides an adequate microbial barrier
- Resists tearing or punctures
- Has proven seal integrity (i.e., does not delaminate when opened and does not allow a reseal after opening)
- Allows for aseptic delivery of package contents
- Is free of toxic ingredients and nonfast dyes
- Is low-linting
- Is cost-effective by cost and value analysis (AORN, 2013h)

Rigid sterilization container systems are one method of packaging instrumentation. Rigid containers can be sterilized, stacked, and stored. Because of the rigid material of the container, they cannot be punctured, abraded, or easily contaminated by environmental microbes. Recommendations and written instructions for sterilizing should be obtained from the container manufacturer. Prior to purchase, performance testing should be carried out in the sterile processing department of the healthcare facility to ensure that all conditions essential for sterilization and drying can be achieved. The container manufacturer should be consulted for information regarding set preparation and the most challenging areas within the container for placement of chemical indicators. Chemical indicators serve to verify that the sterilant has reached the interior of the container and is evidence that one or more of the parameters of the sterilization process were sufficient to cause a color change (see Quality Monitoring Practices). Many in-hospital packaging materials—woven and nonwoven, reusable and disposable—are marketed and should be evaluated carefully before a product is chosen.

If textile wrappers are used, they must be laundered between sterilization exposures to ensure sufficient moisture content of the fibers. This prevents superheating, which can result in a process failure during steam sterilization. Rehydrated materials also deteriorate at a slower rate. All wrappers must be checked for holes or tears before use for packaging. Manufacturer's instructions for use should be consulted to determine acceptable size, weight and density of textile packs. Instrument sets, including the packaging should not exceed 25 pounds (AAMI 2010; 2012).

Wrappers should be held at room temperature (68° to 73° F [20° to 23°C]) at least 2 hours prior to sterilization. Temperature and humidity equilibration of packaging materials are needed to prevent superheating and possible sterilization failure. When textiles are used for wrapping, the items should be wrapped sequentially in two barrier-type wrappers, which may be disposable or reusable. A single-textile reusable wrapper is defined as one layer of 270- to 280-thread count woven fabric. Sequential double-wrapping creates a package within a package, providing for ease in presenting the wrapped item to the sterile field. A commonly used envelope wrap is made by placing the article diagonally in the center of the wrapper. The near corner, which should point toward the worker, is brought over the item, and the triangular tip is folded back to form a cuff. The two side flaps are folded to the center in like manner. The far corner of the wrapper is then folded on top of the other three. Careful wrapping to prevent tenting and gapping of the package is essential (Figure 4-4). The process is repeated with the second wrapper, and the package is secured with autoclave indicator tape.

When the pack is opened for use, the flaps at the corners are used to form a protective cuff over the person's hands during dispensing of the sterile contents.

Single-use disposable nonwoven wrappers made of synthetic materials have largely replaced textiles for wrap. These wrappers are available in a variety of sizes and may be supplied as a single sheet or a double wrap that is bonded together. Double-wrap sheets provide a bacterial barrier at least equivalent to the sequential double wrap and allow for safe and easy presentation of the package contents to the sterile field, providing an alternative to the sequential double-wrapping procedure. Wrapping technique is the same as when using a textile wrapper. Nonwoven, single-use wrappers should not be reused (AAMI, 2012).

Sterilization process (chemical) indicator tape should be used to hold wrappers in place on packages and to indicate that the packages have been exposed to the physical conditions of a sterilization cycle. When packages are opened, these tapes should be first torn so that the package cannot be retaped and then removed from reusable wrappers because they create laundry problems, such as occluding screens and filters. Tapes also may leave an adhesive residue that can interfere with future sterilization of the fabric.

Sterilization pouches, commonly manufactured from a combination of paper or Tyvek and plastic films, provide an option for the

FIGURE 4-4 Envelope-style wrapping.

packaging of single (or small groups) or lightweight instruments or other objects (e.g., medicine cups). Pouches are selected based on material compatibility with the intended sterilization technology. Single or double pouching may be used; however, the pouch manufacturer's instructions for use should be followed to determine if double pouching is acceptable. A chemical indicator appropriate to the sterilization method is placed in the pouch, which is sealed either with heat lamination or with a self-adhesive strip (Figure 4-5). Unless validated by the pouch manufacturer, pouches should not be placed within sets because they cannot be positioned to ensure adequate air removal, steam penetration, or drying (AAMI, 2012). Any writing on the pouch should be done on the plastic side.

Every package intended for sterile use should be imprinted or labeled with a load-control number that identifies the date of sterilization, the sterilizer used, and the cycle or load number. Load-control numbers facilitate identification and retrieval of supplies,

inventory control, and appropriate rotation to ensure that dated packages are used first (AAMI, 2012). Some instruments or packaging systems may present challenges to the sterilization process. Special preparation or loading procedures may be necessary to meet these challenges. Hinged instruments must be arranged so that the sterilant can contact all surfaces of the instrument, including the tips, hinged surfaces, and ratchets. To accomplish this, these instruments must be sterilized in the open position. If the instruments have ringed handles for the fingers, the instruments may be placed on a "stringer," which is a U-shaped metal rod made especially for this purpose. When using container systems for sterilization, basket attachments may be used to immobilize instruments in the proper position for sterilization. Instruments with concave or other surfaces that can hold water must be carefully placed on edge to facilitate removal of air, which may become trapped in the concave surface. Placing the package on edge also facilitates drainage of condensate.

FIGURE 4-5 Sterilization pouch.

Items should be positioned with sufficient space between all surfaces so that the sterilant can contact all surfaces (AAMI, 2012; CDC, 2008a).

When packaging is complete and the sterilizer chamber is loaded, the bundles and packages should be arranged to minimize resistance to sterilant contact or penetration and to enhance air removal. Items capable of holding water, such as basins or medicine cups, should be positioned, usually arranged on their sides, so that condensate can drain.

Rigid container systems should be placed flat on the sterilizer shelf. These containers should not be stacked during sterilization unless the container manufacturer specifically recommends this practice and then should only be stacked in the manner recommended by the manufacturer's written instructions. Stacking may interfere with air removal and sterilant penetration. In addition, during steam sterilization condensation from upper containers may drip down and contaminate lower containers when the sterilizer door is opened and the cooler room air contacts the containers (AAMI, 2012; CDC, 2008a).

When combining containers and pouches and or packs in a sterilizer load, hard goods should be placed on the bottom to prevent condensation from dripping onto lower packs.

Pouches should be positioned on edge in a rack. They should be placed paper to plastic, all facing in the same direction.

The Spaulding Classification System. Items to be sterilized or high-level disinfected are classified as critical, semicritical, and noncritical, based on the risk of infection for the patient. This classification system, known as the *Spaulding classification system* and named for its developer, Earle Spaulding (Banerjee et al, 2008), has withstood the passage of time and continues to be used today to determine the correct processing method for preparing instruments and other items for patient use. According to the Spaulding system, the level of disinfection required is based on the nature of the item and the manner in which it is to be used.

Critical items are those that enter sterile tissue or the vascular system. These items should be subjected to a sterilization process and be sterile at the time of use. Examples of critical items include surgical instruments, needles, and implants (CDC, 2008a). Unsterile critical items may be sterilized using a variety of sterilization technologies. Examples of sterilization technology include steam,

ethylene oxide, and hydrogen peroxide vapor. Many critical items are purchased from the manufacturer as sterile.

Semicritical items contact but do not penetrate mucous membranes. Examples include anesthesia breathing circuits, thermometers, GI endoscopes, and laryngoscopes. Semicritical instruments require high-level disinfection; that is, these items must be free of microorganisms other than bacterial spores. Examples of high-level disinfecting agents include glutaraldehyde, ortho-phthalaldehyde (OPA), stabilized hydrogen peroxide, peracetic acid, and chlorine or chlorine compounds (Banerjee et al, 2008).

Noncritical items are items that come into contact only with intact skin. Because skin is an effective barrier to most microorganisms, most noncritical, reusable items can be cleaned at the point of use. Intermediate-level or low-level disinfectants may be used to process noncritical items. Examples of noncritical items include blood pressure cuffs, bedpans, linens, utensils, furniture, and floors. Examples of low-level disinfectants include alcohols, sodium hypochlorite, phenolic solutions, iodophor solutions, and quaternary ammonium solutions (Banerjee et al, 2008).

Sterilization. *Sterilization* is defined as the complete elimination or destruction of all forms of microbial life. The concept of what constitutes "sterile" is measured as the *probability* of sterility for each item to be sterilized. This probability is known as the *sterility assurance level* (SAL). For terminal steam sterilization processes, 10^{-6} is the recommended probability of survival for microorganisms on a sterilized device. A probability of microorganism survival of 10^{-6} means that there is less than or equal to a 1 in 1 million chance that any viable microorganisms remain after sterilization. The SAL of 10^{-6} is considered appropriate for items to be used on compromised body tissue. For items not intended to come into contact with compromised tissue, an SAL of 10^{-3} is sometimes accepted. An SAL of 10^{-3} represents a 1 in 1000 chance of a surviving microorganism (AAMI, 2012).

Steam Sterilization. Steam sterilization is the oldest, safest, most economical, and most commonly used method of sterilization available in healthcare. It is the preferred method of sterilization for items that are heat and moisture tolerant. The efficacy of steam sterilization depends on lowering and limiting the bioburden on the item to be sterilized, using effective sterilization cycles, and preventing recontamination of sterile items before delivery to the point of use (AAMI, 2009a).

Theory of Microbial Destruction. Microorganisms are believed to be destroyed by moist heat through a process of denaturation and coagulation of the enzyme-protein system within the bacterial cell. Microorganisms are killed at a lower temperature when moist heat is used as opposed to when dry heat is used. This fact is based on the theory that all chemical reactions, including coagulation of proteins, are catalyzed by the presence of water.

Principles and Mechanisms. At standard atmospheric pressure (sea level) when water is heated, the water temperature increases as heat energy is added. After the boiling point of 212° F (100° C) is reached, additional heat energy evaporates the water to form steam. At this point, the steam and the water are at the same temperature, but the steam has more energy than the water. This difference in energy is known as the *latent heat of vaporization.* When a cold item is introduced into the steam, some of the steam releases its latent energy to the object and changes back to liquid water. This phenomenon allows items to be heated much more rapidly in steam than in dry heat. The phenomenon of steam changing to liquid water is called *condensation,* and the steam and the liquid water are at a

TABLE 4-4

Common Time-Temperature Parameters for Steam Sterilization

Type of Sterilization Cycle	Load Configuration	Temperature, in °F (°C)	Time, in Minutes
Gravity displacement	Porous or nonporous	250-254 (121-123)	15-30
		270-275 (132-135)	10-25
Prevacuum	Porous or nonporous	270-275 (132-135)	3-4 or manufacturer's instructions
Steam flush/pressure pulse	Porous or nonporous	250-254 (121-123)	20
		270-275 (132-135)	3-4

temperature of 212° F (100°C) when this occurs. At this point, the steam is said to be saturated. This 212°F (100°C) temperature is insufficient to kill microorganisms, however. To achieve a saturation temperature sufficient to kill microorganisms (250°F [121°C]), it is necessary to have a sealed container. When water is boiled in a vessel from which the steam cannot escape, a higher temperature is reached. As more steam is generated with no escape route, pressure in the vessel increases. The higher the steam pressure, the higher the temperature. The steam is the sterilizing agent. Any compressed air remaining in the vessel mixes with the steam and lowers the steam temperature. This reduced-temperature steam is incapable of sterilization. Air acts as a barrier to steam sterilization (AAMI, 2009b).

Steam entering the sterilizer chamber should contain little or no trapped liquid water. The term *steam quality* describes the amount of steam vapor and liquid water in the mixture. A steam quality of 100% indicates that no liquid water is present in the steam. A steam quality of 97% or greater (i.e., <3% of the mixture is liquid water) is recommended to achieve an efficient sterilization process. Common causes of poor steam quality include improper boiler operation and inadequate or poorly maintained steam distribution lines to the sterilizer (AAMI, 2009b).

Sterilizing. When steam enters the autoclave, it is at the same pressure as the atmosphere. As the valves and doors to the outside close, steam pressure rises inside the chamber, increasing the temperature of the steam. Evacuation of air from the sterilizer is necessary to permit proper permeation of steam. If a sterilizer is improperly loaded, mixing of air with steam acts as a barrier to steam penetration and prevents attainment of the sterilization temperature.

The three factors necessary to achieve steam sterilization are *time, temperature,* and *saturated steam.* The microbial destruction period is based on the known time and temperature necessary to accomplish sterilization in saturated steam. Authorities have shown that definite laws determine the order of death in a given bacterial population subjected to a sterilizing process. If the temperature is increased, the time may be decreased.

To provide a safety margin, the minimum estimated exposure is extended to cover the lag between the attainment of the selected temperature in the chamber and the temperature of the load. The length of exposure varies with the type of sterilizer; cycle design; altitude; bioburden; packaging; and size, design, and composition of items to be sterilized. Written instructions for sterilization parameters should be obtained from the device and the sterilizer manufacturer. If a closed container system is used as packaging for items to be sterilized, the container manufacturer's written instructions for exposure times should be consulted and reconciled with those of the sterilizer and the device manufacturer (AAMI, 2012).

Sterilizers vary in design and performance characteristics. Use of rigid container systems may alter the come-up and exposure times

in steam sterilizers. The configuration of some instruments or medical devices may hinder air removal and steam penetration, making sterilization more difficult. In such circumstances the device manufacturer must be able to specify the necessary parameters to achieve sterility. Typical minimum cycle times for gravity-displacement steam sterilization and typical minimum cycle times for dynamic air-removal steam sterilization are provided in Table 4-4. Certain instruments, instrument sets, and implants require extended time cycles, however. The manufacturer's written instructions for extended cycle times must be followed.

The recording mechanism on the sterilizer gives information about the run of the load and to what temperature the goods were exposed and the exposure time. To achieve sterilization the temperature inside the chamber must be maintained throughout the determined time of exposure. The sterilizer recording device (e.g., printout) documents the come-up time, exposure time, and exhaust time (AAMI, 2012).

Drying, Cooling, and Storing. On completion of the sterilization exposure time, the steam inside the chamber is exhausted immediately so that it does not condense and produce wet packs. When the chamber has been exhausted and the pressure reduced, the door may be opened slightly to permit vapor to escape. Drying time can vary according to load contents. The minimum drying time is approximately 15 to 20 minutes.

After removal from the sterilizer, freshly sterilized packs should be left untouched on the loading carriage until they have cooled to room temperature. This is usually accomplished in 30 to 60 minutes but may take up to 2 hours, depending on the load contents (AAMI, 2012). If freshly sterilized packages are placed on cool surfaces such as metal tabletops, vapor still inside the essentially dry package may condense to water. This water may dampen the package from the inside to the outside. When the outside is wet, bacteria may follow the moist tract into the contents of the package. Because bacteria are capable of passing through layers of wet material, any packages that are wet must be considered unsterile.

A written record of existing conditions during each sterilization cycle should be maintained. It should include the sterilizer number, the cycle or load number, the time and temperature of the cycle, the date of sterilization, the contents of the load, and the initials of the operator. These records should be retained for the length of time designated by the statute of limitations in each state.

Sterile packages must be handled carefully and only as necessary. They should be stored in clean, dry, limited-access areas that are well ventilated and have controlled temperature and humidity. Closed cabinets are preferred to open shelves for sterile storage. If open shelves must be used, the lowest shelf should be 8 to 10 inches from the floor to avoid floor contamination. The highest shelf should be at least 18 inches from the ceiling or the sprinkler head to allow for circulation around the stored items. All shelves should be at least 2 inches from outside walls to facilitate air circulation and avoid any condensation that might accumulate on the walls during periods of severe temperature change (AAMI, 2012). Shelving should be smooth and well spaced, with no projections or sharp corners that might damage the wrappers. Sterilized packs should never be stacked in contact with each other and should only be stacked if the packaging instructions for use indicate this is acceptable. Their arrangement on the shelves should provide for air circulation on all sides of each package. Excessive handling, crowding, dropping, and stacking of sterile packs tend to force particles through the mesh or matrix of the wrapping material, which might contaminate the contents. Sterile items should not be stored in any area where they can become wet.

Shelf life refers to the length of time a pack may be considered sterile. Loss of package sterility is event related as opposed to time related; that is, what happens to the package after sterilization determines its continued sterility—not the length of time the package remains on the shelf ready for use. Variables that must be considered in determining shelf life are the type and number of layers of packaging material used, the presence or absence of impervious protective covers, the number of times a package is handled before use, and the conditions of storage. Impervious protective covers known as *dust covers* may extend shelf life by protecting the sterile package from a contaminating event. When used to protect sterilized items, impervious covers should be designated as such to prevent their being mistaken for a sterile wrap. They should be applied only to thoroughly cooled, dry packs at the time of removal from the sterilizer cart, after the required cooling period (AORN, 2013h).

A large number of commercially sterilized packages carry an expiration date after which the product should not be used. Expiration dating in these instances typically has to do with degradation of the product rather than sterility.

Supply standards should be planned to maintain adequate stock with prompt turnover. Appropriate volume and proper rotation of supplies reduce the need for concern about shelf life. The longer an item is stored, the greater the chances of contamination. For proper rotation, the most recently dated sterile packages should be placed behind those already on the shelves.

Quality Monitoring Practices. Physical, chemical, and biologic monitors are used for quality monitoring of the sterilization process. These monitors assist in identifying process failures that may be a result of equipment malfunction or operator errors. Physical monitoring is accomplished with pressure recorders, digital printouts, and gauges. All mechanical parts of sterilizers, including gauges, steam lines, and drains, should be checked periodically by the engineering department within the facility. The individual responsible for the sterilizers should keep reports of these inspections. Temperature, humidity, and vacuum should be measured with control equipment, independently of the fixed gauges. The methods of keeping a constant check on the proper functioning of a sterilizer and ensuring the efficiency of the sterilizing process are described in Table 4-5.

Most sterilizers provide a digital readout or printout. The readout records the time the sterilizer reaches the desired temperature and the duration of each exposure. It can be determined if a decrease in temperature occurred, warning of sterilizer failure. These recordings verify that the exposure time of loads has been correct and proper temperature limits have been maintained. The daily record should show the number of the sterilizer, the number of cycles run, the

---

TABLE 4-5

Physical, Chemical, and Biologic Sterilization Monitors

Type	Classification	Application
Temperature and pressure recording devices	Physical monitors	Steam EO Low temperature: • Low-temperature H_2O_2 • Ozone • Peracetic acid
Time recording devices		
Digital recording devices		
External trips/tape	Chemical monitors	Used on outside of packages
Bowie-Dick type indicators		Used for dynamic air removal in steam sterilizers
Internal chemical indicator (CI) strips		Used for: • Steam • EO • Low-temperature H_2O_2 • Ozone
Geobacillus stearothermophilus	Biologic monitors (indicator)	Used for routine load release, efficacy monitoring, qualification testing, product quality assurance, etc. Used for: • Steam • Low-temperature H_2O_2 • Ozone sterilizers • Liquid peracetic acid sterilant systems (spore strip only) Should be done weekly, preferably daily, and according to sterilizer manufacturer's written instructions Each load that contains implantable devices should be monitored with a biologic indicator (BI); load should be quarantined until BI test results are obtained
Bacillus atrophaeus (formerly *Bacillus subtilis*)	Biologic monitor	EO monitoring Should be performed on every load to be sterilized

EO, Ethylene oxide.
Modified from Association for the Advancement of Medical Instrumentation (AAMI): *Sterilization in healthcare facilities,* Arlington, VA, 2009, The Association, available at www.aami.org. Accessed June 28, 2013; Association of periOperative Registered Nurses (AORN): Recommended practices for sterilization in the perioperative practice setting. In *Perioperative standards and recommended practices,* Denver, 2013, The Association.

time, and the date. Physical monitoring devices provide real-time assessment of sterilizer-cycle conditions and permanent records. This evidence can be used for detection of malfunctions as soon as possible so that alternative procedures can be implemented while the cause of the malfunction is identified and corrective action is taken. Recordings cannot detect air pockets within the load or pack, however. Air is a poor conductor of heat; it is one of the most common causes, other than human error, of sterilization failure (AAMI, 2009b).

Chemical controls, also known as *chemical indicators,* integrators, or emulators include devices such as pellet-containing, sealed glass tubes; sterilizer indicator tapes; color-change cards or strips. Chemical indicators are used to detect exposure to the sterilant, failures in packaging, loading, or sterilizer function, such as presence of cool air pockets inside the sterilizing chamber. Chemical indicators, such as tape or labels that are impregnated with a material that changes color when steam initiates a chemical reaction, are placed on the outside of instrument trays or other packages and indicate contact with the sterilant. Chemical integrators are so named for their ability to integrate time, temperature, and the presence of steam. Chemical integrators are placed inside every package. They indicate that one or more of the parameters necessary for sterilization have been achieved. Chemical indicator color changes and wording vary for each type of sterilization modality to denote that an instrument set or other item is acceptable for use. As a result, perioperative nurses and scrub persons should always refer to the manufacturer's written instructions when relying on indicators and integrators (AORN, 2013h).

An external chemical indicator should be used on all packages to be sterilized except those that allow direct visualization into the package, where an internal indicator is used (e.g., paper or plastic pouches). The primary purpose of the external indicator is to differentiate between processed and nonprocessed packages. This indicator should be checked after the sterilization process and before a package is opened to determine that the package has been exposed to a sterilization process.

Each package requiring sterilization should have one or more internal chemical indicators, integrators, or emulators placed within the area of the package believed to be least accessible to steam penetration. The chemical indicator should be located and interpreted by the user at the time the package is opened and before use of the contents (AORN, 2013h).

A biologic indicator (BI) is the most accurate method of checking sterilization effectiveness. Commercially prepared BIs should be stored and used according to the manufacturer's written instructions. BIs used for monitoring steam sterilization contain a known population of *Geobacillus stearothermophilus* spores. *G. stearothermophilus* is a spore-forming microorganism that does not produce toxins, is nonpathogenic, and is resistant. Some BIs contain spores with an enzyme-based early readout capability. These indicators provide an enzymatic reaction that is highly correlated to biologic kill. Reaction times range from 1 to 3 hours. The length of time necessary for an initial reading depends on the type of sterilization cycle and the type of indicator used. Because these indicators do contain spores, it is possible, if desired, to incubate them for a longer time to demonstrate actual spore growth and to verify the enzyme-based result.

Biologic testing should be done after initial installation of steam sterilizers, after any major repair of the sterilizer, and with all loads of implantable devices. Except in defined emergencies, implantable devices should be quarantined until the results of the biologic testing are available.

Sterilizer efficacy testing using a BI should be conducted weekly and preferably daily. The BI should be placed in a process challenge device (PCD), sometimes referred to as a test pack, that is positioned in the most challenging location within the sterilizer. The most challenging location is usually the front bottom over the drain. Except with immediate use steam sterilization, the BI test should be run with a full load. Although users may make the PCD using towels according to AAMI instructions (AAMI, 2012), commercially prepared test packs are more commonly used. For immediate use steam sterilization, the PCD is the "flash" container itself, and testing is done in an empty chamber.

After the sterilization cycle, the BI is removed from the PCD and incubated according to the manufacturer's instructions. Negative reports (failure to recover any spores from the indicators in the test pack) indicate that the sterilizer is functioning properly. Results of these tests should be filed as a permanent record. A positive report does not indicate sterilizer failure because false-positive results

FIGURE 4-6 General-purpose steam sterilizer. This type of sterilizer has gravity or dynamic air removal cycles and can be used for terminal or immediate use steam sterilization of instruments and utensils, linen packs, and solutions in specially designed vented flasks. These units are available in several sizes, from small less than 2 cubic feet or tabletop sterilizers, to large floor-loading units. A large unit is pictured here. Some units have sophisticated microprocessor controls that allow maximum flexibility in selecting sterilization and drying times and help in troubleshooting if a problem occurs during a cycle.

sometimes occur. If the cause for the failure is immediately identified or confined to an item in the load, the cause should be corrected and the load reprocessed. If a sterilizer malfunction is found, all items prepared in the suspect load should be considered unsterile. They should be retrieved if possible and cleaned, repackaged, and resterilized in another sterilizer. All items in any load processed since the last negative result also should be considered suspect and should similarly be retrieved if possible (AAMI, 2012). A malfunctioning sterilizer should be repaired and the sterilizer retested. AAMI ST79 should be consulted to determine appropriate testing protocol.

When a dynamic air removal sterilizer (see Types of Steam Sterilizers) is used, a test designed to detect residual air in the chamber should be run daily before the first load of the day. The test, generally known as a *Bowie-Dick* test, is run with an otherwise empty chamber. The Bowie-Dick test determines the efficacy of the air removal system of the sterilizer. Air that is not removed can prevent contact of the sterilant with an item.

Types of Steam Sterilizers. For sterilization to occur, steam must contact all surfaces of the item to be sterilized. To accomplish this, the air in the sterilizer chamber must be evacuated. The terms *gravity displacement* and *dynamic air removal* describe the methods by which air leaves the sterilizer chamber. Dynamic air removal sterilizers use preconditioning techniques to remove air from the sterilizing chamber. This may be through a vacuum pump (prevacuum) or by an above atmospheric pressure process, such as the steam-flush pressure-pulse process. In a gravity displacement cycle the air is removed by the force of gravity.

At the beginning of the cycle in a gravity displacement sterilizer, steam enters the chamber after the door is closed and locked (Figures 4-6 and 4-7). An initial burst of steam enters the chamber and forces out much of the free air in the chamber. Air is heavier than steam, and the two do not mix well. As more steam enters the chamber, the air that is held by gravity at the bottom of the chamber exits through the drain, which is at the bottom of the sterilizer, hence the name *gravity displacement sterilizer.*

In a dynamic air removal (e.g., prevacuum) cycle, rather than passive air removal as is the case with the gravity sterilizer, air is actively removed from the sterilizer (Figure 4-8). When the cycle is initiated, steam is injected with force into the chamber. At the same time, the drain at the bottom of the chamber is automatically closed. As more steam enters the chamber, pressure increases, and the steam and air form a turbulent mixture. When a specific pressure is reached, the drain opens, and the pressurized steam and air rush from the chamber, aided by a water ejector or a vacuum pump. This sudden exit of gas from the chamber creates a vacuum within the chamber. This is the basis for the name *prevacuum sterilizer.* The sterilizer repeats this injection and vacuum process four times in succession in an effort to evacuate all air from the chamber (AAMI, 2009b; CDC, 2008a).

Some dynamic air removal sterilizers have the capability of providing an *abbreviated prevacuum cycle.* In this cycle are two rather than four pulses of the steam injection–vacuum process. This cycle may be used only for simple metal or glass instruments. No instruments with a lumen should be sterilized using this cycle (AAMI, 2009b; CDC, 2008a). Some sterilizers can run only gravity displacement cycles. These sterilizers are referred to as gravity displacement sterilizers. Other sterilizers can run either a dynamic air removal cycle or a gravity displacement cycle. Device manufacturer's instructions should be consulted to determine the preferred or required cycle.

Immediate Use Steam Sterilization. Immediate-use steam sterilization (IUSS) (formerly known as flash sterilization) is a process used to sterilize items that are not intended to be stored for use at a later time. The cycle used for IUSS has a very minimal or no dry time, which decreases the total time for of the processing. Items processed using IUSS should be used as soon as possible after they are removed from the sterilizer. They should not be stored for later use or held for a later procedure (AAMI, 2011). IUSS sterilization

FIGURE 4-7 A, Adjustable racks used within sterilizers are designed to permit maximum loading efficiency. **B,** Instrument baskets or trays should have either wire-meshed bottoms or a sufficient number of perforations in the sheet metal to allow for air removal and drainage of condensate during the sterilization cycle.

FIGURE 4-8 Dynamic air removal/prevacuum steam sterilizer. This type of sterilizer features active, aggressive removal of air rather than relying on the passive action of gravity. When the cycle is initiated, steam is injected with force into the chamber. At the same time, the drain at the bottom of the chamber is automatically closed. As more steam enters the chamber, pressure increases and the steam and air form a turbulent mixture. When a specific pressure is reached, the drain opens, and the pressurized steam and air rush from the chamber, aided by a water ejector or a vacuum pump. This sudden rush of gas from the chamber creates a vacuum within the chamber. This process is repeated several times and deepens the level of vacuum drawn with each pulse. The effect of this pulsing cycle is to displace any air in the load and rapidly increase the chamber and load temperatures. At the conclusion of this conditioning phase, steam flows into the chamber and raises the temperature to sterilization levels, usually 270° to 275°F (132° to 145°C). Steam is removed from the chamber to draw a partial vacuum again. Heated, filtered air is introduced into the chamber to dry the load. Drying times are selected and set by the user, depending on the nature of the load. Some units have a special cycle designed for rapid sterilization of an instrument tray in a single wrapper. This express cycle has fewer conditioning pulses, a 4-minute exposure time, and 1 or 2 minutes of dry time, for a total cycle time of approximately 12 minutes. Although the wrapper feels warm and dry to the touch, the contents may not be totally dry. This package should be handled by individuals wearing sterile gloves and using sterile towels for protection from burns. The instruments sterilized in this express cycle must be used immediately. Because the contents are not dry, the package is not suitable for storage.

can be accomplished in either a gravity displacement or a dynamic air removal sterilizer. IUSS is most frequently used in the OR for sterilizing urgently needed instruments. AORN's *Recommended Practices for Sterilization in the Perioperative Practice Setting* recommend that use of IUSS should be kept to a minimum and should be used only in selected clinical situations and in a controlled manner. Containers specific to IUSS should be used for this process. Items/instruments should not be sterilized in an open pan or tray.

IUSS should not be used for implantable devices except in cases of emergency when no other option is available. In an emergency, when IUSS of an implant is unavoidable, an early readout BI and a chemical integrating indicator should run with the load (AORN, 2013g). Results of the BI may not be known until after completion of the surgery. Documentation should reflect patient follow-up if the BI result indicates a failure. Appropriate perioperative planning along with communicating and working with implant manufacturers may help decrease unplanned IUSS (AORN, 2013g). Devices subject to IUSS should be meticulously cleaned in a dedicated decontamination area. IUSS containers should be used, cleaned, and maintained according to the manufacturer's written instructions. Containers intended only for IUSS should be differentiated from other types of containers (AORN, 2013g). Routine cycle parameters for IUSS sterilization are shown in Table 4-6. Meticulous recordkeeping must be implemented for IUSS. At a minimum, facilities should document the date and time, patient's name, surgery or procedure performed, item(s) cycle parameters (the printout), and the name of the sterilizer operator. Additional information to document includes the reason IUSS was necessary. Analysis of the frequency of and the reasons for IUSS can be used as an impetus for process improvements (i.e., reducing the incidence of IUSS).

Chemical Sterilization. Devices developed with materials that cannot tolerate heat and or moisture are continually being introduced for use in healthcare. These devices require the use of sterilization methods other than steam. Chemical agents provide an effective alternative to steam sterilization. Chemical sterilization is frequently referred to as *low-temperature sterilization.*

Ethylene Oxide. *Ethylene oxide (EO)* is an alkylating agent that results in microbial death under controlled parameters. EO has had application for heat-labile and moisture-sensitive items, such as flexible endoscopes, lensed instruments, delicate surgical instruments, and electrical devices. EO should be used if alternate methods of sterilization are not available or compatible with the medical devices being processed. EO is colorless at ordinary temperatures, has an odor similar to that of ether, and has inhalation toxicity similar to that of ammonia gas. EO is a known carcinogen and must be used carefully because of its toxicity. It is highly explosive and very flammable in the presence of air.

Destruction of microorganisms takes place by alkylation whereby the DNA of the microorganism is destroyed, inactivating the reproductive process of the cell. As with all sterilization and disinfection processes, items to be sterilized with EO must be thoroughly cleaned and dried. Drying inhibits the formation of ethylene glycol (antifreeze) during the sterilization cycle. Items should be disassembled prior to placement within sets or trays and should be configured to permit the gas to circulate throughout the items. The packaging material used should possess the characteristics described previously in this chapter and should be compatible with EO.

Proper loading of the sterilizer is essential to ensure adequate gas circulation and penetration. Distribution and arrangement of items should be in accordance with the sterilizer manufacturer's instructions. An excessively large load or a load that is tightly packed interferes with proper air removal, load humidification, sterilant penetration, and sterilant evacuation at the conclusion of the cycle. An EO-sensitive chemical indicator should be used with each package to indicate that the package was exposed to the gas. The chemical indicator does not indicate achievement of sterility (AORN, 2013g).

Factors affecting sterilization with EO are time of exposure, gas concentration, temperature, humidity, and penetration. The

TABLE 4-6

Time-Temperature Parameters for Immediate-Use Steam Sterilization

Type of Sterilizer/Cycle	Load Configuration	Temperature, in °F (°C)	Time, in Minutes
High-speed gravity displacement	Metal or nonporous items only (no lumens)	270-272 (132-135)	See device, container, and sterilizer manufacturer instructions for use (follow manufacturer's instructions for express cycle to determine number of items permitted and cycle time)
	Metal items with lumens and porous items (e.g., rubber, plastic), which are sterilized together	270-272 (132-135)	See device and container manufacture instructions for use
Prevacuum (dynamic air removal)	Metal or nonporous items only (no lumens)	270-272 (132-135)	See device and container manufacture instructions for use
	Metal items with lumens and porous items, which are sterilized together	270-272 (132-135)	See device and container manufacture instructions for use
Pulsing gravity	All loads	Manufacturer's instructions	See device and container manufacture instructions for use; also see sterilizer manufacturer's instructions

TABLE 4-7

Common Parameters for Ethylene Oxide Sterilization

Time, in Minutes	Temperature, in °F (°C)	Humidity, in %	Gas Concentration, in mg/L
105-300	99-145 (37-63)	45-75	450-1200

exposure time required depends on temperature, humidity, gas concentration, the ease of penetrating articles to be sterilized, and the type of microorganisms to be destroyed (Table 4-7). Gas concentration is affected by the temperature and humidity inside the sterilizing chamber. If the concentration of gas is doubled, the exposure time may be shortened. Temperature and humidity have a pronounced influence on the destruction of microorganisms. They are important in gaseous sterilization with EO because they affect penetration of the gas through bacterial cell walls and through wrapping and packaging material. Dry spores are the most difficult to kill, but when such spores are moistened their resistance to gas penetration is lowered. Dehydration makes some microorganisms nearly immune to EO sterilization, whereas droplets of moisture can inhibit the action of the gas by protecting the organism. EO sterilizers with automatic controls provide for moisture injection to increase the relative humidity within the chamber. Manufacturers of gas sterilizers have developed recommended exposure periods for various EO concentrations in relation to the material to be sterilized. Exposure time is set for absolute destruction of the most resistant microorganisms, which is a very slow process. The adequacy of every EO cycle should be verified using a PCD containing a biologic indicator consisting of a known population of *Bacillus atrophaeus* spores.

EO-sterilized items must be aerated to make them safe for personnel handling and patient use. The length of aeration for each item should be based on the device and the sterilizer manufacturer's written recommendations. Aeration is a lengthy process and may take up to 8 hours or more.

Older ethylene oxide sterilizers, because they did not include an aerator, required transfer of items after sterilization into a separate aerator. This process put personnel at risk of exposure. The EPA no longer permits this process and requires that sterilization and

aeration take place in a single chamber. EO sterilizers sold today sterilize and aerate in the same chamber (EPA, 2010). The EPA also requires that hospitals without a pollution control device must run a full load when using EO sterilization (EPA, 2007).

Because of the highly explosive and flammable nature of EO, it may be supplied in large tanks mixed with an inert gas to render it nonflammable and nonexplosive. It is also, and more commonly, supplied in small cartridges that contain enough gas to sterilize a single load. The sterilizer should be installed in a well-ventilated room and be vented to the outside atmosphere as recommended by the manufacturer and by the requirements of the National Institute for Occupational Safety and Health (NIOSH). Only authorized personnel are allowed access, and hazard signs should be posted. Compliance with other administrative controls to ensure safety is essential.

Excessive exposure to EO represents a health hazard to personnel. It is a known carcinogen and has been linked to reproductive problems and other disorders in animals. Inhalation of, and exposure to, EO should be avoided. OSHA has issued standards regulating personnel exposure to EO (OSHA, 2010). These standards set the permissible exposure level (PEL) (the amount of EO in the air) at 1 part per million (ppm) and the action level (AL) (monitored value at which corrective action should occur) at 0.5 ppm. These are calculated as time-weighted averages (TWAs) over an 8-hour period. OSHA requires that monitoring and surveillance be performed to ensure that exposure levels do not exceed 1 ppm over an 8-hour period (OSHA, 1988). In addition, occupational exposure level to EO may not exceed 15 ppm in any 15-minute period. This is known as the *excursion level* (EL).

Personnel with the potential for EO exposure should wear an EO-monitoring badge that meets the NIOSH accuracy standards.

FIGURE 4-9 Low-temperature gas plasma sterilizers. **A,** Tabletop model. **B,** Floor standing model.

Butyl rubber, nitrile, or neoprene gloves should be worn if it becomes necessary to handle items that have not been fully aerated (AORN, 2013g).

In general, EO sterilization should be used *only* if the materials are heat sensitive and unable to withstand sterilization by saturated steam under pressure. EO's advantages are that it is easily available; it is effective against all types of microorganisms; it easily penetrates masses of dry material; it does not require high temperatures, humidity, or pressure; and it is noncorrosive and nondamaging to items. Sterilization with EO also has numerous disadvantages. The long exposure and aeration periods make it a lengthy process. Liquid EO may produce serious burns on exposed skin if not immediately removed; insufficiently aerated materials can cause skin irritation, burns of body tissue, and hemolysis of blood; and diluents used with EO cause damage to some plastics (AAMI, 2009b; OSHA, 1984).

Low-Temperature Hydrogen Peroxide Gas Plasma Sterilization. Low-temperature hydrogen peroxide gas plasma sterilization should be used for moisture- and heat-sensitive items and when indicated by the device manufacturer. Plasma is the fourth state of matter, the sequence being solid, liquid, gas, and plasma. Gas plasmas are highly ionized gases composed of ions, electrons, and neutral particles. To create gas plasma for sterilization, a precursor solution, such as hydrogen peroxide, is introduced into a closed area in the sterilizer under low-vacuum conditions. Hydrogen peroxide vapor is charged with radiofrequency, and a plasma is created. In this process, microbial life is disrupted when hydrogen peroxide vapor and the free radicals created from hydrogen peroxide gas plasma interact with microbial cell membranes, enzymes, or nucleic acids. The byproducts of this process are oxygen and water (in the form of humidity). Packages are dry at the end of the cycle (AAMI, 2009c; AORN, 2013g).

Low-temperature hydrogen peroxide gas plasma sterilization is replacing ethylene oxide sterilization for most applications. It is designed to provide nontoxic, dry, low-temperature sterilization in a shorter turnaround time than that of ethylene oxide. Cycle times for gas plasma sterilization vary; depending on the model of sterilizer, the cycle time can be as short as just less than 30 minutes. At the completion of the sterilization process, no toxic residues remain on the sterilized items and no aeration is necessary. Device manufacturer's instructions should be consulted to determine compatibility of devices with sterilization in hydrogen peroxide gas plasma. Instrumentation preparation for sterilization includes cleaning and decontaminating procedures, drying, reassembly, and wrapping with nonwoven polypropylene wraps, Tyvek/Mylar pouches, or containers validated for use with hydrogen peroxide gas plasma (Figure 4-9). Cellulosic-based products, such as paper and linen, are not recommended for use with plasma systems because they tend to absorb the vapor and cause the sterilization cycle to abort. Manufacturer's written instructions for use should always be followed (AAMI, 2009c; AORN, 2013g).

Biologic and chemical indicators for process verification are used in the same manner as indicators for steam and ethylene oxide sterilization procedures. Plasma sterilization processes should be tested with biologic indicators containing *G. stearothermophilus* spores. These spores show the greatest resistance to kill in hydrogen peroxide gas plasma. Efficacy testing of the sterilization cycle should be performed daily, preferably with every load (AAMI, 2009b; AORN, 2013g).

Hydrogen Peroxide Vapor. Low-temperature hydrogen peroxide vapor is suitable for devices that cannot tolerate high temperature or moisture and that are indicated as compatible by the device manufacturer. In this process hydrogen peroxide vapor is the sterilant. This is an oxidative process that inactivates microorganisms. The byproducts at the end of the cycle are oxygen and water vapor. Packages are dry at the end of the cycle. The process is nontoxic and no aeration is required.

Items must be cleaned, dried, and packaged as with other sterilization processes. Compatible packaging includes nonwoven polypropylene wraps, Tyvek/Mylar pouches, trays, and containers validated for use with hydrogen peroxide sterilization; cellulose-based products are not recommended. One or more chemical indicators should be placed within each package to be sterilized. Sterilizer efficacy monitoring with a BI containing *B. atrophaeus* spores should be performed with every load.

Dry Heat Sterilization. Dry heat sterilization should be used only when the materials cannot be sterilized by other methods, when the moisture of other processes would damage the materials, or when the materials are impermeable to the process. These materials include grease, anhydrous oils, powders, and some glassware. Anhydrous oils and powders are commercially available, and as a result, dry heat is rarely used in healthcare facilities today. Dry heat is not a suitable sterilization method for fabrics and rubber goods because the high temperatures necessary for sterilization cause deterioration of these materials. There are two kinds of dry heat (also known as *hot air*) sterilizers—the gravity convection type and the mechanical convection type. Both heat by electricity to achieve accurate and dependable temperature control.

In a *gravity convection sterilizer* convection is created by the temperature differences within the sterilizing chamber. The heating apparatus present in the bottom of the chamber warms the air within the chamber. The warmed air rises, contacting the items in the chamber to be sterilized. At contact, heat is transferred from the air to the items. With this loss of heat, the cooled air descends toward the bottom of the chamber, where it is warmed again by the heating coils.

In a *mechanical convection sterilizer* the heating apparatus is outside the chamber, in a compartment separated from the chamber by a diffusing wall placed in front of a motor-driven turbine blower. Through an internal process, air is heated and forced into a chamber on the opposite wall. From this chamber the air is discharged into the chamber uniformly over the vertical plane of the chamber. This system provides for uniform delivery of heated air and equal transfer of heat to all regions of the chamber. This system offers the maximum functional efficiency at a minimum cost and is the system most often used in hospitals (AAMI, 2009b).

Because of the variation in items to be sterilized and packaging methods and materials, parameters for dry heat sterilization vary. Temperature parameters refer to the temperature of the load, not sterilizer chamber temperature.

Spore tests may be used with dry heat sterilization. *B. atrophaeus* is the most commonly used challenge microorganism. The sterilizer manufacturer's instructions should be carefully followed for sterilizer monitoring (AAMI, 2009b).

Liquid Peracetic Acid Sterilant Systems. Many facilities use a liquid peracetic acid sterilant processing system. Liquid peracetic acid systems are used for devices that are heat sensitive, can be immersed, and have been validated by the device manufacturer for use in these systems. It is suitable for devices that cannot be sterilized with terminal sterilization methods. Terminal sterilization includes packaging and a sterilization process that permits storage of the package for an indefinite period. A liquid peracetic acid processing system is a just-in-time process. At the end of the process items are wet, are not wrapped or containerized, and cannot be stored for use at a later time. Peracetic acid is an oxidizing agent—its formula is acetic acid plus an extra BI for monitoring these systems; however, parameters are measured with microprocessors and a printout is provided. A chemical indicator is available and should be used with each cycle. A spore strip is used to test the sporicidal activity of the sterilant dilution. Items processed in these systems should be taken to the point of use and used immediately.

Disinfection. High-level disinfectants play a key role in the processing of semicritical medical devices. Appropriately cleaning, disinfecting, and sterilizing reusable devices are crucial to ensure their safe use and to maintain equipment integrity.

Disinfection is defined as the process that kills all microorganisms with the exception of high numbers of bacterial spores. In contrast, sterilization is a process that kills all microorganisms including high numbers of spores. In healthcare facilities, an item is usually soaked in a liquid chemical for a specified period to achieve disinfection of the item. The disinfection process may destroy tubercle bacilli and inactivate hepatitis viruses and enteroviruses but usually does not kill resistant bacterial spores. The term *disinfection* also may refer to treatment of body surfaces that have been contaminated with infectious material. Chemicals used to disinfect inanimate objects are referred to as *disinfectants*. Chemicals used for body surfaces are known as *antiseptics*. The term *germicide* refers to any solution that destroys microorganisms. Some germicides are disinfectants and antiseptics.

Disinfectants are categorized as high level, intermediate level, or low level, depending on their disinfecting capability.

- High-level disinfectants kill all microorganisms except high numbers of bacterial spores.
- Intermediate-level disinfectants may kill tubercle bacilli, vegetative bacteria, and most viruses and fungi but not bacterial spores.
- Low-level disinfectants kill most vegetative bacteria and some viruses and fungi.

As with sterilization, an item must be cleaned properly before it can be disinfected. Thorough cleaning removes all foreign substances, such as soil or organic material, from a device. This is usually accomplished with an enzymatic detergent.

Types of Disinfectants. Many disinfectants are used alone or in combination, such as hydrogen peroxide and peracetic acid, in healthcare settings. These include alcohols, chlorine and chlorine compounds, glutaraldehyde, OPA, hydrogen peroxide, iodophors, peracetic acid, phenolics, and quaternary ammonium compounds. In healthcare the commercial products are considered unique and must be registered with the EPA or in the case of high-level disinfectants, cleared by the U.S. Food and Drug Administration (FDA). FDA-cleared high-level disinfectants include glutaraldehyde solutions, OPA, hydrogen peroxide, peracetic acid, and hydrogen peroxide solutions. A complete listing may be found on the FDA website (FDA, 2009a). In most cases a given product is designed for a specific purpose and should be used accordingly. Disinfectants are not interchangeable, and incorrect use can cause occupational-associated illness among personnel who use them. Written instructions for use should be followed and precautions should be taken to minimize exposure to these products.

Chemical disinfectants can irritate skin and mucous membranes. High-level disinfection should be performed in a well-ventilated area. A vapor control system can help to protect personnel from irritation.

The following are various types of disinfectants used in healthcare facilities (CDC, 2008a).

High-Level Disinfectants Commonly Used for Instrument Processing

Glutaraldehyde Solutions. Glutaraldehyde is a saturated dialdehyde that has gained wide acceptance as an overall effective high-level disinfecting agent and chemical sterilant. Aqueous solutions of glutaraldehyde are acidic and in this state not sporicidal. The solution is said to be "activated" when alkalizing agents are added to make the solution alkaline. Glutaraldehyde is widely used for high-level disinfection of semicritical items. Glutaraldehyde is actually a chemical sterilant because it is capable of sterilization at extended contact times of up to 10 hours immersion. Because of the lengthy time required to achieve sterilization, and because the device is wet at the end of the process, is unpackaged, and cannot be stored in a sterile state, it is rarely, if ever, used for sterilization. However, depending on the formulation and temperature, high-level disinfection with glutaraldehyde can be achieved in many cases in 10 minutes or less. Immersion times of 20 to 45 minutes may be found on some glutaraldehyde instructions. Glutaraldehyde products are more commonly used in the GI lab for processing GI endoscopes than in the OR or sterile processing department. Glutaraldehyde is not corrosive to endoscopes and has a wide range of materials compatibility. Glutaraldehyde can irritate skin and mucous membranes and has been associated with asthma symptoms. It should be used in a well-ventilated area or under a fume hood. NIOSH has established a recommended exposure limit of 0.2 ppm (CDC, 2012c). Personnel working with glutaraldehyde should wear PPE, which may include nitrile gloves, eye protection, masks, and moisture-repellent gowns. To achieve high-level disinfection, instruments must be free from bioburden and completely immersed in activated aqueous glutaraldehyde solution. During immersion all surfaces of the instrument must be in contact with the liquid chemosterilant. After immersion, instruments must be rinsed thoroughly with sterile water before being used. The minimum effective concentration (MEC) of the solution should be tested with a specific chemical indicator prior to each use. Documentation should include the date when the solution is first opened and put into use and the date the solution will expire according to the label. Results of the MEC should be documented. If the MEC falls below the acceptable level prior to the expiration date, the solution should be discarded. The solution should be discarded at the end of is use life as indicated on the label even if the MEC is still acceptable.

Ortho-phthalaldehyde (OPA). Ortho-phthalaldehyde is a 0.55% OPA solution in an aqueous buffer with a pH of 7.5 and is considered a high-level disinfectant. It is tuberculocidal at a minimum exposure time of 12 minutes at room temperature. It has excellent stability over a wide pH range, is odorless, and is not known to irritate the eyes or nasal passages.

As with any high-level disinfectant, PPE should be used with OPA. It should be used in a well-ventilated area and start of use date and expiration date should be documented. The expiration date of the solution remaining in the bottle differs from the expiration date once it is put into use. Both expiration dates should be noted and documented. OPA can be used for most applications for which glutaraldehyde is used and has broad materials compatibility. The manufacturer's written instructions should be read before use (AORN, 2013g; CDC, 2008a). As with glutaraldehyde, the MEC should be tested and results documented. OPA should not be used beyond its expiration date or if the MEC falls below acceptable levels.

Peracetic Acid Solutions. Peracetic acid is rapid acting and has excellent antimicrobial activity. Automated systems using peracetic acid are commonly used in the GI lab for processing flexible endoscopes. Users should check the endoscope manufacturer's written instructions for use to determine compatibility with peracetic acid. Peracetic acid in combination with hydrogen peroxide is commonly used to disinfect hemodialyzers.

Other Disinfectants

Alcohols. For disinfection in healthcare, the term *alcohol* refers to either 70% or 90% isopropyl alcohol. Both of these compounds are water soluble and have a high degree of germicidal activity. They are bactericidal as opposed to bacteriostatic against vegetative forms of bacteria. They also are tuberculocidal, fungicidal, and virucidal. Isopropyl alcohol (*n*-propanol) and ethyl alcohol (*n*-ethanol) at concentrations of 60% to 80% are potent virucidal agents that can inactivate lipophilic viruses such as herpes and the influenzavirus along with many hydrophilic viruses such as rhinovirus and rotaviruses. Studies have demonstrated the ability of ethyl and isopropyl alcohol to inactivate HBV and to inactivate HIV (CDC, 2008a). The alcohols do not destroy spores or kill certain hydrophilic viruses. Alcohols are flammable and must be stored in a well-ventilated area. Because they evaporate rapidly, extended contact time is difficult to achieve unless items are immersed. Alcohols lack residual effect and are easily inactivated by protein material. Alcohols tend to damage the coating on lensed instruments and may cause hardening of certain rubber and plastic tubing after repeated exposure to the compound. Alcohols are considered intermediate-level disinfectants. They are often used to disinfect thermometers and rubber stoppers on medication vials. Alcohol also is used in processing flexible endoscopes. After high-level disinfection and a tap water rinse, alcohol is effective in inactivating water contaminants. Its speed of evaporation also assists in rapid drying of the endoscope channels. Guidelines from the Association of Practitioners in Infection Control (APIC) should be followed (AORN, 2013i; CDC, 2008a).

Chlorine Compounds. In healthcare facilities, hypochlorites are the most widely used of the chlorine compounds. Hypochlorites are available in a liquid form (sodium hypochlorite [liquid household bleach]) and in a solid form (calcium hypochlorite). Hypochlorites have a broad spectrum of antimicrobial activity. They are inexpensive and fast acting. Low concentrations of free chlorine (50 ppm) are effective against vegetative bacteria and *Mycoplasma*. Free chlorine at 50 ppm inactivates HIV, whereas a 500-ppm concentration is needed to inactivate HBV. Concentrations of 1000 ppm are recommended for inactivation of bacterial spores. Household bleach contains 5.25% sodium hypochlorite. A dilution of 1:1000 provides 50 ppm of available chlorine. A dilution of 1:50 provides 1000 ppm of available chlorine, which is considered adequate to achieve high-level disinfection. The CDC recommends a 1:10 solution, which provides 5000 ppm of available chlorine. Hypochlorite solutions are stable for 30 days in opaque containers. Beyond that time a new solution should be prepared. Hypochlorites are inactivated in the presence of organic matter. All organic material should be removed before application of the disinfecting solution. Hypochlorites are not routinely used for disinfection of surgical instruments because of the corrosive action of the compound. Hypochlorites are most often used for countertops, floors, and other surfaces to be disinfected. Hypochlorites are recommended for environmental disinfection of surfaces suspected of being contaminated with *Clostridium difficile* (Macleod-Glover et al, 2010). Other chlorine compounds that may be used include chlorine dioxide and chloramine-T. Chlorine compounds are the preferred disinfectant in water treatment (AORN, 2013i; CDC, 2008a).

Hydrogen Peroxide. Hydrogen peroxide is active against a wide range of microorganisms, including bacteria, yeasts, fungi, viruses, and spores (CDC, 2008a). Unstable and low concentrations of hydrogen peroxide (<3% solution) may be used as low-level disinfectant for work-surface cleaning and disinfection. Stabilized 6%

hydrogen peroxide is sporicidal and can be used as a liquid sterilant with sufficient exposure time. The solution is corrosive, however, to copper, zinc, and brass. It also can damage rubber and plastic. As with other chemicals, dilution of hydrogen peroxide must be monitored by regularly testing the minimum effective concentration. Hydrogen peroxide is not used widely as a disinfectant in today's healthcare environment (AORN, 2013g; CDC, 2008a).

Iodine and Iodophors. Iodine solutions have been used widely by health professionals, primarily as antiseptics on skin or tissue. An iodophor is a water-soluble combination of iodine and a solubilizing agent or carrier that allows for a slow but continuous release of free iodine over time. Iodophors may be used as disinfectants or antiseptics, depending on the concentration of free iodine. The most widely used iodophor is povidone-iodine, although its use as a skin cleanser or surgical scrub agent has largely been replaced with chlorhexidine gluconate, an antibacterial agent with efficacy against a wide range of pathogenic microorganisms. As disinfectants, iodophors have the advantage of having the germicidal efficacy of iodine without the disadvantages of toxicity and surface irritation. Iodophors are usually nonstaining and effective against vegetative bacteria, *M. tuberculosis,* and most viruses and fungi. Iodophors are not considered suitable for high-level disinfection or for use as hard-surface disinfectants because they have no sporicidal capability (CDC, 2008a).

Phenolics. Phenol (carbolic acid) was first used by Lister in the mid-1800s. Since then, many phenol derivatives (phenolics) have been developed. Phenolics are assimilated by porous material, making their removal difficult. Residual disinfectant can cause tissue irritation. Most phenolic formulations are tuberculocidal, bactericidal, virucidal, and fungicidal. Certain viruses, including echovirus, are resistant to phenolics. Phenolics are not sporicidal, and they are not considered effective as high-level disinfectants. They are used primarily as intermediate-level and low-level disinfectants for environmental cleaning. They are known to have toxic effects, however, and their use has been associated with depigmentation and hyperbilirubinemia in newborns. Because of this, phenolics are not recommended for cleaning incubators or infant bassinets (CDC, 2008a).

Quaternary Ammonium Compounds. Quaternary ammonium compounds ("quats") have been used for many years as a result of a reputation for microbicidal activity, good detergent action, and low-level toxicity. In more recent times, it has been noted that environmental factors, such as hard water, soap residues, and protein soils, reduce or nullify the efficacy of these compounds. Quaternary ammonium compounds are ineffective against *M. tuberculosis* and lipophilic viruses. These compounds are not considered to be sporicidal. Quaternary ammonium compounds are not recommended for high-level, intermediate-level, or low-level disinfection. They are good cleaning agents and are used most often for noncritical surfaces such as floors, walls, and furniture (AORN, 2013d; CDC, 2008a).

Cleaning and Processing Endoscopes and Accessories.
Flexible fiberoptic endoscopes and their associated instrumentation allow for myriad minimally invasive surgical procedures. The list of these procedures grows daily. Current technology allows not only for direct visualization of internal structures, but also for diagnostic biopsies and therapeutic procedures to be performed with reduced pain and shorter recovery time and hospital length of stay. Along with advances in technology, complications also have occurred. Some complications, such as bleeding or tissue perforation, are immediately obvious; infectious complications may be more difficult to identify.

Infections can be caused by organism transmission from an improperly or inadequately cleaned endoscope introduced into the patient via the endoscope. Because of following guidelines for cleaning and disinfection, the incidence of infection transmission in GI procedures is now estimated to be 1 in 1.8 million procedures (Banerjee et al, 2008). Although a number of organisms have been implicated in infection transmission, the organisms of most concern are the viruses hepatitis B, hepatitis C, and HIV, although there have been no reported cases of HIV related to GI endoscopes. High-level disinfection readily kills these viruses and transmission of infection has been associated with a breach in processing protocols.

HBV transmission via a contaminated GI endoscope and tuberculosis transmission via a bronchoscope have been reported (CDC, 2008a). Although the incidence of transmission is low, the risk of a breach or lack of adherence to established processing standards is high. Since 2004 thousands of GI endoscopy patients have had to be notified that they may have been exposed to a risk of infection due to a breach or error during reprocessing of an endoscope (Dept. of Veterans Affairs, 2009).

For an endoscope to be thoroughly disinfected, the disinfecting agent must contact all internal and external surfaces of the endoscope for the prescribed length of time. Organic soil, such as blood, feces, or respiratory secretions, harbors embedded microorganisms and prevents penetration of the disinfecting agent. Some disinfectants are inactivated by organic material. Rigorous cleaning is essential to remove soil and debris from the outside of the scope and from the lumens of all accessible channels (CDC, 2008a). Following is a brief summary of the process for cleaning and disinfecting GI endoscopes. For a more in-depth guideline the reader should refer to the *Multisociety Guideline on Reprocessing Flexible Gastrointestinal Endoscopes* (ASGE, 2011).

Endoscopes and their accessories should be cleaned immediately after use to prevent drying of secretions or other organic soil. They should be cleaned with a nonabrasive enzymatic detergent as recommended by the endoscope manufacturer and in accordance with the detergent manufacturer's written instructions for use (AORN, 2013j; CDC, 2008a). To soften, moisten, and dilute organic debris, endoscope channels should be flushed with copious amounts of water and detergent. The external surfaces of the endoscope should be washed with a detergent solution and rinsed. Internal channels should be brushed to loosen and remove organic matter. The detergent solution should be suctioned or pumped through all channels to remove loosened debris. Special attention should be given to convoluted areas and crevices where contaminated organic material may lodge. The tip of the endoscope should be gently wiped or brushed to remove any debris or tissue that may be lodged around the air and water outlets. Brushes used for cleaning should be disposable or be thoroughly cleaned and sterilized daily. Detachable parts of the endoscope, such as hoods and suction valves, should be removed and soaked in a detergent solution. They should be thoroughly cleaned with a detergent, using a brush to remove any organic material (AORN, 2013j; CDC, 2008a).

Before immersion in any liquid, endoscopes should be pressure tested (leak tested) to determine the integrity of seals and minimize the potential for damage to the head of the scope. If damage is detected, the scope should not be immersed or reused. The endoscope should be removed from service and returned to the manufacturer for repair. An endoscope sent for repair is considered a contaminated item and must be labeled as such for shipping.

After endoscopes are cleaned they should undergo high-level disinfection using either an automated or a manual process. Following disinfection endoscopes should be rinsed, the internal channels flushed with water, and the channels then flushed with 70% to 90% ethyl or isopropyl alcohol (AORN, 2013j). Alcohol inactivates organisms normally found in tap water and helps dry the internal channels of the scope. Care must be taken to dry internal channels of the scopes after being processed and before being stored. Endoscopes should be stored in a vertical position in an area in which recontamination is unlikely. The length of time an endoscope may be stored before it is reprocessed before use is unresolved; however, available data suggest 7 to 10 days (ASGE, 2011). GI endoscopes are semicritical items and therefore require a minimum of high-level disinfection; however, they may also be sterilized using a low-temperature sterilization technology as described previously. The endoscope manufacturer's instructions for use should be consulted to determine scope compatibility with the sterilization technology (AORN, 2013j; CDC, 2008a). Glutaraldehyde, OPA, and peracetic acid solutions are commonly used for processing flexible GI endoscopes.

The facility should maintain a log for each procedure with the patient's name, medical record number (if available), and type of procedure being performed; the endoscopy physician's name; and the serial number or other identifier of the scope. If an automatic endoscope reprocessor is used, identification of this device should be included in the record. This documentation assists in the tracking and investigation in the event of an outbreak or safety concern (AORN, 2013g).

Pasteurization. Pasteurization is a process that uses hot water at a temperature generally at 158° F (70° C) for 30 minutes to achieve high-level disinfection. The actual time/temperature relationship depends on the items to be disinfected. Contact time is inversely related to temperature. For equivalent microbial destruction, longer exposure times are required when the temperature is decreased. Controversy exists as to whether pasteurization results in high-level or intermediate-level disinfection. The CDC definition of high-level disinfection requires destruction of all microbial life except for large populations of bacterial spores. Because pasteurization, by definition, does not kill bacterial spores, some would consider the process to result in only intermediate-level disinfection. Some semicritical items, such as respiratory therapy and anesthesia devices, are ready for patient use after cleaning and pasteurization. High numbers of bacterial spores are not found often on these devices after use. Cleaning before pasteurization reduces the bioburden, and the low number of spores that might be present on a properly pasteurized device of this type would not represent an infective dose when contacting intact mucous membranes. Advantages of pasteurization include absence of toxic residues and the associated need for postprocess rinsing. Disadvantages of pasteurization include the lack of sporicidal activity and the potential for splash burns to personnel involved with the process (AAMI, 2012).

Reprocessing/Reuse of Items Labeled for Single Use Only.
Devices that are labeled as single use should not be reprocessed unless the FDA guidelines for reprocessing can be met. The guidelines are the same as those for the original device manufacturer, and most healthcare facilities cannot meet them (FDA, 2009b). Reprocessing can, however, offer an opportunity for reduced costs. Facilities considering reprocessing of single-use devices should investigate the feasibility of contracting with a commercial reprocessing company that can meet these requirements. Requirements include

registration as a reprocessing firm, listing all devices reprocessed, submitting reports of device adverse events, tracking devices, correcting or removing unsafe devices from the market, and compliance with all manufacturing and labeling FDA requirement (FDA, 2009b) (Patient Safety).

PATIENT SAFETY

Considerations for Reprocessing of Single-Use Devices

The practice of reprocessing single-use, disposable devices has been controversial since the 1970s. According to the *AORN Guidance Statement: Reuse of Single-Use Devices*, it is noted that this process may realize some operational savings. The authors further elaborate on the fact that a cost-benefit ratio analysis should be completed before any unit or organization enters into this practice.

In the May 2009 issue of *OR Manager*, the author discusses the reprocessing debate as it affects ambulatory surgery centers (ASCs). Although the article targets ASCs, this also applies to all healthcare facilities that use single-use devices for patient care. The three ways to handle used single-use medical and surgical devices are identified in the following manner:

- Dispose of them after use.
- Reprocess the device according to the stringent U.S. Food and Drug Administration (FDA) guidelines.
- Contract with a reprocessing specialty company to collect, reprocess, and reship the product to the center.

The FDA publishes an extensive listing of single-use devices that have been identified for reprocessing. The FDA has been monitoring this situation since 2001, with vigorous oversight as well as the development of stringent guidelines and their subsequent enforcement. They have clearly identified those devices that penetrate the mucosa as high risk and do not endorse reprocessing these devices. The FDA became involved in the debate when they were alerted by the original manufacturers of devices that facilities were reprocessing without ensuring the efficacy, effectiveness, and sterility of the original product. The end result was the FDA publication in 2000 of *Enforcement Priorities for Single-Use Devices Reprocessed by Third Parties and Hospitals*.

These guidelines for reprocessing single-use devices include processes that almost no healthcare facility is able to comply with. For example, required validation studies necessitate the use of equipment not found in healthcare facilities. This does not mean that certain single-use devices cannot be effectively and safely reprocessed by commercial enterprises engaged in this activity or more commonly referred to as third-party reprocessors. FDA requirements include:

- Submitting documents for premarket notification of approval
- Registering reprocessing firms and listing all products
- Submitting adverse event reports
- Tracking devices whose failure could have serious outcomes
- Correcting or removing from the market unsafe devices
- Meeting manufacturing and labeling requirements (FDA, 2009)

Many of these requirements are beyond the capabilities of healthcare facilities. Facilities that are considering contracting for reprocessing of single-use devices should thoroughly access the quality of services of third-party reprocessors they are considering.

Modified from DeJohn P: Device reprocessing makes inroads in ASCS, *OR Manager* 25(5):28–29, 2009; Association of periOperative Registered Nurses: AORN guidance statement: reuse of single-use devices. In *Perioperative standards and recommended practices*, Denver, 2012, The Association. FDA: *Reprocessing of single-use devices*, May 2009, available at www.fda.gov/MedicalDevices/DeviceRegulationandGuidance/Reprocessingof Single-UseDevices/default.htm. Accessed November 14, 2012.

Each requirement has associated resource needs. An in-depth discussion of these requirements is beyond the scope of this textbook. Details of the FDA requirements for reprocessors can be found in the *Code of Federal Regulations* (FDA, 2000).

If a user facility chooses to engage a third-party reprocessor it is the facility's responsibility to assess the quality of the services provided under the contractual arrangement with the third-party reprocessor. The user facility must review the processes used by the contracted agency and determine whether correct procedures are being followed (AORN, 2013b; CDC, 2008a).

Aseptic Practices to Prevent Infection

Surgical Aseptic Principles

Asepsis has been defined as the absence of infectious organisms. Surgical aseptic practices are based on the premise that most infections are caused by organisms exogenous to the surgical patient's body. To avoid infection, surgical procedures must be performed in a manner that minimizes or eliminates the patient's exposure to exogenous pathogenic organisms. Opening sterile supplies as close to the time of their use as possible, using sterile drapes to create a sterile field around the incision site, using sterile instruments for the surgical procedure, and placing the operative team in sterile attire after their hands and arms have been cleansed of surface bacteria are examples of means to aid in avoiding infection.

Aseptic technique stems from the principles of asepsis derived over time from microbiologic and epidemiologic concepts. Although some investigators may believe that current aseptic practices and techniques have become too ritualistic or lack scientific research to support their use, present-day infection-control statistics support the application of aseptic principles for safe perioperative nursing practice. Until empiric research shows that a technique is unnecessary or ineffective, the basic aseptic principles should be followed. These principles are as follows:

1. Only sterile items are used within the sterile field. Individuals dispensing sterile items to the sterile field must look at the sterilization indicator on or visible in the package, check for package integrity, and check for the package expiration date (or appropriate marking for event-related shelf life) before dispensing the item to the field.

2. Items of doubtful sterility must be considered unsterile. Examples include sterile items found in unsterile work areas, sterilized packages wrapped in pervious materials that have become wet, sterilized items without an integrator or other internal chemical indicator, or packages in which integrity has been compromised.

3. Whenever a sterile barrier is permeated, it must be considered contaminated. This principle applies to packaging materials and to draping and gowning materials. Obvious contamination occurs from direct contact between sterile and unsterile objects. Other less apparent modes of contamination are the filtration of airborne microorganisms through materials, passage of liquids through materials, and undetected perforations in materials. Moisture soaking through a drape, gown, or package is considered a strikethrough, and the item must be considered contaminated.

4. Sterile gowns are considered sterile in front from the chest to the level of the sterile field and at the sleeves from 2 inches above the elbow to the cuff (Bible et al, 2009). The cuff should be considered unsterile because it tends to collect moisture and is not an effective bacterial barrier. The sleeve cuffs should always be covered by sterile gloves. Other areas of the gown that must be considered unsterile are the neckline, shoulders, axillary area, and back. These areas may become contaminated by perspiration or by collar and shoulder surfaces rubbing together during head and neck movements. Wraparound gowns that completely cover the back may be sterile when first put on. The back of the gown must not be considered sterile, however, because it cannot be observed and protected from contamination. The sterile area of the front of the gown extends to the level of the sterile field because most scrub personnel work adjacent to a sterile table. For this reason the scrub person should avoid changing levels, as would occur while moving from footstool to floor. To maintain sterility, scrub persons should not allow their hands or any sterile item to fall below the level of the sterile field. Scrub persons should neither sit nor lean against unsterile surfaces because the threat of contamination is great. The only time scrub persons may be seated is when the entire surgical procedure is performed at that level. Self-gowning and gloving should be done from a sterile surface separate from the sterile field. This method eliminates reaching over the sterile field to retrieve the sterile towel and then the sterile gown. It also eliminates the potential for water to be dripped on sterile items or on any part of the sterile field, preventing inadvertent contamination. When prepared, the scrub person's hands should be kept in sight at or above waist level. Elbows should be kept close to the body, and the hands should be kept away from the face. Hands should not be folded under the arms because axillary perspiration may permeate the bacterial barrier of the gown.

5. Sterile drapes are used to create a sterile field. When placed, a drape should not be shifted or moved. Items should be dispensed to a sterile field by methods that preserve the sterility of the items and the integrity of the sterile field. Good judgment must be used when dispensing items by presenting them to the scrub person or by placing them securely on the sterile field. A sterile field should be created as close as possible to the time of use. Sterile drapes also are used to create a sterile field when placed over the patient and operative bed. Any item that extends beyond the sterile boundary is considered contaminated and cannot be returned to the sterile field. Interpretation of sterile areas versus unsterile areas on a draped patient requires astute observation and use of good judgment. When contamination of the sterile field occurs, corrective action should immediately be taken unless this will put the patient at risk (AORN, 2013l). A contaminated item must be lifted clear of the operative field without contacting the sterile surface and must be dropped with minimal handling to a nonscrubbed surgical team member, an unsterile area, or a designated receptacle.

6. Items should be dispensed to the field in a manner that preserves the sterility of the item and the integrity of the sterile field. When opening a sterile wrapper, the top flap is first opened away from the operator; the side flaps then follow. The inside or proximal flap is opened last. All flaps are secured in the hand by the operator, so as not to dangle and contaminate other items. When removing an item from a sterile package, the scrub person should lift it straight up from the package. Peel pouches should be presented to the scrub person so as to maintain sterility. The edges of peel pouches have a tendency to curl so that care must be taken to prevent the contents from sliding across an unsterile edge. Interpreting sterile boundaries requires good judgment based on an understanding of aseptic principles.

7. Sterile individuals touch only sterile items or areas; unsterile individuals touch only unsterile items or areas. All members of

the surgical team must understand which areas are considered sterile and which are considered unsterile. All must maintain a continual awareness of these areas. Scrubbed individuals must guard the sterile field to prevent any unsterile item from contaminating the field or the individuals themselves. Unsterile individuals must not touch or reach over a sterile field or allow any unsterile item to contaminate the field. When a perioperative nurse opens a package, hand and arm motions are always from unsterile to sterile objects. The nurse avoids contact with the sterile area by placing the hands under the cuff to provide a protected wide margin of safety between the inside of the pack (sterile) and the hands (unsterile) (Figure 4-10). As the unsterile nurse opens a sterile article that is wrapped sequentially in two wrappers with the corners folded toward the center of the article, the corner farthest from the body is opened first and the corner nearest the body opened last. When a scrub person opens a sterile wrapper, the side nearest the body is opened first. This portion of the wrapper then protects the gown and enables the individual to move closer to the table to complete opening of the wrapper (Figure 4-11). If a solution must be poured into a sterile receptacle on a sterile table, the scrub person holds the receptacle away from the table or sets it near the edge of a waterproof-draped table (Figure 4-12). This procedure eliminates the need for the unsterile nurse to reach over the sterile field. Maintaining a safe margin of space can reduce accidental contamination when items are passed between sterile and unsterile fields.

8. Movement within or around a sterile field must not contaminate the field. The patient is the center of the sterile field during an operative procedure; additional sterile areas are grouped around the patient. If contamination is to be prevented, patterns of movement within or around this sterile grouping must be established and rigidly practiced. Scrub persons stay close to the sterile field. If they change positions, they turn face to face or back to back with another individual while maintaining a safe distance between themselves and other objects. Accidental contamination is a threat to any scrub person who wanders into a

traffic pathway or out of the clean area of the OR. Perioperative nurses approach sterile areas facing them and do not walk between two sterile fields. Keeping sterile areas in view during movement around the area and maintaining a safe distance from the sterile field assist in preventing accidental contamination. Bacterial fallout from the body or clothing is a source of potential contamination when an unsterile individual leans over a

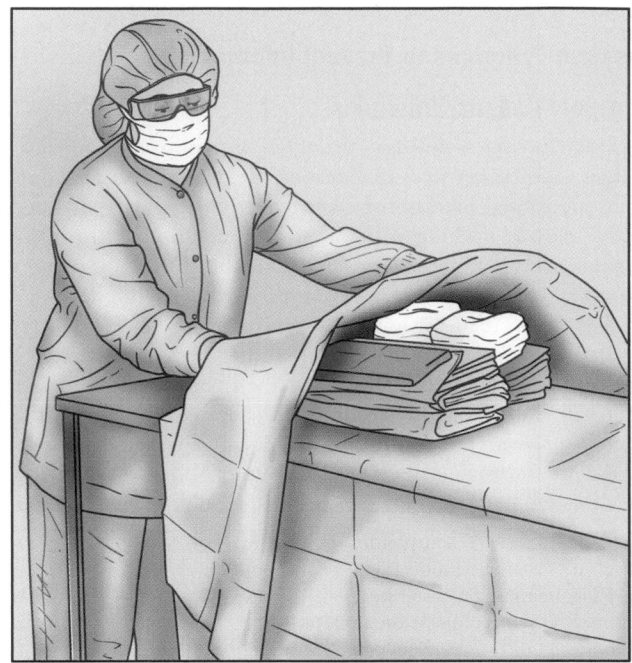

FIGURE 4-10 The perioperative nurse is shown opening the cover of a pack containing sterile drapes for surgery. The cover is cuffed to provide protection for the sterile contents. The nurse avoids contact with the sterile area by keeping all fingers under the cuff as the cover is drawn back over the table to expose the pack contents.

FIGURE 4-11 The circulator creates a sterile field opening on one side of the drape. Then the nurese walks around the table to open the opposite side while taking care not to contaminate the drapes.

FIGURE 4-12 A, When pouring solution into the receptacle held by the scrub person, the perioperative nurse maintains a safe margin of space to avoid contamination of sterile surfaces. **B,** Care must be used when pouring solution into a receptacle on a sterile field to avoid splashing fluids onto the sterile field. Placement of the receptacle near the edge of the table permits the nurse to pour solution without reaching over any portion of the sterile field.

sterile field. All perioperative personnel must maintain vigilance over sterile areas and identify contamination immediately. All personnel moving within or around the sterile field should do so in a manner that prevents contamination of the sterile field (AORN 2013s).

Close adherence to principles of asepsis and consistent observance of the boundaries established in the principles provide protection against infection. Application of the basic principles of aseptic technique depends primarily on the individual's understanding and conscience. Every person on the surgical team must share the responsibility for monitoring aseptic practice and initiating corrective action when a sterile field is compromised.

Traffic Control

The surgical suite should be designed to minimize the spread of infectious organisms and to facilitate movement of patients and personnel within that framework (AORN, 2013m). Ideally, the suite is divided into three areas, each defined by the activities occurring within the area. The *unrestricted* area includes areas outside of the surgical suite and a control point to monitor the entrance of patients, personnel, and materials. Street clothes are appropriate attire in this area, and traffic is not limited, but provisions must be made for isolation of patients with communicable conditions. The *semirestricted* area comprises the peripheral support areas within the surgical suite. These may include storage areas, work areas, and

corridors leading to restricted areas of the surgical suite. Traffic in the semirestricted area is limited to appropriately attired personnel and patients. Personnel must wear surgical attire and cover all head and facial hair when in this area. Patients should have their hair covered, wear clean hospital attire, and be covered with clean hospital linens. The *restricted* area includes the OR, procedure rooms (if any), the central core, and the scrub sink area. Personnel must wear surgical attire including hair coverings when in the restricted area. Masks are worn where open sterile supplies or scrub persons may be present. Except for patients on droplet precautions masks are not required for patients entering this area because a mask could hinder access to the patient's face and airway and cause additional patient anxiety (AORN, 2013m).

Personnel entering semirestricted or restricted areas of the surgical suite should do so through prescribed routes. These routes contain vestibular areas, which serve as transition zones between the outside and inside of the suite. Offices, holding rooms, and locker rooms act as transition zones. Personnel entering the OR should access the locker room via the unrestricted area. After donning clean, hospital-laundered surgical attire, personnel should exit directly into the OR suite without retracing steps through the unrestricted area.

Air is a potential source of pathogenic microorganisms. Airborne contamination increases with movement of the surgical team. This movement should be kept to a minimum during operative procedures. Each OR door should remain closed except during movement of patients, personnel, supplies, and equipment. The positive-pressure gradient of air in the OR is disrupted if the door remains open. The turbulent flow occurring as the pressure equalizes can increase airborne contamination (Anderson et al, 2008; AORN, 2013m).

Surgical equipment and supplies also are potential sources of contamination. Clean and sterile supplies should be separated from contaminated items by space, time, or traffic patterns. Clean and sterile items delivered to the surgical suite should be transported in a manner that preserves package integrity and protects the packaged items from contamination along the travel route. Because external shipping containers may collect dust, debris, and insects during shipment, contents should be removed in the unrestricted area before delivery to the surgical suite. External shipping containers should be removed in the unrestricted area. Within the suite, supplies should move from the clean core or storage area through the OR to the peripheral or semirestricted corridor. Soiled instruments, supplies, and equipment should not reenter the clean core. Instead, soiled items should be covered or contained in closed carts or containers, labeled as biohazard, and transported to an area designated for decontamination. This decontamination area, as well as the soiled linen and trash collection areas, should be separate from personnel and patient traffic areas (AORN, 2013m).

Surgical Attire

Every surgical department should have a written policy and procedure regarding proper attire in the surgical suite. According to OSHA regulations and institutional policy and to prevent transmission of organisms from the patient to personnel, personnel are required to wear PPE when it can be reasonably anticipated that the individual may come into contact with blood or other potentially infectious materials. PPE—which includes protective eyewear; gloves; and fluid-resistant gowns, aprons, and shoe covers—must be included as part of the surgical attire policy as determined by OSHA regulations (AORN, 2013b; OSHA, 1991).

FIGURE 4-13 Proper surgical attire consists of a two-piece pantsuit, a scrub dress, or a one-piece coverall suit. Shoe covers should be worn when it is reasonably anticipated that spills or splashes will occur. If worn, they should be changed whenever they become wet, torn, or soiled. In semirestricted and restricted areas, all head and facial hair should be covered. In restricted areas, all personnel should wear masks. Jewelry should be removed or totally confined. Artificial nails should not be worn. **A,** When a two-piece scrub suit is worn, loose-fitting scrub tops should be tucked into pants. **B,** Tunic tops that fit close to the body may be worn outside of pants. **C,** Nonscrubbed personnel should wear long-sleeved jackets that are buttoned or snapped closed.

People are a major source of bacteria in the surgical setting. To reduce bacterial and skin shedding (scurf) and promote environmental control and cleanliness, all persons entering the semi-restricted and restricted areas of the surgical suite should wear clean, facility-laundered, surgical attire (Figure 4-13) made of multiuse fabric or limited-use nonwoven material (AORN, 2013b). Multiuse surgical attire should be laundered in a healthcare-accredited laundry facility (AAMI, 2012). Controlled laundering of surgical attire, also known as scrub attire, can reduce the risk of spreading contamination to the home environment if laundered at home (AORN, 2013b). Surgical attire should be constructed of a low-linting material that minimizes bacterial shedding, is comfortable, and provides a professional appearance. If a two-piece pantsuit is worn, the top of the pantsuit should be tucked into the trousers or fit close to the body. Care should be taken when donning scrub pants to avoid dragging the pant legs on the floor. A head cover, mask, and, if required, shoe covers complete the surgical attire ensemble. Shoe covers are required if there is a risk of blood or body fluid contamination, as described in OSHA regulations (OSHA, 1991). To protect the patient and the healthcare worker, surgical attire must be changed whenever it becomes soiled or wet with blood; any body fluid, including perspiration; or food. Non-scrubbed personnel should wear long-sleeved freshly laundered or disposable warm-up jackets that are buttoned or snapped closed during wear. These jackets help decrease bacterial and skin shedding from bare arms. Closing the jackets helps prevent inadvertent contamination, which can occur if the loose fabric brushes against a sterile area. All jewelry should be confined within scrub attire or removed when personnel enter the semirestricted or restricted areas of the surgical suite. This includes any visible jewelry associated with body piercing. Confinement reduces the possibility of jewelry

falling or shedding bacteria into a sterile field or wound. Before handwashing, rings, watches, and bracelets should be removed because organisms can be harbored beneath these pieces of jewelry (AORN, 2013b).

Individuals entering the restricted or semirestricted area of the surgical suite should wear a clean, lint-free surgical hat or hood that completely covers all head and facial hair. Hair acts as a filter when left uncovered and collects bacteria, which are released into the air during activity. Hair attracts, harbors, and sheds bacteria in proportion to its length, curliness, and oiliness. A head cover eliminates the possibility of hair or dandruff being shed onto the scrub attire. The design and composition of the hat or hood should minimize dispersal of bacteria, be comfortable to wear, and confine and contain all hair. Head covers should always be worn in areas where equipment and supplies are processed and stored. Disposable bouffant and hood types of head covers are preferred. Disposable head covers are discarded in a designated receptacle immediately after use. Skullcaps that fail to cover the side hair above the ears and hair at the nape of the neck should not be worn in the OR. If reusable hats or hoods are worn, they should be laundered daily. If they become contaminated with blood or body fluids, they must be laundered according to OSHA (1991) regulations.

For personnel safety, shoes that provide protection should be worn. Cloth shoes provide little protection against spilled liquids or sharp items that may be accidentally dropped to the floor. Shoes with enclosed toes and heels help minimize injury. Shoe covers may be worn to help keep shoes clean and may decrease the amount of soil and bacteria tracking throughout the suite. It is easier to change a shoe cover than to stop to clean or change a shoe that has become soiled. If it is reasonably expected that the feet may become contaminated with blood or body fluids, shoe covers are required as part of personal protective attire. Shoe covers should be kept in an area adjacent to the semirestricted area entrance. They should be removed and discarded in the appropriate receptacle when leaving the restricted area (AORN, 2013b). Handwashing should follow removal of shoe covers.

A single surgical mask is worn to reduce the dispersal of microbial droplets expelled from the mouth and nasopharynx of personnel and to protect healthcare workers from aerosolized pathogenic organisms and particles from the surgical environment. Single, high-filtration surgical masks are worn in ORs and other designated areas where open sterile supplies or scrub persons may be located. A single mask provides a filter; double-masking creates an impediment to breathing and does not increase filtration. Masks should cover the nose and mouth and should be secured so as to prevent

venting (AORN 2013b). OSHA regulations mandate the use of surgical masks as part of personal protection. Individual practice settings need to develop polices based on OSHA (1991) and state-mandated recommendations on mask use. Masks with a microbial filtration efficiency of 95% or greater should be selected. The filtration efficiency of masks should ensure protection against aerosol particles that are 0.1 μm or larger. These masks, however, should not be used as protection against surgical smoke or as protection from chemical or particulate contaminants smaller than 0.1 micron as may be found in surgical smoke plume, such as during a laser procedure (AORN, 2013r). Mask selection should be based on the anticipated contaminants (AORN, 2013f). The most effective filter mask is relatively useless if worn incorrectly. Figure 4-14 illustrates the proper application and removal of a surgical mask.

FIGURE 4-14 Proper handling of a mask. **A,** Edges of a properly worn mask conform to facial contours when the mask is applied and tied correctly. **B** and **C,** Personnel should avoid touching the filter portion of the mask when removing it. **D,** Masks should be discarded on removal.

The mask must cover the mouth and nose entirely and have facial compliance, fitting comfortably around the contours of the nose and cheeks. The mask is tied securely without crossing the strings. Crossing strings allows the sides of the mask to gap (tenting) and consequently permits nonfiltered air to escape through venting. Air should pass only through the mask's filtering system (the faceplate). A pliable metal or adhesive strip in the top hem of some masks provides a firm, contoured fit over the bridge of the nose. This strip may help prevent fogging of protective eyewear. Masks should be either on (properly) or off. They should not be reused for different procedures (e.g., by allowing the mask to hang from the neck or by tucking it into a pocket). Bacteria that have been filtered by the mask become dry and airborne if the mask is worn necklace fashion. Touching only the strings during removal of the mask reduces contamination of the hands. Masks should be changed between procedures and sometimes during a procedure if they become wet or soiled. The faceplate, which is contaminated with droplet nuclei, should not come into contact with the hands of personnel. Immediately after removal, masks should be discarded directly into a designated covered waste receptacle. After discarding the mask, the wearer must wash and dry the hands thoroughly (AORN, 2013b).

Gloves should be selected according to the task to be completed: sterile gloves for sterile procedures, and medical, unsterile gloves for nonsterile activities. Gloves should be changed between patient contacts and after contact with any infectious material. Hands should be washed thoroughly after gloves are removed. To reduce the risk of mouth, nose, and eye mucous membrane exposure, protective eyewear, masks, or face shields are worn whenever there is opportunity for contamination by splash or aerosols. When the protective devices become contaminated, they should be discarded or decontaminated as soon as possible to prevent contamination to the wearer. Other protective equipment such as liquid-resistant attire, including gowns and shoe covers, should be worn whenever there is a reasonable expectation of exposure to infectious materials (AORN, 2013b).

Surgical Hand Hygiene

Skin is a major source of microbial contamination in the surgical environment. Although members of the surgical team at the sterile field wear sterile gowns and gloves, the skin of their hands and forearms should be cleaned preoperatively to reduce the number of microorganisms in the event of glove failure. The purposes of surgical hand hygiene are as follows: to remove dirt, skin oil, and transient microorganisms from the nails, hands, and forearms; to reduce the resident microbial count to as near zero as possible; and to leave an antimicrobial residue on the skin to prevent regrowth of microbes for several hours (AORN, 2013n). Hand hygiene has been recognized as a primary method of decreasing healthcare-associated infections (Haas et al, 2008). The skin can never be rendered sterile, but it can be made surgically clean by reducing the number of microorganisms present.

The term *hand hygiene* is used to describe measures related to the physical hand condition and decontamination. Hand decontamination can be done by a variety of the following methods:

- Handwashing using soap and water, antiseptic and water, or antiseptic hand rub if visible soil is not present
- Surgical hand scrub using water-aided brushless surgical antiseptics; waterless, brushless surgical antiseptics; or traditional surgical hand scrub using a sponge (AORN, 2013n; WHO, 2009)

A standardized procedure for handwashing should be established and followed within the healthcare setting.

Scrub persons should be in good health and possess healthy, intact skin. Healthcare personnel with cuts, abrasions, weeping dermatitis, or fresh tattoos on exposed skin should not provide direct patient care because of the potential risk for infection (AORN, 2013n). The AORN's *Recommended Practices for Hand Hygiene in the Perioperative Setting* (2013a) provide guidance for healthcare personnel in relation to direct patient care.

Because microorganisms may be protected and harbored by rings, watches, body-piercing jewelry, and bracelets, these items should be removed before scrubbing (AORN, 2013n). Fingernails of scrub persons should be short, clean, and healthy. The subungual region of the nails harbors most microorganisms on the hands. Soap, running water, and a nail-cleaning device are necessary to clean under the fingernails. Nails that extend beyond the tips of the fingers may be more difficult to clean and can increase the risk of glove tears. Longer nails also may scratch patients during the positioning or transfer process. Artificial nails or synthetic nails should not be worn by personnel in the perioperative environment. Higher numbers of gram-negative organisms have been cultured, both before and after handwashing, from the nails of individuals wearing artificial nails or nail additives than from individuals with natural nails. Fungal growth also occurs under artificial nails as a result of trapped moisture between the natural and artificial nail. The length of artificial nails may interfere with effective hand scrubs and handwashing. Chipped nail polish should be removed because it may harbor large numbers of pathogens. Studies have shown the positive correlation between the number of microorganisms present on healthcare personnel's hands to the number of patients who have surgical site infections (Anderson et al, 2008; AORN, 2013n).

Facility infection control procedures govern the selection of materials and the methods used for surgical hand hygiene. This may be accomplished by a surgical scrub or with the use of an approved hand rub agent.

Surgical Hand Rubs. Alcohol-based hand rubs are easy to use and fast acting, and they provide activity against most bacteria, viruses, and fungi. All hand rub products that are alcohol based are not indicated for use in place of the traditional hand scrub. Rubs come in many forms, combinations, and concentrations of alcohols, which may influence the antimicrobial strength and kill factor. Surgical hand hygiene products should be selected following a thorough analysis of each product's efficacy, effectiveness, application processes, cost-to-benefit ratio analysis, and acceptance by its users. When hand rubs are used for surgical hand antisepsis, the only acceptable products are alcohol-based antiseptic surgical hand rubs with documented persistent and cumulative activity that have met FDA regulatory requirements for surgical hand antisepsis. The manufacturer's written instructions for product use, including time and amount, should be followed. The basic steps of a surgical rub are as follows:

1. Review the manufacturer's written directions for use of the product.
2. Use the recommended amount of hand rub product.
3. Rub hands and cover all surfaces, including the backs of hands, fingertips, inner webs, and palms.
4. Rub hands until they are dry.

A sufficient amount of product is required to ensure the antimicrobial effect of the rub (AORN, 2013n).

Surgical Hand Scrub. A surgical hand scrub should be performed by healthcare personnel before donning sterile gloves for surgical or other invasive procedures (AORN, 2013n). For the traditional, standardized surgical scrub, individually packaged disposable brushes and sponges or synthetic sponges without a brush may be used. The use of synthetic sponges in place of brushes has gained wide acceptance, especially when long and repeated scrubbing may be traumatic to the skin. Disposable brushes or sponges are available with a variety of antimicrobial soap or antiseptic solutions impregnated into the sponge (AORN, 2013n; TJC, 2009).

Surgical hand scrub agent selection should be based on the efficacy and effectiveness of the product, application requirements, contact time, and user friendliness. Surgical hand scrub products should have the following attributes:

• Reduce microorganisms on the skin
• Be fast acting
• Have a broad range of activity
• Not depend on cumulative action
• Have a minimally harsh effect on skin
• Inhibit regrowth of microorganisms

Agents commonly used for surgical hand scrubs include povidone-iodine complex and chlorhexidine gluconate (CHG). These agents are broad-spectrum, rapid-acting antimicrobials that are effective against many gram-positive and gram-negative microorganisms. Moisturizing agents are often incorporated into various surgical scrub agents to reduce the potential of skin irritation resulting from multiple scrubs.

An anatomic scrub, using a prescribed amount of time or number of strokes plus friction, is used to effectively cleanse the skin. The fingers, hands, and arms should be visualized as having four sides; each side must be scrubbed effectively. Individual attention to detail is essential. When using the timed approach, the product instructions for use and the institution's policies and procedures should be followed. Surgical hand scrub procedures should be documented and available within the perioperative practice setting.

Scrub Procedure. Before beginning the surgical hand scrub, members of the surgical team should inspect their hands to ensure that their nails are short, their cuticles are in good condition, and no cuts or skin problems exist. The procedure may include but not be limited to the following steps:

1. Remove all jewelry, including rings, watches, and bracelets, from the hands and forearms.
2. Cover all head and facial hair. Don a surgical mask. If other personnel are at the scrub sink, a surgical mask should be worn in the presence of hand scrub activity. Protective eyewear, such as goggles with side shields or a full-face shield, should be adjusted to ensure clear vision and to avoid lens fogging. Scrub shirts are tucked into the trousers to prevent potential contamination of the scrubbed hands and arms from brushing against loose garments.

The basic steps of the scrub procedure follow:

1. Wash hands and forearms with soap and running water immediately before beginning the scrub procedure, if visibly soiled. Bring water to a comfortable temperature. Most scrub sinks have automatic or knee controls for the faucets.
2. Moisten hands and forearms with water. Using a foot control, dispense the manufacturer's recommended amount of the antimicrobial agent into the palms, adding small amounts of water to create lather if necessary.
3. Wash hands and forearms using the antimicrobial soap or detergent. Rinse before beginning the surgical hand scrub. The amount of time needed varies with the amount of soil and the effectiveness of the cleansing agent.

This may be followed with a surgical hand scrub using either an antimicrobial surgical scrub agent or an alcohol-based antiseptic surgical hand rub.

For a surgical hand scrub:

1. Open the scrub brush/sponge package, remove the brush and nail cleaner, and discard the package. Hold the brush in one hand; clean the subungual areas of both hands under running water, and then complete the nails on the other hand (Figure 4-15).
2. Rinse the hands and arms thoroughly, exercising care to hold the hands higher than the elbows. Avoid splashing water onto the surgical attire because this moisture may cause subsequent contamination of the sterile gown.
3. Moisten the brush or sponge (if the brush or sponge is impregnated with antimicrobial soap) and begin scrubbing. (The use of a brush is not necessary and has been associated with skin cell shedding.) A sponge or soft brush is preferred to reduce damage to the epidermis (AORN, 2013a). If the brush or sponge is not impregnated with soap, apply antimicrobial soap or detergent solution to hands according to the manufacturer's written instructions. Starting at the fingertips, scrub the nails vigorously, holding the brush perpendicular to the nails. Scrub all sides of each digit, including the connecting webbed spaces. Next scrub the palm and back of the hand. Repeat on the other hand and arm.
4. Scrub each side of the forearm with a circular motion (see Figure 4-15) up to the elbows.
5. Hold the hands and arms away from the body, with the hands above the level of the elbows while scrubbing, allowing the water and detritus to flow away from the first-scrubbed and cleanest area. Add small amounts of water during the scrub to develop suds and remove any excess debris.
6. Rinse the hands and arms thoroughly.
7. Turn off the faucet by using the knee control or by using the edge of the brush on a hand control. Discard the brush or sponge.
8. Hold the hands and arms up in front of the body with elbows slightly flexed, and enter the OR.

If the timed method is used, the policies and procedures of the facility should be followed.

If using an alcohol-based surgical hand rub following handwashing, apply the product to hands and forearms according to the manufacturer's instructions.

Drying the Scrubbed Area. Moisture remaining on the cleansed skin after the scrub procedure should be dried with a sterile towel before donning a sterile gown and gloves. The gown and gloves should be opened on a flat surface before the surgical scrub is completed. A small sterile field is created by the gown wrapper, which is opened over the flat surface. The gown and gloves should not be opened on the sterile back table because of the increased chance of contamination to the field. The towel must be used with care to avoid contaminating the clean skin. The folded towel is grasped firmly near the open corner and lifted straight up and away from the sterile field without dripping contaminated water from the skin onto the sterile field. The person steps away from the sterile field and bends forward slightly from the waist, holding the hands and elbows above the waist and away from the body. The towel is allowed to unfold downward to its full length and width (Figure 4-16).

The top half of the towel is held securely with one hand and the opposite fingers and hand are blotted dry, ensuring that they are thoroughly dry before moving to the forearm. A rotating motion is used while moving up and down the arm to avoid contamination;

FIGURE 4-15 Traditional surgical scrub technique. **A,** Cleaning nails with plastic nail cleaner. **B,** Holding brush/sponge perpendicular to nails facilitates thorough scrubbing of underside of nails. **C,** Holding brush/sponge lengthwise along arm covers maximum area with each stroke.

areas are not retracted. The lower end of the towel is grasped with the dried hand, and the same procedure is used for drying the second hand and forearm. Care must be taken to prevent contamination of the towel and hands. On completion, the towel is discarded without dropping the hands below waist level.

Gowning

Before scrub personnel touch sterile equipment or the sterile field, they must put on sterile gowns and surgical gloves to prevent microorganisms on their hands and clothing from being transferred to the patient's wound during surgery. The sterile gowns and gloves also protect the hands and clothing of personnel from microorganisms present in the patient or in the atmosphere. The surgical gown should be made of a combustion-resistant material that establishes an effective barrier to minimize the passage of microorganisms, particulate matter, and fluids between unsterile and sterile areas. Reusable fabrics must allow complete penetration of steam during the sterilization process and should withstand multiple launderings and other processing. Tightly woven textiles eventually lose their barrier quality when subjected to multiple laundering and sterilizations. Users should follow the manufacturer's instructions to determine the useful life of the barrier material. The manufacturer must provide the facility with instructions for testing the material at periodic intervals during the life cycle of the product to ensure continued barrier quality. The particular item should be removed from circulation when the maximum number of processing cycles has been reached. A heat seal patch of the same material as the item being patched may be used or the material may be removed from use. Before each use reusable materials must be examined to determine their integrity. To reduce particle dissemination into the wound and the environment, materials used for surgical gowns and drapes should be resistant to penetration by blood and other body fluids as necessitated by their use (AORN, 2013o). Regardless of the gown material, the shape and size should fit personnel and allow freedom of movement. To provide extra protection, the gown's front from the waist upward and the forearms of the sleeves can be reinforced with additional or different water-repellent material. Each sleeve should be finished with a tight-fitting cuff that prevents the inner side of the sleeve from slipping down onto the outer side of the sterile glove. Cotton tapes, snaps, or Velcro fasteners are attached to the back of the gown to hold it closed. A wraparound gown may be used to achieve better coverage of the back. Once donned, however, the back of the gown is never considered sterile.

Because the outer side of the front and sleeves of the gown come into contact with the sterile field during surgery, the gown must be folded so that the scrub person can put it on without touching the outer side with bare hands. For in-house wrapping and sterilization, the gown is folded with the inner side out and the back edges together. The sleeves are not turned inside out; consequently, they remain within the folded gown. The side folds of the gown are folded lengthwise toward the center back opening, overlapping slightly at the center. With the open edges of the gown remaining on the inside, the bottom third of the gown is folded upward and the top third of the gown is folded over the bottom portion. The gown is then folded in half widthwise so that the inside front

neckline of the gown is visible on top. Gowns with wraparound backs are prepared in the same manner, with care taken to tie the tape securely on the wraparound back flap to the external side tie of the gown before initial folding. A folded hand towel with its free corners facing up is usually placed on top of the folded gown before the gown is wrapped and sterilized. Surgical gowns should be selected for use according to the barrier quality of the item and the wearers' anticipated exposure to blood and body fluids in accordance with OSHA's guidelines for the use of PPE as found in the OSHA Bloodborne Pathogens Standard (OSHA, 1991).

Self-Gowning Procedure. The procedure for donning a wraparound sterile surgical gown is as follows (Figures 4-17 and 4-18). The scrub person should do the following:

1. Grasp the sterile gown at the neckline with both hands and lift from the wrapper. Step into an area where the gown may be opened without risk of contamination.
2. Hold the gown away from the body, and allow it to unfold with the inside toward the wearer.
3. Keep hands on the inside of the gown while it completely unfolds.
4. Slip both hands into the open armholes, keeping the hands at shoulder level and away from the body.
5. Push the hands and forearms into the sleeves of the gown, advancing the hands only to the proximal edge of the cuff.

The perioperative nurse in the circulating role should then do the following:

1. Pull the gown over the scrub person's shoulders, touching only the inner shoulder and side seams.
2. Tie or clasp the neckline and tie the inner waist ties of the gown, touching only the inner aspect of the gown. The gown should be completely fastened by the perioperative nurse before the scrub person dons gloves, to prevent contamination from flapping of the gown.

To secure the gown, the scrub person and the perioperative nurse do the following:

1. Take the tab (which is attached to the back tie of the gown) from the gloved scrub person. The scrub person then makes a three-quarters turn to the left while the perioperative nurse

FIGURE 4-16 Drying hands and forearms. Fingers and hand are dried thoroughly before forearm is dried. Extending arms reduces possibility of contaminating towel or hands.

FIGURE 4-17 Gowning procedure. **A,** Scrub person keeps hands on inside of gown while unfolding it at arm's length. **B,** Circulating nurse reaches under flap of gown to pull sleeves on scrub person. **C,** Circulating nurse snaps neckline of gown, touching only snap section of neckline.

FIGURE 4-18 Methods of tying a wraparound gown. **A,** After handing tab on back tie of gown to perioperative nurse, scrub person makes a three-quarters turn toward the left. **B,** Sterile back panel now covers previously tied unsterile ties; scrub person retrieves back tie by carefully pulling it out of the tab held by the nurse and ties it securely with other tie. **C,** For gowns having no tab on back tie: using sterile inner glove wrapper, scrub person places the end of the back tie in the crease of the wrapper. **D,** After closing the wrapper, scrub person hands tie to the nurse, who grasps it carefully, touching neither the tie nor the gloved hand of the scrub person. The scrub person makes a three-quarters turn to the left, carefully pulls back tie from wrapper, and ties it to other tie.

extends the back tie to its full length. This action effectively wraps the back panel of the gown around the scrub person and covers the previously tied inner waist ties. The scrub person retrieves the back tie by carefully pulling it out of the tab held by the nurse and ties it to the other tie, which had been secured to the front top of the gown.

When a reusable gown is used, the absence of a tab on the back tie necessitates use of an alternative procedure for securing the gown (see Figure 4-18, *C* through *D*). If the closed-gloving technique and commercially prepared, double-wrapped gloves are used, the inner wrap can be used as a protective extension for the gown tie when the perioperative nurse assists with tying a wraparound gown. After gloving, the scrub person unties the exterior gown ties (which were tied at the front of the gown before it was folded, wrapped, and sterilized) and holds both ties. The end of the back tie is placed in the center crease of the empty glove wrapper, approximately two thirds of the way up to the edge of the opened wrapper. The glove wrapper is then closed so that the tie is concealed. The closed wrapper is handed to the perioperative nurse, who firmly grasps the folded edge of the wrapper without touching the tie. The scrub person pivots in the opposite direction from the nurse, who extends the back tie to its full length. The scrub person grasps the exposed portion of the back tie, pulls it out of the glove wrapper while taking care to avoid touching the glove wrapper or the perioperative nurse, and ties both ties. If a sterile glove wrapper is unavailable, a sterile hemostat or ringed forceps may be clamped to the back tie and used in the same manner as a glove wrapper. After the gowning procedure

has been completed, the perioperative nurse retains the instrument in the room to avoid problems with the subsequent instrument count.

If another scrub person is gowned and gloved, that individual, instead of the perioperative nurse, may assist with the wraparound procedure. The assisting individual must extend the back tie to its fullest length before the scrub person turns, to avoid any potential contamination.

Assisted-Gowning Procedure. A gowned and gloved individual may assist another individual in donning a sterile gown (Figure 4-19). The gown is opened in the manner previously described. The inner side with the open armholes is turned toward the individual who is to be gowned. A cuff is made of the neck and shoulder area of the gown to protect the gloved hands. The gown is held until the person's hands and forearms are in the sleeves of the gown. The perioperative nurse assists in pulling the gown onto the shoulders, adjusting the back, and tying the tapes. The wraparound back of the gown is fixed into position by the scrub person after gloving is completed.

Gloving

Scrubbed personnel wear sterile surgical gloves to provide a protective barrier between the patient and healthcare personnel to decrease the probability of exposing the patient to exogenous organisms with a resulting surgical site infection. Gloves also decrease the chance of the healthcare provider being exposed to blood or other potentially

FIGURE 4-19 Gowning another person. Gowned and gloved scrub person cuffs neck and shoulder area of gown over gloved hands to prevent contamination as scrub person puts hands and forearms into sleeves.

infectious material. Nonetheless, many surgeons, first assistants, and perioperative scrub personnel have encountered blood on their hands at the conclusion of a surgical procedure without being aware of any breech in the glove barrier (glove puncture, tear, or rip). Increasing evidence supports and recommends the practice of double-gloving to offer a degree of protection from this and other common events. The evidence for wearing two pairs of gloves during surgical procedures is compelling. According to Copeland (2009, p. 325), "Two layers of surgical gloves can reduce the number of breaks to the innermost glove that might allow cross-infection between the surgical team and patient. ... A second pair of gloves does protect the first set, without apparently lessening surgical skill." Two gloves are better than one, and although this may be considered optional, all evidence points to double-gloving as being the best practice that can protect both the healthcare provider and the patient (Copeland, 2009). Although a breech may occur in the outer glove, the inner glove remains intact and continues to serve as a barrier. Some surgeons who work in areas where perforation risk is high, such as orthopedics or thoracic surgery, opt to wear double-layer gloves, with the inside glove being a colored glove, which allows the wearer to recognize perforations to the outer glove. In orthopedic surgery, surgeons may wear a glove liner between two layers of gloves to reduce perforations to the inner glove. On completion of the case, both pairs of gloves should be discarded, and hand antisepsis should be performed (Copeland, 2009).

Using powder as a glove lubricant is not recommended because of three primary hazards: the potential for postoperative complication of powder granulomas; powder fallout from hands and gloves, which provides a convenient vehicle for dissemination of microorganisms throughout the OR; and the ability of powder to carry and disperse latex proteins, contributing to an increased latex sensitivity among healthcare workers and others. Powder-free gloves are widely available. If powdered gloves are chosen, any glove film or powder must be removed. The gloves must be wiped thoroughly after they are put on and before approaching the sterile field.

Latex Allergies and Sensitivities. The increased reporting of latex sensitivity continues to be a concern among perioperative personnel. Individuals can experience three types of reactions to latex. *Irritant contact dermatitis* is the most common type of reaction and is characterized by dry, reddened, itchy, or cracked hands. Irritant contact dermatitis is not a true allergic reaction. *Allergic contact dermatitis* is considered a type IV allergic reaction and is an allergic response caused by chemicals used in the manufacture of gloves. Allergic contact dermatitis is a delayed reaction, usually appearing 6 to 48 hours after exposure. Symptoms are similar to those of irritant contact dermatitis except that the reaction may extend beyond the actual point of contact. *True latex allergies* are classified as type I allergic responses. This is an allergy to water-soluble natural rubber latex (NRL) proteins. True latex allergies are usually seen within minutes of contact with the proteins. Symptoms range from skin redness and itching to hives, dyspnea, GI upset, hypotension, tachycardia, and anaphylaxis. Reactions to latex rarely progress to anaphylaxis because the wearer is treated with appropriate drugs to interrupt the allergic response. Appropriate latex-free gloves should be provided for healthcare workers with known latex sensitivity or for procedures in which patients have known sensitivity or allergy. Some personnel claim allergy to the starch powder in latex gloves. Although this is possible, it is more likely that individuals are allergic to the latex proteins that bind with the starch powder and become aerosolized (AORN, 2013p).

Closed-Gloving Technique. The closed method of gloving (Figure 4-20) is the technique of choice when initially donning a sterile gown and gloves. When using this technique, the gloves are handled through the fabric of the gown sleeves. The hands are not extended from the sleeves and cuffs when the gown is put on. Instead, the hands are pushed through the cuff openings as the gloves are pulled into place. The woven cuff should remain in the natural wrist area. Because the cuffs of a sterile gown collect moisture, become damp during wearing, and are considered unsterile, the closed-gloving technique can be used only for initial gloving. Cuffs may not be pulled down over the wearer's hand for subsequent gloving. For subsequent gloving, an alternative technique must be used, such as assisted gloving or open gloving.

Open-Gloving Technique. With the open-gloving technique, the everted cuff of each glove permits a gowned individual to touch the glove's inner side with ungloved fingers and to touch the glove's outer side with gloved fingers (Figure 4-21). Keeping the hands in direct view, no lower than waist level, the gowned individual flexes the elbows. Exerting a light, even pull on the glove brings it over the hand, and using a rotating movement brings the cuff over the wristlet. Extreme caution is necessary when using the open method to prevent contamination by the exposed hands. This gloving technique can be used by individuals not wearing a gown.

Assisted-Gloving Technique. A gowned and gloved individual may assist another gowned individual with gloving. To assist another

FIGURE 4-20 Closed-gloving procedure. **A,** When donning gown, scrub person does not slip hands through gown cuffs. Hands are not extended from sleeves. **B,** First the glove is lifted by grasping it through the fabric of the sleeve. The glove's cuff facilitates easier handling of the glove. The glove is placed palm down along the forearm of the matching hand, with thumb and fingers pointing toward elbow. Glove cuff lies over gown cuff. If the scrub person is double-gloving, the larger size gloves are donned first. **C,** The glove cuff is held securely by the hand on which it was placed, and with the other hand the cuff is stretched over the opening of the sleeve to cover the gown cuff entirely. **D,** As the cuff is drawn back onto the wrist, fingers are directed into their cots in the glove, and the glove is adjusted to the hand. **E,** Gloved hand is used to position remaining glove on opposite sleeve in the same fashion. Glove cuff is placed around gown cuff. The second glove is drawn onto the hand, and the cuff is pulled into place. **F,** Fingers of gloves are adjusted, and gloves are wiped with wet gauze sponge or commercially prepared sterile, disposable glove wipe to remove any powder that may be on them.

individual, grasp the glove under the everted cuff. Ensure the palm of the glove is turned toward the ungloved individual's hand with the thumb of the glove directly opposed to the thumb of the individual's hand. Using fingers, stretch the cuff to open the glove. The ungloved individual can insert his or her hand into the glove. Repeat the procedure for the other hand (Figure 4-22).

Removing Soiled Gown, Gloves, and Mask

To protect the forearms, hands, and clothing from contacting bacteria on the outer side of the used gown and gloves, members of

the scrub surgical team should use the following procedure to remove soiled gowns, gloves, and masks (Figure 4-23):

- Wipe gloves clean with a wet, sterile towel.
- Untie surgical gown; the perioperative nurse must unfasten back closures.
- Grasp gown at one shoulder seam without touching scrub clothing.
- Bring the neck and sleeve of the gown forward, over, and off the gloved hand, turning the gown inside out and everting the cuff of the glove.

FIGURE 4-21 Open-gloving procedure. **A,** Scrub person takes one glove from the inner glove wrapper by placing the thumb and index finger of the opposite hand on the fold of the everted cuff at a point in line with the glove's palm and then pulls the glove over the hand, leaving the cuff turned back. If the scrub person is double-gloving, the larger size gloves are donned first. **B,** Scrub person takes the second glove from the inner glove wrapper by placing gloved fingers under the everted cuff. **C,** Scrub person, with arms extended and elbows slightly flexed, introduces free hand into glove and draws it over gown cuff by slightly rotating arm externally and internally. **D,** To bring turned-back cuff on other hand over cuff of gown, scrub person repeats step **C.**

FIGURE 4-22 Gloving another person. Gowned and gloved scrub person places fingers of each hand beneath everted cuff, keeping thumbs turned outward and stretching cuff as gowned person slips hand into sterile glove, using firm downward thrust. If other person is double-gloving, the larger size gloves are donned first.

• Repeat the previous two steps for the other side.
• Keep arms and gown away from body while turning the gown inside out and discarding carefully in the designated receptacle.
• Using the gloved fingers of one hand to secure the everted cuff, remove the glove, turning it inside out. Discard appropriately.

• Using the ungloved hand, grasp the fold of the everted cuff of the other glove and remove the glove, inverting the glove as it is removed. Discard appropriately.
• After leaving the restricted area, remove the mask by touching the ties or elastic only.
• Discard in the designated receptacle.
• Wash hands and forearms.

Patient Skin Antisepsis

To prevent bacteria on the skin surfaces from entering the surgical wound, the skin area at and around the proposed incision site must be cleaned and disinfected. Skin preparation methods vary, but all are based on the same principles and share the same objectives: to remove dirt and transient microbes from the skin, to reduce the resident microbial count as much as possible in the shortest time and with the least amount of tissue irritation, and to prevent rapid rebound growth of microbes. Factors to be considered in skin disinfection are as follows:

1. Condition of the involved area
2. Number and kinds of contaminants
3. Characteristics of the skin to be disinfected
4. General physical condition of the patient

Many soaps and detergents are available for skin cleansing. Although most of them produce similar results for the immediate removal of soil and microorganisms, certain factors require further consideration in selecting a product for surgical use. Most soaps and

FIGURE 4-23 Removing soiled gown and gloves. **A,** To protect scrub suit and arms from bacteria that are present on outer side of soiled gown, the gown is grasped without touching the scrub clothes. **B,** Scrub person turns outer side of soiled gown away from body, keeping elbows flexed and arms away from body so that soiled gown will not touch arms or scrub suit. **C,** To prevent outer side of soiled gloves from touching skin surfaces of hands, the scrub person places gloved fingers of one hand under everted cuff of other glove and pulls glove off hand and fingers. **D,** To prevent ungloved hand from touching outer side of soiled glove, the scrub person hooks bare thumb on inner side of glove and pulls glove off.

detergents emulsify and peptize waste products and oils that are absorbed in surface soil and permit the debris to be rinsed off the skin with running water. The product selected should become hydrolyzed in the presence of water and yield a pH that corresponds to that of average, normal skin. An odorless agent that produces a good lather for easy, comfortable use is usually preferred. It should not irritate the skin or in any way interfere with normal functioning. Equally important, an effective antimicrobial agent should be used to achieve skin antisepsis; it should be selected according to its ability to decrease the microbial count of the skin rapidly, be applied quickly, and remain effective throughout the operation. The agent should not cause irritation or sensitization or be incompatible with or inactivated by alcohol, organic matter, soap, or detergent (AORN, 2013n).

Patients should be instructed to bathe with an antibacterial soap the night before elective surgery (Mangram et al, 1999). More recent recommendations include two preoperative showers with CHG. The process of washing and rinsing repeatedly removes microorganisms from the skin. Some organisms may be difficult or virtually impossible to kill with CHG alone. A recent study, however, suggests that there is no benefit to two preoperative CHG showers to reduce incidence of surgical site infection (Chlebicki et al, 2012). Additional research into the benefits of two chlorhexidine showers is needed) (Research Highlight).

Hair should not be removed from the surgical site unless it is required. The necessity for hair removal depends on the amount of hair, the location of the incision, and the type of surgical procedure to be performed. Preoperative shaving of the surgical site increases the risk of surgical site infection (Anderson et al, 2008; AORN, 2013n). If hair is to be removed, clipping with an electric or battery-operated clipper, or using a depilatory is recommended. Shaving is not recommended. Clipping immediately before surgery is the simplest and least irritating method of hair removal. Use of a depilatory requires a pretest to ascertain that the patient is not sensitive to the depilatory product. The specific manufacturer's written instructions should be carefully followed. If a shave is desired by the surgeon, some institutions require a written order. The patient should be shaved as close to the time of surgery as is possible. The shave should be performed in an area within the surgical suite that affords privacy and is equipped with good lighting. Clipping the morning of surgery as opposed to the day before may reduce the incidence of surgical site infection (Tanner et al, 2011). Hair removal should be performed by skilled personnel, with great care taken to avoid scratching, nicking, or cutting the skin because cutaneous bacteria proliferate in these areas and increase the chances of infection. The method of hair removal and the condition of the skin before and after removal should be documented.

RESEARCH HIGHLIGHT ||

Preoperative Chlorhexidine Shower or Bath for Prevention of Surgical Site Infections

The recommendation to have patients shower or bathe with chlorhexidine preoperatively to reduce skin microbial colony counts is included as a risk prevention measure in the CDC *Guidelines for Prevention of Surgical Site Infection*. Although studies do show that the practice decreases bacterial colony counts as much as ninefold (2.83102 to 0.3) and that the antibacterial effect is cumulative, the evidence does not support whether the practice actually reduces the rate of surgical site infections (SSIs).

In this study the authors undertook a meta-analysis of published, controlled clinical trials to evaluate the efficacy of preoperative showers or baths with chlorhexidine for preventing SSIs. The authors chose to review prospective randomized controlled trials and quasi-randomized trials as well as before/after trials comparing preoperative whole-body chlorhexidine showers or baths with nonantiseptic soap or no bath and reporting SSI as an outcome. Ultimately, 16 studies with a total of 17,932 patients were included in their analysis. Within the group, 7952 received a preoperative chlorhexidine shower or bath and 9980 received a preoperative shower with nongermicidal soap ($n = 5696$) or placebo ($n = 2207$) or nonpreoperative shower/noncompliance with regimen ($n = 2077$).

Three trials showed a significant reduction in the incidence of SSIs; however, no evidence supported significant reduction of SSIs using chlorhexidine when compared with soap, placebo, or no shower or bath. Overall, 6.8% of patients in the chlorhexidine group developed SSIs compared with 7.2% in the other groups.

The authors note that it is possible that chlorhexidine may not have been used as recommended; in all trials, patients were instructed to bathe or shower with the agent, but were not instructed to leave the chlorhexidine on their skin for several minutes before rinsing, and that the application of the agent was unsupervised. They postulate that the duration of the application did not provide enough time for adequate, effective cutaneous antisepsis.

This analysis did not support the routine use of whole-body chlorhexidine showering or bathing for the prevention of SSIs. The authors suggest additional studies using standardized application techniques and a prolonged duration of chlorhexidine with assessment of SSI outcomes are needed.

CDC, Centers for Disease Control and Prevention.
Modified from Chlebicki M et al: Preoperative chlorhexidine shower or bath for prevention of surgical site infection: a meta analysis, *Am J Infect Control* 41(2):167–173, 2013; Centers for Disease Control and Prevention (CDC): *Guidelines for prevention of surgical site infection,* available at www.cdc.gov/hicpac/SSI/001_SSI.html. Accessed December 16, 2012.

FIGURE 4-24 Principles of starting at the intended incision site and working toward the periphery are illustrated on this example of an abdominal prep. Shaded areas indicate the area to be cleaned with antiseptic; arrows show direction of motion for the prep. (Always refer to manufacturer's instruction for prep application. Some instructions may indicate a different pattern to follow.)

The surgical principle followed when preparing the patient's skin for surgery ("prepping") is to prepare ("prep") the cleanest area first and then move to the less clean areas (clean to dirty). The skin at the surgical site should be exposed and inspected before beginning the skin prep. Patients should have been instructed to remove any body jewelry before cleansing the site. Jewelry harbors microorganisms and traps them in adjacent skin. Jewelry should also be removed to reduce the risk of injury when positioning the patient or from using electrical devices. Surgical departments often stock snap-ring pliers to remove jewelry from piercings for emergency situations or when a patient has neglected to remove body jewelry. A variety of skin prepping products are available. A two-step product will include a scrub (clean) and paint and others are one step only.

The skin prep usually begins at the point of the incision and continues to the periphery of the area (Figure 4-24). When prepping the surgical site, the nurse dons sterile gloves and applies the antimicrobial agent using commercially prepared devices or applicators that have handles to provide distance between the nurse's hand and the area being prepared. A soiled applicator is never brought back over a previously prepped surface. On completion of the skin prep, the nurse may or may not, depending on manufacturer's instructions, blot the area with dry, sterile sponges or a sterile towel. Depending on the surgeon's preference, a topical antimicrobial solution or "paint" may be carefully applied to the prepped area, using care to avoid any solution pooling beneath the patient. All wet drapes should be removed from the patient area after the skin preparation is complete (AORN, 2013n).

When an intestinal or urinary stoma or other contaminated area is involved within the surgical field and during the prep procedure, a sponge soaked in the antimicrobial agent of choice is placed over the stoma when the prep is initiated. The area should be cleansed separately from the rest of the prepped area. At the completion of the prep, the sponge is discarded. Sponges used to cleanse or disinfect an open wound, sinus, ulcer, intestinal stoma, the vagina, or the anus are applied once to that area and discarded. In contrast to the principle of working from the proposed incision to the periphery, open wounds and body orifices are potentially contaminated areas and as such are prepared after the peripheral intact skin is cleansed. The surgical principle is to work from the cleanest to the least clean area (AORN, 2013n).

The nurse should document the area prepped and the antiseptic solution used in the perioperative record. Documentation is an effective way to promote safe, continuous patient care. Although at times it may seem time-consuming, periodic audits of the documentation of skin preparation help the perioperative nurse assess the effectiveness of the process, while protecting patients from possible surgical site infections (AORN, 2013n).

Creating the Sterile Field with Surgical Drapes

To create a sterile field, sterile sheets and towels, known as surgical drapes, are strategically placed to provide a sterile surface on which sterile instruments, supplies, equipment, and gloved hands may rest. The patient and OR bed are covered with sterile drapes in a manner that exposes the prepared incision site and isolates it from surrounding areas. Objects normally draped and composing the sterile field include instrument tables, trays, basins, the Mayo stand, some surgical equipment, and the patient. Within this defined sterile area the actual operative procedure takes place.

Today, reusable and single-use (disposable) drapes are widely used. There are advantages and disadvantages for reusable (fabric) and single-use (disposable, nonwoven) drapes. Regardless of the type of material used, surgical drapes should have the following characteristics (AORN, 2013n):

- Create an appropriate barrier to microorganisms, particulate matter, and fluids
- Withstand methods of sterilization
- Maintain integrity
- Sustain durability
- Withstand physical conditions
- Resist tears, punctures, fiber strains, and abrasions
- Be free of toxic ingredients
- Be low linting
- Be free of holes or other defects
- Achieve positive cost-to-benefit ratio

In addition, draping materials should meet or exceed the current requirements of the National Fire Protection Association.

Reusable Drapes. Chemically treated cotton or cotton-polyester fabrics provide a barrier to liquids and are abrasion-resistant. Quantitative data verifying the barrier quality of any textile drape must be provided by the manufacturer. Care should be taken with reusable drapes to eliminate pinholes caused by towel clamps, needles, or other sharp objects. Only nonpenetrating towel clamps should be used. Should breaks in the fabric occur, a heat-sealed patch may be used for repair after laundering. An abundance of heat-sealed patches on any surgical drape may interfere with the sterilization process and render the barrier ineffective. Manufacturer's written instructions on the use of patching should be followed. The exact percentage of any item that may be successfully patched is unknown. As with reusable gowns, laundering eventually impairs the barrier quality of the drape. Most manufacturers report a loss of barrier quality after 75 to 100 laundry or sterilization cycles. The process of laundering and steam sterilization swells the fabric fibers, whereas drying and ironing shrink the fibers. Over time these processes loosen fabric fibers, altering the fabric structure and decreasing the barrier properties and fluid impermeability of the fabric. As with surgical gowns, a system to monitor the number of times an item has been processed is essential for quality control of the barrier and fluid impermeability.

Single-Use (Disposable) Drapes. Commercially packaged and sterilized synthetic single-use disposable drapes are widely used. They reduce the hazards of contamination in the presence of known infectious microorganisms from body fluids and excretions and in situations in which laundering of grossly contaminated textiles may be problematic. They prevent bacterial penetration and fluid breakthrough, also known as *strikethrough*. When considering the purchase of single-use drapes, the perioperative team must determine whether the drapes will meet the needs of the surgical procedure, be acceptable to the perioperative team, and be cost-effective (versus laundering and processing of reusable drapes). A cost-to-benefit ratio analysis may warrant their use in the healthcare facility. Availability of items, storage facilities, and disposal methods must be analyzed (AORN, 2013q).

The environmental effect of disposable items can be only roughly estimated. Each facility must carefully evaluate its capabilities and restrictions for handling single-use and reusable supplies and equipment to make an informed decision about the products it will use in the practice setting.

Compactors provide a relatively inexpensive method of discarding disposable drapes. They accept any material and reduce its volume substantially. Storage, collection, and transportation of compacted waste materials can be a problem. Hospital engineers must establish methods of controlling odor and maintaining sanitation in the compactor area. Because a portion of the compacted material may be grossly contaminated, city or county codes may prohibit transporting this potentially infectious material through city streets or dumping it at landfills. Incineration is an alternative method for destroying waste disposables. If hospital incinerators are used, they must be managed properly to prevent environmental contamination. Facilities choosing to incinerate must follow specific state and local guidelines established for medical waste incinerators and must meet federal standards (EPA, 2012).

In addition to commercially prepared drapes, commercially prepared preassembled sterile, disposable custom packs are used in many healthcare facilities. These packs are specific to a surgical procedure and contain the items needed for a particular procedure. The contents of the pack are determined by the surgeon/facility. Advantages of these packs include reduced setup and room-turnover times resulting from fewer individually wrapped items that must be opened. Other advantages include less waste resulting from fewer individually wrapped items, improved inventory control, and fewer lost charges. Although custom packs may be more expensive than multiple separate items, indirect savings related to increased efficiency can offset those costs.

Drape Configurations. Careful planning by perioperative personnel helps determine the desired types and sizes of surgical drapes required for groups or individual surgical procedures. Standardized draping methods provide management control that ensures patient safety, simplifies staff education, and conserves human and material resources.

A whole, or plain, sheet is used to cover instrument tables, operating tables, and body regions. The sheet should be large enough to provide an adequate margin of safety between the surrounding physical environment and the prepared operative field. Surgical towels should be available in several sizes to drape the operative site. Four surgical towels of woven or nonwoven material are usually sufficient (Figure 4-25).

Fenestrated, or slit, sheets are used for draping patients. They leave the operative site exposed. A typical fenestrated (laparotomy) sheet is large enough to cover the patient and operating bed in any position, extend over the anesthesia screen at the head of the bed, and extend over the foot of the bed (Figures 4-26 to 4-28). The typical fenestrated laparotomy sheet can be used for most procedures on the abdomen, chest, flank, and back. Other types of fenestrated sheets with small or split fenestrations may be used for

FIGURE 4-25 Abdomen may be draped with four sterile towels, which are secured with nonperforating towel clamps. Standard method of placement of disposable towels is used.

FIGURE 4-26 Placement of laparotomy sheet. Identification of top portion of laparotomy sheet helps the scrub person readily determine correct placement of the drape. After placing the folded laparotomy sheet on the patient, with fenestration of sheet directly over site of incision outlined by sterile towels, the scrub person unfolds drape over sides of patient and bed.

FIGURE 4-27 Laparotomy draping continued. Scrub person protects gloved hands under cuff of fan-folded laparotomy sheet and draws the upper section above fenestration toward the head of the bed, draping it over the anesthesia screen. The bottom portion of the fan-folded sheet is extended over the foot of the bed in a similar manner.

FIGURE 4-28 Laparotomy draping completed. Fenestration provides exposure of prepared operative site. **>a,** Reinforced area around drape fenestration provides greater protection and fluid control. **>b,** Built-in instrument pad prevents instrument slippage. **>c,** Perforated tabs provide means of controlling position of cords and suction tubes.

the limbs, head, and neck when the patient is in the supine or prone position. The size of the fenestration is determined by the use for which the sheet is intended. The fenestrated sheet is fan-folded and handled as a typical laparotomy sheet. A perineal drape is needed for procedures on the perineum and genitalia when the patient is in the lithotomy position. A lithotomy drape consists of a fenestrated sheet and two triangular leggings.

Several types of impermeable polyvinyl chloride (PVC) sheeting are available in the form of sterile, prepackaged surgical drapes. Plastic, adherent incisional drapes are available as a plain impermeable drape or impregnated with an antimicrobial. These plastic drapes are useful adjuncts to the conventional draping procedure. They can be applied after the fabric drape, alleviating the need for towel clamps. They obviate the need for skin towels and sponges to separate the surgeon's gloves from contact with the patient's skin. Skin color and anatomic landmarks are readily visible, and the incision is made directly through the adherent plastic drape. These materials facilitate draping of irregular body surfaces, such as neck and ear regions, extremities, and joints (Figure 4-29).

Draping Procedure. Drapes should be folded so that the gowned and gloved members of the team can handle them with ease and safety. The larger, regular sheet is usually fan-folded from bottom to top. The bottom folds may be wider than the upper ones. The small sheet is folded in half and quartered, with the top corners of the sheet turned back or marked for easy identification and handling. To provide for safe, easy handling and a wide margin of safety between the unsterile item and the scrub person's gloved hands, the open end of the Mayo stand cover should be cuffed or folded back on itself (Figure 4-30). Most fenestrated sheets are fan-folded to the

FIGURE 4-29 Sterile, impermeable adhesive drape. For maximum sealing to prevent wound contamination, prepared skin must be dry, and the drape must be applied carefully, preventing wrinkles and air bubbles. **A,** Surgeon and assistant hold plastic drape taut while another assistant peels off back paper. **B,** Surgeon and assistant may apply plastic drape to operative site and, using folded towel, apply slight pressure to eliminate air bubbles and wrinkles. **C,** Surgeon would then make incision through plastic drape.

FIGURE 4-30 Draping Mayo stand. Folded cover is slipped over frame. Scrub person's gloved hands are protected by cuff of drape. Cover is unfolded to extend over upright support of stand.

opening from the top and the bottom, and the folds are rolled or fanned toward the center of the opening. The drape fenestration is place over the incision site and the fan folds are drawn away from the incision site. The edges of the top and bottom folds of the sheet are fanned to provide a cuff under which the perioperative scrub person may place his or her gloved hands. The top and lower sections should be identified by markings to facilitate easy handling.

When applying drapes to create the sterile field, these principles should be followed:

- Allow sufficient time and space to permit careful draping and proper aseptic technique.
- Handle sterile drapes as little as possible. Rapid movement of draping materials creates air currents on which dust, lint, and other particles can migrate (AORN, 2013l).
- Carry the folded drape to the operative site. Carefully unfold the drape, and place it in the proper position. Do not move the drape after it has been placed. Shifting or moving the drape may transport bacteria from an unprepared area of the patient's skin into the surgical field.
- Hold the sterile drape above the level of the OR bed and place it moving from the surgical site to the periphery. Do not allow the drape to fall below the level of the waist as this may increase the risk of contamination. A drape should be carefully unfolded and allowed to fall gently into position by gravity.
- Consider the drape contaminated any time the sterility is questionable and immediately discard a drape that becomes contaminated during the draping procedure.
- Protect the gown by distance. During draping, gloved hands should be protected by cuffing the draping material over the gloved hands to reduce potential contamination. Control all parts of the drape at all times during placement, using precise and direct motions.
- Drape the incisional area first and then the periphery. Always drape from a sterile area to an unsterile area by draping the near side first. Never reach across an unsterile area to drape. When draping the opposite side of the OR bed, go around the bed to drape. The low portion of a sheet that falls below the safe working level should never be raised or lifted back into the sterile area.
- Use nonperforating towel clamps or devices to secure tubing and other items on the sterile field.

After the patient is positioned, prepared, and draped, a time-out is conducted to verify patient identification, correct position, and correct surgical site (and side if applicable) and that required equipment is available.

Environmental Cleaning

Contamination in the OR can occur from various sources. The patient, healthcare workers, and inanimate objects are all capable of introducing potentially infectious material onto the surgical field. The patient should be provided a clean, safe, environment. Techniques have been established to prevent the transmission of microorganisms into the surgical area, such as wearing proper surgical attire and establishing controlled traffic patterns in the surgical suite. During the surgical procedure, traffic within and through the room should be kept to a minimum to reduce air turbulence and to minimize human shedding. All doors in and out of the OR should be kept closed to decrease air turbulence and the potential for contamination. HEPA filters placed between outside air processing and the OR vents are used in many facilities and are recommended for newly constructed systems/facilities. HEPA filters are capable of screening out particles larger than 0.3 μm (AORN, 2013d; CDC, 2008a). The perioperative registered nurse should assess the perioperative environment frequently for cleanliness and take action to implement cleaning and disinfection procedures if needed (AORN, 2013d).

All surgical patients should be considered to be potentially infected with bloodborne or other infectious material. For patient and personnel safety, cleaning procedures should be uniform throughout the OR and for all patients. Using a uniform procedure designed to protect persons from visible or invisible contamination eliminates the need for special cleaning procedures for so-called dirty cases. Cleaning procedures should be carried out in a manner that protects patients and personnel from exposure to potentially infectious microorganisms. Cleaning measures are needed before, during, and after surgical procedures and at the end of each day. A safe, clean environment should be reestablished after each surgical or invasive procedure. Overall housekeeping procedures, such as wall and ceiling washing, should be completed on a defined, regular basis and terminal cleaning and disinfection of operating and invasive procedure rooms should be performed when scheduled procedures are completed for the day or each regular 24-hour period (AORN, 2013d).

Transmission-Based Precautions, as described earlier, are designed for patients who have a documented infection or who are suspected to be infected with a highly transmissible pathogen for which additional precautions are necessary. The CDC (2008a) guidelines should be followed when all facility policies and guidelines for cleaning are developed.

Before beginning the first procedure of the day, horizontal surfaces in the ORs should be dusted with a cloth dampened with a facility-approved disinfecting agent. Dust and lint deposited on horizontal surfaces during the night can become airborne vectors for organisms if not removed. During surgery, efforts should be made to confine contamination to as small an area as possible around the patient. Sponges should be discarded in plastic-lined containers. As they are counted, they should be contained in an impervious receptacle. The perioperative nurse must use protective eyewear and gloves, instruments, or both when collecting and counting sponges or handling contaminated items. Spills should be cleaned immediately, and the cleaned area should be disinfected with a broad-spectrum disinfectant or germicide. Specimens of blood or other potentially infectious tissues or materials should be placed in a container that prevents leakage. The container must be color-coded or labeled using the biohazard symbol (see Figure 4-2). If the outside of the container becomes contaminated, the primary container must be placed within a second container that prevents leakage and is labeled or color-coded. Some facilities use biohazard-labeled impervious bags to transport blood or other potentially infectious material (AORN, 2013d; CDC, 2008a).

On completion of the surgical procedure, soiled linens should be discarded in fluid-impervious bags to eliminate potential contamination from wet linen soaking through to the outside of the bag. Contaminated items should be placed in leakproof, color-coded, or labeled containers. Sharps (e.g., needles, scalpels, electrosurgical tips) are considered infectious and should be placed in special puncture-resistant containers (OSHA, 2001). Bulk blood or suctioned fluid may be poured carefully down a drain connected to a sanitary sewer unless prohibited by environmental regulations. Local and state environmental regulations may exist and should be consulted before establishing guidelines for waste disposal. Wall suction units should be disconnected to eliminate contamination of the wall outlet. Suction contents should be disposed as soon as possible on completion of the procedure. Depending on local and state regulations, powder treatments of a chlorine compound are available to solidify liquid material before transport. This chemical also may be tuberculocidal, virucidal, and bactericidal. Suction tubing should be discarded. Personnel should remove their gowns and gloves and place them in the proper receptacles before leaving the OR, and then perform handwashing. Instruments and supplies should be contained, labeled with a biohazard label, and taken to the decontamination area, where personnel wearing personal protective attire begin the instrument decontamination process. Care should be taken to arrange sharp instruments in such a manner that personnel need not reach into basins where sharp instruments are unexposed and could cause injury. Equipment and furniture in the OR should be cleaned with an EPA-approved hospital disinfectant. It is important to follow manufacturers' instructions. Some disinfectants may require and extended contact time. If the disinfectant dries quickly, meeting the contact requirements may require several applications. The floor should be cleaned as necessary and should be wet-vacuumed with an EPA-registered disinfectant after scheduled cases are completed (AORN, 2013d). A standard practice of cleaning helps prevent surgical site infections and maintains a clean and safe environment (AORN, 2013d; CDC, 2008a).

At the end of each day's operative schedule, all rooms where procedures may be performed should be cleaned by qualified, trained, supervised personnel. Areas to be cleaned include the following:

- Surgical lights and external tracks
- Fixed and ceiling-mounted equipment
- All furniture and equipment including wheels and casters
- Equipment
- Handles of cabinets and push plates
- Ventilation faceplates
- Horizontal surfaces (e.g., countertops, fixed shelving, autoclaves)
- Floor
- Kick buckets
- Scrub sinks

If refillable liquid soap dispensers are used, they should be disassembled and cleaned before being refilled because they can serve as reservoirs for microorganisms. At the conclusion of the housekeeping protocol, cleaning equipment and supplies should be properly cleaned, disinfected, and stored. If a wet vacuum has been used, it should be disassembled and thoroughly washed with a disinfectant before being stored (AORN, 2013d).

KEY POINTS

- Perioperative patient care is based on surgical aseptic principles. Careful adherence to these principles supports infection prevention and control and ultimately improves surgical patient safety and outcomes.
- Infection may be caused by bacteria, viruses, or prions.
- Infection control practices should focus primarily on prevention. Transmission of infection involves a chain of events, including the presence of a pathogenic agent, reservoir, portal of exit, transmission, and portal of entry, and host susceptibility. Prevention occurs when there is a break in the chain of transmission.
- Standard Precautions are intended to reduce the transmission of microorganisms from recognized and unrecognized sources of infection. Standard Precautions should be applied to all patients receiving care regardless of their diagnosis or presumed infection status.
- Preparing items for use in surgery and other invasive procedures requires thorough cleaning and drying of the items followed by either sterilization or high-level disinfection process.
- *Sterilization* is defined as the complete elimination or destruction of all forms of microbial life.

- Disinfection is defined as the process that kills all microorganisms with the exception of high numbers of bacterial spores.
- A variety of methods are available for sterilization. Perioperative personnel choose the appropriate method based on the item to be sterilized and manufacturer's recommendations.
- Aseptic technique stems from the principles of asepsis derived over time from microbiologic and epidemiologic concepts.

CRITICAL THINKING QUESTION

A 42-year-old female is scheduled for an outpatient wound debridement to her right ankle. The perioperative nurse phones the patient the day before her procedure to begin the preoperative assessment. During the course of the assessment the patient tells the nurse that her surgeon called and told her that her recent wound culture was positive for methicillin-resistant *Staphylococcus aureus* (MRSA). Why is this information important for the perioperative nurse to consider in planning care? What nursing interventions should the nurse plan for after the patient arrives?

℮volve *The answers to the Critical Thinking Question can be found at http://evolve.elsevier.com/Rothrock/Alexander.*

REFERENCES

American Institute of Architects Academy of Architecture for Health (AIA): *FGI guidelines for design and construction of hospital and outpatient facilities*, Washington, DC, 2010.

American Society for Gastrointestinal Endoscopy (ASGE): Multisociety guideline in reprocessing of flexible gastrointestinal endoscopes, *Gastrointest Endosc* 73(6):1075 1084, 2011.

Anderson DJ et al: Strategies to prevent surgical site infections in acute care hospitals, *Infect Control Hosp Epidemiol* 29(1):S51–S61, 2008.

Association for the Advancement of Medical Instrumentation (AAMI): *Industrial process control*, Arlington, VA, 2009a, The Association.

Association for the Advancement of Medical Instrumentation (AAMI): *Sterilization equipment design and use*, Arlington, VA, 2009b, The Association.

Association for the Advancement of Medical Instrumentation (AAMI): *Containment devices for reusable medical device sterilization*, Arlington, VA, 2010, The Association.

Association for the Advancement of Medical Instrumentation (AAMI): *Comprehensive guide to sterilization and sterility assurance in health care facilities*, Arlington, VA, 2012, The Association.

Association for the Advancement of Medical Instrumentation, et al: Multidisciplinary position paper on immediate use steam sterilization, February 2011.

Association of periOperative Registered Nurses (AORN): Recommended practices for hand hygiene in the perioperative setting. In *Perioperative standards and recommended practice*, Denver, 2013a, The Association.

Association of periOperative Registered Nurses (AORN): Recommended practices for surgical attire. In *Perioperative standards and recommended practices*, Denver, 2013b, The Association.

Association of periOperative Registered Nurses (AORN): Recommended practices for prevention of transmissible infections in the perioperative practice setting. In *Perioperative standards and recommended practices*, Denver, 2013c, The Association.

Association of periOperative Registered Nurses (AORN): Recommended practices for environmental cleaning in the perioperative setting. In *Perioperative standards and recommended practices*, Denver, 2013d, The Association.

Association of periOperative Registered Nurses (AORN): Recommended practices for the cleaning and care of surgical instruments and powered equipment. In *Perioperative standards and recommended practices*, Denver, 2013e, The Association.

Association of periOperative Registered Nurses (AORN): Recommended practices for a safe environment of care. In *Perioperative standards and recommended practices*, Denver, 2013f, The Association.

Association of periOperative Registered Nurses (AORN): Recommended practices for sterilization in the perioperative practice setting. In *Perioperative standards and recommended practices*, Denver, 2013g, The Association.

Association of periOperative Registered Nurses (AORN): Recommended practices for selection and use of packing systems for sterilization. In *Perioperative standards and recommended practices*, Denver, 2013h, The Association.

Association of periOperative Registered Nurses (AORN): Recommended practices for high level disinfection. In *Perioperative standards and recommended practices*, Denver, 2013i, The Association.

Association of periOperative Registered Nurses (AORN): Recommended practices for cleaning and processing flexible endoscopes. In *Perioperative standards and recommended practices*, Denver, 2013j, The Association.

Association of periOperative Registered Nurses (AORN): Recommended practices for maintaining a sterile field. In *Perioperative standards and recommended practices*, Denver, 2013l, The Association.

Association of periOperative Registered Nurses (AORN): Recommended practices for traffic patterns in the perioperative practice setting. In *Perioperative standards and recommended practices*, Denver, 2013m, The Association.

Association of periOperative Registered Nurses (AORN): Recommended practices for Perioperative skin antisepsis. In *Perioperative Standards and recommended practices*, Denver, 2013n, The Association.

Association of periOperative Registered Nurses (AORN): Recommended practices for selection and use of surgical gowns and drapes. In *Perioperative standards and recommended practices*, Denver, 2013o, The Association.

Association of periOperative Registered Nurses (AORN): AORN latex guideline. In *Perioperative standards and recommended practices*, Denver, 2013p, The Association.

Association of periOperative Registered Nurses (AORN): Recommended practices for product selection in the perioperative practice setting. In *Perioperative standards and recommended practices*, Denver, 2013q, The Association.

Association of periOperative Registered Nurses (AORN): Recommended practices for laser safety in the perioperative setting. In *Perioperative standards and recommended practices*, Denver, 2013r, The Association.

Association of perioperative Registered Nurses (AORN) Recommended practices for sterile technique. In *Perioperative standards and recommended practices*. Denver, 2013s, The Association.

Banerjee S et al: Infection control during GI endoscopy, *Gastrointest Endosc* 67(6):781–790, 2008.

Bible J et al: Which regions of the operating gown should be considered most sterile? *Clin Orthop* 467(3):825–830, 2009.

Centers for Disease Control and Prevention (CDC): Guidelines for preventing the transmission of Mycobacterium tuberculosis in health-care settings, 2005, available at www.cdc.gov/mmwr/preview/mmwrhtml/rr5417a1.htm. Accessed December 9, 2012.

Centers for Disease Control and Prevention (CDC): Management of multidrug resistant organisms in healthcare settings, 2006a, Atlanta, 2006, available at www.cdc.gov/ncidod/dhqp/pdf/ar/mdroguideline2006.pdf. Accessed December 9, 2012.

Centers for Disease Control and Prevention (CDC): *HIV/aids surveillance supplemental report-vol. 14, No. 1, HIV/AIDS data through December 2006*, Atlanta, 2006b, available at www.cdc.gov/hiv/surveillance/resources/reports/2009supp_vol14no1/. Accessed December 9, 2012.

Centers for Disease Control and Prevention (CDC): *Investigation and control of vancomycin intermediate and resistant* Staphylococcus aureus *(VISA/URSA): a guide for health departments and infection control personnel*, 2006c, Atlanta, 2006c, available at www.cdc.gov/ncidod/ dhqp/pdf/ar/visa_vrsa_guide.pdf. Accessed December 9, 2012.

Centers for Disease Control and Prevention (CDC): Overview of healthcare-associated MRSA in healthcare settings, 2007a, Atlanta, 2007, available at www.cdc.gov/ncidod/dhqp/ar_MRSA.html. Accessed December 9, 2012.

Centers for Disease Control and Prevention (CDC): 2007 *Guideline for isolation precautions: preventing transmission of infectious agents in healthcare settings*, 2007b, available at www.cdc.gov/ncidod/dhqp/pdf/guidelines/Isolation 2007.pdf. Accessed December 9, 2012.

Centers for Disease Control and Prevention (CDC): *Guideline for disinfection and sterilization in healthcare facilities,* 2008, Atlanta, 2008a, available at www.cdc.gov/ncidod/dhqp/pdf/guidelines/Disinfection_ Nov_2008.pdf. Accessed December 9, 2012.

Centers for Disease Control and Prevention (CDC): About CJD, 2008b, Atlanta, 2008, CDC, available at www.cdc.gov/ncidod/dvrd/cjd/. Accessed December 9, 2012.

Centers for Disease Control and Prevention (CDC): *Frequently asked questions about* Clostridium difficile *for healthcare providers,* Atlanta, 2010a, available at www.cdc.gov/HAI/organisms/cdiff/Cdiff_faqs_HCP.html#a1. Accessed October 28, 2012.

Centers for Disease Control and Prevention (CDC): Klebsiella *pneumonia in healthcare settings,* Atlanta, 2010b, available at www.cdc.gov/HAI/organisms/klebsiella/klebsiella.html#a4. Accessed October 30, 2012.

Centers for Disease Control and Prevention (CDC): *Antibiotic resistance questions and answers,* Atlanta, 2012a, available at www.cdc.gov/getsmart/anribiotic.use/antibiotic-resistance-faqs.html#g. Accessed November 1, 2012.

Centers for Disease Control and Prevention (CDC): *CJD (Creutzfeldt-Jakob disease classic),* Atlanta, 2012b, available at www.cdc.gov/ncidod/dvrd/cjd. Accessed October 20, 2012.

Centers for Disease Control and Prevention (CDC): *NIOSH Pocket guide to chemicals,* Altanta, 2012c, available at www.cdc.gov/niosh/npg/npgdo301.html. Accessed October 18, 2012.

Centers for Disease Control and Prevention (CDC): Bioterrorism overview, 2007, available at http://emergency.cdc.gov/bioterrorism/overview.asp. Accessed December 9, 2012.

Chlebicki M et al: Preoperative chlorhexidine shower or bath for prevention of surgical site infection: a meta analysis, *Am J Infec Control,* June 2012. In press corrected, available at www.ajicjournal.org. Accessed December 16, 2012.

Cohen S et al: Clinical practice guidelines for *Clostridium difficile* infection in adults, *Infect Contr Hospit Epidemiol* 31(5):431–455, 2010.

Copeland JT: Do surgical personnel really need to double-glove? *AORN J* 89(2):322–330, 2009.

Davenport A, Myers F: How to protect yourself after body fluid exposure, *Nursing* 39(5):23–28, 2009.

Department of Veterans Affairs Office of the Inspector General: Use and reprocessing of flexible endoscopes at VA medical facilities, June 2009, available at www.va.gov/oig/54/reports/VAOIG-09-01784-146.pdf. Accessed October 10, 2012.

Droboni M et al: Vancomycin-resistant enterococci, Point Barrow, Alaska, USA, *EID J,* 15(5):838–839, 2009, available at www.cdc.gov/eid/content/15/5/838.htm. Accessed December 9, 2012.

Environmental Protection Agency (EPA): National emission standards for hospital ethyleneoxide sterilization, *Fed Regis* 72(248), 2007, available at www.epa.gov/ttn/atw/area/fr28de07b.pdf. Accessed October 22, 2012.

Environmental Protection Agency (EPA): Ethylene oxide (ETO): hospitals must use a single chamber when sterilizing medical equipment with ETO, *Pesticide Reregistration,* EPA March, 2010, available at www.epa.gov/oppsrrd1/reregistration/ethylene_oxide/ethylene_oxide_fs.html. Accessed October 4, 2012.

Environmental Protection Agency (EPA): Hospital/medical/infectious waste incinerator, *Technol Transf,* 2012, available at www.epa.gov/ttn/atw01/129/hmiwi/rihmiwi.html. Accessed November 1, 2012.

Geipl U: Pathogenic organisms in joint infections, *Int J Med Sci* 6(5):234–240, 2009.

Gould V et al: Bench-to bedside-review: *Clostridium difficile* colitis, *Crit Care* (12):203, 2008, available at http://ccforum.com/content/12/1/203. Accessed October 28, 2012.

Haas JP et al: Compliance with hand hygiene guidelines: where are we in 2008? *AJN* 108(8):40–44, 2008.

Ignatavicius DD: Care of patients with infection. In Ignatavicius DD, Workman ML, editors: *Medical-surgical nursing: patient-centered collaborative care,* ed 7, St Louis, 2013, Saunders.

Macleod-Glover N et al: Efficacy of cleaning products for *C. difficile*: environmental strategies to reduce the spread of *Clostridium difficile* associated diarrhea in geriatric rehabilitation, *Can Fam Physician* 56(5):417–423, 2010.

Mangram AJ et al: Guideline for prevention of surgical site infection 1999, *Infect Control Hospital Epidemiology* 20:250–278, available at www.cdc.gov/ncidod/dhqp/pdf/guidelines/SSI.pdf. October 26, 2007. Accessed December 9, 2012.

Mitchum R: Unlocked mystery will help target insidious bacterial infection *Clostridium difficile* in hospitals, *Chicago Tribune,* 2009, available at http://articles.chicagotribune.com/2009-03-06/news/0903050516_1_difficile-toxin-clostridium. Accessed December 9, 2012.

Neil JA: Perioperative care of the patient with tuberculosis, *AORN J* 88(6):942–958, 2008.

Occupational Safety and Health Administration (OSHA): Occupational exposure to ethylene oxide, final standard, *Fed Regist* 49(122):25737–25768, 1984, available at www.osha.gov/pls/oshaweb/owadisp.show_document?p_table=FEDERAL_REGISTER&p_id=12438. Accessed December 9, 2012.

Occupational Safety and Health Administration (OSHA): *Ethylene oxide.*29 CFR 1910.1047. July1, 2010, available at www.osha.gov/pls/oshaweb/owadisp.show_document?p_table=STANDARDS&p_id=10070. Accessed November 1, 2012.

Occupational Safety and Health Administration (OSHA): Occupational exposure to ethylene oxide, final standard, *Fed Regist* 53(66):11414–11438, 1988, available at www.osha.gov. Accessed December 9, 2012.

Occupational Safety and Health Administration (OSHA): Occupational exposure to bloodborne pathogens: final rule, *Fed Regist* 56(235):64175–64182, 1991, available at www.osha.gov. Accessed December 9, 2012.

Occupational Safety and Health Administration (OSHA): Occupational exposure to bloodborne pathogens: needlestick and other sharps injuries: final rule, *Fed Regist* 66:5317–5325, 2001, available at www.osha.gov. Accessed December 9, 2012.

Pynnonen M et al: Hemoglobin promotes *Staphylococcus* nasal colonization, *PLoS Pathogens* 7:2011, available at www.plospathogens.org/article/info%3Adoi%2F10.1371%2Fjournal.ppat.1002104. Accessed December 9, 2012.

Ramirez J et al: Changing needs of community-acquired pneumonia, *J Antimicrob Chemother* (Suppl. 3):iii, 3–9, 2011.

Sampson JG, Workman ML: Care of patients with HIV disease and other immune deficiencies, In Ignatavicius DD, Workman ML, editors: *Medical-surgical nursing: patient-centered collaborative care,* ed 7, St Louis, 2013, Saunders.

Sandlin D: Unlocking the mystery of MRSA, *J Perianesth Nurs* 23(2):137–139, 2008.

Scheithauer S et al: The current pathogen spectrum—what are we fighting against? *Orthopade* 41(1)6–12, 2012.

Tanner J et al: Preoperative hair removal to reduce surgical site infection, *Cochrane Database Syst Rev* 9(11), 2011.

The Joint Commission: *Measuring hand hygiene adherence: making the what, why and how decisions,* Oakbrook, IL, 2009, The Joint Commission, available at http://indianahealthcarequality.blogspot.com/2009/04/tjc-measuring-hand-hygiene-adherence.html. Accessed December 9, 2012.

U.S. Food and Drug Administration (FDA) Enforcement priorities for single-use devices reprocessed by third party and hospitals, 2000.

U.S. Food and Drug Administration (FDA): *FDA cleared sterilants and high level disinfectants* with *general claims for reprocessing reusable medical and dental devices,* March 2009a, available at www.fda.gov/MedicalDevices/DeviceRegulationandGuidance/ReprocessingofSingle-UseDevices/ucm133514.html. Accessed October 22, 2012.

U.S. Food and Drug Administration (FDA): *Reprocessing of single-use devices,* 2009b, available at www.fda.gov/MedicalDevices/DeviceRegulationand Guidance/Reprocessingofsingle-.

Widerstrom M et al: Coagulase-negative staphylococci: update on the molecular epidemiology and clinical presentation, with a focus on *Staphylococcus epidermidis* and *Staphylococcus saprophyticus, Eur J Clin Microbiol Infect Dis* 31(1):7–20, 2012.

World Health Organization: *WHO guidelines on hand hygiene in health care,* 2009, available at www.who.int/patientsafety/information_centre/ghhad_download_link/en. Accessed December 9, 2012.

CHAPTER 5

Anesthesia

BRIAN D. CAMPBELL

The first medical report of anesthesia was announced to the world on November 18, 1846, by Henry J. Bigelow in the *Boston Medical and Surgical Journal*. An era had ended during which successful surgery depended largely on the surgeon's speed while working on a struggling, distressed patient. Anesthetic techniques gave the surgeon more time to operate and permitted new procedures to be undertaken that would have been impossible before. Many modern surgical techniques since have become feasible because advances in the art and science of anesthesia have occurred.

The word *anesthesia* is derived from the Greek word *anaisthesia,* which literally means "no sensation." Anesthesia was listed in *Bailey's English Dictionary* in 1721. When the effects of ether were discovered, Oliver Wendell Holmes suggested *anesthesia* be used as a name for the new phenomenon. Some believed that he coined this term; others believed that he knew of the Greek word that Plato had used. In any case, anesthesia was, in the memorable phrase of S. Weir Mitchell, the "death of pain." From these early beginnings anesthesia has developed into a sophisticated science and "clinical art" that interfaces with many other medical specialties.

Without anesthesia most modern surgical procedures would not be feasible. As integral members of the patient care team in operative and other invasive procedure settings, perioperative nurses need to be familiar with the principles and practices of anesthesia and the perioperative functions of the anesthesia provider. This chapter presents an overview of the modern practice of anesthesia, the factors involved, and the interrelationship with the perioperative nurse. It discusses major types of anesthesia, introduces the more commonly used modern medications, reviews standards of anesthesia care, and summarizes problems that can occur during the perioperative period. The anesthesia machine and monitoring equipment also are described so that perioperative nurses can become familiar with their basic functions because the nurse may use them during local anesthesia or conscious sedation/analgesia procedures.

The sections of this chapter are organized so that they can be referred to independently without reading the entire chapter. Experienced perioperative nurses are familiar with the commonly used abbreviations used in this chapter. To provide a single reference source for the student or novice perioperative nurse, most abbreviations are defined in Box 5-1.

Anesthesia Providers

In the United States anesthesia care usually is provided in one of three ways: (1) by an anesthesiologist; (2) by a certified registered nurse anesthetist (CRNA) working alone, in collaboration with, or under the direction of an anesthesiologist or a physician; or (3) by an anesthesiologist's assistant (AA) working under direct supervision of an anesthesiologist.

An anesthesiologist is a licensed physician with 4 or more years of specialty training in anesthesiology. Nurse anesthesia programs last a minimum of 2 years and require a bachelor of science (BS) degree in nursing or other appropriate field and a minimum of 1 year of critical care experience before acceptance. All nurse anesthesia programs are at the master's degree level at a minimum. On completion, graduates must successfully complete a national certification examination. Several programs have already advanced to the doctoral level and by 2025, it is projected that all CRNAs will graduate with a doctor of nursing practice (DNP) degree.

Since 1969 AAs also have been used as assistants to anesthesiologists. Acceptance into an AA program requires a BS degree that includes college-level "premed" education. AAs are graduate students within a medical school and typically receive a master of medical science (MMS) degree from the medical school. They also take a national certification examination administered by the National Commission on Certification of Anesthesia Providers' Assistants under the supervision of the National Board of Medical Examiners.

In this chapter the term *anesthesia provider* denotes the individual *providing* the continuous anesthesia care for the patient. Depending on the practice in a given hospital or surgical setting, this may be an anesthesiologist, a CRNA, or an AA. In many settings an *anesthesia care team* includes CRNAs, with or without AAs supervised by anesthesiologists. In small rural hospitals in many states, an anesthesiologist may not be present, and a CRNA may be the sole anesthesia provider.

The anesthesia provider is the patient's advocate in the perioperative period; as such, he or she must be concerned with many divergent factors when the patient's own sensory and cerebral functions are obtunded by anesthesia. The field of anesthesia has become so complex that in many large hospitals an anesthesia provider may specialize further in obstetric, neurosurgical, pediatric, cardiovascular, regional, or ambulatory anesthesia. The anesthesia provider also may subspecialize in acute and chronic pain management or in critical care medicine.

Patient Safety

Patient safety is always a primary concern during surgery and anesthesia. About 32 million anesthetics are administered each year in the United States. Of these, data from several sources indicate a death rate ranging from 1 per 35,000 to about 1 per 40,000. These rates represent a significant decline during the past 30 years, despite surgical procedures being performed on increasingly higher risk patients than in the past. A study from Germany showed an increase in death rates within 1 year post general anesthesia and as high as 1 in 10 for the population age 65 or more. The authors concede

AANA: American Association of Nurse Anesthetists

ABG: Arterial blood gas; usually includes pH, PaO_2, $PaCO_2$, HCO_3^-, K^+, and ionized Ca^{++}

ACLS: Advanced cardiac life support, a protocol for resuscitation from the American Heart Association

APL: Adjustable pressure-limiting valve; a valve on anesthesia machines that limits the maximum pressure in the patient breathing circuit; frequently referred to as the "pop-off valve"

ASA: American Society of Anesthesiologists

cm: Centimeter; 1×10^{-3} m; 2.54 cm = 1 inch

CRNA: Certified registered nurse anesthetist

CSF: Cerebrospinal fluid; the fluid surrounding the brain and spinal cord; for spinal anesthesia, local anesthetics are injected into the CSF

EGTA: Esophageal (gastric tube) airway; a cuffed tube that is inserted blindly into the esophagus and connected to a mask; this permits ventilation through the mask and gastric suctioning through the cuffed tube

ETCO₂: End-tidal carbon dioxide reported as a partial pressure; see Capnography section

ETT: Endotracheal tube

FIO₂: Fraction of inspired oxygen; this is a fraction (0.00 to 1.00) that corresponds to the percent (0% to 100%) of inspired oxygen

FO: Fiberoptic

mcg: Microgram

kg: Kilogram; 1 kg = 2.2 lb

LED: Light-emitting diode; an electronic device that emits light at a predetermined frequency

LMA: Laryngeal mask airway or laryngeal airway

MAC: Monitored anesthesia care; see Monitored Anesthesia Care section

mg: Milligram; 1×10^{-3} g

MH: Malignant hyperthermia; see Malignant Hyperthermia section

MHAUS: Malignant Hyperthermia Association of the United States

MMS: Master of medical science degree

MRI: Magnetic resonance imaging

NIOSH: National Institute for Occupational Safety and Health

nm: Nanometer; 1×10^{-9} m

NMS: Neuroleptic malignant syndrome; see Malignant Hyperthermia section

N₂O: Nitrous oxide

NSAID: Nonsteroidal antiinflammatory drug

PA: Pulmonary artery

PaCO₂: Partial pressure of arterial carbon dioxide; lowercase "a" denotes "arterial"; an uppercase "A" denotes "alveolar"

PaO₂: Partial pressure of arterial oxygen; lowercase "a" denotes "arterial"; an uppercase "A" denotes "alveolar"

PCA: Patient-controlled analgesia; see Pain Management section

PNB: Peripheral nerve block

ppm: Parts per million; 1 ppm = 1×10^{-6}

psi: Pounds per square inch; a measurement of pressure

QA: Quality assurance; this function also may be identified as quality improvement (QI), continuous quality improvement (CQI), or similar names

RSI: Rapid-sequence induction

SGA: Supraglottic airway device

SpO₂: Saturation (pulse) of oxygen or in a pulsating vessel, expressed as a percentage; see Pulse Oximetry section

SvO₂: Saturation of mixed venous oxygen in percentage; this measurement is made from a special pulmonary artery catheter

torr: A unit of pressure, being the pressure necessary to support a column of mercury one millimeter high at 0 degrees centigrade and standard gravity

that the anesthesia death rate has not declined, but patients are now older and sicker (Gottschalk et al, 2011).

The general public still considers anesthesia to be a major risk of surgery. This attitude may be attributable to sensationalized reports in the news media, magazine articles, and in movies. In addition, people may have a heightened awareness of anesthesia-related deaths because these often occur acutely in the perioperative period, whereas surgical or medical problems unrelated to anesthesia may not result in death until days after the procedure.

Environmental Noise

Many studies demonstrate the effects that noise has on humans. Multiple conversations, loud music, and other noises can create or worsen patient anxiety, as well as make communication difficult among team members and between the patient and team members. Noise can also cause distraction, increasing the potential for miscommunication and errors (AORN, 2013). Patients recovering during the immediate postoperative period have expressed dissatisfaction with high noise levels and overhearing staff member conversations. Improvement in patient satisfaction can be achieved when the noise level lessens in the postanesthesia care unit (PACU) (Smykowski, 2008). While the patient is in the operating room (OR), *especially* during induction and emergence, every effort should be made to maintain a calm, quiet environment. This is especially true when caring for the pediatric patient. Hearing multiple voices can create patient anxiety and confusion.

Awareness During Anesthesia

Remaining conscious during anesthesia is a concern of both patients and anesthesia providers. Some patients are so anxious about being aware of anything during surgery that it may affect their reasoning when discussing the options for anesthesia. Many procedures, such as biopsies, inguinal hernias, or procedures on the lower extremities, can be done under regional anesthesia or monitored anesthesia care (MAC). These patients may want general anesthesia, however, because they do not want to be aware of anything during the procedure. In rare cases, during general anesthesia for emergent procedures or trauma, the patient may be paralyzed, aware of what is occurring but unable to tell anyone.

Intraoperative awareness (IOA) is reported with multiple and differing anesthetic techniques. Several factors may contribute to its occurrence. Overall, 20,000 to 40,000 patients each year experience awareness during general anesthesia (Bazzell et al, 2008). The incidence of awareness may increase to 1% to 1.5% in higher risk patient populations, such as patients requiring anesthesia for obstetrics, major trauma, and cardiac surgery (Ghoneim et al, 2009).

For many years, the electroencephalogram (EEG) was the standard for assessing a person's hypnotic and sleep state. However, using an EEG for all surgical procedures is unrealistic. The late 1990s saw development of the bispectral index system (BIS), which analyzes the relationship and frequency of brain signals using an algorithm to generate a composite, numeric value that seems to correlate with the cerebral state. Four electrodes, positioned across the forehead, connect to a monitor that gives an index (0 to 100) of the patient's hypnotic state or sedation level; an index of 40 to 60 is considered optimal anesthesia. The system monitors the effects of anesthetics and sedatives on the hypnotic status of the brain, but is less informative about the level of analgesia. Motion artifacts and mental changes cause erratic changes under lighter levels of sedation commonly used with MAC. The BIS monitor is not a predictor of motor depression; it also lags by 3 to 5 seconds, leading to a potential for the anesthesia provider not anticipating a sudden rise in the depth of anesthesia. Nonetheless, use of the BIS monitor to alert the anesthesia provider to intraoperative awareness with recall (AWR) using a BIS-based protocol can be effective (Avidan and Mashour, 2013).

Preoperative Preparation

Patient Evaluation

Preoperative evaluation is done in advance of the scheduled surgical procedure, often 1 or more days before the procedure, in a preadmission clinic (sometimes called *preadmission testing, preanesthesia clinic,* or *anesthesia-assessment unit*). Preadmission staff secure admission data, appropriate consent forms, and a preoperative history; they also perform a physical examination, complete a preanesthesia evaluation and examination, obtain an airway history and patient's weight, and process appropriate diagnostic or laboratory tests. Numerous studies have shown only limited benefits from extensive routine preoperative testing (Chung et al, 2009). Patients with higher than average risk based on history are those who usually require more extensive testing. Preoperative care based on careful preanesthesia evaluation can result in significant reduction in costs (Issa, 2011). After assessing the patient's physical status, the anesthesia provider in the preadmission setting selects the most appropriate anesthetic technique. Resolving the patient's questions and concerns follows, as well as instructions aimed to expedite admission on the day of surgery. Prior to elective surgery, the patient should be in optimal medical condition. A primary benefit of preoperative testing is to identify patients at risk for perioperative complications so that appropriate perioperative therapy can foster a return to functional status. Morbidly obese patients present

technical and clinical challenges during anesthesia management (Ortiz and Wiener-Kronish, 2010).

Anesthesia, even in healthy patients, presents particular risks. Risk associated with anesthesia is unique in that rarely does the anesthetic itself offer benefit; rather, it allows performing surgical interventions and procedures that may benefit the patient enormously. Another goal in risk assessment is to inform patients so that they can weigh options and identify opportunities to alter that risk. Analysis of the first 2000 reports submitted in the Australian Incident Monitoring Study (AIMS) found a sixfold increase in mortality in patients who were inadequately assessed preoperatively. In a different study of anesthetic-related perioperative deaths, nearly 40% of deaths involved inadequate preoperative assessment and management (Miller, 2010). If it is determined that the patient's physical status should improve so as to reduce the risks involved, the patient's primary physician or surgeon discusses this with the patient, and, if necessary, elective surgery is deferred until the patient's condition optimizes. In emergent surgery, however, any benefits gained from a delay must be weighed carefully against the hazards of deferral.

The assignment of a physical status classification depends on the patient's physiologic condition independent of the proposed surgical procedure. The physical status classification was developed by the American Society of Anesthesiologists (ASA) to provide uniform guidelines. It is an evaluation of the severity of systemic diseases, physiologic dysfunction, and anatomic abnormalities. The ASA classification system is widely used to estimate perioperative risk (Table 5-1).

Although many hospitals and ambulatory surgery centers commonly use preadmission clinics, nurses may conduct preoperative telephone interviews with patients in reasonably good health. Such

TABLE 5-1

ASA Physical (P) Status Classification

Status*†	Definition	Description and Examples
P1	Normal healthy patient	No physiologic, psychologic, biochemical, or organic disturbance
P2	Patient with mild systemic disease	Cardiovascular disease with minimal restriction of activity; hypertension, asthma, chronic bronchitis, obesity, diabetes mellitus, or tobacco abuse; mild asthma or well-controlled hypertension. No significant impact on daily activity. Unlikely impact on anesthesia and surgery.
P3	Patient with a severe systemic disease that limits activity, but is not incapacitating	Cardiovascular or pulmonary disease that limits activity; severe diabetes with systemic complications; history of myocardial infarction, angina pectoris, poorly controlled hypertension, or morbid obesity; renal failure on dialysis or class 2 congestive heart failure. Significant impact on daily activity. Likely impact on anesthesia and surgery
P4	Patient with a severe systemic disease that is a constant threat to life or requires intensive therapy	Severe cardiac, pulmonary, renal, hepatic, or endocrine dysfunction, acute myocardial infarction, respiratory failure requiring mechanical ventilation. Serious limitation of daily activity. Major impact on anesthesia and surgery
P5	Moribund patient who is not expected to survive 24 hr with or without operation	Surgery is done as last recourse or resuscitative effort; major multisystem or cerebral trauma, ruptured aneurysm, or large pulmonary embolus
P6	Patient declared brain dead whose organs are being removed for donor purposes	

*In statuses 2, 3, and 4, the systemic disease may or may not be related to the reason for surgery.
†For any patient (P1 through P5) requiring emergency surgery, an E is added to the physical status, such as P1E, P2E. ASA 1 through ASA 6 or I to VI is often used for physical status.
Modified from American Society of Anesthesiologists (ASA): *Manual for anesthesia departments,* Park Ridge, IL, 1997, The Association, available at www.asahq.org/Home/For-Members/Clinical-Information/ASA-Physical-Status-Classification-System. Accessed February 3, 2013

nurses pose questions relating to pulmonary and cardiac disease; medication (prescription, over-the-counter, herbal and homeopathic remedies) and alcohol use; medication, latex, or anesthetic allergies; pregnancy; and personal or family history of anesthetic reactions. The preadmission interview, whether by phone or in person, provides an opportunity for patient education as it relates to the proposed procedure (Patient and Family Education).

On the day of surgery, patients arrive 1 to 2 hours before the scheduled surgery to complete other preoperative processes. In some facilities certain ambulatory patients are evaluated further just before surgery. These are usually healthy patients having minor procedures or patients with stable, chronic conditions about to undergo a procedure (e.g., cataract removal, skin lesion excision) under MAC. These preadmission processes reduce costs of healthcare, decrease risk of healthcare-associated infections associated with longer hospital admissions, increase use and efficiency of healthcare resources, improve patient relations, and enhance the chances of having a well-informed patient in optimal health status both before and after the proposed procedure.

In larger hospitals and ambulatory surgery centers the patient evaluator in the preanesthesia clinic is often not the anesthesia provider for the patient's surgical procedure. Immediately before surgery, therefore, the anesthesia provider (1) reviews the patient's chart, laboratory data, and diagnostic studies, such as electrocardiogram (ECG) and chest x-ray if ordered and necessary; (2) confirms that the appropriate consent forms (surgery, anesthesia, use of blood products) have been signed; (3) identifies the patient; (4) verifies the surgical procedure; (5) reviews the choice of anesthesia; (6) examines the patient; and (7) administers preoperative medications as indicated (Miller, 2010). As ambulatory surgery becomes increasingly common, other factors are taken into consideration (Ambulatory Surgery Considerations).

Choice of Anesthesia

The patient, anesthesia provider, and surgeon make the choice of anesthesia for a given surgical procedure. Many factors influence this choice, including the following:

1. Patient's wishes and understanding of the types of anesthesia that could be used
2. Patient's physiologic status
3. Presence and severity of coexisting diseases
4. Patient's mental and psychologic status
5. Postoperative recovery from various kinds of anesthesia
6. Options for management of postoperative pain
7. Type and duration of surgical procedure
8. Patient's position during surgery
9. Surgeon's particular requirements

Premedication

The primary purpose of premedication before anesthesia is to sedate the patient and reduce anxiety. Medications that may be given preoperatively include sedatives and hypnotics, anxiolytics, amnestics, tranquilizers, narcotics or other analgesics, antiemetics, and anticholinergics. A single medication may possess the properties of several medication classes. Midazolam (Versed) is administered frequently to relieve apprehension and to provide amnesia. An analgesic or narcotic may be ordered if preoperative discomfort is anticipated during invasive procedures or during the administration of a regional anesthetic. An anticholinergic, such as atropine or glycopyrrolate, may be used to prevent bradycardia in pediatric

---

PATIENT AND FAMILY EDUCATION
Preanesthesia Preparation

During preoperative assessment the patient is interviewed, and it is important to discuss the following topics:

Preoperative fasting: Explain why it is important, namely, to prevent possible vomiting and gastric aspiration.

Medications: Patients should take necessary medications (such as antihypertensive, cardiac, seizure, and asthma medications) with sips of water, preferably before they leave their homes to come to the facility. Patients with diabetes should continue taking oral hypoglycemic agents until the evening before surgery. If the patient takes insulin, it is common to administer a fraction (one fourth to one half) of the usual morning dose. Aspirin and aspirin-containing products should be discontinued 1 week before surgery. Nonsteroidal antiinflammatory drugs should be discontinued 4 days before surgery. If the patient is taking warfarin, it is usually discontinued 3 days before surgery, if appropriate. The prescribing clinician may need to be consulted to ensure it is safe to discontinue these medications or switch to alternative medications, especially if the patient has recently undergone heart valve replacement surgery or has other serious conditions that must be taken into consideration.

Herbal supplements: Many herbal supplements can interact with anesthetics. It is important to ask about any supplements the patient is taking (see Chapter 30).

Recent upper respiratory tract infections: A patient with a reactive airway has an increased risk of respiratory complications (e.g., bronchospasm, laryngospasm).

Family-centered preanesthesia preparation for children and their families includes treatment options for anxiety, such as administering sedatives, having a parent present during induction, and providing hospital-based preparation programs (Kain et al, 2007). Preanesthesia patient and family education may also include postoperative care instructions and information about pain control, both nonpharmacologic (e.g., distraction, progressive muscle relaxation, diaphragmatic breathing [Roy-Byrne et al, 2009], ice, elevation) and pharmacologic (e.g., how pain will be assessed, when and how medication will be administered). A study by Kastanias and colleagues (2009) determined that information about pain management strategies and medication side effects was extremely important to patients ready to be discharged. Because patients place high importance on information about pain, anesthesia providers and perioperative nurses include discussion of after-discharge pain management plans as part of patient and family education.

An anesthesia provider will also discuss the anesthesia options appropriate for that patient/procedure after reviewing pertinent history and physical information as provided, along with any pertinent diagnostic studies and consultations. The American Association of Nurse Anesthetists (AANA) has a number of patient education brochures available on its website. These brochures can be printed and offered to patients and their families, or the perioperative nurse can simply direct the patient and family to the appropriate website, namely, to www.aana.com/forpatients/pages/Brochures-and-Resources.aspx (accessed April 29, 2013).

Modified from Kain ZN et al: Family-centered preparation for surgery improves perioperative outcomes in children, *Anesthesiology* 106:65–74, 2007; Kastanias P et al: What do adult surgical patients really want to know about pain and pain management? *Pain Manag Nurs* 10(1):22–31, 2009; Roy-Byrne P et al: Brief intervention for anxiety in primary care patients, *J Am Board Fam Med* 22(2):175–186, 2009.

AMBULATORY SURGERY CONSIDERATIONS

Patient Selection

Ambulatory surgery is increasingly common. About 75% of procedures performed in this country are done on an ambulatory basis. Ambulatory surgery may be a "same day" procedure in the hospital, in an office, or in an ambulatory surgery center (ASC). Patients usually enjoy an earlier return to their preoperative physiologic state and fewer complications with ambulatory surgery compared with surgery performed on an inpatient basis in the hospital setting. When performed on an ambulatory basis, procedures also offer a reduced chance of healthcare-associated infections (HAIs). Technologic and medical advances, such as improved administration of anesthesia and development of minimally invasive or noninvasive procedures, have also driven the observed increase in outpatient procedures. For example, minimally invasive arthroscopic procedures require smaller incisions, less cutting of soft tissues, less blood loss, and shorter recovery times as compared to less advanced surgical procedures. Advances in medical devices and pharmaceuticals have also contributed to reduced recovery times, furthering the preference for outpatient surgery. One study of community hospitals in 28 states found that the mean charge for outpatient surgery was $6,100, as compared to the mean cost of inpatient surgery at $39,900. Cost savings have influenced growth in the number of free-standing ASCs: they increased more than 10-fold, from 239 in 1983 to more than 3300, about two decades later (Sharamitaro and Seiler, 2010).

Surgical procedures performed in ambulatory settings continue to grow and broaden in number. Procedures with prolonged immobilization, parenteral pain management, and/or increased incidence of complications, however, continue generally to be performed on an inpatient basis (Marley and Calabrese, 2014).

Patient selection for ambulatory procedures is extremely important. The procedure should have neither a significant incidence of perioperative or postoperative problems, nor require intensive postoperative management (Marley and Calabrese, 2014). The patient should be in general good health or have well-managed existing illnesses. Patients with a significant history should be interviewed before the day of surgery to determine how well coexisting diseases are controlled and what tests or consultations may be needed before the day of surgery.

The following are some patient conditions for which ambulatory surgery is unacceptable:

- Premature infants (gestational age 37 weeks or less at birth)
- Infants with a history of respiratory difficulties, apneic episodes, or feeding difficulties
- Unstable physical status (ASA classification III or IV) (see Table 5-1)
- Active substance or alcohol abuse
- Poorly controlled seizures
- Previously unevaluated and unmanaged obstructive sleep apnea
- Uncontrolled diabetes
- Infectious process requiring isolation
- Anticipation of postoperative pain not controllable with oral analgesics
- Inability to care for self and without access to assistance
- Noncompliance (Marley and Calabrese, 2014)

Anesthetic technique is based on the surgical procedure, surgeon and patient preference, and skill of the practitioner. Goals for anesthesia in an ambulatory setting include minimal physiologic changes secondary to the anesthetic, fast induction, rapid emergence while maintaining patient comfort, intraoperative amnesia and analgesia, suitable operating conditions, minimal perioperative side effects, and minimized postoperative side effects, such as nausea (Marley and Calabrese, 2014). Use of a laryngeal mask airway (LMA), awareness monitoring, and certain anesthetics (such as propofol, sevoflurane, and desflurane) contribute to attaining these goals.

Modified from Marley RA, Calabrese T: Outpatient anesthesia. In Nagelhout JJ, Plaus KL, editors: *Nurse anesthesia*, ed 5, St Louis, 2014, Saunders; Sharamitaro A, Seiler R: Outpatient surgeries show dramatic increase, *Health Capital Topics* 3(5), 2010, available at www.healthcapital.com/hcc/newsletter/05_10/Outpatient.pdf. Accessed February 3, 2013.

---

patients, to control secretions in patients undergoing oropharyngeal procedures, or to control cardiac reflex that may cause bradycardia (e.g., during ophthalmic procedures) (Miller, 2010).

To decrease the risk of aspiration, metoclopramide (Reglan) may be given to empty the stomach and to reduce nausea and vomiting. In addition, an antacid or an H_2-receptor–blocking medication, such as cimetidine (Tagamet), ranitidine (Zantac), or famotidine (Pepcid), may be included to decrease gastric acid production or the acidity of the gastric contents, or both. Chemoprophylaxis, with medications such as these, is part of safe airway management.

Before administering premedication, the anesthesia team answers any last-minute questions from the patient concerning surgery and anesthesia, and completes the preoperative verification process, or "anesthesia time-out," to ensure that all relevant documents (e.g., the history and physical examination, surgical consent) and imaging studies (properly labeled and displayed) are available before the start of the procedure. The anesthesia team reviews these documents, which must be consistent with the patient's stated expectations (when the patient is awake and aware, the patient should actively participate in the verification process). The surgical team must agree that this is the correct patient and the correct procedure on the correct side and site. Any additional special equipment, supplies, or implants also are confirmed as correct and available. Team members must also mark the surgical site before administering premedication.

Administration of premedication(s) may be intramuscular (IM), intravenous (IV), intranasal, or oral (PO) with 15 to 30 mL of water. Patients usually prefer oral premedication, and the small amount of water is readily absorbed directly across the gastric mucosa. Except for the small amount of water needed to swallow any medications, adult patients traditionally must maintain a nothing-by-mouth (NPO) status for a minimum of 4 to 6 hours before elective surgery. More recent data suggest, however, that clear liquids are acceptable up to 2 hours before surgery (ASA, 2011) (Table 5-2). Alternatively, IV premedication is administered 30 to 90 minutes before surgery in preoperative holding or after the patient arrives in the surgical suite. Medication shortages in the United States have had an effect on the preoperative medication chosen (Research Highlight).

Although premedication use is common, studies have shown that visits before surgery by the anesthesia provider and the perioperative nurse are similarly important to relieve patient anxiety and concern. Major patient concerns include fear of the unknown, relinquishing control of one's life to someone else, being awake during surgery, and not awakening from anesthesia, as well as concerns related to the surgery itself (e.g., diagnosis, prognosis).

TABLE 5-2

NPO Fasting Guidelines*

Ingested Material Allowed	Minimal Fasting Period Recommended
Food and fluids as desired	Up to 8 hours
Light meal (e.g., toast and clear liquids, infant formula, and non-human milk)	Up to 6 hours
Breast milk	Up to 4 hours
Clear liquids only, NO solid food or foods with fat content†	Up to 2 hours
No solids or liquids	During the 2 hours until surgical time

*These guidelines are recommended for healthy patients undergoing elective procedures. They are not intended for women in labor. They do not guarantee complete gastric emptying. The fasting periods noted above apply to patients of all ages.

†Clear liquids include water, fruit juices without pulp, black coffee, clear tea, and carbonated beverages. Patients should also be instructed not to chew gum or eat any candies or mints. The type of fluid is more important than the amount and should never include alcohol.

Modified from The American Society of Anesthesiologists: *Practice guidelines for preoperative fasting and the use of pharmacologic agents to reduce the risk of pulmonary aspiration: application to healthy patients undergoing elective procedures,* an updated report, *Anesthesiology* 114(3):495–511, 2011.

Premedication may be unnecessary for older patients because their anxiety levels are lower, their responses to medications are unpredictable, and IV sedation can be given in the OR if required.

Types of Anesthesia Care

TJC has issued its *Comprehensive Accreditation Manual for Hospitals,* which includes anesthesia care standards that apply when patients receive, in any setting, moderate or deep sedation or general, spinal, or other major regional anesthesia. Descriptions of frequently used classifications of anesthesia care follow.

General Anesthesia

General anesthesia is a reversible, unconscious state characterized by amnesia (sleep, hypnosis, or basal narcosis), analgesia (freedom from pain), depression of reflexes, muscle relaxation, and homeostasis or specific manipulation of physiologic systems and functions. Most patients think of general anesthesia when they are scheduled to have a surgical procedure; that is, they expect to be "put to sleep." As such, they experience a medication-induced loss of consciousness during which they are not arousable. Their ability to maintain ventilatory function is often impaired, requiring assistance maintaining a patent airway. Positive-pressure ventilation may be required, given the possibility of decreased spontaneous ventilation or medication-induced depression of neuromuscular function.

RESEARCH HIGHLIGHT

Medication Shortages and Long-Term Implications

Since 2006 there has been a fourfold increase in the number of medications involved in a decreased availability or "shortage," with about 65% being injectables. This has placed a heavy burden on hospitals, infusion clinics, and anesthesia sites that offer invasive procedures and surgery. The largest categories of medications undergoing shortages are those that affect the central nervous system, with an average length of delay consisting of 286 days.

The question is often asked, why are medications of any type in short supply in a modern era of healthcare? It is reported that 54% of medication shortages in 2011 alone had no identified reason for disruption of supply. There are multiple reasons, however, that can explain a medication being in short supply:

1. Manufacturing difficulties: equipment issues that cause contamination of product
2. Lack of raw materials: 80% comes from outside the United States
3. Lack of U.S. Food and Drug Administration (FDA) staff to do timely inspections
4. Sole manufacturers unable to meet supply demands
5. Lack of notice and limited time to prepare for medication's unavailability
6. Facilities' use of lean and efficient inventory policies that promote a "just in time" response to resupply to keep costs down and increase cash flow
7. A manufacturer that changes focus of a medication (e.g., formulation or changing emphasis on a product line for financial reasons)
8. A new indication for a specific medication
9. A sudden outbreak of disease and increased demand for preventive or treatment medications

The short-term implication of all these reasons collectively is of course the unavailability of a certain medication to treat a specific disease process or of one to use as part of a therapeutic treatment regimen. This could delay or cancel a therapeutic treatment or surgical procedure with possible adverse outcomes for the patient. Many facilities seek alternative medications in order to continue to provide services for patients. The FDA has allowed several medications to be marketed in the United States that did not have its approval in the past. The long-term issues of these alternative medications are the possible adverse events that can arise when providers use unfamiliar medications, as well as the subtle differences between new and old medications. For example, substitutes may require changes in delivery protocols in which, instead of mcg/kg/min, the substitute medication must be delivered in mcg/kg/hr. As well, there may be incorrect dosing due to changes in concentration of similar medications, such as having in stock previously 0.4 mg/mL atropine and the newer supply comes in 1 mg/mL, whereas both are found in similar 1-mL vials. Also departments may split-dose medications from larger quantity vials into smaller, more appropriate volumes for multiple patient dose delivery. These actions, although well intentioned, as they aim to increase the length of time a medication is available, directly violate The Joint Commission (TJC) standards that require strictly sterile conditions, usually only available in a pharmacy department, to break up what are single-dose, single-patient supplies into multiple-dose medications for multiple patients. Until resolution of these multiple safety issues, perioperative nurses must remain vigilant as to what medications are affected in their facility and what measures are used to secure substitutes.

Modified from Meyer T: *The anatomy of the drug shortages,* available at www.apsf.org/newsletters/html/2012/spring/04_shortage.htm. Accessed January 23, 2013.

Regional Anesthesia

Regional anesthesia is defined broadly as a reversible loss of sensation in a specific area or region of the body when a local anesthetic is injected to block or anesthetize nerve fibers in and around the operative site. Common regional anesthesia includes spinal (also called "subarachnoid block" or SAB), epidural, caudal, and major peripheral nerve blocks. Although ultrasound guidance has been reviewed as a technique to enhance regional anesthesia and analgesia, it may not eliminate complications such as blood vessel puncture or inadvertent intraneural or intravascular injections. Nonetheless, in some healthcare facilities, ultrasound-guided regional anesthesia and analgesia is used to reduce time or number of attempts to perform blocks (Liu et al, 2009).

Monitored Anesthesia Care

MAC is infiltration of the surgical site with a local anesthetic and is performed by the surgeon (note that "*local standby*" and "*anesthesia standby*" are older, less accurate terms frequently used interchangeably with MAC). The anesthesia provider then supplements the local anesthesia with IV medications that provide sedation and systemic analgesia, monitors the patient's vital functions, and may use additional medication to optimize the patient's physiologic status. MAC is often used for healthy patients undergoing relatively minor surgical procedures. It also may be used for some procedures for critically ill patients who may tolerate a general anesthetic poorly.

Moderate Sedation/Analgesia

Moderate sedation/analgesia (conscious sedation) is administered for specific short-term surgical, diagnostic, and therapeutic procedures performed within a hospital or ambulatory center. As early as 2003, the ASA updated its *Practice Guidelines for Sedation and Analgesia by Non-Anesthesiologists*. The Association of periOperative Registered Nurses (AORN) went on to define moderate sedation/analgesia as "a drug-induced, mild depression of consciousness achieved by the administration of sedatives or the combination of sedatives and analgesic medications, most often administered intravenously, and titrated to achieve a desired effect" (2013, p. 411). Patients can maintain a patent airway and require no interventions; spontaneous ventilation remains adequate. Cardiovascular function is usually maintained. Patients whose only response is reflex withdrawal from a painful stimulus are sedated to a greater degree than that encompassed by conscious sedation/analgesia.

The demand for appropriate providers to administer and monitor the patient receiving conscious sedation/analgesia has grown and now exceeds the supply of anesthesia providers. This demand has resulted in increased use of professional registered nurses with additional training in administering moderate sedation/analgesia medications and monitoring these patients. Various medications and techniques are used to achieve conscious sedation/analgesia, each with advantages and disadvantages. Competency-based education programs and assessment should be established for nurse-monitored sedation. AORN publishes recommendations for managing patients undergoing moderate sedation/analgesia that should be used by healthcare facilities to develop such programs (AORN, 2013).

Local Anesthesia

Local anesthesia refers to the administration of an anesthetic agent to one part of the body by local infiltration or topical application, usually administered by the surgeon. Local anesthesia is used (1) for minor procedures, (2) if the patient's cooperation is necessary for the procedure, or (3) if the patient's physical condition warrants its use. An anesthesia provider is not involved in the patient's care. A perioperative nurse monitors the patient's vital signs, observes for symptoms of toxicity (Wolfe, 2011), and provides supportive care during the procedure. AORN (2013) recommendations for managing patients undergoing local anesthesia and documenting patient care should be used to establish policies and procedures in operative and other invasive settings.

Perioperative Monitoring

Significant advances continue in perioperative monitoring. Among medical specialties, anesthesiology has been a pioneer in review and analysis of perioperative mishaps and implementation of improved monitoring techniques and guidelines. These monitors include pulse oximetry, which measures oxygen saturation in a pulsating vessel (SpO_2), and capnography, which measures end-tidal carbon dioxide ($ETCO_2$) level (Kossick, 2014). These advances have resulted in significant decreases in morbidity and mortality (Matten and Deshur, 2012).

The ASA (2011) amended its Standards for Basic Anesthetic Monitoring (Patient Safety) as guidelines for patient care. Perioperative nurses should be familiar with these standards and understand their significance in patient safety. If routine or frequent deviations from such standards occur, a performance assessment and improvement (also known as *quality assurance* [QA]) review along with a risk management analysis should be considered to ensure safe and high-quality patient care (ECRI Institute, 2009).

Monitors and basic anesthetic monitoring include the following:

- Inspired oxygen analyzer (FIO_2), which is calibrated to room air on a daily basis
- Low-pressure disconnect alarm, which senses pressure in the expiratory limb of the patient circuit
- Inspiratory airway pressure
- Respirometer (these first four devices are an integral part of most modern anesthesia machines)
- Electrocardioscope
- Blood pressure (usually measured with a noninvasive automated unit)
- Heart rate
- Precordial or esophageal stethoscope
- Temperature
- Peripheral nerve stimulator if muscle relaxants are used
- SpO_2
- $ETCO_2$

Newer models of anesthesia machines have basic monitors integrated into a computerized system. These generally include FIO_2; inspired and expired CO_2; inspired and expired volatile agents; airway pressure and disconnect alarms; tidal volume, respiratory rate, and minute ventilation; noninvasive blood pressure (systolic, diastolic, and mean); SpO_2 and pulse rate; temperature; and an event marker. A sophisticated, prioritized system displays caution or alarm conditions in one location, making it unnecessary to scan numerous individual monitors with a variety of displays when an alarm sounds. Perioperative nurses ensure that all appropriate monitor alarm systems are on and active, and that issues of "alarm fatigue" (Welch, 2012) have not induced the anesthesia provider to shut off these alarms.

Based on the cardiovascular and pulmonary status of the patient, scheduled surgical procedure, and the chance of significant physiologic changes, additional invasive monitors may prove necessary.

PATIENT SAFETY

Standards for Basic Anesthetic Monitoring

These standards apply to all anesthesia care, although in emergency circumstances appropriate life support measures take precedence. These standards may be exceeded at any time based on the judgment of the responsible anesthesiologist. They are intended to encourage quality patient care, but observing them cannot guarantee any specific patient outcome. They are subject to revision from time to time, as warranted by the evolution of technology and practice. They apply to all general anesthetics, regional anesthetics, and monitored anesthesia care. This set of standards addresses only the issue of basic anesthetic monitoring, which is one component of anesthesia care. In certain rare or unusual circumstances, some of these methods of monitoring may be clinically impractical, and appropriate use of the described monitoring methods may fail to detect untoward clinical developments. Brief interruptions of continual monitoring may be unavoidable. These standards are not intended to apply to the care of the obstetric patient in labor or in the conduct of pain management.

Standard I

Qualified anesthesia personnel shall be present in the room throughout administration of all general anesthetics, regional anesthetics, and monitored anesthesia care.

Objective

Given the rapidity of possible changes in patient status during anesthesia, qualified anesthesia personnel shall be continuously present to monitor the patient and to provide anesthesia care. In the event there is a direct known hazard (e.g., radiation to anesthesia personnel that might require intermittent remote observation of the patient), some provision for monitoring the patient must be made. In the event that an emergency requires the temporary absence of the person primarily responsible for the anesthetic, the best judgment of the anesthesiologist will be exercised in comparing the emergency with the anesthetized patient's condition and in the selection of the person left responsible for the anesthetic during the temporary absence.

Standard II

During administration of all anesthetics, patient oxygenation, ventilation, circulation, and temperature shall be evaluated continually.

Oxygenation

Objective

To ensure adequate oxygen concentration in the inspired gas and the blood during all anesthetics

Methods

1. *Inspired gas:* During every administration of general anesthesia using an anesthesia machine, the concentration of oxygen in the patient breathing system shall be measured by an oxygen analyzer with a low oxygen concentration limit alarm in use.*
2. *Blood oxygenation:* During all anesthetics, a quantitative method of assessing oxygenation such as pulse oximetry shall be used.* When the pulse oximeter is used, the variable pitch pulse tone and the low threshold alarm shall be audible to the anesthesiologist or anesthesia care team personnel.* Adequate illumination and exposure of the patient are necessary to assess color.*

Ventilation

Objective

To ensure adequate ventilation of the patient during all anesthetics

Methods

1. Every patient receiving general anesthesia shall have the adequacy of ventilation continually evaluated. Qualitative clinical signs such as chest excursion, observation of the reservoir breathing bag, and auscultation of breath sounds are useful. Continual monitoring for the presence of expired carbon dioxide shall occur unless invalidated by the nature of the patient, procedure, or equipment. Quantitative monitoring of the volume of expired gas is strongly encouraged.*
2. When an endotracheal tube or laryngeal mask is inserted, its correct positioning must be verified by clinical assessment and by identification of carbon dioxide in the expired gas. Continual end-tidal carbon dioxide analysis, in use from the time of endotracheal tube/laryngeal mask placement, until extubation/removal or initiating transfer to a postoperative care location, shall be performed using a quantitative method such as capnography, capnometry, or mass spectroscopy.* When capnography or capnometry is used, the end-tidal CO_2 alarm shall be audible to the anesthesiologist or anesthesia care team personnel.*
3. When a mechanical ventilator controls ventilation, there shall be in continuous use a device capable of detecting disconnection of components of the breathing system. The device must sound an audible signal when it exceeds the alarm threshold.
4. During regional anesthesia (with no sedation) or local anesthesia (with no sedation), the adequacy of ventilation shall be evaluated by continual observation of qualitative clinical signs. During moderate or deep sedation, the adequacy of ventilation shall be evaluated by continual observation of qualitative clinical signs and monitoring for the presence of exhaled carbon dioxide unless precluded or invalidated by the nature of the patient, procedure, or equipment.

Circulation

Objective

To ensure the adequacy of the patient's circulatory function during all anesthetics

Methods

1. Every patient receiving anesthesia shall have an electrocardiogram continuously displayed from beginning of anesthesia to preparing to leave the anesthetizing location.*
2. Every patient receiving anesthesia shall have arterial blood pressure and heart rate determined and evaluated at least every 5 minutes.*
3. Every patient receiving general anesthesia shall have, in addition to the above, circulatory function continually evaluated by at least one of the following: palpation of a pulse, auscultation of heart sounds, monitoring of a tracing of intra-arterial pressure, ultrasound peripheral pulse monitoring, or pulse plethysmography or oximetry.

Body Temperature

Objective

To aid in the maintenance of appropriate body temperature during all anesthetics

Methods

Every patient receiving anesthesia shall have temperature monitored when clinically significant changes in body temperature are intended, anticipated, or suspected.

Note that "continual" is defined as "repeated regularly and frequently in steady rapid succession," whereas "continuous" means "prolonged without any interruption at any time."
*Under extenuating circumstances, the responsible anesthesiologist may waive requirements marked with an asterisk (*); it is recommended that when this is done, it should be so stated (including the reasons) in a note in the patient's medical record.
Modified from the American Society of Anesthesiologists (ASA), Park Ridge, IL. Approved by the ASA House of Delegates on October 21, 1986, and last amended on October 20, 2010 with an effective date of July 1, 2011.

These include direct arterial and venous pressure measurements, a pulmonary arterial catheter (PAC), and continuous mixed venous O_2 saturation (SvO_2) measured with a special PAC. One type of PAC provides a continuous measurement of cardiac output, using pulsed thermodilution to provide intermittent heat along a distal segment of the catheter. Small changes in the temperature of the blood are proportional to blood flow (cardiac output). These changes are sensed by a thermistor on the tip of the catheter (Contrera et al, 2014).

For certain conditions, equipment such as transcutaneous O_2 and CO_2 monitors, transesophageal echocardiography (TEE), evoked potentials, EEG, and cerebral or neurologic function monitors may be required. An indwelling urinary catheter is frequently inserted to provide a useful indication of renal function and hemodynamic status.

For procedures posing a risk of venous air embolism, a Doppler probe may be used. A central venous catheter is inserted, and the probe is placed over the right side of the heart, along the right sternal border between the third and sixth intercostal spaces. Positioning is confirmed if there is a change in Doppler signal after a 10-mL bolus of saline is rapidly injected through the catheter. The signal is monitored for the sound of a "mill-wheel" murmur. TEE is the most sensitive method of detection, but may also be the most expensive (Ranalli and Taylor, 2014).

Somatosensory evoked potential (SEP) monitoring may be used during some neurosurgery procedures (Chawla, 2012). It is used widely to assess the integrity of the spinal cord during surgery in which the spinal cord is manipulated. Upper and lower extremities may be monitored. Electrodes are usually placed preoperatively, but occasionally may be placed in the OR, before administration of anesthesia. Ischemia of ascending somatosensory pathways produces a drop in amplitude or loss of waveforms, thus warning the surgeon to take corrective action. Ischemic changes are usually widespread; rarely, however, is motor function lost when somatosensory pathways have not been affected.

Despite some controversy, most anesthesia providers believe that the monitoring used depends on the physiologic status and stability of the patient, the surgical procedure planned and its potential for sudden changes in cardiopulmonary functions, the anticipated blood loss and major fluid shifts, and the anticipated monitoring needs for postoperative management. Although not yet a standard of care, many facilities use the BIS monitor. This monitoring modality is a processed EEG obtained noninvasively from scalp electrodes. It provides a measure of the sedative and hypnotic effects of anesthetic medications on the central nervous system (CNS). Monitoring of some parameters may be negated by the anesthetic technique selected (Clark and Curdt, 2014).

Pulse Oximetry

Pulse oximetry works by analyzing the pulsatile arterial component of blood flow, thereby ensuring that arterial saturation (SpO_2) rather than venous saturation is being measured. Two wavelengths of light are used, usually 660 nm (red) and 940 nm (infrared), because oxygenated and deoxygenated blood absorbs light quite differently at these wavelengths. At 660 nm, HbO_2 (oxygenated hemoglobin) absorbs less light than HbR (reduced hemoglobin, or deoxyhemoglobin) does, whereas the opposite is observed with infrared light. Two diodes emitting light of each wavelength are placed on one side of the probe and a photo diode that senses the transmitted light on the opposite side. The amount of light absorbed at each wavelength by the pulsatile arterial component (AC) of blood flow

differentiates itself from baseline absorbance of the nonpulsatile component and surrounding tissue (DC) (Miller, 2010). Given that absorption by other tissue components is essentially constant, the major variable is saturation of hemoglobin with O_2. An internal microprocessor analyzes variations in absorption of light emitted from both light-emitting diodes (LEDs) and provides a readout of the percent saturation of hemoglobin with O_2. Pulse rate also is given. The pulse oximeter converts the detected light to a plethysmographic signal that measures the drop in light intensity with each beat (Bozimowski, 2014).

The O_2 dissociation curve indicates the percentage of totally saturated hemoglobin with O_2. The following values are approximations (the O_2 saturation [SpO_2] values are percentages and the PaO_2 levels are in torr): 98% to 100% ($\geq$95 torr), 90% (60 torr), 75% (39 torr), 50% (26 torr), and 25% (16 torr). Most pulse oximeters are accurate to within ±2% greater than 70% and ±3% from 50% to 70% but correlate poorly at less than 50%. When breathing room air, the SpO_2 for a young, healthy individual should be 98% to 100%; the SpO_2 percentage for an elderly patient may be in the low 90s, whereas the percentage for a heavy smoker or a patient with severe lung disease may be in the 80s. It is wise to establish a baseline SpO_2 value of a patient before any O_2, medications, or stimulation is introduced. Maintenance of SpO_2 levels greater than 90% corresponds to a PaO_2 value of 60 torr or greater.

The pulse oximeter reading (often referred to as "pulse ox") can be adversely affected by any event that significantly reduces vascular pulsations, such as hypoperfusion, hypotension, hypovolemia, vasoconstriction, or hypothermia. Electrosurgery, motion, or ambient light may also cause artifacts that will decrease the readout falsely. Carboxyhemoglobin (carbon monoxide bound to hemoglobin) falsely elevates indicated SpO_2 saturation, whereas methemoglobin (hemoglobin that has an oxidized iron molecule and cannot reversibly combine with O_2) falsely lowers SpO_2 measurements. IV dyes may affect the pulse oximeter. Methylene blue may cause a drop to 65% for 1 to 2 minutes; indigo carmine, a very slight decrease; and indocyanine green, a slightly greater decrease. Nail polish also can decrease SpO_2 values. Blue, black, or green polish significantly decreases the SpO_2 value, whereas red polish has only a slight effect. Opaque, acrylic nail coverings may block the light beam. Some studies suggest the more advanced monitors have virtually eliminated these effects (Bozimowski, 2014). If nail polish or coverings seem to cause problems, the sensor can be turned sideways so that the fingernail is parallel to the light path.

The sensor usually is placed on a finger or a toe. Some manufacturers have sensors for the earlobe and the bridge of the nose, as well as smaller ones for soles and palms of infants and children. Modern devices are calibrated against laboratory SaO_2 down to 70% saturation, and lower saturations are determined by extrapolation of the curve. Thus the user cannot calibrate pulse oximeters, and their reliability is dependent on the quality of signal processing and the stored calibration curve. Care must be taken to prevent localized neurovascular or ischemic damage. For example, a hard-cased sensor placed on a finger may cause ischemia when the arms are tightly secured at the patient's side during a long procedure.

If trouble with the pulse oximeter arises with use of a local anesthetic, the perioperative nurse should evaluate the patient's ventilatory status, verify proper placement of the sensor, and rule out the factors just listed that may adversely affect operation of the unit. Pulsatile blood flow in the extremity may be inadequate because of hypovolemia, decreased cardiac output, malpositioning, constriction by the blood pressure cuff, or hypothermia. As a final step the nurse can place the sensor on his or her own finger to verify satisfactory function of the pulse oximetry unit, cable, and sensor.

Capnography

A capnometer measures CO_2 concentration; it produces a capnograph that displays the CO_2 waveform. The capnograph provides a continuous display of the CO_2 concentration of gases from the airways. CO_2 concentration at the end of normal exhalation ($ETCO_2$, $P_{ET}CO_2$) is a reflection of gas from the distal alveoli; it therefore represents an estimate of alveolar concentration ($P_A CO_2$). When ventilation and perfusion are well matched, the $P_A CO_2$ closely approximates the $PaCO_2$, and $P_A CO_2 \cong PaCO_2 \cong PetCO_2$ (where $PaCO_2$ is partial pressure arterial, $P_A CO_2$ is alveolar partial pressure, and $P_{ET}CO_2$ is end-tidal partial pressure). The normal gradient between $PaCO_2$ and $P_{ET}CO_2$ is more than 6 mm Hg. The gradient between $PaCO_2$ and $P_{ET}CO_2$ increases when pulmonary perfusion is reduced or ventilation is maldistributed (Hagberg, 2013). Under general anesthesia the gas is sampled at the point where the endotracheal tube (ETT) connects to the patient breathing circuit. During other types of anesthesia, in which oxygen is administered via a nasal cannula, a small-bore tube is connected to the cannula, which is then attached to the anesthesia machine so that $ETCO_2$ levels can be measured. CO_2 analyzers use various principles to measure CO_2 in the inspired and exhaled gases on a breath-to-breath basis and display the CO_2 waveform by mass spectrometry, infrared absorption spectrometry, or Raman scattering. Although capnography typically distinguishes tracheal from esophageal intubation, false-negative results (i.e., ETT in trachea, absent waveform) and false-positive results (i.e., ETT in esophagus or pharynx, present waveform) have been reported (Hagberg, 2013).

Compact units that provide a continuous indication of the $ETCO_2$ level are the most widely used. These units measure the amount of infrared light absorbed by CO_2 in the sample of gas. Two types of monitors are in use. In the *mainstream* unit, all respired gas passes through the detector, whereas in the *sidestream* unit, a portion of the gas is aspirated at a constant rate (50 to 250 mL/min) through small-bore tubing into the unit. Each design has advantages. Most units display a waveform of expiratory CO_2 partial pressure relative to time after a short sampling and processing delay. The waveform is important to interpret output data correctly. Digital readouts usually give $ETCO_2$ and respiratory rate. Daily user calibration is rarely required with newer units. The units confirm proper endotracheal intubation and are useful to detect anesthesia circuit disconnection, alveolar ventilation, early return of respiratory function after muscle relaxants are used, and acute alterations in metabolic functions, such as malignant hyperthermia (MH) or thyrotoxicosis (Bozimowski, 2014).

Anesthesia Machines and Anesthetic Gases

The first apparatus resembling an anesthesia machine was used in 1905. Since then innumerable changes and improvements have been made. Anesthesia machines look complicated, but the basic functions are similar and simple to understand. Perioperative nurses should be familiar with the basic function of anesthesia machines (Figure 5-1) because they may need to administer O_2 during procedures with local anesthesia or conscious sedation/analgesia.

Facility pipelines usually supply oxygen, N_2O, and air to the anesthesia machine at pressures of 50 to 55 pounds per square inch (psi). Gas hoses connected to the machine are color-coded: green (O_2); blue (N_2O); and yellow (medical air). Connectors are specific

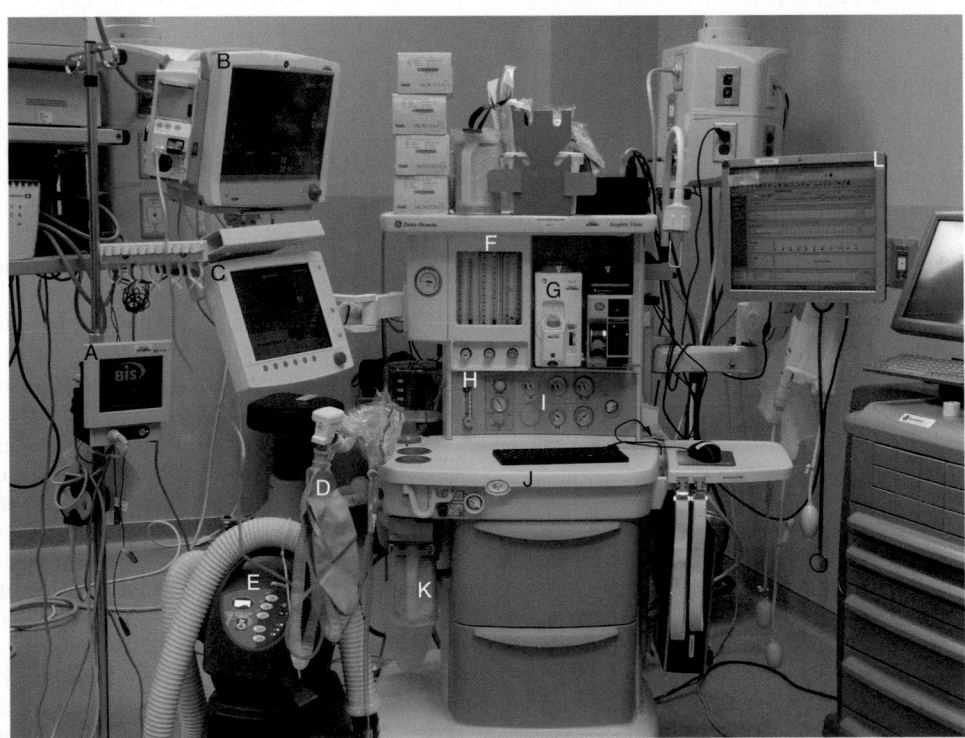

FIGURE 5-1 Modern anesthesia machine. **A,** Bispectral index system (BIS) monitor. **B,** Patient vital signs display monitor. **C,** Ventilator display monitor. **D,** Patient breathing circuit. **E,** Bair Hugger patient warmer. **F,** Gas flowmeters. **G,** Anesthetic vaporizers. **H,** Supplemental oxygen supply. **I,** Oxygen, air, and nitrous oxide gauges. **J,** Oxygen flush valve. **K,** Carbon dioxide absorber. **L,** Electronic record keeping screen.

for each gas so that they cannot be inadvertently cross-connected. If a central gas supply is not available or the hospital piping system fails, machines are equipped with E-size cylinders of O_2 and N_2O. One or two cylinders of each gas are connected to yokes on the machine. These yokes are pin-indexed so that only the correct gas can be connected in that position. In the pin-indexing safety system, two steel pins are in a unique location on the yoke assembly. The mating gas cylinder (e.g., the O_2 tank) has two matching holes in the same locations so that cylinders must be mounted correctly and cannot be mounted in the wrong place (Dosch, 2014).

O_2 stores as a compressed gas in cylinders. A full E-size cylinder contains about 660 L of O_2 at approximately 2000 psi. As the O_2 is used, the pressure decreases in direct proportion to the remaining volume. Because the E-size cylinder is used to provide O_2 while patients are being transported, one must know how much O_2 remains in a partially used tank; 1000 psi indicates 330 L remaining, and 500 psi indicates 165 L remaining or sufficient O_2 at 5 L/min flow for about 30 minutes. When pressure decreases to about 250 psi, the cylinder should not be used because it no longer has an adequate reserve (Dosch, 2014).

N_2O stores as a liquid in cylinders, and pressure above the liquid is 745 psi. A full E-size cylinder contains about 1600 L of N_2O. As the N_2O is used, the pressure above the liquid remains constant. Only when the liquid has been completely vaporized does pressure begin to decrease. The N_2O cylinder can be nearly empty but still show the same pressure. In contrast to O_2, the amount remaining in the N_2O tank cannot be readily determined (Dosch, 2014).

Gases in the cylinders flow through regulators that reduce pressure to about 45 psi as gas enters the machine. Hoses from the hospital gas sources are connected to the machine at the outlet of these regulators. A safety interlock device either shuts off the N_2O flow if O_2 pressure is not present or proportionally lowers the O_2 and N_2O flow rates to maintain 30% O_2. The gases flow through individual flowmeters (or rotameters) on the front of the machine so that the anesthesia provider can select gas flows and the ratio of O_2 to N_2O or air. From the top of the flowmeters, the gases are mixed and then flow through a vaporizer in which the inhalational anesthetic of choice is vaporized and added to the gas mixture. The total gas flow is delivered from the machine to the patient. With a flow-through vaporizer, all the fresh gas moving from the anesthesia machine to the patient flows through the vaporizer. The control dials usually are located on top of these vaporizers and are calibrated in percentages. The filling ports on the vaporizers are usually key-indexed so that personnel can use only the appropriate volatile agent. Newer vaporizers are flow and temperature compensated, meaning that they are reasonably accurate at all flow rates and temperatures (Dosch, 2014).

Desflurane (Suprane) is a unique inhalational anesthetic because it boils at 22.8°C, near room temperature, and its vapor pressure (669 mm Hg) approximates atmospheric pressure (760 mm Hg). The vaporizer for desflurane is pressurized and contains an electric heater. Desflurane also has several other unique characteristics: (1) its solubility in blood (blood-gas partition coefficient) is lower (0.42) than those of N_2O (0.47), sevoflurane (0.63 to 0.69), isoflurane (1.41), and halothane (2.30), which means that it has a faster "wash-in" (induction) and "wash-out" (emergence) than the other agents; (2) metabolism is far less (0.02%) than that of isoflurane (0.2%), sevoflurane (5%), and halothane (15 to 20%); (3) emergence and recovery from general anesthesia and discharge from PACU are significantly faster than when other agents are used; (4) the cardiovascular effects are similar to those of isoflurane; and

(5) muscle relaxation is similar to that which occurs with other inhalational agents. Because desflurane is pungent, it is not used as an induction agent.

Sevoflurane (Ultane) is the most recent volatile agent available in the United States. Its pleasant odor and low solubility in blood make it a popular volatile agent for inhalational induction in pediatric patients. In contrast to any of the other volatile agents, it also can provide a rapid, pleasant mask induction in adults.

Another important feature of the anesthesia machine is the O_2 flush valve. Pushing the O_2 flush valve allows 100% O_2 from the 50 psi line to flow directly to the *fresh gas outlet* on the machine and to the patient. This O_2 flow completely bypasses flowmeters and vaporizers. *Caution must be exercised, however, when using the O_2 flush valve because the pressure is 35 to 50 psi, and the flow rate is 35 to 75 L/min.*

In most hospitals and ambulatory surgery centers in the United States, a semiclosed-circle system (circle system) is used to deliver fresh gas flow (including anesthetic gases) to patients. The circle system is composed of a container filled with a CO_2-absorbing material (e.g., soda lime or calcium hydroxide lime), two one-way (unidirectional) valves, an adjustable pressure-limiting (APL) valve, a reservoir bag, an inlet connection for fresh gas flow, and two connections to the patient through corrugated breathing (or anesthesia circuit) tubing. As the patient inhales, gases are drawn through the CO_2 absorber and from the fresh gas supply through the inspiratory limb of the corrugated tubing. As the patient exhales, the one-way valve on the inspiratory limb prevents backflow, and the exhaled gases flow into the expiratory limb and through the expiratory one-way valve. The expiratory limb and valve are easily identified by the condensation of water vapor along this portion of the circuit. The reservoir bag absorbs the peak flow of expired gases and allows the anesthesia provider to force gas through the CO_2 absorber, along the inspiratory limb of the circuit, and to ventilate the patient. The expired gases flow through the CO_2 absorber, where CO_2 is removed. Substances used in the CO_2 absorbent include an indicator that changes color as exhaustion of the soda lime or calcium hydroxide lime occurs. The soda lime may turn from white to blue, indicating a required change of the absorbent material to prevent a buildup of CO_2 in the patient. Any excess gas vents through the APL valve into the gas-scavenging system. The APL valve usually mounts just ahead of the CO_2 absorber (Dosch, 2014).

The fraction of inspired O_2 (FIO_2) sensor usually is mounted in the inspiratory limb just after the one-way valve. It measures the FIO_2 and can be set to alarm if a low concentration is detected. A low-pressure sensor usually is mounted in the expiratory limb near the one-way valve to detect a ventilator malfunction or a circuit disconnection.

On current machines, volumeters are mounted in the inspired and expired limbs where the patient breathing circuit is connected. When using the ventilator, electronic circuitry measures inspiratory and expiratory volumes to ensure that they correspond with tidal volume and respiratory rate selected. With a cuffed ETT, the ventilator compensates for changes in fresh gas flow or small leaks in the breathing circuit and alarms if a disconnection or inadequate flow occurs (Dosch, 2014).

The advantage of the circle system is that it enables the use of much lower flows of O_2, N_2O, and anesthetic gases; this conserves the patient's body heat and respiratory moisture, and reduces the cost of expensive, volatile agents. A *semiclosed-circle system* typically is used when fresh gas flows into the system (flow rate ranges from 0.5 to 6 L/min). During exhalation some of the expired gases are recycled through the CO_2 absorber, and excess gas is scavenged or eliminated. With a *closed-circle system,* all CO_2 is absorbed. No gas vents from the system, and only enough O_2 is added to meet the basal requirements of the patient (approximately 3.5 mL/kg/min). A *semiopen circuit* (e.g., Ayres T-piece, Magill, Bain T-piece circuits) uses a relatively high flow of fresh gas, and most exhaled gas vents from the circuit. The fresh gas flow rate per minute varies from about two thirds of the patient's minute volume with the Magill circuit to at least 100 mL/kg with the Bain T-piece circuit. The semiopen circuit system is commonly used for newborns, infants, and small children (Dosch, 2014). With all these circuits, the final connection to the patient is by mask, ETT, or laryngeal mask airway (LMA).

General Anesthesia

Mechanism of Action

Along with progress in identifying the molecular mechanisms of anesthesia, our understanding of the nature of the anesthetic state continues to evolve. Whereas the anesthesia provider can induce a coma-like state of general anesthesia by inhaled anesthetics administered at appropriate concentrations (approximately 1.3 times MAC, equivalent to the EC_{95} of a volatile anesthetic), use of such high concentrations is fraught with short- and possibly long-term side effects. It is now clear that anesthesia consists of separable and at least partially independent components or substrates, each of which involves distinct, but possibly overlapping, mechanisms at different sites in the CNS and with variations in relative potencies between specific agents. Immobilization, the core measure of the anesthetic state, is mediated largely at the level of the spinal cord by inhaled anesthetics but not by barbiturates. The spinal cord, however, is unlikely to be the major site of other anesthetic actions, which produce phenomena such as amnesia, sedation, and unconsciousness; these are associated with cerebral cortical function. A functional separation between amnesia and sedation has been demonstrated for IV anesthetics and is likely for inhaled anesthetics as well. These and similar findings have led to the concept that general anesthesia consists of multiple independent components that are experimentally and clinically identifiable. Theoretically, each component can be preferentially induced in a concentration and agent-specific manner using individual cellular/molecular pathways in various regions of the CNS. For example, injections of pentobarbital into discrete sites in the mesopontine tegmentum induce an anesthetic state, whereas sedation induced by systemic administration of propofol can be reversed by microinjections of gamma-aminobutyric acid (GABA$_A$) receptor antagonists into the tuberomammillary nucleus, a sleep-regulating nucleus in the hypothalamus. Thus general anesthetics produce separate identifiable anesthetic substrates via agent-specific actions at discrete anatomic sites in the CNS by different molecular targets. An important consequence of this complexity is that the anesthetic state, based exclusively on the motor response, might not proportionately reflect other components of anesthesia. Although this heterogeneity of anesthetic action complicates a mechanistic understanding, it does open the possibility of developing substrate-specific medications.

Numerous proposed theories explain the action of general anesthetics. Investigations have involved inhalation anesthetics (*volatile anesthetic, potent agent,* and *inhaled* or *inhalational anesthetic* are virtually synonymous with *inhalation anesthetic* and used interchangeably). Evidence suggests that synaptic transmission of nerve impulses is reversibly inhibited in several areas of the CNS. The extent of inhibition and consequent progressive depression of function correlate with partial pressure of the inhaled anesthetic at various sites. Inhibition is believed to occur at a lipophilic site on the biologic membrane of synapses and possibly on small, unmyelinated nerve fibers. Suppression of spinal reflex activity is believed to produce some relaxation of skeletal muscles. Although no single theory explains all phenomena, a few theories explain many of the actions (Miller, 2010). The following theories are some of those more widely accepted.

Protein Receptor Theory. This theory proposes that hydrophobic areas of specific proteins in the CNS act as receptor sites. The steep, dose-response curve of inhaled anesthetics seems to support this theory by suggesting that a critical number of receptor sites must be occupied before patient movement in response to noxious stimuli is deadened sufficiently (Miller, 2010).

Meyer-Overton Theory. This correlation suggests that anesthesia is produced by the volume of anesthetic molecules present (dissolved) at the site, not by the type of inhaled agent present. Nevertheless, continued research on the mechanism of action of inhalation anesthetics has mitigated the utility of this theory (Kossick, 2014).

Endogenous Endorphins. Endogenous endorphins, or opiate-like substances, suppress various pain pathways. Several classes of endorphins have been identified. The action of β-endorphins is antagonized by naloxone or nalmefene, specific narcotic antagonists, but the relative potency of inhaled anesthetics remains unaltered. Although this mechanism explains some degree of analgesia, it does not correlate well with the level of anesthesia achieved by inhaled anesthetics.

IV anesthetics also may function using some of the same mechanisms proposed for inhaled anesthetics. Factors involved in the pharmacokinetics of IV anesthetics include the volume of distribution, biotransformation, and clearance of the medication by metabolism, excretion, or elimination of the medication and its metabolites (Miller, 2010).

No single theory posited to explain the mechanism of anesthetic action explains all effects observed with anesthetic agents. The range of anesthetic activity varies with different anesthetics; the effects on the CNS and skeletal muscles are similar but not identical, structural and spatial differences exist among agents, changes at the membrane and cellular levels occur, and optical isomers produce different responses. Although similar in many respects, anesthetic agents are individually unique and probably work through numerous mechanisms and at multiple sites to produce their multiple effects. Readers interested in further reading can search the *Canadian Journal of Anesthesia* published in 2011 where a special issue specifically addresses "Mechanisms of Anesthesia" (vol 58[2]) (Kossick, 2014).

Levels of General Anesthesia

Guedel integrated the signs and stages of ether anesthesia into a system that was used clinically for more than 60 years. This system applied only to unpremedicated patients breathing spontaneously during ether anesthesia, a technique that is rarely used today except in developing countries. By evaluating physiologic changes and reflex responses, one can estimate a staged depth of anesthesia. Stage 1 is from initial administration of anesthetic agents to loss of consciousness. Stage 2 is from loss of consciousness to onset of regular breathing and loss of eyelid reflex. Stage 2 also is called the *delirium* or *excitement* stage, and thrashing movements may occur. No auditory or physical stimulation should occur during this stage, especially in children. Stage 3, which begins with the onset of a regular breathing pattern and lasts until cessation of respiration, is divided into four planes and is the stage of surgical anesthesia. Stage 4 is from cessation of respiration to circulatory failure that leads to death (Nagelhout and Plaus, 2014).

Although Guedel's system gives us an appreciation for the interrelationships of numerous signs during anesthesia, the variety of medications and anesthetic techniques used today do not provide uniform responses suitable to estimate the exact depth of anesthesia. Premedications such as narcotics and anticholinergic medications alter pupillary responses. Evaluation of respiratory responses and muscle tone is not valid when controlled ventilation and muscle relaxants are used. Today general anesthesia usually is induced with IV injection of a rapid-acting medication, such as propofol (Diprivan) (as of 2011 thiopental is no longer manufactured in the United States), which takes the patient rapidly to stage 3 and eliminates the untoward responses often seen during stage 2.

For optimal anesthesia and good surgical conditions, several different but interrelated factors occur. These include hypnosis (sleep); analgesia (freedom from pain); amnesia (lack of recall or awareness); appropriate surgical conditions, including muscle relaxation and positioning of the patient; and continued homeostasis of the patient's vital functions. Different medications and anesthetic agents possess various properties that facilitate these factors. Combinations of medications are used to obtain the desired effects. Hypotensive or hypertensive medications and cardioactive agents also may be used to achieve optimal depth of anesthesia while affecting physiologic homeostasis as little as possible. The Surgical Pharmacology box briefly describes medications commonly used in anesthesia.

Phases of General Anesthesia

General anesthesia consists of three phases: *induction, maintenance,* and *emergence. Induction* begins with administration of anesthetic agents and continues until the patient is ready for positioning or surgical prepping (surgical prep), surgical manipulation, or incision. Surgical prep often starts after administration of induction medications. This endpoint of induction may vary with the surgical procedure. *Maintenance* continues from this point until near completion of the procedure; the anesthesia provider achieves this phase either with inhalation agents, with IV medications given in titrated doses, or by continuous infusion. *Emergence* varies in length and depends on the patient's state and the depth and duration of anesthesia. Emergence starts as the patient begins to "emerge" from anesthesia and usually ends when the patient is ready to leave the OR. Intubation occurs during the induction phase, and extubation usually is performed during emergence. Recovery from anesthesia amounts to a fourth phase of general anesthesia.

Types of General Anesthesia

The type of general anesthesia used often is described as IV technique, inhalation technique (with a volatile anesthetic agent), or a combination of IV and inhalation techniques. IV technique traditionally includes (1) an induction agent such as propofol, combined with 30% to 40% O_2 and N_2O; (2) an amnestic/anxiolytic, such as midazolam or diazepam; (3) an analgesic such as fentanyl or morphine sulfate; and (4) a muscle relaxant.

In contrast, an inhalation technique may use propofol to facilitate rapid induction or patients may "breathe themselves down" with a potent agent, such as sevoflurane, plus N_2O and O_2.

Inhalation induction is often used with children to avoid inserting an IV catheter while they are awake. Depending on the kind of surgical procedure, maintenance of anesthesia may be accomplished with only inhalation agents and spontaneous, assisted, or controlled ventilation. Effects of volatile agents are dose related and provide differing levels of anesthesia, amnesia, analgesia, muscle relaxation, and hemodynamic responses. If supplemental muscle relaxation is needed, the relaxant dose required is significantly less than the dose necessary during IV anesthesia.

In the past, the term *balanced anesthesia* was used when various combinations of IV medications were "balanced" to provide complete anesthesia. Today the term is often used to describe a combination of IV medications and inhalation agents used to obtain specific effects tailored to each patient and procedure.

Anesthesia providers also may use *total IV anesthesia* (TIVA). They may use this technique in the OR, but they more commonly use it for pediatric, uncooperative, or trauma patients in remote locations, such as in magnetic resonance imaging (MRI), radiology, or surgical laser suites, where waste-gas evacuation systems are not available. TIVA use also occurs in the expanding area of office-based surgical procedures. With TIVA, providers use short-acting medications such as propofol with remifentanil or alfentanil for induction. These medications may be administered by continuous infusion. Anesthesia providers maintain anesthesia by infusion plus O_2 alone or with N_2O. They may also give an intermediate-acting muscle relaxant (cisatracurium, atracurium, rocuronium, or vecuronium). As surgery nears completion, the anesthesia provider titrates off the maintenance medications, and emergence from anesthesia follows.

Muscle Relaxants

Muscle relaxants (also referred to as neuromuscular blocking drugs [NMBDs]) are used to facilitate intubation and provide good operating conditions at lighter planes of general anesthesia. These medications may be used elsewhere for emergency intubation or, less frequently, when a patient is being mechanically ventilated. Muscle relaxants affect skeletal muscle and have little effect on cardiac or smooth muscle. Although not always dose dependent, many of these medications have adverse side effects. The route of metabolism and elimination varies, and this may be important for patients with hepatic or renal disease. Muscle relaxants are classified as *depolarizing* or *nondepolarizing.*

The standard *depolarizing* agent is succinylcholine (Anectine), which was introduced in 1952. It has a chemical structure similar to that of acetylcholine (ACh) and depolarizes the postjunctional neuromuscular membrane. Administration is followed by a brief period of muscle fasciculations that corresponds to initial membrane depolarization and muscle fiber activation. Unlike ACh, which is released in minute amounts and hydrolyzed in milliseconds, succinylcholine requires several minutes for breakdown to occur. During this time the neuromuscular junction remains depolarized, but the muscles relax and will not contract again until the neuromuscular endplate and adjacent sarcoplasmic reticulum return to the resting state and are again depolarized. Relaxation proceeds from the small, distal, rapidly moving muscles to the proximal, slowly moving muscles. The diaphragm is one of the last muscles to relax. To prevent these fasciculations and associated postoperative myalgias, a dose of a nondepolarizing relaxant (such as rocuronium 0.03 mg/kg) (Fukano, 2011) is given 3 to 5 minutes before administering the intubating dose of succinylcholine. Onset of paralysis (30 to 90 seconds) is faster and duration of action (5 to 10 minutes)

Text continued on p. 140

SURGICAL PHARMACOLOGY

Commonly Used Anesthetic Gases and Drugs

	Common Usage	Advantages	Disadvantages	Comments
Inhalation Gases				
Air	Maintenance with O_2; laser surgery near airway	Less support of combustion than N_2O	No anesthetic qualities	Possibly less nausea than N_2O (Miller, 2010)
Oxygen (O_2)	Essential for life	Can slightly ↑ O_2 available to tissues in low cardiac output states	Can cause retinopathy in premature infants	High concentrations hazardous with lasers in surgery of head, neck, and pulmonary areas (Miller, 2010)
Nitrous oxide (N_2O)	Maintenance; frequently for induction	Rapid induction and recovery; additive effects to other anesthetics	No relaxation; can depress myocardium; expands within closed spaces	Hypoxia if overdose given; ↑ uptake of other volatile agents (Miller, 2010)
Desflurane (Suprane)	Maintenance in surgical cases	Rapid emergence; good relaxation; 0.02% metabolized	May cause transient ↑ HR and ↓ BP; airway irritation; requires heated vaporizer	Rapid recovery phase; can use for emergence after maintenance with another volatile agent (Miller, 2010)
Isoflurane (Forane)	Maintenance	Good relaxation; maintains cardiac output; 0.2% metabolized	↑ HR; slightly irritating odor	Isomer of enflurane; commonly used agent (Miller, 2010)
Sevoflurane (Ultane)	Induction and maintenance	Rapid induction and emergence; good relaxation; ≈5% metabolized	Metabolite requires increased fresh gas flow (compound A); is nephrotoxic in rats; effect in humans unknown	Rapid and smooth mask induction in children and adults (Miller, 2010)
Opioid Analgesics				
Morphine sulfate	Perioperative pain; premedication	Inexpensive; duration of action 4-5 hr; euphoria; good cardiovascular stability	Nausea and vomiting; histamine release; postural ↓ BP (↓ SVR); caution with renal failure patients	Used intrathecally and epidurally for postoperative pain; elimination half-life 3 hr (Nagelhout, 2014)
Alfentanil (Alfenta)	Surgical analgesia in ambulatory patients	Duration of action 0.5 hr; used as bolus or infusion	—	Potency: 750 mcg = 10 mg morphine sulfate; elimination half-life 1.6 hr (Nagelhout, 2014)
Fentanyl (Sublimaze)	Surgical analgesia; epidural infusion for postoperative analgesia; add to SAB	Good cardiovascular stability; duration of action 0.5 hr	—	Most commonly used opioid; potency: 100 mcg = 10 mg morphine sulfate; elimination half-life 3.6 hr (Nagelhout, 2014)
Remifentanil (Ultiva)	0.25-1 mcg/kg/min infusion for surgical analgesia; small boluses for brief, intense pain	Easily titratable; metabolized by blood and tissue esterases; short duration; good cardiovascular stability	Requires mixing; increased cost	Potency: 25 mcg = 10 mg morphine sulfate; 20-30× potency of alfentanil; elimination half-life 3-10 min (Nagelhout, 2014)
Sufentanil (Sufenta)	Surgical analgesia	Good cardiovascular stability; duration of action 0.5 hr; prolonged analgesia	Prolonged respiratory depression	Potency: 15 mcg = 10 mg morphine sulfate; elimination half-life 2.7 hr (Nagelhout, 2014)
Hydromorphone (Dilaudid)	Surgical and postoperative pain relief	Long duration of action 3-5 hr; can switch to PO form for postoperative pain management	Caution with seizure history and biliary tract surgery; addiction potential	Reduce dose for patients with hepatic impairment (Duke, 2011)
Morphine liposomal (DepoDur)	For epidural use only	Single dose provides analgesia for up to 48 hr. Decreased requirements for supplemental opioids	Potential for respiratory depression Avoid other epidural medications ≈48 hr	10-15 mg epidural, 1 dose (Duke, 2011)

Continued

Commonly Used Anesthetic Gases and Drugs—cont'd

	Common Usage	Advantages	Disadvantages	Comments
Depolarizing Muscle Relaxants				
Succinylcholine (Anectine, Quelicin)	Intubation; short cases	Rapid onset; short duration	Requires refrigeration; may cause fasciculations, postoperative myalgias, and dysrhythmias; ↑ serum K^+ with burns, tissue trauma, paralysis, and muscle diseases; slight histamine release	Prolonged muscle relaxation with serum cholinesterase deficiency and certain antibiotics; trigger agent for MH (Nagelhout, 2014)
Nondepolarizing Muscle Relaxants—Intermediate Onset And Duration				
Atracurium (Tracrium)	Intubation; maintenance of relaxation	No significant cardiovascular or cumulative effects; good with renal failure	Requires refrigeration; slight histamine release	Breakdown by Hofmann elimination and ester hydrolysis (Nagelhout, 2014)
Cisatracurium (Nimbex)	Intubation; maintenance of relaxation	Similar to atracurium	No histamine release	Similar to atracurium (Nagelhout, 2014)
Rocuronium (Zemuron)	Intubation; maintenance of relaxation	Rapid onset (dose dependent); elimination via kidney and liver	Vagolytic; may increase HR	Duration similar to atracurium and vecuronium (Nagelhout, 2014)
Vecuronium (Norcuron)	Intubation; maintenance of relaxation	No significant cardiovascular or cumulative effects; no histamine release	Requires mixing	Mostly eliminated in bile, some in urine (Nagelhout, 2014)
Nondepolarizing Muscle Relaxants—Longer Onset and Duration				
Pancuronium (Pavulon)	Maintenance of relaxation	—	May cause ↑ HR and ↑ BP	Mostly renal elimination (Nagelhout, 2014)
Intravenous Anesthetics				
Etomidate (Amidate)	Induction	Good cardiovascular stability; fast, smooth induction and recovery	May cause pain with injection and myotonic movements	Administer through large vein to decrease pain on injection. (Duke 2011)
Diazepam (Valium, Dizac)	Amnesia; hypnotic; preoperative medication	Good sedation	Prolonged duration	Residual effects for 20-90 hr; increased effect with alcohol (Duke, 2011)
Ketamine (Ketalar)	Induction, occasional maintenance (IV or IM)	Short acting; patient maintains airway; good in small children and burn patients, hypovolemic shock; bronchospastic disease	Large doses may cause hallucinations and respiratory depression; not indicated in patients with increased ICP	Need darkened, quiet room for recovery; often used in trauma cases (Miller, 2010)
Midazolam (Versed)	Hypnotic; anxiolytic; sedation; often used as adjunct to induction	Excellent amnestic; water soluble (no pain with IV injection); short acting	Slower induction than propofol	Often used for amnesia with insertion of invasive monitors or regional anesthesia (Duke, 2011)
Propofol (Diprivan)	Induction and maintenance; sedation with regional anesthesia or MAC	Rapid onset; awakening in 4-8 min	May cause pain when injected; lipid based can support bacterial growth if aseptic technique is broken	Short elimination half-life (34-64 min) (Miller, 2010)
Sodium methohexital (Brevital sodium)	Induction	Ultrashort-acting barbiturate; low cardiac toxicity; minimal anticonvulsant properties	May cause hiccups	Can be given rectally (Duke, 2011)

SURGICAL PHARMACOLOGY

Commonly Used Anesthetic Gases and Drugs—cont'd

	Common Usage	Advantages	Disadvantages	Comments
Local Anesthetics				
Bupivacaine (Marcaine, Sensorcaine)	Epidural, spinal, or local infiltration; Good wound infiltration	Good relaxation; long acting; can constrict blood vessels to reduce bleeding at site	Overdose can cause cardiac collapse	Epidural or caudal: 2.5 mg/kg; duration: 120-240 min (Nagelhout, 2014)
Chloroprocaine (Nesacaine)	Epidural anesthesia	Ultrashort acting; good relaxation	May cause neurotoxicity if injected into CSF unless preservative free	Maximum dose 600 mg; with epinephrine 14 mg/kg, maximum dose 1000 mg, duration 30-45 min (Miller, 2010)
Lidocaine (Xylocaine)	Epidural, spinal, peripheral, IV anesthesia, and local infiltration	Short acting; good relaxation; low toxicity	Overdose can cause convulsions; possible transient neurologic changes with spinal anesthesia	Also used for ventricular dysrhythmias; maximum dose 7 mg/kg and 5 mg/kg with and without epinephrine; duration 60-120 min (Nagelhout, 2014)
Ropivacaine (Naropin)	Local infiltration, peripheral nerve block Epidural	Fast Slow Moderate	≈30-40% less cardiotoxic than bupivacaine (Duke, 2011)	200-300 mg single doses for duration up to 5 hr achieved by various regional techniques (Miller, 2010)
Tetracaine (Pontocaine)	Spinal anesthesia	Long acting; good relaxation	—	Maximum dose 1-1.5 mg/kg (epinephrine rarely used but 3 mg/kg if used); duration 60-180 min (Miller, 2010)
Anticholinergics				
Atropine	Blocks effects of acetylcholine; ↓ vagal tone; reverse muscle relaxants; treat sinus bradycardia	↑ HR; suppresses salivation, bronchial and gastric secretions	Depresses sweating; may cause dry mouth, flushing, dizziness, CNS symptoms	Quite selective at muscarinic receptors in smooth and cardiac muscle and exocrine glands (Nagelhout, 2014)
Glycopyrrolate (Robinul)	Similar to atropine	Slightly ↑ HR; does not cross blood-brain barrier; can increase gastric pH more than atropine	Prolonged duration of effects	Lower incidence of dysrhythmias than atropine (Nagelhout, 2014)
Cholinergic Agent				
Neostigmine (Prostigmine)	Reverses effects of nondepolarizing neuromuscular blocking agents	Prevents breakdown of acetylcholine by inhibiting acetylcholinesterase	—	Given with either atropine or glycopyrrolate (Nagelhout, 2014)
Other				
Sugammadex* (Bridion)	First selective relaxant binding agent (SRBA) to antagonize a muscle relaxant's effects	Rapidly terminates the neuromuscular block of rocuronium, vecuronium, and pancuronium by diffusion of medication away from neuromuscular junction; choice of anesthetic does not affect efficacy of sugammadex	No effect on succinylcholine or benzylisoquinolinium relaxants	If the need to re-establish muscle relaxation arises after administration of sugammadex, then using a benzylisoquinolinium or succinylcholine is recommended (Naguib and Lien, 2010; Miller, 2010)
Dexmedetomidine (Precedex)	Selective α_2-agonist	Produces centrally mediated sympatholytic, sedative, and analgesic effects	Provides hemodynamic stability, potentiates intraop anesthetics, reduces anesthetic requirements, less respiratory depression than opioids (Duke, 2011)	Its cost relative to other sedative medications has probably limited greater use (Duke, 2011)

BP, Blood pressure; *CNS*, central nervous system; *CSF*, cerebrospinal fluid; *EEG*, electroencephalogram; *HR*, heart rate; *IM*, intramuscular; *IV*, intravenous; *MAC*, monitored anesthesia care; *MH*, malignant hyperthermia; *PO*, oral; *PVC*, premature ventricular contraction; *SAB*, subarachnoid block; *SVR*, systemic vascular resistance.
*Not FDA approved at time of publication.

is shorter than with other relaxants. The speed of onset makes it a preferred medication for rapid-sequence inductions. Adverse side effects associated with use of succinylcholine include cardiac dysrhythmias, hyperkalemia, myalgias (particularly in young and muscular patients), and increases in intraocular, intracranial, and intragastric pressures. It also can trigger MH in susceptible patients. It can be infused for longer procedures, but an excessive dose may cause prolonged relaxation (known as *phase II blockade*). Succinylcholine is hydrolyzed by plasma cholinesterase, and the rare patient with an abnormal or absent enzyme (plasma cholinesterase) has prolonged muscle paralysis (Miller, 2010).

Nondepolarizing muscle relaxants competitively block the depolarizing action of acetylcholine at the neuromuscular junction, which results in skeletal muscle paralysis. Fasciculations do not occur. Nondepolarizing agents can be subdivided by duration of action into intermediate-acting (atracurium, cisatracurium, rocuronium, and vecuronium) and long-acting (pancuronium, pipecuronium, and doxacurium) (Fuhrman, 2011; Nagelhout, 2014). The potency, duration (metabolism and elimination), and side effects of these medications vary and may be individually altered in patients with hepatic or renal dysfunction, electrolyte imbalance, or hypothermia or when used in combination with other perioperative medications (inhalation and local anesthetics, aminoglycoside antibiotics, calcium-entry blockers, magnesium, and cardiac antidysrhythmics). Generally, nondepolarizing relaxants can be used for patients with MH or plasma cholinesterase deficiencies. Side effects vary with individual medications, are dose dependent, and include alterations in blood pressure (BP) and heart rate. The neuromuscular blockade of muscle relaxants can be monitored with a peripheral nerve stimulator. Paralysis caused by nondepolarizing relaxants may be antagonized (reversed) by IV anticholinesterases, such as edrophonium, neostigmine, or rarely pyridostigmine. Sugammadex (Bridion) is a selective relaxant binding agent (SRBA) that encapsulates the steroidal neuromuscular agents and is excreted in the urine (at the time of publication, this drug was not yet FDA-approved). Antagonism occurs even with deep block due to the rapid fall of muscle relaxant concentration, and appropriate doses can antagonize within 3 minutes. Antagonists allow acetylcholine to accumulate and compete for receptor sites at the neuromuscular junction and may be associated with bradycardia, arrhythmias, hypotension, bronchoconstriction, and hypersalivation for which atropine or glycopyrrolate is routinely given (Nagelhout, 2014).

Typical Sequence of General Anesthesia

After arriving in the preoperative area or OR suite, the anesthesia provider again identifies the patient; verifies consent or secures a signed operative permit; reviews current laboratory tests, diagnostic studies, and pertinent medical history; and confirms there have been no interval changes in the patient's status. Depending on the practice of the anesthesia department and institutional policy, an IV infusion may be started in the preoperative area or after the patient is transferred to the OR because nearly all anesthesia-related medications are given IV except inhalation agents. After the patient arrives in the OR and is transferred to the OR bed, monitors are connected.

Before induction the anesthesia provider usually preoxygenates (i.e., denitrogenates) the patient using a mask with 100% O_2 for 3 to 5 minutes. This practice permits washout of most gaseous nitrogen from the body and provides a large reserve supply of O_2 in the lungs. Administration of opioids and benzodiazepines usually follows at this time. If succinylcholine is to be used for intubation,

a small pretreatment dose of a nondepolarizing muscle relaxant (e.g., 0.03 mg/kg of rocuronium [Fukano, 2011], or 0.5 to 1 mg of pancuronium or vecuronium [Abraham et al, 2008]) usually occurs next. If the patient can be safely ventilated with a mask, the anesthesia provider may opt to avoid the adverse effects of succinylcholine and use a nondepolarizing muscle relaxant to intubate the patient.

To induce anesthesia, a short-acting barbiturate, such as propofol (1.5 to 2.5 mg/kg), is given. When the patient becomes apneic and the eyelash reflex is absent, the anesthesia provider checks the airway for patency by ventilating the patient with a mask. Depending on several factors, such as the airway, and type and duration of surgery, O_2 and anesthetic gases may be delivered to a spontaneously breathing patient through a mask held in place with a head strap. Repositioning of the head or insertion of an oral or nasal airway may help to maintain a patent airway. If spontaneous or assisted ventilation is planned, an LMA may be inserted without a muscle relaxant. The anesthesia provider may use a mask or LMA for a patient with a good airway, at minimal risk of aspiration, and undergoing a relatively short procedure, so long as the surgical site is not compromised in the head or neck area.

If mask anesthesia or an LMA is inappropriate, an ETT may be used to facilitate ventilation and to prevent aspiration. Typical equipment for intubation, and airway control and monitoring, appear in Figure 5-2. An "intubating dose" of a muscle relaxant is administered, resulting in temporary paralysis. When the patient is paralyzed, ventilation is controlled during the procedure.

To facilitate intubation, the patient's head is placed in a "sniffing" position. The laryngoscope is held in the left hand. The clean laryngoscope blade (Evidence for Practice) is inserted into the right side of the mouth and moved to the midline, "sweeping" the tongue to the left. The ETT is introduced on the right side of the mouth and gently inserted into the trachea so that the cuff is approximately 1 cm below the vocal cords. The cuff is inflated just enough to occlude any air passage with the peak pressures used for ventilation. Location of the ETT in the trachea is verified by an appropriate level and waveform of $ETCO_2$, bilaterally equal breath sounds and absence of sounds over the stomach (determined using a stethoscope), symmetric movement of the thorax with positive-pressure ventilation, and condensation of moisture from expired air in the ETT and breathing circuit. Proper placement of the ETT appears in Figure 5-3. The vocal cords are the narrowest portion of an adult trachea; however, the smallest portion of a child's airway is below the vocal cords at the cricoid cartilage. Uncuffed ETTs have been traditionally selected for children up to age 8; newer designs for ETTs with microcuffs, however, allow use of cuffed tubes down to age 1 (Miller, 2010). After initial paralysis from the muscle relaxant has worn off, the patient may be allowed to breathe spontaneously with intermittent assistance, or additional muscle relaxant is given and ventilation controlled mechanically.

If the procedure is emergent or the patient is at risk for aspiration (as in cases of a full stomach, intestinal obstruction, hiatal hernia, or significant esophageal reflux), a rapid-sequence induction or an "awake" fiberoptic intubation may be planned. In these instances and in routine intubation, the perioperative nurse must be ready to assist by applying cricoid pressure (Figure 5-4). The nurse exerts downward pressure on the cricoid cartilage with the thumb and index finger of one hand (Sellick maneuver). The cricoid cartilage is the only complete ring in the trachea. Correctly applied downward pressure occludes the esophagus, which lies immediately posterior (or dorsal) to the trachea, enhancing the view required for intubation (Patten, 2007). The pressure should not be released until

FIGURE 5-2 Commonly used anesthesia equipment. **A,** Scissors. **B,** Supplemental oxygen mask. **C,** Nasal trumpet airway. **D,** Guedel oral airway. **E,** Supraglottic airway i-gel laryngeal mask airway (LMA) "Unique." **F,** Cook intubating LMA. **G,** Endotracheal tube. **H,** Long- and short-handled laryngoscopes with curved Macintosh and straight Miller blades. **I,** Nasogastric/orogastric tube. **J,** Peripheral nerve stimulator. **K,** Elastic bougie endotracheal tube (ETT) introducer. **L,** ETT malleable stylet. **M,** Skin temperature probe.

EVIDENCE FOR PRACTICE

High-Level Disinfection for Reusable Anesthesia Equipment

In continuing efforts to reduce surgical site infections (SSIs) and improve patient safety, procedures for storing and processing durable anesthesia equipment are being reviewed. More than 30 years ago, Earle H. Spaulding devised a rational approach to disinfection and sterilization of patient care items and equipment (CDC [Centers for Disease Control and Prevention] Guidelines, 2008). The Spaulding system continues to be used and refined when professionals in infection control plan methods of disinfection and sterilization by classifying items into three categories: critical, semicritical, and noncritical. Spaulding based classification of items on risk of infection according to use. *Critical* items confer a high risk for infection if contaminated with any microorganisms as they enter the vascular system or sterile tissue. *Semicritical* items contact mucous membranes or nonintact skin but do not penetrate the blood barrier. This category includes reusable anesthesia equipment such as laryngoscope blades, esophageal probes, airways, breathing circuits, laryngeal mask airways (LMAs), and fiberoptic endoscopes. *Noncritical* items are those that come in contact with intact skin, but not mucous membranes.

Focusing on the semicritical anesthesia items, the CDC classifies these as minimally requiring high-level disinfection using chemical disinfectants. The U.S. Food and Drug Administration (FDA) approves the use of clear glutaraldehyde, hydrogen peroxide, ortho-phthalaldehyde (OPT), and peracetic acid with hydrogen peroxide, as dependable high-level disinfectants, provided the factors influencing germicidal procedures are met. Meticulous cleaning of disassembled rigid laryngoscopes and all components followed by high-level disinfection using appropriate chemicals should eliminate enough pathogens to prevent transmission of infection (AORN, 2013). Items can be rinsed and flushed using sterile water after high-level disinfection to prevent contamination with organisms in tap water, such as nontuberculous mycobacteria, legionella, or gram-negative bacilli such as pseudomonas. Alternatively, a tap water or filtered water (0.2 m filter) rinse should be followed by an alcohol rinse and forced air-drying. Items should then be stored (e.g., packaged) in a manner that prevents recontamination while in storage. Check with your hospital department, along with your facility's designated infection control personnel, for their approved methods.

Modified from Association of periOperative Registered Nurses (AORN): *Perioperative standards and recommended practices,* Denver, 2013, The Association; CDC: *Guidelines for disinfection and sterilization in healthcare facilities,*2008, available at www.cdc.gov/hicpac/pdf/guidelines/disinfection_nov_2008.pdf. Accessed January 23, 2013.

proper placement of the ETT has been confirmed and the cuff inflated. This procedure has gained wide acceptance among anesthesia providers. Research suggests, however, that this maneuver is difficult to do correctly and effectively (Beavers et al, 2009; Heiner and Gabot, 2014).

The perioperative nurse provides additional assistance if an unexpected difficult intubation occurs or the patient cannot be ventilated adequately via mask (Research Highlight). The difficult-airway cart should be brought into the room immediately. The perioperative nurse should be familiar with the location of the various pieces

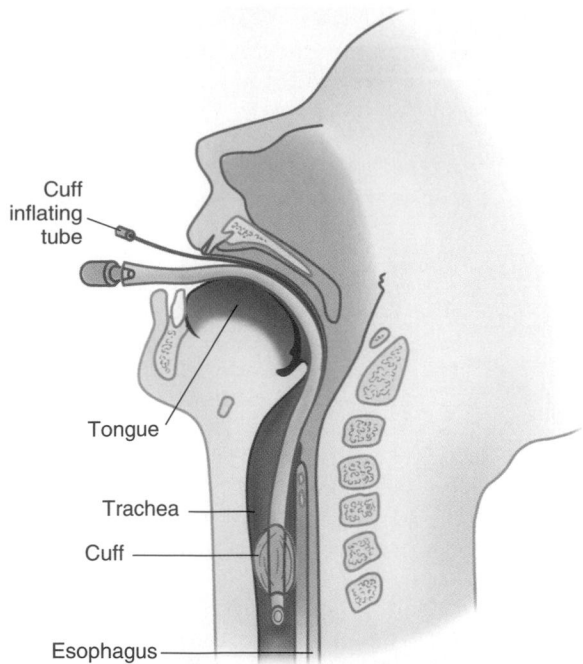

FIGURE 5-3 Endotracheal tube in position.

FIGURE 5-4 Applying cricoid pressure.

RESEARCH HIGHLIGHT

Obstructive Sleep Apnea and the Difficult Airway

Obstructive sleep apnea (OSA) is a common health problem, present in 2% to 4% of the general population. Several factors describe this condition: loud disruptive snoring, either with or without snort or gasping arousals; witnessed apneic periods during sleep; and daytime drowsiness. It is closely associated with hypertension, coronary artery disease, cerebrovascular disease, atrial fibrillation, obesity, and metabolic syndrome (Bope and Kellerman, 2013). Previous studies showed OSA is associated with increased risk among patients less than 50 years of age, with excessive risk declining after age 50. Therefore, the diagnosis of OSA in the younger population carries a higher mortality and should be diagnosed as soon as possible (Marin and Carrizo, 2007). Men with untreated, severe OSA (defined as an apnea-hypopnea index [AHI] of >30 in which AHI is the number of apneas and hypopneas [partial obstructions] per hour of sleep) have greater risk of death than the general population or men with mild OSA.

Polysomnography (PSG) (i.e., a sleep study) is the gold standard for in-laboratory formal assessment of suspected sleep disorders. PSG measures several polygraphic physiologic variables, including electroencephalography (EEG), electro-oculography (EOG), and chin electromyography (EMG), to allow determination of sleep staging; limb EMG leads analyze leg and arm movement. Also measured are oronasal airflow, respiratory effort, body positions, and electrocardiography (ECG). Several out-of-lab devices are available to screen for or to validate existing treatment (Bope and Kellerman, 2013). The presence of OSA is associated with a higher incidence of postoperative hypoxemia, overall complications, intensive care unit (ICU) transfer, and longer length of stay in the hospital (Kaw, 2013). Increased incidents of AHI and oxygen desaturation may occur as late as the third postoperative night versus either preoperative or first night postoperative (Kaw, 2013).

Studies have also linked OSA to difficult airway and possible failed intubations. Airway emergencies can occur at any time during the perioperative period. Serious airway problems can result in adverse outcomes, including death, brain injury, myocardial injury, and airway trauma. It is critical that the perioperative nurse be aware of the patient's status regarding OSA and the anesthesia provider's preplanned strategy for intubation and his/her preformulated strategy for extubation of the difficult airway. Most institutions have a difficult-airway cart (see Box 5-2), centralizing items and supplies necessary to manage airway emergencies. The ASA *Practice Guidelines* (2013) suggest contents for this cart, but anesthesia providers may add or modify preference items.

Follow-up care includes both documentation of the difficult airway and informing and advising the patient (or responsible person) of is occurrence. Patients who experience a difficult-airway are recommended to wear a MedicAlert bracelet. The National Medic Alert Registry for Difficult Airway/Intubation can be contacted. Information regarding why it was difficult to secure an airway and what technique finally worked is recorded in the registry's data bank and can be accessed by future anesthesia providers. It is also important to note two studies from Spain that showed reduction in mortality rates at both 5- and 14-year follow-up for patients treated with (and who comply with) continuous positive airway pressure (CPAP) therapy. The authors concluded that the risk of death from all causes, and particularly from cardiovascular causes, increases in patients with untreated OSA. Effective treatment with CPAP significantly reduces this risk.

Modified from American Society of Anesthesiologists: Practice guidelines for management of the difficult airway, *Anesthesiology* 118(2):1269–1277, 2013; Bope ET, Kellerman RD: *Conn's current therapy 2013*, Philadelphia, 2013, Saunders; Kaw R: Perioperative complications in patients with obstructive sleep apnea, *Sleep Med Clin,* 8(1):129–134, 2013; Marin J, Carrizo S: Mortality in obstructive sleep apnea, *Sleep Med Clin* 2(4):593–601, 2007.

of equipment on the cart, know how to assemble the equipment for use, and assist the anesthesia provider in securing the airway. Securing the airway in an emergency situation requires a concerted team effort. The contents of a typical difficult-airway cart are listed in Box 5-2. If invasive monitors (e.g., an arterial line) are to be placed after induction, the perioperative nurse may assist by properly positioning the patient or extremity; prepping the area or areas with antimicrobial solution; and assisting with placement, connection, and calibration of the monitors. If the procedure is emergent, the perioperative nurse also may assist by obtaining additional IV

BOX 5-2

Typical Contents of a Difficult-Airway Cart

Fiberoptic (FO) Equipment
Flexible FO bronchoscopes (adult and pediatric); FO light source (newer models have their own battery-powered source); Bullard scope (FO); and siliconized spray

Laryngoscope Equipment
Assorted pediatric and adult laryngoscope handles and blades; extra alkaline batteries, or chargers for FO handles; and video laryngoscope (Glidescope, etc.)

Endotracheal Tubes (ETTs)
Regular ETT: uncuffed, 2.5-6 mm; regular ETT: cuffed, 5-9 mm; oral RAE ETT: uncuffed, 3-7 mm; oral RAE ETT: cuffed, 6-8 mm; nasal RAE ETT: uncuffed, 3-7 mm; nasal RAE ETT: cuffed, 6-8 mm; reinforced ETT: cuffed, 7-8 mm; controllable-tip ETT (Endotrol); Combitube

Airways
Regular oral: assorted pediatric and adult; regular nasal: assorted adult; intubating airways: assorted (e.g., Ovassapian, Williams); nasopharyngeal airway with inflatable introducer; assorted sizes of supraglottic airways (e.g., laryngeal mask airways [LMAs], intubating LMA [ILMA]; tongue blades; and water-soluble lubricant (K-Y)

Intubating Equipment
Intubating stylets; McGill forceps: pediatric and adult; esophageal (gastric tube) airway (EGTA); hollow ETT changers with removable Luer-Lok connectors for O_2 insufflation

Suction Equipment
Assorted flexible suction catheters to fit ETT and LMA as well as stiff suction catheters (Yankauer)

Topical Anesthesia Equipment
Atomizers and pressurized topical anesthetic spray; long cotton-tipped swabs; lidocaine 4%; lidocaine 4% with phenylephrine; lidocaine 2%—viscous; lidocaine 5%—ointment; lidocaine 10%; tetracaine 1%

Transtracheal Airway Equipment
Transtracheal O_2 jet ventilator with pressure regulator, manual control valve, and Luer-Lok male connector; assorted large IV catheters; and assorted long guidewires, epidural needles, and epidural catheters (for retrograde intubation)

Miscellaneous
Safety glasses; heat-moisture exchanger (Humidivent); assorted facemasks with port for FO scope; right-angled connector (for facemasks) with port for FO scope; exhaled carbon dioxide detector; $ETCO_2$ chemical indicators (Easy Cap); twill tape (to secure ETT); skin adhesive (Mastisol)

---

access, connecting fluid-warming or patient-warming units, double-checking blood products, and "pumping" IV fluids as needed. If the anesthesia provider faces a critical procedure, such as a difficult airway/airway emergency, the perioperative nurse can perform a valuable service by ensuring provision of 100% O_2, having suction available, observing monitors, recording data (SpO_2 and $ETCO_2$ values), and communicating significant changes to the anesthesia provider.

The LMA (also called "supraglottic airway," or SGA) is a major advancement in airway management (Bosson, 2012). Placement is relatively simple and does not require laryngoscopy or muscle relaxation. When comparing ease of use, invasiveness, and airway protection, the LMA ranks between the facemask and an ETT. It is ideal for a supine patient under general anesthesia with spontaneous ventilation. The LMA also may be useful in a difficult-airway situation in which tracheal intubation cannot be achieved. Multiple companies produce various forms of SGAs, in multiple sizes and configurations that allow for gastric access, and are capable of functioning with positive pressure ventilation. These devices are also available as one-time disposable items.

The recommended technique for insertion of the LMA appears in Figure 5-5, and correct placement in Figure 5-6. Placement of other devices is similar and, in all cases, the manufacturer's instructions and recommendations should be followed. For adults, it is recommended that a 2.5- to 3-cm diameter roll of gauze sponges be used as a "bite block" and inserted beside the LMA tube. The LMA and gauze roll can be secured with tape. Some, like the LMA Supreme, have a bite block integrated within the device (The LMA Instruction Manual, 2011).

The anesthesia provider achieves anesthesia maintenance with IV or inhalational anesthetic techniques, or a combination of both, with or without additional muscle relaxation, and considers a variety of factors when selecting the anesthesia technique for each patient.

Whichever technique is selected for general anesthesia (or for any other anesthesia types discussed subsequently), the entire surgical team participates in a time-out just after the patient is anesthetized, positioned, prepped, and draped, and before starting the surgical procedure. The entire surgical team ceases other activity and verifies the patient's identity; the procedure to be done; operative side and site; and correct surgical position. The patient must be positioned such that the marking of the operative site (e.g., with the word "yes" or the surgeon's initials) is visible on the patient's skin. Implants, special equipment, and any other requirements (e.g., blood or blood products, if ordered) are verified. Any special concerns about the patient or procedure are shared by team members. When complete, the procedure can begin. The time-out is documented according to institutional protocol.

Many factors influence emergence. The objective is to move the patient from the OR bed to the PACU bed as soon as the dressing is applied. During emergence, the anesthesia provider suctions the oropharynx before extubation to decrease the risk of aspiration and laryngospasm after extubation, reverses any residual neuromuscular blockade, and allows the washout of N_2O and volatile agents by giving 100% O_2 for several minutes before extubation. After extubation the patient is transported to the PACU to awaken. In some situations the patient may be transferred to the PACU before extubation and the ETT removed when the patient is fully awake.

Untoward events that can occur with general anesthesia include hypoxia; respiratory, cardiovascular, or renal dysfunction; hypotension; hypertension; fluid or electrolyte imbalance; residual muscle

FIGURE 5-5 Insertion of the laryngeal mask airway (LMA). Select the appropriate-size LMA (1, neonates ≤5 kg; 1.5, infants 5 to 10 kg; 2, infants and children 10 to 20 kg; 2½, children 20 to 30 kg; 3, children and small adults >30 kg; 4, normal size to large adults; 5, large adults). **A,** Carefully deflate the LMA as flat as possible so that the rim faces away from the mask aperture as shown. There should be no folds near the tip. **B,** Under direct vision, press the tip of the LMA cephalad against the hard palate to flatten it out. Using the index finger, continue pressing the LMA against the palate as the LMA is advanced into the pharynx to ensure that the tip remains flattened and avoids the tongue. **C,** Keeping the neck flexed and the head extended, use the index finger to press the LMA into the posterior wall. **D,** Continue pushing with the ball of the index finger, guiding the LMA posteriorly into position. By withdrawing the other fingers and slightly pronating the forearm, it is usually possible to push the LMA fully into position in one fluid movement. **E,** Firmly grasp the tube with the other hand; then withdraw the index finger from the pharynx. Gently press the LMA posteriorly to ensure that it is fully inserted. **F,** Carefully inflate the LMA with the recommended volume of air for size (1, 2 to 4 mL; 2, ≤10 mL; 2½, ≤14 mL; 3, ≤20 mL; 4, ≤30 mL; 5, ≤40 mL). Do not overinflate. Do not touch the LMA tube while inflating, unless it is obviously unstable (as with elderly edentulous patients with loose oropharyngeal tissues). Usually the LMA moves slightly forward out of the hypopharynx as it is inflated. Insert a bite-block (roll of gauze) alongside the LMA tube to minimize occlusion of the tube as the patient is awakening.

FIGURE 5-6 Sagittal views of insertion and proper placement of the laryngeal mask airway (LMA). **A,** Insertion of LMA. **B,** Proper location of LMA (deflated). **C,** Properly placed and inflated LMA.

paralysis; dental damage; neurologic problems; hypothermia; and MH. The anesthesia provider usually directs the treatment and management of such events.

Regional Anesthesia

Regional anesthesia (also called *conduction anesthesia*) can be accomplished by injecting a local anesthetic anywhere along the pathway of a nerve from the spinal cord. This injection provides anesthesia to a region of the body. Preoperative preparation for regional anesthesia is essentially the same as that for general anesthesia. Preoperative medication frequently is ordered before regional anesthesia to ease any discomfort that may be experienced during placement of the block. The criteria for monitoring during regional anesthesia are similar to those during general anesthesia. Whenever regional anesthesia is performed, resuscitative equipment and medications must be immediately available. During preparation and placement of the regional anesthetic, the perioperative nurse can provide valuable assistance. This assistance may include placing appropriate monitors, such as pulse oximetry, ECG, and blood pressure; providing supplemental O₂ if indicated; reassuring the patient; administering sedation, such as midazolam, as directed; and properly positioning the patient, which is crucial for a successful block.

Peripheral blocks on the lower or upper extremities or on the head frequently occur in a preoperative holding area to allow adequate time for the local anesthetic to penetrate the peripheral nerve before the patient is transferred to the OR. For peripheral blocks the perioperative nurse may need to perform aspiration during needle placement (to detect vascular puncture) and inject the local anesthetic while the anesthesia provider stabilizes the needle in the precise location. After an initial period of evaluation by the anesthesia provider, the nurse monitors the patient for any substantial change in vital signs or untoward reactions until transfer of the patient to the OR and hand-off to the perioperative nurse.

Spinal Anesthesia

A local anesthetic (usually lidocaine, tetracaine, or bupivacaine) injected into the cerebrospinal fluid (CSF) in the subarachnoid space is termed a *spinal anesthetic* or a *subarachnoid block (SAB)*. To provide additional analgesia, fentanyl or preservative-free morphine often is added to the local anesthetic. The anesthesia provider inserts a spinal needle into a lower lumbar interspace with the patient either lying on one side or in a sitting position. The local anesthetic, generally mixed with a dextrose solution for a total of 1 to 4 mL, results in a *hyperbaric* (heavier than the CSF) solution. These hyperbaric mixtures settle in a gravity-dependent manner after injection into the CSF. By changing the patient's position, the block can be directed up, down, or to one side of the spinal cord. With prostate surgery, the patient may remain in the sitting position for about 1 minute after injection of the local anesthetic to achieve a bilateral block of the S1-S5 dermatomes.

For surgery in the upper abdomen, the patient may be placed in a slight 5- to 10-degree head-down position to allow the anesthetic to move cephalad while the anesthesia provider carefully checks the level of sensory block. After reaching an adequate level, personnel level the bed to minimize further extension of the sensory block. After 10 to 15 minutes, the block usually "sets" or stabilizes, and does not extend farther. The sympathetic nervous system usually is blocked two dermatomes higher and the neuromuscular system two dermatomes lower than the sensory block. The patient is then positioned as necessary for surgery.

If the local anesthetic is mixed with a larger volume of sterile water, the solution is *hypobaric,* and the medication moves to the nondependent area. Hypobaric spinal anesthesia usually is done after the patient is positioned and the surgical site exposed (with the site of injection above the surgical site, as in perianal surgery in the prone position).

By mixing the local anesthetic with some CSF withdrawn from the subarachnoid space, the solution becomes *isobaric.* Distribution of this solution is minimally affected by gravity.

Spinal anesthesia may cause several physiologic responses, outlined immediately below, that can result in major problems if not properly managed.

Hypotension. Hypotension may occur rapidly after an SAB. It results from vasodilation because the sympathetic nerves that control vasomotor tone are blocked. Peripheral pooling of blood occurs, resulting in reduced venous return to the heart and decreased cardiac output. A hypotensive response usually can be avoided by infusing 750 to 1500 mL of balanced salt solution immediately before the block and placing the patient in a 5-degree head-down position to improve venous return to the heart. A vasopressor, such as ephedrine, also may be appropriate.

Total Spinal Anesthesia. Total spinal anesthesia (or inadvertent high spinal block) may cause paralysis of the respiratory muscles and necessitate immediate intubation and ventilation. Any sign or symptom of respiratory distress occurring shortly after instituting spinal anesthesia should alert the anesthesia provider to the possibility of a high spinal block.

Positioning Problems. Positioning problems can occur because pain and sensory inputs to a portion of the patient's body are blocked. Care must be taken to position the patient intraoperatively to avoid neurologic damage, burns, loss of skin integrity, or other trauma. Positioning the surgical patient is a collaborative effort among the anesthesia provider, surgeon, assistant, and perioperative nurse.

Postdural Puncture Headache. Postdural puncture headache (PDPH) (also called *postspinal cephalgia* or *spinal headache*) is a frequent postoperative complaint after spinal anesthesia. It occurs more commonly in young parturients (new mothers) or other patients younger than 40 years. With use of a 25- or 27-gauge blunt-bevel needle, incidence is about 1% (Olson et al, 2014). PDPH is unrelated to how soon the patient ambulates postoperatively. Current belief suggests the headache results from leakage of CSF through the hole in the dura and typically occurs when the patient assumes an upright position. Incidence, severity, and duration of the headache appear to correlate with the size of the hole left in the dura. The headache usually occurs in the occipital area and generally resolves over 1 to 3 days but may last 2 weeks. Several treatments have been used to relieve the headache: strict bed rest for 24 to 48 hours, vigorous hydration, abdominal binders, PO or IV caffeine, and injection of 5 to 20 mL of autologous blood into the epidural space at the puncture site ("blood patch"). Although rare, a repeat dose can be given within 24 hours (Olson et al, 2014).

Many anesthesia providers use different spinal needles that have a tip shaped like a sharpened wood pencil with the holes on the side of the needle. These 24- to 26-gauge spinal needles (e.g., Whitacre, Sprotte, Gertie Marx) presumably separate or go between the dural fibers as opposed to cutting the fibers, which may occur when a blunt-bevel spinal needle is used. With these "pencil-point" needles, the incidence and severity of PDPH lower substantially (Olson et al, 2014).

Epidural and Caudal Anesthesia

The epidural space is between the ligamentum flavum and the dura, and extends from the foramen magnum to the sacrococcygeal membrane. In it are epidural veins, fat, and loose areolar tissue. For *epidural* anesthesia, the anesthesia provider usually injects local anesthetic through the intervertebral spaces in the lumbar region (lumbar epidural), although injection also can be into the cervical or thoracic regions. The anesthetic spreads cephalad and caudad from the site of injection. A comparative location of the needle points and injected anesthetic appears in Figure 5-7.

For *caudal* anesthesia, the local anesthetic also is injected into the epidural space, but the approach is through the caudal canal in the sacrum. Compared with a lumbar epidural, this approach requires a greater volume of anesthetic to fill the epidural space. Caudal anesthesia has a 5% to 10% technical failure rate. Given its ease of administration, however, it is often used for perineal procedures or pediatric surgery on the lower extremities along with a light general anesthetic (Olson et al, 2014).

Several techniques may be used for epidural or caudal anesthesia. A "single-shot epidural" involves administration of a local anesthetic through the needle before its removal. For intermittent injections or continuous infusions, a small catheter is inserted into the epidural space for administration of local anesthetic.

For combined spinal and epidural anesthesia, the anesthesia provider first inserts the epidural needle (dual-conduit needles now are available to reduce possible complications from a one-channel Tuohy needle) into the epidural space, and then inserts a special, long 25-, 27-, or 29-gauge spinal needle through the epidural needle into the CSF. A small amount of fentanyl or preservative-free morphine may be injected and provides good analgesia for several hours. Removal of the spinal needle follows, and an epidural catheter inserted. When the dual-channel needle is used, the epidural catheter is inserted first, and then the spinal needle is placed. This technique is especially useful for obstetric anesthesia (Olson et al, 2014).

Techniques to identify the epidural space include the "hanging drop" and the "loss of resistance" to injection of either air or liquid (saline or local anesthetic) as the needle is advanced slowly through the ligamentum flavum. With the hanging-drop technique, the needle is filled with liquid to form a meniscus at the needle hub. As the needle is slowly advanced into the epidural space, negative (less than atmospheric) pressure draws the liquid inward toward the epidural space. Location of the needle tip within the epidural space is verified by injection of an additional 1 to 2 mL of air or saline.

When local anesthetics are injected into the epidural space, the major sites of action are the nerve roots as they leave the spinal cord and proceed out the intervertebral foramina beyond the meningeal sheath. Some anesthetic diffuses into the subarachnoid space to the spinal cord. As local anesthetics diffuse away from the site of injection, segmental anesthesia is possible in specific areas. In contrast to spinal anesthesia, much larger volumes of local anesthetic are needed with epidural anesthesia; the head-up, head-down, or lateral position of the patient does not affect the level of the epidural anesthetic as much, and onset of anesthesia is much slower with epidural anesthesia. As with spinal anesthesia, hypotension can occur with epidural anesthesia, but onset is much slower and usually can be managed with rapid IV infusion of balanced salt solution or repositioning of the patient (Sawhney, 2012).

Local anesthetics most frequently used for epidural anesthesia are lidocaine, bupivacaine, and chloroprocaine. Ropivacaine and levobupivacaine are newer local anesthetics that may prove to be less cardiotoxic than bupivacaine and possess a larger therapeutic ratio. Although much of their pharmacologic profile is similar to that of bupivacaine, levobupivacaine and ropivacaine seem to possess more selective action for neural blockade (Olson et al, 2014). Depending on the concentration of the anesthetic agent, effects can range from loss of sensory input to complete motor blockade. To verify that the anesthetic is not being injected into the subarachnoid space or into an epidural vein, a test dose of 3 to 5 mL of lidocaine with a 1:200,000 concentration of epinephrine is frequently used. Injected intravascularly, this test dose causes a transient tachycardia. If injected into the subarachnoid space, it produces a low level of spinal anesthesia.

Complications associated with the use of local anesthetics in the epidural and subarachnoid spaces are unique to the agent used. Permanent neurologic sequelae have been reported when chloroprocaine with a preservative was injected into the subarachnoid space. Bupivacaine is associated with pronounced cardiac toxicity if injected intravascularly (Olson et al, 2014). With epidural anesthesia several complications can occur, including inadvertent dural puncture, subarachnoid injection, and vascular injection.

Inadvertent Dural Puncture. Inadvertent dural puncture with the epidural needle (a wet tap) can cause a PDPH. This headache is significant in about 50% of patients, and its intensity can incapacitate. Treatment is essentially the same as that discussed under Spinal Anesthesia earlier in this chapter.

FIGURE 5-7 Location of needle point and injected anesthetic relative to dura. **A,** Epidural catheter. **B,** Single injection epidural. **C,** Spinal anesthesia. (Interspaces most commonly used are L4-L5, L3-L4, and L2-L3.)

Subarachnoid Injection. Subarachnoid injection occurs if the needle or catheter is unintentionally inserted into the subarachnoid space. If a large volume of local anesthetic is injected as a bolus, it causes "total spinal" anesthesia. This condition is associated with a rapid onset of hypotension caused by vasodilation and profound bradycardia as the sympathetic nerves to the heart are blocked, causing a totally paralyzed patient. Treatment includes intubation, control of ventilation, support of blood pressure and the cardiovascular system, and administration of amnestic medications until the block resolves. If properly managed this problem is not life threatening, but use of the test dose described previously and injection of only 3 to 5 mL at a time usually avoids this problem. With patient movement over time, the epidural catheter can migrate through the dura. Therefore, a small test dose should be given each time additional local anesthetic is injected through the catheter. In addition, each subsequent dose should be injected in increments of 3 to 5 mL each.

Vascular Injection. Injection of local anesthetic into an epidural vein may occur inadvertently with the initial dose or with subsequent injections. Intravenously injected bupivacaine is associated with cardiac arrest (Research Highlight). Toxicity from other local anesthetics can cause sudden and profound hypotension, convulsions from effects on the CNS, and tachycardia if the solution contains epinephrine. The airway is supported/managed for oxygenation and ventilation, seizures are treated, then lipid emulsion infusion is begun to reverse signs and symptoms of toxicity. Basic life support, including chest compressions is used when indicated in order to ensure tissue perfusion and circulation of resuscitation medications, including lipid emulsion (Weinberg, 2012).

Convulsions usually dissipate rapidly as local anesthetic redistributes throughout the body. An IV benzodiazepine may be given to reduce these effects. A vasopressor (e.g., ephedrine or phenylephrine) can be used to restore blood pressure. If the patient becomes paralyzed, intubation and ventilation are required until the toxic effects are gone. Use of a test dose with each injection usually prevents these problems.

Peripheral Nerve Blocks

Peripheral nerves can be blocked effectively by injecting local anesthetic around them to provide adequate surgical anesthesia. Onset and duration of the block depend on the medication used and its concentration and volume, addition of epinephrine, and site of injection. Complications usually arise from an inadvertent intravascular injection or an overdose of the local anesthetic. Rarely, trauma caused by the needle or compression from the volume of local anesthetic injected may cause nerve damage.

Peripheral nerve blocks (PNBs) are an effective method to deliver analgesia and anesthesia, and have been used by surgeons and anesthesia providers since the late 1800s. However, in the twentieth century, PNBs were replaced with general anesthetics, which produce a desired effect of total body anesthesia and analgesia. Ironically, the burgeoning of ambulatory surgery created renewed interest in the use of PNBs.

With that exponential growth of ambulatory surgery and the current demand for time and cost consciousness, the benefits of PNBs can be many. Local anesthetics have quick onset of action, provide prolonged analgesia, and often do not require administration of powerful anesthetics that have undesired side effects. Patients often leave with less pain, and less nausea and vomiting, report greater satisfaction with the quality of care received, and avoid the

---

RESEARCH HIGHLIGHT ❚❚

Lipid Infusion for Local Anesthetic Systemic Toxicity (LAST) and Cardiac Resuscitation

IV local anesthetics work by blocking voltage-gated sodium ion channels that are essential for normal nerve impulse conduction. The result impedes transmission of pain stimuli. However, voltage-gated sodium ion channels are found in cardiac nerve cells. Bupivacaine, a commonly used local anesthetic agent, has been implicated as a causative agent for patients experiencing cardiac arrest following accidental intravascular injection during a peripheral nerve block (PNB). Research findings and case reports suggest that lipid infusion is an effective adjunct to standard cardiac resuscitation procedures for bupivacaine toxicity. A bolus of a 20% lipid emulsion, such as Intralipid (Baxter Pharmaceuticals, Deerfield, IL), that is followed immediately by a continuous infusion (approximately 0.25-0.5 mL/kg/min) for roughly 10 minutes has been shown to help with successful cardiac resuscitation and returning patients to normal cardiac rhythm.

Although the exact mechanism is unknown, Sandlin-Leming (2010) suggests that lipids appear to pull the toxic medication away from cardiac tissue like a sponge and reduce its harmful effects on the heart. Monitor the patient during and after completing injection because clinical toxicity can be delayed up to 30 minutes. Weinberg suggests making a lipid rescue kit for every area in a facility where regional anesthesia blocks are administered. He suggests a box or bag containing a 500-mL bag of 20% lipid solution, IV tubing, 60-mL syringes (2), and needles. A treatment protocol and LAST checklist should be included in the kit. The American Society of Regional Anesthesia and Pain Medicine has a practice advisory for managing LAST which can be accessed via their website at www.asra.com. Weinberg also recommends ready availability of 20% lipid emulsion in any site where local anesthetics are administered.

Modified from Neal JM et al: ASA practice advisory on local anesthetic systemic toxicity, *Reg Anesth Pain Med* 35:152–161, 2010; Sandlin-Leming DC: Resuscitation of local anesthesia-induced cardiac arrest: lipids to the rescue, *J Perianesth Nurs* 25(6):418–420, 2010; Sirianni AJ et al: Use of lipid emulsion in the resuscitation of a patient with prolonged cardiovascular collapse after overdose of bupropion and lamotrigine, *Ann Emerg Med* 51(4):412–415, 2008; Warren JA et al: Intravenous lipid infusion in the successful resuscitation of local anesthetic-induced cardiovascular collapse after supraclavicular brachial plexus block, *Anesth Analg* 106(5):1578–1580, 2008; Weinberg G: Lipid emulsion infusion: resuscitation for local anesthetic and other drug overdose, *Anesthesiology* 117(1): 180–187, 2012.

---

undesirable side effects of excess opioids. PNBs are an essential part of contemporary multimodal anesthesia.

Peripheral Nerve Anatomy and Physiology. The peripheral nervous system consists of 31 pairs of spinal nerves that exit between the vertebrae on each side of the body. These spinal nerves traverse the torso and innervate specific regions in order to coordinate within the CNS our ability to perceive cutaneous sensation and respond with synchronized motor reflexes. Peripheral sensory nerve impulses initiate by noxious stimuli, such as surgical incision. This stimulus creates an "action potential" that changes the electrical voltage traveling across the axonal membrane of the nerve by allowing an influx of sodium ions (referred to as cellular depolarization). This creates a propagating electrical wave that conducts a sensory nerve impulse to the brain, which interprets it as pain. Local anesthetics work by blocking the opening of these sodium ion channels so that the patient perceives no pain (Cousins and Bridenbaigh, 2009).

Common Peripheral Nerve Blocks

Upper Extremity—The Brachial Plexus. Spinal nerves leaving the cervical vertebrae, C5-T1, converge to form a bundle of nerves known as the brachial plexus. Each bundle of nerves innervates the right and left side of the neck and axilla. The brachial plexus divides further into branches that eventually terminate in the radial, ulnar, and median nerves. For example, the median nerve is released from impingement when a carpal tunnel procedure is performed.

PNBs of the brachial plexus are therefore performed for surgery of the shoulder, forearm, or hand. The different anatomic landmarks that anesthesia practitioners use to perform a brachial plexus nerve block are the interscalene, supraclavicular, infraclavicular, or axillary sites. The choice of anatomic site for PNB depends on (1) the area of the arm undergoing surgery and (2) the specific surgical procedure. As an example, a shoulder arthroscopy dictates an interscalene brachial plexus block as appropriate, whereas for carpal tunnel surgery, an infraclavicular or axillary block is proper.

Lower Extremity. Lumbar and sacral spinal nerves, also exiting through each side of the vertebrae, eventually separate into the sciatic, femoral, popliteal, and tibial nerve roots that innervate the lower extremities. PNBs for the lower extremities are often performed for knee and foot procedures. For example, a femoral nerve block is effective for a knee arthroscopy or for pain management after total knee arthroplasty, whereas an ankle block (essentially a block of the deep and superficial peroneal, tibial, and sural nerve branches of the sciatic nerve) is appropriate for podiatric procedures (Brown, 2010).

Peripheral Nerve Block Equipment.

To identify the correct injection site for the PNB, the anesthesia provider typically uses a nerve stimulator, now more often with ultrasound guidance (Vacchiano and Biegner, 2014). The nerve stimulator creates an electrical current. The goal is to elicit a motor response from the nerve while applying the correct amount of voltage. Once the anesthesia provider isolates the desired nerves to be "blocked," the appropriate local anesthetic is carefully injected into tissue close to the nerve. The local anesthetic then inhibits the propagation of nerve impulses to the CNS by blocking sodium ion channels. Depending on the desired site of action, PNBs can take from a few minutes to as long as an hour to achieve complete effect. The duration of the nerve block depends on the local anesthetic used.

Important Nursing Considerations

Expected Side Effects and Special Care Concerns. PNBs often have side effects. For example, with an interscalene block, patients may experience Horner syndrome (miosis, ptosis, and increased salivation) and may also have a unilateral phrenic nerve paralysis that causes breathing difficulty. These side effects may need special anesthesia attention depending on severity. All perioperative staff must remember that the patient with a PNB has lost the protective reflex of pain sensation. Therefore, special care is required for proper patient positioning and properly padded pressure points, as well as for postoperative patient education regarding the risk of burns or falls.

Preparation for Adverse Events. PNB is a safe method of anesthesia and analgesia delivery. It does, however, pose serious potential complications that all perioperative staff must anticipate in advance of emergencies.

Local anesthetic systemic toxicity (LAST) results when a patient absorbs an unsafe amount of a local anesthetic into the bloodstream (see Research Highlight: Lipid Infusion for Local Anesthetic Systemic Toxicity [LAST] and Cardiac Resuscitation). This can occur either slowly from systemic absorption of a local anesthetic correctly injected into tissue, or immediately and catastrophically if injected accidentally directly into a blood vessel. Signs of systemic local anesthetic toxicity often progress in a stepwise manner. Patients may initially report perioral numbness, a metallic taste in the mouth, ringing in the ears, visual disturbances, and/or dizziness. If toxicity progresses, or is immediate, the patient will likely have seizures, respiratory arrest, and/or cardiac arrest.

Performance of PNB is appropriate only in areas well equipped to handle emergencies—that is, areas having access to an external oxygen source, vacuum suction, ventilation bag and mask, laryngoscope, ETT tubes, monitoring equipment, and resuscitation medications to treat hypotension, bradycardia, and seizures. The increased use of PNB has occasioned increased reports of cardiac arrest from accidental intravascular injection; however, the incidence has dropped dramatically, noted by the occurrence of LAST to be 4 per 10,000 epidurals, down from 100 per 10,000 epidurals (Nagelhout, 2014).

Intravenous Regional Anesthesia

IV regional anesthesia was first described by Bier in 1908 and is frequently called a *Bier block*. Although it can be used on a lower extremity, it is used more often on the upper extremities. It is highly reliable and straightforward to accomplish.

A small IV catheter is inserted as distal to the surgical site as feasible, and a single-cuffed or double-cuffed pneumatic tourniquet is placed around the limb proximal to the surgical site. The limb is raised and exsanguinated by wrapping it with an Esmarch bandage. The tourniquet is inflated to approximately 100 mm Hg above the patient's systolic blood pressure, and the Esmarch bandage removed. About 50 mL of 0.5% lidocaine is injected through the catheter. Onset of anesthesia is rapid and lasts until the tourniquet is deflated (Vacchiano and Biegner, 2014).

When a double-cuffed pneumatic tourniquet is used, the proximal cuff is initially inflated. When the patient experiences discomfort from the cuff pressure (usually about 35 to 40 minutes after cuff inflation), the distal cuff, which is located over an anesthetized area, is inflated and the proximal cuff deflated. The proximal cuff remains inflated until the distal cuff has been inflated to prevent loss of the IV anesthetic from the limb. Two single-cuffed tourniquets can substitute for a double-cuffed tourniquet. If the patient experiences pain from the tourniquet, an IV analgesic or sedative can supplement the block, and ketorolac (15-30 mg in the local anesthetic) has been found to provide a degree of postoperative analgesia without increased risk of bleeding (Vacchiano and Biegner, 2014).

Although problems can occur from an overdose or toxic reaction to lidocaine, these are rare if tourniquet inflation lasts more than 20 minutes. Intermittent cuff deflation for a few seconds at a time for several cycles when the surgical procedure concludes minimizes the risk of overdose or toxic reaction. This reduces the transient peak blood level of local anesthetic in the CNS and heart. Conversely, loss of pneumatic pressure in the tourniquet can cause a toxic reaction and loss of anesthesia (New York School of Regional Anesthesia, 2009).

Monitored Anesthesia Care

Surgeons can safely undertake minor and even some major procedures with a peripheral nerve block or when the surgical site is infiltrated with a local anesthetic. These techniques are appropriate for normal, healthy individuals as well as for sicker, unstable patients who otherwise would require more extensive, invasive monitoring and pharmacologic management if general anesthesia were used. For sicker, unstable patients, surgeons and anesthesia providers must weigh the relative risks and benefits of MAC versus general anesthesia.

During MAC, the anesthesia provider usually supplements the local anesthetic with an IV analgesic (e.g., fentanyl) and with sedative and amnestic medications (e.g., midazolam or propofol). Vital signs, respiratory and cardiovascular status, and positioning are carefully monitored, and supplemental low-flow O_2 often administered. Depending on the clinical situation, the anesthesia provider may have to induce general anesthesia or use one of the regional techniques described previously if a greater degree of anesthesia becomes necessary.

Moderate Sedation/Analgesia

Moderate sedation/analgesia refers to IV administration of certain sedatives and analgesics that produces a condition in which the patient exhibits a depressed level of consciousness but retains the ability to maintain a patent airway independently and respond appropriately to verbal commands or physical stimulation. It is also referred to as conscious sedation. The anesthesia provider is not involved in the patient's care. Perioperative nurses who have additional training and demonstrated competencies in (1) administering medications to achieve moderate sedation/analgesia and (2) patient monitoring perform these functions (AORN, 2013). Objectives for a patient receiving moderate sedation/analgesia include mood alteration, continued consciousness, enhanced cooperation, elevated pain threshold, minimal variation of vital signs, some degree of amnesia, and rapid and safe return to activities of daily living.

Selection of patients for moderate sedation/analgesia depends on established criteria developed by an interdisciplinary team. Patients undergo thorough assessment physiologically and psychologically before the procedure. Assessment includes a review of physical examination findings; current medications; existing allergies; current medical problems; history of smoking, alcohol intake, or substance abuse (Tonnesen et al, 2009); current chief complaint; baseline vital signs, height, and weight; age; emotional state; any communication deficits; and patient perceptions of moderate sedation/analgesia. Monitoring methods for patients receiving moderate sedation, medications administered, and interventions initiated must be within the scope of nursing practice as defined by the respective state board of nursing. If the nurse does not feel comfortable managing the care and monitoring of a particular patient, the attending physician and an anesthesia provider should be consulted. During the past few years, advocates have supported propofol administration by nurses. The U.S. Food and Drug Administration (FDA) continues, however, to include a "black box" warning that only trained anesthesia providers should administer propofol. The American Association of Nurse Anesthetists (AANA) and the ASA continue to support the FDA view for patient safety reasons. Even in the hands of an anesthesia provider, propofol can affect respirations, possibly requiring advanced airway management.

When monitoring a patient receiving moderate sedation/analgesia, the nurse should have no other responsibilities that would leave the patient unattended or compromise continuous patient monitoring. The nurse must be clinically competent in the use of monitoring equipment and oxygen-delivery devices, medications used for moderate sedation/analgesia and resuscitation, and airway management. Advanced cardiac life support (ACLS) certification of nurses responsible for monitoring patients receiving moderate sedation/analgesia is usually required. If not, health care professionals with ACLS skills should be readily available to render support if needed in an emergency (AORN, 2013).

The nurse who administers moderate sedation/analgesia medications should know usual dosages, contraindications, interactions with other medications, onset and duration of action and desired effects, adverse reactions, and emergency management techniques. Benzodiazepines (e.g., diazepam, midazolam) and opioids (e.g., fentanyl, meperidine hydrochloride) are used for moderate sedation/analgesia (AORN, 2013). Equipment in the room where moderate sedation/analgesia is administered includes a noninvasive blood pressure device, an ECG, a pulse oximeter, oxygen-delivery devices, and suction. An emergency cart with appropriate resuscitative medications and equipment (e.g., a defibrillator) should be immediately available.

An IV access line is established to administer medications, along with any emergency medications and fluids if needed. Parameters monitored during moderate sedation/analgesia are respiratory rate, cardiac rate and rhythm, blood pressure, oxygen saturation, level of consciousness, and skin condition.

Nursing documentation should include preprocedure assessment; dosage, route, time, and effects of all medications administered; type and amount of fluids administered; physiologic data from continuous monitoring at 5- to 15-minute intervals and on significant events; level of consciousness; nursing interventions initiated and patient responses; and any untoward significant patient reactions and their resolution (AORN, 2013).

Postprocedure monitoring should be provided until the patient has returned to preprocedure baseline parameters. Patients and family members or significant others should receive appropriate, health-literate oral and written discharge instructions and be able to verbalize understanding (i.e., teach back in their own words).

Discharge criteria should be established by an interdisciplinary team and should include adequate respiratory function, stable vital signs, return to preprocedure level of consciousness, intact motor reflexes, return of motor and sensory control, absence of protracted nausea, acceptable skin color and condition, absence of significant pain, and satisfactory surgical site and dressing condition (when present). A responsible adult must accompany and drive the patient home.

Local Anesthesia

The terms *local anesthesia, local,* and *straight local* are used interchangeably to describe the administration of an anesthetic agent to a specific area of the body by topical application, local infiltration, regional nerve block, or "field" block. The surgeon administers local anesthetics. In addition, other physicians, such as cardiologists, pulmonologists, proctologists, and gastroenterologists, may perform local procedures in the OR suite. No anesthesia provider is involved.

Hospitals and ambulatory surgery centers establish interdisciplinary guidelines for selecting patients who are appropriate for local anesthesia procedures and for patient monitoring criteria. Decisions to monitor the patient receiving local anesthesia, parameters that need to be monitored, and the frequency of observation and monitoring are tailored to the patient, the surgical procedure, and medications used. Patients receiving local anesthetics require preoperative assessment and continual monitoring by the perioperative nurse during the procedure.

Local anesthesia usually is used for minor, short-term surgical, diagnostic, or therapeutic procedures. Because the patient does not lose consciousness, local anesthesia is frequently preferred when the patient's cooperation is necessary for the procedure. Local anesthesia is economical and eliminates the undesirable effects of general anesthesia. Adverse reactions, however, may occur from large doses of local agents. If the agent enters the bloodstream directly, convulsions, circulatory and respiratory distress, cardiovascular collapse, or even death can result.

The surgeon chooses local anesthetics based on desired duration of action, surgery site, potency potential, and the patient's physical status. Topical agents, such as cocaine hydrochloride, tetracaine, or lidocaine, may be applied to mucous membranes of the nose, throat, trachea, and urethra. Lidocaine 0.5% to 2%, with or without epinephrine, is the medication most commonly used for local anesthesia, although bupivacaine (Marcaine) may also be selected. Epinephrine may be added to the local anesthetic agent for its vasoconstricting properties in the area injected, slower rate of absorption of the local anesthetic agent, and lower incidence of toxicity. Adding epinephrine allows longer duration of action for the local agent by reducing blood flow to the area injected. Epinephrine must be used with caution in patients with hypertension, diabetes, or heart disease. A general recommendation for a local anesthetic such as lidocaine is that no more than 50 mL of a 1% solution, or 100 mL of a 0.5% solution, should be injected per hour. (For maximum adult dosages, see the Surgical Pharmacology box on pp. 137-139.) All local anesthetic containers or syringes should be clearly labeled, both on and off the sterile field.

Preoperatively, the perioperative nurse reviews the patient's history, physical examination findings, and results of any ordered laboratory or other diagnostic tests. Patients undergo careful assessment to determine physiologic baselines, any allergies (to medications, latex, adhesive tape, or other substances), and emotional status. IV infusion begins before the procedure because adequate venous access is crucial in life-threatening emergent situations, when resuscitative medications must be given immediately (see Research Highlight box on p. 147).

The perioperative nurse must be clinically competent to use monitoring equipment, to make equipment connections, and to interpret data. Most often minimum intraoperative monitoring includes heart rate and regularity, respiratory rate, and mental status. Additional monitoring parameters depend on the patient's condition and include blood pressure, skin condition, and oxygen saturation status (AORN, 2013). Any changes in the patient's condition should be communicated immediately to the surgeon.

The perioperative nurse also must be familiar with the medications administered during the procedure, usual dosages, limits on rate of injection and maximum dosage (usually stated on a per-kilogram basis), duration of action, physiologic and psychologic changes expected, normal and abnormal reactions, and appropriate action to take if untoward reactions occur. The nurse observes the patient for side effects such as CNS disturbances, cardiovascular problems, hypersensitivity to medication, and toxic reaction resulting from high levels of local anesthetic. Emergency medications, suction apparatus, and resuscitation equipment should be readily available. Symptoms of adverse medication reactions include restlessness, unexplained anxiety or fearfulness, diaphoresis, nausea, palpitations, disturbed respiration, pallor or flushing, syncope, and convulsive movements. Signs and symptoms of allergic reaction include urticaria, tachycardia, laryngeal edema resulting in breathing difficulties, nausea, vomiting, and elevated temperature. In some instances, anaphylactoid symptoms, including severe hypotension,

can occur. If any significant change occurs in the patient's physiologic or psychologic status, the nurse should notify the physician immediately. Good communication is essential for optimal patient care (National Quality Forum, 2012). Because the patient is awake during the procedure, extraneous or irrelevant conversation and noise must be minimal.

Documentation of care provided to a patient receiving a local anesthetic should be consistent with the AORN's evidence-based recommendations (AORN, 2013). This includes all medications administered, including their dosages, routes, and times of administration; patient monitoring performed; and results of patient care procedures.

After the procedure the patient's postoperative status undergoes careful assessment. This evaluation and any special patient needs are documented on the chart, and the receiving unit receives a report before the patient's transfer (if the patient is going to a recovery area). The hand-off report should include type and amount of medications given and any adverse reaction noted, site and condition of the IV infusion (if applicable), type and amount of solution infused in the OR, range of intraoperative vital signs, surgical procedure performed, and condition of any dressing. Included are any special postoperative orders, allergies, and a general statement of the patient's tolerance of the procedure. The patient may transfer to the day-surgery and discharge area or return directly to a hospital room. Transfers of local anesthesia patients to PACU for recovery or observation are rare.

Pain Management

Many anesthesia providers have applied their expertise in analgesia and regional anesthesia to acute and chronic pain management. Chronic pain is often multifactorial and may occur after a discrete injury (or trauma), amputation, laminectomy, or other surgical procedure. It also may result from prolonged repetitive stress, such as "low back pain." Chronic pain frequently has complex psychologic components unrecognized by patients or by individuals closely associated with them. Diagnosis and treatment of such chronic pain usually involve multiple medical disciplines and prolonged management.

Acute perioperative pain is a different problem. Traditionally, postoperative pain has been treated with IM narcotics every 3 to 6 hours as needed. This treatment is often associated with undesirable side effects, including oversedation, respiratory depression, deep vein thrombosis (DVT) secondary to decreased mobility, and variable degrees of pain relief. Use of pain management modalities are now successful. Patient-controlled analgesia (PCA) uses a programmable electronic pump that can continuously infuse a small amount of IV narcotic (at a basal rate); in addition, the patient can administer a predetermined bolus "on demand." Safety interlocks limit the frequency of boluses and total dose per hour (Bordi, 2014).

When using spinal or epidural anesthesia for a surgical procedure, a small amount of preservative-free narcotic, such as fentanyl, sufentanil, or morphine, may be added to the local anesthetic mixture. The narcotic acts via central opiate receptors and provides analgesia for 24 to 36 hours.

Continuous epidural analgesia also may be appropriate for prolonged postoperative pain management. Physicians may use this technique for extensive procedures, including total hip or knee replacements; knee reconstruction; and major abdominal, thoracic, or gynecologic operations. In addition, it can be useful for acute trauma, such as multiple rib fractures.

Typically a lumbar or thoracic epidural catheter is inserted before surgery, covered with a transparent occlusive dressing, and injected with local anesthetic. Given the duration, manipulation, or positioning required for the operative procedure, general anesthesia is often used for patient comfort. The epidural greatly reduces analgesic requirements of general anesthesia. This allows for the avoidance of systemic opioids, making regional anesthesia a superb method of pain control (Rieker, 2014). A small dose of preservative-free narcotic, such as fentanyl, sufentanil, or morphine, is usually added to enhance analgesia. After surgery the infusion rate is adjusted to provide analgesia during early recovery. As the level of pain decreases over time, reduction of the infusion rate follows. Catheter removal occurs after 2 to 5 days to minimize infection risk. Benefits of epidural analgesia for acute postoperative pain include good analgesia with minimal sedation, early ambulation and physical therapy, and excellent patient satisfaction. Possible side effects include nausea, pruritus, and areas of slight numbness. These are controlled by using medications such as diphenhydramine (Benadryl) or naloxone (Narcan) and by adjusting the infusion rate. A nonsteroidal antiinflammatory drug (NSAID), such as ketorolac (Toradol), is given for any "breakthrough pain" instead of increasing the epidural infusion (Rieker, 2014).

A single caudal injection is often used in pediatric patients who have surgery of the lower abdomen, pelvis, or lower extremities. It usually follows induction of general anesthesia, with selection typically of a long-acting local anesthetic such as bupivacaine with epinephrine. This injection provides good analgesia for 8 to 24 hours postoperatively and greatly decreases intraoperative requirements for general anesthesia. If the procedure requires prolonged recovery, a lumbar epidural catheter can be placed intraoperatively. Postoperatively, management is similar to that with an epidural catheter (Olson et al, 2014).

Epidural infusions also may be appropriate for patients experiencing the intense pain of terminal malignancies. These patients may experience pain that is so severe that parenteral analgesics fail to provide adequate pain relief and produce deep respiratory depression. Epidural infusions for prolonged periods have succeeded in providing relief for these patients. Transdermal fentanyl patches also may prove successful both for these patients and for patients experiencing chronic pain.

Temperature Control

Monitoring body temperature is an important part of anesthesia monitoring, and standards of care for both the AANA and ASA support the ability to monitor a patient's temperature as essential (Bozimowski, 2014). Increased attention toward intraoperative maintenance of normal temperature ranges (normothermia) for pediatric and adult patients has followed. Hypothermia is the most common disorder of temperature homeostasis and may be intentional or unintentional. Unintentional hypothermia can cause patient discomfort, untoward cardiac events, adrenergic stimulation, impaired platelet function, altered medication metabolism, delayed emergence from anesthesia, and impaired wound healing (Odom-Forren, 2014).

Risk factors for developing inadvertent hypothermia include age extremes (elderly and pediatric patients), comorbidity, surgical duration, cachexia, fluid shifts, cold irrigating fluids, and general and regional anesthesia. Agents such as skeletal muscle relaxants interfere with shivering mechanisms. Agents that depress the CNS decrease autonomic reflexes that ordinarily autoregulate body temperature. Vasodilation, which accompanies use of various anesthetic agents, including inhalation agents, enhances heat transfer from the core to the periphery, where it is lost to the atmosphere. Cold, unhumidified inhalation gases further promote hypothermia through convection and evaporation.

Room temperature can be increased and infrared warming lamps used for pediatric patients. Fresh-gas flow rates of cool, dry anesthetic gases can be lowered. A heat and moisture exchanger (e.g., Humidivent) helps maintain the heat and moisture of inspired gases. A variety of IV fluid warmers are available to warm crystalloid solutions or refrigerated blood products. Some warmer units, originally designed for major trauma procedures, heat fluids at flow rates of 500 mL/min. Forced-air warming devices that blow heated air onto the upper or lower body surface are commonly used to keep patients warm and maintain normothermia. These units are effective in maintaining body temperature even during a long abdominal procedure and can be used later in the PACU. Forced-air warming devices must be used according to manufacturers' instructions. They must be used with an appropriate disposable blanket and should *not* have the hose inserted under surgical drapes to warm the patient (this directs the heat on the patient, with the risk of a burn, rather than filtering it through the blanket). The blanket air temperature is typically a couple of degrees lower than that coming directly from the hose because heat dissipates as it moves through the blanket (Chapter 10 discusses thermoregulation in the PACU).

Malignant Hyperthermia

First identified in the late 1960s, MH is a rare, life-threatening complication that may arise from medications commonly used in anesthesia. Inhalational anesthetics and succinylcholine are the most frequently implicated triggering agents. Trauma, strenuous exercise, or emotional stress also may induce MH. It is multifactorial and genetically transmitted as an autosomal dominant trait with variable expression in affected individuals (Hernandez et al, 2009). The incidence of MH increases in patients with central core disease (a congenital myopathy) and some muscular dystrophies (Karlet and Cahoon, 2014; Malignant Hyperthermia Association of the United States [MHAUS], 2011).

The MH syndrome begins with a hypermetabolic condition in skeletal muscle cells that involves altered mechanisms of calcium function at the cellular level. Characteristics include cellular hypermetabolism resulting in hypercarbia, tachypnea, tachycardia, hypoxia, metabolic and respiratory acidosis, cardiac dysrhythmias, and elevation of body temperature at a rate of $1°$ to $2°C$ every 5 minutes. Increase in body temperature is a late manifestation of MH. These signs may occur during induction or maintenance of anesthesia, although MH can occur postoperatively or even after repeated exposures to anesthesia. It is seen most frequently in children and adolescents (Karlet and Cahoon, 2014; MHAUS, 2011). The signs and symptoms associated with MH appear in Box 5-3.

It is important to remember that MH is a rare, multifaceted syndrome and can have variable clinical presentations. Many of the signs and symptoms associated with MH can have other causes. Other disorders, such as neuroleptic malignant syndrome (NMS), may have similar presentations. NMS occurs after use of neuroleptic medications, such as haloperidol, and is characterized by muscular rigidity, akinesia, hyperthermia, and autonomic dysfunction. Because MH is such a life-threatening disorder, many anesthesia providers initiate a treatment protocol when some of these early signs and symptoms occur that cannot otherwise be readily explained.

BOX 5-3

Signs and Symptoms Often Seen with Malignant Hyperthermia

- Hypercarbia
- Tachycardia
- Tachypnea (may not be seen in a paralyzed patient)
- Muscle stiffness or rigidity
- Hypoxia and dark (desaturated) blood in operative field
- Unstable or elevated blood pressure
- Cardiac dysrhythmias
- Changes in CO_2 absorbent (temperature, color)
- Metabolic and respiratory acidosis
- Peripheral mottling, cyanosis, or sweating
- Rising body temperature (1° to 2°C every 5 minutes)
- Myoglobinuria
- Hyperkalemia, hypercalcemia, lactic acidemia
- Pronounced elevation in creatine kinase level

PATIENT-CENTERED CARE

"Today I will be the nurse taking care of you in the operating room during your shoulder arthroscopy. I see on your anesthesia consent form that you are having a general anesthetic and an interscalene nerve block (ISB). In your own words, can you tell me what you understand will happen? Your experience with us today will be easier if you know what usually happens and what you should expect. If you have questions, we want to answer them clearly and completely."

The patient should be able to relate that the anesthesia provider will inject medication in an area by the neck to help with pain, both during and after the procedure. Because the surgery is in the shoulder, the ISB is an excellent procedure to achieve decreased pain postoperatively. It will also diminish overall requirements for general anesthesia; this may allow the patient to wake up more quickly and to experience possibly less or no nausea and vomiting. The patient should also be able to state that he or she will be sedated lightly during placement of the block and will need to position the head to the side opposite the block site.

Time is crucial when MH is diagnosed. All OR and anesthesia personnel should be familiar with the protocol for its management. In the past mortality ranged up to 80%, but the immediate infusion of dantrolene (Dantrium) and proper treatment have reduced mortality to about 7%. Dantrolene is a hydantoin skeletal muscle relaxant that also has effects on vascular and heart muscle. In addition to dantrolene, the major modalities of treatment include cooling the patient with ice packs and cold IV solutions, administering diuretics, treating cardiac dysrhythmias, correcting acid-base and electrolyte imbalances, and monitoring fluid intake and output and body temperature.

Many hospitals maintain an emergency MH kit or cart that contains the medications, laboratory tubes, other supplies, and instructions to treat MH in the OR area. The location of the iced or cold saline and other equipment also should be listed with the emergency kit. Chilled saline is often kept in the refrigeration unit for blood products (Karlet and Cahoon, 2014; MHAUS, 2011). The Malignant Hyperthermia Association of the United States (MHAUS) has names of on-call physicians available for consultation in MH emergencies at 1-800-MH-HYPER (1-800-644-9737). For patient-referral or nonemergency calls, 1-607-674-7910 should be used.

Patients known or suspected to have MH can be anesthetized with minimal risk if appropriate precautions are taken. If the syndrome is suspected, a muscle biopsy specimen is obtained to make a diagnosis before the patient is electively anesthetized. For their own safety, relatives of persons with MH should be evaluated for the presence of the syndrome (AORN, 2013; MHAUS, 2011).

Perioperative Nursing Considerations

Care of the surgical patient is a cooperative effort, and perioperative personnel should function as a smooth, well-coordinated team. As part of conducting the preoperative patient assessment and developing the plan of care, the perioperative nurse participates with the anesthesia provider in the preoperative verification process. As part of this process, the nurse checks the chart to verify the patient, the surgeon, and the scheduled procedure; confirms that the operative and anesthesia consents are properly signed; identifies and communicates any patient allergies; ensures that the surgical site is marked; and ensures that current reports of laboratory tests and diagnostic studies are complete and in the chart (Patient-Centered Care).

In many OR suites a preoperative preparation or *holding area* is used for insertion of arterial, central venous, or PACs and placement of epidural catheters or PNBs. Nursing personnel from the OR, PACU, or anesthesiology department may staff this area. The purpose of this area is to improve patient care delivery, optimize flow of patients, and provide supportive patient care.

A patient should never be left alone in the OR. When an anesthetized patient is in the OR, a perioperative nurse should always be immediately available to provide assistance if needed. During insertion of IV, arterial, central venous, or pulmonary arterial catheters, the nurse assists as required.

During induction of anesthesia, particularly with urgent and emergency surgical procedures, the patient presumptively has a "full stomach." The perioperative nurse should be ready to apply cricoid pressure to prevent regurgitation of stomach contents and to assist the anesthesia provider in visualizing the vocal cords. When cricoid pressure is used to prevent aspiration, it should not be released until completion of intubation, inflation of the cuff on the ETT, and proper placement of the ETT. When two anesthesia providers are present, one usually provides this support.

OR personnel should never move an unconscious patient without first coordinating the positioning or move with the anesthesia provider. When the patient is positioned for surgery, the perioperative nurse collaborates with the anesthesia provider to check the arms and legs to ensure that no pressure points exist and that the extremities are appropriately positioned and padded (see Chapter 6). After positioning, prepping, and draping, the time-out is conducted and documented.

Before transporting the patient from the OR to the PACU, the circulating nurse, in most institutions, calls the PACU to give a preliminary status report of the patient's condition. This report, like the anesthesia provider's hand-off report, includes the surgical procedure performed, type of anesthesia provided, information specific to the patient's preoperative diagnosis and subsequent outcome(s) related to intraoperative intervention, and any special equipment required (e.g., ventilator, T-piece, arterial pressure monitor). Postanesthesia recovery care and functions are described in Chapter 10.

KEY POINTS

- Without anesthesia, most modern surgical procedures would not be feasible.
- In the United States, anesthesia care may be provided: (1) by an anesthesiologist; (2) by a certified registered nurse anesthetist (CRNA) working alone, in collaboration with, or under the direction of an anesthesiologist or a physician; or (3) by an anesthesiologist's assistant (AA) working under direct supervision of an anesthesiologist.
- Patient safety is always a primary concern during anesthesia.
- Intraoperative awareness (IOA) has been reported with multiple and differing anesthetic techniques.
- Preoperative evaluation for anesthesia is done in advance of the scheduled surgical procedure.
- The patient, anesthesia provider, and surgeon make the choice of anesthesia for a given surgical procedure. Many factors influence this choice.
- Premedication is given before anesthesia to lightly sedate the patient and reduce anxiety.
- Patients may receive, in any setting, moderate sedation/analgesia, general, spinal, major regional anesthesia, or local anesthesia.
- There are many theories as to how general anesthesia works.
- Patients are monitored with various devices during anesthesia.
- Muscle relaxants (also referred to as neuromuscular blocking drugs [NMBDs]) are used to facilitate intubation and provide good operating conditions at lighter levels of general anesthesia.
- Patients with OSA who are undergoing procedures that require sedation, anesthesia, and/or analgesia are at higher risk for complications than patients who do not have OSA.
- Perioperative nurses have many important responsibilities when assessing and monitoring patients undergoing any type of anesthesia.

CRITICAL THINKING QUESTION

Your next patient for surgery is listed as a 67-year-old male for laparoscopic-assisted sigmoid resection for diverticulitis. He has a history of obstructive sleep apnea and prior difficult intubation noted in his medical record, and your preoperative interview reveals that he has not been compliant with his CPAP therapy. You also elicit information that he finds himself sleeping a lot during the day, has trouble focusing on his work, and is more forgetful than before. He is 5'9" and weighs 265 lb for a BMI of 39. What factors would you consider in your plan of care that is influenced by this history? How will your plan address the potential issues that the anesthesia provider will face when inducing this patient prior to attempting an intubation? What equipment and supplies will be needed in the OR and on an on-call basis to prepare for this case? What other nursing interventions will you consider and how will the actual surgical procedure affect your patient's care?

evolve *The answers to the Critical Thinking Question can be found at http://evolve.elsevier.com/Rothrock/Alexander.*

REFERENCES

Abraham V et al: Evaluation of post succinylcholine myalgia and intubation conditions with rocuronium pretreatment: a comparison with vecuronium, *Indian J Anesth* 52(5):551–555, 2008.

American Society of Anesthesiologists (ASA): practice guidelines for management of the difficult airway, *Anesthesiology* 118(2):1269–1277, 2013.

American Society of Anesthesiologists (ASA): Practice guidelines for preoperative fasting and the use of pharmacologic agents to reduce the risk of pulmonary aspiration: application to healthy patients undergoing elective procedures: an updated report by the American Society of Anesthesiologists Committee on Standards and Practice Parameters, *Anesthesiology* 114(3):45–511, 2011.

Association of periOperative Registered Nurses (AORN): *Perioperative standards and recommended practices*, Denver, 2013, The Association.

Avidan MS, Mashour GA: Prevention of intraoperative awareness with explicit recall: making sense of the evidence, *Anesthesiology* 118(2):449–456, 2013.

Bazzell L et al: Consciousness monitoring: a standard for the future? *OR Nurse* 2(7):36–38, 2008.

Beavers RA et al: Analysis of the application of cricoid pressure: implications for the clinician, *J Perianesth Nurs* 24(2):92–102, 2009.

Bope ET, Kellerman RD: *Sleep-related breathing disorders,* Conn's current therapy 2013, Philadelphia, 2013, Mosby.

Bordi SK: Pain management. In Nagelhout JJ, Plaus KL, editors: *Nurse anesthesia*, ed 5, St Louis, 2014, Saunders.

Bosson N: *Laryngeal mask airway*, Medscape, 2012, available at emedicine.medscape.com/article/82527-overview. Accessed February 2, 2013.

Bozimowski G: Clinical monitoring II respiratory and metabolic systems. In Nagelhout JJ, Plaus KL, editors: *Nurse anesthesia*, ed 5, St Louis, 2014, Saunders.

Brown DL: *Atlas of regional anesthesia*, ed 4, Philadelphia, 2010, Saunders.

Chawla J: *Clinical applications of somatosensory evoked potentials*, Medscape, 2012, available at emedicine.medscape.com/article/1139393-overview. Accessed February 2, 2013.

Chung F et al: Elimination of preoperative testing in ambulatory surgery, *Anesth Analg* 108:467–475, 2009.

Clark GD, Curdt NC: Clinical monitoring III: neurologic system. In Nagelhout JJ, Plaus KL, editors: *Nurse anesthesia*, ed 5, St Louis, 2014, Saunders.

Contrera MA et al: Anesthesia for cardiac surgery. In Nagelhout JJ, Plaus KL, editors: *Nurse anesthesia*, ed 5, St Louis, 2014, Saunders.

Cousins MJ, Bridenbaigh PO: *Neural blockade in clinical anesthesia and pain medicine*, Philadelphia, 2009, Lippincott Williams & Wilkins.

Dosch M: Anesthesia equipment. In Nagelhout JJ, Plaus KL, editors: *Nurse anesthesia*, ed 5, St Louis, 2014, Saunders.

Duke J: *Anesthesia secrets*, ed 4, St Louis, 2011, Mosby.

ECRI Institute: Risk management, quality improvement, and patient safety, *Risk Manage Rep* 2:1–15, 2009.

Fuhrman BP: *Pediatric critical care*, ed 4, Philadelphia, 2011, Mosby.

Fukano N: A randomized trial to identify optimal precurarizing dose of rocuronium to avoid precurarization-induced neuromuscular block, *J Anesth*—01-APR-2011; 25(2): 200-204.

Ghoneim MM et al: Awareness during anesthesia: risk factors, causes and sequelae: a review of reported cases in the literature, *Anesth Analgesia* 108:527–535, 2009.

Gottschalk A et al: Is anesthesia dangerous? *Deutsches Arzteblatt Int* 108(27):469–474, 2011.

Hagberg CA: *Benumof and Hagberg's airway management*, ed 3, Philadelphia, 2013, Elsevier Saunders.

Heiner JS, Gabot MH: Airway management. In Nagelhout JJ, Plaus KL, editors: *Nurse anesthesia*, ed 5, St Louis, 2014, Saunders.

Hernandez JH et al: Scientific advances in the genetic understanding and diagnosis of malignant hyperthermia, *J Perianesth Nurs* 24:19–34, 2009.

Issa, MR, Revista brasileira de anesthesiologia; "Preanesthesia evaluation and reduction of preoperative care costs." *Medline* 61(12):60-71, 2011. Accessed November, 2012.

Kain ZN et al: Family-centered preparation for surgery improves perioperative outcomes in children, *Anesthesiology* 106:65–74, 2007.

Karlet MC, Cahoon TM: Musculoskeletal system anatomy, physiology, pathophysiology, and anesthesia management. In Nagelhout JJ, Plaus KL, editors: *Nurse anesthesia*, ed 5, St Louis, 2014, Saunders.

Kossick MA: Clinical monitoring I: cardiovascular system. In Nagelhout JJ, Plaus KL, editors: *Nurse anesthesia*, ed 5, St Louis, 2014, Mosby.

Liu SS et al: Ultrasound-guided regional anesthesia and analgesia: a qualitative systematic review, *Reg Anesth Pain Med* 34(1):47–59, 2009.

LMA airway instruction manual, 2011, available at www.lmana.com. Accessed February 23, 2013.

Malignant Hyperthermia Association of the United States: 2011, available at www.mhaus.org. Accessed February 3, 2013.

Matten EC, Deshur MA: Monitoring in anesthesia and perioperative care, *Anesthesiology* 117(3):688, 2012.

Miller RD: *Miller's anesthesia*, ed 7, Philadelphia, 2010, Churchill Livingstone.

Nagelhout JJ: Neuromuscular blocking agents, reversal agents and their monitoring. In Nagelhout JJ, Plaus KL, editors: *Nurse anesthesia*, ed 5, St Louis, 2014, Saunders.

Nagelhout JJ, Plaus KL: *Nurse anesthesia*, ed 5, St Louis, 2014, Saunders.

Naguib M, Lien C: Pharmacology of muscle relaxants and their antagonists. In Miller RD: *Miller's anesthesia*, ed 7, Philadelphia, 2010, Churchill, Livingstone.

New York School of Regional Anesthesia: Intravenous regional block (Bier block), 2009, available at www.nysora.com/peripheral_nerve_blocks/intravenous_regional_blocks/3009-bier_block.html. Accessed February 3, 2013.

Odom-Forren J: Postanesthesia recovery. In Nagelhout, JJ, Plaus, KL, editors: *Nurse anesthesia*, ed 5, St Louis, 2014, Saunders.

Olson RL et al: Regional anesthesia: spinal and epidural. In Nagelhout JJ, Plaus KL, editors: *Nurse anesthesia*, ed 5, St Louis, 2014, Saunders.

Ortiz VE, Wiener-Kronish J: Perioperative anesthetic care of the obese patient, *Anesthesiology* 115(4):906–907, 2011.

Patten SP: Apply cricoid pressure correctly, *OR Nurse* 1(3):72, 2007.

Ranalli LJ, Taylor GA: Neuroanatomy, neurophysiology and neuroanesthesia. In Nagelhout JJ, Plaus KL, editors: *Nurse anesthesia*, ed 5, St Louis, 2014, Saunders.

Rieker M: Anesthesia for thoracic surgery. In Nagelhout JJ, Plaus KL, editors: *Nurse anesthesia*, ed 5, St Louis, 2014, Saunders.

Sawhney M: Epidural anesthesia: what nurses need to know, *Nursing* 42(8):36–41, 2012.

Smykowski L: A novel PACU design for noise reduction, *J Perianesth Nurs* 23(4):226–229, 2008.

The National Quality Forum: Endorsement Summaries, Surgery, available at www.qualityforum.org, Accessed April 29, 2013.

Tonnesen H et al: Smoking and alcohol interventions before surgery: evidence for practice, *Br J Anaesthesia* 102(3):297–306, 2009.

Vacchiano A, Biegner A: Regional anesthesia: upper and lower extremity blocks. In Nagelhout, JJ, Plaus, KL, editors: *Nurse anesthesia*, ed 5, St Louis, 2014, Saunders.

Weinberg G: Lipid emulsion infusion: resuscitation for local anesthetic and other drug overdose, *Anesthesiology* 117(1):180–187, 2012.

Welch J: *Alarm fatigue hazards: the sirens are calling*, Patient Safety & Quality Healthcare, May/June 2012, available at www.psqh.com/mayjune-2012/1291-alarm-fatigue-hazards-the-sirens-are-calling.html. Accessed February 2, 2013.

Wolfe JW: Local anesthetic systemic toxicity: update on mechanisms and treatment, *Curr Opin Anesthesiol* 24(5):561–566, 2011.

CHAPTER 6

Positioning the Patient for Surgery

PAULINE ANNE HEIZENROTH

Proper patient positioning is essential for safe, successful surgery procedures. The surgical team ensures uncompromised and physiologically safe patient positioning by understanding the systems affected by positioning and their associated risks. Given that surgery may be performed on all anatomic areas, body positioning may result in multiple and sometimes unnatural configurations in order to expose a surgical site. Positioning, combined with anesthesia and its physiologic effects, can yield harmful changes if safety factors are not considered as a paramount patient safety outcome. This chapter discusses some of the risks and prevention strategies associated with standard surgical positions.

The goals of surgical positioning include providing optimal exposure and access to the surgical site, maintaining body alignment, supporting circulatory and respiratory function, protecting neuromuscular and skin integrity, and allowing access to intravenous (IV) sites and anesthesia support devices. Meeting these goals while simultaneously maintaining patient comfort and safety is the responsibility of every member of the surgical team.

Anatomic and Physiologic Considerations

The perioperative nurse must understand thoroughly the anatomic and physiologic changes associated with positioning the patient. These changes are affected by numerous factors, such as the type of surgical position; the length of time the patient is in that position; the operating room (OR) bed, padding, and positioning devices used; the type of anesthesia given; and the operative procedure. These changes most frequently affect: (1) the skin and underlying tissue; (2) the musculoskeletal system; (3) the nervous system; (4) the cardiovascular system; (5) the respiratory system; and (6) other vulnerable areas, such as the eyes, breasts, perineum, and fingers.

Skin and Underlying Tissue

Physical forces used to establish and maintain a surgical position can injure the skin and underlying tissue. These forces include *pressure, shear,* and *friction.* Additionally, OR conditions such as *moisture, heat, cold,* and *negativity* further increase the vulnerability of the skin and underlying tissues to injury.

- *Pressure* is the force placed on underlying tissue. Pressure comes from the weight of the body as gravity presses it downward toward the surface of the bed. Pressure also comes from the weight of equipment resting on or against the patient, such as drills, Mayo stands, surgical instruments, rigid edges of the OR bed or its attachments, or vertical posts for self-retaining retractors. Positioning devices, such as stirrup bars, leg or arm holders, and edges of laminectomy frames, can rest or press against the patient under tension. Surgical team members can also lean on the patient and cause various degrees of pressure.

- *Shear* is the folding of underlying tissue when the skeletal structure moves while the skin remains stationary. A parallel force creates shear compared with a perpendicular force created by pressure (Figure 6-1). This happens when the head of the bed is raised or lowered and when the patient is placed in Trendelenburg (head down, supine) or reverse Trendelenburg (head up, supine) position. As gravity pulls the skeleton down, the stretching, folding, and tearing of the underlying tissues as they slide with the skeleton occlude vascular perfusion, which leads to tissue ischemia.

- *Friction* is the force of two surfaces rubbing against one another. Friction on the patient's skin occurs when the body is dragged across bed linen instead of being lifted. Friction can denude the epidermis and make the skin more susceptible to higher stages of pressure ulcer formation, pain, and infection.

- *Moisture,* in excess, worsens the effects of pressure, shear, and friction. Maceration occurs when prolonged moisture on the skin saturates the epidermis to the point that the connective tissue fibers dissolve and can be easily torn apart. The skin weakens and is more vulnerable to the detrimental effects of external forces. In surgery, skin maceration occurs if the patient perspires or is allowed to lie in a pool of prep solution, blood, irrigation solution, urine, or feces. If this moisture also is located in an area of high pressure, the risk of pressure ulcer increases. If friction occurs on macerated skin, it becomes more vulnerable to denuding into the dermal layer. Every effort should be made to avoid pooling of fluids under the patient. Prolonged exposure to chemicals in the skin prep solution under the pressure area also can increase the likelihood of chemically induced contact dermatitis.

- *Heat* on the body surface increases metabolism of tissue and increases its oxygen and nutritional demands. If tissue is also under pressure, constriction of vessels tends to impede blood flow enough that those demands are not met. Preexisting vascular impairment and the hypotensive effects of anesthesia may harm tissue further and lead to cellular tissue damage. This is especially true when the heated surface is under the weight of the body. Excessive heat can cause thermal damage as well, resulting in burns.

- *Cold* environmental conditions, such as those found in the OR, can lead to hypothermia. Major surgery can cool the patient further by exposing the core of the body to cold air. A cold core temperature can reduce peripheral circulation, thereby reducing oxygen delivery to the skin and underlying tissue.

- *Negativity* occurs when layers of materials, such as extra sheets or blankets, are placed over the OR mattress or padding. Extra linen can add rigidity and diminish the pressure-reducing properties of the mattress or padding. Such linen is absorbent and abrasive and can produce high and inconsistent pressure. Eliminating extra layers of material between the patient and the OR bed can reduce sacral pressure readings.

Pressure Ulcers. The National Pressure Ulcer Advisory Panel (NPUAP) defines a pressure ulcer as "a localized injury to the skin

FIGURE 6-1 Shearing force. As gravity forces the vertebral column downward, skin adhering to surface counters and resists that force. The result is folding and compression of tissue in between.

and/or underlying tissue, usually over a bony prominence, as a result of pressure or pressure in combination with shear and/or friction" (NPUAP, Pressure Ulcer Stages/Categories, 2013). In 2007 the NPUAP revised its Guidelines for Staging Pressure Ulcers to include two additional stages: "deep tissue injury" and "unstageable." Table 6-1 reviews current NPUAP Guidelines for Staging Pressure Ulcers.

In 2008 the Centers for Medicare & Medicaid Services (CMS) decided to end reimbursement to hospitals for many preventable hospital-acquired conditions, which it called "never events." Among these conditions were stage III or IV pressure ulcers that develop after admission (CMS, 2008). This highlights the need to assess the skin thoroughly before surgery. Proper skin assessment includes temperature, color, moisture level, turgor, and integrity. Inarguably, the costs of treating pressure ulcers are far more than the costs of preventing them. Hospitals must therefore focus on preventive strategies that take into account the *extrinsic* and *intrinsic* factors that interact to contribute to the overall risk of developing pressure sores.

Extrinsic Factors. Pressure is the major physical force responsible for pressure ulcer formation. Its intensity and duration affect the ultimate outcome of whether the tissue suffers damage. An inverse relationship exists between pressure and time: the greater the pressure, the shorter time it takes to cause ischemic changes. Pressures greater than 32 mm Hg (capillary interface pressure) can occlude flow of the arterioles, which nourish and oxygenate the tissue at the capillary level. An individual can endure relatively large amounts of pressure for a short time or smaller amounts of pressure

TABLE 6-1

NPUAP Guidelines for Staging Pressure Ulcers

Stage/Category	Definition
Deep tissue injury	Purple or maroon localized area of discolored intact skin or blood-filled blister due to damage of underlying soft tissue from pressure and/or shear. The area may be preceded by tissue that is painful, firm, mushy, boggy, warmer or cooler as compared to adjacent tissue. Deep tissue injury may be difficult to detect in individuals with dark skin tones. Evolution may include a thin blister over a dark wound bed. The wound may further evolve and become covered by thin eschar. Evolution may be rapid, exposing additional layers of tissue even with optimal treatment.
Stage I	Intact skin with nonblanchable redness of a localized area usually over a bony prominence. Darkly pigmented skin may not have visible blanching; its color may differ from the surrounding area. The area may be painful, firm, soft, warmer or cooler as compared to adjacent tissue. Stage I may be difficult to detect in individuals with dark skin tones. May indicate "at risk" persons.
Stage II	Partial-thickness loss of dermis presenting as a shallow open ulcer with a red-pink wound bed, without slough. May also present as an intact or open/ruptured serum-filled or serosanguineous-filled blister. Presents as a shiny or dry shallow ulcer without slough or bruising.* This category should not be used to describe skin tears; tape burns; incontinence associated dermatitis, maceration, or excoriation.
Stage III	Full-thickness tissue loss. Subcutaneous fat may be visible, but bone, tendon, or muscle is *not* exposed. Slough may be present but does not obscure the depth of tissue loss. *May* include undermining and tunneling. The depth of a stage III pressure ulcer varies by anatomic location. The bridge of the nose, ear, occiput, and malleolus do not have (adipose) subcutaneous tissue, and stage III ulcers can be shallow. In contrast, areas of significant adiposity can develop extremely deep category/stage III pressure ulcers. Bone/tendon is not visible or directly palpable.
Stage IV	Full-thickness tissue loss with exposed bone, tendon, or muscle. Slough or eschar may be present. Often includes undermining and tunneling. The depth of a category/stage IV pressure ulcer varies by anatomic location. The bridge of the nose, ear, occiput, and malleolus do not have (adipose) subcutaneous tissue, and these ulcers can be shallow. Stage IV ulcers can extend into muscle and/or supporting structures (e.g., fascia, tendon, or joint capsule) making osteomyelitis or osteitis likely to occur. Exposed bone/muscle is visible or directly palpable.
Unstageable	Full-thickness tissue loss in which actual depth of the ulcer is completely obscured by slough (yellow, tan, gray, green, or brown) and/or eschar (tan, brown, or black) in the wound bed. Until enough slough and/or eschar is removed to expose the base of the wound, the true depth cannot be determined, but it will be either a stage III or IV. Stable (dry, adherent, intact without erythema or fluctuance) eschar on the heels serves as the body's natural (biologic) "cover" and should not be removed.

*Bruising indicates deep tissue injury.

Modified from National Pressure Ulcer Advisory Panel (NPUAP): NPUAP Pressure ulcer stages/categories, 2013, available at www.npuap.org/resources/educational-and-clinical-resources/npuap-pressure-ulcer-stagescategories/. Accessed April 27, 2013. Used with permission of the National Pressure Ulcer Advisory Panel.

for a longer time without sustaining tissue damage. A time limit can be reached, however, when the tissue no longer can withstand the pressure (especially >32 mm Hg) and cells die from lack of oxygen and nutrients. Such prolonged pressure can result in tissue ischemia manifested as a pressure ulcer.

The intensity of pressure depends on the size of the surface area being compressed. The smaller the surface area in which pressure is applied, the greater the force (pressure per surface area). Compression of tissue between an external surface and a bony prominence of the body tends to create high forces of pressure in the local tissue surrounding that bone. Pressure ulcers most often develop around bony prominences such as the heels, elbows, and sacrum in the supine position. Often the tissue injury is most severe in deep areas immediately adjacent to bone. As deeper ischemia progresses outward toward the skin, the damage may not be visible for several days. Theoretically, if pressure could be distributed more evenly over other surfaces of the body, the force of pressure in those vulnerable areas would lessen. This theory fuels manufacturers to create OR mattress overlays and padding materials designed to distribute forces of pressure more evenly.

The greater the amount of time a patient is on the OR bed, the higher the risk of OR-acquired pressure ulcer development when combined with the multiple variables of the intraoperative experience. Duration is considered more of a causative factor than is the intensity of pressure. Healthy individuals may tolerate high external pressures (e.g., 100 mm Hg) over bony prominences for short periods, but longer, constant, unrelieved pressure tends to cause microscopic necrosis. Lowered pressures over extended periods also may cause tissue damage, particularly if tissue tolerance is diminished. Frequent repositioning of an immobilized patient can protect against or lessen adverse effects of pressure. Repositioning a patient every 2 hours has long been the standard for lessening the negative effects of pressure on the immobile patient. However, OR patients cannot be repositioned without jeopardizing access to the operative site and the integrity of the sterile field. Case-based exceptions might include limited repositioning of extremities and/or the head when such movement would not interfere with the surgical procedure or the sterile field. The perioperative nurse should plan ahead to ensure that preventive measures are taken to reduce pressure ulcer risks. Pressure-relieving OR mattresses or overlays may reduce pressure in dependent areas. Padding applied around rigid surfaces in contact with the patient and suspending vulnerable areas off the OR bed can reduce localized pressure.

Patients undergoing regional or general anesthesia are at increased risk because normal muscle tone and pain sensations that enable the body to adjust itself in response to excessive pressure are disabled. Patients often are placed in positions that they would not be able to tolerate comfortably if they were awake or even asleep without the use of anesthetics. Anesthesia also causes hypotension, which can reduce tissue perfusion and thus reduce the exchange of oxygen and carbon dioxide. Connor and colleagues (2010) found that prolonged hypotension is a valid predictor of pressure ulcer risk in the OR. All these anesthetic effects can heighten the effect of pressure forces, particularly if other comorbid conditions are present.

A study by Fred and colleagues (2012) shows that patients with at least a 1°F (1.8°C) drop in temperature may be at increased risk for intraoperatively acquired pressure ulcers. Hypothermia is the frequent result of the cooler OR environment, exposure of external and internal body surfaces, and infusion and irrigation with unwarmed solutions. This causes peripheral vessels to constrict to conserve core temperature and increases the patient's heat metabolism. This increased metabolism leads to increased tissue needs for oxygen, nutrients, and metabolic waste-product removal. When tissue is under pressure, these needs are not easily met. When hypothermic patients later emerge from general anesthesia, they often shiver, which further increases their oxygen requirements and may increase their risk for pressure ulcers as well as myocardial infarction. Minimizing intraoperative hypothermia thus is imperative.

Ways to offset hypothermia in the OR and to reduce its detrimental effects include using forced-air warming therapy *over* the patient. Avoid placing a warming blanket *under* the patient in the area where pressures are greatest because tissue requirements tend to increase there and the effect of tissue ischemia may be more profound. Minimize unnecessary skin exposure and use warm irrigation fluids, especially deep inside the body cavity. To warm IV fluids, insert a fluid-warming coil or place most of the IV fluid tubing under the forced-air warming blanket.

The type of surgery performed can affect pressure ulcer development. Patients who undergo cardiac, general, thoracic, and vascular procedures tend to be at greater risk, possibly because these cases immobilize patients for long periods (Denholm, 2008). In addition, procedures that involve significant blood loss, extracorporeal circulation, and clamping of major vessels can contribute to the lack of blood flow to tissue under pressure.

The type of positioning devices used can increase pressure ulcer development risk as well. Rigid, unpadded objects that press against a body surface, such as stirrup bars, compressed beanbags, or rolled sheets, can cause tissue injury if pressure is not relieved periodically.

Negativity, as explained earlier, can override the pressure-relieving capabilities of mattresses and padding. Placing a warm blanket under a patient may be soothing initially, but if a surgical procedure is long, pressure to the bony prominences resting on the blanket will be greater than if only a sheet and drawsheet are used. Additionally, wrinkles and folds can cause further pressure points.

When a patient is moved into a shear-producing position (e.g., from supine to semi-Fowler) before being prepped and draped, the OR team can take measures to reduce shear forces. One technique is to slightly move the patient's back away from the mattress momentarily to allow the skin to realign with its surrounding skeletal structures. When the patient is placed in these positions *during* a surgical procedure, however, interventions to reduce shear forces are limited. Reducing the time that shear forces are in place is the best measure to reduce tissue injury.

Intrinsic Factors. Intrinsic factors lower a patient's tissue tolerance to pressure and decrease the time and pressure required for tissue breakdown. Certain preexisting conditions are regarded as intrinsic risk factors for OR-induced pressure ulcer development. These conditions include diabetes mellitus, smoking, peripheral vascular disease, cerebral vascular disease, urinary or fecal incontinence, anemia, malignancy, sepsis, steroid use, morbid obesity, malnutrition (serum albumin levels less than 3.5 g/dL), advanced age, body size (obesity as well as thin, frail build), and impaired mobility (Connor et al, 2010; Cox, 2011; Denholm, 2008; Lyder and Ayello, 2008; Munro, 2010; Primiano, 2011; Walton-Geer, 2009).

Various scales exist to determine pressure ulcer potential. One widely used is the Braden Scale, which scores a patient's potential for pressure sore development based on various intrinsic factors. It is valid and reliable in acute care and long-term care settings and has been used for many years to guide nursing interventions. It does not take into account, however, various extrinsic factors patients are subjected to in critical care areas such as the OR or the intensive care unit (ICU), in both of which immobile patients are completely dependent on caregivers to sustain their fragile hemodynamic status and where routine, timely repositioning may be contraindicated.

Recent studies have tested the relevance of the Braden Scale in the perioperative setting (Connor et al, 2010; Galvin and Curley, 2012) and the medical-surgical ICU setting (Cox, 2011, Suriadi et al, 2008). These studies concluded that not all Braden Scale risk factors are predictable in these patients and that other significant risk factors are not identified on Braden or other pressure ulcer predictive scales used in hospital settings. The Braden score may be used as a preoperative baseline, but the OR is unique when compared with other areas of the hospital. Typical predictors of pressure ulcer risks may not work once anesthetized, immobile patients are put in atypical positions for varying lengths of time, which may disrupt their cardiovascular, hemodynamic, and thermoregulation statuses. This potential disruption underscores the suggestion by Walton-Geer (2009) and others that all surgical patients should be considered at risk to develop pressure ulcers. Some patients are at a higher risk than others, and risk assessment scales need to be developed specific to the perioperative patient. Several nursing studies (Connor et al, 2010; Galvin and Curley, 2012; Primiano et al, 2011) have yielded perioperative variables usable to predict pressure ulcer development (Research Highlight). Some OR teams have developed their own perioperative risk assessment tools (Mathias, 2008; Munro, 2010), but these have not as yet been widely tested for validity and reliability.

Over the past decades multiple other studies with surgical patients have attempted to determine risk factors specific to this patient population. The problem with attempting to draw out distinct perioperative risk factors for pressure ulcer development that would apply on a general scale is that so many exist; risk factors vary substantially from hospital to hospital as to type and length of procedures, types of anesthesia, positions, positioning devices, mattress surfaces, patient warming methods, and unplanned surgical and anesthetic events, along with multiple and varying intrinsic factors such as age, weight and comorbidities. Even so, given our extant knowledge coupled with future research, a baseline perioperative pressure ulcer risk scale that could be individualized for each patient and situation would serve as a useful guide to perioperative nurses to plan and care for this patient population. Development of such a prospective scale, particularized for each surgical patient, remains an incomplete goal and unmet need of perioperative nursing.

Assessment for pressure ulcer risk factors and development nevertheless should be done consistently and aimed at three periods: *preoperative, intraoperative,* and *postoperative.* Such assessments should accompany the hand-off report to the nurse in the postanesthesia care unit (PACU) receiving the patient (see Chapter 10). Included in postoperative assessment is inspection for changes in skin temperature, color, moisture level, turgor, and integrity. These inspections start in the preoperative area and OR, continue in the PACU, and go beyond to discharge. It is in the early postoperative phase that many small problems picked up by astute assessments can be treated to avert bigger problems.

Stage I or stage II pressure ulcers (Figures 6-2 and 6-3) may be evident immediately after surgery. These areas must be kept free from additional pressure for healing to occur and to keep them from advancing to higher stages. Such ulcers are sometimes misidentified and treated inappropriately. Stage I pressure ulcers can look like normal erythema, a reaction to pressure in which the healthy tissue blanches when compressed and generally fades on its own in half

RESEARCH HIGHLIGHT

Perioperative Variables Predictive of Pressure Ulcer Development

Conner and colleagues studied 498 patients over 17 months to identify perioperative variables that predict pressure ulcer formation among patients undergoing urologic surgical procedures. A secondary intent was to determine if the Braden Scale was able to detect intraoperative occurrences of pressure ulcers. Some 25 patients (5%) showed evidence of a stage I pressure ulcer in the postanesthesia care unit (PACU). The two variables found to be statistically significant predictors were anesthesia duration and total time of diastolic blood pressure less than 50 mm Hg. The average preoperative Braden score of those who developed pressure ulcers was 22.63 (a score of 18 or lower is considered at risk). The authors did not find the Braden score a reliable predictor of pressure ulcers during the intraoperative phase of surgery.

In other research, Primiano and colleagues studied 258 patients undergoing surgical procedures lasting longer than 3 hours to identify whether certain factors led to the development of pressure ulcers. Their findings revealed that the type of positioning device (pillows under knees), type of mattress material (closed cell foam pad less than 2 inches thick), and male gender related to pressure ulcer development. After surgery, in the PACU, low Braden scores and assessments of major skin abrasions were predictors. One interesting finding in this study was that many (23%) of the patients who developed sacral pressure ulcers had their heels elevated during surgery. The researchers suggested that although this was done to prevent heel ulcers, heel elevation may actually have contributed to the development of sacral pressure ulcers by redistributing weight onto the sacrum.

Galvin and Curley developed a Braden Q+P tool to assess risk factors for pediatric surgical patients at Boston Children's Hospital. They constructed a scale for pediatric patients using Braden and Bergstrom's conceptual framework (Braden Q Scale). This scale was then modified to reflect the unique characteristics of ORs and called the Braden Q+P tool. The OR Skin Care Task Force at the hospital championed implementation of the tool along with supportive nursing education on increased awareness of pressure ulcer prevention. During the 2 years the tool has been used, the incidence of pressure ulcers decreased.

Modified from Connor T et al: Identification of pre-operative and intra-operative variables predictive of pressure ulcer development in patients undergoing urologic surgical procedures, *Urol Nurs* 30(5):289–295, 305, 2010; Primiano M et al: Pressure ulcer prevalence and risk factors during prolonged surgical procedures, *AORN J* 94(6):555–566, 2011; Galvin PA, Curley MAQ: The Braden Q+P: a pediatric perioperative pressure ulcer risk assessment and intervention tool, *AORN J* 96(3):261–270, 2012.

to three quarters of the time that the area was under pressure, with little or no permanent tissue damage. Stage I pressure ulcers do not blanch when compressed. Failure to blanch is a serious sign, indicating that the compromised tissue is not receiving adequate oxygen and nutrients. The blistering or partial dermal loss that occurs in stage II pressure ulcers is often misidentified as a chemical or thermal burn. The lack of contact with a chemical or thermal agent in that area and its location under a bony prominence or near where a hard surface had been during surgery can help distinguish it as a serious stage II pressure ulcer.

Full manifestation of pressure ulcers may not occur from hours to days after the triggering injury. Given such delayed manifestation, the connection to the triggering event (the surgical experience) may be overlooked. Lack of awareness of an early pressure injury can lead to a delay of pressure relief and treatment. Inappropriate

FIGURE 6-2 Stage I pressure ulcer. Skin is intact with localized nonblanchable redness over bony prominence (sacrum).

FIGURE 6-3 Stage II pressure ulcer. Note shallow open ulcer with red-pink wound bed showing partial thickness loss of dermis.

FIGURE 6-4 Deep tissue injury. **A,** Note intact discolored skin localized over bony prominence (sacrum); skin color, however, is deep purple or maroon compared to reddened color in stage I pressure ulcer. **B,** Deep tissue injury over bony prominence (heel) presenting as a blood filled blister.

treatment can contribute to avoidable advancing stages of pressure ulcers.

Deep tissue injury (DTI) (Figure 6-4) must also be differentiated from a stage I or II pressure ulcer. Stage I ulcers present with discolored, nonblanchable, but intact skin, which is also true of a DTI. Instead of pink or red, however, the DTI is purple or maroon in appearance, like that of a deep bruise. Stage II ulcers present as an intact or open/ruptured serum filled blister, whereas a DTI blister fills with blood. The NPUAP added the DTI category to help identify a dangerous form of pressure ulcer in which deeper tissues are subjected to such a long duration of ischemia that reperfusion causes additional microvascular injury (reperfusion injury). What began in appearance as a closed discolored area rapidly deteriorates to a full-thickness stage III or IV pressure ulcer, even with optimal

treatment. The epidemiology, clinical course, and efficacious treatment of DTIs require more research (NPUAP, Deep Tissue Injury, 2013).

Pressure alopecia (pressure-induced hair loss on the scalp) is a complication not typically classified as a pressure ulcer, but can result from prolonged local pressure to the scalp during and after surgery. Symptoms can occur between postoperative days 3 and 28. Occipital scalp pain, swelling, exudate, crusting, or focal ulceration may precede the actual loss of hair. Pressure alopecia most commonly occurs in procedures that require prolonged intubation and head immobilization. In cardiac surgery, for example, the anesthesia induction-to-extubation time may extend more than 24 hours. The longer the time, the greater the risk that alopecia may be permanent. Repositioning the patient's head every 30 minutes using soft, contoured head padding can reduce the potential for pressure alopecia.

Musculoskeletal System

The musculoskeletal system may be subjected to unusual stress during operative positioning. Ordinarily the alert patient maintains normal range of motion by pain and pressure receptors that warn against overstretching and twisting of ligaments, tendons, and muscles. The tone of opposing muscle groups also acts to prevent strain and stretch to muscle fibers. In surgery, however, when pharmacologic agents such as anesthetics and muscle relaxants depress pain and pressure receptors, and muscle tone, a patient's normal defense mechanisms cannot guard against joint damage and muscle stretch and strain. A patient safety goal is to maintain the body's natural alignment as much as possible, while still providing adequate access to the surgical site. The perioperative team needs to be aware of the limits to range of motion, refraining from joint extension beyond what is necessary.

Every time a patient is transferred to or from the OR bed, alignment of the patient's body needs to be maintained. This is especially true when transfer involves moving the patient from a supine position to lateral or prone. During positional changes, extremities must be gently supported; quick, jerky movement of unsupported limbs can cause strain to the muscles and ligaments.

Nervous System

Nervous system depression accompanies the administration of anesthetic agents and other drugs. The degree of depression depends on the type of regional anesthesia or the level of general anesthesia. Pain and pressure receptors may be affected regionally or systemically. The most important factor for perioperative nurses to remember is that when nervous system depression occurs, the body's communication and command system becomes totally or partially ineffective. Compensatory reactions to changes in physical status no longer respond normally. Lifesaving, physiologic adaptive mechanisms are altered. The body can no longer compensate for the stresses of surgical positioning.

Peripheral Neuropathies. Peripheral nerves can suffer injury during positioning, resulting in impaired sensory function or motor function, or both. The mechanisms for nerve injuries include compression (pressure), stretch, direct trauma, laceration, ischemia, and metabolic derangement (Prielipp and Warner, 2009; Saidha et al, 2010). Stretching and compression tend to be the main culprits in position-induced nerve injuries. Prolonged stretching from hyperabduction of an extremity or compression from pressure results in ischemia, which can progress to necrosis. In addition, collateral damage to the surrounding tissue and capillaries can affect circulation and nourishment to nerves. These pathologic forces combine to result in structural or functional damage to the nerves.

There are three degrees of nerve injury. Depending on degree, subsequent injuries may be temporary or permanent. The first degree of injury, neuropraxia, is a response to compression and has the best prognosis. There is only slight demyelination and no axonal degeneration. Full recovery can be expected within 6 weeks without residual loss of function. The second degree of injury, axonotmesis, manifests as the destruction of the axons within a nerve sheath that remains intact. The distal axons degenerate, but proximal axons are able to use the intact sheath to guide regeneration at a rate of 1 mm per day. The third and most severe degree of injury is neurotmesis in which disruption to the axon, sheath, and connective tissue covering are disrupted. Again, the distal axon degenerates. Without an intact sheath to guide regeneration, regrowth is disorganized, sometimes forming painful neuromas. Surgical resection of the axon ends with reapproximation is the only way to help regain function (Ellsworth et al, 2009).

During surgery all patients are at risk for nerve injury if sustained compression is placed on nerves. Numerous patient characteristics have been identified, however, that potentially increase the risk for intraoperatively acquired neuropathies. These include diabetes mellitus, peripheral vascular disease, electrolyte imbalances, vitamin B_{12} deficiency, alcoholism, smoking, malnutrition, advanced age, previous nerve injuries or neuropathies (e.g., carpal tunnel syndrome, thoracic outlet syndrome), arthritis, obesity, thin body habitus, and male gender (for ulnar nerve injuries) (Edgecombe et al, 2008; Renter and Beissel, 2013; Shveiky et al, 2010; Uribe et al, 2010; Welch et al, 2009). Possible risk factors associated with the patient's surgical experience include lengthy surgical procedures, the use of abdominal pelvic self-retaining retractors, long duration in the lithotomy position, sternal retraction from a median sternotomy, surgical procedures in which shoulder braces are used for support while the patient is in steep Trendelenburg, improper arm placement, tight arm restraints, improperly placed blood pressure cuff, prolonged hospitalization, hypotension, hypothermia, and prolonged bed rest postoperatively (Akhavan et al, 2010; ASA, 2011; Cassorla and Lee, 2010; Shveiky et al, 2010; Warner, 2009). Damage usually remains undiscovered until the patient reaches the PACU or even days or weeks after the suspected insult. This delay can lead to some confusion as to whether the injury occurred during surgery or convalescence. Although the incidence is relatively low, claims of peripheral nerve injuries are a significant source of professional liability claims.

Upper Extremity Neuropathies. Upper extremity neuropathies generate from lesions to the brachial plexus and the nerves that emerge from it. The brachial plexus consists of a bundle of nerve cords that run through the shoulder and innervate the lower shoulder, arm, and hand (Figure 6-5). This bundle originates from cervical spinal nerves C5-C8. The nerve cords emerge to form peripheral nerves. The axillary nerve innervates the deltoid muscle. The musculoskeletal nerve innervates the biceps muscle. Three main peripheral nerves run down the arm to the fingers: median, radial, and ulnar (Figure 6-6).

The *median nerve* runs through the antecubital space to the fingers and provides sensory and motor ability to the distal and palmar surfaces of the thumb and adjacent two fingers. A normally perceived pinprick to the palmar surface of the distal index finger generally would show that the median nerve was intact (Figure 6-7).

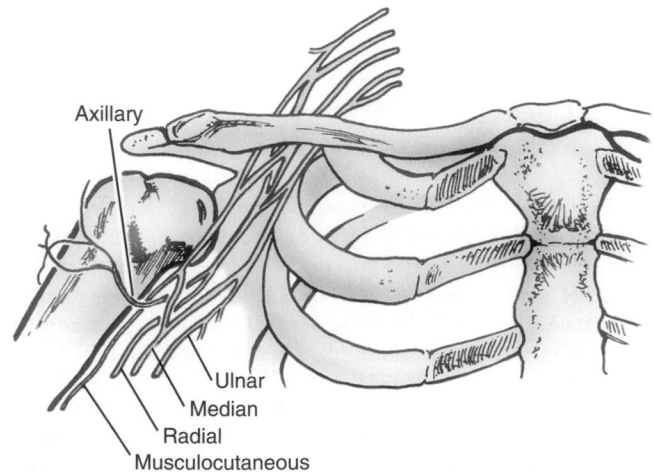

Axillary

Ulnar
Median
Radial
Musculocutaneous

FIGURE 6-5 Brachial plexus on right with associated bone structures and nerve branches that extend down right arm.

Median nerve   Radial nerve   Ulnar nerve

FIGURE 6-6 Median, radial, and ulnar nerves and nerves of right arm with areas of sensory distribution shaded.

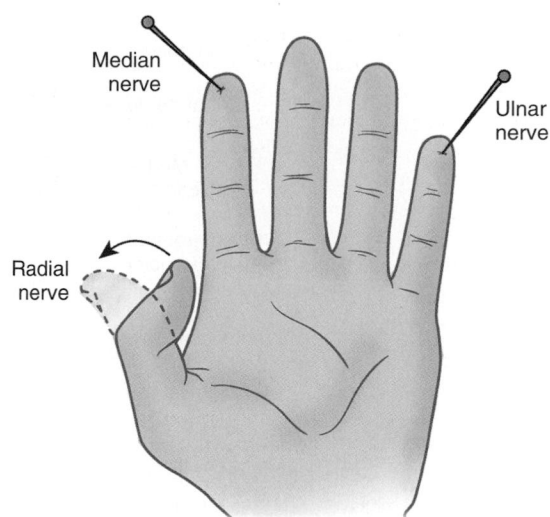

Median nerve

Ulnar nerve

Radial nerve

FIGURE 6-7 A quick way to check for injuries to major peripheral nerves of the upper extremity. Ability to actively extend the thumb indicates an intact radial nerve. A normally perceived pinprick to distal palmar surface of the index finger indicates an intact median nerve. A normally perceived pinprick to distal palmar surface of fifth finger indicates an intact ulnar nerve.

The *radial nerve* loops around the posterior humerus before it runs through the antecubital space to the fingers. It provides motor and sensory function to the triceps and the muscles of the posterior forearm and hand. Injury to this area can cause difficulty extending the wrist and thumb. If the distal thumb can be actively extended, this generally indicates an intact radial nerve (see Figure 6-7).

The *ulnar nerve* runs behind the elbow and innervates the third, fourth, and fifth fingers and the muscles of the medial forearm. It is responsible for wrist flexion and, along with the radial nerve, enables the thumb to oppose the other four fingers. A normally perceived pinprick over the plantar surface of the distal fifth finger generally indicates an intact ulnar nerve (see Figure 6-7).

The most common OR-related nerve injuries are to the ulnar nerve and brachial plexus. There is a good reason for this. As the ulnar nerve circles behind the elbow, it lies superficially in the shallow cubital tunnel of the humerus, where it is subject to pressure and to stretching from flexion of the elbow (Figure 6-8). The brachial plexus resides in the shoulder, which is subject to abduction, manipulation, and sometimes pressure, depending on position. The use of shoulder braces, to reduce sliding while in Trendelenburg position, should be avoided because braces can compress proximal nerve roots and stretch the brachial plexus. Arm abduction on armboards should be limited to 90 degrees or less. Avoid excessive head rotation, especially away from the abducted arm because doing so can stretch and compress the nerves between the clavicle and the first rib (Figure 6-9).

The brachial plexus can also suffer injury by the separation of the sternum during open cardiac procedures that require a median sternotomy. When splitting the sternum, a retractor is used to separate it, allowing access to the heart. This separation forces the ribs to move laterally. If internal mammary artery dissection occurs as part of the procedure, there is additional asymmetric retraction of the rib cage. The first rib compresses the brachial plexus nerve bundles and, in particular, the nerve cord that emerges into the ulnar nerve. If brachial plexus and ulnar neuropathies develop as a result, they generally are not preventable by proper positioning of the patient's arm (Warner, 2009). Improper arm positioning, however, may worsen the insult of the injury.

Isolated ulnar nerve injuries arise primarily from pressure on the vulnerable location of that nerve. The ulnar nerve becomes superficial as it runs behind the elbow, nesting in the epicondyle groove of the humerus, which makes up the cubital tunnel. Ulnar nerve injuries occur primarily in male patients. Warner (2009) offers three anatomic differences between the elbows of men and women, which probably account for this gender anomaly:

1. The tubercle of the coronoid process is 1.5 times larger in men than in women, creating a smaller cubital tunnel around the ulnar nerve.

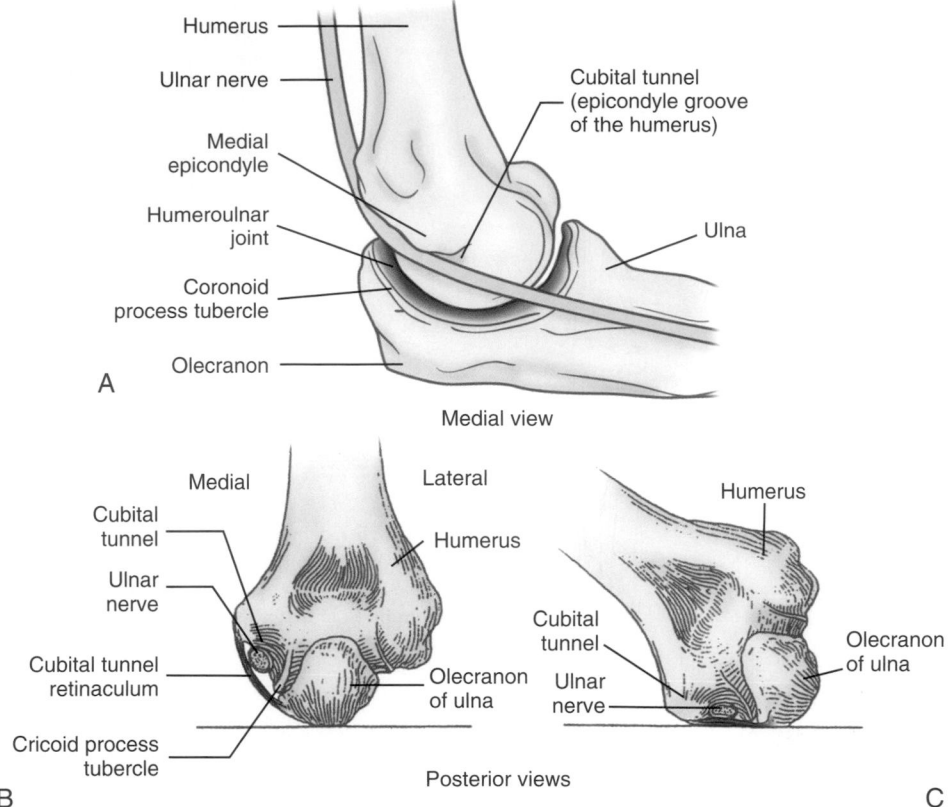

FIGURE 6-8 Ulnar nerve at cubital tunnel. **A,** Medial view. **B,** Posterior view. Note cubital tunnel retinaculum over ulnar nerve in the cubital tunnel. **C,** Posterior view with elbow tilted on medial side. Note compressed ulnar nerve.

2. Men generally have less adipose tissue over the medial aspect of the elbow compared with women with similar body fat composition; this results in less natural padding to that area.

3. Men likewise have a thicker, more developed cubital tunnel reticulum, which can reduce further the space for the ulnar nerve in the cubital tunnel; this increases the risk of injury when the elbow is flexed.

The main goal in protecting the ulnar nerve is to eliminate pressure on it. Pressure on the medial aspect of the elbow may compress the ulnar nerve (see Figure 6-8, *C*). Figure 6-10 illustrates ways to prevent this pressure. Supination (palms up) of the forearms on an armboard (see Figure 6-10, *A*) places the olecranon of the elbow on the flat surface instead of the cubital tunnel, which contains the ulnar nerve. When the arm of a supine patient rests on the trunk, direct trauma can occur to the ulnar nerve as the weight of the arm presses the flexed elbow against the surface of the bed. Padding placed under the upper arm, proximal to the elbow, leaves a free space under the elbow, eliminating pressure on the nerve (see Figure 6-10, *B*). When a patient is prone (abdomen facing down) with arms pronated on armboards, the ulnar nerve is vulnerable to pressure from the elbow. Padding placed proximal and distal to the elbow frees the nerve from pressure (see Figure 6-10, *C*).

Ulnar neuropathy symptoms may manifest in the immediate postoperative period. Sometimes symptoms are delayed until 2 to 7 days after surgery, however, which makes it difficult to isolate the exact event that triggered the complication. The postoperative course cannot be completely ruled out as a possible cause or contributing factor. Some patients are forced to lie on their backs for prolonged periods postoperatively because of devices such as

FIGURE 6-9 Vertical compression on shoulder can injure the brachial plexus. Rotating the head away from an abducted arm can stretch brachial plexus between clavicle and first rib.

endotracheal tubes and abdominal drains. Often they rest with elbows flexed and hands on their chest. This may place pressure on that superficial section of the ulnar nerve under the elbow, which may in turn cause or contribute to injury to the nerve during the postoperative period.

FIGURE 6-10 Three ways to protect ulnar nerve. **A,** Arm of supine patient on armboard with palms up. **B,** Elbow lifted free from bed surface by padding upper arm when arm is resting on trunk. **C,** Arm of prone patient pronated on armboard. Padding above and below elbow frees ulnar nerve from pressure of armboard surface.

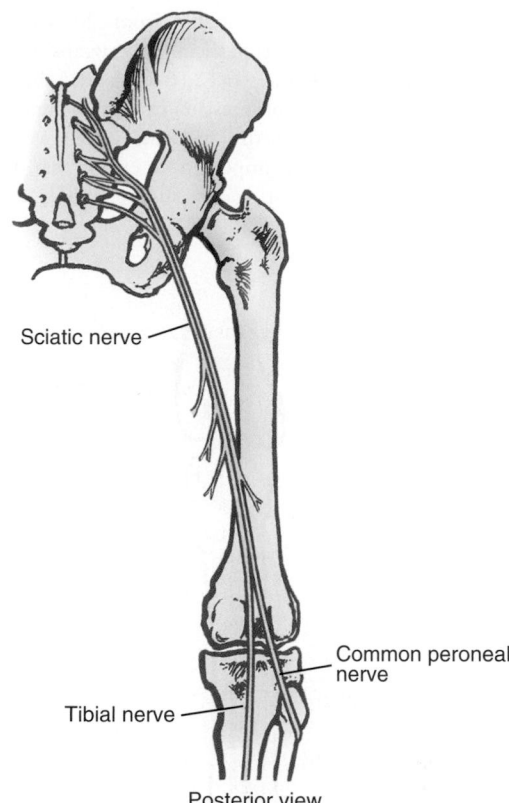

Posterior view

FIGURE 6-12 Right sciatic nerve and right thigh and upper leg, posterior view. Note division of sciatic nerve into the tibial and common peroneal nerves.

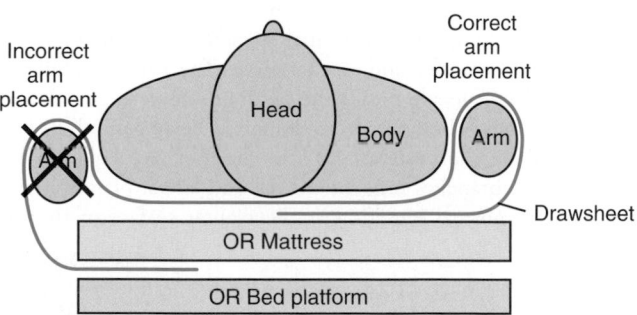

FIGURE 6-11 Correct method for tucking arms in at patient's side.

Many OR-induced peripheral upper extremity nerve injuries can be avoided by properly securing the arms when they are tucked at the patient's side. The arms should be tucked in a way that prevents them from sliding down the side of the OR bed and contacting the bed edge or rigid bed attachments. An effective technique to prevent arm slippage during surgery is to wrap the drawsheet smoothly around the arm and then tuck the drawsheet under the patient's body instead of under the mattress (Figure 6-11). This technique is useful in the supine and prone positions. It is best accomplished with an assistant on the other side of the OR bed, who rolls the patient's body over enough to tuck the drawsheet underneath it. Care should be taken to ensure that the drawsheet is not tucked too tightly as to cause pressure to the arms. A tight fold pressing on the elbow could cause an isolated ulnar nerve injury.

Complete and thorough documentation of intraoperative measures taken to protect vulnerable nerves should include the following:

- How the arms were secured and by whom
- The location of padding
- The angle of armboards (approximate degree of extension from body), the position of the palms, and the location of arm straps
- Times and type of repositioning or passive range of motion done
- Presence of distal pulses, color, and temperature of arms and hands when procedure is long or extremity is compressed, or both

The upper extremities should be evaluated postoperatively. Any changes from the preoperative condition should be verbally reported and documented.

Lower Extremity Neuropathies. Lower extremity neuropathies result most frequently from prolonged lithotomy positioning and tend to manifest symptoms within hours after surgery. The common peroneal, sciatic, and femoral nerves are most frequently implicated.

Intraoperative risk factors include the length of time in lithotomy, high or exaggerated lithotomy, and positioning the extremities beyond their comfortable range of motion when awake. Different types of stirrups vary in the degree to which they control hip flexion. Hip extension should be limited to the minimum amount required for adequate access to the surgical site.

The *common peroneal nerve* branches from the sciatic nerve behind the knee and becomes superficial as it wraps around the lateral head of the fibula (Figures 6-12, 6-13, and 6-14). At this level, it is vulnerable to direct compression by stirrup bars. This risk may be increased in extremely thin patients who have minimal overlying tissue in this area. It is important to ensure that the lateral head of the fibula does not rest against stirrup bars or any other rigid surface. Compressive leg wraps (i.e., intermittent pneumatic compression devices, graduated compression stockings) also can put pressure on this nerve if the wrapping is too tight in this area. In addition, pressure behind the knee can compress the common peroneal and tibial nerves where they run through the popliteal fossa, so only *soft* padding or pillows should be used for knee support. The patient's ability to dorsiflex the great toe (point it upward) indicates that the common peroneal nerve is intact.

The *sciatic nerve* originates from the L4-S3 spinal nerve roots and travels down the buttock and posterior thigh before it divides into the common peroneal and tibial nerves (see Figure 6-12). The stretching that occurs during hyperflexion of the hip may injure it. A patient who has had a total hip replacement may have some preexisting sciatic nerve damage as a result of the excessive rotation of the femur that is part of that operative procedure. Additionally, patients with a history of hip trauma who have required surgery such as open reduction and internal fixation may be at increased risk for sciatic neuropathy because of the potential presence of scar tissue around the nerve area. Because the branches of the sciatic nerve run from the thigh to the hamstring, the patient's ability to flex the thigh generally indicates an intact sciatic nerve.

The *femoral nerve* arises from the L2-L4 spinal nerve roots and runs through the medial thigh. Injury to the deep femoral nerve may occur more as a result of inappropriate placement of abdominal pelvic retractors and vaginal retractors in the pelvic cavity than by virtue of inappropriate positioning (Cassorla and Lee, 2010). The femoral nerve and obturator nerve can be subjected to excessive stretching and injury, however, as a result of inappropriate lithotomy positioning (see Figure 6-14). The patient's ability to flex the thigh to the trunk generally indicates an intact femoral nerve.

The *obturator nerve* originates from the L2-L4 nerve roots. It runs through the obturator foramen of the ischium to innervate the adductor group of muscles in the inner thigh (see Figure 6-14). It can be subjected to excessive stretching when the patient is in lithotomy position. Scrubbed personnel may lean against the inner thigh while holding vaginal or anal retractors, causing additional stretching and compression of the nerve. The patient's ability to adduct the leg generally means the obturator nerve is intact.

The *tibial nerve* branches from the sciatic nerve behind the knee and runs along the posterior tibia to the foot (see Figure 6-12). From there it branches into the medial and lateral plantar nerves. The patient's normal sensation at the plantar surface of the foot

FIGURE 6-13 Right leg, lateral view. Note common peroneal nerve pathway around lateral fibular head. The nerve is very susceptible to injury when patient is in lateral position. Also note sural nerve in heel area. This nerve is susceptible to injury from stirrup straps.

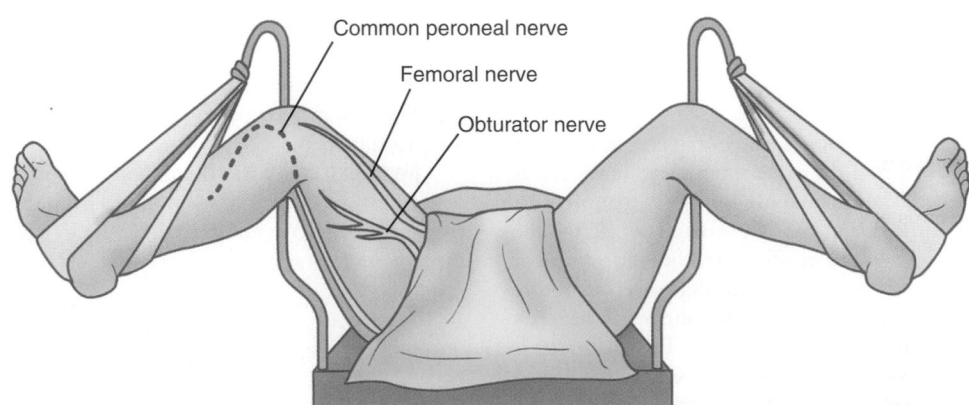

FIGURE 6-14 Nerves of inner thigh. Femoral and obturator nerves can be overstretched by hyperextending hips or by team members leaning against thighs. If lateral knee rests against a stirrup bar, common peroneal nerve can be compressed.

and ability to curl the toes downward generally indicate an intact tibial nerve.

The perioperative nurse should document measures taken to protect the lower extremities from injury, such as:

- Location and type of padding used (i.e., pillow to support knees or calves, padding under heels)
- Type of stirrups used; names of persons placing legs in stirrups
- Type of lithotomy position (low, standard, high, or exaggerated)
- Presence of distal pulses, color, and temperature of legs and feet
- Use of intermittent pneumatic compression devices or graduated compression stockings

The lower extremities should be evaluated postoperatively. Any changes from the preoperative condition should be verbally reported and documented.

The use of intraoperative neurophysiologic monitoring is demonstrably an effective method to prevent peripheral nerve injuries in the upper and lower extremities during procedures in which there is otherwise a high risk of such injuries. A common method of monitoring in the OR is somatosensory-evoked potential (SSEP). Its goal is to establish a baseline of the patient's normal nerve function along selected pathways and then to monitor those pathways at continual intervals during the procedure. Any emerging insult to these nerve structures or pathways will appear and corrective measures taken before permanent nerve injury occurs (Chung et al, 2009).

The Association of periOperatve Registered Nurses (AORN, 2013) offers specific recommendations to prevent nerve injuries during surgery. They are listed in the Evidence for Practice box.

Vascular System

General anesthesia causes peripheral vessels to dilate by depressing the sympathetic nervous system. This dilation decreases overall blood pressure because blood pools in dependent areas of the body. In general anesthesia these effects are systemic, whereas in regional anesthesia, such as spinal and epidural, these effects are more limited to the areas anesthetized.

Position changes affect where blood pooling occurs. Muscle tone and peripheral vascular resistance are no longer as effective in counteracting the forces of gravity on blood pooling. Blood pools to whatever part of the body is lowest. If the head of the OR bed is

---

EVIDENCE FOR PRACTICE

Prevention of Perioperative Peripheral Neuropathies

- When arms are tucked at side of body, the palms and wrists should be in neutral position (facing inward).
- Armboards for a supine patient should be at less than a 90-degree angle on the OR bed with palms facing up or in neutral position.
- Unless contraindicated by the surgical procedure, the patient's head should be placed in a neutral position.
- Avoid positioning arms above the patient's head.
- Prevent the lateral aspect of the knee from resting on the vertical post of a candy cane stirrup when patient is in lithotomy position.
- Avoid using shoulder braces to prevent patient from sliding in Trendelenburg position.

Modified from Bouyer-Ferullo S: Preventing perioperative peripheral nerve injuries, *AORN J* 97(1):111–121, 2013; AORN: Recommended practices for positioning the patient in the perioperative practice setting, *Perioperative standards and recommended practices*, Denver, 2013, The Association, Inc.

raised, the lower torso has increased blood volume, and the upper torso becomes more compensated. Hypovolemia and cardiovascular disease may compromise the patient's status further.

The anesthesia provider can treat some of the hypotensive effects of positioning through pharmacologic agents and increased IV infusion. Vital signs, IV intake, and urinary output need to be monitored closely. Position changes may need to be delayed until blood pressure stabilizes.

Deep vein thrombosis (DVT) is a serious complication of surgical positioning. Compression to deep and peripheral vessels (e.g., resulting from tight safety strap or wrist restraints) may predispose the patient to venous thrombosis. When the legs are in a dependent position (i.e., legs lowered during knee arthroscopy, sitting position, reverse Trendelenburg), venous return slows and thrombosis can occur (Pannucci et al, 2011). Thrombosis also can occur as a result of hyperabduction of the arms beyond 90 degrees. Subclavian and axillary vessels pass through the brachial plexus, and vessel constriction can occur by compression between the clavicle and the first rib. Radial pulses require monitoring whenever arms are extended to ensure that the radial pulse is not obliterated. Graduated compression stockings or intermittent pneumatic compression devices can reduce this risk.

Vascular assessment of upper and lower extremities should occur preoperatively. Document measures taken to reduce assessed risks and evaluate vascular status intraoperatively and postoperatively. Any changes from the preoperative condition require verbal reports and documentation.

Acute compartment syndrome is a serious complication that may arise from excessive constriction to, or improper positioning of, extremities. It is characterized by ischemia, hypoxic edema, and elevated tissue pressure within the fascial components of the extremity, leading to further damage to the muscles and nerves. This process occurs at a cellular level, and distal pulses and capillary refill may initially appear normal; then, however, the process may rapidly escalate to a dangerous condition. The syndrome may progress to rhabdomyolysis with resulting renal damage, permanent nerve damage, loss of limb, or even death. The most effective means to end this syndrome is a decompressive fasciotomy.

Respiratory System

Positioning can compromise the respiratory system. In almost all types of positions, except semi-Fowler, sitting, and reverse Trendelenburg, the abdominal viscera shift upward toward the diaphragm. Subsequently, the diaphragm shifts upward and outward such that it contributes only about two thirds of the ventilatory force and significantly reduces tidal volume. Obese or pregnant patients or those who have pulmonary disease have additional respiratory compromise in these positions. Any patient who experiences dyspnea should have the head of the bed elevated during transport and during local, regional, or spinal anesthesia if this does not interfere with surgical access. During general anesthesia the anesthesia provider normally ventilates these patients mechanically.

External chest movement during surgery needs to be as unrestricted as possible to avoid further reduction in tidal volume. Avoid placement of arms across the chest because arms resting on the chest not only restrict chest expansion, but also add pressure on the ulnar nerve at the elbow area. Some positions (e.g., lateral, fracture bed) require the placement of straps or tape around the chest area to secure the patient to the OR bed without obstructing the surgical site. Such strapping or taping requires efforts to ensure against excessive tightness. These positions are not maintained any longer than necessary. Anesthesia personnel closely monitor the respiratory status of these patients.

Positioning also affects the portions of the lungs perfused with blood. As blood pumps into the lungs, the areas of the lung that are most dependent have a greater pulmonary arterial pressure as the blood pools. The greater the pressure, the greater is the perfusion. The alveoli in the bases of the lungs are more compliant; ventilation is generally highest in those areas. An even distribution of ventilation and perfusion (ventilation-perfusion ratio) is needed for efficient gas exchange. If the position causes a pathologically compromised area of the lung to be dominant and more perfused, the balance between perfusion and ventilation may be disrupted and respiratory status may diminish. The rest of the lung fields may or may not have the capacity to compensate. Oxygen therapy or mechanical ventilation may help compensate, but the amount of time a patient can tolerate a certain position and maintain adequate gas exchange may be limited.

Monitoring of respiratory status should always include pulse oximetry. In some cases, intraoperative arterial blood gas monitoring is also necessary.

Obesity

Obesity is an important consideration in the perioperative environment because its incidence has been steadily rising over the past decades. The upward trend exists among children, teens, and adults. The degree of obesity is based on body mass index (BMI). Obesity and morbid obesity are considered to be BMI of $\geq$30 kg/m^2 or $\geq$40 kg/m^2 (weight)/m^2(height), respectively (Ogunnaike and Whitten, 2009). Morbid obesity is a complex medical disorder that frequently coexists with numerous other medical problems. These include arthritis and degenerative joint disease, sleep apnea (Ambulatory Surgery Considerations), hypertension, type 2 diabetes, and esophageal reflux. The incidence of these conditions increases with the age of the patient and the duration of severe obesity (Richards, 2012). Morbid obesity is associated with some considerable perioperative risks (Patient Safety). Obese patients have a diminished respiratory reserve and become distressed quickly and easily when lying flat in supine. Trendelenburg is even more poorly tolerated and should be avoided until the patient is intubated and mechanical ventilation can assist with breathing (Ide et al, 2008). With excess fat distribution around the patient's back, neck and shoulders, positioning interventions are necessary to gain control of the patient's airway in the supine position. This is done by what has been called "ramping," that is, building a ramp of cushioning materials (e.g., pillows, linens, foam wedges) in order to elevate the head, neck, and shoulders above the chest into alignment with the airway. To create the correct plane, an imaginary horizontal line can be drawn between the earlobe and the sternum as noted in Figure 6-15. This ramped position enables the anesthesia provider to gain control of the patient's airway by aligning the oral, laryngeal and pharyngeal axes. It has also been called the head-elevated laryngoscopy position (HELP) because it facilitates laryngoscopy and intubation (Ogunnaike and Whitten, 2009).

Obese patients are at a high risk for DVTs, and sudden death from pulmonary embolism (Graham et al, 2011). Thromboembolism prophylaxis is imperative in these patients especially if their lower extremities will be bent or in a dependent position. When applying graduated compression stockings or intermittent pneumatic compression devices, they must be large enough so as not to restrict circulation, which might otherwise risk compartment syndrome development.

FIGURE 6-15 This figure illustrates "ramping" obese patient's torso to facilitate optimal airway alignment. Imaginary horizontal line between earlobe and sternum *(dashed line)* references proper position.

AMBULATORY SURGERY CONSIDERATIONS

Patients with Obstructive Sleep Apnea

The Society for Ambulatory Anesthesia published its 2012 consensus statement for selecting patients with obstructive sleep apnea (OSA) who are scheduled for ambulatory surgery. Being obese with positioning precautions in and of itself does not affect candidacy for ambulatory surgery. The suitability of ambulatory surgery for a patient with OSA remains controversial because of concerns of increased risk of serious complications due primarily to airway difficulties.

Among the Society's recommendations are the following:
- Patients with known diagnosis of OSA and optimized comorbid medical conditions may be considered for ambulatory surgery if they are able to use a continuous positive airway pressure (CPAP) device postoperatively.
- Patients with presumed diagnosis of OSA (based on screening tools) and with optimized comorbid conditions may be considered for ambulatory surgery if it is anticipated that their postoperative pain can be managed predominantly with nonopioid analgesics.
- Patients with OSA and nonoptimized comorbid medical conditions may not be good candidates for ambulatory surgery. Consideration should therefore be given to admitting these patients.

Modified from DeJohn P: Sleep apnea: identifying patients at risk in the ASC, *OR Manager* 28(8):26–29, 2012; Joshi GP et al: Society for ambulatory anesthesia consensus statement on preoperative selection of adult patients with obstructive sleep apnea scheduled for ambulatory surgery, *Anesth Analg* 115:1060–1068, 2012.

In addition to being at higher risk for pressure ulcers from long periods of immobility during surgery, obese patients are also at risk for rhabdomyolysis. Pressure from their large body mass can crush dependent tissue causing muscle fiber breakdown, releasing myoglobin into the bloodstream. If not diagnosed early and treated with aggressive IV fluid hydration and diuretics, renal failure can result (Graham et al, 2011).

Beds and accessories must accommodate the width and weight of morbidly obese patients. Available products specifically enhance the safety of the obese patient in surgery. They are discussed in the Operating Room Beds and Accessories section of this chapter.

PATIENT SAFETY

Key Considerations in Positioning Morbidly Obese Patients

The following complications may occur more frequently in surgery patients who are morbidly obese:

- Deep vein thrombosis (DVT) and pulmonary embolism
- Pressure ulcers and rhabdomyolysis
- Ventilation impairment with diminished pulmonary functional residual capacity in all surgical positions except sitting
- Higher rates of perioperative ulnar nerve palsies and brachial plexus neuropathies
- Lower limbs falling off bed causing lateral femoral cutaneous nerve injuries
- Sciatic nerve palsies from tilting the bed sideways
- Postoperative back pain from buttocks acting as a fulcrum for legs, extending the lumbar spine

The following interventions may enhance the morbidly obese patient's safety:

- Provide an OR bed made to accommodate patient's size and weight.
- Use mattress padding and positioning accessories (stirrups, safety straps, etc.) specifically designed and sized for bariatric patients.
- Numerous staff members should assist in transferring patient using transfer aids such as rollers or backboards.
- Elevate the head, upper body, and shoulders to facilitate the airway when supine.
- Have difficult-airway cart immediately available.
- Pad armboards to match the higher elevation of the shoulders to avoid stretching of the brachial plexus.
- As directed by anesthesia provider, apply cricoid pressure to facilitate intubation and prevent aspiration from esophageal reflux.
- Support the knees with pillows to reduce strain on back.
- Use graduated compression stockings or intermittent compression devices on lower extremities.
- Use appropriate transfer devices (air-cushioned transfer pads, pneumatic lifts, etc.) to reduce friction and shear in patients and protect team members from injury.

Modified from Graham D et al: Preventing intraoperative complications in the patient with a high body mass index, *AUHN J* 94(4):334–344, 2011; Bennicoff G: Perioperative care of the morbidly obese patient in the lithotomy position, *AORN J* 92(3):297–312, 2010; Ogunnaike BO, Whitten CW: Anesthesia and obesity. In Barash PG et al, editors: *Clinical anesthesia*, ed 6, Philadelphia, 2009, Lippincott Williams & Wilkins.

Eye Injuries and Perioperative Vision Loss

Perioperative vision loss (PVL), although rare, has become the subject of a substantial number of medical publications because it is so devastating to the patient and has become an important medical-legal issue. Direct pressure on the eye, especially coupled with systemic hypotension, may cause central retinal artery occlusion, which in turn may result in temporary or permanent blindness. Direct pressure can also displace the intraocular lens in a patient who has had cataract surgery. Care needs to be taken to constantly monitor the eyes when using any prone head positioner, especially the horseshoe type (Figure 6-16) because poor placement can put direct pressure on the globe of the eye (ASA Task Force on Perioperative Visual Loss, 2012; Newman, 2010; Warner, 2009). The prone position itself, even without pressure on the eyes, may increase intraocular pressure, which may then lead to ischemic optic neuropathy, particularly with prolonged prone Trendelenburg

FIGURE 6-16 Horseshoe head positioner must be carefully adjusted to avoid putting pressure on eyes.

position or any position that brings the head lower than the heart (e.g., prone on a Wilson frame). Additional risk factors identified include male gender, obesity, long anesthetic duration, high blood loss, low percent of colloid fluid replacement, decreased systemic blood pressure, anemia, diabetes, chronic hypertension, and use of vasopressors (Research Highlight) (Edgecombe et al, 2008; Newman, 2010; Pierce and Kendrick, 2010; Postoperative Visual Loss Study Group, 2012; Warner, 2009).

PVL may be complete or partial, unilateral or bilateral. It is typically painless and noticed by the patient on wakening from general anesthesia or soon afterward. However, sometimes it can take a day or more for the patient to notice vision changes and the optic nerve can slowly atrophy over a period of several weeks (Pierce and Kendrick, 2010). Regardless of onset of symptoms, presently there is no cure and no effective treatment. The emphasis, therefore, is on prevention and continued research on this traumatic phenomenon.

Perioperative Nursing Considerations

Assessment

Assessment for positioning needs should be made before the patient transfers to the OR bed. The perioperative nursing assessment includes a patient interview, physical examination, and review of medical records. Key points of assessment that are related to surgical positioning include age, height and weight, skin condition, nutritional status, preexisting conditions (e.g., conditions of the vascular, respiratory, circulatory, neurologic, or immune system), and physical/mobility limits (e.g., prostheses, implants, range of motion). It also should be determined if there are any particular areas of discomfort that a particular position may cause and what

RESEARCH HIGHLIGHT ▌▌

Risk Factors Associated with Ischemic Optic Neuropathy After Spinal Surgery

In this research, 80 cases of the rare, but devastating complication of perioperative vision loss were reviewed by compiling data from the American Society of Anesthesiologists' (ASA) Postoperative Visual Loss Registry from 17 medical centers. The patients in the study all had spinal fusions in prone position lasting 4 or more hours. When they were compared with 315 matched control patients, six independent risk factors associated with ischemic optic neuropathy (ION) emerged. These were male gender, obesity, Wilson frame use, longer anesthetic duration, greater estimated blood loss, and lower percent colloid administration for non–blood fluid replacement therapy. In their discussion the authors speculated on some of the reasons for their findings. They felt that estrogen might play a protective role in ION, because 69% of the blindness occurred in men, an area that needs further research. Increased abdominal girth of obese patients placed in prone position increases the venous pressure in the head, leading to interstitial edema and reduced perfusion to the optic nerve. Similarly, the Wilson frame causes the head to be lower than the heart, increasing venous pressure to the orbit. Higher blood loss with less colloid non–blood volume replacement for longer periods further compromised optic nerve perfusion. The authors suggest that anesthesia providers use colloid along with crystalloid fluid replacement for high blood loss procedures. They also stress the importance of informing patients of the risk of ION when undergoing lengthy spine surgery in a prone position. Surgeons and patients, being better informed, can share in the decision making between conservative management and various surgical options.

Modified from The Postoperative Visual Loss Study Group: Risk factors associated with ischemic optic neuropathy after spinal fusion surgery, *Anesthesiology* 116(1):15–24, 2012.

interventions might alleviate or reduce that discomfort (AORN, 2013).

The assessment should alert the perioperative nurse to patients and situations that could worsen problems caused by positioning. Vulnerable patients include the following:

- Geriatric patients, whose thin skin layer and increased arteriosclerosis make them more prone to skin breakdown because of pressure
- Pediatric patients, whose size and weight must be considered when selecting positioning aids
- Patients who have respiratory and circulatory disorders, diabetes mellitus, malnutrition, advanced age, and anemia because they are more prone to skin breakdown caused by pressure
- Patients with limited mobility because of congenital anomalies, preexisting injuries, arthritis, or prosthetic implants, who need special considerations during positioning
- Patients with edema, infection, cancer, or conditions of lowered cardiac or respiratory reserves and who have poor general health, making them vulnerable to tissue injury
- Patients with demineralizing bone conditions, such as malignant metastasis or osteoporosis, putting them at higher risk for skeletal fractures
- Patients who will be subjected to anticipated high-risk surgical situations, such as:
  - Lengthy surgical procedures (≥2 hours) because of an increased risk of pressure-related injuries

  - Lengthy time in the lithotomy position because of increased risk of lower extremity nerve injury
  - Vascular surgery because optimal blood perfusion already may be compromised as a result of the patient's disease process
  - Excessive sustained pressure to certain body areas due to the surgical procedure or retraction
  - Cool environment or exposure of large body surfaces, or both, because of the risk of hypothermia and its related complications

Nursing Diagnosis

The encompassing nursing diagnosis related to the care of the patient during surgical positioning is the risk for perioperative positioning injury. Other potentially applicable nursing diagnoses are:

- Impaired Comfort
- Impaired Transfer Ability
- Risk for Falls
- Risk for Impaired Skin Integrity
- Risk for Impaired Tissue Integrity
- Hypothermia
- Impaired Spontaneous Ventilation
- Impaired Physical Mobility
- Risk for Peripheral Neurovascular Dysfunction

Outcome Identification

The outcome identified for safe surgical positioning may be stated as "the patient is free from signs and symptoms of perioperative positioning injury." Primary outcome indicators mandate a review of the skin condition and cardiovascular and neuromuscular status, along with other considerations. The perioperative nurse may define freedom from injury, noting that the patient will:

- Experience a safe transfer to and from the OR bed.
- Be warm and comfortable.
- Experience no tingling, numbness, or pain unrelated to the surgical procedure.
- Maintain skin and tissue integrity consistent with preoperative status.
- Maintain a respiratory status consistent with preoperative status.
- Regain normal physical mobility postoperatively.
- Maintain normal peripheral neurovascular function.

Planning

The perioperative nurse plans activities that will protect the patient from injury and provide physiologic support and comfort, while allowing for optimal exposure and access to the surgical site. Although safe surgical positioning involves all members of the surgical team, the circulating nurse plans and coordinates this teamwork. Knowledge of any preexisting risk factors that may affect positioning strategies (e.g., obesity, diabetes, paralysis, advanced age) should be considered when planning for additional staff assistance for positioning and support devices or padding needed.

It is imperative that the exact location of the operative site be identified so that access to that site is not obstructed. If a secondary surgical procedure is involved, such as a graft donor site, that area needs to be exposed and accessible as well. On occasion, all anticipated incision sites cannot be exposed during initial positioning. Plans need to be made for repositioning an anesthetized patient (i.e., assisting personnel, additional padding devices, additional sterile drapes) so that repositioning occurs quickly and smoothly without unnecessarily prolonged anesthesia time.

Planning for physiologic support involves collaborating with the anesthesia provider. Sometimes chest rolls are needed for adequate lung expansion while the patient is in the prone position. Supports and padding for the head, arms, hands, and axilla should be anticipated and easily accessible.

Planning for the patient's comfort can involve communicating with the patient as to potential areas for discomfort and possible remedies. An awake patient receiving local anesthesia can give feedback on the comfort of the position before, during, and immediately after the procedure. In some cases, all or part of the positioning for a patient who is to undergo general anesthesia can be done before induction if it does not interfere with the anesthesia process. A patient could be placed in the lithotomy position before induction if he or she has a history of discomfort with leg abduction or lower back pain (Patient-Centered Care). If this is done, privacy must be ensured by covering the patient with a sheet or blanket and covering or pulling the blinds on room windows. A Sample Plan of Care for the patient undergoing surgical positioning is shown below.

Implementation

Nursing actions involved in positioning should reflect an individualized plan of care designed to prevent injury while maintaining

PATIENT-CENTERED CARE

Perioperative nurses have a long tradition of providing patient-centered care. The perioperative patient cannot speak for himself or herself. Thus the nurse attends to and engages with the patient to be able to "speak for them." With simple words and actions, the nurse listens, interprets, and makes meaning valuable.

You are doing your preoperative interview with a 72-year-old woman who will be undergoing a uterine dilation and curettage (D&C) for postmenopausal bleeding. As part of your interview, you assess her mobility and flexibility for lithotomy positioning.

Nurse: "Mrs. Smith, we plan to place your legs into stirrups after you get medicine that makes you sleepy so that you will be in a similar position as you were during your gynecology exam in your doctor's office. Did that position cause you any discomfort?"

Mrs. Smith: "Well, like I told my doctor, my legs aren't what they used to be. I'm not doing too well on stairs these days. She helped me get up into those stirrups, but I can't bend my knees very far or it hurts."

Nurse: "Would it be OK with you if we help you get into our stirrups before you get the medicine that makes you sleepy? We will keep your lower body completely covered with a blanket. You can let us know how much we can bend your knees so that you will be comfortable."

SAMPLE PLAN OF CARE

Nursing Diagnosis
Risk for Perioperative Positioning Injury

Outcome
The patient will be free from injury related to perioperative positioning.

Interventions
- Identify surgical site and determine appropriate position.
- Identify and document specific risk factors that may predispose the patient to position-related injuries.
- Identify areas of potential discomfort/limitations in mobility and possible remedies. Note condition of patient's skin and presence of peripheral pulses, as applicable.
- Check OR bed for proper functioning.
- Obtain needed positioning aids, OR bed attachments, and padding materials; verify these are clean and in working order.
- Ensure a safe transfer from the transport vehicle to OR bed and document mode of transfer.
- Safely secure the patient to the OR bed without compromising circulation underneath restraining straps.
- Provide the patient with warmth, privacy, and reassurance.
- If the patient is repositioned after being anesthetized, support all body parts and maintain body alignment throughout the move.
- Use slow, smooth movements in making all position changes, using a team approach.
- Avoid pulling or dragging the patient; use lifting techniques instead.
- Pad or suspend bony prominences and all pressure-prone areas in contact with a solid surface.
- Protect the eyes and anatomic areas containing superficial vessels and nerves.
- Secure the patient to the OR bed to prevent falls or slippage of extremities over the OR bed's edge.
- Monitor physiologic effects of position changes, and be prepared to intervene when necessary.

- Ensure access to airway, intravenous catheters, and monitoring devices.
- Prevent pooling of fluids under dependent areas or any area under pressure by placing towels, impervious pads, or an impervious barrier under or around area to be prepped.
- During long procedures periodically do passive range of motion on accessible extremities if it does not interfere with the surgical procedure, sterile integrity of drapes, or anesthesia administration.
- Maintain normothermia without placing a warming blanket underneath the patient's body.
- Ensure that no equipment or personnel create or impose pressure on the patient throughout the procedure.
- Periodically recheck position, straps, and padding to ensure that nothing has slipped or moved.
- Document all pressure and injury prevention interventions and intraoperative assessments.
- At the end of the procedure, reposition slowly to allow for patient's hemodynamic accommodation.
- Secure patient and remain at patient's side when emerging from anesthesia.
- Transfer patient using a team approach with a secured transport vehicle.
- Reassess tissue integrity; document and verbally communicate any changes during hand-off report.
- Document in detail patient position, including the following:
  - Position of extremities
  - Type and location of restraints, positioning aids, and padding materials
  - Frequency of passive range of motion and other injury prevention interventions
  - Use and location of warming or cooling blankets or devices
  - Positional changes made during procedure (e.g., supine to lithotomy to supine)
  - Adverse physiologic responses to positions and interventions taken

PATIENT AND FAMILY EDUCATION
The Importance of Removing Jewelry and Body Piercings

Perioperative nurses strive to ensure that patients they care for are free from signs and symptoms of a positioning injury. Assessment combined with patient and family education assist in achieving this outcome. During assessment, perioperative nurses routinely ask patients if they have removed all of their jewelry and explain the risk of catching a piece of jewelry or body piercing on equipment as the patient is transferred and positioned. A more difficult issue is dealing with dermal implants. Transdermal and microdermal implants may have posts on them that protrude from the skin. In addition to getting caught on equipment, these posts create a risk for pressure at the site of the implant from the position or positioning accessories.

Educate the patient and family about the reasons you are inquiring about dermal implants. Ask them to be frank with you about their location. Jewelry like this that cannot be removed should be identified and documented; noting the presence of all dermal implants becomes part of the hand-off report and intraoperative plan of care. Part of that plan ensures that prolonged pressure against the implant is avoided by using supportive foam or other devices and that external transdermal and microdermal implant pins are protected with gauze or tape.

Modified from Wanzer LJ, Hicks RW: Identifying and minimizing risks for surgical patients with dermal implants, *OR Connections* 96(4), C5–C6, 2012.

optimal surgical access, patient comfort, and physiologic support. Patient comfort measures need to include physical and emotional aspects. Patient safety measures include verifying that the patient has removed all jewelry, including body piercings (Patient and Family Education). Direct communication with the patient about positioning concerns can help reassure the patient and provide the nurse with insight into possible comfort strategies. Providing the patient warmth and privacy may help the patient feel more comfortable and relaxed and feel respected and cared for.

Assemble all necessary positioning aids, such as padding, pillows, bed accessories, and stirrups, before induction because the patient is generally positioned immediately after anesthesia is administered. Ensure that all positioning devices are clean and in proper working order. Ensure extra staff members are available if needed to lift or turn the patient.

When the patient enters the OR suite, the circulating nurse identifies the patient, using two identifiers, and verifies the correct person, procedure, and operative site. Institutional procedures to prevent wrong-site, wrong-procedure, and wrong-person surgery must be followed. The patient is prepared for transfer onto the OR bed, which should be positioned in the room in such a way that relocation after the patient is anesthetized is kept to a minimum. During transfer the OR bed and transport vehicle should be next to each other and locked. At least one individual should stand on either side to assist the patient in the transfer. If the patient is unable to assist in the transfer, perform a four-person lift using a drawsheet and supporting the head and feet.

Falls are an important consideration during all stages of patient transfer and positioning. Falls can occur during transfers if the two beds are not locked. Falls also can occur while the patient is on the OR bed, whether awake or anesthetized. An awake patient may not fully appreciate the narrowness of the OR bed and can continue to move beyond the bed edges. Someone needs to stand on either side

of the patient until a safety strap is applied. Falls also are a risk during induction and emergence from anesthesia. Lighter stages of anesthesia can result in patient movement. Often the movement is strong enough that safety straps alone do not offer adequate security. Infants and toddlers are particularly at risk because standard safety straps frequently are not used on them because of their small stature. Other means to secure a pediatric patient may be used, depending on the area needed for surgical access. Constant personnel presence immediately at the patient's side and the use of safety straps or portable cushioned side rails minimize the risk of patient falls during vulnerable times.

When the patient is on the OR bed, the safety strap is placed 2 inches above the knees. The strap should be snug but not so tight as to place pressure on nerves or restrict venous return. To ensure snugness without tightness, you should be able to slide two fingers comfortably beneath the strap. The patient's ankles must not be crossed because vessel and nerve constriction and skin pressure may result. The patient should be reminded of this because many patients automatically cross their ankles while lying down.

Movement of the patient should be slow and smooth, ensuring that the whole body is supported during movements. Quick, jerky movements can cause musculoskeletal injury and put the patient at risk for bruises, pinches, abrasions, fractures, or falls. Any lateral, anterior, or posterior movement of the patient on the OR bed should be done by lifting the patient with the drawsheet rather than by pulling or dragging the patient. Vulnerable areas, such as the eyes, breasts, perineum, and fingers, should be protected during all movement.

When in the desired position, the patient should be secured so that movement off the OR bed cannot occur from any direction. Check safety straps and other support accessories for pressure against the patient, particularly in areas adjacent to bony prominences. Padding or adjustment needs to happen at this point because it is the last opportunity before prepping and draping. In addition, consider how the position may cause certain body parts to sustain more gravitational weight. If a pillow elevates the knees, the heels bear additional weight from the calves. Heel padding may be needed to help dissipate this additional pressure. Placing the pillow under the calves elevates the knees and lifts the heels off the surface of the OR bed at the same time.

During the procedure the circulating nurse monitors and assists with any modification to the position that is required. Periodically, the circulator checks pressure points that are accessible and adjusts the patient or padding as needed. Passive range of motion can be done to accessible extremities. This is particularly important during long procedures (≥2 hours). The position, all padding, positioning devices, and methods used to secure the patient to the OR bed are documented. If the patient needs to be repositioned during the procedure, the circulating nurse coordinates the move by calling additional personnel to the OR to assist, ensuring additional positioning devices and padding are available, and protecting the patient from injury as the move commences. All interventions for the repositioning are documented.

Evaluation

After the surgical procedure ends, check all pressure sites, especially those under bony prominences, before transfer to the PACU. Document any changes in skin integrity, mode of transfer, time of discharge, and patient status on discharge as well as actions, observations, and patient responses to treatment. The evaluation of the plan of care should be ongoing during the procedure and conclude with a written and verbal hand-off report to the PACU nurse. The outcome of successful implementation of the plan of care may be measured by the positive patient outcomes listed in Outcome Identification (p. 168).

OR Beds and Accessories

OR Beds

As designed, modern OR beds support and accommodate various anatomic configurations required in surgical positioning. Their height is adjustable, they can tilt laterally, and they adjust to Trendelenburg or reverse Trendelenburg position. Generally OR beds operate electrically or by battery with manual, mechanical backup. They have roller wheels to allow them to move easily and brakes to lock them in place. They consist of a flat platform divided into three major sections: head, torso, and leg sections. Each section has a corresponding removable mattress pad, which usually attaches to the main platform by Velcro or straps. The area between each section is called a "break." Raising or lowering sections is called "breaking the bed."

Along the edges are side rails that separate at each break and run horizontally along both sides of the entire OR bed. Armboards lock directly onto the side rails at any level of the OR bed. The side rails also accommodate sockets, and clamps that can secure a multitude of attachments, including stirrups, anesthesia screens, armboards, and various retractors. Underneath the OR bed platform is a tunnel that runs under the entire body and leg sections to support x-ray cassettes. In addition, in newer models, the entire OR bed platform is radiopaque to accommodate the use of intraoperative fluoroscopy.

The typical OR bed width is relatively narrow to allow easy access to the operative site. Wider beds or side extensions that lock into the side rails of the bed are available for obese patients. All OR beds have weight limitations. Many modern beds are designed to accommodate more weight than earlier models, given the increase in the bariatric patient population. Some can hold up to 1000 pounds. The weight limitations should be marked on the bed. Make sure that the bed you use accommodates your patient's weight.

The torso section is attached to the base of the OR bed because this section supports the heaviest parts of the body: the chest, abdomen, and pelvis. This section also has a break in the center at the hip level that can be flexed or lowered to allow the head and chest areas to be elevated or lowered. At this central break in the torso section is a crossbar, called a *kidney bridge* (body elevator), that can be raised or lowered for kidney or gallbladder exposure. The kidney bridge is concave and can accommodate lateral braces that slide vertically onto the bridge to maintain the patient in a lateral position. The distal portions of the torso section's platform and mattress have a concave perineal cutout to accommodate access to the perineum when the patient is in the lithotomy position. Drainage trays may be fitted into this section for gynecologic, urologic, and proctologic procedures.

The head section of the OR bed can be flexed, lowered, or removed. It connects to the bed by two horizontal posts that fit into corresponding grooves in the front of the torso section as well as the bottom of the leg section. Special headrests, such as a craniotomy or ophthalmic headrest, substitute for the head section and slide into these grooves for specific procedures.

Switching the head section to the leg section allows for movement of C-arm fluoroscopy around the patient's chest and abdomen because the leg section protrudes farther away from the base than the head section does. This configuration can also provide support for the feet when a patient is positioned low on the bed for lithotomy. Once the patient's legs are placed in stirrups that are connected to the side rails of the torso section, the head section (now supporting the feet) can be removed and the leg section lowered to give the surgeon direct access to the perineal area.

The grooves at the bottom of the leg section can also accommodate a distal platform that can be used as a foot extension for tall patients or folded up at 90 degrees to support the feet and ankles when the patient is in steep reverse Trendelenburg.

Additional specialty beds are available for specific types of procedures. The orthopedic fracture bed (Figure 6-17) has multiple movable and removable parts and suspended frames. Special orthopedic extensions and accessories that duplicate the functions of the features on traditional orthopedic fracture beds are available for

FIGURE 6-17 Model on fracture bed. Unaffected leg may be also raised, abducted, and supported in a padded leg rest.

FIGURE 6-18 Axis Jackson system uses hinged technology to position patient in various prone and semi-kneeling positions for spinal surgery.

FIGURE 6-19 Various positioning pads and supports made with dry visco-elastic gel. *Left to right*, Chest rolls for prone positioning, small flat bottom roll used as a bolster or axillary roll (two could be used as pediatric chest rolls), donut head rest, arm sled/toboggan, small pad *(right front)*.

some OR beds. Although urologic procedures can be done on a general OR bed set up in the lithotomy position, specialty urology beds remain useful in the OR because they have built-in drainage trays and radiologic equipment. Special beds are made specifically for spinal procedures (Figure 6-18). These beds support the prone patient's torso so that the abdomen falls freely. This prevents the abdominal contents from compressing the aorta, inferior vena cava, and diaphragm. This allows for better circulation and ventilation and reduces venous constriction, which in turn reduces bleeding during spinal surgery. The leg supports are open at the knees, thus eliminating pressure on them.

Multiple positioning accessories help to achieve desired positions and cushion pressure points. Examples include various headrests, stirrups, arm supports, hand tables, and footboards. Foam and gel pads, and overlays, come in various shapes and sizes for specific areas of the body (Figure 6-19).

Mattress Materials and Their Pressure-Reducing Properties

OR mattresses should meet certain basic requirements. They should be durable, versatile for many uses, nonflammable, resistant to bacterial growth, radiolucent with low x-ray attenuation, compatible with warming and cooling devices, and covered with flexible nonallergenic antistatic fabric. Many mattress pads are now made without latex. OR mattresses should also have pressure-reduction capabilities.

Pressure-reduction and pressure redistribution are primary considerations in OR mattress pads. When neither the position of the patient nor time spent on the OR bed can be altered easily during surgery, using effective pressure-reducing mattresses and positioning devices along with initial and ongoing perioperative assessment of the patients' tissue integrity may be the most appropriate methods to prevent pressure ulcers. With more attention being directed toward optimal pressure relief, manufacturers are improving OR mattresses to be more protective of tissue integrity.

As mentioned earlier, distributing pressure over a larger surface of the body decreases the force of that pressure. Overall interface pressure can be reduced by providing even pressure distribution without "bottoming out" (i.e., flattening or collapsing such that parts of the body rest on the underlying hard surface, defeating the purpose of the mattress). Generally the thinner the foam, the easier it is to "bottom out." Mattress materials vary in their pressure-reducing characteristics. Following are some examples of materials on the market.

Standard Foam OR Mattress Pads. Standard foam OR mattress pads have greatly improved in quality over the years. They are usually purchased with OR beds, or replacement pads can be purchased. Years ago these mattresses used to be about 2 inches thick, made of standard foam, and covered with a relatively rigid vinyl covering. Many of today's mattresses are more than 2 inches thick and have greater protection against the effects of pressure. They have a soft, pliable waterproof cover. The more pliable the cover, the greater the patient benefit from the pressure-reducing properties of the foam or other material inside the mattress. Many pads are made with new advanced foam technology that reduces bottoming out. Higher specification foams should be used whenever possible (Stannard, 2012); they have contouring properties, which allow the bony prominences to sink into the surface of the foam so that they no longer are the sole "landing gear." As other body surfaces also contact the resting surface, overall interface pressures lower. By allowing more body surfaces to make contact with the foam, these pliable covers also help to reduce shear. The many benefits of these newer products have allowed manufacturers to offer them as their new "standard" OR pads.

Bariatric OR Bed Pads. Some OR bed pads are made for bariatric patients. These pads are 4 or more inches thick, and manufacturers claim the foam contours to the patient's body in all areas it contacts to "immerse" the patient in the foam, thereby distributing pressure forces over more of the body surface. Various products accommodate patients of varying weight with side attachments that also accommodate varying widths.

Gel Products. Gel products made of viscoelastic polymer are generally used as overlays to mattress segments and positioning devices. Some OR bed mattress pads are made with a layer of gel over the foam and under a pliable cover. Gel products seem to reduce the effects of shear forces because they are pliable and have qualities similar to body fat. They support weight and prevent shearing and "bottoming out" (Walton-Geer, 2009).

Positioning Accessories. Various accessories are available to achieve and maintain certain surgical positions. Many are made of viscoelastic polymer gels (see Figure 6-19). Some have specific uses; others can be used in multiple ways. Table 6-2 provides a list of some common positioning devices and their typical uses.

Transfer devices enable perioperative staff to perform lateral transfers ergonomically and to protect patients from the effects of shear and friction. Slide boards and rollers are the most often used lateral transfer devices (Figure 6-20). However, bariatric patients present a higher risk of injury to both patient and staff during transfers. Special air assisted transfer devices (Figure 6-21) enable the patient to "float" on a small cushion of forced air. These devices may be placed deflated under the patient on the OR bed. After the

procedure they can be inflated and used to transfer the patient onto the PACU bed. This prevents friction on the patient's skin as well as injury from a fall or trauma from a rough move. The healthcare team is also protected from back and muscle injuries. Thus lateral moves of even morbidly obese patients can be smoother and safer for everyone. (Chapter 3 has a full discussion of patient transfers and workplace safety.)

Standard Surgical Positions

This section discusses standard positions and variations for certain surgical procedures, unique risks, and nursing interventions that diminish patient risks.

Supine

The supine (dorsal recumbent) position is most common. The patient lies with the back flat on the OR bed. The arms may be tucked at the side or placed on armboards. This is the most natural position of the body at rest and is the position in which the patient usually undergoes anesthesia.

FIGURE 6-20 Lateral transfer devices. *Front,* roller; *back,* low friction slide board.

A   B

FIGURE 6-21 HoverMatt air transfer system allows for easy lateral transfers of bariatric patients because patient floats on a small cushion of air.

TABLE 6-2

Positioning Accessories: Their Purpose and Uses

Accessory Device	Purpose	Types of Procedures	Corresponding Figure
Head rests; donut, contoured	Used to support head in alignment with body	Most general and plastic procedures, ear, nose, and throat (ENT), vascular, orthopedic in all positions except prone	Figures 6-19, 6-22, 6-37
Prone head positioners	Support head in prone, enabling space for and support to endotracheal tube	Spinal, posterior craniotomies, anal/rectal, Achilles tendon surgery	Figures 6-16, 6-32, 6-35
Mayfield head device	Totally immobilizing head without putting pressure on facial structures	Craniotomies, spinal surgery	Figures 6-31, 6-36
Pillow	Used for a variety of padding needs, including under knees to reduce back strain in supine, supporting head in supine, between knees, ankles, and arms in lateral positions	Most general and plastic supine procedures Lateral kidney, chest, shoulder and craniotomies	Figures 6-31, 6-36
Heel pads	Used to protect heels from pressure in supine and dependent foot in lateral positions	Most lengthy general and plastic supine procedures, especially when pillow is placed under knees Lateral kidney, chest, shoulder, and craniotomies	Figure 6-25
Wedge	Placed under right flank in supine to shift weight of pregnant uterus or abdominal panniculus off vena cava	C-section, general or plastic surgery done on bariatric patient; for prone and semilateral positions	Not pictured
Chest rolls	Used to provide space for diaphragm and chest expansion and to ↓ compression on abdominal cavity while in prone	Posterior craniotomies, anal/rectal, Achilles tendon, liposuction of flank and hips	Figures 6-19, 6-33, 6-34
Axillary roll	Placed under dependent lateral ribs to create enough space to prevent compression of vessels and nerves in the brachial plexus	Procedures on kidney, chest, shoulder, and craniotomies in lateral position	Figure 6-38A, B
Shoulder roll	Placed horizontally under shoulder blades to hyperextend the neck	Tonsillectomy, bronchoscopy, esophagoscopy, thyroid procedures in supine	Figure 6-25
Wilson frame	To arch back in order to separate and expose vertebrae during laminectomies and to allow for diaphragm and chest expansion and to ↓ compression on abdominal cavity while in prone	Posterior cervical, thoracic, and lumbar laminectomy procedures in prone	Figure 6-32
Perineal post	To counteract the tension on tibia, femur, or hip during open reduction and internal fixation (ORIF); also to stabilize patient on fracture bed	ORIF of lower extremity fractures in modified supine on fracture bed	Figure 6-17
Stirrups	To support legs while providing access to the perineal and rectal area	Gynecologic, obstetric, urologic, and rectal procedures in lithotomy	Figures 6-14, 6-23, 6-28, 6-29
Beach chair attachment	To provide access to the shoulder and upper chest while in semi-Fowler position	Shoulder, posterior arm, and anterior chest surgery in Fowler or semi-Fowler	Figure 6-30
Bean bag	Support chest and trunk in lateral position; prevents sliding in steep Trendelenburg	Kidney, lateral chest, hip, elbow, shoulder procedures	Figures 6-23, 6-36
Lateral braces	Used as support in lateral position; one round pad placed at abdomen, and vertical pads placed at lumbar area and buttocks	Kidney, lateral chest, hip, elbow, shoulder procedures	Figure 6-37
Foam and/or folded linen	To elevate or pad selected areas of the body in order to provide support and/or protection from pressure	Any procedure	Figures 6-10, 6-15, 6-22, 6-24, 6-31, 6-32, 6-34, 6-35, 6-36, 6-38

The supine position allows access to the major body cavities (peritoneal, thoracic, pericardial). It also allows access to the head, neck, and extremities. Vulnerable pressure areas in the supine position are the occiput, scapulae, olecranon, thoracic vertebrae, sacrum, coccyx, and calcaneus (Figure 6-22).

A safety strap is placed 2 inches above the knees, with a sheet or blanket placed between the safety strap and the patient's skin. The strap, applied with enough tension to secure the patient to the OR bed, must not compromise circulation underneath the strap.

The patient's head generally rests on a small pillow or head cushion to support cervical alignment, reduce occipital pressure, and minimize neck muscle strain.

Tuck arms at the side only when necessary for surgical reasons. Arm tucking subjects the patient to the risk of pressure injury to the tissue and nerves of the arms, hands, and fingers from scrubbed team members leaning against the arms or being tucked too tightly against the body, further risking compartment syndrome. An infiltrated IV may not be recognized (AORN, 2013; Denholm, 2009). If the arms

FIGURE 6-22 Potential pressure areas: supine position. Pillow under calves frees popliteal areas and heels from pressure.

FIGURE 6-23 Model demonstrates proper positioning in a vacuum-packed positioning device (i.e., beanbag) for lithotomy position with steep Trendelenburg.

must be tucked, follow the safety steps discussed in the Upper Extremity Neuropathies section and illustrated in Figure 6-11.

Place arms palms up on padded armboards that are at the same level as the OR bed. Abduction should be less than a 90-degree angle to prevent stretching and compression of the brachial plexus. Wrist restraints should be soft and nonocclusive.

Sometimes the patient's legs need to be flexed in a frog-leg fashion to provide access to the groin, perineum, and medial aspects of the lower extremities. To accomplish this, externally rotate the thighs, and flex the knees, which are supported with a pillow under each leg. Use of this position occurs when access to the genitals is required for abdominal gynecologic and urologic procedures. During coronary artery bypass graft procedures, this position allows access to harvest the saphenous vein. Sometimes, instead of pillows, the surgical team may use a special contoured positioning pad.

In the supine position, blood volume to the heart and lungs increases compared to the erect position because venous blood from the lower body flows back to the heart without the counterforce of gravity. This increased blood volume increases cardiac output and workload. The weight of the chest in obese patients can cause increased intrathoracic pressure and increase cardiac workload further. If a patient has cardiovascular deficiencies, supine position can further increase risk for cardiac failure.

Increased pressure on the inferior vena cava from abdominal viscera, abdominal masses, or a fetus in a pregnant woman may decrease blood return to the heart; blood pressure would then lower. The inferior vena cava lies slightly to the right of the vertebral column. Tilting the patient slightly to the left by placing a small roll or wedge under the right flank can divert the weight away from the vena cava. An example is tilting a supine cesarean section patient slightly to the left until the fetus delivers.

The supine position can compromise respiratory function because tidal volume is less than that in the erect posture. The position does allow a more even distribution of ventilation from the apex to the base of the lungs. Anterior and upward excursion of the chest during inspiration is not greatly impeded except in an obese patient, whose chest wall weight significantly compresses the rib cage. The abdominal viscera lessen diaphragmatic excursion, particularly when an abdominal retractor is used and packs are placed toward the diaphragm.

Trendelenburg

Trendelenburg position is a variation of supine in which the upper torso is lowered and the feet are raised. This position facilitates pelvic organ visualization during open or laparoscopic surgeries in the lower abdomen or pelvis. Trendelenburg position can be used

to improve circulation to the cerebral cortex and basal ganglia when blood pressure suddenly lowers. In this position the knees are often bent by flexing the leg section of the bed to keep the patient from sliding. The patient's knees must be over the break in the bed to maintain safe anatomic positioning.

Sometimes the legs are placed in stirrups during steep Trendelenburg, frequently used during laparoscopic gynecology or urology procedures (Figure 6-23). Shearing is a significant risk in this position. The skeletal structure slides up toward the head of the bed. If the patient is draped, lifting the patient to realign the tissue cannot be done. Shoulder braces historically were used to limit upward sliding; however, such braces pose a risk to the brachial plexus (as described in the Upper Extremity Neuropathies section earlier in this chapter) and should not be used. In robotic-assisted laparoscopic procedures, even the slightest movement due to sliding can negatively affect delicate steps of such procedures done under high magnification. To prevent sliding while protecting the nerves of the brachial plexus, Chitlik (2011) suggests using a vacuum-packed positioning device (i.e., beanbag) that is approved for use in lithotomy position with steep Trendelenburg (see Table 6-1). Another method described by Shveiky and colleagues (2010) is to place the patient directly on a gel overlay (without a sheet) to create a high friction coefficient and to counteract some of the effects of shear and pressure. Additionally, padded cross-chest straps secured to the bed after the arms have been padded and tucked at the sides (Figure 6-24) can further secure the patient. Some manufacturers offer Trendelenburg positioning kits with padded cross-chest straps and arm padding.

Any variation of Trendelenburg position should continue only as long as necessary. In this position, blood pools in the upper torso, increasing blood pressure and intracranial pressure. Although the head-down position facilitates drainage of secretions from the bases of the lungs and the oropharyngeal passages, the weight of the abdominal viscera further impedes diaphragmatic movement; as abdominal viscera push the diaphragm up and compress the lung bases, pulmonary compliance and tidal volume diminish. Fluid shifts into the alveoli, causing edema, congestion, and atelectasis. Slow, smooth postural transitions allow sufficient time for the body to adjust to physiologic changes. Hypotension may result if the patient is not returned slowly to the supine position.

FIGURE 6-24 Cross-chest strap stabilization technique for steep Trendelenburg.

FIGURE 6-25 Reverse Trendelenburg position with soft roll under shoulder for thyroid, neck, and shoulder procedures.

Reverse Trendelenburg

Reverse Trendelenburg position is described as the head-up, feet down, supine position (Figure 6-25). It is frequently used to provide access to the head and neck and to facilitate gravitational pull on the viscera away from the diaphragm and toward the feet. When the foot of the bed tilts toward the floor, a padded footboard supports the patient's body.

For thyroid, neck, or shoulder surgery, a pillow or soft roll is placed horizontally under the patient's shoulders to hyperextend the neck. Flex the knees slightly to counteract sliding forward and minimize shearing. Tuck the arms at the side to allow for closer access to the surgical site.

In reverse Trendelenburg position, respiratory function is similar to that in the erect position. Venous circulation may be compromised by extended time in the legs-downward position. When this is anticipated, preoperative application of graduated compression stockings, elastic bandages, or intermittent pneumatic compression devices can aid superficial venous return. If the legs are wrapped, avoid compression of the common peroneal nerve at the head of the fibula. Return to the supine position from reverse Trendelenburg slowly and smoothly to avoid overload to the cardiovascular system.

Fracture Bed Position

The orthopedic fracture bed allows the patient to be positioned for hip fracture surgery or closed femoral nailing (see Figure 6-17). The patient may be brought into the OR in the hospital bed with traction applied. Before transfer the patient can be anesthetized. During

transfer to the fracture bed, manual traction to the injured leg can be applied. Distal lower extremity pulses should be evaluated before, during, and after this position.

The fracture bed stabilizes the pelvis by use of a vertical post placed close to the perineum. This post should be placed between the genitalia and the uninjured leg so that pressure is not directly on the genitalia. If the post is not well padded, the intense pressure placed on the pelvis during traction of the injured leg can crush and severely injure the genitalia and pudendal nerve. Injury to the perineal and pudendal nerves can cause fecal incontinence and loss of perineal and penile sensation (Warner, 2009).

Traction occurs by securing the foot of the injured leg in a well-padded bootlike device connected to the traction bar so that the leg may be rotated, pulled into traction, or released, as surgery requires. One method to secure the foot in this device is use of a boot-shaped cuff that wraps around the entire foot and connects to the traction device. It is inflated with air to secure the foot. Another method is to cushion the foot and secure it to the device with restraining straps, Ace bandages, or a self-adhering wrap. Whatever method is used, excessive pressure on the foot and ankle, especially while traction is being applied, must be avoided and adequate padding must be used. If the boot-shaped cuff is used, do not inflate it beyond the manufacturer's recommendations. The unaffected leg rests on a well-padded, elevated leg holder or is secured in a well-padded bootlike device. C-arm fluoroscopy examinations can be done during surgery because the unaffected leg is abducted out of the field of the x-ray machine.

The arm on the operative side is generally secured over the patient's body in a padded sling or a post-supported arm holder to reduce obstruction of the operative area. Avoid pressure on the ulnar nerve. The edges of the sling should not be right on the bend of the elbow. If a post supports the arm holder, the post and arm holder should be distal to the elbow, freeing the cubital tunnel from pressure.

Lithotomy

The lithotomy position is used for gynecologic, rectal, and urologic procedures. With the patient supine, the legs are raised and abducted to expose the perineal region. The legs are placed in stirrups to maintain this position. There are four levels of lithotomy: low, standard, high, and exaggerated (Figure 6-26). *Low lithotomy* is used for most urologic procedures and for procedures that require access to the perineum and abdomen simultaneously. The thighs are elevated approximately 30 to 45 degrees. *Standard lithotomy* is the most commonly used position for gynecologic procedures. The thighs are flexed approximately 90 degrees from the trunk, and the calves remain horizontal. For improved perineal access, some surgeons prefer a *high lithotomy* position. The hips are often flexed beyond 90 degrees, and the legs are suspended high toward the ceiling. The *exaggerated lithotomy* position is sometimes used for transperineal access to the retropubic area. This extreme position moves the legs completely out of the way of the surgical field. The thighs are flexed toward the abdomen; the calves are suspended vertically; and the pelvis is flexed vertically at the spine, propped upward on a pillow or pad. Compartment syndrome is a more likely complication of the high and exaggerated lithotomy positions. Although the hips must be flexed beyond 90 degrees, care should be taken that the knees are not flexed beyond 90 degrees as well. No pressure should be placed on the legs from stirrup edges or leaning scrubbed surgical staff. The amount of time in these positions should be as limited as possible. If the patient will be in this

FIGURE 6-26 Four basic types of lithotomy position with progressively increasing leg elevation. **A,** Low. **B,** Standard. **C,** High. **D,** Exaggerated.

position for longer than 2 hours, graduated compression stockings/intermittent pneumatic compression devices should be applied to the patient's legs.

The stirrups should be checked before use so that they are securely fastened to the side rails of the OR bed. Slippage of the stirrups or dropping of the legs during stirrup adjustments could cause hip dislocation, muscle or nerve injury, or bone fractures. Both stirrups should be at equal height and attached to the OR bed at the same level. The legs should be raised simultaneously to prevent strain on the patient's lower back; this requires two people to accomplish so that both legs are totally supported throughout the move. Each person grasps the sole of a foot with one hand and supports the calf near the knee with the other. They then raise the legs and flex the knees in slow, smooth movements.

When the legs are secured in the stirrups, the mattress of the leg section of the OR bed is removed, and the leg section platform is lowered. The buttocks should be even with the edge of the perineal cut out section of the OR bed, not hanging beyond the edge, to reduce the risk of lumbosacral strain.

Arms are supported on armboards, placed across the trunk, or tucked at the patient's side. If tucked, extreme caution should be taken when the leg section of the bed is elevated back to a horizontal position at the conclusion of the procedure. The hands and fingers can be caught in the break of the bed and crushed (Figure 6-27).

Several stirrup types are used for lithotomy positioning (Figure 6-28). The most common include posts with knee crutches, candy cane–shaped bars with straps that wrap around the ankles and plantar surface of the foot, and boot-type stirrups that cradle the lower foot and heel and extend to the midcalf area. Each type can create unique hazards.

Knee crutch stirrups (see Figure 6-28, *B*), in which the weight of the leg rests solely on the knee supports, may put pressure on the posterior tibial and common peroneal nerves, and the popliteal artery, in the popliteal fossa. This pressure predisposes the patient to complications, such as neuropathies and compartment syndrome.

When using candy cane stirrups (see Figure 6-28, *C*), the knees can drop close enough to the vertical stirrup bars that the lateral or medial side of each knee or calf may rest against the bars. This can

Incorrect hand position

FIGURE 6-27 Improper placement of arms puts fingers at risk for crush injuries when lower section of bed is raised.

put pressure on the common peroneal nerve as it curves laterally over the fibula, which may cause footdrop and a lack of sensation below the knee. If the medial aspect of the knee or calf rests against a stirrup bar, the saphenous branch of the femoral nerve may compress against the tibia. Padding the stirrup bars softens the rigidity of the bars, but will not eliminate pressure totally if the legs rest against the stirrup bars.

Hips should not be flexed more than 90 degrees. When the legs of an anesthetized patient hang freely in candy cane stirrups, the relaxed hips may separate further than they comfortably would if the patient were awake. There is a risk of hyperabduction of the hips, which can stretch the sciatic and obturator nerves as well as strain the hip joint and muscles.

When relatively thin ankle straps support the weight of the entire leg, such straps put pressure on the ankles and distal sural and plantar nerves. Neuropathies of the foot and pressure ulcers of the ankle support sites may result. Heavier leg weight in obese patients adds to the pressure on the ankle supports. Using wide

A

B   C

FIGURE 6-28 A, Lithotomy position using boot-type stirrups. **B,** Knee crutch stirrup. **C,** Candy cane stirrup.

FIGURE 6-29 Securing morbidly obese patient's legs in lithotomy using pneumatic lifts.

straps or cradling the feet with gel or foam padding before placing them in the stirrup straps reduces localized pressure to the nerves in the foot. This is especially important when legs are highly elevated and so maintained for a long time. Compartment syndrome may be an undesired outcome of a patient kept in high or exaggerated lithotomy for many hours.

Boot-type stirrups (see Figure 6-28, *A*) allow for controlled and limited abduction, support the foot and calf, and distribute pressure more evenly, reducing the risk of extreme localized pressure on any one area of the foot or leg. The foot and calf must be well cradled in the padding of the stirrup. Slightly angle each stirrup outward to align with the shoulder. Ensure that the upper edge of the boot puts no pressure on the lateral and medial aspects of the calf and knee.

Special care is needed for the patient who has a limited range of motion attributable to a hip prosthesis. Avoid severe hip flexion and abduction of the joint. The stirrup should be as low as possible.

Preexisting lumbar backache may worsen in lithotomy position if the buttocks or lower back are not adequately supported. Likewise, elevating the legs may aggravate the pain of a herniated nucleus pulposus. Such a patient may be placed in lithotomy position before anesthesia induction to assess areas of discomfort and to implement therapeutic measures (e.g., additional padding under the lumbar area).

The weight of the legs in the morbidly obese patient may be too great for safe use of any stirrups discussed here. The thighs need to separate enough for surgical access to the perineum while safely supporting the weight of the legs. Bennicoff (2010) describes using two pneumatic lifts, with pillows placed in the slings to reduce their concave shape and thick gel pads extending beyond the sling edges to cradle the feet, calves, and knees (Figure 6-29). Egg crate foam further protects any additional pressure areas on the legs.

Lithotomy position poses significant risk for respiratory and circulatory compromise. Risks increase as the position is exaggerated for radical surgery of the groin, vulva, or prostate. Extreme flexion of the thighs impairs respiratory function by increasing intra-abdominal pressure against the diaphragm, decreasing tidal volume. Interference with gravity flow of blood from the elevated legs causes pooling in the trunk of the body during the operative procedure. This effect is greater when hip and knee flexion is extreme, as in high or exaggerated lithotomy positions. This increased trunk volume may mask blood loss during surgery. When the legs are lowered, however, trunk volume returns to the general circulation, circulating volume reduces, and blood pressure may decrease. Effects of anesthesia on the nervous system depress normal compensatory mechanisms, and hemodynamic adjustment may not be achieved easily.

Arms must not impede chest movement and respiration. The weight of the limbs on the chest, especially in infants and children, may fatigue the muscles used in respiration and induce respiratory problems. In addition, elevating the legs pushes abdominal viscera toward the diaphragm. Lowering the head of the bed can exaggerate this shift further as diaphragmatic excursion lessens.

Releasing the patient from lithotomy position must be done slowly and with adequate assistance. Both legs are taken out of stirrups and lowered simultaneously, giving support to the joints to prevent strain on the lumbosacral musculature. Lower the legs slowly to allow for gradual hemodynamic adjustment as more blood shifts into the lower extremities. Distal lower extremity pulses should be evaluated before, during, and after this position.

Semi-Fowler

Semi-Fowler (beach chair) position may be used for some cranial, shoulder, nasal, abdominoplasty, or breast reconstruction procedures. This position begins with the patient first in supine position. The upper body section of the bed is flexed 45 degrees, and the leg section is lowered slightly, flexing the knees. The arms may rest on a pillow in the lap or be secured on armboards parallel to the OR bed. A footboard may be flexed at the bottom of the OR bed to act as a footrest and prevent footdrop. The entire OR bed is tilted so that the head of the bed is not so erect. This can reduce sliding and shearing effects and diminish the hemodynamic effects of anesthesia.

FIGURE 6-30 Shoulder chair with drop-away shoulder support panels to allow surgical access to shoulder while maintaining torso support. Padded U-shaped head restraint with adjustable Velcro straps holds head secure and reduces undue stress on neck when back section is positioned.

FIGURE 6-31 Model demonstrates sitting position, head secured with Mayfield pin device.

When using semi-Fowler for shoulder surgery, a shoulder chair attachment placed at the patient's torso allows for a segment of the back support to be removed on the affected side to expose the entire shoulder area (Figure 6-30). A head holder wraps around the head, supports it in neutral position, and moves vertically as the head of the bed is raised and lowered. The affected arm and shoulder are prepped and draped to allow for intraoperative shoulder manipulation. They can then be placed in a sterile draped pneumatic arm holder that the surgeon repositions as needed throughout the procedure. The opposite arm is bent at about 90 degrees and rests in an arm holder secured to the bed. A large padded bolster placed under the patient's legs allows the knees to bend and secures the patient in position.

Diaphragmatic excursion improves in this position compared with supine. Although pressure points remain similar to those of the supine position, additional pressure occurs on the ischial tuberosities, calcanei, and coccyx. The risk of shear increases as the head of the bed is raised and lowered.

Fowler

Fowler (sitting) position is used for some ear and nose procedures as well as craniotomies involving a posterior or occipital approach (Figure 6-31). This position begins initially with the patient supine. Slowly, the upper body section of the OR bed is raised 90 degrees, while the knees are slightly flexed and the legs lowered. A footrest is used to prevent footdrop. The arms either rest in the lap on a pillow with elbows flexed 90 degrees or less or remain at the sides on padded armboards. The cervical, thoracic, and lumbar sections of the spine should be in alignment when the position is established. When this position is used for posterior fossa craniotomy or cranial ventricular procedures, a special craniotomy headrest secures and immobilizes the head.

The main pressure points in Fowler position include the scapulae, ischial tuberosities, calcanei, and coccyx. Also, pressure increases on the sciatic nerve. Padding should be adequate at the lumbar area and under the elbows, knees, buttocks, and heels. The popliteal

space requires checking to ensure that the edge of the mattress imposes no pressure at the bottom of the torso section.

This position poses significant circulatory compromises and risks. Blood pooling occurs in the lower torso and legs, which in turn causes significant orthostatic hypotension and diminished perfusion to the brain. Venous return from the lower extremities also lessens, and such hindrance increases the threat of venous thrombosis. Graduated compression stockings or pneumatic compression devices assist in supporting venous return.

With the operative site elevated as compared to the heart, gravity causes a negative venous gradient between the operative site and the right atrium; this negative gradient creates the potential for an air embolism if a venous sinus is opened. During a craniotomy this potential increases when the surgeon dissects tissue free from the cranium, removes bone, tacks up the dura, or enters a highly vascular tumor bed. Monitoring for venous air embolism includes central venous catheter insertion into the pulmonary artery or right atrium, and placement of a Doppler probe over the chest wall. If air embolism is diagnosed, the scrub person irrigates the area quickly with normal saline to prevent further aspiration of air into the vein. The exposed area is then packed with saline-soaked sponges or cottonoids. If air embolism occurs during bone entry, bone wax placed immediately over the exposed bone seals it. The anesthesia provider may aspirate air from the right atrium through the central venous line. The circulator assists and supports the anesthesia provider and scrub team.

Respiration is probably least impeded in Fowler position compared with other surgical positions. It is important to ensure that if arms are resting on a pillow in the lap and secured with tape, they do not restrict chest movement. Avoiding head and neck flexion prevents kinking of the endotracheal tube and airway obstruction.

When the procedure concludes, repositioning the patient back to supine happens slowly so that the patient can make hemodynamic adjustments gradually. Evaluate distal lower extremity pulses before, during, and after Fowler position.

Sometimes Fowler position is used intermittently in short durations during breast augmentation to check the size and symmetry of the breasts under gravity and in an upright position. Although these short intervals carry none of the risks of longer durations in this position, care is taken to ensure that the arms do not fall off the armboards when raising the head of the bed. Wrapping the arms

FIGURE 6-32 Prone position using Wilson laminectomy frame for spinal procedures and face pillow head support.

loosely, but securely, in Webril prior to draping keeps them in place during position changes.

Prone

In prone position, the patient lies with the abdomen toward the surface of the OR bed (Figure 6-32). Modifications of the position allow approaches to the posterior cranium, posterior spine, rectal area, and dorsal areas of the extremities. Pressure points include the cheeks, eyes, ears, female breasts, male genitalia, knees, and toes. Range of arm and cervical motion, as well as positional neck and arm pain, should be assessed before anesthesia induction.

Anesthesia is induced with the patient in supine position, usually on the transport vehicle. Before the patient is turned, the anesthesia provider secures the endotracheal tube with tape, applies eye ointment in each eye, and tapes the eyelids closed to prevent corneal abrasions. The transport vehicle is locked adjacent to the locked OR bed. Four people using the log-roll technique accomplish turning the supine patient to prone position safely, smoothly, and gently. The anesthesia provider supports the head and neck during the turn. A second person stands at the side of the transport vehicle with hands at the patient's shoulders and buttocks to initiate the roll of the patient. A third person stands at the opposite side of the OR bed, with arms extended to support the chest and lower abdomen as the patient is rolled laterally onto the abdomen. The fourth person stands at the foot of the transport vehicle to support and turn the legs. At the completion of the turn, the transport vehicle is removed.

The respiratory system is most vulnerable in prone position because normal anterior lateral respiratory movement is restricted, and the compressed abdominal wall and rib cage inhibit normal diaphragmatic movement. This position generally requires ventilator assistance.

Prone position presents unique hazards and potential complications. As the anesthetized patient is turned from supine to prone, endotracheal tubes, IV lines, and monitoring devices can dislodge easily. In prone position, normal compensatory mechanisms are depressed, and the patient cannot readily adjust to imposed hemodynamic changes and resulting hypotension. Crush injuries can occur to the extremities during the roll from supine to prone and back. Pressure necrosis can injure the skin, peripheral nerves, and brachial plexus. Pressure on the eyes can cause blindness. Venous air embolism can occur when the surgical site is above the level of the heart. If an airway problem occurs as a result of a kinked, dislodged, or obstructed endotracheal tube, reintubation, and emergency airway management are extremely difficult from this position.

Also, the position can result in swelling of the tongue, causing macroglossia.

Arm Support. Proper arm placement requires due care to avoid injury: the arms may be secured alongside the torso, placed on armboards, or brought alongside the head in a "surrender" pose. If the patient has symptomatic thoracic outlet syndrome, the arms are best placed alongside the torso (Warner, 2009). Arms need to be secured so that they do not hang over the edge of the OR bed; if allowed to do so, the weight of the humerus against the OR bed side rails can compress the radial nerve quickly. Arms and palms should be neutral, close to the body, and secured with the drawsheet pulled smoothly around the arms and tucked under the patient's body. The elbows are facing outward in this position, so there is less risk of pressure on the ulnar nerve from the mattress; however, compression still can occur from a too-tight drawsheet or from scrub personnel inadvertently leaning on the elbow. Padding the elbow minimizes this risk. An alternative is to wrap foam padding around the arms and secure them to the sides of the OR bed with arm sleds.

If the arms are to be placed on armboards, bring the arms down and forward slowly, with minimal abduction to prevent shoulder dislocation and brachial plexus injury. Armboards should be at the same height as the OR bed or at a lower line parallel to the OR bed, arms resting with elbows flexed 90 degrees or less and hands pronated. Pads are placed distal and proximal to the elbow so that the ulnar nerve cannot contact with the armboard (see Figure 6-10, *C*). If using the "surrender" position, abduct the arms less than 90 degrees without tension to the musculature of the shoulders, and pad the elbows. The wrist pulses should be strong and full (Warner, 2009).

Chest and Trunk Support. If a patient were to lie flat on the OR bed surface in prone, blood return from the inferior vena cava would be impaired between the compressed abdomen and the weight of the spine and back structures. This could cause decreased cardiac output, venous stasis, and thrombotic complications (Edgecombe et al, 2008). Blood return would divert through the epidural plexus, increasing the potential for bleeding during spinal surgery (Drummond and Patel, 2010). Allowing the abdomen to hang free by using a ventral support or frame can counteract this. These devices also raise the chest and permit the diaphragm to move more freely and the lungs to expand. The choice of support depends on the requirements of the procedure, the physique of the patient, and the availability of the equipment (Warner, 2009). One type of ventral support consists of two parallel rolls of linen or cylindric flat-bottomed gel pads (see Figure 6-19) extending lengthwise from the clavicle to the iliac crest; these are often called "chest rolls." The Wilson laminectomy frame (see Figure 6-32) also uses two parallel pads, but they are on an arched frame to facilitate spinal access. With both of these supports, female breasts may suffer compression between the weight of the body and the ventral chest supports. If the breasts displace laterally, their medial borders can be stretched and injured. If the patient has a mammary prosthesis, direct pressure can rupture the implant. Diverting the breasts inward, toward the midline (Figure 6-33), tends to be better tolerated (Warner, 2009).

A bolster or pillow under the pelvis can further decrease abdominal pressure on the inferior vena cava, especially in obese patients with large abdominal girths. Care should be taken, however, that a bolster rests at the iliac crest, and not at the lower anterior groin,

FIGURE 6-33 Breasts diverted inward toward midline while on chest rolls in prone position (posterior view).

where it can compress femoral nerves and vessels or crush male genitalia. Female breasts and male genitalia should be checked after final positioning to ensure freedom from pressure. A cushion or pillow is placed under the ankles to prevent pressure on the toes.

Another type of ventral support uses four pillar-type padded frames, two to support the chest and two to support the hips (Relton-Hall frame) or a single horizontal pad on the superior chest at the sternum and two pads supporting each side of the hip (Jackson spinal bed or Axis Jackson system, pictured in Figure 6-18). The legs are either supported with thigh pads and a padded foot support or are placed in a padded suspension sling.

Head Support. Protection of the head and neck while positioning in prone is extremely important in order to prevent serious complications. The head of the anesthetized patient should be kept in a neutral position. Inadvertent rotation of the head and neck may lead to mechanical stress on the carotid and vertebral arteries that supply blood to the brain and spinal cord, possibly leading to a cerebrovascular accident (Akhavan et al, 2010, Ellsworth et al, 2009). Hyperextension, hyperflexion, lateral flexion or rotation should be avoided: any one of these can lead to brainstem and cervical spine ischemia, which in turn may cause quadriparesis or quadriplegia (Edgecombe et al, 2008).

Face pillows and facial helmet devices enable positioning with the head facing straight down while in the prone position, thus establishing natural spinal alignment. Such devices consist of foam or gel contoured to reduce pressure to the eyes, nose, and mouth (see Figures 6-18 and 6-32). Openings on the side of the devices allow access to the ETT. Some come with mirrors to enable the anesthesia provider to see the facial structures during surgery. The weight of the head is supported by the foam or gel at the forehead, cheeks, and chin. These areas require monitoring for signs of pressure. Studies show that interface pressures are lower on such contoured devices (Grisell and Place, 2008).

A horseshoe headrest is another device used to stabilize the head in prone position (see Figure 6-16). It attaches to the OR bed and replaces the removable head section. It stabilizes the head by supporting the cheeks and forehead. Its advantage is that the anesthesia provider can access and observe the entire head, face, and airway without obstruction by the OR bed. Its disadvantage is that the head is not fixed in place, so it can move. The head may become unstable during adjustments to the OR bed, which can make it difficult to keep pressure off the eyes.

Pin fixation of the head (e.g., Mayfield head device for sitting patient, as in Figure 6-31) is frequently used for craniotomies in the prone position (as well as other positions). Three pins are tightened into the skull to support the head. This has the advantage of providing complete access to the head, face, and airway, yet, unlike the horseshoe headrest, allows for complete stabilization of the head without the risk of pressure to the eyes or other facial structures. Goodwin and associates (2011) describe one patient who had a chin ulcer and another with forehead and cheek ulcers from resting too long on a face cushion in prone. They turned to the use of Mayfield pin positioning to eliminate incidences of facial pressure ulcerations.

Tightening of the pins on the scalp, however, has a profound stimulating effect and may cause tachycardia and hypertension. Such a hemodynamic effect could be detrimental to the patient with increased intracranial pressure or a cerebral aneurysm. For these patients, a local anesthetic is injected into the skin before pin fixation (regardless of whether the patient is awake or anesthetized). Patients under general anesthesia should have their anesthesia deepened prior to the application of pins. Additional complications include entering veins within the skull during placement causing an air embolism; therefore, the pin sites should be lubricated. Perforation of the skull can occur in patients with thin skulls (especially children) or if overtightening occurs. Special pins are be used for children. Perforation of the skull can injure the middle meningeal artery, which can cause an epidural hematoma or a middle meningeal arteriovenous fistula. In patients who have had previous cranial surgery or shunts, care is required so as to not to reenter previous pin or burr hole sites, strike craniotomy plates, or puncture a shunt valve or tubing.

Use of both the horseshoe headrest and pin fixation device risks dropping the head before it is stabilized in these devices. One designated team member must hold the head until it is secured into the device. Dropping the head at this point would be catastrophic. This team member should have no other responsibility but to support the head until it is safely secured in the head-positioning device.

After completion of a procedure done in prone, returning the patient back to supine position onto the transport vehicle requires a four-person log-roll technique. If a laminectomy frame was used, it can be tilted in the direction of the transport vehicle to initiate the move. Skin integrity is checked over all pressure-point areas. Distal extremity pulses should be evaluated before, during, and after prone position.

Prone Jackknife. The jackknife (or Kraske) position is a modification of the prone position often used for hemorrhoidectomy or pilonidal sinus procedures (Figure 6-34). The patient's hips are placed on a bolster or pillow over the break in the lumbar section of the OR bed, and the bed is flexed at a 90-degree angle, raising the hips and lowering the head and trunk. The patient's head, chest, and feet need the usual prone supports in this position. Chest rolls

FIGURE 6-34 Jackknife (Kraske) position.

FIGURE 6-35 Kneeling position with pressure points highlighted in red.

placed from under each shoulder to the iliac crest relieve pressure on the brachial plexus from the clavicle. A pillow should be placed under the lower legs to prevent pressure on the toes. The restraint strap is placed across the posterior thighs.

For anal procedures the buttocks may be separated with strips of 3-inch tape secured firmly at the level of the anus a few inches from the midline on either side. These strips are pulled tight simultaneously and are fastened to the underside of the bed surface. The strips are released at the end of the procedure to facilitate approximation of the wound edges.

Jackknife position causes circulatory changes because the head and feet are in dependent positions, causing cephalad and caudad venous pooling. Graduated compression stockings/intermittent pneumatic compression devices assist in venous return and decrease the risk of venous thrombosis.

This position also severely compromises respirations because it restricts anterior lateral chest movement. In addition, it allows the abdominal viscera to exert pressure on the diaphragm, and that stress further exacerbates the pressure from the flexed OR bed.

When the procedure is completed, the patient is placed on the transport vehicle in supine position. The OR bed is first straightened very slowly so that the body can adjust hemodynamically. Four people using the log-roll technique turn the patient. Distal lower extremity pulses should be evaluated before, during, and after the prone jackknife position.

Prone Kneeling. Use of the kneeling modification to the prone position occurs primarily for spinal surgeries such as thoracic and lumbar laminectomies and diskectomies, but can also be used for adrenal or rectal surgery (Figure 6-35). The prone kneeling position requires the hips and knees to be flexed approximately 90 degrees. A padded platform supports the legs, and the feet and toes are supported so they remain free of pressure. Either lateral supports on both sides of the hip or a posterior support at the back of the buttocks stabilizes the hips and buttocks. Place a safety strap around the posterior area of the thighs, avoiding compression of the nerves and vessels in the popliteal fossa. If a female patient's breasts are large, a flat-bottomed gel bolster placed above the breasts supports the chest. If the breasts are small, the bolster is placed immediately below the breasts. Male genitalia are checked to ensure that they are not compressed between the pelvis and OR bed. The head is supported in a neutral position with a head positioner. The arms are supported on armboards placed parallel to the OR bed (St-Arnaud and Paquin, 2008; Warner, 2009). The prone kneeling position can be achieved on a regular OR bed with the support accessories described here or on a spinal surgery bed (Andrews) designed specifically for this position.

Pressure points are a vital consideration for this position. They include the eyes, ears, chin, anterior rib cage, female breasts, anterior iliac crests, male genitalia, anterior tibial aspects of the calves, dorsal feet, toes, and especially the knees. These areas need to be well padded and supported. Pedal and radial pulses should be assessed before, during, and after prone kneeling positioning to ensure adequate perfusion of all four extremities.

The advantage of this position is that it enables the abdomen to hang free, reducing pressure on the abdomen and the inferior vena cava. This eases ventilation and reduces bleeding by minimizing pressure on the epidural veins. It also provides good exposure and access to the posterior spine. Complications associated with this position are similar to those of prone, but also raise concern for the effects of legs being lower than the body and the weight of the hips and thighs resting on bent knees. The knees sustain significantly more pressure than in any other position. Injury to the knee joint and necrosis to the skin and muscles around the knee may result. Hypotension occurs due to the pooling of blood into the lower extremities. This can be somewhat counteracted by the use of graduated compression stockings/intermittent compression devices placed on the patient prior to anesthesia induction. However, the longer this position continues, the greater the risk for thrombosis and pulmonary embolism. Also, the literature contains reports of compartment syndrome and rhabdomyolysis as complications of prone kneeling position, particularly when the knees and hips are flexed beyond 90 degrees (the tuck or knee-chest position). These risks are increased in the obese patient (Edgecombe et al, 2008; Warner, 2009). A 45/45 suspended position (i.e., hips and knees flexed at 45 degrees and legs suspended in a sling) could reduce the risk of compartment syndrome for procedures that require a kneeling or knee-chest position. Some newer specialty spinal bed systems use a hinged frame to place the patient in a 45/45 suspended prone position (see Figure 6-18), accomplishing the surgical access benefits of the prone kneeling position while limiting some of the associated risks.

Lateral

In the lateral (lateral recumbent, lateral decubitus, or Sims) position, the patient lies on the nonoperative side, providing access to the upper chest, the kidney, or the upper section of the ureter (Figure 6-36). Reference to right or left lateral position depends on the side on which the patient lies: in right lateral position, the

FIGURE 6-36 Lateral position with Mayfield pins and beanbag positioner. Pressure points highlighted in red.

FIGURE 6-37 Maintaining lateral position with three lateral braces positioned at abdomen, lower back, and upper posterior thighs.

patient lies with the right side down; in left lateral, the patient lies with the left side down.

After induction of anesthesia and with the patient in supine position on the OR bed, the patient is turned to the side. A four-person team uses a prepositioned lift-sheet under the patient to facilitate a safe, smooth, gentle turn.

A pillow, cushion, or other head positioner (the Mayfield pin device is pictured in Figure 6-36), is placed under the patient's head to maintain good alignment with the cervical spine and the thoracic vertebrae; good alignment also helps to minimize stretching on the dependent brachial plexus. Bottom leg flexion at the knee and hip stabilizes the patient on the OR bed. The top leg is straight or slightly flexed. A pillow is placed lengthwise between the patient's legs. Padding at the lateral aspect of the bottom knee and ankle prevents pressure on the common peroneal nerve and distal fibula. Designated team members remain at the patient's front and back to steady and support the torso during positioning of the lower extremities.

Pillows, rolled blankets, padded lateral braces (Figure 6-37), or a surgical positioning system, (sometimes referred to as a "vac-pac," or "beanbag" as shown in Figure 6-36), support the torso. A beanbag

is a soft pad filled with tiny beads. When suction is attached to a port on the pad, it conforms to the shape of whatever it is wrapped around. A valve closes to maintain the vacuum. The beanbag acts as an immobilizer until air is reintroduced, and then softens back into its original shape. During the time it is rigid, the beanbag increases the interface pressures on all the tissue it contacts, and risk of pressure ulcer development increases. Some manufacturers offer beanbag positioners with a layer of gel on the surface to reduce interface pressures.

Wide tape fastened to the platform of the OR bed secures the shoulders, hips, and legs. The upper arm is placed on an elevated armboard or rests on a pillow in front of the patient. The lower arm is flexed and rests on an armboard. The lower shoulder should be brought slightly forward, and an axillary roll is placed under the rib cage of the down chest, posterior to the axilla (Figure 6-38). This places the weight of the chest on the rib cage instead of compressing the down shoulder and axilla, which could lead to injury to the brachial plexus of the dependent arm. An axillary roll is typically made of rolled linen or a cylindric gel pad. IV bags should not be used for this purpose (Denholm, 2010) because they are not designed to redistribute pressure. They can roll and leak, saturating the area with electrolyte solution. This increases the risk of tissue trauma, pressure ulcers, and electrosurgical burns. After the patient is positioned, radial pulses are checked to confirm adequate circulation in the dependent hand and arm.

Systolic and diastolic pressures decrease in the lateral position because pharmacologic agents and pathophysiologic processes depress normal compensatory mechanisms. The patient may not readily compensate for abrupt postural changes. Respiratory function is compromised by the weight of the body on the lower chest. Chest movements are limited, and the chest size may be decreased. Distal extremity pulses should be evaluated before, during, and after lateral position and all of its modifications.

Lateral Chest. The lateral chest position is a modification that allows an operative approach to the uppermost part of the thoracic cavity. A variation in upper arm placement occurs when the arm is flexed slightly at the elbow and raised above the head to elevate the scapula. This provides access to the underlying ribs and widens the intercostal spaces. A raised armboard or pillow supports the uppermost arm. Slanting the upper section of the bed downward places the trachea and mouth at a level lower than the lungs, a position that enables bronchial secretions and fluids from the lung bases to drain into the mouth and not pass into the unaffected side of the chest.

A respiratory effect of lateral chest position is that the dependent lung is more perfused because of gravitational pooling of blood. The nondependent lung is more easily ventilated, however, because it is less compressed. This results in a ventilation-perfusion mismatch. The anesthesia provider applying positive end-expiratory pressure (PEEP) to both lungs helps to compensate for this decrease in functional lung capacity. When the nondependent lung is the site of the operation and decompressed, however, functional lung capacity worsens further.

Lateral Kidney. The lateral kidney position allows approach to the retroperitoneal area of the flank. While being turned from supine to lateral kidney position, the anesthetized patient is positioned so that the lower iliac crest is just below the lumbar break on the OR bed where the kidney bridge is located. For torso stabilization, well-padded lateral braces can support the abdomen, back, and hips. To

FIGURE 6-38 Proper placement of axillary roll in lateral position. **A,** Note the placement of arms with additional padding under the head to maintain alignment. Dependent eye is clear of the headrest. **B,** The roll is placed under the chest wall, caudal to the axilla, leaving the axilla area free to prevent compression of the brachial plexus.

render the kidney region readily accessible, the kidney bridge is raised, and the bed flexed so that the area between the twelfth rib and the iliac crest elevates. Raising the kidney bridge depends on the cardiovascular response of the body to increased pressure transmitted from this area. It should be raised slowly and the anesthesia provider should monitor blood pressure frequently. The OR bed is flexed to lower the patient's head and legs. The patient's affected side thus presents a straight horizontal line from shoulder to hip. In this position the gravitational force on the head and torso opposes that on the extended limb to facilitate operative exposure.

Increased intra-abdominal pressure evoked by the kidney bridge and by flexion of the lower limbs toward the abdomen limits diaphragmatic movement. The acute angulations of the body in the lateral kidney posture and the effect of gravity also may decrease blood return to the right side of the heart.

Before wound closure the kidney bridge is lowered and the bed is straightened to facilitate approximation of wound edges.

KEY POINTS

- In order to ensure the safety of patients undergoing surgery, perioperative nurses need to understand the physiologic effects of placing anesthetized patients in their intended positions and take preventative measures to safeguard them from complications that may arise from those positions.
- Physical forces during lengthy surgical procedures predispose patients to skin and tissue injuries related to pressure, shear, friction, moisture, and heat. Perioperative nurses need to identify and pad pressure points, avoid shear and friction producing movement, keep the skin dry, and prevent thermal injuries.
- Nerve injuries are an avoidable surgical complication. Perioperative nurses must know the location of commonly injured nerve sites (such as the ulnar nerve and brachial plexus) and use positioning strategies to safeguard nerves in these areas.
- Severely and morbidly obese patients present unique challenges and risks during surgical positioning. Perioperative nurses need to properly prepare for these patients in order to ensure their safety during transfer and positioning without causing injury to them or OR personnel. The OR bed and accessories need to provide an adequate surface with appropriate padding to protect patient tissue and nerves. Perioperative nurses need to understand and accommodate for respiratory and vascular challenges in any intended position.

CRITICAL THINKING QUESTION

A 35-year-old woman is scheduled for an open reduction internal fixation (ORIF) of a fractured distal fibula. She weighs 305 pounds and is 5'5" tall. She was recently diagnosed as having type 2 diabetes. You interview her in the preoperative area and note that the head of her bed is elevated about 60 degrees. She is alert and oriented and states she broke her ankle while walking on an uneven sidewalk. What factors would you incorporate in your perioperative plan of care? What critical assessment factors would you include? What perioperative nursing interventions would you use to address them?

Ⓔvolve   *The answers to the Critical Thinking Question can be found at http://evolve.elsevier.com/Rothrock/Alexander.*

REFERENCES

Akhavan A et al: Complications associated with patient positioning in urologic surgery, *Urology* 76(6):1309–1316, 2010.

American Society of Anesthesiologists: Practice advisory for prevention of perioperative peripheral neuropathies, *Anesthesiology* 114(4):741–754, 2011.

American Society of Anesthesiologists Task Force on Perioperative Visual Loss: Practice advisory for perioperative visual loss associated with spine surgery, *Anesthesiology* 116(2):2745–2785, 2012.

Association of periOperative Registered Nurses (AORN): Recommended practices for positioning the patient in the perioperative practice setting. In *Perioperative standards and recommended practices*, 425-444, Denver, 2013, The Association.

Bennicoff G: Perioperative care of the morbidly obese patient in the lithotomy position, *AORN J* 92(3):297–312, 2010.

Centers for Medicare & Medicaid Services: *Hospital-acquired conditions*, 2008 (present on admission indicator), available at www.cms.gov/Medicare/ Medicare-Fee-for-Service-Payment/HospitalAcqCond/Hospital-Acquired_ Conditions.html. Accessed January 21, 2013.

Cassorla L, Lee JW: Patient positioning and anesthesia. In Miller RD, editor: *Miller's anesthesia*, vol 1, ed 7, Philadelphia, 2010, Churchill Livingstone.

Chitlik A: Safe positioning for robotic-assisted laparoscopic prostatectomy, *AORN J* 94(1):37–45, 2011.

Chung I et al: Upper-limb somatosensory evoked potential monitoring in lumbosacral spine surgery: a prognostic marker for position-related ulnar nerve injury, *Spine J* 9(4):287–295, 2009.

Connor T et al: Identification of pre-operative and intra-operative variables predictive of pressure ulcer development in patients undergoing urologic surgical procedures, *Urol Nurs* 30(5):289–295, 305, 2010.

Cox J: Predictors of pressure ulcers in adult critical care patients, *AJCC* 20(5):364–375, 2011.

Denholm B: Perioperative pressure ulcers, *AORN J* 87(2):430–432, 2008.

Denholm B: Tucking patients' arms and general positioning, *AORN J* 89(4):755–757, 2009.

Denholm B: Using IV bags to position patients, *AORN J* 92(1):106–107, 2010.

Drummond JC, Patel PM: Neurosurgical anesthesia. In Miller RD, editor: *Miller's anesthesia*, vol 2, ed 7, Philadelphia, 2010, Churchill Livingstone.

Edgecombe H et al: Anaesthesia in the prone position, *Br J Anaesth* 100(2):165–183, 2008.

Ellsworth WA et al: Perioperative considerations for patient safety during cosmetic surgery–preventing complications, *Can J Plast Surg* 17(1):9–16, 2009.

Fred C et al: Intraoperatively acquired pressure ulcers and perioperative normothermia: a look at relationships, *AORN J* 96(3):251–260, 2012.

Galvin PA, Curley MAQ: The Braden Q+P: a pediatric perioperative pressure ulcer risk assessment and intervention tool, *AORN J* 96(3):261–270, 2012.

Goodwin CR et al: Prevention of facial pressure ulcers using the Mayfield clamp for sacral tumor resection, *J Neurosurg* 14(1):85–87, 2011.

Graham D et al: Preventing perioperative complications in the patient with a high body mass index, *AORN J* 94(4):334–344, 2011.

Grisell M, Place H: Face tissue pressure in prone positioning: a comparison of three face pillows while in prone position for spinal surgery, *Spine J* 7(5):84S–85S, 2008.

Ide P et al: Perioperative nursing care of the bariatric patient, *AORN J* 88(1):30–53, 2008.

Lyder C, Ayello E: Pressure ulcers: a patient safety issue. In Hughes RG, editor: *An evidence based handbook for nurses*, Rockville, MD, 2008, Agency for Healthcare Research and Quality, available at www.ahrq.gov/qual/ nurseshdbk/nurseshdbk.pdf. Accessed January 21, 2013.

Mathias JM: Save our skin: periop teams rally to prevent pressure ulcers in OR, *OR Manager* 24(3):1, 11–13, 2008.

Munro CA: The development of a pressure ulcer risk-assessment scale for perioperative patients, *AORN J* 92(3):272–287, 2010.

National Pressure Ulcer Advisory Panel: *Pressure ulcer stages/categories*, available at http://www.npuap.org/resources/educational-and-clinical-resources/ npuap-pressure-ulcer-stagescategories. Accessed April 27, 2013.

National Pressure Ulcer Advisory Panel: *Deep tissue injury*, available at http:// www.npuap.org/resources/white-papers/Accessed April 27, 2013.

Newman NJ: Perioperative visual loss after nonocular surgeries, *Am J Ophthalmol* 145(4):604–610, 2010.

Ogunnaike BO, Whitten CW: Anesthesia and obesity. In Barash PG et al, editors: *Clinical anesthesia*, ed 6, Philadelphia, 2009, Lippincott Williams & Wilkins.

Pannucci CJ et al: The effect of increased hip flexion using stirrups on lower-extremity venous flow: a perspective observational study, *Am J Surg* 202(4):427–432, 2011.

Pierce V, Kendrick P: Ischemic optic neuropathy after spine surgery, *AANA J* 78(2):141–145, 2010.

Postoperative Visual Loss Study Group: Risk associated with ischemic optic neuropathy after spinal fusion surgery, *Anesthesiology* 116(1):15–24, 2012.

Prielipp RC, Warner MA: Perioperative nerve injury: a silent scream? *Anesthesiology* 111(3):464–466, 2009.

Primiano M et al: Pressure ulcer prevalence and risk factors during prolonged surgical procedures, *AORN J* 94(6):555–566, 2011.

Renter T, Beissel D: *Proper positioning helps avoid nerve damage during surgery*, available at ce.nurse.com/PrintTopic.aspx?TopicId=744. Accessed January 21, 2013.

Richards WO: Morbid obesity. In Townsend CM et al, editors: *Sabiston textbook of surgery*, ed 19, Philadelphia, 2012, Saunders.

Saidha S et al: Spectrum of peripheral neuropathies associated with surgical interventions: a neurophysiological assessment, *J Brachial Plex Peripher Nerve Inj* 5(9):1–4, 2010.

Shveiky D et al: Brachial plexus injury after laparoscopic and robotic surgery, *J Minim Invasive Gynecol* 17(4):414–420, 2010.

St-Arnaud D, Paquin MJ: Safe positioning for neurosurgical patients, *AORN J* 87(6):1156–1168, 2008.

Stannard D: Support surfaces for pressure ulcer prevention, *J Perianesth Nurs* 27(5):341–342, 2012.

Suriadi SH et al: Development of a new risk assessment scale for predicting pressure ulcers in an intensive care unit, *Nurs Crit Care* 13(1):34–43, 2008.

Uribe JS et al: Brachial plexus injury following spinal surgery—a review, *J Neurosurg* 13(4):552–558, 2010.

Walton-Geer PS: Prevention of pressure ulcers in the surgical patient, *AORN J* 89(3):538–548, 2009.

Warner MA: Patient positioning and related injuries. In Barash PG et al, editors: *Clinical anesthesia*, ed 6, Philadelphia, 2009, Lippincott Williams & Wilkins.

Welch MB et al: Perioperative peripheral nerve injuries, *AORN J* 111(3):490–497, 2009.

Sutures, Needles, and Instruments

JIM MCCARTHY

Sutures, needles, and instruments are the tools of the surgical team that are necessary to successfully complete a surgical procedure. It is the responsibility of the perioperative nurse to understand these tools and be proficient with their preparation for surgery. Although there are many other aspects of the perioperative registered nurse (RN) role that ensures the expected outcome of a surgical intervention, these items are the basis for surgical procedures. This chapter describes and illustrates a basic knowledge for the perioperative RN, but as the surgical arena continues to evolve, especially technologically, the perioperative RN should be receptive to change and develop proficiencies in new surgical devices and techniques.

Suture Materials

The development of surgical sutures has been closely associated with the development of the art and science of surgery. Medical writings of ancient Egyptian and Assyrian cultures dating back to 2000 BC mention the various materials used, to a limited extent, for suturing and ligating. The concept of suturing and ligating also is recorded in the writings of the father of medicine, Hippocrates, born 460 BC. Gut of sheep intestines was first mentioned as suture material by the ancient Greek physician Galen. The Persian physician and philosopher Rhazes is credited with using surgical gut, or catgut, in AD 900 for suturing abdominal wounds. However, the word *catgut* is a misnomer, and its use is inappropriate. According to the *Oxford English Dictionary,* it refers to the Dutch word *kattedarm,* "cat-intestine." Use of the term *catgut* was adopted by the English around 1560 to 1600 under obscure conditions, possibly connected humorously with caterwauling.

Suture is a generic term for all materials used to repair and reapproximate incised or torn tissues. The primary goal is to encourage wound healing of the injured tissue to reduce the risk of infection. To *suture* is to stitch together cut or torn edges of tissue (*Mosby's Dictionary,* 2012). A *ligature* is a strand of suture material used to tie off or occlude blood vessels to prevent bleeding, or to isolate a mass of tissue for excision. A variety of suture materials are available for ligating, suturing, and closing the wound. The choice of suture takes into consideration several characteristics, such as the following: absorbable versus nonabsorbable, tensile strength, monofilament or multifilament (braided), ease of knot tying, and the inflammatory response of the tissue. An understanding of the characteristics of suture materials, knowledge of the risk factors of wound healing, and awareness of the interactions between tissues and suture materials for proper wound healing is essential for the perioperative nurse, as well as all members of the surgical team.

Characteristics of Suture Material

Key features used to evaluate the general properties of suture material are (1) physical characteristics, (2) handling characteristics, and (3) tissue-reaction characteristics (Box 7-1).

The ideal suture material is one that causes minimal inflammation and tissue reaction while providing maximal strength during the lag phase of wound healing (see Chapter 9). There is no ideal suture for every application, and even the best application presents risks of individual suture failure. Perioperative nurses should evaluate the characteristics of sutures to determine the ideal choice for surgical patient care and incorporate research findings into their clinical practice.

Physical Characteristics. Physical characteristics of sutures are defined and described by the *United States Pharmacopeia (USP),* which is the official compendium for suture manufacture. Characteristics can be measured or visually determined and include the following properties:

- *Physical configuration:* Suture material can be single-strand (monofilament) or multistrand (multifilament), containing numerous fibers rendered into a single thread by twisting or braiding (Figure 7-1).
- *Capillarity:* The ability to transmit fluid along the strand.
- *Diameter (size):* Size is measured in millimeters, and expressed in USP sizes with zeros. That is, the smaller the cross-sectional diameter, the more zeros; sizes range from #7, the largest, to 11-0, the smallest. Suture sizes 0 to 4-0 are the most commonly used in general surgery. (The surgeon usually selects the finest suture possible for the tissue being closed. The finer diameter [smaller size] provides better handling qualities and small knots. Improved suturing techniques are possible with sutures of finer diameter.)
- *Tensile strength:* The amount of weight (breaking load) necessary to break a suture (breaking strength); it varies according to the type of suture material (Table 7-1)
- *Knot strength:* The force necessary to cause a given type of knot to slip, either partially or completely
- *Elasticity:* The suture's inherent ability to regain original form and length after having been stretched
- *Memory:* The capacity of a suture to return to its former shape after being re-formed, as when tied; high memory yields less knot security

Handling Characteristics. Handling characteristics of suture material are related to pliability (e.g., how easily the material bends) and the coefficient of friction (e.g., how easily the suture slips through tissue and can be tied). A suture with a high friction coefficient tends to drag through tissue. It is more difficult to tie because its knots do not set easily. Some suture materials are coated to reduce their coefficient of friction. This coating not only improves the way they pull through tissue on insertion but also lessens the force needed to remove the suture after the wound is healed. The coefficient of friction should not be too low, however, because then knots will be loosened too easily.

Tissue-Reaction Characteristics. Because it is a foreign substance, all suture materials cause some tissue reaction. Tissue reaction begins when the suture inflicts injury to the tissue during insertion. In addition, tissue reacts to the suture material itself (Table 7-2). This reaction begins with an infiltration of white blood cells into the area; macrophages and fibroblasts then appear; and by about the seventh day, fibrous tissue with chronic inflammation is present. The reaction persists until the suture is encapsulated (nonabsorbable material) or absorbed (absorbable material) by the body.

Types of Suture Material

Suture materials are classified into two main groups: absorbable and nonabsorbable. The suture may then be divided into two subgroups: braided and monofilament. Absorbable sutures have varying lengths of absorption time, which affects healing time and strength of the closure.

Absorbable Sutures. The USP defines an absorbable surgical suture as "sterile, flexible strand prepared from collagen derived from healthy mammals, or from a synthetic polymer...." It is capable of being absorbed by living mammalian tissue but may be treated to modify its resistance to absorption. It may be modified with respect to body or texture. It may be impregnated with a

---

BOX 7-1

Characteristics of Suture Material

Physical Characteristics
- Physical configuration
- Capillarity
- Fluid absorption ability
- Diameter (caliber; also referred to as size)
- Tensile strength
- Knot strength
- Elasticity
- Plasticity
- Memory

Handling Characteristics
- Pliability
- Tissue drag (related to the coefficient of friction)
- Knot tying (related to the coefficient of friction)
- Knot slippage (related to the coefficient of friction)

Tissue-Reaction Characteristics
- Inflammatory and fibrous cell reaction
- Absorption
- Potentiation of infection
- Allergic reaction

Modified from *Ethicon wound closure manual*, available at http://academic departments.musc.edu/surgery/education/resident_info/supplement/suture_manuals/ethicon_wound_closure_manual.pdf. Accessed March 10, 2013.

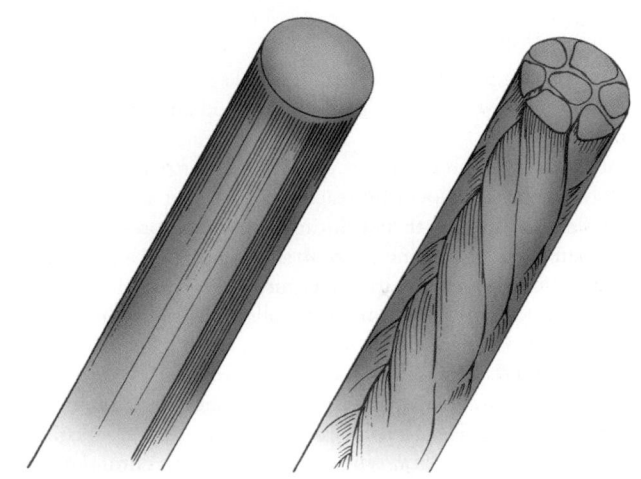

FIGURE 7-1 *Left*, Monofilament suture; *right*, multifilament (braided) suture.

TABLE 7-1

Relative Straight-Pull Tensile Strength of Suture Materials

	Greatest → Least				
Nonabsorbable	Steel	Polyester (Mersilene)	Nylon (monofilamentous)	Nylon (braided)	Polypropylene (Prolene)	Silk
Absorbable	Polyglycolic		Polyglactin 910 (Vicryl)		Polydioxanone (PDS)	Poliglecaprone (Monocryl)	Catgut

Modified from *Ethicon wound closure manual*, available at http://academicdepartments.musc.edu/surgery/education/resident_info/supplement/suture_manuals/ethicon_wound_closure_manual.pdf. Accessed March 10, 2013.

TABLE 7-2

Relative Tissue Reactivity to Sutures

	Greatest → Least			
Nonabsorbable	Silk, cotton	Polyester coated	Polyester uncoated	Nylon	Polypropylene (Prolene)
Absorbable	Catgut	Polyglactin 910 (Vicryl)	Polyglycolic acid	Poliglecaprone (Monocryl)	

Modified from *Ethicon wound closure manual*, available at http://academicdepartments.musc.edu/surgery/education/resident_info/supplement/suture_manuals/ethicon_wound_closure_manual.pdf. Accessed March 10, 2013.

TABLE 7-3

Comparison of Absorbable Sutures

Ethicon	Covidien	Configuration	Tensile Strength	Absorption Rate
Surgical gut (plain)	Plain gut	Twisted	0% at 2-3 wk	Unpredictable (12 wk)
Surgical gut (chromic)	Chromic gut	Twisted	0% at 2-3 wk	Unpredictable (12 wk)
Polyglactin 910 (Vicryl Rapide)		Braided	0% at 14 days	Complete at 42 days
Poliglecaprone (Monocryl)		Monofilament	20%-30% at 2 wk	Complete in 91-119 days
	Polyglycolic acid (Dexon S)	Braided or monofilament	20% at 3 wk	Complete in 60-90 days
	Polyester (Polysorb)	Braided	30% at 3 wk	Complete in 56-70 days
	Polycaprolate (Dexon II)	Braided	35% at 3 wk	Complete in 60-90 days
	Polydioxanone (Biosyn)	Monofilament	40% at 3 wk	Complete in 90-110 days
Polyglactin (Vicryl 910)		Braided or monofilament	50% at 3 wk	Complete in 56-70 days
Polydioxanone (PDS)		Monofilament	60% at 3 wk	Complete within 6 mo
	Polyglyconate (Maxon)	Monofilament	Excellent until 6 wk	Complete within 6 mo

Modified from *Ethicon wound closure manual*, available at http://academicdepartments.musc.edu/surgery/education/resident_info/supplement/suture_manuals/ethicon_wound_closure_manual.pdf. Accessed, March 10 2013; *Covidien suture catalog*, available at www.covidien.com/campaigns/pagebuilder.aspx?topicID=181589&page=SPC:Main. Accessed March 10, 2013.

suitable coating, softening, or antimicrobial agent. It may be colored by a color additive approved by the U.S. Food and Drug Administration (FDA).

Absorbable sutures can be digested (by enzyme activity) or hydrolyzed (broken down by reaction with water in tissue fluids) and assimilated by the tissues during the healing process. Absorbable sutures vary in treatment, color, size, packaging, and resistance to absorption, according to their purpose. Types of absorbable suture include plain or chromic surgical gut, collagen, and glycolic acid polymers (Table 7-3).

Surgical Gut. Surgical gut is obtained from the collagen of the submucosal layer of the small intestine of sheep or the intestinal serosa of cattle or hogs. The processed strands or ribbons of collagen are either untreated (plain, type A) or treated with chromium salts (chromic, type C).

Chromatization delays absorption of the suture in living mammalian tissue. The strength of the chromium salt content and the duration of the chromatizing process are accurately controlled and tested. Proper chromatizing of gut ensures the integrity of the suture and maintenance of its strength during the early stages of wound healing. It enables a wound with slow healing power to heal sufficiently before the suture is entirely absorbed.

The elaborate processes of mechanical and chemical cleaning of the raw gut are followed by sterilization, usually with ionizing radiation, and storage in hermetically sealed packages. Modern manufacturing processes also ensure tensile strength, more controlled absorption, and more predictable results.

Absorption occurs by digestion of the gut by tissue enzymes. The absorption rate of surgical gut is influenced by the type of body tissue it contacts and, to some extent, by the patient's general physical condition. Studies also show that surgical gut is absorbed faster in serous or mucous membranes than in muscular tissues. When fine chromic gut is properly buried in successive layers of the gastrointestinal tract, it retains its strength long enough for primary union to take place.

Surgical gut suture is wet-packaged in an alcohol solution to provide maximal pliability and should be used immediately after removal from the packet. When a gut suture is removed from its packet and is not used at once, the alcohol evaporates, which causes the strand to lose its pliability. If required, the strand's pliability may be restored just before use by immersing it in sterile water or normal saline solution, preferably at body temperature, for only a few seconds. This immersion is recommended only for eye sutures; in other areas, tissue fluids moisten the gut sufficiently as it passes through the tissue when the surgeon sews. Excessive moisture reduces tensile strength.

Collagen Sutures. Collagen sutures are derived from cattle tendons. They are chemically treated to remove noncollagenous material, purified, and processed into strands that have physical properties superior to those of surgical gut. Collagen suture is used most often as a fine suture material for the eye.

Synthetic Absorbable Sutures. To produce synthetic absorbable sutures, specific polymers are extruded into suture strands. The base material for synthetic absorbable sutures is a combination of lactic acid and glycolic acid polymers (Vicryl, Dexon, and Polysorb). The molecular structure of these products has a tensile strength sufficient for approximation of tissues for 2 to 3 weeks, followed by rapid absorption.

Other synthetic polymers (PDS, Maxon, and Monocryl) provide wound support for longer periods (3 months). They are used when prolonged support for wound healing is desired, as with fascial closure or for elderly or oncology patients. They combine the desirable qualities of extended wound support and eventual absorbability.

An additional type of synthetic absorbable suture approved by the FDA is MonoMax. Recombinant deoxyribonucleic acid (DNA) technology is used to produce this poly-4-hydroxybutyrate suture. This suture has a high degree of flexibility and maneuverability, but may have limitations for use in patients who are allergic to the cells or the growth medium used for its production. The suture is not indicated for use in cardiovascular or neurologic tissues or for microsurgery or ophthalmic surgery. It has been used in laparotomy closure (Research Highlight).

Synthetic absorbable sutures are absorbed by slow hydrolysis in the presence of tissue fluids. Hydrolysis is the chemical process whereby the polymer reacts with water to cause an alteration of breakdown of the molecular structure. These sutures are degraded in tissue by this process at a more predictable rate than surgical gut (or collagen) and with less tissue reaction. These sutures are dry-packaged in sizes 10-0 to #3. They should not be dipped in solutions because moisture reduces their tensile strength. Some polymers have additional coatings to reduce drag in tissue.

RESEARCH HIGHLIGHT

Evaluation of Bioengineered Ultra–Long-Term Absorbable Suture in Abdominal Wall Closure

Abdominal wounds are particularly vulnerable to complications such as dehiscence and infection in the short term and hernia formation in the longer term. Different techniques and sutures have been developed to provide closure of abdominal wounds with the goal of preventing complications. Slowly absorbable suture is often used in abdominal wound closure because research has found it to be superior to nonabsorbable suture in preventing incisional hernias. Absorbable sutures must be capable of supporting tissue layers through the critical healing process until the wound is able to withstand normal stress. The tensile strength of the suture should never exceed the tensile strength of the tissue. As the wound heals, the relative loss of suture strength over time should be slower than the gain of tissue tensile strength.

This study sought to evaluate the use of a poly-4-hydroxybutyrate suture (P4HB) for abdominal wound closure. P4HB is a synthetic suture that uses a genetically engineered *Escherichia coli* K12 microorganism that incorporates new biosynthetic pathways to produce the homopolymer. It is an ultra–long-term absorbable monofilament suture material with high elasticity and flexibility, high knot tensile strength retention, and long-lasting linear tensile strength.

The study was a single-arm multicenter prospective study comparing MonoMax (P4HB) suture for abdominal wound closure against PDS (polydioxanone) and MonoPlus (polydioxanone) suture closure used in a previous study (Seiler et al, 2009) as historical controls. All sutures had similar tensile and knot pull strength, but degradation rates and mass absorption rates for P4HB suture versus the polydioxanone sutures differed significantly (e.g., 100 days for degradation for P4HB suture versus 42 and 35 days for the polydioxanone sutures and 390 days for absorption for P4HB suture versus 180 to 210 days for the polydioxanone sutures).

Researchers hypothesized that the combined frequency of wound infection and reoperation due to dehiscence would be equal to or lower in their study compared with the control group study (Seiler et al, 2009). They also evaluated the incidence of incisional hernias 12 ±1 months after surgery, the length of postoperative stay, wound infection rate, and complicated wound healing. There were 140 patients in the control group and 150 patients in the study group.

Results showed that 11 patients in the study group using the P4HB (MonoMax) suture experienced wound dehiscence or infection compared to 16 patients in the control group using polydioxanone (PDS and MonoPlus) suture. The length of stay was comparable for both groups. Follow-up 1 year later observed incisional hernias in 21 of the study patients treated with P4HB compared with 30 patients in the control group who were treated with polydioxanone. Researchers concluded that the P4HB suture was effective but recommend additional studies using the randomized controlled trial methodology to better evaluate and validate effectiveness.

Modified from Albertsmeier M et al: Evaluation of the safety and efficacy of MonoMax suture material for abdominal wall closure after primary midline laparotomy—a controlled prospective multicentre trial: ISSAAC [NCT005725079], *Langenbecks Arch Surg* 397: (3):363–371, 2012; Odermatt EK et al: MonoMax suture: a new long-term absorbable monofilament suture made from poly-4-hydroxybutyrate, *Int J Polym Sci*, 2012, available at www.hindawi.com/journals/ijps/2012/216137/cta/. Accessed March 12, 2013; Seiler CM et al: Interrupted or continuous slowly absorbable sutures for closure of primary elective midline abdominal incisions: a multicenter randomized trial (INSECT: ISRCTN24023541), *Ann Surg* 249:576–582, 2009.

Nonabsorbable Sutures. Nonabsorbable sutures are strands of material that effectively resist enzymatic digestion in living animal tissue. The USP classifies nonabsorbable surgical suture as follows:

- *Class I* suture is composed of silk or synthetic fibers of monofilament, with a twisted or braided construction.
- *Class II* suture is composed of cotton or linen fibers or coated natural or synthetic fibers, in which the coating significantly affects thickness but does not contribute significantly to strength.
- *Class III* suture is composed of monofilament or multifilament metal wire.

The strand of suture material may be uncoated or coated with a substance to reduce capillarity and friction when passing through the tissue. Several products are used for coating, including silicone, polytef (Teflon), and various polymers. Fibers may be uncolored, naturally colored, or impregnated with a suitable dye.

Nonabsorbable suture material is encapsulated or walled off by the tissues around it during the process of wound healing. Skin sutures, for which nonabsorbable materials are often the choice, are removed before healing is complete. The most common nonabsorbable suture materials are silk, nylon, polyester fiber, polypropylene, and stainless steel wire (Table 7-4).

Silk. Silk is prepared from thread spun by the silkworm larva while making its cocoon. Top-grade raw silk is (1) processed to remove natural waxes and gum, (2) manufactured into threads, and (3) colored with a vegetable dye. The strands of silk are twisted or braided to form the suture, which gives it high tensile strength and better handling qualities. Silk handles well, is soft, and forms secure knots.

Because of the capillarity of untreated silk, body fluid may transmit infection along the length of the suture strand. For this reason surgical silk is treated to eliminate its capillarity properties (able to resist the absorption of body fluids and moisture). It is available in sizes 9-0 to #5, in sterile packets or precut lengths, and with or without attached needles. Silk should be kept dry. Wet silk loses 20% of its original strength. Silk is not a true nonabsorbable material. When buried in tissue, it loses its tensile strength after about 1 year and may disappear after several years.

Cotton. Surgical cotton sutures are made from individual cotton fibers that are combed, aligned, and twisted to form a finished strand. Because new types of fibers have been introduced, cotton suture is rarely used. Some companies no longer manufacture it.

Umbilical tape, although not used for suturing, is produced by suture manufacturers and packaged in the same way as suture. It consists of long woven ribbons of cotton, $\frac{1}{16}$ to $\frac{1}{8}$ inch wide, and is used for retraction or suspension of small structures and vessels. (Other soft, pliant products, such as vessel loops, are available and more commonly used for this purpose.)

Nylon. Surgical nylon (Dermalon, Ethilon, Surgilon, Nurolon, Bralon, Monosof) is a synthetic polyamide material. It is available in two forms: multifilament (braided) and monofilament strands. Multifilament nylon is relatively inert in tissues and has a high tensile strength. It is used in conditions similar to those in which silk and cotton are used. Monofilament nylon is a smooth material that is particularly well suited for closing skin edges and for tension sutures. Because of its poor knot security, the surgeon usually ties three knots in small sutures and a double square knot in large sutures. It is used frequently in ophthalmology and microsurgery because it can be manufactured in fine sizes. Size 11-0 nylon is one of the smallest suture materials available.

Polyester Fiber. Surgical polyester fiber (polyethylene terephthalate, polyester/Dacron) is available in two forms: an untreated

TABLE 7-4

Comparison of Nonabsorbable Suture

Sutures	Materials	Construction
Pronova Poly	Polymer blend of poly (vinylidene fluoride) and poly (vinylidene fluoride-co-hexafluoropolypropylene)	Monofilament
Ethibond Excel polyester	Polyester/Dacron	Braided
Mersilene polyester suture	Polyester/Dacron	Braided
Ethilon nylon suture	Nylon 6	Monofilament
Nurolon suture	Nylon 6	Braided
Permahand silk suture	Silk	Braided
Prolene polypropylene suture	Polypropylene	Monofilament
Surgical stainless steel suture	316L stainless steel	Monofilament
Vascufil	Butylenes terephthalate and polyteramethylene ether glycol	Monofilament
TiCron	Polyethylene terephthalate	Braided
Monosof	Nylon 6 and nylon 6.6	Monofilament
Dermalon		
Surgilon	Nylon 6.6	Braided
Silk	Silk	Braided
Surgipro II	Polypropylene	Monofilament
Surgipro		
Steel	316L stainless steel	Stainless steel

Modified from *Ethicon product catalog, suture/adhesives, drains, hernia repair*, 2009, available at www.akinglobal.com.tr/medikal/tr/dokumanlar/JHONSON&JHONSON/SUTURES.pdf. Accessed March 10, 2013; *Covidien suture catalog* 2013, available at www.covidien.com/campaigns/pagebuilder.aspx?topicID=181589&page=SPC:Main. Accessed March 10, 2013.

polyester fiber suture and a polyester fiber suture that has been specifically coated or impregnated with a lubricant to allow smooth passage through the tissue. Polyester fiber is available in fine filaments that can be braided into various suture sizes to provide good handling properties.

Polybutester (Novafil) is a special type of polyester suture that possesses many of the advantages of polyester and polypropylene. Because it is a monofilament, it induces little tissue reaction.

Polyester material has many advantages over other braided, nonabsorbable sutures. It has greater tensile strength, minimal tissue reaction, and maximal visibility and does not absorb tissue fluids. It is used frequently as a general-closure fascia suture and in cardiovascular surgery for valve replacements, graft-to-tissue anastomoses, and revascularization procedures.

Polypropylene. Polypropylene is a clear or pigmented polymer. This monofilament suture material (Prolene, Surgilene, Surgipro, Dermalene) is used for cardiovascular, general, and plastic surgery. Because polypropylene is a monofilament and is extremely inert in tissue, it may be used in the presence of infection. It has high tensile strength and causes minimal tissue reaction. Sizes range from 10-0 to #2.

Stainless Steel. Surgical stainless steel is formulated to be compatible with stainless steel implants and prostheses. This formula, 316L (L for "low carbon"), ensures absence of toxic elements, optimal strength, flexibility, and uniform size. Monofilament and multifilament surgical stainless steel sutures are known for their strength, inert properties, and low tissue reaction. Stainless steel suturing technique is very exacting, however. Steel can pull or tear out of tissue, and necrosis can result from a suture that is too tight. Barbs on the end of steel can traumatize surrounding tissue or tear gloves. Torn or cut gloves fail to provide an adequate and effective barrier for the patient or the surgeon and assistant and can remain undetected. Kinks in the wire can render it practically useless. For this reason, packaging has played an important part in the

TABLE 7-5

Steel Suture Comparison

Size (USP)	B&S Gauge	Size (USP)	B&S Gauge
6-0	40	0	26
6-0	38	1	25
5-0	35	2	24
4-0	34	3	23
4-0	32	4	22
000	30	5	20
00	28	7	18

B&S, Brown and Sharp; *USP*, United States Pharmacopeia.

development of surgical stainless steel sutures. Surgical stainless steel is available in packets on spools or in packages of straight, precut, sterile lengths, with or without attached needles. This packaging affords protection to the strands and delivery in straight, unkinked lengths.

Before surgical stainless steel was available from suture manufacturers, it was purchased by weight with the Brown and Sharp (B&S) scale for diameter variations. Today the B&S gauge, along with USP size classifications, is used to distinguish diameter ranges. Table 7-5 compares steel suture sizes.

Barbed Suture. Barbed suture is a lesser known suture type. The suture has many small barbs cut into its monofilament core along its length, and is available in several absorbable and nonabsorbable polymers, including polydioxanone, PGA-PCL, and polypropylene. The barbs ensure that the suture stays in place and approximates the tissue without the need to tie knots, ensuring even distribution wound tension and decreased closure time. It is used extensively in plastic surgery and also has applications in other specialties as well such as orthopedics and general surgery (Lombardi et al, 2011) (Figure 7-2). If the suture breaks during suturing, the surgeon leaves it in place and begins again rather than removing it to prevent tissue damage.

Surgical Needles

Surgical needles vary in shape, size, point design, and wire diameter (Figure 7-3). Needle selection is determined by the type of tissue, suture material, and action to be performed. Surgical needles are made from stainless steel or carbon steel. Various metal alloys used in manufacturing surgical needles determine their basic characteristics. They must be strong, ductile, and able to withstand the stress imposed by tough tissue. Stainless steel is the most popular, not only because it provides these physical characteristics, but also because it is noncorrosive. The three basic parts of a surgical needle are the *eye,* the *body,* and the *point* or *tip*.

Eye

The eye of the surgical needle falls into the following three general categories:

1. Eyed needles, in which the needle must be threaded with the suture strand, and two strands of suture must be pulled through the tissue (Figure 7-4, *A*)
2. Spring, or French, eyed needles, in which the suture is placed or snapped through the spring (see Figure 7-4, *B*)
3. Eyeless needles, a needle-suture combination in which a needle is swaged (permanently attached) onto one or both ends of the suture material (see Figure 7-4, *C*)

The use of eyed needles has all but been eliminated in current surgical practice. The swaged needle is universally available and the preferred method of suture application. The swaged suture is a single strand of suture material that when drawn through the tissue is less traumatic to the tissue than is an eyed needle and suture. The swaged needle may need to be cut off with suture scissors or swaged for controlled release of the suture (semi-swaged), commonly referred to as a "pop off." With semi-swaged suture, the needle remains attached until the surgeon releases it with a straight tug of the needle holder.

Body

The body, or shaft, of the needle may be round, triangular, or flattened. Surgical needles also may be straight or curved; the curve is described as part of an imaginary circle (see Figure 7-3). As the radius of the imaginary circle increases, the size of the needle also increases. The body of a round needle gradually tapers to a point.

Point

Taper needles, which are round with a point, are the most common needles used and are provided as swaged sutures in many sizes for both absorbable and nonabsorbable materials. Blunt needles are generally indicated for organ biopsy or repair and very delicate tissue that may be torn or injured when penetrated by a sharp

FIGURE 7-2 Barbed suture.

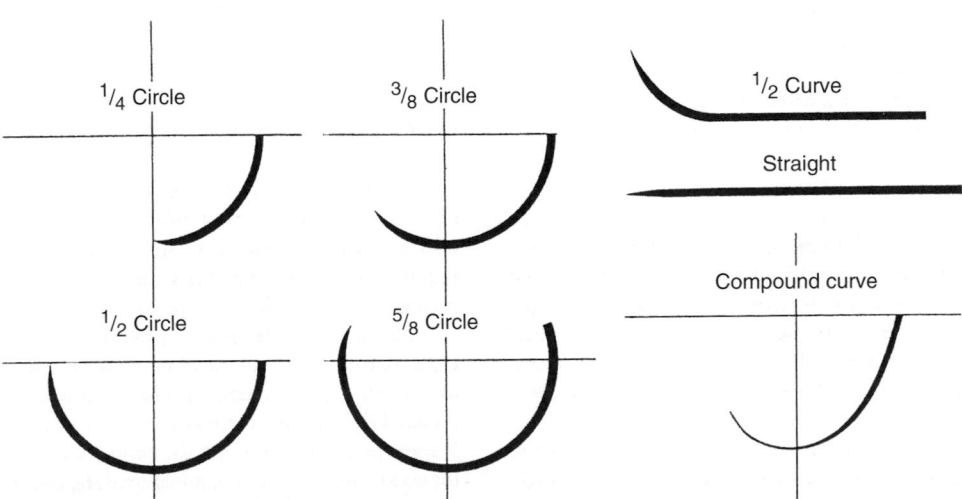

FIGURE 7-3 Surgical needles vary in shape, size, type of point and body, and how the suture is attached.

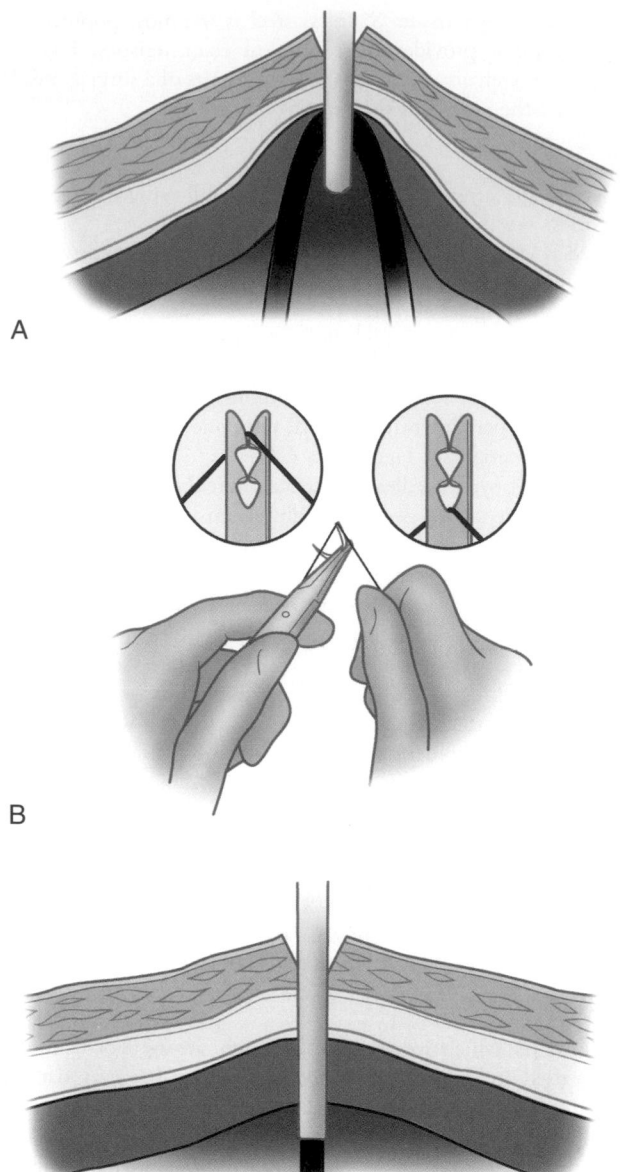

FIGURE 7-4 Types of needles. **A,** Eyed needle. Greater tissue trauma is caused by the double suture strand threaded through eyed needles. **B,** Spring eye. Holding suture strand taut with left hand, bring strand down over top and spring into eye. **C,** Atraumatic (eyeless) needle causes minimal tissue trauma by eliminating the double suture strand.

needle. The cutting needle, which is round with sharp triangular edges at the objective end of the needle, is most often used for dense or tough tissues such skin closure, thick scar, or bone (Table 7-6).

Available blunt protect-point needles have been recommended as an alternative to taper point needles. Interest in blunt needles has evolved because of the risk of bloodborne exposure from percutaneous injuries (PIs).

The use of blunt needles represents a key strategy to reduce risk to the surgical team. Blunt needles are associated with a statistically significant reduction in PIs and can be substituted for conventional curved needles in a variety of surgical procedures.

Triangular needles have cutting edges along three sides. The cutting action may be conventional or reverse. The cutting edge of the conventional cutting needle is directed along the inner curve of the needle, facing the wound edge when suturing is performed.

The reverse cutting needle is preferred for cutaneous suturing. When it transects the skin lateral to the wound, the outside cutting edge is pointed away from the wound edge, and the inside flat edge is parallel to the edge of the wound. This cutting action reduces the tendency for suture to tear through tissue.

For certain types of delicate surgery, needles with exceptionally sharp points and cutting edges are used. Microsurgery, ophthalmic surgery, and plastic surgery require needles of this type; special honing wheels provide needles of precision-point quality for surgery in these specialties. In some instances the application of a microthin layer of plastic to the needle surface provides for easier penetration and reduces drag of the needle through tissue.

Suture Packaging, Storage, and Selection

Types of Packaging

For packaging, the suture material is sealed in a primary inner packet, which may or may not contain fluid; placed inside a dry outer peel-back packet; and sterilized. This method permits easy dispensing onto the sterile field. Various forms of foil, plastic, and special paper are used for the inner and outer packets.

Each primary suture packet is self-contained, and its sterility for each patient is ensured as long as the integrity of the packet is maintained. Some suture packets have expiration dates that relate to stability and sterility. Packages should be stored in moisture-proof and dust-proof containers in units of one size and type.

Suture without needles are packaged as multiple strands and in reels for delivery as free ties. Suture with swaged needles can be packaged as single stitches or as multipacks containing several of the same sutures commonly used for the planned procedure. Multipacks may be permanently swaged needles that require being cut for tying or control-release (pop-off) for easy needle detachment. Some sutures may be double-armed, with a needle at each end of the strand. Double-armed sutures are most commonly used for vascular procedures such as anastomoses and vessel repairs.

Color Codes. Color-coded packaging based on suture fiber is used by most companies to make identification quicker and easier. Each individual packet is color-coded, as is the dispenser box. Although most color codes are universal across companies, there are some exceptions. Ethibond, a coated polyester, is coded orange, whereas most polyesters are coded in shades of green. Dexon, a glycolic acid polymer, is gold, whereas Vicryl, a comparable polymer, is violet.

Suture Selection

The choice of suture material, size, needle, and type depends on the procedure, the tissue being sutured and type of reapproximation required by the general condition of the patient, and the surgeon's preferences. A surgical services committee or project team may be responsible for establishing standard suture uses for various operations. Current guides published by suture manufacturers should be consulted. These guides list the specific suture materials recommended for various wounds and are based on current clinical practice and research. Although the perioperative nurse is not responsible for choosing the suture material used, he or she must be knowledgeable of the suture properties to ensure the best possible outcome for the surgical patient.

TABLE 7-6

Atraumatic Needles

Needle Type	Description of Body	Use
Taper point	Round shaft, straight or curved, taper point, no cutting edge	Soft tissue closure, such as gastrointestinal, fascial, vascular, and most soft tissues below skin surface
Penetrating point	Taper body with finely sharpened point; optimal penetration with less tissue wound	Ligaments, tendons, and calcified, fibrous, and cuticular tissue; mostly used for vascular, thoracic, plastic, obstetrics/gynecology, and orthopedic surgery; excellent penetration through synthetic grafts and scar tissue during repeat surgeries
Blunt point	Taper body with rounded point, no cutting edge	Friable tissue, fascia, liver, intestine, kidney, muscle, uterine cervix (note recommendations regarding use of blunt needles, p. 192)
Protect-point	Taper body with blunted point, no cutting edge	Primarily in fascia and mass closure to minimize potential of needlesticks
Reverse cutting	Triangular point with cutting edge on outer curvature	Skin closure; retention sutures; subcutaneous, ligamentous, or fibrous tissues
Cutting taper	Reverse-cutting tip with taper shaft	In microsurgery for excellent penetration through tough tissue, such as vasovasostomy, tuboplasty
Hand-honed reverse cutting	Same as reverse cutting but hand-honed for added sharpness	Primarily in plastic surgery for delicate work and where good cosmetic result is priority
Spatula side cutting	Two cutting edges in horizontal plane	Ophthalmic surgery for muscle and retinal repair; also for delicate eyelid or plastic surgery; cutting edges "ride" along scleral layers
Regular cutting	Triangular point with cutting edge on outer curvature	General skin closure, subcutaneous tissue; sometimes for ophthalmic surgery, plastic, or reconstructive surgery
Lancet, inverted lancet	Spatula needle with cutting edge (lancet) or outer (inverted lancet) curvature	Ophthalmic surgery and microsurgery

Modified from *Ethicon product catalog, suture/adhesives, drains, hernia repair*, 2009, Available at www.akinglobal.com.tr/medikal/tr/dokumanlar/JHONSON&JHONSON/SUTURES.pdf. Accessed March 10, 2013.

FIGURE 7-5 Primary suture line on the abdominal wall, midline incision.

Suturing Techniques/Wound Closures

Surgeons may use suture or other devices to accomplish wound closure. The *primary suture line* refers to sutures that obliterate dead space, prevent serum from accumulating in the wound, and hold the wound edges in approximation until healing takes place (Figure 7-5).

The *secondary suture line* refers to sutures that supplement the primary suture line. They are placed on each side of the primary suture line, passing through several layers of tissue at once. A secondary suture line helps eliminate tension on the primary sutures and reduces the risk of evisceration or dehiscence. Retention sutures are a type of secondary suture line.

An *interrupted suture* is inserted into tissues or vessels in such a way that each stitch is placed and tied individually. This type of suture is widely used and generally considered the strongest and most secure (Figure 7-6, *A*). Although wound closure with interrupted technique is more time consuming, it is intended to distribute stress uniformly along the incision/wound as well as improve strength and encourage better healing. Interrupted closure should be considered when significant preoperative wound healing comorbidities exist, such as COPD, diabetes, infection, and steroid dependence. The interrupted technique is routinely used for bowel and vascular anastomoses and vascular repairs.

A *continuous suture* consists of a series of stitches, of which only the first and last are tied (see Figure 7-6, *B*). With this type of suture, a break at any point may mean a disruption of the entire suture line. It is used to close tissue layers where there is little tension but tight closure is required, such as the peritoneum, to prevent the intestinal loops from protruding, or on blood vessels to prevent leakage.

Retention (or *stay*) sutures are placed at a distance from the primary suture line to provide a secondary suture line (see Figure 7-6, *C*), relieve undue strain, and help obliterate dead space.

These sutures are placed in such a way that they include most if not all layers of the wound. A simple interrupted or figure-of-eight stitch is used. Usually heavy, nonabsorbable suture materials, such as silk, nylon, polyester fiber, or wire, are used to close long, vertical abdominal wounds and lacerated or infected wounds. To prevent the suture from cutting into the skin surface, a small piece of rubber tubing (bumper, bolster, bootie) or other type of device (bridge, button) is passed over or through the exposed portion of the suture. The bridge device allows the surgeon to adjust tension over the wound postoperatively.

Subcuticular sutures, sometimes referred to as *buried*, are sutures placed completely under the epidermal layer of the skin (see Figure 7-6 *D*). This technique is often used to achieve a cosmetic closure.

FIGURE 7-7 Straightening the suture material.

FIGURE 7-6 Types of stitches. **A,** Interrupted. Each stitch is made with a separate piece of suture material, which is tied separately. **B,** Continuous or "running." A stitch is made with one uninterrupted length of suture material. **C,** Retention. Stitches are used to reinforce the primary suture line; heavy, strong suture material is used. **D,** Subcuticular. Stitch is placed completely under the epidermal layer of the skin. **E,** Purse-string. A stitch runs parallel to the edge and encircles a circular wound.

A *purse-string suture* is a continuous circular suture placed to surround an opening in a structure and cause it to close (see Figure 7-6, *E*). This type of suture may be placed around the appendix before its removal, or it may be used in an organ such as the cecum, gallbladder, or urinary bladder before it is opened so that a drainage tube can be inserted; then the purse-string suture is tightened around the tube. It may also be used in plastic surgery for periareolar reduction.

The Nursing Interventions Classification (NIC) lists suturing as a nursing intervention, defined as "approximating edges of a wound using sterile suture material and a needle" (Bulechek et al, 2013). The NIC was developed to classify nursing interventions so that the work of nursing could be documented and nursing knowledge improved through the evaluation of patient outcomes. In perioperative nursing practice, the act of suturing is considered part of the education and subsequent role of the registered nurse first assistant (AORN, 2012).

General Considerations

In the preparation and use of sutures in surgery, every precaution must be taken to keep the sutures sterile, to prevent prolonged exposure and unnecessary handling, and to avoid waste. Before perioperative personnel prepare any suture materials, they should review the sutures listed on the physician's preference card or in the computerized data/preference sheets. Care should be taken to ensure fiscal responsibility by minimizing the number of sutures on the field when the initial count is performed. The perioperative nurse should have an adequate supply of sutures available for immediate dispensing to the sterile instrument table as needed throughout the procedure.

Customized suture kits that contain a designated number and variety of sutures for particular procedures, surgeons, or both are available for use when suture preferences are consistently the same. These kits may be more economical than individually packaged sutures because of reduced packaging costs, decreased gathering and dispensing times, and less capital outlay for inventory.

Opening Primary Packets

The scrub person tears the foil packet across the notch near the hermetically sealed edge and removes the suture. Some sutures may be packaged for delivery to the field in their inner folders, ready to load, with no foil wrapper.

Handling Suture Materials

To remove suture strands to be used for ties when they are not on a reel or disk, the user pulls the loose end out with one hand while grasping the folder with the other hand. To straighten a long suture, the free end is grasped (using the thumb and forefinger of the free hand) and the kinks, caused by package memory, are removed by gentle pulling with the free ends secured, one in each hand, and then the arms are slowly abducted to straighten the strands (Figure 7-7).

The scrub person should never remove kinks from suture by running gloved fingers over the strand because this action causes fraying. The tensile strength of a gut suture should not be tested before it is handed to the surgeon. Sudden pulls or jerks may damage the suture so that it will break when in use.

To remove a suture-needle combination from the package, the scrub person grasps the needle with a needle holder and gently pulls (Figure 7-8). To straighten the suture in a suture-needle combination, the scrub person grasps the suture 1 to 2 inches distal to the needle and pulls gently on the other end of the strand with the other hand to remove kinks. The jaws of the needle holder grasp the flattened surface of the needle to prevent breakage and bending.

To facilitate suturing, the needle is secured about $\frac{1}{8}$ inch distal from the tip of the needle holder (Figure 7-9). The holder is placed on the needle about one third of the distance distal from the eye or swaged end.

A suture or free ligature should not be too long or too short. A long suture is difficult to handle and increases the possibility of contamination because it may be dragged across the sterile field or

FIGURE 7-8 Loading a suture directly from packet.

FIGURE 7-9 Loading a needle holder. Clamp needle holder approximately one third the distance from the swaged end or eye to point of needle.

fall below it. A short suture makes tying difficult. The depth and distance to the site of tying or suturing guide the scrub person in preparing ties or sutures of the correct length.

For general surgery, a continuous suture swaged on a needle is usually about 24 inches long, and its short end is 3 to 4 inches long (half lengths). An interrupted suture is 12 to 14 inches long, with 2 or 3 inches threaded through the needle (quarter lengths). To ligate a vessel in the epidermal and subcutaneous layers, the ligature may be quarter lengths. Vessels or structures deep in the wound are ligated with a suture or ligature that is 24 to 30 inches long (third lengths to half lengths). Sutures also are provided in 12- to 60-inch precut lengths by the manufacturer. Also supplied are the more commonly used 54-inch lengths on reels or disks and labyrinth packs, where precut strands may be removed one at a time from the package rather than all at once.

Threading Surgical Needles

Free needles, packaged separately, must be threaded by the scrub person. A curved needle is threaded from within its curvature so that the short end falls away from the outside curvature (Figure 7-10). This practice helps to prevent accidental pullout. The scrub person pulls the suture about 4 inches through the eye of the needle to prevent the suture from being pulled out of the eye during suturing.

Knot-Tying Techniques

The successful use of the many varieties of suture materials depends, in final analysis, on the skill with which the surgeon or first assistant ties the knot. The completed knot should be firm to prevent

FIGURE 7-10 Eyed needle is threaded from inside curvature, taking care to avoid pricking glove on sharp needle point.

slipping and should be small, with ends cut short, to minimize the bulk of suture material in the wound. The suture may be weakened by inappropriate handling (Research Highlight). Excessive tension, sawing, friction between the strands, and inadvertent crushing with clamps or hemostats should be avoided.

Endoscopic Suturing/Minimally Invasive/Robotic Surgical Knot Tying. Suturing through an endoscope is a learned skill, not an innate talent. An array of needles and suture materials are available for endoscopic suturing, and research and development of techniques, instruments, needles, and suture materials continue to evolve as the types of procedures done endoscopically, minimally invasive, and robotically assisted increase and methods are perfected. Knot tying is one of the most challenging aspects of endoscopic surgery. Preformed ligature loops are used in ligating the appendix or blood vessels. Extracorporeal knots are tied outside the abdomen and slid into the abdomen using a knot pusher. They can be tied rapidly and securely; the square knot is commonly tied with braided suture and slip, or granny knot, is tied when monofilament suture is used. Intracorporeal knotting is done completely within the abdominal cavity whenever fine sutures are being placed in tissues for reconstruction purposes. When the intracorporeal method is required, the suture is generally precut to a significantly shorter length permitting adequate view and easy access of the suture ends for tying. All suturing and knot-tying techniques performed through the endoscope require excellent hand-eye coordination, practice, and the ability to perform these techniques while the operative site is being viewed on a television monitor. Competency in performing surgical tasks that require the surgeon or surgical assistant perform tasks originating from a three-dimensional (3-D) visual field (extracorporeal) to a two-dimensional (2-D) visual field (intracorporeal via monitor) requires practice, preparation, and focus. Robotic surgical procedures are exceptional examples of these skills. The surgeon performs much of the surgery from a computer console (Figure 7-11) that provides a 3-D visual field, which is possible through the innovation of the bi-ocular telescope. The console also provides the surgeon with control of the robotic instruments and enables him or her to manipulate, dissect, and suture tissue in a similar manner as done in an open surgical procedure. The endoscopic instrumentation is designed to mimic the motion of the human wrist, with 90 degrees of articulation, fingertip control, and intuitive motion. The scrubbed surgical assistant views from a 2-D monitor and performs extracorporeal tasks such as passing suture and implants and using the knot pusher for placing and setting intracorporeal knots.

Skin Staples. Skin staples are one of the most frequently chosen methods of skin closure and can be used on many types of surgical

RESEARCH HIGHLIGHT

Surgical Knot Tensile Strength

Many factors influence the strength of a surgical knot, including suture type, gauge, and the techniques used to tie it. The ability to tie a strong knot is a critical skill for medical personnel because loosening of a surgical knot before or after completion could compromise the intended outcome.

Square knots are the most commonly used in surgery because they are more secure when a risk of the knot tearing through tissue is present. The term "throw" is used in conjunction with knot tying and refers to the action of making a loop and passing it (as if throwing a lariat) around an object to begin a knot. Ching and colleagues sought to evaluate a small group of surgical trainees' knot-tying techniques to determine the knot security.

In the study, 25 participants with up to 5 years of surgical experience, tied 40 knots each, using polyglactin 910 and polypropylene suture. They tied knots in four different series: 4 knots as they would normally in surgery, 4 knots with three throws, 4 knots with 5 throws, and 4 knots with 6 throws. Knots were tied over a metal rod with a smooth surface. The rod was removed from its holder at the end of each series and the knots were collected.

Each knot was visually inspected and then photographed with a digital microscope to determine the knot type (e.g., square knot or slip knot). Slip knots were defined as knots in which the throws were formed in alternating fashion causing one strand within the knot being straight. All knots were then measured with a tensiometer.

Tensile strength was defined as the force required to cause knot failure by slippage or breakage. Each of the 1000 knots tied in the study were tested for type and tensile strength. The rate of knots slipping and untying were greater in slip knots than in square knots, and the overall rate of knot strength was greater in square knots than in slip knots. The overall rate of slippage decreased if the number of throws were increased for both suture types. When square knots and slip knots were evaluated separately the researchers found that the polyglactin 910 had the greatest tensile strength at 4-throw square knots and that the polypropylene had the greatest tensile strength at 6-throw square knots.

Researchers considered 63 out 500 of the polyglactin 910 knots and 28 out of 500 polypropylene knots dangerous in that they could slip or break (all dangerous knots were slip knots). They concluded that the human element in knot tying, when the participants failed to reverse the direction of their hands during the placement of each throw, resulted in slip knots and noted that their testing methodology could be used as an objective measurement tool for knot tying competency in healthcare personnel.

Modified from Ching SS et al: Assessment of surgical trainees' quality of knot tying, *J Surg Educ* 70:48–54, 2013.

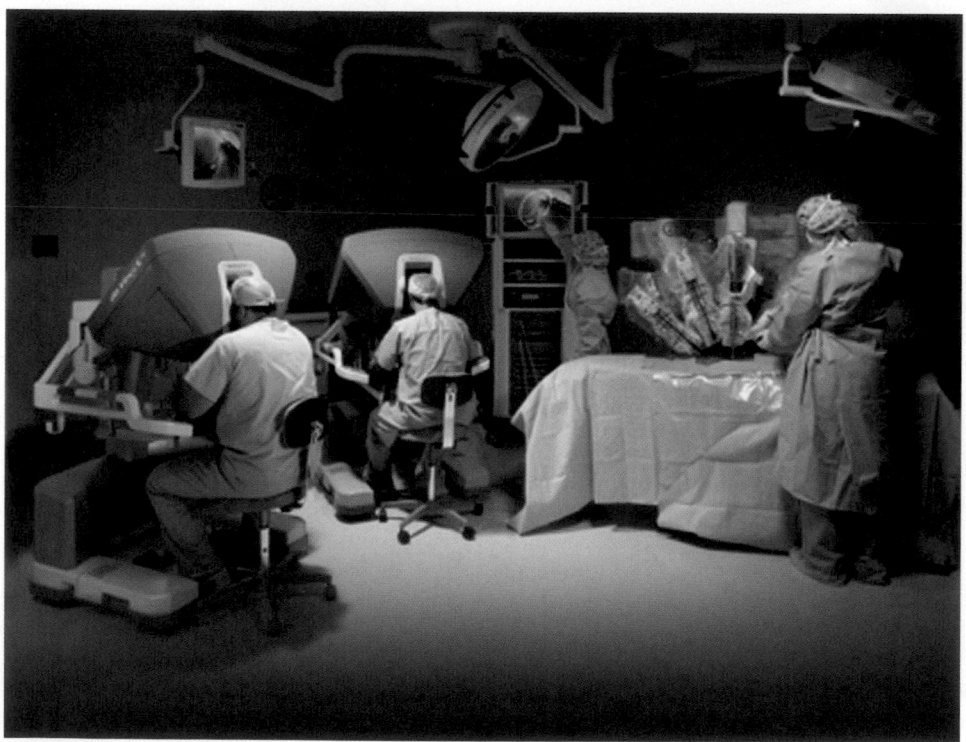

FIGURE 7-11 Surgeon operates while seated at the robotic console.

incisions. The staple appliers are easy to use. They reduce operating time and tissue trauma, allowing uniform tension along the suture line and less distortion from the stress of individual suture points. When properly applied (Figure 7-12), they provide excellent cosmetic results. Some staplers use bioabsorbable staples that are placed under the skin and then absorbed similar to suture. Others use stainless steel staples. With these, the length of time the staples stay in place depends on the part of the body affected; they are usually removed within 5 to 7 days. An extractor is required for their removal.

Most staplers use a similar anvil-type mechanism for forming the staple, but the application device varies from company to company. Device choice usually is determined by the weight, handling characteristics, ease of application, and unobstructed view of

FIGURE 7-12 Application of skin staples. The stapler is lightly positioned over everted skin edges. It is not necessary to press the staple, or stapler anvil, into the skin to get a proper "bite" (just "kiss" the skin). Center the staples over the incision line, using the locating arrow or guideline, and place staples approximately ¼ inch apart.

the site during application. Staplers are packaged in various assortments of numbers and types of staples, depending on the length of the incision and the type of tissue encountered.

Wound Closure Strips. Wounds that are subjected to minimal static and dynamic tension are easily approximated with skin tape. The selection of surgical tape for skin closure is based on the tape's adhesive ability, tensile strength, and porosity. The tape must provide a firm tape-to-skin bond to keep the wound edges closely adhered. The tensile strength must be sufficient to maintain wound approximation. A tape that is too occlusive limits moisture or vapor transmission; fluid may accumulate under the tape and lead to maceration and bacterial growth. Microporous tapes prevent this problem. The surgeon must apply the tape to dry skin; an adhesive adjunct (e.g., tincture of benzoin or other skin barrier) may be applied in a thin film to the skin at the wound edges before tape application. If an alcohol-based adhesive adjunct is used, care must be taken to prevent inadvertent surgical fires (e.g., electrosurgery unit [ESU] must be shut off before the agent is delivered to the field by the perioperative nurse). Edema at the surgical site may cause taped wound edges to invert; supplemental skin sutures may be used to enhance closure. Tapes may be cut to accommodate smaller incisions. Tapes are applied perpendicularly to the wound edge, first on one side and then the other, so that the edges can be pulled together (Figure 7-13).

FIGURE 7-13 Application of skin tapes. **A,** Perforated tab is bent and removed. **B,** Tape is peeled from the card. **C,** Tape is applied to wound. **D,** Completed application.

FIGURE 7-14 Surgical skin adhesive. Ampule is crushed and adhesive applied to skin edges.

Surgical Adhesives. Tissue adhesives, such as cyanoacrylate, may be used for skin closure by applying on approximated and dry skin edges (Figure 7-14). Cyanoacrylate tissue adhesives combine cyano-acetate and formaldehyde in a heat vacuum along with a base to form a liquid monomer. When the monomer comes into contact with moisture on the skin's surface, it chemically changes into a polymer that binds to the top epithelial layer. Some tissue adhesives include an initiator, which speeds up polymerization.

Topical skin adhesives are best used in areas not subject to high skin tension or across areas in which tension may increase (such as knuckles, elbows, or knees) and can be used to replace subcuticular sutures that are 4-0 or smaller in diameter, as long as the skin edges are tension free and well approximated. They provide a flexible water-resistant protective coating that naturally sloughs off the incision in 7-10 days and may offer equivalent wound cosmesis to sutures.

The surgeon manually and evenly apposes the wound edges, then crushes the vial of adhesive and, depending on the product being used, inverts it or holds it straight up. Next, the adhesive is applied with a gentle brushing motion, while avoiding pressing the applicator tip into the wound. If the adhesive enters the wound it could cause a foreign body reaction and prevent wound healing. The surgeon maintains manual approximation of the wound edges for approximately 60 seconds after applying the adhesive. Multiple layers may be required to be applied based on the product being used. Full polymerization is expected when the adhesive is no longer tacky. No topical liquid or ointments should be applied to the closed wound because they can weaken the polymerized film, causing early peeling and skin separation (Ethicon, 2011).

Hemostasis

Hemostasis is an ongoing process during surgery. In addition to the damaging physiologic effects of blood loss for the patient, bleeding from cut vessels obscures visualization of the operative site for the surgeon and must be controlled. Hemostasis may be accomplished from direct pressure applied with surgical soft goods (e.g., radiopaque sponges or towels) or by the use of suture materials, electrosurgical devices, lasers, and chemical agents. Before wound closure the surgeon carefully checks the operative site to ensure that all active bleeding has been stopped.

Methods of Ligating Vessels

A ligature is a strand of suture material used to encircle and obstruct the lumen of a vessel to affect hemostasis, block a structure, or prevent leakage of materials. Ties may be on a reel (i.e., a spool or disk containing a long length of suture) that the surgeon may use to ligate several superficial vessels, or they may be free ties (i.e., precut lengths of suture) handed to the surgeon one at a time, usually for bleeders in deeper tissues.

Following are several techniques used to secure a ligature in deep tissues:
- A hemostat is placed on the end of the structure; the ligature is then placed around the vessel. The knot is tied and tightened with the surgeon's fingers or with the aid of forceps.
- A slipknot is made, and its loop is placed over the involved structure by means of a forceps or clamp.
- In deeper cavities, ties are often placed on clamps with the long end extending from the tip. These are sometimes called *ties on a pass* or *bow ties*. The extending long end is held tightly against the rings by the surgeon (creating the bow), who then passes the tip of the clamp under the vessel or duct to be ligated. The first assistant grasps the extending tie with a forceps, the surgeon releases it, and the tie is pulled under and up to the wound surface and tied.
- A forceps or a clamp is applied to the structure, and transfixion sutures are applied and tied. A *suture ligature, stick tie,* or *transfixion ligature* is a strand of suture material threaded or swaged on a needle. This is usually placed through the vessel and around it to prevent the ligature from slipping off the end.
- When two ligatures are used to ligate a large vessel, usually a free ligature is placed on the vessel and a suture ligature is placed distal to the first ligature. To ligate a blood vessel situated in deep tissues, the strand must be of sufficient strength and length to allow the surgeon to tighten the first knot.

Ligating Clips

Ligating clips are small V-shaped staple-like devices that are placed around the lumen of a vessel or structure to close it. They may be made of one of several metals, such as stainless steel, tantalum, or titanium. Stainless steel clips are the most economical to use. Although more expensive, titanium clips are used frequently in specific surgical procedures because the starburst reflection on postoperative radiographs is less with titanium than with other metals. Absorbable clips made of synthetic absorbable suture material also are available.

Ligating clips are available in several sizes. These clips are available in individual sizes that must be loaded by the scrub person or as preloaded, disposable, prepackaged units. (NOTE: The scrub person may be a surgical technologist or RN. He or she is referred to in this chapter as "scrub person.") Multiple sizes and lengths of clips can be used in both open and endoscopic procedures. Ligating clips afford a rapid and secure method of achieving hemostasis when arteries, veins, nerves, and other small structures are ligated. Since the introduction of minimally invasive endoscopic surgery, the need for ligating clips that can be applied through a trocar has emerged. These clips are changing frequently and no one standard has emerged. Regardless of the type of clip, the surgeon applies them similarly. The surgeon often follows the application of a clip with a request for scissors (Figure 7-15).

Instruments

Historical Perspective

The history of surgical instruments dates back to 2500 BC. The first instruments were sharpened flints and fine animal teeth. Ancient Greek, Egyptian, and Hindu instruments are amazing in their resemblance to contemporary instruments.

To be equipped for the practice of surgery in the late 1700s, the surgeon had to use various skilled artisans, such as coppersmiths; steelworkers; needle grinders; turners of wood, bone, and ivory; and

FIGURE 7-15 Laparoscopic instrumentation. **A,** Endoclip being applied to proximal end of gallbladder duct. **B,** Gallbladder duct being cut with endoscopic scissors. **C,** View of severed duct with artery behind it.

silk and hemp spinners. The surgeon had to explain the mechanisms of the instruments and supervise their manufacture. The resulting instruments were crude, expensive, and time consuming to make. Each artisan used hand labor exclusively and devoted time to making only one type of instrument, thus gaining proficiency in the manufacture of a certain kind of instrument. For example, a cutter would keep a small supply of surgical knives. Thus began physicians' supply houses and surgical instrument making.

In the mid-1800s, physicians' principal tools were their eyes and ears. Official records show that amputation, the trademark of the Civil War, was the end result in three of four operations performed. Surgeons were scarce, and medical instruments were almost nonexistent. Kitchen knives and penknives, carpenter saws, and table forks did the job. After the Civil War the advent of the administration of ether and chloroform brought a demand for new ideas and methods in surgery and instruments. The division of general surgery into specialties occurred in the late 1800s and early 1900s. Delicate instruments were seen as more useful than the force of crude and heavy instruments. So that instruments could withstand repeated sterilization, handles of wood, ivory, and rubber were discontinued.

The development of stainless steel in Germany ensured a better material for surgical instruments and other equipment. Today, surgeons and perioperative nurses assist manufacturers in research, design, and development of new and better instrumentation. Most instrument companies design an instrument to a physician's specifications. Advancement in endoscopic surgery continually requires the development of instrumentation specifically designed for this type of surgery.

Throughout the history of surgery, the tools of the surgeon and the manual aspects of the surgical technique have influenced the evolution of practice. Along with innovative wound closure materials and tools in recent decades, there have been unprecedented developments of new and improved instrumentation. The benefits of minimally invasive surgery are well documented, especially in surgical procedures that typically required lengthy hospital stays, required long and sometimes difficult postoperative recovery or rehabilitation, and exposed the patient to increased risk of surgical infection.

Composition of Surgical Instruments

Successful management of instrumentation requires a continual partnership between surgeons, perioperative nurses, surgical technologists, and central processing personnel, each of whom shares responsibility for the use, handling, and care of surgical instruments. A basic knowledge of how these instruments are manufactured can help in their selection and maintenance. Surgical instruments are expensive and represent a major investment for every institution.

Instruments used today are made in the United States, Germany, France, and Pakistan. The United States does not have an agency that reviews or sets standards for surgical instruments. The quality is set by the individual manufacturer. A reputable company endorses its product. An instrument that receives proper care should last 10 years or more.

Most instruments are manufactured from stainless steel. Stainless steel is a compound of iron, carbon, and chromium, which means that stainless steel can have varying qualities. These qualities are designated by grading the steel into series by the American Iron and Steel Institute (AISI). The 400 series stainless steel has some noncorrosive characteristics and good tensile strength. It resists rust, produces a fine point, and retains a keen edge. Handheld ringed

FIGURE 7-16 Basic cutting instruments. *1,* Knife handle; *2,* Mayo scissors, straight; *3,* Mayo scissors, curved; *4,* Metzenbaum scissors, curved; *5,* suture scissors, straight.

instruments, such as scissors and clamps, should be 400 series stainless steel.

For ringed instruments, the raw steel is converted into instrument blanks by a machinist making an impression of the piece in a stainless steel blank. These blanks are die-forged into specific pieces—male and female halves. The excess metal is trimmed away, and the instrument parts are ready for the final steps.

The two halves are milled to prepare the box lock fittings, jaw serrations, and ratchets, and the jaws and shanks are properly aligned. After this is completed, the halves are assembled by hand. A hole is drilled through the box lock, and a pin or rivet is inserted through the hole. Final grinding and hardening, accomplished by heat-treating, permit the object to attain proper size, weight, spring temper, and balance.

The last part of the process is called *passivation.* The instruments are submerged into nitric acid to remove any residue of carbon steel. The nitric acid also produces a surface coating of chromium oxide. Chromium oxide is important because it produces a resistance to corrosion in the stainless steel instrument. The instrument is then polished.

There are three types of instrument finishes. The first is the bright, highly polished mirror finish, which tends to reflect light and may interfere with the vision of the surgeon. The second is the satin or dull finish, which tends to eliminate glare and lessen eyestrain for the surgeon. The third finish is ebonized, which produces a black finish. Ebonized instruments are used during laser surgery to prevent deflection of the laser beam.

The final inspection and testing are for hardness, proper jaw closure, and smooth lock-and-ratchet action. The instrument is then ready for sale.

Instrument Categories

Although there is no standard nomenclature for specific instruments, there are four main categories: *cutting instruments* (also called *dissectors*), *clamps, retractors,* and *accessory* or *ancillary* instruments.

Cutting Instruments (Dissectors). Dissectors, which may be sharp or blunt, are instruments used to cut or separate tissue. The largest categories of sharp dissecting instruments are scalpels and scissors (Figure 7-16). Scalpels are probably the oldest of all surgical

FIGURE 7-17 Scalpel/knife blades. From left to right: blade sizes 10, 11, 12, 15, and 20, respectively (actual size).

instruments. Most scalpels are handles (knife handle) with one end suited to the attachment of disposable blades (Figure 7-17). Safety scalpels have been modified to provide an engineering control in sharps injury prevention strategies. During an operation, the blades may be conveniently changed by the scrub person as often as necessary. The blades are available prepackaged and sterile and are passed onto the sterile field as needed by the perioperative nurse. Careful handling of blades during the procedure and disposal of blades at the end of a procedure are important in the implementation of Standard Precautions.

Scissors are designed in various shapes and sizes for different purposes in cutting body tissues and surgical materials. The basic design consists of two blades, each having a chisel-shaped edge with the bevel consistent with the structure or material it has to cut. Scissor tips may be blunt or sharp, and the blades may be straight or curved. Conventional scissors require two movements in use: one to open and another to close the jaws. Other scissors may have a spring action in the body design that holds the jaws in an open position. A single movement pressing the spring together closes the jaws to cut. Scissors designed for delicate plastic and eye surgery are often of the latter type. A basic instrument set usually includes a curved Mayo scissors for dissection of heavy tissues, a Metzenbaum scissors for dissection of delicate tissues, and a straight

FIGURE 7-18 Anatomy of a clamp.

Tips

Jaws

Box lock pin
Box lock

Shanks

Ring handles

Ratchet

1   2   3

FIGURE 7-19 Basic clamping instruments. *1,* Crile hemostatic forceps; *2,* Rochester-Péan forceps; *3,* Ochsner or Kocher hemostatic forceps

scissors for cutting suture. For surgery in deep areas of the body, scissors with long handles and short blades are used for better control and easier use.

Other sharp dissectors include drills, saws, osteotomes, rongeurs, and other instruments such as adenotomes and dermatomes. Some instruments in the dissecting category are produced in sharp or blunt form, such as curettes and periosteal elevators. Instruments or devices used for blunt dissection include gauze dissectors (e.g., peanuts, pushers, kitners), a sponge on a stick, the back of a knife handle, and the surgeon's finger or hand.

Clamps. Clamps are instruments specifically designed for holding tissue or other materials, and most have an easily recognizable design (Figure 7-18). They have finger rings, for ease of holding; shanks, whose length is appropriate to the wound depth; ratchets on the shanks near the rings, which allow for the distal tip to be locked on the tissue or object grasped; a joint, which joins the two halves of the instrument and allows opening and closing of the instrument. Instruments made up of two halves have one of three types of joints.

- The most common joint is the box lock, where one arm has been passed through a slot in the other arm and is riveted or pinned. This joint is needed where accurate approximation of the tips is necessary, and it is basic to most ringed instruments.
- The second type is the screw joint. The two halves are aligned and placed on top of each other, connected only by a screw. The joint must be checked and tightened periodically because the screw may become loose. Screw-joint instruments are easy to make and comparatively inexpensive.
- The final and least common type is the semibox, or aseptic, joint. It has the advantage that the two halves can be separated for easy cleaning.

Clamps also have a jaw, which is the working portion of the instrument and defines its use (Figure 7-19). Clamps are divided into the following categories.

Hemostats are used to close the severed ends of a vessel with a minimal amount of tissue damage. They prevent the excessive loss of blood in the course of dissection. The jaws have deep transverse cuts so that the bleeding vessels may be compressed with sufficient force to stop bleeding. The serrations must be cleanly cut and perfectly meshed to prevent the tissue from slipping free from the jaws of the clamp.

Occluding clamps usually have vertical serrations or special jaws that have finely meshed, multiple rows of longitudinally arranged teeth to prevent leakage and to minimize trauma when clamping bowel, vessels, or ducts that are to be reanastomosed.

Graspers and *holders* are used for tissue retraction and generally have jaws of specific design based on their use. The Kocher (also referred to as an Ochsner) clamp has transverse serrations and large teeth (1×2) at its tip to grasp tightly on tough, slippery tissue such as fascia. The Allis clamp has multiple, interdigitating short teeth on the tip, minimizing crushing or damaging tissue. The Babcock clamp has broad, flared ends with smooth tips, and it atraumatically grips or encloses delicate structures, such as bowel, ureters, or fallopian tubes. Other holding forceps have handles like clamps with specialized tips or jaws, which may be triangular, straight, angular, or T-shaped (Figure 7-20).

Non-clamp graspers and holders are known as *forceps* or *pickups* because they are used to lift and hold tissue (see Figure 7-20). Often, while the surgeon is cutting with scissors or sewing with a needle, forceps are used in the other hand. Forceps are held like a pencil. The most common kinds are the various two-arm spring forceps. Forceps resemble tweezers, vary in length and thickness, and are available with and without teeth. Non-toothed forceps create minimal damage and hold delicate, thin tissues. Toothed forceps hold thick or slippery tissues that need extra grip. Toothed forceps ("rat tooth") have interdigitating teeth that hold tissue without slipping; these are used to hold skin or dense tissue. Adson tissue forceps have small, serrated teeth on the edge of the tips; these are designed for light, careful handling of tissue and are commonly used during skin closure.

Grasper and holder clamps may hold objects as well. Sponge-holding forceps with ring-shaped jaws (see Figure 7-20) are available in 7- and 9-inch lengths. They can be used to grasp or handle tissue but are commonly used to hold soft goods. The soft good is folded and placed in the jaws and is used to retract tissue, to absorb blood in the field, and occasionally to perform blunt dissection.

Needle holders (Figure 7-21), because they must grasp metal rather than soft tissues, are subject to greater damage. As a result, needle holders must be repaired and replaced regularly. For maximal usage, needle holders must retain a firm grip on the needle. Many

FIGURE 7-20 Basic holding instruments. *1*, Tissue forceps, smooth; *2*, tissue forceps with teeth; *3*, Adson tissue forceps; *4*, sponge-holding forceps; *5*, towel clamp; *6*, Allis forceps; *7*, Babcock intestinal forceps.

FIGURE 7-21 A, Needle holders. **B,** Fine. **C,** Regular. **D,** Heavy.

types of jaws have been designed to meet this need. The so-called *diamond jaw* needle holder has a tungsten carbide insert designed to prevent rotation of the needle. In needle holders of standard design, a longitudinal groove or pit in the jaw releases tension, prevents flattening of the needle, and holds the needle firmly. Needle holders may have a ratchet similar to that of a hemostat, or they may have a spring action that may or may not lock.

Towel clamps also are considered holding instruments. Of the two basic types, one is a nonpenetrating towel clamp used for holding draping materials in place. The other has sharp tips used to penetrate drapes and tissues, and it is damaging to both. The use of sharp towel clamps to secure drapes is highly discouraged because they penetrate the sterile field.

Retractors. Retractors are used to hold back the wound edges, structures, or tissues to provide exposure of the operative site. A surgeon needs the best exposure possible that inflicts a minimal degree of trauma to the surrounding tissue. Retractors are

FIGURE 7-22 Basic retractors. *1,* Malleable retractor; *2,* vein retractor; *3,* Parker retractor; *4,* army-navy retractor; *5,* Richardson retractor; *6,* Volkmann rake retractors; *7,* Deaver retractors; *8,* Weitlaner retractor; *9,* Balfour retractor with blades.

self-retaining or manually held in place by a member of the surgical team (Figure 7-22). The two types of self-retaining retractors are (1) retractors with frames to which various blades may be attached, and (2) retractors with two blades held apart with a ratchet. An example of the latter is a Weitlaner retractor. Other very large self-retaining retractors, such as the Omni or Bookwalter, are equipped with multiple blades and attachments of varying lengths and sizes. With handheld retractors, the handles may be notched, hook-shaped, or ring-shaped to give the holder a firm grip without tiring. The blade is usually at a right angle to the shaft and may be a smooth blade, rake, or hook. A malleable (ribbon) retractor is a flat metal ribbon that may be shaped at the field.

Accessory and Ancillary Instruments. Accessory and ancillary instruments are designed to enhance the use of basic instrumentation or to facilitate the procedure (Figure 7-23). These include suction tips and tubing; irrigators-aspirators; electrosurgical devices;

and special-use devices, such as probes, dilators, mallets, and screwdrivers.

Many miscellaneous instruments or specialty items are particular to a certain specialty but generally fall into one of the categories just mentioned. Microsurgical instruments are delicate and expensive. They are extremely fine and should be handled separately from other instruments. Instruments used in specialty surgery are discussed in each of the chapters under Surgical Interventions.

When perioperative members can analyze the planned surgical procedure and approach and identify each instrument and its specific function, they are able to select instrument sets without omitting necessary items and without including items that will not be used. This intelligent, planned approach ensures economy of time and motion, protects instruments from misuse, and prevents unnecessary handling. During the operation the informed scrub person who anticipates instrument needs becomes a more valuable member of the surgical team.

FIGURE 7-23 Accessory items. *1,* Frazier suction; *2,* Poole suction; *3,* Yankauer suction; *4,* silver probe; *5,* grooved director.

FIGURE 7-24 Internal staplers. **A,** Terminal end stapler, designed for closing the end of a hollow organ, such as the stomach, with a double staggered line of staples. **B,** Internal anastomosis stapler, designed to connect hollow organ segments to fashion a larger pouch or reservoir. **C,** End-to-end stapler, designed to staple two hollow tubelike organs, such as bowel, to create a continuous circuit.

Endoscopic Instrumentation

Laparoscopy has introduced new equipment and instrumentation to the surgical suite. In addition to insufflation equipment, an optical system, and a documentation system, perioperative personnel must be familiar with the instrumentation used by the surgeon when performing a surgical procedure through the endoscope. Basic instrumentation, which may be disposable or reusable, includes trocars, forceps or graspers, clip appliers, stapling devices, scissors, needle holders, and aspiration-irrigation systems.

Verres needles and trocars provide access to the peritoneal and thoracic cavities. A retractable safety shield protects abdominal structures from being inadvertently punctured during insertion. Forceps or graspers are available in 3-, 5-, and 10-mm sizes. Atraumatic graspers provide appropriate retraction and little risk to tissues. Bipolar coagulation forceps are used to control bleeding. The forceps are available with different tips, including ring, paddle, dolphin nose, claw, spoon, DeBakey, Allis, Pollack, Pennington, Glassman, Maryland, Reddick-Saye, Duval, and Babcock. Some dissectors are available with coagulation capability. Scissors also come with different tips: hook, straight and microtipped, serrated, and curved. Also, several disposable instruments coagulate and cut the tissue.

Needle holders have a hinged-jaw tip to allow easy positioning of the needle before intracorporeal suturing and using the sliding sheath. The sliding sheath holds the needle in a distal notch and

inner spring-loading mechanism. To aid with extracorporeal knot tying, the surgeon may use a knot pusher (e.g., a Clarke-Reich) to deliver tied knots into the abdomen. A slide and cinch pusher (Gazayerli) also is used to deliver and secure the preformed knot. Intra-abdominal stapling devices have been modified to fit and function through the endoscope. The development and introduction of robot-assisted surgery has produced a new generation of multiarticulating instruments.

Stapling Instruments

Instrumentation for internal stapling, first introduced in 1908, has been refined and is now widely used (Figure 7-24). Various instruments to suture tissue mechanically are used for ligation and division, resection, anastomoses, and skin and fascia closure. In general, these instruments may be classified as follows (Neumayer and Vargo, 2012):

* Ligating and dividing staplers (LDSs)
* Gastrointestinal anastomosis (GIA) staplers
* Thoracoabdominal (TA) staplers
* End-to-end anastomosis (EEA) staplers
* Laparoscopic hernia mesh staplers
* Open hernia mesh staplers
* Endo-GIA devices

Used in many surgical specialties, the mechanical application of these instruments reduces tissue manipulation and handling. The edema and inflammation that usually accompany anastomoses are

FIGURE 7-25 Using the gastrointestinal anastomosis (GIA) stapler to staple and join stomach and jejunum. At the same time, the blade in the GIA cuts between double staple lines, creating a stoma for a gastrojejunostomy.

minimized because the noncrushing B shape of the staples allows nutrients to pass through the staple line to the cut edge of the tissue (Figure 7-25).

Mechanical staplers (both nondisposable and disposable) use cartridges of tiny stainless steel staples or absorbable nonmetallic staples that are commercially preloaded, prepackaged, and presterilized. The staples are essentially nonreactive; metal staples remain permanently in the tissue. The staplers may fire individually or lay down multiple rows in a straight or circular pattern. Devices to cut or anastomose bowel and other structures are available for open-wound use or through endoscopic cannulae. The use of staplers significantly decreases operating time and may shorten postoperative stays.

Selecting and Preparing Instruments for Patient Use

Designated OR or central supply personnel arrange the various instruments into trays or sets. The trays are named according to their functions. Tray/set names and instrument composition vary by institution, but three basic OR instrument sets are the minor/plastic, the basic laparotomy, and the dilation and curettage (D&C). A minor (or plastic surgery) set includes instruments needed for simple superficial incision, excision, and suturing. A basic laparotomy set includes instruments to open and close the abdominal cavity and repair any gross defects in the major body musculature. A D&C set, in addition to its use for dilation and curettage, is often used as the basic instrumentation for vaginal surgery.

According to each procedure's needs, more individualized instruments or specialty sets, such as an intestinal set or a vascular set, may be added. In the same way, basic instrument sets may be selected for opening other body cavities, such as the skull, chest, and pelvis.

Instruments are selected according to the size of the patient's body structures and the nature of the organs involved. Proper selection requires a general understanding of surgical procedures and approaches and knowledge of anatomy, possible pathologic conditions, and the design and purpose of instruments.

Basic Table Setups. In most ORs the instruments are set up on Mayo stands and back tables in a planned, standardized, organized, functional manner to maintain continuity when the original scrub person is replaced by another. Care is taken on all sterile fields to

ensure that all solutions, syringes, and medication cups are clearly labeled to guarantee patient and staff safety. Each facility should create tools as a part of a comprehensive orientation process to ensure standardization of setups.

A proficient scrub person must know the instrument inventory of the department; the instruments routinely needed for each type of operation; the individual surgeon's preferences; and the correct use and handling, method of preparation, and postoperative care of the instruments. A file of preference cards or computerized data/preference sheets usually lists the procedures each surgeon performs, the surgeon's glove size, the preferred skin prep solution, specific draping instructions, and instruments required for the procedure.

Before an operative procedure, the scrub person may assist the perioperative nurse in gathering the needed supplies, equipment, and sutures. The scrub person scrubs; dons gown and gloves; and begins to set up the sterile tables with drapes, instruments, supplies, and sutures. Instruments are arranged with those most frequently used on the Mayo stand.

One or two back tables, according to the number of instruments and supplies, also are set up. The scrub person prepares the sutures and ligatures and places the knife blades on the handles. Other supplies needed are suction tubing and tips, electrosurgical cord and tip, drains, basins, gowns, gloves, drapes, sponges, and needles, all of which are sterile and set up on the back table according to standardized institutional policy (Figure 7-26). During the final "time-out" before incision, the scrub person has the responsibility to articulate instrument and equipment readiness to the team to enhance a safe, seamless procedure. When the patient is on the OR bed and is draped, the Mayo stand, set up for instrument use at the immediate operative site, is brought across the lower part of the patient's legs (Figure 7-27).

The scrub person must be attentive to the sterile field to anticipate the surgeon's needs. Instruments should be passed in a positive and decisive manner. Each instrument is placed or slapped firmly into the surgeon's palm in such a manner that it is ready for immediate use with no wasted motion. When a curved instrument is passed to the surgeon, the curve should be pointing in the direction of intended use; there should be no need for readjustment. It is necessary to know if a surgeon or assistant is left-handed or right-handed to pass instruments efficiently and in the correct position.

Often the surgeon or assistant uses hand signals for the type of instrument desired, to eliminate unnecessary talking. Scrub persons should become familiar with the basic signals for knife, scissors, suture, forceps, and clamp.

Care and Handling of Instruments. An instrument should be used only for the purpose for which it is designed. Proper use and reasonable care prolong its life and protect its quality. Scissors and clamps, which are most frequently misused, can be forced out of alignment, cracked, or broken when used improperly. Tissue scissors should not be used to cut suture or gauze dressings. Hemostatic clamps should not be used as towel clamps or to clamp suction tubing.

Each instrument should be inspected before and after each use to detect imperfections. An instrument should function perfectly to prevent needlessly endangering a patient's safety and increasing operative time because of instrument failure.

Forceps, clamps, and other hinged instruments must be inspected for jaw and teeth alignment. Instrument jaws and teeth should meet perfectly so that blood flow is occluded without damaging the vein or artery. Ratchets should hold firmly yet release easily. Instrument joints should work smoothly.

FIGURE 7-26 A, Back table setup. **B,** Labeled medications and sharps on table setup.

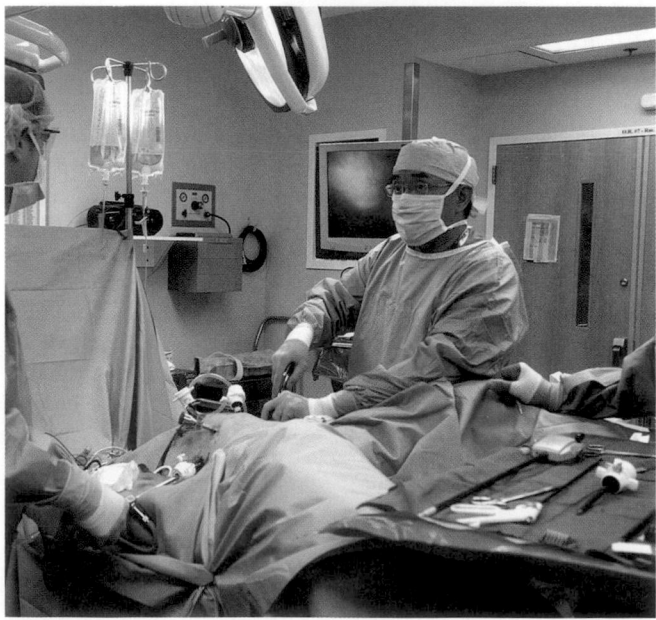

FIGURE 7-27 Mayo stand, with instruments required for start of surgical procedure, is moved into place across the lower part of the draped patient.

All instruments should be checked for worn spots, chips, dents, cracks, or sharp edges. Damaged instruments should be set aside and sent for repair or replacement. An instrument repair service should be selected carefully and used for regular maintenance, such as sharpening and realignment.

Instruments must be handled gently. Bouncing, dropping, and setting heavy equipment on top of them must be avoided. During the procedure the scrub person should wipe the used instruments with a damp sponge or place them in a basin of sterile water to prevent blood from drying on the surfaces and in the box locks. Saline solution should never be used on instruments because the salt is corrosive and accelerates rusting or deterioration of the metal. As time allows during the procedure, the scrub person should rinse and dry the used instruments and replace them on the back table to facilitate closing counts.

At the end of a procedure, during the table breakdown process, the scrub person must handle the instruments in a logical organized fashion, either individually or in small groups. Sharp and delicate instruments should be set aside for individual handling and cleaning to avoid damage and accidental injury. Surgeon-specific instrumentation should be isolated to prevent loss or damage in the cleaning and reassembly process. Standard Precautions should be applied as dictated by institutional policy. All instruments set up for the procedure should be terminally sterilized or disinfected before reassembly. Instruments must be completely clean to ensure effective sterilization. Refer to Chapter 4 for information on instrument decontamination and sterilization.

With today's focus on cost containment, perioperative nurses must assess the care and handling of instrumentation carefully. Instrument sets can be monitored for use, and instruments that are used infrequently can be removed and packaged separately to prevent continued wear from unnecessary resterilization.

Storing Instruments. Instruments should be stored in a manner that keeps them safe and supports the maintenance of the container's integrity (see Chapter 4). Cabinet shelving should be adjustable and properly spaced for storage of various sizes and types of instruments. Most institutions store instruments in presterilized trays or containers. Attached labels and diagrams in cabinets assist personnel. An inventory of all instruments should be taken at periodic intervals.

Perioperative Nursing Considerations

Surgical Counts

Retained foreign bodies after surgery are a complication with serious potential consequences for the people involved. The surgical count process is undertaken to ensure that needles, sharps, soft goods, and instruments are not retained in the patient. Soft goods are defined as radiopaque sponges, towels, and textiles (Box 7-2).

One of the patient outcomes identified in the Perioperative Nursing Data Set (PNDS) is that "the patient is free from signs and symptoms of injury due to extraneous objects" (Petersen, 2010). One of the many perioperative nursing activities undertaken to achieve this patient outcome is the performance of counts to ensure that the patient is free from injury related to retained soft goods, sharps, or instruments. Institutions vary in their policies regarding

---

BOX 7-2

Surgical Soft Goods

Surgical soft goods (e.g., radiopaque sponges, towels, and other textiles) are used to effect hemostasis via direct pressure, absorb intraoperative blood loss and drainage, act as aids to blunt dissection, pack the viscera from the field, and keep areas of the wound moist. Surgeons may also use sponges as a filter between a suction tip and delicate tissue. A variety of surgical sponges are available commercially packed in increments of 5 or 10. Any sponge used during a surgical procedure must contain an x-ray–detectable element to facilitate location of the item if a count discrepancy occurs.

The following is a list of the types of surgical sponges:

- *Radiopaque 4 × 4s:* Commonly referred to as a Ray-Tec or 4 × 4, this sponge is composed of loosely woven gauze folded into a 4-inch square. A radiopaque thread, which may change to a darker color when exposed to fluid, is integrated into the sponge. This type of sponge is useful for superficial small incisions, and may be folded into thirds and mounted onto a sponge stick for use in deeper incisions. Other sizes such as 4 × 8 may also be available.
- *Laparotomy sponges.* Also referred to as "laps," "lap pads," or "tapes," these sponges are either square or oblong and have a loop of colored twill tape with a radiopaque marker sewn to one corner. Used for major surgical procedures with large incisions, laparotomy sponges are presented to the surgeon either moist or dry.
- *Dissectors:* Dissecting sponges have the radiopaque element incorporated into the weave of the material and are generally composed of very tightly rolled cloth tape. They may be referred to as "peanuts," "pushers," or "kitners." Dissecting sponges are *always* presented to the surgeon mounted on a clamp because of their small size.
- *Round sponges:* Often known as "tonsil" or "cherry" sponges, round sponges are gauze-covered cotton balls with strings attached. The radiopaque element is woven into the gauze covering. These sponges are often used in the oropharynx and are presented on the tip of a clamp or sponge stick.
- *Flat neurosurgical patties:* Flat sponges are composed of soft compressed cotton or rayon with an embedded radiopaque element and string attached. Often used in neurosurgical procedures, these sponges are available in a multitude of sizes and widths. They may be used as a filter for a suction tip to prevent damage to the underlying tissue, or as a vehicle for the application of topical anesthetic to the nasal mucosa.

---

needle and sharps counts during operative procedures, but most follow established procedures based on the Association of periOperative Registered Nurses (AORN) *Recommended Practices for Prevention of Retained Surgical Objects* (AORN, 2013a). Initial counts before the start of the procedure provide the basis for subsequent counts. All items that have the potential to be retained in a cavity or large wound should be included in the initial count and added as necessary. Policies should be established to determine when and what items may be excluded from counts for less invasive procedures. Trauma centers should have specific policies to account for purposely retained objectives when secondary procedures will be necessary.

The documentation of counts should include the items on the instrument table at the beginning of the procedure as well as those added during the procedure. The counts should be performed audibly and with each sharp, soft good, and instrument visualized by both the scrub person and the perioperative nurse. The number of needles, soft goods, and instruments should be recorded.

During the procedure the scrub person should be aware of the location of items on the sterile field. Needles should be accounted for by the scrub person as they are placed in the neutral zone on a one-for-one exchange basis when possible. The scrub person places soiled soft goods in a designated container off the sterile field (such as a sponge bucket at the end of the OR bed) for retrieval by the circulating nurse. To facilitate counting, the circulating nurse places the soft goods in visible pocketed bags. Needles are retained on the sterile field and counted according to the number indicated on the package; the scrub person verifies this number with the perioperative nurse when the package is opened. Used needles should be kept on a needle pad or counter on the scrub person's table. Broken or missing needles must be reported to the surgeon and accounted for in their entirety. Instruments that break during the procedure or are disassembled (e.g., certain retractor systems) must be accounted for in their entirety. Subsequent counts should be performed by the scrub person and perioperative nurse before closure of a body cavity or deep, large incision; after closure of a body cavity; and at skin closure. Additional counts should be an element of the hand-off process when either the scrub person or the perioperative nurse is permanently relieved by other personnel. In situations in which personnel may be relieved on a temporary basis, the verbal hand-off should include a discussion about counted items. In all situations it is imperative that two individuals be involved in the count—one counting and the other witnessing that the count is correct. Rushing at the end of a surgical procedure can result in incorrect or incomplete counts. When the scrub person and perioperative nurse are rushed, it may be necessary to call for a "pause for the count," enabling counts to be carried out in an orderly manner. All counted items are retained in the OR during the surgical procedure. Many institutions have printed forms to keep track of routinely counted items. Others use erasable count boards visible to all personnel. Recording the count is the responsibility of the perioperative nurse. Depending on institutional policy and practices, the count sheet may become part of the patient's record.

Each institution should have established policies for dealing with incorrect counts. As institutions move toward electronic and paperless documentation, count sheets may be used only as worksheets. Policies and procedures must be revised to account for these changes in practice and a method for documentation and electronic signatures be implemented. Unintentional retention of objects during surgery has been identified as a "never event"; institutions need to adopt a comprehensive strategy to manage the complexity of this

EVIDENCE FOR PRACTICE

Use of Blunt-Tip Suture Needles to Decrease Percutaneous Injuries to Surgical Personnel

The U.S. Food and Drug Administration (FDA), in conjunction with the Occupational Safety and Health Administration (OSHA), Department of Labor, and the National Institute for Occupational Safety and Health (NIOSH), Centers for Disease Control and Prevention (CDC), and the Department of Health and Human Services strongly recommend using blunt-tip suture needles as an alternative to standard suture needles when suturing fascia and muscle to decrease the risk of needlestick injury.

Blunt-Tip Suture Needles

Blunt-tip suture needles, which are not as sharp as standard (sharp-tip) suture needles, are designed to penetrate muscle and fascia and reduce the risk of needlesticks. Blunt-tip suture needles are regulated by the FDA and have been marketed in the United States for more than 25 years.

Summary of Problem and Scope

Needlestick injuries continue to occur in surgical settings when suturing muscle and fascia, despite the availability of safety-engineered devices, such as blunt-tip suture needles, and the endorsement of their use by professional organizations.

Sharp-tip suture needles are the leading source of percutaneous injuries to surgical personnel, causing 51% to 77% of these incidents. Sharp-tip suture needles not only injure surgical staff but also present a risk to patients from potential exposure to injured staff's blood. Suture needle injuries can occur when surgical personnel:

- Load or reposition the needle into the needle holder
- Pass the needle hand-to-hand between team members
- Sew toward the surgeon or assistant while the surgeon or assistant holds back other tissue
- Tie the tissue with the needle still attached
- Leave the needle on the operative field
- Place needles in an overfilled sharps container
- Place needles in a poorly located sharps container

Needlestick injuries have the potential to expose healthcare personnel to bloodborne viruses, such as hepatitis B virus (HBV), hepatitis C virus (HCV), and human immunodeficiency virus (HIV). Of the estimated 384,000 needlestick injuries that occur in hospitals each year, 23% occur in surgical settings. Published literature indicates that although needlestick injury rates have been decreasing among nonsurgical healthcare providers, this has not been the case among those who work in surgical settings. According to a 2010 article published in the Journal of the American College of Surgeons and citing data from a 1998 study, more than half of needlestick injuries involving suture needles occur during the suturing of fascia or muscle.

Benefits of Using Blunt-Tip Suture Needles

Published studies show that using blunt-tip suture needles reduces the risk of needlestick injuries from suture needles by 69%. Other trials and reports have shown that blunt-tip suture needles are technically satisfactory when used appropriately and that their use results in substantial reduction or elimination of injuries to surgical personnel. Although blunt-tip suture needles currently cost about 70 cents more than their standard suture needle counterparts, the benefits of reducing the risk of serious and potentially fatal bloodborne infections for healthcare personnel support their use when clinically appropriate.

A 2007 report suggests that the slight difference in costs of blunt-and sharp-tip suture needles is balanced by the economic savings associated with needlestick injury prevention. This report, which assessed the costs of managing occupational exposures to blood and body fluids, concluded that the cost of managing a needlestick injury can range from $376 to $2,456 per reported incident. In addition, personnel who receive needlestick injuries may experience anxiety and a loss of productivity as they await the results of blood tests.

Government Agencies and Professional Organizations Endorse the Use of Blunt-Tip Suture Needles

The OSHA Bloodborne Pathogens standard, revised on January 18, 2001, in response to the Needlestick Safety and Prevention Act of 2000, requires the use of safer devices, such as blunt-tip suture needles, when clinically appropriate, to reduce the risk of needlestick injury and subsequent pathogen transmission to personnel. The revised standard requires employers, with input from non-managerial direct patient care employees, to consider and implement available appropriate and effective safer medical devices designed to eliminate or minimize occupational exposure.

In 2007, OSHA and NIOSH issued a joint Safety and Health Information Bulletin emphasizing OSHA's requirement and NIOSH's recommendation to use blunt-tip suture needles, when clinically appropriate, to decrease needlestick injuries to surgical personnel.

The American College of Surgeons (ACS) recommends the universal adoption of blunt-tip suture needles as the first choice for the closure of fascia and muscle. This statement is endorsed by the Association of periOperative Registered Nurses, American Association of Nurse Anesthetists, American Association of Surgical Physician Assistants, American Society of Anesthesiologists, American Society of PeriAnesthesia Nurses, and Association of Surgical Technologists.

Recommendation

The FDA, NIOSH, and OSHA strongly encourage healthcare professionals in surgical settings to use blunt-tip suture needles to suture muscle and fascia, when clinically appropriate, to reduce the risk of needlestick injury and subsequent pathogen transmission to surgical personnel. Employers in workplaces that use suture needles have the responsibility under the Bloodborne Pathogens standard to evaluate the use of blunt-tip suture needles as well as other appropriate safer medical devices. After this evaluation, which must include input from non-managerial employees responsible for direct patient care [29 CFR 1910.1030(c)(1)(v)] (e.g., in this case surgical personnel), employers must use safer devices to replace corresponding conventional sharp-tip suture needles in their workplaces when clinically appropriate. The introduction of any device must include training staff in its proper use and follow-up to ensure a successful transition from conventional to safer devices. When an employer has determined that the use of available safer devices is not feasible, the clinical justification for this determination must be documented in the facility's exposure control plan and the employer must implement alternative means of protecting surgical personnel from percutaneous injuries.

Modified from FDA, NIOSH and OSHA Joint Safety Communication: *Blunt-tip surgical suture needles reduce needlestick injuries and the risk of subsequent bloodborne pathogen transmission to surgical personnel,* 2012, available at www.fda.gov/MedicalDevices/Safety/AlertsandNotices/ucm305757.htm. Accessed March 12, 2013; *Use of blunt-tip suture needles to decrease percutaneous injuries to surgical personnel safety and health information bulletin* SHIB 03–23–2007, DHHS (NIOSH) Publication No. 2008–101 (supersedes 2007–132), available at www.cdc.gov/niosh/docs/2008-101/pdfs/2008-101.pdf. Accessed March 12, 2013.

issue. Strategies include several elements, such as emphasizing forced communication, standard processes, and checklists. In general, the surgeon is immediately notified of an incorrect count, and a recount is initiated. Sterile team members and the perioperative nurse initiate a search of the sterile and unsterile fields. If the missing item is not revealed after a recount and search, the surgeon is asked to explore the wound. If the missing item is still not found, agency policy may dictate that an x-ray film be taken. Documentation of these activities should be completed according to institutional policy and procedure.

Sharps No-Touch Technique

Because sharp instruments used in surgery are a frequent cause of injury, recommendations for eliminating hand-to-hand passing have been established, and numerous engineering controls, such as safety scalpels and blunt suture needles, have been developed (Patient Safety). AORN and the American College of Surgeons (ACS) have made statements and recommendations for the adoption of a hands-free technique (HFT), and use of engineered sharps injury prevention (ESIP) devices along with double-gloving and

PATIENT SAFETY

Neutral/Safe Zone Procedures

Creating a neutral or safe zone for passing sharps is an important action the scrub person undertakes to minimize the risk of injury by sharps (e.g., hypodermic needles, suture needles, sharp trocars, blades on knife handles, etc.) for the scrubbed perioperative team members. To create the safe zone the scrub person:

- Sets up the surgical field with the appropriate neutral zone or sharps receptacle, communicates its location, and, if necessary, orients the surgeons to the procedure for using it. The neutral zone should be as flat and level as possible, within easy arm's reach of the surgeon.
- Passes all sharp instruments and other items requested by the surgeon to the designated neutral zone. The surgeon picks up the item and replaces it after use to the same area. Examples of neutral zones include:
  - A designated area on a Mayo tray
  - A metal or heavy plastic passing basin
  - A magnetic mat, needle magnet pad, or nonslip pad

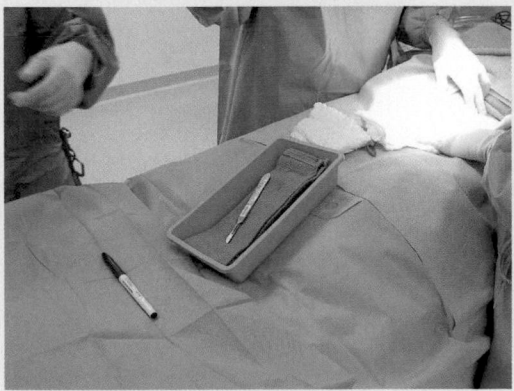

Puncture-proof container used as safe zone device.

Modified from *AORN sharps safety tool kit: policies, procedures and plans*, 2012, available at www.aorn.org/Secondary.aspx?id=20948. Accessed March 10, 2013; photo courtesy William P. Schecter, MD.

blunt needles (ACS, 2007; AORN, 2013b) (Evidence for Practice, p. 208). AORN has developed the Sharps Safety Tool Kit, which incorporates the recommendations of the ACS and other healthcare organizations that provides educational information, policy recommendations, and plans to implement an improved culture of sharps safety in the perioperative setting (AORN, 2013c).

KEY POINTS

- Suture is the generic term used for materials used to repair and reapproximate incised or torn tissues.
- Suture choice is determined by characteristics such as absorbable versus nonabsorbable, strength, braided or monofilament, ease of knot tying, and the inflammatory response of the tissue.
- Absorbable sutures include gut, collagen, synthetics such as polyglactin, and bioengineered substances such as poly-4-hydroxybutyrate.
- Nonabsorbable sutures include silk, cotton, nylon, polyester fiber, polypropylene, and stainless steel.
- Suture may be packaged as strands or in reels or used with needles.
- Needles may be eyed (and need to be manually threaded) or swaged onto suture.
- Stainless steel is most common material used to create surgical instruments.
- Instruments are broadly categorized into cutting instruments, clamps, retractors, and accessory instruments.
- The surgical count process is undertaken to ensure that needles, sharps, soft goods, and instruments are not retained in the patient.

CRITICAL THINKING QUESTION

You are the circulating nurse for a patient undergoing an open hemicolectomy. Per your facility policy you conducted a soft good, sharps, and instrument count before bringing the patient to the OR. The surgeon begins to close the patient's wound and you and a scrub person begin your counts. During the sharps count you note a one-needle discrepancy in the needle count. What are the possible causes of the incorrect count?

⊖volve *The answer to the Critical Thinking Question can be found at http://evolve.elsevier.com/Rothrock/Alexander.*

REFERENCES

American College of Surgeons (ACS): *Statement on sharps safety*, 2007, available at www.facs.org/fellows_info/statements/st-58.html. Accessed March 10, 2013.

Association of periOperative Registered Nurses (AORN): *Position statement on RN first assistants*, 2012, available at www.aorn.org/Clinical_Practice/Position_Statements/Supporting_documents/PosStat_RNFA-2012.aspx. Accessed March 9, 2013.

Association of periOperative Registered Nurses (AORN): Recommended practice for prevention of retained surgical items. In *Perioperative standards and recommended practices*, Denver, CO, 2013a, The Association.

Association of periOperative Registered Nurses (AORN): Guidelines and Guidance Statement: Sharps injury prevention. In *Perioperative standards and recommended practices*, Denver, CO, 2013b, The Association.

Association of periOperative Registered Nurses (AORN): *Sharps safety tool kit*, 2013c, available at www.aorn.org/Secondary.aspx?id=20852. Accessed March 10, 2013.

Bulechek G M et al: *Nursing interventions classification (NIC)*, ed 6, St Louis, 2013, Mosby.

Ethicon: *Dermabond, instructions for use*, 2011, available at www.dermabond.com/sites/all/files/uploads/EPI.pdf. Accessed March 10, 2013.

Lombardi AV et al: Advancing suture technology: a stitch in time, *Semin Arthro* 22:179–181, 2011.

Mosby's dictionary of medical, nursing, and health professions, ed 9, St Louis, 2012, Mosby.

Neumayer L, Vargo D: Principles of preoperative and operative surgery. In Townsend C M et al, editors: *Sabiston textbook of surgery*, ed 19, Philadelphia, 2012, Saunders.

Petersen C: *Perioperative nursing data set*, Denver, 2010, Association of periOperative Registered Nurses.

CHAPTER 8
Surgical Modalities

KAY A. BALL

Surgery continues to evolve as less-invasive procedures and instrumentation are adopted. Modalities have been developed that enhance and advance surgical procedures. This chapter provides information about the evolution of some widely used surgical modalities, including laparoscopy (sometimes referred to as endoscopy), other minimally invasive surgery (MIS) technologies, video technology, and energies used during surgical intervention.

Minimally Invasive Surgery Overview

In the late 1980s the "laparoscopy revolution" began in the United States. General surgeons developed techniques to perform procedures using the laparoscope, eliminating the need for a large incision. As surgeons and perioperative nurses accessed evolving knowledge and information, the surgical industry worked to accommodate a rapid change from open surgical procedures to newer techniques of MIS. Perioperative nurses and surgical technologists experienced the opportunity to acquire new competencies. Since the 1990s, equipment, instrumentation, surgical skills, and perioperative nursing knowledge have markedly expanded as MIS has become a safe approach for many surgical interventions. Ongoing changes in surgery that aim to incorporate MIS procedures present complex challenges for the surgical team while offering patients potentially shorter hospital stays (Sajid et al, 2009), reduced postoperative pain, lower rates of surgical site infections (Poon et al, 2009), and faster recuperation (Schmock, 2009) (Table 8-1). A keen understanding of the goals of endoscopic MIS, clinical competence, and preoperative patient assessment establish the basis for the perioperative plan of care.

Endoscopes

An endoscope is a tube inserted into a natural body orifice or through a small incision to access internal organs or structures. Endoscopes are flexible, rigid, or semirigid. Flexible endoscopes include angioscopes, bronchoscopes, choledochoscopes, colonoscopes (Figure 8-1), cystonephroscopes, hysteroscopes, mediastinoscopes, ureteroscopes, and ureteropyeloscopes. Rigid endoscopes include cystoscopes, laparoscopes, sinuscopes, arthroscopes, bronchoscopes, laryngoscopes, and hysteroscopes (Figure 8-2). Some endoscopes are manufactured in flexible and rigid forms. A semirigid endoscope, such as the deflectable-tip video laparoscope, allows movement through a deflectable tip to provide a complete field of view from different angles (Figure 8-3).

Endoscopes are diagnostic or operative. *Diagnostic* scopes are for observation only and have no operating channels. The system is sealed at both ends. A diagnostic scope can be used, however, when multiple access sites are planned for the introduction of other instrumentation to perform a surgical procedure. *Operative* endoscopes are channeled to irrigate, suction, insert, and connect accessory instrumentation (Figure 8-4). For example, when a potassium titanyl phosphate (KTP) laser is used, the laser fiber is inserted into the operating port of the laparoscope. Advanced laparoscopic techniques may include the use of a flexible endoscope to check for anastomotic leaks, identify bleeding sites, or detect other problems before, during, or immediately after the laparoscopic procedure.

Endoscopes are available in various diameters and lengths, depending on access to the area being visualized and the requirements of the procedure. Optical capability through a rigid scope is controlled by a lens system and can be direct (0-degree angle) or angled (e.g., 30, 70, 120 degrees) (Figure 8-5). Some rigid endoscopes integrate a distally mounted camera chip inside the scope with a rotation dial for proper orientation of the target site. Because flexible scopes are able to be angulated, they allow for a more panoramic view.

There are two types of flexible endoscopes: fiberoptic endoscopes and videoscopes. Fiberoptic endoscopes have an eyepiece with a lens for visualization; the image is carried through the endoscope via a bundle of tiny glass fibers. Videoscopes have, at their distal end, a video chip that provides an image that is directly viewed on a monitor; a videoscope does not have an eyepiece for direct viewing.

Flexible endoscopes have four distinct components:
1. Control body (e.g., angulation knobs, air-water channels, biopsy port, eyepiece for fiberoptic endoscopes)
2. Insertion tube (e.g., flexible tube containing channels for suction, biopsy, irrigation, air and water, image bundles for the fiberscope, light bundles)
3. Bending section at distal tip (e.g., bending rubber, lenses, air-water nozzle, C-cover, charge-coupled device [CCD] chip for videoscopes)
4. Light-guide connector unit (e.g., suction, air-water channel)

Flexible endoscopes also have three different systems that include some of the various components within the endoscope:
1. Mechanical system (provides ports to introduce accessories to perform treatments and procedures)
2. Angulation system (allows the endoscope's distal tip to be moved in different directions)
3. Illumination system (provides light to view internal structures)

Rigid endoscopes also have four distinct components:
1. Eyepiece (e.g., ocular lenses; rigid videoscopes are also available without an eyepiece)
2. Body (e.g., light-guide connector, valves)
3. Shaft (e.g., rod lenses, spacers)
4. Distal end (e.g., objective lens, negative lens)

Understanding the parts of an endoscope can help assess technical problems that can occur during any endoscopic procedure.

TABLE 8-1

Advantages of Minimally Invasive Surgery Over Open Surgery

Minimally Invasive	Open
Ambulatory or shortened length of stay (LOS)	Hospital admission
Short postoperative recuperation	4- to 6-week recuperation
Decreased postoperative pain; decreased need for pain medications	Postoperative pain related to surgical site; more analgesics required
Earlier return to normal activities and lifestyle	Return to normal activities and lifestyle varies with recuperation period

FIGURE 8-1 Flexible colonoscope.

FIGURE 8-2 Rigid endoscope.

FIGURE 8-3 Semirigid ureteroscope.

FIGURE 8-4 Operative laparoscope.

FIGURE 8-5 The lenses inside the endoscope determine the angle of view.

FIGURE 8-6 Dissected flexible endoscope, showing the complexity of the internal structure and design.

FIGURE 8-7 Light source with universal light cable adapter.

FIGURE 8-8 Universal light cable with interchangeable light source connectors and endoscope adapters.

Internal components are complex, sophisticated, and sometimes delicate (Figure 8-6) and the endoscope must be treated with care.

Light Sources and Fiberoptic Cables

Endoscopic light is often referred to as *cold light,* meaning that the heat from the light source is not transmitted through the length of the scope. Therefore, tissue damage from heat at the distal tip of the endoscope is minimized. When the ends of the fiberoptic cables are disconnected from the scope, however, they may be very hot. The surgical team uses extreme caution to ensure the ends of the cables do not contact the patient's skin or any flammable materials or liquids. If the fiberoptic cable is disconnected from the endoscope during surgery, the scrub person ensures that the cable end is held away from drapes or placed on a moist towel to prevent burns and fires. Ideally the light should be turned off whenever disconnected from the endoscope. ECRI Institute (formerly, the Emergency Care Research Institute) recommends labeling all fiberoptic light sources with a warning to prevent fires from the hot light source energy. High-intensity fiberoptic light sources and cables can ignite drapes and other materials. To prevent a fire, all cable connections must be completed before activating the light source. The light source must be placed on standby when the cables are disconnected.

Light sources should have adjustable manual and automatic brightness modes. The automatic mode adjusts brightness according to the video image. When the light source is set in this mode, the circulating nurse need not constantly make adjustments.

When selecting a light source, certain options are considered. A light source that can adapt to several rigid endoscopic systems is desirable, such as one with a universal light cable adapter, which enhances flexibility and usage (Figure 8-7). If a previously purchased unit does not provide this feature, universal light cables with

FIGURE 8-9 Inside the light cable are hundreds of glass fibers that transmit light.

connectors to an interchangeable light source and endoscope adapters are available (Figure 8-8). A generic cord can be used with most scopes and light sources, but some light cables can only be used with specific sizes of endoscopes. For example, a 2.5-mm cable is used with a scope less than 4 mm and a 4.5-mm cable is used with a 10-mm scope. Using the incorrect light cable with an endoscope may overheat or damage the optics. Color-coding different cable sizes helps differentiate them. Light sources also must have connection capability with different camera units.

Handle fiberoptic light cables with extreme care. They consist of hundreds of glass fibers that transmit light (Figure 8-9) and the tiny

FIGURE 8-10 The light cable can be checked for broken fibers by holding one end toward a bright light while looking at the other end.

FIGURE 8-11 Disposable endoscopic instruments are designed to meet procedural needs during endoscopic surgery.

fibers can be broken easily if kinked or dropped. Cables are loosely coiled, never bent, when not in use. After multiple uses, fibers can break. Cables must therefore be checked after each use. To do this, hold one end of the cable pointing toward a bright light while the opposite end is observed for light transmission (Figure 8-10). Do not test the cable by looking into the end while it is attached to the light source. The visible light and ultraviolet light produced by the light source may harm the eye if directly viewed for extended periods. "Peppering" on the light cable end indicates broken fibers. When approximately 20% of the fibers are broken, the cable is replaced because adequate light for visualization cannot be transmitted through fractured fibers.

Bulbs within the light source usually are easy to replace. Extra bulbs are stored in lamp-assembly drawers, which are readily accessible. The bulb itself is not touched because (1) it may be very hot and (2) the oils on an individual's hands and fingers can adhere to the bulb, causing the bulb to burn out more quickly. Nonmetal handles usually are built into the light source for bulb removal and replacement.

Three popular types of light sources are available today: xenon, metal halide, and halogen. Advantages and disadvantages are associated with each. Xenon bulbs are more expensive, but last longer. Xenon light is better for smaller-diameter endoscopes (≤2 mm) because the light can be focused to a smaller spot size. Xenon light also is a preferred light for video or picture taking. Metal halide bulbs have a shorter life span (about 250 hours) and are less expensive. These bulbs are easier than others to handle and replace, and do not require large fans for cooling. Halogen light sources are used for office and some hospital applications. They do not, however, offer the light intensity required for many endoscopic and video applications. Personal preference and conditions for use are two key factors in choosing an appropriate light source for endoscopy. A light source that incorporates a lamp-life status–testing mode is desirable so that bulb replacement can be anticipated.

Given that light sources produce different colors of light whenever a camera is used, *white balancing* must be performed during each procedure. White balancing adjusts the camera to all other optical components (endocoupler, light cable, laparoscope). This method enables the camera to reference white so that it can identify all primary colors properly. White balancing is performed once the scope and light cable are connected, the light source turned on, and the lens held close to a white gauze or white drape (for white color referencing).

Endoscopic Minimally Invasive Surgery Instrumentation

Endoscopic MIS instrumentation is designed to correspond with the surgical site and the technique used while functioning as an extension of the surgeon's hand. The length and working end of the instrument must be adequate to perform surgery at the target site. The hand control is ergonomically designed for the operator's maximum comfort and reduced fatigue. Graspers and other instrumentation used by the assistant in surgery often are built for a shorter hand span because many women function in this role.

Because endoscopic MIS and robotic approaches differ from traditional open equivalents, modifications of existing instruments have been made. Some basic patterns have been used for years and continue to be popular, whereas others have been designed to accommodate newer MIS and robotic approaches. This new era in surgery began in the 1990s, and some instrument designs are now in their sixth and seventh generations. As surgery becomes ever more sophisticated, so do the instruments required for successful, less-invasive techniques (Figure 8-11). MIS instrumentation is discussed in more detail in the next sections, and insufflation safety and MIS complications and considerations are addressed in Practices and Potential Risks During MIS.

Trocar System. When a natural orifice does not exist for diagnostic or operative procedures, one or several orifices are created. To do so, a trocar system is used, consisting of an obturator and a sleeve (also known as a cannula or sheath). The trocar system provides a mechanism to insert and remove instruments while MIS is performed. The obturator and sleeve are inserted to access the operative site. When the port of entry has been made, the obturator is removed, and the sleeve is left in place. More complex laparoscopic procedures may require a greater number of trocar systems and puncture sites.

If a reusable trocar system is used, the obturator tip must be sharpened routinely. The stopcock and trumpet valves are inspected before and after each use to ensure proper functioning. Internal gaskets may need occasional replacement. The obturator and sleeve must fit properly and may not always be interchangeable. Component parts are kept together, but are disassembled completely for cleaning and sterilization.

Disposable trocar systems offer several advantages (Figure 8-12). One is that the obturator is always sharp. When multiple ports of the same size are used, the same obturator is reused on the same patient. Some manufacturers also package one obturator and two

FIGURE 8-12 Disposable trocars and cannulae.

FIGURE 8-13 A close-up view of the trocar safety shield in place.

FIGURE 8-14 Blunt-tipped trocars can be used to minimize injuries during insertion.

or more sleeves of the same size. The same obturator is used to establish multiple access ports. Disposable units also may provide siliconized obturator tips and safety features when entry has been made. Systems are available that both engage a safety shield to advance automatically over the obturator tip (Figure 8-13) and provide retraction of the obturator tip when entry is made.

Many disposable sleeves have gripping devices that can reduce the risk of accidental sleeve removal during repeated advancement and withdrawal of the instruments. Grippers are incorporated into the sleeve or as separate entities. Grippers can be used with reusable sleeves as long as the fit is appropriate.

Disposable sleeves have a stopcock assembly for insufflation gas, similar to the reusable system. One-way flapper valves in disposables provide leakproof protection and operate automatically for instrument insertion, specimen removal, or rapid desufflation. Because instrument diameters vary with design and use, different sizes of obturator and sleeve units may be required for one procedure. Reusable and disposable trocar systems are available in a variety of diameters and lengths. To increase flexibility, converters and reducers are used to adapt the size of the instrument. Converters can be separate or built into the sleeve as a diaphragm seal. Both systems are designed to reduce the chance of carbon dioxide (CO_2) leaks so that the pneumoperitoneum can be maintained. Radiolucent disposable sleeves offer the ability to visualize tissue and lesions without obstruction. This feature may be crucial during an endoscopic

cholangiogram to avoid obstructing the view during fluoroscopy. During other procedures this design may not be necessary.

Radially expanding dilator systems, consisting of a cannula with blunt obturator and an insufflation/access needle with a radially expandable sleeve, have been shown to cause less traumatic abdominal wall entry and yield smaller fascial defects. Intra-abdominal entry is accomplished using an access needle with a radially expandable sleeve. When insufflation is achieved, the needle is withdrawn, leaving the expandable sleeve in place. While the sleeve and tissue are expanded, a tapered, blunt-tipped dilator is inserted, providing a large working channel for an access port. Because a sharp-tipped obturator is not used, the muscles are spread, not cut, and the risk of abdominal wall or vascular damage is minimized. Bladeless obturators, which separate tissue in a sequential fashion rather than cut or stretch tissue, also are available in an optical version that allows the surgeon to visualize all tissue layers being separated.

Occasionally a procedure is scheduled as an *open laparoscopy.* Patients who have had multiple surgeries or who have developed adhesions, and pediatric patients, can present an added risk and may be candidates for open laparoscopy. A small paraumbilical incision is made and tissues dissected. The peritoneum is opened and a large blunt-tipped obturator-sleeve assembly is inserted (Figure 8-14). The sleeve is designed to fit snugly against the peritoneum from underneath and against the skin from above. Stay sutures are used to close any excess incision. Wafer seals reduce further loss of CO_2 gas. Pneumoperitoneum is then created and maintained. If a reusable system is used, stay sutures also are used to stabilize the system. Sealed system devices have been developed to introduce not only instrumentation but also the surgeon's hand when direct surgical approaches are necessary during laparoscopy.

When extracorporeal surgery is performed during laparoscopy (i.e., when tissue undergoing surgery is brought outside the body through a small hole), a larger diameter port is used. During certain bowel resections, loops of bowel are brought through a larger port to be resected or sutured. When the chest is entered, shorter blunt obturators are used with grippers that provide stabilization while in the pleural cavity. This type of obturator does not have insufflation ports (Figure 8-15). If insufflation is required to assist the anesthesia provider in collapsing the lung, regular obturators with insufflation ports are used.

Single-incision laparoscopic surgery (SILS), in which the surgeon operates through a single entry port, usually the umbilical area, leaves only a single small scar (Patient-Centered Care). There are

FIGURE 8-15 Thoracic blunt trocar and gripper assembly. Notice absence of stopcock insufflation capability.

FIGURE 8-16 Single entry access platform that facilitates triangulation of laparoscopy instruments.

PATIENT-CENTERED CARE

Promoting patient (and family engagement) is in the interest of perioperative patient care and it is becoming an expectation in healthcare settings as well. Two simple and straightforward tenets of patient-center care are empowerment and health literacy. As this model for care becomes more powerful, perioperative nurses are increasingly interested in soliciting and sharing patient perspectives, asking questions, offering information, and inviting the patient to express confusion or misunderstandings. For a patient scheduled for a single-incision laparoscopic surgery (SILS) procedure, an invitational introduction by the perioperative nurse might go like this:

"Today I will be the nurse taking care of you during your surgical procedure. I see you have signed a consent form for Dr. Brown to perform a *single port access laparoscopic procedure for a hysterectomy*. I know those words can be very confusing. Can you tell me in your own words what this means? I want to answer any questions you may have about this procedure."

single port platforms that provide an airtight fulcrum that assists with access and the triangulation of standard or articulating instrumentation (Figure 8-16). Single port laparoscopy is associated with minimal postoperative pain and scarring. Advancements in this type of laparoscopic technique have been made not only in adult but also pediatric laparoscopy (Research Highlight).

Dissecting Instruments. Dissecting instruments are used to cut, divide, or separate tissue. Scissors and dissectors that are similar to their open-procedure counterparts have been designed for use in MIS procedures.

Scissors are available for blunt or sharp dissection. They can be straight or curved (including hook scissors), depending on the location of the target tissue and technique used (Figure 8-17). Scissors usually have a rounded tip when closed so that they also can be used to manipulate tissue without trauma. When open, both blades of the scissors should be visualized to prevent inadvertent injury. Some scissors are designed to be connected to an electrosurgical energy source so that coagulation can be provided during cutting.

Dissectors are used to separate or divide tissue. Many different tip shapes are available to dissect, spread, divide, grasp, retract, and coagulate structures (Figure 8-18). Other dissecting instruments, such as balloon dissectors, have been developed for blunt dissection

RESEARCH HIGHLIGHT

Single Incision Laparoscopic Surgery

Single-incision laparoscopic surgery (SILS) has become more widespread as industry has introduced instrumentation and devices to facilitate this technique. In adults, procedures accomplished via a single incision include a wide variety of specialties and procedures such as cholecystectomy, hernia repair, hysterectomy, oophorectomy, and bariatric weight loss surgery. In this research, a mini-series study was conducted on the use of SILS to treat correctable biliary atresia (BA) in pediatric patients. Four correctable BA patients were included. The study authors reviewed operative time, patient age, postoperative length of hospital stay, resumption of full diet, postoperative complications, and perioperative laboratory tests. Different postoperative tests, such as ultrasonography, upper GI contrast studies, and blood analyses, were performed as follow-up. Importantly, results revealed that median operative time was 2 hours and blood loss was minimal. No mortality or surgical complications were evident, leading the authors to conclude that SILS for treatment of correctable biliary atresia is safe and effective when performed by an experienced surgeon.

Modified from Mei Diao et al: Initial experience of single-incision laparoscopic hepaticojejunostomy using conventional instruments for correctable biliary atresia, *J Laparoendosc Adv Surg Tech* 22(6):615–620, 2012.

or creation of a space so that surgery can be performed. A balloon dissector may be used to create a preperitoneal space during laparoscopic herniorrhaphy (Figure 8-19).

Clamping and Grasping Instruments. Clamping instruments are used to grasp and hold tissue or other materials. Ratchets are used in the instrument design to allow the distal tip to be locked onto the tissue being grasped. Graspers, forceps, and biopsy forceps are classified as clamping instruments.

Graspers and forceps can be (1) traumatic, with sharp teeth, or (2) atraumatic, with a smooth, serrated jaw surface (Figure 8-20). Traumatic graspers and forceps customarily are used to hold tissue that will be excised, whereas the atraumatic versions are used to gently hold structures, such as the bowel or liver. Some clamping instruments are insulated so that electrosurgical energy can be transmitted to provide coagulation.

FIGURE 8-17 Straight and curved endoscopic scissors.

FIGURE 8-18 Dissector with jaws open to divide and separate tissue.

FIGURE 8-19 Balloon dissecting instrument.

Suturing and Stapling Instruments. Suturing or stapling instruments deliver sutures, staples, or clips to join, hold, and secure tissue. Needle holders, clip appliers, and staplers are in this category.

Needle holders are designed to deliver and place sutures within body cavities during MIS procedures. Tungsten carbide jaw inserts on needle holders are used to prevent rotation of the suture needle.

FIGURE 8-20 Endoscopic grasping instruments.

FIGURE 8-21 Endoscopic needle holder that transfers the needle from one prong of the jaw to the other.

These inserts can be replaced when they become worn. Some needle holders are designed to transfer the needle from one jaw to the other during suturing (Figure 8-21). Suture passers and curved needle holders also are available.

A clip applier is used to provide hemostasis and tissue security. Its use represents the safest, easiest, and quickest way to occlude small vessels and structures. Reusable appliers exist, but many must be removed from the cannula each time to be reloaded. This process adds time, contributes to loss of pneumoperitoneum (if used), and causes frustration when the clip is dislodged on reinsertion. For this reason, automatic-feed, reloadable, disposable versions are more desirable (Figure 8-22).

Staplers provide cutting and stapling during MIS resections (Figures 8-23 and 8-24). Certain structures can be easily resected intracorporeally (i.e., within the abdominal cavity), such as the ovary or appendix. Others may necessitate extracorporeal resection (outside the body) or reanastomosis; if this is necessary, traditional stapling devices are used.

FIGURE 8-22 Disposable endoscopic rotating clip applier.

FIGURE 8-23 Disposable linear cutter with reloading unit.

FIGURE 8-24 Disposable endoscopic stapling device.

The evolution of more complex MIS techniques has challenged traditional suturing and ligation methods. As a result, several devices and techniques have been developed for laparoscopic tissue suturing. When surgical clips and staples cannot be used, a laparoscopic suture may be substituted. Conditions that preclude the use of clips include large arteries and edematous or inflamed ducts. Most general surgeons prefer to use nonabsorbable sutures and ligation materials to prevent rapid absorption. Three basic types of laparoscopic suturing materials are *loop ligatures, extracorporeal sutures,* and *intracorporeal sutures.*

Loop Ligatures. Preknotted suture loops (loop ligatures) are used to ligate pedicle tissues. The suture loop is packaged with an introducer sleeve, which is inserted through one of the obturator sheaths. The loop is passed over the target tissue or pedicle using a grasping forceps to assist. When the loop is in position, the existing suture knot is pushed down the introducer sleeve until it is cinched tightly around the tissue. The suture is cut with endoscopic scissors (Figure 8-25).

Extracorporeal Sutures. Tissue can be approximated intra-abdominally when the knot is tied extracorporeally (i.e., outside the body). To accomplish this, endoscopic swaged sutures are used. The suture is grasped proximally to the needle, and both are inserted through one of the obturator sleeves into the abdomen. The needle is held with the grasper or laparoscopic needle holder and driven through the desired tissue. A second grasper or needle holder inserted through a second obturator sleeve is used to assist. The needled end of the suture is pulled through the tissue and out through the sleeve. The needle is removed, and a knot tied extracorporeally. The knot is advanced down the sleeve and onto the tissue. The suture is cut with laparoscopic scissors (Figure 8-26). The three types of knots tied extracorporeally are the *slip knot,* the *fisherman's knot,* and the *surgeon's knot.*

Intracorporeal Sutures. A suture ligature also can be passed through the obturator sleeve to be tied while it is inside the body. The tissue is approximated in the same fashion but tied intracorporeally (i.e., inside the abdomen) using grasping forceps or laparoscopic needle holders.

Retractors and Accessory Instruments. Retractors are used to hold tissue and expose the operative target site (Figure 8-27). Retractors can be traumatic to some structures, such as the bowel and liver, and are used with caution. Mini-retractors and balloon retractors have been designed for use on delicate structures. A miniature version of a surgical clamp with blades that splay the incision open beneath the tissue is available. Other accessory instruments have been designed to enhance the use of basic MIS instruments, provide exposure, and facilitate the procedure. Probes used to manipulate tissue are blunt to minimize tissue trauma. Some probes have centimeter gradations to measure structures within the body. Irrigation-aspirator probes enhance visualization of internal structures, and electrosurgical probes provide hemostasis. Endoscopic specimen bags contain specimens in order to minimize cross-contamination. Special accessory instruments are continually being designed to enhance MIS procedures.

Care and Handling of Endoscopes and Instrumentation. Endoscopes and instruments must be clean and free from all bioburden (contaminating organisms) before sterilization or high-level disinfection. During routine use, bioburden accumulates in channels, ports, crevices, and other movable parts of scopes and instruments. Periodically throughout the procedure, gross blood and bioburden must be removed by flushing the channels and wiping the surfaces with sterile water. Saline is never used routinely to remove gross debris during the procedure because this salt solution can leave mineral deposits on or in the device. Keeping instruments and endoscopes relatively clean during the procedure helps prevent debris from drying, thus facilitating the cleaning process and protecting the instrument.

After each procedure all instruments and devices are decontaminated thoroughly. Immersible equipment is cleaned or flushed with an enzymatic or other appropriate detergent solution; this loosens organic material and makes it easier to remove. Instruments that can withstand cavitation or ultrasonic cleaning (processes whereby high-frequency energy causes microscopic bubbles to assist with

FIGURE 8-25 Surgitie ligating loop. **A,** Back-load loop into introducer completely. **B,** Insert introducer into trocar, all the way down. **C,** Push suture loop through introducer. Grasp desired tissue with grasping forceps (passed through another trocar), and maneuver loop over tissue. **D,** Push down knot by advancing nylon carrier all the way until knot is cinched. Cut suture.

debris removal) can be placed in an ultrasonic device. Fiberoptics and endoscopes usually cannot be placed in an ultrasonic machine because the vibratory motion can damage tiny fiberoptic bundles.

Selection of appropriate cleaning solution or detergent is critical. Detergents consist of various formulations that may include pH builders, buffers, surfactants, and chelants that provide the chemical compositions that clean devices. The amount of cleaning power within a solution is determined by the pH of the formulation. The "potential for hydrogen" is the meaning of pH, which represents the degree of acidity (more hydrogen ions present), neutrality (equal hydrogen and hydroxyl ions), and alkalinity (more hydroxyl ions present). A detergent with a very low pH can cause staining and pitting on the surfaces of stainless steel instruments because they are more susceptible to damage during prolonged exposure of acidic solutions. When detergents are combined with the mechanical or automatic force of a cleaning spray, removal of bioburden is easier.

A low-sudsing detergent is recommended so that the detergent can be completely removed. Cleaning solutions with surfactant are less desirable because they are more difficult to rinse. If surfactant is left on the surface, the device may feel sticky or gummy, which could affect the electrical conductivity of the instrument. Careful attention is paid to the solution used as well as the type of device being cleaned. Certain detergents are not appropriate for cleaning both endoscopes and endoscopic instruments.

Careful rinsing and flushing with copious amounts of water follows the cleaning process. Often deionized or demineralized water is recommended for the final rinse to minimize mineral buildup from tap water. The manufacturer's written recommendations for cleaning and processing always should be followed. After the final rinse, instruments are be dried before disinfection or sterilization.

Automatic cleaning devices that flush the ports of instruments provide an economic and effective way to clean reusable channeled instruments (Figure 8-28). Although instruments have flush ports, debris can become lodged distally. Some automatic systems provide a means to flush in a retrograde fashion, forcing debris from the larger proximal port. Sealed instruments also can be tested for seal integrity using this system.

After the device has been thoroughly cleaned, rinsed, and dried, its integrity and functionality are assessed. Personnel involved with reprocessing MIS devices must be aware of instrument composition, design, and use. Any device with electrosurgical capabilities is checked to ensure that the length of the insulation sheath has not been compromised. Equipment is available that scans these instruments for electrical leakage through breaks in insulation.

Often new MIS accessories are purchased and used without educating the staff responsible for their reprocessing. Staff members cannot understand design and use of a device without proper

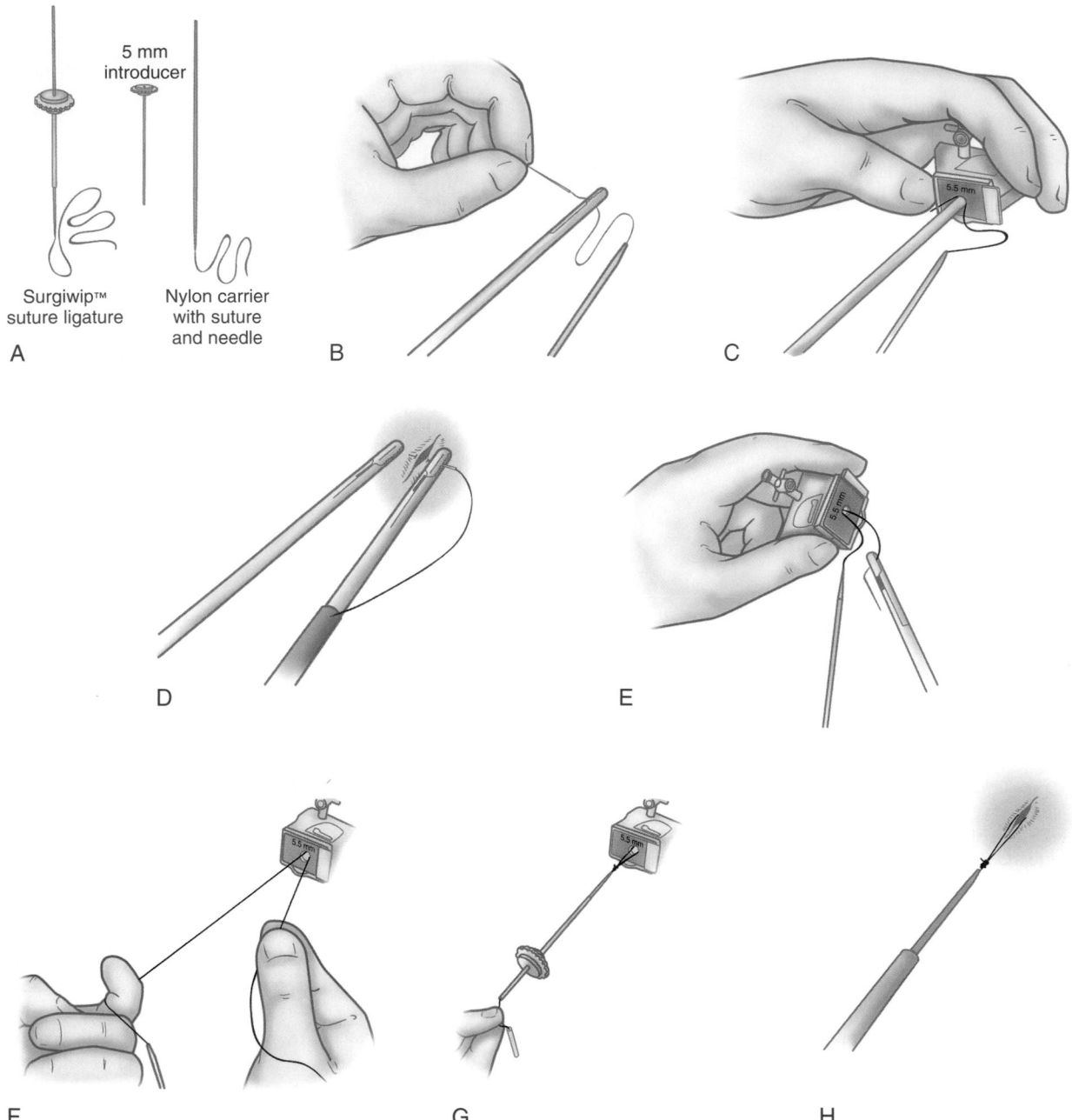

FIGURE 8-26 Surgiwip suture ligature application for approximating tissue intra-abdominally by extracorporeal knot tying (outside body). **A,** Component pieces. **B,** Grasp suture behind swage of needle with tissue grasper or needle holder. **C,** Introduce grasper or needle holder and suture through trocar into abdomen. **D,** Drive needle through tissue to be approximated. Place instrument close to center of needle for control. Pull needle through tissue using second grasper (introduced through another trocar). **E,** Regrasp needle behind swage intracorporeally, and pull it through and out the same trocar. (Allow for slack of suture to avoid tissue tears.) **F,** Remove needle. Tie knot. **G,** After knot is tied, break end of nylon carrier. **H,** Push knot down with nylon carrier and out onto tissue. Cut suture. For additional suturing, repeat steps **B** through **H** until tissue is satisfactorily approximated.

instruction. The U.S. Food and Drug Administration (FDA) requires that any device purchased as reusable must have written instructions for reprocessing. Staff must understand how the instrument works to ensure that functionality of the device has not changed during reprocessing. Compliance with federal, professional, and regional standards for reprocessing is mandatory.

Instruments and devices that contact sterile tissues and the vascular system must be sterile. Instruments contacting intact mucous membranes can be processed using high-level disinfection (Figure 8-29). This means that sterility is required for all laparoscopy, angioscopy, thoracoscopy, and arthroscopy procedures. High-level (cold-soak) disinfection may be acceptable for colonoscopy, laryngoscopy, bronchoscopy, cystoscopy, and other diagnostic procedures in which surgical devices touch intact mucous membranes. Invasive procedures that access the vascular system (biopsies) are performed during many endoscopy procedures. The adequacy of high-level

FIGURE 8-27 Endoscopic fan retractor with five fingers.

FIGURE 8-28 Endoscope lumen instrument cleaner used by a reprocessing company.

FIGURE 8-29 High-level disinfection reprocessor that handles two scopes at one time.

rises to approximately 0.4 ppm, which is double the recommended maximum exposure level. The odor of glutaraldehyde becomes an irritant at 0.3 ppm, causing tearing, nausea, and other effects. Hooded systems to house glutaraldehyde solutions are designed to remove odor and fumes. When using this or any other chemical germicide, the device must be totally immersed and soaked for the specified contact time, following the manufacturer's recommendations for cleaning protocols, preparing the solution, maintaining contact time, and calculating expiration dates. Other solutions are available for high-level disinfection without the hazards that glutaraldehyde presents.

Institutional policy sets the guidelines from which practitioners work. Insight and coordination are required to provide comparable levels of care when there are too few instruments for the number of scheduled procedures. If sterile instruments are required for a particular procedure, they should be used for all patients undergoing that procedure. Sufficient instruments, accessory items, and equipment must be purchased to accommodate patient volume, or other reprocessing measures must be implemented.

When sterile devices and instruments are needed, multiple options for sterilization include steam, ethylene oxide, gas-plasma, peracetic acid, and ozone sterilization methods (Association of periOperative Registered Nurses [AORN], 2013). Often steam cannot be used on delicate endoscopes, but accessory instruments may withstand the heat produced during steam sterilization. Some arthroscopes and laparoscopes have been designed to withstand high temperatures of steam sterilization. For items that cannot withstand high temperatures, options include the following (see Chapter 4 for a more thorough discussion):

- *Ethylene oxide sterilization*—This process has been used for many years to sterilize endoscopes and instruments. Past decisions to

disinfection must be evaluated for these procedures. Viruses and microorganisms, such as human immunodeficiency virus (HIV), hepatitis B and C viruses, *Mycobacterium* (tuberculosis bacteria), and antibiotic-resistant organisms, are not easily destroyed during high-level disinfection. Even though high-level disinfection has been the accepted primary standard of reprocessing for some endoscopic instrumentation, the concern over viruses and microorganisms has caused debate about the adequacy of using high-level disinfection. Therefore, sterilization is quickly becoming the standard for reprocessing endoscopes and endoscopic instruments.

Thermal pasteurization, using a washer/pasteurizer, may be chosen for thermal high-level disinfection. An FDA-approved chemical germicide is selected for chemical high-level disinfection. Glutaraldehyde, used for many years, has hazards for staff that must be considered when this agent is selected for high-level disinfection. The maximum recommended exposure level of glutaraldehyde determined by the Occupational Safety and Health Administration (OSHA) is 0.2 parts per million (ppm). When solution is being poured after mixing or when devices are being submerged, the level eliminate agents that were combined with ethylene oxide to decrease flammability, such as chlorofluorocarbon (CFC) and halogenated CFC (HCFC), have led to the use of 100% ethylene oxide for safe and effective sterilization. Limitations of ethylene oxide sterilization are the prolonged time needed for aeration of ethylene oxide and the installation and monitoring requirements for this type of sterilizer.

• *Plasma sterilization system*—This system uses hydrogen peroxide gas plasma, which sterilizes within 24 to 75 minutes (depending on the system) and dissociates into nontoxic byproducts. Understanding the advantages and limitations (e.g., lumen restrictions) of this system is important when determining if it would meet the needs of endoscope or instrument sterilization.

• *Liquid chemical sterilization*—Powerful chemicals, such as 35% peracetic acid, can provide sterilization for cleaned, immersible, reusable, and heat-sensitive devices. The pH-neutral chemical solution eliminates all microbial life and then can be safely rinsed down the drain. The use-dilution is gentle on delicate surgical instruments, including flexible endoscopes with multiple channels.

• *Ozone sterilizer*—Oxygen is used in a natural process to produce ozone. When oxygen is exposed to an intense electrical field, the oxygen molecule separates into atomic oxygen (O). Atomic oxygen combines with other oxygen molecules (O_2) to create triatomic oxygen (O_3), which is ozone. Ozone reverts quickly back to its oxygen state while producing no toxic residuals. Ozone is a powerful sterilizing agent because it oxidizes organic matter (fungi, bacterial spores, viruses). Key features of ozone sterilization include ease of use, low-temperature sterilization, cost-effectiveness, and compatibility with anodized aluminum containers. The manufacturer's instructions must be followed regarding operation of the sterilizer, instrument and device preparation, and device limitations.

Single-Use Versus Reusable Instrumentation. Many facilities use a combination of reusable and single-use laparoscopic instruments. Advantages of single-use items include sharpness, reliability related to function, guaranteed sterility, and safety. Indirect advantages include no reprocessing, no repair costs, and comparable levels of patient care. Upgraded designs are more easily brought to market when the device is labeled for single use. Disadvantages include the need for increased storage space, budgetary implications, and environmental concerns related to disposal of biohazardous waste.

Advantages of reusable instruments include less storage space, reduced costs (except for initial purchase and repair), and minimal waste. With reusable instruments, decontamination and reprocessing systems must be reliable, compatible with the devices being processed, and monitored for effectiveness.

Above all, safe and effective patient outcomes should be the major criteria considered when comparing single-use with reusable instrumentation. Advantages and disadvantages of reusable versus single-use devices must be explored, using a risk-to-benefit analysis, before purchasing decisions can be made. Institutional policy may dictate whether reusable or single-use items are chosen. The choice between single-use and reusable instrumentation and equipment must be evaluated thoroughly in each individual practice setting and justified accordingly.

Reprocessing Single-Use Devices (SUDs). Reprocessing SUDs is a practice that has grown in acceptance. In the United States the practice of reprocessing SUDs is highly regulated by the FDA. The

first FDA guidance document was published in 2000. The document was updated and published in 2006, titled *Guidance for Industry and FDA Staff: Medical Device User Fee and Modernization Act of 2002, Validation Data in Premarket Notification Submissions (510[k]s) for Reprocessed Single-use Medical Devices* (FDA, 2006). The document outlines regulatory requirements, enforceable by the FDA, for reprocessing previously used SUDs. The FDA continues to provide prescriptive guidelines to control this industry. In 2008 the Government Accounting Office (GAO) published a document stating that there was no elevated risk with reprocessing SUDs (GAO, 2008).

A "reprocessor" is usually a third-party reprocessing company that reprocesses single-use devices. Hospitals rarely pursue the challenges of becoming listed as a reprocessor, given the expense involved with this activity. Reprocessing organizations are considered manufacturers, are subject to the same regulatory requirements as the original device manufacturer, and must comply with the original 2000 document guidelines (FDA, 2000):

1. *Registration and listing with the FDA*—Any organization reprocessing single-use devices must register with the FDA and provide a comprehensive list of all single-use medical devices that it reprocesses.

2. *Medical device reporting (MDR)*—Any organization reprocessing single-use devices must comply with the FDA's manufacturer reporting requirements and report not only all patient injuries from device malfunctions or failures but also any event that could have led to patient injury or death.

3. *Device tracking*—The FDA can issue a tracking order for any specific device, if applicable. These devices are typically high-risk, class III medical devices, such as implants. Reprocessing companies usually refrain from reprocessing class III devices.

4. *Corrections and removals*—Every reprocessor must have a formal procedure in place to recall or correct affected devices.

5. *Quality system regulation (QSR)*—Every reprocessor must develop and maintain comprehensive quality system controls that comply with the FDA's requirements for all aspects of their reprocessing operation.

6. *Labeling requirements*—Every reprocessor must provide instructions-for-use documents (IFUs) with reprocessed medical devices and must comply with specific requirements for what appears on the device label. Any reprocessed single-use device must be labeled "prominently and conspicuously," with the following statement: "Reprocessed device for single use. Reprocessed by (name of manufacturer that reprocessed the device)."

7. *FDA premarket submission of a premarket notification (510[k]) or premarket approval (PMA)*—Every reprocessor is required to register each device to be reprocessed by submitting a 510(k) or PMA. The specific FDA requirements for the regulation of devices are based on the criticality (critical, semicritical, or noncritical) and the risk category/class of the device.

Reprocessors also repackage and resterilize items with an expired shelf life date or when sterility of the outer packaging has been compromised. Single-use devices that are reprocessed are segregated into two categories for reprocessing: *open/not used* and *open/used*. The devices that have been used are grossly decontaminated before they are sent for reprocessing. If devices are not grossly decontaminated, they are collected in approved containers and transported by a licensed biohazardous material hauler using appropriate packaging materials and labeling.

Liability is an important concern for those engaged in reprocessing single-use items. A hospital or surgery center may be liable if

FIGURE 8-30 Single-use device is carefully sharpened during reprocessing at a third-party company.

reprocessing occurs within the confines of the facility. If a third-party company provides this service, it may likewise be liable and must document liability insurance coverage for this service. Although the original manufacturer of a device warrants a disposable product for one use, a reprocessing company also warrants the reprocessed device for one additional use.

Questions to ask when determining whether to reprocess SUDs include the following:

- Can the disposable device be adequately cleaned?
- Can the device withstand disinfection or sterilization? Can it be adequately aerated if ethylene oxide sterilization is used?
- Is the device tested and checked for proper form and function after cleaning has been completed?
- Has device integrity been destroyed during reprocessing or is equipment available to test the integrity of the device? How is the integrity of insulation checked on an electrosurgical instrument?
- Can the device be returned to its original intended use (Figure 8-30)?
- Will cost savings be passed on to the patient, if appropriate?
- What is the maximum number of safe reuses, as determined through comprehensive testing? How is the number of reuses indicated on the device?
- Should the patient be informed that a reprocessed device may be used? The FDA does not require informed consent for the use of reprocessed SUDs. Many providers contend that because reprocessing is so highly regulated and the risk of using a reprocessed device is the same as using the device for the first time, there is no need to seek informed consent.

No matter where reprocessing is performed, appropriate equipment must be available to ensure that the form and function of the device have not been compromised. Customers should inquire about reprocessing and quality assurance practices if dealing with a third-party reprocessor. Usually these companies have appropriate equipment to perform comprehensive device and validation testing. They must register with the FDA and comply with the QSR (FDA,

2000). Reprocessors should provide documentation of FDA registration, any reports of FDA inspection, such as an establishment inspection report (EIR), FDA warning letters, all-important 510(k) or PMA documentation, and the limited number of uses for each specific device.

The practice of reprocessing SUDs continues to grow in popularity as significant cost savings are realized by all sizes and types of healthcare facilities. Surgical team members must work closely with their purchasing agent, infection control officer, financial administrator, and others to decide if reprocessing SUDs is an appropriate option for their facility.

Video Technology

Evolution of Video Technology

A basic standard medical video system includes the scope, light cable, light source, camera head, camera cord, camera-scope coupler, camera control unit, and video monitor. Additional peripheral equipment is necessary for specific surgical procedures and is discussed later. Given the complexity of video technology, a glossary of terms is provided in Box 8-1.

Setting up a video system in surgery begins with the image source—the camera. A camera control unit (CCU) is needed to convert the image signal from the camera into viewable format. The monitor is then connected as the display device that shows the image signal. Options can be added to this setup to record the surgical procedure or to take still images. The image recorder and/or printer is positioned before the display device.

Video systems use light energy from a source, convert it into electrical energy, and then convert it back into light energy to provide pictures. The camera head contains a sensor, which is light sensitive. The sensor may be a solid-state unit or chip, called a *charge-coupled device (CCD),* which produces the unprocessed video signal, or the sensor may be a high-definition (HD) system.

The CCD is composed of small picture elements called *pixels,* which in the presence of light are conductive and in the absence of light remain nonconductive. Each pixel can sense red, blue, or green light. The picture is transformed into a matrix made up of the conductive and nonconductive pixels. This matrix will scan at an extremely rapid rate that generates the signal frequency.

The National Television Standards Committee (NTSC) sets the standard analog video format in the United States, Canada, Japan, and most of South America and Asia. It was established for broadcast purposes. Even though the NTSC format has been used for more than 50 years, most transmissions in the United States were replaced with the Advanced Television Systems Committee (ATSC) format in 2009, and by August 31, 2011, the ATSC format began to be used in Canada.

The three most commonly used video formats are S-Video, HD-SDI, and Digital Visual Interface (DVI). S-Video is short for Super-Video and is a technology used for analog video signals. The information of S-Video is divided into two separate signals, one for color (chroma) and one for luminance (brightness), and carries standard definition video. Standard definition displays 720 lines vertically (side to side) and 480 lines horizontally (from top to bottom). This is usually designated as 720 × 480 resolution, which produces 345,600 pixels. An S-Video cable is needed to support this transmission.

For medical imaging, the two most widely used systems are High-Definition Serial Digital Interface (HD-SDI) and DVI. The HD-SDI system was engineered for the highest picture quality (and

---

BOX 8-1

Video Glossary

Autoexposure: An electronic circuit built into cameras to eliminate electronically (within the camera) excess light from the picture; sometimes referred to as electronic shutter.

Automatic gain control: Ability to increase or decrease video output levels depending on the average light level of the viewed object.

Blooming: A glaring effect on the monitor caused by excessive light.

Boost: The ability to increase the signal strength of the camera. When used under low light conditions, boost provides increased sensitivity.

CCD: Charge-coupled device.

CCU: Camera control unit.

Chroma: Saturation of a color.

Chromiance: Defines the video camera's ability to handle the color red, the most difficult color to reproduce. The more accurate the color reproduction, the higher the chromiance.

C-mount: Standard thread size and diameter for a standard video camera lens.

Color bars: A test pattern used to adjust controls on the monitor for color, brightness, and contrast.

Color reproduction: Ability of an imaging device to reproduce colors exactly as the human eye perceives them.

Composite video output: Most commonly used video signal; the typical television video signal.

DICOM: Digital Imaging and Communications in Medicine; format for images in healthcare.

DVI: Digital Visual Interface, a popular system for medical imaging.

Electronic shutter: Ability of a camera to freeze image information within fractions of a second (1/60, 1/125, 1/1000, 1/10,000).

Foot-candle: Standard measure of luminance; the amount of light emitted by a standard candle at a distance of 1 foot from the flame; 10 luxes equals 1 foot-candle.

HD-SDI: High-Definition Serial Digital Interface; a popular medical imaging system.

High-definition television (HDTV): A digital broadcasting system with higher resolution capabilities than traditional television systems, such as standard-definition TV (SDTV). Less bandwidth is needed for transmission because of digital video compression.

Light gain: Another circuit within the camera that amplifies the picture electronically to show a brighter image; sometimes referred to as automatic gain control (AGC), or boost circuit.

Luminance: Intensity or effectiveness of a given light on the eye.

NTSC: National Television Standards Committee; also a designation for a television signal used in the United States.

Orientation: A mark or ridge on the camera head to orient the top portion of the video monitor.

PACS: Picture Archiving Communication System.

Pixel: A signal-sensor element on a solid-state video chip; most solid-state chips used in medical videography have about 400,000 pixels on their surface. Each pixel is light-sensitive and sees its own small part of the total picture.

Resolution: An optical device's ability to separate fine detail; usually expressed in TV lines. Resolution traditionally is measured by aiming the camera at a target chart with squares of fine lines. The maximum resolution of the optical device is determined at the point where it begins to blur the lines together. If a box showing 400 lines per inch is still clear with spaces between the lines, the optical device has at least 400 lines-per-inch resolution.

Sensitivity: The response to low light levels by a video system.

S-Video: Super-Video, used to designate analog video signals.

S-VHS output: Super-Video Home System (Japan Victor Co.), a signal from the camera that splits the chroma and luminance, allowing for a richer resolution recording.

White balance: Different light sources produce different temperatures of light and different colors of light. White balancing is an adjustment of the camera for various sources of light.

---

is most widely used for endoscopic systems), whereas DVI was engineered for copy-protected distribution.

HD systems that produce ultrasharp images with increased levels of contrast have replaced many standard analog video systems. HD systems offer picture quality almost equivalent to what one experiences with the naked eye.

An HD video system refers to a system that has higher resolution (greater numbers of lines of resolution) than with the standard-definition analog systems. The HD visual image is much sharper because gaps between the scan lines are either narrower or invisible to the naked eye. This improvement is most evident with larger screens, but on smaller screens there is no noticeable improvement in picture quality. With a higher number of pixels, as compared to the old standard analog video signal, HD results in a much clearer picture, with higher quality and greater detail.

Vertical lines are also described with a lowercase "i," meaning interlaced, or lowercase "p," meaning progressive (which also describes the picture refreshment rate). An interlaced scanning format divides the 1080 lines of resolution into pairs, with the first 540 alternate lines on one frame, then another 540 lines on a second frame. The progressive scanning method displays all 1080 lines simultaneously on every frame, which then requires a greater bandwidth. Today's highest achievable resolution is 1920 × 1080p. HD video systems that use 1080i resolution are appropriate for

endoscopy because this procedure targets small areas and uses slow-moving videos.

Visualization Systems

Endoscopes are used to offer visualization only to the operating physician. The introduction of the teaching arm provided direct visualization not only for the physician but also for the assistant, perioperative nurse, and other surgical team members. Often, however, images seen through the teaching arm were not identical to the images seen through the primary optics. The inability to interact effectively with the physician or to anticipate surgical needs was frustrating and time-consuming.

In the late 1960s and early 1970s, medical video and still cameras were continually being introduced to the marketplace; this allowed for still photography and video documentation of select surgical procedures. Tube-style cameras were large, bulky, and heavy—inadequately meeting the video needs of surgery. Video technology rapidly changed with the introduction of the chip TV camera. Its lightweight, low-profile design triggered the era of video-guided surgery. Cameras that previously weighed several pounds now weigh only a few ounces (Figure 8-31).

Rapid developments in video imaging resulted in higher-resolution monitors. Today's integrated video systems provide increased visual capabilities. This leads to enhanced participation by

FIGURE 8-31 Evolution of medical video cameras.

assistants and promotes accurate assessment and planning by perioperative staff. Video technology has evolved to the point of being almost mandatory during MIS procedures. All surgical disciplines have been enhanced by the availability and capability of video systems.

Camera, Cable, and Control Unit. The video camera represents the beginning of the optical-electronic chain of the video system. The camera cable transfers the signal frequency from the camera to a camera control unit (processor), which modifies the signal and then transmits the image to a video monitor, recorder, or hard copy picture, or all three. The camera, being the first in the video chain, is the most important component of the video system. Camera options vary widely according to available technology, specialty, and personal preference.

Cameras have either one or three CCD chips. Three-chip cameras provide enhanced color and image quality, but are larger, can cost three times that of a single-chip camera, and are not as light sensitive. Color and the resulting image are enhanced because each chip is dedicated to one of the primary colors—red, green, or blue. For this reason three-chip cameras are often used with microscopes when higher magnification requires increased resolution.

Newer single-chip cameras are available with digital processing in their control units, which boosts resolution. In essence, this technology incorporates three-chip quality in a single chip. Although signal processing in the control unit may be digital, the video output from most cameras is still an analog signal.

Digital processing refers to the way information is delivered through the various components of the control unit. This processing format allows for image enhancement and manipulation of the video image. It also allows multiple video signals to be shown on one monitor and has electronic zoom capability. Digital processing also provides the user with freeze-frame capability when using video printers and when using picture-in-picture systems.

Most cameras also feature the ability to adjust to changes in light intensity while in use. This adjustment is done by an automatic shutter (iris), which measures the availability of light and adjusts accordingly. Automatic shutter activation also helps reduce glare from light reflected off instruments and moist viscera. The ability for continuous variable shutter speeds (rather than discrete speeds) allows for instruments to be brought into the field without glare, while still maintaining adequate illumination of background objects. The shutter's response should be rapid, without perceptible stepping of image intensity.

Camera heads have buttons to control certain functions, such as white balancing; light-sensitivity boosting (ability to provide a

FIGURE 8-32 Microdigital I RGB color video camera with fingertip control.

FIGURE 8-33 Camera control unit.

brighter picture when the image requires more light, especially when a scope less than 3 mm is used during sinusoscopy); starting and stopping the recorder; and taking hard copy prints. The surgeon controls these functions at the camera head instead of requesting the circulating nurse to do so each time at the recording device or with a remote; therefore, the surgeon also has the ability to capture events exactly as and when they occur (Figure 8-32).

White balancing is performed by turning on the light source, holding the camera about 2 inches away from a white surface, and pressing the white balance button, usually found on the camera head or camera control unit. By sensing pure white, the primary colors of red, green, and blue are controlled so that a white image is created without a visible tint or color cast.

All cameras have focusing capability at the camera-coupler interface. Some also have zoom capability, allowing for closer visualization of specific structures or pathologic conditions. A camera cable connects the camera head to the camera control unit (Figure 8-33). Most camera malfunctions are cable related, not camera related. For this reason a system that provides field-replaceable cables is optimum (Figure 8-34). If wires in the cable break, a new cable can be quickly exchanged, reducing downtime from having to ship the camera and cable for repair. Because wires in the flexible cable can break, the cable must be handled with care. Cables should never be twisted, crimped, or kinked. They also must be long enough to allow sufficient space between the sterile field and the visualization system.

Couplers (Adapters). Endocouplers are optical coupling devices used to connect cameras to various endoscopes. They are usually available in 22- to 35-mm focal lengths, with different optical magnifications.

FIGURE 8-36 This camera can be directly attached to the endoscope for viewing on the monitor.

FIGURE 8-34 Camera and field-replaceable cable. *1,* Camera head; *2,* O-ring; *3,* knurled ring; *4,* cable connector; *5,* replaceable cable; *6,* camera connector; *7,* soak cap.

FIGURE 8-37 The camera adapter with a beam splitter allows the physician to look through the eyepiece while others view the procedure on the monitor.

FIGURE 8-35 This camera adapter provides a direct link from the camera to the monitor when eyepiece viewing is not desired.

The specific coupler required depends on the surgery or diagnostic procedure to be performed and endoscope to be used. When the surgeon will view only on a monitor, a direct-link coupler between the telescope and camera head is required (Figures 8-35 and 8-36). For the surgeon to look directly through the endoscope and have monitor-viewing capability, a beam-splitter coupler is necessary (Figure 8-37). Beam splitters often are used with flexible endoscopes. There are rotating beam splitters designed for the surgeon who operates in a sitting position. Zoom couplers provide variable focal lengths, with ranges from 18 to 50 mm.

A videoscope is a camera-to-scope connection designed without using a coupler (Figure 8-38). As a coupler adds one more link to the chain, coupler connections can cause loss of light and lens fogging. Connecting the camera and scope with a screw-in design instead of a coupler clamp achieves a tighter fit. This design, however, requires that the camera and scope be purchased as a unit; there is no interchangeability between systems. It does not allow for sterile bagging of the camera because the camera is part of the endoscope.

Lens fogging can be frustrating. It occurs because a cool metal scope is introduced into a warm body. There are several ways to

FIGURE 8-38 A one-piece design with a camera incorporated into the endoscope provides consistent, superior image quality.

address this problem. Elimination of a coupler has been discussed. Sterile defogging solutions can be applied to the endoscope and coupler lenses. These provide a coating and reduce the incidence of fogging. Other options on the market include O-ring seals at connections, sapphire lenses, and various water seals. Warming the endoscope before insertion also may reduce fogging. The endoscope can be warmed by wrapping it with lap sponges that have been soaked in warm, sterile water. Also available are scope warmers, such

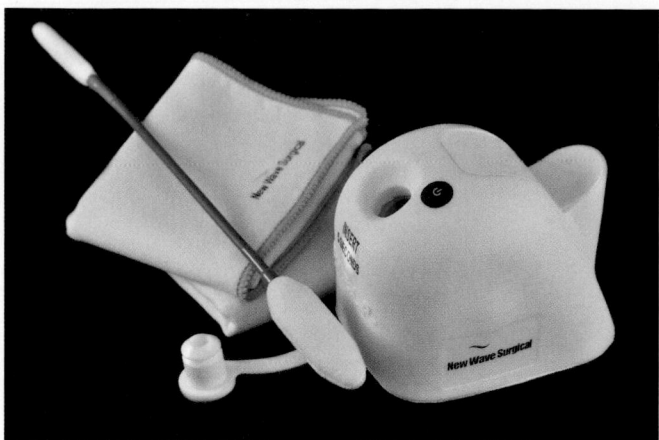

FIGURE 8-39 Scope warmer used to decrease lens fogging during laparoscopy.

as wraps, sleeves, thermos jugs, and other devices that warm the scope while maintaining sterility (Figure 8-39).

Another method is to use a CO_2 insufflator that warms the gas (if used) before it enters the body. It may be sufficient to change the insufflation site to a secondary port, after the initial pneumoperitoneum has been achieved. The surgeon also may opt to warm the lens of the endoscope by gently touching an intra-abdominal structure that requires visualization, obviating the need to withdraw the scope to wipe or defog the outer lens.

An advanced video system has been developed that uses the "chip on a tip" technology. This innovative digital imaging system positions a video chip at the distal tip of the endoscope so that the target is clearly and consistently visualized. The seamless one-piece design eliminates couplers that join together the camera head, telescope, and light cable. The distal end can have either a rigid or flexible tip to access hard-to-reach areas. This unique videoscope minimizes problems encountered by other video systems, such as fogging and faulty connections.

Video Monitor. High-resolution video monitors are the end of the chain in video endoscopy. They have become the "windows of observation" during MIS. Monitors should match closely the resolution quality of the camera used. A high-resolution monitor that meets or exceeds the horizontal resolution of the camera is required for optimum visualization. By definition, the camera-monitor system will always have the resolution of the least-detailed element. Determining picture quality of monitors is difficult unless the monitors are side by side. Picture-tube design is the component that alters a monitor's picture quality. Monitors must be able to handle the camera/recorder format (standard analog or HD).

Many operative procedures require two video monitors, one placed on each side of the patient so that the primary surgeon and assistant can view the screen simultaneously. The second monitor is called the *slave monitor.* Abdominal and thoracic procedures are performed in this manner. Certain procedures can be performed with only one monitor. Whenever the monitor can be placed comfortably in a position of visibility to both the surgeon and assistant, only one is necessary. This is usually the method of choice for urologists, endoscopists, gynecologists, and otorhinolaryngologists. Most general surgeons require only one monitor whenever they perform surgery with the endoscope directed toward the patient's feet (as in laparoscopic herniorrhaphy).

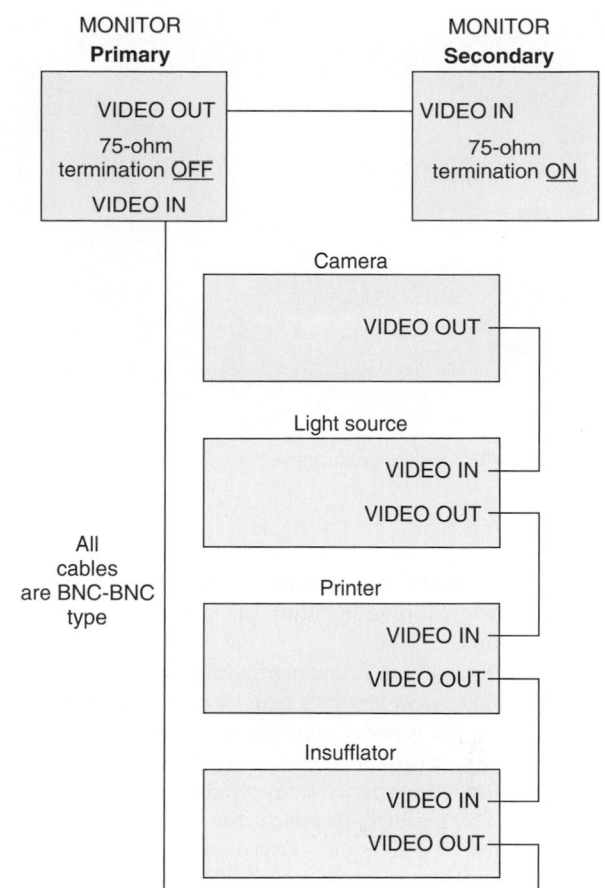

FIGURE 8-40 Basic wiring configuration. *BNC,* Bayonet Neill-Concelmen (type of connection).

Monitors should be at least 19 inches (diagonal measurement of screen) for adequate visualization. When the endoscopic revolution began, most institutions purchased 19- or 20-inch main monitors and 13-inch slave monitors. Today many institutions purchase mainly 24- to 32-inch monitors. This size increases flexibility in usage and provides excellent visibility from most observational angles and distances.

When only one monitor and a composite signal are used, the 75-ohm termination on-off switch must be in the *on* position. When multiple monitors are used, the switch on the last monitor in line to receive the video signal should be in the *on* position, and all others should be in the *off* position to enhance picture quality. Some monitors are self-terminating and do not have termination switches (Figure 8-40), an electronic wiring design known as a "daisy chain."

Recording Systems. Some recording devices allow for archiving the surgical procedure or selected portions of it. The most commonly used is the video printer (Figure 8-41), similar to a Polaroid camera in that it takes still pictures instantly. The printer stores the selected image and prints it onto special paper. Many units can be programmed to print 1, 4, 9, or 25 pictures on one piece of $5\frac{1}{2} \times$ 8-inch paper in split-screen fashion. Comparisons can then be made as the pathologic condition changes. Information such as patient name, date, time, and operating surgeon usually can be superimposed on top of the print. These prints can be used both

FIGURE 8-41 Video printer producing a picture of the endoscopic image.

FIGURE 8-42 Video laparoscopy cart.

for teaching purposes and as part of the permanent record. Some patients are interested in seeing prints of "before and after" images of their condition.

Video disc recorders store and permit easy access to video information. Video disc recorders are a popular documentation format. To use a video disc recorder, one also must use a video printer because the images stored are limited to video. HD recorders with touchscreen monitors are available; they record on an internal hard drive (usually 250 gigabytes or more). The images and videos can then be exported via a USB port, burned on a DVD, or sent to the hospital's server. The optical disc standard, known as Blu-ray, can provide digital storage for up to 10 hours of HD, depending on the encoder settings used.

If a picture or video is sent to the hospital's server, Health Insurance Portability and Accountability Act (HIPAA) regulations must be met. The digital images must be saved in a Digital Imaging and Communications in Medicine (DICOM) format as opposed to JPG or MPG formats used in the consumer market. The digital images are exported from the camera to the hospital's server system, the Picture Archiving Communication System (PACS).

Storage Systems. Space, storage capability, security, and required components determine the type and size of video storage carts needed. Purchasing a cart that can house multiple components of the video system is optimum (Figure 8-42). Such carts eliminate the clutter of multiple smaller carts and tables. They also eliminate the number of cord connections to wall outlets because most carts have power strips incorporated in their electrical setup. If a cart has a power strip, an on-off main switch usually is located near its base. The power switch must be in the *on* position for the equipment that is plugged into the strip to work. Given the location of the switch, it can be turned off easily during transport and cleaning. Time and embarrassment can be avoided if this switch position is routinely checked before each use.

Articulating arms can be used as monitor mounts. Surgeon preference and room space determine if this option is necessary or possible. If a surgical or treatment room has been designated for endoscopy, the monitor can be suspended from the ceiling on a swivel mount. The mount should be placed in a location where the monitor can be easily and comfortably viewed and cleaned. Care must be taken to ensure the swivel mount can support the weight of the monitor and other equipment.

Carts have either a locked or an open shelf design. Institutional security determines this configuration. Storage, tampering, and key availability are important issues. A locked drawer may be ideal to store HD recording devices, printing paper, and other valuable video supplies. Carts also should be selected for ease of movement, component accessibility, and cleaning. Carts may also include an optional storage bracket for E-cylinders when insufflation is required. Secondary (slave) monitor carts usually do not contain multiple shelving and cabinet components.

Robotics

Research and experimentation continue to advance robotic technology to assist with more delicate and precise procedures, such as laparoscopic surgeries. Basic robotic devices are used to assist with holding and maneuvering a laparoscope, thus freeing team members to perform other roles and attend to other duties. A robotic arm that holds a laparoscope minimizes shaky video images and reduces miscommunications between surgeon and assistant. The robot's movement can be controlled directly by foot pedals, handheld control panels, and voice activation. Advantages of a robotic device for laparoscope positioning include minimizing fatigue associated with holding and moving the scope, returning scope control to the physician, accommodating quick scope movements through a computerized memory, minimizing scope-positioning time, providing a steady image that enhances video quality ensuring consistent scope positioning and movement (not always possible with human assistants), and freeing the surgeon's hands to perform other tasks (Dziedzic, 2013). Advances in laparoscope stabilization and movement facilitate the procedure, promote safety, and sometimes minimize the time to perform the procedure.

Computer-assisted surgery (CAS) (also called image-guided surgery, surgical navigation, and three-dimensional [3-D] computer surgery) complements robotic procedures. CAS is any computer-based surgery that uses high technology, such as 3-D computer imaging and real-time sensing, to provide ultimate visibility and site targeting in the performance of surgical procedures. Image-guided surgery was first developed to assist with the treatment of brain tumors but has expanded greatly to other services. An image-guided system tracks the position of a surgical probe and displays the anatomy near it. Today's image-guided systems can use different tracking techniques, such as mechanical, optical, electromagnetic, and ultrasonic.

When CAS is combined with robotics, great precision is realized. To use both of these technologies during a robotic laparoscopic procedure, small incisions are made into the abdomen to insert three to four robotic arms. One arm serves as the camera, two of the arms act as the surgeon's hands, and a fourth may be used to retract structures that are in the way. The surgeon is seated at a nearby console and through the viewfinder sees a 3-D image of the surgical site. The surgeon manipulates the robotic arms through special devices that direct the instrumentation. Any tremors in the surgeon's hands are filtered out so delicate procedures can be expertly performed. The type of robotic procedure is a "shared-control system" because the procedure is performed by the surgeon through the use of a robot. Robot technology continues to evolve as research demonstrates improved patient outcomes.

Videoconferencing

Videoconferencing is a method to reach distant sites through two-way interactive communications using live audio and video signals. Communications between two or more sites may be live, or one site may play a videotape for the other sites connecting to the videoconference. This technology requires basic videoconferencing equipment and a network mode to transmit the communication signal to multiple sites. The higher the network bandwidth used by the participating sites, the better are audio and video motion-handling capabilities, and the resolution of the video signal that can be transmitted to each. A videoconference can be held between two sites or dozens of sites simultaneously. Videoconferencing applications in healthcare include education, remote assessments and consultation, administrative meetings, and product development.

Formal education and continuing education are the foundations of quality healthcare, and providing education to and from distant sites has gained tremendous popularity. Healthcare workers practicing in remote areas do not feel as isolated because educational videoconferencing is widely available. Distant preceptorships also have been offered as one physician monitors and oversees another physician learning a new surgical technique or using advanced surgical instruments.

Remote consultation to evaluate patients at remote sites has been used as assessment technology has been introduced and accepted. A physician or nurse practitioner (depending on state regulations) can assess heart sounds of a patient located at a distant location through the use of a telemedicine stethoscope. The retina of a diabetic patient can be viewed from afar by use of a special remote-assessment ophthalmoscope. A perioperative nurse practitioner located in a rural area can consult with a specialty physician located in a large urban teaching institution regarding treatment of a patient (Figure 8-43).

Videoconferencing can also be conducted for administrative and other meetings to minimize travel expenses and time away from

FIGURE 8-43 A nurse practitioner can consult with a physician at a remote location about a patient's treatment.

work. Product development also can be enhanced using videoconferencing. A company that manufactures surgical devices can communicate on a regular basis with key customers who are conducting trials of its devices. Device malfunctions and limitations can be assessed easily through real-time audio and video communication.

Some issues remain with videoconferencing. Standardization must be followed so that videoconferencing equipment can communicate and be compatible with each other. Some governmental and professional organization recommendations and mandates have guided manufacturers to meet approved criteria so that global interconnectivity can occur more easily. Because patient information, assessment data, and treatment results are being shared among providers by means of videoconferencing, patient confidentiality and privacy must be maintained. HIPAA compliance is vital when transmitting patient records. Private networks, advanced coding systems, and other technology can help address this issue. Practicing across state lines is a concern as videoconferencing in healthcare evolves. A state board of nursing, through the Nurse Licensure Compact (NLC), enables multistate licensure for nurses, providing the ability to practice across state lines physically and electronically. In 2013, there were 24 NLC states (NCSBN, 2013). Reimbursement for remote consultation and assessment is being analyzed by many insurance carriers. Pilot project sites have been established by the Centers for Medicare & Medicaid Services (CMS, formerly the Health Care Financing Administration) to study reimbursement practices. When reimbursement is consistently provided, more healthcare providers and facilities will embrace videoconferencing.

Practices and Potential Risks During MIS

Insufflation

To help visualize abdominal structures and enhance safety during laparoscopic procedures, a pneumoperitoneum is created. The surgeon makes a paraumbilical incision and inserts an insufflation (Verres) needle into the abdomen (Figure 8-44). To decrease the risk of bladder perforation when the needle is inserted, the bladder must be empty. Preoperatively the patient is told to empty his or her bladder. A straight catheter is used intraoperatively to ensure the bladder is empty. Trendelenburg position is used to reduce the risk of visceral perforation (see Chapter 6). As the surgeon inserts the needle, he or she lifts up the patient's abdomen by grasping and lifting a fold of tissue on either side of the umbilicus. Preoperative

FIGURE 8-44 Verres needle insertion into abdomen.

FIGURE 8-45 A smoke evacuator that can manually remove the insufflation gas using a closed system.

FIGURE 8-46 Disposable insufflation tubing with two-way filter.

patient education includes the possibility of finger-pinched bruising at the site where the abdominal tissue is grasped.

The needle safely enters the peritoneum positioned at a 45-degree angle. Placement is confirmed by negative bowel and blood return on aspiration and by saline instillation that meets no resistance. This is a relatively blind procedure because no scope can be introduced until the pneumoperitoneum is established. Newer laparoscopic trocar systems use the obturator tip instead of a needle. When this is inserted, there is less penetration into the peritoneum; then rapid insufflation is provided.

After needle confirmation, insufflation tubing is connected and the process begun. CO_2 gas is used to insufflate because it does not support combustion, can be absorbed at large volumes per minute without serious side effects, and is fairly inexpensive. The peritoneal cavity is filled, first at a low flow rate that is increased to a high flow rate of at least 9 L/minute ideally. Flow rate refers only to how quickly a predetermined intra-abdominal pressure can be reached. Intra-abdominal pressure is the actual measure that must be closely monitored and should be maintained between 14 and 16 mm Hg. High flow rates are important because during the procedure, the insufflation CO_2 gas can escape through smoke evacuation, instrument changes, and other practices. The more quickly the gas can be replaced, the less time is spent waiting for the abdomen to be redistended. Perioperative nurses must demonstrate competence in insufflation, and understand and manage its potential risks.

Insufflator control panels monitor and display the variables of flow rate, volume delivered, and intra-abdominal pressure. Selection of an insufflator that accommodates a high flow rate is important. Insufflators delivering 15 to 20 L/minute are much more effective than those delivering gas at slower rates. The insufflator must monitor insufflation pressure continuously, stop the insufflation process when the predetermined set pressure has been reached, and release pressure if there is an inadvertent pressure increase (called "taking a breath"). Intra-abdominal pressure can be increased for reasons other than CO_2 insufflation; leaning on the abdomen and additional gas introduction from other sources, such as an argon-beam coagulator or a CO_2 laser with a purge gas system, can inadvertently increase intra-abdominal pressure.

Overpressurization can be extremely hazardous to the patient. Excess pressure can force CO_2 to diffuse into the blood, resulting

in hypercarbia. End-tidal CO_2 monitoring becomes a crucial assessment parameter to detect increased CO_2 absorption. Excess pressure also increases diaphragmatic pressure, which can cause gastric regurgitation and aspiration of stomach contents. It also can reduce intrathoracic space, resulting in decreased respiratory effort and cardiac output. The phrenic nerve innervates the diaphragm and is responsible for some motor activity associated with respiration. CO_2 gas can irritate this nerve, causing postoperative pain in the shoulder and neck. Excessive pressure could cause tremendous postoperative discomfort and severe nerve damage. The surgeon or assistant should press on the patient's abdomen to release as much residual CO_2 gas as possible before removal of the last trocar sheath when the procedure is completed. Insufflators that automatically vent excess CO_2 gas into the air ensure that many potential complications can be avoided. A special smoke evacuator provides a safe and quick method to manually remove the insufflated gas using a closed system so that no gas escapes into the environment when the surgeon is releasing the insufflated gas (Figure 8-45). This minimizes contaminated air that could be inhaled by the surgical team.

A two-way, single-use disposable filter should be incorporated into the insufflation tubing (Figure 8-46). This hydrophobic filter provides patient protection from harmful gas-tank contamination, such as chromium particles. It also provides protection from the colonization of organisms in the insufflator itself. Without a filter, when the insufflator is turned on, organisms such as *Klebsiella,* *Pseudomonas,* and *Staphylococcus aureus* can be blown into the

FIGURE 8-47 Computerized high-flow insufflator with CO_2 warmer.

patient. This contamination could be deadly for a very ill, elderly, or immunocompromised patient. The manufacturer's written instructions must be followed when performing CO_2 insufflation. Perioperative nurses should consider the following steps to reduce cross-contamination of the patient and insufflator during CO_2 insufflation:

1. *Before* the procedure, verify that the cylinder is medical-grade CO_2; note the level of gas in the cylinder.
2. Flush insufflator and tubing with CO_2 gas before attaching to patient.
3. Use a disposable hydrophobic filter on insufflation tubing. Discard after procedure.
4. *During* the procedure, monitor level of CO_2 remaining in cylinder; have second cylinder readily available.
5. Keep insufflator elevated above the patient to prevent fluid backflow.
6. At end of the procedure, disconnect tubing from insufflator before turning off.

An insufflator capable of warning the team of insufflation problems throughout the procedure is vital. Alarms that sound when there is a deviation from predetermined parameters call attention to the need for immediate intervention, such as an alarm ringing and a monitor blinking "Gas supply low." An alarm sounding when overpressurization occurs from a secondary source (e.g., by leaning on the abdomen) also alerts the team to take corrective action.

Insufflators are also available with CO_2 warming devices (Figure 8-47). Cylinder CO_2 is a liquid, and as it is released, it expands into a gas. During conversion from liquid to gas, energy is lost, and the gas becomes colder. The higher the flow, the colder the gas. Some warming occurs as the gas travels through insufflation tubing. Use of cold CO_2 can cause a decrease in patient temperature, especially with prolonged laparoscopy. Many factors contribute to reduced body temperature during laparoscopic procedures (e.g., cold irrigation, room temperature, surface exposure, length of the procedure, patient's age and medical history, anesthetic choice); cold CO_2 represents an additional one. The best way to reduce patient heat loss and the risk for hypothermia is to address all variables and intervene wherever possible.

Anesthetic Considerations and Potential Complications During Minimally Invasive Surgery

Although anesthetic technique and delivery are the responsibility of the anesthesia provider, perioperative nurses must anticipate and respond appropriately to associated risks during MIS procedures. Many formerly performed open surgical procedures are now performed as MIS procedures in ambulatory surgery. With this change, anesthetic technique also has changed. Today emphasis is on

minimal anesthesia during surgery. Short-acting drugs are used so that the patient awakens quickly and experiences far fewer side effects (see Chapter 5).

Three major goals of the anesthesia provider during MIS procedures are: *respiratory stability, appropriate muscle relaxation,* and *hemodynamic stability.* In addition, during many laparoscopic and pelviscopic procedures, it is necessary to control diaphragmatic excursion. Patient monitoring includes an electrocardiogram (ECG) and assessment of end-tidal CO_2, blood pressure, oxygen saturation, and temperature.

When Trendelenburg position is used, intra-abdominal pressure increases, and this can cause respiratory complications, including hypoxia. CO_2 absorption from the peritoneal cavity can aggravate this situation. Reverse Trendelenburg position, on the other hand, can cause decreased venous return, reduced cardiac output, and hypotension. CO_2 insufflation in this position can also cause an increase in total peripheral resistance, especially if intra-abdominal pressure is high and the aorta compressed. The perioperative nurse must be prepared to quickly change the position of the OR bed, decrease the CO_2 flow rate of the insufflator, and assist the anesthesia provider with medications and extra supplies.

CO_2, highly soluble in blood, generally is not hazardous when used during laparoscopic insufflation because it is rapidly absorbed in the splanchnic vascular region. Excessive intra-abdominal pressure or any anesthetic technique that reduces splanchnic blood flow, however, could increase the potential for CO_2 gas emboli. This in turn could lead to circulatory collapse. CO_2 also could advance from the heart to pulmonary circulation, causing acute pulmonary hypertension with right-sided heart failure. If these effects are undetected and CO_2 insufflation continues, cardiac arrest and death may occur. If there are signs of CO_2 embolus, and there is not sufficient assistance, it may be necessary to call a rapid response team.

Intraoperative hypotension can result from excessive bleeding, excessive intra-abdominal pressure, and hypoxia. CO_2 insufflation rates may need to be reduced. Extra intravenous fluids may be needed. Likewise, intraoperative hypertension can result from increased intra-abdominal pressure, and increased CO_2 gas absorption also may be evident. Increased bleeding may result. The perioperative nurse may need to decrease CO_2 insufflation flow rates. Additional hemostatic agents and endoscopic clips may be required.

Gastric reflux may occur if the patient is obese, a hiatal hernia is present, or excessive pneumoperitoneum occurs. A nasogastric or orogastric tube may be inserted after general anesthesia is induced. Postoperative discomfort is less if an orogastric tube is used. During epidural and regional anesthesia, patients are usually awake, and insertion of a gastric tube may be poorly tolerated. For this reason the tube is not inserted unless gastric distention occurs. The perioperative nurse must be quick to respond if assistance is required during gastric tube insertion. Intercostal nerve blocks offer surgical pain relief and abdominal muscle relaxation when the patient is awake during MIS surgery. The perioperative nurse's role during intercostal nerve block induction is to remain at the patient's side and help reduce anxiety. Other risks during MIS procedures include hypercarbia, subcutaneous emphysema, and pneumoscrotum.

The surgical team must always be ready to rapidly convert an endoscopic procedure into an open procedure. Appropriate equipment and instruments must be readily available to provide a seamless transition. Many facilities require nurses to perform counts during the MIS procedure just in case there is a chance the procedure is converted to open. Those policies are followed for counting soft goods, instruments, and sharps to prevent a retained surgical item.

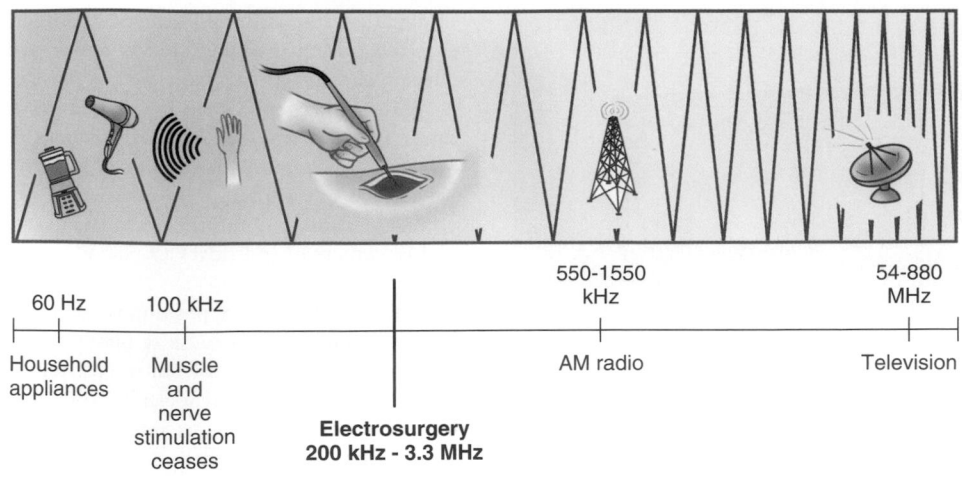

FIGURE 8-48 Frequency spectrum.

Energies Used During Surgery

Electrosurgery

Electrosurgical units (ESUs) have been used for many years to cut and coagulate tissue, but ESU use also has been associated with numerous patient injuries and accidents. The same laser safety measures used to prevent surgical fires and to evacuate surgical smoke are also used for electrosurgery (see Laser Safety for detailed information). Education is vital to ensure safe use of electrosurgery by understanding the principles and actions of this surgical energy.

Physics of Electrosurgery. The basic principles of electricity underpin electrosurgery. Electricity involves the motion of subatomic particles that behave in a consistent and predictable manner. Electrons orbit the nucleus of an atom. Once electrons are charged, they jump from one atom to the orbit of another, creating a charged particle or ion, and an electrical current is generated.

Three terms describe the properties of electricity—current, voltage, and impedance. *Current* is the flow of electrons measured in amperes or amps. *Voltage* is the force or push that moves the electrons from one atom to another and is measured in volts. *Impedance* is the opposition to the flow of current and is measured in ohms. As electrons encounter impedance, heat is produced, and a tissue effect results.

Electricity must have a complete circuit or pathway so that electrons can flow. That is, if an electrical current originates from earth, the electricity must be returned to ground to complete the circuit. Two forms of electrical current are used today—direct current (DC) and alternating current (AC). With DC the electrons flow in only one direction, whereas with AC the electrons flow back and forth as polarity changes. During electrosurgery, AC enters the patient's body, causing the patient to become part of the circuit as the energy is returned to the source of the energy.

Frequency is the number of waves passing through a given point over a specified time. This is measured in hertz (Hz) or cycles per second. Electrosurgical systems operate at frequencies greater than 100,000 Hz, which also is the frequency at which nerve and muscle stimulation ceases. In comparison, the electrical current in a normal household wall outlet in the United States alternates at 60 cycles per second, or 60 Hz. An ESU generator takes the 60-cycle current and increases its frequency to greater than 200,000 Hz so that it

FIGURE 8-49 Monopolar electrosurgical circuit.

can pass through the patient's body without muscle or nerve stimulation and with no risk of electrocution (Figure 8-48).

"Electrocautery" often is misused as a reference for electrosurgery. Electrocautery devices use direct current because electrons flow in one direction through a wire. The wire provides resistance and becomes hot. As the hot wire is held in contact with tissue, coagulation results. Electrocautery units are usually battery operated, such as the small disposable units used during ophthalmic procedures to coagulate small blood vessels.

Electrosurgical Modes. The two modes used for electrosurgical cutting or coagulation are *monopolar* or *bipolar*. In a monopolar system, electrical energy flows from the generator through an active electrode to the patient (Figure 8-49). If energy is concentrated in a small area, and the tissue provides increased impedance, controlled heat is generated and cutting or coagulation is achieved. Electrical energy passes through the patient to a dispersive electrode (pad) or patient return electrode (PRE) placed on the patient's body. The dispersive electrode surface area is large enough that energy is not concentrated enough to generate significant heat. Energy is then returned to the generator as the circuit is completed. If the dispersive electrode is tented, or only a small part of the pad is in contact

FIGURE 8-50 Bipolar electrosurgical circuit (ESU).

FIGURE 8-51 Electrosurgery waveforms: typical examples.

with the patient's body, electrical energy becomes concentrated, and a burn can result. With monopolar electrosurgery, the patient completes the electrical circuit; it is the most common mode of electrosurgery used today.

In a bipolar system a dispersive electrode is not needed because electrical energy flows from one tine (or prong or blade) of the bipolar instrument to the other tine as it passes through the tissue located between the tines (Figure 8-50). Energy returns directly through the instrument to the generator to complete the circuit, eliminating flow of current through the patient. During bipolar electrosurgery, the flow of electricity stops if a certain impedance level is reached. This is frequently 100 ohms but may differ for various bipolar generators available today. Although the ESU seems to be activated because an audible sound is heard while the pedal is depressed, the flow of current significantly decreases when the specified impedance is met. Impedance meters (or ammeters) are often used to alert the physician when tissue desiccation is occurring or when complete desiccation has occurred.

Tissue Effects. As electrosurgery variables change, different tissue effects can be achieved. Electrosurgery variables, explained below, include the following:
- Waveform
- Power setting
- Length of exposure
- Active electrode size
- Type of tissue
- Eschar presence

As waveform changes, so does tissue effect. Waveforms range from pure cut to pure coagulation. To produce a pure-cut mode, the generator must be on a 100% duty cycle, meaning that the electrical flow is continually applied, and heat is quickly generated for cutting and tissue vaporization (Figure 8-51). Current is high, but voltage is low. As less force (voltage) is used to push the current, the cut mode may be considered safer than other modes. As the cut mode produces a constant bombardment of electrons on the tissue, heat is produced, cells rupture, and the tissue is cut. For maximum activity the active electrode used to deliver the current should be held slightly above the tissue so that the electrons have to jump through the impedance of the air to reach the target site. This generates even more heat. Most of the heat dissipates as steam as tissue cells vaporize.

In pure coagulation mode, current is decreased but voltage is increased. The duty cycle is on only about 6% of the time, leaving 94% of the time with no flow of electrons to the surgical site (see Figure 8-51). To compensate for this "off" duty cycle, the voltage, or force of the push, must be increased to produce the desired wattage. During coagulation this intermittent delivery of electrons causes cells to heat and then cool, producing a coagulative effect. Higher voltage allows the active electrode to be held over the area while a fulguration or spraying effect delivers the electrical energy to coagulate a larger area. The tissue effect is superficial, collapsing the cells and producing a coagulum.

Most ESUs have a blend mode that allows the operator to achieve different levels of simultaneous coagulation in the cut mode. Increasing voltage and decreasing the duty cycle provide increased coagulation effects (see Figure 8-51).

The power setting also influences tissue effect. Higher power settings produce more extensive tissue effects. Long activation of electrical current increases thermal effects in tissue. Thermal energy can spread from the target site, causing damage to adjacent tissue. Smaller active electrodes concentrate electrical energy and require lower power settings; larger electrodes disperse electrical energy and require higher power settings.

Tissue type also influences tissue effect. Tissue that is not well vascularized, such as adipose tissue, offers more impedance. As a result, electrical energy is not conducted as well, and higher power settings may be required. Muscle tissue is well vascularized and requires less power to achieve a tissue effect. Electrosurgical tips on the active electrode must be kept clean and free from debris (eschar) to function properly. Eschar is less conductive and impedes the flow of electrons, requiring more power to be used to achieve the desired tissue effect. Electrode tips with nonstick coating make removal of eschar easier.

Electrosurgical Units. Four ESU systems have evolved over the years: grounded, isolated, dispersive electrode monitoring, and tissue response monitoring.

Grounded ESU. The grounded ESU system was the first ESU introduced to the surgical market during the late 1920s. The grounded ESU delivers electrical energy from the generator to the patient and returns energy to ground, which is intended to be the generator. As electricity takes the path of least resistance, current can flow or divide through any grounded alternative path, such as an ECG pad or an intravenous pole that touches the patient, as it returns to a grounded site. Patients have sustained burns at these alternative path sites as the electricity searches for the most conductive object or path to return to ground. When an alternate path is chosen, the current may not be dispersed over a large area, so an alternate site burn may result as current concentrates.

Isolated ESU. During the late 1960s the isolated ESU was introduced. An isolated ESU has a transformer that causes current to return only to the generator and not use alternate pathways to return to its source. Current flows through the patient's body and must return to the generator to complete the circuit. If this is not possible, the generator shuts down, adding to the safety of this type of unit. An isolated ESU prevents alternative site burns, but not PRE burns. The function of a PRE is to remove electrical current from the patient safely, but this may not always happen. If the PRE is tented, the electrical current arcs from the patient's skin to the pad to complete the circuit. The current concentrates in the reduced PRE-patient interface surface area and may cause a burn at this site. With experience, surgical teams became more focused on proper PRE placement by choosing a well-vascularized site with a secure PRE-patient interface. Monitoring PRE placement with an isolated ESU is a crucial responsibility of the perioperative nurse.

Dispersive Electrode Monitoring. In the 1980s different dispersive electrode monitoring systems were introduced, using a variety of names: dispersive pad monitoring, return electrode monitoring (REM), return electrode contact quality monitoring system (RECQMS), contact quality monitoring system, and patient safety system. Dispersive monitoring protects the patient from dispersive electrode site burns caused by inadequate contact of the dispersive electrode. The system continually monitors impedance under the split pad as it transmits an interrogation circuit to measure impedance levels (Figure 8-52). The system deactivates current flow when impedance under the pad increases to an unsafe level, thus preventing a burn.

Placement of a dispersive electrode pad is crucial to prevent patient injuries. The pad should be placed over an area that is well vascularized, such as a muscle mass. Sites with excessive hair, bony prominences, excessively dry skin, or adipose tissue should be avoided. When a patient is repositioned after the pad has been placed, the pad site must be inspected again to ensure proper adherence.

A capacitance pad working on the principle of "bulk resistivity" and "capacitive coupling" is an advanced technology. A capacitor is defined as two conductors separated by an insulator. With an ESU the patient is one conductor (plate), and the conductive mesh (plate) inside the pad is the other conductor. The ability for current flow to be induced from one plate of the capacitor to the other is affected by three primary variables: (1) frequency of current, (2) size of the plates, and (3) distance between the plates. Higher-frequency large plates and less distance between plates lead to better current flow. One small low-frequency plate or a great distance between the plates yields decreased current flow.

The large capacitive pad, approximately 2 feet by 3 to 4 feet, consists of a flexible conductive fabric surrounded by a nonlatex urethane insulating material. The pressure reduction version of this pad is composed of a dry, viscoelastic polymer.

This large reusable pad is placed on the OR bed (Figure 8-53) with a linen sheet and drawsheet placed on top of it. When the

FIGURE 8-52 Split pad for dispersive (return) electrode monitoring.

FIGURE 8-53 Capacitance pad that provides pressure reduction to prevent skin breakdown.

patient is lying on the OR bed, the electrode pad forms a large capacitor with the patient that capacitively couples or connects the patient into the ESU circuit. When in place, this dispersive electrode completes the circuit by capacitive reactance, allowing the ESU to function. The amount of current transmitted into the pad is directly proportional to the amount of contact with the pad. The pad serves as the gatekeeper for this current. With too little current, there is very little current flow, too low to cause burns.

The capacitive pad can be used for patients in all types of positions. A positioning chart is available from the manufacturer to

FIGURE 8-54 Pediatric capacitive dispersive pad for infants weighing from 0.8 to 50 pounds.

assist the surgical team with safe and appropriate positioning. This larger pad is inappropriate for patients weighing less than 25 pounds because adequate contact (weight-bearing area) cannot be achieved. Pediatric capacitive pads are available for patients between 0.8 and 50 pounds (Figure 8-54).

The large capacitive pad eliminates the need for an individual adhesive dispersive electrode pad, which is problematic if an ESU is used without dispersive electrode monitoring capabilities and the pad tents during a procedure. The bulk resistivity of this unique capacitive pad ensures that current densities are kept to a clinically safe level such that pad site burns rarely occur. Adhesive pads also can irritate sensitive skin, may require a shaved area for placement, or may become a hazard if not placed on the patient appropriately. As surgical teams learn more about the use and safety features of the capacitance pad, its acceptance continues to grow.

Tissue Response Monitoring. This system represents a substantial advancement in ESU generator technology. It uses a computer-controlled tissue feedback system that senses impedance of the tissue and automatically adjusts current and voltage output to maintain a constant surgical effect. This feedback system eliminates the need to adjust power settings for different tissue types. In addition, improved performance at lower power settings and voltages reduces the risk of patient injury.

Another advanced feedback–controlled generator has been combined with a bipolar instrument to seal vessels and tissue bundles reliably for surgical ligation during open and laparoscopic procedures. The feedback system helps to achieve a reliable tissue seal in less time, reducing thermal spread compared with traditional bipolar systems. With a single activation this system combines uniform compression and heat to provide stable seals on tissue bundles or on vessels up to 5 to 7 mm in diameter (Figure 8-55). The surgeon is able to assess the level of hemostasis at the seal site before cutting. The strength of the seal compares favorably to mechanical ligation methods, such as suture or clips, and is significantly stronger than standard bipolar coagulation. It is important to note that tissue response systems use the cut mode, and the new tissue sensing systems give feedback when implementing the coagulation mode of ESU generators.

Special Electrosurgery Considerations During Endoscopic MIS. Three unique problems can occur during MIS procedures involving electrosurgery: direct coupling, insulation failure, and capacitive coupling (Spruce and Braswell, 2012).

FIGURE 8-55 Advanced bipolar vessel sealing instrument that controls the temperature and provides uniform compression.

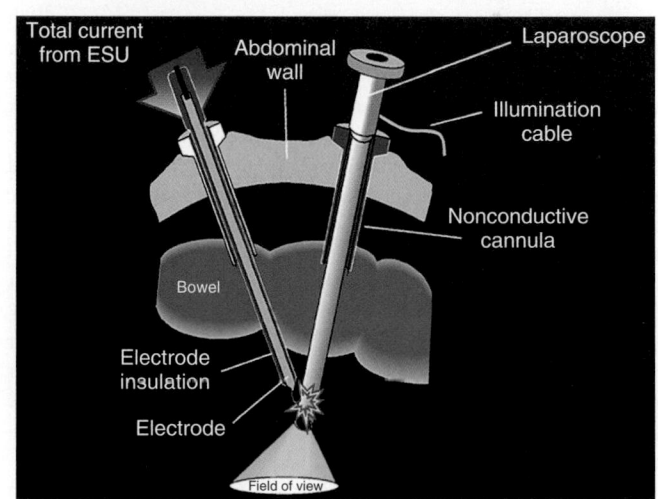

FIGURE 8-56 Direct coupling during laparoscopy. *ESU,* Electrosurgical unit.

Direct Coupling. Direct coupling occurs when the active electrode accidentally touches a noninsulated metal instrument, allowing the electrical energy to flow from one to the other (metal-to-metal sparking) (Figure 8-56). Direct coupling may also occur if an active electrode is activated while in contact with a clip. When the metal instrument or clip receives electrical energy, a burn can easily result. This coupling is often called "pilot error" because it is within the surgeon's control to avoid. The surgeon should not activate the active electrode until the target site is within the field of vision and the active electrode is in proximity or direct contact with target tissue and not a metal object.

Insulation Failure. Insulation failure occurs when the insulation coating of an endoscopic instrument has been compromised. If a crack or break occurs in the insulation along the shaft of the

FIGURE 8-57 Insulation failure during laparoscopy.

FIGURE 8-58 Capacitive coupling occurs when electrical energy flowing from an instrument charges a nearby metal trocar sheath or laparoscope.

instrument, electrical energy can escape at the point of the defect and burn untargeted tissue (Figure 8-57). Insulation must be inspected before, during, and after each use of the instrument. A scanning device can be used to ensure that insulation is not compromised during reprocessing. Even an area of insulation that is merely weakened may be penetrated by electrical flow if high voltage, or pure coagulation mode, is being used. Given that the force (or voltage) of electrons is greater in coagulation mode, any weakened area may become an actual break along the insulation sheath. Insulation failure presents the greatest risk to the patient because the full energy output can be delivered to nontargeted tissue. Insulation failure may result in instantaneous, irreversible death to tissue as a result of the high power density that insulation failure creates on the instrument shaft. The resulting tissue burn may not be observed or realized by the surgeon because it may not be within the field of vision.

Laparoscopic instruments may be purchased with a dual layer of insulation. The outer black insulation layer lies on top of a bright yellow insulation layer. When the top black layer is penetrated, the bright yellow layer can be seen easily and alerts the user that insulation failure may be imminent.

Capacitive Coupling. Capacitive coupling is a natural radio frequency (RF) electrosurgical energy phenomenon that occurs when energy is transferred through intact insulation on the laparoscopic instrument shaft to nearby conductive materials (Figure 8-58). A capacitor consists of *two conductors* separated by an *insulator*. The metal active electrode is one conductor, and an adhesion, an adjacent organ, or a conductive trocar/suction irrigation cannula can act as the second conductor. The primary insulation on the instrument represents the insulator. When an electrode is activated within a narrow suction irrigator, the RF energy can flow from the active electrode through the intact insulation and transfer 20% to 80% of the power displayed on the ESU to the metal suction irrigator. The induced current on the suction irrigator can cause a burn even though the outer insulation on the first instrument has been inspected and determined to be intact.

Monopolar ESUs used in concert with metal suction irrigators or shafts increase the risk of visceral burns through capacitive thermal energy. The laparoscope also can cause alternate-site burns if the ESU electrode is used through a narrow-lumen scope. In

Primary insulation layer   Protective shield

Active electrode element   Outer insulation

FIGURE 8-59 Cross section of active electrode monitoring instrument.

addition, long and narrow instruments with thin insulation, combined with high voltage, increase the incidence of capacitive coupling.

An electrical charge remains in the second metal instrument until it finds a path to the dispersive electrode to complete the circuit. Usually this energy disperses safely through the large surface of the abdominal wall from the conductive cannula. However, if a nonconductive device, such as a plastic stability collar, is in this path, energy cannot be safely discharged and will burn any tissue touched by the metal instrument. These burns often are undetected by the surgeon, and the problem is not diagnosed until the patient presents with complications after surgery. Accordingly, surgeons avoid hybrid instruments (combination of plastic and metal) during laparoscopy to minimize capacitive coupling.

To eliminate the hazard of capacitive coupling and insulation failure, special instruments that provide active electrode monitoring (AEM) are available to capture stray energy that is transferred from one conductive device to another (AORN, 2013). AEM laparoscopic instruments are shielded and monitored to detect stray RF current and prevent ESU burns. The protective shield built within an AEM instrument provides the neutral path for capacitive-coupled energy and returns it to the ESU (Figure 8-59). These safety devices also detect insulation failure and provide a path for stray current back to the generator. AEM is the only fail-safe technology currently designed to address insulation failure and capacitive coupling. AEM ensures that 100% of electrosurgical energy is delivered at the intended site.

Many hospitals that have implemented AEM technology require documentation of its use on the patient's perioperative chart for liability and risk management, much like rationales for documenting needle and soft good counts.

Electrosurgery Safety. Misuse of electrosurgery devices is often the cause of surgical accidents today. *AORN Perioperative Standards and Recommended Practices* note that the electrosurgery pencil should be placed in a safety holster when not in use (AORN, 2013). This prevents the device from being inadvertently activated. Longer electrosurgical devices used during laparoscopic procedures require special attention to ensure that they are safely secured on the sterile field when not in use. Electrosurgical devices that are controlled with a foot pedal require the foot pedal to be identified and the handpiece given to the practitioner who will deliver the electrosurgical energy to the tissue during the procedure.

Electrosurgery devices (along with other surgical energy sources) must not be used near flammable liquids (such as alcohol), instruments, and other supplies. The electrosurgery device can serve as an ignition source for a fire if flammables and an oxygen-enriched environment are present. A hot electrosurgery blade after activation can provide the heat source to ignite a flammable material, such as a surgical drape, radiopaque sponge, or plastic instrument.

The size of the electrosurgery blade often determines the amount of energy delivered to the surgical site. The manufacturer often sets cutting and coagulation limits depending on the electrosurgery blade to tip size. For example, an insulated needle tip can only conduct limited amounts of energy to tissue. The power settings for cut and coagulation on the electrosurgical unit are thus adjusted accordingly.

Many physicians have power settings listed on their preference cards depending on the type of procedure to be performed. These power settings must be verbalized to the surgeon at the beginning of each procedure. Before power settings are increased, other factors must be reviewed that could affect these settings (such as the presence of eschar on the blade, the size of the electrosurgery blade, the type of tissue being treated, etc.). The surgical team must always react to an electrosurgical unit alarm because this indicates that safety parameters are being compromised.

The scrub person removes any charred material from the electrosurgery pencil blade or tip so that the electrical energy can be efficiently delivered to the surgical site. Residual debris on an electrosurgical blade obstructs the delivery of the electrons and can cause an increased heat buildup, thus causing an unwarranted need to increase the electrosurgical power. Cleaning pads are available to scrape off any charred debris. Some manufacturers provide a coated blade tip for easy cleaning because the coating prevents debris accumulation.

Argon-Enhanced Electrosurgery. An argon-enhanced ESU device combines argon gas with electrosurgical energy to improve the effectiveness of the electrosurgical current. Because argon gas is heavier than air, inert, and noncombustible, it creates an efficient pathway for electrosurgical energy to travel from electrode to target tissue. The flow of argon gas also clears the surgical site of blood and fluids, allowing for greater visibility of the bleeding site or target area, and disperses oxygen, decreasing the chance of combustion and formation of surgical smoke.

Benefits of argon-enhanced electrosurgery include:
- Rapid coagulation of diffuse bleeding site with reduced blood loss
- Reduced risk of rebleeding
- Noncontact tissue coagulation

- Reduced depth of penetration by electrical energy and less adjacent tissue damage (Dooley and Braghieri, 2008)

When an argon-enhanced ESU is used during laparoscopic procedures, care must be taken not to overinsufflate (or overpressurize) the abdomen because the constant flow of argon gas could cause formation of a gas embolism. Often another port is left open during activation of argon-enhanced ESUs to allow excess gas to escape. An insufflator with an audible alarm indicating overpressurization should be used. The patient should be monitored closely so that early symptoms of an embolism can be detected and treated.

Laser

A healthcare revolution occurred with the birth and evolution of the laser. Perioperative nurses must be aware of expanded responsibilities associated with laser applications. The laser has significantly affected surgery by making possible less-invasive procedures, decreasing inpatient hospitalization, diminishing postoperative complications, and saving healthcare dollars.

Laser Biophysics

Principles of Light. *LASER* is an acronym that describes a process in which light energy is produced—*l*ight *a*mplification by *s*timulated *e*mission of *r*adiation. The term also refers to the device that generates laser energy.

Light is a form of electromagnetic energy that can be graphically illustrated on a continuum known as the electromagnetic spectrum (Figure 8-60). The unit of measurement for this continuum is called a wavelength, the distance between two successive peaks of a wave. Wavelength determines color and usually is measured in nanometers (10^{-9} m) or micrometers (1000 nm). Various wavelengths of light extend from the shorter waves in the ultraviolet area to the longer waves in the infrared region (Table 8-2). Visible laser wavelengths occupy only a small portion of this continuum. Radiation used in laser technology in healthcare is nonionizing in that it does not present the hazard of cellular deoxyribonucleic acid (DNA) disruption with continual tissue exposure. Pregnant women, for example, can work with lasers because laser energy produces no harmful ionizing radiation.

Briefly, the laser functions in the following way. A negatively charged electron orbits a positively charged nucleus while the atom is in its ground or resting state, its lowest energy level. An outside source of energy (e.g., electricity, flash lamps, other lasers) can excite the atom and cause an electron to jump to a higher, less stable orbit.

FIGURE 8-60 Electromagnetic spectrum.

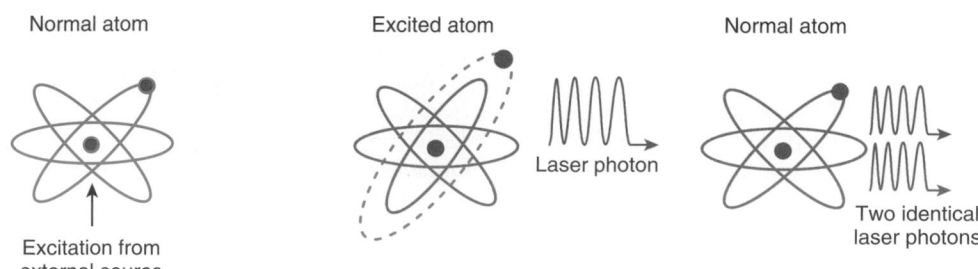

FIGURE 8-61 Laser energy is produced when an external source excites the atom to emit a photon spontaneously. This photon can "stimulate" the emission of two identical photons.

TABLE 8-2
Electromagnetic Spectrum Wavelengths

Type of Light	Wavelength (nm)
Ultraviolet (UV)	100-400
Visible	400-750
Near-infrared (NIR)	750-3000
Mid-infrared (MIR)	3000-30,000
Far-infrared (FIR)	30,000 nm-1 mm

The electron almost immediately returns to its stable orbit, and the atom resumes its normal resting state. As the unstable electron returns to its ground state, it spontaneously releases a tiny packet of light energy known as a photon, which travels away from the source in the form of waves. If the photon is close to another similar atom while it is still in the excited state, it interacts with this atom. The photon triggers the excited second atom to return to its resting state, and in this process another photon of laser light is emitted. These two photons of identical energy travel together. The process of stimulated emission has occurred, and laser energy initiated (Figure 8-61). This process repeats itself over and over again, creating more photons of laser energy.

This activity occurs in the resonating chamber of the laser, where the lasing medium is contained. The name of the laser usually is derived from the actual medium that causes the lasing action. The photons generated during the stimulated emission process are reflected back and forth between mirrors at each end of the resonating chamber as the process is amplified, until the number of excited atoms surpasses the number of resting atoms. This is known as population inversion. One of the mirrors in the chamber is partially reflective and, when activated, allows a stream of laser photons to escape the unit. These photons are introduced to the target area by means of a specific delivery system.

Characteristics of Laser Light. Three distinct characteristics distinguish laser light from ordinary light. Laser light is monochromatic, collimated, and coherent.

1. *Monochromatic light* is composed of photons of the same wavelength or color. In contrast, ordinary light consists of many different colors or wavelengths. When white light is passed through a prism, an array of different colors is displayed. White light is the presence of all colors, whereas laser light consists of one color or wavelength.
2. A *collimated* laser beam consists of waves parallel to each other that do not diverge significantly, minimizing any loss of power.

When a collimated beam is passed through a lens, the light pattern is changed, allowing the light to be focused into a tiny spot that highly concentrates the energy. In comparison, the light waves from a flashlight are not parallel and lose intensity as they travel away from the source. A lens cannot easily focus these noncollimated waves to concentrate the light into a small area.

3. Laser light is *coherent*—all the waves are orderly and in phase with each other as they travel in the same direction. All peaks and troughs of the waves are opposite each other in time and space. This property provides an additive effect that gives the laser beam power. Ordinary light is incoherent because the waves radiate away from the source without being in phase or in an orderly pattern.

Laser Power. The power, or energy, of a laser beam is measured in watts. An important factor in laser applications is the concept of power density, or irradiance of the beam. *Power density* is the amount of power that is concentrated within an area and is described by the following formula:

$$\text{Power density} = \text{watts/spot size (cm}^2)$$

The spot size of the laser beam can be controlled when the beam is passed through a special lens that causes the beam to converge. The focal configuration of the lens determines at what distance from the lens the beam would be most intense; this is called the *focal point*. If the beam is defocused into a larger spot size, the laser energy is spread over a greater area, decreasing the intensity or power density of the beam. In contrast, a small spot size of the beam concentrates the laser energy into a smaller area, increasing the intensity or power density of the beam. When power density is increased, the beam has a greater depth of penetration into the tissue.

A *joule* is the unit of measure used to describe total energy used. A joule is expressed by the power multiplied by the time duration of the beam exposure (expressed in the equation joule = watts × time). Often the laser energy used during ophthalmic procedures is expressed in millijoules.

Fluence is a term that expresses the power and duration of exposure of the beam and measures the specific amount of energy delivered to tissue. Fluence is also known as energy density or radiant exposure. The following equation calculates fluence:

$$\text{Fluence} = \text{watts} \times \text{duration time/spot size (cm}^2)$$

Tissue Interaction. When laser energy is delivered to a target site, four different interactions can occur: reflection, scattering, transmission, or absorption (Figure 8-62). The extent of reaction of

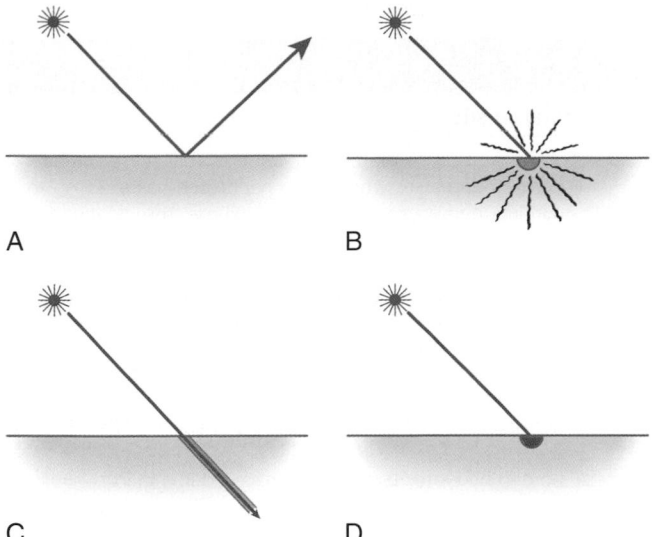

FIGURE 8-62 Laser-tissue interaction. **A,** Reflection. **B,** Scattering. **C,** Transmission. **D,** Absorption.

Tissue Changes with Temperature Increases

Temperature °F (°C)	Visual Change	Biologic Change
98.6-140°F (37-60°C)	No visual change	Warming, welding
140-149°F (60-65°C)	Blanching	Coagulation
149-194°F (65-90°C)	White/gray	Protein denaturization
194-212°F (90-100°C)	Puckering	Drying
>212°F (>100°C)	Smoke plume	Vaporization, carbonization

the beam on the target depends on laser wavelength, power settings, spot size, length of contact time with target tissue, and tissue characteristics.

Reflection of the laser beam occurs when the direction of the beam is changed after it contacts an area. Specular reflection occurs when the angle of the incoming light is equal to the angle of the reflected light. Laser light can be intentionally reflected in this manner off a reflective mirror to contact hard-to-reach areas. Such reflection also can pose safety problems by inadvertently striking untargeted areas if it is not controlled at all times. The CO_2 laser beam can be reflected off of the surface of a shiny instrument and impact a surgery team member's mask, causing it to ignite. Accordingly, eye and fire safety measures are mandatory when the potential for laser beam reflection is high.

Scattering of laser light occurs when the beam spreads over a large area as tissue causes the beam to disperse. The intensity of the beam decreases as the waves travel in different directions. The Nd:YAG laser beam can backscatter up an endoscope and cause damage to the end of the scope, the optics, or the operator's eye. The noncontact Nd:YAG beam also can scatter through tissue, causing penetration of 3 to 5 mm.

Transmission of the laser beam occurs when the beam passes through fluids or tissue without thermally affecting the area. The argon beam can be transmitted through clear fluids and structures of the front part of the eye and the vitreous to cause thermal photocoagulation on the retina, whereas the cornea, lens, and vitreous are unaffected by transmission of this beam.

Absorption of laser light results when tissue is altered from the absorption of the beam. As the amount of energy delivered to tissue (fluence) increases, different tissue effects can be produced. The lowest level of energy produces a photochemical reaction. Then as fluence increases, a photothermal reaction occurs. With the highest level of fluence, a photoacoustic effect occurs. Reactions from the lowest to highest level of energy occur as follows:

- *Photochemical effect*—laser energy is selectively absorbed by tissue containing a light-sensitive dye, leading to a chemical change that produces singlet oxygen, which ultimately causes tissue destruction.

- *Photothermal effect*—laser energy is absorbed by tissue, heating it.
- *Photoacoustic effect*—laser energy is absorbed, creating kinetic energy that produces a snapping sound, disrupting the tissue without significant thermal effect.

Consistency, color, and water content of the target tissue often determine the rate of absorption of laser energy. Laser wavelength also affects absorption of the beam. Certain laser light, such as that from the argon laser, is highly absorbed by pigmented tissues. The CO_2 laser, however, is independent of color-selective absorption. CO_2 laser light is absorbed superficially by tissue to a shallow depth of approximately 0.1 to 0.2 mm, whereas the holmium laser beam is absorbed to about 0.4 to 0.6 mm. Argon laser light is readily absorbed by pigmented tissue to a depth of approximately 1 to 2 mm, whereas that of the noncontact Nd:YAG laser beam is more readily absorbed by darkened tissue to a depth of 3 to 5 mm.

Photothermal tissue reaction becomes more pronounced as the temperature of the target area increases during absorption of the laser beam (Table 8-3). As laser energy is absorbed, the water within each cell is heated. As temperature increases, intracellular protein is destroyed and water inside the cell turns to steam. Eventually the cellular membrane ruptures from increased pressure, spewing cellular debris and plume (smoke) from the tissue. The surrounding tissue also is heated through conduction because it borders the impingement site. The degree of adjacent tissue damage depends on the duration of laser-beam exposure that causes the intended thermal destruction of target tissue.

Laser Systems. New laser systems are introduced into healthcare regularly. Constant efforts by researchers and physicians to explore the use of different wavelengths frequently change surgical approaches in a variety of specialties. Some of the most common lasers are described in Table 8-4, beginning with lasers in the infrared region with long wavelengths, through visible wavelengths, and finally to short ultraviolet wavelengths.

Laser System Components. Five major components of a laser system are the laser head, excitation source, ancillary components, control panel, and delivery system. When a laser malfunctions, an organized investigation of each of these parts (Figure 8-63) usually can determine the source of the problem.

The *laser head,* or resonating chamber, is the component in which laser energy is generated and amplified. The laser head contains the active medium or substance that actually produces the photons that generate laser light. The active medium can be a gas (CO_2 or argon), a solid crystal (Nd:YAG), a liquid (tunable dye), or a semiconductor crystal (diode). As technology continues to advance, laser wavelengths are being combined into a single unit so that a selection of wavelengths, such as the Nd:YAG, erbium:YAG, or holmium:YAG, can be offered easily during a procedure.

TABLE 8-4

Description of Common Lasers Used

Active Medium	Wavelength	Delivery System	Penetration	Characteristics
CO_2 laser (gas laser)	10,600 nm, infrared	Articulated arm, waveguide, scanner, microscope via microslad	Shallow penetration (0.1-0.2 mm), photothermal effect	Highly absorbed by water. Not color selective. Helium-neon aiming beam. Sometimes the handpiece has a tubing to conduct compressed air to keep plume from coating the lens. CO_2 energy can be delivered in a continuous wave or pulsed mode. When delivery system is attached, the laser must be test fired to ensure the aiming beam is aligned with CO_2 beam. Used on soft tissue, ablations, cutting, coagulation, vaporization.
Erbium:YAG laser (solid crystal laser)	2940 nm, infrared	Fiber (handpiece, microscope)	Shallow penetration, photothermal effect	Highly absorbed by water. Delivered in pulsed mode. Helium-neon aiming beam. Frequently used in dermatology for skin resurfacing and ablation. Also used in dentistry.
Holmium:YAG laser (solid crystal laser)	2140 nm, infrared	Fiber (handpiece, microscope)	Shallow penetration (0.4-0.6 mm), photothermal effect	Absorbed by water but can be delivered in a fluid environment within a vapor bubble if fiber is within 55 mm of target site. Helium-neon aiming beam. Pulse mode. Used for sculpting and ablating soft tissue. Has also been used on cartilage. Also used to fragment urinary or biliary stones with photo-acoustical effect.
Neodymium:YAG laser (Nd:YAG) (solid crystal laser)	1064 nm, infrared	Contact and noncontact fibers, contact tips, handpiece for dermatology, slit lamp for ophthalmology, microscope	Scatters in tissue (3-5 mm) for noncontact fiber. Shallow penetration (<1 mm) for contact delivery	Transmitted through clear solutions. Highly absorbed by pigmented tissue. Helium-neon aiming beam usually used. Used in continuous or pulsed modes. Ophthalmology Nd:YAG lasers (class 3B lasers) use special pulsed mode delivery (Q-switched) to provide photo-acoustical effect within the eye to rupture the secondary membrane.
KTP (potassium titanyl phosphate) laser (solid crystal laser)	532 nm, visible (frequency doubled YAG)	Fiber (handpiece, microscope)	1-2 mm depth of penetration	An Nd:YAG incident beam (1064 nm) is passed through a KTP crystal which doubles the frequency and halves the wavelength (532 nm). Aiming beam can be a low power KTP beam or helium-neon beam. Highly color selective. Transmitted through clear solutions. Often used in dermatology, urology, general surgery, gynecology.
Argon laser (gas laser)	Blue-green light of 488 and 514.5 nm (or 457 and 528 nm), visible	Fiber (handpiece, microscope, slit lamp)	1-2 mm depth of penetration	Intense visible blue-green laser light. Aiming beam can be a low power argon beam or a helium-neon beam. Highly color selective. Transmitted through clear solutions. Often used in ophthalmology, dermatology, and soft tissue procedures.
Tunable dye laser (liquid laser)	Range of 400-900 nm visible	Fiber (handpiece, microscope, slit lamp)	Depends on wavelength	Can dial in desired wavelength within limited range of visible light. By changing dyes and other parameters, the wavelength can be altered. Laser energy formed by exposing a liquid dye to an intense light source, such as an argon beam. The dye absorbs the laser light and fluoresces over a broad spectrum of colors and with special prisms, diffraction gratings or filters, a specific wavelength is produced. Some wavelengths are highly absorbed by pigmented tissues. Can be delivered in continuous or pulsed modes. Often used in dermatology, ophthalmology, urology (fragment stones).
Diode laser (semiconductor crystal laser)	Varies (i.e., 532-910 nm), visible	Fiber (handpiece, microscope, slit lamp)	Depends on wavelength	Compact, reliable laser system. Often used for ophthalmology and dermatology.
Excimer laser (gas laser)	Ultraviolet (wavelength depends on chemical composition of active medium)	Fiber (handpiece, microscope, slit lamp)	Depends on wavelength (mostly <1 mm). Acts by disassociating cellular molecular bonds	"Excited dimer" laser. Most popular excimer lasers are argon fluoride (ArF) at 193 nm, krypton fluoride (KrF) at 248 nm, xenon chloride (XeCl) at 308 nm, and xenon fluoride (XeF) at 351 nm. Appropriate protective housing needed for laser needed because gases are extremely toxic. Extremely effective ablative capabilities. Used for corneal sculpting. Also used for other ablative procedures. Used experimentally to treat psoriasis and vitiligo.

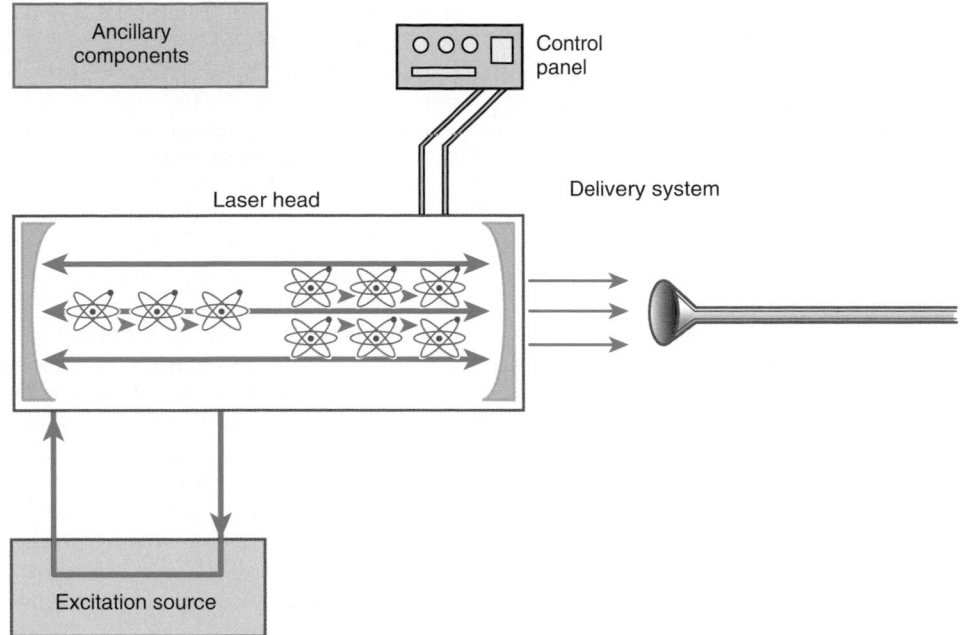

FIGURE 8-63 Parts of a laser system.

The *excitation source* supplies the energy to excite the active medium in the laser head. Different sources include flash lamps, electricity, radio waves, batteries, chemicals, and other laser systems. The CO_2 laser gas mixture is excited by electrical current or radio waves, and the Nd:YAG laser crystal is excited by flash lamps. Diode lasers, such as the gallium arsenide laser, are solid-state lasers that are excited by electrical energy.

Ancillary components are other laser parts needed to help produce laser energy. A cooling system maintains the appropriate temperature of the laser head and keeps the unit from overheating. Usually lasers are air cooled or water cooled. A vacuum pump may be required in a CO_2 free-flowing laser to pull the gas mixture from an external cylinder into the laser head for laser light production. Current sealed-tube CO_2 lasers do not require a vacuum pump because the laser gas mixture is catalyzed to regenerate itself for the lasing action to continue, using the same gas mixture over and over again.

The *control panel* consists of a board that regulates delivery of laser energy. Various power settings, modes, durations, and other parameters can be selected. Most laser panels are computerized, allowing the laser to be controlled quickly and accurately.

The *delivery system* is the device or accessory that conducts laser energy from the laser head to the target area. CO_2 laser energy usually is delivered to tissue through an articulated arm (hollow tube) with a series of special mirrors at each joint to reflect the laser energy forward. Care must be taken when moving the laser so that mirrors are not jarred out of alignment. The articulated arm can be attached to a microscope, a special handpiece, or a scanner for the most precise energy delivery. A lens system within these attachments causes the beam to converge at the focal point. A special coating on the lens maintains the beam's integrity and intensity, and must be carefully maintained, following manufacturer's instructions, so that the coating is not disrupted. The focal length of the lens is the distance from the lens to the focal point where the beam converges and is most concentrated and intense within a small spot. The size of the spot can be changed by focusing or defocusing the lens to allow the spot to become larger or smaller. When the CO_2 handpiece is moved toward and then away from the tissue, the spot size changes.

The articulated arm is connected to a microscope through the use of a microslad (or micromanipulator). Laser energy is conducted through the articulated arm to a mirror within the microslad that directly reflects the beam to tissue. The position of the beam is controlled by moving a joystick. When connected to a scanner, a specific geometric pattern of laser pulses can be delivered to the tissue during ablation (dermatologic) or vaporization (gynecologic) procedures.

The CO_2 laser beam also can be conducted through a narrow wave guide, which consists of a hollow, semiflexible tube that allows energy to "wiggle" down its path by being reflected off the surface of the inner lumen. With this reflection some beam power is lost as it exits the delivery device. Solid fibers that will conduct the CO_2 wavelength to target sites are being developed.

The commonly used argon, KTP, Nd:YAG, and holmium lasers deliver energy through a fiber system. The core fiber, usually made of quartz, is surrounded by a polytetrafluoroethylene (Teflon) silicone coating or cladding that retains the light. This is known as a bare fiber. If the bare fiber is encased by a catheter sheath, a purge gas, air, or fluid can be conducted down the length of the fiber. This purge is used to cool the fiber tip and keep debris from accumulating.

Most laser fibers deliver the laser energy to the tissue in a *noncontact mode,* meaning that the fiber does not touch the tissue. If the noncontact fiber contacts the tissue, any debris on the end of the fiber can cause the fiber to heat to the point of destroying the tip. Some fibers can deliver the laser energy to the tissue using the *contact method*. For example, a synthetic sapphire contact probe or scalpel that is attached to the end of a fiber with a special connector can deliver Nd:YAG laser energy directly to the tissue in a more concentrated manner. These contact tips are available in a variety of configurations. Depending on the desired tissue effects, the appropriate contact tip is chosen. A scalpel is used to cut; a rounded probe is used to vaporize. A flat probe may be used to coagulate tissue. The end of the quartz fiber also may be sculpted into a configuration that can be used in direct contact with the tissue. Contact technology provides precision because the power output of the beam is confined to a small area and less wattage is needed. It causes less thermal buildup, so adjacent tissue is relatively unaffected.

Benefits of Laser Technology. Laser technology evolves as more surgical applications are explored and introduced. As physicians become more adept in laser applications, use continues to grow. The laser has fostered the development of new minimally invasive procedures and endoscopic techniques along with ophthalmic and dermatologic applications. The true potential of the laser has yet to be realized as healthcare practitioners explore different procedures that can benefit from its use. Following are some advantages that have been associated with laser technology, depending on the procedure performed:

- Seals small blood vessels (less intraoperative and postoperative blood loss)
- Seals lymphatics (decreases postoperative edema and potential spread of malignant cells in the lymphatic system)
- Seals nerve endings (on selective procedures, decreases postoperative pain)
- Sterilizes tissue (from the heat generated at the laser-tissue impact site)
- Decreases postoperative stenosis (by decreasing the amount of scarring that could lead to stenosis)
- Produces minimal tissue damage (from precision of the laser beam)
- Reduces operative and anesthesia time
- Allows a shift to more ambulatory surgery procedures
- Allows more use of local anesthetics instead of general anesthetics
- Provides quicker recovery and return to daily activities

Laser Safety. Because laser systems are capable of concentrating high amounts of energy within very small areas, they present hazards. Safe and appropriate use of lasers is the responsibility of the entire healthcare team. Each member must be acutely aware of the many controls needed to prevent accidental injury. The laser team member must be given the responsibility and authority to shut down the laser system if safety policies are not being followed.

The laser is a class III medical device that is subdivided into four subclasses. Lasers designated as subclasses 3 and 4 have the potential to cause injury. Some ophthalmic Nd:YAG lasers that cause a photoacoustic, instead of a photothermal, reaction are classified in the subclass 3B category and can cause injury with sustained interaction. Most of the lasers used in surgical applications are subclass 4 lasers and can cause photothermal reactions that may lead to fire, skin burns, and optical damage by either direct or scattered radiation. Specific safety precautions must be followed to prevent injury from these lasers.

Many agencies address laser safety. Healthcare facilities must develop safety protocols in anticipation of mandates by regulatory agencies as technology advances and grows.

The American National Standards Institute (ANSI), a nongovernmental organization of experts, first published standards (Z136.1—American National Standard for Safe Use of Lasers) in 1973 as safety guidelines for laser use in warfare, industry, and healthcare with a subsequent revision published in 2007. The

standards were expanded and ANSI Z136.3 (American National Standard for Safe Use of Lasers in Health Care) was published to provide specific recommendations for laser use in healthcare environments (ANSI, 2011). The appendix of ANSI Z136.3 discusses a consensus on laser safety in each of the special areas of medicine and surgery. These standards are reviewed periodically and revised as surgical trends change. The most current versions of both ANSI standards are recommended to be available for referencing because the Z136.3 document often refers to the Z136.1 publication.

Other guidelines have been introduced by the Center for Devices and Radiological Health (CDRH), AORN, American Society for Laser Medicine and Surgery (ASLMS), Laser Institute of America (LIA), FDA, OSHA, and individual state and local regulatory bodies.

Hospitals and other healthcare delivery facilities need to create laser safety policies and procedures using these expert references as resources. In developing safety guidelines for a facility, protocols should address various situations while being neither too general nor too specific. A policy or procedure must be general enough to address the need, but not so detailed that the surgical team cannot follow it consistently. Staff must realize that they are accountable for following their own safety policies and procedures. Basic education on written laser policies and procedures for all personnel in the surgical environment (including orderlies, aides, and housekeeping personnel) should be mandatory. Topics for policy and procedure development for laser safety should include the following areas, each of which is addressed in more detail below:

- Eye protection
- Controlled access
- Fire safety
- Smoke (plume) evacuation
- Documentation
- Laser team responsibilities
- Skin/tissue protection
- Electrical safety
- Education/training
- Credentialing

Eye Protection. The eye is extremely sensitive to laser radiation and great care must be taken to protect eyes during laser intervention. Even low levels of laser radiation can lead to permanent optical damage. Possible ophthalmologic injuries depend on laser wavelength (Figure 8-64). The CO_2 laser can damage the cornea because this beam is absorbed readily by water within surface cells, causing a burn. Immediate pain is associated with this corneal injury. Lasers, like the argon and Nd:YAG, in contrast, are transmitted through clear optical structures and fluids and can be refocused by the eye's lens. The beam's intensity after refocusing can permanently damage the retina. No pain may be felt during this injury (Patient Safety).

Adequate eye protection requires understanding the two concepts of maximum permissible exposure (MPE) and nominal hazard zone (NHZ). According to the ANSI Z136.3 standards, the MPE is the level of laser radiation to which a person may be exposed without hazardous effects to the eye or skin. MPE levels are determined through consideration of laser wavelength, power, exposure time, and pulse repetition.

The NHZ is the space where the level of direct, reflected, or scattered radiation during normal laser operation exceeds MPE; eye, skin, and fire safety precautions must be followed while one is working within this hazard zone. The NHZ can be calculated mathematically to determine the distance from the laser beam emission in which the beam can cause skin and eye damage. With power, operating modes, and other parameters changing frequently during a procedure, this calculation is not always possible. Therefore, the area inside the surgical room usually is considered to be within the NHZ so that consistency and simplicity can be maintained when lasers are used.

Protective goggles and glasses must be inscribed with the appropriate filtering capabilities and adequate optical densities for the

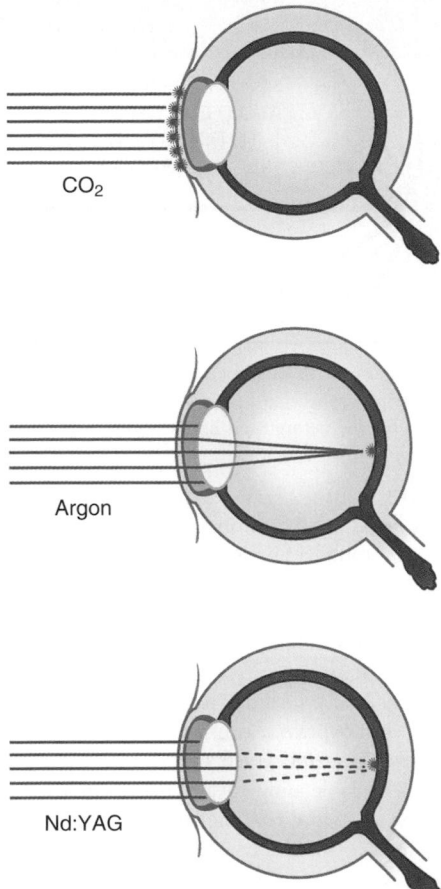

FIGURE 8-64 The CO_2 laser beam can damage the cornea; the argon and Nd:YAG beams can injure the retina.

specific wavelength being used (Figure 8-65). For example, a pair of Nd:YAG goggles may be inscribed "1064 nm, optical density 5." The optical density of the lens is the capability of the lens material to absorb a specific wavelength. Darker lens shades do not indicate higher optical density, nor do they give more protection than lighter ones. There are lighter lens shades with high optical densities that provide adequate safety. Laser team members must ensure that eyewear is properly labeled, handled, and stored so that hazards are minimized, and scratching and damage of the eyewear avoided.

During surgical procedures using multiple wavelengths, protective eyewear must change as wavelengths change. Some eyewear protects against a limited range of wavelengths. If the range is expanded to block a greater variety of wavelengths, the transparency of the eyewear is reduced.

Controversy exists as to the appropriateness of using personal prescription eyeglasses as CO_2 laser eye protection when the wearer is not in the immediate vicinity of the laser beam emission (e.g., the circulating nurse). Prescription eyeglasses do not have wavelength protection inscribed on them and have not been tested to

FIGURE 8-65 The frame of the protective eyewear displays wavelength and optical density information.

PATIENT SAFETY

Eye Safety During Laser Surgery

- Ensure that everyone in the laser room is wearing the appropriate eye protection with side shields before activating the laser. The eyewear should have the laser wavelength protection and optical density of the lens material inscribed on it.
- Place a special lens cover over the eyepiece of an endoscope to protect the physician's eye from laser backscatter. Remember that the physician's other eye is unprotected.
- Ensure that everyone in the laser room is wearing eye protection during laser endoscopic procedures.
- Connect an automatic lens shutter to a microscope head, if needed, to provide eye protection for individuals viewing the procedure through the microscope.
- When general anesthesia is used, cover the patient's closed eyes with moistened gauze pads. When the patient is awake, place the appropriate glasses or goggles on the patient. Explain the need for eye protection to the patient.

- During laser surgery near the eye, place a special laser eye shield directly on the anesthetized eye surface.
- Ensure that the appropriate protective eyewear is available at all entrances to the laser room for anyone entering this area.
- Cover windows in the laser treatment area appropriately, depending on the wavelength of the laser used.
- To prevent reflection of the laser beam, follow special precautions (i.e., using anodized or ebonized instruments near the laser-tissue impact site, covering large reflective retractors with wet towels or sponges).
- When storing protective eyewear, guard against scratches and mishandling. Scratches on the lenses may decrease their effectiveness. Inspect the eyewear regularly to ensure the integrity of the eyewear lenses has not been compromised.

Modified from AORN: *Perioperative standards and recommended practices,* Denver, 2013, The Association.

determine the protective ability of the lens; therefore, adequate protection cannot be guaranteed. Proponents state that the NHZ is so limited when the CO_2 beam is passed through the focusing lens that individuals who are not close to the laser emission port are not at high risk for eye damage. Facilities must address this controversy and develop a policy for the surgical team. Contact lenses and half glasses do not offer adequate protection against CO_2 laser energy and should not be used.

During a microscopic procedure, the optics of the microscope provide eye protection against CO_2 laser energy for the operative physician. When other wavelengths are used, such as argon or Nd:YAG, an automatic lens shutter can be connected to the microscope head. During laser activation the shutter allows a lens filter to drop into place to provide a shield from any laser backscatter, protecting the laser operator's eyes. When this device is attached to the microscope head, any observer tube being used also must be placed above the filter so that all portal optics offer protection. Others involved with the procedure must wear appropriate eyewear.

A lens filter can be placed over the eyepiece of a rigid or flexible endoscope. The lens must offer appropriate protection for the specific laser being used. Guidelines recommend that other surgical team members also wear eye protection, even though laser energy seems confined within an enclosed cavity. Optical injury is always possible if a fiber or articulated arm separates from the endoscope while the laser is activated, or if a fiber fractures and the beam escapes at the fracture site.

For healthcare professionals who routinely work with laser systems, a baseline eye exam is sometimes recommended, including visual acuity and an assessment of retinal health. Another eye exam can be performed after any ophthalmic accident or on termination of employment. The baseline exam provides a foundation for comparison with abnormal findings from subsequent exams. Performing baseline eye exams merely documents the ocular health of laser team members so that it can be used during a potential workers' compensation claim for retinal damage from accidental beam exposure. Some facilities opt not to follow this expensive and difficult-to-monitor guideline of performing baseline eye exams. Instead they strictly enforce their eye safety policy, minimizing the chance of ophthalmic injury. These facilities state in their eye safety policy that an eye exam will be performed if an ocular accident occurs.

The patient's eyes also must be protected during laser intervention. When general anesthesia is used, patients' eyes are covered with wet gauze, eye pads, or a towel; the eyelids are taped closed. If awake or under local anesthesia, the patient wears appropriate eye protection. Explanations about this eye protection should be provided. If the laser is to be used in the immediate vicinity of the eye, such as to lighten a port-wine stain on the eyelid, a special laser eye shield can be placed on the eye's surface after instilling a drop of ophthalmic local anesthetic. If the laser eye shields are sterilized with steam, these devices must be cooled completely before being placed on the cornea to prevent burns.

Controlled Access. Inadvertent access to rooms where laser treatments are being performed should be prevented. Laser warning signs must be placed at all entrances to the treatment area so that access is granted only to individuals who have been appropriately educated in laser safety. The word "Danger" and the universally accepted laser symbol should be present on laser warning signs to indicate the possibility of hazards (Figure 8-66). Laser signs should be removed when the procedure has been completed.

Windows and ports into rooms where lasers are used must be covered with appropriate protection for the specific laser being used.

FIGURE 8-66 Warning signs should be placed at all entrances to the surgical room to notify personnel that a laser is being used, and that appropriate eye protection is needed before entering the room.

The CO_2 laser beam, passed through a lens, and the holmium laser beam, delivered through a fiber, provide a limited NHZ, so window coverage is not required. Argon, Nd:YAG, and certain other laser wavelengths can be transmitted through window glass and have longer NHZs. Windows and ports must be covered with a blocking barrier that stops transmission of specific wavelengths with more extensive NHZs. Many facilities require window coverage for all laser procedures just to provide consistency within the laser program.

The laser key must not be left in the laser during storage. The key should be available only to authorized personnel who have appropriate education and training to operate the laser. Laser keys can be stored in the narcotics cabinet or in a special key lockbox to control access.

Fire Safety. An awareness of laser biophysics and tissue interaction is necessary to understand actions needed to prevent laser fires. A fire can be started by a reflected beam as easily as from direct impact. The laser team responds quickly if a fire occurs. Immediate action is key to minimize injury to the patient and the surgical team. The Patient Safety box on page 245 provides important detailed measures for fire safety during laser surgery.

Sterile water or saline solution should be readily available to douse a small fire on the patient. A laser-appropriate fire extinguisher should be available to control a fire within the laser system. During surgery, combustibles, such as any soft goods near the laser target site, should be kept wet to prevent ignition. The surgical team should monitor constantly the moisture level of sponges and other materials to prevent drying, which eventually could support a fire.

A laser beam can ignite flammable draping material easily. Some water-repellent drapes and other laser-safe materials are able to withstand laser impact because the flammability of the material is minimal. If the flammability of draping material or any other supplies is questionable (e.g., plastic tooth protectors), the suspect item can be tested in the manufacturer's or researcher's laboratory.

Instruments used in the immediate vicinity of the laser target site should be nonreflective to decrease the chance of the laser beam bouncing off the surface and accidentally impacting another area. The laser beam can easily be reflected off shiny instrument surfaces

FIGURE 8-67 A polyvinyl chloride endotracheal tube can become a blowtorch if ignited by a laser beam.

and can cause skin or eye injury or ignite flammable materials. To decrease reflectivity, an instrument may be ebonized by coating it with a special substance (usually black). The instrument should be inspected regularly to ensure integrity of the coating. Any scratched surface where ebonization has worn off should be recoated.

Instruments also may be anodized or surfaced with a matte finish to decrease reflectivity. Other coatings and surfaces that cause laser light to scatter and diffuse on impact are being introduced. Large retractors can be covered with wet sponges or towels so that the laser beam cannot accidentally reflect off a shiny surface.

Special instruments have been designed to provide backstops for laser energy to decrease adjacent tissue damage and fire risk. Titanium rods are effective backstops. Quartz rods often are used as backstops for the CO_2 laser beam, but argon and Nd:YAG beams may be transmitted through them. Wet sponges also can be used as backstop material. Glass rods are never to be used with a CO_2 laser because glass material heats and shatters after continuous impact by a laser beam. Teflon backstops are not to be used because they can melt when heated and produce toxic fumes.

Special laser mirrors that directly reflect the beam onto hard-to-reach areas are available. Mirrors may be made of rhodium or stainless steel. Glass-surface mirrors do not withstand laser impact and heat and shatter instead. Using a laser mirror requires skill because the beam must be focused on the target area and not on the mirror to deliver the full impact of laser energy. A laser beam that is misdirected off a mirror can easily cause a fire.

Flammable skin preparations should not be used for laser procedures. During skin cleansing, prep solution can pool underneath a patient, and ethanol vapors from alcohol-based preparations can be trapped beneath drapes. The volatility of these vapors increases the risk of a surgical drape fire. If flammable skin preps are used, then the drying must be adequate to allow the flammable vapors to dissipate. Iodophor or any other tinted prep solution should be wiped before argon or Nd:YAG lasers are used because the tint may increase laser absorption by the skin.

When a laser is used in the rectal area, a wet pack may be used to tamponade the bowel to prevent the escape of methane gas, which could enter the surgical area from the colon and cause an explosion. Wet sponges used for the pack must be counted so that packing is not inadvertently left in place after surgery. Some practitioners disagree with this practice, stating that inserting wet sponges may stretch the colon walls, increasing peristalsis and the movement of methane gas into the surgical area. Whatever method is chosen, a cleansing bowel prep before surgery also helps decrease this potential hazard.

Airway explosion caused by the laser beam igniting the endotracheal tube (ETT) can cause a potentially lethal accident for the patient. A polyvinyl chloride (PVC) ETT is highly flammable, especially when a high concentration of oxygen flows through it during anesthesia administration (Figure 8-67). Specific laser-retardant ETTs should be used during oral, tracheal, or esophageal laser procedures that require general anesthesia. The laser power limitations of a commercially manufactured ETT must be followed closely to ensure proper protection. The cuff of the ETT should be inflated with sterile saline to provide a heat sink and retard a fire if perforated by the laser beam. Saline may be tinted with methylene blue to note a cuff rupture more quickly as the blue dye escapes. A protocol should be developed to describe the emergency steps needed to control an endotracheal fire. Immediate considerations include the following:

- Stop ventilation (disconnect gas flow).
- Remove the ETT, ensuring entire tube is removed.
- Extinguish all flames with saline.
- Ventilate the patient by mask or reintubate immediately to prevent laryngospasm.
- Examine the airway (mouth, oral cavity, bronchial tree) for burns, foreign bodies, or both.
- Decide on the next course of action (anesthesia provider and surgeon), that is, cancel or continue with procedure.

A nonintubation technique involving jet ventilation also may be used during laser microlaryngoscopy. A jet ventilator is a mechanical ventilation unit that delivers oxygen through a small metal needle used with a rigid laryngoscope. Under pressurization, the jet ventilator is set to deliver a predetermined amount of oxygen with a set rate, pressure (in pounds per square inch [psi]), and percentage of inspiratory time. The needle is positioned between the vocal cords on the side opposite the lesion. The needle extends into the trachea so that the proper amount of oxygen is easily delivered. After surgery the patient may be intubated to maintain an open airway if postoperative edema or tracheal spasm is anticipated.

Other nonintubation techniques, such as apneic methods, can be used to avoid intubation. The patient's oxygen saturation must be monitored closely when these techniques are used.

Endoscope Safety. Special precautions should be followed when using the laser during an endoscopic procedure. When a laser fiber is introduced through the biopsy port of a flexible or rigid endoscope, the operator must view at least 1 cm of the tip of the fiber before activating the laser (Figure 8-68). If the end of the fiber is still within the sheath of the endoscope and the laser is fired, the heat from the laser energy quickly damages the optics and channel of the endoscope.

When a "bare" fiber is placed down the biopsy channel of a flexible endoscope, the sharp tip can tear the inside lumen of the channel. A length of medical-grade tubing can be placed over the fiber with the tip recessed within the sheath. The entire unit is then passed through the endoscope. When the end of the tubing is observed, the medical-grade tubing is withdrawn sufficiently to expose the end of the fiber. This procedure effectively protects the inside lumen of the endoscope channel during fiber insertion.

Smoke Evacuation. Smoke evacuation and odor control must be adequate whenever a plume is generated, whether it is from the laser, ESU, or other energy devices being used in surgery. When "hot" tools such as these are used to cut, excise, ablate, or coagulate tissue, cells of the target tissue are heated to the point of boiling. This causes cellular membranes to rupture, spewing cell contents into the air and producing surgical smoke.

One of the crucial elements of adequate smoke evacuation is to determine the method of smoke evacuation. The method selected depends on the amount of plume produced.

An *in-line smoke evacuation filter* is appropriate only for small amounts of plume generation, similar to what is produced during microlaryngoscopy vaporization of vocal cord polyps. The in-line filter connects to the existing suction line by positioning it between the wall connection and suction canister (Figure 8-69). If the filter becomes wet, it loses its effectiveness.

FIGURE 8-68 The laser fiber should extend past the end of the endoscope before the laser is activated.

To Wall Suction   To Patient

FIGURE 8-69 An in-line filter is placed between the suction canister and the wall outlet and is used to evacuate small amounts of surgical smoke.

If an in-line filter is not used, particulate matter from surgical smoke can occlude and corrode suction pipes and contaminate the building. Also suction flow may not be forceful enough to capture the plume adequately. Wall suction usually generates 2 cubic feet per minute (cfm) of air movement, whereas an individual smoke evacuator may move air at 35 to 50 cfm. An in-line filter is changed after each procedure (or according to the manufacturer's instructions).

When greater amounts of surgical smoke are generated, an *individual smoke evacuator* is used. Individual smoke evacuators have filtration systems that include a charcoal filter and an ultra–low-penetration air (ULPA) filter (Figure 8-70). The charcoal filter removes toxic gases and odor, whereas the ULPA filter removes small particulates with filtration of 0.12 micron size matter at 99.9999% efficiency (Ball, 2010a).

Maintenance of a smoke evacuator requires changing the filter per the manufacturer's written instructions (Figure 8-71). Standard Precautions should be used when changing a contaminated filter because of the possibility of bacterial and/or viral contamination (AORN, 2013). Many manufacturers recommend that the contaminated filter be treated as infectious and disposed of as regulated medical waste (biohazardous).

Centralized smoke evacuation systems provide smoke evacuation for several surgical rooms at the same time. The smoke evacuation line needs to be routinely flushed and cleaned to prevent debris buildup and pathogen growth within the system. A central system is convenient because it is always available; however, if it malfunctions, smoke evacuation is not available to multiple surgical areas.

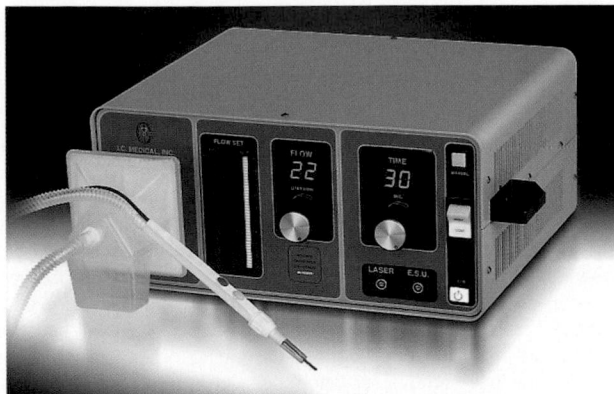

FIGURE 8-70 Individual smoke evacuator.

FIGURE 8-72 Electrosurgery pencil with the smoke evacuation system built into the device.

FIGURE 8-71 Contaminated filter being removed from smoke evacuator.

Contamination by surgical plume and tissue splatter is decreased when the surgical team wears gloves, gowns, and masks. The surgical team must ensure that the smoke evacuation wand or suction device is close to the target site so that all plume is evacuated. Devices are available that attach or are built into the ESU or laser delivery system that effectively evacuate surgical smoke as it is generated (Figure 8-72). Using appropriate smoke evacuation methods (Evidence for Practice) to ensure that all plume is eliminated is the only practice that protects the surgical team from exposure to hazardous surgical smoke. The Research Highlight box on page 248 describes a comparative study on methods to control surgical smoke by perioperative nurses.

Compliance studies have been performed to note the acceptance and implementation of smoke evacuation recommendations. Education has clearly been the reason for compliance with using appropriate smoke evacuation practices. The main barriers to compliance have been that the equipment and supplies are not available, the surgeon refuses to allow smoke evacuation to be performed during the procedure, the smoke evacuator is too noisy, and the staff is complacent and just won't use available smoke evacuation equipment and devices (Ball, 2010a, 2010b; Edwards and Reiman, 2012).

Surgical smoke that arises during flexible endoscopic or laparoscopic procedures impairs visibility. Hand control suction devices and valve filters provide gentle movement of plume during laparoscopy without destroying the pneumoperitoneum.

A high-flow insufflator is recommended for continual replacement of CO_2 gas. A special smoke evacuator may be used that automatically provides slow evacuation of plume without destroying the pneumoperitoneum.

Other Safety Measures. Foot pedals present safety problems if mistakenly activated. Multiple foot pedals placed on the floor can be confusing and lead to accidents. The laser pedal should be identified clearly and used only by the physician delivering laser energy to the target area.

Laser team members must appreciate potential electrical hazards because the laser, similar to the ESU, is high-voltage equipment. Water and other solutions should not be placed on the laser unit, and the components of the laser should be protected against spills or splatter, which could cause short-circuiting. The outside housing of the laser should never be removed by unauthorized personnel because of the potential for electrical shock or electrocution.

Transportation hazards are always a threat because some laser systems are quite heavy. When these units need to be moved, proper body mechanics must be used to prevent injury to the transporter. The laser unit should be pushed instead of pulled to provide less stress on the transporter's back muscles. The laser should not be bumped against a wall because its internal components can be damaged or become misaligned.

Documentation. Closely following written laser safety procedures is crucial for safety and legal reasons, as with any hazardous equipment. Specific notes about laser safety can be written on a laser log form or as part of the intraoperative nursing note. Either record should be placed in the patient's medical record so that safety activities can be recorded. Safety measures may not be specifically documented if already described and mandated in the facility's policies and procedures. This is referred to as "documentation by exception."

Smoke Evacuation During Laser Surgery

- Use the appropriate smoke evacuation system, depending on the amount of plume generated. If small amounts of plume are generated and room suction is to be used, an in-line suction filter is positioned between the suction canister and the wall outlet to capture surgical smoke particulate. An individual smoke evacuation system is used if larger amounts of plume are generated.
- Change the smoke evacuation filter(s) according to the manufacturer's written instructions.
- Hold the smoke evacuation suction tube close (<1 inch away) to the tissue interaction site to remove as much plume (odor and particulate matter) as possible.
- Smoke evacuation tubing should have a smooth inner lumen to eliminate any whistling.
- Use a reducer fitting to adapt a large smoke evacuation tube to a smaller suction or evacuation tube.
- The scrub person or first assistant can operate the smoke evacuation foot pedal (if available) to minimize wear and tear on the smoke evacuator motor and to decrease noise. Some smoke evacuators have sensing mechanisms that automatically activate the smoke evacuator when plume is generated.
- Evacuate surgical smoke generated during endoscopic or laparoscopic procedures. Endoscopic smoke evacuation instruments, such as suction tubes, help decrease the presence and retention of plume inside a body cavity or organ. A low-pressure suction valve can be used to remove plume gently during a laparoscopic procedure without destroying the pneumoperitoneum. A high-flow insufflator is recommended to replace any lost insufflation gas quickly. A special smoke evacuator that provides automatic plume removal also can be used to evacuate the intra-abdominal smoke without destroying the pneumoperitoneum.
- Wear a surgical mask that provides adequate filtration (0.1-µm filtration) to protect against residual smoke particulate that has not been evacuated. The high-filtration mask must fit snugly around the face. Wearing a high-filtration mask does not replace the use of a smoke evacuation system to remove surgical smoke from the environment.
- Continuing education helps healthcare personnel to understand the hazards of surgical smoke and encourages the use of appropriate methods for evacuation.

Modified from AORN: *Perioperative standards and recommended practices*, Denver, 2013, The Association; Ball K: Compliance with surgical smoke evacuation guidelines: implications for practice, *AORN J* 92:142–149, 2010; Ball K: Surgical smoke evacuation guidelines: are you compliant? *OR Nurse 2011* 5(6):40–44, 2011a; Ball K: Surgical smoke evacuation recommendations, *Hosp Healthc Eur*, 2011b; Ball K: 14 irrefutable reasons to eliminate surgical smoke, *Outpatient Surg* XII (7):46–51, 2011c.

Comparison of Current and Past Surgical Smoke Control Practices

After teaming with AORN in 2007 to conduct a survey on practices to control surgical smoke, the authors teamed with AORN 3 years later to repeat the survey to note any practice changes in compliance with established smoke evacuation recommendations throughout North America. The 2010 survey resulted in 1356 responses, representing about 14% of the population of perioperative nurses who received the email solicitation in all 50 states and Canada. There was a clear preference for using the wall suction with an in-line filter for all smoke-producing procedures except during laser hair removal or laser-assisted in situ keratomileusis (LASIK) surgery. An individual smoke evacuator was used more frequently for laser procedures than for procedures using other energies, like electrosurgery or ultrasonic energy, which is similar to the 2007 results. The number one reason for noncompliance with smoke evacuation recommendations was surgeon resistance or refusal to let smoke evacuation devices be used. Other reasons included cost, bulkiness of smoke collection devices, and smoke evacuator noise. Some comments noted that the only way to overcome noncompliance would be a clear regulation (from an agency like the Occupational Safety and Health Administration [OSHA]) to overcome resistance within their facility. In summary, the 2010 survey noted that smoke evacuation practices continue to be very mixed with some increase in use of wall suction for smoke evacuation. Smoke evacuation continues to be a practice not well established despite aggressive programs to provide education on the negative consequences of exposure to surgical smoke.

Modified from Edwards BE, Reiman RE: Comparison of current and past surgical smoke control practices, *AORN J* 95:337–350, 2012.

A special laser log can be designed to be a permanent part of the patient's record and might include information such as the laser used, power, pulse duration, and other laser parameters. The use of smoke evacuation, fibers, and contact tips also may be documented, especially if specific charges for these items are made. A sample laser log is shown in Figure 8-73.

Role of the Laser Team Member. As the use of laser technology grows, the role of the laser team member becomes more important. The backbone of a progressive and successful laser program is the enthusiastic and dedicated laser team. Expanded responsibilities are being assumed by the laser team member to provide consistency and promote a safe environment for the patient and the surgical team. Some roles of the laser team member may include serving as the laser safety officer, serving on the laser committee, becoming actively involved with laser procurement, and promoting the laser program through marketing.

According to ANSI Z136.3 (2011), the definition of the laser safety officer (LSO) is "the one person in each facility or organization responsible for the laser safety program ... [who] has the training and experience to administer a laser safety program ... is authorized by the health care facility administration and is responsible for monitoring and overseeing the control of laser hazards" (p. 7). Following are some of the duties of the LSO:

- Ensures all lasers have been labeled by manufacturer with appropriate hazard classification
- Evaluates potential hazards of the laser
- Serves on laser committee
- Enforces standard operating procedures (e.g., maintenance, service, perioperative checklists, policies)
- Ensures protective equipment and devices are in good working order (e.g., protective eyewear)
- Ensures laser installation and maintenance are carried out by qualified individuals, documented, and performed regularly
- Ensures appropriate training and education on laser safety are conducted and documented
- Documents incidents with lasers that could cause or have caused harm to patients or healthcare providers
- Delegates duties within the laser program as appropriate

```
Date _____ OR Room No. _____

PATIENT INFORMATION:
Name _____ Patient ID No. _____
Zip Code _____ Sex: M F Age _____
Status: IP OP

SURGERY INFORMATION:
Physician _____ Anesthesia: General MAC Local
Procedure _____

LASER INFORMATION:
Laser and wavelength_____
Power _____ Duration _____
Total spots _____ Total energy _____
Laser time on _____ Laser time off _____

DELIVERY SYSTEM:
Laser fiber _____ _
Contact tip _____ _
Microscope handpiece _____

LASER SAFETY:
Eye protection_____
Smoke evacuation _____
Fire safety_____
Other safety measures _____
_____

COMMENTS:
_____
_____

Laser team member _____
```

FIGURE 8-73 Sample laser log.

Perioperative nurses who are part of the laser team are often involved with patient education. The perioperative nurse reinforces what the physician has described to the patient before a laser procedure. When told that surgery is needed, the patient is often anxious because of the unknown. Anxiety may be compounded because the patient is confronted with two alarming unknowns. Many patients develop uneasiness about laser procedures based on information from science-fiction movies, talk shows, and other such sources. The patient always should have the opportunity to discuss a proposed procedure to allay any worries. The perioperative nurse may provide additional information if the patient has further questions about laser technology. After the physician has explained the procedure, a surgical consent is signed, timed, and dated. Sometimes the consent form reflects that a laser will be used during surgery. Some physicians, however, suggest that a laser is merely a tool used during surgery and do not believe it is necessary to list laser use on the consent form.

Adequate time should be allotted for patient questions before the procedure. If a local anesthetic is used, the patient should understand what to anticipate during surgery, what sounds or odors will arise, why eye protection is needed, and what the patient's role is during the procedure. If the patient understands the application, the role of the laser, and his or her responsibility during and after the procedure, the perioperative nurse can expect better compliance and less anxiety in the patient.

Discharge instructions are required for any ambulatory procedure; laser discharge instructions may be preprinted for each surgical application. These written instructions should be reviewed and given to the patient on discharge. A follow-up phone call helps the perioperative nurse evaluate the care delivered during the laser intervention and the patient's compliance with postoperative instructions.

Sometimes the perioperative nurse is placed in a compromising position by being expected to circulate during the surgical procedure as well as operate the laser. This nurse has the tremendous responsibility of being accountable for two crucial roles in the OR; the risk of a laser incident may increase. In the traditional setting one nurse circulates while another nurse or a technologist, a member of the laser team, operates the laser. The healthcare facility must determine which procedures require more staffing to deliver safe patient care.

Ultrasonic Device Surgery

Vibrating mechanical energy devices provide a safe option for cutting and coagulation. High-frequency sound waves are propagated to a blade tip to produce ultrasonic energy. These ultrasonic waves have a frequency of greater than 20,000 Hz and cannot be sensed by the human ear.

Production of ultrasonic energy begins with electrical current that generates an electrical signal sent through a coaxial cable to a transducer in a handpiece. The transducer converts electrical energy to mechanical motion through contraction and expansion of piezoelectric ceramic elements (Figure 8-74). A longitudinal vibratory response that moves the tip at the end of the handpiece from 23,000 Hz to greater than 55,000 Hz is produced. As the power increases, the frequency remains the same, but longitudinal excursion of the tip lengthens.

Because the tip is in contact with tissue, mechanical motion causes tissue protein to denature as hydrogen bonds are broken. As protein molecules become disorganized, a sticky coagulum forms

FIGURE 8-74 Mechanical motion is created in the ultrasonic handpiece.

FIGURE 8-75 Energy system with different handpieces.

that welds and coagulates smaller bleeding vessels. Aerosolization occurs during cellular destruction, consisting of a small amount of water vapor that usually dissipates quickly. Only a small amount of thermal energy is produced and any adjacent tissue damage is minimal.

Different tip configurations include a blade, ball, and hook (Figure 8-75). To obtain optimal tissue response, countertraction must be applied to the structure being treated. A shear-grasper to hold the tissue between a blade and tissue pad can be used to eliminate the need for countertraction.

The following are advantages of using an ultrasonic device to cut and coagulate:

- No surgical plume or odor is generated; only a small amount of aerosolization is created.
- Less adjacent tissue is damaged compared with laser and ESU devices.
- Tactile feedback is retained.
- No nerve or muscle stimulation occurs because no electrical current is delivered to the target area.
- No stray electrical or laser energy is produced.
- Precise cutting and control are offered.

Neutral Plasma Coagulation. A neutral plasma coagulator is an energy source that produces pure plasma to provide coagulation.

Plasma is created when a low flow of argon gas is excited within the handpiece, consisting of an anode (where current enters) and cathode (where current exits). The gas, in the plasma state, emerges from the handpiece tip as an electrically neutral pale blue jet stream that coagulates tissue. When the plasma reaches bleeding tissue, it releases its kinetic energy as heat and causes coagulation of the bleeding surface as well as cutting capabilities. Because the electrodes are contained within the handpiece, no dispersive pad is used. Patient risk is reduced because no electrical current passes through the patient. Thermal conductivity is very limited, so the depth of tissue damage is minimized. This energy can be used near pacemakers, metallic implants, and defibrillators because it is electrically neutral. The plasma flow helps to remove liquid from the target site, so the surgeon's visibility is not compromised. The neutral plasma jet can cut all tissues, including bone, while simultaneously providing coagulation. The system consists of a range of disposable handpieces.

Microwave Ablation. Microwave ablation uses frictional heat generated from rotation of water molecules that creates an ablation zone with simultaneous application of one or more antennas. When the antennas are close to each other (i.e., 1.5 to 2 cm apart), one combined ablation zone is created. No electrical current flows through the patient and no dispersive pad is required. The system automatically shuts off when the set ablation time is achieved. The advantage of microwave ablation is that the desired level of soft tissue coagulation can be reached more quickly compared to other radiofrequency ablation devices.

Microwave ablation can be used for treatment during percutaneous, laparoscopic, or open access procedures to treat primary and secondary diseases, such as liver disease, lung malignancies, renal and adrenal tumors, and even bone metastases. Tumor boundaries have been successfully treated using microwave energy. Research in this technology may confirm microwave ablation as a new era in tumor ablation.

Hydrodissection and Irrigation

Hydrodissection and irrigation are essential during most open and endoscopic procedures to provide a clear field of view and even release structures. Hydrodissection is used routinely for cataract extraction through a process called phacoemulsification. Nerve hydrodissection, such as carpal tunnel release, is a relatively new technique performed by using ultrasound guidance to inject a small amount of fluid around the affected nerve. The nerve is then released by using a hydrodissection process, thus allowing the nerve to glide easier within surrounding structures.

Irrigation is accomplished with irrigation probes for open procedures; via irrigating channels built into endoscopes; or by irrigating systems inserted through an operating port, cannula sheath, or operative endoscope. For endoscopic procedures, irrigating fluid can be introduced manually using a syringe and stopcock attached to irrigation tubing on one end and an irrigation bag and tubing assembly on the other. Fluid flows by gravity and is manually forced through the distal tubing.

A pressure bag can be used to increase flow, if desired. Irrigation through a flexible endoscope also can be delivered directly by a syringe attached to the irrigation port. Fluid travels through a specific channel built into the scope. Rigid scopes, such as ureteroscopes, cystoscopes, and hysteroscopes, also have this capability, as do operative laparoscopes.

Pumps are used for large quantities of fluid and when manual operation is cumbersome and time consuming. Pumps are beneficial when irrigation is used for hydrodissection because more fluid can be introduced to the surgical site under pressurization. More force can be exerted over longer periods, and the pressure is adjustable.

A common pump irrigation system includes the irrigation pump (CO_2 or electric), irrigation bottle caps, irrigation probe with dual trumpet valves, and Y-tubing irrigation set. When a CO_2-controlled system is in use, an E-cylinder of CO_2 gas is attached by means of a tank yoke and input hose. A wrench must be available to turn off the tank when not in use. It is important to check tank pressure before and after each use. The pump usually has an adjustable pressure on-off capability and dual irrigation bottle selection. As one bottle empties, a flip of the switch redirects CO_2 flow to the second bottle. Bottles can be replaced as needed. The system operates by displacement of water or saline with CO_2 gas.

When an electric setup is used, a carrier bag with an inflatable bladder surrounds the solution bag. When the bladder inflates, adequate pressure can be achieved and controlled to provide irrigation and hydrodissection. Distal tubing attaches directly to an irrigation probe. The length of time and volume of irrigation are controlled by a trumpet valve (Figure 8-76). Probes are available as reusable, disposable, or a combination of both. All three types incorporate a second trumpet valve for suctioning.

FIGURE 8-76 A trumpet valve controls the flow of irrigant and suction.

If reusable probes are used, they are completely disassembled for cleaning and sterilization or disinfection. Each trumpet valve has a spring mechanism (similar to that of a ballpoint pen). These springs are under pressure when the trumpet valve is inserted. During disassembly it is important to hold a hand over the valve so that the spring cannot eject, disappear, or cause eye injury. Protective eyewear is worn during disassembly, and extra springs should be available.

Completely disposable units are available; other systems incorporate disposable with reusable components. In the latter, tubing and pistol-grip handles containing the trumpet valves are disposable, but suction and irrigation probes are reusable. The disposable and disposable-reusable units may also incorporate electrosurgical capability, allowing the device to be used for three separate functions.

Choice of irrigation fluid depends on surgeon preference. Traditionally, normal saline has been used. Because saline is a conductive fluid, use of a monopolar ESU presents a safety hazard relating to potential for transfer of heat and current to adjacent tissues. As a result, sterile water or other nonconductive solutions should be considered to prevent ESU energy from transferring to alternative sites when extensive use of a monopolar ESU is anticipated. Sorbitol, also used for irrigation during hysteroscopy, can be absorbed rapidly into the vascular system, especially during excessive venous bleeding. The patient must be monitored carefully because of the potential for congestive heart failure from fluid overload.

Cryosurgery

Cryosurgery is used to destroy small quantities of unwanted tissue, such as skin tumors, and to ablate larger tissue targets, such as liver tumors, prostatic cancer, and cervical dysplasia. Cryosurgery causes tumor death by freezing. When internal tumors (e.g., liver cancer) are treated, dead tumor cells eventually are absorbed into surrounding tissue. Cryosurgery often involves cycles or steps during treatment as a tumor is frozen, allowed to thaw, and then refrozen.

To freeze tissue properly a cooling device or cryosurgical probe must produce an ice ball capable of destroying tissue at approximately $-122°$ F ($-50°$ C) and colder. Some devices produce temperatures as low as $-464°$ F ($-240°$ C). The cooling source is usually gaseous nitrogen or supercooled liquid nitrogen.

For external tumors, liquid nitrogen is applied directly to the dysplastic tissue either with a cotton swab or with a spraying device. For internal tumors, liquid nitrogen is circulated through the length of a cryoprobe with an insulated shaft to confine freezing to the distal tip. Ultrasound imaging often is used to guide the cryoprobe and monitor tumor freezing. By localizing the freezing effects, nearby healthy tissue is spared. Smaller cryoprobes can be inserted through small trocar sites.

Cryosurgery may be used to treat early-stage skin cancers (basal and squamous cell carcinomas) and retinoblastoma (a childhood cancer that attacks the retina of the eye). Precancerous lesions, such as actinic keratosis and cervical intraepithelial neoplasia, may also be treated with this therapy. Cryosurgery has been used to treat a variety of cancers, including prostate, liver, breast, bone, brain, spinal, lung, and tracheal. It may be used in combination with other cancer treatments, such as radiation, hormone therapy, chemotherapy, and surgery. Cryosurgery has also been found useful in ophthalmology to reattach detached retinas and to treat other eye problems, such as retinoblastoma.

The primary advantage of cryosurgery over other therapies for cancer treatment is that it is less invasive. Only a small incision is needed to introduce the cryoprobe through the skin, and less bleeding, pain, and other complications occur. Cryosurgery is also less expensive compared with other treatments and often requires shorter hospital stays and recovery time. The main disadvantage of cryosurgery is the uncertainty of its long-term effectiveness because microscopic cancer cells can spread easily if they are missed during the freezing application. Cryosurgery continues to evolve as new techniques are explored for treatment and palliative therapy.

KEY POINTS

- The perioperative nurse is responsible and accountable for the safe use of a variety of different devices and pieces of equipment.
- The main components of a flexible endoscope include the control body, insertion tube, bending section with distal tip, and light-guide connector that form the foundation of the mechanical system, angulation system, and illumination system.
- The main components of a rigid endoscope include the eyepiece, body, shaft, and distal end.
- To check the transmission of light within a fiberoptic cable, one end of the cable is held pointing toward a bright light while the other end is checked for any peppering, which indicates broken fibers. When approximately 20% of the fibers are broken, the cable must be replaced.
- White balancing allows the camera to adjust to white light so all primary colors appear properly.
- Instrumentation and port access devices have been introduced to allow single-entry laparoscopic procedures because there is less scarring and increased recovery with this technique.
- Endoscopes and instrumentation must be reprocessed following the manufacturer's written instructions. Devices must be thoroughly cleaned so that sterilization by steam, ethylene oxide, plasma, liquid chemical, or ozone can be accomplished.
- The FDA closely monitors the practice of reprocessing single-use devices, enforcing the regulatory guidelines that have been published.
- Nurses must understand the technical components of a video system that include the camera, cable, control unit, couplers (adapters), monitors, recording systems, and storage systems.
- Nurses must be aware of insufflation hazards and closely monitor the rate of flow and the volume of gas delivered while also monitoring the patient's intra-abdominal pressure.
- Electrosurgery is the most common energy source used in surgery today; therefore, nurses must understand the difference between coagulation and cutting settings, monopolar and bipolar systems, and dispersive pad considerations.
- The three hazards associated with electrosurgery used during laparoscopy are direct coupling, insulation failure, and capacitive coupling.
- Laser energy can cause photothermal, photoacoustic, or photochemical reactions.
- When laser energy impacts tissue it can be reflected, scattered, transmitted, or absorbed depending on the laser wavelength.
- Complying with laser safety guidelines is mandatory when laser energy is used during a surgical procedure. Some of these protocols include smoke evacuation, eye safety, fire safety, and controlled access.
- Nurses must be educated on different energies used during surgery to provide a safe environment for the patient and staff.

CRITICAL THINKING QUESTION

You are the team member assigned to operate the CO_2 laser during a laser ablation of rectal condyloma. You have received the specialized laser education required to serve on the laser team. You understand the hazards associated with laser technology when using a laser in the rectal area. What devices would you gather to provide a safe laser environment for the patient and the surgical team during this procedure? What critical assessment factors would you consider and what would you include as intraoperative nursing interventions as the laser team member?

evolve *The answers to the Critical Thinking Question can be found at http://evolve.elsevier.com/Rothrock/Alexander.*

REFERENCES

American National Standards Institute, Inc: *American national standard for the safe use of lasers in health care facilities, ANSI Z136.3,* New York, 2011, ANSI.

Association of periOperative Registered Nurses (AORN): *Perioperative standards and recommended practices,* Denver, 2013, The Association.

Ball K: Surgical smoke evacuation guidelines: compliance among perioperative nurses, *AORN J* 92:e1–e23, 2010a.

Ball K: Compliance with surgical smoke evacuation guidelines: implications for practice, *AORN J* 92(2):142–149, 2010b.

Ball K: Surgical smoke evacuation guidelines: are you compliant? *OR Nurse 2011,* 001-005, November 2011a.

Ball K: Surgical smoke evacuation recommendations, Hospital Healthcare Europe, *The Official Hope Reference Book,* 001-005, 2011b, Brussels.

Ball K: 14 irrefutable reasons to eliminate surgical smoke, *Outpatient Surg* 46–51, 2011c.

Dziedzic ME: *Nursing challenges in the care of patients who undergo minimally invasive surgery—are you prepared?* 2013, available at www.nursingconsult.com/nursing/clinical-updates/full-text?clinical_update_id=198886. Accessed February 8, 2013.

Dooley MM, Braghieri T : Take the path of least resistance with ESUs, *OR Nurse* 2(2):37–39, 2008.

Edwards BE, Reiman RE: Comparison of current and past surgical smoke control practices, *AORN J* 95:337–350, 2012.

Government Accounting Office, *Reprocessed single-use medical devices: FDA oversight has increased, and available information does not indicate that use presents an elevated risk,* 2008, available at www.gao.gov/new.items/d08147.pdf. Accessed February 9, 2013.

National Council of State Boards of Nursing: *Nurse licensure compact,* 2013, available at www.ncsbn.org/nlc.htm. Accessed February 8, 2013.

Poon JT et al: Impact of laparoscopic colorectal resection on surgical site infection, *Ann Surg* 249:77–81, 2009.

Sajid MS et al: Laparoscopic versus open repair of incisional/ventral hernia: a meta-analysis, *Am J Surg* 197:64–72, 2009.

Schmock BA: Technological advances in the operating room, *Pa Nurse* 64(1):13, 28, 2009.

Spruce L, Braswell ML: Implementing AORN recommended practices for electrosurgery, *AORN J* 95:373–384, 2012.

U.S. Food and Drug Administration (FDA): *Enforcement priorities for single-use devices reprocessed by third parties and hospitals,* Rockville, MD, 2000, U.S. Department of Health and Human Services.

U.S. Food and Drug Administration (FDA): *Guidance for industry and FDA staff: medical device user fee and modernization act of 2002, validation data in premarket notification submissions (510(k)s) for reprocessed single-use medical devices,* Rockville, MD, 2006, U.S. Department of Health and Human Services, available at www.fda.gov/MedicalDevices/DeviceRegulationandGuidance/GuidanceDocuments/ucm071434.htm. Accessed February 9, 2013.

CHAPTER 9

Wound Healing, Dressings, and Drains

JACQUELINE R. BAK

The ability to heal wounds is one of the most powerful defensive properties humans possess. Wound healing is a complex, highly organized response by an organism to tissue disruption caused by injury. This process is highly reliable in the absence of endogenous and exogenous infection, mechanical interference, or certain disease processes. Apposition and maintenance of the edges of a cleanly incised wound almost always result in prompt healing. A primary goal of perioperative patient care is the prevention of surgical site (wound) infections. Surgical site infections (SSIs) are a significant cause of illness, death, and excessive healthcare costs. Surgical wounds have the potential for infection from strains of antibiotic-resistant bacteria, such as methicillin-resistant *Staphylococcus aureus* (MRSA) and vancomycin-resistant enterococci (VRE) (Research Highlight).

Postoperative SSIs are a major complication for approximately 30 million individuals undergoing surgery annually in the United States, with an estimated 20% acquiring a healthcare-associated infection (HAI). SSIs are the third most commonly reported HAI, resulting in a complication rate of 1% to 12% of all surgical procedures, with an estimated cost of $12,000 to $30,000 per infection (Peterson, 2009). Although many surgeries are performed on an ambulatory basis and the average number of admissions to hospitals and length of stay have decreased since the 1980s, the incidence of HAIs has increased (Ambulatory Surgery Considerations). In response to the Deficit Reduction Act of 2005, the Centers for Medicare & Medicaid Services (CMS) have modified payment for selected reasonably preventable complicating conditions that have evidence-based prevention guidelines. Examples of these conditions are catheter-related infections and infections associated with coronary artery bypass grafts, certain orthopedic procedures, and certain bariatric surgery procedures (CMS, 2012). Actions taken by perioperative personnel sometimes can mean the difference between developing an SSI and normal healing. A clear understanding of these actions along with a solid knowledge of wound healing and factors adversely affecting healing are essential to the appropriate management of patients undergoing surgery. It is also imperative in light of the evolving CMS-implemented reduction in payment for an expanding array of avoidable conditions that include wound-related infections.

Anatomy

The skin is the largest organ of the body and acts as the first line of defense against infection. It provides protection and sensation, regulates fluid balance and temperature, and produces vitamins (e.g., vitamin D) and immune system components. The skin of the average adult covers about 3000 square inches, weighs about 6 pounds, and receives one third of the body's circulating blood volume. It varies in thickness from 0.5 mm in the tympanic membrane to 6 mm on the soles of the feet and the palms of the hands. Key structures of the skin are the primary layers of the epidermis, the dermis, and the subcutaneous. The *epidermis* is the outermost layer of the skin, lines the ear canals, and is contiguous with the mucous membranes. The epidermis is composed of several layers consisting of keratin and lipids. Keratin is the primary substance that hardens nails and hair and protects the body from fluid loss and invasion by pathogens. The epidermis is supported by the *dermis,* which is thicker than the epidermis and composed of collagen. The dermis is the largest portion of the skin, providing strength and structure. Contained within the dermis are blood vessels, lymph ducts, hair roots, nerves, and sebaceous and sweat glands. The dermis is vascularized and innervated (Figure 9-1). The innermost *subcutaneous* layer is composed of adipose tissue that merges with the deepest layer of the dermis to provide insulation, shape, and support. Any wound or disruption of the skin can provide a portal for bacteria and possible infection.

Etiology of Wounds

The causes of wounds can be described as follows:
- *Surgical*—caused by an incision or excision
- *Traumatic*—caused by mechanical, thermal, or chemical destruction
- *Chronic*—caused by an underlying pathophysiologic condition (e.g., pressure ulcers or venous stasis ulcers) over time

The amount of tissue loss, the existence of contamination or infection, and the degree of damage to tissue are some factors that determine the type of wound closure selected by the surgeon. The healing process is inherently related to whether the wound is closed or left open. This process occurs in one of three ways: primary intention, second intention (granulation and contraction), and third intention (delayed closure) (Figure 9-2).

Types of Wound Closure

Primary Intention

Healing through primary intention occurs when wounds are created aseptically, with a minimum of tissue destruction and postoperative tissue reaction. Wounds closed with sutures, staples, tape, or surgical adhesive applied as soon after the time of injury as possible fall into this category. When wounds are created under sterile conditions, healing is optimized and begins almost immediately. This type of healing is known as primary intention and occurs under the following conditions:
- Edges of an incised wound in a healthy individual are promptly and accurately approximated.
- Contamination is held to a minimum by rigid adherence to aseptic technique.

RESEARCH HIGHLIGHT

Epidemiology of Surgical Site Infections

Surgical site infections have an economic impact and are likely to increase hospital stay, affect admission to the intensive care unit, and impact multiple readmissions. With this in mind it is important to understand and identify the causative pathogens associated with surgical site infections and the outcomes. The purpose of this multicenter study was to investigate the current epidemiology of surgical site infections (SSIs) that require the patient's readmission to the hospital. The study was conducted over a 4.5-year period and had a total of 8302 patients who met the selection criteria, with a median age of 58 years; 45.6% were male. The principal diagnosis was postoperative infection with a positive surgical wound culture.

The most common isolated pathogen was *Staphylococcus aureus,* with methicillin-resistant *S. aureus* (MRSA) infections increasing significantly among the patients with positive culture SSI during the study period (16%-20%). MRSA infection had higher raw mortality rates (1.4% vs. 0.8%), longer hospital stays (6 vs. 5 days), and higher hospital costs ($7,036 vs. $6,134). The researchers noted that MRSA infection risk-adjusted attributable length of stay increase was 0.93 days and the cost increase of $1,157. The other significant risk factors that contributed to the patient's length of stay and increasing cost included illness severity, transfer from another facility, and previous admission within 30 days. Study results revealed that SSIs caused by MRSA significantly increased during the 4.5-year study and were independently associated with both clinical and economic burden.

Modified from Weigelt JA et al: Surgical site infections: causative pathogens and associated outcomes, *Am J Infect Control* 38:112–120, 2010.

AMBULATORY SURGERY CONSIDERATIONS

Post-Discharge Follow-up About Wound Management

Most postoperative superficial surgical site infections (SSIs) occur within 28 days of surgery. Infection control practitioners often use 30 days as the accepted length of surveillance for infections after procedures that do not involve prosthetic implants. Post-discharge surveillance methods have been used with varying degrees of success for different procedures and different hospitals. The methods include direct examination of patients' wounds during follow-up visits with the surgeon, nurse practitioner, physician assistant, or a clinic; review of medical records; and mail or telephone surveys with patients. As integrated health information systems become widespread, tracking surgical patients throughout their care may become easier, more practical, and more effective. There is currently no consensus on which post-discharge surveillance methods are the most sensitive, specific, and practical. The method chosen will reflect the facility's mix of surgical procedures, personnel resources, and data needs. Some questions to consider in a post-discharge telephone call to determine presence of an SSI are:

- Are you having any difficulty following the instructions you were given?
- Have you noticed any of the warning signs we talked about (list these, such as redness, swelling, pain, hot to the touch)?
- Have you taken your temperature? Is it more than 100 degrees?
- Do you have chills?
- Is there anything I can help you with?

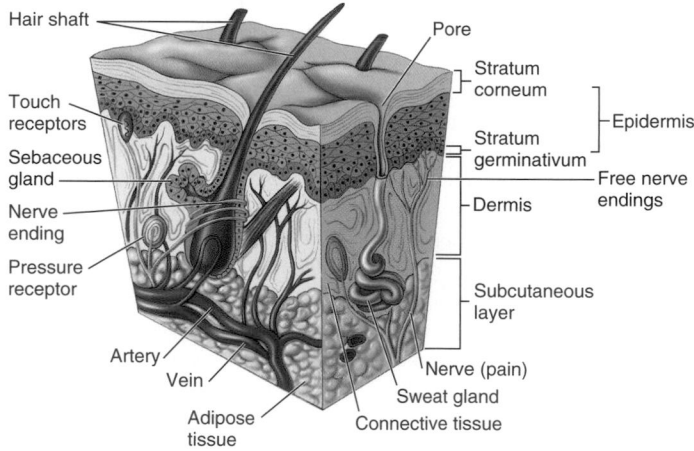

FIGURE 9-1 The skin.

- Trauma is minimal.
- No tissue loss occurs.
- On completion of closure, no dead space remains to become a potential site of infection.
- Drainage is minimal.

Second Intention (Granulation and Contraction)

When surgical wounds are characterized by tissue loss with an inability to approximate wound edges, healing occurs through second intention (see Figure 9-2). This type of wound is usually not closed; instead, it is allowed to heal from the inside toward the outer surface. In infected wounds this process allows the proper cleansing and dressing of the wound as healthy collagen tissue expands from the inside. The area of tissue loss gradually fills with granulation tissue, comprising fibroblasts and capillaries. Scar tissue is extensive because of the size of the tissue gap that must be closed. The scar is referred to as a *cicatrix*. Contraction of surrounding tissue also occurs. Consequently this healing process takes longer than primary intention healing. Healing by second intention is often seen in chronic wounds, dirty wounds, and traumatic wounds in which large areas of tissue are lost.

▶ Healing by First Intention

| Clean incision | Early suture | "Hairline" scar |

An aseptically made wound with minimal tissue destruction and minimal tissue reaction begins to heal as the edges are approximated by close sutures or staples. No open areas or dead spaces are left to serve as potential sites of infection.

▶ Healing by Second Intention (Granulation) and Contraction

  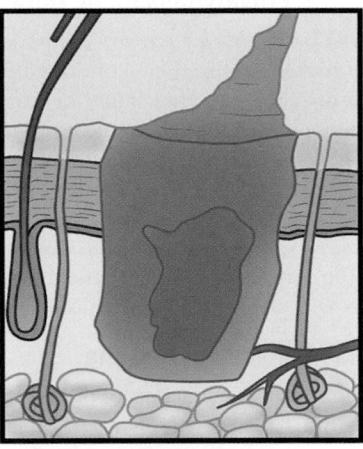

| Gaping, irregular wound | Granulation and contraction | Growth of epithelium over scar |

An infected or chronic wound or one with tissue damage so extensive that the edges cannot be smoothly approximated is usually left open and allowed to heal from the inside out. The nurse periodically cleans and assesses the wound for healthy tissue production. Scar tissue is extensive, and healing is prolonged.

▶ Healing by Third Intention (Delayed Closure)

| Infected wound | Granulation | Closure with wide scar |

A potentially infected surgical wound may be left open for several days. If no clinical signs of infection occur, the wound is then closed surgically.

FIGURE 9-2 Processes of wound healing.

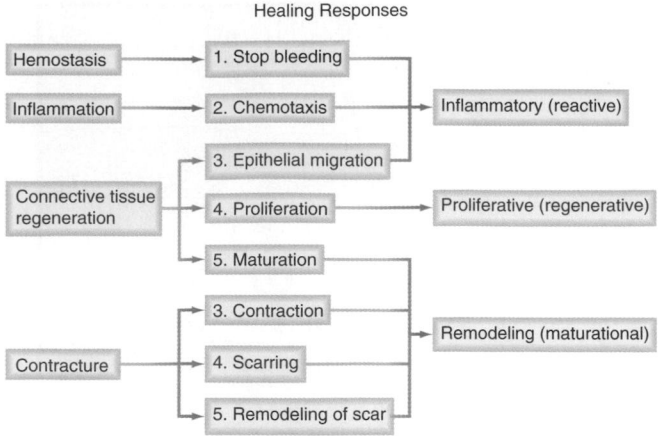

Healing Responses

FIGURE 9-3 Schematic diagram of the wound-healing continuum.

Delayed Primary Closure or Third Intention

As the name *delayed primary closure* implies, this healing process occurs when approximation of wound edges is intentionally delayed by 3 or more days after injury or surgery (see Figure 9-2). These wounds may require debridement and usually require a primary and secondary suture line, such as when retention sutures are used. The conditions leading to a decision to delay closure are as follows:

- Removal of an inflamed organ
- Heavy contamination of the wound
- The critical nature of the patient's intraoperative condition, such as with hemodynamically unstable trauma patients

Phases of Wound Healing

Wound healing is the effort of the injured tissue to return to normal integrity after injury. It is an intricate biologic process that occurs in three simultaneous yet overlapping phases: (1) inflammatory (also known as the reactive stage), (2) proliferative (also known as the regenerative stage), and (3) remodeling (also known as the maturational stage) (Leong and Phillips, 2012) (Figure 9-3).

Inflammatory Phase

In the inflammatory phase, an exudate containing blood, lymph, and fibrin begins to clot and loosely binds the cut edges together. Blood supply to the area increases, and the basic process of inflammation begins. Inflammation is a prerequisite to wound healing and is a vascular and cellular response to dispose of bacteria, foreign material, and dead tissue. Leukocytes increase in number to fight bacteria in the wound area and by phagocytosis help to remove damaged tissues. The severed tissue is quickly glued together by strands of fibrin and a thin layer of clotted blood, forming a scab. Plasma seeps to the surface to form a dry, protective crust. This seal helps to prevent fluid loss and bacterial invasion. During the first few days of wound healing, however, the seal has little tensile strength. The inflammatory phase normally lasts 1 to 4 days. The skin edges may appear mildly swollen and slightly red in this phase as a result of the inflammatory processes at work. Many chronic wounds "stall" at this phase.

Proliferative Phase

The proliferative phase, beginning within hours of the injury, allows new epithelium to cover the wound. Epithelial cells migrate and proliferate to the wound area, covering the surface of the wound to close the epithelial defect. Epithelialization also provides a protective barrier to prevent fluid and electrolyte loss and to reduce the incidence of infection. While reepithelialization takes place collagen synthesis and wound contraction are occurring. Contraction begins approximately 5 days after the wound onset and peaks at 2 weeks, gradually shrinking the entire wound. Granulation tissue forms under the edges of the incision and can be palpated as a hard ridge, which eventually resolves during the remodeling phase. Epidermal migration is limited to about 3 cm from the point of origin. Larger wounds may require skin grafting because of this limited epidermal migration. Collagen synthesis produces fiber molecules that crosslink to provide strength to the wound.

Remodeling Phase

Remodeling begins after approximately 2 to 4 weeks, depending on the size and nature of the wound. It may last 1 year or longer. During the remodeling phase, scar tissue formed during fibroplasia changes in bulk, form, and strength. Throughout normal wound healing, new collagen is produced while old collagen breaks down in a balanced fashion. This collagen turnover allows randomly deposited connective tissue to be arranged in linear and lateral orientation. As the scar ages, fibers and fiber bundles become more closely packed and form a crisscross pattern, ultimately creating the final shape of the wound. At best, the tensile strength of scar tissue is never more than about 80% of the tensile strength of nonwounded tissue.

Factors Affecting Wound Healing

Patients should be assessed for factors that may impair wound healing. Important factors in tissue repair and healing to consider are the patient's age, physical status, preexisting conditions, nutritional status, oxygenation level, and overall recuperative power. The inflammatory response and oxygen tension depend on microcirculation to deliver components to the wound. Decreased oxygen tension to the wound area inhibits fibroblast migration and collagen synthesis, resulting in decreased tensile strength of the wound. Nutritional status also has a profound effect on healing because of the need for an adequate supply of protein necessary for the growth of new tissues. Protein also is required for the regulation of the osmotic pressure of blood and other body fluids and the formation of prothrombin, enzymes, hormones, and antibodies. Other nutritional essentials are water; vitamins A, C, B$_6$, and B$_{12}$; iron; calcium; zinc; and adequate calories. It is also important to maintain body temperature (normothermia) (Schwulst and Mazuski, 2012).

The most common cause of delayed wound healing in a surgical patient is SSI. Box 9-1 lists types of SSIs and defines criteria for classification. There are many possible causes of SSIs, including patient susceptibility to and severity of illness, microbial contamination by the patient's microflora, and exogenous wound contamination from the operating room (OR) environment and personnel. Adherence to strict aseptic principles, careful observation of sterile technique, and thorough antimicrobial preparation of the patient and operative site are essential to minimize the risk of postoperative SSI. Perioperative personnel who are not scrubbed at the sterile field must maintain meticulous hand hygiene during the procedure to decrease the transmission of bacteria to the surgical field or the patient (Patient Safety).

Wound healing also can be impaired by poor surgical technique. Rough handling of tissue may cause trauma that can lead to bleeding and other conditions conducive to infection. Examples of surgical technique promoting wound healing include adequate hemostasis, precise cutting and suturing techniques, efficient use of time to minimize wound exposure to air, elimination of dead spaces, and minimal pressure from retractors and other instruments.

BOX 9-1

Criteria for Defining a Surgical Site Infection (SSI): Reportable Infections

Superficial Incisional SSI

- Infection occurs within 30 days after the procedure.
- Involves only skin or subcutaneous tissue of the incision *and* at least *one* of the following:
  1. Purulent drainage, with or without laboratory confirmation, from the superficial incision
  2. Organisms isolated from an aseptically obtained culture of fluid or tissue from the superficial incision
  3. At least one of the following signs or symptoms of infection: pain or tenderness, localized swelling, redness, or heat *and* superficial incision is deliberately opened by surgeon, *unless* incision is culture-negative
  4. Diagnosis of superficial incisional SSI by the surgeon or attending physician

Deep Incisional SSI

- Infection occurs within 30 days after the procedure if no implant* is left in place or within 1 year if implant is in place and the infection appears to be related to the procedure.
- Infection involves deep soft tissues (e.g., fascial and muscle layers) of the incision *and* at least *one* of the following:
  1. Purulent drainage from the deep incision but not from the organ/space component of the surgical site
  2. A deep incision spontaneously dehisces or is deliberately opened by a surgeon when the patient has at least one of the following signs or symptoms: fever greater than 100.4°F (>38°C), localized pain, or tenderness, unless site is culture-negative

3. An abscess or other evidence of infection involving the deep incision is found on direct examination, during reoperation, or by histopathologic or radiologic examination
4. Diagnosis of a deep incisional SSI by a surgeon or attending physician

Note:

- Report infection that involves both superficial and deep incision sites as deep incisional SSI.
- Report an organ/space SSI that drains through the incision as a deep incisional SSI.

Organ/Space SSI

- Infection occurs within 30 days after the procedure if no implant* is left in place or within 1 year if implant is in place and the infection appears to be related to the procedure.
- Infection involves any part of the anatomy (e.g., organs or spaces), other than the incision, which was opened or manipulated during a procedure *and* at least *one* of the following:
  1. Purulent drainage from a drain that is placed through a stab wound† into the organ/space
  2. Organisms isolated from an aseptically obtained culture of fluid or tissue in the organ/space
  3. An abscess or other evidence of infection involving the organ/space that is found on direct examination, during reoperation, or by histopathologic or radiologic examination
  4. Diagnosis of an organ/space SSI by a surgeon or attending physician

*National Nosocomial Infection Surveillance definition: a nonhuman-derived implantable foreign body (e.g., prosthetic heart valve, nonhuman vascular graft, mechanical heart, or hip prosthesis) that is permanently placed in a patient during surgery.
†If the area around a stab wound becomes infected, it is not an SSI. It is considered a skin or soft tissue infection, depending on its depth.
Modified from Mangram AJ et al: *Special report: guideline of surgical site infection,* 1999, available at www.cdc.gov/hicpac/SSI/table1-SSI.html. Updated May 2011. Accessed January 23, 2013.

PATIENT SAFETY

Perioperative Handwashing

The Joint Commission (TJC) has made patient safety a priority through annual National Patient Safety Goals (NPSGs). One NPSG is reducing the risk of healthcare-associated infections (TJC, 2013). One of the criteria for meeting this goal is for organizations to comply with the current hand hygiene recommendations from the Centers for Disease Control and Prevention (CDC) or the World Health Organization (WHO). Perioperative nurses are especially vigilant about complying with hand hygiene guidelines. Patients are vulnerable whenever their intact skin barrier is breached. Activities that are not properly conducted in a sterile fashion, such as application of surgical dressings to a fresh incision, provide an opportunity for entry of pathogens. Healthcare workers (HCWs) often have a false sense of security about the protection that gloves offer and may think that frequent hand hygiene is unnecessary. Use of gloves cannot replace routine, faithful adherence to effective hand hygiene. Effective hand hygiene is the easiest, least expensive, and most effective tool that perioperative nurses have when acting as patient advocate. The goal of hand hygiene is a sufficient reduction of microbial counts on the skin to prevent cross-contamination of pathogens. Good hand hygiene practices also provide safety and protection to the HCW.

After extensive research, the WHO along with the CDC have published guidelines for hand hygiene. The guidelines are ranked by category ratings, which provide direction to facilities for implementation.

Category I rankings (IA and IB) are applicable to all settings and should be adopted; they are listed here.

Rankings
Indications for Hand Hygiene
Category IA

- If hands are not visibly soiled, use an alcohol-based hand rub for routinely decontaminating hands.
- Perform hand hygiene after contact with body fluids or excretions, mucous membranes, nonintact skin, and wound dressings.

Category IB

- Perform hand hygiene:
  - Before and after having direct contact with patients
  - Before handling an invasive device for patient care; gloved or ungloved
  - When moving from a contaminated body site to another body site during care of the same patient
  - After removing nonsterile gloves
  - After contact with inanimate surfaces, objects, medical equipment in immediate vicinity of patient

Continued

PATIENT SAFETY

Perioperative Handwashing—cont'd

- If alcohol-based hand rub is not obtainable, wash hands with soap and water.
- Wash hands with soap and water when visibly dirty or visibly soiled with blood or other body fluids.
- Handwashing with soap and water is the preferred method if exposure to potential spore-forming pathogens is strongly suggested or proven, including outbreaks of *Clostridium difficile*.
- Use an alcohol-based hand rub or wash hands with either plain or antimicrobial soap and water before handling medication or preparing food.

Hand Hygiene Techniques
Category IB
- Apply a palmful of alcohol-based hand rub and cover all surfaces of hands. Rub hands until dry.
- When washing hands with soap and water, wet hands first with water, then apply an amount of product necessary to cover all surfaces. Rinse hands with water and dry thoroughly with a single-use towel. Use clean, running water whenever possible. Avoid using hot water, because repeated exposure to hot water may increase the risk of dermatitis.
- Use a towel to turn off tap/faucet.
- Dry hands thoroughly using a method that does not recontaminate hands. Make sure towels are not used multiples times or by multiple people.

Recommendations for Surgical Hand Preparation
Category IB
- Artificial nails are prohibited.
- Brushes are not recommended for surgical hand preparation.
- Surgical hand antisepsis should be performed using either a suitable antimicrobial soap or suitable alcohol-based hand rub, preferably with a product ensuring sustained activity, before donning sterile gloves.
- When performing surgical hand antisepsis using an antimicrobial soap, scrub hands and forearms for the length of time recommended by the manufacturer, typically 2 to 5 minutes. Long scrub times (e.g., 10 minutes) are not necessary.
- When using an alcohol-based surgical hand rub product with sustained activity, follow the manufacturer's instructions for application times. Apply the product to dry hands only.
- When using an alcohol-based hand rub, use sufficient product to keep hands and forearms wet with the hand rub throughout the surgical hand preparation procedure.
- After application of the alcohol-based hand rub as recommended, allow all hands and forearms to dry thoroughly before donning sterile gloves.

Selection of Hand Hygiene Agents
Category IA
- Do not add soap to a partially empty soap dispenser. If soap dispensers are reused, follow recommended procedures for cleaning.

Category IB
- Provide HCWs with efficacious hand hygiene products that have low irritancy.
- To maximize acceptance of hand hygiene products by HCWs, solicit their input regarding the skin tolerance, feel, and fragrance of any products under consideration.
- When selecting hand hygiene products:
  - Solicit information from manufacturers about the risk of product contamination.
  - Ensure that dispensers are accessible at the point of care.
  - Elicit and evaluate information from manufacturers regarding any effects that hand lotions, creams, or alcohol-based hand rubs may have on the efficacy of antimicrobial soaps being used in the institution.

Skin Care
Category IA
- Provide HCWs with hand lotions or creams to minimize the occurrence of irritant contact dermatitis associated with hand antisepsis or handwashing.

Category IB
- Include information regarding hand-care practices designed to reduce the risk of irritant contact dermatitis and other skin damage in education programs for HCWs.

Use of Gloves
Category IB
- Using gloves does not replace the need for hand hygiene by either hand rubs or handwashing.
- Remove gloves after caring for a patient. Do not wear the same pair of gloves for the care of more than one patient.
- Reusing gloves is not recommended.

Other Aspects of Hand Hygiene
Category IA
- Do not wear artificial fingernails or extenders when having direct contact with patients.

Category	Ranking System for Evidence
IA	Strongly recommended for implementation and strongly supported by well-designed experimental, clinical, or epidemiologic studies
IB	Strongly recommended for implementation and supported by some experimental, clinical, or epidemiologic studies and a strong theoretic rationale

Modified from The Joint Commission: *National patient safety goals for hospitals*, 2013, available at jointcommission.org/assets/1/18/NPSG_Chapter_Jan2013_HAP.pdf. Accessed January 23, 2013; *WHO guidelines on hand hygiene in healthcare*, 2009, available at www.cdc.gov/Handhygiene. Updated May 2011. Accessed January 23, 2013.

Additional factors affecting wound healing are the patient's age, stress level, immunologic status, and smoking history. Preexisting conditions, such as diabetes, anemia, malnutrition, cancer, obesity, certain drug therapies (e.g., steroid therapy), and cardiovascular or respiratory impairments, also contribute to poor wound healing. Additional terms used in connection with wound healing are shown in Box 9-2.

Wound Classification

The Centers for Disease Control and Prevention (CDC) have long recommended four surgical wound classifications: clean wounds, clean contaminated wounds, contaminated wounds, and dirty or infected wounds. This classification scheme reflects the probability of infection and enables appropriate preventive measures to be

---

BOX 9-2

Additional Terms Used in Connection with Wound Healing

Adhesions: Adherence of serous membranes to one another, causing fibrous tissue to form; sometimes occur in healing and inflammatory processes; commonly occurs in or around gastrointestinal tract, where adhesions may form bands and cause obstructions and subsequent surgical emergencies.

Chemotaxis: A cellular function, particularly of neutrophils and monocytes, whose phagocytic activity is influenced by chemical factors released by invading microorganisms.

Dead space: Air or empty space between layers of tissue or beneath wound edges that have been approximated.

Dehiscence: Separation of layers of surgical wound (Figure 9-4).

Evisceration: Extrusion of internal organs or viscera through gaping wound (see Figure 9-4).

Gangrene: Anaerobic infection process that may occur instead of healing; implies necrosis (death of tissue) and putrefaction (decomposition); usually caused by failure of nutriment or blood to reach a part.

Keloid: Dense, unsightly connective tissue or excessive scar formation that is often removed surgically.

"Proud flesh": A mass of excessive granulation formed when a wound shows no other sign of healing or excessive cicatrization.

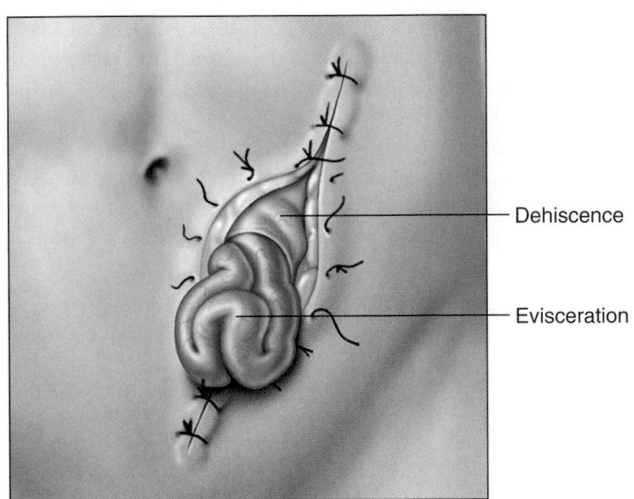

— Dehiscence

— Evisceration

FIGURE 9-4 Complications of wound healing.

taken. The AORN *Recommended Practices for Prevention of Transmissible Infection* note the importance of documenting the wound classification in the patient record (AORN, 2013). Following are descriptions of each classification.

Clean Wounds (Class I)

Clean wounds are uninfected wounds in which no inflammation is encountered, and the respiratory, alimentary, and genitourinary tracts are not entered. They are closed with a primary suture line. If required, they can be drained using a closed wound drainage system. Clean wounds show no sign of infection. Examples are breast biopsy, total hip replacement, and open heart surgery.

Clean Contaminated Wounds (Class II)

Clean contaminated wounds are those in which the respiratory, alimentary, or genitourinary tract is entered under controlled conditions. There is no sign of infection and no break in surgical aseptic technique. Examples of clean contaminated wounds are nonperforated appendectomy, hysterectomy, and thoracotomy.

Contaminated Wounds (Class III)

Contaminated wounds are open, fresh, accidental wounds, such as penetrating trauma, open fractures, or operations with major breaks

in aseptic technique, such as the inadvertent intraoperative use of nonsterile instruments or supplies. Incisions with signs of infection or gross spillage from the gastrointestinal tract also are included. Examples are a penetrating abdominal trauma involving bowel and a gunshot wound to the abdomen.

Dirty or Infected Wounds (Class IV)

Infected wounds include old, physically induced (traumatic) wounds with retained devitalized tissue and wounds that involve an existing clinical infection or perforated viscera. Examples are excision and drainage of abscess and delayed primary closure of a wound after appendectomy for ruptured appendix.

Antimicrobial Prophylaxis

The most effective course of action in dealing with SSI is prevention. Appropriate antimicrobial prophylaxis (antibiotic administration) also is an important factor in the prevention of SSI (Evidence for Practice). Major considerations in administering prophylactic antimicrobial therapy include selecting the appropriate agent, properly timing the administration of the agent, and limiting the duration of therapy.

Proper selection of the prophylactic antimicrobial agent is based on clinical efficacy, safety, cost, and whether the agent is broad spectrum. The surgeon commonly considers the nature of the surgical procedure, noting the most common pathogens associated with it (e.g., common pathogens of the small bowel in undertaking a small-bowel resection). Cephalosporins often are used for elective clean or clean contaminated surgical procedures. For these procedures a single dose usually is administered during the immediate preoperative period. It is important to carefully evaluate the need for antibiotics with the emergence of antibiotic-resistant microorganisms.

To enhance the effectiveness of prophylactic antimicrobial therapy, it is necessary for the optimal level of the antibiotic to be present in the tissue at the time of the incision. Equally important is the need to maintain circulating blood levels throughout some procedures. The antibiotic of choice should be administered within 1 hour before the skin incision. The anesthesia provider usually administers the antibiotic intravenously. If the surgical procedure is longer than the half-life of the antibiotic, another dose usually is administered intravenously during the procedure. Antibiotic therapy is usually discontinued within 24 hours; there is little evidence that ongoing administration contributes to decreased SSI rates in clean or clean contaminated procedures.

Antimicrobial Prophylaxis

According to the Institute for Healthcare Improvement an estimated 40% to 60% of surgical site infections (SSIs) are preventable with appropriate use of prophylactic antibiotics. Overuse, underuse, improper timing, and misuse of antibiotics occurs in 25% to 50% of operations. A large number of hospitalized patients develop infections caused by *Clostridium difficile,* and 16% of this type of infection in surgical patients can be attributed to inappropriate prophylaxis use alone. Inappropriate use of broad-spectrum antibiotics or prolonged courses of prophylactic antibiotics puts all patients at even greater health risks due to the development of antibiotic-resistant pathogens. Suggestions for the appropriate use of prophylactic antibiotics are described:

- Designate responsibility and accountability for preoperative prophylactic antibiotic administration (e.g., preoperative nurse, circulating nurse, anesthesia provider) connected to key point in process.
- Standardize administration process to occur with commonly performed activity within 1 hour prior to incision.
- Through the use of antibiotic standing orders specific to surgical site, administer prophylactic antibiotics according to guidelines based on local consensus.
- Make agreed-on antibiotics available in the operating room (OR).
- Standardize delivery process to ensure timely delivery of preoperative antibiotics to the holding area.
- Provide visible reminder or checklist to give antibiotics on each procedure (e.g., brightly colored sticker).
- Ensure systematic documentation of antibiotic administration on every patient chart (paper or electronic).
- Develop system in which antibiotic is hanging at head of patient's bed ready for administration.
- Design protocols to deliver antibiotic to OR with patient.
- Educate OR staff regarding the importance and reasoning of antibiotic timing, selection, and duration.
- Provide feedback on prophylaxis compliance and infection data monthly.
- Involve pharmacy staff to ensure that timing, selection, and duration are maintained.
- Institute a computerized physician order entry system with procedure-specific fields for antibiotic selection, timing, and duration.
- Improve screening for allergies to beta-lactam antibiotics to eliminate false-positives.
- Consider weight-based antibiotic dosing (higher dose for larger patients). Because this may be cumbersome, may want to increase cephalosporins from 1 to 2 g for all patients because of minor issues around toxicity.
- Re-dose for longer surgeries (e.g., after 3 hours for short half-life cephalosporin).

Modified from the Institute for Healthcare Improvement: Changes to Prevent Surgical Site Infection, available at www.ihi.org/knowledge/Pages/Changes/ChangestoPreventSurgical SiteInfection.aspx. Updated April 26, 2011. Accessed January 24, 2013.

Nursing Diagnoses

The nursing diagnoses—Risk for Infection, Risk for Impaired Skin Integrity, Imbalanced Nutrition, Ineffective Peripheral Tissue Perfusion, and Hypothermia—point the perioperative nurse toward strategies that can be used to prevent wound infections and promote healing.

The World Health Organization (WHO) provides SSI prevention guidelines for consideration in planning and implementing nursing interventions to optimize successful patient outcomes (Box 9-3). The nurse assesses the patient's susceptibility for infection, classifies the wound on the intraoperative record, implements sterile technique, protects the patient from cross-contamination, collaborates in administration of antibiotic prophylaxis, and performs other responsibilities to create and control the environment of care (Petersen, 2011). Attention is also given to controlling perioperative serum glucose levels in major surgical procedures, to maintaining skin integrity through proper positioning and the use of pressure-reducing mattresses as needed (see Chapter 6), and to using safe practices during electrosurgery (see Chapter 8). The perioperative nurse plays an essential role in preventing adverse events and patient injury by using critical thinking, clinical reasoning, and technical knowledge.

Patient and Family Education and Discharge Planning

Given that more patients are discharged from the acute care setting to the home care setting much earlier in their recovery, more surgical wound care is delivered by patients, their families, and home care providers instead of by the hospital nurse. Early planning and teaching about wound care, Standard Precautions, and medical waste disposal have become a vital part of preparing the patient to continue to manage the wound after discharge (Patient-Centered Care). Chassin also reports that calling patients within a week after discharge to review wound care management is significant in reducing surgical site infections (Hospitals Cut Colorectal Surgical-Site Infections by a Third, 2012).

Wound Management

A variety of treatments exist for acute and chronic wound management. Perioperative nurses often care for patients with infected wounds and are familiar with surgical wound debridement and sterile dressing changes performed under anesthesia. Patients also may come to the OR with chronic wounds being managed with a combination of surgical interventions and other treatment modalities. An understanding of adjunct wound therapies is essential to planning perioperative nursing care. These therapies include hyperbaric oxygenation (HBO), negative pressure therapy, hydrotherapy, use of engineered living skin substitutes, and the topical application of growth factors.

Debridement

Debridement is the act of removing dead and devitalized tissue from a wound. It is necessary because dead tissue in the wound provides a nidus for wound infection. Perioperative nurses often care for patients scheduled for surgical wound debridement (i.e., the sharp excision of dead or devitalized tissue). Debridement also can be accomplished through mechanical means (forceful irrigation), enzymatic action (application of chemical agents), and biologic methods (sterile maggot debridement therapy) (Ebner and Maytin, 2009). There are advantages and disadvantages to each method. Surgical debridement may not always be precise and healthy tissue may be sacrificed. Additionally, the act of surgical debridement may shower organisms into the bloodstream, resulting in bacteremia. Mechanical debridement is painful and nonselective in the tissue it removes. Enzymatic debridement may be uncomfortable for the patient and may macerate surrounding tissue. Biologic debridement, also referred to as biosurgery, may not be accepted by most patients. However, the nonsurgical options may be alternatives for patients who are not candidates for general anesthesia. Patients with chronic, nonhealing wounds may become well known to the perioperative

---

BOX 9-3

Guidelines for Prevention of Surgical Site Infections from the World Health Organization

Surgical site infections (SSIs) account for 14% to 16% of all hospital-acquired infections. An understanding of the guidelines for preventing SSIs enables perioperative nurses to weigh factors that are viewed as effective in preventing SSIs. The following guidelines from the World Health Organization (WHO) are based on a review of evidence and research. They focus on hand hygiene, appropriate and judicious use of antibiotics, antiseptic skin preparation at the surgical site, wound care, and instrument decontamination and sterility. As with many of the recent AORN Recommended Practices (RPs), these potentially beneficial practices are classified into categories on the basis of clinical evidence or expert opinion as to their ability to reduce the likelihood of serious, avoidable surgical harm. If adherence was unlikely to introduce injury, was only to "be considered" for surgical procedures, or was of unmanageable cost, it is not included here.

Highly Recommended (Practice That Should Be in Place in Every Procedure)

- Prophylactic antibiotics should be used routinely in all clean–contaminated surgical procedures and considered for use in any clean surgical procedure. When antibiotics are given prophylactically to prevent infection, they should be administered within 1 hour of incision (this is also a SCIP infection measure) at a dosage and with an antimicrobial spectrum that is effective against the pathogens likely to contaminate the procedure. During the time-out, and before skin incision, the team should confirm that prophylactic antibiotics were given within the past 60 minutes. (When vancomycin is used, infusion should be completed within 1 hour of skin incision.)
- Every facility should have a routine sterilization process that includes means for verifying the sterility of all surgical instruments, devices, and materials. Indicators should be used to determine sterility and checked before equipment is introduced onto the sterile field. Before induction of anesthesia, the nurse or other person responsible for preparing the surgical trays should confirm the sterility of the instruments by evaluating the sterility indicators and should communicate any problems to the surgeon and anesthesia provider. (See Chapter 4 for a full discussion of sterilization processes and indicators.)
- Re-dosing with prophylactic antibiotics should be considered if the surgical procedure lasts more than 4 hours or if there is evidence of excessive intraoperative bleeding. (When vancomycin is used as the prophylactic agent, there is no need for re-dosing in operations lasting less than 10 hours.)

- Antibiotics used for prophylaxis should be discontinued within 24 hours of the procedure.
- Hair should not be removed unless it will interfere with the procedure. If hair is removed, it should be clipped less than 2 hours before the procedure. Shaving is not recommended because it increases the risk for SSI.
- Surgical patients should receive oxygen throughout the perioperative period according to individual requirements and intraoperative fire safety precautions.
- Measures to maintain core normothermia should be instituted throughout the perioperative period.
- The skin at the surgical site should be prepared with an appropriate antiseptic agent before surgery. The antimicrobial agent should decrease the microbial count of the skin rapidly and have persistent efficacy throughout the procedure.
- Surgical hand antisepsis (rub or scrub) should be performed with an antimicrobial agent approved by the facility. The hands and forearms should be scrubbed for 2 to 5 minutes. If the hands are physically clean, an alcohol-based hand antiseptic agent can be used for antisepsis as long as manufacturer's instructions are followed.
- The OR team should cover all hair and wear sterile gowns and sterile gloves during the procedure.

Recommended (Practice That Is Encouraged for Every Procedure)

- "On call" orders for administration of antibiotic prophylaxis should be discouraged.
- If hair is to be removed, the use of depilatories is discouraged.
- Tobacco use should be stopped at least 30 days before elective surgery if possible.
- Patients should take up to three preoperative showers or baths with antiseptic soap such as CHG.
- Prior infections should be eliminated before a scheduled procedure.
- The operating team should wear masks during the procedure.
- Surgical drapes should be effective barriers to the transmission of microorganisms.
- Sterile dressings should be applied over the surgical wound and maintained for 24 to 48 hours.
- Active surveillance for SSIs should be conducted prospectively by trained infection control practitioners.
- Information on the surgical site infection rate should be provided to surgeons and appropriate administrators.

CHG, Chlorhexidine gluconate; *SCIP*, surgical care improvement project.
Modified from Hicks RW, Hernandez J: Perioperative pharmacology: a focus on vancomycin, *AORN J* 93(5): 593–596, 2011; The Joint Commission: *Surgical care improvement project*, available at www.jointcommission.org/surgical_care_improvement_project. Accessed January 24, 2013; World Health Organization: *The WHO guidelines for safe surgery*, 2009, available at http://whqlibdoc.who.int/publications/2009/9789241598552_eng.pdf. Accessed January 23, 2013.

---

staff as they are scheduled for procedures such as debridement, grafting, flaps, and other wound coverage. Perioperative nurses play a key role in wound care and must be familiar with various wound care treatments in order to support patients throughout the course of their recovery.

Hyperbaric Oxygenation (HBO)

Some form of HBO treatment for medical disorders has been used since 1662. HBO increases the capacity of blood to carry oxygen to the tissues. The increased oxygenation assists in cellular

restoration, is directly bactericidal to anaerobes, and improves leukocyte migration and phagocytosis to the wound bed (Van Hoesen, 2012). HBO therapy is administered in a pressurized chamber with the patient breathing 100% oxygen. Chambers may be monoplace to accommodate a single patient or multiplace to allow simultaneous treatment of multiple patients. Patients who undergo HBO therapy may require the insertion of myringotomy tubes to manage pressure changes while in the chamber. Perioperative nurses may be involved in the placement of the tubes and may be involved in wound debridement procedures for these patients.

Patients or their designated support person need to demonstrate knowledge of wound management. In a patient-centered care framework, that involves knowledge (the patient repeats the instructions correctly), skills (the patient demonstrates wound care measures), and affect (the patient cooperates and verbalizes ability to cope with managing the surgical wound). To facilitate this, use simple, easy-to-understand words. Obtain an interpreter if necessary. Be culturally sensitive, individualize information to the patient's lifestyle, and provide necessary time for questions about instructions. An example follows:

Wound Care Helps Prevent Pain and Infection
Home Care
- Only take medicine as told by your physician.
- Clean the wound daily with mild soap and water.
- Change any bandages (dressings) as told by your physician.
- Put medicated cream and a bandage on the wound as told by your physician.
- Change the bandage if it gets wet, dirty, or starts to smell.
- Take showers. Do *not* take baths, swim, or do anything that puts your wound under water until your physician says you may.
- Rest and raise (elevate) the wound until the pain and puffiness (swelling) are better (as applicable).
- Keep all physician visits as told.

Get Help Right Away if:
- Yellowish white fluid (pus) comes from your wound.
- Medicine does not lessen your pain.
- There is a red streak going away from your wound.
- You cannot move your finger or toe (if an extremity is the surgical site).
- You have a fever.

Make Sure You:
- Understand these instructions.
- Will watch your condition.
- Will get help right away if you are not doing well or get worse.

Modified from ExitCare Patient Information ©2012 ExitCare, LLC document released: 09/26/2009, document revised: 08/29/2012, document reviewed: 04/22/2012; AORN: *Perioperative nursing data set*, ed 3, Denver, The Association, 2011.

Negative-Pressure Wound Therapy

Also known as vacuum-assisted closure (VAC), negative-pressure wound therapy (NPWT) is used for difficult to manage wounds that do not respond to traditional wound care methods. NPWT works by using a device to apply constant controlled negative pressure to a wound that is filled with a drainage sponge (polyurethane foam) and sealed with an occlusive dressing. The VAC system has three main mechanisms of action that promote wound healing. First, the negative pressure results in mechanical tension on the tissues, causing a reduction in edema and fluid removal. The second action is macro-deformation and wound contraction, and the third action is micro-deformation and mechanical stretch perfusion (Netsch, 2012). VAC therapy may be used for acute and traumatic wounds, subacute wounds, pressure ulcers, chronic open wounds, meshed skin grafts, and skin flaps. The incidence of abdominal compartment syndrome decreases with the use of NPWT in open abdominal wounds, because it protects and contains the abdominal contents, avoiding the need for fascial sutures, and exerts a mechanical pull on the wound edges (Park et al, 2010). NPWT must be

FIGURE 9-5 The VAC pump.

used carefully and monitored frequently and evaluated to avoid complications such as bacterial colonization and biofilm generation, which may result in increased wound exudate that is not well managed with the NPWT system. Other potential complications while NPWT is in use include significant pain, particularly during dressing changes, and problems obtaining an adequate seal in irregularly shaped wounds (Marston, 2010). Gauze-based NPWT may accelerate granulation tissue formation and promote closure in a number of wound types while reducing pain during dressing changes (Tuncel et al, 2012).

According to a report published by the Pennsylvania Patient Safety Authority (2011), contraindications to NPWT therapy for chronic wounds include, but may not be limited to, exposed vital organs (until the organ has been covered by Vicryl absorbable mesh), inadequately debrided wounds; granulation tissue that will not form over necrotic tissue; untreated osteomyelitis or sepsis within the vicinity of the wound; presence of untreated coagulopathy; necrotic tissue with eschar; malignancy in the wound (NPWT may lead to cellular proliferation); and an allergy to any component required for the procedure.

The negative pressure unit may be applied in the OR after wound debridement. All nonviable tissue is first removed to reduce bacterial load in the wound bed. The skin area around the wound is dried and specialized reticulated foam is cut to fit the wound bed, including all tunnels and tracks. The surgeon takes care not to overfill the wound with the sponge because this could cause further mechanical trauma. When the sponge is in place, the surgeon covers the entire sponge, wound bed, and surrounding skin with a transparent occlusive drape, taking care to seal the edges completely. A 2-cm or greater edge of intact periwound skin is left available to ensure an airtight seal of the dressing. A 2-cm cut is made through the occlusive dressing into the sponge for insertion of the drainage tube, which has side and end ports. The tubing is connected to a VAC pump (Figure 9-5). A portable, battery-operated unit also is available for ambulatory patients. A canister collects the fluid and exudate. The NPWT acts to reduce edema, promote granulation tissue perfusion and formation, and remove exudate and infectious materials. The vacuum pump creates an intermittent or continuous subatmospheric pressure in the range of −50 mm Hg to –125 mm Hg. The need for suction should be assessed at least every 20 hours of use. The unit should be in continuous use with a disruption of no more than 2 hours at a time (Netsch, 2012).

When working with a NPWT system, the perioperative nurse protects patients by not cutting the foam sponges directly over the wound, keeping track of the number of sponge pieces and sizes placed in the wound, and following institutional protocol for implementing NPWT, including using correct pressure ranges and conducting patient assessments (Steelman and Graling, 2012).

Hydrotherapy and Hydrosurgery

Traditionally, hydrotherapy is undertaken via immersion in a whirlpool tank or tub. The mechanism of agitated water and injected air is thought to dilute bacterial loads and remove debris while increasing circulation to the area. Because immersion in a tank is not practical from an intraoperative perspective, the hydrotherapy method most frequently used in the OR is pulsatile lavage. Manufacturers provide a variety of systems to deliver pulsatile lavage. Most systems consist of a motor that creates pressure within tubing set to allow the delivery of fluid at 10 to 15 pounds per square inch (psi) through a handpiece to the wound bed. The handpiece is equipped with a splash shield to help concentrate the spray and minimize droplet aerosolization of the irrigant. While the system is delivering the fluid, it simultaneously suctions it to remove debris and bacteria. Standard Precautions are implemented by all healthcare team members while using pulsatile lavage, and the patient is also protected from aerosolization.

Hydrosurgery is a form of wound debridement and irrigation that uses a powered handpiece system with a narrow nozzle through which pressurized saline (up to 15,000 pounds psi) is used to excise necrotic tissue. The highly pressurized stream creates a vacuum effect that allows the surgeon to remove devitalized tissue from the wound bed while preserving healthy tissue (Graybill et al, 2012) (Research Highlight).

Skin Substitutes

An evolving technology for the treatment of wounds is the use of an engineered skin substitute. The skin substitute stimulates wound epithelialization and is capable of producing growth factors. The skin substitute may be used in lieu of a split-thickness skin graft for wound coverage. Skin substitutes are not permanent solutions in most cases, but are a bridge to permanent closure with skin grafts or granulation tissue. Skin substitutes are formed by placing human cells onto matrices that are collagen or synthetic based. As the cells grow and divide, they secrete growth factors and other useful substances to help build a foundation for healing. The substitutes are formed into a variety of shapes and sizes to facilitate wound coverage. They also may be used to cover donor sites from skin graft harvesting. Table 9-1 summarizes the description and indications for some commercially available skin substitutes. Advantages to using skin substitutes are increasing as are the wide variety and availability of these wound treatment products.

Growth Factors

Growth factors are naturally occurring proteins (cytokines and peptides) that are "signaling molecules." They stimulate cycles of mitosis of fibroblasts and epidermal cells, smooth muscle cells, and vascular endothelial cells. Human or recombinant growth factors may be applied to wounds in the OR, but are more typically administered in the clinic setting. Growth factors initiate wound healing by accelerating the formation of granulation tissue and work most

---

RESEARCH HIGHLIGHT

Hydrosurgical Wound Debridement

Surgeons use many techniques to manage wounds and to prepare wound beds for healing or closure, including the use of pressurized fluid delivered via a bulb syringe or pulsed lavage. These hydrosurgery methods have limitations in terms of effectiveness of tissue removal and increased exposure of the patient and surgical team to droplet aerosolization or splashing from irrigant use. Newer hydrosurgery technology allows surgeons to remove devitalized tissue via the Versajet, a commercially available system that pressurizes an irrigant via a disposable handpiece. As the irrigant is forced through the handpiece, a localized vacuum is created and the dissected tissue is suctioned.

Surgeons used the Versajet hydrosurgery system to prepare wound beds in 16 patients ages 35 to 80 years with a variety of wounds (e.g., necrotic, burns, traumatic, diabetic). The authors reported that the system was more selective in tissue removal and allowed them to perform a single wound debridement in many cases instead of multiple debridement sessions using traditional sharp dissection. Although a comparative analysis was not conducted, the authors stated anecdotally that the speed of the system over traditional methods saved operating time, and they estimated the time per debridement procedure was approximately 15 minutes. Other advantages included decreased bleeding (which decreased the need for electrocoagulation and thermal tissue damage), improved wound visibility, decreased tissue edema, removal of tissue in layers, and subjective patient reports of decreased pain. Formalized studies remain necessary to substantiate the authors' findings.

Modified from Pascone M et al: Use of a novel hydrosurgery device in surgical debridement of difficult-to-heal wounds, *Wounds* 20(5):139–146, 2008.

---

effectively in the proliferative phase of wound healing. They improve the cellular or molecular environment of the wound and signal target cells to begin tissue repair. Growth factors generally are categorized by their source (i.e., if obtained from platelets, they are designated as platelet-derived growth factors [PDGFs]; from the epidermis, epidermal growth factor [EGF]). To obtain PDGFs, typically 50 to 200 mL of venous blood is withdrawn. The platelets are separated and activated with thrombin to make a gel that is applied to a clean wound bed. The wound is covered with a nonadherent gauze dressing. Debridement may help to speed the wound healing process by exposing viable receptors for proper growth factor–receptor interaction (Robinson et al, 2010).

Wound Scaffolds

Acellular matrix products are used in a wide variety of applications, including burns and reconstructive surgery, soft tissue and abdominal wall repair, and even as internal implants for orthopedic use in joint resurfacing and tendon repair. They are frequently used as scaffolds in hard-to-heal wounds such as diabetic foot ulcers, venous leg ulcers, and pressure ulcers (Table 9-2) (International Consensus, 2010). Work goes on in research labs to develop extracellular matrix (ECM) from native cardiac tissue (potential use of acellular cardiac ECM as a biomaterial for heart regeneration), and in tissue engineering of the esophagus.

Dressings

Application of surgical dressings is often the responsibility of the perioperative nurse. The dressing may serve one or more of the following purposes:

TABLE 9-1

Dermal and Bilayered Skin Substitutes

Category	Trade Name	Description	Indications
Allogeneic dermal	Dermagraft (Advanced Biohealing, Westport, CT)	Fibroblasts seeded and cultured on bioabsorbable mesh, then cryopreserved; delivered on dry ice. 5 × 7.5 cm. Apply to either side of wound.	Nonhealing full-thickness diabetic foot ulcers >6 weeks' duration, extending through dermis, but without tendon, muscle, joint, or bone exposure
Allogeneic bilayered	Apligraf (Organogenesis, Canton, MA)	Fibroblasts mixed with bovine collagen gel and cultured. Keratinocytes seeded and cultured on gel. 44 cm². Delivered fresh. Apply dermal side toward wound.	Venous ulcers >1-month duration Full-thickness diabetic neuropathic foot ulcers >3 weeks' duration but without tendon, muscle, capsule, or bone exposure
Cadaver skin	GammaGraft (Promethean LifeSciences, Pittsburgh, PA)	Gamma-irradiated human cadaver skin. Stored at room temperature up to 2 years. May stay in place until wound heals if it remains adherent to wound bed. Left in place while new host skin grows in under dressing. Gradually dries out and edges peel away.	Chronic wounds and burns
Cadaver skin	TheraSkin (Soluble Systems, Newport News, VA)	Cryopreserved human cadaver skin. Delivered on dry ice. Available in 2 sizes and meshed.	Chronic wounds and burns

Modified from Seaman S: Skin substitutes and extracellular matrix scaffolds. In Bryant RA, Nix DP, editors: *Acute and chronic wounds: current management concepts*, ed 4, St Louis, 2012, Mosby.

TABLE 9-2

Acellular Extracellular Matrix Scaffolds

Category	Trade Name	Description	Indications
Allogeneic	AlloDerm (LifeCell, Branchburg, NJ)	Derived from cadaveric human skin from tissue banks. Epidermis and all cellular components removed, leaving dermal matrix. Freeze-dried; rehydrate to use. Contains intact collagen fibers to support ingrowth of new tissue, elastin filaments to provide strength, and hyaluronan and proteoglycans for cell attachment and migration.	Burns, traumatic or oncologic wounds with deep structure exposure, hernia repair, breast and other tissue reconstruction
Allogeneic	Cymetra (LifeCell)	Injectable micronized particulate form of AlloDerm. Dry form, packaged in syringe, rehydrated prior to use with either normal saline or lidocaine for injection.	Cosmetic soft tissue augmentation and treatment of vocal cord paralysis by injection laryngoplasty
Allogeneic	GraftJacket Regenerative Tissue Matrix (Wright Medical Technology, Arlington, TN)	Same as AlloDerm, but meshed 1:1 to allow wound exudate to pass through. Available in two sizes (4 × 4 cm and 4 × 8 cm) and one thickness (0.4-0.8 mm) for chronic wound care. Available nonmeshed and thicker for tendon and ligament repair.	Diabetic foot ulcers and other chronic wounds, ligament and tendon repair
Allogeneic	GraftJacket Xpress (Wright Medical Technology)	Same as Cymetra. Available in a prefilled 5-mL syringe. Once rehydrated, is injected to fill the entire dead space of a sinus tract or deep wound.	Deep wounds, tunnels or sinus tracts
Allogeneic	DermaMatrix (Synthes CMF, West Chester, PA)	Cadaver human skin from tissue banks. Donor skin is processed to remove all cellular components, including epidermis, and then is freeze-dried. Rehydrate to use.	Similar to indications for AlloDerm: soft tissue repair, breast reconstruction, abdominal hernia repair, head and neck reconstruction
Biosynthetic	Biobrane (UDL Laboratories, Sugar Land, TX)	Very thin sheet of semipermeable silicone bonded to a knitted trifilament nylon fabric. Nylon coated with type 1 porcine collagen, which creates hydrophilic coating that facilitates adherence to wound. Silicone membrane has water vapor loss rate similar to that of intact skin; once Biobrane has adhered to a wound, it provides moist, protected environment that minimizes water loss.	Partial-thickness burns, skin graft donor sites, superficial wounds after surgery, laser resurfacing, dermabrasion. Lesions secondary to toxic epidermal necrolysis and pemphigus, as coverage for chronic wounds.

TABLE 9-2

Acellular Extracellular Matrix Scaffolds—cont'd

Category	Trade Name	Description	Indications
Biosynthetic	Biobrane-L (UDL Laboratories)	Same as Biobrane, except monofilament nylon is used instead of knitted trifilament nylon, which renders it less adherent to wound bed.	Indicated where less adherence is desired (e.g., over meshed autografts)
Biosynthetic	Integra Dermal Regeneration Template (IDRT) (Integra Life Sciences, Plainsboro, NJ)	Bilayered product composed of outer semipermeable silicone sheet (functions as epidermal substitute) and inner ECM scaffold containing bovine crosslinked collagen and chondroitin-6-sulfate. Inner layer facilitates cell migration and tissue ingrowth, which leads to formation of neodermis, usually within 2 to 3 weeks of application. As neodermis is formed, ECM matrix degrades. Silicone covering is then removed.	Deep partial- or full-thickness burns, contracture release procedures, reconstructive surgery of complex wounds and surgical defects
Biosynthetic	Integra Bilayer Matrix Wound Dressing (BMWD) (Integra Life Sciences)	Same product as IDRT but repackaged for chronic wound care. Available meshed or unmeshed in multiple sizes.	Chronic wounds of various etiologies, surgical wounds, traumatic wound; can be placed over deep structures
Biosynthetic	Integra Matrix Wound Dressing (Integra Life Sciences)	The ECM scaffold of the BMWD without silicone membrane. Can be used alone or with BMWD for deeper wounds (Matrix Wound Dressing first, then covered with BMWD).	Same indications as BMWD
Biosynthetic	Integra Flowable Wound Matrix (Integra Life Sciences)	Same ingredients (minus silicone layer) as other Integra products. ECM matrix is provided in syringe as dry granules that are rehydrated with saline prior to one-time use. Injected directly into wound until filled.	Same indications as BMWD but use focuses on application to wounds with deep tunnels or undermining
Synthetic	Suprathel (PolyMedics Innovations, Denkendorf, Germany)	Synthetic epidermal substitute composed of copolymer of polylactide, trimethylene carbonate and ε-caprolactone. Completely dissolves within 4 weeks.	Used in Germany since 2004 for deep partial-thickness burns, superficial full-thickness burns, skin graft donor sites, abrasions, scar revision
Xenographic porcine	Oasis Wound Matrix (Healthpoint, Fort Worth, TX)	Porcine small intestinal submucosa (SIS) with complex matrix of collagen, glycosaminoglycans, proteoglycans, cell adhesive glycoproteins, and growth factors. Freeze-dried. Available multiple sizes, fenestrated, or meshed.	Partial- and full-thickness wounds, chronic ulcers, traumatic wounds, superficial and second-degree burns, surgical wounds
Xenographic porcine	MatriStem (Medline Industries, Mundelein, IL)	Derived from porcine urinary bladder matrix (UBM) with intact basement membrane. Composed of collagen matrix, glycosaminoglycans, glycoproteins, and proteoglycans. Available as fenestrated sheets of variable sizes or as powder. Must be rehydrated prior to use and cut to size of wound.	Partial- and full-thickness wounds, traumatic wounds, surgical wounds, chronic wounds
Xenographic equine	Unite Biomatrix (Synovis Orthopedic and Woundcare, Irvine, CA)	Derived from decellularized equine pericardium. Available fenestrated, in three sizes. Must be rehydrated. Apply 2-4 mm larger than wound and staple in place.	Partial- and full- thickness wounds, chronic wounds, traumatic wounds, surgical wounds
Xenographic bovine	PriMatrix (TEI Biosciences, Boston, MA)	Derived from fetal bovine dermis, which has been decellularized, freeze-dried, and sterilized. Must be rehydrated. Available nonfenestrated in various sizes and thicknesses. Must fenestrate for high-exudating wounds.	Skin ulcers, second-degree burns, surgical wounds
Xenographic porcine	Mediskin and E-Z Derm (Brennan Medical, St. Paul, MN)	Porcine skin with epidermis and dermis. Mediskin is frozen and irradiated, with shelf life of 24 months; stored in a standard freezer. E-Z Derm is chemically crosslinked for durability; stored at room temperature up to 18 months. Both are available in multiple sizes, perforated or nonperforated.	Temporary coverage of burns, surgical wounds, partial- and full-thickness wounds of variable etiologies

ECM, Extracellular matrix.

NOTE: The products included in this list are representative of what is available, and are not meant to be inclusive.

Modified from Seaman S: Skin substitutes and extracellular matrix scaffolds. In Bryant RA, Nix DP, editors: *Acute and chronic wounds: current management concepts,* ed 4, St Louis, 2012, Mosby.

- Cushioning and protection of the wound from trauma and gross contamination
- Absorption of drainage
- Debridement of the wound
- Support, splinting, or immobilization of the body part and incisional area
- Assistance in hemostasis and minimization of edema and dead space, as in a pressure dressing
- Promotion of the patient's physical comfort and aesthetic appearance
- Maintenance of a moist environment and prevention of cell dehydration
- Application of medications

Dressings are selected based on the characteristics of the surgical site, depth, and area, and the patient's overall condition (Table 9-3). Questions to ask when choosing a dressing are as follows:

- What does the wound need?
- What is the purpose of the product?
- How well does the product function? Is there evidence to support use of this product?
- What does the patient need?
- What is available?
- What is practical? Is it also cost-effective?

Dressings can be grouped into two main categories: primary and secondary dressings. *Primary* dressings are placed directly over or in the wound. A variety of primary dressing materials are available on the market. Their function is to absorb drainage and then wick it away from the wound edge. Cotton gauze or synthetic dressings may be used for this purpose. The layer of primary dressing directly contacting the wound should be nonadherent, unless debridement is desired.

Secondary dressings are placed directly over the primary dressing. These function to absorb excessive drainage, provide hemostasis by compression, and protect the wound from further trauma. These functions usually are accomplished with a bulky dressing, such as an abdominal pad. These pads have a cotton filling that provides extra absorbency.

Dressings may be secured with a variety of products, including tape, Elastoplast, ACE bandages, or soft roll products. Tape is available with a variety of backing materials (cloth, paper, taffeta, plastic) and with regular or nonallergenic adhesive. The strength and elasticity required, patient allergies, the condition of the patient's skin,

TABLE 9-3

Wound Dressing Formulary

Product and Examples	Description	Indications for Use	Instructions for Use
Antimicrobial: Antiseptics, cadexomer iodine, honey, Hydrofera blue, mupirocin ointment, silver cream, silver dressings	Inhibits growth and replication of microorganisms	Partial- or full-thickness wound Critical colonization, infection, or biofilms Odorous wound	Cleanse wound Avoid saline in nanocrystalline silver products Apply to wound Apply appropriate secondary dressing as needed and secure in place
Calcium alginate: Restore CalciCare (Hollister), SeaSorb (Coloplast), Algisite (Smith & Nephew)	Polysaccharide derived from brown seaweed Highly absorbent Converts to viscous, hydrophilic gel Provides moist environment Hemostatic properties	Partial- or full-thickness wound with or without depth Moderate to heavily exudative wound Contraindicated in third-degree burns	Cleanse wound base Place or lightly pack into wound Apply appropriate secondary dressing and secure in place Change as needed, usually every 24 to 48 hours
Charcoal: CarboFlex odor control (ConvaTec), Lyofoam C (Molnlycke, ConvaTec)	Activated carbon (charcoal) Absorbs toxins and wound degradation products Absorbs volatile amines and fatty acids responsible for odor	Malodorous wound (e.g., infected, fungating) Fecal fistula Pressure ulcer	Apply as a "filter" for odor control If absorbing exudate, may need to be changed daily; weekly if no exudate Can be reused if filter only
Collagen: Puracol collagen (Medline), Biostep (Smith & Nephew), Cellerate gel (Hymed Group), CollaSorb (Hartmann)	May enhance deposition of organized collagen fibers Chemoattractant to granulocytes and fibroblasts Bioresorbable Hemostatic properties Most processed from bovine or porcine sources	Full-thickness wound with or without depth Noninfected wound Minimal to moderate drainage Contraindicated in bovine sensitivities and third-degree burns	Packaged as gels, alginates, sheets, powders Cleanse wound as appropriate Apply to wound base Apply appropriate secondary dressing Secure as necessary
Promogran (Systagenix Wound Management)	Some collagens also inactivate matrix metalloproteinases	Chronic wound free of necrotic tissue	Read manufacturer's instructions carefully; some may need to be moistened with saline if wound bed dry
Composite: Tegaderm absorbent clear acrylic dressing (3M), Alldress (Molnlycke), Covaderm Plus (DeRoyal)	Combine physically distinct components into single dressing Functions as bacterial barrier Absorptive layer distinct from alginate, foam, hydrocolloid, hydrogel Semiadherent or nonadherent	Partial- or full-thickness wound without depth Dry to heavy exudate (depends on dressing components) Product selection varies based on wound characteristics	Cleanse wound as appropriate Dressing application dependent on product selected Can function as either primary or secondary dressing May be used with topical medications

TABLE 9-3

Wound Dressing Formulary—cont'd

Product and Examples	Description	Indications for Use	Instructions for Use
Contact layer: Restore TRIACT technology (Hollister), Mepitel (Molnlycke)	Protects wound bed from direct contact with other agents and dressings Conforms to wound shape Porous to allow exudate to pass or medication to absorb into wound	Partial- or full-thickness wounds with or without depth Infected wounds Donor sites Split-thickness skin grafts	Cleanse wound as appropriate Line wound bed Apply topical agent over contact layer *or* apply secondary dressing for absorption Not intended to be changed with each dressing change
Fiber gelling: Aquacel Hydrofiber (ConvaTec)	Carboxymethylcellulose Absorbs heavy exudate Converts to a gel Keeps wound base moist	Partial- or full-thickness wound with or without depth Moderate to heavily exudative wound	Cleanse wound base Place or lightly pack into wound Apply appropriate secondary dressing and secure in place Change every 24 to 48 hours
Foam: Biatain (Coloplast), Hydrocell (Derma Sciences), PolyMem (Ferris Mfg Corp)	Absorptive and nonadherent Consists of hydrophilic polyurethane or film-coated layer	Partial- or full-thickness wound without depth (sheets) or with depth (fillers) Moderate to heavily exudative wound Contraindicated in ischemic wound with dry eschar and third-degree burns Frequently a secondary dressing	Cleanse wound base and dry well Apply topical agent or primary dressing to wound base Place foam dressing in wound Apply appropriate secondary dressing and secure in place Change every 24 hours or as needed
Gauze: Hypertonic saline Curasalt (Tyco Healthcare/Kendall), Mesalt (Molnlycke Health Care)	Gauze impregnated with dry sodium chloride by the manufacturer	Full-thickness, heavily exudating wound and nonviable wound base with or without infection	Cleanse wound, apply to the wound dry, cover with secondary dressing
Hydrocolloid: DuoDERM (ConvaTec), Exuderm (Medline), Replicare (Smith & Nephew)	Contains gel-forming agents (gelatin, pectin, carboxymethylcellulose) Forms gelatinous mass Impermeable to contaminants, reducing risk of infection Promotes autolysis Reduces pain and protects Promotes moist wound Molds to body contours Adhesive	Partial- or full-thickness wound without depth Minimal to moderately exudative wound Avoid acutely infected wound Avoid dry eschar Use with caution in persons with diabetes Contraindicated in third-degree burns	Cleanse wound and dry periwound area well Select dressing 1 to 2 inches larger than wound Apply light pressure to allow body heat to promote adhesion Change every 3–5 days as needed Use periwound skin preparation product
Hydrogel: Skintegrity (Medline), Elasto-Gel (Southwest Technologies), Vigilon (Bard)	Maintains clean, moist wound Nonadherent Little or no absorption Various formulations: amorphous gel, sheet, impregnated gauze Cool and soothing Decreases pain Aggressive autolytic debridement by autolysis	Partial- or full-thickness wound without depth (sheet or gel) or with depth (impregnated gauze) Dry to minimally exudative wound Sterile gel for every 3-day dressing changes Nonsterile gel can be used for daily dressing changes Contraindicated in third-degree burns	Cleanse wound Apply to cover wound base Do *not* use as wound filler Use appropriate secondary dressing Secure as necessary Change daily
Transparent film: Tegaderm (3M) Suresite (Medline), Opsite (Smith & Nephew)	Permeable to oxygen and water vapor Protects from environmental contaminants—good shield Maintains moist wound Creates "second skin" Reduces friction Nonabsorbent Promotes autolysis	Shallow partial-thickness wound Dry to minimally exudative wound Not recommended for acutely infected wound Contraindicated in third-degree burns	Cleanse wound and dry periwound area Allow for 1- to 2-inch border around wound Apply without stretching or tension Change every 4 to 7 days *or* as needed Use skin sealant around wound edges
Wound fillers: Flexigel strands (Smith & Nephew), Multidex maltodextrin (DeRoyal)	Pastes, granules, powders, beads, gels	Full-thickness wound with depth Minimal to moderate exudate Infected or noninfected	Cleanse wound as appropriate Apply directly to wound Use appropriate secondary dressing to optimize moist wound environment Change every 1 to 2 days

NOTE: Examples of product brand names within this formulary are neither inclusive nor intended as a product endorsement.
Modified from Rolstad BS et al: Topical wound management. In Bryant RA, Nix DP, editors: *Acute and chronic wounds: current management concepts,* ed 4, St Louis, 2012, Mosby.

and anticipated frequency of dressing change determine which type is selected. When applying tape to the dressing, the perioperative nurse applies pressure evenly from both sides of the tape and away from the direction of the incision. Applying tape with excessive pressure may result in stretching and trauma to the skin. The tape covers the edges of the dressing and is placed at right angles to the direction of motion when applied over a joint. When frequent dressing changes are anticipated, Montgomery straps can be selected to secure the dressing (Figure 9-6). When compression of the wound for hemostasis or reduction of edema is desired, a polyurethane dressing, elastic tape, or elastic bandage may be used to secure the secondary dressing. Immobilization is accomplished with the addition of soft padding, elastic bandages, splints, and casting materials (splints and casts are discussed in greater detail in Chapter 20).

In some situations, the wound is not dressed at all. An undressed wound that heals by exposure to air has the following advantages: (1) allows for optimal observation of the incisional area, (2) aids bathing, (3) prevents possible adhesive-tape reactions, (4) increases comfort and maneuverability for many patients, and (5) seems to minimize adverse responses by the patient to the operation.

Drains

Drains control ecchymosis and provide exits through which air and fluids, such as serum, blood, lymph, intestinal secretions, bile, and pus, can be evacuated from the operative site. Drains also may be used to prevent the development of deep wound infections. They

usually are inserted at the time of surgery, primarily through a separate small incision known as a *stab wound*, close to the operative site. Drains may or may not be sutured to the skin.

In some instances (e.g., chest, common bile duct, bladder), drainage is directly through the lumen of the tube (as with a Foley

FIGURE 9-6 Montgomery straps.

FIGURE 9-7 Drains are available in a variety of styles. Pictured are Penrose (**A**) and T-tube (**B**), which drain by gravity, and Jackson Pratt (**C**) and Hemovac (**D**), which represent closed foundainage systems.

retention catheter) or via perforations or fenestrations in the tubing into a closed drainage system. In other instances (e.g., peritoneal cavity or skin wound), drainage of pus or blood is primarily along the outside surface of the drain by capillary action and gravity (as with the simple Penrose drain) into a dressing. The selection of a simple versus a closed drainage system depends on the needs of the site to be drained, patient activity, and overall healing capability. Many types of drains are available. The most common are made of latex, polyvinyl chloride (PVC), silicone, or silver coated (Figure 9-7). Particular care should be taken to ensure that the patient is not allergic to latex when considering any latex drain. For many wounds, a portable, self-contained closed wound suction unit is selected. These units create a negative pressure in a reservoir attached to the drain. Fluid is gently drawn out of the wound and collected in the reservoir.

The perioperative nurse documents the location and type of drain and ensures the drain is working properly before the patient leaves the OR. This information is important for the hand-off report to nurses caring for the patient in the postanesthesia care unit (PACU) and postoperative nursing units. Some wounds yield significant drainage and must be monitored closely during the postoperative course. A disadvantage of wound drains is that they create a portal for entry and exit of infectious microorganisms. Extreme care must be taken in emptying drain reservoirs to avoid contamination. Closed autologous drains allow for collection of blood from a surgical wound and the return of that blood to the patient; this minimizes the need for transfusion of blood from outside donors, reducing the risk of bloodborne pathogen transmission.

KEY POINTS

- Wound healing and the final surgical result depend on anatomic location, structure of the skin, and functional interaction with underlying elements of the operative region.
- The skin, with its multilayer organization of the epidermis, dermis, and appendages, has unique healing properties.
- In surgical procedures, there are four potential sources of contamination: the surgical team, the surgical environment, the patient, and the instruments/supplies. The patient's normal flora is the most common reservoir of microorganisms.
- Preoperative assessment should include a review of the medical, surgical, and social history; list of current medications; and results of physical examination.
- Wound healing occurs in overlapping phases: the inflammatory, the proliferative, and the remodeling phases.
- Dressings cover the wound, absorb drainage, apply pressure, and provide a moist environment for healing.

CRITICAL THINKING QUESTION

The perioperative nursing assessment is essential to individualizing your plan of care and communicating information to the surgical team. With surgical infection prevention (SIP) a priority initiative to reduce SSIs, what risk factors would place a patient at an increased risk for a SSI? What nursing interventions would you include in your perioperative plan of care that pertain to antibiotic prophylaxis?

⊖volve *The answers to the Critical Thinking Question can be found at http://evolve.elsevier.com/Rothrock/Alexander*

REFERENCES

Association of periOperative Registered Nurses (AORN): *Perioperative standards and recommended practices,* Denver, 2013, The Association.

CMS hospital-acquired conditions, available at www.cms.gov/Medicare/Medicare-Fee-for-Service-Payment/HospitalAcqCond. Last modified 9/30/2012. Accessed January 24, 2013.

Ebner JA, Maytin EV: Cutaneous wound healing. In Vidimos AT et al, editors: *Dermatologic surgery,* St Louis, 2009, Mosby.

Graybill JC et al: Traumatic wounds: bullets, blasts, and vehicle crashes. In Bryant RA, Nix DP, editors: *Acute and chronic wounds: current management concepts,* ed 4, St Louis, 2012, Mosby.

Hospitals Cut Colorectal Surgical-Site Infections by a Third, *Medscape,* Nov 28, 2012, available at www.medscape.com/viewarticle/775225. Accessed January 23, 2013.

International Consensus: *Acellular matrices for the treatment of wounds. An expert working group review.* London, 2010, Wounds International, available at: www.woundsinternational.com/pdf/content_9732.pdf. Accessed January 30, 2013.

Leong M, Phillips LG: Wound healing. In Townsend CM et al, editors: *Sabiston textbook of surgery: the biological basis of modern surgical practice,* ed 19, Philadelphia, 2012, Saunders.

Marston WA: Wound care. In Cronenwett JL, Johnston KW, editors: *Rutherford's vascular surgery,* ed 7, Philadelphia, 2010, Saunders.

Netsch DS: Negative pressure wound therapy. In Bryant RA, Nix DP, editors: *Acute and chronic wounds: current management concepts,* ed 4, St Louis, 2012, Mosby.

Park H et al: Complex wounds and their management, *Surg Clin North Am* 90:1181–1194, 2010.

Pennsylvania Patient Safety Authority: *Improving the safety of negative-pressure wound therapy,* 2011, available at http://patientsafetyauthority.org/ADVISORIES/AdvisoryLibrary/2011/mar8(1)/Pages/18.aspx. Accessed January 24, 2013.

Petersen C: *Perioperative nursing data set,* ed 3, Denver, CO, 2011, The Association.

Peterson SL: Surgical wound infection. In Harken AH, editor: *Abernathy's surgical secrets,* ed 6, Philadelphia, 2009, Mosby.

Robinson JK et al: *Surgery of the skin: procedural dermatology,* ed 2, St Louis, 2010, Mosby.

Schwulst SJ, Mazuski JE: Surgical prophylaxis and other complication avoidance care bundles, *Surg Clin North Am* 92(2), 2012.

Steelman V, Graling P: Three top emerging patient safety issues, *Periop Insider* April 25, 2012, available at www.informz.net/admin31/content/template.asp?sid=6634&ptid=410&brandid=436&uid=91094496&mi=1412123. Accessed January 24, 2013.

Tuncel U et al: Clinical experience with the use of gauze-based negative pressure wound therapy, *Wounds* 24(8):227–233, 2012.

Van Hoesen KB: Hyperbaric medicine. In Auerbach PS, editor: *Wilderness medicine,* ed 6, Philadelphia, 2012, Mosby.

CHAPTER 10

Postoperative Patient Care and Pain Management

JAN ODOM-FORREN

The postoperative phase of care begins as soon as the surgical procedure concludes and the patient is transferred to the postanesthesia care unit (PACU). The PACU, in the past, was called the *recovery room* or *postanesthesia room.* Florence Nightingale (1863) first described a postanesthesia area this way: "It is not uncommon, in small country hospitals, to have a recess or small room leading from the operating theater in which the patients remain until they have recovered, or at least recovered from the immediate effects of the operation."

An assigned area for the care of the postoperative patient is a relatively recent addition to surgical patient care. Although surgical procedures have been performed for thousands of years, and general anesthesia has been available for almost 150 years, PACUs became common only in the second half of the 20th century. A few recovery rooms were opened in the 1920s and 1930s. In the 1940s numerous PACUs opened because of the shortage of nurses during the war years and the need to centralize patients, equipment, and personnel for postoperative care. Hospitals soon realized that use of the PACU decreased patient morbidity and mortality and shortened the stays of some patients. When researchers reported that as many as a third of perioperative deaths examined over an 11-year period could have been prevented by improved postoperative nursing care (Odom-Forren and Clifford, 2010; Ruth et al, 1947), many hospitals opened PACUs.

PACUs have since flourished. Technologic innovation has profoundly affected PACUs, as in other critical care areas. The complexity of anesthesia management demands specially trained nurses who have expertise in prompt recognition and management of postoperative complications. Most patients who receive general anesthesia, major regional anesthesia, or monitored anesthesia care are transferred to the PACU. PACU is considered postanesthesia phase I, in which basic life-sustaining needs are of the highest priority. Patients then transition to phase II (preparation for discharge home), an inpatient setting, or a critical care unit (CCU, or intensive care unit [ICU]) (ASPAN, 2012). In some PACUs, because of space constraints and cost containment, PACU nurses also manage the care of overflow ICU or telemetry patients or provide space for managing pain or inserting central lines, for example.

PACUs are adjacent to the surgical suite with easy access for patient transport. The patient's status is assessed for needs during transfer (e.g., oxygen, manual positive-pressure ventilation device, a patient hospital bed). A perioperative nurse accompanies the patient to the PACU with an anesthesia provider and gives a hand-off report on the status of the patient to a perianesthesia nurse. A PACU nurse assumes care of the patient after initial assessment of the patient and report from the transferring team.

Perianesthesia Considerations

Assessment

Admission to the PACU. Initial assessment of the postoperative patient begins with an immediate determination of airway and circulatory adequacy. The airway is assessed for patency, humidified oxygen applied, and respirations counted. Pulse oximetry is initiated on all patients, and the quality of breath sounds determined. The PACU nurse connects the patient to the cardiac monitor, and evaluates rate and rhythm. Blood pressure is measured by means of a manual cuff or an automatic cuff. If the patient has an arterial line, the PACU nurse connects it to the monitor.

After the PACU nurse assesses the *ABCs* (*a*irway, *b*reathing, *c*irculation), the perioperative nurse and anesthesia provider give a comprehensive hand-off report. A patient hand-off is defined by the Joint Commission Center for Transforming Healthcare (2010) as a transfer and acceptance of patient care responsibility achieved through effective communication. It is a real-time process of passing patient-specific information from one caregiver to another or from one team of caregivers to another for the purpose of ensuring continuity and safety. Standardization of how information is communicated ensures that the information will be accurate and complete. The perioperative nurse collaborates by adding and verifying important patient information. Box 10-1 includes suggestions on what each surgical team member reports.

The patient's American Society of Anesthesiologists (ASA) physical classification status (see Chapter 5) also is provided during the hand-off report. Useful information that the perioperative nurse also provides includes airway status and presence of tubes, drains, catheters, and intravascular lines. Any postoperative orders to be initiated in the PACU are discussed at this time.

The anesthesia provider should not leave the patient until the PACU nurse accepts responsibility for the patient's care. Standard III-3 of the ASA's *Standards for Postanesthesia Care* (ASA, 2009) states that "the member of the anesthesia care team shall remain in the PACU until the PACU nurse accepts responsibility for the nursing care of the patient."

Initial Assessment. After immediate assessment of the ABCs and completion of the hand-off report, the PACU nurse begins a more thorough postanesthesia assessment. The assessment is performed quickly and is specific, in part, to the type of operative procedure. Recommended elements of an initial assessment in the PACU are presented in Box 10-2.

BOX 10-1

Suggestions for Hand-off Report from Anesthesia Provider and Perioperative Nurse to PACU Nurse

Anesthesia Provider May Report:
- Patient name, allergies, surgical procedures performed
- Pertinent medical and/or surgical histories
- Current medications
- Anesthetic delivered
- Medications administered
- Regional anesthetic used
- Intraoperative course (anesthesia related)
- Lines, fluids, losses; the anesthesia provider may include estimated blood loss (EBL) in the hand-off report to the PACU nurse. In some institutions a surgical Apgar score is calculated at the end of the surgical procedure from the EBL, lowest mean arterial pressure (expressed in mm Hg), and lowest heart rate rhythm recorded on the anesthesia record during the procedure. The score may be used to identify patients with a higher likelihood of developing complications after surgery (Wuertz et al, 2011).
- Anesthesia complications
- Pain and comfort management
- PACU orders

- Questions and answers

Perioperative Nurse May Report:
- Identity of patient
- Preoperative diagnosis
- Procedure performed
- Location of incision(s), dressings, drains, catheters, tubes, packing, stomas
- Surgical complications
- Allergies and reactions
- Medications, fluids, irrigations delivered by surgeon or RN
- Positioning during surgery
- Communication of other pertinent issues:
  - Location/presence of family or significant others
  - Special requests verbalized by the patient preoperatively
  - Special devices
  - Patient deficits
- Questions and answers

PACU, Postanesthesia care unit.
Modified from American Society of PeriAnesthesia Nurses: 2012-2014 *Perianesthesia nursing standards, practice recommendations and interpretive statements*, Cherry Hill, NJ, 2012, ASPAN; Chard R: Care of postoperative patients. In Ignatavicius DD, Workman ML, editors: *Medical-surgical nursing: patient-centered collaborative care*, ed 7, St Louis, 2013, Saunders; Odom-Forren J: *Drain's perianesthesia nursing: a critical care approach*, ed 6, St Louis, 2013, Saunders; Wuertz TH, et al: The surgical Apgar Score in hip and knee arthroplasty, *Clin Orthop Relat Res* 469(4):1119-26, 2011.

BOX 10-2

Initial Assessment in the PACU

Initial assessment in the PACU includes documentation of the following:
1. Integration of data received at hand-off report for transfer of care
2. Vital signs
   a. Respiratory status—airway patent, breath sounds, type of artificial airway, mechanical ventilator settings, oxygen saturation, and end tidal CO_2 monitoring if indicated
   b. Blood pressure—cuff or arterial line
   c. Pulse—apical, peripheral
   d. Cardiac monitor, rhythm documented
   e. Temperature/route
   f. Hemodynamic pressure reading if indicated (central venous, arterial blood, pulmonary artery wedge, and intracranial pressure)
3. Pain/sedation/comfort assessment (including emotional comfort)
4. Neurologic function including level of consciousness

5. Position of patient
6. Condition and color of skin
7. Patient safety needs
8. Neurovascular—peripheral pulses and sensation of extremity or extremities as applicable
9. Condition of dressings or suture line, drains, tubes, receptacles
10. Amount and type of drainage
11. Muscular response and strength/mobility status
12. Pupillary response as indicated
13. Fluid therapy—location of lines, condition of IV site, and security and amount of solution given and infusing (including crystalloid, colloid, and blood component therapy)
14. Intake and output
15. Postanesthesia score (if scoring system used)
16. Procedure-specific assessment

IV, Intravenous; *PACU*, postanesthesia care unit.

Some PACUs use a head-to-toe assessment to organize the data obtained (Figure 10-1). Other PACUs take a major body systems approach (Figure 10-2). In any case, the PACU nurse assesses admitting vital signs and the ABCs, beginning with the respiratory system. Respiratory assessment comprises rate, rhythm, auscultation of breath sounds for ventilatory adequacy, oxygen saturation level, and end-tidal CO_2 level if applicable. Any artificial airway and type of oxygen delivery system are noted.

The PACU nurse next assesses the cardiovascular system by monitoring heart rate and rhythm. The patient's initial blood pressure is compared with one or more preoperative readings. Body temperature is obtained, skin condition examined, and peripheral pulses checked, if indicated. Next, the PACU nurse assesses neurologic function by asking the following: Has the patient reacted (awakened from anesthesia)? Can the patient follow commands? Is the patient oriented, at least to name and hospital? Can the patient move all extremities and lift the head? Are there deviations from preoperative neurologic functioning? Some operative procedures require a more detailed assessment.

To assess renal function, the PACU nurse measures intake and output. Total intraoperative fluid intake and estimated blood loss are reviewed. Intravenous (IV) lines, infusions, and irrigation

FIGURE 10-1 Head-to-toe assessment.

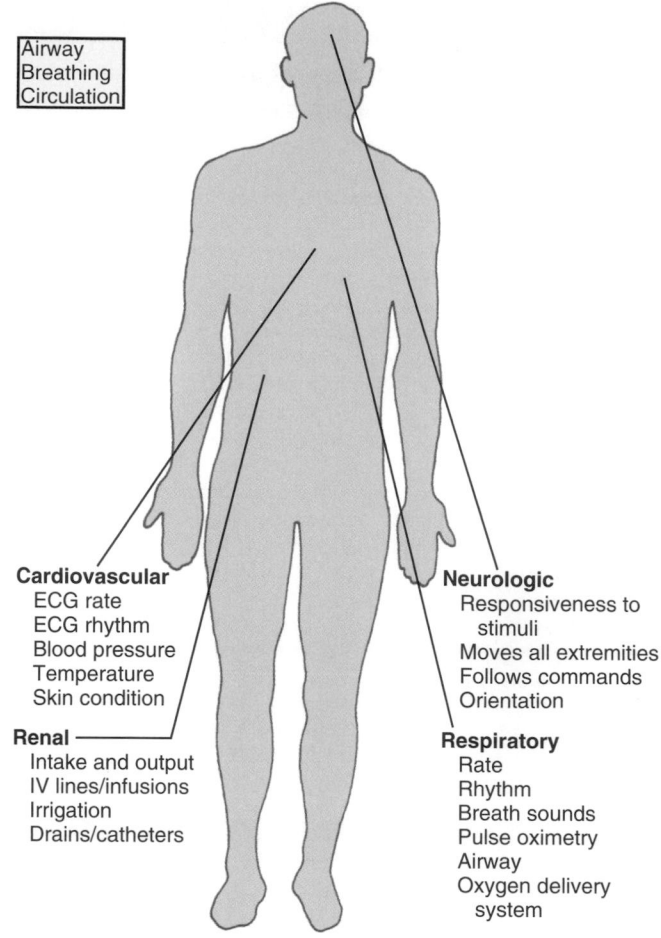

FIGURE 10-2 Postanesthesia care unit (PACU) major body systems assessment. *ECG,* Electrocardiogram; *IV,* intravenous.

solutions are noted and recorded. Any drains or catheters are listed; their output is noted for color, amount, and consistency.

The surgical site is checked, noting any drainage on the bandage, including amount and color. The area around the incision is inspected so that any future changes may be compared. Patients undergoing vaginal hysterectomy require that the abdomen be assessed for firmness. A rigid abdomen may indicate hemorrhage. Noting firmness of the abdomen on admission and later findings of a rigid abdomen leads to important comparisons. The patient is also assessed for signs or symptoms of pain, discomfort, or nausea, and medicated appropriately.

Information obtained from the admission assessment is documented in the PACU record.

Nursing Diagnosis

Common nursing diagnoses related to the care of postanesthesia patients include the following:
- Ineffective Breathing Pattern
- Decreased Cardiac Output
- Ineffective Thermoregulation
- Acute Pain

Outcome Identification

Outcomes identified for the selected nursing diagnoses can be stated as follows:

- The patient will demonstrate adequate ventilation, perfusion, and expansion of the lungs on discharge from the PACU.
- The patient will achieve and maintain adequate cardiac output on discharge from the PACU.
- The patient will attain a normal body temperature (96.8° to 100.4° F [36° to 38° C]) on discharge from the PACU.
- The patient will exhibit 4 or less on a numeric pain rating scale of 0 to 10 (or a pain/comfort level established by the patient as "acceptable") on discharge from the PACU.

Planning

When nursing diagnoses and desired outcomes are identified for the postoperative patient, a plan of care is designed that considers specific patient needs. Some nursing diagnoses are appropriate for all postanesthesia patients. A Sample Plan of Care for a patient in PACU is on p. 273.

Implementation

The nurse in the PACU continually assesses the patient and implements interventions for care. In addition to constant vigilant monitoring discussed under assessment, the perianesthesia nurse often begins a stir-up regimen that helps minimize complications. The stir-up regimen includes deep breathing exercises, coughing, positioning, mobilization, and pain management to facilitate respiratory function (O'Brien, 2013a). Oxygen delivery is monitored and

SAMPLE PLAN OF CARE

Immediate Postoperative Patient Care in the PACU

Nursing Diagnosis

Ineffective Breathing Pattern related to medications associated with anesthesia, type of surgical procedure, pain, tracheobronchial obstruction

Outcome

The patient will demonstrate adequate ventilation, perfusion, and expansion of lungs on discharge from the PACU as evidenced by regular respiratory rate and pattern, clear and equal bilateral breath sounds, blood pressure and pulse within preoperative range, oxygen saturation at least 92% or equal to preoperative status, patent airway, and control of pain.

Interventions

- Determine need for chin tilt or jaw thrust if patient is nonreactive without patent airway. Insert artificial airway if needed. Call anesthesia provider for further assistance.
- Assess respiratory status on admission to the PACU and at intervals until discharge.
- Determine level of consciousness (to assess for need to reverse opioid, benzodiazepine, or muscle relaxant).
- Administer humidified oxygen; assess need for continued oxygen after discharge.
- Elevate head of bed (if not contraindicated).
- Encourage patient to take deep breaths or sustained maximal inspiration.
- Note preoperative assessment for sleep apnea. Have patient's own equipment available if applicable.
- Assess patient for level of comfort. Administer pain medication as needed, per order or protocol.

Nursing Diagnosis

Decreased Cardiac Output related to anesthetic agents and other medications, fluid or blood loss or replacement, peripheral pooling of blood, alteration in preload or afterload, alterations in rate or rhythm

Outcome

The patient will maintain adequate cardiac output on discharge from the PACU as evidenced by blood pressure within preoperative range, skin warm and dry, oriented to person and place, and pulse strong and regular.

Interventions

- Monitor vital signs, electrocardiogram, and central venous pressure, with or without pulmonary artery catheter.
- Assess level of consciousness to determine effect of medication still in circulation.
- Monitor and record any drainage from surgical site.
- Monitor and record intake and output.
- Administer fluid or blood products if indicated.
- If hypotensive, elevate legs unless contraindicated; increase rate of fluid administration.
- Maintain patency of intravenous lines.
- Administer medication if needed to improve depressed myocardial contractility, increase cardiac output, and promote diuresis.
- Administer vasodilators, vasoconstrictors, or antidysrhythmics as ordered.
- Warm patient to 96.8° F (36° C).
- Administer humidified oxygen.

Nursing Diagnosis

Ineffective Thermoregulation related to surgical procedure: anesthetic agents, length of surgery, age of patient, OR environment, irrigation, type of surgery, or genetic predisposition to malignant hyperthermia

Outcome

The patient will attain a normal body temperature (96.8° to 100.4° F [36° to 38° C]) on discharge from the PACU.

Interventions

- Measure body temperature on admission; document temperature and route of measurement.
- Use same route of measurement for each temperature documented.
- Assess peripheral circulation.
- Monitor vital signs and oxygen saturation.
- Observe for shivering.
- Initiate measures to warm patient if hypothermic: place warmed blankets on patient's body and head; use forced-air warming device to rewarm patient.
- Initiate appropriate measures for malignant hyperthermia, if indicated (see Chapter 5).
- Maintain ongoing temperature monitoring until discharge.

Nursing Diagnosis

Acute Pain related to operative or other invasive procedures

Outcome

The patient will exhibit a 4 or less on a numeric pain rating scale of 0 to 10 (or a pain/comfort level established by the patient as tolerable) on discharge from the PACU.

Interventions

- Assess for subjective signs of pain: patient reports to the PACU nurse that he or she is in pain; patient is given a visual analog or numeric scale to rate pain level.
- Assess for objective signs of pain: protective guarding behavior, moaning, crying, whimpering, restlessness, irritability, diaphoresis, dilated pupils, facial expression of pain, and changes in vital signs (blood pressure, respiratory rate, or pulse).
- Refer to agency protocol for assessing and treating pain based on patient's pain rating.
- Monitor for pain relief and adverse reactions (respiratory depression, oversedation), and document.
- Administer pain medication as prescribed: titrate intravenous doses; initiate patient-controlled analgesia (PCA) or patient-controlled epidural analgesia (PCEA) as applicable.
- Encourage use of a multimodal approach to pain management including nonopioid analgesics.
- If epidural analgesia (EA) is used, assess for numbness, leg weakness, pruritus, and respiratory depression. Document findings and notify physician if findings are positive.
- If patient is intubated but conscious, collaborate in pain rating scale by pointing to a number or face and having patient indicate yes or no. If patient is unconscious, be especially attentive to signs such as grimacing.
- Initiate alternate methods of pain relief: transcutaneous electrical nerve stimulation (TENS), music, massage, relaxation, guided imagery.
- Reposition patient for comfort if not contraindicated.
- Assess causes of pain (e.g., surgical site versus chest pain).
- Document medications administered, dose, route, time, and effectiveness of pain relief.

decreased as per patient condition and PACU orders. In some cases, the patient may have entered the PACU with a capnograph in place, so the nurse monitors end-tidal CO_2 and intervenes when ventilation is inadequate.

The PACU nurse monitors blood pressure and heart rate to assess cardiovascular function and cardiac output throughout the patient stay. The nurse will also provide interventions to maintain adequate normothermia and pain management. Throughout post-anesthesia care, dangerous and life-threatening changes can occur rapidly (see Perianesthesia Complications).

Evaluation

The PACU nurse evaluates the identified patient outcomes prior to discharge from PACU. For the outcomes presented previously in this chapter, these might be stated as follows:

- The patient demonstrated adequate ventilation, perfusion, and expansion of lungs on discharge from the PACU. Oxygen saturation was adequate while receiving room air.
- The patient maintained adequate cardiac output; blood pressure and heart rate were within normal range.
- The patient was normothermic at discharge from the PACU.
- The patient's pain was 4 or less (on a scale of 0 to 10) or at a pain/comfort level established as acceptable by patient. The patient was relaxed and slept at intervals. The patient verbalized satisfactory pain relief.

Perianesthesia Complications

The following complications are pertinent to the care of all patients during the immediate postoperative period. Three of the most common complications in the PACU are upper airway obstruction, hypotension, and nausea and vomiting (Nicholau, 2009). Prompt recognition and immediate intervention are imperative for the well-being of PACU patients.

Respiratory

Airway Obstruction. The first priority in the care of the postanesthesia patient is to establish a patent airway. A common cause of airway obstruction is the tongue, which is relaxed because of anesthetic agents and muscle relaxants used during surgery (Nicholau, 2009) (Figure 10-3). The patient may present with snoring, little or no air movement on auscultation of the lungs, retraction of intercostal muscles, asynchronous movements of the chest and abdomen, and a decreased oxygen saturation level. The nursing action taken may be simple, such as stimulating the patient to take deep breaths, positioning the patient on the side, or providing supplemental oxygen. If the patient is still unresponsive, the nurse may need to open the airway with a chin tilt or jaw thrust. A chin tilt is accomplished by lifting the chin with one hand while tilting the forehead back with the other. A jaw thrust is accomplished by displacing the temporomandibular joint forward bilaterally. The patient also can be repositioned on the right side. This position is called the recovery position. Placing the patient in this position allows the tongue to move forward and the airway to remain open.

If these actions do not open the airway, an artificial airway may need to be inserted. An oral or nasal airway may be used. An oral airway is used with an unresponsive patient (Figure 10-4). A nasal airway, better tolerated by an awake patient, is indicated for patients who are arousable.

Hemorrhage after neck surgery or carotid endarterectomy also can cause acute obstruction of the airway. The PACU nurse assesses such patients carefully for bleeding. In situations such as apnea,

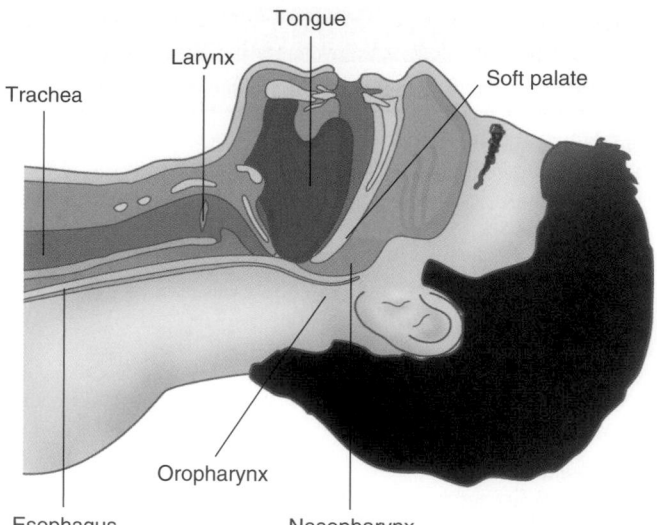

FIGURE 10-3 Obstruction of airway by tongue.

FIGURE 10-4 Oropharyngeal airway in place.

intubation with ventilation may be required. If intubation is impossible, the patient may require a tracheostomy, although this rarely is needed.

Laryngospasm. A serious PACU complication is laryngospasm, usually the result of an irritable airway. Laryngeal obstruction may occlude the airway as a result of partial or complete spasm of the intrinsic or extrinsic muscles of the larynx. The muscles of the larynx contract and the vocal chords either partially or completely obstruct the airway; the patient can become hypoxemic quickly (Drain, 2013). With laryngospasm, remove the irritating stimulus, suction secretions that may be triggering a glottic response, hyperextend the patient's neck, oxygenate the patient, and prepare to administer an aerosol with racemic (optically inactive) epinephrine. An awake patient experiencing a laryngospasm is terrified and needs reassurance and a calm demeanor from nurses and physicians. In many cases, positive-pressure ventilation is delivered by mask and bag. If symptoms last longer than 1 minute and are unrelieved by positive pressure, administration of a muscle relaxant, such as succinylcholine, by the anesthesia provider is required to relax the muscles of the larynx (Drain, 2013). Reintubation is undesirable and used only as a last resort.

Bronchospasm. Bronchospasm is a lower airway obstruction caused by spasms of the bronchial tubes. These spasms can cause complete airway closure because of lack of cartilaginous support in the bronchioles. The patient presents with wheezing, dyspnea, use of accessory muscles, and tachypnea (Odom-Forren, 2014). Bronchospasm can result from aspiration, pharyngeal suctioning, or histamine release secondary to allergic response or related to medication use. Inhaled bronchodilators are the first choice of therapy for these patients, followed by IV aminophylline. Both IV and inhaled lidocaine can ease bronchospasm induced by histamine (Benca, 2007). If bronchospasm becomes life threatening, epinephrine may be administered. Steroids, such as methylprednisolone, also may be administered if the underlying cause is inflammatory disease (e.g., asthma).

When obstruction occurs, partial pressure of arterial carbon dioxide ($PaCO_2$) increases significantly and quickly. With obstruction, the PACU nurse makes a quick assessment, rapidly intervenes with airway assistance, and calls for help from the anesthesia provider.

Cardiovascular

Cardiovascular system instability is a frequent finding after surgery because many anesthetic agents exert a depressive effect on the heart and vascular system. Common problems include hypotension, hypertension, and dysrhythmias. A rare complication in the PACU is cardiopulmonary arrest. Essential components of competent nursing care in the PACU includes early clinical response to signs and symptoms of complications and maintenance of resuscitation skills (Tallman et al, 2011).

Hypotension. Hypotension has been defined as a blood pressure reading that is 20% less than baseline or preoperative blood pressure measurement; it indicates either relative or absolute hypovolemia (O'Brien, 2013b). Clinical signs of hypotension include a rapid, thready pulse; disorientation; restlessness; oliguria; and cold, pale skin. Because hypovolemia is the most common cause of postoperative hypotension, the initial intervention is to administer IV fluids (physiologic saline or lactated Ringer's solution) at a maximum rate while making a specific diagnosis.

Cardiac output and vascular resistance determine blood pressure. Hypotension may be caused by cardiac dysfunction (such as myocardial infarction, tamponade, embolism, ischemia, dysrhythmias, congestive heart failure, valvular dysfunction) or by medications (including anesthetic agents). In such cases, the heart no longer pumps effectively. Hemodynamic monitoring, supplemental oxygen, and cardiac stimulants are used as needed.

Hypovolemia. Hypovolemia reduces cardiac output and may be caused by hemorrhage, dehydration (inadequate fluid replacement),

or increased positive end-expiratory pressure (PEEP). Fluid or blood replacement is used to treat hypovolemia. If the patient is hemorrhaging at the surgical site, a return to the operating room (OR) is indicated.

Decreased vascular resistance, which causes relative hypovolemia (interference with venous return to the heart), can be related to medications, general and regional anesthesia, or anaphylaxis (Odom-Forren, 2014). Vasodilation can be treated with fluids, vasopressors, or by elevating the patient's legs. Anaphylactic reactions are treated with epinephrine, antihistamines, and additional fluids.

Hypertension. The normal ranges for systolic and diastolic blood pressures are generally accepted as 100 to 140 mm Hg and 60 to 95 mm Hg, respectively, although these ranges vary. Hypertension has been defined as a 20% to 30% increase above baseline blood pressure measurement or persistent elevation of systolic blood pressure greater than 140 or diastolic pressure greater than 90 (O'Brien, 2013b; Odom-Forren, 2014). Hypertension is among the most common postoperative complications and often occurs early in the recovery phase. Blood pressure must be verified and rapidity of its change noted. Clinical signs and symptoms are the most important indicators of the severity of the hypertension. Headache, mental status changes, and substernal pain are all indicators of end-organ damage. Hypertension may be caused by volume overload or pulmonary edema, which causes an increase in the cardiac output. In this case the patient is given diuretics, placed on fluid restriction, and hemodynamically monitored. The patient with a history of cardiac disease is more at risk for adverse results.

Asymptomatic hypertension commonly occurs in the PACU and is usually considered harmless. The solution usually is determined by the cause. Patients with a history of essential hypertension are more likely to experience systemic hypertension in the PACU (Nicholau, 2009). Pain is one of the most common causes of hypertension. Other causes of hypertension are anxiety, reflex vasoconstriction from hypothermia, hypoxemia, hypercapnia, and viscus distention, all of which cause increased vascular resistance. Patients in pain are medicated, and patients with hypothermia are warmed. Patients are oxygenated and ventilated if necessary to improve hypoxemia or hypercapnia. Patients are encouraged to void or are catheterized to empty a full bladder.

Antihypertensive drugs are used as necessary to control blood pressure. Beta-blockers and α_2-agonists may be used postoperatively when needed. Other agents are available and may include the patient's usual prescription for hypertension (Odom-Forren, 2014). Patients who were on beta-blockers prior to surgery should be given a beta-blocker the day of surgery. Surgery patients receiving a beta-blocker during the perioperative period is one of the Surgical Care Improvement Project (SCIP) measures evaluated during the perioperative period (TJC, 2013). Patients should resume taking prescribed preoperative antihypertensives as soon as possible after surgery. Ambulatory surgery patients and inpatients usually are directed to take their prescribed antihypertensives on the day of surgery.

Dysrhythmias. Most dysrhythmias seen in the PACU have an underlying cause that is unrelated to myocardial injury (Odom-Forren, 2014). A common dysrhythmia after surgery is sinus tachycardia (rate >100 beats/min in an adult). Frequent causes include pain, hypoxemia, hypovolemia, increased temperature, and anxiety. The underlying cause of the dysrhythmia is treated. Propranolol, metoprolol, or esmolol may be given. Sinus bradycardia (heart rate <60 beats/min in an adult) also is a common dysrhythmia in the PACU. Causes include hypoxemia, hypothermia, high spinal anesthesia, vagal stimulation, and some medications commonly given during or after surgery. The underlying cause of the bradycardia is treated. Atropine is the drug of choice to increase heart rate, and usually no other treatment is required. Temporary or permanent pacemakers sometimes are required.

Premature ventricular contractions (PVCs) are represented by wide, bizarre-looking QRS complexes. The most common causes in the postoperative period are hypoxemia and hypokalemia, which are treated. Often, if cardiac disease or hypotension is not present, PVCs do not require medication.

Treatment of dysrhythmias begins with determining and removing the source of the problem. The urgency of treating cardiac dysrhythmias depends on the patient's underlying condition; dysrhythmias are most harmful in patients who have a history of coronary heart disease (Nicholau, 2009). Antidysrhythmic drugs, resuscitation equipment, and monitoring equipment should be immediately available.

Thermoregulation and Temperature Abnormalities

Hypothermia. Postoperative hypothermia, defined as a temperature less than 96.8°F (36°C) (Hooper et al., 2010), continues to be a widespread PACU problem. While hypothermia may not be life threatening, it does cause physiologic stress. Hypothermia can prolong recovery time and contribute to postoperative morbidity. Especially vulnerable to the effects of hypothermia are the elderly and children 2 years old or younger. Other risk factors include female gender, burn patients, patients who received general anesthesia with neuraxial anesthesia, low ambient temperature of the OR, length and type of surgical procedure, cachexia, significant fluid shift, and use of cold irrigants. The prevention and management of unplanned perioperative hypothermia remain a national priority in preventing surgical site infection, and it has been designated as an SCIP quality measure (Langham et al, 2009; TJC 2013).

Assessing the need for prewarming begins preoperatively. Preventive warming measures are begun for normothermic patients and active warming measures instituted for hypothermic patients (Hooper et al, 2010).

Prevention of heat loss continues in the OR. Under general anesthesia patients do not produce heat and depend on ambient temperature. Prevention of heat loss includes increasing the ambient temperature in the OR, providing the patient with warm blankets on arrival in the OR, and using draping techniques that minimize exposure during the procedure. Heated humidifiers and fluid warmers add heat. A common device to prevent hypothermia in the OR is a forced-air warming device (Figure 10-5).

In the PACU tremendous demands are made on the body when the patient shivers. Shivering can increase the need for oxygen by 300% to 400%. Hypothermic patients should have oxygen therapy initiated immediately on admission. For a patient with a healthy heart, there may be no harmful effects. For a patient with coronary artery disease or cardiomyopathy, however, decompensation can occur. Perioperative hypothermia has been associated with increased incidence of cardiac incidents including myocardial ischemia and myocardial infarction (Nicholau, 2009).

Other problems associated with hypothermia include intravascular volume loss attributable to a fluid shift from the extracellular space, probably related to vasoconstriction (Reynolds et al, 2008).

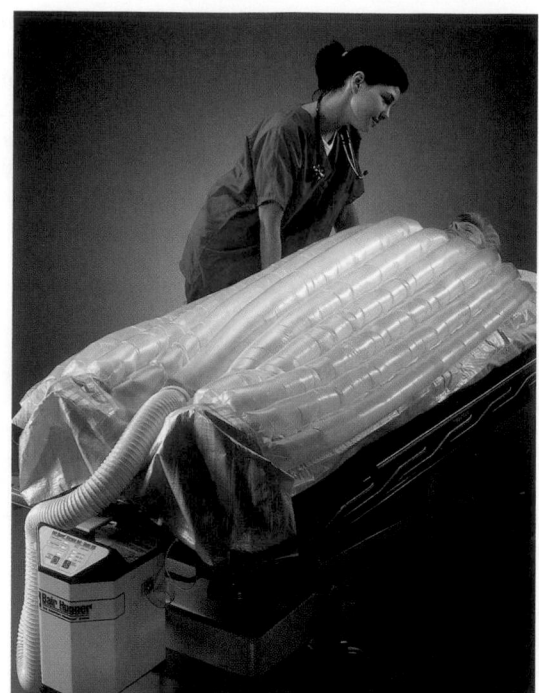

FIGURE 10-5 Bair Hugger: focused thermal environment.

As the patient begins to rewarm, vasodilation follows, and the patient can require large amounts of IV fluids to avoid hypovolemia. The central nervous system is depressed by hypothermia. A cold postanesthesia patient remains more anesthetized than a warm patient while recovering. Nitrogen loss and hypokalemia can cause a predisposition to wound infection. Impaired wound healing and surgical site infection have been linked to hypothermia (Paulikas, 2008).

Hypothermia slows metabolism and alters the effects of some anesthetic drugs. Of special interest is the prolonged elimination of muscle relaxants in hypothermic patients. Clotting abnormalities can occur. Platelet activity declines, and fibrinolysis increases with hypothermia; both conditions enhance the tendency to bleed (Hooper, 2013).

Rewarming is a priority for the postoperative patient. Wet and cold gowns and blankets are removed, and warm, dry gowns and blankets are applied to the head and body. Several external rewarming techniques are available. Application of warm cotton blankets has been a PACU tradition. Warm blankets are applied every 5 to 10 minutes until the patient is normothermic. Cotton blankets gradually increase the patient's temperature. They do not actively heat patients, however, and warming can be a slow process. Forced-air warming devices are effective in rewarming patients. They produce a thermal-focused environment that transfers heat by blowing warm air through a plastic and tissue paper blanket that covers the patient. Forced-air warming devices are standard hypothermia treatment in PACU settings. This is an evidence-based nursing initiative that actively decreases hypothermia (Hooper et al, 2010).

There is some evidence that continuous fluid-circulating blankets or warm-water mattresses, radiant heat lamps, gel pads, and resistive heating work (Hooper et al, 2010). Continuous fluid-circulating blankets may not work as well because the size of the surface area in contact with the heat source is limited. Radiant heat lamps depend on exposure of large areas of body surface and are of limited use to adult patients. Fluid and blood warmers are useful for large volumes of cool fluids, but not to reverse hypothermia. Single strategies such as forced-air warming were more effective at increasing temperature than passive warming as determined by one systematic review; however, combined strategies, including use of preoperative prewarming, use of warmed fluids, forced-air warming, and other active strategies were more effective in vulnerable groups (Moola and Lockwood, 2011).

Studies have explored the best method to obtain accurate temperatures in the PACU when invasive core temperature measures (e.g., pulmonary artery, distal esophagus, nasopharynx, and tympanic membrane) are unavailable. A study comparing eight noninvasive techniques to bladder temperature (Langham et al, 2009) concluded that the most accurate method for routine postoperative temperature monitoring was via electronic oral temperature devices.

Hyperthermia. Hyperthermia may indicate an infectious process, sepsis, or a serious hypermetabolic process—malignant hyperthermia (MH). MH is a life-threatening emergency that is genetic in origin (Rosero et al, 2009). It is triggered by volatile anesthetic agents and the depolarizing muscle relaxant *succinylcholine.* Death may ensue unless MH is immediately recognized and treated (see Chapter 5 for a discussion of MH). Some institutions have crisis checklists in the PACU and OR to guide staff step by step thorough emergencies such as MH (Arriaga et al, 2012).

Disturbances in Cognitive Function

PACU patients may be disoriented, drowsy, confused, or delirious. Attempts have been made to differentiate emergence delirium from agitation, with agitation defined as mild restlessness and mental distress. Causes of agitation range from residual effects of anesthetics to pain and anxiety. Hypoxemia is ruled out first; it remains the most common cause of postoperative agitation. Chemically dependent patients often awaken in an agitated state. Viscus distention also can contribute to agitation in a drowsy, confused patient. The PACU nurse should identify and eliminate the cause of the agitation or confusion, if possible. The patient can be engaged in short conversations and reoriented to place and person. Baseline preoperative data are important to determine the cause of agitation. Persistent changes from preoperative status require thorough assessment and possible intervention by the physician.

McGuire and Burkard (2010) identified pain and trauma, both physical and psychologic, as potential risk factors for emergence delirium in military personnel. In another study, patients who were less than 75 years of age and had a pain level of less than 4 were more likely to recover from delirium (Decrane et al, 2011). These authors point out that aggressive pain management may be the key in facilitating early recovery from delirium. Figure 10-6 provides a summary of factors contributing to emergence delirium and treatment options.

Nausea and Vomiting

Postoperative nausea and vomiting (PONV) is a problem that affects approximately 30% of PACU patients (Fetzer, 2010). Primary risk factors associated with PONV are female gender, nonsmoker, history of PONV or motion sickness, use of volatile anesthetics, use of nitrous oxide, postoperative use of opioids, duration of surgery, and type of surgery (Gan et al, 2007). Patients with four or more risk factors have a higher incidence of PONV. Management of nausea and vomiting begins preoperatively and continues into the intraoperative period. Preventive therapy for patients at high risk of PONV is effective in reducing its incidence. There is no

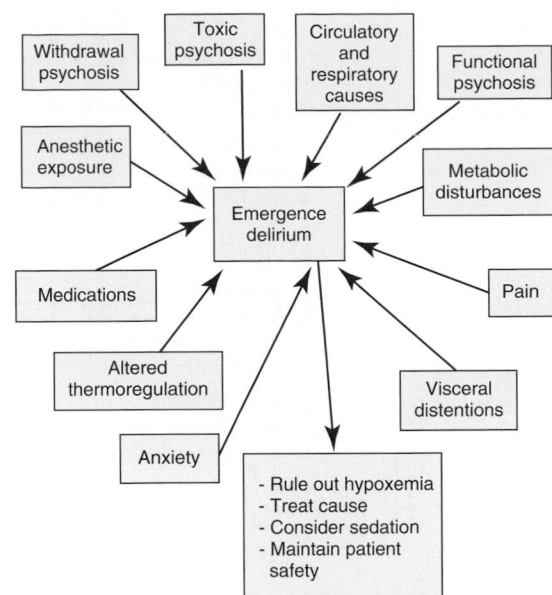

FIGURE 10-6 Emergence delirium in the postanesthesia care unit: contributing factors and treatment.

single method to prevent or treat PONV. Many causative factors relate to anesthesia and surgery. Pharmacologic prophylaxis improves patient comfort, readiness for discharge, and satisfaction with care (Practice Guidelines, 2013).

Risk factors for PONV should be assessed preoperatively and care planned accordingly. Two risk assessment tools commonly are used. Apfel and colleagues (1999) developed their risk assessment tool based on four risk factors: female gender, smoking status, history of PONV or motion sickness, and postoperative use of opioids. Koivuranta and colleagues (1997) identified five risk factors: surgery lasting more than 60 minutes, female gender, history of motion sickness, history of PONV, and nonsmoking status. Figure 10-7 lists guidelines regarding preoperative management and prophylaxis of PONV.

Receptors that can cause nausea and vomiting when triggered are dopamine type-2, serotonin type-3, histamine type-1, muscarinic cholinergic type-1, and neurokinin type-1. Patients at risk for PONV receive either one or a combination of agents that block one or more of these receptor sites (Surgical Pharmacology). Effective medications are aprepitant (Emend), ondansetron (Zofran), dolasetron (Anzemet), granisetron (Kytril), promethazine (Phenergan), prochlorperazine (Compazine), dexamethasone, palonosetron (Aloxi), and transdermal scopolamine. Other medications that can be considered are metoclopramide (Reglan) at a dosage of at least 25 to 50 mg IV, dimenhydrinate (Dramamine), diphenhydramine (Benadryl), or droperidol (Inapsine). Droperidol has a black box warning; the patient must be monitored for QT prolongation/torsades de pointes after administration (U.S. Food and Drug Administration, 2001). If the patient is hypotensive with nausea and vomiting, ephedrine and additional fluids may be administered. PONV rescue medication administered in the PACU should be an antiemetic from a different pharmacologic class than medication given for prophylaxis (Apfel, 2009). Figure 10-8 reviews postoperative management of the patient with PONV.

Patients may also experience nausea and vomiting after discharge home from ambulatory surgery. Apfel and colleagues (2012) determined that predictors for postdischarge nausea and vomiting

FIGURE 10-7 Preoperative patient management of PONV/PDNV. *NSAIDs,* Nonsteroidal antiinflammatory drugs.

SURGICAL PHARMACOLOGY

Antiemetic Pharmacology

Agent	Receptors Affected	Route and Dosage	Comments
Aprepitant (Emend)	NK₁	40 mg PO	Patient should receive 1-3 hours before surgery.
Dexamethasone (Decadron)	?	4 mg IV	Administer before induction.
Dimenhydrinate (Dramamine)	H₁, M₁	50-100 mg IV, IM	Side effects include dry mouth, urinary retention.
Diphenhydramine (Benadryl)	H₁, M₁	12.5-25 mg IM, IV	Side effects include dry mouth, urinary retention.
Dolasteron (Anzemet)	5-HT₃	12.5 mg IV	
Droperidol (Inapsine)	D₂	0.625-1.25 mg IV	Use requires ECG monitoring for 3 hours after dose.
Graniseteron (Kytril)	5-HT₃	5 mcg/kg-1 mg IV	
Metoclopramide (Reglan)	D₂	10 mg IV	Increases GI motility; no effective prophylaxis.
Ondansetron (Zofran)	5-HT₃	4 mg IV or ODT	Give 15-30 minutes before end of surgery.
Prochlorperazine (Compazine)	D₂	5-10 mg IV, IM	Side effects include dry mouth, urinary retention.
Promethazine (Phenergan)	D₂, H₁, M₁	6.25 mg-12.5 mg IV; 12.5-25 mg IM; PR	Extrapyramidal symptoms possible.
Scopolamine (Transderm Scōp)	H₁M₁	1.5-mg transdermal patch	Apply 4 hours before end of surgery; anticholinergic effects.

D_2, Dopamine receptor blocker; *ECG,* electrocardiogram; *GI,* gastrointestinal; *IM,* intramuscular; *IV,* intravenous; *5-HT₃,* serotonin receptor blocker; *H₁,* histamine blocker; *M₁,* muscarinic receptor blocker; *NK₁,* NK receptor blocker; *ODT,* ondansetron dissolving tablet; *PO,* per os, orally; *PR,* per rectum.
Modified from Fetzer SJ: Postoperative nausea and vomiting. In Schick L, Windle P, editors: *Perianesthesia nursing core curriculum: perioperative, phase I and phase II PACU nursing,* ed 2, St Louis, 2010, Saunders; Odom-Forren J: *Drain's perianesthesia nursing: a critical care approach,* ed 6, St Louis, 2013; Odom-Forren J: Postoperative and postdischarge nausea and vomiting. In Stannard D, Krenzischek DA, editors: *PeriAnesthesia nursing care: a bedside guide for safe recovery,* Sudbury, CT, 2012, Jones & Bartlett.

(PDNV) were female gender, age less than 50 years, a history of nausea or vomiting, opioid administration, or nausea in the PACU (Research Highlight). Depending on the number of factors present, the patient's risk for PDNV can be predicted as 10%, 20%, 30%, 50%, 60%, or 80%. Less research is available to direct the care of these patients, but use of transdermal scopolamine, promethazine (suppositories or oral), or ondansetron dissolving tablets (ODTs) is supported by small studies. Longer-acting antiemetics may be needed (DeJohn, 2013). Figure 10-9 reviews management of patients with PDNV.

FIGURE 10-8 Postoperative patient management of postoperative nausea and vomiting (PONV). *VAS*, Visual analog scale; *VDS*, verbal descriptor scale.

RESEARCH HIGHLIGHT ‖

Patients at Risk for Postdischarge Nausea and Vomiting After Ambulatory Surgery

Apfel and colleagues conducted a study to determine risk scores for postdischarge nausea and vomiting (PDNV). For those patients who suffer from postoperative nausea and vomiting, risk scores have been developed to better manage this outcome in hospitalized patients. However, there has been no risk score for PDNV in ambulatory surgical patients. The authors conducted a prospective multi-center study of 2170 adults undergoing general anesthesia at ambulatory surgery centers in the United States. PDNV was assessed from discharge until the end of the second postoperative day. The overall incidence of PDNV was 37%. Logistic regression analysis of the development dataset (n = 1,913) identified five independent predictors (odds ratio; 95% CI): female gender (1.54; 1.22 to 1.94), age less than 50 years (2.17; 1.75 to 2.69), history of nausea and/or vomiting after previous anesthesia (1.50; 1.19 to 1.00), opioid administration in PACU (1.93; 1.53 to 2.43), and nausea in PACU (3.14; 2.44 to 4.04). In the validation dataset (n = 257), zero, one, two, three, four, and five of these factors were associated with a PDNV incidence of 7%, 20%, 28%, 53%, 60%, and 89%, respectively.

Four of the five predictors are identifiable before surgery and the fifth predictor is identifiable in the PACU. Perianesthesia nurses and their perioperative nurse colleagues can use this simplified risk score to identify patients who would benefit from long-acting prophylactic antiemetics and other nonpharmacologic methods of management at discharge from the ambulatory care center.

Modified from Apfel C et al: Who is at risk for postdischarge nausea and vomiting after ambulatory surgery? *Anesthesiology* 117:475–486, 2012.

Aspiration

Aspiration, the passage of regurgitated material into the lungs, occurs most often during tracheal intubation or extubation. The PACU nurse protects the airway of unconscious or semiconscious patients to prevent aspiration of gastric contents. Prevention of aspiration postoperatively includes responding quickly to reports of nausea and vomiting, avoiding conversations that could elicit nausea and vomiting, and preventing rapid movement and head elevation of the patient. Nonreactive patients can be placed on their sides in the recovery position (ASA, 2011).

Volume and acidity of the aspirate determine the extent of damage to the lungs. The most severe damage seems to be in cases in which the pH is less than 2.5 or the volume greater than 25 mL. Preoperatively, patients may receive clear, nonparticulate antacids, such as sodium citrate (Bicitra), to raise the gastric fluid pH (Fowler and Spiess, 2009). Histamine H_2-receptor antagonists, such as cimetidine, ranitidine, or famotidine, decrease gastric acid

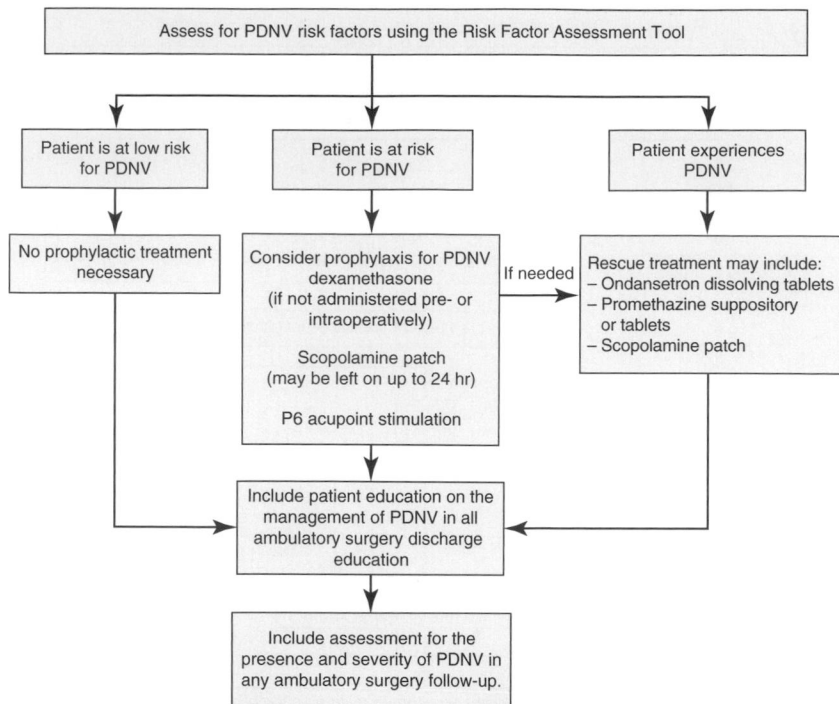

FIGURE 10-9 Management of postdischarge nausea and vomiting (PDNV).

production. Metoclopramide speeds gastric-emptying time. Aspiration does not occur in patients with normal protective reflexes. Risk factors can be divided into general and specific (Table 10-1).

Signs and symptoms of aspiration include tachypnea and hypoxemia attributable to a decrease in lung compliance. Wheezing, coughing, dyspnea, hypotension, apnea, and bradycardia may occur. Treatment focuses on promoting tissue oxygenation. Supplemental oxygen is given. Positive pressure applied by use of a mask or an endotracheal tube may be needed to maintain arterial oxygenation, and a chest x-ray may be performed. If intubated, the trachea can be suctioned. Bronchoscopy is performed if aspirated particles are large and cause airway obstruction. Neither steroids nor antibiotics are warranted. Tracheal secretions can be cultured, and if the results are positive, appropriate antibiotic therapy is started (Fowler and Spiess, 2009). Bronchodilators are used as required. Patient recovery depends on recognition of the problem, quantity and pH of aspirate, physical condition before the event, and speed with which medical intervention begins.

Acute Pain

Pain is a subjective experience and may or may not be verbalized. Often healthcare providers require objective signs of discomfort in addition to subjective reports of pain from the patient, which can lead to undertreatment of pain. The guiding principle in pain care is that pain is whatever the patient says it is; the most reliable indicator of the existence and intensity of pain is the patient's self-report (Pasero, 2009; Pasero and McCaffery, 2011). All patients should be assessed for pain severity using a verbal descriptor rating scale, numeric rating scale, or a visual analog scale (Flaherty, 2008) (Figures 10-10 and 10-11).

Pain management is one of the highest priorities of postanesthesia care. Patients should be assessed for pain on admission to the PACU and at frequent intervals (Box 10-3). It is important to remember that not all patients respond to pain in the same manner,

TABLE 10-1

Risk Factors for Pulmonary Aspiration

General Risk Factors	Specific Risk Factors
Age (older > younger)	Emergency
Gender (female > male)	Pregnancy
Comorbid diseases	Recent oral intake
Type 1 diabetes	Opioid administration
CNS deficits	Increased gastric residual volume, as with gastrointestinal obstruction or delayed gastric emptying
Peripheral vascular disease	Obesity
Hepatobiliary or gastrointestinal diseases	Difficulty in protecting airway, as with depressed level of consciousness
Renal dysfunction	Previous esophageal dysfunction
	Head injury or neurologic dysfunction
	Lack of coordination of swallowing and respiration
	Procedures that increase intra-abdominal pressure (e.g., upper abdominal surgery, straining with ETT)
	Difficult intubation/airway

CNS, Central nervous system; *ETT,* endotracheal tube.
Modified from King W: Pulmonary aspiration of gastric contents, March, 2011, available at http://update.anaesthesiologists.org/wp-content/uploads/2011/03/Pulmonary-aspiration-of-gastric-contents.pdf. Accessed March 25, 2013; Schick L: Perianesthesia complications. In Schick L, Windle P, editors: *Perianesthesia nursing core curriculum: perioperative, phase I and phase II PACU nursing,* ed 2, St Louis, 2010, Saunders.

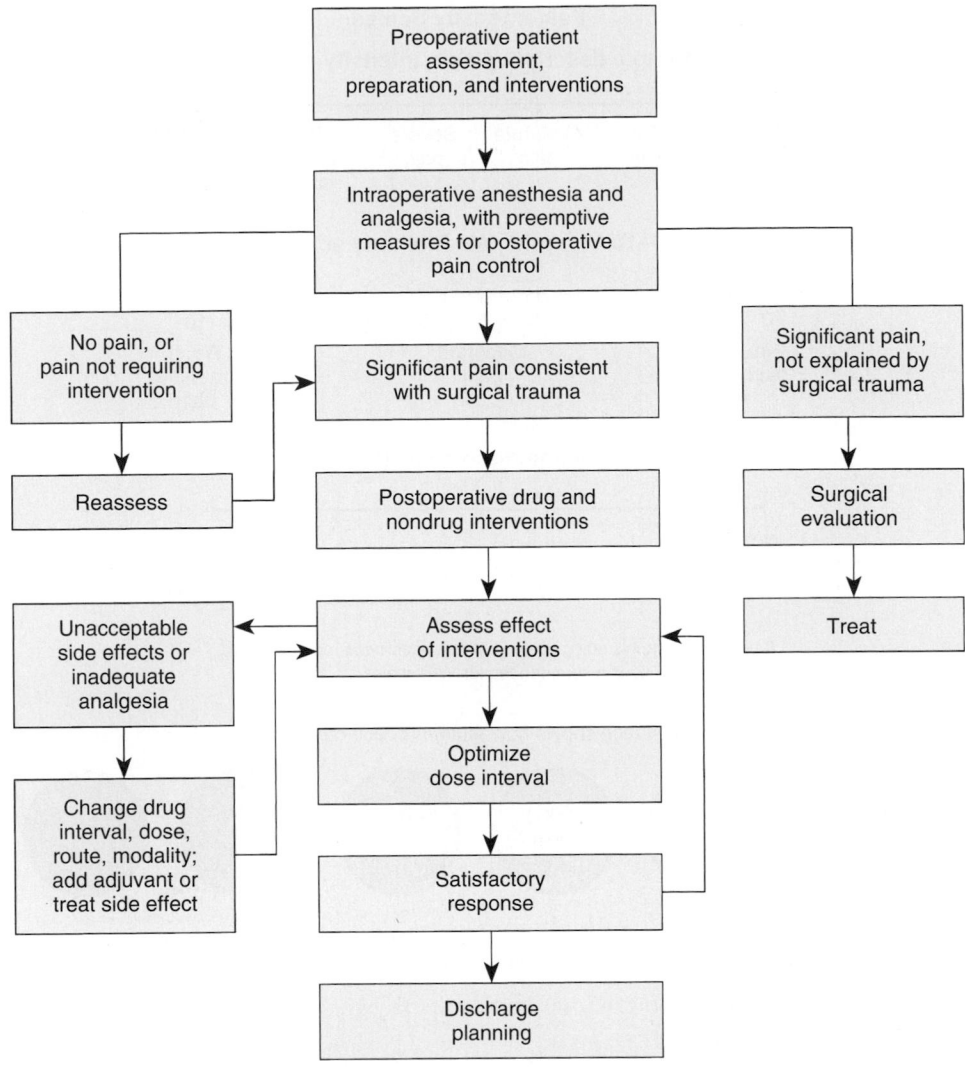

FIGURE 10-10 Acute pain management in adults.

despite comparable surgical procedures. Measures of pain assessment should be correlated with the patient's self-report as the most important measure of intensity. Measures to determine pain intensity in a patient who cannot self-report include exposure to a painful procedure or underlying painful conditions; behavioral signs, such as crying or restlessness; using valid and reliable behavioral pain assessment tools; a proxy pain rating by someone who knows the patient well; and physiologic indicators, such as elevated vital signs (Makic, 2013; Pasero, 2009). An analgesic trial can be attempted as a final measure in the hierarchy of importance in assessing the nonverbal patient. Improvement in behaviors after the analgesic trial indicates that pain was the likely underlying cause (Pasero, 2009).

Evidence indicates that early analgesia reduces postoperative problems. Nonopioids such as acetaminophen, nonsteroidal antiinflammatory drugs (NSAIDs), or cyclooxygenase type 2 (COX-2) inhibitors for patients who have experienced adverse effects from conventional NSAID use, and opiates are the analgesics of choice. Newer nonopioids available in IV format are acetaminophen (paracetamol) and ibuprofen (Groudine and Fossum, 2011; Pasero and McCaffery, 2011). Onset of analgesia occurs within 5 to 10 minutes of IV administration, with peak analgesic effect occurring within 1 hour and duration of 4 to 6 hours. Availability of these

IV nonopioids for postoperative patients adds an option when developing a multimodal plan of pain management in the PACU (Surgical Pharmacology: Dosing Data for Nonopioid Analgesics, p. 283 and Surgical Pharmacology: Dosing Data for Opioid Analgesics, p. 284). Multimodal pain techniques that use nonopioids as well as opiates can reduce opioid requirements significantly (Pasero and Stannard, 2012). The ASA recommends the use of multimodal pain management therapy including central regional blockade with local anesthetics, and unless contraindicated, patients should receive an around-the-clock regimen of COX-2 inhibitors, NSAIDs, or acetaminophen with treatment individualized to each patient. It also suggests that gabapentin and pregabalin can be beneficial in some patients as part of a multimodal therapy (ASA Task Force, 2012).

Inadequate pain relief experienced by postoperative patients using intramuscular (IM) injections is attributable to varying blood levels and is no longer a supported method of analgesic delivery. A common opioid-delivery system is patient-controlled analgesia (PCA), which allows patients to control their analgesic administration. Dosage, time between doses, and the maximum allowable dosage are programmed into the PCA pump. This form of analgesia also allows for a basal rate of opioids to infuse continuously, if

Text continued on p. 285

Pain Intensity Scales

Simple descriptive pain intensity scale*

A — No pain | Mild pain | Moderate pain | Severe pain | Very severe pain | Worst possible pain

0–10 Numeric pain intensity scale*

B — 0 1 2 3 4 5 6 7 8 9 10
No pain | Moderate pain | Worst possible pain

Visual analogue scale (VAS)†

C — No pain | Pain as bad as it could possibly be

* If used as a graphic rating scale, a 10-cm baseline is recommended.
† A 10-cm baseline is recommended for VAS scales.

Which face shows how much hurt you have now?

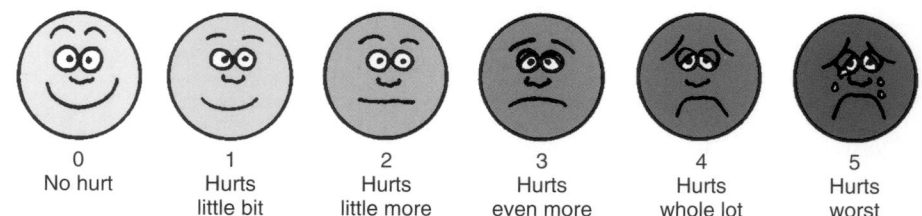

D
0 No hurt | 1 Hurts little bit | 2 Hurts little more | 3 Hurts even more | 4 Hurts whole lot | 5 Hurts worst

FIGURE 10-11 A-C, Examples of pain intensity and pain distress scales. **D,** FACES pain rating scale. *VAS,* Visual analog scale.

BOX 10-3

Pain Assessment and Reassessment

Principles
- Pain is multidimensional. Patients experience its aspects in different, personal ways. Comprehensive pain assessment considers the physical, sensory, behavioral, sociocultural, cognitive, affective, and spiritual dimensions of pain.
- Patients who have difficulty communicating their pain require particular attention. This includes patients who are cognitively impaired, psychotic, or severely emotionally disturbed; children; the elderly; patients who do not speak English; and patients whose level of education or cultural background differs significantly from that of the healthcare team.
- Unexpectedly intense pain, particularly if sudden or associated with altered vital signs, such as hypotension, tachycardia, or fever, is reported and evaluated immediately; diagnoses, such as wound dehiscence, infection, or deep vein thrombosis, should be considered.
- Family members should be involved when appropriate.

Pain Assessment Tools
- The most reliable indicator of the existence and intensity of pain and any resultant distress is the patient's self-report.

- Self-report measurement includes numeric or verbal descriptor ratings and visual analog scales.
- Tools should be reliable, valid, and easy for the patient and nurse or physician to use. One may use these tools by showing a diagram to the patient to indicate the appropriate rating. One may also simply ask the patient for a verbal response: "On a scale of 0 to 10 with 0 as no pain and 10 as the worst pain possible, how would you rate your pain?" or "Please describe your pain for me, from no pain to mild, moderate, severe, or pain as bad as it could be."
- Tools must be appropriate for the patient's gender and age, developmental, physical, emotional, cognitive, and cultural status.

Preoperative Preparation
- Discuss the patient's previous experiences with pain and beliefs about and preferences for pain assessment and management.
- Give the patient information about pain management therapies and the rationale underlying their uses.
- Develop with the patient a plan for pain assessment and management.
- Select a pain assessment tool and teach the patient to use it.

BOX 10-3

Pain Assessment and Reassessment—cont'd

- Provide the patient with education and information about pain control, including nonpharmacologic options, such as relaxation, distraction, imagery, and massage.
- Inform patients that it is easier to prevent pain than to attempt to reduce it after it is established, and that communication of unrelieved pain is essential for its relief. Emphasize the importance of a factual report of pain, avoiding stoicism or exaggeration.

Postoperative Assessment

- Assess the patient's perceptions, along with behavioral and psychologic responses. Observations of behavior and vital signs should not be used instead of a self-report, unless the patient is unable to communicate.
- Assess and reassess pain frequently during the immediate postoperative period. Determine frequency of assessment based on the procedure performed and severity of pain. Assess pain every 2 hours during the first postoperative day after major surgical procedures (assess for procedure-specific pain).
- Increase frequency of assessment and reassessment if pain is poorly managed.
- Record pain intensity and response to intervention in an easily visible and accessible place, such as a bedside flow sheet or in the electronic health record.
- Revise the management plan if pain is poorly controlled.
- Review with the patient before discharge the interventions used and their efficacy, and provide specific discharge instructions regarding pain and its management. Have patient "teach back" or repeat instructions in his or her own words.

Modified from Bai J et al: Validation of the COMFORT behavior scale and the FLACC scale for pain assessment in Chinese children after cardiac surgery, *Pain Manag Nurs* 13(1):18–26, 2012; Edwards RR, Berde CB: Pain assessment. In Benzon H et al, editors: *Essentials of pain medicine*, ed 3, St Louis, 2011, Saunders; Flaherty E: Using pain-rating scales with older adults, *AJN* 108(6):40–47, 2008; Lee H et al: Postoperative pain assessment for upper lid blepharoplasty in Asians, *Ann Plast Surg* 69(3):244–246, 2012; Pasero C, McCaffery M: *Pain assessment and pharmacologic management*, St Louis, 2011, Mosby.

SURGICAL PHARMACOLOGY

Dosing Data for Nonopioid Analgesics

Drug	Usual Adult Dose	Usual Pediatric Dose*	Comments
Oral			
Acetaminophen (OFIRMEV)	Oral: 650-975 mg q4hr IV per 15-min infusion: 1000 mg maximum single dose q6hr to maximum total dose of 4000 mg/24 hr	Oral: 10-15 mg/kg q4hr IV per 15-min infusion: 15 mg/kg q6hr to maximum total dose of 75 mg/kg per 24 hr	Acetaminophen lacks peripheral antiinflammatory activity of NSAIDs. Do not exceed the maximum daily dose of acetaminophen or hepatic injury may result, including risk of severe hepatotoxicity and death. Available also in liquid and suppository.
Aspirin	650-975 mg q4hr	10-15 mg/kg q4hr[†]	The standard against which other NSAIDs are compared. Inhibits platelet aggregation; may cause postoperative bleeding.
Choline magnesium trisalicylate (Trilisate)	1000-1500 mg bid	25 mg/kg q12hr	May have minimal antiplatelet activity; also available as oral liquid.
Diflunisal (Dolobid)	1000 mg initial dose followed by 500 mg q12hr	—	—
Etodolac (Lodine)	200-400 mg q6hr	—	—
Fenoprofen calcium (Nalfon)	200 mg q4-6hr	—	—
Flurbiprofen	100 mg bid, tid, qid	—	—
Ibuprofen (Motrin, Caldolor, others)	Oral: 400 mg q4-6hr IV: 400 mg to 800 mg q6hr to maximum of 3200 mg; dilute in 100 mL normal saline or 5% dextrose and infuse over 30 min	Oral: 10 mg/kg q6-8hr IV formulation for adults only	IV ibuprofen is contraindicated for the treatment of perioperative pain for coronary artery bypass graft (CABG) surgery.
Ketoprofen (Orudis)	25-75 mg q6-8hr	—	—
Magnesium salicylate	650 mg q4hr	—	Many brands and generic forms available.
Meclofenamate sodium (Meclomen)	50 mg q4-6hr	—	—
Mefenamic acid (Ponstel)	250 mg q6hr	—	—
Naproxen (Naprosyn)	500 mg initial dose followed by 250 mg q6-8hr	5 mg/kg q12hr	Also available as oral liquid.

Continued

Dosing Data for Nonopioid Analgesics—cont'd

Drug	Usual Adult Dose	Usual Pediatric Dose*	Comments
Naproxen sodium (Anaprox)	550 mg initial dose followed by 275 mg q6-8hr	—	—
Oxaprozin	600 mg q24hr	—	Long half-life, so can be given once daily.
Salsalate (Disalcid, others)	500 mg q4hr	—	May have minimal antiplatelet activity.
Sodium salicylate	325-650 mg q3-4hr	—	Available in generic form from several distributors.

Selective COX-2 Inhibitor

Celecoxib (Celebrex)	100-200 mg q12-24hr; maximum of 400 mg	—	Reduces risk of GI side effects and renal toxicity. No effects on platelet aggregation. May have a higher risk of having heart attack or stroke.

Parenteral NSAID

Ketorolac	30 or 60 mg IM initial dose followed by 15 or 30 mg q6hr Oral dose after IM dose: 10 mg q6-8hr IV dose: 30 mg for healthy adults and 15 mg for adults >65 years	—	IM dose not to exceed 5 days; IV administration comparable to 10 mg IM morphine.

NOTE: Only the above NSAIDs have U.S. Food and Drug Administration approval for use as simple analgesics, but clinical experience has been gained with other drugs as well.
bid, Twice daily; *COX-2*, cyclooxygenase type 2; *IM*, intramuscular; *IV*, intravenous; *NSAID*, nonsteroidal antiinflammatory drug; *qid*, four times daily; *tid*, three times daily.
*Drug recommendations are limited to NSAIDs for which pediatric dosing experience is available.
†Contraindicated in presence of fever or other evidence of viral illness.
Modified from Acute Pain Management Guideline Panel: *Acute pain management in adults: operative procedures. Quick reference guide for clinicians,* AHCPR pub. no. 92-0019, Rockville, Md, 1992, Agency for Health Care Policy and Research, U.S. Public Health Service, U.S. Department of Health and Human Services; Odom-Forren J: *Drain's perianesthesia nursing: a critical care approach,* ed 6, St. Louis, 2013; Pasero C, McCaffery M: *Pain assessment and pharmacologic management,* St. Louis, 2011, Mosby.

Dosing Data for Opioid Analgesics

Drug	Approximate Equianalgesic Oral Dose	Approximate Equianalgesic Parenteral Dose	Recommended Starting Dose (Adults >50 kg Body Weight)		Recommended Starting Dose (Children and Adults <50 kg Body Weight)*	
			Oral	Parenteral	Oral	Parenteral
Opioid Agonist						
Morphine†	30 mg q3-4hr (around-the-clock dosing) 60 mg q3-4hr (single dose or intermittent dosing)	10 mg q3-4hr	30 mg q3-4hr	10 mg q3-4hr	0.3 mg/kg q3-4hr	0.1 mg/kg q3-4hr or 0.05-0.1 mg/kg IV q1-2hr
Codeine§	130 mg q3-4hr	75 mg q3-4hr	60 mg q3-4hr	60 mg q2hr (IM/SubQ)	1 mg/kg q3-4hr¶	NR
Hydromorphone† (Dilaudid)	7.5 mg q3-4hr	1.5 mg q3-4hr	6 mg q3-4hr	1.5 mg q3-4hr	0.06 mg/kg q3-4hr	0.015 mg/kg q3-4hr
Hydrocodone (in Lorcet, available as Lortab, Vicodin, others)	30 mg q3-4hr	NA	10 mg q3-4hr	NA	0.2 mg/kg q3-4hr¶	NA
Levorphanol (Levo-Dromoran)	4 mg q6-8hr	2 mg q6-8hr	4 mg q6-8hr	2 mg q6-8hr	0.04 mg/kg q6-8hr	0.02 mg/kg q6-8hr
Meperidine (Demerol)†	300 mg q2-3hr	100 mg q3hr	NR	100 mg q3hr	NR	0.75 mg/kg q2-3hr
Methadone (Dolophine, others)	20 mg q6-8hr	10 mg q6-8hr	20 mg q6-8hr	10 mg q6-8hr	0.2 mg/kg q6-8hr	0.1 mg/kg q6-8hr

Dosing Data for Opioid Analgesics—cont'd

Drug	Approximate Equianalgesic Oral Dose	Approximate Equianalgesic Parenteral Dose	Recommended Starting Dose (Adults >50 kg Body Weight)		Recommended Starting Dose (Children and Adults <50 kg Body Weight)*	
			Oral	Parenteral	Oral	Parenteral
Oxycodone (Roxicodone, also in Percocet, Percodan, Tylox, others)	30 mg q3-4hr	NA	10 mg q3-4hr	NA	0.2 mg/kg q3-4hr[¶]	NA
Oxymorphone[‡] (Numorphan)	NA	1 mg q3-4hr	NA	1 mg q3-4hr	NR	NR
Opioid Agonist-Antagonist and Partial Agonist						
Buprenorphine (Buprenex)	NA	0.3-0.4 mg q6-8hr	NA	0.4 mg q6-8hr	NA	0.004 mg/kg q6-8hr
Butorphanol (Stadol)	NA	2 mg q3-4hr	NA	2 mg q3-4hr	NA	NR
Nalbuphine (Nubain)	NA	10 mg q3-4hr	NA	10 mg q3-4hr	NA	0.1 mg/kg q3-4hr
Pentazocine (Talwin, others)	150 mg q3-4hr	60 mg q3-4hr	50 mg q4-6hr	NR	NR	NR

*CAUTION: Dosages listed for patients with body weight <50 kg cannot be used as initial starting doses in infants <6 months of age. Consult the Agency for Healthcare Research and Quality *Clinical practice guideline for acute pain management: operative or medical procedures and trauma* on management of pain in neonates for recommendations.

†Meperidine is not typically used for long-term pain management due to breakdown into neurologic stimulant, normeperidine.

‡For morphine, hydromorphone, and oxymorphone, rectal administration is an alternate route for patients unable to take oral medications, but equianalgesic doses may differ from oral and parenteral doses because of pharmacokinetic differences.

§CAUTION: Codeine doses >65 mg often are inappropriate because of diminishing incremental analgesia with increasing doses but continually increasing constipation and other side effects.

¶CAUTION: Doses of aspirin and acetaminophen in combination opioid/nonsteroidal antiinflammatory drug preparations also must be adjusted to the patient's body weight.

NOTE: Published tables vary in the suggested dosages that are equianalgesic to morphine. Clinical response is the criterion that must be applied for each patient; titration to clinical response is necessary. Because there is not complete cross-tolerance among these drugs, it is usually necessary to use a lower equianalgesic dose when changing drugs and to retitrate to response.

CAUTION: Recommended dosages do not apply to patients with renal or hepatic insufficiency or other conditions affecting drug metabolism and kinetics.

NA, Not available; *NR*, not recommended; *SubQ*, subcutaneous.

Modified from Acute Pain Management Guideline Panel: *Acute pain management in adults: operative procedures. Quick reference guide for clinicians,* AHCPR pub. no. 92-0019, Rockville, MD, 1992, Agency for Healthcare Research and Quality, U.S. Public Health Service, U.S. Department of Health and Human Services, available at http://books.google.com/books?id=xrzWIu RnmJcC&printsec=frontcover&source=gbs_ge_summary_r&cad=0. Accessed March 16, 2013; Odom-Forren J: *Drain's perianesthesia nursing: a critical care approach,* ed 6, St Louis, 2013, Saunders; Pasero C, McCaffery M: *Pain assessment and pharmacologic management,* St Louis, 2011, Mosby; Schick L, Windle P, editors: *Perianesthesia nursing core curriculum: perioperative, phase I and phase II PACU nursing,* ed 2, St Louis, 2010, Mosby.

ordered. The PCA pump also can be set to deliver continuous infusion and patient boluses. This setting allows the patient to use the bolus function to premedicate before an activity or for breakthrough pain. When PCA devices are started in the PACU, delays in preventing pain are avoided, effectiveness of the PCA in managing pain can be evaluated, and the patient's understanding and ability to use PCA can be monitored.

Other forms of postoperative pain relief may involve use of spinal analgesia, usually in the form of epidural opioid or local anesthetic administration. Patients who have had extensive procedures, including total hip or knee replacements, knee reconstruction, and major abdominal or thoracic operations, have been shown to profit from this method of pain control. Benefits of epidural analgesia for acute postoperative pain include good analgesia with minimal sedation, early ambulation and physical therapy, and excellent patient satisfaction. An extended-release epidural morphine (DepoDur) that provides pain relief for 48 hours after a single bolus injection is available. Side effects of intrathecal administration of opioids include nausea, pruritus, urinary retention, areas of slight numbness, and respiratory depression. These side effects can be controlled by adjusting the infusion rate or by adding drugs such as diphenhydramine, ondansetron, or naloxone.

Naloxone is the opioid antagonist used most frequently to reduce opioid-induced respiratory depression. It is administered slowly, never as a bolus, while the nurse observes the patient's response. The patient should be able to open his or her eyes and

talk to the nurse within 1 to 2 minutes of administration; naloxone is discontinued when the patient can take deep breaths on instruction and respond to physical stimulation.

Other techniques that have been shown to reduce the level of pain for the surgical patient include infiltration of the incision site with a local anesthetic in the OR before the initial incision and use of a long-acting local anesthetic at the incision site at the conclusion of the surgical procedure. Local anesthetics as part of a multimodal approach to pain management can contribute to a considerable decrease in opioid dosage with minimal side effects (ASA Task Force, 2012; Pasero and McCaffery, 2011). One option is perineural local anesthetic infusion, in which a catheter is threaded along or into the wound. A diluted concentration of a long-acting local anesthetic is delivered to the surrounding nerves by a mechanical infusion pump for inpatients or a disposable infusion pump for ambulatory surgery patients. Thorough patient education is imperative, including removal of the catheter for patients who will be discharged home with the pump. It also is important to know the type of anesthetic the patient received during surgery and the type of local anesthetic in the pump to prevent overdose of local anesthetic. Multimodal analgesia allows a smaller dose of each component, which helps to minimize adverse effects.

Nonpharmacologic interventions used to relieve pain include positioning for comfort, verbal reassurance, touch, applications of heat or cold, massage (Research Highlight), transcutaneous electrical nerve stimulation (TENS), relaxation, imagery, music, distraction,

RESEARCH HIGHLIGHT

Effect of Foot and Hand Massage in Post-Cesarean Birth Pain Control

The aim of this randomized, controlled trial was to determine the effect of hand and foot massage on post-cesarean birth pain in 80 pregnant women who underwent elective cesarean birth and met inclusion criteria for study. A visual analog scale was used to determine pain intensity before, immediately after, and then 90 minutes after conducting 5 minutes of foot and hand massage. Pain intensity was reduced after the intervention compared with the intensity before the intervention (p <0.001). There was also a significant difference between groups in terms of pain intensity and request for an analgesic (p <0.001). According to these findings, foot and hand massage can be considered a nurse-initiated integrative therapy (also referred to as complementary or alternative therapy) to effectively reduce the pain of cesarean birth and decrease the amount of medications and their side effects.

Although other integrative therapies for pain relief are available, massage therapy in particular appears to be a reasonable choice in postoperative settings. Massage skills do not require extensive training, and they can easily be used. Massage may be a beneficial, noninvasive, cost-effective pain management strategy for patients whose pain is not adequately controlled by medication. It is possible that findings from this study are generalizable to other postoperative patient cohorts.

Modified from Abbaspoor Z et al: Effect of foot and hand massage in post–Cesarean section pain control: a randomized control trial, *Pain Manag Nurs*; 2013, in press.

and biofeedback. Nonpharmacologic interventions are designed to supplement, not substitute, pharmacologic interventions.

The physiologic effects of pain can be harmful to postoperative patients (Patient Safety). Such effects include decreased thoracic movement, increased splinting, reduced lung compliance and volume (leading to atelectasis), decreased mobility, increased risk of thromboembolism, exaggerated catecholamine response (which increases cardiac work and myocardial oxygen demand), increased risk for myocardial ischemia, impaired immune system, and delayed return of bowel and gastric function. Physiologic responses to acute pain include increased blood pressure and heart rate, dilated pupils, perspiration, increased respiratory rate, and decreased respiratory excursion (Dunwoody et al, 2008).

Psychologically, patients in pain may display fear, helplessness, anxiety, anger, or frustration (Krenszichek, 2010). There is also an association between poorly controlled postoperative pain and the risk of developing chronic pain, which emphasizes the importance of pain control in the perioperative period (Dunwoody et al, 2008). Patients of differing cultures respond to and communicate pain differently. A patient may believe that nonverbal communication expresses the pain to the nurse, but the nurse may not recognize the clues. Common misconceptions about pain also abound. These misconceptions must be recognized and corrected. A summary of misconceptions is listed in Table 10-2.

Guidelines to address management of acute postoperative pain are available from specialty organizations such as the American Society of Pain Management Nurses, American Society of Anesthesiologists (ASA), and American Society of PeriAnesthesia Nurses (ASPAN). Procedure-specific and evidence-based pain management guidelines are available through a web-based program called PROSPECT (Procedure Specific Postoperative Pain Management) (PROSPECT, 2013). These clinical practice guidelines and

recommendations were developed by consensus of an international group of surgeons and anesthesia care providers who reviewed pain research and graded the evidence (Figure 10-12).

Unfortunately, patients who are managed with opioids as part of their analgesic program can have adverse events related to the medication. Two of the most serious opioid-related adverse events are unintended advancing sedation (which generally precedes respiratory depression) and respiratory depression. Education of the perioperative health care team and use of multimodal pain management are of utmost importance in decreasing these events (Jarzyna et al, 2011). Perianesthesia nurses work diligently to identify patients who are at risk for unintended sedation and respiratory depression, assess and monitor patients who are using opioids for pain management, and intervene appropriately to prevent the deterioration of the patient's condition (Jarzyna et al, 2011). Pasero (2013) offers detailed strategies to prevent opioid-related sentinel events after discharge from the PACU that include (1) changing the way pain is managed—from opioid only; (2) establishing patient monitoring practices that enhance nurse decision making; (3) providing comprehensive education; and (4) evaluating personal practice.

Obstructive Sleep Apnea

Patients in the PACU sometimes present with obstructive sleep apnea (OSA), exhibiting a period of partial or complete obstruction of the upper airway. These patients may have a history of OSA or may be previously undiagnosed. Airway obstruction may cause episodic oxygen desaturation and hypercarbia, and may lead to cardiac dysfunction. It is estimated that 9% of women and 24% of men in the United States show disordered breathing while asleep, and 2% of women and 4% of men show overt symptoms of OSA (Fowler and Spiess, 2009). These numbers are likely to increase as the population ages and becomes increasingly obese. Perioperative patients with undiagnosed OSA have an increased incidence of morbidity, complications, longer length of stay in the hospital, and a higher rate of admission to the ICU (ASPAN, 2012).

Assessment and screening of patients for risk factors should occur preoperatively using standardized screening tools (ASPAN, 2012). Postanesthesia management concerns with OSA patients include use of analgesia, appropriate oxygenation, patient positioning, and monitoring. Supplemental oxygen should be used immediately postoperatively. Patients who use continuous positive airway pressure (CPAP) or noninvasive positive-pressure ventilation at home should continue to use these therapies during the post-surgery stay. The patient's position can be changed based on the type of surgery to decrease the chance of airway obstruction. Lateral, prone, and sitting positions result in better airway management for the OSA patient compared to supine. Use of telemetry for monitoring pulse oximetry, electrocardiogram (ECG), or ventilation can be beneficial in reducing adverse postoperative events and should be used on a patient-need basis (Fowler and Spiess, 2009). Patients with OSA may require extended monitoring in the postoperative period (ASPAN, 2012) (Evidence for Practice).

Discharge from the PACU

The PACU nurse completes a final assessment immediately before the patient's discharge and transfer to the surgical unit. The nurse assesses vital signs, level of consciousness, condition of the operative site, pain and comfort level, intake and output, respiratory function and oxygen saturation, and mobility. If the patient requires ongoing oxygen therapy, a transport oxygen canister is provided, and oxygen supply is prepared in the hospital room.

PATIENT SAFETY

Educating Patients About Medications for Pain Management

- Explain the purpose, dosage, schedule, and route of administration of any prescribed medications and side effects to report to the physician or nurse.
- Give the patient general guidelines for the use of pain medications.
- Explain that a variety of pain relief measures may be necessary for some types of pain.
- Instruct the patient to use pain relief measures before pain becomes severe. Determine the patient's ability or willingness to participate actively in the use of pain relief measures, and suggest measures the patient believes would be helpful.
- Encourage the patient to try a pain relief measure at least twice before abandoning it as ineffective. Instruct the patient to keep an open mind as to what may relieve pain.
- Urge the patient to keep trying to relieve the pain and not become discouraged.
- Discuss the use of nonopioid analgesics.
  - Inform the patient that nonopioid analgesics include acetaminophen, aspirin, and nonsteroidal antiinflammatory drugs, such as ibuprofen, indomethacin, and naproxen.
  - Explain that these medications are generally well tolerated, but have the potential to cause gastrointestinal ulceration, renal and hepatic toxic effects, and inhibition of platelet aggregation.
  - Tell the patient that if the nonopioid drug does not have a therapeutic effect initially, the dosage should be increased before another type of drug is tried.
- Discuss the use of opioids, which are indicated for severe postoperative pain or intractable pain such as that associated with cancer.
  - Inform the patient that opioids include morphine, hydromorphone, and methadone, and that these may be administered by oral route, intravenous drip, intrathecally, or epidurally to enhance the analgesic effect.
  - Explain that fixed dosage schedules with adequate doses for pain relief provide more constant blood levels and predictable pain relief. Suggest that additional doses may be needed for breakthrough pain.
- Discuss the side effects of opioid analgesics, including constipation, vomiting, and respiratory and central nervous system depression.
- Review the use of opioid agonists and antagonists, including nalbuphine (Nubain), butorphanol (Stadol), pentazocine (Talwin), and buprenorphine (Buprenex).
- Explain the use of analgesic potentiators.
  - Inform the patient that these drugs include hydroxyzine (Vistaril); diazepam (Valium); lorazepam (Ativan); diphenhydramine (Benadryl); and phenothiazine derivatives, such as promethazine (Phenergan), prochlorperazine (Compazine), and chlorpromazine (Thorazine).
  - Discuss the use of stimulants.
  - Inform the patient that these drugs include cocaine, methylphenidate (Ritalin), dextroamphetamine, and caffeine.
- Discuss other types of drugs used in pain control, including tricyclic antidepressants, such as amitriptyline (Elavil), imipramine (Tofranil), and doxepin (Sinequan); and butyrophenones, such as droperidol (Inapsine) and haloperidol (Haldol).
- Discuss and demonstrate the use of equipment for administering pain-relief medications.
  - External and implantable pumps for intravenous, epidural, and intrathecal administration of opioid analgesics
  - Patient-controlled analgesia (PCA) or patient-controlled epidural analgesia (PCEA), particularly for the management of acute pain, such as postoperative pain
  - Continuous wound infiltration with an ambulatory infusion pump
  - Transcutaneous electrical nerve stimulation (TENS)
- Discuss the side effects of opioids. For example, constipation requires the use of laxatives and stool softeners (e.g., senna [Senokot]).

TABLE 10-2

Misconceptions About Pain

Misconception	Correction
Best judge of the existence and severity of patient pain is the physician or nurse caring for the patient.	The patient is the authority about his or her pain. The patient's self-report is the most reliable indicator of the existence and intensity of pain.
Clinician must believe what the patient says about pain.	The clinician must accept and respect the patient's self-report of pain and proceed with an appropriate assessment and treatment. The clinician is entitled to a personal opinion but should not allow it to guide practice.
Patients should not receive analgesics until the cause of pain is diagnosed.	Symptomatic relief of pain should be provided while the investigation of cause proceeds.
Visible signs, either physiologic or behavioral, accompany pain and can be used to verify its existence and severity.	Even with severe pain, periods of physiologic and behavioral adaptation occur, leading to periods of minimal or no signs of pain.
Pain never killed anyone.	Unrelieved pain may be dangerous and is unacceptable. Postoperative pain can delay healing and contribute to complications that can be life threatening. Acute pain warns of actual or potential tissue damage and resolves when healing has occurred. Unrelieved postoperative pain is a complication or risk, not an acceptable consequence of surgery.
If the patient requires higher doses of opioids than other patients, "he's hitting the PCA button too often."	There is no set dose of opioid that is effective for all patients. Even an opioid-naive patient may require 6× more opioid than another patient. A patient who is opioid-tolerant may require 100× the opioid of an opioid-naive patient.

Modified from Edwards RR, Berde CB: Pain assessment. In Benzon H et al, editors: *Essentials of pain medicine*, ed 3, St Louis, 2011, Saunders; Pasero C, McCaffery M: *Pain assessment and pharmacologic management*, St Louis, 2011, Mosby.

FIGURE 10-12 Algorithm for the management of postoperative pain—total knee arthroplasty (TKA). *COX-2*, cyclooxygenase type 2; *GA*, general anesthesia; *IV*, intravenous; *LA*, local anesthesia; *NSAID*, nonsteroidal antiinflammatory drug; *PCA*, patient-controlled analgesia; *VAS*, visual analog scale.

EVIDENCE FOR PRACTICE

Obstructive Sleep Apnea (OSA) in the Adult Patient: Recommended Practice

The purpose of this practice recommendation developed by the American Society of PeriAnesthesia Nurses (ASPAN) is to promote perianesthesia patient safety in the care of adult patients with known or suspected OSA who have received opioids, procedural sedation, general, or regional anesthesia. The strategic work team proposed seven recommendations to promote patient safety in this population of patients:

1. Assess and screen patients for risk factors associated with OSA. Examples in the guideline include but are not limited to obesity, cardiovascular disease, and age.
2. Assess and screen undiagnosed patients for signs of OSA such as daytime sleepiness, observed snoring, and apnea reported by the sleeping partner.
3. Incorporate the use of a standardized screening tool to identify patients at risk for OSA.

4. Postanesthesia care unit (PACU) management of the patient with OSA includes monitoring, positioning, individualized pain management plan, and possible extended monitoring needs.
5. Develop a plan for discharge from PACU for the patient with OSA.
6. Develop a plan for discharge from phase II PACU for the patient with OA.
7. Provide discharge education for the patient with OSA.

OSA is associated with airway obstruction during sleep. In the United States, approximately 3% to 7% of males and 2% to 5% of females have OSA. The risk increases in obese individuals and further increases for surgical patients who are at risk for decreases in oxygen saturation and increases in carbon dioxide during sleep. This practice recommendation offers strategies that improve care and safety of diagnosed and undiagnosed perioperative patients with OSA who have increased morbidity and complications, increased length of stay, and increased intensive care unit (ICU) admission.

Modified from ASPAN OSA PR Strategic Work Team: The ASPAN obstructive sleep apnea in the adult patient evidence-based practice recommendation, *J Perianesth Nurs* 27:309–315, 2012.

The patient usually is discharged from the PACU by an anesthesia care provider, who may be present and write a discharge order. Alternatively, a numeric scoring system approved by the department of anesthesia may be used to determine if the patient is ready for discharge. The most common scoring system in use is the Aldrete score. Activity, respiration, circulation, consciousness, and oxygen saturation level are scored from 0 to 2. A total score of 8 to 10 is generally acceptable for PACU discharge, with exceptions made by physician order.

A hand-off report on the patient's condition is given to the nurse who will assume care for the patient on the surgical or short procedure unit. This report may be given by telephone before the patient leaves the PACU or in person after the patient reaches the unit. The report should include a preoperative history, pertinent information regarding the patient's surgery and recovery, medications the patient was given, physician's orders, and all other appropriate information.

Admission to the Ambulatory Surgery Phase II Unit

When the patient has had an ambulatory surgery procedure, the next step after discharge from phase I PACU care is transfer to phase II PACU care (Ambulatory Surgery Considerations). The nursing role in phase II PACU typically focuses on preparation for care at home. The patient is transitioned to oral analgesics, and discharge instructions are provided to the patient and caregiver in preparation for discharge to home. The length of time required for phase II care is directly related to the type of procedure and readiness for discharge status of patient.

Fast-Tracking the Ambulatory Surgery Patient

In some instances the surgeon and anesthesia provider may determine that the patient is a candidate for "fast-tracking." In fast-tracking the patient bypasses PACU phase I and goes directly to PACU phase II care. The patient must meet phase I discharge criteria prior to leaving the OR. Each healthcare facility must have criteria in place to safely, appropriately, and effectively use fast-tracking. At the very least, discharge criteria from the OR should include awake or easily arousable, hemodynamically stable, breathing effectively on room air, minimal pain and nausea, and stable condition of surgical site (ASPAN, 2012).

Admission to the Surgical Unit

The patient's room is prepared for admission, and any necessary equipment is obtained. The patient is assisted into the bed. To

---

AMBULATORY SURGERY CONSIDERATIONS

Important Education and Information for Patients Who Are Discharged from Phase II Recovery to Home

Anesthesia
- Advise patient of common side effects: dizziness and drowsiness, have assistance if needed; sore throat; postdischarge nausea and vomiting.
- For the next 24 hours the patient should not drive or operate machinery, drink alcohol, or sign important papers, and a responsible adult should stay with the patient.

Activity limitations
- Advise patient to go home and rest for next 24 hours.
- Inform patient of any limits to activity because of procedure (e.g., no sexual activity for 4 weeks, no lifting of objects that weigh more than 10 pounds).

Diet
- Instruct patient how to progress to regular diet, or give instructions to patient detailing specific diet required because of procedure.

Safety concerns
- Review preparation of home for patient return (e.g., removal of rugs that increase fall risk, sleeping area close to bathroom).

Medications
- Discuss new take-home medications or prescriptions. Document last dose of medication on patient's written instructions if given before discharge. Confirm that patient has prescription or that it has been electronically sent to patient pharmacy.
- Discuss resumption of home medications. Physician should have noted which home medications the patient is to continue after discharge (medication reconciliation).
- Instruct the patient to take the medication with food (unless contraindicated) to decrease stomach irritation.
- Discuss the use of acetaminophen or ibuprofen if the patient has no pain medication ordered (unless contraindicated).
- Advise patient not to take acetaminophen if taking other pain medications that include acetaminophen as an ingredient.

Surgical procedure
- Discuss any information that pertains to specific procedure (e.g., when to remove dressing, when to resume showers or baths, ice at site, weight-bearing restrictions). Confirm that patient can state correct name of procedure performed.

Bowel habits
- Increase dietary fiber and fluids.
- Use stool softener if needed.

When to call the healthcare provider
- Fever greater than 101°F (38°C) orally
- Pain that becomes worse or is not relieved by pain medication
- Bleeding that is unexpected
- Warmth, redness, or swelling at the operative site
- Evidence of pus from the surgical incision
- Inability to eat or drink by day after discharge
- Persistent nausea and vomiting
- Inability to void

Follow-up care
- Instruct patient about next appointment with physician or ascertain that appointment is already scheduled.
- Give patient telephone number for physician's office.
- If applicable, give patient telephone number of ambulatory surgery center.

Home procedures
- If patient requires procedures at home such as dressing change or emptying drainage reservoir, ascertain that responsible adult has received instructions and given a return demonstration of action.

Written instructions
- All discharge instructions should be in writing and given to the patient, including all the pertinent information included above, specific information about any new medication, and a list of home medications that physician requests be continued or discontinued.

BOX 10-4

Patient Assessment on Admission to Postoperative Unit from the PACU

- Respiratory status
  - Patency of airway
  - Respirations—depth, rate, character
  - Breath sounds—presence, character
- Circulatory status
  - Pulse, blood pressure
  - Skin color, temperature
  - Capillary filling
- Neurologic status
  - Level of consciousness
  - Ability to move extremities, peripheral pulses (as applicable)
- Dressing
  - Presence of drainage
  - Presence of tubes to be connected to drainage systems
- Comfort
  - Presence of pain, nausea, vomiting

- Pain score
- Patient positioned for comfort and to facilitate ventilation
- Other comfort measures as determined by patient preference (e.g., warm blanket, music, massage)
- Safety
  - Use of two patient identifiers
  - Necessity for side rails
  - Call cord within reach and instructions on operation reviewed
- Equipment
  - Monitors connected and functioning
  - IV fluids—location of insertion site, type and size of IV device, type of infusion, rate, amount in bag, patency of tubing, assessment of site
  - Drainage systems (e.g., nasogastric, chest, urinary)—type, patency of tubing, connection of appropriate container, character and amount of drainage

IV, Intravenous; *PACU*, postanesthesia care unit.

---

prevent falls the bed rails are raised until the patient is fully awake. The patient is informed to call the nurse for assistance to ambulate. Family members also are instructed and enlisted to maintain safety for the patient. Equipment and the patient's condition should be explained to family members present. A special concern is the use of PCA. Family members should be instructed that the PCA is for the patient's use only and that pushing the PCA button for the patient can have a detrimental effect on the patient's well-being.

Postoperative Nursing Considerations

Assessment

The nurse in the receiving unit makes an immediate assessment as soon as the patient transfers to the bed. The nurse may choose a head-to-toe or systems assessment. Parameters include respiratory, cardiovascular, and neurologic status. The condition of the dressing and surgical site and patient comfort and safety also are assessed (Box 10-4).

Nursing Diagnosis

Nursing diagnoses related to the care of the postoperative patient include the following:
- Risk for Infection
- Ineffective Breathing Pattern
- Acute Pain
- Imbalanced Nutrition: Less Than Body Requirements
- Impaired Physical Mobility

Outcome Identification

Outcomes identified for the selected nursing diagnoses could be stated as follows:
- The patient will be free from infection as indicated by normal vital signs; temperature within normal range; normal white blood cell count; clear breath sounds; clear, yellow urine; and warm, dry skin.
- The patient's respirations will be easy, unlabored, and adequate in rate and depth.
- The patient will verbalize subjective assertions of comfort: "I am in no pain." "My pain is a 2 on the scale of 0 to 10." The patient

will have no objective signs of discomfort (e.g., grimaces, tachycardia).
- The patient will eat well from prescribed diet; weight loss will be minimal.
- The patient will ambulate at an appropriate level and carry out other activities appropriate for condition.

Planning

Planning for the postoperative patient requires knowledge of surgical procedures and underlying medical conditions. Throughout the patient's stay, planning involves the patient and family or significant others (as appropriate and desired by the patient) with setting measurable goals to be achieved by discharge. A Sample Plan of Care for the postoperative patient is on p. 291.

Implementation

Wound Healing. Nursing care of the postoperative patient includes assessment of wound healing. Nursing interventions focus on preventing and monitoring wound complications. The nurse uses strict aseptic technique when placing a new dressing. Monitoring for signs and symptoms of infection includes noting any of the following: elevated body temperature; red, swollen, warm area surrounding the incision; elevated white blood cell count; tachycardia; or purulent drainage from the wound (Hoch, 2011). For a detailed discussion of the pathophysiology of wound healing, see Chapter 9.

Adequate Respirations. Postoperative patients are at risk for pulmonary complications because of increased respiratory secretions, decreased lung expansion, depression of the respiratory center, and the possibility of aspiration of gastric contents. These complications can be minimized by appropriate nursing management, including elevating the head of the bed whenever possible; encouraging coughing, turning, and deep breathing every 2 hours; ambulating the patient as soon as possible; and encouraging hydration (Hoch, 2011).

Circulation. Venous stasis in the postoperative patient can lead to thrombophlebitis, which is usually a preventable complication. Platelets adhere to the venous wall and form a thrombus, with

SAMPLE PLAN OF CARE

Admission to the Postoperative Patient Care Unit

Nursing Diagnosis
Risk for Infection related to altered skin integrity, compromised aseptic technique, or malnutrition

Outcome
The patient will be free from infection, as indicated by normal vital signs; temperature within normal range; normal white blood cell count; clear breath sounds; clear, yellow urine; and warm, dry skin.

Interventions
- Monitor vital signs every 4 hours or as prescribed.
- Monitor temperature every 4 hours as needed; document and report increased temperature.
- Monitor laboratory values for evidence of infection; report variance from normal.
- Encourage patient to take deep breaths or sustained maximal inspiration or use respiratory aids.
- Preserve closed urinary system and provide catheter care. Remove catheter as soon as possible.
- Encourage patient to eat foods high in protein and vitamin C.
- Avoid antiinflammatory drugs such as steroids to facilitate healing.
- Use aseptic technique when changing dressings and change soiled dressings immediately.
- Monitor contents of wound drainage catheters.
- Teach patient and family members how to care for surgical site, what to expect, and when and who to call if drainage at incision or drain sites increases or if other symptoms develop, such as fever, increased pain at site, and redness and swelling of incision.

Nursing Diagnosis
Ineffective Breathing Pattern related to postoperative pain, decreased energy, fatigue, decreased lung expansion, surgery

Outcome
The patient's respirations will be easy, unlabored, and adequate in rate and depth.

Interventions
- Monitor respirations and chest expansion frequently for 24 to 48 hours after the surgical intervention.
- Place the bed in high-Fowler position if possible.
- Auscultate lungs and evaluate productiveness of cough; document any adventitious breath sounds and nature and amount of sputum associated with cough (as appropriate).
- Have patient cough and deep breathe at regular intervals; collaborate with patient to identify cues to remember to undertake these activities or recommend 10 deep breaths each hour.
- Encourage use of respiratory aids (e.g., incentive spirometry, if appropriate).
- Treat underlying conditions, such as pain.
- Demonstrate splinting incisional area with pillow before cough.
- Encourage patient to turn and change positions at least every 2 to 3 hours.
- Encourage early and regular ambulation and explain importance to patient.

Nursing Diagnosis
Acute Pain

Outcome
The patient will verbalize subjective assertions of comfort: "I am in no pain." "My pain is a 2 on a scale of 0 to 10." The patient will have no objective signs of discomfort (e.g., grimaces, tachycardia).

Interventions
- Discuss the concept of pain and what it means for patient (e.g., throbbing, aching, stabbing, burning, tight).
- Educate patient and family members on the use of pain rating scale:
  - Show pain rating scale and explain its purpose.
  - Explain the components of the scale (if numeric scale used, explain what the numbers mean).
  - Set realistic comfort goals (pain rating score should be ≤4).
- Encourage patient to report pain, emphasizing that this is an important part of his or her care.
- Consider personal, cultural, spiritual, and ethnic beliefs in developing a pain management plan with patient.
- Document assessment of pain (intensity, duration, location, frequency) and response to pain management therapies.
- If patient has continuous local anesthetic infusion therapy (also known as site-specific infusion therapy) (common with select orthopedic procedures, abdominal hysterectomy, mastectomy, or hernia repair):
  - Assess site to ensure dressing is intact and catheter site is clean and dry.
  - Query patient to determine if symptoms of local anesthetic toxicity are present (dizziness, ringing in the ears, metallic taste, tingling or numbness of lips, slowed speech); contact physician to initiate immediate treatment if assessment is positive.
- If patient is to be discharged with infusion therapy, provide verbal and written instructions.
- Support patient in the use of personally effective nonpharmacologic pain management strategies (e.g., relaxation techniques, distraction, massage, biofeedback, music, guided imagery, meditation).

Nursing Diagnosis
Imbalanced Nutrition: Less Than Body Requirements related to surgery

Outcome
The patient will exhibit adequate nutritional intake from prescribed diet; weight loss will be minimal.

Interventions
- Encourage patient to eat foods high in protein and vitamin C.
- Offer frequent, small amounts of food or high-protein liquids to patient with little or no appetite.
- Encourage ambulation (improves appetite).
- Schedule procedures not to conflict with mealtime.
- Administer medication for pain as needed.

Continued

SAMPLE PLAN OF CARE

Admission to the Postoperative Patient Care Unit—cont'd

- Determine patient's previous history of nausea and vomiting after surgery; consult with physician regarding preventive measures for discharge if history is positive.
- Refer to nutritional support team if appropriate; dietary consultation may be important for patient with cultural or ethnic food preferences.

Nursing Diagnosis
Impaired Physical Mobility related to surgical procedure or pain

Outcome
The patient will ambulate at an appropriate level and carry out other activities appropriate for condition.

Interventions
- Encourage muscle-strengthening exercises before ambulation. Encourage ambulation or position changes and extremity exercises at least every 8 hours.
- Encourage leg exercises in bed.
- Before attempting to ambulate, have patient dangle legs over side of bed until pulse rate has stabilized and patient is not dizzy.
- Have two people help ambulate if patient is weak or obese.
- Encourage patient to walk further with each ambulation.
- Teach proper use of appropriate assistive devices (e.g., crutches, slings, walkers) and observe return demonstration.

---

resultant potential for deep vein thromboembolism (DVT) or pulmonary embolus (PE).

Prevention may include administration of prophylactic heparin, aspirin, dextran, or warfarin. Application of an intermittent pneumatic compression device (IPCD) or graduated compression stockings may be ordered. Nursing measures that prevent formation of a thrombus include applying the stockings whether the patient is in or out of bed, teaching the patient not to cross the legs, having the patient perform isometric leg exercises, and encouraging early ambulation.

If thrombophlebitis is suspected (pain or tenderness, erythema, localized area of warmth, swelling), the patient should return to bed and the physician notified. Treatment consists of rest, heat, graduated compression stockings, and anticoagulant therapy.

Urinary Function. One of the priorities during surgery and immediately afterward is to keep the patient well hydrated so that voiding occurs 6 to 8 hours after surgery. Usually intake is greater than output for 48 hours, as fluid and electrolyte balance returns to normal. Every effort is made to refrain from use of a catheter to avoid the risk of urinary tract infection. Measures to help the patient void include warming the bedpan, letting water run, applying warm water to the perineum, and allowing the patient to use the bathroom when possible. If discomfort is present and the bladder is palpable, catheterization becomes necessary. A portable bladder ultrasound may be used to assess the volume of urine in the bladder. A straight catheter is preferred, but in the event that several catheterizations are required, an indwelling catheter is inserted. Hydration of the patient becomes a priority. Intake and output are recorded accurately. A urine output of less than 0.5 mL/kg/hr is reported to the physician (Hoch, 2011).

Bowel Elimination. The postoperative patient who undergoes abdominal or pelvic surgery may have decreased peristalsis for at least 24 hours; this may persist for several days for the patient who has gastrointestinal (GI) surgery (Hoch, 2011). Increased fluid intake and early ambulation promote return of peristalsis. Bowel sounds are auscultated with a stethoscope to ensure that peristalsis has returned, and the abdomen assessed for distention.

Constipation occurs frequently after surgery because of the effects of the anesthetic agents and opioids, immobility, and decreased GI motility. Fluids, roughage, and bulk laxatives can

FIGURE 10-13 Benefits from early postoperative ambulation.

relieve constipation. Occasionally a suppository or an enema is needed to empty the lower bowel.

Early Ambulation. Early ambulation expedites recovery and prevents complications. Early ambulation increases muscle tone, improves GI and urinary tract function, stimulates circulation, and increases vital capacity (Hoch, 2011). Benefits are shown in Figure 10-13. Ambulation usually is postponed if severe infection or thrombophlebitis is present.

Evaluation

Evaluation of the postoperative patient outcomes on the surgical unit might be stated as follows:
- The patient's vital signs, temperature, urinary output, breath sounds, and laboratory values were within normal limits; the surgical site showed no signs or symptoms of infection.
- The patient's breathing was easy and unlabored, at a normal rate and of adequate depth.

- The patient verbalized freedom from pain and was free from facial grimaces, moaning, and other evidence of pain or discomfort.
- The patient was eating well; there was no weight loss or complaints of nausea or vomiting.
- The patient ambulated regularly and was assessed as capable of performing appropriate activities.

Patient and Family Education and Discharge Planning

Ideally, patient and family education and discharge planning begin before the patient's admission for surgery. The patient and family are prepared to assume any care that may be needed after discharge (Patient-Centered Care). If needed, community resources are used. Home healthcare is a valuable resource for patients with treatment needs after discharge. The nurse responsible for the patient's care in the acute care setting collaborates and communicates with the home health team as soon as the need is identified so that the patient's care will be consistent.

The patient and family members are instructed in the proper care of the wound or incision and signs and symptoms of a wound infection. They should know how to take a temperature and when the physician should be notified for elevated temperature. They should be knowledgeable about medication that the patient will be using at home, including analgesics. Appropriate nonpharmacologic methods of pain control, such as imagery, distraction, massage, music therapy, and relaxation, also can be taught. An appointment for a return visit with the surgeon should be scheduled. The patient resumes normal activities gradually according to the physician recommendations.

The chapters on surgical interventions in Unit II have incorporated important elements for patient and family education and discharge planning. These elements assist the perioperative nurse in identifying and teaching what patients need to know and facilitate safe self-care during recovery from operative and other invasive procedures.

KEY POINTS

- Immediate postoperative patient care includes basic life-sustaining needs (airway, breathing, circulation) and are of the highest priority.
- Hand-off reports for postoperative patients are a critical time that require clear, focused communication. Times that are at risk for communication problems are transfer from OR to PACU, from PACU to phase II PACU, from PACU to inpatient bed. Try to have no interruptions or distractions during hand-offs and care transitions.
- Continuous assessment of postoperative patients in PACU includes assessment of vital signs, including pulse oximetry and

end-tidal CO_2, wound, pain and comfort, and other appropriate parameters (these are often procedure-specific).
- Complications can occur quickly in the PACU, including airway obstruction, laryngospasm, bronchospasm, aspiration, cardiac dysrhythmias, delirium, excessive pain, and nausea and vomiting.
- The function of phase II PACU is to assist the patient in discharge and home readiness.

CRITICAL THINKING QUESTION

Your new patient in the PACU is a 46-year-old male who presented with ruptured diverticula. He weighs 320 pounds and is 5 feet 10 inches tall. He underwent general anesthesia for a colon resection. He was given hydromorphone 4 mg, ondansetron 8 mg, and midazolam 4 mg during surgery. The nursing and anesthesia history include type 2 diabetes, 1 ppd smoker × 30 yrs, and osteoarthritis. He is married and has three children. He has limited insurance and wants to go back to work as soon as possible. He has never had surgery, and only takes ibuprofen and metformin. His initial vital signs (VS) are 170/110, 120, 32, 89% O_2 saturation on room air, T 100.5°F, pain level 8 (0-10), some nausea. What are your major concerns about this patient? What are his risk factors? List the components of your nursing assessment in priority order. Address each of the assessment findings and discuss your interventions for each finding.

℮volve *The answers to the Critical Thinking Question can be found at http://evolve.elsevier.com/Rothrock/Alexander*

REFERENCES

American Society of Anesthesiologists: *Standards for postanesthesia care* (amended by House of Delegates, October 21, 2009), Park Ridge, IL, The Society, available at www.asahq.org/For-members/-/media/For%20Members/documents/Standards%20Guidelines%20Stmts/Postanesthesia%20Care%20Standards%20For.ashx. Accessed January 28, 2013.

American Society of Anesthesiologists: Practice guidelines for preoperative fasting and the use of pharmacologic agents to reduce the risk of pulmonary aspiration: application to healthy patients undergoing elective procedures: an updated report by the American Society of Anesthesiologists Committee on Standards and Practice Parameters, *Anesthesiology* 114: 495–511, 2011.

American Society of Anesthesiologists Task Force on Acute Pain Management: Practice guidelines for acute pain management in the perioperative setting: an updated report by the American Society of Anesthesiologists Task Force on Acute Pain Management, *Anesthesiology* 116:248–273, 2012.

American Society of PeriAnesthesia Nurses: *2012-2014 Perianesthesia nursing standards, practice recommendations and interpretive statements*, Cherry Hill, NJ, 2012, ASPAN.

Apfel CC et al: A simplified risk score for predicting postoperative nausea and vomiting, *Anesthesiology* 91:693–700, 1999.

Apfel CC: Postoperative nausea and vomiting. In Miller R, editor: *Anesthesia*, ed 7, New York, 2009, Churchill Livingstone.

Apfel C et al: Who is at risk for postdischarge nausea and vomiting after ambulatory surgery? *Anesthesiology* 117:475–486, 2012.

Arriaga AF et al: Simulation-based trial of surgical-crisis checklists, *N Engl J Med* 368:246–253, 2012.

Benca J: Bronchospasm. In Atlee JL, editor: *Complications in anesthesia*, ed 2, Philadelphia, 2007, Saunders.

Decrane SK et al: Factors associated with recovery from early postoperative delirium, *J Perianesth Nurs* 26:231–241, 2011.

DeJohn P: Helping to avoid postdischarge nausea and vomiting, *OR Manager* 29(1):28–29, 2013.

Drain C: The respiratory system. In Odom-Forren J, editor: *Drain's perianesthesia nursing: a critical care approach*, ed 6, St Louis, 2013, Saunders.

Dunwoody CJ et al: Assessment, physiological monitoring, and consequences of inadequately treated acute pain, *J Perianesth Nurs* 23:S15–S17, 2008.

Fetzer SJ: Postoperative nausea and vomiting. In Schick L, Windle P, editors: *Perianesthesia nursing core curriculum: perioperative, phase I and phase II PACU nursing*, ed 2, St Louis, 2010, Saunders.

Flaherty E: Using pain-rating scales with older adults, *AJN* 108(6):40–47, 2008.

Fowler MA, Spiess BD: Post anesthesia recovery. In Barash PG et al, editors: *Clinical anesthesia*, Philadelphia, 2009, Lippincott.

Gan TJ et al: Society for Ambulatory Anesthesia guidelines for the management of postoperative nausea and vomiting, *Anesth Analg* 105:1615–1628, 2007.

Groudine S, Fossum S: Use of intravenous acetaminophen in the treatment of postoperative pain, *J Perianesth Nurs* 26:74–80, 2011.

Hoch CR: Nursing management: postoperative care. In Lewis SM et al, editors: *Medical-surgical nursing: assessment and management of clinical problems*, ed 8, St Louis, 2011, Mosby.

Hooper VD: Care of the patient with thermal imbalance. In Odom-Forren J, editor: *Drain's perianesthesia nursing: a critical care approach*, St Louis; 2013, Saunders.

Hooper VD et al: ASPAN's evidence-based clinical practice guideline for the promotion of perioperative normothermia: second edition, *J Perianesth Nurs* 25:346–365, 2010.

Jarzyna D et al: American Society for Pain Management Nursing guidelines on monitoring for opioid-induced sedation and respiratory depression, *Pain Manag Nurs* 12(3):118–145, 2011.

Joint Commission Center for Transforming Healthcare: *Improving transitions of care: handoff communication*, available at www.centerfortransforming healthcare.org/assets/4/6/CTH_Hand-off_commun_set_final_2010.pdf. Accessed March 16, 2013.

Koivuranta M et al: A survey of postoperative nausea and vomiting, *Anaesthesia* 52(5):443–449, 1997.

Krenszichek DA: Pain and comfort management. In Schick L, Windle P, editors: *Perianesthesia nursing core curriculum: perioperative, phase I and phase II PACU nursing*, St Louis, 2010, Saunders.

Langham GE et al: Noninvasive temperature monitoring in postanesthesia care units, *Anesthesiology* 111:90–96, 2009.

Makic MBF: Pain management in the non-verbal critically ill patient, *J Perianesth Nurs* 28(2):98–101, 2013.

Moola S, Lockwood C: Effectiveness of strategies for the management and/or prevention of hypothermia within the adult perioperative environment, *Int J Evid Based Health* 9(4):337–345, 2011.

McGuire JM, Burkard JF: Risk factors for emergence delirium in U.S. military members, *J Perianesth Nurs* 25:392–401, 2010.

Nicholau D: The postanesthesia care unit. In Miller R, editor: *Anesthesia*, ed 7, New York, 2009, Churchill Livingstone.

Nightingale F: *Notes on hospitals*, ed 3, London, 1863, Longman, Green, Roberts, Longman & Green.

O'Brien D: Patient education and care of the perianesthesia patient. In Odom-Forren J, editor: *Drain's perianesthesia nursing: a critical care approach*, ed 6, St Louis, 2013a, Saunders.

O'Brien D: Postanesthesia care complications. In Odom-Forren J, editor: *Drain's perianesthesia nursing: a critical care approach*, ed 6, St Louis, 2013b, Saunders.

Odom-Forren J, Clifford T: The evolution of perianesthesia nursing. In Schick L, Windle P, editors: *Perianesthesia nursing core curriculum: perioperative, phase I and phase II PACU nursing*, ed 2, St Louis, 2010, Saunders.

Odom-Forren J: Postanesthesia recovery. In Nagelhout JJ, Plaus KL, editors: *Nurse anesthesia*, ed 5, St Louis, 2014, Saunders.

Paulikas CA: Prevention of unplanned hypothermia, *AORN J* 88(3):358–364, 2008.

Pasero C: Challenges in pain assessment, *J Perianesth Nurs* 24:50–54, 2009.

Pasero C: The perianesthesia nurse's role in the prevention of opioid-related sentinel events, *J Perianesth Nurs* 28:31–37, 2013.

Pasero C, McCaffery M: *Pain assessment and pharmacologic management*, St Louis, 2011, Mosby.

Pasero C, Stannard D: The role of IV acetaminophen in acute pain management, *Pain Manag Nurs* 13:107–124, 2012.

Practice guidelines for postanesthetic care: An update report by the American Society of Anesthesiologists task force on postanesthetic care, *Anesthesiology* 118(2):291–307, 2013.

PROSPECT: *Procedure-specific postoperative pain management*, available at www.postoppain.org. Accessed February 7, 2013.

Reynolds L et al: Perioperative complications of hypothermia, *Best Pract Res Clin Anaesthesiol* 22:645–657, 2008.

Rosero EB et al: Trends and outcomes of malignant hyperthermia in the United States, 2000 to 2005, *Anesthesiology* 110:89–94, 2009.

Ruth HS et al: Anesthesia study commission, *JAMA* 35:881–884, 1947.

Tallman K et al: Cardiac arrest in the PACU: an analysis of evolving challenges for perianesthesia nursing, *J Perianesth Nurs* 27:4–8, 2011.

The Joint Commission: *Surgical care improvement project core measure set*, available at www.jointcommission.org/assets/1/6/Surgical%20Care%20Improvement%20Project.pdf. Accessed January 31, 2013.

U.S. Food and Drug Administration: *Droperidol (Inapsine)*, available at www.fda.gov/Safety/MedWatch/SafetyInformation/SafetyAlertsforHuman MedicalProducts/ucm173778.htm. December 16, 2001. Accessed February 2, 2013.

CHAPTER 11

Gastrointestinal Surgery

DENISE JACKSON

Surgeons embark on surgery of the gastrointestinal (GI) system to diagnose, remove, or prevent the progression of pathologic conditions. When cure is not possible, palliative measures to relieve symptoms can provide comfort and nutrition, and promote quality of life and dignity in death. Advances in technology and the science of human digestion, metabolism, immunology, and inflammatory responses to illness and injury have greatly broadened the spectrum of possible modalities and approaches to manage and treat patients with GI disorders. Clinical research uses patient outcomes to compare the effectiveness of new approaches and innovative methods to more traditional methods of GI procedures; that research continues to grow rapidly, providing new evidence for practice and decision making (Anderson et al, 2012; Cone et al, 2011; DeMaria et al, 2011; Fried, 2012; Mason, 2012).

GI surgery comprises the surgical management of pathologic conditions of the esophagus, stomach, and small and large intestines. Gastroenterology is a medical specialty that uses endoscopy to locate, identify, mark, and sometimes treat intraluminal pathology in the GI tract. Endoscopic procedures are a critical component of surgical diagnosis, staging of disease, and postoperative evaluation. Although general surgeons and surgical teams may specialize in laparoscopy, surgical endoscopy, bariatrics, surgical oncology, or colorectal surgery, perioperative nurses and scrub personnel must be familiar with the fundamentals of GI surgery and common patient care requirements.

Surgical Anatomy

The GI tract, or alimentary canal, is a continuous, tubelike structure that spans the human torso (Figure 11-1). It includes the mouth; pharynx; esophagus; stomach; small intestine, consisting of the duodenum, jejunum, and ileum; and large intestine. The large intestine consists of the cecum, ascending colon, transverse colon, descending colon, sigmoid colon, rectum, and anus. The length of the GI tract is about 6 meters (20 feet). Basic functions of the GI tract are ingestion, secretion, mixing, digestion, propulsion, absorption, and elimination by defecation. The GI tract is a complex microbiologic ecosystem that supports and maintains essential digestive and protective functions vital to life. Substantial populations of microorganisms—both obligate anaerobes and facultative bacterial spores—exist in the intestinal lumen. The organisms of the upper tract differ from those of the lower tract, with the highest concentration in the distal bowel. These organisms can contribute to contamination and disease processes within the intestinal tract and throughout the body.

The esophagus is a collapsible musculomembranous tube through which ingested material moves, by peristalsis, from the pharynx to the stomach. After exiting the pharynx, the esophagus passes through the neck, posterior to the trachea and anterior to the vertebral column. The mediastinal portion of the esophagus enters the thoracic cavity at the level of the first thoracic vertebra where it lies posterior to the heart. The esophagus enters the peritoneal cavity through the esophageal hiatus of the diaphragm, where it joins the cardia of the stomach. The lower esophageal sphincter (LES) is at the terminal end of the esophagus; its function is to prevent reflux of gastric contents. Blood supply to the esophagus originates from branches of the inferior thyroid arteries, bronchial arteries, the thoracic aorta, and branches of the left gastric and inferior phrenic arteries. The venous drainage from the esophagus empties into the subclavian veins, the azygos vein on the right, the hemiazygos vein on the left, and through the coronary vein in the portal circulation. The nerve supply is from branches of the vagus nerve and the sympathetic nervous system.

The stomach lies in the upper abdominal cavity, to the left of the midline, inferior to the diaphragm and anterior to the pancreas. It is attached to the spleen on the left by the gastrosplenic ligament, the liver on the right by the hepatogastric ligament, the duodenum on the right by the gastroduodenal ligament, and the transverse colon inferiorly by the posterior layer of the greater omentum. Physiologically cells in different regions of the stomach have unique functions related to digestion. Description of the stomach is by names related to each region, such as the cardia, fundus, body, antrum, and pyloric canal (Figure 11-2). The fundus lies inferior to the left lobe of the liver and medially adjacent to the spleen. Inferior to the fundus the body and antrum curve obliquely to the right, before terminating at the pylorus. The concave, or medial, margin of the stomach is referred to as the lesser curve and the convex, or lateral, margin of the stomach is known as the greater curve.

The omentum is a double layer of fatty peritoneum attached along the greater curve of the stomach. It drapes down loosely over the intestines and then folds posteriorly on itself before sweeping upward to attach along the transverse colon. The mesentery is also a double layer of peritoneum, but it differs from the omentum in that it connects the small bowel and parts of the colon to the posterior abdominal wall and contains the blood supply, nerves, and lymphatics of the intestines within its layers.

The blood supply to the stomach originates at the celiac trunk of the aorta, which branches into the left gastric, splenic, and common hepatic arteries. The right gastric and gastroduodenal arteries are branches of the common hepatic artery. The left and right gastric arteries supply the lesser curve of the stomach; the stomach's greater curve receives its supply from the right gastroepiploic artery, a branch of the gastroduodenal artery, and the left gastroepiploic artery, which originates from the splenic artery. Additional blood supply comes from the inferior phrenic arteries and

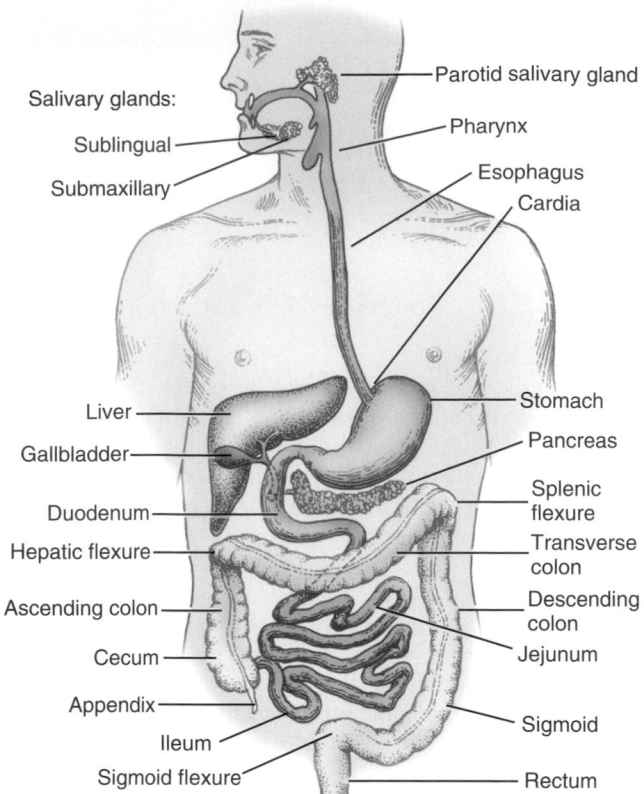

FIGURE 11-1 Alimentary canal and its appendages.

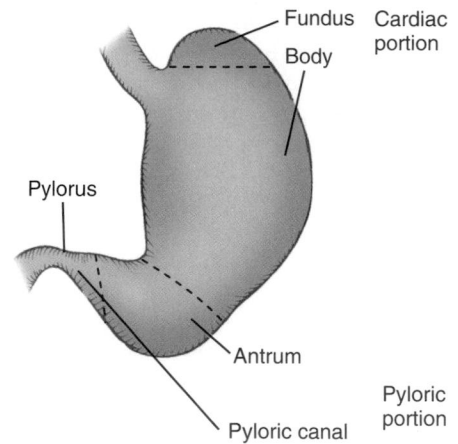

FIGURE 11-2 Regional anatomy of stomach.

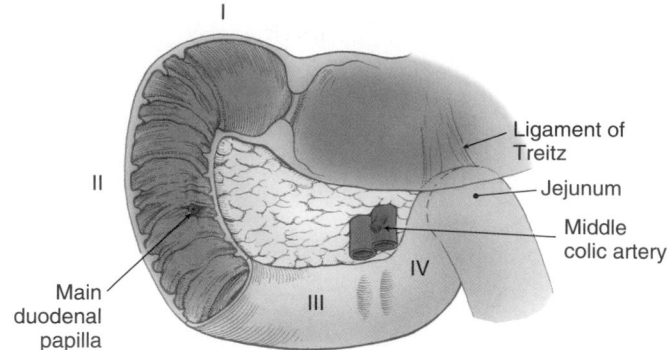

FIGURE 11-3 The duodenum consists of four portions, as illustrated.

the short gastric arteries located between the greater curve and the spleen. The gastric veins follow the same pathways as the arteries and drain into the portal vein. The right gastroepiploic vein drains into the superior mesenteric vein and the left gastroepiploic vein drains into the splenic vein. Regional lymph nodes are located at the gastroesophageal junction, the splenic hilum, and the pylorus; they receive gastric lymphatic drainage, all of which empties into the celiac nodes and ultimately into the cisterna chyli and thoracic duct. The autonomic, sympathetic, parasympathetic, and enteric nervous systems regulate gastric function.

The stomach receives ingested food from the esophagus to begin the digestive process; it then propels partially digested food, or

chyme, into the duodenum through the pylorus. In anticipation of receiving ingested material, the stomach prepares for its role in digestion by increasing motility, producing gastric acid, and releasing pepsinogen, intrinsic factor, gastric fluids, and mucus. Peptide hormones in the stomach (gastrin, somatostatin, and ghrelin) function directly and indirectly to regulate gastric secretions and motility. Gastrin causes enterochromaffin-like (ECL) cells in the body of the stomach to release histamine, thereby stimulating gastric acid secretion from the parietal cells. Somatostatin inhibits gastrin, histamine, and acid secretion. Production of ghrelin, a peptide hormone discovered in 1999, occurs in the fundus. It stimulates gastric motility as well as the appetite, regulates hunger and satiety during meals, and plays a role in long-term body weight regulation (King and Hines, 2013). Research regarding ghrelin's role in obesity and potential medications for the treatment of obesity is ongoing (Mahvi and Krantz, 2010).

The small intestine is the longest part of the digestive tract. It begins at the pylorus and ends at the ileocecal valve. The adult small intestine varies in length but is usually about 3 meters long with a diameter of approximately 2.5 cm. It has three parts: the duodenum, the jejunum and the ileum. The length of the duodenum is about 20 cm; the jejunum, approximately 110 cm; and the ileum, on the order of 155 cm long.

The first portion of the small intestine is the duodenum. Its proximal 2 cm are mobile and considered to be intraperitoneal, whereas the remaining duodenum is retroperitoneal and fixed posteriorly by peritoneal attachments. The first part of the duodenum, called the duodenal bulb, dilates. Characteristic circular folds of the small intestinal mucosa begin in the duodenum, continue through the jejunum, and become less prominent in the ileum. The purpose of these folds, called plicae circulares of Kerckring, is to provide greater mucosal surface area for absorption of nutrients. The duodenum forms a C-shaped curve around the head of the pancreas. The common bile duct and the main pancreatic duct enter the posteromedial wall of the duodenum at the ampulla of Vater (also referred to as the main duodenal papilla) within this curve (Figure 11-3). The duodenum continues in a medial direction along the inferior border of the body of the pancreas before it ascends slightly to the duodenojejunal flexure, at which point it becomes the jejunum.

The blood supply to the duodenum comes from the gastroduodenal artery, located behind the duodenal bulb (Figure 11-4). At the inferior margin of the bulb, the gastroduodenal artery divides into the right gastroepiploic and superior pancreaticoduodenal arteries to supply the proximal duodenum and head of the pancreas.

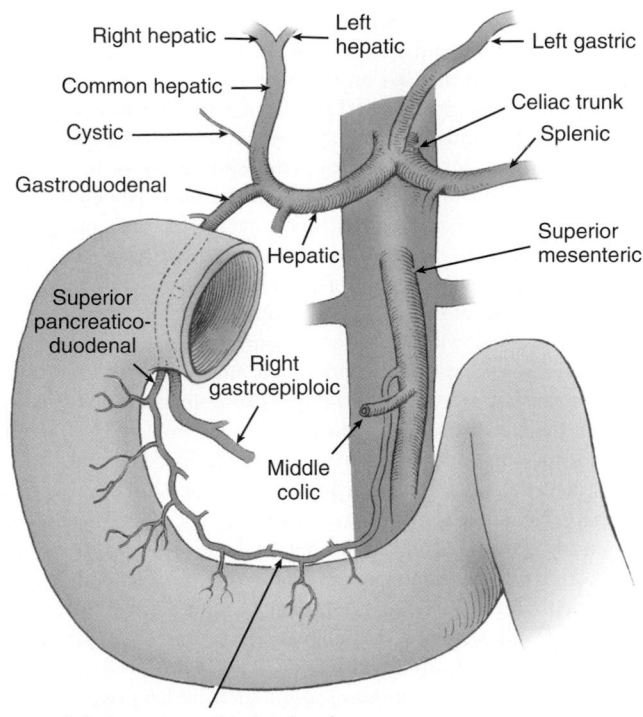

FIGURE 11-4 Arterial blood supply of the duodenum.

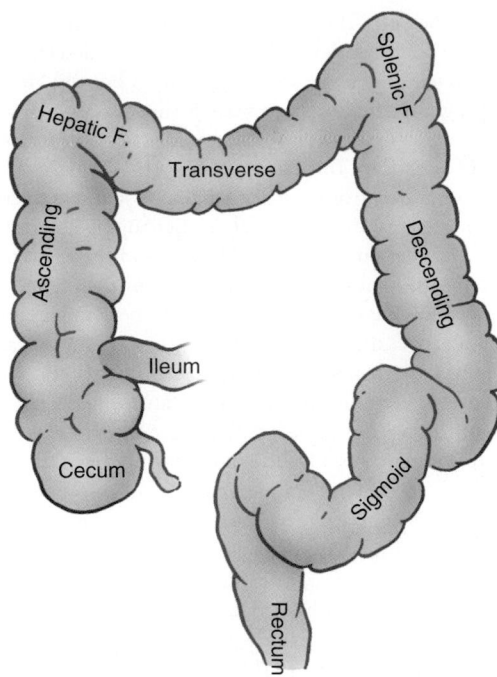

FIGURE 11-5 Anatomic division of large intestine, showing locations of hepatic flexure and splenic flexure. *F*, Flexure.

The inferior pancreaticoduodenal artery, a branch of the superior mesenteric artery, supplies the transverse and ascending portions of the duodenum, as well as the head and body of the pancreas.

In the left upper quadrant, the ligament of Treitz supports the duodenojejunal flexure and serves as a landmark to identify the beginning of the jejunum. The jejunum continues for about 2.5 meters (8 feet) before it transitions into the ileum in the right lower quadrant. The ileum continues for about another 3.5 meters (12 feet) before it ends at the ileocecal junction.

The blood supply to the jejunum and ileum comes entirely from their respective branches of the superior mesenteric artery. The mesentery of the jejunum and ileum is about 5.5 meters (18 feet) long, accounting for its mobility within the abdominal cavity. Along its antimesenteric, or opposite, border, the mucosa of the ileum contains major deposits of lymphatic tissue, known as Peyer patches. The rich lymphatic drainage of the small bowel plays a major role in fat absorption. Lymphatic drainage from the mucosa proceeds through the wall of the small intestine to lymph nodes adjacent to the mesentery. It then proceeds to larger lymphatics that communicate with the retroperitoneal cisterna chyli and from there to the thoracic duct, where it terminates in the internal jugular vein. The lymphatics of the intestine play a major role, both in the body's immune defense and in the distribution of cells arising from intestinal neoplasms.

The large intestine (Figure 11-5) consists of the cecum, colon, rectum, and anal canal (not illustrated). The cecum attaches to the lateral abdominal wall by peritoneal attachments called cecal folds. The terminal branch of the superior mesenteric artery, the ileocolic artery, supplies blood to the cecum.

The appendix is a 7- to 10-cm wormlike structure that arises from the posteromedial wall of the cecum, below the ileocecal junction, and attaches to the cecum by the mesoappendix. The blood

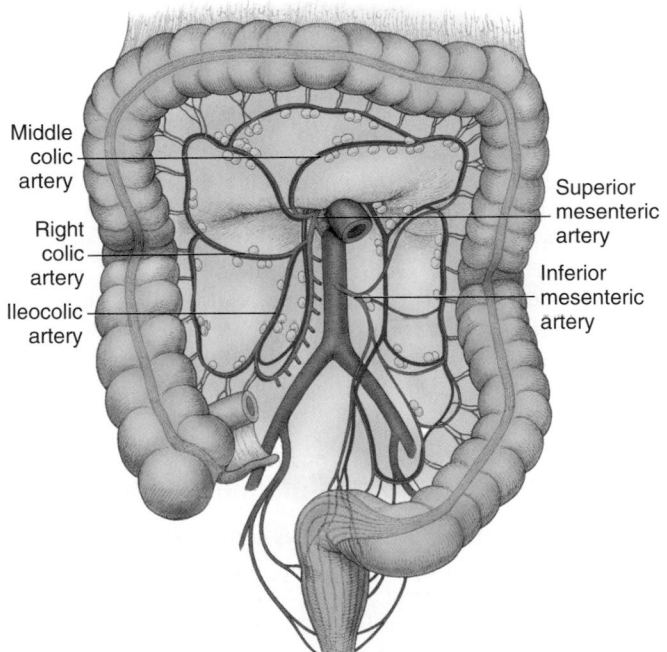

FIGURE 11-6 Blood supply of the colon.

supply to the appendix comes from the appendicular artery, which branches from the terminal part of the ileocolic artery.

The ascending colon extends upward from the cecum to the hepatic flexure, where it lies behind the right lobe of the liver and in front of the anterior surface of the right kidney. It receives its blood supply from the ileocolic and middle colic arteries (Figure 11-6). The transverse colon begins at the hepatic flexure and ends at the splenic flexure. It lies below the stomach, suspended by the transverse mesocolon. The blood supply to the transverse colon is via the middle colic artery (see Figure 11-6). The descending colon extends downward from the splenic flexure to become the sigmoid colon. The sigmoid colon makes an S-shaped curve toward the midline, where it descends to transition into the rectum at the rectosigmoid junction. The arterial supply to the descending and sigmoid colon comes from the left colic and sigmoid arteries. The superior, middle, and inferior rectal arteries supply the rectum and anal canal. The marginal artery of Drummond forms an arcade of collateral circulation along the inner border of the colon.

Distinguishing physical characteristics of the colon are the teniae coli, epiploic appendices, and haustra. The teniae coli are three separate, longitudinal bands of muscle distributed along the length of the colon. The epiploic appendices are fatty appendages attached to the colon along the teniae and have no particular function. Haustra are sacculations of the colon wall along the contracted teniae, giving it a segmented appearance.

The rectum begins at the rectosigmoid junction, where the teniae coli merge at the level of the sacral promontory. The absence of distinct teniae serves as a visual landmark for the upper margin of the rectum. The rectum has three characteristic lateral curves, or flexures, that coincide internally with transverse rectal folds called valves of Houston (Fry et al, 2010). The rectum lies on the sacrum posteriorly. As it descends into the pelvis, the posterior rectum attaches to the anterior surface of the sacrum by the rectosacral fascia. It also attaches to the pelvis by fascia extending from the right and left pelvic sidewalls. In the male, the rectovesical fascia, also called Denonvilliers fascia, separates the anterior rectum from the seminal glands, prostate, bladder, ureters, and ductus deferens. In the female the rectovaginal fascia separates the anterior rectum from the vagina. The terminal rectum, or ampulla, dilates to receive and hold feces prior to passage into the anal canal. The anal canal is the most distal portion of the GI tract. It is a 3- to 5-cm funnel-like passage that begins at the anorectal junction, lies between the internal and external anal sphincters, and ends at the anal verge.

The large intestine recovers water, electrolytes, and nutrients from succus entericus, a mixture of undigested fluids, starches, proteins, and bile salts received from the ileum. The remaining waste product descends toward the rectum, solidifies into feces, and stores in the rectal ampulla until its expulsion through the anal canal, or, commonly, defecation.

Perioperative Nursing Considerations

GI surgery and endoscopic procedures vary widely, depending on the patient's medical diagnosis, the purpose of the intended procedure, the surgical approach, and the involved anatomic structures. Other influencing factors include the patient's goals and desire for treatment, the surgeon's preferred approach based on training and experience, and the availability of advanced technologies in imaging, access, and instrumentation.

Assessment

Patient-centered care begins with an assessment that integrates information about the physiologic and psychosocial status of the patient into an individualized plan of care. Key sources of information that facilitate and guide the assessment process include medical history, physical examination, physician orders, and results from laboratory and other diagnostic studies. Laboratory studies might include a complete blood count, as well as a complete metabolic panel to measure serum glucose, serum electrolytes, kidney function, liver function, and serum proteins. Coagulation studies such as international normalized ratio (INR) and prothrombin time or partial thromboplastin time (PT/PTT) may be appropriate if indicated (Mehrdad and Marks, 2011; Stonemetz, 2011). Abnormal values require specific notation and communication to the surgeon and anesthesia provider (lab values are presented in Appendix A).

Diagnostic procedures, determined by the patient's presenting signs and symptoms, the location of suspected pathology, and the potential sites of metastasis may include esophageal manometry, pH monitoring, and motility studies. Additional tests may include radiologic studies, with or without contrast markers, endoscopic examinations, abdominal or endoscopic ultrasound (EUS), computed tomography (CT) imaging scans, magnetic resonance imaging (MRI), or positron emission tomography (PET). Technologic advances in endoscopic imaging include EUS, chromoendoscopy, confocal laser endomicroscopy, endocystoscopy, optical coherence tomography (Friedland and Van Dam, 2012), magnification endoscopy (Guelrud, 2012), narrow band imaging (Bergman, 2012), and wireless video capsule endoscopy (Cave, 2012). These provide enhanced details of GI anatomy and are essential tools in identifying and staging GI malignancies in order to determine surgical options and other treatments.

Barriers to patient communication such as language, sensory deficits, altered cognitive function, and distractors, such as pain or emotional stress, require assessment throughout the preoperative interview. The perioperative nurse needs to acknowledge tearfulness, as well as expressions of fear, anger, denial, depression, nervousness, and anxiety, as legitimate, and to encourage the patient to verbalize his or her concerns.

After confirming the patient's identity, the perioperative nurse asks the patient to verify, in his or her own words, an understanding of the scheduled procedure, the planned approach, and laterality if applicable (Patient-Centered Care). Due to the nature and unpredictability of GI surgery, if a minimally invasive approach is planned, the patient must understand the possibility of the need to convert to a laparotomy. If intestinal diversion (ileostomy, colostomy) is a possibility, the perioperative nurse determines if a wound ostomy continence nurse (WOCN) has marked the site of the stoma and assesses the patient's understanding and acceptance of this part of the procedure. Individualized ostomy site selection by a WOCN helps prevent appliance leaks and peristomal skin complications (Maidl and Ohland, 2012). Optimally, the site of the ostomy is within the rectus muscle to decrease risk of peristomal hernias; is not placed in or across a skinfold, crease, or at the belt line; and is visible and easily accessible to enable the patient to perform self-care postoperatively. A WOCN's preoperative counseling and education, aimed at assisting the patient and family to adapt to expected lifestyle changes, to accept altered body image, to address sexuality concerns, and to understand elements of ostomy self-care, have demonstrated a positive effect on long-term outcomes (Doughty and Landmann, 2012).

The perioperative nurse checks the review of systems (Table 11-1) in the medical record to identify and confirm patient conditions that can increase the risks of perioperative complications.

Current medications, including use of supplements, require review with the patient. Verify the last dose taken on all medications. Conditions of the GI tract requiring surgical intervention are often accompanied by alterations in nutritional status, which can cause increased risk for infection, poor wound healing, incidence of pressure ulcers, and overgrowth of bacteria in the GI tract (Tess

PATIENT-CENTERED CARE

Patient-centered communication demonstrates an understanding and respect for patient values, preferences, and needs. When patients understand their diagnosis, treatment options, risks, and expected outcomes, they are more likely to participate in decisions about their care. Concerns about functional disability, relief from pain, and self-care needs after discharge are common and should be addressed using clear everyday language that the patient understands.

Mrs. Kipton is scheduled for a low anterior colon resection, possible end-to-end anastomosis, or a possible abdominal perineal resection (APR) with a permanent colostomy. When Karla, the RN, meets Mrs. Kipton in the preoperative holding area, patient-centered communication might sound like the following:

"Good morning, my name is Karla. I am a registered nurse and I will be taking care of you during your surgery." Mrs. Kipton introduces Karla to her daughter. Karla gets permission to continue the patient interview in the daughter's presence and then says, "Can you tell me what procedure you are having today?" Mrs. Kipton replies, "Yes, there is a cancer near the end of my colon that has to be removed. My surgeon told me I might need to have a colostomy if the cancer is too big for him to put me back together." To confirm that Mrs. Kipton understands the significance of having a colostomy and an APR, Karla says,

"Yes, that is what it says here on your surgical consent form. The end of your colon is called the rectum. If the cancer is too low in your rectum, making it unsafe for the surgeon remove all of the cancer and still reconnect your healthy bowel to your remaining rectum, the entire rectum will be removed and a colostomy made. Your surgeon will bring the end of the healthy bowel up through a small hole in your abdominal wall, where it will be secured with stitches. The surgeon will then make another incision all of the way around the opening where your bowel movements come out and finish removing the rectum from the outside. If you do need to have a colostomy, instead of having bowel movements like you do now, your colon will empty into a small plastic bag that snaps onto a ring that is part of a pad that adheres to your skin. Unfortunately, we do not know exactly what the surgeon will find until he gets inside. If you do need a colostomy, the bag will be located there, on the left side of your abdomen, where Jan, the nurse who will teach you all about caring for your colostomy, put a mark yesterday. Is this what you understand?" Mrs. Kipton replies, "Yes, I do understand and thank you for describing things so that my daughter and I could understand what you were saying. I was having difficulty explaining all of this to her and now I think she understands it, too."

Modified from Bertakis KD, Azari R: Patient-centered care is associated with decreased health care utilization, *J Am Board Fam Med* 24(3):229–239, 2011; Delbanco T, Gerteis M: A patient-centered view of the clinician-patient relationship. In Basow DS, editor: *UpToDate*, Waltham, MA, UpToDate, 2012; Hassilgren P et al: Perioperative management: practical principles, molecular basis of risk and future directions. In Fischer JE, editor: *Fischer's mastery of surgery*, Philadelphia, 2012, Lippincott Williams & Wilkins; Mulsow JJ: Beyond consent—improving understanding in surgical patients, *Am J Surg* 203(1):112–120, 2012.

TABLE 11-1

Preoperative Nursing Review of Systems

System	Condition	Increased Risk	Relevant Assessment Data
Cardiovascular	Ischemic heart disease	Cardiac death, nonfatal MI	Recent MI, cardiac surgery, cardiac stents, nitrate use for angina, abnormal ECG (pathologic Q waves)
	Heart failure	Respiratory complications, fluid imbalances	Pulmonary edema-bilateral rales, S_3 gallop, shortness of breath, peripheral edema
	Hypertension BP >180/110	BP instability, arrhythmias, myocardial ischemia	Beta-blockers, ACE inhibitors, ARBs, calcium channel blockers
Endocrine	Insulin-dependent diabetes uncontrolled	Postoperative infections, cardiac complications	HgA_{1c} >7% Serum glucose ≥200
	Obesity	DVT, pneumonia, wound infection, UTI	BMI >20
Immune	Malignancy, HIV, rheumatoid arthritis, systemic lupus erythematosus (SLE)	Infection, difficult intubation and IV access, risk of aspiration, pulmonary embolism	Malnourished, recent treatment with chemotherapy, chronic use of glucocorticoids (Prednisone), renal insufficiency
Pulmonary	COPD, asthma, respiratory infection	Postoperative respiratory complications	Abnormal chest x-ray, poor pulmonary function, inhaler use, cough, breathlessness
Renal	End-stage renal disease	Altered medication metabolism	Azotemia, abnormal serum potassium
Liver	Hepatitis, cirrhosis	Altered medication metabolism; bleeding	Malnutrition, vitamin K deficiency, ascites
GI	Malnutrition	Poor wound healing	Decreased albumin, transferrin, pre-albumin
Anticoagulant therapy	Atrial fibrillation, coronary stents, recent DVT	Intraoperative and postoperative bleeding	Prolonged bleeding times, epistaxis, bruising Medication list includes aspirin, clopidogrel,
Coagulopathy	von Willebrand disease		dabigatran, warfarin, NSAIDs, cyclooxygenase-2 (COX-2) inhibitors, dipyridamole

ACE, Angiotensin-converting enzyme; *ARBs,* angiotensin receptor blockers; *BMI,* body mass index; *BP,* blood pressure; *COPD,* chronic obstructive pulmonary disease; *DVT,* deep vein thrombosis; *ECG,* electrocardiogram; *GI,* gastrointestinal; *HIV,* human immunodeficiency virus; *IV,* intravenous; *MI,* myocardial infarction; *NSAIDs,* nonsteroidal antiinflammatory drugs; *UTI,* urinary tract infection.
Modified from Hassilgren P et al: Perioperative management: practical principles, molecular basis of risk and future direction. In Fischer J, editor: *Fischer's mastery of surgery*, Philadelphia, 2012, Lippincott Williams & Wilkins.

Calculating a Patient's Body Mass Index

A patient's body mass index (BMI) is an estimate of total body fat. BMI is a weight-to-height ratio that is used to determine if an individual is underweight, at a healthy weight, overweight, or obese. BMI is expressed as kilograms per square meter and calculated by the following formula:

$$BMI = (\text{weight in pounds} \div \text{height in inches}^2) \times 703$$

Calculated BMI	Meaning
25-29.9 kg/m^2	Overweight
30-34.9 kg/m^2	Obese—Class I
35-39.9 kg/m^2	Moderately Obese—Class II
40-49.9 kg/m^2	Severely or extremely obese—Class III
>50 kg/m^2	Super obese—Class IV

Modified from Andrews RA, Lim RB: Surgical management of severe obesity. In Basow DS, editor: *UpToDate*, Waltham, MA, UpToDate, 2012; Gagnon LE, Karwacki EJ: Outcomes and complications after bariatric surgery: five of the most common procedures and nursing implications for pre- and postoperative care, *Am J Nurs* 112(9):26–36, 2012.

and Fairfield, 2012). Assessment of the patient's nutritional status includes determining the patient's body mass index (BMI) (Box 11-1), history of recent weight loss or gain, difficulty swallowing, nausea, vomiting, diarrhea, constipation, and NPO status.

Components of a nursing physical assessment include notation of general appearance and body-mass distribution. Assessments of skin integrity, quality of peripheral pulses, presence of neuropathies, and physical limitations help determine baseline data for evaluation of outcomes related to positioning and hydration status. Focused examination of the patient's abdomen includes inspection for skin integrity, hair distribution, scars, and distention. Palpation to assess for rigidity, referral and/or localization of pain, masses, and unusual pulsations may follow if indicated.

Relevant social assessment includes use of tobacco, alcohol, or recreational drugs. Inquiries about the patient's ability to perform activities of daily living, circumstances of the patient's home situation, and availability of family, friends, or other support systems during hospitalization and after discharge play an important part of discharge planning.

Nursing Diagnosis

Nursing diagnoses related to the care of patients undergoing GI surgery might include the following:

- Anxiety related to perioperative events
- Deficient Knowledge related to impending surgery
- Disturbed Body Image related to intestinal diversion (when diversion possible or planned)
- Risk for Imbalanced Body Temperature
- Risk for Infection at the surgical site
- Risk for Perioperative Positioning Injury
- Impaired Tissue Integrity related to lasers, thermal devices, electrosurgery, radiation, or chemical solutions
- Risk for Injury from retained surgical items, wrong procedure, wrong site, or administration of wrong or incorrect medications
- Risk for Imbalanced Fluid Volume

Outcome Identification

Outcomes identified for selected nursing diagnoses could be stated as follows:

- The patient will demonstrate or verbalize decreased anxiety and ability to cope throughout the perioperative period.
- The patient will verbalize understanding of the surgical procedure, expected responses, and postoperative self-care requirements.
- The patient will demonstrate acceptance of expected changes in appearance.
- The patient will be at, or returning to, normothermia at the conclusion of the immediate postoperative period.
- The patient will be free from signs and symptoms of surgical site infection.
- The patient will be free from perioperative positioning injury.
- The patient will be free of evidence of impaired tissue integrity.
- The patient will be free from injury related to retained surgical items, wrong procedure, wrong site, and medication errors.
- The patient's fluid volume, electrolyte levels, and acid-base balance will be consistent with or improved from preoperative baseline levels.

Planning

The preoperative assessment provides the perioperative nurse with critical information to develop an individualized plan of care. Analysis of patient-specific physiologic and psychosocial data assist in identifying nursing interventions to comfort patients, mitigate risks for complications, prevent injury and infection, and help the patient to achieve the best possible outcomes. Planning for optimal patient care also includes ensuring that necessary instruments, supplies, and equipment are at hand for the planned procedure. A Sample Plan of Care for patients undergoing GI surgery can be found on p. 301.

Implementation

The perioperative nurse implements the plan of care throughout all phases of the patient's surgical experience. Communication and cooperation between all members of the surgical team, working together to help the patient achieve identified outcomes, is essential. There is strong evidence that preoperative checklists prevent a number of surgical safety events (Shekelle et al, 2013).

Most patients undergoing open and laparoscopic GI surgery require general endotracheal anesthesia. A midthoracic epidural, placed preoperatively as an adjuvant to general anesthesia, can decrease postoperative pain, increase adherence to pulmonary exercises, and promote early ambulation. Intravenous (IV) moderate sedation is appropriate for outpatient endoscopic procedures, such as esophagogastroduodenoscopy (EGD) or colonoscopy. Monitoring devices and parameters typical to general and epidural anesthesia techniques appear in Chapter 5.

Fluid management during significant blood loss may require arterial monitoring and frequent intraoperative sampling of hemoglobin and hematocrit (H&H), arterial blood gases (ABGs), electrolytes, and coagulation studies. Preoperatively the physician may order a type and screen or type and crossmatch in anticipation of intraoperative blood/blood component transfusion. Replacement fluids include packed red blood cells (PRBCs), albumin, platelets, fresh frozen plasma, electrolytes, and colloids or crystalloids.

Prior to elective surgery, patients may choose to donate 1 or 2 units of autologous blood for use at surgery. Friends and family members may also donate donor-directed, compatible blood.

SAMPLE PLAN OF CARE

Nursing Diagnosis
Anxiety related to perioperative events

Outcome
The patient will demonstrate or verbalize decreased anxiety and ability to cope throughout the perioperative period.

Interventions
- Explain preoperative activities and expectations (e.g., IV lines, skin preparation, positioning), sequence of sensory experiences and activities in the OR, and postoperative expectations (e.g., postanesthesia care unit [PACU], drains, catheters, dressings).
- Provide time for patient and family members to ask questions.
- Determine effective coping strategies used by patient in the past; support these as appropriate.
- Minimize stimuli in the OR that can contribute to anxiety (e.g., high noise levels, excessive talking, music that is not the patient's preference).
- Remain with the patient during induction; convey caring behaviors (e.g., appropriate touch; a soft, reassuring voice; warm blankets).
- Maintain the patient's dignity and privacy.
- Encourage expression of feelings and concerns.
- Communicate unresolved or excessive anxiety to team members.

Nursing Diagnosis
Deficient Knowledge related to impending surgery

Outcome
The patient will verbalize understanding of the surgical procedure, expected responses, and postoperative self-care requirements.

Interventions
- Verify information the patient and family need and want to know. Determine current knowledge level and perceptions of surgery. Take into consideration language, culture, hearing or visual impairment, health literacy, cognitive impairments, and any relevant disability.
- Initiate preoperative education and discharge planning early in the perioperative process.
- Assess readiness to learn and patient's preferred learning style.
- Include family or patient's accompanying responsible adult in teaching. Use simple language. Present information in the patient's dominant language (use an interpreter if necessary). Note any sensory impairments and accommodate for them. When possible, provide written information that replicates verbal education.
- Verify patient's understanding of material presented by having the patient repeat back, in his or her own words, information that has been presented. Correct misunderstandings.
- Communicate patient or family concerns to appropriate surgical team members or make appropriate referral.

Nursing Diagnosis
Disturbed Body Image related to intestinal diversion (when diversion possible or planned)

Outcome
The patient will demonstrate acceptance of expected changes in appearance and self-care.

Interventions
- Encourage verbalization of feelings about anticipated alterations in body function if diversion procedure planned.
- Elicit the patient's and family's (if appropriate) perceptions of planned surgical intervention.

- Identify effective sources of support.
- Encourage patient to implement cultural, religious, ethnic, or social customs associated with perceived loss.
- Provide accurate information relevant to patient's postoperative expectations (general principles of ostomy care and solutions to concerns that may worry patient).
- Refer patient to wound, ostomy, and continence nurse (WOCN) if this has not already been done.

Nursing Diagnosis
Risk for Imbalanced Body Temperature

Outcome
Patient will be at or returning to normothermia at the conclusion of the immediate postoperative period.

Interventions
- Determine patient's risk to develop inadvertent hypothermia.
- Regulate ambient room temperature in range between 68° and 78°F (20° and 25.6°C) as appropriate.
- Monitor patient temperature during surgery.
- Minimize unnecessary patient exposure. Keep patient covered with warm blankets before induction. Ask patient if he or she is comfortable and warm enough.
- Use effective skin-surface warming methods (e.g., forced-air warming, circulating water garment, energy transfer pads) preoperatively, intraoperatively, and in PACU as needed.
- Use warmed irrigating solutions and fluid replacement therapy (e.g., IVs) as appropriate. Follow manufacturer's recommendations when using warming equipment.
- Cover patient with a warm blanket before transport to the PACU.

Nursing Diagnosis
Risk for Infection at the surgical site related to operative or other invasive procedure

Outcome
Patient will be free from signs and symptoms of surgical site infection.

Interventions
- Identify patient-specific risk factors for infection (e.g., altered nutritional status, chronic diseases, preoperative chemotherapy, radiation therapy).
- Follow institutional protocol for perioperative skin preparation (patient bath or shower preoperatively with prescribed antimicrobial agent; intraoperative skin preparation with antimicrobial agent).
- Initiate practices required to create and maintain a sterile field.
- Protect the patient from cross-contamination—use bowel/GI technique as appropriate.
- Designate appropriate wound classification (clean, clean-contaminated, contaminated, dirty/infected) at end of procedure.
- Initiate traffic control measures/protocols.
- Administer medication as prescribed (e.g., antibiotic prophylaxis), using safe medication practices.

Nursing Diagnosis
Risk for Perioperative Positioning Injury

Outcome
Patient will be free from signs of perioperative positioning injury.

Interventions
- Assess patient for physical alteration, prosthetics, or corrective devices requiring modifications to procedure-specific position.

Continued

SAMPLE PLAN OF CARE—cont'd

- Position patient in body alignment with attention to possible modifications of surgical position, patient limitations, and safety.
- Use adequate body supports, restraints, and padding of pressure sites specific to planned position and patient body mass. Reassess position status throughout procedure.
- Lift and transport patient carefully with sufficient assistance and lifting aids as needed.
- Reassess patient for signs and symptoms of injury at conclusion of procedure.

Nursing Diagnosis
Risk for Impaired Tissue Integrity related to lasers, thermal devices, electrosurgery, radiation, or chemical solutions

Outcome
The patient will be free of evidence of impaired tissue integrity.

Interventions
- Inspect skin condition and determine patient's risk factors related to skin injury.
- If hair must be removed from surgical site, select removal method most likely to preserve skin integrity.
- Protect patient from thermal, electrical, laser, and chemical injury by following institutional practice guidelines. Implement fire precautions with skin prep solution.
- Before applying dressings, clean and dry skin at incision site or sites.
- Prevent stretching of the skin when securing dressings with tape.
- Reassess patient for signs of skin injury at conclusion of procedure and document findings.
- Wash patient of blood and body fluids and cover with clean gown and blankets before transfer to PACU.

Nursing Diagnosis
Risk for Injury from retained surgical items, wrong procedure, wrong site, or medication administration

Outcome
The patient will be free from injury related to retained surgical items, wrong procedure, wrong site, or administration of wrong or incorrect medications.

Interventions
- Confirm patient identity.
- Initiate preoperative verification process. Verify surgical procedure, and involve patient in marking surgical site.
- Identify any allergies to medications.
- Perform and document required counts. If necessary, take a "pause for the count" to avoid distractions.
- Administer medications and solutions as prescribed. Label all medications and solutions on and off the sterile field.
- Verify and record implants.
- Follow protocols to contain, identify, label, preserve, transfer, and transport surgical specimens.

Nursing Diagnosis
Risk for Imbalanced Fluid Volume

Outcome
The patient's fluid volume, electrolyte levels, and acid-base balance will be consistent with or improved from preoperative baseline levels.

Interventions
- Review baseline laboratory data; confer with surgeon or anesthesia provider regarding deviations from normal.
- Assess nutritional status, skin turgor, renal status, and other conditions or medications affecting fluid, acid-base, and electrolyte balance.
- Collaborate with surgeon and anesthesia provider in accurately estimating fluid and blood loss and maintaining or correcting losses (administration of fluid replacement therapies, electrolytes, or medications).
- Record all solutions administered from the surgical field.
- As appropriate, include estimated blood loss (EBL) in hand-off report to receiving unit. In some institutions, calculation of a surgical Apgar score occurs at the end of the surgical procedure, based on the EBL, lowest mean arterial pressure (expressed in mm Hg), and the lowest heart rate rhythm recorded on the anesthesia record during the procedure. The score helps identify patients with a higher likelihood to develop complications after surgery.

Autotransfusion, or cell salvage, of the patient's blood during surgery may not be appropriate, given potential contamination from bowel contents or from malignant GI tumors. A nasogastric (NG) tube, inserted to decompress the stomach, suctions gastric secretions as well. Insertion of a urinary catheter decompresses the bladder and provides accurate measurement of urinary output and renal function.

Administration of IV antibiotics occurs before the incision and repeats as needed to maintain adequate levels throughout the procedure (Surgical Pharmacology). Antibiotic solutions may be used for irrigation during the procedure and before closure. Additional intraoperative medications may be appropriate per institutional standard or surgeon preference. Use of hemostatic agents, anticoagulants, steroid preparations, and local anesthetics is possible also. The best guide for planning medications, therefore, is a comprehensive and frequently updated pick-list, or surgeon/procedure preference sheet.

Chapter 6 thoroughly discusses safely positioning the patient for surgery. Common positions for patients undergoing GI procedures include supine position, low modified lithotomy position, and jackknife position. In the supine or modified lithotomy position, the patient's arms are secured on armboards or tucked at the sides. When there are surgical reasons to tuck the arms at the side, pad the elbows to protect the ulnar nerve, turn the palms inward, and maintain the wrist in a neutral position (Association of periOperative Registered Nurses [AORN], 2013). When the patient is in modified lithotomy position with arms secured on armboards, the perioperative nurse ensures there is adequate space between the base of the armboards and the stirrup holders for the surgeon and first assistant to stand. This can be challenging with patients of short stature. If necessary, tucking the arms at the patient's sides is an option; it is imperative, however, to ensure the hands and fingers are protected when raising or lowering the foot of the OR bed. Exposure of key anatomy may require frequent intraoperative changes in the orientation of the OR bed. Common positions used to shift abdominal organs away from the operative site to optimize visualization include Trendelenburg, reverse Trendelenburg, and tilting of the OR bed from side to side into a lateral position. The

SURGICAL PHARMACOLOGY

Commonly Administered Antibiotics in GI Surgery

Medication/Category	Dosage/Route	Purpose/Action	Adverse Reactions	Nursing Implications
Cefazolin (first-generation cephalosporin)	<80 kg: IV 1 g 81-160 kg: IV 2 g >160 kg: IV 3 g	Enteric gram-negative bacilli, gram-positive cocci		Administer within 1 hr of incision
Cefoxitin (second-generation cephalosporin)	IV 1-2 g	Enteric gram-negative bacilli, enterococci, clostridia		Administer within 1 hour of incision
Ampicillin sulbactam (aminopenicillin and beta-lactamase inhibitor)	IV 1.5-3 g q6hr	*Enterococcus faecalis,* gram-negative bacilli	Diarrhea, nausea	Administer within 1 hr of incision
Clindamycin	<80 kg: IV 600 mg 81-160 kg: IV 900 mg >160 kg: IV 1200 mg	Aerobes, anaerobes, enteric gram-negative bacilli	Nausea	Dilute each 300 mg in 50 mL D_5W and give over 10-60 min
Ertapenem/carbapenem	IV 1 g	Enterobacter, *Escherichia coli*		Adjust dose for renal impairment
Metronidazole hydrochloride	<80 kg: IV 500 mg 81-160 kg: IV 1000 mg >160 kg: IV 1500 mg	Anaerobes	Headache, nausea, vaginitis, candida	Infuse over 1 hr Do not give IV push Incompatible with aztreonam and ceftriaxone
Vancomycin (glycopeptide)	IV 1000 mg or 10-15 mg/kg over 1 hr	MRSA, *Staphylococcus aureus, Enterococcus*	Erythematous rash on face and upper body, hypotension	Infuse over 1 hr
Ciprofloxacin (fluoroquinolone)	IV 400 mg	Gram-negative bacilli, *Streptococcus pneumoniae,* gram-positive cocci, mycobacterial species	Rash, anorexia, nausea, vomiting, headache, dizziness, phototoxicity	Administer within 1 hr of incision
Levofloxacin (fluoroquinolone)	IV 750 mg	Gram-negative bacilli, *S. pneumoniae,* gram-positive cocci, mycobacterial species		Administer within 1 hr of incision
Aztreonam (miscellaneous)	IV 1-2 g	Gram-negative bacteria		Administer within 1 hr of incision
Gentamicin	IV 1-2.5 mg/kg	Gram-negative bacteria		Administer within 1 hr of incision

MRSA, Methicillin-resistant *Staphylococcus aureus.*
Modified from Anderson DJ, Sexton DJ: Overview of control measures to prevent surgical site infection. In Basow DS, editor: *UpToDate,* Waltham, MA, UpToDate; Solomkin J, Fischer JE: *Nursing 2011 drug handbook,* Philadelphia, 2011, Lippincott Williams & Wilkins Mobile; Solomkin J: Perioperative antimicrobial prophylaxis and treatment of surgical infection. In Fischer JE, editor: *Fischer's mastery of surgery,* ed 6, Philadelphia, 2012, Lippincott Williams & Wilkins.

surgical team collaboratively positions the patient and ensures that the patient is secured properly to the OR bed before draping. Special considerations to address the unique challenges of positioning the morbidly obese patient also appear in detail in Chapter 6. Measures for safe patient handling and lifting appear in Chapter 3.

GI surgery patients are at increased risk for venous thromboembolism (VTE) events such as deep vein thrombosis and pulmonary embolism. Mechanical VTE prevention includes the use of graduated compression stockings and intermittent pneumatic compression devices (IPCDs) on the lower extremities. An IPCD has an electrically operated pump that intermittently inflates sleeves wrapped around the lower legs or the lower legs and thighs, compressing the veins and increasing venous blood flow toward the heart (Elpern et al, 2013). This should be applied and turned on before induction of anesthesia. Wrap the sleeves around the legs smoothly to prevent folds when the legs are positioned in stirrups. Ensure that there are no pressure points from the hose connections. The unit is hung on the OR bed or an IV pole or is placed on the floor under the OR bed in an area away from team members' feet and areas that may be wet. A blanket or mat placed under the unit can lessen vibration noise (AORN, 2013).

Patients having GI surgery are also at risk for hypothermia. A mechanism to measure core body temperature throughout the procedure should be available. The four most reliable sites for core monitoring of temperature are the tympanic membrane, distal esophagus, nasopharynx, and pulmonary artery. Risk factors for unplanned hypothermia include extremes of age, low body weight, open-cavity surgery, thyroid disorders, diabetic neuropathy, peripheral vascular disease, a cold OR, infusion of cold fluids, and irrigating the abdomen with cold normal saline or other solutions (AORN, 2013). Warming the patient before induction of anesthesia may help reduce redistribution of core body heat to the periphery (AORN, 2013) and contribute to normothermia in PACU (Nicholson, 2013). To prevent thermal injury all devices for warming patients and solutions should be used according to the manufacturer's instructions (Wu, 2013).

Hair removal at the operative site, per surgeon order, occurs in the preoperative holding area as close as possible to the time of surgery. Hair removal is usually accomplished with clippers.

Antimicrobial skin preparation and draping receive extensive coverage in Chapter 4. Abdominal skin preparation follows general protocols for laparotomy, with generous borders should the surgeon extend the incision or need to accommodate the creation of stomas and drain placement. The perioperative nurse takes precautions to prevent accumulation or pooling of prep solutions under the patient or in the patient's hair in order to prevent chemical skin injury and surgical fires (risk management strategies for preventing surgical fire and chemical injury are discussed in Chapter 2). Sites within the prepped area with high concentrations of microorganisms, such as an existing stoma, draining fistula, or the rectum, are prepped last. Before surgical skin prep, cover and protect existing stomas with an occlusive sterile clear plastic dressing or a collection appliance or isolate them with a plastic drape secured with adhesive strips.

Draping the abdomen follows standard draping process as for laparotomy, discussed in Chapter 4. If the patient is in modified lithotomy position, extra drapes are needed to put under the buttocks and to cover the stirrups. Plan for additional drapes, towels, gowns, and gloves for the surgical team to implement proper techniques to keep clean and dirty items separate during open bowel procedures (often referred to as "bowel technique" or "GI technique") (AORN, 2013).

The surgeon may request placement of ureteral catheters by a urologist before a GI procedure begins. The catheters may be lighted and inserted to enable the surgeon to see and palpate the ureters during the GI procedure. A basic cystoscopy setup includes sterile ureteral catheters, two of each size (see Chapter 15).

If transabdominal intraoperative endoscopic examination of the bowel lumen is necessary, endoscopes of an appropriate length should be sterile and set up on a separate sterile table. Consider this table contaminated after removal of the scope. Ensure availability of endoscopic accessories such as a light source, a mechanism to insufflate the bowel, and a suction device for intraluminal secretions. Team members who have participated directly in the endoscopic procedure change gown and gloves before proceeding with the remainder of the surgical intervention.

Additional accessory instruments or devices may include a sterile plastic drawstring intestinal bag to confine loops of normal bowel from the operative segment or sterile radiopaque surgical towels. If planning intraoperative ultrasound, ensure the components of a high-resolution ultrasound system are available, including necessary sterile probes or transducers.

GI linear and circular stapling devices streamline resection and approximation of GI viscera. These instruments deliver double or triple rows of closely spaced, staggered inert staples, and are designed for both open or laparoscopic use. The staples are designed to approximate tissue while preserving blood supply to tissue edges. Stapling devices typically accept multiple cartridges for successive use. They can be straight or curved, linear or circular; they also can apply staples only, or they can apply staples and cut tissue between the staple lines. Stapling devices for laparoscopic use have longer shafts, have articulating heads, use triple staple technology, provide for tissue compression before staples are fired, and accommodate larger bites of tissue. Personnel must be familiar with types of available stapling instruments, applications, assembly if indicated, and proper loading of cartridges. A variety of staplers and reloads should be available for GI procedures.

Common suture materials used in GI procedures include permanent silk sutures, and absorbable polyglycolic acid and polydioxanone sutures. Generally, surgeons use 3-0 and 4-0 sutures on a semicircular intestinal (tapered) needle on intestinal tissues. Ligatures for small vessels usually require a 3-0 or 4-0 suture, whereas larger vessels may require a size 0 or 2-0. For closure of enterotomies or hand-sewn anastomosis of the bowel, surgeons commonly use size 3-0 or 4-0 absorbable suture on the mucosa and seromuscular layers. Some surgeons may also want controlled-release 3-0 or 4-0 silk sutures available. For abdominal closure, the fascia and peritoneum are closed as one layer using a running suturing technique with a number 1 or 0 slow absorbing suture (e.g., polydioxanone) on a large tapered needle. The surgeon's preference will dictate which skin staples or suture should be available for skin closure.

Bowel technique (also referred to as GI, contamination, or isolation technique) prevents cross-contamination of the wound or abdomen with bowel organisms. Surgeons also use this technique during cancer procedures to prevent mechanical metastasis, or "seeding" of malignant cells, throughout the abdomen. Bowel technique begins as soon as the GI tract is clamped and transected, and proceeds through wound irrigation, before wound closure. Instruments used for bowel resection and anastomosis are kept separate from the rest of the sterile back table. Contaminated GI tract instruments are handed off or left on a separate Mayo stand. After wound irrigation, the surgical team dons fresh gowns and gloves. Clean instruments are used for closure. Planning during preoperative setup includes having the necessary extra instruments to accommodate bowel technique. Surgeon preference and institutional protocol determine the details of bowel technique (AORN, 2013).

Surgical specimens may be contaminated with microorganisms or malignant cells. Careful handling of the specimen, therefore, to prevent cross-contamination of instruments and the sterile field is important. The surgeon determines how the specimen is to be labeled and prepared for transfer to pathology. Accuracy is verified with the surgeon by reading back (referred to as "write down, read back") the label and pathology form before removing the specimen from the room or before the surgeon leaves the room, and documented according to institutional protocol. Specimens may be sent fresh, in saline, or in a preservative solution. Tissue may be sent for frozen-section examination to verify pathologic condition and to determine if tissue margins are free of malignant cells. Specimens to be entered into research protocols may require further special handling, storage, transport, and documentation.

Closed suction drains evacuate fluids from the abdominal cavity. A variety of catheters (e.g., Malecot, Pezzer) are inserted into the stomach as a gastrostomy tube, decompressing the stomach until normal bowel peristalsis returns. A red rubber catheter may be used as a jejunostomy tube to deliver postoperative enteral nutrition. Most drains and feeding tubes secure to the skin with a nonabsorbable suture. Gastrostomy tubes and jejunostomy tubes require appropriately sized catheter plugs or must be connected to a drainage bag before patient transfer from the OR. All tubes and drains require labeling and documentation according to type and location.

Determination and documentation of wound classification occur at the end of the procedure. Controlled entries into the GI tract without spillage of gastric or bowel contents are classified as "clean-contaminated." Gross contamination from the GI tract, major breaks in sterile technique, or visible presence of acute infection changes the classification to "contaminated."

Evaluation

Evaluation of patient care continues throughout the procedure and through patient transport to the postanesthesia care unit (PACU) or surgical intensive care unit (SICU). Accounting for all sharps, instruments, and soft goods is mandatory and accords with hospital policy and procedure.

Secure the dressing, drains, and any pain management pump tubing to prevent dislodging or damage during transfer from the OR bed. Assess the skin for redness or bruising. Remove the ESU dispersive pad, inspect the site, and document skin condition. Ensure that the patient is covered with a clean, warm blanket before being transported to the PACU or SICU. Any variances require reporting to the surgeon, documentation in the patient's record, and inclusion in the hand-off report to the nurse in the PACU, SICU, or nursing unit. Patient outcomes, based on the perioperative nursing diagnoses, undergo review. Postoperative documentation reflects and measures how each outcome was met and notes significant variations from desired results.

Patient and Family Education and Discharge Planning

Patients undergoing surgical intervention for GI disorders vary greatly in length of time and complexity of recovery. Recovery and convalescence depend on the procedure, surgical approach, site of surgery, anesthesia, pain management, and health of the patient. Teach patients that coughing and deep-breathing exercises will be necessary after surgery to prevent pneumonia by opening alveoli and removing pooled excretions. Coughing can be uncomfortable after abdominal surgery. Show the patient how to splint the incision by holding a small pillow or folded blanket firmly over the incision while coughing. Incentive spirometry provides a way to visibly measure inspiratory effort and is a helpful tool to encourage deep breathing. When possible, provide preoperative instructions for use with return demonstration and allow the patient to practice with the machine. Inform the patient that early ambulation helps regain overall muscle tone and strength, supports cardiac and pulmonary function, reduces or prevents the risk of deep vein thrombosis (DVT) in lower extremities, and boosts a sense of well-being. Preventing pulmonary and vascular complications also helps reduce hospital readmission rates (Research Highlight).

Pain management is critical for recovery. Explain the methods of pain control that might be available after surgery. For example, placing an epidural catheter immediately before surgery for postoperative pain control is possible. For most major GI procedures, patient-controlled analgesia (PCA) provides consistent pain control in the first 1 to 3 postoperative days of hospital recovery. Surgeons often order additional medication for breakthrough pain.

Inform patients that narcotics may delay return of normal bowel peristalsis. Most patients experience a temporary decrease in bowel activity for about 3 days after GI surgery, called "postoperative ileus." Activity (or motility) of the small intestine usually returns to normal within a few hours after surgery. Stomach motility returns to normal within 24 to 48 hours, and the large intestine returns to normal within 48 to 72 hours (Litkouhi, 2012).

Consider postoperative ileus prolonged when it lasts beyond the expected 3 days. Signs and symptoms of prolonged ileus are absence of bowel sounds, abdominal distention, diffuse abdominal pain, nausea, and vomiting (Doorly and Senagore, 2012). Causes of prolonged ileus vary and can arise from neurogenic, inflammatory, hormonal, pharmacologic, or mechanical effects of surgery, including overmanipulation of the intestines during surgery. Identifying early bowel sounds through abdominal auscultation may signal

RESEARCH HIGHLIGHT

Risk Factors for 30-day Hospital Readmission

Patient readmissions within 30 days of discharge are a measure of quality patient care for hospitals. The Centers for Medicare & Medicaid Services (CMS) began decreasing payments to hospitals with excessive readmission rates in April 2012. With the focus on 30-day readmissions for surgical patients, hospitals are actively looking at ways to decrease unnecessary surgical readmissions. In this exploratory study to identify factors associated with readmission after a general surgical procedure, the investigators reviewed data related to 163 patients readmitted to their hospital within 30 days of discharge after a general surgery procedure and found that the most common reasons for readmission were nausea/vomiting, bowel obstruction, surgical site infections, and failure to thrive or malnutrition. The procedures associated with readmissions were pancreatectomy, colectomy, small bowel resection, gastrectomy, and ventral hernia repair.

Data elements such as age, sex, race, and transfer status were not associated with an increased risk of readmission; patients with an American Society of Anesthesiologists (ASA) score of 4 and 5 and patients who were inpatients at least 24 hours prior to surgery, however, were at increased risk. Comorbidities most associated with readmissions were widespread cancer, preoperative history of shortness of breath, and the presence of an open wound. Interestingly, diabetes, smoking, chronic obstructive pulmonary disease (COPD), preoperative ventilator dependence, ascites, hypertension, chronic steroid use, unintended preoperative weight loss, and renal failure did not have a statistically significant effect on readmission risk.

Patients who were readmitted had one or more of the following complications during their hospital stay: wound complications; blood transfusion within 72 hours of surgery; urinary tract infection; pulmonary complications; sepsis or septic shock; or vascular complications such as deep vein thrombosis or pulmonary embolism.

The investigators found that postoperative complications were the most significant independent risk factor leading to hospital readmissions. They concluded that allocating institutional resources to focus on preventing and appropriately managing postoperative complications in high-risk patients could reduce readmissions. Additionally, spending extra time and effort to educate high-risk patients about their wound care, antibiotic regimens, and general rehabilitation prior to discharge may help prevent readmissions.

Modified from Kassin MT et al: Risk factors for 30-day hospital readmission among general surgery patients, *J Am Coll Surg* 215(3):322–330, 2012.

return of small intestine motility; only the passage of flatus or stool, however, indicates full return of bowel function and resolution of ileus (Ricciardi and MacKay, 2012).

Many lifestyle changes occur for patients with a new ostomy. A WOCN helps patients to learn how to care for their stoma and surrounding skin. They also learn from the WOCN about proper appliance selection and application, stoma irrigation, diet, and bowel training. A WOCN consultation assists the patient to consider quality-of-life strategies to deal with key issues such as clothing selection, self-esteem, body image, sex and intimacy, travel, public toileting, and odor control (Doughty and Landmann, 2012). An excellent patient resource for learning about living with an ostomy is the United Ostomy Associations of America at www.uoaa.org.

After some GI surgeries, patients may require prolonged nutritional support with total parenteral nutrition (TPN) or with enteral feedings. Obtaining referral and consultation for home care support and nursing care to administer TPN or enteral feedings are an essential part of discharge planning for this patient population. General discharge instructions for the patient undergoing GI surgery include both verbal and written instructions (Patient and Family Education).

Ambulatory surgery considerations and education are based on patient, procedure, and anesthesia selection. Patient instructions before and at discharge are critical, and depend on the patient's ability, self-efficacy, and family support for home care.

PATIENT AND FAMILY EDUCATION

General Discharge Instructions for GI Surgery Patients

Prior to discharge patients should receive verbal and written detailed information about postoperative activity, diet, wound care, when and with whom to make follow-up appointments, and what to do and who to call if they experience problems at home. All discharge medications are reviewed to ensure the patient understands the purpose of the medication, when to take it, and possible side effects.

Written instructions may include the following:

- Walking is good for you. Start with short walks. Gradually increase your physical activity as you grow stronger.
- Avoid lifting heavy items (greater than 10 pounds) until cleared to do so by your surgeon.
- Continue with deep-breathing exercises every 2 hours throughout the day.
- Avoid sitting for prolonged periods (greater than 1 hour) without getting up and walking around. This will help prevent blood clots from forming in your legs.
- Expect to get tired easily. Plan for several periods of rest throughout the day.
- Expect changes in appetite and alterations in how food tastes. You may find that you get full faster and eat less than you did before surgery. Eat four to six small frequent meals throughout the day rather than three large meals. Follow all dietary restrictions your surgeon has prescribed for you. If there are no restrictions, gradually work up to your preoperative dietary habits. If you are on a liquid diet, avoid caffeine, carbonated beverages, and drinks high in sugar content. It is important to drink plenty of water to stay hydrated.
- Keep your incision(s) clean and dry. A small amount of clear or pink drainage from your incision may occur for a few days after you go home. You can use a gauze pad to cover your incision to protect your clothes until the drainage stops.
- Take the pain medicine you have been prescribed if you need it.
- Do not drive or operate heavy equipment while taking pain medication.
- Take only the medications that are listed in your written discharge instructions.
- Call your surgeon if you experience any of the following symptoms:
  - Temperature greater than 101°F (38.4°C)
  - Increasing abdominal pain
  - Persistent nausea or vomiting
  - Persistent diarrhea or absence of bowel movements
  - Sudden pain, swelling, or warmth in one or both of your legs
  - Shortness of breath or difficulty breathing
  - Redness, bright red bleeding, or yellow foul-smelling drainage at the incision site(s)

Modified from Dziedzic ME: Nursing challenges in the care of patients who undergo minimally invasive surgery—are you prepared? *Mosby's Nursing Consult Clinical Updates,* 2010.

Surgical Interventions

Laparotomy

Laparotomy is surgical entrance into the abdominal cavity. The purpose of laparotomy may be to explore the abdomen to make a diagnosis or as a means to perform a planned surgical procedure. Surgeons access the abdominal cavity by a variety of incisions, described next.

Open Abdominal Incisions

Various incisions to enter the abdominal cavity appear in Figure 11-7. Key elements in planning the location and length of surgical incisions are access, preserving abdominal wall function, and the ability to securely close the wound. An optimally placed incision provides adequate access to the targeted pathology, provides sufficient visualization and room to complete the procedure without undue trauma to surrounding structures, can be extended if unexpected findings require additional exposure to complete the procedure, and can be closed securely with minimal risks for disruption (Evans and Bhanot, 2012; Mizell, 2012a). Other factors considered are the patient's condition and need for fast abdominal entry, uncertainty of diagnosis and need for flexibility, previous surgical scars, potential need for future abdominal surgery or ostomy, body habitus (physique), risk for bleeding, postoperative pain, and cosmetic results.

The layers of the abdominal wall appear in Figure 11-8. In the midline, the abdominal wall consists of the skin, subcutaneous fat, the linea alba, preperitoneal fat, and peritoneum. At the midline, the anterior and posterior rectus sheaths fuse together to form the linea alba, an avascular nerve-free structure that vertically divides the right and left rectus muscles from the xiphoid process to the symphysis pubis. Lateral to the linea alba, the anterior and posterior rectus sheaths cover the rectus muscles (Figure 11-9). On the lower abdominal wall, the arcuate line is a landmark located about one third of the distance between the umbilicus and the symphysis pubis. Above this imaginary line, the aponeurosis of the internal oblique muscle splits and joins the aponeuroses of the external

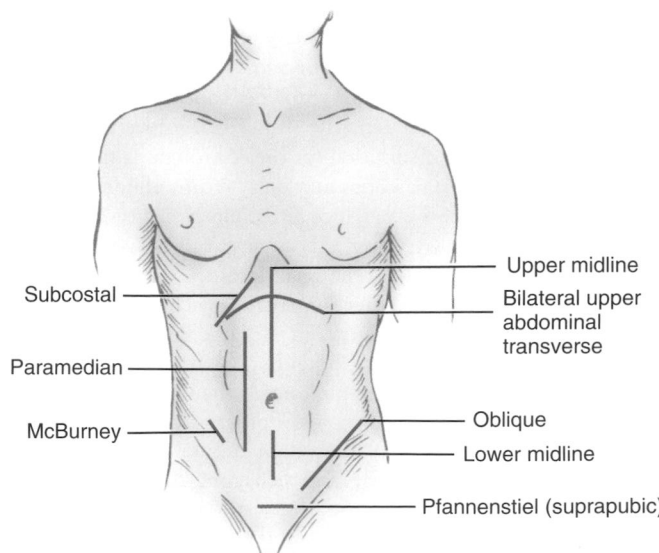

FIGURE 11-7 Incisions made through the abdominal wall.

oblique muscle anteriorly and the transversalis fascia posteriorly to form the anterior and posterior rectus sheaths. Below the arcuate line there is no posterior rectus sheath.

Procedural Considerations: Open Laparotomy.

A basic laparotomy set includes instruments for sharp and blunt dissection, clamping tissue, grasping tissue, suturing, cutting suture, and retracting tissue. An instrument list may include Metzenbaum scissors, curved Mayo scissors, straight Mayo scissors (also called suture scissors), tissue forceps with teeth, Adson tissue forceps with teeth, Russian tissue forceps, DeBakey tissue forceps, Ferris Smith tissue forceps, Crile or Kelly hemostats, mosquitos, Péan clamps, Allis clamps, Babcock clamps, right-angle clamps, assorted needle holders, ringed forceps, and towel clips. The following retractors are usually included in various sizes: Deaver, Richardson, Harrington, Army Navy,

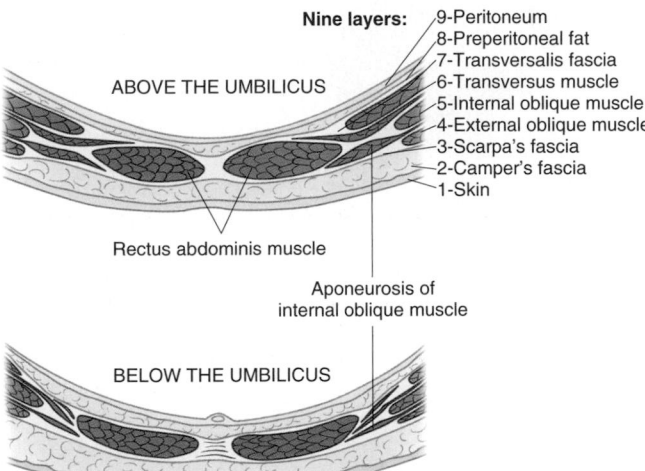

Nine layers:
9-Peritoneum
8-Preperitoneal fat
7-Transversalis fascia
6-Transversus muscle
5-Internal oblique muscle
4-External oblique muscle
3-Scarpa's fascia
2-Camper's fascia
1-Skin

ABOVE THE UMBILICUS

Rectus abdominis muscle

Aponeurosis of internal oblique muscle

BELOW THE UMBILICUS

FIGURE 11-8 Horizontal section of abdominal wall. Aponeurosis of internal oblique muscle splits into two sections, one lying anterior and the other posterior to rectus abdominis muscle, thereby forming an encasing sheath around muscle above the umbilicus. Below the umbilicus, aponeuroses of all muscles pass anterior to rectus sheath.

malleable, and abdominal wall. Additional instruments to have available might include self-retaining retractors such as a Balfour, or Bookwalter set; atraumatic intestinal clamps; Yankauer and Poole suction tips; and longer versions of basic instruments for procedures in the pelvis, in obese patients, or in thoracoabdominal procedures. An electrosurgical unit, smoke evacuator, and suction machine are basic to performing laparotomy.

Before any incision all surgical team members pause for a time-out briefing that includes the components of The Joint Commission's (TJC) Universal Protocol for preventing wrong site, wrong procedure, wrong person surgery. This is a TJC National Patient Safety Goal (NPSG) and is discussed in Chapter 2.

Vertical Incisions

Midline Incision.

A midline incision offers fast entry into the abdomen, provides excellent exposure to any part of the abdominal cavity, can be closed securely and rapidly, and is the standard incision for exploratory laparotomy (Evans and Bhanot, 2012). The incision starts above the umbilicus and is carried down through the subcutaneous layer to the linea alba. At the umbilicus the surgeon diverts the incision from the midline, around rather than through the umbilicus (Figure 11-10, *A*). Incision of the linea alba exposes the peritoneum (see Figure 11-10, *B*). To prevent injury to underlying structures, before incising the peritoneum, surgical assistants use hemostats or smooth forceps to lift the peritoneum away from the intestines or other structures. The surgeon lifts the abdominal wall to protect underlying structures and extends the peritoneal incision in either direction as needed (see Figure 11-10, *C*), and can carry the extension of the incision cephalad to just below the xiphoid process. Taking culture samples may occur at this point. If extensive exposure of the liver is needed, the surgeon can divide and ligate the falciform ligament between two clamps. The surgeon also can extend the incision caudad, down to just above the symphysis pubis, taking care not to injure the bladder. Use of laparotomy pads and suction is needed for exposure. The abdominal wall is often retracted with large Richardson retractors during initial exploration. Once the affected organs are identified, a self-retaining retractor, such as a Balfour or Bookwalter retractor system, is used to establish hands-free exposure.

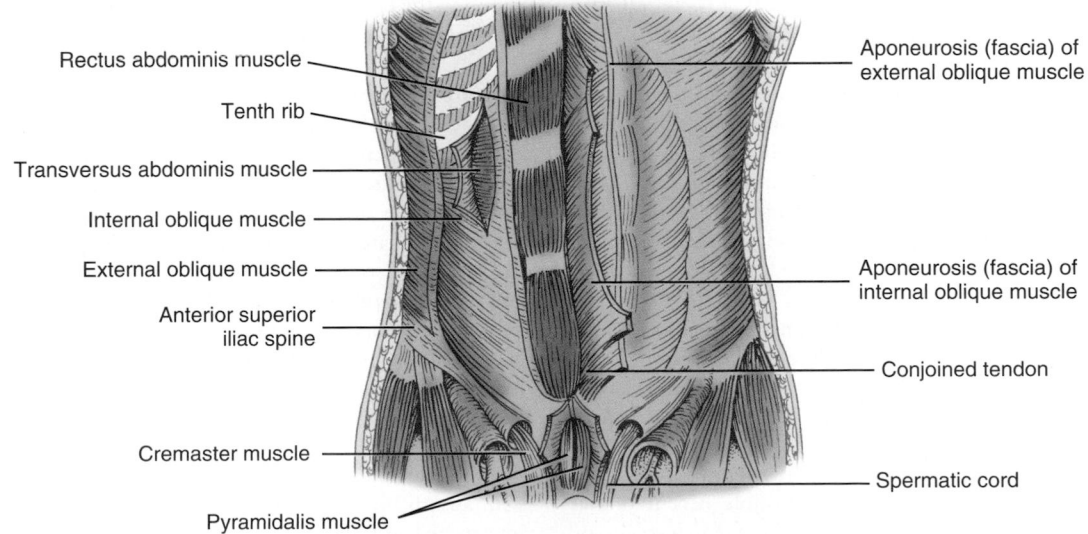

Rectus abdominis muscle
Tenth rib
Transversus abdominis muscle
Internal oblique muscle
External oblique muscle
Anterior superior iliac spine
Cremaster muscle
Pyramidalis muscle

Aponeurosis (fascia) of external oblique muscle
Aponeurosis (fascia) of internal oblique muscle
Conjoined tendon
Spermatic cord

FIGURE 11-9 Superior muscles of abdominal wall.

FIGURE 11-10 A, Midline laparotomy incision around the umbilicus. **B,** External fascia is incised. **C,** Entry into the peritoneal cavity.

Current literature states that closure of midline incisions should incorporate all layers of the abdominal wall except the skin. Closure entails use of a running suturing technique (see Chapter 7). A large-gauge, delayed absorbing suture about four times longer than the length of the incision is required for this running suturing technique. During skin closure using an interrupted suturing technique, stitches are placed at least 1 cm from the wound edge with at least 1 cm between sutures (Mizell, 2012a). Closure of the skin can also occur with skin staples, absorbable subcuticular sutures, adhesive skin tapes, or dermal glue. Surgeons seldom use internal or external retention sutures for primary abdominal closure. This is because there is little evidence to support their effectiveness in preventing wound disruption and there is an association between them and increased incisional pain and wound complications (Evans and Bhanot; 2012; Mizell, 2012a). If retention sutures are needed, #1 or #2 nonabsorbable suture material is appropriate, coupled with prepackaged retention bridges or flexible tubing bolsters to protect the incision site.

Paramedian Incision. Surgeons place paramedian incisions about 2 to 5 cm lateral to either side of the midline on the upper or lower abdomen. Incision of skin and subcutaneous tissue exposes the anterior rectus sheath, which in turn is incised vertically. Lateral retraction of the rectus muscle exposes the posterior rectus sheath, also then incised vertically. Entry into the peritoneum occurs in the same fashion as the midline incision. A possible benefit of the paramedian incision is potential decreased risk for dehiscence or hernia; disadvantages include risk of injury to the epigastric vessels

and risk of nerve injury resulting in paralysis of the rectus muscle. Closure is similar to the midline incision.

Oblique Incisions

The oblique inguinal incision is between the pubic tubercle toward the anterior iliac crest, slightly above and parallel to the inguinal ligament. This is the standard incision for open inguinal herniorrhaphy. The incision through the external oblique muscle provides access to the cremaster muscle, inguinal canal, and cord structures. This incision typically does not interrupt major abdominal arteries.

McBurney Incision. Use of the McBurney muscle-splitting incision is common for open appendectomy. In the lower right abdomen the surgeon incises the skin along the skin tension lines at a point one third of the distance between the anterior iliac spine and the umbilicus. Electrosurgical dissection of the subcutaneous layer and Scarpa fascia carries down to the external oblique fascia. The surgeon then sharply divides the fascia along its fibers. The internal oblique and transversus abdominis muscles are split in the direction of their fibers and retracted to expose the transversalis fascia and peritoneum. The surgeon then incises the fascia and peritoneum together, in the same direction as the incision (Mizell 2012a). This incision is quick and easy to open, close, and extend if additional exposure is necessary. The incision can extend medially or laterally. The surgeon can close the transversalis fascia and peritoneum together with absorbable suture and loosely approximate the muscles with interrupted absorbable sutures. The external oblique fascia is closed with interrupted or continuous absorbable suture. In large patients with a subcutaneous layer less than 2 cm, Scarpa fascia may be approximated. Closure of the skin is according to surgeon preference. A transverse modification of a McBurney incision is the Rocky-Davis or Elliot modification.

Subcostal Incision. A subcostal (Kocher) incision begins approximately 3 cm below the xiphoid process and extends laterally, staying 2.5 to 3 cm below and parallel to the costal margin. The incision descends through the subcutaneous layer. The surgeon identifies and divides the anterior fascia of the rectus muscle; division of the rectus, external oblique, internal oblique, and transversalis muscles follows. Electrocoagulation of the superior epigastric vessels in the rectus muscle may follow or they may undergo division between clamps and ligation. The surgeon lifts the peritoneum from the underlying viscera and sharply opens it. A right subcostal incision is appropriate for open procedures of the gallbladder, biliary system, and pancreas (Figure 11-11), as is a left subcostal incision for open access to the spleen.

Joining of the right and left subcostal incisions in the midline is appropriate to make a "chevron" incision. Chevron incisions provide excellent exposure for gastric, duodenal, pancreatic, and portal system procedures. Closure of the subcostal incision is in layers. The surgeon approximates the falciform ligament if divided. Closure of the peritoneum, posterior rectus fascia, and anterior rectus fascia is with absorbable, running or interrupted sutures. Skin closure is with absorbable, subcuticular sutures or skin staples. Disadvantages of this incision include poor cosmesis and increased postoperative pain (Mizell, 2012a).

Thoracoabdominal Incision. The thoracoabdominal incision joins the thoracic and abdominal cavities together. It provides exposure to the esophagus, cardia of the stomach, liver, spleen, kidneys, adrenal glands, lungs, aorta (left side), inferior vena cava (right side), and esophagus. The patient is in a semilateral position with the torso rotated 45 degrees and both hips on the OR bed (Evans and

Bhanot, 2012) (Figure 11-12). Entry into the abdomen is first through a subcostal or midline incision. Entry into the thoracic cavity occurs by extending the incision in a posterolateral direction. The surgeon carries the thoracic incision down through the latissimus dorsi, serratus anterior, and external oblique muscles. The intercostal muscles undergo division in the eighth intercostal space; the surgeon then lifts the pleural cavity to protect the lung and opens it sharply. Removal of a short piece of costal cartilage can

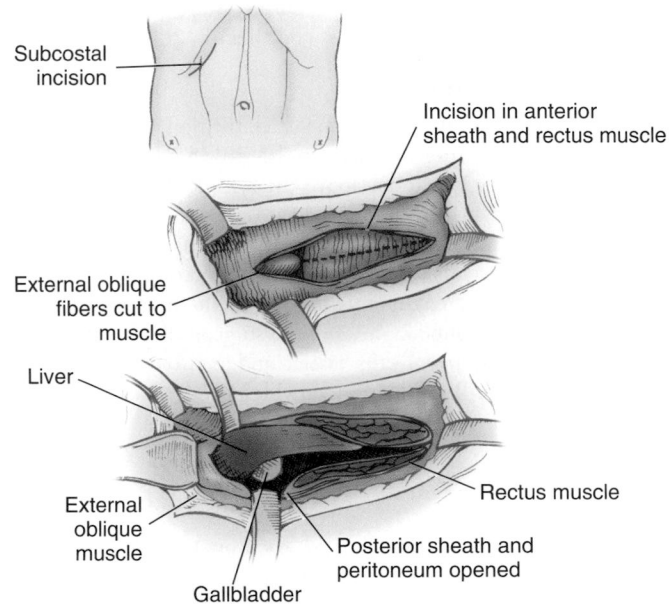

FIGURE 11-11 Subcostal incision in upper right quadrant. Anterior sheath has been divided transversely, and muscle is exposed. Posterior sheath and peritoneum have been opened transversely.

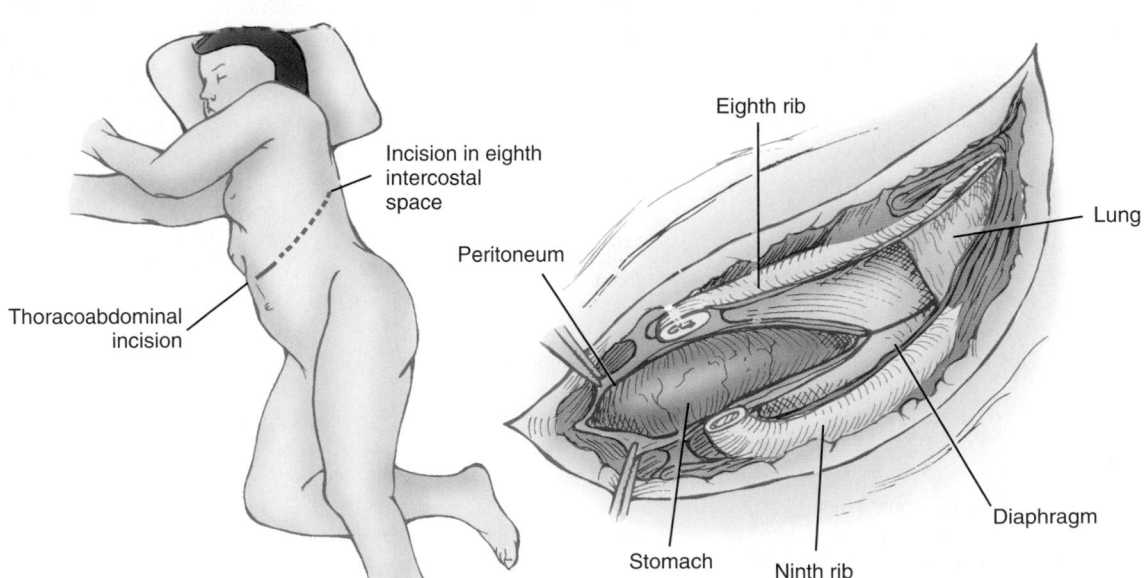

FIGURE 11-12 Thoracoabdominal incision. Patient is placed on unaffected side. Incision is usually made from a point midway between the xiphoid process and the umbilicus to the costal margin at the site of the eighth costal cartilage. Dissection is carried down to the peritoneum and pleura. Costal cartilage and diaphragm are divided, and the stomach is exposed.

provide additional exposure before insertion of a self-retaining rib retractor, slowly opened to expand the intercostal space. Division of the diaphragm is next, after which division of the phrenic vessels between clamps and ligation follows. Before closing, team members insert chest tubes into the pleural cavity through separate stab incisions. The surgeon closes the diaphragm using two layers of non-absorbable suture via an interrupted vertical mattress technique, approximates the divided ribs with heavy sutures, and closes the chest wall and abdominal muscles in layers. Absorbable suture is appropriate to close the chest muscles, as is a delayed absorbing suture for closure of the abdomen. The surgeon approximates the skin edges and secures them with suture, staples, skin-bonding adhesive, or skin tape strips (Evans and Bhanot, 2012).

Transverse Incisions

Pfannenstiel Incision. The Pfannenstiel incision is optimal for pelvic surgery. The surgeon makes a 10- to 15-cm skin incision transversely, about 3 to 5 cm above the symphysis pubis, usually within the pubic hairline (Figure 11-13). Opening the anterior rectus fascia transversely occurs next. Elevation of the fascial edges with heavy clamps follows, as does blunt separation of the fascia from the underlying rectus muscle. The rectus muscles undergo separation at the midline raphe, and the surgeon divides the transversalis fascia, posterior rectus fascia, and peritoneum vertically along the midline. This incision provides good exposure, secure closure, and acceptable cosmesis. Closure of the peritoneum is with continuous absorbable suture. Approximation of the rectus muscles is with interrupted absorbable suture. The anterior fascia is closed with slow-absorbing continuous suture.

Incision Complications

Dehiscence and Evisceration. Wound *dehiscence* is a risk of abdominal surgery and constitutes a disruption or separation of the wound edges that occurs when tension of the abdominal wall overcomes the tensile strength of the suture or integrity of the surgical knot. *Evisceration* occurs when bowel or other abdominal structures protrude through the open wound. Prolonged hypothermia with decreased tissue oxygenation, bleeding, devitalized or strangulated tissue, and excessive dead space in the subcutaneous layer can lead to seroma formation, wound infection, and disruption of a surgical wound. Other risk factors for dehiscence include obesity, advanced age, male gender, chronic pulmonary disease, coughing, malignancy, previous radiation, trauma, poor nutritional status, and chronic steroid use (Mizell, 2012b). Additional risk factors associated with wound dehiscence include excessive tension on the wound edges, incisions longer than 18 cm, and improper surgical technique such as placing sutures too close to the wound edges; placing sutures too close to each other; strangulating tissue by pulling or tying sutures too tightly; or surgical knots that are insecure or cut too short, causing unraveling.

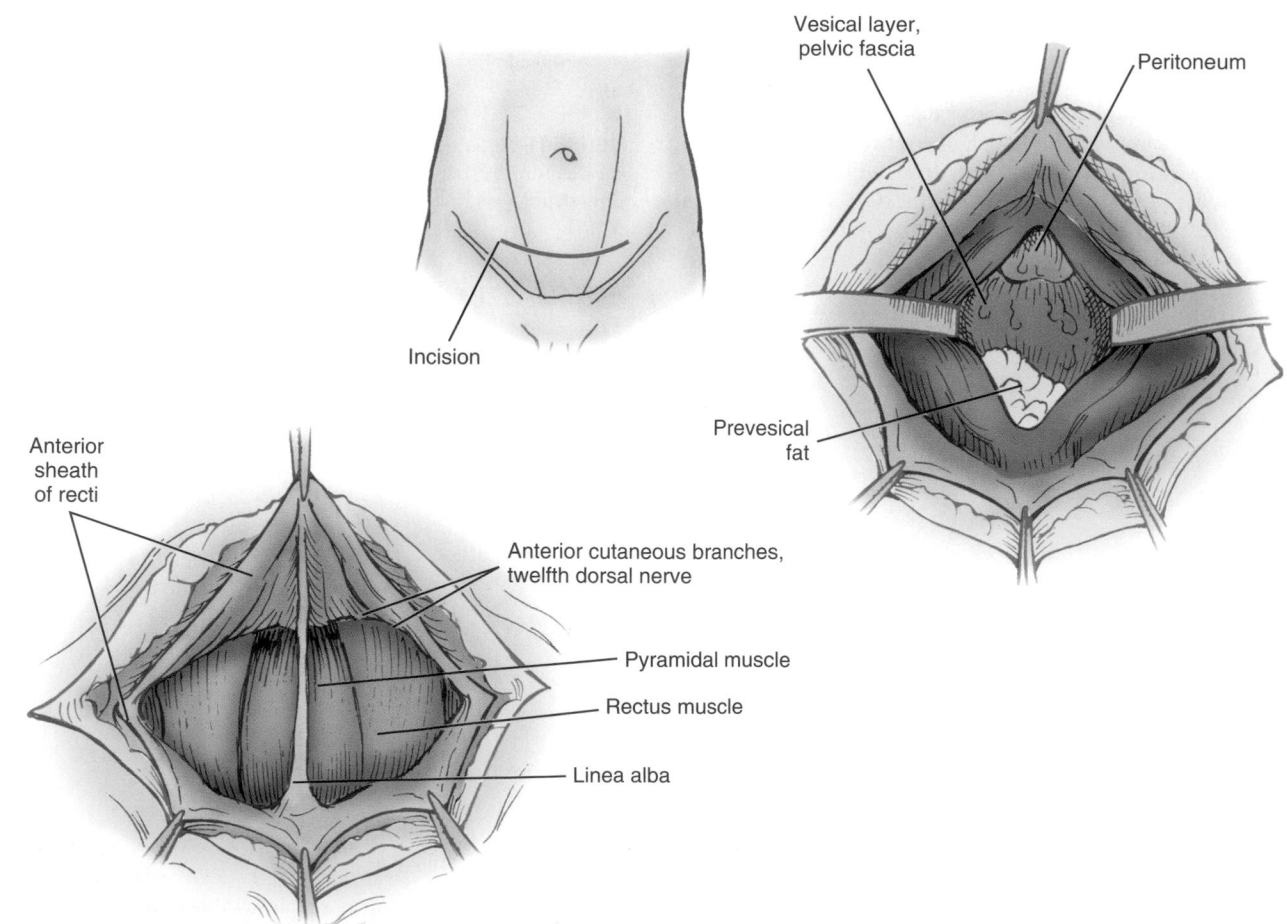

FIGURE 11-13 Pfannenstiel incision (suprapubic).

Nerve Injury. Injury to abdominal wall nerves can cause chronic pain, loss of sensation, or abdominal wall weakness. Nerve injuries occur when nerves are severed during incision, entrapped with suture during closure, or compressed or stretched with retractors or instruments (Mizell, 2012b).

Minimally Invasive Surgery—Laparoscopy

From its origins in gynecologic surgery, laparoscopy has evolved from a minimally invasive technique used primarily for sterilization and diagnostic purposes into a surgical approach adopted by many surgical specialties to perform major resection, extraction, and repair of intra-abdominal organs (Box 11-2).

Procedural Considerations

Most laparoscopic procedures progress in similar fashion and require the same basic equipment, instruments, and supplies. Mentally organizing laparoscopic procedures into common components of progression facilitates the planning process. The general progression of a laparoscopic procedure includes: (1) gaining abdominal access, (2) establishing pneumoperitoneum, (3) exposing the targeted organ, (4) completing the critical steps of the procedure, (5) extracting a specimen, (6) irrigating the wound, and (7) closing the incisions.

General equipment for laparoscopic procedures includes a variety of access port devices: visualization and insufflation equipment; energy devices for coagulating, sealing, and dissecting tissue; and devices or equipment to evacuate surgical smoke. Instruments

---

BOX 11-2

Minimally Invasive Approaches to GI Surgical Procedures

Robotic GI Procedures
- Nissen and Toupet fundoplication
- Gastric bypass
- Sleeve gastrectomy
- Colectomy
- Rectal resection
- Small bowel resection
- Gastrectomy
- Esophagectomy

SILS GI Procedures
- Appendectomy
- Right hemicolectomy
- Proctocolectomy

NOTES GI Procedures
- Transvaginal appendectomy
- Transgastric appendectomy
- Transgastric gastrojejunostomy (animal studies only)
- PEG tube salvage
- Transrectal colectomy (animal studies only)
- Transesophageal Heller myotomy

GI, Gastrointestinal; *NOTES,* natural orifice transluminal endoscopic surgery; *PEG,* percutaneous endoscopic gastrostomy; *SILS,* single-incision laparoscopic surgery.
Modified from Chambers WM, Bicsak M et al: Single-incision laparoscopic surgery (SILS) in complex colorectal surgery: a technique offering potential and not just cosmesis, *Colorectal Disease* 13:393–398, 2011; Reider E, Swanstrom LL: NOTES: What is currently possible? In Cameron JL, Cameron AM, editors: *Current surgical therapy,* ed 10, Philadelphia, 2011, Mosby.

---

may include laparoscopic dissectors, graspers, scissors, needle holders, knot pushers, suction/irrigator, and endoscopic staplers.

Any laparoscopic procedure has the potential need for conversion to an open procedure; it is prudent therefore to have a laparotomy instrument set readily available. If not specified by institutional policy or protocol, the decision to have laparotomy instruments opened and counted *before* the procedure begins depends on patient assessment, experience of the surgical team, and expected technical difficulty of the intended procedure. If anticipated, the possibility or probability of converting to an open procedure should be part of the preoperative team briefing. Sharps and soft goods opened on the field require counting before the procedure begins, regardless of approach or incision size. Reasons to convert to an open approach may include abdominal adhesions that prevent abdominal access (Evidence for Practice); significantly distorted anatomy that precludes safe dissection; gross fecal contamination or infection; uncontrollable bleeding; or pulmonary or cardiac changes related to the patient's inability to tolerate pneumoperitoneum or extreme positioning required for exposure.

Operative Procedure

1. The surgical team positions, preps, and drapes the patient as appropriate for the intended procedure. Common patient positions for laparoscopic procedures are supine, lithotomy, and modified lithotomy.
2. Insufflation tubing, camera cord, light cord, and cords for energy devices are secured to the sterile drapes; ends are passed off the sterile field for connection to the appropriate control units. To lessen the risk of fire, ensure the light cord does not rest on sterile drapes when attaching it to the light source and before turning on the light source.
3. The surgeon enters the abdomen by a variety of techniques. The three discussed here are common GI laparoscopy techniques.

Abdominal Access: Closed Technique

1. The surgeon makes an infraumbilical skin incision with a #11 or #15 blade. The length of the skin incision must accommodate the size of the access port intended for this site.
2. One or two towel clips are used to elevate the abdominal wall before insertion of the Veress needle through the linea alba and peritoneum.
3. To verify correct positioning of the tip of the Veress needle, a 10-mL syringe, partially filled with normal saline, is attached to the Veress needle. Gentle aspiration on the syringe will yield bloody fluid or intestinal content if the needle has entered a vessel or the intestine. No aspirate appears if the needle tip is clear. A "saline drop test," performed by injecting a small amount of saline into the clear chamber located just below the hub of the Veress needle, follows. If the Veress needle has entered the abdominal cavity, the saline in the chamber will quickly drop into the abdomen.
4. Insufflation tubing, attached to the Veress needle, enables insufflation of the abdomen. It is important to position the insufflator to enable the surgeon to visualize insufflation pressures and flow rate.
5. After establishing pneumoperitoneum, the Veress needle is removed and the surgeon blindly inserts a 5- or 10-mm access port. The insufflation tubing is then transferred to the access port. The size of the laparoscope typically determines the size of the access port at this site. An alternate site to gain initial access to the abdomen is in the upper right quadrant, about three fingerbreadths

EVIDENCE FOR PRACTICE

Preventing Abdominal Adhesions

The incidence of abdominal adhesions after GI surgery is high. Adhesions are fibrous bands of tissue between abdominal structures that are normally not connected. They can be very thin and avascular or they can be very thick and contain blood vessels and nerves. Injury or inflammation of the peritoneal surface triggers the body's natural healing process that begins with an inflammatory response at the site of the injury. In the final stages of this process, fibrin deposits, degrades, and reabsorbs at the site of injury. Interruption or disturbance of this final phase of healing by the presence of foreign bodies, drugs, blood, bacteria, or devitalized tissue can result in adhesion formation.

Adhesions can form between the peritoneal surfaces of the abdominal wall and its underlying abdominal structures, or they can form between adjacent structures within the abdomen such as the omentum, small bowel, and colon. Adhesions may be asymptomatic, but often result in complications that can occur in the early postoperative stage or years after an abdominal surgery. Complications include small bowel obstruction, abdominal/pelvic pain, and infertility.

Methods that have been used to prevent or minimize the formation of postoperative adhesions fall into one of the following categories: surgical technique, physical barriers, and pharmacologic agents. Recommended surgical techniques to prevent adhesions include gentle handling of tissue to minimize trauma, meticulous hemostasis, minimizing tissue ischemia, keeping tissues moist, and limiting the introduction of foreign materials, such as talc from surgical gloves, lint from sponges, excess suture material, and char from cauterized tissue. For long laparoscopic procedures, it has been shown that the use of heated and humidified CO_2 to insufflate the abdomen can decrease the incidence of peritoneal adhesions. Physical barriers may prevent or minimize the incidence of adhesions by keeping peritoneal surfaces separated during the healing process.

Examples and characteristics of solid physical barriers are as follows:
- Oxidized regenerated cellulose (Interceed; Ethicon, Inc.)
  - Absorbable, flexible, knitted fabric
  - Indicated for open and laparoscopic procedures
  - Available in 1.5 × 2- or 3 × 4-inch sheets
  - Excess fluid must be removed from injured tissue before placement
  - Injured tissue must be completely covered by the product

- Moisten lightly with irrigation to keep in place after positioning
- Will absorb in 2 weeks
- Hyaluronic acid sheets with carboxymethylcellulose (Seprafilm; Genzyme Biosurgery)
  - Transparent, brittle filmlike material that breaks easily when bent
  - Indicated for open procedures that do not involve bowel anastomosis. It cannot be passed through a trocar without breaking into pieces.
  - Material readily adheres to moist surfaces, including surgical gloves and surgical instruments. Handle with dry instruments. When it comes into contact with wet surfaces, it forms a sticky gel that is difficult to reposition.
  - Product comes out of the sterile package positioned between two sheets of paper to facilitate handling and proper positioning the film. Do not remove the paper.
  - Available in 5 × 6-inch sheets
  - Will absorb in 7 days
- Expanded polytetrafluorethylene (Preclude Peritoneal Membrane; Gore-Tex Surgical Membrane)
  - Flexible, nonabsorbable fabric sheet
  - Can be cut to size. It should extend 1 cm beyond the injured tissue to facilitate anchoring it in place with suture.
  - Nonabsorbable monofilament suture such as nylon or polypropylene used to suture in place
- Polyethylene glycol (SprayGel; Confluent Surgical Inc.)
  - Comes in two syringes full of polyethylene glycol–based solutions that are simultaneously dispensed onto the injured tissue
  - Spray forms an adherent gel-like barrier
  - Components of the gel break down in 5 to 7 days and are absorbed by the kidneys
  - Currently available in Europe; awaiting FDA approval in the United States

Liquid physical barriers include:
- Hyaluronic acid (Sepracoat; Genzyme Corporation)
- Cross-linked hyaluronic acid (Intergel; Hyalobarrier gel; Baxter Healthcare Corporation)
- Icodextrin 4% (Adept; Baxter Healthcare Corporation)

Several systemic pharmacologic agents have been studied as a means to prevent abdominal adhesions, but to date there has been no evidence demonstrating effectiveness in humans.

FDA, U.S. Food and Drug Administration.

Modified from Arung W et al: Pathophysiology and prevention of postoperative peritoneal adhesions, *World J Gastroenterol* 17(41): 4545–4553, 2011; DeCherney A, Senthil K: Preventing postoperative peritoneal adhesions. In Basow DS, editor: *UpToDate*, Waltham, MA, UpToDate, 2012.

---

below the right costal margin in the midclavicular line. Surgeons often select this site when they suspect lower abdominal wall adhesions due to previous surgery.

Abdominal Access: Cutdown or Hasson Technique

1. The surgeon makes an infraumbilical skin incision as described previously for the closed technique. Blunt dissection of subcutaneous tissue with a tonsil clamp follows.
2. The linea alba is exposed using small handheld retractors to retract the subcutaneous tissue.
3. The surgeon then places stay sutures (heavy absorbable suture on a small, heavy, curved needle) through the fascia on each side of the midline. Using two hemostats to elevate the abdominal

wall, the loose ends of the sutures are clamped (referred to as "tagged") while the surgeon incises the fascia and peritoneum vertically to accommodate the access port.
4. Insufflation of the abdomen is with CO_2 as previously described.

Abdominal Access: Direct Visual Entry

Another common technique for laparoscopic access to the abdomen uses an optical view access port to visualize layers of the abdominal wall as they are entered.

Insufflation of the abdomen may occur before or after insertion of the access port.

1. The surgeon makes the incision as previously described for open entry techniques.

2. A laparoscope inserts into the center of the access port's trocar. The trocar has a clear, nonbladed tip for visualization. The camera focuses on the inside tip of the trocar.

3. The trocar and port lock onto the shaft of the laparoscope; with a twisting motion, combined with controlled downward pressure, the access port, trocar, and laparoscope advance as one unit through the abdominal wall. The surgeon visualizes each layer of the abdominal wall as the trocar passes through.

4. With pneumoperitoneum established, the surgeon visually explores the abdomen to verify that the procedure can proceed laparoscopically as planned.

5. Additional access ports are inserted under direct visualization provided by the laparoscope. The size, number, and position of these ports must be well planned, based on the surgical procedure and anticipated use of instruments, stapling devices, and size of the specimen to be extracted. For example, certain instruments, such as endoscopic staplers, will pass only through 11- or 12-mm access ports. When expecting a large specimen, the surgeon may position access ports so that they can be joined together at the end of the procedure to accommodate extraction of the specimen. The laparoscope generally remains in the infraumbilical port, and the first assistant or scrub person operates it. The surgeon will use at least two additional ports to perform the procedure and may insert additional ports if needed for instruments used by the first assistant.

6. At the end of the procedure removal of access ports is under direct visualization. Removal of the laparoscope from the umbilical port follows, as does evacuation of the pneumoperitoneum into a smoke evacuation system. Next is removal of the umbilical port. The midline fascial incision is closed with a size 0 absorbable suture on a taper needle if the incision is greater than 5 mm.

7. Skin incisions are closed according to surgeon preference and may include a subcuticular technique with a 3-0 or 4-0 absorbable sutures. The application of dressings ends the procedure.

Single-Incision Laparoscopic Surgery

Procedural Considerations

Single incision laparoscopic surgery (SILS) is a modification of the traditional laparoscopic approach in which introduction of the laparoscope and all instruments into the abdomen is through multiple channels of a single access port. The surgeon makes a single abdominal incision to accommodate the size of the access port. Various single access port systems with different numbers and sizes of channels are commercially available. The location and orientation of the incision for the access port depend on patient anatomy and the procedure being performed. The umbilicus is a common site for port placement.

Before development of modified laparoscopes and instruments, surgeons used standard rigid laparoscopes and laparoscopic instruments to perform single-incision procedures. The proximity and parallel orientation of these instruments often resulted in instrument "sword-fighting/collisions" within the abdomen and "clashing hands" conflicts outside the abdomen. In addition, the small working space of a single port inhibited the ability to place the laparoscope and instruments in the traditional and familiar laparoscopic "triangular" orientation. Visual perspective of the anatomy and working space significantly changed for the better as laparoscopes with flexible rotating tips developed to enhance visualization. Likewise, instruments with bendable rotating tips and curved flexible shafts have increased maneuverability. The VeSPA instrument line (Intuitive Surgical, Inc.), coupled with its multiple-channel access port, is available for robotic-assisted SILS. The access port has an 8.5-mm channel for the endoscope, a 12-mm channel for the assistant, and two 5-mm crossing curved channels for the surgeon's instruments. The VeSPA line uses special da Vinci software that recognizes the crossing of instruments.

Reported benefits of SILS are improved cosmesis (Pryor and Yoo, 2012), reduced surgical trauma, less postoperative pain, and shorter hospital stays. Many traditional laparoscopic procedures have adopted the single-incision approach. The following GI-specific, single-incision laparoscopic procedures appear in the surgical literature: appendectomy, right hemicolectomy, extended right hemicolectomy, proctocolectomy and ileostomy for ulcerative colitis, high anterior colon resection, and restorative proctocolectomy with ileoanal pouch (Chambers et al, 2011).

Robotic-Assisted Laparoscopy

Robotic assistance enhances numerous laparoscopic GI procedures. Examples include Nissen fundoplication, bowel resection, Heller myotomy, and gastric bypass. The da Vinci surgical system (Intuitive Surgical, Inc.) is the only robotic system approved by the U.S. Food and Drug Administration (FDA) for commercial use in the United States (Zender and Thell, 2010). As robotic technology develops, new systems and platforms will become available. Robotic instruments that provide haptic (tactile) and force feedback or are controlled by the surgeon's voice, eyes, or head movements, are already in development (Jayne et al, 2011). As healthcare systems assess the need to start a robotics program, advantages and disadvantages of owning and using a surgical robotic system require serious evaluation (Box 11-3).

Procedural Considerations

Patient safety in robotic surgery is a collaborative effort involving the entire surgical team, which must acquire education and training specific to patient care and all technical aspects of the robotic system. The team must be knowledgeable about the physical configuration of the system components. The perioperative nurse and scrub personnel need to be competent in assembly, disassembly, and proper shutdown of all equipment; in the calibration and configuration of the system; in troubleshooting the system; in draping the robotic arms, endoscope, and other related equipment; in docking the robot to the patient; in disconnecting the arms from the trocars; in removing instruments from the trocars; and in undocking and disconnecting the components of the system (Zender and Thell, 2010).

Three mobile carts house the components of the da Vinci surgical system. These include the surgeon's console, where the surgeon sits to control the robotic arms; the patient cart, which holds four robotic arms and a touch screen monitor; and the vision cart, which holds the camera control unit, light source, insufflator and electrosurgical unit (ESU). The vision cart may hold other laparoscopic accessory items as well.

Equipment used with the da Vinci system is specific to the system and includes a 0- and 3-degree high-definition endoscope system with three-dimensional technology; a camera, light cord, monopolar hook cautery, sterile drapes for the robotic arms, and special access ports designed to connect or dock with the robotic arms. The access ports come in three sizes: 8.5 mm for the endoscope, two 5-mm ports for the surgeon's instruments, and a 10-mm port for other instruments if needed. The "wristed" da Vinci instruments are unique in that they are capable of a wide range of motion

BOX 11-3

Robotics and Robotically Assisted Surgery: Advantages and Disadvantages

Advantages

- Binocular, three-dimensional real-time visual feedback
- High-definition technology
- Hand controls at surgeon's console are ergonomically positioned
- Scaled adjustment of movement allows for very fine precision dissection and suturing capabilities with no tremor
- Articulating robotic arms mimic full rotation of wrists giving surgeon better range of motion, dexterity, and control
- Stability of camera
- Four operating arms: one for an instrument in each of the surgeon's hands, one for the scope, and one for an assistant's instrument
- Surgeon sits at a console outside of the sterile field rather than stands
- Assistant and scrub person are in the sterile field
- The assistant may use an instrument to retract or provide suction, pass suture, pass clips as needed, or may exchange instruments

Disadvantages

- Large bulky equipment
- Limited field of view
- Surgeon not at the field; depends on someone else to insert instruments
- Increased distance from the field increases time delay in movement (more of a consideration for telesurgery across long distances)
- Initial cost of equipment
- Cost of yearly maintenance of equipment and software upgrades
- Increases the length of procedures
  - Setup time
  - Steep learning curve
- Requires specialized training and a dedicated surgical team
  - Calibration of instruments
  - Care and handling of instruments
- Emergent access to the abdomen takes more time due to the need to undock the robot

RESEARCH HIGHLIGHT

Assessing Patient Risk Factors Associated with Complications in Robotic Surgery

To identify risks related to robotic surgery, investigators at a large university hospital analyzed mortality and morbidity rates, rate and reason for conversion to an open procedure, reoperation rate, and average length of stay for 884 patients who had undergone general surgery robotic procedures.

Risk factors identified for morbidity and mortality were grouped in terms of the patient's condition, the degree of surgical stress or complexity of procedure, and quality of surgical performance, which included surgeon skill, experience of the surgical team, and volume of procedures performed.

Patient Risk Factors

- Cardiovascular disease
- Hypertension
- Renal comorbidities
- ASA score ≥3
- BMI <30
- Age ≥70
- Malignant disease

Procedure-Related Risk Factors

- Technically difficult, complex
- Location of procedure—multiquadrant surgery
- Intraoperative blood loss ≥500 mL
- Blood transfusion

ASA, American Society of Anesthesiologists; *BMI,* body mass index.
Modified from Buchs NC et al: Perioperative risk assessment in robotic general surgery, *Arch Surg* 147(8):701–708, 2012.

---

similar to that of the surgeon's wrist. An instrument set may include a Cadiere forceps, clip applier, curved dissecting scissors, Maryland dissector, various graspers, and needle holders for suturing.

Depending on the experience of the surgeon and the robotic team, robotic-assisted laparoscopic procedures can last for several hours. Individual patient risk factors are assessed (Research Highlight). During the procedure there is heightened awareness of increased risk for hypothermia, DVT, surgical site infection, pressure ulcers, and position-related injuries or complications. This is an important part of nursing care for patients undergoing longer robotic-assisted procedures (Zender and Thell, 2010).

Operative Procedure

1. The surgeon places access cannulae into the abdomen, using one of the techniques previously described for laparoscopy.
2. To calibrate the system and prepare for docking the arms to the access ports, the cart with the robotic arms is positioned over the patient with guidance from the surgeon.
3. The surgeon then "scrubs in," attaches the robotic arms to the trocars, and inserts the camera and instruments into the abdomen.

4. The surgeon leaves the sterile field to perform the planned procedure from the surgeon console.
5. A scrub person and a first assistant remain in the sterile field. The first assistant's role may include exchanging instruments for the surgeon, retracting tissues, instilling irrigation, suctioning, or cutting suture.

Natural Orifice Transluminal Endoscopic Surgery (NOTES)

NOTES appears to be a promising alternative approach for GI surgery in the future. When compared with open and laparoscopic techniques, the potential benefits of NOTES include no visible scars, possibly less pain, and potentially shorter hospital stays (Rieder and Swanstrom, 2011). Disadvantages are that the surgeon must open a closed viscera intentionally to access the abdomen; complications related to failure of that opening to heal after closure can result in peritonitis; and male gender limits the vaginal approach.

Procedural Considerations

Surgeons perform NOTES procedures by entering the abdominal cavity through an incision created in the wall of a natural orifice such as the stomach (peroral transgastric), rectum (transanal), or the vagina (transvaginal). Instruments are in development to overcome the challenges related to closing the defect created in the natural orifice to gain abdominal access.

Pure NOTES procedures are transluminal procedures performed using flexible endoscopes and instruments passed through the scopes' working channels. Many surgeons use a hybrid NOTES technique that combines laparoscopic visualization with natural orifice access.

Using a transvaginal hybrid NOTES technique, the surgeon inserts a 3- or 5-mm access port at the umbilicus to create a pneumoperitoneum (Garud and Willingham, 2012). The surgeon next inserts a rigid laparoscope into the abdominal access port to visualize entry of the vaginal access port from inside the abdomen and then moves the laparoscope to the vaginal access port. It is possible to insert a grasper through the umbilical port to use as a retractor to facilitate the NOTES procedure. GI procedures modified for a NOTES or hybrid NOTES approach include transvaginal appendectomy (Roberts et al, 2012); transgastric appendectomy; transvaginal and transgastric cholecystectomy; full-thickness resection of gastric cancer with laparoscopic lymph node dissection; percutaneous endoscopic gastrostomy (PEG) tube salvage; and transesophageal Heller myotomy (Rieder and Swanstrom, 2011).

Gastrointestinal Endoscopy

GI endoscopy permits visual inspection of the mucosal lining of the esophagus, stomach, duodenum, colon and rectum; its performance is for a wide range of screening, surveillance, diagnostic, and therapeutic procedures. Table 11-2 includes common therapeutic and diagnostic endoscopic procedures.

Performance of GI endoscopy is via flexible video endoscopes. Ancillary equipment includes a light source, suction, irrigation, air source, ESU, video processor, camera for photo documentation of findings, and a monitor (Ponsky and Pearl, 2012). Containers with saline for biopsy specimens and water-soluble lubricating jelly should also be available.

Flexible endoscopes are semicritical patient care devices that must undergo high-level disinfection before each use (see Chapter 4). They are easily damaged by misuse and must be cleaned, disinfected, and stored according to the manufacturer's recommendations. Flexible endoscopes vary in length and diameter, depending on intended use. Using wheeled knobs and buttons on the handle of the scope, the endoscopist can deflect the tip of the scope up and down, left and right, instill air or water, and activate suction. Diagnostic endoscopes can be as small as 9 mm. For planned therapeutic procedures, the endoscope will have a larger diameter to accommodate the working channel through which endoscopic instruments pass. Specialized endoscopes with over tubes and balloons enable examination of the small bowel. Because instrumentation for endoscopic procedures may penetrate the intestinal mucosa, instruments are considered critical devices that must be sterilized before each use.

Endoscopy instruments and accessories include cytology brushes, snares, biopsy forceps, specimen retrieval nets, long-needle injection/aspiration catheters, and hydrostatic balloons. Instruments for hemostasis may include appliers for clips, bands, and loops; monopolar or bipolar electrocoagulation probes; and argon plasma coagulation probes. Radiofrequency ablation balloons, removable stents, and permanent stents may also be necessary for some therapeutic procedures.

Pre-procedure preparation for EGD (sometimes called "upper GI endoscopy") includes limiting ingestion of solid foods and liquids for prescribed periods before the procedure. Preparation for colonoscopy may include preprocedure limitation of oral intake, as well as bowel cleansing preparations and enemas (Ponsky and Pearl, 2012).

Endoscopic procedures most commonly occur with moderate sedation/analgesia to ensure patient comfort, cooperation, and a safe and complete examination. Medications and safety measures for moderate sedation appear in Chapter 5. Monitoring the patient's airway, vital signs, oxygenation, level of consciousness, and comfort continues throughout the procedure and postprocedure recovery.

Esophagogastroduodenoscopy

Procedural Considerations. Esophagogastroduodenoscopy (EGD) affords visualization of the oropharynx, esophagus, stomach, and

TABLE 11-2

Endoscopic Procedures

Procedure	Indications (Diagnostic/Screening/Surveillance)	Indications (Therapeutic)
Esophagogastroduodenoscopy	• Abnormal upper GI x-ray • Upper GI bleeding • Dysphasia • Persistent heartburn • Persistent epigastric pain • Persistent vomiting • GERD • Odynophagia • Pyrosis • Ingestion of caustic substance • Gastric polyposis • Surveillance (Barrett's esophagus, gastric ulcers)	• Endoscopic mucosal resection (EMR) • Endoscopic submucosal dissection (ESD) • Foreign body retrieval • Sclerosing of esophageal varices • Stricture dilation • Ablation of tumors • Palliative stenting of tumors • Control of bleeding • Placement of percutaneous endoscopic gastrostomy (PEG) tube • Polypectomy • Radiofrequency ablation (RFA) • Endoscopic 270-degree fundoplication
Colonoscopy	• Screening (cancer) • Diagnosis (inflammatory colitis) • Surveillance (ulcerative colitis) • GI bleeding	• Polypectomy • Decompression • Hydrostatic balloon dilatation of strictures • Palliative dilation of obstructions with self-expanding metal stents • Detorsion of volvulus

GERD, Gastroesophageal reflux disease; *GI,* gastrointestinal.

proximal duodenum. The procedure begins with the patient in left lateral decubitus position with neck flexed forward (Greenwald and Cohen, 2012). To enhance passage of the endoscope for better visualization, the endoscopist may direct or use other positions such as supine, semi-Fowler, or sitting.

Procedure

1. The endoscopist or anesthesia provider may anesthetize the posterior pharynx with a topical agent such as benzocaine spray or gel.
2. A bite-block, positioned over the shaft of the endoscope and placed between the patient's upper and lower teeth, prevents the patient from accidentally biting down on the shaft of the endoscope during the procedure.
3. The endoscopist gently advances the tip of the lubricated gastroscope through the mouth and esophagus, and into the stomach and duodenum.
4. Visual inspection of the target organ follows.
5. Biopsies or brushings are obtained as needed; safe specimen handling practices are initiated (see Chapter 2).
6. Indicated therapeutic procedures follow.
7. While visualizing the mucosa, the endoscopist slowly withdraws the endoscope.
8. Once the patient's gag reflex returns, the patient is moved to a monitoring area and offered fluids.

Deep Small Bowel Enteroscopy

Procedural Considerations. The small bowel can be difficult to view endoscopically due to its length and contractility. Although video capsule endoscopy (discussed below) allows for visualization of the small bowel, therapeutic procedures cannot follow. Double balloon enteroscopy (DBE) is a technique that provides both visualization and the capability to perform therapeutic procedures in the small bowel (Kita, 2012). Other techniques include single balloon enteroscopy and spiral enteroscopy. Before the procedure patients receive instruction to fast after midnight the day of the procedure. They must also undergo a bowel prep to empty the colon. DBE commences from the mouth or the anus, or both, depending on the location of the suspected lesion. Due to longer procedure times, general anesthesia is frequently used for the oral approach (Kita, 2012).

Procedure

1. The balloon-tipped endoscope inserts (back-loaded) through a soft overtube, which also has a balloon.
2. The endoscope inserts orally, through the esophagus and stomach, into the duodenum.
3. When the scope will not advance any more, the operator inflates the balloon on the endoscope.
4. The overtube advances over the endoscope to the first balloon, and the balloon on the overtube inflates.
5. With both balloons inflated, the operator withdraws the endoscope slightly to pleat the small bowel on the overtube, providing a straight pathway to advance the endoscope.
6. After deflating the endoscope balloon, the operator advances the scope.
7. The cycles of inflation and deflation, and advancement and withdrawal, repeat until the endoscope cannot advance farther.
8. The team marks the most distal location reached by the scope with a tattoo for later identification with capsule endoscopy.
9. The process reverses as the operator withdraws the scope.

Capsule Endoscopy

Procedural Considerations. Capsule endoscopy is a noninvasive diagnostic test that uses a small wireless camera in the shape of a capsule about the size of a large vitamin. It is swallowed with a few sips of water and propelled along the GI tract by normal peristalsis. The capsule glides down the esophagus, taking two color digital pictures per second, which it transmits to a recording device worn by the patient. This device is suitable for imaging the mucosal surface of the esophagus, stomach, and small intestine. The battery power of the capsule lasts about 8 hours. The capsule eventually passes naturally within 24 to 72 hours. The wireless capsule dramatically enhances the ability to visualize the mucosal surface of the small intestine. The small bowel, about 90% of the mucosal surface of the entire GI tract, formerly suffered constraints within the limits of traditional diagnostic modalities.

The only preparation for capsule endoscopy is an 8-hour fast. Contraindications to the procedure include inability to swallow a large capsule; small bowel strictures, narrowing, or fistulas; swallowing disorders; suspected intestinal obstruction; and pacemakers. Patient instructions include no MRI for at least 30 days to ensure that the capsule has passed and therefore cannot cause internal thermal injury. All reports and images of capsule endoscopy results should be available at the time of any surgery (Cave, 2012).

Colonoscopy

Procedural Considerations. Colonoscopy provides endoscopic visualization of the colon from the rectum to the ileocecal valve. The clinician inspects the mucosa for abnormalities such as sites of bleeding, polyps, inflammation, ulceration, or tumors during both insertion and withdrawal of the colonoscope. Colonoscopy can be diagnostic and therapeutic (see Table 11-2). Performance of colonoscopy also is possible through an ostomy stoma to inspect an anastomosis site or identify recurrence of disease or bleeding. Likewise, reservoir pouches can undergo inspection postoperatively for anastomosis integrity, inflammation, bleeding, and other abnormalities. Tattooing lesions found during colonoscopy that will require surgical removal is common. Such tattooing assists with localization of the lesion during a later operative procedure. However, an intraoperative colonoscopy may be necessary to verify location of a colon lesion that is difficult to identify otherwise.

Procedure. Positioning of the patient is on the left side with knees bent. The operator passes a well-lubricated colonoscope slowly into the anal canal and advances it continually until it reaches the cecum. The endoscopist or surgeon may ask for a repositioning of the patient to prone position or may ask the perioperative or endoscopy nurse to apply gentle abdominal pressure or to lift the patient's left side to assist advancement of the scope. With sigmoidoscopy, examination extends only to the left colon. Flexible sigmoidoscopy is achievable without sedation with a cooperative patient. After endoscopic examination, the patient is observed for bleeding, pain, signs of perforation, or reaction to medications.

Endoscopic Ultrasound

Endoscopic ultrasound (EUS) combines endoscopy and ultrasound, using sound waves to generate an image of the histologic layers of the esophageal, gastric, and intestinal walls. EUS is critically important in staging GI malignancies and determining surgical options and potential for therapeutic resection. The frequencies used, higher than those used in traditional ultrasound, provide highly accurate depths of any mucosal invasion. Endoscopic image-enhancement techniques include high-resolution endoscopes with narrow-band imaging and magnification to identify mucosal surface details; narrow-band filters to see capillary patterns, pits, and villi; and chromoendoscopy (staining techniques) and fluorescence to differentiate between normal and dysplastic tissue.

Endoscopic Procedures for Gastroesophageal Reflux Disease

Gastroesophageal reflux disease (GERD) is a condition in which the LES is incompetent and allows stomach contents to reflux into the esophagus. GERD symptoms include heartburn, regurgitation, and dysphagia. Less common GERD-related symptoms include chest pain, hypersalivation, and painful swallowing.

Complications of GERD are esophagitis and Barrett's esophagus (BE) due to repeated or prolonged exposure to gastric acid. Endoscopic procedures to treat GERD by improving the gastroesophageal flap valve, improving function of the LES, or tightening the tissue at the gastroesophageal (GE) junction are available for patients who are unresponsive to or cannot take GERD medications, or who do not wish to have a surgical procedure.

Endoscopic procedures to treat GERD include radiofrequency ablation, intraluminal endoscopic sewing devices, transmural fasteners, and staplers. The Stretta (Mederi Therapeutics, Greenwich, CT) procedure delivers controlled amounts of radiofrequency heat energy through a balloon catheter positioned endoscopically in the distal esophagus, creating thermal lesions that tighten the tissue at the lower esophageal sphincter (Nikfarjam and Ponsky, 2011) (Ambulatory Surgery Considerations).

The EndoCinch (C.R. Bard, Inc.) device endoscopically places sutures in mucosal folds at a location distal to the "Z" line of the GE junction. The EsophyX technique (EndoGastric Solutions) endoscopically creates a 260-degree internal plication of the gastric fundus to create a neogastroesophageal valve. The SRS endoscopic stapling system staples the gastric fundus to the esophagus to create a neogastroesophageal flap valve (Rothstein and Swain, 2012).

Endoscopic Procedures for Barrett's Esophagus

BE entails the presence of metaplastic changes to the cells lining the esophagus as a result of chronic exposure to gastric acid. BE can progress to dysplasia, or precancerous changes, increasing the risk of the development of adenocarcinoma of the esophagus. The goal of the treatment for BE is to prevent progression to dysplasia by minimizing or eliminating acid reflux through diet, lifestyle changes, and antireflux medications. When BE progresses to a high-grade dysplasia, endoscopic treatment options include radiofrequency ablation (RFA), endoscopic mucosal resection (EMR), and photodynamic therapy.

Radiofrequency Ablation. Radiofrequency ablation (RFA) of BE involves application of radiofrequency (RF) energy to the abnormal cells using the HALO 360 or HALO 90 systems by the Covidien subsidiary, BÂRRX Medical. The HALO 360 system consists of a generator, a guidewire, a sizing catheter with a 4-cm-long balloon used to measure the inner diameter of the esophagus, and various sizes (18, 22, 25, 28, 31 mm) of HALO 360+ ablation catheters. The ablation catheters are 165 cm long, with a balloon tip that contains a bipolar electrode with 60 tightly coiled electrode rings that wrap around the balloon. The clinician introduces the appropriately sized ablation catheter, inflates the balloon, applies RF energy, repositions the balloon and endoscope, and repeats the process along the length of abnormal tissue. The clinician then

---

The Stretta Procedure

When medications used to treat symptoms of gastroesophageal reflux disease (GERD) are not effective, or when side effects or the cost of long-term use of these medications becomes a problem, a new option for patients is to have a radiofrequency (RF) treatment for GERD, also known as the Stretta procedure. The following is information the nurse may offer the patient:

The Stretta procedure is an ambulatory surgery procedure. Your experience will be very similar to the upper GI endoscopy you have already had as part of your preoperative testing. Before the procedure begins, a nurse will apply monitoring devices and start an IV. You will be given medication to sedate you. Your throat will be numbed with a special spray. When you are ready, the doctor will insert a flexible scope through your mouth and down your throat to look inside your esophagus, or swallowing tube. The scope does not interfere with your ability to breathe. After the doctor takes measurements, the scope will be removed and replaced with a special endoscopic instrument that will be used to apply a controlled amount of RF energy to the lower end of your esophagus. The RF energy produces heat that will cause a superficial burnlike reaction of the tissue. When it heals, the scarring of the tissue helps the barrier in the lower esophagus prevent acid reflux from your stomach. You may feel a little discomfort during the application of the RF energy, but the medication should help with that. Let the doctor or nurse know if you are too uncomfortable.

Instructions
- Do not eat or drink anything for at least 8 hours before you arrive.
- Wear comfortable clothing.
- Leave your valuables at home.
- You will be sedated so you will need an adult to drive you home. Do not drive or operate heavy equipment for at least 24 hours after your procedure.
- The procedure will take about 1 hour.
- You may have a mild sore throat after the procedure. Drink liquids and eat soft foods until the soreness goes away.
- You can expect to return to normal activity and diet the day after the procedure.
- Contact your doctor immediately if you have severe throat pain, shortness of breath, cough or spit up blood, have a fever, or continue to feel sedated after 24 hours.

Modified from Triadafilopoulos G: Radiofrequency treatment for gastroesophageal reflux disease (the Stretta procedure). In Basow DS, editor: *UpToDate*, Waltham, MA, UpToDate, 2012; Stretta Procedure: *Patient education, ExitCare patient information*, 2012, ExitCare, LLC, accessed March 29, 2013 from www.mdconsult.com/das/patient/body/385222491-3/1385502358/10089/57317.html; Upper GI Endoscopy: *Patient education, ExitCare patient information*, 2012, ExitCare, LLC, accessed March 29, 2013 from www.mdconsult.com/das/patient/body/385222491-8/1385509719/10089/56129.html

---

removes the ablation catheter, cleans the electrode, irrigates and cleans the esophagus, and repeats the process. After 12 weeks, if residual abnormal tissue remains, repetition of the original procedure is possible or small focal ablation can follow with the HALO 90 electrode, which has a flat panel electrode to apply RF energy to smaller areas than the HALO 360+ electrode (Bergman, 2012).

Endoscopic Mucosal Resection. Endoscopic mucosal resection (EMR) is the excision of dysplastic lesions related to BE.

Prior to EMR, endoscopic ultrasound may help determine the depth of invasion into the esophageal wall. The lesion or dysplastic tissue receives injected saline to separate the superficial mucosa from deeper submucosal and muscular layers. Separation of these tissue planes facilitates snare resection. Using suction attached to the endoscope, the clinician pulls the elevated lesion into a cap secured to the end of the scope and resects it with a rigid wire snare. This technique offers the added advantage of submitting a tissue specimen for histologic examination (Bergman, 2012).

Photodynamic Therapy. Photodynamic therapy (PDT) is a laser ablation technique. Dysplastic tissue uptakes a photosensitizer drug, Photofrin II (sodium porfimer), activated by the laser. IV administration of the drug occurs 48 hours before the procedure to allow for tissue uptake. Normal tissue excretes the drug sooner than abnormal or dysplastic tissues. The mucosal layer retains the drug, limiting the depth of the laser effect. After 48 hours the procedure commences. The clinician introduces the laser fiber through the endoscope channel and directs laser light toward the mucosa, causing tissue destruction and cell death of those areas identified by the uptake of the photosensitizer drug. The patient may continue to be light sensitive for 60 to 90 days after the injection and must take precautions to prevent cutaneous burns. Unlike EMR, PDT does not provide a tissue specimen. Clinicians often combine PDT with endoscopic resection.

Percutaneous Endoscopic Gastrostomy Tube Insertion

A percutaneous endoscopic gastrostomy (PEG) procedure involves percutaneous insertion of a uniquely designed gastrostomy tube into the stomach under endoscopic visualization. A PEG tube provides a means to provide enteral feedings to patients unable to ingest food orally, but who have a normally functioning GI tract. This procedure may occur in the endoscopy suite under IV sedation/analgesia or in the OR under general anesthesia in conjunction with another surgical procedure.

Procedural Considerations. Supplies include a prepackaged PEG tube kit. The contents of the kit vary depending on the technique used. Three techniques are the pull method (Ponsky technique), push method (Sacks-Vine technique), and the sheath method (Russell technique, which is rarely used and not described). Kits for the Ponsky and Sacks-Vine techniques contain a knife handle with a #11 blade, a 14- to 18-gauge trocar needle, a long silk suture, a guidewire, a gastrostomy tube, and a skin disk to secure the tube to the skin. A gastroscopy setup with a flexible scope, a wire snare, light source, air source, suction, and monitor are required. This procedure requires an endoscopist and an assistant. The patient is positioned supine. The monitor is positioned so that the endoscopist/surgeon and assistant can see it during tube insertion. The abdomen is prepped and preoperative antibiotics administered. If the patient is awake, a bite-block is inserted into the patient's mouth.

Procedure (Ponsky Technique)

1. The gastroscope is inserted and advanced into the fundus of the stomach. Insufflation of the stomach with air through the gastroscope follows. The flexible tip of the scope is angled anteriorly to provide transillumination through the anterior stomach and abdominal wall. Using transillumination, the physician confirms there are no abdominal viscera between the stomach and the anterior abdominal wall.
2. The physician injects local anesthetic at the site of the intended gastrostomy site if the patient is awake.
3. The physician then makes a small stab wound with a #11 blade.

4. As the 14- to 18-gauge trocar needle inserts through the abdominal wall and the anterior wall of the stomach, entry of the needle into the stomach is visualized with the gastroscope.
5. The long silk suture passes through the trocar needle into the stomach, where a wire snare that has been passed through the working channel of the gastroscope entraps it.
6. After removal of the trocar needle, a hemostat is clamped to the end of the suture that remains outside the abdomen.
7. The gastroscope and snare are removed together, pulling the suture out of the patient's mouth.
8. The suture is attached to the tapered distal end of the gastrostomy tube and then guided into the patient's oral cavity, down the esophagus and into the stomach, and pulled out through the abdominal wall.
9. Reinsertion of the gastroscope follows to confirm correct positioning of the feeding tube.
10. The gastrostomy tube is secured in place against the abdominal wall using the disk.
11. The distal end of the tube is plugged, the stomach deflated, and the procedure ends.

Procedure (Sacks-Vine Technique). Steps 1 through 4 are identical to the Ponsky technique (the pull method) just described. Instead of passing a long silk suture as mentioned in step 5, a guidewire is passed, ensnared, and pulled through the mouth where a feeding tube threads over the guidewire and then is "pushed" through the mouth, into the stomach, and through the skin, where the assistant grabs the feeding tube as it exits. The remainder of the procedure is the same as the pull method.

Surgery of the Esophagus

Esophagectomy

Esophagectomy is indicated for cancer, dysplastic mucosal changes, and stricture of the esophagus due to injury or benign disease. Most malignant tumors of the esophagus and gastroesophageal junction (GEJ) are squamous cell carcinoma (SSC) or adenocarcinoma (Saltzman and Gibson, 2012). Adenocarcinoma has steadily increased in prevalence over the past few decades. It occurs at the GEJ and is associated with BE, GERD, obesity, and smoking (Swanson, 2012).

Determination of the treatment and prognosis for patients with esophageal cancer is based on the cancer cell type, tumor location, depth of invasion, involvement of lymph nodes or spread to other structures, and overall physical condition of the patient. Preoperative evaluation involves many medical disciplines and often includes endoscopic examination and biopsy, endoscopic ultrasound, and a PET scan with or without CT scan to assess for metastasis. Patients may also undergo diagnostic laparoscopy, thoracoscopy, mediastinoscopy, or bronchoscopy before proceeding with esophagectomy (Saltzman and Gibson, 2012). Some patients receive chemotherapy and radiation prior to esophagectomy.

The approach to esophagectomy depends on location and size of the tumor in the esophagus, the extent of planned lymph node dissection, the type of conduit used to replace the esophagus, and surgeon preference. Open approaches include transhiatal esophagectomy (THE), transthoracic esophagectomy (TTE or Ivor Lewis), and en bloc, or "tri-incisional" esophagectomy.

Reestablishing continuity of the GI tract after esophagectomy occurs by performing an anastomosis between the proximal esophagus and a variety of esophageal replacement conduits. The surgeon can create the anastomosis through a cervical incision or a chest incision; its location depends on location of the esophageal tumor and the approach used for esophagectomy. The anastomosis is either hand sewn or endostapled. A cervical anastomosis requires linear cutting staplers, whereas a thoracic anastomosis requires an end-to-end or circular stapling device. The most common conduit to replace the transected esophagus is the stomach. Other conduits include the jejunum and colon, both of which may require microvascular anastomosis. Additional supplies such as microvascular instruments, a microscope, and related supplies are then required.

Procedural Considerations. Instrumentation includes a thoracotomy set, laparotomy set, long and short vascular instruments, GI instruments, long versions of basic instruments, deep retractors, self-retaining abdominal and rib retractors, linear and circular stapling devices, and long vascular ligating clip appliers and clips in a variety of sizes. Additional supplies to have available include short and long silk sutures and ties in a variety of diameters according to surgeon preference; one or two long ½- or 1-inch Penrose drains, one or two chest tubes (sized according to surgeon preference) with appropriate 5/1 connector(s) and a closed chest drainage system; and a closed suction drain(s) with suction bulb(s). If planning for resection of cervical esophageal cancer, instruments and supplies for pharyngectomy, laryngectomy, thyroidectomy, neck dissection, and tracheostomy should be available as well.

Minimally invasive esophagectomy (MIE) requires laparoscopic and thoracoscopic instruments, video and insufflation equipment, and energy sources. If the surgeon plans to perform an EGD, a mediastinoscopy, or a bronchoscopy immediately before the procedure, additional equipment is necessary. Postoperatively, patients are NPO for an extended time while the esophagogastric anastomosis heals. Additional supplies, therefore, for insertion of a feeding jejunostomy should be available in the OR.

Esophagectomy requires general anesthesia with endotracheal intubation. A double-lumen endotracheal tube provides the option for single-lung ventilation if thoracic exposure is needed. A radial artery catheter for blood pressure monitoring is inserted as is an indwelling urinary catheter. The patient's position on the OR bed depends on the planned surgical approach. Appropriate measures to prevent hypothermia and pressure ulcers are initiated.

If needed, a pathologist renders intraoperative histologic confirmation of tumor-free margins. An intraoperative EGD may be done to confirm location of the tumor. A thoracic epidural or interscalene perineural blockade can augment postoperative pain management. Patients undergoing esophagectomy may transfer to the intensive care unit (ICU) after surgery.

Transhiatal Esophagectomy

The transhiatal approach requires an upper midline abdominal incision and an incision in the left neck. The preferred left-side-of-the-neck approach decreases the risk of injury to the recurrent laryngeal nerve, because it descends and recurs lower, around the aortic arch rather than the subclavian artery as it does on the right side (Loran and Zwischenberger, 2010).

Operative Procedure

1. The patient is supine. Skin prep includes the neck, chest, and abdomen.
2. The surgeon makes an upper midline incision, extends it cephalad to the xiphoid process, and explores the abdomen, after

which a self-retaining retractor is positioned. Removal of the xiphoid process may achieve better access to the hiatus.
3. The liver is retracted to the right and the stomach mobilized to expose the esophageal hiatus. A Penrose drain encircles the esophagus for manipulation and retraction.
4. Performance of a pyloromyotomy facilitates postoperative gastric drainage into the duodenum.
5. The esophageal hiatus is enlarged, facilitating mobilization of the thoracic esophagus.
6. The surgeon makes a left neck incision just above the clavicle and exposes the cervical esophagus, taking care not to injure the recurrent laryngeal nerve with excessive lateral retraction.
7. A second Penrose drain is passed around the cervical esophagus, and mobilization of the cervical and upper thoracic esophagus using blunt finger dissection follows.
8. The cervical esophagus is divided with a linear stapler; it is then pulled through the mediastinum into the abdomen.
9. A linear cutting stapler is used to resect the esophagus, cardia, and part of the lesser curve of the stomach. This "tubularizes" the stomach, preparing it for the cervical esophagogastric anastomosis.
10. The stomach "tube" is pulled through the esophageal hiatus and posterior mediastinum into the neck.
11. Closure of the crura is with interrupted 2-0 nonabsorbable sutures; fixation of the stomach to the diaphragm is with a 3-0 silk suture.
12. A feeding jejunostomy tube is placed.
13. The anastomosis between the stomach and cervical esophagus is created through the neck incision.
14. Closure of the abdomen is with a running 0 polydioxanone (PDS) suture; skin closure is with staples.
15. A second stab incision is made and a closed suction drain (Jackson-Pratt) placed in the neck wound.
16. Closure of the neck incision in two layers follows, according to surgeon preference.
17. A chest x-ray taken in the OR ensures there is no pneumothorax or hemothorax.

Transthoracic Esophagectomy—Ivor Lewis

The TTE entails both an upper midline abdominal incision and a right thoracotomy incision. If the surgeon performs the procedure in one stage, the patient is in supine position with a roll under the torso on the side of the planned thoracotomy. Elevation of the arm on the side of the thoracotomy can be on an over armboard, draped out of the surgical field, or the arm may be prepped and draped into the surgical field. The neck, chest, and abdomen are prepped.

Alternatively, for a two-stage technique, patient placement position is supine for the abdominal portion of the procedure and then repositioned on the left side for the thoracic portion. Before repositioning, the abdomen is closed and dressed. Positioning aids (beanbag, over armboard, etc.) and supplies for reprepping and redraping are available.

Operative Procedure

1. The surgeon makes an upper midline abdominal incision, retractors are positioned, and mobilization of the stomach follows, as described above for the transhiatal approach.
2. The surgeon next makes a separate thoracotomy incision in the sixth or seventh intercostal space on the intended side. The anesthesia provider may clamp the double-lumen endotracheal

tube on the affected side to deflate the lung for better visualization. Gentle retraction of the lung with a handheld retractor exposes the pleura overlying the esophagus. The surgeon lifts and incises the pleura over the esophagus.

3. A long Penrose drain encircles the esophagus for manipulation. Mobilization of the esophagus is circumferential, proximal, and distal to the tumor, ensuring tumor resection achieves clear margins.

4. Transection of the esophagus is proximal to the tumor, using a linear cutting stapling device.

5. The surgeon pulls the previously mobilized stomach into the chest through the esophageal hiatus of the diaphragm and fires a linear cutting stapling device across the proximal fundus and cardia of the stomach to complete the esophageal resection.

6. To reconnect the proximal esophagus to the stomach, placement of the anvil of a circular stapling device such as an EEA is in the proximal esophagus. The EEA stapler inserts into the stomach and connects to the anvil through an opening made in the stomach. Firing of the stapler follows and the anastomosis between the remaining esophagus and stomach is complete. Closure of the opening in the stomach is with nonabsorbable suture. Alternatively, the surgeon may hand sew the end-to-end anastomosis between the proximal esophagus and stomach in two layers, using interrupted 3-0 nonabsorbable sutures.

7. To decrease tension on the staple line of the anastomosis, the stomach can be tacked to the prevertebral fascia and to the esophageal hiatus with interrupted 3-0 nonabsorbable sutures.

8. A 36-French (F) chest tube is inserted through a separate stab wound and the thoracotomy incision closed in layers, according to surgeon preference.

9. Closure of the abdominal incision is as described above for the transhiatal approach.

En Bloc (Tri-incisional) Esophagectomy

This technique is the most radical approach to esophagectomy.

Operative Procedure

1. Through a right thoracotomy, the surgeon removes the esophagus and surrounding healthy tissues en bloc. The venous and lymphatic vessels are also ligated, divided, and removed with the specimen. Radical thoracic and mediastinum lymph node dissection follows.

2. Through an upper midline incision, stomach mobilization through the abdominal incision is as described in the transhiatal approach, and a radical upper abdominal lymph node dissection follows.

3. Preparation of the gastric conduit is as previously described; its delivery to the neck is through the posterior mediastinal space.

4. The surgeon creates a cervical esophagogastric anastomosis through the neck incision (Maish, 2010; Swanson, 2012).

5. The incision is closed and dressings applied.

Minimally Invasive Esophagectomy

Minimally invasive modifications to open esophagectomy are common (Maish, 2010). Any of these procedures may also occur with robotic assistance. Team communication regarding the intended approach for esophagectomy is an essential part of preoperative planning, should be discussed either during the briefing or time-out, and ensures that all necessary equipment and supplies will be readily available.

Laparoscopic Esophageal Myotomy (Modified Heller Myotomy)

Esophageal myotomy treats achalasia, a condition in which degeneration of the nerves to the lower esophagus results in inability of the LES to relax with swallowing. Normally the LES, a circular band of muscle encircling the esophagus, relaxes to allow ingested food and liquids to pass into the stomach. After swallowing, the LES contracts to prevent gastric reflux into the esophagus. Patients with achalasia have difficulty swallowing because the LES is in a state of constant contraction. Over time, the peristaltic function of the esophagus may decrease and the proximal esophagus becomes dilated. Due to prolonged mucosal irritation of the esophagus, untreated achalasia increases the risk of esophageal cancer. Symptoms include difficulty swallowing, regurgitation of undigested food and liquids, heartburn, difficulty burping, hiccups, choking after meals, nighttime cough, and weight loss (Maish, 2010). Achalasia is not curable, but esophageal myotomy can alleviate its symptoms. The goal of myotomy is to relieve the obstruction caused by the contracted LES while preventing postoperative gastric reflux, scarring, and subsequent stricture (Spechler, 2012).

The most common approach to esophageal myotomy is the laparoscopic modified Heller myotomy combined with partial gastric fundoplication to prevent gastric reflux (Eakin and Melvin, 2011).

Procedural Considerations.
The procedure requires general anesthesia with endotracheal intubation. The patient is in modified lithotomy or split-leg position. The OR bed will be in a steep reverse Trendelenburg position. Setup includes standard laparoscopy equipment, instruments, and supplies. The surgical team will use five access ports: two ports are for the surgeon, the third port is for the 30-degree laparoscope, the fourth is for a liver retractor, and the fifth is for the first assistant to use. Laparoscopic instruments include fine curved or right-angled dissectors, a hook dissector, clip appliers, liver retractor, atraumatic graspers or Babcock, ultrasonic shears, needle holders, and suture to close the crura and perform the antireflux procedure.

Use of intraoperative gastric endoscopy is common to confirm location of the Z-line at the GEJ and to inspect for unintended perforations of the mucosa. A flexible gastroscope, light source, video camera and monitor, suction, air source, and other related equipment are ready on a separate nonsterile table or cart.

Operative Procedure—Laparoscopic Technique

1. Abdominal access is obtained according to surgeon preference, and pneumoperitoneum then established.

2. Insertion of the liver retractor to retract the left lobe of the liver follows.

3. The surgeon identifies the right and left crura and opens the retroesophageal space.

4. A Penrose drain passes around the esophagus and its ends are secured together. The Penrose drain is used to manipulate the esophagus during mobilization.

5. Using blunt dissection, the distal esophagus is mobilized circumferentially.

6. A curved dissector is used to develop the plane between the esophageal mucosa and the inner muscular layer. A hook dissector can be used to divide the muscle. The myotomy begins about 2 cm proximal to the GEJ, extends proximally for about 8 cm, and then extends distally to a point approximately 2 to 3 cm below the GEJ on the anterior stomach.

7. Endoscopy is performed.
8. The antireflux procedure follows.
9. Instruments and access ports are removed and the incision closed according to surgeon preference.

Excision of Pharyngoesophageal (Zenker) Diverticulum

Pharyngoesophageal diverticula are the most common type of esophageal diverticula (Maish, 2010). Zenker diverticulum is considered "false diverticulum" because it involves only two layers of the esophageal wall, the mucosa and submucosa. Zenker diverticula herniate through the thyropharyngeus and cricopharyngeus muscles, forming a sac where food can lodge. As the diverticulum enlarges, symptoms develop: a persistent cough, excessive salivation, regurgitation of undigested food, halitosis, voice changes, retrosternal pain, and intermittent dysphasia. Repair of Zenker diverticulum occurs through an incision in the neck or endoscopically.

Procedural Considerations. Instrumentation includes a thyroid set with fine dissecting hemostats, 5-inch Adson or other fine-toothed forceps, and lateral retractors. The procedure requires general anesthesia or a cervical block. Positioning of the patient is supine with a shoulder roll to extend the neck. The head may be turned away from the operative side. Skin prep extends from the mandible to the nipples and includes the neck and anterior chest. If using an alcohol-based prep solution, team members assess fire risk and take appropriate action to prevent surgical fires. Results of a preoperative barium esophagram can confirm location of the diverticulum (or diverticula, if there is more than one).

Operative Procedure

1. The surgeon makes a vertical incision parallel to the inner border of the sternocleidomastoid muscle (SCM), between the level of the hyoid bone and a point 2 cm above the clavicle; an alternative is a transverse incision centered over the middle third of the SCM.
2. Handheld retractors are used to retract the SCM and carotid sheath laterally and the thyroid gland and larynx medially. Care is taken to not stretch the recurrent laryngeal nerve with excessive medial retraction. The surgeon may divide the omohyoid muscle with electrosurgery or retract it superiorly to expose the diverticulum.
3. The sac of the diverticulum is grasped with an Allis clamp and dissected from surrounding tissue. The anesthesia provider then may insert an esophageal dilator into the esophagus.
4. Performance of an 8- to 10-cm esophageal myotomy above and below the extruding diverticulum follows to expose its base.
5. If larger than 2 cm, resection of the diverticulum follows. Resection can be with a linear cutting and stapling device or with a scalpel, followed by closure of the mucosal defect with a running 4-0 absorbable suture.
6. Removal of the esophageal dilator is next and an NG tube replaces it. Saline is poured into the wound and a small amount of air instilled through the NG tube to test the staple line or suture closure for any leaks.
7. A closed suction drain is placed in the wound through a separate stab incision.
8. After removal of the retractors, closure of the platysma is done with interrupted stitches using a 4-0 absorbable suture.
9. Closure of the skin follows according to surgeon preference, and a nonabsorbable suture secures the drain to the skin. Dressings are applied.

Paraesophageal Hiatal Hernia Repair

The esophageal hiatus is the opening in the diaphragm through which the esophagus enters the abdominal cavity. Normally the phrenoesophageal membrane anchors the distal esophagus and the GEJ to the diaphragm. With a type I, or "sliding," hiatal hernia, widening of the esophageal hiatus and relaxation of the phreno-esophageal membrane allows the GEJ to migrate into the thoracic cavity, often resulting in the development of GERD. Types II, III, and IV hiatal hernias are "paraesophageal" hiatal hernias, which have a true hernia sac. In type II hernias, the GEJ remains fixed in its abdominal position while the fundus of the stomach migrates into the chest next to the esophagus through a localized defect in the phrenoesophageal membrane. As the defect enlarges, more of the stomach moves into the thoracic cavity, rotating around the fixed GEJ. Type II paraesophageal hernias progress to type III hernias as the hernia defect continues to enlarge and the GEJ itself begins to migrate into the chest along with the rest of the stomach. When other organs such as the colon, spleen, pancreas, and small bowel enter the hernia sac, the paraesophageal hiatal hernia becomes a type IV hiatal hernia.

Symptoms of hiatal hernia may include epigastric or chest pain, heartburn, chronic cough, regurgitation of undigested food, dysphasia, early satiety, vomiting, aspiration, and iron deficiency anemia. Possible complications of paraesophageal hiatal hernias include esophageal reflux gastritis; gastric ulceration; gastric volvulus with risk of strangulation, necrosis, and perforation; gastric outlet obstruction; hemorrhage; and pneumonia.

Surgical repair can be via laparotomy, thoracotomy, or laparoscopy. Some surgeons reserve an open approach for patients who have had previous abdominal surgeries and a thoracotomy approach when an open abdominal approach has failed (Rosen and Blatnik, 2012).

Procedural Considerations. For an open abdominal approach, instrumentation and supplies include the following: a laparotomy set; long instruments, a self-retaining retractor; and a long ½- to 1-inch Penrose drain. Thoracic instruments should also be available if an open thoracic approach is possible. The laparoscopic approach is the most common technique and is described below.

Basic laparoscopy instruments and video equipment are needed. Additional laparoscopic instruments include a 30-degree laparoscope, two Babcock graspers, clip applier, ultrasonic shears, fan liver retractor, and a laparoscopic needle holder and knot pusher or other suturing device. Nonabsorbable suture is required to close the diaphragmatic defect and perform the fundoplication. Specialized long suture is needed for extracorporeal tying with a knot pusher and standard 18-inch suture is used for intracorporeal tying techniques.

This procedure requires general anesthesia. Arrangement of Bougie or Maloney esophageal dilators in a variety of sizes (32F to 60F) is in ascending order on a nonsterile table for the anesthesia provider to insert during the procedure. Ensure water-soluble lubricant is on the table to facilitate passage of the dilators. Stomach decompression with an NG tube may be needed as may be insertion of a urinary bladder catheter. Patient placement is in supine or low modified lithotomy position, depending on surgeon preference. Arms may be padded and tucked at the patient's sides if necessary. The abdomen is prepped from nipple line to the pubic symphysis.

Operative Procedure—Laparoscopic Approach

1. Abdominal access and establishment of pneumoperitoneum depend on surgeon preference.

2. Retraction of the left lobe of the liver exposes the esophageal hiatus.

3. The surgeon gently reduces the hernia sac and stomach, opens the hernia sac, dissects it free, and excises it.

4. A Penrose drain passes behind and around the distal esophagus, enabling manipulation of the esophagus during dissection.

5. Using laparoscopic Babcock graspers or other nontraumatic graspers, the surgeon pulls the stomach and at least 2.5- to 3-cm of the distal esophagus into the abdominal cavity.

6. The anesthesia provider inserts the appropriately sized esophageal dilator (56F to 60F). Insertion of the dilators requires critical coordination with the surgeon to ensure the stomach's retraction at the appropriate angle to facilitate smooth passage and to prevent perforation of the esophagus or stomach.

7. The surgeon approximates the crural fibers with interrupted size 0 nonabsorbable sutures to close the crura posterior to the esophagus. The esophageal dilator acts as a stent to ensure closure of the defect is not too tight around the esophagus. Note: If the hiatal defect is extremely large, use of a piece of biologic mesh to reinforce the repair is likely.

8. An antireflux procedure follows, using a 360- or a 270-degree posterior fundoplication. Fundoplication is described below.

9. Removal of the esophageal dilator and Penrose drain is next.

10. The surgeon may suture the stomach to the anterior abdominal wall to keep it from sliding back into the chest.

11. Removal of the liver retractor, instruments, and trocars is under direct visualization, followed by removal of the laparoscope. After release of pneumoperitoneum, removal of the final access port follows.

12. Closure of all incisions ends the procedure.

Laparoscopic Nissen Fundoplication

Recurrent or persistent reflux of gastric contents into the esophagus or mouth constitutes GERD. A defective or incompetent LES fails to prevent gastric reflux. In addition to an incompetent LES, patients simultaneously may have a hiatal hernia. In the presence of a hiatal hernia, the LES migrates into the thoracic cavity, altering the normal pressure gradient between the abdominal cavity and the thoracic cavity. The resulting increase in abdominal pressure can alter the LES's ability to adequately prevent reflux. If a hiatal hernia is present, it is repaired along with Nissen fundoplication.

Symptoms of GERD include heartburn, regurgitation of gastric contents, chest pain, and difficulty swallowing. Diagnostic studies include EGD, barium swallow, 24-hour esophageal pH monitoring, and esophageal manometry to rule out other causes of gastric reflux such as esophageal motility disorders. Complications of GERD include esophagitis, ulcers, stricture, aspiration pneumonia, BE, and esophageal cancer. Initial treatment for GERD includes dietary changes, weight loss, lifestyle changes, and medications such as antacids, histamine antagonists, and proton pump inhibitors. When these treatments fail to relieve symptoms, or if patients cannot tolerate or comply with prescribed medication regimens, consideration shifts to surgical intervention. A description of the most common surgical procedure performed for GERD, laparoscopic Nissen fundoplication, follows.

Procedural Considerations. Basic setup includes laparoscopy instruments and video equipment. Additional laparoscopic instruments include a 30-degree laparoscope, two Babcock graspers, clip appliers, ultrasonic shears; fan liver retractor, and a laparoscopic needle holder and knot pusher or other suturing device. Nonabsorbable suture is used to close the diaphragmatic defect and perform the fundoplication. Specialized long suture for extracorporeal tying with a knot pusher and standard 18-inch suture for intracorporeal tying techniques should be available.

This procedure requires general anesthesia. Bougie or Maloney esophageal dilators in sizes 32F to 60F are arrayed in ascending order on a nonsterile table for the anesthesia provider to insert during the procedure. Ensure water-soluble lubricant is also on the table to facilitate passage of the dilators. If there is need for stomach decompression, an NG tube is required. An indwelling urinary catheter is often required. Patient placement is in supine or low modified lithotomy position per surgeon preference. The abdomen is prepped from nipple line to the pubic symphysis.

Operative Procedure

1. The surgeon gains abdominal access and pneumoperitoneum follows. The laparoscope is inserted in the umbilical access port.

2. Two trocars are placed under direct visualization to the right and left of the midline above the umbilicus and below the xiphoid process. These two ports are used for dissection and suturing. Additional ports are placed in the left and right lower abdomen.

3. A fan-shaped retractor, used to lift and retract the left lobe of the liver to expose the GEJ, inserts through the right lower port.

4. A Babcock grasper, inserted through the left lower port, is positioned on the fundus of the stomach, enabling the first assistant to provide lateral and downward traction.

5. The surgeon identifies the right and left crura and opens the retroesophageal space, creating a window through which the fundus will pass.

6. A Penrose drain is passed around the esophagus and its ends are secured together; the drain enables manipulation of the esophagus (Figure 11-14).

7. The surgeon then mobilizes the cardia, fundus, and upper portion of the greater curvature of the stomach. This may include ligation and division of the short gastric vessels between the fundus and the spleen. Division of the short gastric vessels occurs either between clips or with ultrasonic shears.

8. The surgeon passes a Babcock from right to left behind the esophagus to grasp the fundus and pull it behind and around the esophagus, creating a 360-degree wrap. Noting any tension on the wrap, the surgeon may extend the stomach mobilization along the greater curve if needed.

9. Before closing the crura or suturing the wrap, the anesthesia provider inserts the appropriately sized esophageal dilator (56F to 60F). Insertion of the dilators requires critical coordination with the surgeon to ensure the stomach retracts at the appropriate angle to facilitate smooth passage and to prevent perforation of the esophagus or stomach.

10. The surgeon approximates the crural fibers with interrupted size 0 nonabsorbable sutures to close the hiatal defect, or crura, posterior to the esophagus. The esophageal dilator acts as a stent to ensure closure of the defect around the esophagus is not too tight.

11. If a hiatal hernia is present, it is repaired by approximating the crura posterior to the esophagus with nonabsorbable interrupted sutures.

12. With the esophageal dilator still in position, the gastric wrap is secured to itself with nonabsorbable interrupted sutures.

13. Removal of the esophageal dilator follows.

14. After release of pneumoperitoneum, the abdomen is inspected for hemostasis.
15. Instruments and ports are removed and incisions closed.

There are common variations of the Nissen fundoplication. The Rossetti-Nissen fundoplication also uses a 360-degree wrap; the procedure, however, does not entail ligation of the short gastric vessels. The Toupet fundoplication uses a partial 270-degree wrap, whereas the Dor fundoplication adopts a partial 180-degree fundal wrap anterior rather than posterior to the esophagus (Schwaitzberg, 2012).

Surgery of the Stomach

Pyloroplasty

A pyloroplasty is a gastric drainage procedure that widens the pylorus to allow greater egress of stomach contents into the duodenum. The most commonly performed technique is the Heineke-Mikulicz pyloroplasty, described here (Angel, 2010).

Procedural Considerations. Instrumentation and supplies include a laparotomy set and a self-retaining retractor. If closure of the pylorus is to be hand sewn, a long 3-0 absorbable suture on a tapered GI needle and several 3-0 silk sutures on the same type of needle are available. If the pyloric closure will be with a stapler, a linear stapler is available. The procedure requires general anesthesia with endotracheal intubation. Patient placement is supine. The abdomen is prepped. Unless gastric distention is present, there is no insertion of an NG tube. A urinary bladder catheter may not be needed because the time needed to complete this procedure is relatively short.

Operative Procedure

1. The surgeon makes a small midline laparotomy incision in the upper abdomen.
2. With the antrum of the stomach and duodenum exposed, the surgeon identifies the pylorus.
3. The surgeon next makes a full thickness 3-cm longitudinal incision between the stomach and the duodenum, parallel to the axis of the pylorus.
4. After placing sutures on the superior and inferior edges of the incision, a hemostat tags the sutures at the halfway point. A team member then applies perpendicular traction to the sutures to facilitate horizontal closure of the incision.
5. The surgeon closes the pylorus incision in two layers, using a running 3-0 absorbable suture on the mucosa followed by interrupted seromuscular stitches with 3-0 nonabsorbable sutures.
6. Alternatively, the surgeon can use a linear stapler (TA 55) to close the pylorus.
7. Closure of the abdomen is in two layers, the standard laparotomy closure. Dressings are applied.

Repair of Perforated Peptic Ulcer

Repair of a perforated peptic ulcer maybe be performed via laparotomy or laparoscopically. The most common site of perforation is the anterior surface of the first portion of the duodenum (Evers, 2010b). The standard procedure for operative management of a perforated peptic ulcer is a Graham patch closure as described on p. 324 (Soll, 2012). Because the physical condition of patients with a perforated peptic ulcer can deteriorate rapidly, the need for surgical intervention can become urgent.

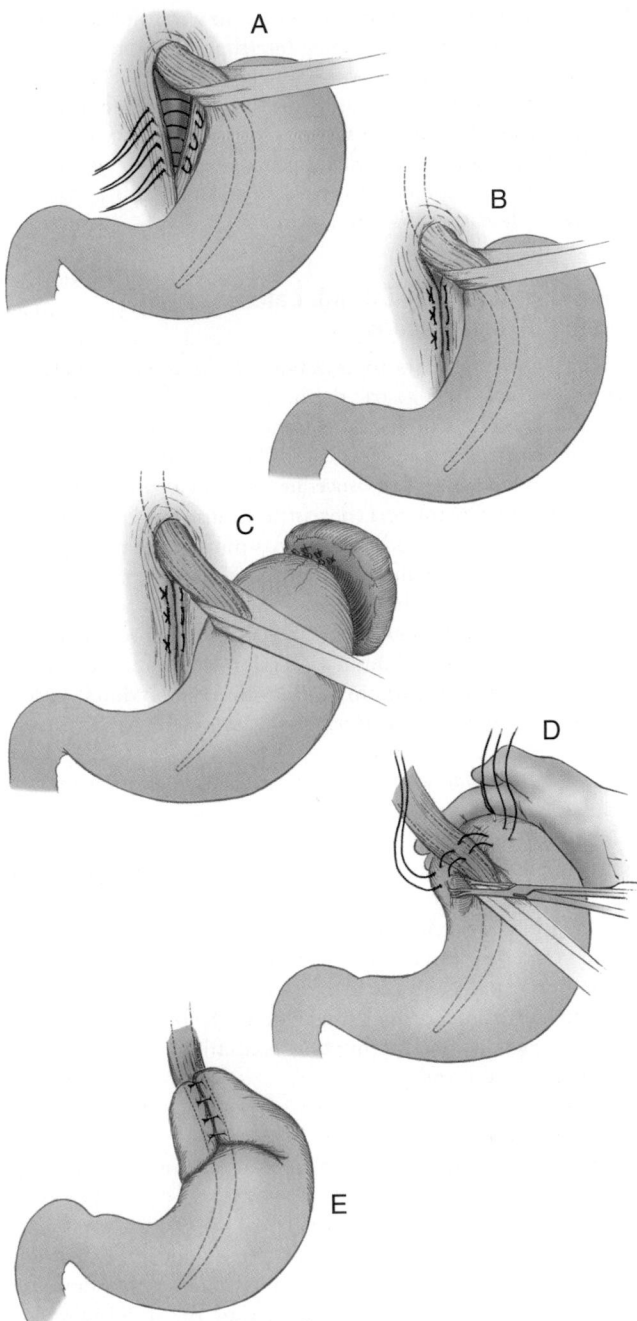

FIGURE 11-14 The Nissen fundoplication procedure begins with complete mobilization of the distal esophagus to create a posterior esophageal window for passage of the fundus of the stomach. **A,** After the esophagus is mobilized, a Maloney or Bougie esophageal dilator (40F to 48F) is passed orally into the stomach. **B,** A Penrose drain around the esophagus retracts the esophagus laterally to expose the esophageal hiatus. **C,** Heavy mattress sutures (0 braided nonabsorbable) are placed in the crura of the diaphragm to narrow the aperture of the hiatus but not so tight as to constrict the esophagus, thus the purpose of stenting the esophagus with the Maloney dilator. **D,** The fundus of the stomach is pulled through the posterior esophageal window and wrapped around the distal esophagus. **E,** The 360-degree wrap is secured with nonabsorbable sutures to complete the procedure.

Procedural Considerations. A standard laparotomy instrument set is needed for an open approach. The laparoscopic technique requires basic laparoscopy instruments and equipment including four trocars, laparoscopic needle holders, dissectors, graspers, and scissors. The technique for closure of the perforated ulcer is the same for laparotomy and laparoscopy with the exception of using intracorporeal suturing techniques for the laparoscopic approach.

Operative Procedure—Open Technique

1. The surgeon makes an upper midline laparotomy incision.
2. Exploration of the upper abdomen to locate the site of the perforation follows.
3. The surgeon performs a tissue biopsy of the ulcer to rule out malignancy.
4. To "close" the perforation, the surgeon places a small pedicle of omentum over the perforation and secures it to the stomach wall with interrupted 3-0 absorbable sutures; the omentum patch is called a Graham patch.
5. The abdomen requires copious irrigation with warm saline.
6. Closure of the abdomen is in two layers. Dressings are applied.

Gastrojejunostomy

A gastrojejunostomy establishes a permanent communication between the proximal jejunum and the stomach as a means to bypass an obstruction of the distal stomach or proximal duodenum resulting from an unresectable gastric tumor or severe stenosis of the pylorus (Evers, 2010a).

Procedural Considerations. Setup includes laparotomy and GI instrument sets. Circular and linear cutting stapling instruments should be available in several sizes. Patient positioning is supine, after which induction of general anesthesia takes place. The anesthesia provider inserts an NG tube after intubation. Placement of an indwelling catheter into the urinary bladder precedes abdominal skin prep.

Operative Procedure

1. The surgeon makes an upper midline abdominal incision, explores the abdomen, and directs placement of warm, moist packs and positioning of a self-retaining retractor.
2. After identifying the ligament of Treitz, the surgeon grasps a loop of proximal jejunum with a Babcock forceps and measures it (Figure 11-15, *A*). The surgeon determines the location of the anastomosis on the stomach and positions the jejunum against the stomach wall several centimeters posterior to the greater curvature.
3. The surgeon next places nonabsorbable 2-0 or 3-0 traction sutures through the seromuscular layer at each corner of the intended anastomosis and then a row of interrupted 3-0 nonabsorbable sutures in the seromuscular layers of the jejunum and stomach to create the back wall of the anastomosis (see Figure 11-15, *B*).
4. The field is now draped for open anastomosis (bowel technique).
5. The surgeon opens the jejunum and stomach along the length of the back wall suture line (see Figure 11-15, *C* through *F*).
6. The surgeon closes the posterior and anterior mucosal layers with two 3-0 running absorbable sutures placed through the full thickness of the jejunum and stomach (see Figure 11-15, *G*).

7. The anastomosis is completed with a row of stitches placed in the anterior serosal layer, using interrupted 3-0 nonabsorbable sutures.
8. After removal of the traction sutures, team members discard contaminated instruments into a basin.
9. The wound is irrigated with warm saline.
10. Sterile members of the surgical team don fresh gowns and gloves, close the abdominal wound in layers, and apply a dressing.

Partial Gastrectomy—Billroth I and Billroth II Reconstruction

Partial gastrectomy refers to resection of the distal stomach for treatment of malignant gastric tumors and complications of peptic ulcer disease such as bleeding, perforation, and obstruction. The extent of gastric resection depends on the type and location of the gastric lesion. The Billroth I procedure is a distal gastrectomy with GI reconstruction to connect the gastric remnant to the duodenum via an end-to-side or end-to-end anastomosis (gastroduodenostomy) (Figure 11-16). Billroth I procedures entail resections at, or distal to, the antrum of the stomach. The Billroth II procedure is a distal gastrectomy combined with GI reconstruction to connect the gastric remnant to the jejunum via end-to-side or an end-to-end anastomosis (gastrojejunostomy). Billroth II procedures address gastric lesions extending proximal to the antrum.

Procedural Considerations. Setup requires basic laparotomy instruments, long instruments, and GI instruments. Also available are long, straight, and angled clip appliers and clips in assorted sizes; a self-retaining abdominal retractor; and a medium length fine right-angle clamp. Linear cutting and end-to-end stapling instruments and cartridges should be available in a variety of sizes. The patient is supine and general anesthesia induced. The anesthesia provider inserts an NG tube after endotracheal intubation. Insertion of an indwelling urinary catheter occurs before abdominal skin prep. Team members take appropriate precautions to prevent DVT, hypothermia, and pressure ulcers.

Operative Procedure—Billroth I

1. The surgeon opens and explores the abdomen through an epigastric midline incision.
2. A self-retaining retractor is positioned to optimize exposure.
3. Mobilization of the greater curvature of the stomach begins with sharp entry into the gastrocolic ligament, midway along the greater curvature. Working toward the duodenum, the surgeon frees the stomach from the gastrocolic omentum by ligating and dividing the gastric branches of the gastroepiploic vessels close to the gastric wall, leaving the gastrocolic omentum. This occurs with clamps and ties, hemostatic clips, ultrasonic shears, or with a sealing bipolar instrument. For malignant tumors, the surgeon leaves the gastrocolic omentum attached to the stomach and resects closer to the transverse colon instead.
4. Mobilization of the greater curve continues, and clamping and division of the right gastroepiploic vessels follow.
5. The surgeon mobilizes the first and second portions of the duodenum to facilitate the gastroduodenostomy.
6. The surgeon next mobilizes the lesser curve of the stomach, and divides and ligates the right gastric vessels between clamps, preserving the left gastric artery if possible.
7. The operative field undergoes preparation for open anastomosis (bowel technique).

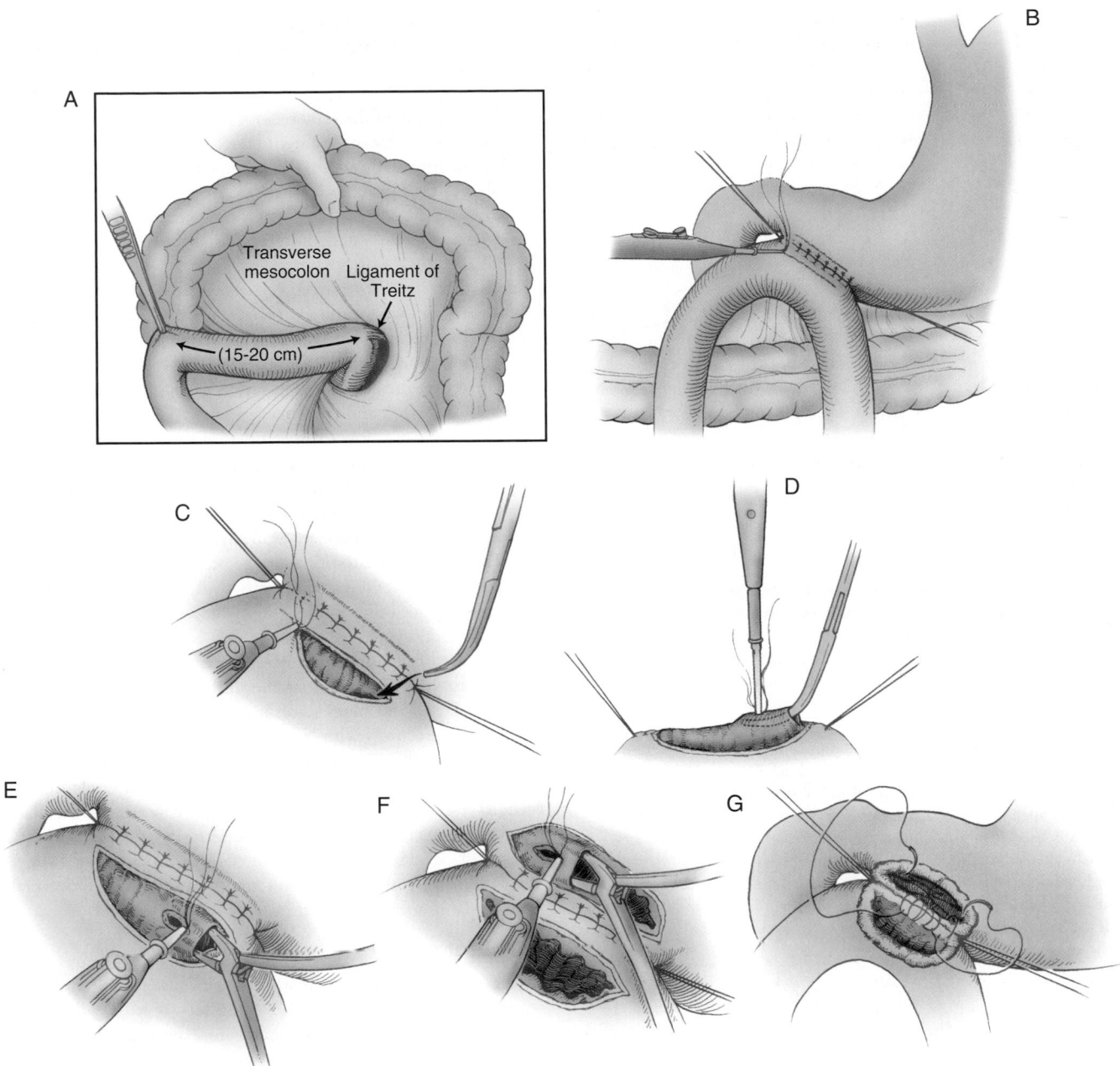

FIGURE 11-15 Gastrojejunostomy. **A,** Selection of a segment of jejunum that will be anastomosed to the stomach; the distance between the ligament of Treitz and the anastomosis should not be excessively long or under any tension. **B,** A posterior row of interrupted sutures is placed between the gastric and jejunal serosae, and the sites of the gastric and jejunal stomas are scored with the electrosurgical pencil. **C,** The jejunal stoma is created by dissecting through the serosa and muscularis with the electrosurgical pencil. An opening is made in the mucosa, and a right-angled clamp is inserted into the lumen. **D,** The clamp is opened and elevated. **E,** Electrosurgery is applied between the two jaws of the clamp. **F,** The procedure is repeated to create the gastric stoma. **G,** Full-thickness anastomosis is begun posteriorly.

8. The distal margin of the gastric resection includes the proximal duodenum. Its division is either between intestinal clamps or with a linear stapler. The surgeon divides the proximal stomach with a large GI stapling device.

9. The gastrectomy is complete. Reinforcement of the staple line of the gastric remnant is possible with a running 3-0 silk suture.

10. Next the surgeon positions the duodenum adjacent to the gastric remnant at the planned anastomosis site and secures it at the corners with nonabsorbable 3-0 traction sutures placed

through the serosa at each corner. A hemostat tags these sutures.

11. The surgeon places a row of interrupted 3-0 nonabsorbable sutures in the seromuscular layer of the duodenum and the stomach to create the back wall of the anastomosis.

12. The surgeon makes matching enterotomies in the duodenum and stomach equidistant from the back wall suture line.

13. Anastomosis of the posterior and anterior mucosal layers of the enterotomies is with two 3-0 running absorbable sutures

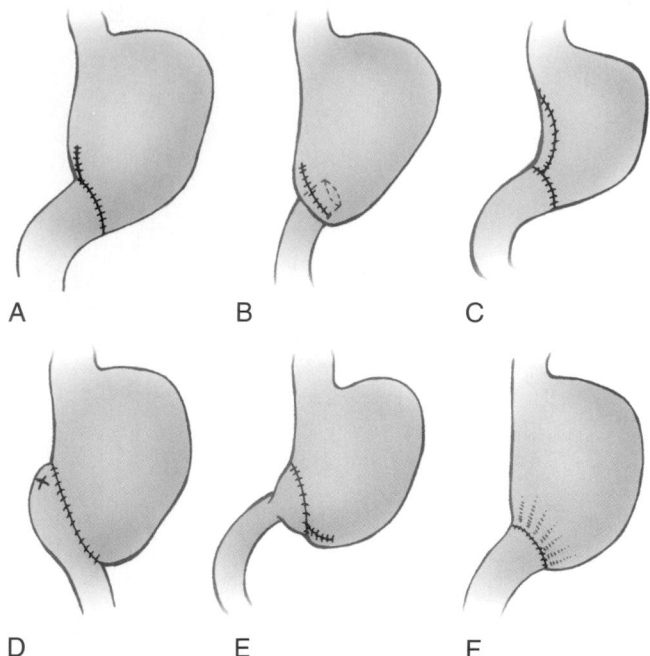

FIGURE 11-16 Diagrams illustrating resections of stomach with anastomosis of stomach and duodenum (gastroduodenal anastomosis). All are modifications of the Billroth I technique, in which the stomach is moved to the duodenum. **A,** Billroth I: after pylorus is removed, lesser curvature is partially closed and duodenum is sutured to open end of stomach at its lower margin. **B,** Kocher: distal end of stomach is closed, and duodenum is transferred up to posterior margin of closed stomach. **C,** Schoemaker: lesser curvature of stomach is sutured closed and brought down to same size as duodenum, and end-to-end anastomosis is done. **D,** von Haberer-Finney: side of duodenum is transferred up to end of stomach so that entire end of stomach is open for direct anastomosis. **E,** Horsley: lesser curvature end of stomach is used to suture to duodenum and closes greater curvature end. **F,** von Haberer: modification of operation shown in **D.** Stomach is narrowed or puckered so that it fits end of duodenum. Modification of this is done by some surgeons as follows: duodenum is split longitudinally and its ends are flared open so that the opening is large enough to fit the open end of the stomach.

placed through the full thickness of the duodenum and stomach walls.

14. Closure of the front wall of the anastomosis is with a row of interrupted 3-0 nonabsorbable sutures placed in the seromuscular layer. The anastomosis is complete.

15. After removal of traction sutures, team members discard contaminated instruments into a basin.

16. Sterile members of the surgical team don fresh gowns and gloves, close the abdominal wound in layers, and apply a dressing.

Operative Procedure—Billroth II. Instruments and supplies for Billroth II (gastrojejunostomy) (Figure 11-17) are the same as described for Billroth I.

1. The surgeon opens and explores the abdomen through an epigastric midline incision.

2. A self-retaining retractor is positioned to optimize exposure.

3. Mobilization of the greater curvature begins with sharp entry into the gastrocolic ligament, midway along the greater curvature of the stomach. Working toward the duodenum, the surgeon frees the stomach from the gastrocolic omentum by

ligating and dividing the gastric branches of the gastroepiploic vessels close to the gastric wall, leaving the gastrocolic omentum. For malignant tumors, resection of the gastrocolic omentum follows.

4. Mobilization of the greater curve continues, after which clamping and division of the right gastroepiploic vessels occur.

5. The surgeon mobilizes the lesser curve of the stomach and divides the right gastric vessels between clamps. The vessels are ligated. The left gastric artery is preserved if possible.

6. Division of the duodenum just distal to the pylorus is with a GI linear stapling device.

7. The surgeon fires a large GI stapler across the stomach and directs removal of the gastric specimen. A bioabsorbable buttressing material can reinforce the staple line.

8. The surgeon mobilizes a loop of proximal jejunum, pulls it up in front of the colon, and positions it adjacent to the posterior wall of the remaining stomach.

9. Placement of a row of interrupted 3-0 nonabsorbable sutures in the seromuscular layer of the jejunum and the stomach creates the back wall of the anastomosis.

10. Creation of matching enterotomies in the jejunum and stomach equidistant from the back wall suture line follows.

11. The surgeon anastomoses the posterior and anterior mucosal layers of the enterotomies with two 3-0 running absorbable sutures placed through the full thickness of the duodenum and stomach walls.

12. Closure of the front wall of the anastomosis is with a row of interrupted 3-0 nonabsorbable sutures placed in the seromuscular layer. The anastomosis is complete.

Distal gastrectomy with laparoscopic Billroth I or II reconstruction is also possible. Standard laparoscopic instruments, equipment, and supplies are needed. Laparoscopic hemostasis energy devices such as a bipolar vessel-sealing instrument or ultrasonic shears should be available along with a wide variety of laparoscopic GI linear and circular stapling instruments. A subtotal gastrectomy, a more extensive gastric resection, removes at least four fifths of the stomach (Bumm and Siewert, 2012).

Total Gastrectomy

As the name implies, total gastrectomy entails complete stomach resection. Reestablishment of GI continuity is with a Roux-en-Y anastomosis between the jejunum and esophagus (esophagojejunostomy) (Figure 11-18). A Roux-en-Y anastomosis is a Y-shaped anastomosis that includes a Roux, or alimentary, limb and a "Y" limb.

Procedural Considerations. Basic laparotomy instruments, long instruments, and GI instruments are required. Also needed are straight and angled clip appliers and clips in assorted sizes, a self-retaining abdominal retractor, and a medium-length fine right-angle clamp. Linear cutting and end-to-end stapling instruments and cartridges should be available. The patient is positioned supine and general anesthesia induced. The anesthesia provider inserts an NG tube after endotracheal intubation. After insertion of an indwelling urinary catheter, abdominal skin prep follows. Observe precautions to prevent DVT, hypothermia, and pressure ulcers according to hospital protocol.

Operative Procedure

1. The surgeon opens and explores the abdomen via a midline or bilateral subcostal incision. A self-retaining retractor is positioned to optimize exposure.

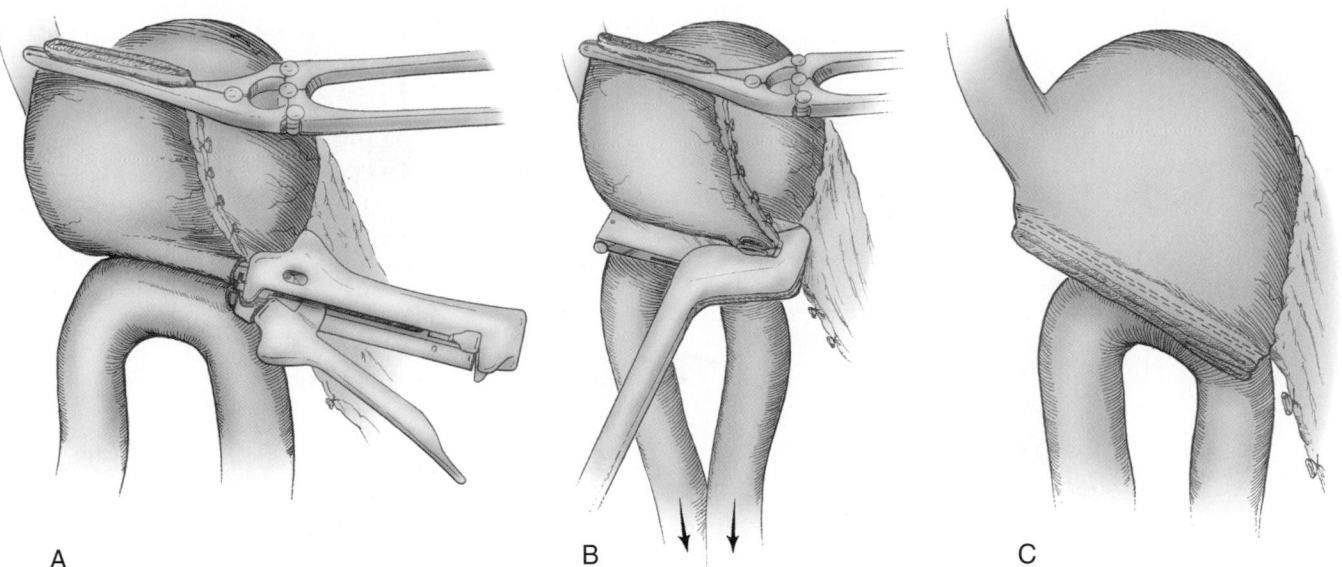

A   B   C

FIGURE 11-17 Subtotal gastrectomy with stapled Billroth II anastomosis. **A,** The distal stomach has been dissected free and resected just distal to the pylorus. A proximal limb of jejunum is transferred up to anastomose to the posterior wall of the stomach with a linear stapling instrument that transects between two parallel staple lines. **B,** The stomach is elevated, and a 90-degree mechanical stapling device is placed across the distal stomach. **C,** Illustration of the completed subtotal gastrectomy with stapled antecolic gastrojejunostomy.

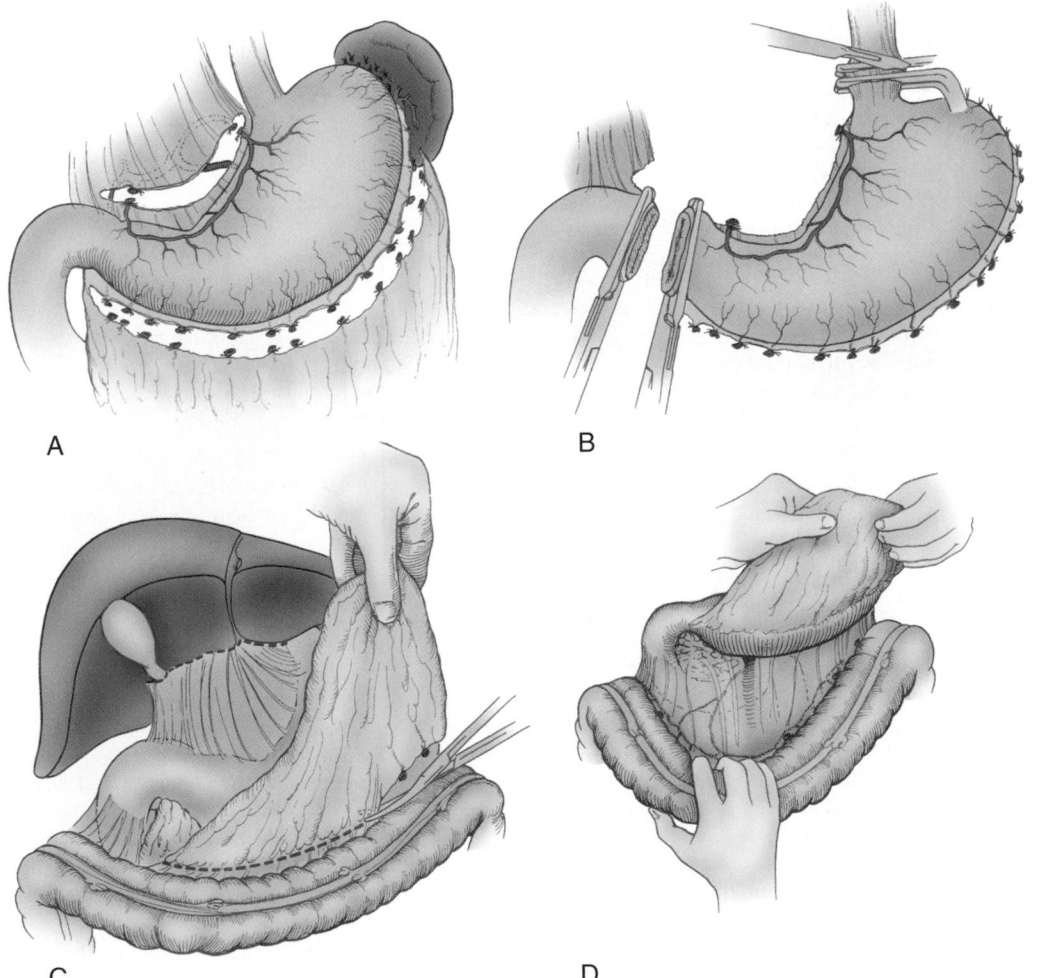

A   B

C   D

FIGURE 11-18 Total gastrectomy. **A,** The mobilization of the stomach for benign disease is demonstrated. Serial division of the vessels in the gastrocolic ligament and gastrohepatic ligament is performed to free the greater and lesser omentum. The short gastric vessels connecting the stomach to the spleen are divided, and the spleen is preserved. **B,** The duodenum is divided distally to the pylorus, and the proximal line of division is at the distal intra-abdominal esophagus. **C,** For malignancies the line of resection includes both the lesser and the greater omentum. **D,** The retrogastric area is inspected for tumor involvement. The spleen and tail of the pancreas may be included in the resection.

Continued

FIGURE 11-18, cont'd **E,** A sizer is inserted into the lumen of the distal esophagus. **F,** The EEA or intraluminal anastomosis (ILA) is inserted into the lumen of the jejunum to facilitate esophagojejunostomy. **G,** The anvil is inserted into the distal esophagus where purse-string sutures will be snugged around the protruding arm of the anvil. **H,** The distal esophagus and the jejunum are united by the mechanism of the stapling device, and the intraluminal anastomosis will be performed. **I,** The "donuts," distal esophagus and jejunal tissues, are examined for integrity and completeness. **J,** Illustration of the esophagojejunostomy completed.

2. For malignant tumors, the gastrocolic omentum along the greater curvature undergoes resection from the transverse colon and removal with the stomach.

3. Clamping and division of the right and left gastroepiploic vessels follow.

4. Mobilization of the fundus requires division of the short gastric vessels located between the spleen and fundus. Care is taken not to tear the splenic capsule with excessive retraction.

5. After mobilization of the lesser curve of the stomach, the left and right gastric vessels are individually clamped, divided, and ligated.

6. Using a GI linear stapler distal to the pylorus, the surgeon divides the first portion of the duodenum. Reinforcement of the staple line on the duodenal stump may be necessary with interrupted or running 3-0 absorbable sutures, to prevent leakage or to control bleeding on the staple line.

7. The left lobe of the liver undergoes mobilization and retraction cephalad to expose the esophageal hiatus.

8. Mobilization and transection of the distal esophagus is with a GI linear stapling device.

9. Using a GI stapler the surgeon divides the jejunum about 40 cm from the ligament of Treitz and creates a Roux limb of approximately 50 cm, to be brought up to the esophageal stump through a hole created in the mesentery of the colon. This is called a retro-colic technique.

10. The surgeon creates a side-to-side jejunojejunostomy between the proximal jejunum and a segment distal to the Roux loop to allow for biliary and pancreatic drainage.

11. Using an end-to-end circular stapling device, the surgeon creates the esophagojejunostomy.

12. The anvil of the stapler either passes down the esophagus through the mouth, or the surgeon makes an enterotomy in order to position the anvil directly in the esophagus (see Figure 11-18, *G*).

13. The stapler passes through an enterotomy made at the staple line of the Roux limb.

14. Once the anvil and the stapler join together (see Figure 11-18, *H*), the surgeon fires the stapler, achieving anastomosis between the esophagus and the Roux limb of the jejunum. Closure of the enterotomies is with a small linear stapling device. After inspection of the donuts (see Figure 11-18, *I*), the anastomosis is complete (see Figure 11-18, *J*).

15. Using a flexible gastroscope, the surgeon inspects the anastomosis.

16. After irrigation of the abdomen with warm saline, closure in layers follows as previously described and a dressing is applied.

Bariatric Surgery

Bariatric surgery, also termed "weight loss" or "weight reduction" surgery, is surgical treatment of obesity. Morbid obesity is a disease affecting more than 35.7% of U.S. adults (Jones and Jones, 2012). More than 200,000 bariatric procedures occur in the United States each year (Scortino et al, 2011). Obesity is defined by BMI, an estimate of total body fat using a height-to-weight ratio (see Box 11-1).

Obese patients typically present with serious coexisting health conditions, such as diabetes, cardiopulmonary disease, obstructive sleep apnea (OSA), gallstone disease, hypertension, hyperlipidemia, and joint disease. Eligibility criteria for patients seeking bariatric surgery have included a BMI of 40 kg/m² or greater without coexisting medical problems or those with a BMI of 35 kg/m² or greater with comorbidities such as type 2 diabetes (T2D), hypertension, hyperlipidemia, or OSA. In recent guidelines, patients with diabetes or metabolic syndrome and a BMI of 30 to 34.9 kg/m² may be offered a bariatric procedure (Mechanick et al, 2013). This underscores evidence that remission of diabetes is durable in a significant proportion of bariatric surgery patients, prompting emergence of the terminology "metabolic surgery" to treat T2D as well as to reduce cardiometabolic risk factors in obese patients (ECRI, 2013; Mechanick et al, 2013). Patients also must demonstrate psychologic stability and motivation to commit to postsurgical lifestyle changes (Patient Safety). Formal mental health evaluations are necessary in patients who actively abuse alcohol or recreational drugs, or who have poorly controlled psychiatric disease; bariatric surgery may be contraindicated for these patients (Scortino et al, 2011).

There are three categories of bariatric procedures: restrictive (such as laparoscopic adjustable gastric banding [LAGB], described following, and laparoscopic sleeve gastrectomy [not described]),

PATIENT SAFETY

Impaired Alcohol Metabolism After Roux-en-Y Gastric Bypass, Laparoscopic Gastric Banding, and Laparoscopic Sleeve Gastrectomy

The investigators in the first study compared preoperative and postoperative differences in the alcohol metabolism of 19 morbidly obese patients using measurements of breath/blood alcohol content (BAC) before and after laparoscopic Roux-en-Y gastric bypass surgery. The same surgeon performed each procedure. The pouch size ranged from 15 to 30 mL, and the length of the Roux limb was 100 cm.

BAC measurements were taken preoperatively and then again at 3 months and 6 months after surgery. At each measurement the patients were asked to drink 5 ounces of red wine in less than 1 minute. BAC was measured 15 minutes after the last sip of wine was taken and subsequently measured every 5 minutes until the BAC returned to 0%. Each patient's preoperative measurement served as the control used for comparisons of the postoperative measurements.

Results showed that postoperatively a smaller volume of ingested alcohol was required before patients began to experience self-identified symptoms of intoxication. For each patient the preoperative BAC measurements increased at 3 months and increased again at 6 months postoperatively and the time it took to return to a BAC of 0% increased at each subsequent measurement. The investigators concluded that Roux-en-Y gastric bypass surgery altered alcohol metabolism.

In a second study of similar design, investigators examined the preoperative BAC levels of patients undergoing either a laparoscopic adjustable band or laparoscopic sleeve gastrectomy procedure and compared them with levels measured at 3 months and 6 months postoperatively. They found there were no significant changes in peak BAC levels or increases in time needed to return to a BAC of 0%. They concluded that these procedures did not alter alcohol metabolism.

Perioperative nurses should counsel patients who have had a Roux-en-Y gastric bypass that their bodies may respond differently to alcohol after surgery and they may not recognize signs of intoxication as they did before surgery. Bariatric patients should be warned not to drink and drive, and if they do choose to drink, they should limit alcohol intake to no more than one 12-ounce beer, 6 ounces of wine, or 2 ounces of liquor every 2 hours.

Modified from Changchien EM et al: Alcohol metabolism after gastric banding and sleeve gastrectomy: a case-crossover trial, *J Am Coll Surg* 215(4):274--279, 2012; Woodard GA et al: Impaired alcohol metabolism after gastric bypass surgery: a case-crossover trial, *J Am Coll Surg* 212(2):209–213, 2011.

malabsorptive, or a combination of both. Restrictive procedures reduce the size of the stomach. When the patient eats, food is digested and absorbed normally, but the smaller capacity of the stomach gives the feeling of fullness, and the patient eats less. In malabsorptive procedures, surgery reduces the absorptive capacity of the small intestine with a bypass of a segment or segments of the proximal small bowel.

Adjustable Gastric Band

Adjustable gastric banding is a restrictive procedure using a silicone strip and adjustable elastic ring called an adjustable gastric band. The band is laparoscopically placed around the top of the stomach. The surgeon sutures a fold of stomach around the band to secure it in place (Figure 11-19). The band has a port, inflated with saline

FIGURE 11-19 Proper position of the Lap-Band. The silicone band around the fundus of the stomach creates a small gastric pouch. The inner lining of the band contains an inflatable balloon connected to a subcutaneous port on the patient's abdomen (not shown). The band can inflate or deflate to adjust stomach size as needed.

4 weeks postoperatively. The constriction created by the inflated band restricts the amount of ingested food that can enter the stomach, preventing overeating. This procedure is adjustable and reversible and has been shown to improve long-term health, including reducing risks of cardiovascular disease and T2D (De la Cruz-Munoz et al, 2011; DeMaria et al, 2011).

Laparoscopic Roux-en-Y Gastric Bypass

Roux-en-Y gastric bypass (RYGB) is a largely restrictive and mildly malabsorptive procedure that reroutes the passage of ingested food and fluid from a small pouch created with surgical staples or sutures in the proximal stomach to a segment of the proximal jejunum. Laparoscopic RYGB is relatively common in the United States.

Procedural Considerations. All patients undergoing bariatric surgery need special consideration because they usually have associated serious comorbidities that place them at heightened risk during the procedure (Research Highlight). A special OR bed that can accommodate patients who weigh more than 350 pounds (159 kg) is required. In addition to laparoscopic instrumentation and accessory supplies, extra-large blood pressure cuffs and extra-long trocars are necessary. Positioning requires additional padded safety restraints, pressure-reduction devices to reduce the risk of pressure injury, and properly fitting IPCDs. The perioperative nurse anticipates the potential for anesthesia assistance during intubation and airway management.

Operative Procedure

1. This surgery requires placement of five trocars above the umbilicus (Figure 11-20): two on the midline, two in the left upper

---

Predicting Risk for Serious Complications After Bariatric Surgery

Using data collected on 25,469 patients who had bariatric surgery at one of the 29 hospitals enrolled in the Michigan Bariatric Surgery Collaborative (MBSC) between 2006 and 2012, investigators developed a risk prediction model to determine the probability of an individual patient developing serious complications after bariatric surgery.

Data used in the development process included the type of bariatric procedure, all postoperative complications, preexisting patient comorbidities, and other patient information such as age, gender, insurance status, mean body mass index (BMI), smoking history, and mobility limitations.

Comorbidities included pulmonary disease, cardiovascular disease, sleep apnea, psychologic disorders, prior venous thromboembolism, diabetes, chronic renal failure requiring dialysis, liver disease, urinary incontinence, gastroesophageal reflux disease, peptic ulcer disease, cholelithiasis, and history of previous ventral hernia repair.

Complications included in the study occurred within 30 days of the surgery, and were classified or graded according to severity. Serious complications were defined as life threatening, or associated with disability or death, and included myocardial infarction; renal failure that required long-term dialysis; respiratory failure that required more than 7 days of mechanical ventilation, or tracheostomy; and death.

The investigators' analysis of the data showed that the most significant risk factors for serious complications were as follows:
- Type of procedure (listed in descending order from most significant risk to least significant risk)
  - Biliopancreatic diversion with duodenal switch
  - Roux-en-Y gastric bypass
  - Sleeve gastrectomy
  - Adjustable gastric band
- History of venous thromboembolism
- Mobility limitations
- Coronary artery disease
- Pulmonary disease
- History of smoking
- Male gender

There was no difference noted in risk for complications between open and laparoscopic approaches.

A calculator to determine risks of severe complications before surgery can be used to determine the best bariatric procedure for each patient, based on existing comorbidities. In addition it can identify modifiable risk factors and comorbid conditions that can be optimized prior to surgery. The risk calculator is at https://michiganbsc.org/Registry/calculator/outcomesCalculator.

Modified from Finks JF et al: Predicting risk for serious complications with bariatric surgery, *Ann Surg* 254(4):633–640, 2011.

---

quadrant, and one in the right upper quadrant. The surgeon also makes an incision for the liver retractor.
2. The surgeon mobilizes the omentum and identifies the ligament of Treitz.
3. Using a vascular stapler the surgeon divides the jejunum 40 cm distal to the ligament of Treitz (Figure 11-21).
4. While the proximal jejunum is left to lie in the patient's right side, the surgeon lifts the Roux limb superiorly and passes it through the transverse colon mesentery (Figure 11-22).
5. With several loads of a linear stapler, the surgeon creates a gastric pouch.

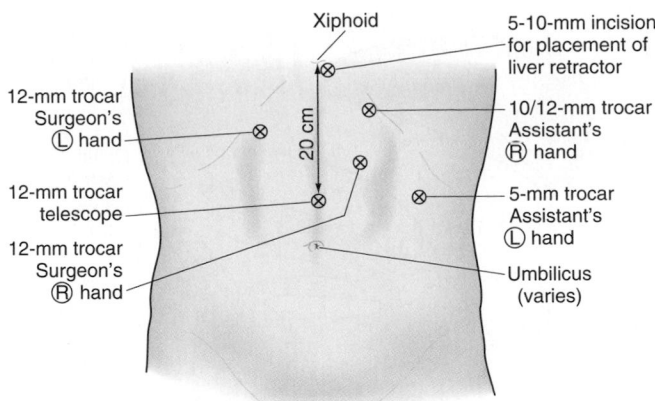

FIGURE 11-20 Trocar configuration for laparoscopic Roux-en-Y gastric bypass.

FIGURE 11-21 Placing stapler to divide jejunum to create roux limb.

6. The surgeon next anastomoses the Roux limb to the proximal gastric pouch. Methylene blue is instilled to check for leaks. The surgeon may perform the gastrojejunostomy with either traditional suturing techniques or a circular EEA stapler.
7. The surgeon closes any mesenteric defects, inspects the abdomen, and directs closure of the port sites.

With RYGB, avoidance of a critical segment of the calorie- and nutrition-absorbing mucosal surface occurs. The gastric pouch is generally less than 30 mL in volume. This procedure results in considerable weight loss for the patient. Serious complications, however, can arise, including hemorrhage, anastomotic leaks, pulmonary embolism, pneumonia, infection, small bowel obstructions or stenosis, and incisional hernia (Table 11-3). Nutritional deficits, nausea, flatus, diarrhea, and dumping syndrome are other common complications.

Biliopancreatic diversion (BPD) (Figure 11-23) and duodenal switch (Figure 11-24) are largely malabsorptive and mildly restrictive procedures. In both, the Roux limb and the biliopancreatic limb are longer, leaving a shortened common channel for digestion and absorption of proteins, fats, and carbohydrates. These procedures present serious risks of complications, nutritional deficiencies, liver abnormalities, anemia, and lactose intolerance.

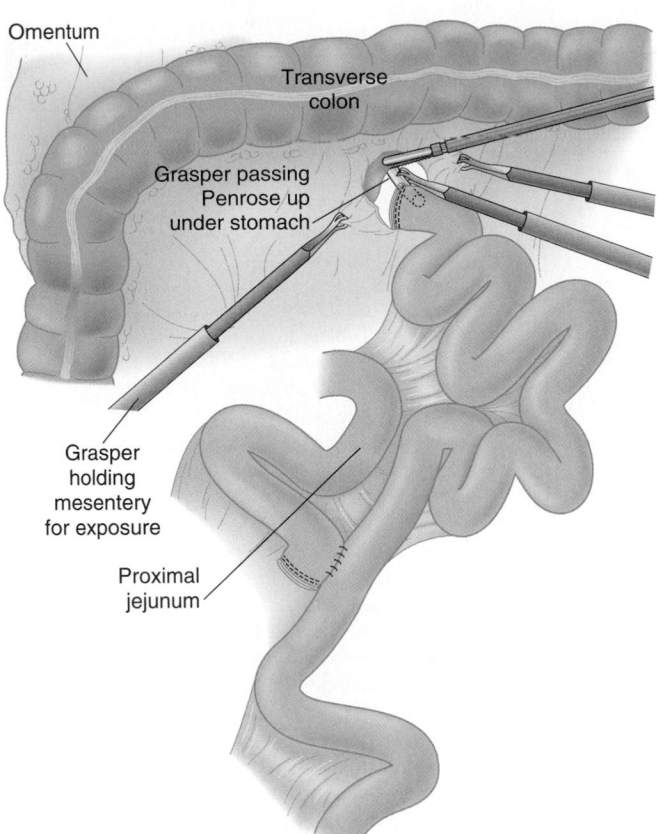

FIGURE 11-22 Passing the Roux limb into a retrocolic and retrogastric position.

Surgery of the Small Bowel

Meckel Diverticulectomy

Meckel diverticulum forms when the vitelline duct fails to close completely by birth. The diverticulum includes all layers of the intestinal wall, and ileal, gastric, or pancreatic mucosa can line it. Meckel diverticulum is uncommon and in most cases does not cause symptoms. The most common complication is GI bleeding, followed by intussusception, obstruction, strangulation, diverticulitis, and volvulus (Vickers et al, 2012).

Procedural Considerations. Laparotomy and GI sets are required. Linear stapling devices should be available. Patient positioning is supine, and general anesthesia is administered. The anesthesia provider may insert an NG tube after intubation. Insertion of an indwelling urinary catheter precedes abdominal skin prep.

Operative Procedure

1. The surgeon opens the abdomen through a low midline or right lower quadrant incision and identifies the diverticulum.
2. If the diverticulum is long and narrow with a narrow base, it is double-clamped and divided at its base.
3. Closure of the bowel beneath the clamp is with full-thickness 3-0 absorbable sutures.
4. A row of inverting sutures using 3-0 or 4-0 nonabsorbable suture is used to close the outer layer.
5. Alternatively, a linear GI stapler may be used to resect the diverticulum.

TABLE 11-3

Complications of Bariatric Surgery

Procedure	Surgery-Related Complications

Adjustable gastric band	• Band
	  • Erosion into the stomach
	  • Slippage with gastric prolapse
	  • Infection
	• Port
	  • Infection
	  • Tubing disconnection
	• Pouch dilation
	• Stomal obstruction
	• Gastric perforation
	• Delayed gastric emptying
	• Bleeding
	• Incisional hernia
	• Esophageal dilatation; esophagitis
	• Hiatal hernia

Vertical banded gastroplasty	• Staple line disruption • Anastomotic stenosis and obstruction • Erosion of mesh band • Gastroesophageal reflux • Vomiting

Sleeve gastrectomy	• Anastomotic leak
	• Gastric leaks
	• Stenosis of gastric outlet
	• Bleeding from mobilization of the greater curve of the stomach
	  • From short gastric vessels
	  • From staple line
	  • From splenic injury

Roux-en-Y gastric bypass	• Gastric remnant distention • Stricture of the gastrojejunal anastomosis • Marginal ulcers • Gallstones • Internal hernia in the mesentery • Ventral hernia • Dumping syndrome • Vitamin deficiency • Renal failure • Postoperative hypoglycemia
Biliopancreatic diversion with duodenal switch	• Anastomotic leak • Loose stools/diarrhea/frequent flatus • Protein calorie malnutrition • Anemia • Metabolic bone disease • Fat-soluble vitamin deficiency; vitamin B_{12} deficiency
Non–procedure-specific complications	• Deep vein thrombosis • Pulmonary embolism • Cardiovascular complications • Pulmonary complications • Addiction transfer (drugs, alcohol) • Depression; suicide • Failure to lose weight or weight regain

Modified from Adair JD, Ellsmere JC: Complications of bariatric surgery. In Basow DS, editor: *UpToDate*, Waltham, MA, UpToDate, 2012; Gagnon LE, Karwacki EJ: Outcomes and complications after bariatric surgery: five of the most common procedures and nursing implications for pre- and postoperative care, *Am J Nurs* 112(9):26–36, 2012.

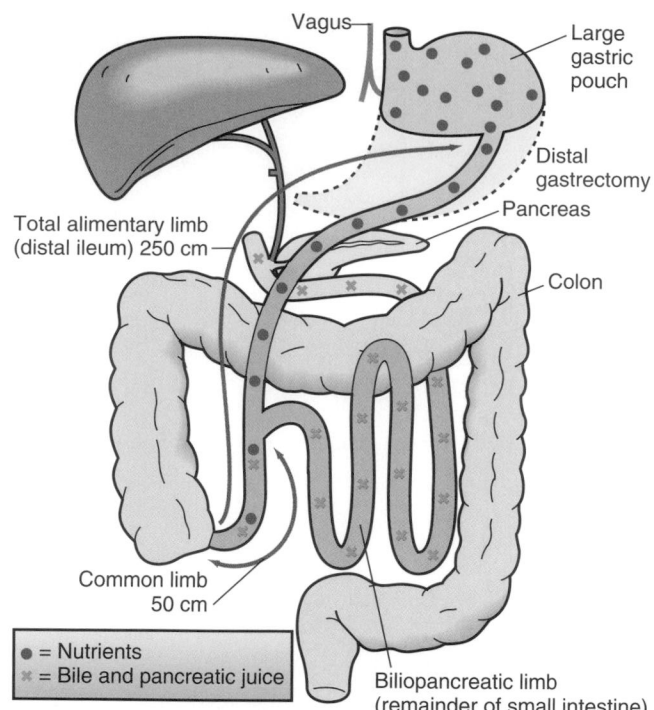

FIGURE 11-23 Configuration of the biliopancreatic diversion (BPD), which is transection of the stomach with anastomosis of the duodenum to the distal ileum. In this malabsorptive procedure, the pancreatic enzymes and bile enter near the ileum, allowing nutrients to pass from the stomach to the distal ileum without being digested. Weight loss occurs because of the partial gastrectomy, which restricts intake, and because of the shortened alimentary canal, which causes malabsorption.

If the base is broad, the surgeon may isolate the loop of bowel containing the diverticulum from the mesentery and perform a limited small bowel resection. Completion of an anastomosis of the divided ends is with an inner continuous layer of 3-0 synthetic absorbable sutures and an interrupted outer layer of 4-0 nonabsorbable sutures. Closure of the abdominal wound follows. This procedure can also be performed laparoscopically using an endoscopic GI linear stapling device.

Appendectomy (Open Approach)

Appendectomy is severance and removal of the appendix from its attachment to the cecum through a right lower quadrant, muscle-splitting incision (McBurney). This procedure removes an acutely inflamed appendix.

Procedural Considerations. Setup requires a basic laparotomy instrument set. Patient positioning is supine, and general anesthesia is administered. Culture tubes and specimen labels are available.

Operative Procedure

1. The surgeon usually makes a right lower quadrant muscle-splitting (McBurney) incision. Retraction of muscles with Richardson or Parker retractors exposes the peritoneum.
2. The peritoneum is lifted and entered. Peritoneal fluid is collected with aerobic and anaerobic culture swabs. Extension of the incision is then done with Metzenbaum scissors.

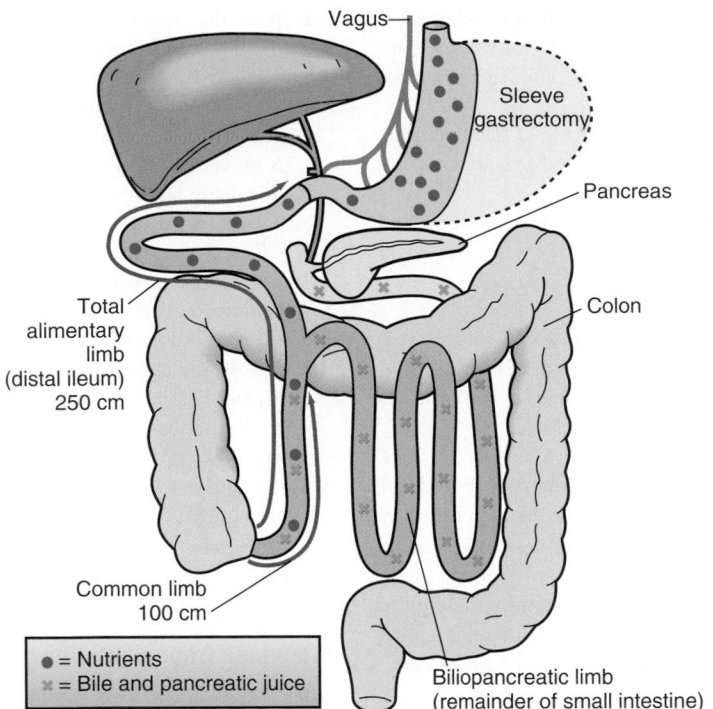

Vagus

Sleeve gastrectomy

Pancreas

Total alimentary limb (distal ileum) 250 cm

Colon

Common limb 100 cm

● = Nutrients
✕ = Bile and pancreatic juice

Biliopancreatic limb (remainder of small intestine)

FIGURE 11-24 Configuration of the duodenal switch, which leaves a larger portion of the stomach intact, including the pyloric valve. This alleviates dumping syndrome.

3. The distal appendix is grasped with Babcock forceps and gently lifted, exposing the mesoappendix containing the appendiceal artery.
4. The mesoappendix is dissected from the appendix and the artery ligated with a 2-0 nonabsorbable suture.
5. The appendix is elevated and a purse-string stitch placed in the cecum around the base of the appendix using an absorbable 2-0 suture.
6. A 3-0 synthetic absorbable suture ligature is tied around the base of the appendix, distal to the purse-string stitch.
7. Bowel technique commences by placing protective gauze sponges over the cecum to protect the wound from spillage. A basin is brought to the field for the specimen and the bowel-contaminated instruments.
8. The appendix is amputated with a scalpel. Soiled instruments are discarded into the basin.
9. After irrigation of the wound with warm saline, the wound is closed in layers.

If the appendix has ruptured, the surgeon irrigates the peritoneal cavity with copious warm fluids and inserts a closed suction drain in the appendiceal bed. Deeper layers of the site are closed; the subcutaneous tissue and skin may remain open. The wound is packed with moist fine-mesh gauze for healing by secondary intention. This healing method may apply in any case in which bowel contamination or abscess formation is present. It allows clean healing and protects against subcutaneous wound infection.

Appendectomy (Laparoscopic)

The laparoscopic approach to appendectomy is appropriate for uncomplicated appendicitis. In the presence of perforation, conversion to an open procedure will likely be necessary.

Procedural Considerations. Setup requires standard laparoscopic instrumentation, equipment, and supplies. The procedure requires placement of three trocars. The patient is positioned supine and general anesthesia induced. Insertion of an indwelling urinary catheter precedes abdominal skin prep.

Operative Procedure

1. Pneumoperitoneum is established. A 5-mm trocar is placed at the umbilicus for insertion of the laparoscope (if a 5-mm laparoscope is not available, use of a larger trocar is an alternative). A 5-mm (or larger) trocar placed in the right upper quadrant (RUQ) serves as the working port. Another 5-mm trocar placed in the midline suprapubic site serves as the traction trocar.
2. A 5-mm laparoscopic Babcock forceps is inserted into the RUQ trocar for grasping and retracting the cecum toward the liver.
3. The surgeon grasps the appendix at its tip with a grasping forceps inserted through the suprapubic trocar and holds it in an upward position.
4. After removal of the Babcock forceps, insertion of a dissecting instrument through the RUQ trocar enables creation of a mesenteric window in the mesoappendix (the peritoneal fold connecting the appendix to the ileum).
5. Dissection, performed in proximity to the appendix, begins directly under the base and progresses 1 to 2 cm in length.
6. Depending on surgeon preference, the appendix may be transected in one of several ways: (a) with an endoscopic linear stapling instrument, (b) with a ligating loop instrument, or (c) with a suturing instrument.
7. In the endoscopic stapling technique, grasping forceps rotate the tip of the appendix so that the surgeon can snug the stapling device to the base of the appendix and close it. The

stapling instrument is fired and withdrawn, after which inspection of the staple line follows. The remainder of the mesoappendix is dissected, hemostasis achieved, and the appendix removed through the RUQ port.

8. It is possible to use a specimen pouch to extract the appendix.
9. The abdomen is irrigated using a suction and irrigation device and pneumoperitoneum released.
10. Closure of trocar sites is with suture; a dressing or skin-bonding sealer is applied.

Resection of the Small Intestine

Small bowel resection removes a segment of diseased, obstructed, or necrotic small intestine. When possible, connecting the distal and proximal segments of the remaining small bowel restores continuity.

Procedural Considerations. Setup requires laparotomy and GI sets. GI linear stapling instruments should be available in a variety of sizes. Patient positioning is supine with general anesthesia. The anesthesia provider may insert an NG tube after intubation. Insertion of an indwelling urinary catheter precedes abdominal skin prep. If the planned procedure is laparoscopic, basic laparoscopic equipment, instrumentation, and stapling devices should be available.

Operative Procedure

1. The surgeon incises the abdominal wall through a midline incision and explores the peritoneal cavity. Wound edges require protection with warm moist packs. Positioning of a self-retaining abdominal retractor optimizes exposure.
2. The surgeon identifies the diseased segment of small intestine.
3. Small mesenteric windows, created at the proximal and distal ends of the diseased small bowel segment, accommodate the arms of the linear staplers.
4. The surgeon positions the staplers across the small bowel and fires them.
5. Using clamps and suture ties with either a bipolar sealing device or ultrasonic shears, the surgeon mobilizes the transected small bowel from its mesentery.
6. Using a two-layer suturing technique or GI linear staplers, the surgeon reestablishes continuity of the GI tract with a functional end-to-end, end-to-side, or side-to-side anastomosis.

End Ileostomy

An end ileostomy entails bringing a transected portion of the ileum through the abdominal wall to divert small bowel content away from the GI tract distal to the ileostomy. An ileostomy can be temporary or permanent.

Procedural Considerations. Laparotomy and GI sets along with linear stapling instruments are required. Patient positioning is supine with general anesthesia. The anesthesia provider may insert an NG tube after intubation. Insertion of an indwelling urinary catheter precedes abdominal skin prep. An ostomy appliance for the stoma is available.

Operative Procedure

1. Through a midline incision the surgeon explores the peritoneal cavity and determines the pathologic condition.
2. Mobilization and resection of the ileum follow, as described in small intestinal resection.
3. The skin is incised at the predetermined site of the ileostomy.

4. Next the surgeon makes a cruciate (cross-shaped) incision in the fascia and peritoneum to accommodate two fingers.
5. The proximal end of the ileum is grasped with a Babcock clamp.
6. The surgeon pulls the ileum through the abdominal wall to the skin, ensuring that it does not stretch or twist, and that there is no compromise of its blood supply.
7. The ileum is secured to the parietal peritoneum on the abdominal wall with interrupted 3-0 nonabsorbable sutures.
8. Closure of the abdomen follows.
9. The stoma is sutured to the skin with everting absorbable sutures to protect the serosal surface against drainage from the stoma (Cima and Pemberton, 2010).
10. An ostomy appliance, cut to fit the diameter of the ileostomy, is placed over the stoma to collect small bowel contents.

An alternative to an end ileostomy is the Kock pouch. This involves creation of an ileal pouch with a nipple valve connected to a stoma on the skin. When working properly the stoma and pouch are continent and do not continually drain stool. A catheter, inserted into the stoma three or four times daily, evacuates the contents, eliminating the need for an external appliance (Cima and Pemberton, 2010).

Intestinal Transplantation

Intestinal failure occurs when there is an inadequate length of healthy small bowel necessary to absorb enough fluids, electrolytes, and other essential nutrients from ingested food to sustain life without the assistance of long-term use of TPN (Buchman, 2010). One cause of intestinal failure is short bowel syndrome (SBS). SBS arises as a result of multiple or extensive bowel resections to treat complications of Crohn's disease, mesenteric infarction, trauma, or malignancies. Complications of long-term TPN include thrombosis of TPN access sites, catheter-related sepsis, and liver failure (Sax, 2011). Intestinal transplantation (ITx) is reserved to treat patients with intestinal failure who otherwise have failed medical management and are no longer candidates for TPN.

Procedural Considerations. As with any transplant procedure, an intestinal transplantation requires a specialized team with coordination between the organ procurement team and the recipient team to minimize the cold ischemia time of the donor organ. Instruments include a laparotomy set, vascular instruments, and any other transplant-related equipment necessary to prepare the graft. Patient positioning is supine with general endotracheal anesthesia. If central venous access is not attainable, the anesthesia provider may request transesophageal Doppler ultrasound to monitor cardiac status of the patient. Insertion of an NG tube and urinary catheter follows. Possible performance of a feeding jejunostomy or gastrostomy requires that additional supplies should be considered (Khan and Selvaggi, 2012).

Operative Procedure

1. The transplant surgeon completes the final visual inspection and assessment of the donor organ. The location of the recipient's incision depends on previous surgical incisions and the location of present or planned stomas.
2. The surgeon dissects the recipient inflow and outflow vessels.
3. An anastomosis is created from the superior mesenteric artery of the donor organ to the recipient's infrarenal aorta.
4. Connecting the donor superior mesenteric vein to the recipient portal vein or vena cava establishes venous drainage of the donor organ.

5. Reperfusion begins with release of venous flow as the clamps open.
6. Release of the arterial clamp follows.
7. Continuity of the intestine returns after establishing vascular supply. Proximal anastomosis joins the donor jejunum to the recipient stomach, duodenum, or proximal jejunum. A side-to-side anastomosis joins the distal ileum with the remaining colon.
8. The surgeon brings up the distal end of the graft as an end or loop ileostomy, usable for later endoscopic evaluation and intestinal biopsies.
9. The surgeon inspects the intact intestine, verifies hemostasis, and closes the abdomen.

Surgery of the Colon

Colostomy

Reestablishing continuity of the GI tract after colon resection sometimes is neither recommended nor feasible. Creation of a colostomy requires bringing the proximal end of the divided colon (or a loop of colon) through the anterior abdominal wall and suturing it to the skin in order to divert the fecal stream. A temporary colostomy, or fecal diversion, may be necessary to allow an abdominal infection to resolve, or to allow a distal anastomosis to heal. A permanent colostomy may be needed after colon resection when the remaining colon is of insufficient length to allow safe reconnection (Francone, 2012).

Procedural Considerations. Setup requires laparotomy instruments and GI instruments. The surgeon may use a GI linear stapler to transect the colon. Several 3-0 absorbable sutures on a controlled-release tapered GI needle are commonly used to sew the colostomy to the skin. A colostomy appliance covers the stoma. If a loop colostomy is planned, additional items may include a colostomy rod, red rubber tubing, or a loop ostomy bridge. Patient positioning is supine with general anesthesia. The anesthesia provider may insert an NG tube after intubation. Insertion of an indwelling urinary catheter precedes abdominal skin prep.

End Colostomy

Operative Procedure (Figure 11-25)
1. The surgeon opens the abdomen, protects the wound edges, retracts the colon, and divides or resects it.
2. Mobilization of the proximal end of the colon ensures that it will reach the anterior abdominal wall without excess tension.
3. A Kocher clamp is placed on the skin at the ostomy site, marked preoperatively. Lifting the Kocher puts traction on the skin while the surgeon uses a knife to cut the lifted skin.
4. Using electrosurgical dissection, the circular incision is carried down to the fascia. A cruciate incision is made in the fascia to accommodate the diameter of the colon. Army Navy retractors are placed.
5. A Babcock is inserted into the abdomen, and the surgeon grasps and pulls the colon through the skin.
6. The surgeon secures the colon internally to the peritoneum of the anterior abdominal wall to prevent it from slipping back into the abdomen during abdominal closure and to prevent future formation of a hernia around the stoma. A handheld retractor is used to lift the abdominal wall slightly during placement of these sutures.
7. After closure of the abdomen, the incision undergoes either dressing with sterile gauze or covering with a sterile towel while the colostomy matures.

8. To mature the colostomy, the surgeon sutures the colon to the skin at evenly spaced intervals around the circumference of the stoma. The colostomy appliance is cut to fit the diameter of the stoma and then secured to the skin. The skin around the stoma should be clean and dry before application of the ostomy appliance.

Loop Colostomy—First Stage. For a temporary loop colostomy, instead of transecting the bowel, the surgeon makes a small opening in the mesentery near the bowel with curved hemostats and Metzenbaum scissors. A Penrose drain is passed around the colon, and a Péan holds the two ends together. Mobilization of the loop of colon is as described for end colostomy. The surgeon uses the Penrose drain to pull the loop of colon through the abdominal wall (Figure 11-26). Closure of the abdominal incision is next. A loop ostomy bridge or a 14F red rubber catheter is used to support and retain the loop of colon in position on the abdominal wall. The loop of intestine is left intact and a petrolatum gauze dressing applied.

Loop Colostomy—Second Stage. After 48 hours the surgeon opens 75% to 80% of the colon loop with the tip of an electrosurgical pencil. Absorbable sutures may secure the colostomy to the skin if the procedure is performed in the OR. If sutures are not used the surgeon can perform this procedure in the patient's room or in a treatment room. Application of an ostomy appliance completes the second stage of loop colostomy.

Closure of a Colostomy

Closure of a colostomy reestablishes GI continuity. Closure of the fascial defect at the ostomy site is with a heavy absorbable suture. The subcutaneous fat and skin may be left open to heal by secondary intention or closure may follow according to surgeon preference. The stoma site is considered contaminated.

Procedural Considerations. Setup requires laparotomy and GI sets. Linear stapling instruments are available. Patient positioning is supine with general anesthesia. Insertion of an indwelling urinary catheter precedes abdominal skin prep. Depending on what portion of the bowel is to undergo reconnection, the patient remains supine or is repositioned in low lithotomy. Low lithotomy is necessary if surgery involves the sigmoid colon or rectum and access to the anus is required to insert a circular stapler to perform an end-to-end anastomosis. If the ileum is to be connected to the transverse or left colon, the patient remains supine.

Operative Procedure
1. A midline laparotomy incision begins the procedure as previously described.
2. The surgeon makes a circumferential incision around the colostomy to free it from the abdominal wall, allowing it to drop back into the abdomen.
3. Resection with a GI linear stapler (or between bowel clamps) of the distal portion of the colon that was attached to the skin follows.
4. Positioning the proximal and distal segments of bowel end to end, the surgeon makes an enterotomy in the proximal end, inserts the anvil of the circular stapler, and secures it with a purse-string stitch using a nonabsorbable suture.
5. An assistant moves between the legs to insert the cutting circular stapler through the anus into the rectum. A separate table for this portion of the procedure must be set up for the assistant performing the "below part." The anvil and the stapler connect

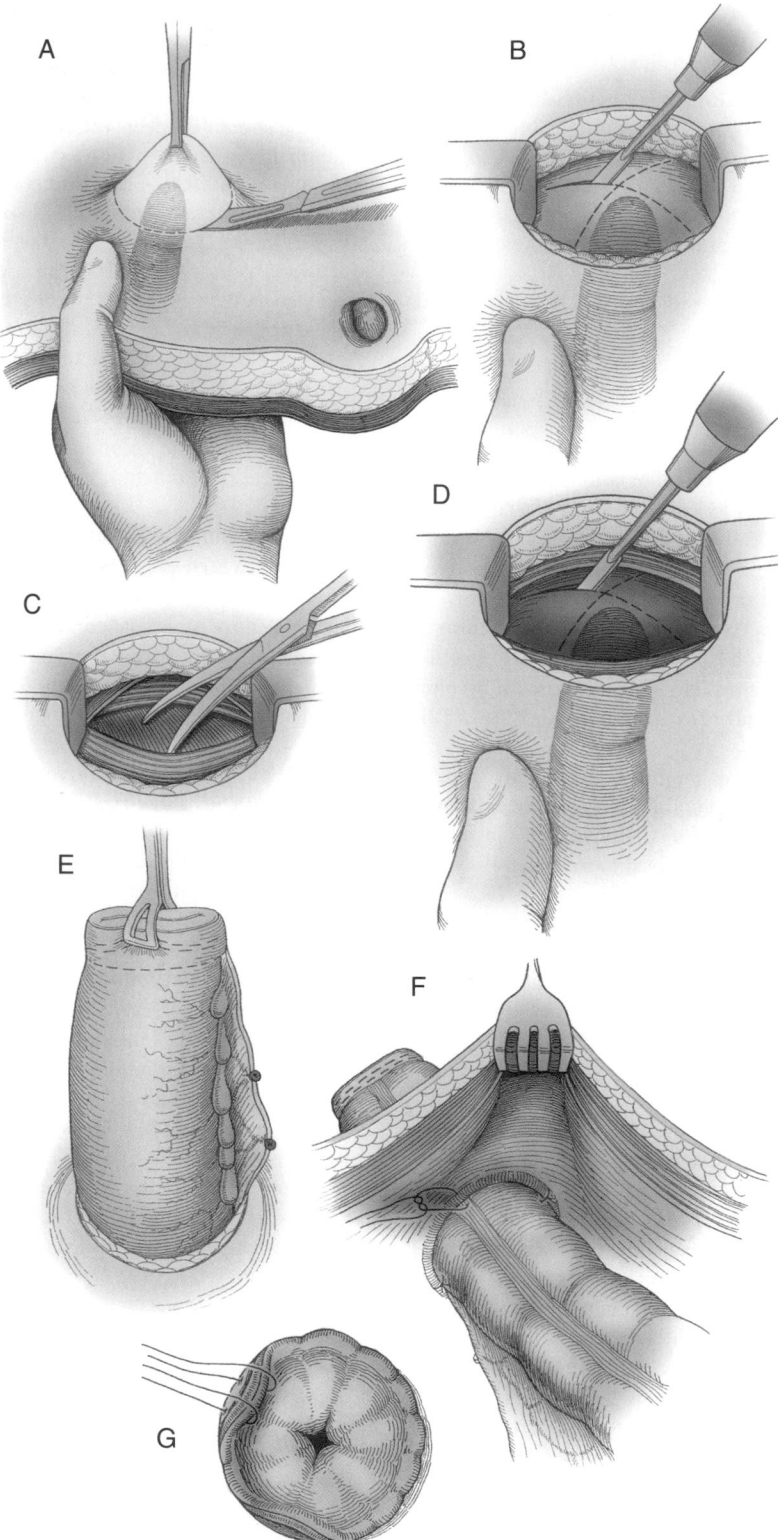

FIGURE 11-25 Construction of a colostomy through the anterior abdominal wall. **A,** A core of subcutaneous tissue is removed after making a circular skin incision with a #10 blade and using an electrosurgical pencil to dissect down to the anterior fascia. **B,** Muscle fibers are split. **C,** Tissues are dissected to the posterior layers, and, **D,** the peritoneum is opened. **E,** The colon is delivered through the abdominal wall so that it extends 2 to 3 cm beyond the skin surface. **F,** The bowel is tacked internally to the peritoneal defect. **G,** Four sutures are placed in each quadrant, incorporating the full-thickness cut end of the colon, the serosal surface approximately 1 to 2 cm below the open end of the colon, and up to the dermis. Additional sutures are used to mature the stoma, which refers to everting the mucosa to create a stable opening through which feces can evacuate.

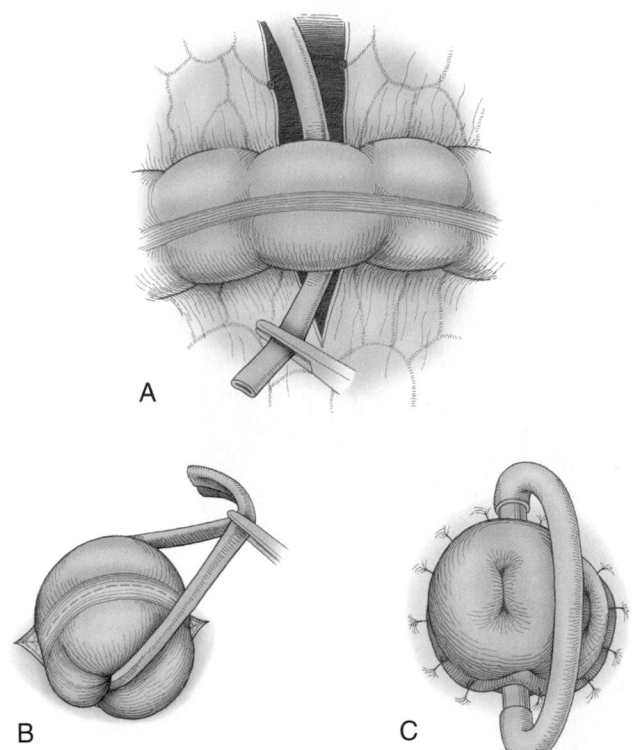

FIGURE 11-26 Transverse loop colostomy. **A,** The mesentery adjacent to the colon is taken down so that a Penrose drain may be passed beneath the colon. **B,** The colon is pulled through the transverse incision and opened longitudinally along the taeniae. **C,** An apparatus or rod is placed underneath the stoma; sutures are used to mature the colostomy. The rod can be removed after the seventh postoperative day.

and tighten, and the stapler fires to connect the bowel to the rectum. Removal of the proximal and distal bowel donuts from the stapler follows; the donuts undergo inspection for completeness; and the surgeon checks the anastomosis for leaks.

6. To check for leaks the proximal colon undergoes occlusion with a bowel clamp. Warm saline is instilled into the abdomen. The assistant instills air gently into the rectum from below while the surgeon observes the abdomen for bubbles. If present, bubbles indicate a leak that must be oversewn with suture. If there are no bubbles, the assistant dons a new gown and gloves before returning to the abdomen. New sterile drapes are placed over the legs.
7. The abdomen is closed in layers and a dressing applied.

Colon Resection

The purpose of colon resection is to remove malignant and nonmalignant lesions, to relieve an obstruction or a stricture, to repair a traumatic injury, or to treat inflammatory diseases of the bowel. The most common colon resections (Figure 11-27) are right hemicolectomy, transverse colon resection, left hemicolectomy, low anterior colon resection (Figure 11-28), and abdominal perineal colon resection (not illustrated). The extent of colon resected depends on the indication. Typically for malignant lesions, the resection includes the affected segment of colon and its regional lymph nodes, with the goal of removing as much tumor as possible at the time of surgery. Optimally the procedure also includes restoration of GI tract continuity, but when restoration is not possible, such as with

abdominal perineal resection for low-lying rectal cancer, a permanent colostomy may be required.

Supplies and instruments are the same for all types of colon resection. Instrumentation required includes a laparotomy set, GI instruments, long instruments, a self-retaining abdominal retractor, and a variety of GI linear and circular stapling devices. EEA sizers should be available. A long electrosurgical pencil tip is often needed and should be available. An extra Poole-type suction tip is kept clean for use when irrigating the abdomen with warm saline at the end of the procedure. Many surgeons perform an intraoperative colonoscopy, sigmoidoscopy, or ultrasound. Endoscopes and related equipment should be readily available along with a sterile ultrasound probe. All bowel resection procedures require use of bowel technique as previously described in order to keep contaminated instruments separate from uncontaminated instruments and supplies.

Open Right Hemicolectomy with Ileocolostomy

Procedural Considerations. Right hemicolectomy involves resection of the terminal ileum, the cecum, the ascending colon, and a portion of the transverse colon. It serves to remove disease of the cecum, ascending colon, or hepatic flexure. Extended right hemicolectomy removes lesions located in the transverse colon. A functional end-to-end, side-to-side, or end-to-side anastomosis creates a connection between the transverse colon and terminal ileum. These anastomosis techniques require one GI linear cutting stapler, three reloads, and one TA stapler. Alternately, the surgeon may hand sew the anastomosis in two layers using 3-0 absorbable and nonabsorbable suture on a tapered GI needle. Patient positioning is supine with general anesthesia. The anesthesia provider may insert an NG tube after intubation. Insertion of an indwelling urinary catheter precedes abdominal skin prep.

Operative Procedure

1. The surgeon opens through a midline incision and explores the peritoneal cavity. A self-retaining retractor is used to optimize exposure. Moist laparotomy sponges protect the wound edges or may pack the small bowel out of the immediate surgical field.
2. The surgeon identifies and confirms the lesion, and determines the extent of the resection.
3. The surgeon creates a mesenteric window for the GI linear stapler at the site of transection of the terminal ileum and divides the ileum.
4. Next the terminal ileum is freed from its mesenteric attachment. The mesenteric vessels undergo clamping, division with Metzenbaum scissors, and ligation with silk ties.
5. Mobilization of the cecum and its retraction medially expose the right peritoneal reflection. The right ureter is identified and protected.
6. Lateral mobilization carries up and around the hepatic flexure, with care taken not to damage the second portion of the duodenum.
7. At the limit of the planned resection, the surgeon creates a window in the mesentery of the transverse colon to allow insertion of the GI linear stapler. The stomach is identified as it lies behind the transverse colon.
8. The surgeon scores the mesentery between the transected ends of bowel with the electrosurgery pencil. Next the mesenteric vessels are isolated, clamped with Péan clamps, divided with Metzenbaum scissors, and ligated with 2-0 nonabsorbable or absorbable suture.

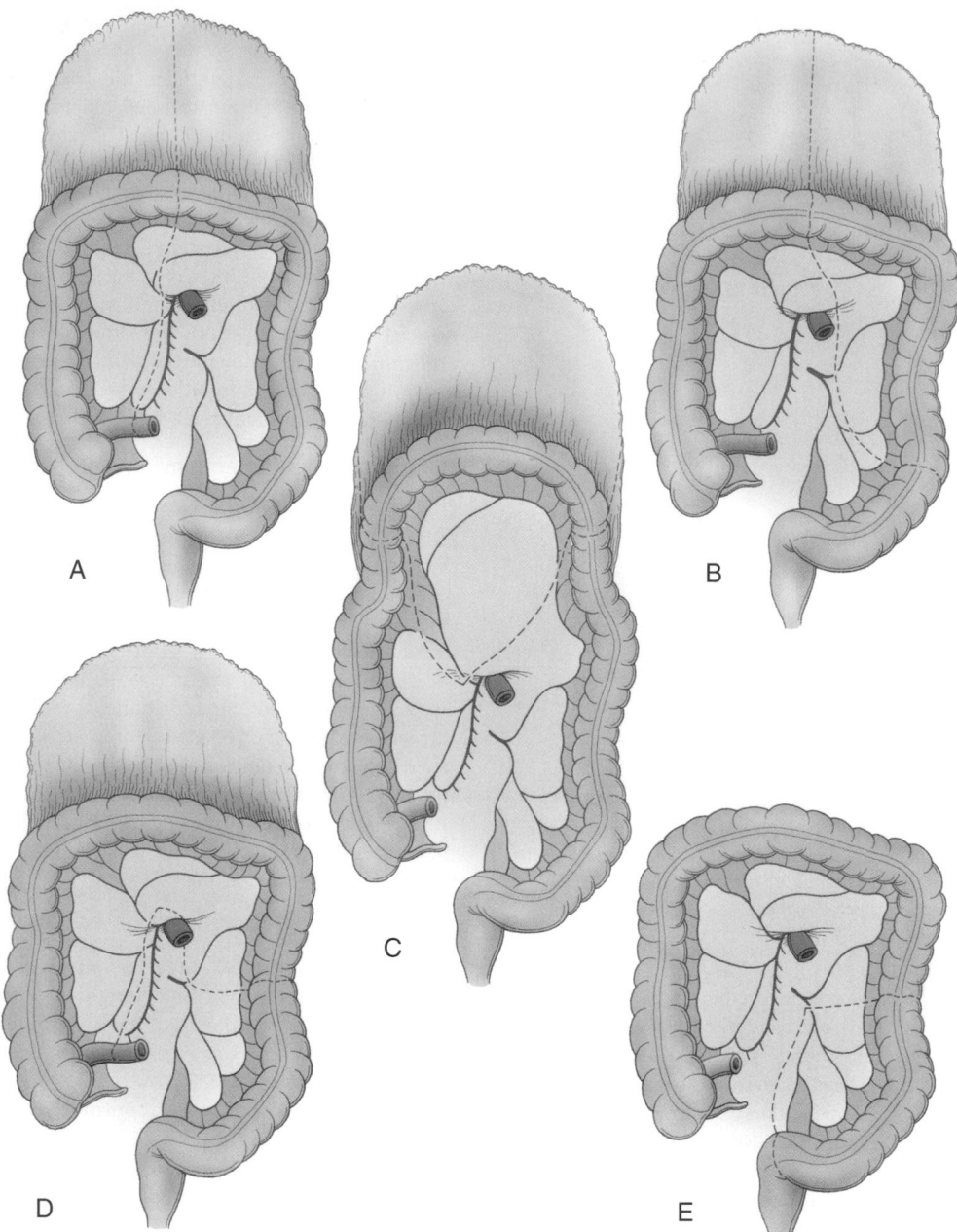

FIGURE 11-27 The resection lines for various types of colon resection. **A,** Right hemicolectomy and ileocolostomy. **B,** Left hemicolectomy. **C and D,** Transverse colectomy. **E,** Anterior resection of sigmoid colon and rectosigmoidostomy.

9. When the mesenteric resection is complete, the freed specimen passes off the field.
10. In preparation for the anastomosis, bowel technique commences.
11. With the stapled ends of the proximal and distal bowel facing the same direction, the transected ends of the bowel are in side-by-side position. The surgeon cuts a small corner of each segment diagonally across the staple line. Four mosquito clamps hold the two holes open to accept one leg each of a GI linear stapler. The stapler closes and fires, creating the anastomosis between the two segments of bowel. Three Allis clamps approximate the remaining enterotomy in a transverse direction and a linear stapler fires along the clamps. Using heavy

Mayo scissors or a knife, the surgeon excises the remnant of tissue held by the Allis clamps.
12. The staple lines undergo inspection for hemostasis. Contaminated instruments are placed in a basin, and the surgical team changes gowns and gloves.
13. The abdomen is irrigated with warm saline, closed in two layers using fresh sterile instruments, and dressings applied.

Laparoscopic Colon Resection

More and more colorectal surgical procedures use the laparoscopic approach, given continuing advances in laparoscopic technologies, acquisition of advanced laparoscopic skills by more surgeons, and growing evidence that laparoscopic surgical outcomes are as good

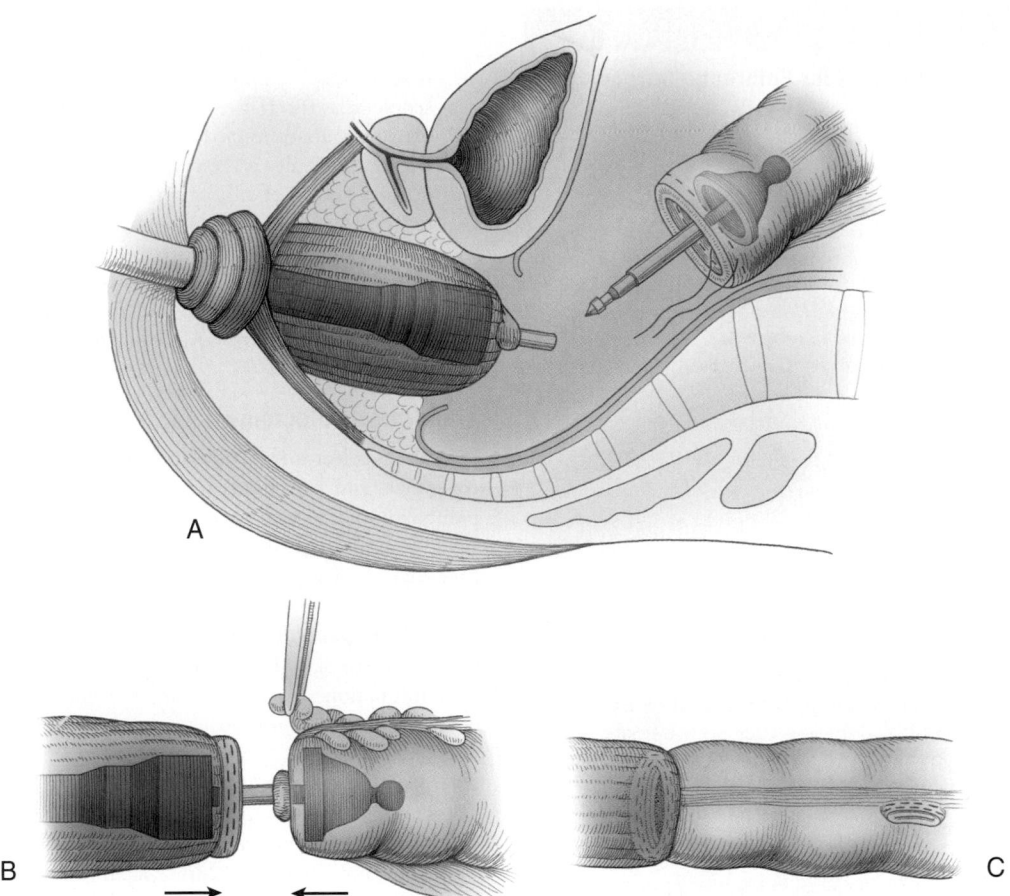

FIGURE 11-28 EEA stapling device, used to perform low anterior anastomosis. **A,** Stapler is introduced into anus, and the anvil is placed into the proximal colon loop. **B,** EEA is advanced to level of the anvil, and the EEA is closed and fired. **C,** Circular double-staggered row of staples joins bowel; simultaneously, circular blade in instrument cuts stoma. Instrument is gently removed. The resulting anastomosis is illustrated with bowel wall transparent to depict reconstruction.

as if not better than open approach surgical outcomes (Lengyel et al, 2010). Benefits of laparoscopic colon resection include less postoperative pain, potential for quicker return of bowel function, shorter hospital stays, and faster return to normal activity after surgery. Multidisciplinary enhanced recovery or "fast track" programs are becoming common for preoperative preparation and postoperative care of patients undergoing laparoscopic colorectal surgery (Evidence for Practice).

Procedural Considerations. Required instruments include a laparotomy set, laparoscopy instruments, and supplies, including a 30-degree laparoscope; a variety of laparoscopic GI linear and circular stapling devices; bipolar tissue sealing forceps; ultrasonic shears; atraumatic grasping forceps to manipulate the bowel; and laparoscopic suturing instruments or devices such as needle holders, knot pushers, and specialized suture.

Depending on the segment of bowel to be removed, patient positioning is supine or modified lithotomy position. Tucking the patient's arms allows for full access to all abdominal trocars by the surgeon and assistants. For sigmoid colectomy or low anterior colectomy, access to the rectum is necessary to perform an end-to-end anastomosis. The surgeon may stand on the patient's right, left, or between the patient's legs. Application of IPCDs minimizes the risk

of DVT. Restraining straps or wide cloth tape secures the patient to the OR bed to prevent shifting during steep position changes. A beanbag device also may aid positioning. Insertion of an NG tube and urinary catheter precede abdominal skin prep. A preoperative or intraoperative sigmoidoscopy or colonoscopy can verify the location of the lesion to be resected.

Operative Procedure (Laparoscopic Right Hemicolectomy)
1. Pneumoperitoneum is established and the surgeon enters the abdomen as described in the section on laparoscopy.
2. Placement of additional access ports (usually 5 mm) depends on the segment of colon being resected.
3. Beginning at the level of the cecum, the surgeon mobilizes the colon from its lateral peritoneal attachments using ultrasonic shears or bipolar vessel-sealing forceps. Some laparoscopic surgeons will mobilize the colon from a medial to lateral direction, taking the mesenteric blood vessels before mobilizing the lateral attachments. The description here is for the lateral to medial approach. Atraumatic graspers provide gentle medial traction on the colon. Patient positioning is as needed to optimize exposure.
4. The surgeon identifies the cecum and terminal ileum. The right ureter is also identified and protected. Mobilization of the

Enhanced Recovery Programs for Colorectal Surgery

Evidence-based strategies to enhance recovery after elective colorectal surgery accelerate a patient's return to preoperative levels of health and functional status and facilitate early discharge by reducing the surgical stress response and organ dysfunction that can occur after major abdominal surgery. Also known as fast track programs, enhanced recovery programs combine individual evidence-based strategies to create standardized preoperative, intraoperative, and postoperative pathways of care that are implemented by multidisciplinary patient care teams to improve patient outcomes and reduce health care costs. Examples of a colorectal fast track program follow:

Preoperative Strategies
- Extensive patient education about ostomy care, what to expect in regard to recovery milestones such as return to regular diet, driving, work, and other activities; addressing self-care needs or challenges, and ensuring patients know what postoperative conditions require them to seek medical attention after discharge
- Preoperative assessment, risk evaluation, and optimization of comorbid conditions
- Limited use or eliminating bowel preparation
- Fasting from meat and fried and fatty food for 8 hours
- Fasting from light meals and unclear liquids for 6 hours
- Fasting from clear liquids for 2 hours

Intraoperative Strategies
- Deep vein thrombosis prophylaxis
- Antibiotic prophylaxis
- High concentration of inspired oxygenation
- Thoracic epidural analgesia
- Anesthesia using rapid-onset, short-acting anesthetic gases and drugs
- Balanced fluid management
- Temperature regulation
- Limited use of nasogastric tubes
- Laparoscopic approach when possible
- Limited use of peritoneal drains

Postoperative Strategies
- Minimized use of opioid analgesia when possible
- Aggressive management of nausea
- Enteral nutrition on day 1
- Liquid diet within a few hours after surgery
- Early mobilization (on day of surgery)
- Early removal of urinary catheter

Modified from Ricciardi R, MacKay G: Fast-track protocols in colorectal surgery. In Basow DS, editor: *UpToDate*, Waltham, MA, 2012, UpToDate.

cecum and ileum follows. The surgeon creates a small mesenteric window and places a GI stapler in the window across the terminal ileum. The stapler fires and transects the bowel.

5. The lateral peritoneal dissection carries up and around the hepatic flexure, as the surgeon takes care not to damage the second portion of the duodenum.
6. At the limit of the planned resection the surgeon creates a window in the mesentery of the transverse colon to allow insertion of the GI linear stapler.
7. Positioned across the transverse colon, the stapler fires, transecting the transverse colon.

8. Division of the mesentery between the transected ends of the bowel follows, using a GI linear stapler, ultrasonic shears, a bipolar vessel-sealing device, or hemostatic clips and laparoscopic scissors. If the surgeon uses the stapler, several staple cartridges are necessary.
9. Bowel continuity is reestablished by intracorporeal or extracorporeal creation of a functional end-to-end or side-to-side anastomosis using GI linear stapling devices.
10. Closure of mesentery defects is with 3-0 nonabsorbable figure-of-eight sutures, according to surgeon preference.
11. The abdomen is irrigated and then inspected for hemostasis. Access ports are removed under direct visualization and port sites closed.

Transverse Colectomy

Transverse colectomy removes malignant lesions of the ascending, transverse, and left colon. The extent of resection depends on the pathology and location of the lesion to be removed (see Figure 11-27, *C* and *D*). A functional end-to-end anastomosis reestablishes bowel continuity.

Procedural Considerations. Patient positioning is supine with general anesthesia. The anesthesia provider may insert an NG tube after intubation. Insertion of an indwelling urinary catheter precedes abdominal skin prep.

Operative Procedure
1. The surgeon opens the abdomen through a midline incision and explores the peritoneal cavity. A self-retaining retractor is placed to optimize exposure. Moist laparotomy sponges protect the wound edges or may pack the small bowel out of the immediate field.
2. The surgeon identifies and confirms the lesion and determines the extent of the resection.
3. Incising the lateral peritoneal attachments mobilizes the hepatic flexure of the colon. Mobilization of the splenic flexure of the colon follows in similar fashion.
4. A mesenteric window is created for the GI linear stapler at the proximal and distal site of transection. The linear stapler divides the bowel. A staple reload achieves the second resection.
5. The surgeon uses hemostats, Metzenbaum scissors, and 3-0 nonabsorbable ligatures on the middle and left colic vessels.
6. Bowel technique commences and creation of a functional end-to-end anastomosis takes place as described for right colectomy.

Low Anterior Resection of the Sigmoid Colon with End-to-End Rectosigmoidostomy

A low anterior resection removes malignant lesions in the sigmoid colon or proximal rectum or treats inflammatory bowel disease of the colon. This resection removes the distal portion of the sigmoid colon and rectosigmoid portion of the rectum (see Figure 11-27, *E*). Surgery can include reestablishment of continuity between the proximal sigmoid colon and the rectum if the distal rectal margin is cancer-free and adequate length remains to create a tension-free well-vascularized anastomosis (Ko, 2010).

Procedural Considerations. Laparotomy and GI sets are required. Linear stapling instruments as well as the end-to-end curved mechanical stapling instruments (EEA) are necessary along with long instruments for dissecting into the pelvis. A rigid sigmoidoscope may be required both before patient preparation and after anastomosis. A self-retaining retractor set is also required. A table with rectal instruments, the rigid sigmoidoscope, an end-to-end circular stapler, and suction tubing should be available for the portion of the procedure performed through the anus. Another table with instruments reserved for closure of the abdomen may also be prepared, according to surgeon preference. Lighted or unlighted ureteral stents help identify the ureters intraoperatively. If requested, equipment and supplies for a cystoscopy and insertion of ureteral stents will be necessary. A urologist will place stents before abdominal prep.

Operative Procedure

1. The surgeon opens the abdomen through a midline incision and explores the peritoneal cavity. A self-retaining retractor is placed to optimize exposure. Moist laparotomy sponges protect the wound edges or may pack the small bowel out of the immediate field.
2. The surgeon identifies and confirms the lesion and determines the extent and feasibility of the resection.
3. Lateral mobilization of the sigmoid colon begins along the avascular peritoneal reflection using sharp and blunt dissection, taking care to protect the left ureter and gonadal vessels as they enter the pelvis.
4. Medial mobilization follows, as the surgeon takes care to visualize and protect the right ureter.
5. The surgeon develops the presacral space and frees the rectum circumferentially from its anterior, posterior, medial, and lateral attachments with blunt and sharp dissection, and bipolar vessel-sealing forceps.
6. Retraction of the uterus or bladder, if needed, is with a lighted retractor, Harrington, Deaver, or other long retractor.
7. The surgeon identifies the distal margin of resection and transects the rectum with a curved articulating GI linear stapler.
8. Resection of the proximal sigmoid colon is with a GI linear stapler.
9. Mobilization of the remaining sigmoid and left colon from their lateral attachments follows as needed to allow for a tension-free anastomosis to the rectum.
10. The proximal and distal segments of bowel are positioned end to end. The surgeon makes an enterotomy in the proximal end, inserts the anvil of the circular stapler, and secures it with a purse-string stitch using nonabsorbable suture.
11. An assistant moves between the legs to insert the cutting circular stapler anally into the rectum. The assistant performing the "below part" requires the previously set up table for this portion of the procedure. The anvil and the stapler connect and tighten; the stapler then fires to connect the bowel to the rectum (see Figure 11-28). Removal of the proximal and distal bowel donuts from the stapler and inspection ensure they are complete circles. The donuts are included as part of the specimen.
12. The anastomosis is checked for leaks. The proximal colon is occluded with a bowel clamp, and warm saline is instilled into the abdomen. The assistant then gently instills air into the rectum from below while the surgeon observes the abdomen for bubbles; bubbles indicate a leak that needs oversewing with suture. If there are no bubbles, the assistant dons a new gown and gloves before returning to the abdomen. A new sterile drape is placed over the legs.
13. The abdomen is closed and dressings applied.

Abdominoperineal Resection

Abdominoperineal resection (APR) (Figure 11-29) is complete excision of the sigmoid colon, rectum, and anus for low rectal or anal cancers, complications of ulcerative colitis or Crohn's disease, or fecal incontinence (Monson and Fleming, 2012).

Procedural Considerations.
The abdominal portion of the procedure occurs with the patient in supine or lithotomy position. If the perineal portion of the procedure requires the jackknife position, the abdominal part will occur with the patient supine. After mobilization and transection of the rectum the abdomen undergoes closure and dressing, and patient positioning changes to jackknife position for perineal dissection. If two teams work simultaneously, patient positioning is modified lithotomy. Two setups are required if two teams are to work at the same time. Insertion of an indwelling catheter into the urinary bladder occurs after induction of anesthesia. Before perineal prep, the rectum may be irrigated with povidone-iodine solution and then sewn closed with a purse-string stitch. A cystoscopy and placement of ureteral stents may follow. The anesthesia provider may insert an NG tube after intubation. A GI instrument set and a colostomy appliance are required for the abdominal portion of the procedure. A rectal set for the perineal portion of the procedure is also required.

Operative Procedure

1. The surgeon opens the abdomen through a midline incision and explores the peritoneal cavity. A self-retaining retractor is used to optimize exposure. Moist laparotomy sponges protect the wound edges or may pack the small bowel out of the immediate surgical field.
2. The surgeon identifies and confirms the lesion and determines the extent and feasibility of the resection.
3. The abdominal portion of the procedure proceeds as described for a low anterior resection.
4. The surgeon mobilizes and resects the proximal colon for creation of a colostomy, completed after closure of the abdomen.
5. The surgeon makes an incision around the anus in an elliptic manner outside the sphincter muscles with a generous margin of perianal skin. A self-retaining rectal retractor is used for exposure.
6. Hemorrhoidal vessels are suture ligated and divided.
7. The surgeon divides the anococcygeal ligament and levator ani muscle to enter the pelvic fossa.
8. Mobilization and removal of the sigmoid and rectal stump are through the perineal incision.
9. Any bleeding points are clamped and tied.
10. Drains are placed and exteriorized through stab wounds in the buttocks.
11. If two teams are not available for synchronous excision of the perineum, the perineal portion of the operation follows completion of the abdominal resection.

Ileoanal Endorectal Pull-Through (Ileal Pouch–Anal Anastomosis)

Ileal endorectal pull-through, also called ileal pouch–anal anastomosis (IPAA), reestablishes GI continuity between the ileum and the rectum after proctocolectomy if the anal sphincter muscles are intact. Proctocolectomy with IPAA is the procedure of choice to treat ulcerative colitis (UC) or familial adenomatous polyposis (FAP), a heredity condition in which patients are at high risk to develop colon cancer at an early age (Cima and Pemberton, 2010;

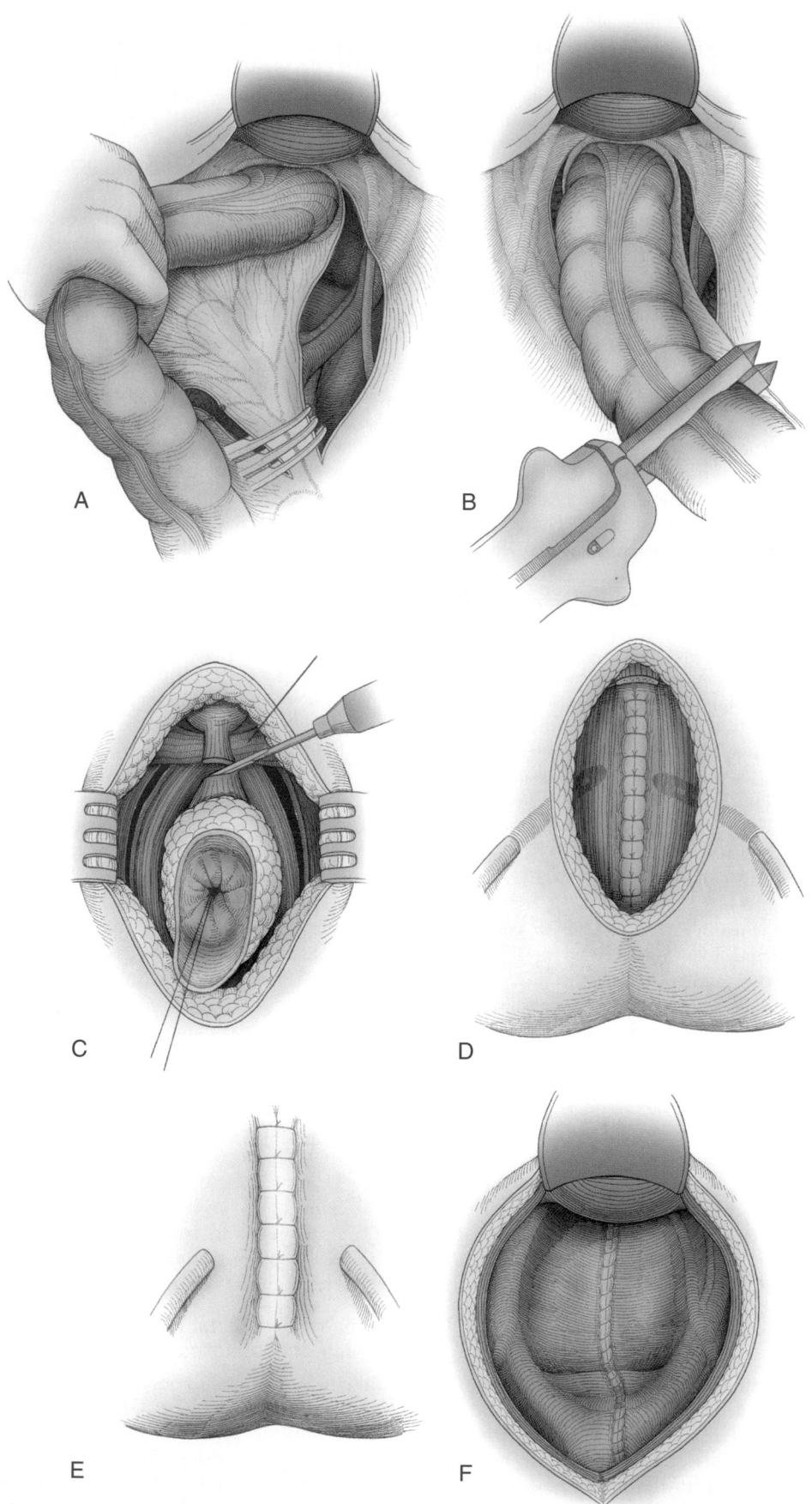

FIGURE 11-29 Abdominoperineal resection for cancer of the rectum. **A,** The sigmoid colon is deflected to the right to complete the rectosigmoid peritoneal detachment. **B,** The distal sigmoid is transected to allow for better access to mobilize the rectum from the sacrum. **C,** The rectal stump is excised from the perineal approach. **D,** Drains are placed and moved through stab wounds; the levator tissues are reapproximated with 2-0 synthetic absorbable sutures. **E,** The perineal skin is closed. **F,** The pelvic peritoneal floor is closed from the abdominal approach.

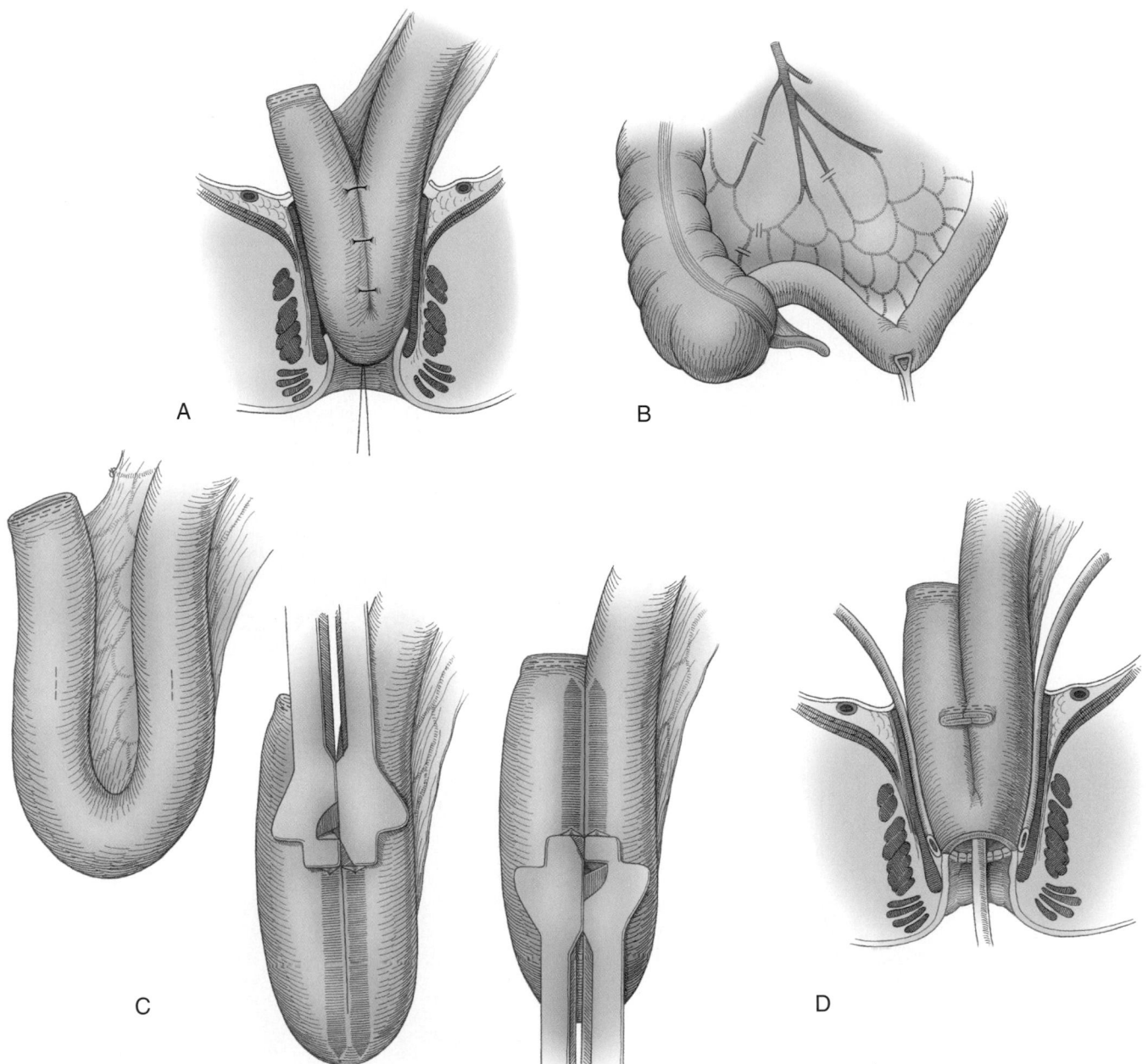

FIGURE 11-30 J pouch for ileoanal endorectal pull-through. **A,** The J pouch is created at terminal ileum by folding two adjacent loops of small bowel, approximately 10 to 15 cm each, parallel to each other. **B,** Mesenteric vascular arcades may need to be divided to provide adequate length for anal anastomosis. **C,** The two loops are anastomosed using a mechanical cutting and stapling device (GIA). **D,** Opening is made at bottom of pouch, and pouch is pulled through rectal stump. Bottom of pouch is anastomosed to anus.

Park et al, 2012). To decrease the frequent number of stools produced after a straight ileoanal anastomosis, the surgeon creates a pouch in the shape of a J, then staples it to the remaining anus (Figure 11-30). IPAA requires two surgical procedures. At the time of the proctocolectomy the surgeon creates the ileoanal J pouch, but to allow the pouch staple lines to heal properly, also creates a diverting ileostomy. At the second operation some 8 to 12 weeks later, closure of the ileostomy follows (Cima and Pemberton, 2010).

Procedural Considerations. Patient positioning is in modified lithotomy. The anesthesia provider inserts an NG tube after intubation. Insertion of an indwelling urinary catheter precedes abdominal

skin prep. Setup includes a laparotomy set, GI instrument set, a perineal set, rectal instrumentation, and a self-retaining retractor system. Preparation of separate instrument tables accommodates the distinct rectal and abdominal approaches. A proctoscope is available for use at the conclusion of the procedure to check for anastomotic leaks. Application of an ileostomy appliance occurs at the end of the procedure.

Operative Procedure

1. The surgeon opens the abdomen through a midline incision and explores the peritoneal cavity. A self-retaining retractor is used to optimize exposure. Moist laparotomy sponges protect the

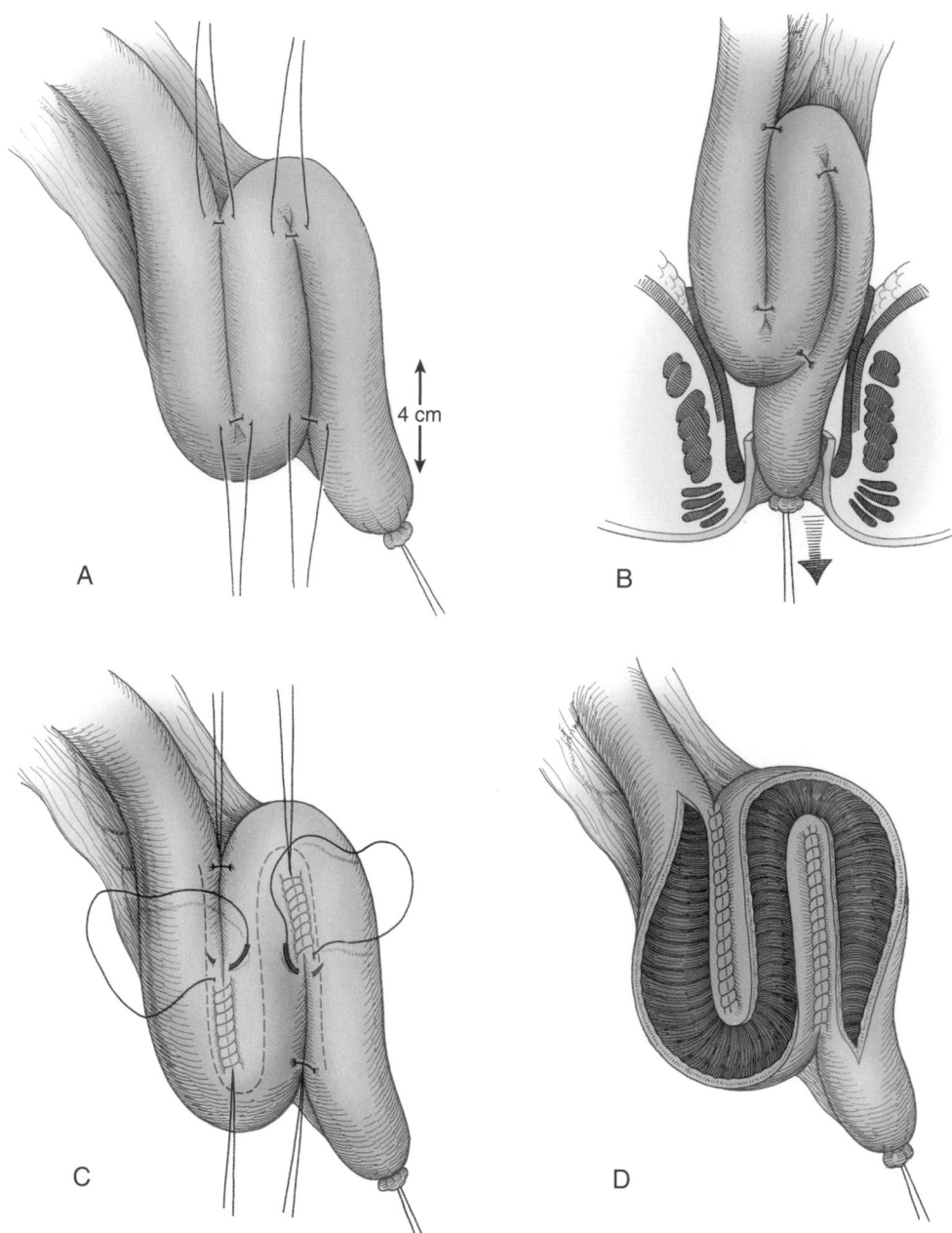

FIGURE 11-31 S pouch for ileoanal endorectal pull-through. **A,** Pouch is created by aligning distal ileum in S configuration with each limb (three in total) approximately 12 cm in length. **B,** The length is measured before anastomosis begins. **C,** Three limbs are incised and anastomosed to create pouch. **D,** Incision is made as illustrated.

E

F

G

H

FIGURE 11-31, cont'd E, The pouch is closed using suture for the formation of the reservoir. **F,** Distal ends of ileum and pouch are pulled through the rectal stump, and the lower outflow tract is trimmed. **G,** With 3-0 absorbable sutures, the outflow tract is anastomosed to the anus at the dentate line. **H,** Drain in place in the lumen of the newly created ileoanal-rectal canal.

wound edges or may pack the small bowel out of the immediate surgical field.

2. Using a GI linear stapler between the cecum and the distal ileum, the surgeon divides the bowel, taking care to preserve the ileocolic vessels.

3. The terminal ileum and an adjacent segment of ileum are placed side by side in the pelvis to create the pouch. A measuring device gauges the distance of the mesenteric pedicle to the apex of the pouch. Preservation of blood supply to the pouch occurs by taking care to prevent tension on the mesentery.

4. Sequential firings of a 75-mm GI stapler in the two limbs of the ileum create the J pouch, after which the surgeon makes an opening in the bottom of the pouch. One surgeon moves between the legs to perform the perineal portion of the procedure while the other surgeon stays "above."

5. A self-retaining rectal retractor (Lonestar) is placed to provide exposure of the anal canal. Injection of about 10 to 20 mL of 0.25% bupivacaine with 1:200,000 epinephrine into the submucosal plane of the anus lifts the anal mucosa off the longitudinal muscle. Next the anal canal mucosa is circumferentially excised.

6. The surgeon hand sews the opening at the bottom of the pouch to the dentate line (also called the pectinate line) in the anal canal with interrupted 2-0 absorbable sutures.

7. After the anastomosis is complete it is tested it for leaks. The abdomen is filled with warm saline. The ileum is occluded with a bowel clamp proximal to the J pouch. Air instillation with a proctoscope follows. Bubbles in the abdomen indicate a leak, which is oversewn with nonabsorbable suture.

8. With the pouch complete, the surgical team dons new sterile gowns and gloves before closing the abdomen and creating a loop ileostomy.

9. Dressings and an ileostomy appliance are applied.

Alternatively, the surgeon may opt to create a Y pouch by aligning the distal ileum in an S configuration (Figure 11-31) with each of the three limbs about 10 cm in length. The most distal 2 cm of the ileum are not incorporated into the pouch, but preserved for anastomosis to the anus. The surgeon manually incises the three limbs and anastomoses them to create a pouch. Mucosal tissue is anastomosed with absorbable suture; nonabsorbable suture is used on the serosal layer. The surgeon pulls the preserved distal end of the ileum and the pouch through the rectal stump and anastomoses it to the anus. This completes the anal portion of the procedure.

The scrub team changes gowns and gloves, redrapes, and completes the abdominal procedure by creating a loop ileostomy through the abdominal wall on a previously designated site.

Surgery of the Rectum

Hemorrhoidectomy

Hemorrhoidectomy, an ambulatory surgical procedure, is excision of internal and external hemorrhoids. Hemorrhoids can cause rectal bleeding, pain, and itching. When hemorrhoids do not respond to conservative medical treatment, surgical excision is appropriate (Gore, 2010).

Procedural Considerations. Preoperative anal dilation helps expose the vessels and contributes to patient comfort in the immediate postoperative period. Many surgeons prefer to perform a rigid proctoscopy to rule out rectal disease before surgery. Spinal, caudal, epidural, and local anesthesia are options. Patient positioning usually is in lithotomy or jackknife with the buttocks taped apart. Required instrumentation is a rectal set.

Operative Procedure

1. The surgeon inserts an anal retractor to expose the hemorrhoid.

2. The hemorrhoid is grasped with an Allis or Babcock clamp and traction applied.

3. The surgeon positions and ties a 2-0 absorbable suture around the apex of the hemorrhoid.

4. Excision of the hemorrhoid is with electrosurgery, a knife blade, or Metzenbaum scissors. Care is required to preserve the rectal sphincter.

5. The anal mucosa is closed with a 2-0 absorbable suture and a petrolatum gauze dressing placed over the wound in the anal canal.

Excision of Pilonidal Cyst and Sinus

Excision of a pilonidal cyst and sinus is removal of the cyst with sinus tracts from the gluteal fold overlying the sacrum (Figure 11-32). Pilonidal cysts and sinuses result from ingrown hairs in the gluteal fold. Pilonidal cysts are more common in men. They rarely become symptomatic until the individual reaches adulthood. Symptoms vary from a mild, irritating, draining sinus tract to a painful, acute abscess that may recur frequently. Treatment consists of drainage in the acute stage and total surgical excision during remission. Complete excision of the cyst and sinus tracts prevents recurrence. The defect resulting from recurrence may be too large for primary closure; if so, the wound is left open to heal by granulation.

Procedural Considerations. Setup includes a minor set and rectal instruments, as well as methylene blue, a 10- or 20-mL syringe, and a blunt-tipped needle. The patient is positioned in jackknife with the buttocks taped open laterally and secured to the sides of the OR bed.

Operative Procedure

1. The surgeon identifies the sinus tract(s) with a probe and makes an incision over the probe.

2. The tract(s) is injected with methylene blue using a blunt needle.

3. The surgeon makes an elliptic incision down to the fascia.

4. With a curette, granulation tissue is removed.

5. The surgeon completes excision of the cyst and sinus tract(s), and any bleeding is controlled.

6. If the surgeon plans to close the skin, extensive "undermining" of the skin may be needed to avoid excessive tension on the wound edges.

KEY POINTS

- GI surgery is a very broad field that encompasses surgical procedures of the esophagus, stomach, small intestine, large intestine, and rectum.
- Many GI surgical procedures have been adapted to accommodate a minimally invasive approach.
- A sound understanding of surgical anatomy and common approaches to the structures of the GI tract is critical to planning surgical care.
- Planning surgical care for patients undergoing GI surgery requires a team approach with clear communication among the entire surgical team.

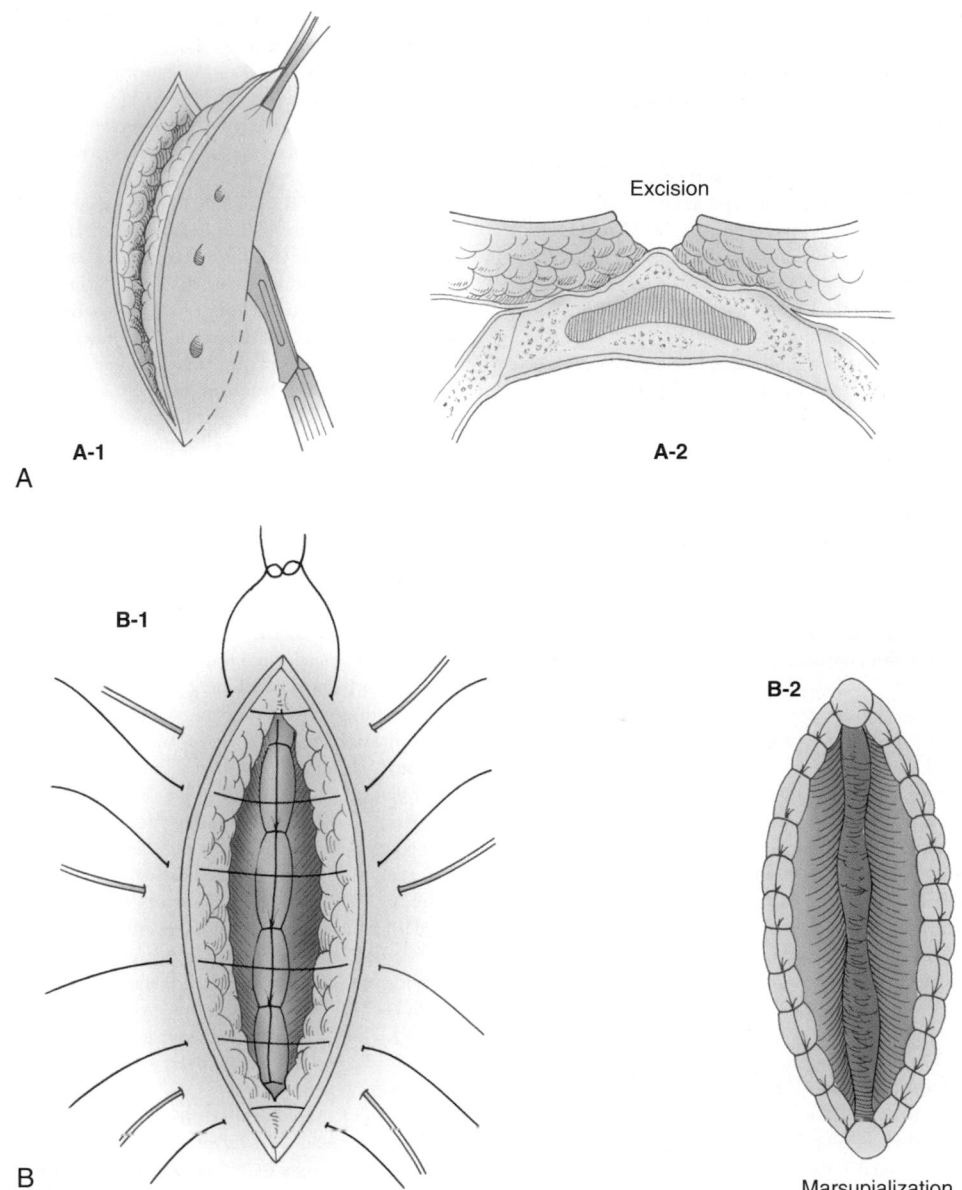

FIGURE 11-32 Pilonidal cyst. The pilonidal sinus tract is identified with injection of methylene blue into the tract. **A,** Wide elliptic incision *(A-1)* is made to include all the subcutaneous tracts and tissue that are part of the fascia overlying the sacrum and coccyx *(A-2)*. **B,** Closure of the wound can be primary *(B-1)* or secondary *(B-2)*.

CRITICAL THINKING QUESTION

Your next patient is scheduled for laparoscopic, possible open, low anterior colon resection with possible end-to-end anastomosis. Knowing that this is a major GI procedure, what are some of the patient care factors that need to be considered in preparing for this patient?

⊖volve *The answer to the Critical Thinking Question can be found at http://evolve.elsevier.com/Rothrock/Alexander.*

REFERENCES

Anderson J et al: The first national examination of outcomes and trends in robotic surgery in the United States, *J Am Coll Surg* 215(1):107–116, 2012.

Angel C: Pyloromyotomy. In Townsend C, Evers BM, editors: *Atlas of general surgical techniques*, Philadelphia, 2010, Saunders.

Association of periOperative Registered Nurses (AORN): *AORN Standards and Recommended Practices*, Denver, 2013, AORN, Inc.

Bergman J: Radiofrequency ablation for Barrett's esophagus. In Basow DS, editor: *UpToDate*, Waltham, MA, 2012, UpToDate.

Buchman AL: Short bowel syndrome. In Feldman M et al, editors: *Sleisenger and Fordtran's gastrointestinal and liver disease: pathophysiology, diagnosis, management*, ed 9, Philadelphia, 2010, Saunders.

Bumm R, Siewert R: Distal gastrectomy with Billroth I or Billroth II reconstruction. In Fischer JE, editor: *Fischer's mastery of surgery*, ed 6, Philadelphia, 2012, Lippincott Williams & Wilkins.

Cave D: Wireless videocapsule endoscopy. In Basow DS, editor: *UpToDate*, Waltham, MA, 2012, UpToDate.

Chambers W et al: Single-incision laparoscopic surgery (SILS) in complex colorectal surgery: a technique offering potential and not just cosmesis, *Colorectal Dis* 13:393–398, 2011.

Cima RR, Pemberton JH: Ileostomy, colostomy, and pouches. In Feldman M et al, editors: *Sleisenger and Fordtran's gastrointestinal and liver disease: pathophysiology, diagnosis, management*, ed 9, Philadelphia, 2010, Saunders.

Cone M et al: Dramatic decreases in mortality from laparoscopic colon resections based on data from the nationwide inpatient sample, *Arch Surg* 146(5):594–600, 2011.

De la Cruz-Munoz N et al: Bariatric surgery significantly decreases the prevalence of type 2 diabetes mellitus and pre-diabetes among morbidly obese multiethnic adults: long term results, *J Am Coll Surg* 212(4):505–511, 2011.

DeMaria EJ et al: Early postoperative outcomes of metabolic surgery to treat diabetes from sites participating in the ASMBS bariatric surgery center of excellence program as reported in the bariatric outcomes longitudinal database, *Ann Surg* 252(3):505–511, 2011.

Doorly MG, Senagore A: Pathogenesis and clinical and economic consequences of postoperative ileus, *Surg Clin North Am* 92:259–272, 2012.

Doughty D, Landmann, MD: Management of patients with a colostomy or ileostomy. In Basow DS, editor: *UpToDate*, Waltham, MA, 2012, UpToDate.

Eakin J, Melvin WS: Achalasia. In Cameron J, Cameron AM, editors: *Current surgical therapy*, ed 10, Philadelphia, 2011, Saunders.

ECRI Institute's top 10 C-suite Watch list: *Hospital technology issues for 2013, ECRI, Plymouth Meeting, PA*, available at www.ecri.org/2013watchlist. Accessed March 12, 2013.

Elpern E et al: Original research: the application of intermittent pneumatic compression devices for thromboprophylaxis, *Am J Nurs* 113(4):30–36, 2013.

Evans S, Bhanot P: Abdominal wall incision and repair including release. In Fischer JE, editor: *Fischer's mastery of surgery*, ed 6, Philadelphia, 2012, Lippincott Williams & Wilkins.

Evers BM: Gastrojejunostomy. In Townsend C, Evers BM, editors: *Atlas of general surgical techniques*, Philadelphia, 2010a, Saunders.

Evers BM: Open and laparoscopic closure of perforated gastric ulcer. In Townsend C, Evers BM, editors: *Atlas of general surgical techniques*, Philadelphia, 2010b, Saunders.

Francone TD: Surgical principles of ostomy construction. In Basow DS, editor: *UpToDate*, Waltham, MA, 2012, UpToDate.

Fried GM: Emerging technology in surgery: informatics, robotics, and electronics. In Townsend CM et al, editors, *Sabiston's textbook of surgery*, ed 19, Philadelphia, 2012, Saunders.

Friedland S, Van Dam J: Optical coherence tomography in the gastrointestinal tract. In Basow DS, editor: *UpToDate*, Waltham, MA, 2012, UpToDate.

Fry RD et al: Colon and Rectum. In Townsend C, Evers BM, editors: *Atlas of general surgical techniques*, Philadelphia, 2010, Saunders.

Garud SS, Willingham FF: Natural orifice transluminal endoscopic surgery, *Gastrointestinal Endoscopy* 76(3):491-495, 2012.

Gore D: Hemorrhoidectomy. In Townsend C, Evers BM, editors: *Atlas of general surgical techniques*, Philadelphia, 2010, Saunders.

Greenwald D, Cohen J: Overview of upper gastrointestinal endoscopy (esophagogastroduodenoscopy). In Basow DS, editor: *UpToDate*, Waltham, MA, 2012, UpToDate.

Guelrud M: Management of benign esophageal strictures. In Basow DS, editor: *UpToDate*, Waltham, MA, 2012, UpToDate.

Jayne D et al: Robotic platforms for general and colorectal surgery, *Colorectal Dis* 13(7):78–82, 2011.

Jones D, Jones S: Perioperative management of morbid obesity. In Fischer JE, editor: *Fischer's mastery of surgery*, ed 6, Philadelphia, 2012, Lippincott Williams & Wilkins.

Khan FA, Selvaggi G: Overview of intestinal and multivisceral transplantation. In Basow DS, editor: *UpToDate*, Waltham, MA, 2012, UpToDate.

King J, Hines O: Anatomy and physiology of the stomach. In Yeo CJ, editor: *Shackelford's surgery of the alimentary tract*, ed 7, Philadelphia, 2013, Saunders.

Kita H: Overview of deep small bowel enteroscopy. In Basow DS, editor: *UpToDate*, Waltham, MA, 2012, UpToDate.

Ko TC: Low anterior resection—total mesorectal excision. In Townsend C, Evers BM, editors: *Atlas of general surgical techniques*, Philadelphia, 2010, Saunders.

Lengyel J et al: Trends towards increased use of the laparoscopic approach to colorectal surgery, *Colorectal Dis* 12:1007–1012, 2010.

Litkouhi B: Postoperative ileus. In Basow DS, editor: *UpToDate*, Waltham, MA, 2012, UpToDate.

Loran D, Zwischenberger J: Esophagectomy—transhiatal. In Townsend C, Evers BM, editors: *Atlas of general surgical techniques*, Philadelphia, 2010, Saunders.

Mahvi D, Krantz SB: Stomach. In Townsend C, Evers BM, editors: *Atlas of general surgical techniques*, Philadelphia, 2010, Saunders.

Maidl L, Ohland J: Care of stomas. In Fischer JE, editor: *Fischer's mastery of surgery*, ed 6, Philadelphia, 2010, Lippincott Williams & Wilkins.

Maish MS: Esophagus. In Townsend C, Evers BM, editors: *Atlas of general surgical techniques*, Philadelphia, 2010, Saunders.

Mason J: Mechanisms of nutrient absorption and malabsorption. In Basow DS, editor: *UpToDate*, Waltham, MA, 2012, UpToDate.

Mechanick JI et al: Clinical practice guidelines for the perioperative nutritional, metabolic, and nonsurgical support of the bariatric surgery patient—2013 Update: Cosponsored by American Association of Clinical Endocrinologists, The Obesity Society, and American Society for Metabolic & Bariatric Surgery, *Endocr Pract* e1–e36, available at http://aace.metapress.com/content/53256517v45810x4. Accessed March 29, 2013.

Mehrdad N, Marks J: Preoperative preparation of the surgical patient. In Cameron J, Cameron AM, editors: *Current surgical therapy*, ed 10, Philadelphia, 2011, Saunders.

Mizell J: Abdominal surgical incisions: prevention and treatment of complications. In Basow DS, editor: *UpToDate*, Waltham, MA, 2012a, UpToDate.

Mizell J: Principles of abdominal wall closure. In Basow DS, editor: *UpToDate*, Waltham, MA, 2012b, UpToDate.

Monson J, Fleming F: Abdominal perineal resection (APR): Open technique. In Basow DS, editor: *UpToDate*, Waltham, MA, 2012, UpToDate.

Nicholson M: A comparison of warming interventions on the temperatures of inpatients undergoing colorectal surgery, *AORN J* 97(3):310–322, 2013.

Nikfarjam M, Ponsky J: Endoluminal approach to gastroesophageal reflux disease. In Cameron J, Cameron AM, editors: *Current surgical therapy*, ed 10, Philadelphia, 2011, Saunders.

Park K et al: Cost-effectiveness of early colectomy with ileal pouch-anal anastomosis versus standard medical therapy in severe ulcerative colitis, *Ann Surg* 256(1):117–124, 2012.

Ponsky J, Pearl JP: Upper and lower gastrointestinal endoscopy. In Fischer JE, editor: *Fischer's mastery of surgery*, ed 6, Philadelphia, 2012, Lippincott Williams & Wilkins.

Pryor A, Yoo J: Abdominal access techniques used in laparoscopic surgery. In Basow DS, editor: *UpToDate*, Waltham, MA, 2012, UpToDate.

Rieder E, Swanstrom L: Natural orifice transluminal endoscopic surgery. In Cameron J, Cameron AM, editors: *Current surgical therapy*, ed 10, Philadelphia, 2011, Saunders.

Ricciardi R, MacKay G: Fast-track protocols in colorectal surgery. In Basow DS, editor: *UpToDate*, Waltham, MA, 2012, UpToDate.

Roberts KE et al: Pure transvaginal appendectomy versus traditional laparoscopic appendectomy for acute appendicitis, a prospective cohort study, *Ann Surg* 255(2):266–269, 2012.

Rosen M, Blatnik J: Paraesophageal hernia: clinical features and surgical repair. In Basow DS, editor: *UpToDate*, Waltham, MA, 2012, UpToDate.

Rothstein RI, Swain CP: Endoscopic therapy for gastroesophageal reflux disease: sewing and full-thickness plication. In Basow DS, editor: *UpToDate*, Waltham, MA, 2012, UpToDate.

Saltzman JR, Gibson, MK: Diagnosis and staging of esophageal cancer. In Basow DS, editor: *UpToDate*, Waltham, MA, 2012, UpToDate.

Sax H: Management of short bowel syndrome. In Cameron J, Cameron AM, editors: *Current surgical therapy*, ed 10, Philadelphia, 2011, Saunders.

Schwaitzberg S: Surgical management of gastroesophageal reflux in adults. In Basow DS, editor: *UpToDate*, Waltham, MA, 2012, UpToDate.

Scortino C et al: Morbid obesity. In Cameron J, Cameron AM, editors: *Current surgical therapy*, ed 10, Philadelphia, 2011, Saunders.

Shekelle PG et al: *Making health care safer ii: an updated critical analysis of the evidence for patient safety practices*, Comparative Effectiveness Review No. 211 (prepared by the Southern California-RAND Evidence-based Practice

Center under contract no. 290-2007-10062-I), AHRQ Publication No. 13-E001-EF, Rockville, MD, Agency for Healthcare Research and Quality, available at www.ahrq.gov/research/findings/evidence-based-reports/ptsafetyuptp.html. Accessed March 28, 2013.

Soll A: Overview of the complications of peptic ulcer disease. In Basow DS, editor: *UpToDate*, Waltham, MA, 2012, UpToDate.

Spechler SJ: Management of Barrett's esophagus. In Basow DS, editor: *UpToDate*, Waltham, MA, 2012, UpToDate.

Stonemetz J: Preoperative preparation of the surgical patient. In Cameron J, Cameron AM, editors: *Current surgical therapy*, ed 10, Philadelphia, 2011, Saunders.

Swanson S: Surgical management of localized esophageal cancer. In Basow DS, editor: *UpToDate*, Waltham, MA, 2012, UpToDate.

Tess A, Fairfield, K: Nutritional issues in the surgical patient. In Basow DS, editor: *UpToDate*, Waltham, MA, 2012, UpToDate.

Vickers SM et al: Adjunctive procedures in intestinal surgery. In Fischer JE, editor: *Fischer's mastery of surgery*, ed 6, Philadelphia, 2012, Lippincott Williams & Wilkins.

Wu X: The safe and efficient use of forced-air warming devices, *AORN J* 97(3):302–308, 2013.

Zender J, Thell C: Developing a robotic surgery program in a rural hospital, *AORN J* 92(1):72–82, 2010.

CHAPTER 12

Surgery of the Liver, Biliary Tract, Pancreas, and Spleen

JANICE A. NEIL

A pathologic condition in the liver, biliary tract, pancreas, or spleen often requires surgical intervention. These organs are highly vascular and control many of the body's metabolic and immune functions. Surgical intervention may be indicated for infection, cystic anomalies, congenital anomalies, metabolic diseases, trauma (see Chapter 28), or malignancy. Many new cases of malignancy of the gallbladder, pancreas, or extrahepatic biliary tract are diagnosed each year and the prognosis for these is often poor (Jackson and Evans, 2012; Jensen et al, 2012). Pancreatic cancer remains the fourth leading cause of death in the United States (National Cancer Institute, 2011). Surgeries of the liver and biliary tract have become more advanced as research and new technology permit more complete diagnoses of pathologic conditions. Resection of the liver for carcinoma has achieved a recognized role for cure or substantial palliation with safety and low morbidity.

Cholecystectomy is the most common, nonemergency abdominal operation performed in the United States (Ingraham et al, 2011). Laparoscopic cholecystectomy is now the gold standard surgical intervention for the treatment of cholecystitis. Compared with open-incision cholecystectomy, laparoscopic cholecystectomy results in reduced trauma to tissues as well as shorter postoperative recoveries, both distinct advantages. About 94% of cholecystectomies are elective surgeries; the remaining 6% are emergencies (Overby et al, 2010). Laparoscopic cholecystectomies were the precursor to numerous abdominal procedures now performed or assisted with the laparoscope.

New diagnostic technology and intraoperative use of ultrasonography, biliary endoscopy, and radiography enable surgeons to better treat diseases of the biliary tract. Solid organ transplantation, such as for the liver and pancreas, is a common means to treat primary hepatic tumors, end-stage liver disease, and insulin-deficient diabetes. Liver transplant procedures include entire organ transplants as well as living-related organ donations.

This chapter explores the most common open and minimally invasive procedures performed on the liver, biliary tract, pancreas, and spleen.

Surgical Anatomy

The liver is in the right upper quadrant of the abdominal cavity, beneath the dome of the diaphragm and directly above the stomach, duodenum, and hepatic flexure of the colon. The external covering, known as *Glisson's capsule,* is composed of dense connective tissue. The visceral peritoneum extends over the entire surface of the liver, except at its posterior attachment to the diaphragm. This connective tissue branches at the porta hepatis into a network of septa that extends into an intrahepatic network of support for the more than 1 million hepatic lobules. The porta hepatis is located on the inferior surface of the liver and provides entry and exit for the major vessels, ducts, and nerves. The hepatic artery maintains the arterial blood supply. Venous blood from the stomach, intestines, spleen, and pancreas travels to the liver by the portal vein and its branches (Figure 12-1), and the hepatic venous system then returns blood to the heart via the inferior vena cava.

Lobules are the functional units of the liver. Each lobule contains a portal triad that consists of a hepatic duct, a hepatic portal vein branch, and a branch of the hepatic artery, nerves, and lymphatics. A central vein is located in the center of each lobule and provides venous drainage into the hepatic veins.

Lobules also contain hepatic cords, hepatic sinusoids, and bile canaliculi. The hepatic cords consist of numerous columns of hepatocytes—the functional cells of the liver. The hepatic sinusoids are the blood channels that communicate among the columns of hepatocytes. The sinusoids have a thin epithelial lining composed primarily of Kupffer cells—phagocytic cells that engulf bacteria and toxins. The sinusoids drain into the central vein.

Bile is manufactured by the hepatocytes. The bile canaliculi are tiny bile capillary vessels that communicate among the columns of hepatocytes. The bile canaliculi collect and transport bile to the bile ducts in the portal triad of each lobule, from which bile then flows into the hepatic ducts at the porta hepatis. These ducts join immediately to form one common hepatic duct that merges with the cystic duct from the gallbladder to form the common bile duct (Figure 12-2). The common bile duct opens into the duodenum in an area called the *ampulla,* or *papilla of Vater,* located about 7.5 cm below the pyloric opening from the stomach.

Bile contains bile salts, which facilitate digestion and absorption, and various waste products. The liver is essential in the metabolism of carbohydrates, proteins, and fats. It metabolizes nutrients into stores of glycogen, used for regulation of blood glucose levels and as energy sources for the brain and body functions.

The liver plays several important roles in the blood-clotting mechanism. It is the organ that synthesizes plasma proteins, excluding gamma globulins but including prothrombin and fibrinogen. Vitamin K, a cofactor to the synthesis of prothrombin, is absorbed by the metabolism of fats in the intestinal tract as a result of bile formation by the liver. Patients with liver disease may have altered blood-coagulation abilities.

The liver also synthesizes lipoproteins and cholesterol. Cholesterol is an essential component of the blood plasma. It serves as a precursor for bile salts, steroid hormones, plasma membranes, and

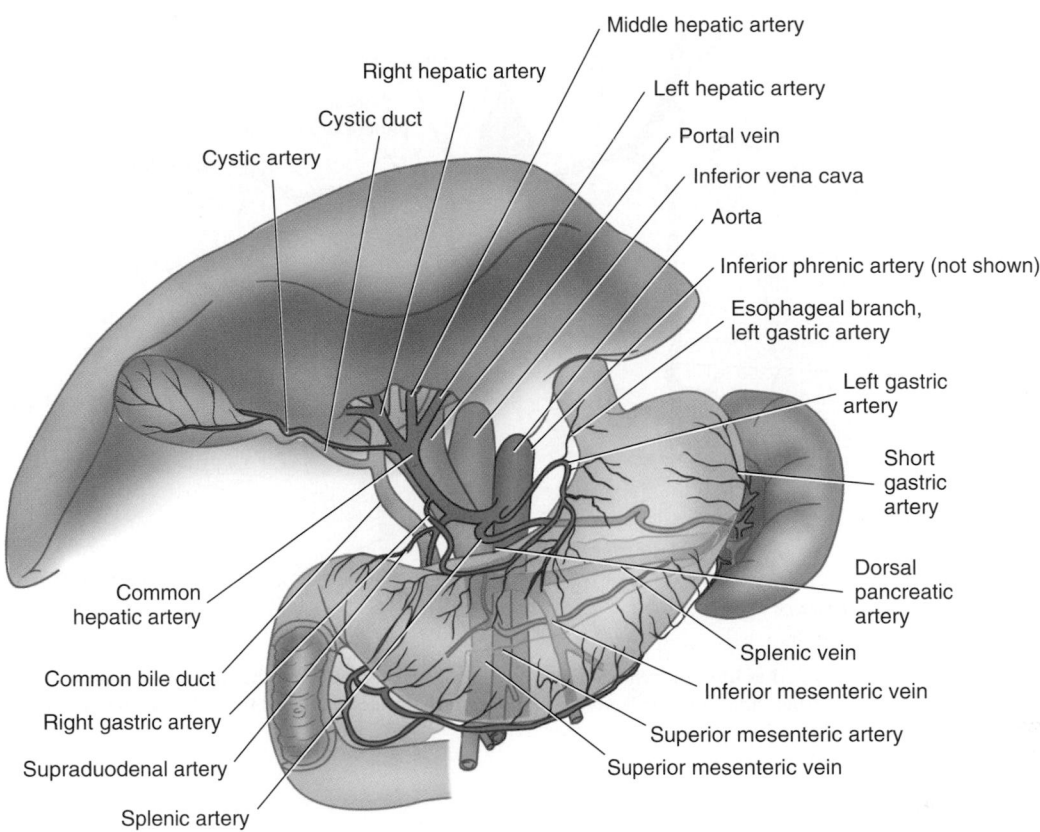

FIGURE 12-1 Intricate relationships of the arterial and venous blood supply of the liver, gallbladder, pancreas, spleen, and the biliary ductal system.

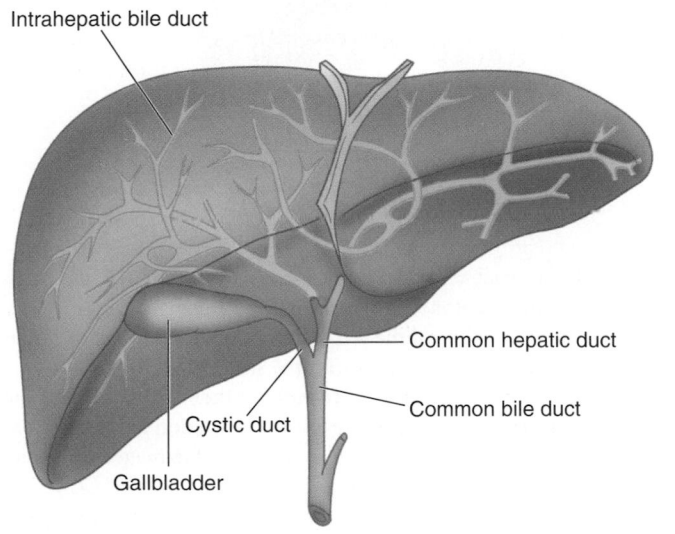

FIGURE 12-2 Biliary system can be divided into three anatomic areas: the intrahepatic bile duct, the extrahepatic bile duct (common hepatic and common bile ducts), and the gallbladder and cystic duct.

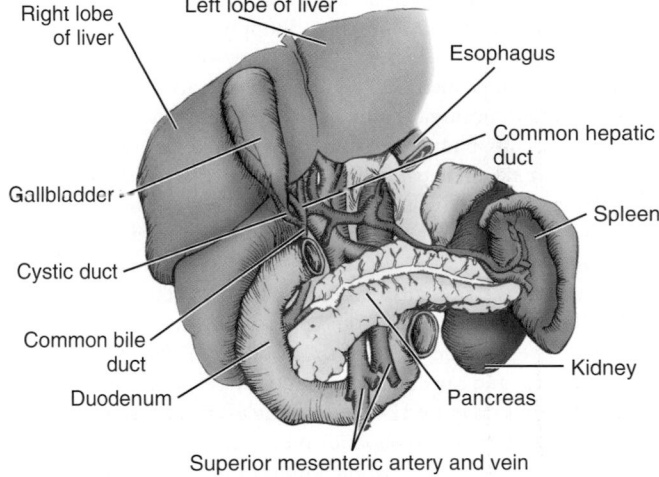

FIGURE 12-3 Gallbladder and surrounding anatomy.

other specialized molecules. A diet high in cholesterol reduces the amount that must be synthesized by the liver. When the diet is deficient in cholesterol, the liver increases synthesis to maintain levels necessary for production of vital chemical molecules.

The liver also functions in the metabolic alteration of foreign molecules or biotransformation of chemicals. The microsomal enzyme system (MES) plays a major role in the body's response to foreign chemicals, such as pollutants, drugs, and alcohol. Patients with liver disease may have an altered response to chemical substances. This consideration is important in the induction and management of general anesthesia for patients with liver disorders.

The gallbladder, which lies in a sulcus on the undersurface of the right lobe of the liver, terminates in the cystic duct (Figure 12-3). This ductal system provides a channel for the flow of bile to the gallbladder, where it becomes highly concentrated during storage. The liver produces about 600 to 1000 mL of bile each day. The gallbladder's average storage capacity is 40 to 70 mL. As foods,

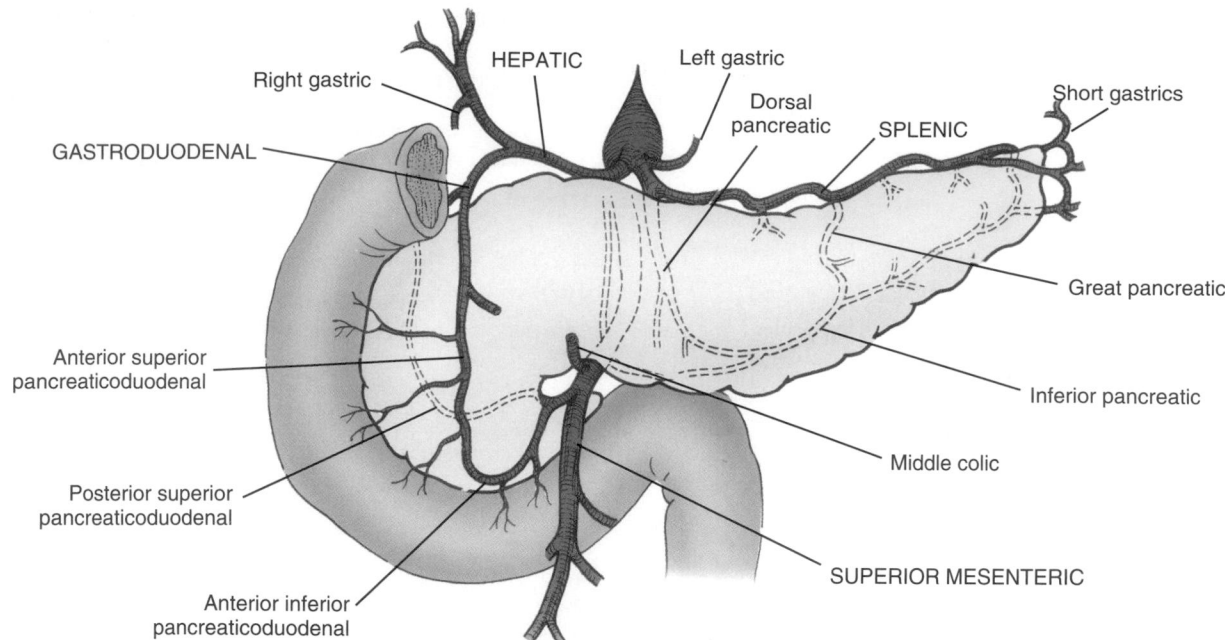

FIGURE 12-4 Arterial supply to the pancreas arises from the celiac axis (hepatic and splenic arteries) and the superior mesenteric artery. The blood supply to the head of the gland is by way of the pancreaticoduodenal (anterior and posterior) arcades that arise from the gastroduodenal artery (superior) and superior mesenteric arteries (inferior).

especially fats, are ingested, the duodenal cells release cholecystokinin. When the musculature of the gallbladder contracts, bile is forced into the cystic duct and through the common duct. As the sphincter of Oddi in the ampulla of Vater relaxes, bile is released, flowing into the duodenum to aid in digestion by emulsification of fats. The gallbladder receives its blood supply from the cystic artery, a branch of the hepatic artery. The triangle of Calot contains the cystic artery (and sometimes the right hepatic artery); it is an anatomic landmark in surgical removal of the gallbladder (Jackson and Evans, 2012). Its boundaries may be remembered as the "3 Cs": *c*ystic duct, *c*ommon hepatic duct, and *c*ystic artery. Innervation for the gallbladder and biliary tree is controlled by the autonomic nervous system. Parasympathetic innervation stimulates contraction, whereas sympathetic innervation inhibits contraction.

The pancreas (see Figure 12-3) is a fixed structure lying transversely behind the stomach in the upper abdomen. The head of the pancreas is fixed to the curve of the duodenum. Blood is supplied to the pancreas and the duodenum from the celiac axis and superior mesenteric artery (Figure 12-4). The body of the pancreas lies across the vertebrae and over the superior mesenteric artery and vein. The tail of the pancreas extends to the hilum of the spleen. In total, the pancreas extends about 25 cm. Pancreatic secretions containing digestive enzymes are collected in the pancreatic duct, or duct of Wirsung, which joins with the common bile duct to enter the duodenum about 7.5 cm below the pylorus. The dilated junction of the two ducts at the point of entry forms the ampulla of Vater.

The pancreas also contains groups of cells, called *islets,* or *islands, of Langerhans,* that secrete hormones into the blood capillaries instead of into the duct. These hormones are insulin and glucagon, and both are involved in carbohydrate metabolism.

The spleen (Figure 12-5) is in the upper left abdominal cavity, with full protection provided by the tenth, eleventh, and twelfth ribs; its lateral surface is directly beneath the dome of the diaphragm. The anterior medial surface is in proximity to the cardiac

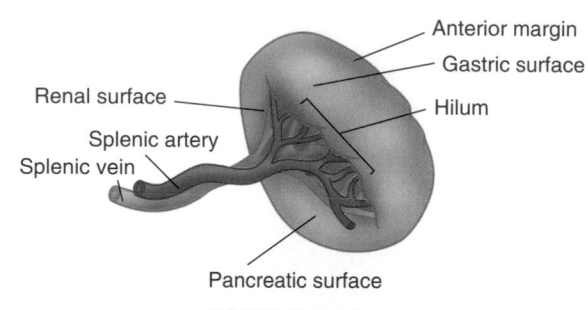

FIGURE 12-5 Spleen.

end of the stomach and the splenic flexure of the colon. The spleen is covered with peritoneum that forms supporting ligaments. The splenic artery, a branch of the celiac axis, furnishes the arterial blood supply. The splenic vein drains into the portal system.

The spleen has many functions. Among them are defense of the body by phagocytosis of microorganisms, formation of nongranular leukocytes and plasma cells, and phagocytosis of damaged red blood cells. It also acts as a blood reservoir.

Perioperative Nursing Considerations

Assessment

The patient with hepatobiliary disease may have extreme jaundice, urticaria, petechiae, lethargy, and irritability. Depending on the extent of the disease, bleeding and coagulation times may increase and the platelet count decrease, contributing to intraoperative concerns with achieving hemostasis. A thorough nursing history is necessary for proper assessment of the health status of patients with dysfunctions of the hepatobiliary system, pancreas, or spleen. Assessment includes data about the patient's history of chronic disease, current medications, perceptions of his or her disease, comfort status, nutritional status, fluid and electrolyte balance, bowel and elimination patterns, energy level and independence, and exposure to toxins. Many industrial compounds are toxic to the liver (Table 12-1).

TABLE 12-1

Common Hepatotoxic Agents and Types of Liver Damage

Toxic Agent	Source	Liver Damage
Aflatoxin B	Moldy foods, rice, corn, cassava, oil, grain dust (during bin clean-out and animal feeding in enclosed buildings)	Jaundice, fatty liver, hepatocellular carcinoma, thromboses
Amanita phalloides	Poisonous mushrooms	Centrilobular and massive necrosis
Benzene	Chemical industry, to make plastics, resins, and nylon and synthetic fibers	Fatty liver, cirrhosis
Beryllium	From x-ray tube and fluorescent lamp manufacture; alloys are used in automobiles, computers, sports equipment (golf clubs and bicycle frames)	Necrosis and granulomas
Boron, cadmium, nickel, chromium, copper	From gold smelting, plating	Liver damage, rise in levels of liver enzymes
Carbon tetrachloride	Propellants for aerosol cans, as a pesticide, cleaning fluid, degreasing agent, fire extinguishers, spot removers (now banned)	Centrilobular necrosis
Kerosene	From fuel handling	Liver damage, rise in levels of liver enzymes
Lead	Environment	Steatosis, hepatitis
Pesticides	Polyvinyl chloride, farming industry	Steatosis, angiosarcoma (liver tumors)
Phosphorus	From poisons and firecrackers	Fatty liver, necrosis, fibrosis
Toluene, xylene	Occurs naturally in crude oil	Fatty liver, fibrosis
Vinyl chloride	Used to make polyvinyl chloride (plastics; also named PVC)	Angiosarcoma (liver tumors), fibrosis

Modified from Orfei L: *Toxic liver injury,* 2012, available at www.meddean.luc.edu/lumen/MedEd/orfpath/toxicinjury.htm. Accessed January 28, 2013; Aflatoxin B1 exposure, 2009, available at www.ncbi.nlm.nih.gov/pubmed/19273485. Accessed January 28, 2013; *Amanita phalloides,* 2012, available at www.ncbi.nlm.nih.gov/pubmed/22811920, accessed January 28, 2013; *Toxic Substances Portal,* available at www.atsdr.cdc.gov/toxicsubstances.html. Accessed January 28, 2013.

Establishing an objective database for a person with hepatobiliary or pancreatic dysfunction requires particular attention to characteristic signs of organ dysfunction (Evidence for Practice). Increased abdominal girth and distention, palmar erythema, distended periumbilical veins, hemorrhagic areas, spider nevi, muscle wasting, and dry mucous membranes are some characteristic signs and symptoms. Vascular volume is assessed by noting vital signs, including any orthostatic changes, skin turgor, temperature, and appearance, as well as weight gain or loss. Physical examination of

EVIDENCE FOR PRACTICE

National Surgical Quality Improvement Project: Hepatic, Pancreatic, and Complex Biliary Surgery

Hepatic, pancreatic, and complex biliary (HPB) surgery can be associated with major morbidity and significant mortality. For the past 5 years the American College of Surgeons (ACS) National Surgical Quality Improvement Program (NSQIP) has gathered a large amount of data on patients undergoing HPB surgery. Improved outcomes result in fewer complications and decreased costs. Using standard reporting systems leads to decreases in morbidity and mortality by improved management. More than 400 academic and community hospitals nationwide participate in reporting to the NSQIP dataset. Standardized reporting of surgeries, complications, and histopathology results are tracked. This tracking allows hospitals to achieve measurable improvements in quality care.

NSQIP findings related to hepatic, pancreatic, and complex biliary surgery include:

- Predictive of adverse outcomes in patients undergoing HPB surgery: Using a sample size of 13,558 patients who underwent an HPB procedure, 7321 (54%) had pancreatic, 4881 (36%) hepatic, and 1356 (10%) biliary surgery. Overall, 70.3% of patients had a cancer diagnosis. Postoperative complications occurred in 3850 patients for an overall morbidity of 28.4%. Serious complications occurred in 2522 (18.6%) patients; 366 patients died for an overall perioperative mortality of 2.7%. Perioperative outcomes were associated with diagnosis and type of procedure.
- Data collected include age, gender, smoking status, body mass index (BMI), and history of recent weight loss.
- Potential preoperative predictive variables include comorbidities of hypertension that requires medication, dyspnea at rest/with moderate exertion, presence of congestive heart failure, previous cardiac intervention(s), history of chronic obstructive pulmonary disease (COPD), preoperative ventilator dependence, emergency admission, presentation with ascites, existing acute renal failure, diabetes mellitus (insulin dependent and noninsulin dependent), chronic steroid use, and sepsis.
- Of the preoperative variables examined, age >74, dyspnea with moderate exertion, steroid use, prior cardiac procedure, ascites, and preoperative sepsis were associated with morbidity and mortality (p <0.05 for all variables).
- The highest 30-day mortality was associated with hepatic trisectionectomy (5.8%) and total pancreatectomy.

An ACS-NSQIP "HPB risk calculator" may be developed to help better risk stratify patients being considered for complex HPB surgery. The large database results also suggest that pancreatic surgery is best performed at large-volume centers by large-volume surgeons.

Modified from Donahue TR, Reber HA: Pancreatic surgery, *Curr Opin Gastroenterol* 26:499–505, 2010; Kneuertz PJ et al: Risk of morbidity and mortality following hepato-pancreato-biliary surgery, *J Gastrointest Surg* 16:1727–1735, 2012.

the patient's abdomen includes palpation and percussion to evaluate tenderness, ascites, and organ enlargement.

Common laboratory tests to assess liver function are those that evaluate fat metabolism, protein metabolism, blood coagulation properties, bilirubin metabolism, and antigens and antibodies of hepatitis (Appendix A). Common tests of pancreatic function also can be found in Appendix A. Radiographic studies commonly used to evaluate function of the liver, pancreas, and spleen include abdominal examination, upper gastrointestinal (GI) series, ultrasound studies, computed tomography (CT) scan, radioisotope scanning, nuclear magnetic resonance (NMR) imaging, angiography, cholecystography, and cholangiography. The hepatic iminodiacetic acid (HIDA) scan can be used to evaluate the physiologic secretion of bile. State-of-the-art imaging includes contrast-enhanced MRI, MR cholangiopancreatography (MRCP), endoscopic ultrasound (EUS), and high-resolution, thin-section spiral CT for imaging pancreatic and biliary structures. In addition, fluorodeoxyglucose positron emission tomography (FDG-PET) is a whole-body technique that can detect metastases, recognition of which may change surgical management (Jackson and Evans, 2012).

Endoscopy and biopsy are more invasive diagnostic procedures. Endoscopic retrograde cholangiopancreatography (ERCP) (Figure 12-6) allows direct visualization of the biliary tract, injection of radiographic dye into the ductal system, and biopsy when indicated. Percutaneous transhepatic cholangiography (PTC) uses percutaneous insertion of a long flexible needle into a bile duct of the liver. Contrast medium is injected and serial x-ray examination is performed. Arteriography of the liver, biliary tree, pancreas, and spleen requires femoral arteriotomy and placement of a catheter into the celiac branch of the abdominal aorta under fluoroscopic visualization. Contrast medium is then injected and serial x-ray examination allows the vessels to be visualized during the perfusion and drainage phases.

Nursing Diagnosis

After reviewing the nursing assessment, the perioperative nurse formulates nursing diagnoses. Nursing diagnoses related to the care of patients undergoing surgery of the liver, biliary tract, pancreas, or spleen might include the following:

- Anxiety related to impending surgical procedure, perioperative events, and surgical outcome
- Risk for Imbalanced Fluid Volume
- Hypothermia related to exposure of body surface or abdominal cavity and effects of anesthesia on thermoregulation
- Risk for Infection related to organ systems involved (portions of the GI tract)
- Risk for Perioperative Positioning Injury
- Risk for Impaired Skin Integrity related to invasion of body structures, disruption of skin surface
- Acute Pain related to surgical procedure

Outcome Identification

Statements about desired outcomes reflect nursing diagnoses identified for a patient population. Nursing diagnoses are also individualized according to cultural, ethnic, religious, and spiritual values, as well as an individual patient's status. From these are derived the outcomes the perioperative nurse wishes to achieve. The best outcome statement has specific criteria by which the perioperative nurse intends to measure whether the outcome has been met. These criteria are more meaningful when they are established in partnership with the patient. Not all outcomes will be planned with the patient, but ones relating to nursing diagnoses such as anxiety and

FIGURE 12-6 A, Endoscopic retrograde cholangiopancreatography demonstrates several calculi within the distal common bile duct. **B,** Stone removal with a Fogarty catheter.

coping can and should reflect patient participation. Outcomes identified for the selected nursing diagnoses might be stated as follows:

- The patient will verbalize management of anxiety and ability to cope, demonstrate knowledge of his or her psychologic responses to the planned procedure, and show an understanding of the planned sequence of perioperative events.
- The patient will maintain fluid volume equilibrium throughout the operative procedure.
- The patient will evidence an intraoperative core body temperature within the normal range (96° to 99° F [35.5° to 37.2° C]).
- The patient will be free of clinical signs and symptoms of surgical site infection (SSI).
- The patient will maintain baseline neuromuscular function and intact skin at positional pressure sites.
- The patient will demonstrate understanding of the plan to heal the incision site.
- The patient will report that the pain management regimen relieves pain to a satisfactory level (Ackley and Ladwig, 2011).

Planning

Planning the patient's care requires knowledge of the anatomy and subsequent physiologic complications that may occur with surgical interruption of tissues. Planning is driven by intended outcomes. The experienced perioperative nurse reflects on those intended outcomes and, using theory, science, and what has been learned through experience, identifies actions required for outcome achievement (Benner et al, 2009). Principles of safe surgical positioning, maintenance of asepsis, prevention of biologic and electrical hazards, and provision of proper instrumentation and equipment are a few constituents of the plan of care that are based on theory and science and augmented by nursing experience.

A review of the nursing assessment and a patient interview provide insights as to the specific needs of the patient. The patient's medical and surgical history, as well as age, size, and nutritional status, will assist the perioperative nurse in developing an effective plan of care. A Sample Plan of Care for a patient undergoing surgery of the liver, biliary tract, pancreas, or spleen is shown below.

SAMPLE PLAN OF CARE

Nursing Diagnosis
Anxiety related to impending surgical procedure, perioperative events, and surgical outcome

Outcome
The patient will verbalize management of anxiety and ability to cope, demonstrate knowledge of his or her psychologic responses to the planned procedure, and indicate an understanding of the planned sequence of perioperative events.

Interventions
- Greet the patient positively; determine the name he or she prefers to be called.
- Introduce the patient to the OR team.
- Avoid hasty movements or gestures of indecision.
- Speak slowly and clearly when addressing the patient, and use terminology the patient can understand.
- Offer emotional reassurance by using touch, assisting the patient to a position of comfort on the OR bed, and offering warm blankets (thermal comfort).
- Classify the patient's level of anxiety (mild, moderate, severe) by asking the patient and observing signs of anxiety (e.g., clenching/unclenching hands, crying, tremors).
- Determine the patient's personally effective coping mechanisms and facilitate use of these.
- Identify the patient's special concerns, values, and wishes concerning his or her care.
- Provide explanations of perioperative events; encourage questions.

Nursing Diagnosis
Risk for Imbalanced Fluid Volume

Outcome
The patient will maintain fluid volume equilibrium throughout the surgical procedure.

Interventions
- Review orders for blood/blood products; have products available in easily accessible, refrigerated storage for timely access.
- Communicate availability of blood/blood products during the preop briefing or time-out.

- Measure, communicate, and record estimated or real fluid volume loss throughout surgical procedure.
- Anticipate and communicate to blood bank personnel the potential need for additional blood and blood products.
- Collaborate with anesthesia provider in fluid replacement therapies using safe blood administration practices.
- Check laboratory values intraoperatively; monitor and note deviations in study results; read back critical lab values; report to surgeon and anesthesia provider.

Nursing Diagnosis
Hypothermia related to exposure of body surface or abdominal cavity and effects of anesthesia on thermoregulation

Outcome
The patient will maintain an intraoperative core body temperature of 96° to 99° F (35.5° to 37.2° C).

Interventions
- Determine thermal comfort: ask the patient if he or she is cold.
- Adjust room temperature and humidity to accommodate preservation of body temperature.
- Provide warm blankets on transfer to OR bed.
- Expose only that part of the body necessary for the surgical prep; cover all other body surfaces to maintain body heat.
- Provide warm irrigation solutions, first ensuring solution temperature is less than 105° F (40.5° C).
- Collaborate with anesthesia provider in warming intravenous (IV) fluids and blood/blood products before infusion.
- Use other active warming measures (such as forced-air warming system) for preventing hypothermia.
- Monitor body temperature to evaluate response to thermoregulation measures.

Nursing Diagnosis
Risk for Infection related to organ systems involved (portions of the gastrointestinal tract)

Outcome
The patient will be free of clinical signs and symptoms of surgical site infection.

Continued

SAMPLE PLAN OF CARE—cont'd

Interventions

- Implement aseptic technique; communicate and correct breaks in asepsis.
- Ensure that preoperative antibiotics are administered as ordered; prophylactic antibiotics should be administered 1 hour before surgical incision is made. Follow guidelines for safe medication practices.
- Contain and confine contaminants appropriately.
- Ensure that all sterilization procedures have been performed properly.
- Ensure the integrity of sterile supply packaging is intact before dispensing items to the sterile field.
- As ordered, verify that patient has performed preoperative showers or baths.
- Perform intraoperative skin preparation with institutionally approved antimicrobial agent.
- Implement measures to prevent cross-contamination.
- Initiate traffic control and environmental measures that reduce risk for infection.
- Use aseptic technique in applying dressings to surgical sites.
- Correctly classify wound according to established wound classification system.
- Manage culture specimen collection according to institutional policy and safe practices for specimen management.

Nursing Diagnosis
Risk for Perioperative Positioning Injury

Outcome
The patient will maintain baseline neuromuscular function and intact skin at positional pressure sites.

Interventions

- Identify any physiologic alterations or mobility limitations that may affect procedure-specific positioning.
- Implement measures to prevent shearing forces during patient transfer to and from OR bed and during positional changes.
- Ensure that all positioning equipment is clean and functioning properly.
- Ensure patient is in optimal anatomic alignment after induction of anesthesia.
- Adequately pad all bony prominences and vulnerable neurovascular areas.

- Secure limbs to ensure position is maintained and to prevent limb from falling from positioning device (as appropriate to procedure-specific position).
- Verify correct position during time-out.
- Ensure that no weight or stress is placed on body parts and structures during the surgical intervention.
- Check protective padding and safety restraints after all positional changes.

Nursing Diagnosis
Risk for Impaired Skin Integrity related to invasion of body structures, disruption of skin surface

Outcome
The patient will regain integrity of skin surface.

Interventions (Postoperative)

- Monitor incision site for color, redness, swelling, warmth, and pain.
- Avoid positioning patient on incision site.
- Individualize plan according to patient's skin condition, needs, and preferences.
- Monitor incision edges for intactness, bleeding, and drainage.
- Maintain a moist wound healing environment that is balanced with the need to absorb exudate.

Nursing Diagnosis
Acute Pain related to surgical procedure

Outcome
The patient will report that the pain management regimen relieves pain to a satisfactory level, using a pain assessment scale.

Interventions (Postoperative)

- Review use of a pain scale with the patient and family before surgery.
- Identify cultural and value components related to pain.
- Provide patient and family with information on pain management.
- Determine whether the patient is experiencing pain at the time of the initial postoperative assessment.
- Assess and document intensity and location of pain.
- Treat pain as ordered; document response to treatment.
- Use a preventive approach to keep pain at or below an acceptable level.

Implementation

Patients having surgery of the liver, biliary tract, pancreas, or spleen are usually given a general anesthetic. The following pertinent factors should be considered in caring for these patients.

Universal Protocol. The Joint Commission (TJC) requires that the "wrong site, wrong procedure, wrong person" prevention protocol be carried out before each surgical procedure (TJC, 2012). This protocol is discussed in Chapter 2.

Positioning the Patient. For biliary surgery the patient is placed in supine position. Arms are placed on padded armboards with the palms up and fingers extended. Armboards are maintained at less than a 90-degree angle to prevent brachial plexus stretch. If there are surgical reasons to tuck the arms at the side, the elbows are padded to protect the ulnar nerve, the palms faced inward, and the

wrists maintained in a neutral position (Phillips, 2013). A drape secures the arms. It should be tucked snuggly, but not tightly, under the patient, not under the mattress. This prevents the arm from shifting downward intraoperatively and resting against the operating room (OR) bed rail. A small positioning aid may be placed under the lower right side of the thorax to elevate the lower rib cage, providing better exposure and access to the viscera in the right upper quadrant of the abdomen. Alternatively, a lateral tilt of the OR bed may be used in combination with reverse Trendelenburg for procedures such as laparoscopic cholecystectomy.

Positioning for laparoscopic procedures requires the perioperative nurse to exercise caution when applying safety straps. Given that the patient may be placed in a severe side tilt or reverse Trendelenburg position, safety or restraining straps must be placed securely, but not too tightly. Attention is given to proper alignment of the patient's body and extremities, and padded footboards are applied to prevent the patient from slipping. Areas of pressure in the selected surgical position (see Chapter 6) and bony prominences are padded well to prevent interruption of circulation and pressure injury to tissues and neurovascular structures. These precautions are especially important for diabetic, circulatory-impaired, immuno-compromised, and elderly patients. Close monitoring of the patient is essential during positional changes, especially in laparoscopic procedures with decreased lighting in the room.

When anticipating an operative cholangiogram, the periopera-tive nurse must ensure that the OR bed has been equipped and positioned so that C-arm image intensification can be accomplished efficiently. Radiation-protection devices for the surgical team and patient should be available and applied/worn as indicated.

Thermoregulation. The risks of intraoperative hypothermia have been well documented (see Chapter 5). When laparotomy is per-formed, patients are at further risk for hypothermia. To prevent unplanned hypothermia, the perioperative nurse takes affirmative measures to maintain body temperature in the OR. Proper environ-mental temperature and humidity prevent body heat loss caused by evaporation and convection. A forced-air warming blanket placed over the patient's upper body, head, and neck assists in maintaining body temperature. Minimizing body exposure to ambient air and using warm irrigating solutions also support thermoregulation. The temperature of irrigating fluids should be no higher than body temperature (98.6° F [37° C]) (AORN, 2013). A blood- and fluid-warming device may be used by the anesthesia provider to deliver intravenous (IV) fluids at a temperature higher than room air tem-perature (see Chapter 5). The anesthesia provider commonly moni-tors the patient's core temperature by use of an esophageal temperature probe when duration and complexity of the surgical procedure place the patient at risk for hypothermia. Additional comfort measures include using warm blankets before and after surgery.

Application of Intermittent Pneumatic Compression Device. Patients undergoing lengthy surgical procedures are at risk for venous dilation and blood pooling in the lower extremities. This may predispose the surgical patient to develop venous thromboembolism (VTE) in the postoperative period. Intermittent pneumatic com-pression devices (IPCDs) in conjunction with graduated compres-sion stockings (referred to as mechanical prophylaxis) are applied in the OR before commencing lengthy surgical procedures in order to prevent or minimize VTE risks (Alexander-Magalee, 2013).

Draping the Patient. After the abdominal prep the surgical team must allow time for the prep solution to dry and vapors to dissipate. This is an essential patient safety precaution when flammable prep solutions are used in conjunction with electrosurgery (or other igni-tion sources, such as a laser). Sterile towels are then arranged to accommodate the intended incision. A sterile drape sheet may be placed over the patient's lower torso and a laparotomy sheet then placed to provide a wide sterile field and to cover all exposed body surfaces except the incision site. Further information on draping can be found in Chapter 4.

Instrumentation. Instrumentation for open (i.e., performed via a laparotomy incision) surgeries of the liver, biliary tract, spleen, and pancreas includes a basic laparotomy set, biliary probes and forceps for dilating and exploring the ducts of the pancreas and biliary tract, vascular clamps, GI clamps, and ligating clips and appliers of all

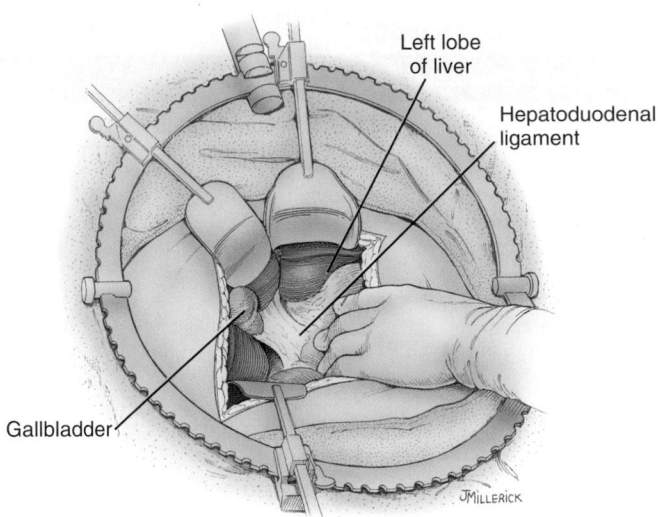

FIGURE 12-7 Bookwalter self-retaining retractor in place to provide optimal exposure to the abdominal viscera.

sizes. Linear stapling instruments also should be available. A self-retaining system such as the Bookwalter retractor set (Figure 12-7) provides excellent exposure of the abdominal viscera. In addition, a flexible choledochoscope, Cavitron ultrasound suction aspirator (CUSA), intraoperative ultrasound, laser, argon beam coagulator, harmonic scalpel, and electrosurgical unit (ESU) may be required to perform certain procedures on the hepatobiliary system. Safe practices when using devices that generate surgical smoke require the use of a smoke evacuation system and accessories in both open and laparoscopic procedures (AORN, 2013).

The basic equipment for minimally invasive surgery (MIS) pro-cedures consists of two high-density monitors, an insufflation unit, ESU, light source, camera, and 0- and 30-degree telescopes in 10- and 5-mm sizes. A printer is optional. An ultrasonic dissecting unit is often used with MIS procedures. Trocars and sleeves are available in reusable, disposable, and reposable designs. Trocars and sleeves are commonly designed to accommodate 10- to 5-mm instruments and 12- to 5-mm accessories and instruments. MIS instruments include scissors and shears, dissecting forceps, atraumatic grasping forceps, hooks, Babcock clamps, retractors, needles, suturing devices, pouches, suction-irrigating devices, and mechanical stapling devices.

Thrombin, Gelfoam, Surgicel, Avitene, and other chemical hemostatic agents (Surgical Pharmacology) should be available in the OR suite. Radiographic dye, supplies, and radiation-protection devices are required if intraoperative radiography or angiography is planned as part of the procedure.

Drainage Materials. Tubes and catheters are selected for the areas to be drained. If a defective drain is used, a free fragment may remain in the wound on removal of the tube. Thus the scrub person should note the condition of all drainage materials and should test them for patency before they are placed in the patient.

Soft rubber or latex tissue drains may be used after an open cholecystectomy or a choledochostomy. Verify that the patient has no latex allergy before using these devices and substitute nonlatex drains if necessary. The surgeon will prepare a latex rubber T-tube drain of suitable size after exploring the duct. The center of the crossbar is notched opposite the junction of the vertical limb so that

SURGICAL PHARMACOLOGY

Chemical Hemostatic Agents

Agent	Chemical Composition	Actions	Perioperative Precautions
Absorbable gelatin: Powder or compressed forms (Gelfoam)	Purified porcine gelatin, beaten, dried, and heat sterilized	On areas of capillary bleeding, deposits fibrin, forming a clot. Absorbs 45 times its own weight.	Dipped in warm saline or soaked in thrombin. Must be squeezed to remove air.
Absorbable collagen (Collastat, Superstat, Helistat, Lyostypt)	Bovine collagen origin	Collagen activates coagulation mechanism, aggregation of platelets.	Must be kept dry and applied with dry gloves. Do not use in infected areas or in pooled blood.
Microfibrillar collagen (Avitene, Surgiflow, Instat)	Hydrochloric acid salt of purified bovine corium collagen	Promotes adhesion of platelets and prompt fibrin deposition.	Applied dry. Use firm pressure against bleeding surface.
Oxidized cellulose (Surgicel, Surgicel Nu-Knit)	Absorbable oxidation product of cellulose	On contact with blood, clot forms. Increases in size and forms gel. Absorbs 10 times its own weight.	Applied dry. May be sutured in place.
Oxytocin	Synthetic pituitary hormone	Injected directly into uterine muscle during cesarean birth to cause contraction after delivery of baby and placenta. Prevents uterine hemorrhage.	Also may be given intravenously to induce labor
Phenol and alcohol	Chemical compounds used to electrocoagulate tissue across lumen of appendix	Phenol coagulates proteins, and 95% alcohol neutralizes phenol.	Phenol is caustic and may cause severe burns.
Epinephrine (Adrenalin)	Adrenal hormone	Powerful vasoconstrictor; prolongs action of local anesthetics to decrease bleeding	Gelatin sponges may be soaked in 1 : 1000 epinephrine; especially useful in ear and microsurgical procedures.
Tannic acid	Powder from astringent plant	Used on nose and throat mucous membranes to stop capillary bleeding	Also used in dental procedures.
Silver nitrate	Crystals of silver nitrate compound mixed with silver chloride and molded onto applicator sticks	Astringent and antimicrobial. Seals areas of surgical incisions.	May also be used in treatment of burns.
Thrombin	Enzyme extracted from bovine blood	Accelerates coagulation of blood. Unites rapidly with fibrin to form clot.	May be used topically as a dry powder or as a solution in which gelatin sponges are dipped. May also be sprayed onto site. Topical use only. Loses potency after 3 hours.
Zeolite beads (QuikClot)	Derived from form of volcanic pumice	Beads cause hemostasis by absorbing water from blood.	Used for emergency hemostasis in uncontrollable bleeding or evisceration, especially in trauma. Causes an exothermic reaction. Must be removed; not biodegradable.
Kaolin-based product	Natural mineral form of hydrated aluminum silicate that is insoluble in water	QuikClot has been incorporated into a new product for hemostasis.	For uncontrolled emergency bleeding. American troops have been deployed for combat with this product.
Zinc chloride paste	Chemical compound	Causes coagulation over a denuded area	Sometimes used after Mohs micrographic surgery.

Modified from Phillips NF: *Berry and Kohn's operating room technique,* ed 12, St Louis, 2013, Mosby.

its ends will bend more readily during removal. The ends are beveled and tailored to fit the duct.

Drains are usually exteriorized through separate stab wounds and anchored to skin edges to prevent their retraction. The perioperative nurse should document the types of drains and reservoirs inserted during the procedure. Depending on institutional protocol, these may be identified with an applied label. All drains and their locations should be included in the perioperative nurse's hand-off report to the nursing unit to which the patient is transferred postoperatively.

Aseptic Considerations. When the common duct is opened or an anastomosis is established between a duct and other parts of the alimentary tract, it may be the institution's policy or the surgeon's preference to isolate contaminated instruments and materials from the remainder of the operative field, as described for GI surgery (see Chapter 11). The wound is classified according to a standard system: any procedure in which the alimentary tract is entered under controlled conditions and without unusual contamination is considered a *clean contaminated wound;* if there is gross spillage, however, the wound is classified as *contaminated.* Proper wound classification is considered an important predictor of post-operative SSI (Phillips, 2013).

Blood Products. During the preoperative verification process the perioperative nurse should ascertain the type and amount of blood and blood products, both requested and available, as well as ensure the patient has a signed consent for transfusion. Constant, ongoing evaluation of blood loss is communicated to the anesthesia provider and surgical team during the procedure. When additional blood or blood products are required, the perioperative nurse communicates with blood bank personnel so that products are readily available and carries out the required steps to verify blood/blood products with the anesthesia provider before transfusion.

Autologous blood or donor-directed blood products may be used in elective procedures involving the liver, pancreas, spleen, and biliary tract. Cell-saver devices may be used when potential contamination of the blood from bile or bowel does not exist.

Evaluation

Evaluation of the patient after surgery includes examination of all skin surfaces and comparison with preoperative assessment data. Abdominal drains, chest drainage systems, urinary drainage systems, and peripheral infusion lines are assessed for patency. Fluid volume use and loss are documented and communicated appropriately. A report of the patient's history, preoperative assessment, intraoperative events, and postoperative evaluation is communicated to the postanesthesia care unit (PACU) or surgical intensive care unit (SICU) nurse during the hand-off.

Evaluation of patient status can be phrased as outcome statements such as the following:

- The patient verbalized management of anxiety and ability to cope, expressed awareness of his or her psychologic responses to the planned procedure, and indicated an understanding of the sequence of perioperative events.
- The patient maintained equilibrium in fluid volume; hematocrit remained in the expected range; vital signs were stable.
- The patient's intraoperative core body temperature remained consistently in the 96° to 99°F (35.5° to 37.2°C) range.
- The patient's surgical incision was dressed aseptically and was dry and intact. There will be no clinical signs or symptoms of infection.
- At the conclusion of the surgical procedure skin surfaces were clean, intact, and free of reddened areas; adequate capillary filling was noted after blanching of tissues. The patient had palpable pulses in all distal extremities and showed no evidence of diminished neuromuscular function.
- The patient will be able to perform activities of recovery with acceptable levels of pain.

Patient and Family Education and Discharge Planning

The length of time and complexity of recovery vary greatly for patients undergoing surgical intervention for disorders of the liver, biliary tract, pancreas, or spleen. Laparoscopic cholecystectomy may be performed on an ambulatory surgery basis with extended recovery and observation of 6 to 8 hours (Ambulatory Surgery Considerations). In contrast, patients undergoing liver transplant or resection may require extensive recovery that includes a stay in the intensive care unit.

Patients undergoing laparotomy for surgical procedures on the liver, biliary tract, pancreas, or spleen may have varying degrees of postoperative edema, decreased GI peristalsis, and alterations in

---

AMBULATORY SURGERY CONSIDERATIONS

Same-Day Surgery Versus Overnight Stay: Laparoscopic Gallbladder Surgery

Many patients have same-day surgery for elective laparoscopic cholecystectomy. As surgical stays for laparoscopic cholecystectomy become shorter, sometimes with a 4- to 8-hour observation before discharge, patient education and discharge planning become even more critical. Control of postoperative pain, nausea, and vomiting is paramount for successful same-day discharge. Before the patient departs the ambulatory surgery center, the nurse verifies that the patient is hemodynamically stable, oriented, and alert; tolerates oral fluids; has voided; has dressings that are clean and dry; and has resolved or controlled postoperative nausea and vomiting (PONV). Important discharge preparation includes information about early and continuing ambulation to decrease venous thromboembolism (VTE) risk, diet, changes in bowel patterns (feces may pass more quickly after cholecystectomy), steps to take if diarrhea is persistent, when to call the surgeon or other healthcare provider (for routine follow-up as well as problems with bleeding, fever, abdominal distention, persistent pain, jaundice, persistent cough, or shortness of breath), and medication management strategies (these are especially important if a bile acid binder has been prescribed). After reviewing this and other important discharge planning information, have the patient and family, if applicable, "teach back" instructions in their own words and allow an opportunity to ask questions.

Modified from Society of American Gastrointestinal and Endoscopic Surgeons (SAGES): *Patient information for laparoscopic gallbladder removal (cholecystectomy) from SAGES,* available at www.sages.org/publications/patient_information. Accessed January 28, 2013; Overby DW et al: SAGES guidelines for the clinical application of laparoscopic biliary tract surgery, *Surg Endosc* 24:2368–2386, 2010.

---

tissue oxygenation and lymphatic drainage, depending on the amount of manipulation, resection, and trauma to the normal anatomic structures of these viscera. General anesthesia is commonly administered. Smooth muscle relaxation is imperative for most major abdominal procedures. The patient usually experiences decreased peristalsis for 2 to 5 days after laparotomy. A nasogastric (NG) tube or gastrostomy tube is inserted during the procedure to evacuate large volumes of gastric juices. Diet is introduced only after bowel sounds return. The patient may experience nausea and vomiting if food or oral fluid is introduced too early for the GI system to function with normal absorption and motility.

Coughing and deep breathing are important for patients recovering from general anesthesia and abdominal surgery. Splinting of the abdominal muscles and use of an incentive spirometer assists the patient in postoperative coughing and deep breathing. Early ambulation assists the patient to regain overall muscle tone and prevents VTE in the lower extremities.

Pain management is very important in the patient's recovery and discharge planning. For most patients undergoing abdominal surgery, patient-controlled analgesia (PCA) or epidural analgesia may be used for better and more consistent control of pain and discomfort in the first 1 to 3 postoperative days. Narcotics may, however, add to the length of time for normal bowel peristalsis to return and their use is monitored closely after the third postoperative day.

General discharge instructions for the patient undergoing surgery for disorders of the liver, biliary tract, pancreas, or spleen might include the recommendations found in the Patient and

PATIENT AND FAMILY EDUCATION

General Discharge Instructions for the Patient Undergoing Surgery for Disorders of the Liver, Biliary Tract, Pancreas, or Spleen

- Keep incision area clean and dry.
- Swelling inside the gastrointestinal tract may produce a feeling of tightness; this should dissipate in 6 to 8 weeks.
- Solid foods should be added to the diet gradually. Chew solid foods well, and avoid gulping or eating fast or swallowing large, bulky portions.
- Avoid carbonated beverages for 3 to 4 weeks to help prevent gas bloating.
- Plan small, frequent meals because the feeling of fullness comes quickly.
- Increase exercise gradually to return to normal activities of daily living. Exercise regularly.
- Make an appointment for follow-up care with the surgeon.

Family Education box. In addition to such general instructions, surgical patients and their family or caregiver should receive surgery-specific special instructions. The discharge nurse should review medications the patient will be taking after discharge (medication reconciliation) along with purposes, dosages, schedules, and routes of administration for each, as well as any side effects to be reported. Both verbal and written instructions are provided, with phone numbers of those to call if questions arise and instructions for emergency situations. Patients should "teach back," in their own words, all instructions and should be able to state the name of their surgical procedure. For most patients, a healthcare provider (such as the surgeon, nurse practitioner [NP] or physician assistant [PA]) should be notified if any of the following develop:

- Persistent fever (body temperature of 101° F [38.3° C] or higher)
- Bleeding
- Increased abdominal swelling or pain
- Chills
- Persistent cough or shortness of breath
- Persistent pain, redness, swelling, or purulent drainage from incision sites

Follow-up care may also require providing referrals for home care (or other) services.

Surgical Interventions

Surgery of the Biliary Tract

Laparoscopic Cholecystectomy

Cholecystectomy is removal of the gallbladder. It is performed for the treatment of diseases such as acute or chronic inflammation (cholecystitis) or stones (cholelithiasis) (Box 12-1). Most of these procedures are done laparoscopically. Laparoscopic cholecystectomy is the surgical treatment of choice for patients with gallbladder disease who meet the appropriate criteria for safe laparoscopic intervention. Preoperative evaluation of patients having laparoscopic cholecystectomy differs little from that for patients scheduled for open cholecystectomy. For patients with a history of peptic ulcer disease, a flexible esophagogastroduodenoscopy (EGD) may be performed to rule out existing disease. For patients with suspected

RESEARCH HIGHLIGHT

Identifying Risk Factors for Complications of Laparoscopic Cholecystectomy

Even though laparoscopic cholecystectomy (LC) is the treatment of choice for cholecystitis, perioperative nurses must anticipate possible conversion to an open procedure and have the necessary equipment and supplies available for a "difficult cholecystectomy." In this study, researchers used a large, prospective database to attempt to accomplish two objectives: (1) identify perioperative risk factors that might be used to predict a difficult cholecystectomy and (2) determine the relationship of the risk factors to perioperative complications for LC. These complications were divided into two categories: (1) local intraoperative and postoperative complications (such as bleeding or bowel injury) and (2) systemic complications (such as myocardial infarction or pulmonary embolism).

There were 22,953 patients in the Giger study database. Their mean age was 54.5 years, there were twice as many males as females, and the majority underwent LC for chronic cholecystitis. Although the overall complication rate was 7%, the rate was higher for patients with acute cholecystitis. Using multivariate analysis, the researchers identified the following associated factors for increased local intraoperative complications:

- Male gender
- Duration of the procedure
- Increased body weight
- Surgeon experience

Postoperative local complications were associated with the following factors:

- Male gender
- Patient age
- Intraoperative complication
- American Society of Anesthesiologists (ASA) class III or IV
- Increased body weight
- Emergency surgery
- Duration of the procedure

Systemic postoperative complications were associated with the following factors:

- Conversion to an open procedure
- ASA class III or IV
- Emergency surgery
- Duration of the procedure

During the OR briefing, perioperative nurses, the anesthesia provider, and the surgeon can use this information to review and communicate possible risks based on assessment findings. Physical characteristics (gender, age, body weight), ASA class, and clinical reason for the procedure (acute or chronic cholecystitis) can be used to estimate the risk of complications. A well-prepared surgical team can lessen the duration of surgery by good planning; complication rates in this study were four times higher for procedures lasting more than 2 hours.

Modified from Giger UF et al: Risk factors for perioperative complications in patients undergoing laparoscopic cholecystectomy: analysis of 22,953 consecutive cases from the Swiss Association of Laparoscopic and Thoracoscopic Surgery database, *J Am Coll Surg* 203:723–728, 2006; Hasbahceci M et al: Laparoscopic cholecystectomy in a single, non-teaching hospital: an analysis of 1557 patients, *J Laparoendosc Adv Surg Tech* 22(6):527–532, 2012.

ductal stones, a preliminary ERCP or other diagnostic evaluation is often done. A laparoscopic procedure always has the potential to be converted to a laparotomy—a potential the patient should be informed about before the surgical procedure (Research Highlight). Laparotomy instrumentation and supplies should be available in the OR.

BOX 12-1

Overview of Cholelithiasis and Cholecystitis

The two most common diseases of the biliary tree are cholelithiasis (stone formation in the gallbladder) and *cholecystitis* (inflammation of the gallbladder). These conditions may occur alone but usually occur simultaneously. Gallstones are becoming more common in the United States, affecting an estimated 8% to 10% of adults. Cholecystectomy is one of the most common surgeries performed. Gallstones are usually found in individuals older than 40 years, with a high incidence in people of Pima and Chippewa descent, white women, and blacks.

Clinical conditions that may predispose one to gallstones include diabetes, obesity, cirrhosis, ileal disease or resection, cancer of the gallbladder, and pancreatitis. Cholecystitis usually results from obstruction of the cystic duct from gallstones (acute calculous cholecystitis); in a few patients, however, it results from stasis, bacteria, or sepsis (acute acalculous cholecystitis).

Pathophysiology

The pathophysiology of gallstones depends largely on the type of stone, the stone's location within the ductal system, and the nature of its occurrence (i.e., acute or chronic). Gallstones form as a result of the imbalance of cholesterol, bile salts, and calcium. The metabolism of cholesterol is often altered so that the bile is supersaturated, leading to precipitation and formation of stones. Cholesterol stones are the most common type and occur more often in women. Mixed stones are a combination of pigment and cholesterol stones. The exact cause of gallstone formation is unclear. Contributing factors include:

- *Supersaturation of bile with cholesterol.* Bile is composed mainly of water, with other components including cholesterol, bile salts, and pigments. Cholesterol alone is insoluble in water; it must be combined with other components (e.g., bile salts) to remain in solution. When bile salts are insufficient to maintain cholesterol in solution, cholesterol crystals form.
- *Bile stasis.* This occurs when the gallbladder has not contracted normally in response to a meal and the bile is stagnant and then becomes thick and concentrated. This occurs in patients receiving total parenteral nutrition (TPN) for a prolonged period. Approximately 50% of these patients develop "sludge" (a mucous gel composed of calcium bilirubinate and cholesterol

crystals) in the gallbladder by week 6 of TPN therapy. Gallstones frequently occur during periods of fasting or dieting, during which there is a lack of stimulus for the gallbladder to contract.

- *Nucleation.* A nucleus (nidus) is formed of agents such as bacteria, bile, pigments, cellular debris, and calcium salts. Additional substances aggregate around this nucleus, forming a stone.
- *Genetics* may be a factor, as evidenced by increased prevalence in people of Pima and Chippewa descent.

Some stones may form and pass through the ducts without causing clinical manifestations (asymptomatic cholelithiasis). Symptomatic cholelithiasis occurs when stones intermittently become lodged in the cystic duct, causing biliary colic (episodic pain in the right upper quadrant or epigastric area). The pain usually occurs after meals, especially high-fat meals, as a result of increased intraluminal pressure when the gallbladder attempts to contract to release bile (a normal response to food entering the duodenum) against the obstructing stone.

Cholecystitis develops as stones become impacted within the cystic duct, causing unyielding obstruction, edema, distention, and inflammation of the gallbladder. In chronic cholecystitis, gallstones remain, causing recurrent obstructions and producing changes in the gallbladder wall from recurrent edema and inflammation. The muscular coat becomes fibrous, and the gallbladder functions less effectively.

Complications

Edema and distention of the gallbladder walls decrease blood supply, resulting in patchy areas of necrosis and gangrene. Perforation of these areas can then occur. Bile leakage through these perforations into the peritoneum results in peritonitis. Abscess formation may occur if secretions from the ruptured gallbladder are confined by the omentum or other adjacent organs (e.g., colon, stomach, duodenum, or pancreas).

Stone migration from the gallbladder to the common bile duct (CBD) may cause cholangitis (acute CBD inflammation). The presence of gallstones in the CBD is called choledocholithiasis. CBD stones are a major source of morbidity in patients with symptomatic gallstone disease. Stone migration to the ampulla of Vater can cause pancreatitis.

Modified from Lewis SL et al, editors: *Medical-surgical nursing: assessment and management of clinical problems,* ed 8, St Louis, 2012, Mosby.

Procedural Considerations. Patients are generally admitted to the ambulatory surgery center (ASC) on the morning of surgery and will commonly require less than a 24-hour stay or admission to an extended recovery unit (ERU). A general anesthetic is used, and antibiotic prophylaxis may be administered in the immediate preoperative period. The following instrumentation, supplies, and equipment are required for laparoscopic cholecystectomy: laparoscope, two 5-mm trocars and sheaths, two 10- or 11-mm trocars and sheaths (trocar size depends on surgeon preference and may vary), a #7 knife handle with a #11 blade, multiple clip appliers, blunt grasping forceps (an assortment of alligator, Babcock, and spatula), and laparoscopic scissors. A laparoscopic video unit and secondary "slave" monitor, laparoscopic camera and control unit, light source, CO_2 source and insufflation unit, ESU, suction-irrigator (disposable), filtered insufflation tubing (disposable), and a pressure bag for IV saline 0.9% are commonly used. Instrumentation and supplies for laparoscopic common bile duct exploration should be available in the room. This may include a balloon-tipped

Fogarty catheter, wire baskets, dilators, a T-tube, and a small, flexible choledochoscope. The patient is positioned supine with the usual comfort and safety measures observed. A Foley catheter (for bladder decompression) and an NG tube (for decompression of the stomach) may be inserted. Anesthesia is administered, the time-out completed, and the patient then placed in reverse Trendelenburg position of 10 to 20 degrees.

Pneumoperitoneum may be accomplished using the closed or open technique. In the closed technique, a special hollow insufflation needle (Veress) with a retractable cutting sheath is inserted into the peritoneal cavity through a supraumbilical incision and used for insufflation. In the open technique, sometimes termed the *Hasson technique,* a small incision is made above or below the umbilicus into the peritoneal cavity. A blunt-tipped cannula (Hasson cannula) with a gas-tight sleeve is inserted, and then insufflation takes place. This approach is used for patients who have had a prior abdominal incision near the umbilicus or for those who have the potential for intraperitoneal adhesions. The Hasson technique may also use sutures, placed on either side of the sleeve, to anchor and hold the sleeve in place.

The gas of choice for pneumoperitoneum is CO_2. Gas flow is initiated at 1 to 2 L/minute. Elevated CO_2 levels and respiratory acidosis may occur because CO_2 diffuses into the patient's bloodstream during laparoscopy. Intra-abdominal pressure is normally between 8 and 10 mm Hg and the surgeon commonly uses that range as an indicator for proper Veress needle placement. If the pressure gauge shows a higher pressure, the needle may be in a closed space (such as fat), be buried in omentum, or be in the lumen of the intestine. The perioperative nurse should set the insufflation unit to a maximum pressure of 15 mm Hg. When intra-abdominal pressure reaches 15 mm Hg, flow will stop. Pressure higher than 15 mm Hg may result in bradycardia or a change in blood pressure, or it may force a gas embolus into an exposed blood vessel during the operative procedure. Most insufflation units are equipped with an alarm to alert the operative team if the intra-abdominal pressure is exceeded. Alarm systems on clinical equipment should be activated and sufficiently audible with respect to competing noise in the OR. The surgeon may frequently ask what the pressure reading is, as may the anesthesia provider.

Operative Procedure

1. A small skin incision is made in the folds of the umbilicus with a #11 blade on a #7 knife handle.
2. Pneumoperitoneum is created using either the open or the closed technique.
3. An 11-mm trocar is inserted through the supraumbilical incision; this becomes the umbilical port.
4. The laparoscope with attached video camera is inserted through the umbilical port, and the peritoneal cavity is examined. The surgeon usually stands on the left side of the patient while the first assistant stands on the right. Video monitors are positioned at eye level at both the right and left sides of the operative field. The patient is then placed in a 30-degree reverse Trendelenburg position and tilted slightly to the left.
5. Three additional trocars are inserted into the peritoneal cavity under direct visualization of the laparoscopic view (Figure 12-8).
6. Blunt grasping forceps are inserted through the medial 5-mm port to grasp the gallbladder.
7. The gallbladder is retracted laterally (Figure 12-9, *A*), exposing the triangle of Calot. The junction of the gallbladder and cystic duct is then identified. The endoscopic dissector, hook, and

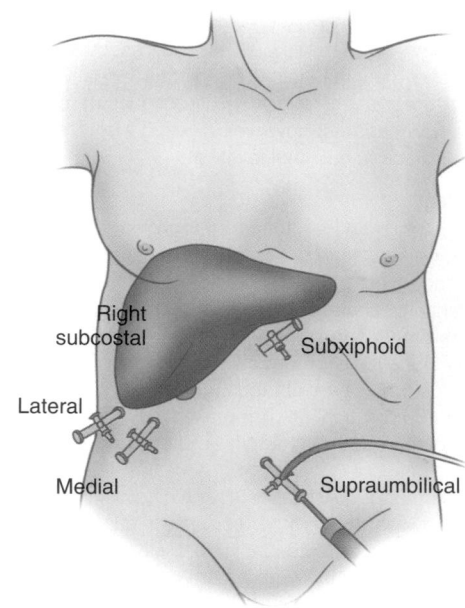

FIGURE 12-8 Trocar placement for laparoscopic cholecystectomy.

A

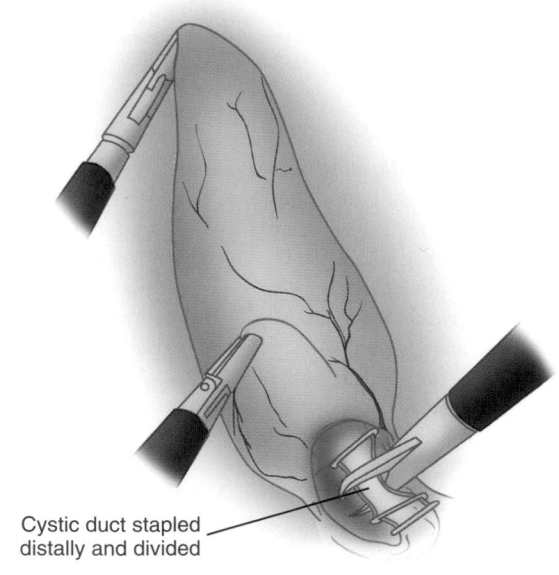

B

FIGURE 12-9 A, The gallbladder is retracted cephalad (using the grasper on the fundus) and laterally at the infundibulum. The peritoneum overlying the gallbladder infundibulum and neck and cystic duct is divided bluntly, exposing the cystic duct. **B,** Once the gallbladder–cystic duct junction has been clearly identified, clips are placed proximally and distally on the duct and it is sharply divided.

scissors are used to partially dissect the base of the gallbladder off the liver bed. Electrosurgery is also used. The electrosurgical instrument (active electrode) may have a channel through which suction can be applied to evacuate smoke plume. Some disposable instruments permit suction, electrocoagulation, and irrigation through the same instrument.

8. Hemoclips are placed proximally and distally on the cystic artery, and the artery is divided. The use of a disposable, pre-loaded, multiple-clip applier assists in the placement of ligating clips in a more efficient manner than a singly loaded, reusable applier.

9. An intraoperative cholangiogram may be performed by placing a hemoclip proximally on the cystic duct, incising its anterior surface, and passing the cholangiogram catheter into the duct. Once the cholangiogram is completed, two clips are placed distally on the cystic duct and it is divided (Figure 12-9, *B*). A pre-tied loop ligature may be used if the duct is large.

10. Attention is then given to dissecting the gallbladder out of its fossa.

11. The surgical site is inspected for hemostasis and the gallbladder dissected off the liver.

12. The gallbladder is then removed through the umbilical port (Figure 12-10). An endobag or similar specimen-retrieval accessory may be used to secure the gallbladder for extraction.

13. The peritoneal cavity is decompressed. The port sites are closed and dressed with Steri-Strips.

Laparoscopic Transcystic Duct Exploration of the Common Bile Duct

1. If the intraoperative cholangiogram indicates stones are present in the common bile duct, exploration can proceed using the same opening created for the cholangiogram.

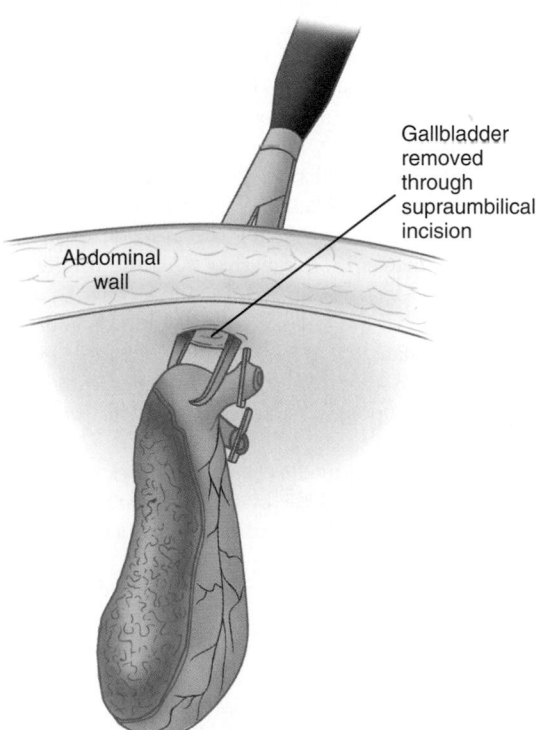

FIGURE 12-10 The gallbladder being removed through a supraumbilical incision.

2. A balloon catheter may be used to dilate the cystic duct enough for the stones to be removed.

3. A choledochoscope can be inserted through the cystic duct incision to visualize stones. The choledochoscope needs to have a working channel of at least 1.2 mm. Saline at body temperature is used to irrigate the common bile duct to aid in visualization.

4. A straight wire basket is threaded past the stone, and opened. When the stone is entrapped the basket is withdrawn. The choledochoscope and basket are removed together as a unit. The process is repeated until all stones are removed.

Laparoscopic cholangiography, choledochotomy, and common bile duct exploration are common procedures; the open approach is limited to extremely rare cases (Antoniou et al, 2011). A single-port access approach is an alternative to the multiport technique in which one incision is made at the umbilicus with trocar insertion at different points of the incision (Rottman et al, 2010; Targarona et al, 2010). Generally this type of approach is used in optimal conditions such as when there is no acute inflammation or gallbladder pathology, because of a higher risk of bile duct injuries (Joseph et al, 2012) (Research Highlight).

RESEARCH HIGHLIGHT

Single-Incision Laparoscopic Cholecystectomy (Single-Incision Laparoscopic Surgery)

Since 2008, single-incision laparoscopic surgery (SILS) for chole-cystectomy has gained popularity. A recent study of 1166 patients reveals a success rate of 90.7% and a complication rate of 6.1%. The mean operative time was 70.2 minutes with a hospital stay of 1.4 days. Complications were more common in patients more than 45 years old and those with higher body mass indexes (>30).

Advantages to the SILS approach are an essentially scarless abdomen with a better cosmetic appearance, less incisional pain, and fewer wound related complications. Most patients are able to resume oral fluid intake in 6 hours.

Common approaches to SILS include an umbilical incision with the use of two ports and anchorage of the gallbladder with two or three percutaneous sutures. Another method uses three umbilical ports and gallbladder suspension with a grasper. Routine intraoperative cholangiography can be performed. Insertion of an endobag can be accomplished by replacing one of the 5-mm ports with a 10- or 12-mm port. Most of the equipment is identical to that used for classic laparoscopy. In some current techniques multiple instruments are placed through a single access point. This allows the surgeon to approach the surgical site from different angles. The SILS port, SILS stitch articulating suturing device, and the new SILS articulating hand instruments (Covidien) offer both precision and maneuverability.

Some reasons for failure of SILS or conversion to a traditional laparoscopic approach are adhesions, acute or chronic inflammation, and inadequate exposure or inability to maintain pneumoperitoneum. Intraoperative complication rates, noted to be about 2.7%, include gallbladder perforation/bile spillage or hemorrhage. Postoperative wound infection and hematoma rates, reported to be about 2.1%, include bile leakage (0.4%), and choledocholithiasis (0.3%). Bile duct injuries may be slightly more common with SILS when compared with traditional laparoscopic approaches. Most of the time, SILS is used most effectively under optimal conditions, such as in the absence of acute inflammation.

Modified from Antoniou SA et al: Single-incision laparoscopic cholecystectomy: a systematic review, *Surg Endosc* 25:367–377, 2011; Joseph M et al: Single-incision laparoscopic cholecystectomy is associated with a higher bile duct injury rate, *Ann Surg* 256(1):1–6, 2012; Vidal O et al: Single-incision laparoscopic cholecystectomy for day surgery procedure: Are we prepared? *Am Surg* 78:436–439, 2012.

Robotic-Assisted Laparoscopic Cholecystectomy

Procedural Considerations. Robotic surgery enables surgeons to perform more advanced and complex procedures. For this surgery the surgeon controls two robotic arms with laparoscopic instruments and cameras while sitting at a console. Surgical assistants are positioned at the field. Many laparoscopic instruments have been developed to facilitate abdominal procedures. These include a bladeless trocar to minimize injury on entry and the ultrasonic shear to facilitate laparoscopic dissection with hemostasis. An endoscopic stapler and suture device may be used to facilitate intracorporeal anastomosis and knot tying (Gomez, 2012). Laparoscopic cholecystectomy was one of the first procedures to demonstrate the utility of surgical robots in general surgery. For cholecystectomies, robotic operative times may be slightly longer because of equipment setup, but clinical outcomes are equivalent. Robotic surgery is arguably superior in cholecystectomy because it offers a magnified three-dimensional picture of ductal anatomy, which may prevent bile duct injuries.

The da Vinci Surgical System (Intuitive Surgical Inc.) and the Zeus Robotic Surgical System (Computer Motion, Inc.) are two robotic systems used for minimally invasive laparoscopic surgery. The Automated Endoscopic System for Optimal Positioning (AESOP) can be "trained" to recognize the surgeon's voice. A CT scan can be imported into the console so that the surgeon can perform preoperative planning and surgical procedure rehearsal. It is even possible to perform telesurgery—the complete separation of the surgeon from the operative field. This has already been accomplished in Canada through a high-speed Internet connection to a remote site 400 miles away. Several operative procedures were performed including fundoplication, sigmoidectomy, right hemicolectomy, and inguinal hernia repair, all without conversion or significant complications derived from the robotic technology itself (Gomez, 2012). For advantages and myths about robotic surgery see Box 12-2 and Table 12-2.

BOX 12-2

Advantages of Robot-Assisted Surgery for the Patient and Surgeon

Advantages for the Patient
- Smaller incisions
- Decreased postoperative pain
- Shorter length of hospital stay
- Reduced blood loss
- Reduced tissue trauma and inflammatory response to surgery
- Improved cosmetic result
- Faster return to work

Advantages for the Surgeon
- Better visualization (higher magnification)
- Hand tremor eliminated, allowing great precision
- Three-dimensional video image of the operative field; view of ductal anatomy enhanced
- Robotic "wrist" more flexible than human wrist, improving maneuverability around organs and vessels
- Movements can be reduced, allowing complex technical tasks.
- Better ergonomic environment (sitting at a console), better levels of concentration

Modified from Gomez G: Emerging technology in surgery: informatics, electronics, robotics. In Townsend CM et al, editors: Sabiston textbook of surgery, ed 19, Philadelphia, 2012, Saunders.

Cholecystectomy (Open Approach)

The few contraindications to the laparoscopic approach to cholecystectomy include patients with suspected or diagnosed cancer of the gallbladder, third trimester of pregnancy, cirrhosis with portal hypertension, generalized peritonitis, septic shock, previous surgery that prevents access, and poor pulmonary or cardiac reserve (Jackson and Evans, 2012; Overby et al, 2010). Such patients may not be able to tolerate the pneumoperitoneum required in laparoscopy. Further, if the surgeon is unable to identify all anatomic structures during a laparoscopic approach, conversion to an open procedure becomes necessary.

Procedural Considerations. A basic laparotomy set and biliary instruments are used when cholecystectomy is performed through an open abdominal incision. The patient is positioned supine and receives a general anesthetic. After the patient is intubated, the anesthesia provider inserts an NG tube. Antibiotic prophylaxis may be administered. When an operative cholangiogram is anticipated, the perioperative nurse must ensure that the OR bed has been equipped and positioned so that C-arm image intensification can be efficiently accomplished. Radiation-protection devices for the surgical team and patient are used during image intensification.

Operative Procedure

1. The abdominal cavity is opened through a right subcostal or upper midline incision.
2. Hemostasis of capillary vessels is achieved with electrocoagulation. Larger vessels are clamped with hemostats and ligated with suture material.
3. Retractors and laparotomy packs are placed as the abdominal cavity is carefully examined.
4. The common duct is palpated for evidence of stones, and pathologic conditions are determined.
5. Harrington, Deaver, or self-retaining retractors, such as an upper-hand or Gomez retractor, are placed to provide exposure. Long tissue forceps and suction are used to manipulate tissues. The surrounding organs are isolated from the gallbladder region by moistened laparotomy packs and deep retractors.
6. To facilitate gentle traction, Péan forceps are usually placed on the body of the gallbladder (Figure 12-11, *A*).
7. The peritoneal fold overlying the junction of the cystic and common duct is incised with a #7 knife handle and a #15 blade, long Metzenbaum scissors, and forceps. Suction is available, and bleeding vessels are clamped and ligated or electrocoagulated.
8. Adhesions are separated by blunt dissection with small, round, dry dissector sponges; sponges on holders; and blunt right-angled clamps.
9. Dissection is continued to expose the neck of the gallbladder, the cystic artery, and the cystic duct. Lateral traction on the gallbladder neck allows incision of the peritoneum overlying the triangle of Calot.
10. Dissection is continued to expose the cystic artery as it enters the wall of the gallbladder.
11. On complete exposure and visualization of the branches, the cystic artery is doubly ligated with silk or clamped with ligating clips and divided (see Figure 12-11, *B*).
12. Occasionally a third ligature or clip may be used. If the cystic artery has more than one branch, each is ligated and divided separately.

TABLE 12-2

Myths About Robotic Surgery

Myth	Reality
Robots do all the work.	A *surgical robot* has been defined as a powered, computer-controlled device that can be programmed to aid in the positioning and manipulation of surgical instruments. The surgeon manages the robot system from a console away from the operative field.
Robotic systems are alike.	There are several types of robots:
	Camera holder robots: System includes control computer, a power system, and an articulated, electromechanical arm for holding and maneuvering the telescope. The arm attaches to the operating table, and its action can be controlled by foot pedals, hand controls, or a voice activation/ recognition system.
	Master-slave robots: Computer-controlled devices governed by the surgeon. The master surgeon is seated at a control console, and the slave robotic arm is located at the surgical field over the patient.
	Neurosurgery robots: Functions under the guidance of a dedicated CT imaging system.
	Orthopedic robots: Designed for orthopedic surgery. Target site can be effectively stabilized. More precise bone drilling, better alignment of fragments and prostheses.
	Passive: The energy to propel the system is provided by the surgeon.
	Semiactive and synergistic robots: Combine the capability of some autonomous function with other actions carried out by the surgeon.
	Urology robots: A powered image-guided, computer-controlled robot for TURP.
Robotic surgery is better than conventional surgery.	Current surgical outcomes are comparable. Surgical robots represent sophisticated powered instruments that enable the surgeon to carry out more complex tasks.
Robotic arms function just like a surgeon's hands.	Robotic arms are better than human hands—steadier and more precise, with no tremor and smaller hand movements, and able to work in a very small space. However, hand dexterity is missing—a human hand can move 20 ways; robotic arm has good but not exactly replicable range of motion.
Robots make surgery simpler, faster, or less expensive.	System setup time can be lengthy. Some surgeries take longer to perform with a robotic system. Robotic systems require larger OR space.
Robotic surgery is limited.	Examples of surgical tasks assigned to robotic systems include percutaneous biopsy of solid organs (e.g., brain, prostate, kidney), high-precision drilling or cutting (e.g., bone), automated resection of solid organs (e.g., prostate), image processing (e.g., magnification); reproduction of 3-D vision, microsurgery (e.g., motion scaling), suturing in MIS, endoscope holding, and surgery under biohazardous conditions.
Robotic surgery is useful only in the OR.	Integrated robotic systems will be capable of assisting in the preoperative, intraoperative, and postoperative management of surgical patients. A surgical robot linked to another robotic system such as a CT or MRI scanner can have access to imaging studies. Robots have the potential to assist not only with preoperative planning but also rehearsal of individualized operations. Purpose-designed robots in surgical simulation may become invaluable tools for surgical training and licensing procedures.

CT, Computed tomography; *MIS,* minimally invasive surgery; *MRI,* magnetic resonance imaging; *TURP,* transurethral resection of the prostate.
From Gomez G: Emerging technology in surgery: informatics, electronics, robotics. In Townsend CM et al, editors: *Sabiston textbook of surgery,* ed 19, Philadelphia, 2012, Saunders.

13. Abnormalities of the arterial and ductal anatomy are common (Figure 12-12), and the surgeon and assistant work with care to identify these structures.
14. The true junction of the cystic duct with the common bile duct is visualized.
15. The cystic duct is identified and carefully dissected down to its junction with the hepatic duct.
16. Any stones in the cystic duct are "milked" back into the gallbladder, and a tie is placed around the proximal part of the cystic duct.
17. If necessary, a cholangiogram is performed at this time (see following procedure, Intraoperative Cholangiogram). If a cholangiogram is not done, the cystic duct is doubly ligated and divided (see Figure 12-11, *C*). A fine, absorbable transfixion suture may be used on the stump of the cystic duct near the common bile duct.
18. The gallbladder is then dissected from the liver bed and removed (see Figure 12-11, *D*).
19. All bleeding is controlled; reperitonealization of the liver bed, if indicated, is accomplished with interrupted or continuous fine absorbable intestinal sutures.

20. A closed suction drain may be inserted near the cystic duct stump. The free end of the drain is exteriorized through a stab wound in the lateral abdominal wall.
21. The wound is closed in layers and a dressing applied.

Intraoperative Cholangiogram

An intraoperative cholangiogram is usually performed with both open and laparoscopic cholecystectomy to visualize the common bile duct and the hepatic ductal branches, and to assess the patency of the common bile duct.

Procedural Considerations. An intraoperative cholangiogram requires fluoroscopy to visualize filling of the ducts. Before the patient's arrival in the OR, the perioperative nurse confirms that a radiolucent bed is available or prepares the OR bed with an image-intensification attachment and ensures that the patient has not had previous allergic reactions to the x-ray medium before dispensing the pharmaceutic agent to the sterile field. Safe medication practices should be followed for labeling and dispensing all medications on and off the sterile field. X-ray aprons or leaded shields are used for all members of the surgical team and the patient.

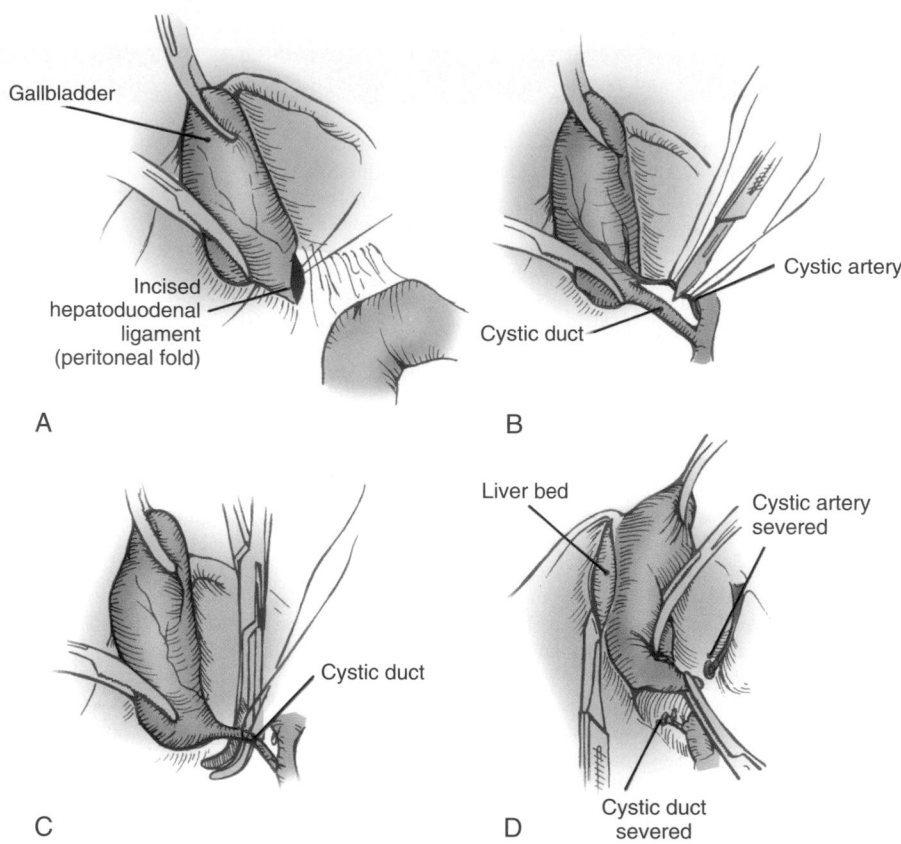

FIGURE 12-11 Cholecystectomy. **A,** With Péan forceps in place, gentle traction is maintained as peritoneum over the triangle of Calot is incised. **B,** Cystic artery is clearly visualized, doubly ligated, and divided. **C,** Cystic duct is carefully dissected and identified before forceps and ligatures are applied. **D,** Dissection of gallbladder from liver bed is completed.

FIGURE 12-12 Arterial blood supply of the liver and biliary system is variable. **A,** The most common anatomic arrangement is a cystic artery arising from the right hepatic artery. **B,** A dual hepatic blood supply is found in 15% to 20% of patients, with the right hepatic artery arising from the superior mesenteric artery in a significant number of patients, as in **C.**

Because the patient's abdomen remains open while the x-ray equipment is positioned directly over the operative site, appropriate draping to maintain asepsis is necessary. Radiopaque sponges and any unnecessary instrumentation are removed from the abdominal site to avoid obscuring the view of the contrast medium filling the ducts.

The scrub person prepares a cholangiocatheter by attaching a stopcock with a 20-mL syringe of saline and a 20-mL syringe of contrast medium to the Luer-Lok ports. All air bubbles are removed because they might be misinterpreted as gall duct stones on the x-ray film.

Intraoperative Procedure

1. The cholangiocath is irrigated with saline before and during its insertion into the cystic and common bile ducts.
2. The cholangiocath is inserted into the duct using atraumatic grasping forceps. Irrigation during insertion facilitates dilation and reduces trauma to the ductal lumen.
3. The cholangiocath is anchored in the lumen of the common bile duct by the surgeon's preferred method. Common methods are applying a Ligaclip proximal to the insertion site; tying or suturing the catheter in place; or using a ring-jawed holding clamp, such as a Swenson clamp, that has been designed specifically for this purpose.
4. With placement of the cholangiocath confirmed and anchored, all radiopaque sponges, instruments, and obstructing equipment are removed from the field.
5. The surgical field is draped with a sterile drape sheet to maintain asepsis of the wound and field. The image-intensifier equipment (C-arm) is positioned as the surgeon redirects the stopcock to allow for injection of the contrast medium. If stones are found, the surgeon removes them under fluoroscopic guidance.

Cholecystostomy

Cholecystostomy establishes an opening into the gallbladder for drainage and removal of stones. The open approach is usually selected for patients with advanced medical problems who cannot tolerate general anesthesia or more extensive surgery. Ultrasound-guided percutaneous cholecystostomy has become an accepted procedure for patients who are not otherwise good candidates for surgery. Because of the high incidence of gangrene, perforation, and empyema, open cholecystostomy is often the preferred approach. Many patients are critically ill. If the diagnosis is uncertain, percutaneous cholecystostomy can be both diagnostic and therapeutic. About 90% of patients improve with percutaneous cholecystostomy (Jackson and Evans, 2012). In the rare situation when interventional radiology is not available, an open procedure may be done, as is described here.

Procedural Considerations. A large Toomey syringe (50 mL) or an Asepto syringe may be needed for irrigation purposes. If a local anesthetic is used, the anesthetic agent, syringes, and needles are assembled. Protocols for safe administration and labeling of all medications/solutions on and off the sterile field must be followed. Specified drainage tubes or catheters should be available. The patient is positioned supine. Although many surgeons prefer a right subcostal incision, when cholecystostomy procedures are performed as emergencies, a quicker midline or transverse incision may be used. Instrumentation includes a basic laparotomy set plus a gallbladder set.

Operative Procedure

1. After incision into the abdominal cavity, the gallbladder is isolated by retraction of the surrounding viscera.
2. The fundus of the gallbladder is grasped with an Allis or Babcock forceps and, if needed, the proposed opening is encircled by means of an absorbable purse-string suture, leaving the ends long.
3. If the gallbladder is distended or tense, it may be isolated with moistened laparotomy packs to protect the abdominal cavity from contamination.
4. If decompression of the gallbladder is required, a large-bore needle (e.g., 18 gauge) may be inserted with suction attached. Gallbladder contents are aspirated and the site closed using surgical clips on a clip applier.
5. If a trocar is used within the purse-string suture, suction tubing is attached to the trocar sheath.
6. As the contents are aspirated, culture specimens may be taken. The contaminated trocar and sheath are removed and isolated in a discard basin.
7. The opening into the gallbladder can be enlarged with Metzenbaum scissors. Gallstones are removed with malleable scoops and stone forceps.
8. Irrigating the gallbladder with isotonic saline solution may be necessary to remove small stones, grit, or pastelike material. A syringe with a catheter or an Asepto syringe is sometimes used for irrigation.
9. Remaining contaminated instruments are placed in a discard basin.
10. A drainage tube is inserted into the gallbladder opening. The purse-string suture is tightened around the catheter, with care taken not to occlude it.
11. The free end of the catheter or tube is exteriorized through a stab wound and then anchored to the skin edges, as described for open cholecystectomy.
12. Drainage of the abdominal cavity is established with the exterior ends of each drain secured.
13. The wound is closed in layers, as described for laparotomy, and dressings applied at the incision and drain sites.

Common Bile Duct Exploration (Open Approach)

With the advent of endoscopic, percutaneous, and laparoscopic techniques (Figure 12-13), open exploration of the common bile duct is rare. However, when these methods are not available, when they are not possible because of prior surgery, or when an open procedure is otherwise necessary, open common bile duct exploration is performed. Intraoperative ultrasound may be used to delineate relevant anatomy, detect bile stones, and decrease the risk of bile duct injury (Overby et al, 2010).

Procedural Considerations. The patient is positioned supine after administration of a general anesthetic. The anesthesia provider inserts an NG tube after intubation. An indwelling urinary catheter may be inserted before the abdominal skin prep. Instrumentation includes a basic laparotomy set with the addition of gallbladder instruments. T-tubes of assorted sizes should be available. Intraoperative cholangiography will most likely be used to confirm that all stones have been removed; radiation-protection devices for the patient and surgical team are required. Culture tubes are needed. Soft rubber catheters for irrigation, balloon-tipped catheters such as the biliary Fogarty catheter, stone baskets, and the surgeon's

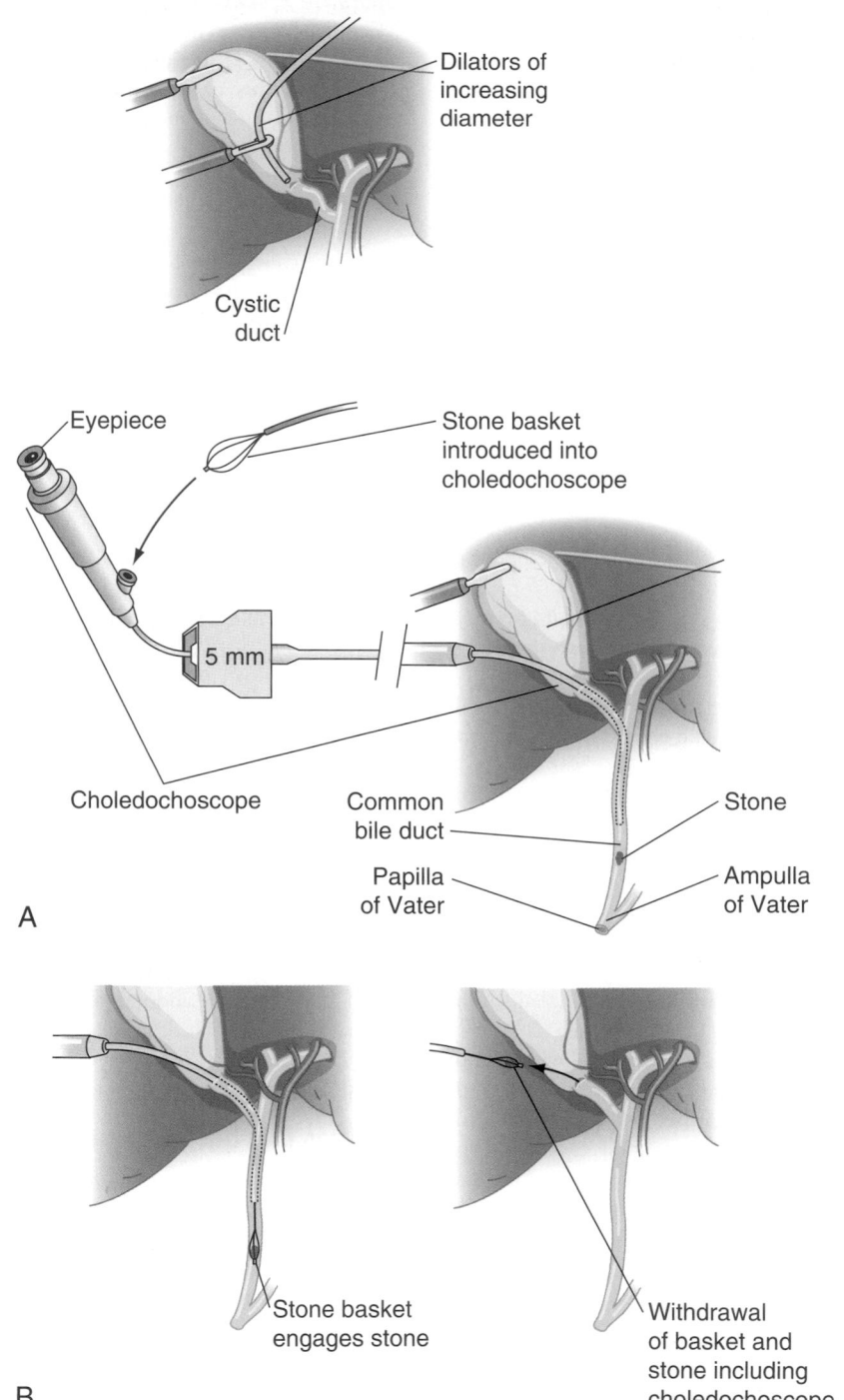

FIGURE 12-13 A, Laparoscopic common bile duct exploration. After dilation of the cystic duct, the flexible choledochoscope is inserted into the abdomen through the small trocar and maneuvered into the distal common bile duct. **B,** A stone basket is passed through the working channel of the choledochoscope and is used to snare a common duct stone. The stone basket and choledochoscope are then withdrawn together.

preferred cholangiocath should be available, as well as both flexible and rigid choledochoscopes. A choledochoscope requires the following:
- Choledochoscope with accessories: biopsy forceps, stone-grasping forceps, and a sheath that can be used to direct other instruments into various portions of the biliary tract

- Video camera and viewing screen
- Light cord
- 0.9% normal saline (1000-mL bag)
- Sterile IV tubing
- Pressure bag
- Light source for the choledochoscope

Distending the common duct is necessary for better visualization and is accomplished by irrigating the duct with copious amounts of sterile saline. A pressure bag is placed around an IV bag of 0.9% saline, and pressure to 300 mm Hg is applied. Sterile tubing is then passed from the sterile field and attached to the saline bag. The scrub person attaches the distal end of the sterile IV tubing directly to the irrigating stopcock on the scope.

Operative Procedure

1. The abdomen is opened through a subcostal incision or midline incision.
2. If the gallbladder has not been previously removed, it is exposed and removed or retracted by means of laparotomy packs and retractors.
3. The common duct may be identified by means of an aspirating syringe and fine-gauge needle to make certain that the suspect duct is not a blood vessel. Culture specimens may be obtained.
4. The common duct region is isolated with moistened laparotomy packs and narrow-blade retractors. A discard basin for contaminated instruments is placed at the lower end of the operative field and suction is prepared for immediate use.
5. Two fine-traction sutures are placed in the wall of the duct, below the entrance of the cystic duct. A longitudinal incision is made in the common duct, between the traction sutures, with a long #3 knife handle and #15 or #11 blade, and enlarged with Potts angled or Metzenbaum scissors.
6. Visible stones are removed with gallstone forceps, after which exploration of the duct is begun with small, malleable scoops, proximal and then distal to the opening. Isotonic solution in an Asepto syringe and a soft, small-lumen catheter or a balloon-tipped catheter are used to facilitate the removal of small stones and debris as well as to demonstrate patency of the common bile duct in its entirety to the duodenum.
7. The choledochoscope may be used to identify additional stones. The scope is inserted into the common duct, which is then flushed with saline. After visualizing the duct to ensure that no stones remain, a T-tube is placed in the common bile duct and the choledochotomy is closed around the tube. A final cholangiogram is performed to be certain all stones have been removed. The wound is closed, the T-tube anchored to the skin, and dressings applied. Sterile tubing is used to connect the T-tube to a small drainage container or bag.

Anastomoses: Cholecystoduodenostomy, Cholecystojejunostomy, Choledochoduodenostomy, Choledochojejunostomy and Transduodenal Sphincteroplasty

There are several types of anastomoses between the gallbladder and the small bowel.

- Cholecystoduodenostomy and cholecystojejunostomy create an anastomosis between the gallbladder and duodenum or the gallbladder and jejunum, respectively, to relieve an obstruction in the distal end of the common duct. An obstruction in the biliary system may be caused by a tumor of the ducts involving the head of the pancreas or the ampulla of Vater, an inflammatory lesion, a stricture of the common duct, or the presence of stones.
- Choledochoduodenostomy is an anastomosis between the common duct and the duodenum, and choledochojejunostomy is an anastomosis between the duct and the jejunum. These procedures (referred to as choledochal drainage procedures) may be necessary in postcholecystectomy patients to circumvent an

obstructive lesion and reestablish the flow of bile into the intestinal tract.
- Transduodenal sphincteroplasty achieves a choledochoduodenostomy between the distal end of the common duct and the side of the duodenum. The sphincters normally affecting the distal common and pancreatic ducts are rendered functionless because the stoma is noncontractile and therefore remains permanently open. An indication for transduodenal sphincteroplasty is sphincter of Oddi dysfunction—a poorly defined clinical syndrome that is characterized by pain characteristic of biliary colic and recurrent acute pancreatitis. Both endoscopic sphincterotomy and transduodenal sphincteroplasty with transampullary septectomy have been used with similar results. The procedure described in the following text has the advantage of including division of the transampullary septum, which promotes pancreatic duct drainage.

Procedural Considerations. Surgical approaches are similar for these anastomoses. Instrumentation for an open procedure includes a basic laparotomy set; gallbladder instruments with two curved Doyen intestinal forceps with guards, or similar atraumatic holding forceps; and a self-retaining retractor system. Linear stapling devices, and T-tubes and stents in varying size should also be available. Fluoroscopy should be anticipated and radiation-protection devices for the patient and the surgical team should be available. The patient is positioned supine after administration of a general anesthetic. The anesthesia provider inserts an NG tube after intubation. An indwelling urinary catheter is inserted before abdominal skin preparation.

Open Operative Procedure: Cholecystoduodenostomy and Cholecystojejunostomy

1. The abdomen is opened, the gallbladder exposed, the contents aspirated, and the pathologic condition confirmed.
2. The anastomosis site is prepared, posterior serosal silk sutures placed, and open anastomosis performed.
3. Anastomosis of the gallbladder to the duodenum or loop of the jejunum is usually performed as a two-layer anastomosis.
4. The serosa of the duodenum or loop of the jejunum is sutured to the full thickness of the fundus of the gallbladder.
5. A 1- to 1.5-cm opening is made into the small bowel and gallbladder in corresponding positions. GI technique (also referred to as bowel technique) (see Chapter 11) is instituted.
6. Interrupted fine monofilament (5-0 or 4-0) sutures are then placed around the entire circumference.
7. Contaminated instruments are placed in the discard basin and the operative field is prepared for closure.

Surgery of the Pancreas

Drainage or Excision of Pancreatic Cysts (Open Method)

Pancreatic pseudocysts are localized collections of pancreatic secretions in a cystic structure. Surgical drainage is indicated for patients with pancreatic pseudocysts that cannot be treated with endoscopic techniques or for patients whose endoscopic treatment fails (Jensen et al, 2012).

The preferred operative therapy in patients with uncomplicated pseudocysts is internal drainage by one of three options: cystojejunostomy (use of a defunctionalized Roux-en-Y jejunal limb) (Figure 12-14), cystogastrostomy (drainage into the stomach), or cystoduodenostomy (drainage into the duodenum) (Jensen et al, 2012). Treatment depends on the location of the cyst. Cystogastrostomy is

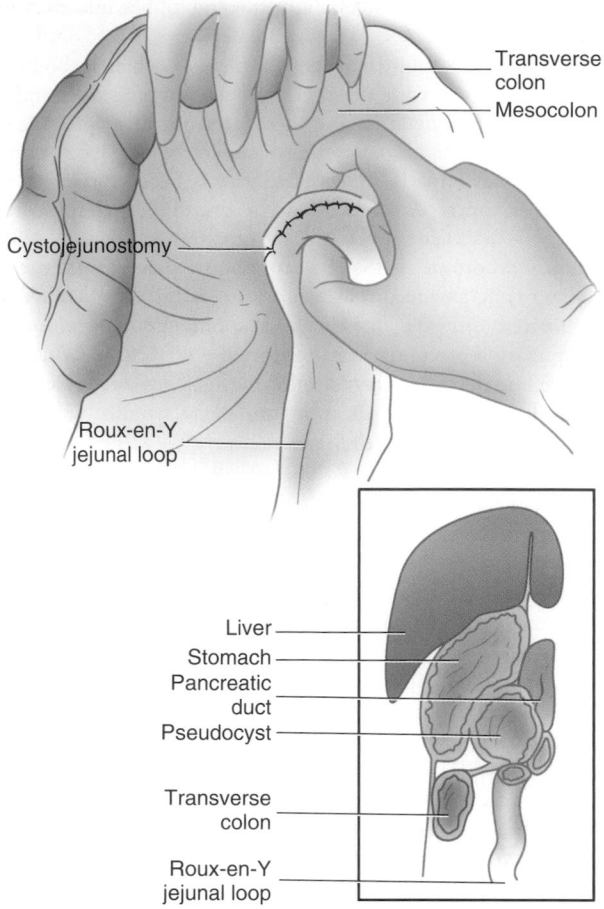

FIGURE 12-14 Internal drainage of a pancreatic pseudocyst by Roux-en-Y cystojejunostomy through the base of the transverse mesocolon.

a faster and technically simpler procedure used when the cyst adheres to the posterior wall of the stomach. Cystojejunostomy is the more versatile drainage procedure. Cystoduodenostomy is used in selected cases, depending on cyst location, but has limited utility.

Procedural Considerations. The patient is positioned supine after administration of a general anesthetic. The anesthesia provider inserts an NG tube after intubation. An indwelling urinary catheter is inserted before abdominal skin preparation. Instrumentation and supplies necessary for this procedure include a basic laparotomy set, gallbladder instruments, a GI set, and a self-retaining retractor system.

Operative Procedure
1. A midline incision is made into the abdomen.
2. A self-retaining retractor system is used to expose the pancreatic area.
3. The pancreatic cyst is examined and the area isolated with moist packs.
4. Internal drainage may be accomplished by an incision into the anterior wall of the stomach, directly opposite the cyst if it adheres to the posterior wall, thereby providing drainage through the GI tract.

5. A fistula is established between the anterior wall of the cyst and the posterior wall of the stomach. Many surgeons prefer an anastomosis between the cyst and a Roux-en-Y loop of jejunum (see Figure 12-14) or into the duodenum directly, depending on the location of the cyst.
6. The anterior gastrostomy is closed and wound closure completed.

Laparoscopic Pancreatic Cyst–Gastrostomy

Laparoscopic techniques may be used for internal drainage procedures for pancreatic pseudocysts. CT imaging is used to diagnose the pancreatic pseudocyst. An EUS may also provide additional information. The location, size, and thickness of the wall of the pseudocyst are all assessed to determine the more appropriate procedure for drainage, either a laparoscopic pancreatic cyst–gastrostomy or a Roux-en-Y pancreatic cystojejunostomy. Endoscopic drainage of pseudocysts may also be done in surgical centers where endoscopists are experienced in percutaneous drainage techniques. Laparoscopic treatment of pancreatic pseudocysts enables definitive drainage with faster recovery (Oida et al, 2011).

Procedural Considerations. General anesthesia is induced and an NG tube inserted. The patient is positioned supine. Equipment and instrumentation are a 30-degree telescope (10 mm or 5 mm); a video camera; two high-density video monitors; a high-flow insufflator with CO_2 tank; an ESU; two 12.5-mm trocar ports; two 5-mm trocar ports; an endodissecting instrument (5 mm) or atraumatic grasping forceps (5 mm); endoshears/scissors (5 mm) with electrocoagulation connection; an endo-Babcock instrument; a mechanical stapling device; a 10-mm endoclip applier; a 10-mm endosuturing instrument (optional); 2-0 suture material, 7-inch length (optional); an electrocoagulation hook; a long 5-mm laparoscopic needle; and an endoretractor.

Operative Procedure
1. Pneumoperitoneum is created and the trocars inserted via port sites as illustrated in Figure 12-15.
2. The pancreatic pseudocyst is located by entering the lesser sac at the greater curvature. Hemostasis is achieved by using the endoclip applier. An endostapling device (gastrointestinal anastomosis [GIA] type) with vascular cartridges is used to dissect the greater curvature.
3. The surgeon assesses the site for entry into the stomach. An endoretractor may be used to retract the left hepatic lobe.
4. Using electrodissection, an incision centered between the lesser and greater curvatures is made on the anterior wall of the stomach and then extended.
5. A long laparoscopic aspiration needle is inserted into the intraabdominal and gastric cavity. The camera is advanced to visualize the posterior wall of the stomach.
6. The needle is inserted into the cyst and its presence is confirmed by aspiration.
7. A small incision is made into the cyst and the pancreatic fluid aspirated.
8. The endostapling device is inserted into the gastric cavity. The smaller jaw of this instrument is inserted into the pseudocyst. The stapling device is closed. It is important that the anastomosis not be under tension. The stapling device is fired and the anastomosis checked for integrity. An endosuturing instrument is used to close any defects in the anastomotic line.
9. An NG tube is directed into the pseudocyst.

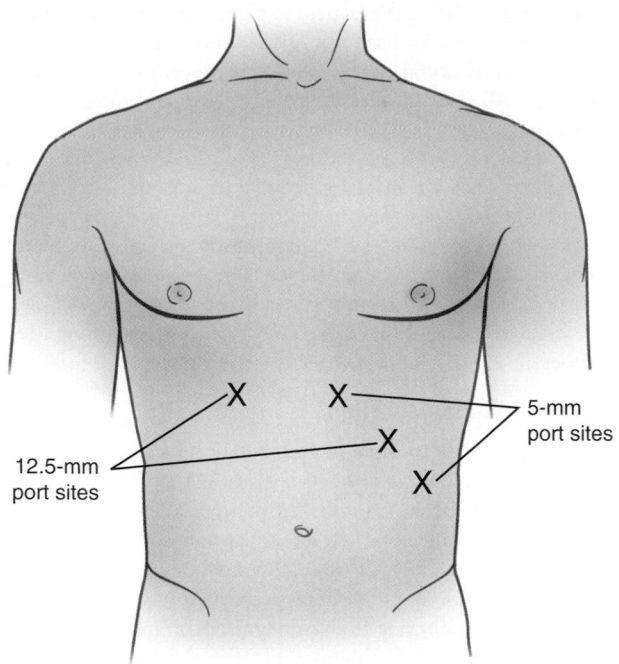

FIGURE 12-15 Port sites for trocar placement in laparoscopic pancreatic cyst–gastrostomy.

10. The two edges of the anterior wall gastrostomy are approximated using endograsping forceps (atraumatic) or an endodissecting instrument. The gastrostomy is then closed using an endostapling device (TA type).
11. A drain is placed, the abdomen deflated, trocar ports removed, and trocar sites closed and dressed.

Other Laparoscopic Pancreatic Procedures

Laparoscopic pancreatic surgery is an emerging approach, but it has not gained wide acceptance due to the complexity of the procedures, the accuracy needed to perform the operation, and the typically steep learning curve required to master the procedures (Giulianotti et al, 2010). Laparoscopic resection of lesions in the body and tail of the pancreas is done in specialized centers. Pancreatic exploration and resections of peri-pancreatic tissue, endocrine tumors, pancreatic carcinomas, and cystic tumors have all been achieved laparoscopically (Rosok et al, 2010). Laparoscopic surgery may be used as an initial step to rule out metastatic disease prior to resection (Baumgartner et al, 2012).

Severe attacks of acute pancreatitis can result in pancreatic necrosis that may require debridement and drainage by surgical or radiologic methods. Minimal access techniques include laparoscopy with necrosectomy (resection of necrotic tissue) (Raraty et al, 2010).

Robotic-Assisted Laparoscopic Pancreatic Procedures

Procedural Considerations. Pancreatic lesions can be resected with robotic-assisted laparoscopy. Pancreaticojejunostomy may be performed following an open pancreaticoduodenectomy. Computer-assisted robotic surgery may be used to resect, drain, and reconstruct the pancreatic duct. Precise tissue manipulation and three-dimensional imaging allow better surgical approaches for reconstruction of the pancreatic or common bile ducts than open techniques. Robotic surgery enables difficult technical maneuvers

with the advantage of minimally invasive techniques, and there may be improved results due to less tissue trauma (Giulianotti et al, 2010).

Pancreaticoduodenectomy (Whipple Procedure)

Pancreatic cancer is treated using a multidisciplinary approach that may include surgeons, gastroenterologists, oncologists, radiologists, nurses, and nutritionists. Tumors arise from the exocrine glands (95%) and endocrine glands (5%) in the pancreas. Ductal adenocarcinoma constitutes 80% of all pancreatic tumors. Most tumors begin in the head of the exocrine gland, obstruct the bile duct, and extend to the duodenum, intestines, and spine. Metastasis occurs to regional lymph nodes, and common metastatic sites include the liver and lungs. Because symptoms most often occur late in the disease, the prognosis is usually poor. Pancreaticoduodenectomy (Whipple procedure) is the removal of the head of the pancreas, the entire duodenum, a portion of the jejunum, the distal third of the stomach, and the lower half of the common bile duct, with reestablishment of continuity of the biliary, pancreatic, and GI tract systems. For patients who have cancer of the ampulla of Vater, newer less invasive pancreatic-sparing duodenectomy techniques are used as an alternative to pancreaticoduodenectomy (Chen et al, 2012).

Procedural Considerations. A basic laparotomy set, a GI instrument set, a self-retaining retractor system (e.g., Bookwalter), linear stapling devices, and appropriate drains and catheters are required. The perioperative nurse should ensure that ordered blood and blood products are available. Pancreaticoduodenectomy may take 5 to 6 hours and require the transfusion of many units of blood or blood products. The patient is positioned supine after administration of a general anesthetic. Attention is paid to padding positional pressure points with gel pads or using a pressure-reducing OR bed mattress. Intermittent pneumatic compression devices (IPCDs) are applied as well as a forced-air warming device and other active warming measures to prevent hypothermia. The anesthesia provider inserts an NG tube after intubation. An indwelling urinary catheter is inserted before abdominal preparation. The abdomen is prepped from nipple line to midthigh.

Operative Procedure
1. The abdomen is entered through either an upper transverse, a bilateral subcostal, or a long paramedian incision. Resectability is assessed, exploring for hepatic metastases, serosal implants of tumor, and lymph node metastases. If these are outside the zone of resection, the disease is unresectable.
2. Laparotomy packs and retractors are used to expose the operative site and protect vital structures.
3. The duodenum is mobilized using the Kocher maneuver (incision of peritoneal reflection lateral to the second portion of the duodenum) with Metzenbaum scissors and subsequent blunt dissection of loose areolar tissue.
4. Mobilization of the duodenum continues and bleeding vessels are ligated with silk.
5. The gastrocolic ligament and the gastrohepatic omentum are divided between curved forceps and are ligated or transfixed.
6. The gastroduodenal and right gastric arteries are clamped, divided, and ligated.
7. The prepyloric area of the stomach is mobilized.
8. The operative field is prepared for open anastomosis by isolating the area with laparotomy sponges.

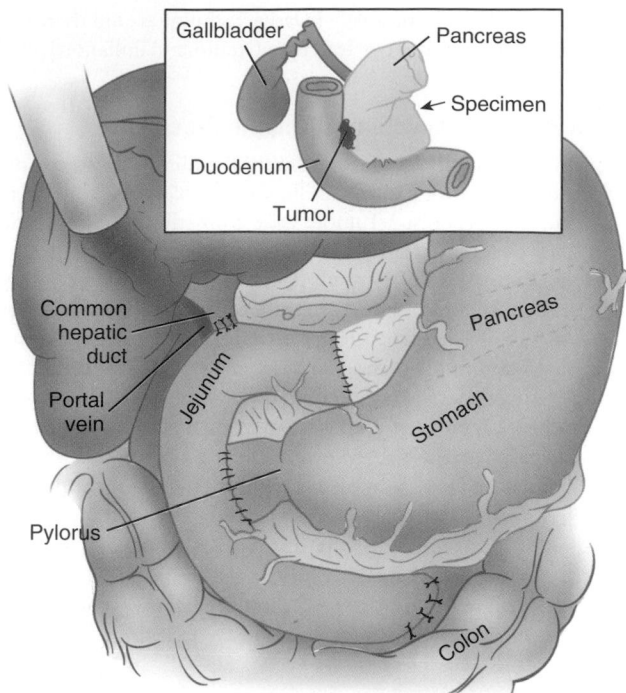

FIGURE 12-16 Illustration of a pylorus-preserving pancreaticoduodenectomy and the subsequent reconstruction. The inset at the top depicts the resected specimen. The jejunal limb is passed through and sutured to the transverse mesocolon.

9. By placing two long Allen or Payr clamps near the midportion of the stomach, the transection is completed.
10. The duodenum is reflected, the common duct is divided, and the hepatic end is marked or tagged for later anastomosis.
11. The jejunum is clamped with two Allen forceps and the duodenojejunal flexure divided.
12. The pancreas is divided and the duct carefully identified.
13. Further mobilization of the duodenum and division of the inferior pancreaticoduodenal artery are done to permit complete removal of the specimen.
14. The most common reconstructive technique is anastomosis of the pancreas to the jejunum first, followed by the bile duct and then the duodenum (Figure 12-16).
15. Drains may be placed, the abdomen closed, and an abdominal dressing applied.

Laparoscopic Whipple Resection

Laparoscopic pancreaticoduodenectomy is challenging and laparoscopic techniques are constantly being developed and refined. Traditional pancreatic surgery requires wide exposure through a large incision, gentle dissection and tissue manipulation, correct interpretation of anatomy and blood supply, and very precise reconstruction of the biliopancreatico-digestive anatomy (Giulianotti, 2010). Dissection of the pancreatic head from the portal vein and superior mesenteric artery is very challenging (Kuroki et al, 2010). Given the complexity of the procedure and the fact that the major morbidities following pancreaticoduodenectomy are not related to the size of the incision, the laparoscopic Whipple procedure has not become widely adopted (Jensen et al, 2012). However, Rosok and colleagues (2010) described the following method.

Operative Procedure. The patient is placed in supine position and in addition to trocars used for distal resection, two additional trocars are placed lateral to the right rectus sheath in the medioclavicular line. All dissection is done with a vessel-sealing device in accordance with standard oncologic surgical principles and identical to those used for open procedures. Anastomosis is done with a 4-cm incision with a minimally invasive laparotomy retractor ring used with specially designed instruments. Hepaticojejunostomy is achieved with an end-to-side anastomosis using monofilament sutures. In addition, the pancreatic anastomosis is made as an end-to-side pancreaticogastrostomy. The gastroenterostomy is stapled as a side-to-side anastomosis using an endoscopic stapling device (Rosok et al, 2010).

Pancreatic Transplantation

Pancreatic transplantation is the implantation of a pancreas from a donor into a recipient for patients with type 1 (formerly known as juvenile-onset) diabetes. Options for pancreatic transplant include a pancreas transplant alone (PTA), an option chosen for patients with functioning kidneys; a simultaneous pancreas-kidney transplant (SPK), because severe diabetes is often associated with chronic renal failure; or a pancreas after kidney (PAK) transplant, in which the pancreas is transplanted sometime after the kidney transplant. Pancreatic transplantation differs from other organ transplants in that it does not have immediate lifesaving results. It is done in the hope of preventing debilitating side effects of diabetes, such as cardiovascular, retinal, and renal disease. For patients, a significant benefit is freedom from dependence on insulin. However, pancreatic transplant in patients with brittle diabetes remains a rare procedure because the trade-off of insulin dependence is lifelong immunosuppression (Boggi et al, 2010). Transplant is most effective in people with few or no secondary diabetic complications and it can reverse or stop the progression of these complications. Another new option on the horizon for persons with diabetes is an implanted micro-electromechanical system (MEMS). This is a technology that could replace injectable insulin and glucose meters. This technology includes an implantable insulin pump that will deliver insulin in response to blood glucose levels (Allen, 2012).

Procedural Considerations. The majority of pancreas transplants performed in the United States are SPK procedures (Figure 12-17). Instrumentation includes a transplant set as described for kidney transplantation in Chapter 15. In addition to the transplant set, vascular instruments and instruments for resection of the duodenal segment and management of the pancreatic duct are required. A linear stapling device may be used.

The patient is positioned supine after administration of a general anesthetic. The anesthesia provider inserts an NG tube after intubation. An indwelling urinary catheter is inserted before the abdominal skin prep and is attached to a urometer. Like other transplant procedures, these procedures are lengthy, lasting 5 to 7 hours. Positional pressure sites must be padded and a pressure-reducing mattress placed on the OR bed. Given the patient's diabetes, maintaining skin and tissue integrity is paramount. IPCDs will likely be used. Careful monitoring of blood glucose level occurs throughout the procedure by the anesthesia provider. Blood and blood products are ordered, and their availability must be verified. Blood-warming devices, a forced-air warming device, warmed irrigating solution (105° F [<40.5° C]), and other measures are used to maintain normothermia. Communication among team members is essential in all transplant surgery. Prevention of technical failure is the main

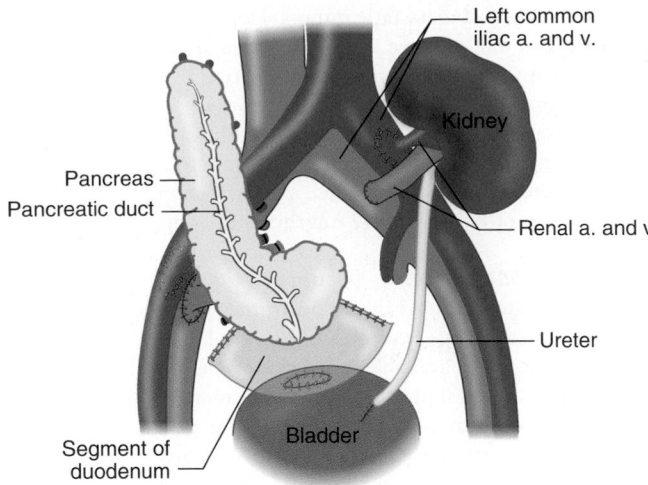

FIGURE 12-17 Transplantation of the pancreas with drainage of the bladder through a pancreaticoduodenocystostomy. A renal transplant is also shown with the common iliac vessels used for vascular anastomoses. *a,* Artery; *v,* vein.

objective for pancreatic transplant. Many variables are associated with the procedure and no single technique is universally used. The patient is usually transferred to the surgical intensive care unit (SICU) on completion of the procedure. Measures to address and reduce patient and family anxiety are part of all transplant programs. At-home rehabilitation is a gradual process, and social services and other resources are part of the transplant team. The patient must take immunosuppressive drugs indefinitely. The verification process for organ transplant, established by the United Network for Organ Sharing (UNOS), must be followed to ensure that the organs of the donor and the recipient are compatible (Patient Safety).

Operative Procedure (Whole-Organ Pancreatic Transplantation)

1. The whole-organ pancreatic transplantation procedure is performed through an oblique incision opposite the side of the renal transplant in the lower abdominal quadrant. A midline incision may also be used for pancreatic transplant.
2. The external iliac artery and vein are skeletonized and lymphatics are tied off with 4-0 nonabsorbable ligatures.
3. The external iliac vein is clamped with noncrushing vascular clamps and a #11 blade used to make a venotomy.
4. The venotomy incision is extended with Potts scissors.
5. An end-to-side anastomosis of the donor portal vein to the recipient's external iliac vein is performed with four double-armed 5-0 polypropylene sutures.
6. The external iliac artery is then clamped and an aortic punch used to make an arteriotomy.
7. An end-to-side anastomosis of the recipient's external iliac artery with the donor aortic patch containing the origin of the superior mesenteric artery and the celiac axis is performed with four double-armed 6-0 polypropylene sutures.
8. Management of the pancreatic duct is then performed, according to the type of en bloc procedure performed.
9. Various enteric procedures for drainage of pancreatic duct secretions have been performed with whole-organ transplants en bloc with a segment of duodenum and the spleen. They include cutaneous jejunostomy, drainage into an ileal loop, and

duodenojejunostomy with end-to-end or side-to-side anastomosis. Direct grafting of the pancreatic duct into the enteric or urinary system is also performed for management of exocrine secretions. Surgical procedures include pancreaticojejunostomy with an established Roux-en-Y loop of jejunum (Figure 12-18), pancreaticoductoureterostomy, and pancreaticocystostomy. The whole-organ pancreas transplant may also be performed as a pancreaticoduodenal transplantation or a pancreaticoduodenalsplenic transplantation.

Surgery of the Liver

Drainage of Abscess

Abscesses of the liver occur primarily by spread of bacteria or other organisms through the portal system (a direct route after trauma),

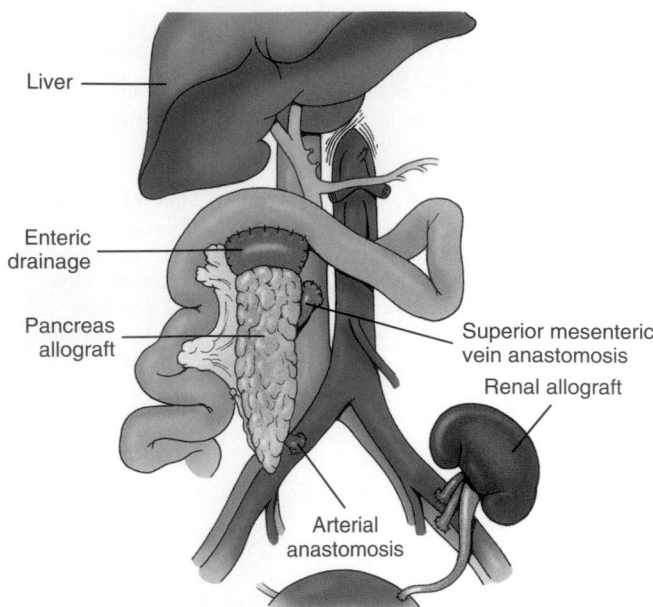

Liver

Enteric
drainage

Pancreas
allograft

Superior mesenteric
vein anastomosis

Renal allograft

Arterial
anastomosis

FIGURE 12-18 Pancreas and kidney transplants (PAK or SKP) with the donor pancreas vascularized to facilitate enteric exocrine drainage to a proximal portion of the jejunum (enteric drainage [ED] technique). The donor kidney is implanted in the left iliac fossa anastomosed to the femoral vessels and a ureteroneocystostomy is performed.

the biliary tract, or the hepatic artery (in generalized septicemia). In addition, direct extension from a subdiaphragmatic or subhepatic abscess can lead to a liver abscess. In most instances percutaneous drainage is effective and safe for hepatic abscesses. Laparoscopic drainage procedures have been reported with some success and are a reasonable option for select patients (D'Angelica and Fong, 2012). Open procedures, however, may be required, often via the transperitoneal route. This approach permits inspection of the abdominal cavity for the underlying source of the abscess.

Procedural Considerations. A basic laparotomy set is used. Biliary instrumentation, drainage materials, and aerobic and anaerobic culture tubes are needed. Safe practices for handling specimens such as cultures are initiated. The patient is positioned supine after administration of a general anesthetic. The anesthesia provider inserts an NG tube after intubation. An indwelling urinary catheter may be inserted before the abdominal skin prep.

Operative Procedure
1. The incision preferred by many surgeons is the transperitoneal route; the surgical approach may be modified, however, according to the location of the abscess (e.g., in a high posterior abscess, the transpleural approach may be selected).
2. The abdomen is opened as described for laparotomy and abdominal inspection carried out.
3. The abscess is mobilized and evacuated, and cultures obtained.
4. Surgical drains are placed and the wound closed.

Hepatic Resection
Anatomically the liver is divided into left and right lobes, with the caudate lobe lying in the dorsal segment. Resection of the liver is undertaken for primary tumors, benign conditions (e.g.,

hepatolithiasis), and metastatic tumors. Hepatic resection is usually approached in one of three ways. The *anatomic* approach is based on the premise that malignant cells distribute along the portal venous segmental supply. In the *enucleation* approach specific benign lesions with limited chance of local invasion are removed. The third approach, the *nonanatomic*, includes resections appropriate for a pathologic process in which a limited margin is acceptable, such as in tumor debulking (D'Angelica and Fong, 2012).

Procedural Considerations. Instruments used are a laparotomy set, biliary instruments, vascular instruments, noncrushing liver clamps, a self-retaining retractor, and a surgical stapler. Supplies and equipment should be available for thermoregulation, electrosurgery, measurement of portal pressure, and replacement of blood loss. For major liver procedures, intraoperative ultrasound (to guide vessel isolation and minimize vascular occlusion), the argon beam coagulator, and the CUSA are used. Special blunt needles for suturing liver tissue are also necessary.

The patient is placed in supine position. Mild Trendelenburg position may be requested by the surgeon. The anesthesia provider inserts an NG tube after induction of general anesthesia and intubation. An indwelling urinary catheter is inserted before abdominal skin preparation. The abdomen is prepped from nipple line to midthigh. Surgeons often use a right subcostal incision, with the ability to extend with a left subcostal if necessary. In some instances a median sternotomy or right thoracotomy incision is required, and chest instruments are then necessary. Liver sutures, absorbable or nonabsorbable according to the surgeon's preference, vessel loops, and umbilical tapes should be available on the sterile field.

Hemostatic material, such as Gelfoam, Surgicel, or Avitene, and absorbable collagen sheets should be readily available when the resection begins. The potential for bleeding exists both intraoperatively and postoperatively because of the high vascularity of the liver. If postoperative bleeding and subsequent hypovolemia occur, it may become necessary to call a rapid response team.

Surgeons use various methods to remove liver tissue. A CUSA allows the surgeon to dissect tissue using ultrasonic waves incorporated with fluid and suction. The ultrasonic waves cut through liver tissue, emulsifying it and diluting the tissue with fluid so that it can be suctioned. The electrosurgical pencil uses electrical current to cut through and desiccate liver tissue. Finger-fracture of the liver tissue is performed by digital pressure against the parenchyma.

Operative Procedure
1. Through a right subcostal incision, the abdominal cavity is opened and examined.
2. Pathologic condition is determined and respectability evaluated.
3. Moist laparotomy packs are inserted and a self-retaining retractor placed.
4. Intraoperative ultrasonography (US) is performed to assess all segments of the liver (Figure 12-19). Ultrasound-guided digital intraparenchymal isolation of vessels is used during resection.
5. Lymph nodes in the porta hepatis and along the gastrohepatic ligament are then assessed by palpation to determine extrahepatic metastasis.
6. The intended resection line is scored with the blade tip of the electrosurgical pencil, and coagulation is set at the surgeon's selected setting (Figure 12-20).
7. The liver parenchyma is then delicately resected using the CUSA handpiece (Figure 12-21).

FIGURE 12-19 Use of intraoperative ultrasound using a 7-MHz T-probe to permit assessment of the liver.

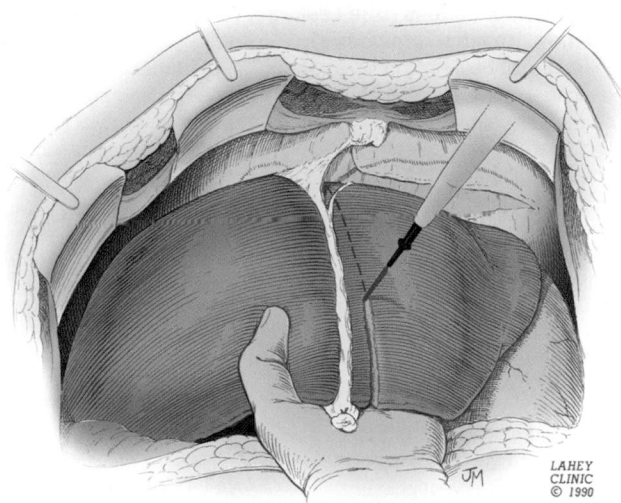

FIGURE 12-20 Use of electrosurgical pencil with blade tip to score the line of resection on the surface of the liver.

8. Once the portion of the liver is resected, the remaining liver resection margins are assessed for bleeding and bile leakage.
9. A laparotomy sponge may be placed against the transected surface for several minutes. The laparotomy sponge is gently rolled from the surface, which is then examined for bile leakage.
10. Areas may then be oversewn with 2-0 or 3-0 absorbable suture, or an intended layer of eschar is applied using electrocoagulation or the argon beam coagulator.

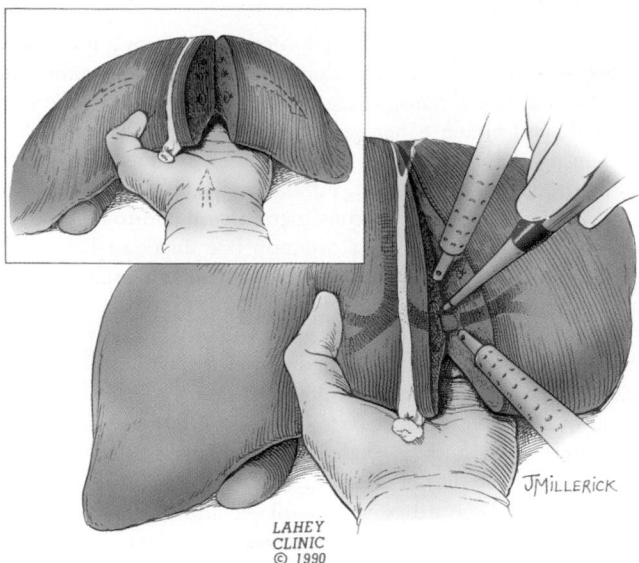

FIGURE 12-21 Use of the Cavitron ultrasonic surgical aspirator (CUSA) handpiece to dissect through the hepatic parenchyma.

11. Abdominal drains may be placed along the liver bed and exteriorized through the abdominal wall through separate stab wounds.
12. The abdominal wound is then closed and dressings applied.

Laparoscopic and Robotic-Assisted Laparoscopic Hepatic Surgery

Procedural Considerations. Laparoscopy for liver resection is a highly specialized field. It can present severe technical difficulties such as control of bleeding (Idrees and Bartlett, 2010; Jones et al, 2011; Reddy et al, 2011). Other limitations relate to inadequate retraction, the inability to assess safe margins of resection with the loss of tactile sense, difficulty with safe parenchymal transection, and the potential for injury of adjacent structures (Idrees and Bartlett, 2010). However, laparoscopic liver surgery has become a safe and effective approach in many institutions to manage liver disease (Gaujoux et al, 2011).

Minimally invasive hepatic resection approaches include pure laparoscopic, hand-assisted laparoscopic and a hybrid approach where the procedure is begun laparoscopically to mobilize the liver and start dissection, followed by a small laparotomy to complete the parenchymal transection (Reddy et al, 2011). Single-incision approaches have also been developed in an attempt to minimize abdominal wall trauma (Gaujoux et al, 2011).

Robotic surgery offers multiple benefits: less blood loss, faster recovery, less scarring, and reduced postoperative pain. The robot extends the surgeon's skills by providing a 360-degree range of motion that is not possible with traditional laparoscopic instruments. It also allows access to all the fine structures of the liver and better visualization of delicate blood vessels (Idrees and Bartlett, 2010).

Laparoscopic ultrasound navigation is often an important element in laparoscopic hepatic surgery as well. It enables determination of tumor location and the relationship to adjacent vascular and biliary structures. At low power it causes no tissue damage and is used mainly for diagnostic purposes. With a high-frequency setting, ultrasound can be used to dissect, cut, and coagulate (Abdalla, 2011; Neumayer and Vargo, 2012).

Liver Transplantation

Liver transplantation is implantation of a liver from a donor into a recipient. The procedure includes retrieving or procuring the liver from a donor, transporting the donor liver to the recipient's hospital, performing a hepatectomy on the recipient, and then implanting the donor liver. Reanastomoses are then undertaken of the suprahepatic vena cava, infrahepatic vena cava, portal vein, and hepatic artery; biliary reconstruction with end-to-end anastomosis of donor and recipient common bile ducts; or Roux-en-Y anastomosis if the recipient's bile duct is absent as a result of biliary atresia.

Liver transplantation is indicated for patients with chronic hepatocellular disease, chronic cholestatic disease, metabolic liver disease, primary hepatic cancer, acute fulminant liver disease, and inborn errors of metabolism. When malignancies are the cause of end-stage liver disease, the right upper quadrant may be radiated intraoperatively—after hepatectomy and before transplantation.

Patients undergo extensive physiologic and psychologic assessment and evaluation by physicians and transplant coordinators before being placed on a national-network waiting list. The potential for postoperative complications (Table 12-3) requires ongoing evaluation.

Procedural Considerations. Successful transplantation requires the cooperative efforts of the organ procurement agency and the staffs of the donor and recipient hospitals. Usually two members of the surgical team from the recipient's hospital travel to the donor's hospital to procure the donated liver. Often multiple transplant teams may arrive at the donor hospital to procure various organs for transplantation. UNOS policies dictate a detailed system for checking and rechecking organs for transplantation to ensure that organs of the donor and recipient are compatible (see Patient Safety, p. 373). These policies must be strictly followed before any transplant can take place. Safe practice further requires that hospital policies are consistent with applicable law and organ donation regulations and should address patient and family preferences for organ donation, as well as specify the roles and desired outcomes for every stage of the donation process (NQF, 2009).

Preparing the OR for the Donor. The donor OR is set up for a major laparotomy procedure. Basic instrumentation and equipment include a basic laparotomy set, cardiovascular instruments, power sternal saw, and nephrectomy instruments. A sterile, draped, medium-size instrument table is needed for preparation of the liver away from the main sterile field and instrument tables. The procurement team provides special Collins solution for flushing the organs, sterile plastic containers and ice chests for organs, and in situ flush tubing. The liver is generally placed in two Lahey bags immediately after procurement.

Preparing the OR for the Recipient. Each transplant surgeon has preferred instruments, supplies, and sutures. In general the following are needed in the recipient's OR: a basic laparotomy set, a cardiovascular instrument set, an assortment of T-tubes, a slush unit or means of providing iced lactated Ringer's solution, two ESUs, a forced-air warming device, a temperature probe, IV volumetric pumps on stands, two blood warmers or water baths, an indwelling urinary catheter, an insertion tray, and a urometer. An argon beam coagulator may be used and should be available. A defibrillator is always located in the room with sterile external paddles available.

Large-bore cannulae for IV monitoring and fluid or blood replacement lines are placed in addition to an arterial line and a central venous line.

TABLE 12-3

Assessment and Prevention of Common Postoperative Complications Associated with Liver Transplants

Assessment	Prevention
Acute Graft Rejection	
Occurs from fourth to tenth postoperative day	Expect prophylaxis with immunosuppressant agents, such as cyclosporine.
Manifested by tachycardia, fever, right upper quadrant (RUQ) or flank pain, diminished bile drainage or change in bile color, or increased jaundice	Diagnose early to treat with more potent antirejection drugs.
Laboratory changes include increased levels of serum bilirubin, transaminases, and alkaline phosphatase and prolonged prothrombin time.	Use antibiotic prophylaxis.
Infection	
Can occur at any time during recovery	Diagnose early and treat with organism-specific antiinfective agents.
Manifested by fever or excessive, foul-smelling drainage (urine, wound, or bile); other indicators depend on location and type of infection.	Perform frequent cultures of tubes, lines, and drainage. Remove invasive line as early as possible. Use good hand hygiene.
Hepatic Complications (Bile Leakage, Abscess Formation, Hepatic Thrombosis)	
Manifested by decreased bile drainage, increased RUQ abdominal pain with distention and guarding, nausea or vomiting, increased jaundice, and clay-colored stools	Keep T-tube in dependent position and secure to patient; empty frequently, recording quality and quantity of drainage.
Laboratory changes include increased levels of serum bilirubin and transaminases.	Report manifestations to physician immediately. May necessitate surgical intervention
Acute Renal Failure	
Caused by hypotension, antibiotics, cyclosporine, acute liver failure, or hypothermia	Monitor all drug levels with nephrotoxic side effects. Prevent hypotension.
Indicators of hypothermia include shivering, hyperventilation, increased cardiac output, vasoconstriction, and alkalemia.	Observe for early signs of renal failure and report them immediately to physician.
Early indicators of renal failure include changes in urinary output, increased blood urea nitrogen (BUN) and creatinine levels, and electrolyte imbalance.	Report manifestations to physician immediately.

Modified from Ignatavicius DD, Workman ML: *Medical-surgical nursing: patient-centered collaborative care*, ed 7, Philadelphia, 2013, Saunders.

Two surgeon headlights and light sources will be necessary to augment visualization of the abdominal site. A venovenous bypass system may be used to support peripheral blood flow. To support the many steps of the transplantation procedure, these additional supplies should be available: extra drape sheets, table covers, gowns, towels, gloves, soft goods such as sponges, gauze dissectors, and laparotomy pads; cold IV Ringer's solution; sterile IV administration set for flushing the new liver; umbilical tape; booties; hemostatic agents; and vessel loops.

A cart containing sutures and the numerous other small items should be arranged and placed in the room for each procedure. This minimizes the need for the circulating nurse to leave the patient and surgical team to obtain extra supplies.

Liver transplantation is a lengthy procedure that takes many hours. The following aspects of implementing a plan of care deserve special attention.

Patient Positioning. The patient is placed supine with knees slightly flexed and padded. An indwelling urinary catheter is inserted after induction of anesthesia. Accurate body alignment is essential. A gel pad that is the length of the OR bed or a pressure-reducing OR bed mattress should be used, with attention to all potential pressure areas. Heel protectors are applied and IPCDs are placed on the patient's legs. The safety strap is placed over the lower part of the thighs and secured. A forced-air warming device is applied over the upper body, neck, and head to assist in maintaining the patient's temperature. Fluid warmers are used to warm blood products and IV solutions.

Skin Preparation. The patient is prepped from the neck to midthigh, bedline to bedline. Prep solution should not pool at the bedline or wet the sheets on the OR bed. Fire safety precautions for prep solutions must be followed.

Blood Loss and Replacement. Blood loss may be extensive and replacement must be timely. The perioperative nurse should confirm that blood products are available at the beginning of the procedure. These include 10 units each of packed red blood cells (RBCs) and fresh frozen plasma (FFP) and 1 unit of pooled donor platelets. The perioperative nurse should be available to assist the anesthesia provider during the insertion of peripheral and arterial lines. An autologous cell saver device may be used to assist in blood replacement by way of autotransfusion.

Intraoperative Laboratory Testing. It is possible that as many as 50 blood specimens will be drawn for analysis during the procedure. Safe specimen collection practices are implemented. These specimens must be recorded on the blood-loss record and calculated into replacement needs. Specimens are delivered to the laboratory immediately. A telephone in the OR is useful for receiving and reading back critical test results/reports directly from the laboratory. Safe practices for reporting of critical test results require the perioperative nurse to verify the critical test results such as these by "reading back" the result (NQF, 2009). Standard Precautions in collection of specimens must be observed.

Length of Procedure. Procedures may last from 6 to 20 hours. Special attention must be paid to maintaining the integrity of the sterile environment, given the length of surgery and number of people entering and exiting the OR.

Communication with Family. Frequent reports to the family are important. Family members often are knowledgeable about liver function tests and laboratory values and want this information in addition to reports on the condition of their loved one (Patient-Centered Care). One person should be assigned in advance to make regular contacts with family and support persons. The UNOS team

---

PATIENT-CENTERED CARE

Patient-centered care is a guiding principle of excellence in perioperative nursing care. Patients and families are increasingly asking to partner with healthcare providers in making decisions that affect their own health or the health of a family member. As these partnerships are formed, perioperative nurses find themselves committing to communicating with words that patients and families can easily comprehend. When speaking with the family of a liver transplant patient, the nurse might say:

"I understand that your family member is having a liver transplant today. The procedure involves getting the liver from a donor, transporting it to this hospital, and putting it in the patient. This requires the cooperative efforts of the organ procurement agency and the staff of the donor and recipient hospitals. Members of the surgical team from our hospital are traveling to the donor's hospital now to get the donated liver. We will be using a detailed system for checking and rechecking to make sure that the liver of the donor and recipient match. Since this is an effort of many people, we will be keeping you informed at each step and give you regular updates as the surgery progresses."

---

also works closely in communicating with the donor's and recipient's families.

Communication Among Teams. The perioperative nurse ensures that communication occurs among teams. Coordination among the procurement team, anesthesia team, and surgical teams is essential for a successful transplantation procedure. Perioperative nursing responsibilities also include monitoring and communicating blood-loss volume in suction canisters and on sponges, the availability of blood and blood products, laboratory results, time of organ arrival, ischemic time, and other events as they unfold in preparation for and during the transplant procedure.

Operative Procedure

1. Bilateral subcostal incisions are made with a midline incision extended toward the umbilicus. If necessary, the xiphoid is removed. The right side of the chest is entered if additional exposure is needed.
2. Initial dissection of the underlying tissues is achieved with electrosurgery and suture ligatures.
3. Isolation of all hilar structures and dissection to mobilize the lobes of the native liver are performed.
4. The retrohepatic vena cava is skeletonized, as are the hepatic artery, portal vein, common bile duct, and inferior vena cava.
5. The donor liver is examined.
6. Preparations may be made at this time for venovenous bypass using an extracorporeal assist device if the patient is unstable.
7. The infrahepatic vena cava and the suprahepatic vena cava are clamped, as are the portal vein, the hepatic artery, and the common bile duct.
8. Native hepatectomy is then performed.
9. The donor liver is placed in the right upper abdomen, and revascularization of the donor organ begins with end-to-end anastomoses in the vena cava and portal vein, with double-armed fine vascular suture.
10. At this point the clamps on the portal vein, suprahepatic vena cava, and infrahepatic vena cava are released slowly, and blood flow through the vena cava and portal vein is restored.
11. The anastomosis sites are then checked for leaks.

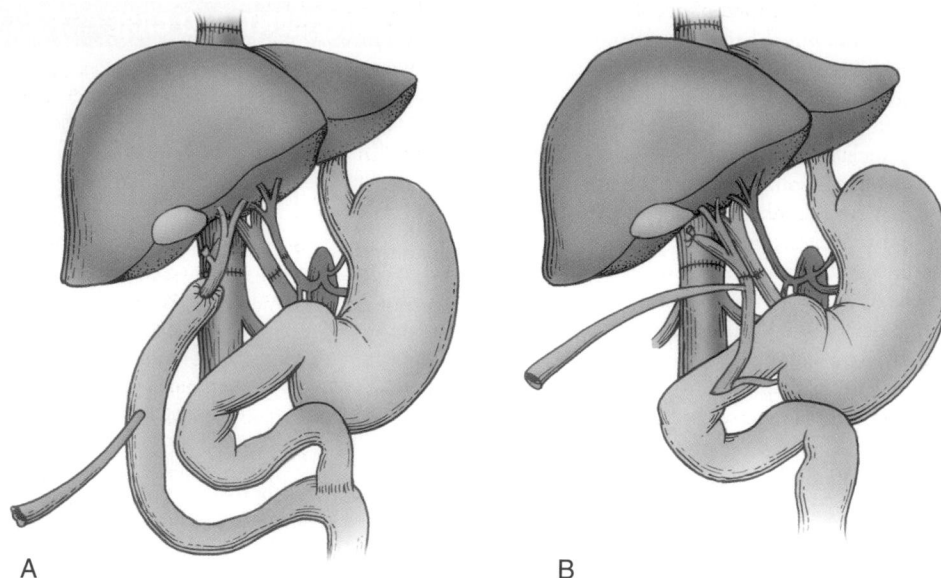

FIGURE 12-22 Completed orthotopic liver transplant with Roux-en-Y biliary reconstruction **(A)** and end-to-end anastomosis of the donor-to-recipient common bile ducts **(B)**.

12. If it was used, venovenous bypass is discontinued, and the cannulation sites are closed.

13. The postrevascularization phase focuses on achieving hemostasis. Complete hemostasis may require extensive time at this point. Bleeding may be exacerbated by a fibrinolytic episode associated with the reperfusion of the donor organ. The liver is monitored for a change in color from dusky to pink. An intraoperative Doppler may be used to confirm patency of the blood supply.

14. The anastomosis of the hepatic artery is then commenced, followed by bile duct reconstruction. This varies with the status of the recipient's biliary tract. If biliary atresia is the cause of the patient's end-stage liver disease, choledochoenterostomy into a Roux-en-Y loop of jejunum is performed (Figure 12-22).

15. The anastomoses are then checked for leaks.

16. Drains are placed behind and in front of the liver and exteriorized. The abdomen is then closed.

Donor Hepatectomy

Donor hepatectomy is performed for procurement of a healthy liver for transplant into a patient who has end-stage liver failure. This procedure occurs only after the donor patient has been determined to be brain dead and family consent for organ donation has been obtained. Donor hepatectomy can be performed at any hospital. Organ procurement agencies arrange contact with transplant centers when a viable organ donor has been identified.

Procedural Considerations. Once the liver transplant candidate has been identified, the procurement team from that transplant center travels to the institution where the organ donor is hospitalized. If multiple organs are being donated, surgeons from several transplant centers may arrive to procure the organs they will be transplanting at their respective centers.

The procedure for procurement of multiple organs differs according to the transplant centers represented. Most commonly, the systemic cooling of the donor's body temperature is started before the procurement of the heart. Cannulation sites also vary according to which organs are procured.

Perioperative nurses at the donor hospital are responsible for supplying a basic laparotomy setup with instrumentation to open the sternum. Basic vascular clamps are also required to clamp the major vascular structures. Cold lactated Ringer's solution for parenteral infusion and cold Ringer's solution for irrigation are usually used in large amounts.

Operative Procedure

1. The donor patient is positioned supine on the OR bed. The skin area from neck to midthigh is prepped and draped.

2. A midline incision is made from the suprasternal notch to the pubis.

3. A subcostal incision is performed bilaterally on the abdomen for better exposure of the abdominal viscera.

4. Retractors are placed to provide optimal exposure of the organs that will be procured.

5. The aorta and vena cava, superior and inferior to the liver and kidneys, are skeletonized by dissection and ligation of the lymphatics and smaller vasculatures.

6. The porta hepatis is dissected; the superior mesenteric artery and celiac trunk are then dissected and delicately exposed as close to the aorta as is convenient.

7. The superior mesenteric vein is dissected and prepared for cannulation. The donor is heparinized and systemically cooled.

8. If the heart is to be procured, removal takes place at this time.

9. Further cooling and flushing of the pancreas, liver, and kidneys are achieved by cannulation and infusion of cold lactated Ringer's solution through the inferior vena cava just superior to the bifurcation.

10. The liver, pancreas, spleen, and a segment of the duodenum harboring the pancreatic duct are procured en bloc by placing clamps on the suprahepatic and infrahepatic venae cavae.

11. The suprahepatic vena cava is transected with a surrounding cuff of diaphragm intact.

12. The infrahepatic vena cava is transected above the level of the renal veins.

13. The celiac axis is detached from the aorta as an aortic patch or taken with a full aortic circumference.

14. The duodenal segment is procured, using a linear stapling device at opposite ends of the segment.

15. The en bloc organs are taken to a back table for further dissection and ligation to separate the liver from the en bloc pancreas, spleen, and duodenal segment graft. Meanwhile, other members of the procurement team continue working to free the kidneys and ureters if they are to be taken.

16. The liver is placed in a basin of cold Ringer's solution, double-bagged in sterile Lahey bags, and placed in an ice chest for transport to the recipient's hospital.

17. The kidneys are placed in sterile cassettes and mechanically perfused.

18. The pancreatic en bloc graft is also placed in a basin of cold Ringer's solution, bagged, and transported in a thermal chest of ice.

19. The abdomen is closed with a single layer of size 1 or 0 non-absorbable suture.

20. Drapes are removed, and the donor patient is cleaned and washed. Tubes and infusion lines are tied off or clamped. Sometimes family members of the donor patient request to view the body after organ donation. This factor may be important in helping them face their loss. Before family viewing, the donor's body is covered with a warm blanket. The perioperative nurse assists the family in their grieving process by providing a quiet and private environment in which to say good-bye to their family member. The nurse should stay with family members to support them.

21. The donor patient is then transported by stretcher to the morgue.

Living-Related Liver Transplantation

Just as kidney transplantation has evolved into living-related donor possibilities, so too has liver transplantation. The capacity of the liver to regenerate provided the scientific basis for development of the living-related donor transplantation procedure. Reduced-size and split-liver transplantations have been performed successfully. Reduced-size liver transplantation has been performed for infants, children, or very small adults with results comparable to those obtained with whole-organ transplantation. Safety issues are of the highest priority for a living donor. Careful selection of the candidate, combined with fastidious surgical technique, minimize any potential complications (Markmann et al, 2012). Minimally invasive techniques (laparoscopic approaches) are used in some institutions (Abdalla, 2011). In addition, the recipient of these grafts may have an increased risk for postoperative complications such as bleeding or bile leakage from the cut surface and potential short- and long-term problems with the biliary-enteric anastomosis (Markmann et al, 2012). Prospective living donors are thoroughly evaluated with a protocol that includes blood group compatibility, a comprehensive history and physical examination, laboratory studies, psychosocial evaluation, independent advocate opinion, anatomic compatibility, review of candidacy with the donor, and presentation to a selection committee. As cloning, biogenetic engineering, and other technologic advances increase the possibilities for organ transplants, society will need to address ongoing debates of ethical dilemmas surrounding transplantation (Research Highlight).

Surgery of the Spleen

Splenectomy (Open Approach)

Splenectomy is removal of the spleen. It is performed for multiple reasons: trauma to the spleen; specific malignant conditions (Hodgkin disease and non-Hodgkin lymphomas; hairy cell, chronic lymphocytic, and chronic myelogenous leukemias); hemolytic jaundice or splenic anemia; idiopathic thrombocytopenic purpura (ITP); tumors, cysts, or splenomegaly; or accidental injury during vagotomy or other procedures involving mobilization of the splenic flexure of the colon. If accessory spleens are present, they are also removed because they are capable of perpetuating hypersplenic function. In most instances patients evaluated for elective splenectomy are considered candidates for laparoscopic splenectomy. Contraindications to laparoscopic splenectomy include severe portal hypertension, uncorrectable coagulopathy, severe ascites, extreme splenomegaly, extensive adhesions, and most traumatic injuries to the spleen. For these patients an open approach is indicated. If splenectomy is required due to trauma and there is massive hemorrhage, a surgical-crisis checklist may be implemented; Arriaga and colleagues (2013) found checklist use was associated with significant improvement in managing OR emergencies.

Procedural Considerations. Instrumentation is as described for a basic laparotomy, plus two large right-angled pedicle clamps, long instruments, and hemostatic materials and devices. Abdominal suction apparatus is available and a cell-saver may be requested. The patient is positioned supine. After induction of general anesthesia and intubation, the anesthesia provider inserts an NG tube. An indwelling urinary catheter may be inserted before the abdominal prep. The abdomen is prepped from nipple line to midthigh. The OR bed is moved to reverse Trendelenburg position with a slight tilt to the right. A midline abdominal incision provides access to the spleen and allows maximal exposure of all abdominal organs. Occasionally a subcostal approach is used for a patient without traumatic injury. Rarely a thoracoabdominal approach is used.

Operative Procedure

1. The abdomen is opened through the selected incision.

2. Retractors are placed over moistened laparotomy packs and exploration is carried out.

3. The costal margin is retracted upward.

4. The splenorenal, splenocolic, and gastrosplenic ligaments are clamped and divided with long dressing forceps, long hemostats, sponges on holders, and long Metzenbaum or Nelson scissors.

5. Adhesions posterior to the spleen are freed.

6. The spleen is delivered into the wound.

7. The short gastric vessels are now easily identified, clamped, divided, and ligated.

8. The cavity formerly occupied by the spleen is packed with moist laparotomy pads, if necessary.

9. The splenic artery and vein are dissected free with fine dissecting scissors and forceps.

10. The artery is clamped and doubly ligated. The artery is ligated first to permit disengorgement of blood from the spleen and facilitate return of venous blood to the circulatory system.

11. The splenic vein is then clamped, divided, and ligated.

12. The specimen is removed, bleeding vessels controlled, and the wound closed in layers, as described for laparotomy. Dressings are applied.

RESEARCH HIGHLIGHT ‖

The Future of Liver Transplantation

Liver transplantation positively affects the survival and quality of life of patients with advanced liver disease. Monumental improvements since the first liver transplants 45 years ago include better knowledge of the natural history of liver diseases; improved recipient selection processes; and the heightened efficacy of new potent antibacterial, antiviral, and antifungal drugs. There are also new immunosuppressive drugs and protocols. Postoperative management has been refined and improved. Some highlights of these improvements and changes include:

- *Immunosuppression:* More selective and less toxic immunosuppressive agents and the application of combination protocols can be more individualized
- *Some immunosuppressive protocols are now obsolete:* Early withdrawal of corticosteroids, application of monoclonal antibodies in the induction phase, and the start of mycophenolate mofetil plus calcineurin inhibitors seek to prevent the effect of post-transplant complications such as renal dysfunction, hepatitis C virus recurrence, metabolic disorders (diabetes mellitus), and cardiovascular risks (arterial hypertension, hyperlipidemia)
- *Immunologic manipulation:* Induced immunologic response without tissue injury
- *Pharmacogenetics and pharmacogenomics:* The investigation of the effects of the drugs based on individual genes or whole genome
- *Bioartificial livers:* These bridge the gap until a new graft is available, using an artificial extracorporeal supportive device for an individual who is suffering from acute liver failure.
- *Bioartificial organs:* These are derived from stem cells are a potential future alternative to solid organ transplant. In addition, regeneration of hepatic cells in the early phase of the disease may avoid the need for a transplant.

Considerations for increasing the pool of liver allograft donors:

- The waiting list for liver transplants steadily grows, but the pool of available grafts does not. Death on the waiting list resulting from a disproportionately lower number of donors is still common. Potential solutions include:

- *Partition of the graft for two recipients* (split liver technique)
- *Domino transplantation:* Sequential liver transplant—an unusual procedure in which one person receives a new liver from a deceased donor to cure a paralyzing disease and then that patient's liver is transplanted into another person with liver failure
- *Use of grafts from asystolic donors:* The donor undergoes cardiac arrest instead of brain death. The donor is then declared dead in the traditional sense. This presents a challenge for those recovering the organs because the organs must be recovered quickly in order for them to remain healthy and function properly once they are transplanted.
- *Xenotransplantation:* The use of non-human species, such as a pig, for human clinical transplantation
- *Use of grafts from marginal (expanded criteria) donors:* Such grafts have evolved as transplant programs have been forced to consider suboptimal donors, including older donors, hepatitis C– and hepatitis B–core antibody-positive donors, and livers with a moderate amount of steatosis (up to 30%)

The following table describes some of the controversies related to the types of hepatic transplants.

Type of Hepatic Transplant	Possible Ethical Issues	Greater Technical Difficulty	Smaller Effect on Donor Pool	Greater Rate of Postop Complications
Living donor	X	X		
Split graft		X	X	X
Domino transplant			X	
Asystolic donors				X
Xenotransplantation	X			
Acceptance of graft from marginal donors	X			X

Modified from Ericzon BG et al: Domino liver transplantation: risks and benefits, *Transplant Proc* 40(4):1130–1131, 2008; Granger DK, Ildstad ST: Transplantation immunology and immunosuppression. In Townsend CM et al, editors: *Sabiston textbook of surgery*, ed 19, Philadelphia, 2012, Saunders; Perez EV, Castroagudin JF: The future of liver transplantation, *Transplant Proc* (42):613–616, 2010; Taner CB et al: Asystole to cross-clamp period predicts development of biliary complications in liver transplantation using donation after cardiac death donors, *Transpl Int* 25(8):838–846, 2012.

13. Drainage is usually required only if extensive adhesions to the diaphragm were divided or if significant clotting abnormalities exist.

Laparoscopic Splenectomy

Laparoscopic splenectomy is standard procedure for surgical treatment of benign hematologic disorders; its benefits include less postoperative pain, decreased intraoperative bleeding, and decreased length of stay (Gelmini et al, 2011; Shelton and Holzman, 2012). Indications are the same as with open procedures, with the exception of the contraindications noted previously. The laparoscopic technique has been successfully used in blunt trauma as well (Carobbi et al, 2010).

Robotic assistance allows for a 3-dimensional view, greater freedom of movement and more accuracy. However, robotic systems often have higher costs and longer operative time. Often the OR bed cannot be repositioned without disconnecting the robotic arms, which can increase operative time (Gemini et al, 2011).

Procedural Considerations. After induction of general anesthesia, an NG tube and indwelling urinary catheter are inserted, and IPCDs applied to the lower extremities. The patient is positioned in right lateral position, with the OR bed flexed and kidney rest raised to increase the distance between the lower rib and iliac crest. The anterior abdomen is brought close to the edge of the OR bed. A beanbag device may be used. Safety restraints must be placed, especially in anticipation of a possible slight backward patient tilt. Alternatively, supine or modified lithotomy position may be used. The surgeon stands on the patient's right side, as does the scrub person, and assistants stand to the left.

Instrumentation and equipment include a 30-degree telescope (10 mm or 5 mm); a camera (triple-chip or single-chip); a high-flow insufflator with tank; a high-resolution monitor (second monitor optional for assistant); a printer (optional); a Surgineedle or Veress needle; four 12-mm trocars (trocar size depends on surgeon preference—some surgeons substitute one or two of the 12-mm trocars with 5-mm trocars or even 3-mm trocars); endoshears/

scissors; ultrasonic endoshears; an endodissecting forceps or endo-grasper (atraumatic); an endoretractor; an endoclip applier; a linear stapling device (GIA type) with vascular cartridges; an endoretrieval pouch; and a suction-irrigation system. As with other laparoscopic procedures, instruments and supplies are available if it becomes necessary to convert to an open approach.

Operative Procedure

1. Pneumoperitoneum is created and the first trocar placed under direct visualization. Three to five 2- to 12-mm operating ports are used, with the camera port at the umbilicus.
2. The laparoscope is inserted through the port and the camera placed.
3. The stomach is retracted to expose the spleen and a search made for any accessory spleens.
4. Initial dissection is begun by mobilizing the splenic flexure of the colon.
5. The splenocolic ligament is divided using sharp dissection, mobilizing the inferior pole of the spleen. The spleen is now retracted cephalad, taking care not to rupture the splenic capsule during retraction.
6. The lateral peritoneal attachments of the spleen are then incised using either sharp dissection or ultrasonic endoshears.
7. The lesser sac is entered along the medial border of the spleen.
8. With the spleen elevated, the short gastric vessels and main vascular pedicle are visualized. The tail of the pancreas is also visualized and avoided.
9. The short gastric vessels are divided by means of an ultrasonic dissector, endoclips, or an endovascular stapling device.
10. After the short gastric vessels have been divided, the splenic pedicle is carefully dissected from both the medial and lateral aspects.
11. After the artery and vein are dissected, the vessels are divided by application of the endovascular stapler. Multiple vascular branches may be encountered and each is taken individually.
12. The spleen is now devascularized and ready for removal.
13. An endobag is introduced through one of the trocar sites, usually the left lateral site.
14. The bag is opened and the spleen placed into it. The drawstring is grasped and the bag closed, leaving only the superior pole attachments, which are now divided.
15. The open end of the bag is exteriorized from the abdomen through the supraumbilical port or epigastric trocar site. The spleen is then morcellated and removed in fragments.
16. The laparoscope is reinserted and the splenic bed is assessed for hemostasis.
17. If necessary a drain is placed in the intra-abdominal cavity, the abdomen deflated, and the trocars removed.
18. The trocar sites are then closed.

A single-port access approach is an alternative to multiport techniques. One incision is made at the umbilicus. Each trocar is inserted through a separate fascial location within the single umbilical incision. A slight extension of the incision may be necessary for the spleen removal from the abdominal cavity. The benefits of this approach include a concealed scar, decreased adhesion formation, less parietal trauma, and faster recovery (Rottman et al, 2010, Targarona et al, 2010).

KEY POINTS

- A pathologic condition in the liver, biliary tract, pancreas, or spleen often requires surgical intervention. Surgeries of the liver and biliary tract have become more advanced as research and technology permit more complete diagnoses of pathologic conditions.
- The nursing process of assessment, outcome identification, planning, implementation, and evaluation is used in every phase of the perioperative experience. Planning for the patient's care patient requires knowledge of the anatomy and subsequent physiologic complications that may occur with surgical interruption of tissues.
- Cholecystectomy is the most common, nonemergency abdominal operation performed in the United States. Laparoscopic cholecystectomy has become the gold standard surgical intervention for the treatment of cholecystitis.
- The patient with hepatobiliary disease may have extreme jaundice, urticaria, petechiae, lethargy, and irritability. Depending on the extent of the disease, bleeding and coagulation times may be increased and the platelet count decreased, contributing to intraoperative concerns with achieving hemostasis.
- Laparoscopic pancreatic surgery is an emerging approach but has not gained wide acceptance due to the complexity of the procedures, the accuracy needed to perform the operation, and the steep learning curve required to master the procedures. Pancreatic cancer is treated using a multidisciplinary approach that may include surgeons, gastroenterologists, oncologists, radiologists, nurses, and nutritionists.
- Pancreaticoduodenectomy (Whipple procedure) is the removal of the head of the pancreas, the entire duodenum, a portion of the jejunum, the distal third of the stomach, and the lower half of the common bile duct, with reestablishment of continuity of the biliary, pancreatic, and GI tract systems.
- Anatomically the liver is divided into left and right lobes with the caudate lobe lying in the dorsal segment. Resection of the liver is undertaken for primary tumors, benign conditions (e.g., hepatolithiasis), and metastatic tumors.
- Liver transplantation is the implantation of a liver from a donor into a recipient. The total procedure involves retrieving or procuring the liver from a donor, transporting the donor liver to the recipient's hospital, performing a hepatectomy on the recipient, and then implanting the donor liver. Successful transplantation requires the cooperative efforts of the organ procurement agency and the staffs of the donor and recipient hospitals.
- Splenectomy is removal of the spleen. It is performed for multiple reasons: trauma to the spleen; specific malignant conditions (Hodgkin disease and non-Hodgkin lymphomas; hairy cell, chronic lymphocytic, and chronic myelogenous leukemias); hemolytic jaundice or splenic anemia; idiopathic thrombocytopenic purpura (ITP); tumors, cysts, or splenomegaly; or accidental injury during vagotomy or other procedures involving mobilization of the splenic flexure of the colon.

CRITICAL THINKING QUESTION

A 45-year-old Latina woman is scheduled for a laparoscopic cholecystectomy for cholelithiasis. When you interview her, you realize her understanding of English is very limited. She wants to know if she will have a big scar from being "cut open." What consequences might result from her limited understanding of English? What factors would you incorporate into your plan of care for this patient?

evolve *The answers to the Critical Thinking Question can be found at http://evolve.elsevier.com/Rothrock/Alexander.*

REFERENCES

Abdalla E: Advances in hepato-pancreato-biliary surgery, *Expert Rev Gastroenterol Hepatol* 5(4):457–460, 2011.

Ackley BJ, Ladwig GB: *Nursing diagnosis handbook: an evidence-based guide to planning care*, ed 9, St Louis, 2011, Mosby.

Alexander-Magalee MA: Mechanical and pharmacologic prophylaxis for DVT, *OR Nurse* 7(1):45–47, 2013.

Allen R: Implant advances enhance the medical market, *Elec Design State Indust* 60(8):48, 2012.

Antoniou SA et al: Single-incision laparoscopic cholecystectomy: a systematic review, *Surg Endosc* 25:367–377, 2011.

Arriaga AF et al: Simulation-based trial of surgical-crisis checklists, *N Engl J Med* 368:246–253, 2013.

Association of periOperative Registered Nurses (AORN): *Perioperative standards and recommended practices*, Denver, 2013, AORN.

Baumgartner J et al: Distal pancreatectomy with en bloc celiac axis resection for locally advanced pancreatic adenocarcinoma following neoadjuvant therapy, *J Gastrointest Surg* 16:1152–1159, 2012.

Benner P et al: *Expertise in nursing practice: caring, clinical judgment, and ethics*, ed 2, New York, 2009, Springer Publishing Co.

Boggi U et al: Surgical techniques for pancreas transplantation, *Curr Opin Organ Transplant* 15:102–111, 2010.

Carobbi A et al: Laparoscopic splenectomy for severe blunt trauma: initial experience of ten consecutive cases with a fast hemostatic technique, *Surg Endosc* 24:1325–1330, 2010.

Chen D et al: Pancreas-sparing duodenectomy with regional lymphadecnectomy for pTis and pT1 ampullary carcinoma, *J Surg* 151(4):510–517, 2012.

D'Angelica M, Fong Y: The liver. In Townsend CM et al, editors: *Sabiston textbook of surgery*, ed 19, Philadelphia, 2012, Saunders.

Gaujoux S et al: Single incision laparoscopic liver resection, *Surg Endosc* 25:1489–1494, 2011.

Gelmini R et al: Laparoscopic splenectomy: conventional versus robotic approach—a comparative study, *J Laparoendosc Adv Surg Tech* 21(5):393–398, 2011.

Giulianotti PC et al: Robot-assisted laparoscopic pancreatic surgery: single-surgeon experience, *Surg Endosc* 24:1646–1657, 2010.

Gomez G: Emerging technology in surgery: informatics, electronics, robotics. In Townsend CM, et al, editors: *Sabiston textbook of surgery*, ed 19, Philadelphia, 2012, Saunders.

Idrees K, Bartlett D: Robotic liver surgery, *Surg Clin North Am* 90(4):761–774, 2010

Ingraham AM et al: A current profile and assessment of North American cholecystectomy: results from the American College of Surgeons National Surgical Quality Improvement Program, *J Am Coll Surg* 211(2):176–186, 2010.

Jackson PG, Evans SRT: Biliary system. In Townsend CM et al, editors: *Sabiston textbook of surgery*, ed 19, Philadelphia, 2012, Saunders.

Jensen EH et al: Exocrine pancreas. In Townsend CM et al, editors: *Sabiston textbook of surgery*, ed 19, Philadelphia, 2012, Saunders.

Jones C et al: Perioperative management of liver resection surgery, *J Perioper Pract* 21(6):198–202, 2011.

Joseph M et al: Single incision laparoscopic cholecystectomy is associated with a higher bile duct injury rate, *Ann Surg* 256(1):1–6, 2012.

Kuroki T et al: Pancreas-hanging maneuver in laparoscopic pancreaticoduodenectomy: a new technique for the safe resection of the pancreas head, *Surg Endosc* 24:1781–1783, 2010.

Markmann JF et al: Transplantation of abdominal organs. In Townsend CM et al, editors: *Sabiston textbook of surgery*, ed 19, Philadelphia, 2012, Saunders.

National Cancer Institute: *Pancreatic Cancer, Incidence and Mortality Trends*, available at: www.cancer.gov/researchandfunding/snapshots/pdf/Pancreatic-Snapshot.pdf, 2011. Accessed January 28, 2013.

National Quality Forum (NQF): *Safe practices for better healthcare, 2009 update: a consensus report*, Washington, DC, 2009, NQF.

Neumayer L, Vargo D: Principles of preoperative and operative surgery. In Townsend CM et al, editors: *Sabiston textbook of surgery*, ed 19, Philadelphia, 2012, Saunders.

Oida T et al: Laparoscopic cystogastrostomy via the posterior approach for pancreatic pseudocyst drainage, *Hepatogastroenterology* 58:1771–1775, 2011.

Overby DW et al: SAGES guidelines for the clinical application of laparoscopic biliary track surgery, *Surg Endosc* 24:2368–2386, 2010.

Phillips NF: *Berry & Kohn's operating room technique*, ed 12, St Louis, 2013, Mosby.

Raraty MGT et al: Minimal access retroperitoneal pancreatic necrosectomy. Improvement in morbidity and mortality with a less invasive approach, *Ann Surg* 251(5):787–793, 2010.

Reddy SK et al: Laparoscopic liver resection, *World J Surg* (35):1478–1486, 2011.

Rosok BI et al: Single-centre experience of laparoscopic pancreatic surgery, *Br J Surg* 97:902–907, 2010.

Rottman SJ et al: Single port access (SPA) splenectomy, *J Soc Laparoendsc Surg* 14:48–52, 2010.

Shelton J, Holzman MD: The spleen. In Townsend CM et al, editors: *Sabiston textbook of surgery*, ed 19, Philadelphia, 2012, Saunders.

Targarona EM et al: Single incision approach for splenic diseases: a preliminary report on a series of 8 cases, *Surg Endosc* 24:2236–2240, 2010.

The Joint Commission (TJC): *Universal protocol for preventing wrong site, wrong procedure and wrong person surgery, October 22, 2012*, available at www.jointcommission.org/standards_information/npsgs.aspx. Accessed January 28, 2013.

CHAPTER 13

Hernia Repair

MAYA N. CLARK-CUTAIA

A hernia is an abnormal protrusion of a peritoneum-lined sac through the musculoaponeurotic covering of the abdomen. The word *hernia* is a Latin term that means "rupture" of a portion of a structure. Descriptions of hernia reduction date back to Hammurabi of Babylon and the Egyptian papyrus. Weakness of the abdominal wall, congenital or acquired, results in the inability to contain the visceral contents of the abdominal cavity within their normal confines. This defect occurs frequently; hernia repair is the most common operation in general surgery. About 10% of the population develops some type of hernia during their lifetime, with more than 800,000 hernia repairs performed each year. About 50% are for indirect inguinal hernias, with a male-to-female ratio of 7:1, and 25% are for direct inguinal hernias. Fourteen percent are umbilical (female-to-male ratio, 1.7:1), 5% are femoral (female-to-male ratio, 1.8:1), and 10% are incisional (female-to-male ratio, 2:1). With aging, the prevalence of all varieties of hernias increases (Erickson, 2011).

Hernias have a tremendous economic significance in the United States. The number of workdays lost is substantial. The increase in ambulatory surgery for hernia repair is one of many attempts to provide cost-effective healthcare that also leads to patient satisfaction.

A hernia can occur in several places in the abdominal wall, with protrusion of a portion of the parietal peritoneum and often a part of the intestine. The weak places or intervals in the abdominal aponeurosis are: (1) the inguinal canals, (2) the femoral rings, and (3) the umbilicus. Any number of conditions causing increased pressure within the abdomen can contribute to the formation of a hernia. Contributing factors to hernia formation include age, gender, previous surgery, obesity, nutritional status, occupation, and pulmonary and cardiac disease. Loss of tissue turgor occurs with aging and in chronic debilitating diseases, perhaps impairing collagen metabolism and weakening fibroconnective tissue in the groin. Successful hernia repair is measured by incidence of complications, total costs, ability to return to work or normal activities (Tolver et al, 2012) and rate of recurrence (Research Highlight).

Surgical Anatomy

A hernia is a sac lined by peritoneum that protrudes through a defect in the layers of the abdominal wall. Generally, a hernia mass is composed of covering tissues, a peritoneal sac, and any contained viscera. Hernias may be acquired or congenital.

Depending on their location, hernias are classified as direct inguinal, indirect inguinal, femoral, umbilical, incisional, or epigastric (Figure 13-1). Hernias in any of these groups are either reducible or nonreducible; that is, the contents of the hernia sac either can be returned to the normal intra-abdominal position or are trapped in the extra-abdominal sac (incarcerated). The conditions preventing the return of the hernia contents to the abdomen can result from: (1) adhesions between the contents of the sac and the inner lining of the sac, (2) adhesions among the contents of the sac, or (3) narrowing of the neck of the sac. Patients with incarcerated hernias may have signs of intestinal obstruction, such as vomiting, abdominal pain, and distention. The greatest danger of an incarcerated hernia is that it may become strangulated. In a strangulated hernia, the blood supply of the trapped sac contents becomes compromised and eventually the sac contents necrose. When bowel is strangulated in such a hernia, resection of necrotic bowel, in addition to the repair of the hernia defect, becomes necessary. This is a surgical emergency.

Inguinal Hernias

The anterolateral abdominal wall consists of an arrangement of muscles, fascial layers, and muscular aponeuroses lined interiorly by peritoneum and exteriorly by skin (Figure 13-2). The abdominal

---

RESEARCH HIGHLIGHT

Congruence of Reoperation Rate with Recurrence Rate After Ventral Hernia Repair

Ventral hernia repair is a common procedure in general surgery. Risk of recurrence is often used as a surgical quality metric and may be estimated by reoperation rates, clinical examination, or both. Yet it remains unclear whether reoperation rates reflect the overall clinical risk for recurrence. This prospective study demonstrated that reoperation rates underestimate the total recurrence rate by as much as 39%.

Participants, recruited from the Danish Ventral Hernia Database and the Danish National Patient Registry from January 2007 to December 2007, were included if they had undergone primary umbilical/epigastric or incisional hernia repair. A total of 646 patients status post umbilical/epigastric hernia repair and 256 patients status post incisional hernia repair were included in the analysis.

The researchers found that after umbilical/epigastric hernia repair, cumulative risks of reoperation and overall recurrence were 4% and 15%, indicating a fourfold underestimation. For the incisional hernia repair group, cumulative risks of reoperation and overall recurrence were 8% and 37%, a fivefold underestimation. This study revealed that reoperation rates for research participants did not reflect recurrence rates after ventral hernia repair and clinical recurrence should be taken into consideration in future calculations of surgical quality metrics.

Modified from Helsgard F et al: Reoperation versus clinical recurrence rate after ventral hernia repair, *Ann Surg* 256(6):955–958, 2012.

FIGURE 13-1 Types of abdominal hernias.

wall in the groin area is composed of two groups of these structures: a superficial group (Scarpa fascia, external and internal oblique muscles, and their aponeuroses) and a deep group (internal oblique muscle, transversalis fascia, and peritoneum).

Essential to an understanding of inguinal hernia repair is an appreciation of the central role of the transversalis fascia as the major supporting structure of the posterior inguinal floor. The inguinal canal, which contains the spermatic cord and associated structures in males and the round ligament in females, is approximately 4 cm long and takes an oblique course parallel to the groin crease. The inguinal canal is covered by the aponeurosis of the external abdominal oblique muscle, which forms a roof (Figure 13-3). A thickened lower border of the external oblique aponeurosis forms the inguinal (Poupart) ligament, which runs from the anterior superior iliac spine to the pubic tubercle. Structures that traverse the inguinal canal enter it from the abdomen by the internal ring, a natural opening in the transversalis fascia, and exit by the external ring, an opening in the external oblique aponeurosis, to go to either the testis or the labium. If the external oblique aponeurosis is opened and the cord or round ligament is mobilized, the floor of the inguinal canal is exposed. The posterior inguinal floor is the structure that becomes defective and is susceptible to indirect, direct, or femoral hernias.

The key component of the important posterior inguinal floor is the transversalis muscle of the abdomen and its associated aponeurosis and fascia. The posterior inguinal floor can be divided into two areas. The superior lateral area represents the internal ring, whereas the inferior medial area represents the attachment of the transversalis aponeurosis and fascia to the Cooper ligament (iliopectineal line). The Cooper ligament is the site of insertion of the transversalis aponeurosis along the superior ramus from the symphysis pubis laterally to the femoral sheath. The inguinal portion of the transversalis fascia arises from the iliopsoas fascia and not from the inguinal ligament.

Medially and superiorly the transversalis muscle becomes aponeurotic and fuses with the aponeurosis of the internal oblique muscle to form anterior and posterior rectus sheaths. As the symphysis pubis is approached, the contributions from the internal oblique muscle become fewer and fewer. At the pubic tubercle and behind the spermatic cord or round ligament, the internal oblique muscle makes no contribution. The posterior inguinal wall (floor of the inguinal canal) is composed solely of aponeurosis and fascia of the transversalis muscle.

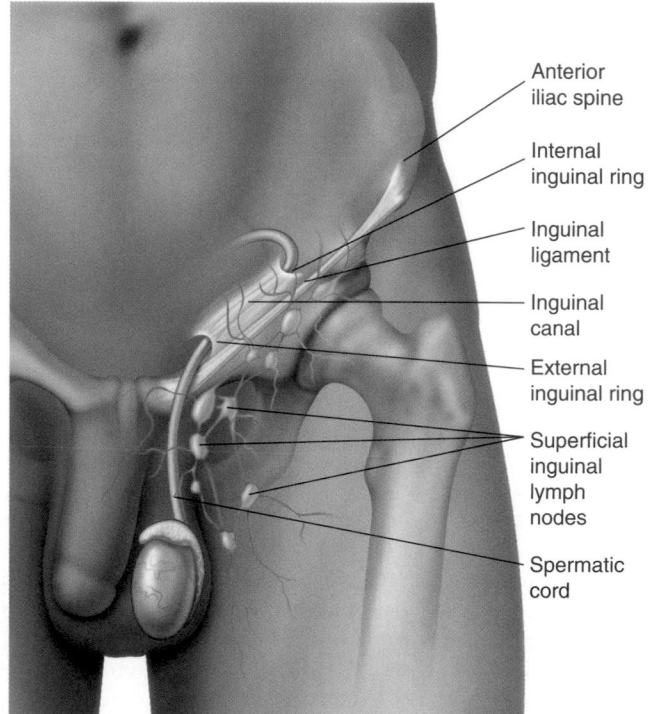

FIGURE 13-2 Structures of the inguinal area.

None of the three groin hernias (direct and indirect inguinal hernias and femoral hernia) develops in the presence of a strong transversus abdominis layer and in the absence of persistent stress on the connective tissue layers. When a weakening or a tear in the aponeurosis of the transversus abdominis and the transversalis fascia occurs, the potential for development of a direct inguinal hernia is established.

Femoral Hernias

When the transversus abdominis aponeurosis and its fascia are only narrowly attached to the Cooper ligament, a femoral hernia may develop. The resultant enlarged femoral ring and canal allows for the prominence of the iliofemoral vessels, giving rise to a femoral herniation.

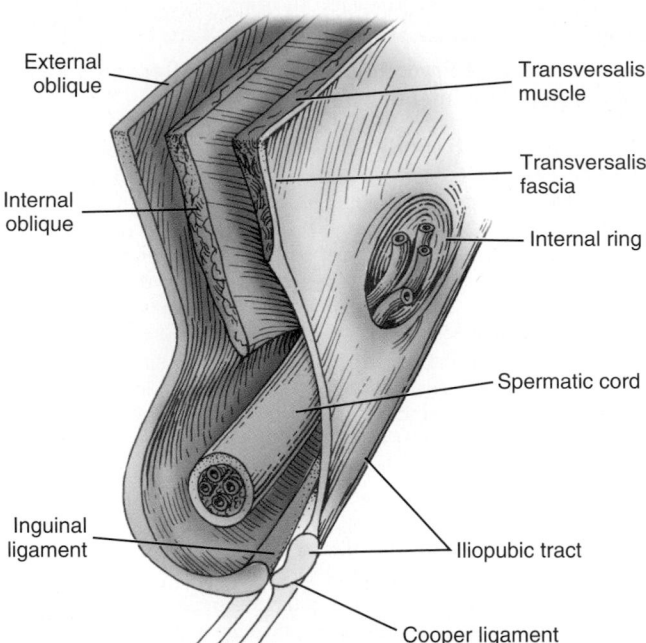

FIGURE 13-3 Right inguinal region, parasagittal section. Roof of inguinal canal is formed by external oblique aponeurosis, and floor is formed by transversalis aponeurosis and fascia.

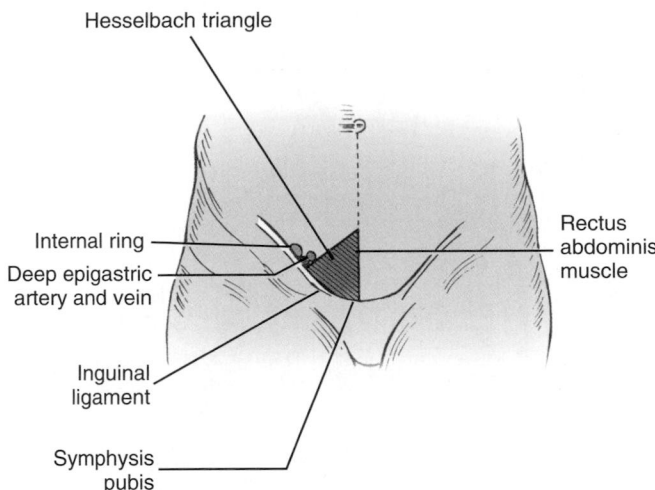

FIGURE 13-4 Schema of the Hesselbach triangle. Boundaries of the Hesselbach triangle are deep epigastric vessels laterally, inguinal ligament inferiorly, and rectus abdominis muscle medially.

The walls of the femoral sheath are formed anteriorly and medially from the transversalis fascia, posteriorly from the pectineus and psoas fascia, and laterally from the iliaca fascia. The pelvis ostium consists of a relatively fixed rim of bone and connective tissue: anteriorly and medially the iliopubic tract, posteriorly the superior ramus, and laterally the iliopectineal arch.

The femoral sheath is subdivided into three compartments. The lateral compartment contains the femoral artery, and the intermediate compartment contains the femoral vein. The medial compartment is the smallest and constitutes the femoral canal, which is formed anteriorly and medially by the iliopubic tract. This opening is bound laterally by the iliofemoral vessels and posteriorly by the superior pubic ramus and pectineus fascia. Superiorly, laterally, and inferiorly the fossa is formed by the falciform margin of the fascia lata. The iliopubic tract forms the superolateral border of the so-called triangle of pain, an area bounded medially by the spermatic vessels. In this area, tacking of surgical mesh (see Surgical Interventions) is avoided because of the risk of injury to the femoral branch of the genitofemoral nerve or the lateral femoral cutaneous nerve (Sherwinter, 2011a).

Abdominal Hernias

The anterior abdominal wall is composed of external abdominal oblique muscles attached to a thick sheath of connective tissue called the *rectus sheath*. The linea alba extends superiorly and inferiorly from above the xiphoid process to the pubis. Beneath the rectus sheath lies the rectus abdominis muscles, laterally to the right and left of the linea alba. Lateral to the rectus abdominis is the linea semilunaris. The transversus abdominis muscles originate from the seventh to the twelfth costal cartilages, lumbar fascia, iliac crest, and inguinal ligament, and insert on the xiphoid process, the linea alba, and the pubic tubercle. The third layer of abdominal wall includes the internal abdominal oblique muscles originating from the iliac

crest, inguinal ligament, and lumbar fascia, and inserting on the tenth to twelfth ribs and rectus sheath.

Direct and Indirect Inguinal Hernias

The deep epigastric vessels (inferior epigastric) arise from the external iliac vessels and enter the inguinal canal just proximal to the internal ring. The triangle formed by the deep epigastric vessels laterally, the inguinal ligament inferiorly, and the rectus abdominis muscles medially is referred to as the *Hesselbach triangle* (Figure 13-4). Hernias that occur within the Hesselbach triangle are called *direct inguinal hernias*. Indirect inguinal hernias occur laterally to the deep epigastric vessels. Both direct and indirect hernias represent attenuations or tears in the transversalis fascia (Figure 13-5).

Direct hernias protrude into the inguinal canal but not into the cord and therefore rarely into the scrotum. Direct inguinal hernias usually result from heavy lifting or other strenuous activities. Indirect hernias leave the abdominal cavity at the internal inguinal ring and pass with the cord structures down the inguinal canal. Consequently, the indirect hernia sac may be found in the scrotum. Indirect hernias may be either congenital, representing a persistence of the processus vaginalis, or acquired. In a congenital hernia the hernia sac has a small neck, is thin-walled, and is closely bound to the cord structures. In an acquired indirect hernia the neck is wide and the sac is both short and thick-walled. When both direct and indirect hernias are present, the defect is called a *pantaloon hernia* after the French word for "pants."

Perioperative Nursing Considerations

Assessment

Assessment begins with a thorough review of the patient's history, which includes previous surgeries related to the herniated area. Information relating to a familial history of hernias, the patient's nutritional status, duration of the symptoms, and a history of obesity, increased intra-abdominal pressure, chronic cough, constipation, benign prostatic hypertrophy, intestinal obstruction, colon malignancy, or pregnancy are noted. A list of the patient's current medications is collected, along with any history of chronic illness

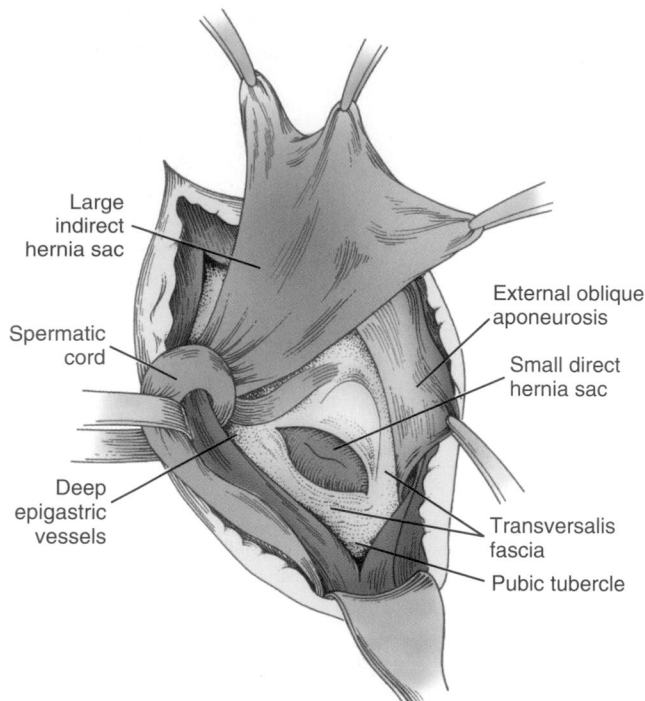

FIGURE 13-5 Defect in transversalis fascia, medial to deep epigastric vessels, results in direct hernia. Defect lateral to deep epigastric vessels results in indirect hernia.

and allergies, including latex allergies (because a Penrose drain may be used during the procedure). The patient's occupation and physical activities are listed. If it is part of institutional protocol, verification of preoperative showering or bathing with an antiseptic agent is done during assessment (Evidence for Practice).

Pain is often a notable symptom for the patient; it may be described as a burning sensation. An accurate description of the type and degree of pain is included in the assessment; obtain general information about onset, duration, severity, and quality of pain and about exacerbating and remitting factors. Patients often describe the feeling of a foreign body, or mass, at the hernia site. This may appear on arising in the morning and disappear while sleeping.

The diagnosis of hernias should be accompanied by clinical physical examination. Palpation of the herniated area reveals the contents of the hernia sac. Fingertip palpation allows the nurse to feel the edges of the external ring or abdominal wall. Having the patient stand and cough during the examination also assists in the evaluation of the herniated area. If a definitive diagnosis is not confirmed, ultrasonic scanning and imaging techniques (e.g., computed tomography [CT], herniography, standard radiography) may be used.

In some patients a hernia may cause no symptoms; its only sign may be a swelling or protrusion in a restricted area of the abdominal wall. If the hernia is unilateral, the patient notes the lack of a protrusion on the other side in comparison. The area may be visible when the patient stands or coughs and may disappear on reclining. Femoral hernias can be difficult to diagnose and may resemble an enlarged lymph node.

Formerly, routine studies (e.g., complete blood count [CBC], chest x-ray, and electrocardiogram [ECG]) were ordered preoperatively as elements in preanesthesia evaluation. It was believed that

EVIDENCE FOR PRACTICE

Effectiveness of Preoperative Showers in Reducing Risk of Surgical Site Infections

First recommended by the Centers for Disease Control and Prevention (CDC) in 1999, preoperative showers have long been considered an important strategy for reducing the risk of surgical site infections. AORN's recommended practice for preoperative patient skin antisepsis states that patients undergoing open class I ("clean") surgical procedures below the level of the chin, such as inguinal hernia repair, have two preoperative showers with chlorhexidine gluconate (CHG) (AORN, 2013).

This study from the Medical College of Wisconsin, Milwaukee, was conducted to validate effective skin surface concentrations of CHG using a standardized, timed protocol. It compared skin surface concentrations of CHG measured after showering with a 4% CHG liquid soap, as recommended by AORN, to those measured after cleansing the skin surface with a 2% CHG-impregnated polyester cloth. Researchers found that a timed, standardized preoperative shower was effective in achieving high skin surface levels of CHG that exceeded the concentration required to inhibit the growth of *Staphylococcus aureus,* the most common organism causing surgical site infections, and *Staphylococcus epidermidis.* Compared with 4% CHG soap, use of 2% CHG-impregnated polyester cloths resulted in considerably higher skin concentrations with no gaps in antiseptic coverage. CHG provides excellent activity against gram-positive organisms, and good antimicrobial activity with gram-negative bacteria and viruses, providing excellent residual activity. The researchers concluded that preoperative antiseptic showers are valuable in reducing surface skin colonization, which can play an important role in reducing the risk of surgical site infections.

In another study that examined multidrug-resistant organisms (MDROs) and use of CHG washcloths, the overall rate of hospital-acquired bloodstream infections was 4.78 cases per 1000 patient days with CHG versus 6.60 cases with nonantimicrobial washcloths, a 28% lower rate with CHG.

CHG-impregnated washcloths significantly reduced the risks of acquiring MDROs and developing hospital-acquired bloodstream infections, these researchers concluded.

To meet the needs of patients, their families, and the healthcare system, perioperative patient care should be based on research and best evidence—national guidelines, such as those promulgated by AORN, are one of the common elements sought in determining evidence-based practice.

Modified from Association of periOperative Registered Nurses: *Perioperative standards and recommended practices,* Denver, 2013, The Association; Climo MW et al: Effect of daily chlorhexidine bathing on hospital-acquired infection, *N Engl J Med* 368:533–542, 2013; Edmiston CE et al: Preoperative shower revisited: can high topical antiseptic levels be achieved on the skin surface before surgical admission? *J Am Coll Surg* 207:233–239, 2008; Makic MB et al: Questioning common nursing practices: What does the evidence show? *Am Nurse Today* 8(3):10–13, 2013.

such studies determined the patient's fitness for anesthesia and surgery. During the past few decades this practice has been a subject of much controversy. It has been somewhat established that performing routine screening tests in patients who are otherwise healthy is of little value in detecting diseases and in changing the anesthetic management or outcome. A thorough history and physical examination of the patient probably is the best method for screening diseases. This may be followed by selective tests based on the patient's health, invasiveness of planned surgery, and potential for blood loss (Kumar and Srivastava, 2011). Thus an otherwise healthy patient presenting for hernia repair will have, in some institutions, only selective testing, which reduces cost without sacrificing safety or quality of surgical care.

Nursing Diagnosis

Nursing diagnoses related to the care of the patient undergoing hernia surgery might include the following:
- Activity Intolerance related to pain
- Risk for Urinary Retention
- Risk for Ineffective Peripheral Tissue Perfusion of the scrotal area
- Deficient Knowledge related to disease process (hernia) and convalescence

Outcome Identification

Outcome measurement and management are important parts of perioperative nursing care. Outcomes identified for the selected nursing diagnoses could be stated as follows:
- The patient will return to his or her previous level of activity.
- The patient will not experience urinary retention.
- The patient will be free of or manage scrotal edema.

- The patient and family or significant others will verbalize knowledge regarding the disease process (hernia) and convalescence.

Planning

The perioperative nurse formulates a plan of care for the patient undergoing herniorrhaphy by assimilating knowledge pertaining to the anatomy involved, principles of asepsis, the planned surgical procedure, and requisite information provided/gained during planning specific to the surgical patient (Patient-Centered Care). Instrumentation, draping, and positioning for the patient's surgery depend on the type of hernia and repair to be performed, for example, open versus laparoscopic.

A Sample Plan of Care for a patient having surgery for hernia repair is shown on p. 388.

Implementation

The patient is identified using two (2) identifiers, such as name and medical record number or date of birth. This should match the ID band. The surgical procedure/procedural consent should match the planned procedure for which the team is preparing. The patient may

---

PATIENT-CENTERED CARE

Regardless of the type of planned hernia repair, discussions between the patient and anesthesia provider, perioperative nurse, and surgeon should cover specific topics to ensure that the patient knows what to expect and what is expected of the patient. Patient-centered care emphasizes involving the patient in selecting the type of anesthesia for surgery and discussion about postoperative pain management before surgery. Online resources for patients such as that found at www.asahq.org/patientEducation.htm introduce types of anesthesia and provide material about different anesthetics and pain-relief techniques. The information can be downloaded so patients and their caregivers can review it together preoperatively.

Topics for Discussion
- Preoperative dietary recommendation
  - Targeted nutritional and dietary advice for obese patients in the weeks before surgery—weight loss may improve anesthetic management and postoperative rehabilitation
- Immediate preoperative preparation
  - Continuation, alteration, or cessation of normal medications
  - Need for fasting (NPO)
- Choice of anesthetic technique
  - General anesthesia (with or without peripheral nerve blocks)
  - Central neuraxial anesthesia (spinal or epidural) with or without sedation
  - Inguinal nerve block/field block/local infiltration with or without sedation
  - Risks and benefits of recommended techniques on an individual patient basis
  - Possibility of converting regional techniques to general anesthesia
- Informed consent
  - Information regarding surgical, anesthetic, and postoperative pain management, including benefits and complications. Allow time for questions/clarifications.
- Potential surgical complications
  - General complications such as deep vein thrombosis (DVT), pulmonary embolism, pneumonia, infection, and seroma
- Information on pain management

If early postoperative pain is intense, rehabilitation and ambulation may be delayed unless pain is appropriately treated. Different techniques may be used to manage different levels of pain immediately following surgery, within the first postoperative day, and thereafter. Thus pain management often involves a "step-down" approach.
- For successful pain management outcomes:
  - Patients need a reasonable expectation of their likely postoperative stay.
  - Information is given on postoperative pain assessment, such as the use of visual analogue scale (VAS).
  - Patients receive realistic expectation of the intensity and duration of postoperative pain.
  - Pain management techniques that require patient involvement (intravenous patient-controlled analgesia [PCA], patient-controlled epidural analgesia [PCEA] pain pumps) are properly demonstrated.
  - Patients receive information about all medications to be taken after discharge (medication reconciliation) as well as medications/strategies for management of pain and postoperative nausea.
- Postoperatively, patients know what to expect with regard to:
  - Location and size of the surgical incision, dressings, and any drains
  - Intravenous (IV) fluids (as appropriate)
  - Possibility of a urinary catheter
  - Associated postoperative symptoms, such as postoperative nausea and vomiting (PONV)
  - When to return to normal oral fluids and nutrition
- Information on their recovery (see Patient and Family Education box on p. 390 for detailed information)
  - Approximate timetable for return to normal activities, personal as well as professional
  - Advice for other postoperative care
  - Contact numbers for use after discharge and information on follow-up calls or appointments with the surgeon

Modified from Hobbs JL: A dimensional analysis of patient-centered care, *Nurs Res* 58(1):52–60, 2009; *PROSPECT (procedure specific postoperative pain management)—herniorrhaphy*, available at www.postoppain.org/frameset.htm. Accessed March 14, 2013.

SAMPLE PLAN OF CARE

Nursing Diagnosis
Activity Intolerance related to pain

Outcome
The patient will return to his or her previous level of activity.

Interventions
- Determine the patient's baseline activity level.
- Encourage early postoperative ambulation and explain reasons for its importance.
- Instruct the patient to use prescribed pain medications before physical activity and as needed.
- Advise the patient to gradually increase activity as tolerated.
- Explain anticipated postoperative activity recommendations and limitations (see Patient and Family Education).

Nursing Diagnosis
Risk for Urinary Retention

Outcome
The patient will not experience urinary retention.

Interventions
- Encourage patient to void before surgery.
- Monitor and record intake and output status.
- Assess bladder postoperatively for signs of urinary retention (palpable bladder or patient discomfort).
- Encourage and assist patient with early ambulation.
- Maintain adequate oral fluid intake without nausea or vomiting before discontinuing IV fluids.
- Catheterize the patient if urinary retention occurs.

Nursing Diagnosis
Risk for Ineffective Peripheral Tissue Perfusion of the scrotal area causing scrotal edema

Outcome
The patient will be free of or manage scrotal edema.

Interventions
- Discuss the possibility of swelling and ecchymosis during preoperative assessment.

- Apply scrotal support intraoperatively.
- Assess scrotum for evidence of swelling, ecchymosis, and redness.
- Apply ice packs as prescribed.
- Elevate the scrotum on a soft pillow to prevent or control swelling.
- Reassure the patient, and instruct him on the importance of wearing the scrotal support.
- Reassure the patient that the swelling and ecchymosis will subside.

Nursing Diagnosis
Deficient Knowledge related to disease process (hernia) and convalescence

Outcome
The patient and family or significant others will verbalize an understanding of the disease process (hernia) and convalescence.

Interventions
- Review possible contributing factors (as individualized for type of hernia and specific patient) to hernia formation.
- Discuss postoperative pain management strategies during recovery at home.
- Describe and verify patient understanding of surgical site or incision care and reportable signs and symptoms (e.g., temperature, wound redness, tenderness at incision site, swelling, drainage). Use language such as, "Can you tell me how you will take care of this at home and when you should call your doctor?"
- Determine patient's dietary habits; discuss importance of fiber (fruits, vegetables, grains) to prevent constipation.
- Provide written discharge instructions. Review these with patient and family or significant others to validate understanding.
- Provide opportunity for "teach back" (see Patient Safety box) by the patient or family. Have them repeat discharge instructions in their own words.
- Allow time for questions; provide (or reinforce) answers and clarification.
- Verify that patient has or knows how to schedule follow-up appointment.

---

receive a general anesthetic, an inguinal nerve block, a field block, a spinal or epidural block, a regional anesthetic with sedation, or a local anesthetic with moderate sedation/analgesia. Chapter 5 describes required monitoring equipment, such as a three-lead or five-lead ECG, oxygen-saturation monitor, and blood pressure cuff, for patients receiving local anesthesia with or without moderate sedation/analgesia. An intravenous (IV) line is inserted for fluid replacement and medication administration. The surgical site is marked as part of the preoperative verification process and rechecked during the time-out; the site mark should be visible after draping. As part of the time-out, all members of the surgical team identify themselves and their roles and ask simple questions such as, "Does everyone agree that this is Patient X, undergoing a right inguinal hernia repair?" The perioperative nursing team reviews critical checklist information (AHRQ, 2013; DeJohn, 2013) such as confirming sterility of the instruments and supplies (including indicator results); discusses any equipment issues or concerns; notes whether antibiotic prophylaxis has been given within the last 30 to 60 minutes (antibiotics should be given as close to the time of incision as possible) and whether re-dosing is anticipated (re-dosing is based on the patient's body mass index [BMI] and whether the

procedure will last for more than 3 hours [Moody and Davis, 2013]); confirms mesh implant/material is available (as appropriate); and verifies whether essential imaging studies are displayed, if applicable. A preop briefing is held in many institutions, during which surgical team members discuss the planned procedure, potential patient needs, and any anticipated problems so they can be resolved prior to the patient being brought in to the operating room (OR) (Braman, 2013) (Research Highlight).

The patient is usually positioned supine (see Chapter 6) following basic prepping and draping procedures (see Chapter 4). As with any surgical procedure, the prep solution must dry before the start of the surgical procedure as part of fire safety measures. To maintain the patient's dignity and modesty, expose only the part of the patient's body necessary for antimicrobial skin preparation. Instruments used for hernia repair are those found in standard laparotomy sets, laparoscopy sets, or minor sets. Additional supplies and anticipatory preparation for other patient care needs depend on the perioperative nurse's knowledge of the planned procedure as well as communication and teamwork. Research suggests that interventions to improve OR teamwork and communication may have beneficial effects on technical performance as well as on patient

RESEARCH HIGHLIGHT ||

Preoperative Team Briefing Improves Clinical Practice

Individual professions play distinct and integral roles in the function of the interprofessional surgical team. Coordinated efforts provided by the team ensure safe, quality patient care. Inadequate team communication can result in adverse patient outcomes. Team briefings, or "huddles," have been associated with improved communication patterns and are an important aspect of ensuring patient safety. In this study, researchers sought to quantify the effect of preoperative team briefings on direct patient care, comparing the timing of preoperative antibiotic administration and accepted treatment guidelines.

The study used a retrospective preintervention/postintervention design to assess the effect of a checklist-guided preoperative briefing on prophylactic antibiotic administration timing in surgical cases across three institutions. The intervention involved the performance of a preoperative team briefing prior to the initiation of the surgical procedure, which allowed team members to share knowledge and voice knowledge deficits. A total of 259 preintervention and 283 postintervention cases were included in the analysis. Analyses focused on whether there were significant differences in timely antibiotic administration between study phases.

The researchers found that antibiotic administration was on time for 77.6% of those cases in the preintervention phase and on time for 87.6% of cases in the postintervention phase. This difference in timeliness was found to be statistically significant ($p < 0.01$). These results indicate that a strong relationship exists between the team's new adoption of a communication routine, and an improvement in the timing of antibiotic prophylaxis. The researchers concluded that the use of a preoperative team checklist briefing was associated with improved physician compliance with antibiotic administration guidelines. They further recommend the use of standardized roles within the healthcare team, specifically, who will administer the antibiotics, when the antibiotics will be administered, and where they will be administered. Lastly, the researchers suggest an identified location for documentation of the antibiotic administration that is clear and consistent.

Preoperative briefings are a common safe surgery practice in many institutions. As illustrated in this study, such a communication model allows the team to discuss the planned procedure, any potential patient needs, and any anticipated problems.

Modified from Braman JP: *Teaching safe surgery: implementing the surgical pause*, AORN Congress Presentation, San Diego, CA, March 4, 2013; Lingard L et al: Evaluation of a preoperative team briefing: a new communication routine results in improved clinical practice, *BMJ Qual Saf* 20(6):475–482, 2008.

outcomes. Improving the effectiveness of communication among caregivers remains a National Patient Safety Goal for The Joint Commission (TJC, 2013).

Self-retaining retractors, such as a Weitlaner, facilitates separation of tissue layers. A moistened Penrose drain is often used to retract the spermatic cord structures for better exposure. Because the peritoneal cavity may be entered in this procedure, soft goods, sharps, and instrument counts are initiated. Different size meshes should be available. There are many brands and types of mesh for the repair of inguinal hernias: absorbable and permanent synthetic meshes; allograft material; and xenograft material, such as sterile lyophilized acellular porcine collagen. Mesh is available in flat sheets, precut segments, and three-dimensional forms. Some mesh products for hernia repair include additional components to resist adhesions, to allow for fixation, or to prevent infection (Pickett, 2013).

The mesh must be large enough to produce a wide overlap beyond the defect's edges. A polypropylene or polyester mesh is often used. There are lighter, more porous meshes that maintain the strength of the repair but are credited by the manufacturer with reducing the inflammatory response. The mesh chosen is primarily based on surgeon preference and training (Sherwinter, 2011b).

With a sliding or an incarcerated hernia, the possibility of having to enter the peritoneal cavity must be considered. If the hernia is strangulated, necrotic bowel is resected and instruments for performing a bowel anastomosis are added. If antibiotics are added to irrigation solution, safe medication practices are followed. All medications and solutions on and off the sterile field are labeled. When the antibiotic solution is passed to the surgeon, the surgical technologist or other scrub person should announce the name and strength of the antibiotic solution to be used for irrigation.

Repair of an inguinal hernia includes approximation of the transversalis fascia with a heavy nonabsorbable type of suture; mesh may also be used. With some indirect hernias, only two or three sutures may be necessary. In other cases, however, up to 10 sutures in succession may be needed. Scarpa fascia is approximated with absorbable sutures, and the skin is closed by one of several methods. Several types of prosthetic mesh are available and often used to support hernia repair.

A laparoscopic hernia repair is technically similar to an open laparotomy, but the instrumentation includes laparoscopic equipment. There is always a possibility that a laparoscopy may become a laparotomy, and instrumentation for this change in procedure is always available.

Evaluation

Evaluation of the patient having repair of a hernia includes examining all skin surfaces to assess variances with preoperative assessment data. The patient should awaken from general anesthesia, if it is used, in a reasonable amount of time without exhibiting signs of anxiety or extreme disorientation. Extubation should be timely to avoid stress on the repaired hernia site. Evaluation of the patient's status can be phrased in outcome statements such as the following:

- The patient will return to his or her previous level of activity.
- The patient will not experience urinary retention.
- The patient will remain free of or manage scrotal edema.
- The patient and family or significant others will verbalize understanding of hernia and recommendations for convalescence and will be able to describe possible complications (infection, seroma formation, hematoma, or postoperative neuralgia) that are to be reported to the physician.

When the patient's care is transferred to the postanesthesia care unit (PACU) nurse, the perioperative nurse gives a hand-off report pertaining to relevant events and patient status during the operative procedure.

Urinary retention may occur after herniorrhaphy, and measures are taken to prevent overdistention of the bladder. Early ambulation is encouraged to facilitate resumption of bladder and bowel functions, as well as lung expansion for patients who were intubated for induction of general anesthesia. If the bowel has been resected because of strangulation, a nasogastric (NG) tube and suction may be required to reduce the incidence of postoperative vomiting and distention with subsequent strain on the suture line.

Patient and Family Education and Discharge Planning

Greater involvement of patients in their care increases the likelihood of achieving the best outcomes and simultaneously supports a quality-improved, cost-conscious environment. For the hernia patient to assume such responsibilities, plans for patient and family education along with plans for discharge and home recovery need to be designed. Issues such as open or laparoscopic repair techniques, surgical and recovery times, analgesic requirements, complication rates, and times for return to full activity become part of informed consent (Patient Safety). Once the patient and surgeon have decided on the surgical approach, perioperative nursing responsibilities for teaching the patient initial postoperative management strategies become crucial. Preferably, discharge planning is begun before admission. This becomes increasingly important because hernia repair is usually performed as an ambulatory procedure. Anticipated postoperative care, including incision care, incisional splinting as appropriate to the repair approach, and the importance of early ambulation and deep breathing, is reviewed. The Patient and Family Education box presents specific home care requirements. Pain management is important as a part of discharge planning; frequently, surgical patients report inadequate pain management during their postoperative recovery and convalescence. The Ambulatory Surgery Considerations box presents information on continuous wound infiltration via use of postoperative pain pumps.

PATIENT SAFETY

Surgical Consent and "Teaching Back"

There is considerable evidence that many patients leave medical encounters with a poor understanding of their disease and the recommended treatment. Informed consent is a central element of safe surgical patient care. The National Quality Forum (NQF) recommends that each patient or legal surrogate "teach back," in his or her own words, key information about the proposed treatments or procedures for which he or she is being asked to provide informed consent. Recommended elements of this safe practice for informed consent include:

- Ask each patient or his or her legal surrogate to recount what he or she has been told during the informed consent discussion.
- Use informed consent forms written in simple sentences and in the primary language of the patient or legal surrogate.
- Engage the patient in a discussion about the nature and scope of the procedure covered by the consent form. For example, when describing hernia surgery the nurse might state the following:

- "Before surgery, you will be given some medicine (sedative) to make you drowsy. A numbing medicine (anesthesia) will be also used so you do not feel pain during the operation. Sometimes the operation is done while you are under general anesthesia (unconscious and pain-free). The surgeon makes a cut over the area of the hernia. The bulging tissue or organ is placed back inside your muscle wall, the muscle tissue is repaired, and the skin is closed. In many inguinal hernia operations, a small piece of plastic mesh is used to make the muscle tissue stronger."
- Provide an interpreter or reader to assist non–English-speaking patients or legal surrogates, vision-impaired or hearing-impaired patients, and low-literacy patients.
- Verify that the patient and/or family member/legal surrogate can state the name of the procedure and, using their own words, describe it.

Modified from Clarke ME, Degannes CN: *Cultural competency in healthcare: a clinical review and video vignettes from the National Medical Association,* available at Cme.Medscape.Com/Viewprogram/12540. Accessed January 28, 2013; Kemp EC et al: Patients prefer the method of "tell back-collaborative inquiry" to assess understanding of medical information, *J Am Board Fam Med* 21(1):24–30, 2008; National Quality Forum: *National Quality Forum safe practices 2009,* Washington, DC, 2009, Author, available at http://Psnet.Ahrq.Gov/Resource.Aspx?Resourceid=9757&Sourceid=1&Emailid=12706. Accessed March 14, 2013.

PATIENT AND FAMILY EDUCATION

Home Care for the Hernia Patient

Home Care
- Give the patient and the caregiver *verbal* and *written* instructions. Provide them with the name and telephone number of a physician or nurse to call if questions arise.
- General information
  - Review/explain procedure and specific follow-up care. Verify that the patient can state name of the procedure performed.
  - Explain and discuss development of hernias, causes or contributing factors, care and treatment, and prevention.
- Wound/incision care
  - Discuss and demonstrate proper wound management and dressing changes: procedures, frequency, and signs to report.
- Warning signs
  - Stress importance of seeking emergency care if bleeding from the incision or wound dehiscence with exposure of deep wound tissue occurs.
  - Review signs and symptoms that should be reported to a physician or nurse.
    - Infection: fever, pain, edema, erythema, warmth, purulent drainage, foul odor from the incision

- Abdominal distention, nausea, vomiting
- Separation of wound edges
- Hernia recurrence: firm, tender, globular, irreducible swelling in the groin or mid-abdomen
- Special instructions
  - Apply and demonstrate to the male patient scrotal support or ice packs to decrease scrotal edema and discomfort. Ice can be placed in a sterile bag. A towel is placed between the skin and ice bag. Ice is usually left on for 15-20 minutes, 3 or 4 times/day for the first 2 days.
  - Assist the patient in obtaining appropriate supplies, such as sterile dressings.
  - Advise the patient with diabetes that optimal glucose level control promotes wound healing.
- Medications
  - Remind patient that it is normal to be sore for a couple of weeks after surgery.
  - Explain purpose, dosage, schedule, and route of administration of any prescribed drugs, as well as side effects to report to a physician or nurse. Review all postdischarge medications.

PATIENT AND FAMILY EDUCATION

Home Care for the Hernia Patient—cont'd

- Activity
  - Discuss allowances and limitations with respect to occupation, recreation, or activities.
  - Instruct the patient to avoid coughing, straining, stretching, constipation, heavy lifting (>10 lb), strenuous exercise, and sports for at least 3 weeks (or as directed).
  - Demonstrate splinting the incision manually or with a pillow during coughing, sneezing, or hiccups.
  - Stress the importance of activity restrictions and splinting the incision for up to 6 weeks after surgery.
  - Demonstrate proper body mechanics for moving and lifting.
  - Advise returning to work in 2 weeks for desk work and 6 weeks for heavy labor.
  - Advise that sexual activity should be avoided for several weeks to avoid strain on the incision and discomfort to the scrotum, if edematous.
- Diet
  - Advise the patient to plan a high-fiber diet to help prevent constipation; provide the patient with a list of high-fiber foods.
  - Advise the patient to drink plenty of fluids, up to 2 to 3 L per day, unless contraindicated.
  - Stress the importance of weight loss if the patient is obese.

Integrative/Alternative Therapy
- Advise the patient to avoid yoga exercises for 6 weeks postoperatively.

- Remind patient and family to refrain from applying lotions and creams to the incision until wound edges are completely closed and healed.
- Discuss options for pain management, including music therapy and guided imagery, to minimize use of narcotics, which can cause constipation.

Elder Care
- The older adult may be at greater risk for delayed wound healing because of preexisting cardiac disease or nutritional deficits.
- Vitamin supplements may promote wound healing, if not contraindicated.

Psychosocial Care
- Encourage the verbalization of fears and concerns about altered sexual function secondary to impaired blood supply to the vas deferens.
- Encourage active participation in plan of care.

Follow-up Care
- Stress the importance of regular follow-up visits. Make sure the patient has necessary names and telephone numbers.
- Stress the importance of smoking cessation to eliminate "smoker's cough" as a contributing factor to hernia development.

Referral
- Provide information and refer the patient to community resources for weight loss and smoking cessation, if indicated.

Modified from Canobbio MM: *Mosby's handbook of patient teaching*, ed 3, St Louis, 2006, Mosby; *Care after surgical hernia repair*, ExitCare patient information, ExitCare, LLC, 2012, available at www.mdconsult.com/das/patient/body/405458046-8/0/10089/57547.html (subscription required). Accessed March 14, 2013.

AMBULATORY SURGERY CONSIDERATIONS

Safe Use of Postop Pain Pumps for Surgical Analgesia

Elastomeric pumps, such as the ON-Q PainBuster, deliver local anesthetic intended to reduce pain after surgery to the tissue around the surgical site. The popular ON-Q PainBuster postop pain relief system provides continuous infusion of a local anesthetic directly into the patient's surgical site for effective, non-narcotic postoperative pain relief for up to 5 days. Four pump models are available with this pain-relief system: one with a fixed flow rate that cannot be changed; one that delivers a basal infusion and also allows delivery of on-demand boluses; one that allows the user to adjust the flow rate within a predetermined range; and one with an adjustable rate controller and bolus device. Various sizes and types of catheters are available to deliver the medication. Pumps such as ON-Q pumps are used in many general surgical procedures. The following safe practice recommendations should be implemented to improve safety when using elastomeric pumps such as ON-Q pumps.

Before Using the Pumps
- Establish protocols for use of ON-Q pumps, including indications; models and tubing to be used for each indication; steps for prescribing, preparing, and dispensing the pump of all associated medications; required testing of knowledge and skills; hand-off communication between providers; patient/family education; and patient monitoring.
- Have a committee, such as the pharmacy and therapeutics committee, approve the drugs that can be administered through the

ON-Q pump, taking into consideration the accuracy of the infusion rate (±15% to 20% of desired rate) and conditions that could influence the rate (e.g., heat and cold).
- Ensure clinical staff education before use. Include the signs of bupivacaine, ropivacaine, and lidocaine cardiotoxicity and risks associated with pump use.

Prescribing the Pumps
- Establish standard order sets for prescribing the pumps and specific medications. Specify any concomitant analgesics that are acceptable or should be avoided. Require activation of the appropriate order set before the patient is transferred from the OR.

Placing the Catheters and Setting Up the Pumps
- Ensure proper insertion of the catheter(s) in the tissue and/or adjacent nerves surrounding a wound. Do not insert the catheter directly into a joint.
- Label the pump with the name of the drug, its concentration, infusion rate (in milliliters per hour and dose per hour), and start date.
- Ensure that the adjustable rate controller (available on some models) is clicked into place under the specified rate of infusion.
- Apply an occlusive dressing over the catheter insertion site.
- Tape the flow restrictor to the patient's skin. Do not tape over the filter.

Continued

AMBULATORY SURGERY CONSIDERATIONS

Safe Use of Postop Pain Pumps for Surgical Analgesia—cont'd

Dispensing Pumps and Medication
- Establish standard concentrations for the local anesthetics (and other drugs, if appropriate) used in the pumps. Also establish pharmacy-compounding procedures for preparing any mixtures of drugs.
- Establish order sets in the pharmacy computer that will facilitate automated screening of the drug(s) being used for appropriate dose, drug interactions, allergies, and duplicate therapy.
- Require pharmacy preparation of the medication reservoir balls following a protocol that specifies the exact amount of solution to instill based on the duration of therapy and expected rate of infusion.

Perioperative Nursing Considerations for Patients with Pumps
- Ensure that all medications administered via the pump are listed on the intraoperative nursing record.

- Ensure the occlusive dressing over the catheter site is intact.
- Check that the flow restrictor is taped to patient's skin for accurate flow rates.
- Include information about the pump in the hand-off report to the postanesthesia care unit (PACU) or other discharge unit.

Educating Patients About Pumps
- Educate patients and caregivers about how the pump works and items to periodically check (e.g., flow restrictor is taped to the skin, medication ball appears to be getting smaller each day, pain is under control).
- Educate patients about the signs of cardiotoxicity, when to call the physician, and how to clamp the tubing to prevent further drug administration, if necessary (Surgical Pharmacology).
- Send the patient guidelines provided by the manufacturer home with patients.

Modified from Institute for Safe Medication Practices (ISMP) Safety Alert: *Process for handling elastomeric pain relief balls (ON-Q PainBuster and others) requires safety improvements,* July 16, 2009, Newsletter, available at www.ismp.org/Newsletters/acutecare/articles/20090716.asp. Accessed March 14, 2013.

SURGICAL PHARMACOLOGY

Bupivacaine, Ropivacaine, and Lidocaine Cardiotoxicity

Lidocaine (Xylocaine), bupivacaine (Marcaine), and ropivacaine (Naropin) all have similar actions. They produce analgesic effects via nerve conduction blockade. They are contraindicated in patients with hypersensitivity to amide local anesthetics (see Chapter 5). Compared with other local anesthetics, bupivacaine is markedly cardiotoxic. However, adverse drug reactions (ADRs) are rare when it is administered correctly. Most ADRs relate to systemic exposure, such as with pain pump failure.

Systemic exposure to excessive quantities of bupivacaine primarily results in central nervous system (CNS) and cardiovascular effects. CNS effects may include CNS excitation (nervousness, tingling around the mouth, tinnitus, tremor, dizziness, blurred vision, or seizures) followed by depression (drowsiness, loss of consciousness, respiratory depression, and apnea). Bupivacaine and ropivacaine are look-alike/sound-alike drugs. Safe medication practices are initiated.

Ropivacaine is found to have less cardiotoxicity than bupivacaine in animal models. Compared with bupivacaine, ropivacaine has similar CNS and cardiovascular effects.

Perioperative nurses providing discharge instructions to patients with pain pumps filled with one of these local anesthetics should be sure the medication is part of discharge medication reconciliation. An information sheet should be printed for patient and caregiver, and they should have one to take to the primary care physician. Be specific and direct in providing information about cardiotoxicity. Use descriptions of signs and symptoms that the patient can understand. For instance, you might tell the patient:

"The following symptoms may represent a serious medical condition. Immediately close the clamp on the pump tubing and call your doctor or 911 if you have any of the following:
- Difficulty breathing
- Dizziness, lightheadedness
- Blurred vision
- Ringing, buzzing in your ears
- Metallic taste in your mouth
- Numbness and/or tingling around your mouth, fingers, or toes
- Drowsiness
- Confusion"

Surgical Interventions

Surgery for Repair of Groin Hernias

Repair of Inguinal Hernias

Several operative procedures for repair of inguinal hernias are used. Approaches that reestablish the integrity of the transversalis fascia and simultaneously reestablish and strengthen the posterior inguinal floor are favored. A surgical repair in which transversalis fascia is sewn to the Poupart ligament accomplishes this goal.

Procedural Considerations. The patient is in supine position for abdominal wall and inguinal or femoral hernia repairs. Arms are placed on padded armboards with the palms up and fingers extended. Armboards are maintained at less than a 90-degree angle to prevent brachial plexus stretch. If there are surgical reasons to tuck the arms at the side, as may occur in laparoscopic hernia repair, pad the elbows to protect the ulnar nerve, face the palms inward, and maintain the wrist in a neutral position (Denholm, 2009). A drape secures the arms. It should be tucked snugly under the patient, not under the mattress. This prevents the arm from shifting downward intraoperatively and resting against the OR bed rail.

The patient's skin from above the umbilicus to mid-thigh is exposed, prepped with antimicrobial solution, and draped with sterile drapes. A sterile drape should be placed under the scrotum if it becomes necessary to enter the scrotum. Safe practices when using devices that generate surgical smoke, such as the electrosurgical unit (ESU), require the use of a smoke evacuation system and accessories in both open and laparoscopic procedures (AORN, 2013) (see Chapter 8).

Operative Procedure

McVay, or Cooper, Ligament Repair. A McVay, or Cooper, ligament repair approximates transversalis fascia superior to the inferior insertion of the transversalis fascia along the Cooper ligament. It is accompanied by a relaxing incision to reduce tension ("tension-free") on the suture line.

1. A transverse suprainguinal skinfold incision is made; some surgeons prefer an oblique incision, made parallel to the inguinal ligament, ending two fingerbreadths lateral to the pubic tubercle (Figure 13-6).
2. The incision is carried through the superficial and deep (Scarpa) fascia to the external oblique aponeurosis. Hemostasis is maintained with fine ties or electrocoagulation.

3. The external oblique aponeurosis is opened by way of a small incision over the inguinal canal, lateral to the inguinal ring and in the direction of its fibers, to the external ring. The aponeurotic flaps are reflected back along the iliohypogastric and ilioinguinal nerves, which are identified and preserved from injury (see Figure 13-6). The ilioinguinal nerve is a sensory nerve that innervates the medial thigh and the scrotum.
4. The cremaster muscles that form an envelope around the spermatic cord and represent the continuation of the internal oblique muscles are opened, and the cord is exposed. The medial fibrous portion of the internal oblique is called the *conjoined tendon.*
5. The cord and surrounding structures are dissected and freed circumferentially from the canal. A moistened Penrose drain is often used to gently retract the vessels and vas deferens. The cord is then examined for an indirect hernia, the sac of which is located adjacent to the cord; the sac originates from the internal ring lateral to the inferior epigastric vessels and is initially adherent to the cord.
6. If an indirect sac is identified, it is carefully dissected away from the cord until the neck of the hernia is clearly delineated (Figure 13-7).
7. The sac is opened, and any abdominal contents are returned to the peritoneal cavity.

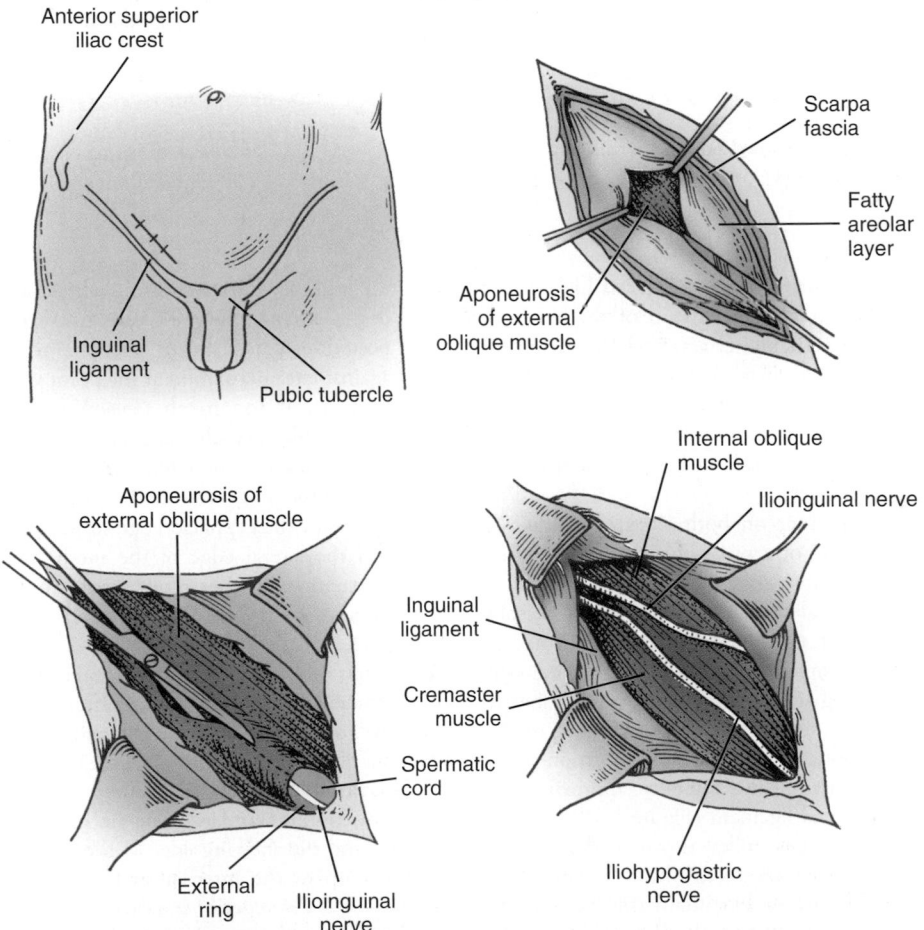

FIGURE 13-6 Skin incision with division of superficial muscle and fascial layers.

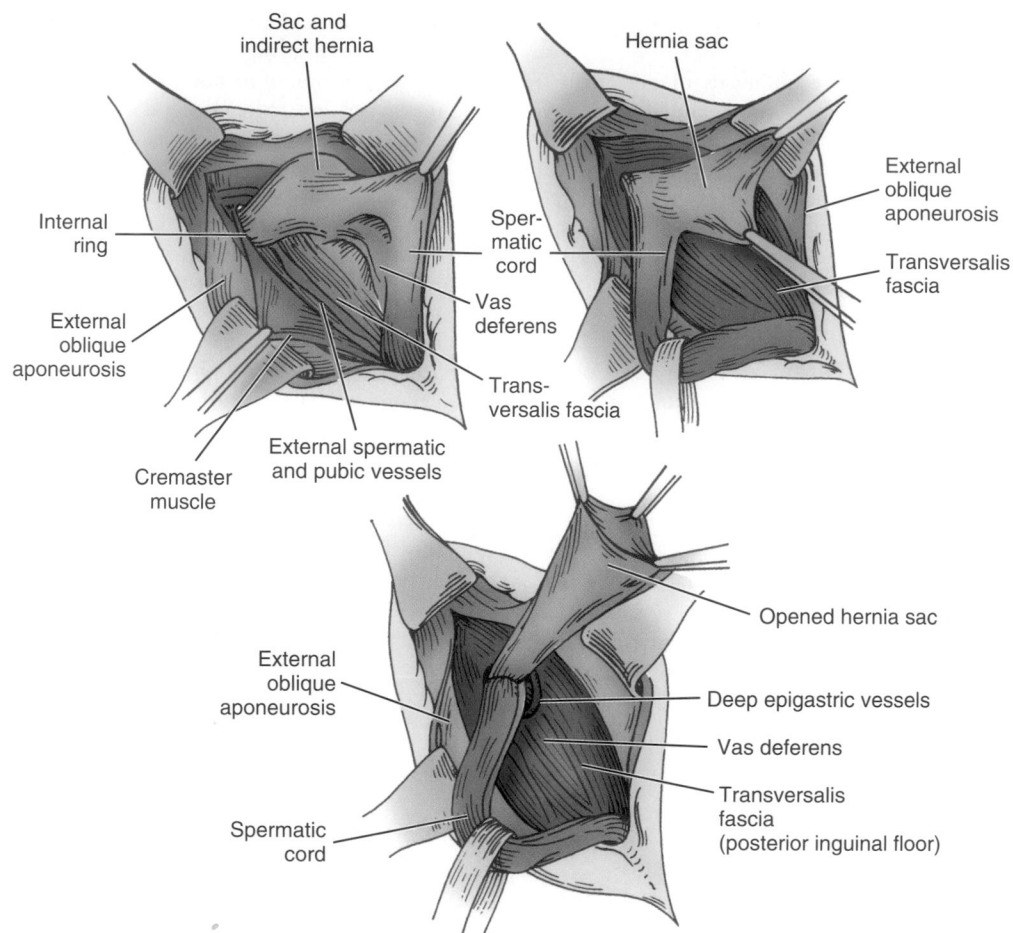

FIGURE 13-7 Indirect hernia sac is identified along with cord structures and dissected away from cord. Neck of hernia sac is clearly delineated, and sac is opened to check for abdominal contents.

8. A suture ligature or purse-string suture is placed high in the neck of the sac, and the excess peritoneum of the hernia is excised. The ligated stump quickly retracts into the peritoneal cavity. (If the sac is long, the distal segment may be splayed open and left in place.) The inguinal floor is then inspected for evidence of a direct hernia. If only a direct sac is present, usually no resection of the hernia is done because the sac easily returns to the abdominal cavity.

9. If transversalis fascia is present on both sides of the hernia defect, it is sutured together or a piece of mesh is interposed (Figure 13-8). Suturing begins at the pubic tubercle and continues laterally to the internal ring. If the inferior transversalis fascia is weak or not present, the superior portion is sutured to the Cooper ligament, the site of insertion of the transversalis fascia. In this case, suturing again begins at the pubic tubercle and is continued laterally along the Cooper ligament to the medial border of the femoral sheath, where a transition stitch is placed. The repair is then carried laterally, approximating transversalis fascia to inguinal ligament (Figure 13-9).

10. When the transversalis fascia is pulled down to the Cooper ligament, a relaxing incision in the rectus sheath is sometimes necessary to relieve excess tension. Essentially this incision is 5 to 7 cm long in the anterior rectus sheath. The incision begins immediately above the pubic crest, approximately 1 cm from

the midline, and extends cephalad, following the line of fusion of the external oblique aponeurosis with the rectus sheath. The posterior rectus sheath and the rectus muscle itself guard against later herniation at the point where the relaxing incision is made. If too much tension makes direct approximation undesirable, a synthetic surgical mesh is sutured in place as the new inguinal floor ("tension-free" mesh repair). The caudad edge of the mesh is sutured to the shelving edge of the inguinal ligament, the cephalad edge sutured to the conjoined tendon, and the lateral edge of the mesh split to accommodate the spermatic cord. Slit mesh versus non-slit mesh is more likely to be used and to result in lower rates of recurrence (Domniz et al, 2011).

11. After the integrity of the posterior inguinal floor has been reestablished, the cremaster muscles are reapproximated around the cord. Repair is completed with approximation of the external oblique aponeurosis, the Scarpa fascia, and the skin.

Bassini Repair. The Bassini repair was introduced in 1887 and was formerly the standard of repair. In this procedure the conjoined tendon and the shelving edge of the inguinal ligament are sutured together up to the internal ring. The major difference with this repair is that the superior transversalis fascia is sutured to the inguinal ligament with no attempt made to approximate it to the inferior portion of the transversalis fascia or the Cooper ligament (pectineal

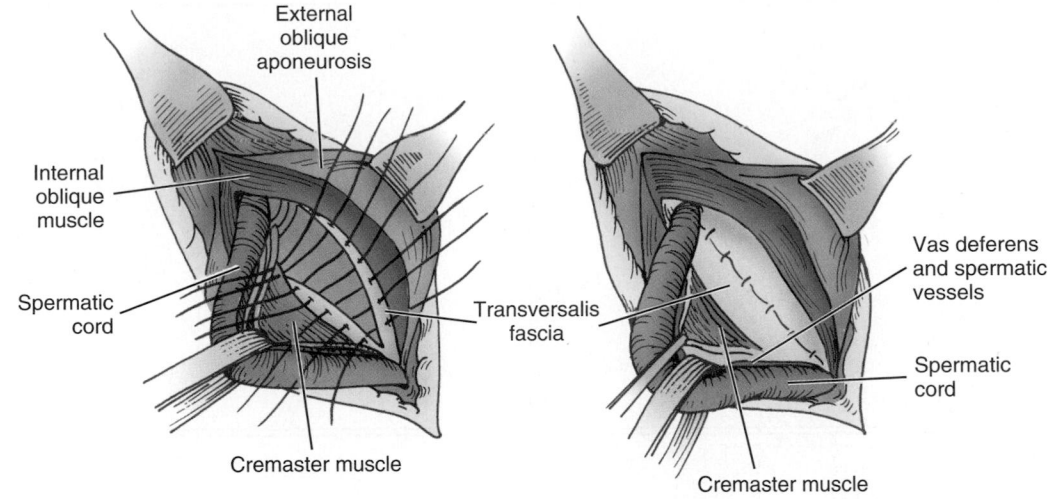

FIGURE 13-8 Transversalis fascia on either side of large hernia defect is approximated.

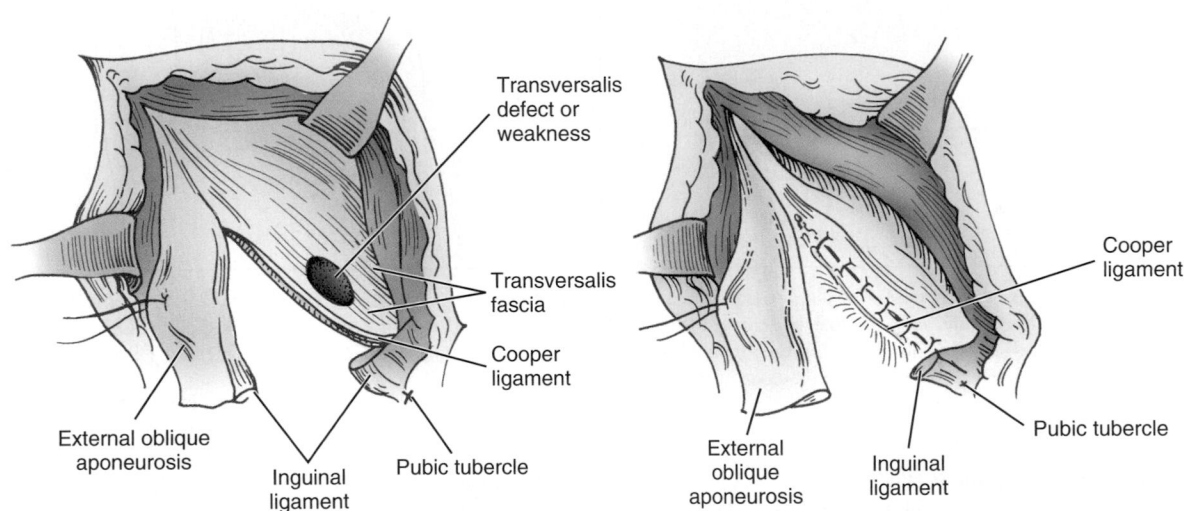

FIGURE 13-9 Defect in transversalis fascia repaired by approximation of fascia to the Cooper ligament.

ligament). Critics of this procedure claim that it is not anatomic because layers that originally are not integrated (transversalis fascia and inguinal ligament) now are approximated. Nonetheless, this repair has been used successfully by many surgeons.

Shouldice Repair. In the Shouldice repair a multilayer imbricated repair of the posterior wall of the inguinal canal with a continuous running suture technique is performed. The posterior wall of the inguinal canal is reconstructed by superimposing running suture lines progressing from deep to more superficial layers. First, the transversus abdominis aponeurotic arch is secured to the iliopubic tract. Next, the internal oblique and transversus abdominis muscles and aponeuroses are sutured to the inguinal ligament. The Shouldice repair is associated with a very low recurrence rate and a high degree of patient satisfaction (Malangoni and Rosen, 2012).

Mesh-Plug Repair. The mesh-plug technique has been recommended for the treatment of primary and recurrent direct and indirect inguinal hernias. Various hernia types have been classified by Gilbert (Kulacoglu, 2011) and have a corresponding relationship to the use of mesh plugs. Types I, II, and III are indirect hernias. Type I is characterized by a tight internal ring through

which any size peritoneal sac can pass. The sac, when surgically reduced, is held within the abdominal cavity by the intact internal ring. Type II hernias have a moderately enlarged internal ring, 4 cm or smaller. Type III hernias have a patulous internal ring larger than 4 cm. In this type the sac can have a sliding component that impinges on the direct space. Type IV and type V hernias are direct hernias. In type IV hernias the defect involves virtually the entire floor of the inguinal canal. Type V is a diverticular defect of the floor and is generally in a suprapubic position, resembling a punched-out recurrent hernia. Type VI includes components of both indirect and direct hernias. Femoral hernias are classified as type VII.

Regardless of the hernia type, the mesh-plug technique is performed on an ambulatory basis, through a small incision, often laparoscopically. Repair of inguinal hernias with the mesh-plug technique provides advantages when compared with conventional suture techniques—a plug repair requires less overall dissection, has a decreased chance of nerve injury, and ensures a tension-free hernioplasty. These factors increase patient comfort, speed rehabilitation, and contribute to a low recurrence rate.

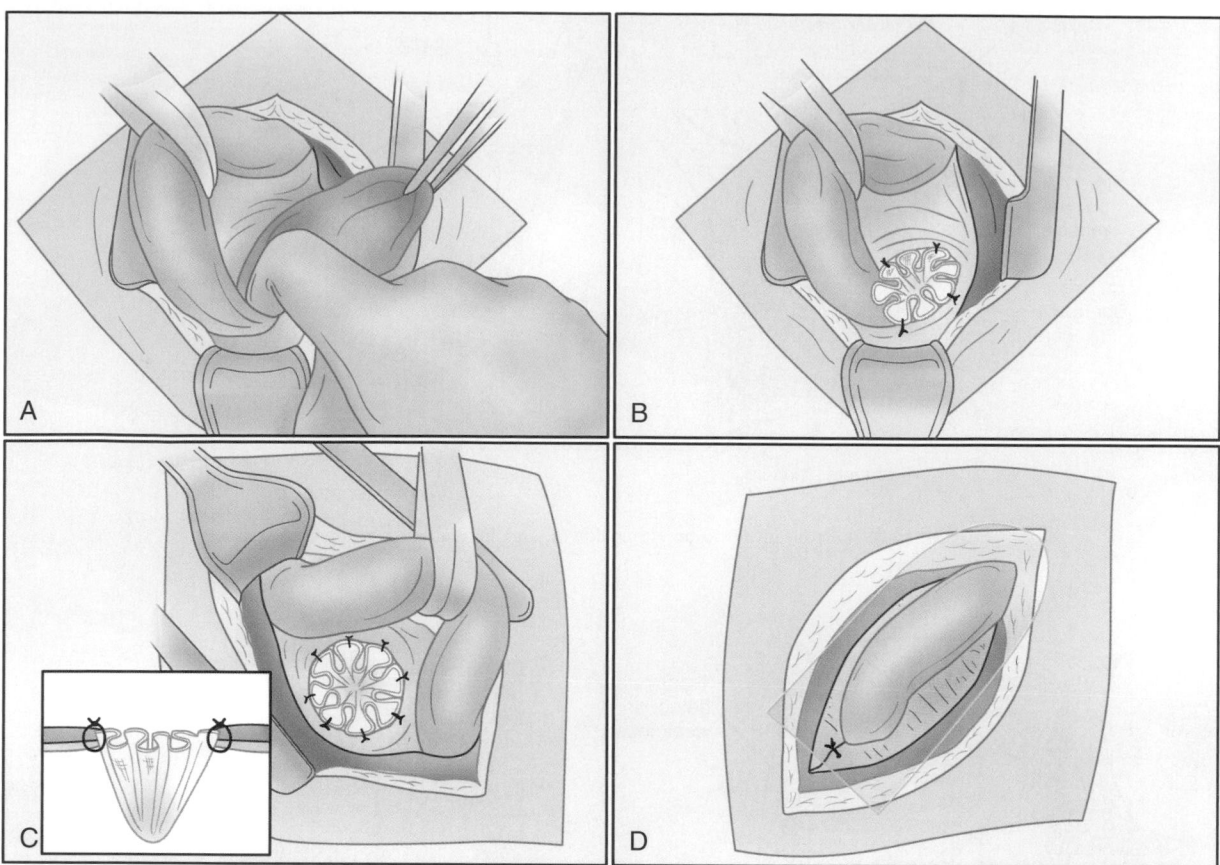

FIGURE 13-10 Mesh-plug repair using the PerFix plug. **A,** The hernia sac is dissected free of the cord structure to the level of the internal ring. **B,** Typically, a large plug is used. Some of the internal petals may be removed if the plug is too bulky. **C,** Large or extra-large PerFix plug is inserted. The plug should not be stretched to fill the defect. Typically, 8 to 10 sutures are used. **D,** Sutureless onlay patch. The tails of the onlay patch are taken around the cord and sutured together. The onlay patch is not sutured to the floor of the inguinal canal.

Surgical Technique Using the PerFix Plug

1. An oblique incision, 6 cm long, is made, and the external oblique fascia is opened through the external ring. Exposure is obtained by using a self-retaining retractor (e.g., a Beckman); a handheld retractor such as a Gouley also may be required. Hemostasis is usually achieved with electrocoagulation, described in the McVay repair. The ilioinguinal and genital femoral nerves are identified and preserved. The medial external oblique fascia is separated from the underlying transversus abdominis aponeurosis with a sweeping motion of the index finger.

2. An indirect sac and any lipoma of the cord are dissected free (Figure 13-10, *A*). The sac and lipoma are allowed to drop back through the internal ring and into the abdominal cavity. Rarely is the sac opened except for incarcerated hernias.

3. Using the Gilbert classification, the internal ring is sized and the tapered end of the mesh plug is inserted through the internal ring and positioned just beneath the crura. The plug is designed such that its fluted outer layer, combined with its inside configuration of eight mesh petals, maintains its overall contour while allowing it to conform tension-free to the configuration of the internal ring (see Figure 13-10, *B*).

4. Repair of indirect hernias. Type I indirect hernias require one or two synthetic absorbable sutures; in type II and type III hernias, more sutures are required because of the increased size of the internal ring.

5. Repair of direct hernias. In direct hernias the fusiform or saccular defect is circumscribed near its base with an electrosurgical device and the hernia is reduced, providing a surrounding margin of intact tissue for securing the plug. The plug is then inserted through the floor of the defect (see Figure 13-10, *C*). With type IV and type V (direct) hernias, the mesh plug is routinely secured with up to 10 interrupted synthetic absorbable sutures. Where there are both indirect and direct hernias (type VI), two mesh plugs may be needed. Type VII defects are treated similarly with mesh plugs.

6. Repair of femoral hernias. In femoral hernias a small or medium-size plug is secured in position after the sac has been reduced.

7. In most types of mesh-plug hernia repairs, a second piece of flat mesh is used for reinforcement. The piece is cut to match the shape of the inguinal canal and then placed without sutures on the anterior surface of the posterior wall of the inguinal canal. The proximal portion is split to provide an opening for the spermatic cord, and the mesh tails are united with sutures to form a new internal ring (see Figure 13-10, *D*).

8. With the spermatic cord structures placed on top of this flat mesh, the external oblique fascia is reapproximated over the structures with a running synthetic nonabsorbable suture.

9. An interrupted suture of a similar size is used to integrate the subcutaneous tissue, and the skin is closed with a subcuticular stitch.

Laparoscopic Hernia Repairs. Ger was the first surgeon to perform a laparoscopic herniorrhaphy. In 1982 he described a laparoscopic transabdominal hernia approach. Variations in techniques for laparoscopic hernia repair continue to develop as surgeons gain experience with these procedures.

Techniques used today for laparoscopic herniorrhaphy include the transabdominal preperitoneal patch (TAPP) repair, the totally extraperitoneal patch (TEP) repair, and the intraperitoneal onlay mesh (IPOM) repair (this repair is done much less frequently). The difference between TAPP and TEP is the manner in which access is gained to the preperitoneal space. The TAPP uses intraperitoneal trocars and the creation of a peritoneal flap over the posterior inguinal region. TEP provides access to the preperitoneal space without entering the peritoneal cavity. Kaul and colleagues performed a meta-analysis that did not show an advantage of staple fixation of mesh over fibrin glue fixation in laparoscopic TEP inguinal hernia repair. Fibrin glue mesh fixation with laparoscopic inguinal hernia repair achieves similar hernia recurrence rates compared with staple/tack fixation. They did, however, note a decreased incidence of chronic inguinal pain, suggesting that the fibrin glue may be the preferred technique (Kaul et al, 2012).

Studies of long-term postoperative hernia recurrence and complication rates with these approaches vary. Average recurrence rates for TAPP range from 2% to 7%; for TEP it approximates 1.8%. Laparoscopic hernia repair purportedly has the advantages of a quicker return to normal activity, less postoperative pain, and some reduction of postoperative adhesions related to the minimal dissection required (Research Highlight). Analysis of postoperative pain and paresthesia associated with laparoscopic hernia repair suggests that most patients experience minimal immediate postoperative pain and, after postoperative day 1, have minimal need for analgesics. In general, the procedure requires placing operative cameras and ports, identifying the inguinal floor, removing an indirect hernia sac, inserting mesh to fit around the spermatic cord and form a new inguinal floor, and closing ports.

A hernia repair device is also available (Rebound HRD, Minnesota Medical Development, Inc.) for the repair and/or reinforcement of hernia or other soft tissue defects where weakness exists and support of a nonabsorbable material is preferred. The device is a self-expanding framed/surgical mesh made of Nitinol, a family of intermetallic materials containing a nearly equal mixture of nickel and titanium that offers both superelasticity and shape memory. The device can be folded and inserted laparoscopically, after which it "rebounds" to its original shape for quick and easy placement over the hernia defect. Although ideally suited for laparoscopic surgery, the device also may be used in open approaches.

Procedural Considerations. After induction of general anesthesia the patient is placed in supine position with the arms tucked at the sides and padded. The anesthesia screen is moved as far to the head of the bed as possible to improve surgeon ability to maneuver the laparoscope. A Foley catheter is used by some surgeons to decompress the bladder and maximize the preperitoneal space. If the patient has voided preoperatively, urinary catheterization can be avoided.

The skin is prepped and draped to include the lower abdomen, genital area (manipulation of the scrotal sac may be necessary), and upper thighs. Following introduction of the laparoscope, the patient is placed in Trendelenburg position (see Chapter 6 for positioning precautions) so that viscera fall away from the inguinal area. The following are needed: appropriately sized trocars and scopes (often a 30-degree laparoscope is used), depending on the type of repair

RESEARCH HIGHLIGHT

Comparative Effectiveness: Surgical Options for Inguinal Hernia Repair

Herniorrhaphy is the most commonly performed general surgical procedure in the United States. Approximately a half-million surgical repairs of inguinal hernias are performed annually. This surgical volume suggests that even modest patient outcome improvement initiatives would have a substantial impact. Surgical inguinal hernia repairs fall into three categories: open repair without the use of mesh implant, open repair with mesh, and laparoscopic repair with mesh. In a study reported by the Agency for Healthcare Research and Quality (AHRQ), investigators set out to perform a systematic review of the existent evidence on comparative effectiveness to improve medical decisions about surgical options for inguinal hernia repair.

The analysis included only full articles published in English, studies with patients randomized to treatments, or use of other methods to address selection bias. Studies were either prospective or retrospective with consecutive enrollment. Additionally, treatments must have been performed during the same time period, and at least 85% of participants enrolled in any given study must have had the condition specific to the question posed by investigators. Literature searches identified 2722 articles, of which 223 publications were eligible for inclusion.

Investigators concluded that the following should influence decisions to undergo herniorrhaphy and type of herniorrhaphy: quality of life at 1 year, risk of recurrence, length of hospital stay if not an ambulatory procedure, recovery time, risk of long-term pain, risk of complications, and long-term patient satisfaction. Additionally, these same factors should be taken into account when considering which type of procedure one should undergo.

Modified from Treadwell J et al: *Surgical options for inguinal hernia: comparative effectiveness review*, No. 70. AHRQ Publication No. 12-EHC091-EF. Rockville, MD, August 2012.

planned, ESU and appropriate smoke evacuation system, blunt graspers, hook electrosurgery, a tacking device (absorbable or nonabsorbable tacks, per surgeon choice) or fibrin glue applicator system (Paajanen et al, 2011), laparoscopic clip applier and suction irrigator (have available), balloon dissector (used by some surgeons to create the preperitoneal space), and the primary monitor and video cart.

Operative Procedure—Totally Extraperitoneal Patch Approach (Figure 13-11)

1. An infraumbilical incision is made. The anterior rectus sheath is incised and the ipsilateral rectus abdominis muscle is retracted laterally.
2. With blunt dissection, a space is created beneath the rectus.
3. A dissecting balloon (preperitoneal distention balloon, PDB) is inserted deep to the posterior rectus sheath, tunneled and advanced to the pubic symphysis, then inflated under direct laparoscopic vision.
4. The space is opened and the PDB removed and replaced with a blunt-tip trocar. The preperitoneal space is insufflated under low pressure. Additional trocars are then placed.
5. Using a 30-degree telescope, the inferior epigastric vessels and lower portion of the rectus sheath are identified and retracted anteriorly.
6. The Cooper ligament is cleared from the pubic symphysis medially to the level of the external iliac vein.

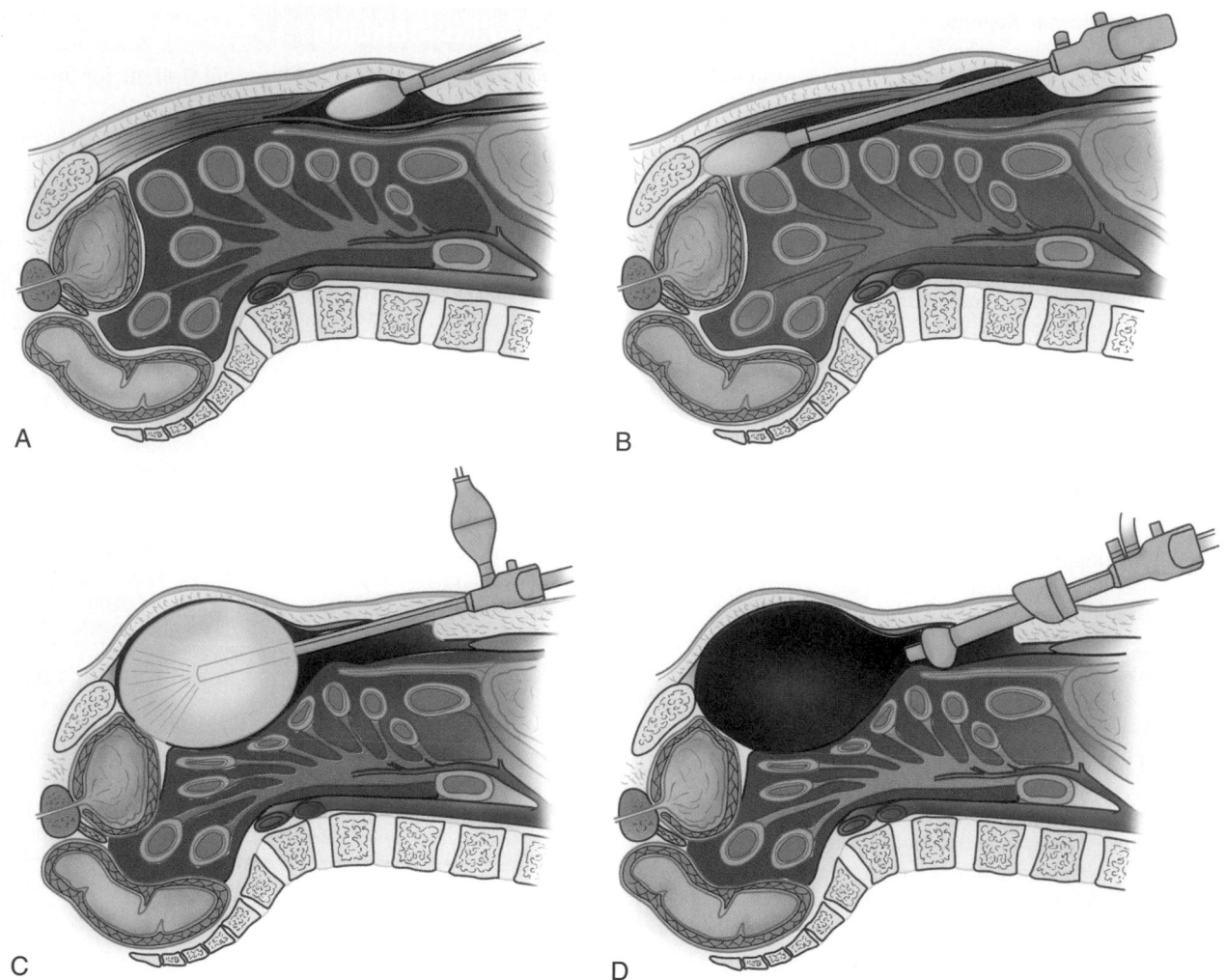

FIGURE 13-11 Totally extraperitoneal patch (TEP) laparoscopic hernia repair. **A,** The TEP approach for laparoscopic hernia repair is demonstrated. Access to the posterior rectus sheath is gained in the periumbilical region. A balloon dissector is placed on the anterior surface of the posterior rectus sheath. **B,** The balloon dissector is advanced to the posterior surface of the pubis in the preperitoneal space. **C,** The balloon is inflated, thereby creating an optical cavity. **D,** The optical cavity is insufflated by carbon dioxide, and the posterior surface of the inguinal floor is dissected.

7. The iliopubic tract is identified. Care is taken to avoid injury to the femoral branch of the genitofemoral nerve and the lateral femoral cutaneous nerve.
8. Lateral dissection is carried out to the anterior superior iliac.
9. The spermatic cord is skeletonized.
10. A *direct hernia sac* is gently reduced by retraction if it has not already been reduced by balloon expansion of the peritoneal space. A *small indirect sac* is mobilized from the spermatic cord and reduced into the peritoneal cavity. *A large sac* may be divided with electrocoagulation near the internal ring. The proximal peritoneal sac is closed with a loop ligature to prevent pneumoperitoneum from occurring. A piece of polypropylene mesh is inserted; unfolded to cover the direct, indirect, and femoral spaces and rest over the cord structures; and carefully secured with a tacking stapler.

Repair of Inguinal Hernias in Females. Regardless of the specific technique used, the initial approach to the repair of a hernia in the female is the same as that used in the male. After the cremaster muscles are opened to expose the round ligament, variations that may be encountered include the following: (1) with the sac exposed and cleared from the round ligament, the round ligament and accompanying vessels are dissected free from the inguinal floor to the labium; (2) at the labium the round ligament is clamped, ligated, and divided; (3) the sac at the internal ring is opened, checked to be sure that no abdominal contents are present, and ligated at its neck, together with the round ligament and associated vessels; or (4) the sac distal to the ligature is removed with the distal round ligament, while the ligated stump retracts promptly into the abdomen. The remainder of the repair is the same as that previously described.

Repair of Femoral Hernias. A femoral hernia protrudes from the groin below the inguinal ligament into the thigh (Figure 13-12). In its most obvious form, a femoral hernia is an inflamed, tender mass below the inguinal ligament. Unfortunately, the presentation is frequently more subtle and the diagnosis is completely missed or confused with enlarged inguinal lymph nodes, a psoas muscle abscess, a saphenous varix, a lipoma, or an indirect or direct inguinal hernia. The defect is usually small and frequently nonreducible.

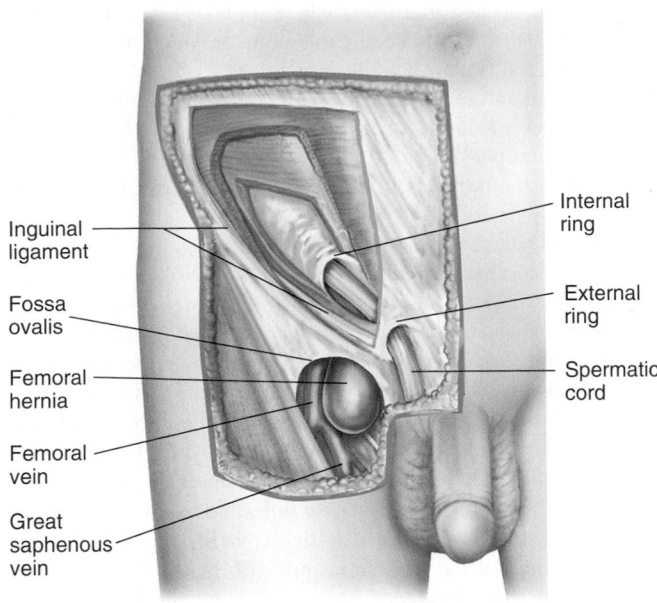

FIGURE 13-12 Bulge from femoral hernia occurring below inguinal ligament.

Femoral hernias are highly likely to become incarcerated and strangulated; elective repair is clearly indicated unless serious contraindications to surgery exist.

Operative Procedure. The general approach is surgical treatment to free the tightly bound hernia, closely examine the contents of the hernia for ischemic change, and repair the hernia defect. The principles for repair of this type of hernia are the same as those described for inguinal herniorrhaphies. Ultimately, the defect must be obliterated. Repair of a femoral hernia requires approximating the aponeurotic margins of the femoral canal. The sutures are placed through the iliopubic tract superiorly and through the Cooper ligament and pectineus fascia inferiorly. Care is taken to not compromise the femoral artery and vein.

Preperitoneal (Properitoneal) Repair—Open Approach. Preperitoneal (properitoneal) repair also is based on the essential role of the transversalis fascia in the cause and subsequent correction of a hernia. This repair is suitable for direct, indirect, and femoral hernias. It is particularly applicable in dealing with recurrent hernias and bilateral hernias, because exposure is obtained by operating through virgin surgical fields rather than through previous scars.

Operative Procedure

1. A transverse incision is made 2 cm above the symphysis pubis, through the rectus abdominis muscle on the affected side (Figure 13-13, *A*).

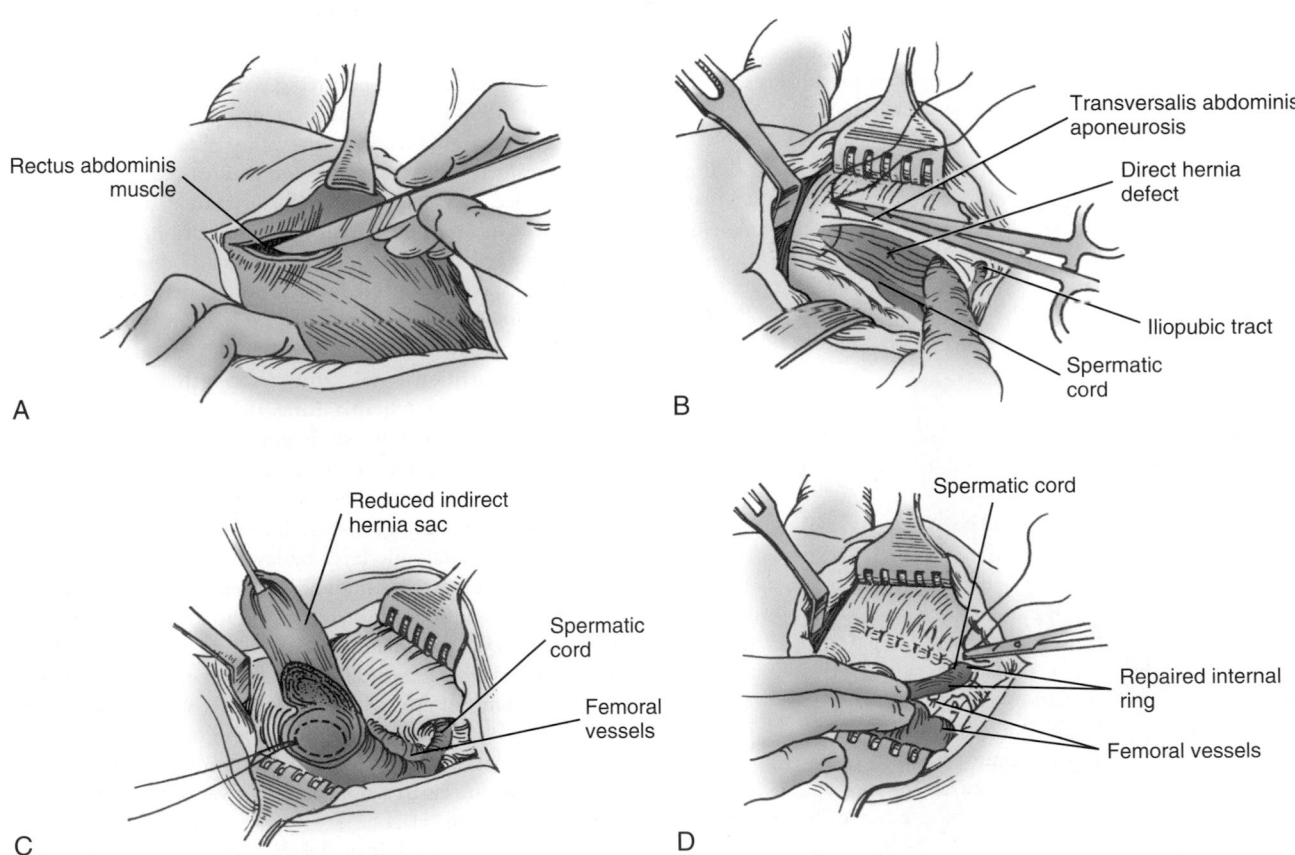

FIGURE 13-13 Preperitoneal repair. **A,** Skin incision starts 2 cm above symphysis pubis and is extended through external oblique, internal oblique, and transversalis muscles. **B,** With finger in direct hernia defect, the surgeon sutures the transversalis abdominis aponeurosis to the iliopubic tract. **C,** In case of indirect defect, the sac is reduced and then excised, with high ligation being achieved by use of a purse-string suture. **D,** Internal ring is tightened after transversus abdominis aponeurosis has been approximated to iliopubic tract.

2. The wound is deepened by cutting the external oblique, internal oblique, and transversalis muscles.

3. The transversalis fascia is then cut, and the preperitoneal space entered. This is the plane of dissection for the remainder of the operation.

4. Retraction on the lower side of the incision reveals the posterior inguinal wall and the hernia defect.

Variations in the procedure are performed for different types of hernias.

1. If the hernia is direct, it can be reduced easily and the superior edge of the defect (the transversalis fascia) sutured to the iliopubic tract (origin of the transversalis fascia) (see Figure 13-13, *B*).

2. In an indirect hernia, the sac is gently retracted from the inguinal canal. A purse-string suture is placed around the peritoneal defect as the sac is excised (see Figure 13-13, *C*). The lateral aspect of the internal abdominal ring is closed, and the posterior wall is reinforced as with the direct hernia.

3. In repair of a femoral hernia, the sac is again reduced by traction. After the sac is inspected for contents, a high ligation is performed. As it approaches the Cooper ligament, the defect in the posterior inguinal floor is clearly identified and is repaired by direct approximation (see Figure 13-13, *D*).

After repair of any of the aforementioned hernias, the preperitoneal space is irrigated with saline solution and the appropriate layers are approximated.

Repair of Sliding Hernias. Direct or indirect hernias may occur as sliding hernias. A sliding inguinal hernia occurs when the wall of a viscus forms a portion of the wall of the hernia. The most common sliding hernias involve the bladder in direct hernias, the sigmoid colon in left indirect hernias, and the cecum in right indirect inguinal hernias (Figure 13-14). This hernia must be recognized early in the repair because attempts at surgical removal of the entire sac will injure the sliding viscus.

Operative Procedure. All operations designed to repair sliding hernias adhere to the basic principle of repairing the defect in the transversalis fascia. To free the bowel from the sac, the following steps must be taken:

FIGURE 13-14 Sliding hernia.

1. The sac is opened in an area where no bowel is present and is excised medially and laterally to a point at which the bowel can be mobilized (Figure 13-15).

2. The lateral and medial peritoneal margins are approximated.

3. The bowel is reduced to the peritoneal cavity, and high ligation of the sac is performed.

4. Repair of the transversalis fascia is done by one of the methods previously described.

Littre, Maydl, and Richter Hernias. An inguinal hernia containing a Meckel diverticulum is called a *Littre hernia,* and one containing two loops of bowel is called a *Maydl hernia.* A special type of strangulated hernia is a *Richter hernia* (Figure 13-16). In this hernia only a part of the circumference of the bowel is incarcerated or strangulated in the hernia. Frequently it is described as a knuckle of bowel that becomes trapped and ischemic. Because initially a very small area is necrotic, diagnosis may be delayed. A Richter hernia most frequently occurs in femoral hernias because of the small size and sharp, relatively inflexible nature of the fascial ring in this area. A strangulated Richter hernia may be reduced spontaneously, and the gangrenous piece of intestine may be overlooked at the time of surgery. Most commonly, the distal ileum is involved in a Richter hernia; however, omentum is frequently encountered in the sac. The favored approach for repair is through the preperitoneal space.

Surgery for Repair of Hernias of the Anterior Abdominal Wall

Ventral or Incisional Hernias

Ventral hernias can appear either spontaneously or after previous operations. Spontaneously occurring ventral hernias include epigastric and umbilical hernias. Advanced age, open repair, large hernia defect, and vertical incision at the primary laparotomy procedure are significant risk factors in development of postoperative ventral hernias, called *incisional hernias* (Helgstrand et al, 2013). Operations that involve a potential for contamination, such as that for acute perforated ulcer or other perforated abdominal viscera, or wounds that become infected, are more prone to developing subsequent ventral hernias. Patients taking steroids or diagnosed with chronic obstructive pulmonary disease (COPD), as well as patients with a poor nutritional state and resulting hypoproteinemia, are predisposed to ventral hernia formation. Finally, faulty surgical technique, such as the choice of inappropriate suture materials, may result in the ultimate appearance of a ventral hernia.

Several methods have been developed for repairing ventral hernias (Research Highlight). If all layers of the abdominal wall are easily identified, anatomic layer-by-layer repair may be done. Frequently a type of overlap method for repair is used. Vertical and transverse overlap procedures are referred to as *vest-over-pants repair.* For large defects, in which approximation of tissue would result in closure with excessive tension or would cause either circulatory or respiratory compromise, synthetic materials such as surgical mesh or patches are used. Long-term follow-up of patients in randomized clinical trials is needed in order to determine effectiveness-based conclusions about laparoscopic repair of ventral/incisional hernias (Sauerland et al, 2011).

When a very large fascial defect is present, a technique that extrapolates on the principles of tissue expansion may be used. A Tenckhoff catheter is placed percutaneously into the peritoneal cavity. Gradual expansion of the abdominal fascia is accomplished by insufflation of the abdomen with 1 to 2 L of carbon dioxide gas,

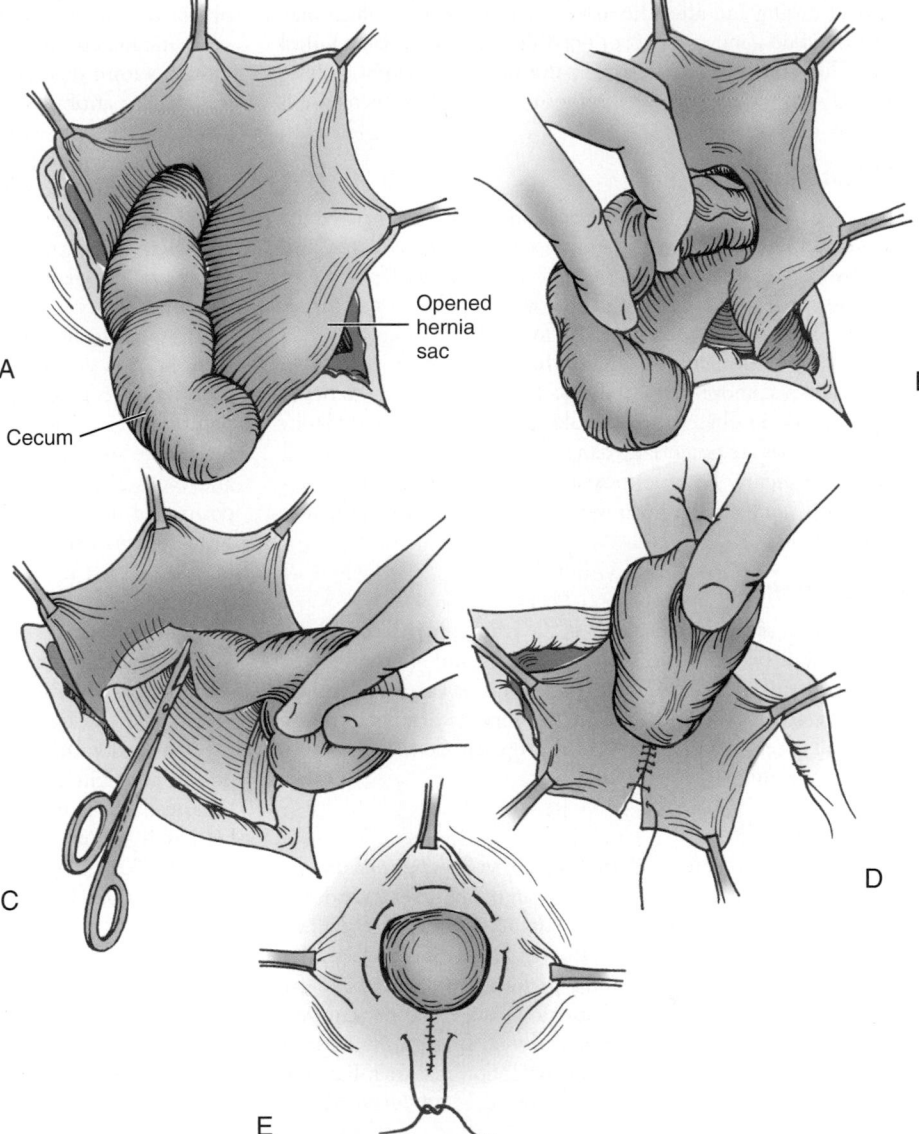

FIGURE 13-15 Right sliding hernia. **A,** Cecum forms posterior wall of hernia sac. **B,** Peritoneum is excised medially (**C**) and laterally (**D**) to allow mobilization of cecum for subsequent reduction to peritoneal cavity. Lateral and medial margins are approximated. **E,** After reduction, high ligation is accomplished using a purse-string suture.

Opened hernia sac

Cecum

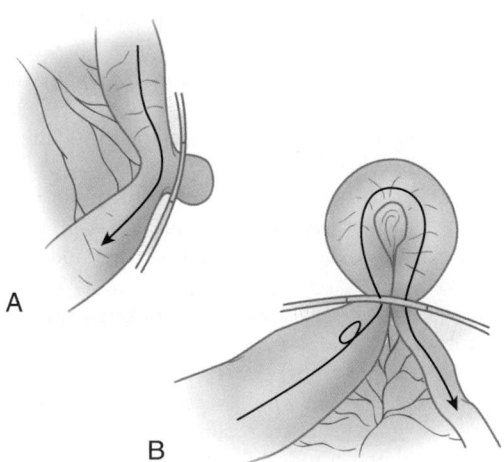

FIGURE 13-16 A, Richter hernia. Only a portion of bowel passes through hernial ring; arrow indicates that bowel need not be obstructed mechanically even with strangulation. **B,** Incarcerated hernia. Distended bowel in hernia cannot return to abdomen through narrow fascial defect.

RESEARCH HIGHLIGHT

Comparison of Laparoscopic Primary Versus Open Primary Repair of Ventral Hernia

The purpose of this study was to compare recurrence rates and operative times for laparoscopic primary repair versus open primary repair of ventral hernias in 51 patients. Results were determined using median follow-up of 33 months. Mean laparoscopic operative time was not determined to be significantly shorter than the open repair group, and only a single patient in each group experienced hernia recurrence. There were, however, advantages to performing laparoscopic repair over open procedures. Surgeons can often obtain better exposure of the defect and patients may experience reduced pain and less morbidity. These procedures can also be performed in conjunction with other laparoscopic procedures. Laparoscopic hernia repair, however, is considered a highly specialized skill and is not recommended, by this group of investigators, for the repair of large ventral hernias.

Modified from Anadol AZ et al: Comparison of laparoscopic primary and open primary repair of ventral hernias, *Surg Laparosc Endosc Percutan Tech* 21(5):301–305, 2012.

similar to the procedure for laparoscopy. The patient's vital signs are monitored during and after the insufflation procedure, which may be performed on a nursing unit or possibly in an outpatient clinical setting. The graduated expansion of the tissues sometimes allows for primary closure of the defect without the use of synthetic mesh or a patch.

Umbilical Hernias

Umbilical hernias are extraperitoneal and occur as small fascial defects under the umbilicus. They are common in children and frequently disappear spontaneously by 2 years of age. If the defect persists, a simple approximation of the overlying fascia is all that is necessary for repair (see Chapter 26 for a description of hernia repair in children). In adults umbilical hernias represent a defect in the linea alba just above the umbilicus. These hernias tend to occur more frequently in obese people, making diagnosis more difficult. Umbilical hernias are potentially dangerous because they have small necks and frequently become incarcerated. Surgical repair is indicated for all adults with both symptomatic and asymptomatic umbilical hernias.

Epigastric Hernias

Epigastric hernias are protrusions of fat through defects in the abdominal wall between the xiphoid process and the umbilicus. Patients with epigastric hernias can have nausea, vague abdominal pain, or epigastric pain similar to that observed with cholecystitis or duodenal ulcers. Surgical repair of epigastric hernias is simple and very successful.

Spigelian Hernias

The linea semilunaris, often referred to as the *Spigelius line,* marks the transition from muscle to aponeurosis in the transversus abdominis muscle. The area of aponeurosis that lies between the linea semilunaris and the lateral edge of the rectus muscle is referred to as the *spigelian zone.* Protrusion of a peritoneal sac, preperitoneal fat, or other abdominal viscera through a congenital or acquired defect in this area is called a spigelian hernia. It is usually located between the different muscle layers of the abdominal wall. For this reason a spigelian hernia may be referred to as an *interstitial* or *intramuscular hernia.*

Spigelian hernias are uncommon and are generally difficult to diagnose. Ultrasound imaging has improved the diagnosis of such hernias. When ultrasound is not conclusive, CT can better visualize the hernia orifice.

Interparietal Hernias

An interparietal hernia lies between the layers of the abdominal wall. These hernias may be classified by dividing them into those that present with ventral swelling and those without ventral swelling. Diagnosis is often made during an exploratory laparotomy for symptoms of intestinal obstruction.

Repair follows the same procedure as that done for a strangulated hernia. The sac contents are closely examined for ischemia, the sac is resected, and the defect is repaired.

Synthetic Mesh and Patch Repairs

An ideal prosthetic mesh should not be physically modified by tissue fluids; be chemically inert, noncarcinogenic, and nonallergenic; resist mechanical strain; be permeable, allowing tissue ingrowth; and be pliable. Synthetic meshes, such as Mersilene, Marlex, Prolene, and Dacron, have been particularly helpful in

repairing recurrent or large ventral hernias. Closure of the defect is obtained with minimal or no tension on the suture line. These synthetic materials are strong and durable, promoting fibrovascular growth within their pores, which lends extra strength to the repair. Single-dose antibiotic prophylaxis may be used to reduce surgical site infection rates with prosthetic hernia repair.

Another synthetic material, the Gore-Tex patch, has become popular for the reconstruction of abdominal wall defects and repair of soft tissue. Gore-Tex soft tissue patches are available in both 1- and 2-cm thicknesses. Impregnation of Gore-Tex patches with an antimicrobial agent has been associated with reduced incidence of infection.

Essential to the use of mesh or patch in a hernia repair are the identification and cleaning of tissue planes to which the mesh or patch will be attached (Figure 13-17, *A*). In a ventral hernia the peritoneum is dissected from the undersurface of the rectus abdominis muscle and the mesh or patch is placed between the peritoneum and the rectus (see Figure 13-17, *B*). After the mesh or patch is positioned, it is sutured in place on one side, using the synthetic suture material compatible with the type of mesh or patch used (see Figure 13-17, *C*).

At this point the peritoneum can be closed, if possible. If the peritoneum cannot be closed, the mesh or patch can be placed directly over the omentum. The mesh or patch is then placed and sutured to the other side of the defect, with moderate tension maintained (see Figure 13-17, *D*). If possible, the mesh or patch is then covered with a fascial or muscular layer before the subcutaneous fat and skin are closed. Closed-wound drainage catheters may be placed in the wound. Using mesh or a patch to repair inguinal hernias is based on the same principles used for closing ventral hernias. With inguinal hernias, the mesh or patch is sutured to transversalis fascia on both sides of the defect.

KEY POINTS

- A hernia is defined as an abnormal protrusion of an organ or tissue through a defect in its surrounding walls.
- Although a hernia can occur at various sites of the body, these defects most commonly involve the abdominal wall, particularly the inguinal region.
- Hernia repair is the most common operation in general surgery.
- Hernias occur most often in males.
- Hernias may be direct, indirect, femoral, umbilical, or occur at previous sites of surgical incisions (incisional hernia). Indirect inguinal hernia is the most common hernia in males and females.
- Hernias can be reducible or nonreducible; the latter requires immediate surgical evaluation.
- Understanding the type and anatomic structures of the hernia guide procedural considerations and surgical approach.
- The tension-free repair is the dominant method of inguinal hernia repair.
- Current practices in hernia management often use a synthetic mesh prosthesis to bridge the defect.
- Laparoscopic inguinal hernia repair is another method of tension-free mesh repair, with several repair options. The most popular techniques include a totally extraperitoneal (TEP) and transabdominal preperitoneal (TAPP) approach.
- Most hernia repairs (herniorrhaphy) are performed on an ambulatory surgical basis.
- The perioperative plan of care includes thorough review of discharge instructions for care at home.

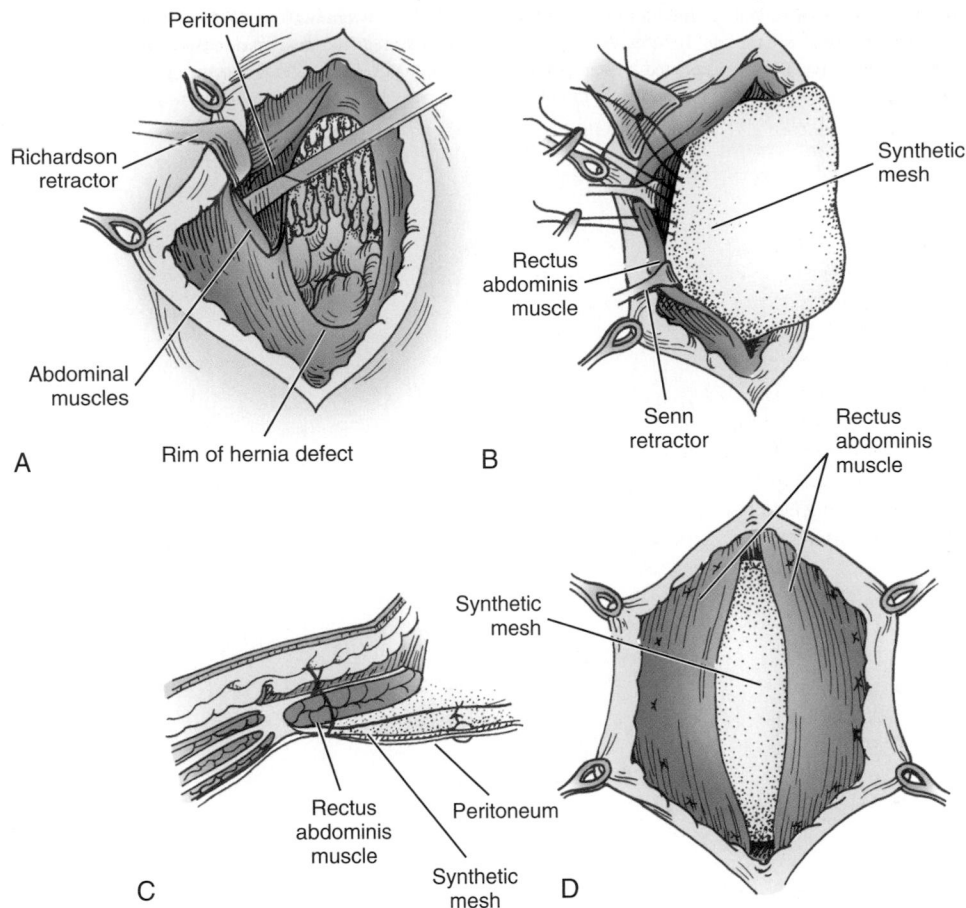

FIGURE 13-17 Use of mesh in hernia repair. After layers of abdominal wall surrounding ventral hernia are identified **(A)**, mesh is inserted between rectus and peritoneum **(B). C,** Mesh is sutured into place on one side. **D,** With moderate tension, mesh is inserted between appropriate layers on opposite side and is sutured into place.

CRITICAL THINKING QUESTION

An elderly male patient presents to the emergency department with complaints of a long history of right inguinal swelling and tenderness. He denies nausea and vomiting. What would the perioperative nurse look for during abdominal assessment? Which factors in the patient's history are considered most relevant to his convalescence? What would be patient and family education priorities for this patient after an inguinal hernia repair?

℮volve *The answers to the Critical Thinking Question can be found at http://evolve.elsevier.com/Rothrock/Alexander.*

REFERENCES

AHRQ Identifies Top 10 Patient Safety Strategies, March 4, 2013, available at www.medscape.com/viewarticle/780237?nlid=29036_785&src=wnl_edit_medp_nurs&uac=19435CR&spon=24. Accessed March 14, 2013.

Association of periOperative Registered Nurses (AORN): *Perioperative standards and recommended practices,* Denver, 2013, The Association.

Braman JP: *Teaching safe surgery: implementing the surgical pause,* AORN Congress Presentation, San Diego, CA, March 4, 2013.

DeJohn P: ASCs jump on the surgical checklist bandwagon, *OR Manager* 29(3):26–29, 2013.

Denholm B: Tucking patient's arms and general positioning, *AORN J* 89(4):755-757, 2009.

Domniz N et al: Slit versus non-slit mesh placement in total extraperitoneal inguinal hernia repair, *World J Surg* 35(11):2382–2386, 2011.

Erickson KM: *Abdominal hernias,* September 19, 2011, available at http://emedicine.medscape.com/article/189563-overview#showall. Accessed March 11, 2013.

Helgstrand F et al: Nationwide prospective study of outcomes after elective incisional hernia repair, *J Am Coll Surg* 216(2):217–228, 2013.

Kaul A et al: Staple versus fibrin glue fixation in laparoscopic total extraperitoneal repair of inguinal hernia: a systematic review and meta-analysis, *Surg Endosc* 26(5):1269–1278, 2012.

Kulacoglu H: Current options in inguinal hernia repair in adult patients, *Hippokratia* 15(3):2230231, 2011.

Kumar A, Srivastava U: Role of routine laboratory investigations in preoperative evaluation, *J Anaesthesiol Clin Pharmacol* 27:174–179, 2011.

Malangoni MA, Rosen MJ: Hernias. In Townsend CM et al, editors: *Sabiston textbook of surgery,* ed 19, Philadelphia, 2012, Saunders.

Moody JA, Davis SS: *Hot topic! CSI: Conquering surgical infections,* AORN Congress presentation, San Diego, CA, March 4, 2013.

Paajanen H et al: Randomized clinical trial of tissue glue versus absorbable sutures for mesh fixation in local anaesthetic Lichtenstein hernia repair, *Br J Surg* 98(9):1245–1255, 2011.

Pickett LC: Prosthetic choice in open inguinal hernia repair. In Jacob BP, Ramshaw B, editors: *The SAGES manual of hernia repair,* New York, 2013, Springer.

Sauerland S et al: Laparoscopic versus open surgical techniques for ventral or incisional hernia repair, *Cochrane Database Syst Rev* (3):1–59, 2011.

Sherwinter DA: *Laparoscopic inguinal hernia repair*, updated September 13, 2011(a), available at http://emedicine.medscape.com/article/1534321-overview#showall. Accessed March 11, 2013.

Sherwinter DA: *Open inguinal hernia repair*, updated September 13, 2011(b), available at http://emedicine.medscape.com/article/1534281-overview. Accessed March 13, 2013.

The Joint Commission: *2013 National Patient Safety Goals*, available at www.jointcommission.org. Accessed March 13, 2013.

Tolver MA et al: Determinants of a short convalescence after laparoscopic transabdominal preperitoneal inguinal hernia repair, *Surgery* 151(4):556–563, 2012.

CHAPTER 14
Gynecologic and Obstetric Surgery

SUSAN A. CARZO AND JOSEPH H. VIVEIROS

At some point in their lives, many women face the prospect of undergoing gynecologic surgery. Surgical procedures on structures of the female reproductive system are performed for diagnostic, therapeutic, or cosmetic purposes. Conditions requiring surgery include abnormal bleeding, benign or suspected malignant neoplasms, infertility, or the need to remove or repair weakened structures. A majority of surgical procedures carried out in the United States are performed on women (Healthcare Cost and Utilization Project [HCUPnet], 2009). With the resurgence of interest in issues and priorities related to women's health (Berg et al, 2013), a holistic approach with sensitivity to the special needs of this population is an essential component of perioperative patient care.

Surgical Anatomy

The female reproductive organs and their relationships are shown in Figures 14-1 and 14-2. The adult female structures associated with the process of reproduction are the external organs (vulva), the associated ligaments and muscles, the soft tissues and contents of the pelvic cavity, and the bony pelvis.

Female External Genital Organs (Vulva)

The external organs, referred to collectively as the *vulva,* include the mons pubis, the labia majora and labia minora, the clitoris, the vestibular glands, the vaginal vestibule, the vaginal opening, and the urethral opening (Figure 14-3).

The mons pubis is a mound of adipose tissue covered by skin and, after puberty, by hair as well. It is situated over the anterior surface of the symphysis pubis.

The labia majora are two folds of adipose tissue covered with skin that extend downward and backward from the mons pubis. Varying in appearance according to the amount of adipose tissue, they unite below and behind the mons pubis to form the posterior fourchette and in front of the mons pubis to form the anterior fourchette. The labia minora are the two hairless, flat, delicate folds of skin that lie within the labia majora. Each labium splits into lateral and medial parts. The lateral part forms the prepuce or hood of the clitoris and the medial part forms the frenulum. The posterior folds of the labia are united by a delicate fold extending between them, forming the fossa navicularis.

The clitoris is the homolog of the penis in the male. It hangs freely and terminates in a rounded glans (small, sensitive vascular body). Unlike the penis the clitoris does not contain the urethra. The vaginal vestibule is a smooth area surrounded by the labia minora, with the clitoris at its apex and the fossa navicularis at its base. It contains openings for the urethra and the vagina.

The urethra, which is about 4 cm long in premenopausal women, is close to the anterior vaginal wall and connects the bladder with the urethral meatus. Two small paraurethral ducts, which are commonly known as *Skene ducts,* lie on either side of the urethral meatus and drain *Skene glands.*

The vaginal opening lies below the urethral meatus. The hymen surrounds the virginal vaginal opening and may be circular, crescentic, or fimbriated. Its remnants after vaginal intercourse are the carunculae hymenales or hymeneal tags.

Bartholin glands and ducts are located on each side of the lower end of the vagina at the 5 and 7 o'clock positions. The narrow ducts open into the vaginal orifice on the inner aspects of the labia minora. The glands secrete mucus and can become infected or inflamed.

Pelvic Cavity

Uterus

The uterus is an inverted pear-shaped organ situated in the pelvic cavity between the bladder and the rectum. It gains much of its support from its direct attachment to the vagina and from indirect attachments to nearby structures, such as the rectum and pelvic diaphragm. The uterus is supported on each side by the broad, round, cardinal, and uterosacral ligaments and levator ani muscles (see Figures 14-1 and 14-2). The upper lateral points, the uterine cornua, receive the fallopian tubes. The fundus of the uterus is the upper, rounded portion positioned above the level of the tubal openings and just below the pelvic brim. Below, the body, or corpus, of the uterus joins the cervix. The corpus is separated from the cervix by a slight constriction (canal) called the *isthmus.* The cervix lies at the level of the ischial spines. The body of the uterus communicates with the cervical canal at the internal orifice, called the *internal os.* The constriction (endocervical canal) ends at the vaginal portion of the cervix at the external orifice, called the *external os.* The external os varies in appearance and is typically round and 2 to 3 mm in diameter in the nulliparous woman; after delivery, it may become oval, round, or wide and slitlike.

The uterine body has three layers: (1) the outer peritoneal, or serous, layer, which is a reflection of the pelvic peritoneum; (2) the myometrium, or muscular layer, which houses smooth muscle, nerves, blood vessels, and lymphatics; and (3) the endometrium, or mucosal layer, which lines the cavity of the uterus.

The ureters descend into the pelvis posteriorly at the level of the ovaries, after which they pass under the uterine arteries and run laterally along the base of the paracervcial ligament, where they connect to the posterior bladder, anterior to the vagina. Because of the proximity of the ureters to the female reproductive organs, it is

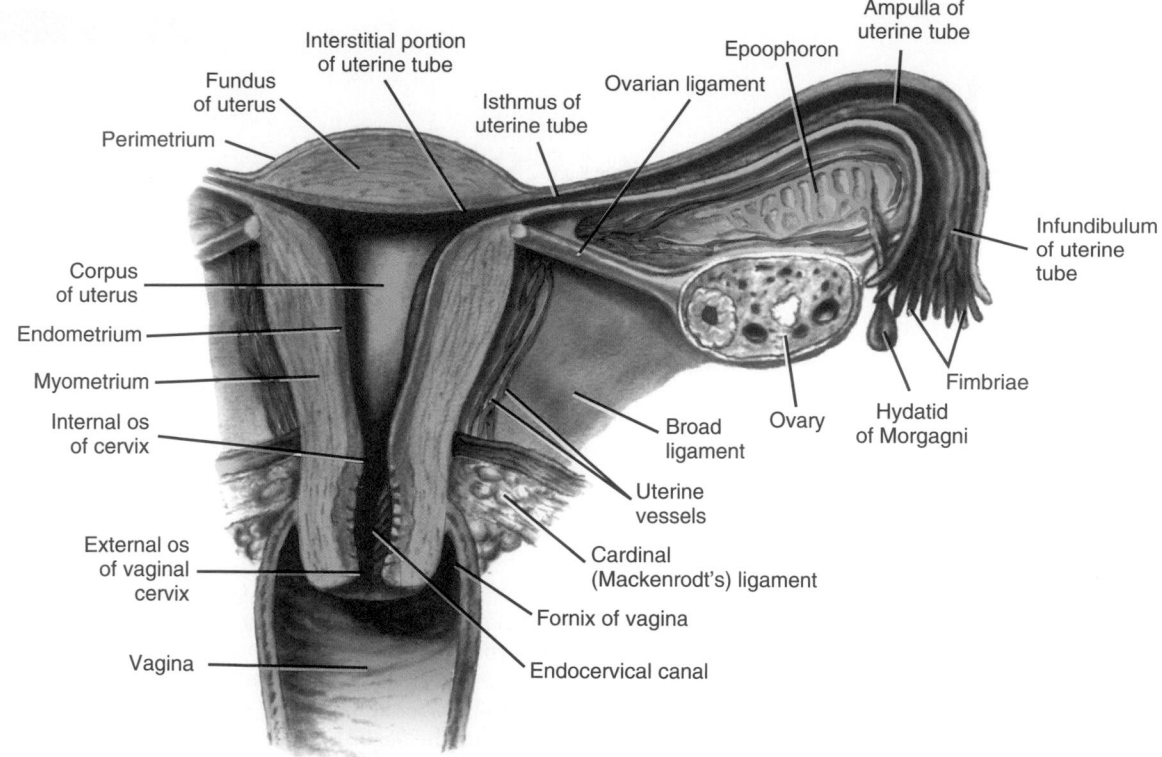

FIGURE 14-1 Female reproductive organs.

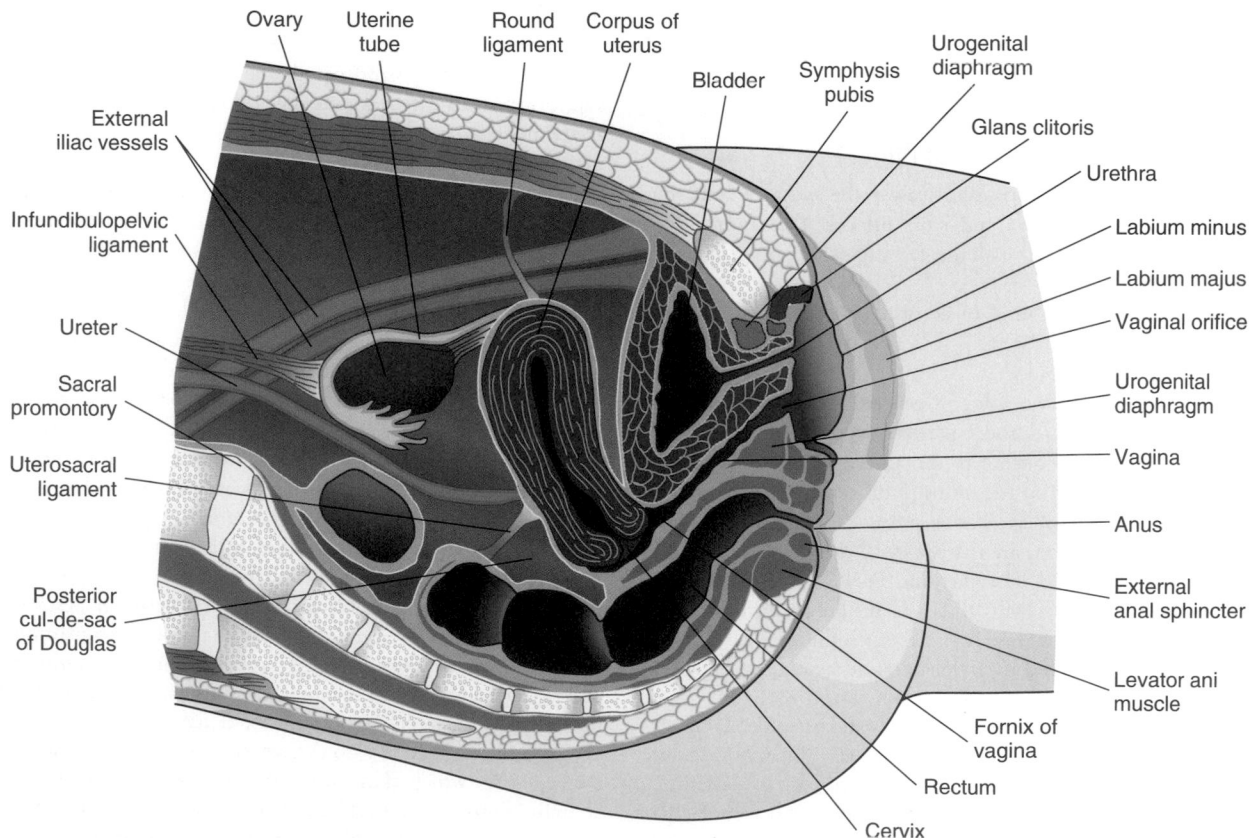

FIGURE 14-2 Female pelvic organs as viewed in midsagittal section.

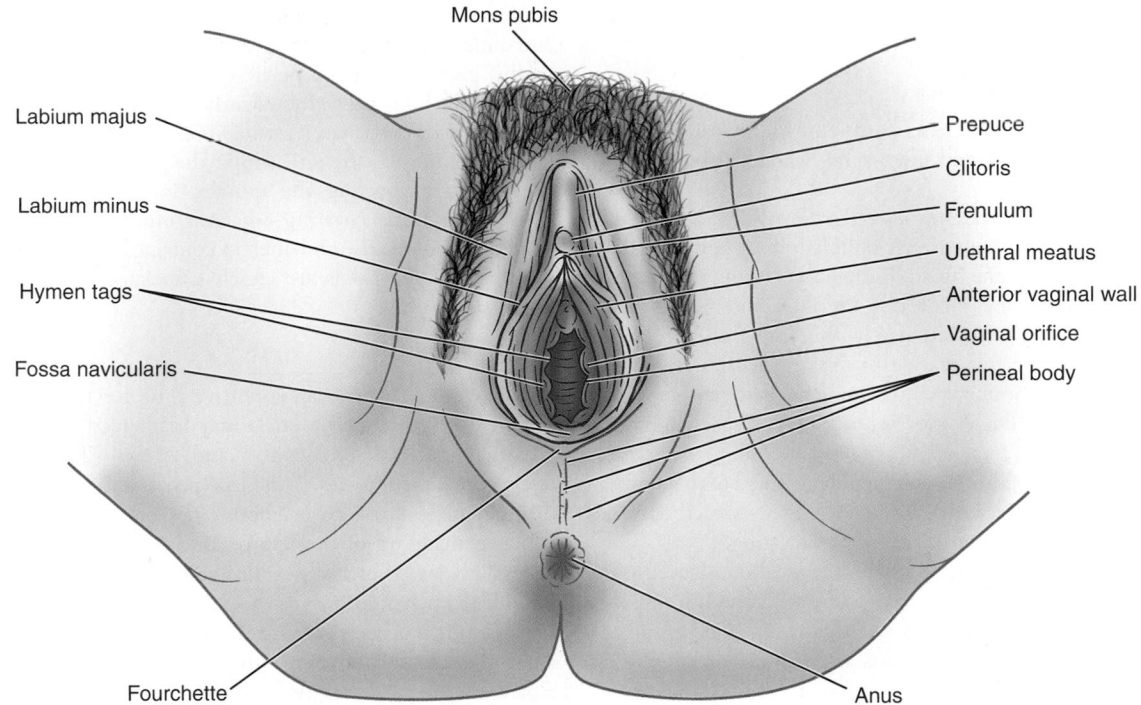

FIGURE 14-3 The structures of the external genitalia that are collectively called the vulva.

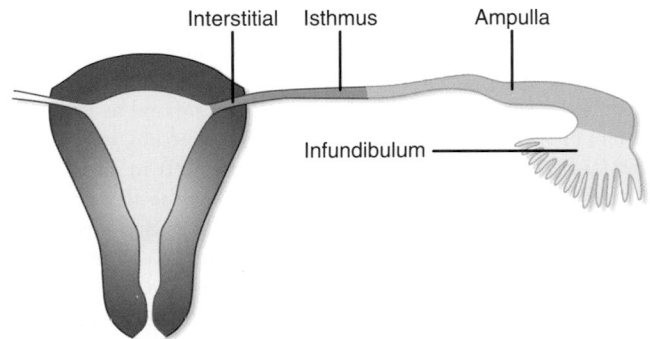

FIGURE 14-4 The anatomic segments of the fallopian tube.

important to identify and understand their anatomic relationship to other structures within the pelvic cavity during gynecologic surgical procedures.

Fallopian Tubes (Oviducts)

The Greek word *salpinx,* meaning "trumpet" or "tube," is used to refer to the fallopian tubes (Figure 14-4). The tubes are paired and consist of a musculomembranous channel about 10 to 13 cm long, forming the canals through which the ova are conveyed to the uterus from the ovaries. The outer surfaces of the tubes are covered by peritoneum. The inner layers are composed of muscular tissue lined with ciliated epithelium. Each tube receives its blood supply from the branches of the uterine and ovarian arteries and has four parts. (1) The infundibulum is trumpet shaped, opens into the abdominal cavity, and has finger-like projections called *fimbriae.* (2) The ampulla forms more than half of the tube and is thin walled and tortuous. (3) The isthmus is cylindric and forms approximately

one third of the tube. (4) The remainder of the fallopian tube is known as both the intramural or interstitial portion. Measuring approximately 1 cm in length, it passes through the wall of the uterus.

It has been theorized that transfer of the ova from the ruptured follicles into the uterus is accomplished through vascular changes that occur during contraction of the smooth muscle fibers of the tube. The peristaltic action of the muscular layer and the ciliary movement propel the ova toward the uterus.

The right tube and ovary are in close relationship to the cecum and appendix; the left tube and ovary are situated near the sigmoid flexure.

Ovaries

The ovaries are located on each side of the uterus. The ovaries and tubes are collectively known as the *adnexa.* Each ovary lies within a depression (ovarian fossa) on the lateral wall of the pelvic cavity and above the broad ligament (see Figure 14-1). The anterior border of each ovary is attached to the posterior layer of the broad ligament by a peritoneal fold (mesovarium) and is suspended by the ovarian ligament.

The ovaries are small almond-shaped organs composed of an outer layer, known as the *cortex,* and an inner vascular layer, known as the *medulla.* The medulla consists of connective tissue containing nerves, blood vessels, and lymph vessels. The ovary is covered by epithelium, not peritoneum. The cortex contains ovarian (graafian) follicles in different stages of maturity. After ovulation the corpus luteum arises from the graafian follicle that expelled the ovum.

The ovaries produce ova after puberty and also function as endocrine glands, producing hormones such as estrogen, secreted by the ovarian follicles. Estrogen controls the development of secondary sexual characteristics and initiates growth of the lining of the uterus during the menstrual cycle. Progesterone, which is secreted by the corpus luteum, is essential for implantation of the fertilized ovum and for the development of the embryo.

Ligaments of the Uterus

The uterus has numerous ligaments to support its structure such as the broad, round, cardinal, and uterosacral ligaments (see Figures 14-1 and 14-2).

The pelvic peritoneum extends laterally, downward, and posteriorly from each side of the uterus. A double fold of pelvic peritoneum forms the layers of the broad ligament, enclosing the uterus. These layers separate, thereby covering the floor and sides of the pelvis. The fallopian tube is situated within the free border of the broad ligament. The free margin of the upper division of the broad ligament, lying immediately below the fallopian tube, is termed the *mesosalpinx.* Each ovary lies behind its respective broad ligament.

Round ligaments are fibromuscular bands attached to the uterus. Each round ligament passes forward and laterally between the layers of the broad ligament to enter the deep inguinal ring.

Cardinal ligaments (also known as paracervical or Mackenrodt ligaments) are composed of connective tissue with smooth muscle fibers and provide strong support for the uterus. They are found at the base of each of the broad ligaments and contain or house the uterine artery and vein.

Uterosacral ligaments are a posterior continuation of the peritoneal tissue. The ligaments pass posteriorly to the sacrum on either side of the rectum.

Vagina

The vagina is a rugated musculomembranous tube. It carries the menstrual blood from the uterus, serves as the organ for sexual intercourse, and is the terminal portion of the birth canal. The anterior wall measures 6 to 8 cm in length and the posterior wall 7 to 10 cm (see Figures 14-1 and 14-2). The anterior wall of the vagina is in proximity to the bladder and urethra. The lower posterior wall is anteriorly adjacent to the rectum. The upper portion of the vagina lies above the pelvic floor and is surrounded by visceral pelvic fascia. The lower half is surrounded by the levator ani muscles.

Cervix

The cervix consists of a supravaginal portion, which is closely associated with the bladder and the ureters, and a vaginal portion, which projects downward and backward into the vaginal vault. The projection of the cervix into the vaginal vault divides the vault into four regions, called *fornices:* anterior, posterior, right lateral, and left lateral.

The posterior fornix is in contact with the peritoneum of the pouch or cul-de-sac of Douglas. The rectovaginal septum lies between the vagina and rectum. The dense connective tissue separating the anterior wall of the vagina from the distal urethra is termed the *urethrovaginal septum.*

Bony Pelvis

The pelvis is the portion of the trunk below and behind the abdomen. The bony pelvis is composed of the ilium, symphysis pubis, ischium, sacrum, and coccyx. The so-called *pelvic brim* divides the abdominal false portion, located above the arcuate line, from the true portion of the pelvis, located below this line. The bony pelvis accommodates the growing fetus during pregnancy and the birth process.

The true pelvis is considered to have three parts: inlet, cavity, and outlet. The muscles lining the pelvis facilitate movement of the thighs, give form to the pelvic cavity, and provide a firm elastic lining to the bony pelvic framework. All organs located in the pelvis are covered by pelvic fascia, which is extremely important in maintaining the normal strength within the pelvic floor.

The fascia covering the muscles is usually dense and firm, whereas the fascia covering organs is often thin and elastic. The nerves, blood vessels, and ureters coursing through the anatomic structures of the pelvis are closely associated with muscular and fascial structures.

Pelvic Floor

The pelvic floor acts as a supportive sling for the pelvic contents (Figure 14-5). The pelvic fascia may be divided into three general groups: parietal, diaphragmatic, and visceral. The parietal pelvic fascia covers the muscles of the true pelvic wall and perineum. The diaphragmatic fascia covers both sides of the pelvic diaphragm, which is made up of the levator ani and coccygeal muscles. The visceral fascia is thin and flexible and covers the pelvic organs. The floor of the pelvis, known as the *pelvic diaphragm,* gives support to the abdominal pelvic viscera in this region. It consists of the levator ani and coccygeal muscles with their respective fascial coverings, separating the pelvic cavity from the perineum.

The levator ani muscles, varying in thickness and strength, may be divided into three parts: the iliococcygeal, the pubococcygeal, and the puborectal muscles. The fibers of the levator ani muscles blend with the muscle fibers of the rectum and vagina. The pubovaginal fibers of the pubococcygeal portion of the levator ani muscles, lying directly below the urinary bladder, are involved in the control of micturition. The pubococcygeal fibers of the levator ani muscles control and pull the coccyx forward and assist in the closure of the pelvic outlet. The fibers pull the rectum, vagina, and bladder neck upward toward the symphysis pubis in an effort to close the pelvic outlet and are responsible for the flexure at the anorectal junction. Relaxation of the fibers during defecation permits a straightening at this junction. During childbirth, the action of the levator ani muscles directs the fetal head into the lower part of the passageway.

Vascular, Nerve, and Lymphatic Supply of the Reproductive System

The blood supply of the female pelvis is derived from the internal iliac branches of the common iliac artery and is supplemented by the ovarian, superior rectal, and median sacral arteries, which are branches of the aorta.

The nerve supply of the female pelvis comes from the autonomic nerves that enter the pelvis in the superior hypogastric plexus (presacral nerve). The lymphatics of the female pelvis either follow the course of the vessels to the iliac and preaortic nodes or empty into the inguinal glands (Figure 14-6).

Perioperative Nursing Considerations

Assessment

Quality perioperative patient care depends on thorough nursing assessment and planning skills. Gynecologic patient information is gathered through nursing and physician interviews, evaluation of the patient's systems, physical examination, collection of medical and surgical histories (Box 14-1), and thorough diagnostic testing.

FIGURE 14-5 Muscles of the female pelvis viewed from above. The sacral nerve roots have been divided close to the sacral foramina. The anorectal junction, vagina, and urethra have been divided at the level of the pelvic floor.

FIGURE 14-6 Major lymphatics of the pelvis. The major lymph nodes of the pelvis follow the major vessels. Each group of nodes receives contributions from multiple organs. The groupings are somewhat arbitrary because there is no distinct separation of individual node groups.

Family history of gynecologic disease, hypertension, diabetes, and heart disease are vital elements to consider when assessing and planning patient care.

Skillful interpersonal communication techniques are essential components to any nursing assessment. Patient interviews are conducted in ambulatory surgical centers, preoperative holding rooms, and on hospital patient care units. During this preoperative period the perioperative nurse provides support and patient education, and obtains information to help prepare for the surgical procedure and

nursing plan of care (Goodman and Spry, 2014). Privacy is provided during the patient's perioperative interview whenever possible, providing a safe environment for sharing information between patient and perioperative nurse. Questions concerning reproduction and gynecologic history may embarrass or be distressful for the patient. Personal values, native language, and cultural beliefs are all considered and respected during the interview process.

Throughout the assessment the perioperative nurse remains open, nonbiased, compassionate, and supportive to assist in establishing a trusting therapeutic relationship. Creating a trusting relationship also facilitates the nurse's assessment for intimate partner violence (IPV). IPV is a major health concern worldwide (Shaver et al, 2013). A World Health Organization (WHO) multi-country study found 15% to 71% of women have reported an experience of IPV in their lifetime (WHO, 2011). The perioperative nurse must identify and understand the warning signs of IPV. The patient's concerns for her own safety during the perioperative period and beyond are also addressed (Patient Safety).

The gynecologic patient's history includes a chronologic listing of each pregnancy, length of gestation, type of delivery, complications during pregnancy, duration of labor, and fetal weight. Her menstrual cycle is discussed and data should include age at onset, length of cycle, amount of flow, duration of bleeding, and any pain or discomfort associated during her menses. The amount of flow is described in relation to number of pads and tampons used during her menstrual cycle. Onset of menopause is also documented when applicable. Additional considerations for the gynecologic assessment are noted in Box 14-1. See the laboratory values in Appendix A for common studies in the reproductive assessment of gynecologic patients.

Gynecologic disorders may be associated with urinary problems. The perioperative nurse inquires about stress incontinence or loss of urine while coughing, sneezing, exercising, or laughing. Getting up at night to urinate may reflect irritative changes in the bladder,

BOX 14-1

Focused Assessment for Gynecologic Patients

Gynecologic History
- Prior Papanicolaou (Pap) smears, human papillomavirus (HPV) testing and results
- Prior abnormal Pap smears, how treated, follow-up
- Recent gynecologic procedures
- Past gynecologic procedures or surgery (e.g., tubal ligation, hysterectomy, oophorectomy, laparoscopy, cryosurgery, conization)
- Sexually transmitted infections (STIs)
- Pelvic inflammatory disease (PID)
- Vaginal infections
- Cancer of reproductive organs or related cancers (breast, colorectal)

Menstrual History
- Age of menarche
- Date of last menstrual period: first day of last cycle
- Number of days in cycle and regularity of cycle
- Character of flow: amount (number of pads or tampons used in 24 hours on heaviest days), duration, presence of clots
- Dysmenorrhea: characteristics, duration, frequency (occurs with each cycle?), relief measures
- Intermenstrual bleeding or spotting: amount, duration, frequency, timing and relation to phase of cycle
- Intermenstrual pain: severity, duration, timing; association with ovulation
- Premenstrual symptoms: headaches, weight gain, edema, breast tenderness, irritability or mood changes, frequency (occur with every period?), interference with activities of daily living, relief measures

Abnormal Bleeding
- Character: shortened interval between periods (<19-21 days), lengthened interval between periods (>37 days), amenorrhea, prolonged menses (>7 days), bleeding between periods; postmenopausal bleeding
- Change in flow: nature of change, number of pads/tampons used in 24 hours (tampons/pads soaked?), presence of clots
- Associated symptoms: pain, cramping, abdominal distention, pelvic fullness, change in bowel habits, weight loss or gain
- Medications: oral contraceptives; hormones; tamoxifen

Pain
- Temporal sequence: date and time of onset, sudden versus gradual onset, course since onset, duration, recurrence
- Character: specific location, type, and intensity of pain
- Associated symptoms: vaginal discharge or bleeding, gastrointestinal symptoms, abdominal distention or tenderness, pelvic fullness
- Association with menstrual cycle; timing, location, duration, changes
- Relationship to body functions and activities: voiding, eating, defecation, flatus, exercise, walking up stairs, bending, stretching, sexual activity
- Aggravating or relieving factors
- Previous medical care for this problem
- Efforts to treat
- Medications: analgesics

Vaginal Discharge
- Character, amount, color, odor, consistency, changes in characteristics
- Occurrence: acute or chronic
- Douching habits
- Clothing habits: use of cotton or ventilated underwear and pantyhose, tight pants or jeans
- Presence of discharge or symptoms in sexual partner
- Use of condoms
- Associated symptoms: pruritus; tender, inflamed, or bleeding external tissues; dyspareunia; dysuria or burning on urination; abdominal pain or cramping; pelvic fullness
- Efforts to treat: antifungal vaginal cream
- Medications: oral contraceptives; antibiotics

Sexual History
- Current sexual activity: number of current and previous partners; number of their partners; gender of partner(s), sexual preference
- Method(s) of contraception: current and past; satisfaction with
- Use of barrier protection for STIs
- Prior STIs
- Problems: pain on penetration (entry or deep); decreased lubrication, lack of orgasm
- Use of recreational drugs

Obstetric History
- G: gravida: total number of pregnancies
- T: number of **t**erm pregnancies
- P: number of **p**reterm pregnancies
- A: number of **a**bortions, spontaneous or induced
- L: number of **l**iving children
- Complications of pregnancy, delivery, abortion, or with fetus or neonate
- Duration of labor, fetal weight
- Diabetes (gestational)

Infertility
- Length of time attempting pregnancy, sexual activity pattern, knowledge of fertile period in menstrual cycle, length of cycle
- Abnormalities of vagina, cervix, uterus, fallopian tubes, ovaries
- Contributing factors: stress, nutrition, chemical substances
- Factors relating to partner's fertility
- Diagnostic evaluation to date

Menopausal History
- Age at menopause or currently experiencing
- Associated symptoms: menstrual changes, mood changes, tension, hot flashes
- Postmenopausal bleeding
- Birth control measures during menopause
- General feelings about menopause: self-image, effect on intimate relationships
- Mother's experience with menopause
- Medications: hormone therapy; dose and duration, related side effects: breast tenderness, bloating, vaginal bleeding; serum estrogen receptor modulators, related side effects: hot flashes, breast tenderness
- Use of complementary and alternative therapies

Modified from Seidel HM et al: *Mosby's guide to physical examination*, ed 7, St Louis, 2011, Mosby.

PATIENT SAFETY

Assessment Techniques for Intimate Partner Violence (IPV)

IPV can be defined as the actual or threatened physical, sexual, psychologic, or emotional abuse by a spouse, ex-spouse, boyfriend, girlfriend, ex-boyfriend, ex-girlfriend, date, or cohabitating partner. IPV may also include rape and stalking. Abuse or violence crosses all ages and segments of society; it is not limited to certain economic groups or educational level.

Nurses and other healthcare providers may represent the first and only contact that an isolated woman will seek outside of the abusive relationship and are a primary source of relief; therefore, screening for IPV should be an integral part of the perioperative assessment. A variety of screening tools is available and summarized in the CDC publication, *Intimate Partner Violence and Sexual Violence Victimization Assessment Instruments for Use in Healthcare Settings.* Characteristics common to the tools include trying to normalize the conversation with neutral opening statements, such as, "In this health service, we are concerned about your health and safety, so we ask all women about violence and safety at home. Are you ever afraid of your partner?" In addition, healthcare providers should use direct questions when violence is suspected, such as, "Have you ever been hit, kicked, or punched by someone close to you?"

Cues to abuse include delay in seeking medical assistance (hours or days), vague explanations of injuries, nonspecific complaints, a partner who seems reluctant to leave the woman alone with the healthcare provider, and substance abuse. Physical signs include new and old injuries to the face, breasts, abdomen, and buttocks; fractures that have a suspicious etiology; injuries at various stages of healing; and patterns that indicate injuries made by biting or fist/hand patterns. Pregnant women have an increased risk for IPV and therefore should be thoroughly assessed by the perioperative nurse.

If the nurse suspects IPV, he or she is mandated in most states to report the abuse. Domestic violence is considered a crime in all states, but the category (e.g., misdemeanor or felony) varies by state definition. Nurses must be aware and knowledgeable of the reporting requirements for the state in which they reside. In addition to reporting the abuse or suspected abuse, the nurse must document the findings in the medical record. If appropriate to the situation, photographs can be taken and included in the record.

Nurses in ambulatory surgery must assess the patient's safety before she is discharged and provide her with written information about her legal options, shelters, crisis intervention services, and counseling. The National Domestic Violence Hotline (1-800-799-SAFE) is available 24 hours a day, 7 days a week. Nurses also facilitate patient safety by providing education to women and empowering their understanding that abuse is a violation of their basic human rights, promoting assertiveness, and recommending resources that enhance their independence.

Modified from Centers for Disease Control and Prevention (CDC): *Intimate partner violence and sexual violence victimization assessment instruments for use in healthcare settings,* available at www.cdc.gov/NCIPC/pub-res/images/IPVandSVscreening.pdf. Accessed February 23, 2013; Esposito N: Violence against women. In Lowdermilk DL et al, editors: *Maternity and women's health care,* ed 10, St Louis, 2012, Mosby; World Health Organization (WHO): *Violence against women fact sheet,* November 2012, available at www.who.int/mediacentre/factsheets/fs239/en. Accessed February 23, 2013.

shifting of extravascular fluids in the recumbent position, or decreased bladder capacity. Any urgency, pain or burning sensations during urination is also assessed.

A medication history includes the use of analgesics, oral contraceptives, estrogen therapy, diuretics, antihypertensives, cardiac medications, and use of herbal supplements or nutraceuticals. Herbal supplements can interfere with the patient's ability to clot effectively during surgery (e.g., vitamins C and E and St. John's wort) (see Chapter 30 for a thorough discussion of integrative therapies). It is essential to note the name, frequency, dose, and duration of all medications in the patient's record during the perioperative assessment. The nurse continues the assessment by reviewing the physician's history and physical examination, lab results, and results of any diagnostic studies. This knowledge assists with planning intraoperative care.

The gynecologic patient may undergo numerous preoperative diagnostic studies. The studies performed depend on the gynecologic problem or disease. Some studies performed as part of preoperative assessment include ultrasonography, computed tomography (CT) scanning, and magnetic resonance imaging (MRI). Each of these studies contributes to the evaluation of patients suspected of having a malignancy and/or possible disease involvement of other surrounding organs. Vaginal and pelvic ultrasonography assists with diagnosing adnexal disease, endometrial hyperplasia, and uterine fibroids, as well as detecting blood or fluid within the pelvis.

Hysterosalpingograms or sonohysterograms are commonly performed in radiology and used to identify abnormalities in the uterine cavity or possible occlusions within the tubal folds. These diagnostic tools are most useful in detecting causes of infertility and identifying intrauterine masses that appear as endometrial thickening on routine ultrasound.

A colposcopy, with binocular magnification, is often performed in the surgeon's office. Patients who have an abnormal Papanicolaou (Pap) smear suggestive of dysplasia undergo this examination. Colposcopy identifies cellular abnormalities involving the vulva, vagina, or cervix and helps to identify localized areas of dysplasia and carcinoma in situ. Endocervical curettage samples can be obtained during the colposcopic procedure to rule out invasive carcinoma or to detect early adenocarcinoma of the cervix.

Gynecologic Carcinoma. Gynecologic cancers commonly occur in the cervix, ovaries, vagina, and endometrial layer of the uterus. Less common sites for gynecologic carcinomas are the vulva and fallopian tubes. Some risk factors associated with gynecologic cancers are human papillomavirus (HPV) infection, inherited familial predisposition to cancer, such as Lynch syndrome (hereditary nonpolyposis colorectal cancer [HNPCC]) and *BRCA* gene mutation carriers. Other risk factors linked with the development of these cancers are noted in Table 14-1.

Endometrial cancer (Figure 14-7) is responsible for the most new cases of gynecologic cancer per year in the United States. This includes uterine sarcomas, which account for approximately 2% of the total number of endometrial cancers. It is estimated 1 in 38 women will be diagnosed with endometrial cancer during their lifetime. Patients with this type of cancer may be asymptomatic or they may experience postmenopausal bleeding as their primary symptom. Most women diagnosed are older than 50 years of age (American Cancer Society [ACS], 2012).

TABLE 14-1

Risk Factors for Cancers of the Reproductive System

Risk Factor	Endometrial Cancer	Cervical Cancer	Ovarian Cancer	Vulvar Cancer	Vaginal Cancer	Fallopian Tube Cancer
Age	Increased with age		Infrequent before 40 yr; range usually is 40-65 yr	After 50 yr; peak is 60-70 yr	Most after 40 yr; most cases are 70 yr or older	Occurs mostly in 50-60 yr of age
Family history	Increased risk	Increased risk	Increased risk	—	DES exposure	Increased risk
Personal history	Diabetes, hypertension, late menopause, women in reproductive years, breast or ovarian cancer may increase risk	Multiple sex partners, first intercourse at younger than 18 yr of age	Breast, bowel, or endometrial cancer, *BRCA1* or *BRCA2* gene, endometriosis, high-fat diet	Cervical cancer, diabetes, vulvar disease	Cervical cancer, alcohol use, multiple sex partners	Ovarian, *BRCA1* gene
Body size	Obese	Obese	Obese	—	Obese	—
Parity	Nulliparity	Multiparity	Nulliparity	—	Multiparity	—
Estrogen use	Prolonged use without shielding effects of progesterone	Possibly long-term birth control pill use	Prolonged use increases risk	—	Oral contraceptive use	—
Smoking	Increased risk	Possibly double the risk	—	Increased risk	Increased risk	—
Infection (STI)	—	Possibly STI (herpes simplex virus type 2 or papillomavirus infection)	—	Possibly (papillomavirus infection), Lichen sclerosus (LSA), HIV	HIV, STI (papillomavirus infection)	—

DES, Diethylstilbestrol; *HIV,* human immunodeficiency virus; *STI,* sexually transmitted infection.
Modified from Ignatavicius DD, Workman ML: Diseases and disorders. In Ignatavicius DD, Workman ML, editors: *Medical-surgical nursing: patient-centered collaborative care,* ed 7, St Louis, 2013, Saunders; American Society of Clinical Oncology (ASCO): *Fallopian tube cancer,* Alexandria, VA, 2012, available at www.cancer.net/cancer-types/fallopian-tube-cancer/risk-factors-and-prevention. Accessed February 23, 2013; American Cancer Society (ACS): *Vulvar cancer,* Atlanta, 2012, The Society, available at www.cancer.org/cancer/vulvarcancer/detailedguide/vulvar-cancer-risk-factors. Accessed February 23, 2013.

FIGURE 14-7 Total abdominal hysterectomy (TAH) and bilateral salpingo-oophorectomy (BSO) showing large polypoid adenocarcinoma of the endometrium with deep myometrial invasion.

Invasive cervical cancer is diagnosed in about 12,000 women a year. HPV is one of the main causative factors of cervical cancer. Increased Pap smear screening provides a means of early detection and aids in cancer treatment and lower mortality rates (Table 14-2). Pap smears detect early changes in cervical cells and thus initiate prompt treatment. In its early invasive stage, cervical cancer may be asymptomatic or associated with painless vaginal spotting, postcoital bleeding, or irregular intermenstrual bleeding. During the early preinvasive stage, the disease may be described as dysplasia. From moderate or severe dysplasia, the disease progresses to carcinoma in situ (CIS). Preinvasive cancers may also be designated as cervical intraepithelial neoplasia (CIN) and classed according to severity (ACS, 2012; Lowdermilk, 2012):

CIN 1: Mild
CIN 2: Moderate
CIN 3: Severe, to carcinoma in situ (Figure 14-8)

Ovarian cancer is the leading cause of death from gynecologic malignancies in the United States, affecting women primarily older than age 50. It is frequently diagnosed in the later disease stages due to the absence of early disease symptoms. Signs and symptoms can

TABLE 14-2

Screening Methods for Cervical Cancer: Joint Recommendations of the American Cancer Society, the American Society for Colposcopy and Cervical Pathology, and the American Society for Clinical Pathology

Population	Recommended Screening Method	Comment
Women younger than 21 years	No screening	
Women ages 21-29 years	Cytology alone every 3 years	
Women ages 30-65 years	HPV and cytology co-testing (preferred) every 5 years	Screening by HPV testing alone is not recommended
	Cytology alone (acceptable) every 3 years	
Women older than 65 years	No screening is necessary after adequate negative prior screening results	Women with a history of CIN 2, CIN 3, or adenocarcinoma in situ should continue routine age-based screening for at least 20 years
Women who underwent total hysterectomy	No screening is necessary	Applies to women without a cervix and without a history of CIN 2, CIN 3, adenocarcinoma in situ, or cancer in the past 20 years
Women vaccinated against HPV	Follow age-specific recommendations (same as unvaccinated women)	

CIN, Cervical intraepithelial neoplasia; *HPV*, human papillomavirus
Modified from Saslow D et al: American Cancer Society, American Society for Colposcopy and Cervical Pathology, and American Society for Clinical Pathology screening guidelines for the prevention and early detection of cervical cancer, *CA Cancer J Clin*, 62:147–172, 2012.

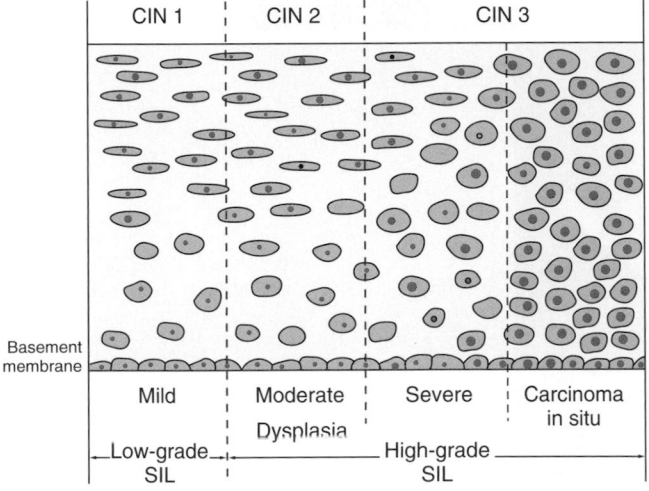

FIGURE 14-8 Diagram of cervical epithelium showing progressive changes and various terms used. *SIL*, Squamous intraepithelial lesion; *CIN*, cervical intraepithelial neoplasm.

FIGURE 14-9 Gross stage IA ovarian cancer. The right ovarian mass is free of adhesions and visible adjacent to a normal fallopian tube and uterine corpus.

be vague and are often accompanied by indicators typically attributable to common gastrointestinal (GI) diseases such as hiatal hernia, diverticular disease, or gallbladder disease. Tumors (Figure 14-9) that are epithelial account for about 95% of ovarian cancers. Germ cell and gonadal stromal cell tumors of ovarian cancer account for 2.5%, respectively, and occur in premenopausal women (ACS, 2012; Fuller, 2011).

Ovarian tumors spread directly to other organs in the abdominal and pelvic cavity because there is approximately 50 mL of normal peritoneal body fluid floating around in these cavities. As the ovary's cells slough off into the abdominal and pelvic cavity, they circulate in the peritoneal fluid and, in turn, continually bathe the abdominal and pelvic cavity organs and the surrounding tissues before being reabsorbed in the right subphrenic space. If an ovary has a cancerous tumor, this "bathing" can promote ovarian cancer seeding

throughout the peritoneum (Fuller, 2011). As expected, early sites of spread are on the right diaphragm or in the right or left paracolic gutters. Seventy-five percent of patients have involvement of their peritoneal organs or omentum when diagnosed (Fuller, 2011).

Vulvar cancer (Figure 14-10) represents about 4% of the gynecologic reproductive cancers and is typically slow growing. It appears most often in women during their middle 60s to 70s. In younger women the incidence is often linked to genital warts (condylomata acuminata) caused by HPV. Symptoms include irritation and pruritus or nonhealing lesions in the perineal area (ACS, 2012; Lowdermilk, 2012).

Vaginal cancer is rare. Approximately 1 out of every 100 women who are diagnosed with a reproductive cancer is diagnosed with vaginal cancer. There are fewer than 1000 deaths per year (ACS, 2012) associated with this disease. Vaginal cancer is usually

FIGURE 14-10 Cancer of the vulva. **A,** T1 lesion on the right side of the vulva. **B,** Defect after excision of the primary lesion. **C,** Postoperative results after closure and node dissection via separate incisions.

associated with previously treated cervical cancer or precancer. It is generally asymptomatic in the early stages and may be accompanied by bleeding after coitus, dyspareunia, and foul-smelling discharge; urinary symptoms develop in the later stages (Lowdermilk, 2012).

Fallopian tube cancer is very rare, with an incidence of less than 1%. Symptoms include vaginal bleeding, vaginal discharge, and lower abdominal pain. This type of cancer is often misdiagnosed as ovarian because of contiguous growth, or endometrial cancer because it may present with postmenopausal bleeding (Lowdermilk, 2012).

Nursing Diagnosis

Perioperative nursing care is a planned process that is implemented to ensure safe, effective, surd efficient patient outcomes. Nursing

diagnoses are formulated after reviewing the patient's record and conducting a patient assessment. All significant data collected are reviewed and prioritized, then incorporated into the perioperative plan of care. The gynecologic patient may have multiple nursing diagnoses that warrant perioperative nursing interventions including the following:

- Anxiety and Disturbed Body Image related to planned surgical intervention
- Risk for Urinary Retention related to edema, anesthesia, opioids, or pain
- Risk for Infection at the surgical site related to operative or other invasive procedures
- Risk for Hypothermia
- Risk for Perioperative Positioning Injury

Outcome Identification

Outcomes identified for the selected nursing diagnoses could be stated as the following:

- The patient will verbalize reduced or controlled anxiety and acknowledge feelings regarding her body image (as applicable).
- The patient will maintain or regain normal patterns of urinary elimination.
- The patient will remain free from a surgical site infection.
- The patient will remain normothermic.
- The patient will be free from injury related to surgical positioning.

Planning

Planning enables the perioperative nurse to provide patient care in an organized and individualized manner. Planning involves preparation for both psychosocial and physiologic needs. Part of planning efficient and effective patient care is gathering the necessary equipment and supplies, positioning accessories, surgical devices, and adjuncts requisite to the specific gynecologic surgical intervention. For example, if the gynecologic patient is undergoing a lengthy surgical procedure, the perioperative nurse has available a forced-air warming device, pressure-reducing positioning devices, graduated compression stockings, and intermittent pneumatic compression devices. Undertaking these actions assists with maintaining the patient's body temperature, promoting skin integrity, and preventing venous stasis, aiding in the prevention of thrombus or emboli formation. Nursing interventions that will help the gynecologic patient reach desired outcomes are identified for each patient. Examples of interventions for the gynecologic patient are shown in the Sample Plan of Care box on page 416.

Implementation

During implementation of the plan of care, the perioperative nurse performs the identified nursing interventions. Implementation includes gathering the appropriate instruments and patient care supplies, positioning the patient on the operating room (OR) bed, performing antimicrobial skin preparation, inserting urinary catheters, draping the patient, creating and maintaining a sterile field, initiating safety measures, and monitoring the patient. Throughout the patient's perioperative experience, data continue to be collected, the plan of care is adjusted, and documentation is updated. Informative comprehensive handoff reports are given to all relief personnel, ensuring continuity with the patient's plan of care.

Instrumentation. The planned gynecologic surgical procedure and any anticipated intraoperative surgical interventions will determine what instrumentation is needed. A basic vaginal instrument tray (also referred to as a "kit" or "tray") is required for vaginal and vulvar surgery. A basic open abdominal gynecologic instrument tray is required for open abdominal gynecologic surgery. Laparoscopic, hysteroscopic, or robotic specialized instruments are used during minimally invasive surgery. Surgeon's instrument preferences as well as each facility's instrument tray components will vary. The instrumentation described in this chapter is not meant to be all-inclusive. For most abdominal gynecologic procedures, a dilation and curettage (D&C) tray is available.

Positioning. Patient positioning principles, methods, and safety measures for different types of surgical procedures are described in Chapter 6. Stirrups for the lithotomy position may support only the patient's feet (canvas, fabric, or gel-pad ankle straps) or may

cradle and support the thighs, popliteal spaces, and lower legs. Padded cradle stirrups promote maintenance of skin integrity and aid in preventing nerve injury (such as peroneal neuropathy). The nurse anticipates that the patient's position may be modified based on the surgical procedure and surgeon's preference. The patient is placed in lithotomy position for most vaginal and vulvar surgery. Careful attention is focused on preventing injury and vascular compression. The patient's legs are supported above and below the knee joint while positioning to prevent hyperextension of the knee. The perioperative nurse seeks assistance during positioning the patient in lithotomy to ensure the legs are raised and lowered simultaneously.

For abdominal gynecologic surgery, Trendelenburg (low or standard) position may be used. This position facilitates access to the pelvic and para-aortic lymph nodes. It further allows access to the sigmoid colon if a sigmoid resection is required due to the involvement of metastatic disease.

Maximum or steep Trendelenburg position is used during robotic surgery for exposure of the pelvic organs. This position allows gravity to assist the bowel in falling back into the abdominal cavity and out of the pelvis, providing optimal exposure.

Patients placed in Trendelenburg position for prolonged gynecologic procedures are at increased cardiovascular risk because of decreased pulmonary compliance and functional residual capacity (FRC) (Cassorla and Lee, 2009). Whenever possible, position the patient's arms on padded armboards with the palms up and fingers extended to prevent ulnar nerve injury. Armboards are maintained at less than a 90-degree angle to prevent stretching of the brachial plexus. If there are surgical reasons to tuck the arms at the patient's side, pad the patient's elbows to protect the ulnar nerve, face the palms inward toward the hip, and maintain the wrists in a neutral position (Cassorla and Lee, 2009; Denholm, 2009). A folded drawsheet under the patient is used to secure the arms. The drawsheet is wrapped over the patient's arms and then snugly tucked directly under the patient, not under the mattress. This prevents the arm from shifting downward intraoperatively and resting against the OR bed rail, where it could be inadvertently injured. Care is taken to protect all patients from integumentary, musculoskeletal, and nerve injury while ensuring adequate circulatory, renal, and respiratory functions.

The bladder is often decompressed at the beginning of the procedure by placing a straight (in and out) or indwelling urinary catheter to monitor urinary output. This practice can also aid in the prevention of bladder injury. The surgeon may request the perioperative nurse to inflate the bladder intraoperatively with normal saline to assist in determining bladder margins.

The size of sutures, needles, and drains also varies depending on the surgical procedure, surgeon preference, and patient needs. The perioperative nurse consults with the surgeon prior to the procedure to ensure all essential items are readily available.

Prepping. Skin preparation and routine draping procedures are described in Chapter 4. Care is taken to prevent cross-contamination and to avoid pooling under the patient when prepping multiple areas, as in an abdominal hysterectomy. Prep the abdomen before beginning the vaginal prep, using the clean to dirty principle. Care is taken to avoid splashing of vaginal prepping solution onto the already prepped abdomen. Two separate prepping setups are used and kept separate. The perioperative nurse takes care when performing vaginal preps on patients who have been experiencing vaginal bleeding and may have clots in the vaginal vault. The clots and any

SAMPLE PLAN OF CARE

Nursing Diagnosis
Anxiety and Disturbed Body Image related to planned surgical intervention

Outcome
The patient will verbalize reduced or controlled anxiety and acknowledge feelings regarding her body image (as applicable).

Interventions
- Determine the patient's previous experience and expectations with surgery as well as her level of knowledge related to the planned surgical intervention (see Patient-Centered Care).
- Assess the patient's level of anxiety and physical reactions to anxiety (e.g., tachycardia, tachypnea, blood pressure elevation, and nonverbal expressions of anxiety); classify her anxiety as low, moderate, or high.
- Use presence and touch (if welcome) to communicate comfort and caring. Acknowledge denial, anger, or depression as normal feelings when adjusting to change in body image or function. Determine and respect her personal space.
- Provide time for and encourage expression of concerns or needs. Clarify and correct any misconceptions she may express about her diagnosis and the effect it will have on her body image.
- Explore coping skills previously used by the patient to relieve anxiety (e.g., relaxation, deep breathing, imagery, or listening to music); reinforce these skills or techniques and facilitate their use.
- Explain the sequence of perioperative nursing activities and procedures, using nonmedical terms and clear, concise language that the patient can understand. Encourage questions and expression of concerns. Reinforce information provided by other healthcare team members.
- Minimize environmental stimuli and noise while maintaining patient's privacy.

Nursing Diagnosis
Risk for Urinary Retention related to edema, anesthesia, opioids, or pain

Outcome
The patient will maintain or regain normal patterns of urinary elimination.

Interventions
- Before surgery, explain that an indwelling or temporary (straight) catheter will be inserted (if applicable).
- Verify the absence of any latex allergy; a latex-free catheter will be required for latex-allergic patients.
- Insert indwelling or straight catheter using aseptic technique.
- Secure tubing to prevent inadvertent stretching or stress on catheter.
- Document size of catheter inserted.
- Keep drainage bag below the level of the bladder.
- Observe and document the color and amount of urine on insertion; report abnormalities preoperatively or postoperatively to the surgeon.
- Check patency of catheter and drainage system whenever patient is repositioned.
- Discuss with the patient the importance of adequate postoperative fluid intake and early ambulation.
- Clarify any patient misconceptions.
- Encourage the patient to verbalize feelings and concerns regarding inability to void postoperatively and discomfort or pain associated with the presence of an indwelling catheter.

Nursing Diagnosis
Risk for Infection at the surgical site related to operative or other invasive procedures

Outcome
The patient will remain free from surgical site infection.

Interventions
- Administer and document antibiotic prophylaxis as prescribed. Follow safe practices for all medications administered.
- Initiate measures to warm patient and maintain normothermia.
- Prepare surgical site with an antiseptic solution; document skin condition at surgical site and solution used.
- Apply dressing to surgical site before sterile drapes are removed to prevent contamination of incision.
- Use infection prevention and control practices.
- Maintain aseptic technique, and monitor members of the surgical team for breaks in technique.
- Correctly classify surgical wound at end of procedure.
- Document presence, location, and type of any drains inserted during surgical intervention.
- Review with patient signs and symptoms of infection at surgical site:
  - Redness
  - Swelling
  - Warmth
  - Tenderness
  - Pain
- Discuss importance of proper handwashing techniques, especially when changing surgical wound dressings, as applicable.

Nursing Diagnosis
Risk for Hypothermia

Outcome
The patient will remain risk free of hypothermia.

Interventions
- Initiate measures to warm patient and maintain normothermia. Begin with preoperative warming and continue intraoperatively.
- Prevent unnecessary skin exposure when prepping, positioning, or moving the patient.
- Place a forced-air warming blanket on patient after transfer to OR bed.
- Use warm IV and irrigating fluids (as applicable).

Nursing Diagnosis
Risk for Perioperative Positioning Injury

Outcome
The patient will be free from injury related to surgical positioning.

Interventions
- Note and document any preexisting patient considerations (e.g., nutritional status, weight, preoperative chemotherapy, limitations in mobility or range of motion, neurovascular impairments) that place the patient at risk for positioning injury.
- Use adequate numbers of personnel to transfer and position the patient.
- Place safety belts and straps on the patient and secure to the OR bed without friction or undo pressure.
- Assess and document condition of dependent skin areas.
- Use pressure-reducing positioning devices.
- Pad and protect bony prominences and dependent pressure sites.
- Maintain proper body alignment.
- Provide graduated compression stockings and intermittent pneumatic compression devices as indicated.
- Reassess padding and protection during any positional changes.

gross blood on the thighs or vulva must be removed before beginning the prep. This practice ensures the prepping solution will come into contact with the skin and all mucous membranes of the perineum and vaginal area. Women who have undergone radiation of the pelvis, as well as younger and older female patients, may have narrow or foreshortened vaginal vaults. Take extra care when prepping these patients.

Examination Under Anesthesia (EUA). Many physicians perform a pelvic examination after the patient is anesthetized and positioned, but before the operative site is prepped. The perioperative nurse anticipates this examination and ensures nonsterile gloves and an appropriate lubricant is available. Culture specimens (e.g., gonococcal, chlamydial, trichomonal) and a Pap smear may be obtained during the examination. Verify with the surgeon that the lubricants used are compatible with cytologic evaluation. Safe specimen practices are initiated.

Dressings, Drains, and Packing. Various dressings are used in gynecologic surgery and may range from simple (e.g., wound closure tapes and surgical skin glue) to complex (e.g., multilayer gauze, ostomy appliances, and abdominal binders). Perineal pads and mesh pants are often used in combination after vaginal surgery.

Closed or open drains may be used with or without a reservoir. Indwelling catheters are also commonly used in gynecologic surgery. All drains and catheters are secured for patient comfort and to avoid dislodgement. Verify the patient does not have a latex allergy because many of these drains contain latex.

Packing may be used in fistulas or other abnormally created cavities, to support and stent the vagina, absorb postoperative drainage, or aid in hemostasis. Products used for vaginal packing can include narrow or large fine-mesh gauze available in various yardages. Vaginal packing is usually moistened with saline or coated with antibiotic, antifungal, or an estrogen cream before insertion. Packing is inserted with care to avoid distention of the vaginal vault and compression of its vascular structures. If the length of packing needs to be cut, then it is documented in the patient's record and communicated during the patient handoff report. This ensures all vaginal packing is accounted for when removed postoperatively.

Evaluation

During evaluation the perioperative nurse determines whether the patient met the previously established outcomes. Some outcomes can be reached during the preoperative and intraoperative phases of care; they are evaluated before the patient's discharge from the OR. Others require ongoing monitoring and measurement in the postoperative phase; these are denoted by the word "will" to indicate their ongoing nature. Part of the perioperative nursing handoff report to the postanesthesia care unit (PACU) includes the outcomes of the nursing plan of care. They can be phrased as follows:

- The patient will effectively cope with her anxiety and disturbance in body image; questions will continue to be answered and misconceptions clarified. Patient's anxiety was reduced; she verbalized concerns and used personally effective coping strategies.
- Urinary elimination patterns and patency were maintained; urinary output was adequate. Color and amount of urine were monitored for any changes, documented in patient record, and communicated with surgeon and the anesthesia provider.
- The patient's skin integrity and surgical asepsis were maintained.
- Normothermia was maintained.
- There was no apparent evidence of injury related to surgical positioning; range-of-motion and neurovascular status were consistent with preoperative levels.

In addition, the perioperative nurse evaluates and reports the patient's alertness and orientation status, pain level, and respiratory status in the perioperative nursing handoff report to the PACU nurse.

Patient and Family Education and Discharge Planning

Patient and family education, along with discharge planning, are critical perioperative nursing activities. Many gynecologic surgical procedures are performed on an outpatient basis, both in hospitals and ambulatory surgical centers. Hospital length of stays for patients requiring admission after their surgical procedure continues to decrease. Therefore, patient education and discharge planning begin before admission in preadmission testing. Regardless of the gynecologic procedure performed, the perioperative nurse begins patient and family education with vital postoperative care information.

The main goal is to restore normal body function and may include early ambulation, prevention of respiratory complications, wound care, anticipated postoperative discomfort, managing postoperative pain, restrictions in activity, diet, and any other patient concerns. Topics such as progression of activities, returning to work, lifting limitations, emotional and physical issues, sexual activity, general nutritional needs, and health maintenance aid in guiding the educational process.

Gynecologic patients are provided with specific information regarding postoperative signs and symptoms to report, especially in relation to vaginal bleeding and the surgical wound, along with restrictions related to douching and vaginal penetration (tampons or sexual intercourse). Today, patients may go home on the same day of their surgical procedure or be admitted for a 23-hour stay (Ambulatory Surgery Considerations). Simple, clear information and instructions such as those presented in the Patient and Family Education box help enhance patient learning and understanding.

Lasers in Gynecologic Surgery

Carbon dioxide (CO_2) and argon lasers are used in gynecology to treat extrauterine disease such as pelvic endometriosis, cervical dysplasia, condylomata acuminata, pelvic adhesive disease, and premalignant diseases of the vulva and vagina. Lasers are generally used in conjunction with the colposcope and operating microscope,

AMBULATORY SURGERY CONSIDERATIONS

Minimally Invasive Gynecologic Surgery

A variety of gynecologic surgical procedures can be performed using minimally invasive techniques. An advantage of minimally invasive surgery (MIS) is that patients can be discharged on the same day of surgery or within 23 hours of admission. Nurses who are involved in MIS gynecologic ambulatory procedures should consider the following factors when planning and implementing perioperative patient care.

Preoperative Care

Preoperative care of patients undergoing MIS focuses on early patient teaching. Provide patients with written and verbal instructions, review preadmission procedures, and alleviate concerns or confusion. Teaching focuses on the following issues:

- Explaining the specifics of the particular surgical procedure: provide educational pamphlets or informative websites such as for robotic surgical procedures. Be sure websites show a Health on the Net (HON) code of conduct seal.
- Alleviating anxiety: ensure the patient understands the surgeon is controlling the robot and the robot is just a surgical tool that aids the surgeon to be more efficient and effective.
- Explaining expectant levels of postoperative pain and any activity limitations: remember that patients and their families will be providing much of the postoperative care at home after surgery.
- Explaining possible complications: review signs and symptoms to watch for and ensure the patient knows when to contact her healthcare provider about problems (e.g., infection).
- Teaching care of the operative site: provide written instructions when teaching because preoperative anxiety may distract the patient's attention and her comprehension of teaching material. These instructions are reviewed postoperatively, prior to discharge.
- Preprocedural screening of patients: aimed at identifying risks for infection, clotting disorders, hypertension, heart or lung disease, and numerous other diseases that may interfere with the patient's care. The patient's general health is assessed to ensure she can tolerate the procedure and the anesthesia plan of care. MIS procedures use gas (usually

CO_2) to create visual space in the peritoneum—a pneumoperitoneum. Insufflation with CO_2 can cause cardiopulmonary and hemodynamic complications.

The following are complications associated with CO_2 insufflation:

- Hyperkalemia
- Pulmonary complications
- Cardiovascular and vascular complications
- Subcutaneous emphysema
- Metabolic inflammatory responses
- Gas embolism (rare)

Intraoperative Care

Intraoperative care is specific to the planned procedure. In robotic procedures the nursing team must know how to set up, calibrate, and operate the robotic system. During surgery, monitoring cues and messages from the robotic system is important. Troubleshooting is critical to ensure patient safety and to avoid prolonging the procedure. Knowing emergency protocols is vital in MIS and robotic procedures. The surgical team may find that developing a checklist for surgical emergencies such as converting to an open procedure assists in efficient care rather than relying on memory alone (Arriaga et al, 2013).

Postoperative Care

Postoperative care of the MIS patient is provided according to the same standards as those of traditional surgery. Early care focuses on stabilizing the patient, maintaining pain control, carefully monitoring the operative site, carefully monitoring vital signs and level of consciousness, and following specific care requisites for the particular procedure.

Because the length of stay for these patients is generally short, keen assessment skills are important to handle issues before discharge. Teaching within the shortened timeframe may be impeded by patients and family who are not ready to learn because of postoperative pain or the effects of anesthesia. The nurse always provides verbal and written discharge instructions, has the patient or family member teach back key points, and, when possible, follows up with the patient and her family after discharge to ensure that complications do not arise and patients are having no problems following instructions.

Modified from Dziedzic ME: *Mosby's nursing consult: clinical updates: nursing challenges in the care of patients who undergo minimally invasive surgery—are you prepared?* January 25, 2013, available at www.nursingconsult.com/nursing/clinical-updates/full-text?clinical_update_id=198886. Accessed February 24, 2013.

or the laparoscope. A laser plume evacuator or suction system is necessary to remove smoke and fumes from the operative field (Association of periOperative Registered Nurses [AORN], 2013). Surgical personnel in the room wear a high-filtration laser mask to prevent exposure from the laser plume and implement laser safety precautions (see Chapter 8 for full discussion of lasers and laser safety).

Surgical Interventions

Vulvar Surgery

A variety of malignant and nonmalignant conditions may affect the vulva. Nonmalignant lesions are generally excised. The treatment of early malignant disease of the vulva is accomplished by a local wide excision, or for more multicentric or extensive lesions, by simple or radical vulvectomy.

Excision of Condylomata Acuminata

Vulvar/perineal condyloma is caused by HPV (Figure 14-11), most commonly the low-risk HPV subtypes, which are transmitted sexually. These warty lesions may extend into the vaginal vault or the anus and may be aggravated by hormonal changes during pregnancy. Depending on the strain of the virus, the condition may be benign or associated with high-risk subtypes of HPV leading to moderate or severe dysplasia and malignancy. Surgical treatment ranges from desiccation of the lesions with a monopolar electrosurgical unit (ESU) to sharp excision or eradication through use of the laser. Surgical intervention is based on the type and extent of the lesions.

PATIENT AND FAMILY EDUCATION

Gynecologic Surgery

Whenever possible, provide the patient and her caregiver with verbal and written instructions. Provide them with the phone number of the physician, nurse practitioner, or physician assistant to call if questions arise. Use visual aids to enhance instruction. Encourage the patient to verbalize any concerns she may have regarding her condition and surgery. Misconceptions about the outcome of gynecologic surgery are common. Patients may believe that undergoing a hysterectomy will cause depression, nervousness, mental instability, weight gain, wrinkles, masculinity, and hirsutism. Provide education to correct any misconceptions, and discuss other concerns, such as fear of death, cancer, loss of femininity and childbearing ability, pain management, and changes in sexuality. Education points for common gynecologic procedures are as follows.

Dilation and Curettage of the Uterus
- Notify physician if an elevated temperature or foul-smelling vaginal discharge develops.
- Clean the perineum after elimination and change perineal pads often.
- Eat foods high in iron and protein to promote tissue repair and red blood cell replacement.
- Avoid sexual intercourse, tub baths, and the use of tampons for 2 weeks to allow healing and prevent infection.
- Slight bleeding is normal. However, if bleeding is as heavy as during your normal menstrual period or if it lasts longer than 2 weeks, call your physician.
- If a procedure was performed for miscarriage, add the following:
  - Mood swings and depression are common after pregnancy loss. It can be helpful to talk to friends, family, or clergy about your loss.
  - Support groups may be helpful in the recovery period.
  - Allow yourself (and your partner) to grieve the loss before becoming pregnant again.
  - Attempts at subsequent pregnancy should be postponed until indicated by your physician.

Endometrial Ablation
- Vaginal discharge is expected for 4 to 6 weeks.
- The next menstrual period may be irregular.
- Analgesics or NSAIDs may be used for pain relief as needed.
- You can return to your normal activities within several days.

- The physician should be called if you have heavy bleeding or signs of infection.
- Avoid sexual intercourse and the use of tampons for 2 weeks to allow healing and prevent infection.

Vulvectomy
- Avoid sexual activity for 4 to 6 weeks or as long as directed by healthcare provider.
- Rest frequently.
- Avoid crossing your legs and sitting or standing for long periods.
- Avoid tight, constricting clothing, and wear cotton underwear.
- Keep your perineal area clean and dry. Rinse perineum after each elimination with warm water, and pat dry.
- Report any temperature greater than 102.2° F (39° C).
- Report any swelling, redness, unusual tenderness, drainage, or foul odor of the incision site to your healthcare provider.
- Eat a well-balanced diet to promote healing.
- Elevate legs periodically to prevent pelvic congestion.

Hysterectomy
- You will no longer have a period, although you may have some vaginal discharge after you go home.
- Eat foods high in protein, iron, and vitamin C to aid tissue healing; include foods with high fiber content, and drink six to eight glasses of water daily.
- Rest when tired; resume activities as comfort level permits. Avoid vigorous exercise and heavy lifting for 6 weeks. Avoid sitting for long periods. Resume driving when comfort allows or on advice from your healthcare provider.
- Avoid tub baths, intercourse, and douching until after your follow-up examination.
- When vaginal intercourse is resumed, use water-soluble lubricants to decrease discomfort.
- Report the following symptoms to your physician: vaginal bleeding, gastrointestinal changes, persistent postoperative symptoms (e.g., cramping, distention, change in bowel habits), and signs of wound infection (e.g., redness, swelling, heat, or pain at the incision site).
- If your ovaries were removed you may experience symptoms of menopause, including hot flashes, night sweats, and vaginal dryness.
- Hormone replacement therapy may be prescribed.

NSAIDs, Nonsteroidal antiinflammatory drugs.
Modified from Lowdermilk DL: Structural disorders and neoplasms of the reproductive system. In Lowdermilk DL, Perry SE, editors: *Maternity and women's health care,* ed 10, St Louis, 2012, Mosby.

Superficial Vulvectomy

Superficial vulvectomy is the removal of the external skin from the affected area, which has been previously identified with a stain such as toluidine blue or acetic acid. The purpose of this procedure is to preserve the underlying structures of the external genitalia. This procedure may be done to treat not only dysplasia but also leukoplakia, intractable pruritus, or other types of skin lesions and chronic venereal granulomas.

Procedural Considerations. The basic vaginal instrument tray is required, plus an ESU, if desired. The nurse assists with placing the patient in the lithotomy position (see Chapter 6 for positioning considerations) and performs a perineal and vaginal prep.

Operative Procedure. The external skin is excised from the affected area (Figure 14-12, *A*).

Simple Vulvectomy

Simple vulvectomy is removal of the labia majora and labia minora, possibly but not preferably the glans clitoris, and occasionally tissue from the perianal area. A simple vulvectomy is usually done to treat carcinoma in situ of the vulva when it is multicentric. Rarely, a simple vulvectomy is necessary for the treatment of either leukoplakia or intractable pruritus.

Procedural Considerations. The instrumentation required and patient positioning is as described for superficial vulvectomy.

FIGURE 14-11 Condylomata acuminata.

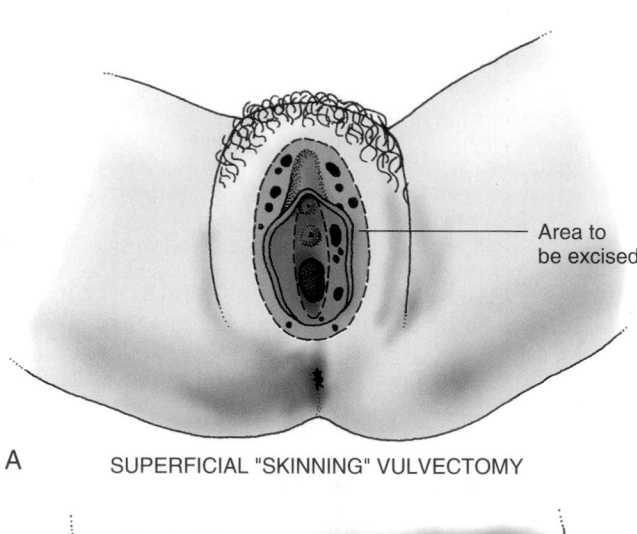

A SUPERFICIAL "SKINNING" VULVECTOMY

Area to
be excised

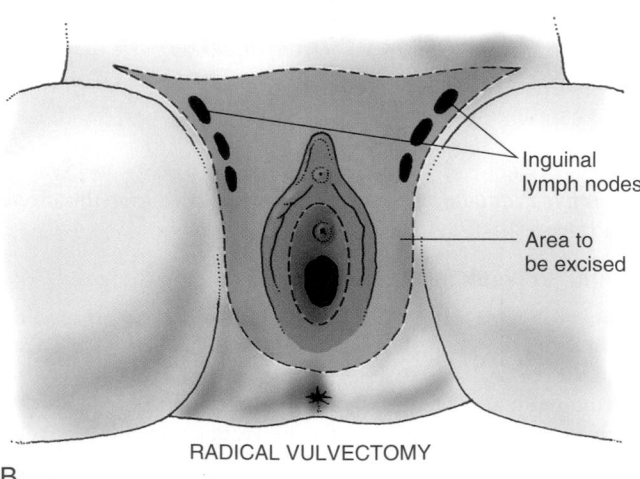

B RADICAL VULVECTOMY

Inguinal
lymph nodes

Area to
be excised

FIGURE 14-12 Outline of incisions used for **(A)** superficial vulvectomy and **(B)** radical vulvectomy.

Operative Procedure

1. The surgeon incises the affected skin, usually starting anteriorly above the clitoris. The incision is continued laterally to the labia majora, to the midline of the perineum, and around the anus, if it is involved. A knife, hemostats, radiopaque gauze sponges on sponge-holding forceps, tissue forceps, and Allis forceps are required. Bleeding vessels are clamped, ligated, or electrocoagulated with the ESU.

2. Periurethral and perivaginal incisions are made. Bleeding of this vascular area can be controlled by means of Kelly or Crile hemostats and electrocoagulation with the ESU. Ligation of blood vessels should be minimal. Allis-Adair forceps are used for holding diseased tissues.

3. Using curved dissecting scissors, tissue forceps, Allis forceps, and sponges on holding forceps, the surgeon undermines and mobilizes the skin and subcutaneous tissues.

4. The wound is closed, usually by simple bilateral Z-plasty. In some cases, the surgeon excises the skin around the anus to accomplish a sliding skin flap.

5. Closed-wound drainage catheters may be placed in the dependent areas, an indwelling urinary catheter is inserted, and vaginal gauze packing may be placed in the vagina. Dressings are applied.

Radical Vulvectomy and Groin Lymphadenectomy

Radical vulvectomy and groin lymphadenectomy involves dissection of the following structures: the labia majora, the labia minora, the clitoris, the mons veneris, and involved terminal portions of the urethra, vagina, and other vulvar organs, as well as the superficial and deep inguinofemoral nodes, portions of the round ligaments, portions of the saphenous veins, and the lesion itself. In the past dissection was carried out en bloc; now as is true with breast surgery and axillary dissection, the procedure is discontinuous, and minimal, if any, skin in the groin is sacrificed. It also may involve reconstruction of the vaginal walls and pelvic floor and closure of the abdominal wounds, if a segment of vagina is resected. A plastic surgeon may complete skin grafts or rotation flaps to cover defects (see Chapter 22).

Radical vulvectomy and groin lymphadenectomy involve abdominoperineal dissection and groin dissection, which may be performed as a one- or two-stage operation. When performed as a one-stage operation, it is optimally done by a four-person perioperative team. The skin prep is extensive, including the abdomen and thighs; if a skin graft is needed, the donor site will be prepped as well. Many such extensive lesions may be alternatively treated with chemoradiation therapy, avoiding loss of intestinal or bladder function. Early lesions may also be treated by sentinel node biopsy (as in breast disease) in order to avoid unnecessary dissection of negative nodes and attendant morbidity, including chronic lymphedema.

Procedural Considerations. The patient lies supine and may be placed in Trendelenburg and low lithotomy positions, as required for the various stages (see Chapter 6 for positioning considerations). The skin prep includes the abdomen, perineum, vagina, and thighs. An indwelling urinary catheter is often inserted to act as a urethral marker and to prevent postoperative urethral trauma. As in other radical surgeries the perioperative nurse is prepared to measure blood loss and anticipates measures to maintain normovolemia (see Chapter 2 for the procedure for weighing sponges to measure blood loss).

For radical vulvectomy the basic vaginal instrument tray is required, with the addition of assorted sizes of Richardson retractors, Volkmann rake retractors, skin hooks, and closed wound drainage systems.

For groin lymphadenectomy the basic abdominal gynecologic instrument tray is required, with the addition of Schmidt tonsil forceps, Kantrowitz right angle thoracic clamps, ligating clips and appliers, suture ties, an ESU, and closed wound drainage systems.

Operative Procedure
Radical Vulvectomy

1. The skin incisions of the abdomen and thigh join with those for vulvectomy. The incisions in the vulva encircle the urethra.
2. In the vulvar dissection the surgeon removes the terminal portions of the urethra and vagina, the mons veneris, the clitoris, the frenulum, the prepuce of the clitoris, Bartholin and Skene glands, and fascial coverings of the vulva with the specimen (see Figure 14-12, *B*).
3. Reconstruction of the vaginal walls and the pelvic floor is completed.
4. An indwelling urinary catheter is inserted, a closed wound drainage system is placed in the denuded area, and pressure dressings are applied.

Groin Lymphadenectomy

1. The surgeon makes the first skin incision on the side of the primary lesion. If nodes on the same side of a lateralized lesion are negative on histologic section, it will not be necessary to carry out the contralateral node dissection. The end of the incised skin is grasped with Allis forceps. The incision is extended to the aponeurosis of the external oblique muscle.
2. The fascia over the inguinal ligament and the fascia lata of the upper thigh are exposed, separated, and freed with retractors, blade, scissors, hemostats, and radiopaque gauze sponges.
3. Bleeding vessels, including the superficial iliac artery and vein, the epigastric artery and vein, and the superficial external pudendal artery and vein, are preserved when possible; otherwise they are clamped and ligated. Smaller bleeding vessels are controlled with the ESU.

4. Using Metzenbaum scissors, tissue forceps without teeth, and retractors, the surgeon excises the nodes most commonly involved with metastatic disease. These nodes are those superficial to the cribriform fascia and medial to the femoral vein. The surgeon pays particular attention to the resection of these nodes and if suspicious they should be submitted for frozen section examination. Involvement of these nodes is indicative of a need for postoperative groin irradiation, and then only grossly involved nodes need be removed.
5. The lymphatic node beds may be identified by placing metal clips in the area during the procedure. Fine, long, sharp tissue dissection scissors are needed.
6. The node-bearing regions are exposed for complete dissection by means of retractors and are protected by warm, moist radiopaque laparotomy pads. The saphenous vein is preserved, if possible, to reduce risk of postoperative lymphedema. If not possible, ligation is performed using scissors, forceps, and hemostats and then doubly tied.
7. The surgeon clears the femoral canal of its lymphatics; the round ligament is clamped, cut, and ligated.
8. The wound is closed using the surgeon's preferred suture material, and dressings applied.
9. An indwelling urethral catheter is inserted before the patient is transferred to the PACU.

Gynecologic Surgery Using Vaginal Approach

Plastic Reconstructive Repair of the Vagina (Anterior and Posterior Repair; Colporrhaphy)

A vaginal repair is done to correct a cystocele or a rectocele, to reestablish the support of the anterior and posterior vaginal walls and restore the bladder and rectum to their normal positions.

A cystocele is a herniation of the bladder that causes the anterior vaginal wall to bulge downward (Figure 14-13). A defect in the anterior vaginal wall is usually caused by obstetric or surgical trauma, advanced age, or an inherent weakness. A large protrusion

FIGURE 14-13 A, Cystocele resulting from unrepaired tears of muscles of pelvic floor and those under bladder, usually resulting from childbirth, surgical trauma, advanced age, or inherent weakness. **B,** Cystocele *(arrow)*.

A   Bulge   B

FIGURE 14-14 A, Rectocele resulting from unrepaired tears of muscles of pelvic floor and those under bladder, usually resulting from childbirth, surgical trauma, advanced age, or inherent weakness. **B,** Rectocele *(arrow).*

may cause a sensation of pressure in the vagina or present as a mass at or through the introitus; it may also cause voiding difficulties.

A rectocele occurs when the anterior rectal wall (posterior vaginal wall) protrudes into the vagina. In general, the anterior rectal wall forms a bulging mass beneath the posterior vaginal mucosa (Figure 14-14). As the mass pushes downward into the lower vaginal canal, the rectum may be separated from the fascial and muscular attachments of the urogenital diaphragm and the pelvic wall. The levator ani muscles become stretched or separated. The patient may present with a mass protruding into the vagina, difficulty in evacuating the lower bowel, hemorrhoids, and a feeling of pressure.

An enterocele is a herniation of the peritoneum through the central portion of the vaginal vault in women who have undergone a prior hysterectomy. If a woman has a uterus, the herniation is between the uterosacral ligaments. An enterocele can contain a loop of the small intestine.

Procedural Considerations. The procedure is done with the patient in the lithotomy position (see Chapter 6 for positioning considerations). The basic vaginal instrument tray is required. Vaginal retractors are used for exposure. The labia may be sutured to the medial thigh on each side to expose the vaginal introitus. A D&C tray should be available.

Operative Procedure
Cystocele Repair
1. The bladder is drained by straight catheterization or insertion of an indwelling urinary catheter (surgeon's preference). Areolar tissue between the bladder and vagina at the bladder reflection is exposed. A mixture of intravenous (IV) normal saline and vasopressin or local anesthetic with epinephrine may be injected into the tissue for hemostasis and to facilitate tissue plane dissection. Full-thickness dissection of the vaginal wall is done up to the bladder neck with a blade, curved scissors, tissue forceps, Allis-Adair or Allis forceps, and radiopaque gauze sponges.

Bleeding vessels are clamped and tied with ligatures or controlled with a bipolar or monopolar ESU.
2. The surgeon mobilizes the urethra and bladder neck with a blade, radiopaque gauze sponges, and curved scissors.
3. Sutures are placed adjacent to the urethra and bladder neck in such a manner that, after they have been tied, the bladder neck and the posterior urethrovesical angle are narrowed (Figure 14-15, *A*).
4. The surgeon sutures the connective tissue on the lateral aspects of the cervix into the cervix to shorten the cardinal ligaments.
5. Allis-Adair forceps are applied to the edges of the incision, and the left flap of the vaginal wall is drawn across the midline. Edges are trimmed according to the size of the cystocele. The surgeon repeats the process on the right flap of the vaginal incision.
6. The anterior vaginal wall is closed in a manner resulting in reconstruction of an anterior vaginal fornix (see Figure 14-15, *B*). Cystoscopy instrumentation may be required to evaluate the integrity of the urethra and ureteral orifices. A perineal pad may be applied.

Rectocele Repair
1. The surgeon places Allis forceps posteriorly at the mucocutaneous junction on each side, at the hymenal ring, and just above the anus (Figure 14-16, *A*). A mixture of IV normal saline and vasopressin may be injected into the tissue for hemostasis and to facilitate tissue plane dissection. Skin and mucosa are incised and dissected from the muscles beneath with a blade, tissue forceps, curved scissors, and radiopaque gauze sponges.
2. Allis-Adair forceps are placed on the posterior vaginal wall, scar tissue (from obstetric trauma) is removed, and the surgeon continues the dissection to the posterior vaginal fornix and laterally, depending on the size of the rectocele (see Figure 14-16, *A* and *B*).
3. The perineum is denuded by sharp dissection, and trimming of the posterior vaginal wall is carried out with Allis forceps and curved scissors (see Figure 14-16, *C*).

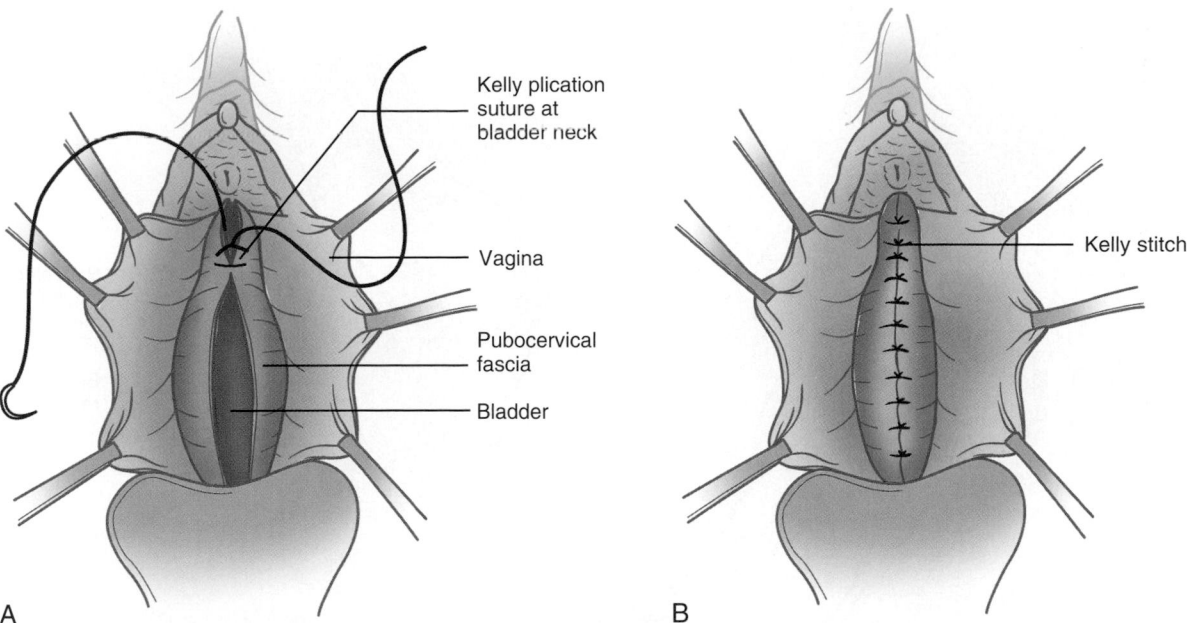

FIGURE 14-15 Cystocele repair. **A,** The placement of a Kelly stitch in the pubocervical fascia at the junction of the urethra with the bladder neck. **B,** The repair of the cystocele as the pubocervical fascia is sutured. Thus the cystocele is plicated.

4. The rectal wall proximal to the puborectal muscle is strengthened by placement of sutures.
5. Bleeding is controlled, and the surgeon closes the vaginal wall from above, downward to the anterior edge of the puborectal muscle. The rectocele is repaired from the posterior fornix to the perineal body. Remains of the transverse perineal and bulbocavernosus muscles are used to augment the perineum. The anterior edge of the levator ani muscle may be approximated (see Figure 14-16, *D*).
6. The mucosa and skin are trimmed, and the remaining closure is performed with interrupted sutures.
7. The vagina may be packed with 2-inch vaginal gauze packing with an added antibiotic, antifungal, or an estrogen cream. An indwelling urinary catheter is inserted and a perineal pad may be applied.
8. The surgeon will require an additional pair of sterile gloves if a rectal digital examination is performed to prevent cross contamination of the vaginal, rectal, and anal tissue flora.

Enterocele Repair. The procedure is illustrated in Figure 14-17. The peritoneal sac is carefully dissected from the underlying rectum, the overlying bladder, or both, so that the peritoneal tissues are completely freed from the surrounding structures. The sac is opened to establish true identification and is then closed as high as possible by permanent purse-string sutures. The portion of peritoneal tissue distal to the purse-string ties is then excised, and the area is reinforced locally by transverse suture closures using any available supportive tissues. This technique is used to prevent recurrence.

Perineal Repair. The procedure is illustrated in Figure 14-18.

Vesicovaginal Fistula Repair. A vesicovaginal fistula (a communication between the urinary bladder and the vagina) is repaired by free dissection of the mucosal tissue of the anterior vaginal wall, closing of the fistula tract, and repair of the fascial attachments between the bladder and vagina, with establishment of urinary

drainage. Fistulas vary in size from a small opening that permits only slight leakage of urine into the vagina to a large opening that permits all urine to pass into the vagina (Figure 14-19). They may result from radiation therapy, radical surgery for the management of pelvic cancer, chronic ulceration of the vaginal structures, penetrating wounds, or obstetric trauma. Vesicovaginal fistulas are repaired either through the vaginal or transperitoneal approach (see Chapter 15 for a description of the transperitoneal approach).

Urethrovaginal Fistula Repair (Vaginal Approach). An urethrovaginal fistula (a communication between the urethra and the vagina) (see Figure 14-19) usually causes constant incontinence or difficulty in retaining urine. This condition occurs after damage to the anterior wall and bladder, radiation therapy, or parturition.

Procedural Considerations. The basic vaginal instrument tray is required, with the addition of Kelly fistula or Metzenbaum scissors, dressing forceps, probes, skin hooks, Frazier suction tips, urethral catheters, and sterile saline for irrigation into the bladder. The patient is placed in the lithotomy position, and the perioperative nurse seeks assistance during positioning to safely raise and lower the patient's legs simultaneously to prevent injury (see Chapter 6 for positioning considerations).

Operative Procedure

1. After traction sutures are placed around the fistulous tract, the surgeon grasps the tissues with Allis-Adair forceps and plain tissue forceps.
2. The surgeon excises scar tissue around the fistula, locates the cleavage between the bladder and vagina, and mobilizes the flaps using scissors, forceps, and radiopaque gauze sponges.
3. The bladder mucosa is inverted toward the interior of the bladder with interrupted sutures. The sutures are passed through the muscularis of the bladder down to the mucosa.
4. A second layer of inverting sutures is placed in the bladder and tied, thereby completely inverting the bladder mucosa toward the interior.

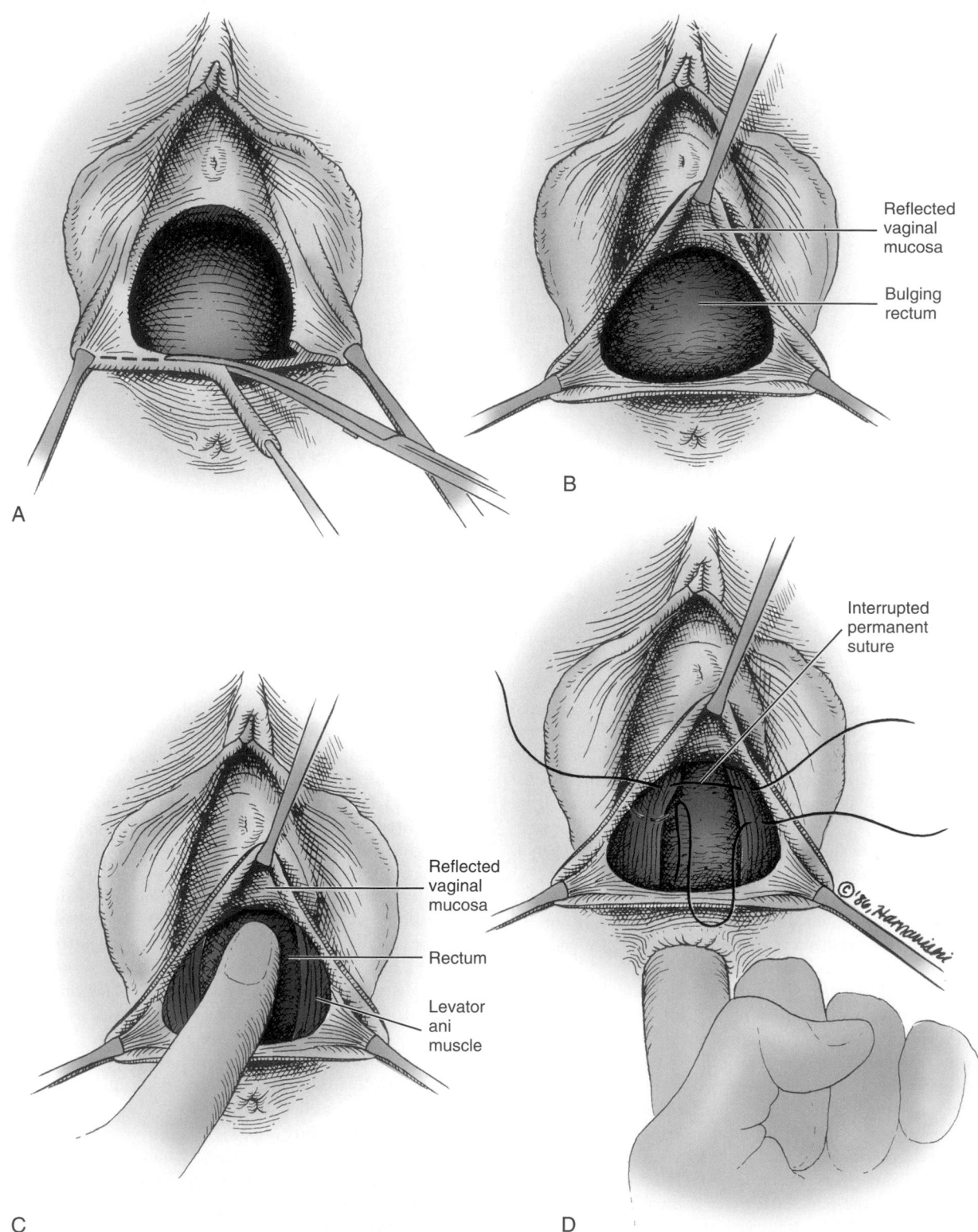

Reflected
vaginal
mucosa

Bulging
rectum

Reflected
vaginal
mucosa

Rectum

Levator
ani
muscle

Interrupted
permanent
suture

FIGURE 14-16 Rectocele repair. **A,** Placement of Allis clamps at margins of perineal incision; perineal incision is being made. **B,** Reflected vaginal mucosa with rectum bulging. **C,** Depression of rectum identifying margins of levator ani muscle. **D,** Placement of sutures in perirectal tissue and levator ani bundles.

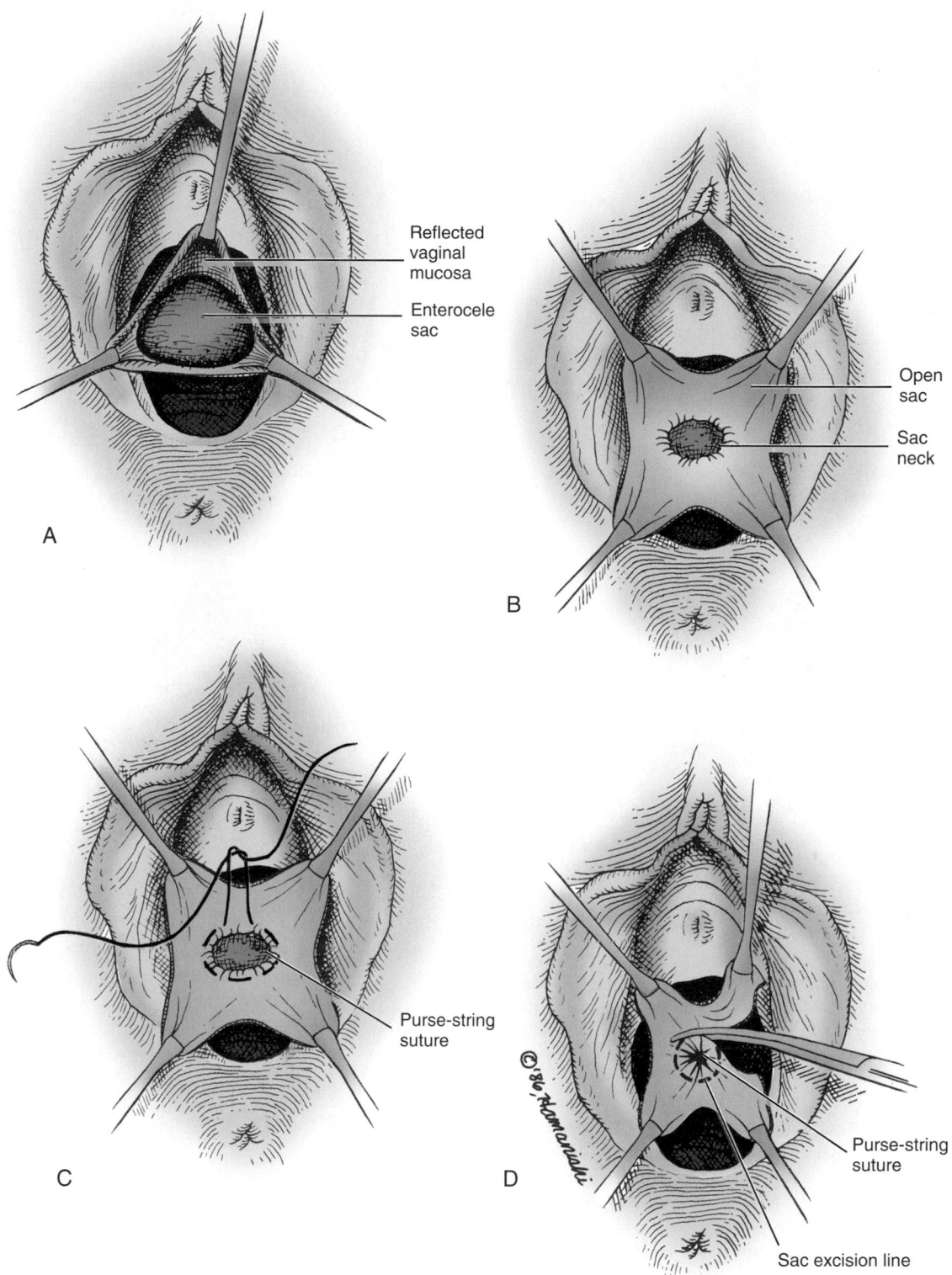

FIGURE 14-17 Enterocele repair. **A,** Appearance of enterocele sac with vaginal wall reflected. **B,** Appearance of open enterocele sac with sac neck identified. **C,** Placement of purse-string suture at neck of enterocele sac. **D,** Excision of enterocele sac.

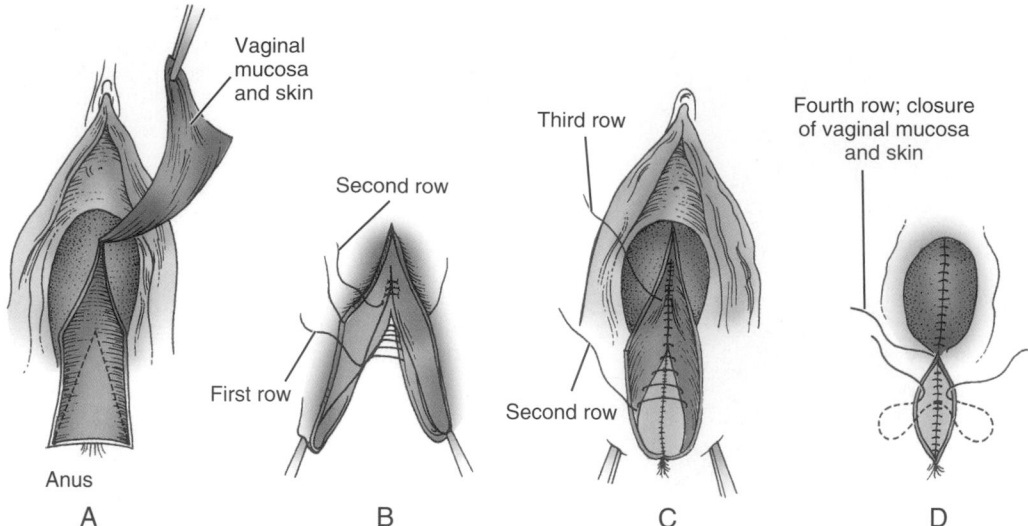

FIGURE 14-18 Repair of complete lacerations of the perineum. **A,** Lower margins of incision. **B,** Placement of first and second rows of sutures. **C,** Second and third rows of sutures. **D,** Fourth row of sutures.

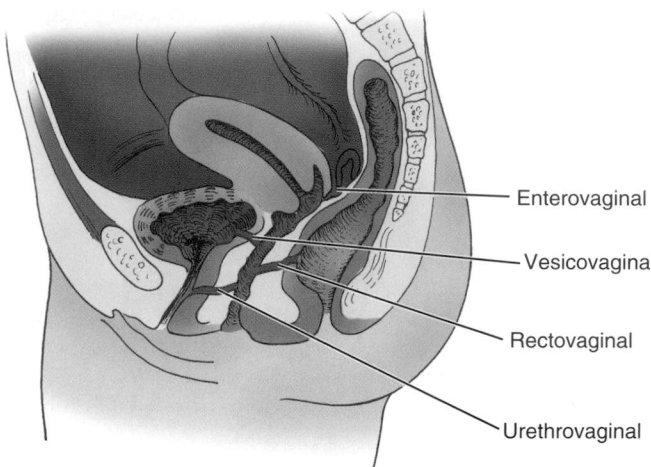

FIGURE 14-19 Genital fistulas may present as communications between the urethra, bladder, one of the ureters, or the bowel and some part of the genital tract. Two of the most common types are urethrovaginal and vesicovaginal, both of which empty into the vaginal canal.

5. The surgeon closes the vaginal wall in multiple layers, approximating the anterior and posterior vaginal walls distal to the closure of the bladder with interrupted sutures in a direction opposite the closure of the bladder wall.
6. The bladder is distended with sterile saline to determine any leaks. An indwelling urinary catheter is inserted and a perineal pad may be applied.

Ureterovaginal Fistula. An ureterovaginal fistula (a communication between the distal ureter and the vagina) develops as a result of injury to the ureter. In some cases reimplantation of the ureter into the bladder or ureterostomy may be done (see Chapter 15 for a description of these procedures).

Rectovaginal Fistula Repair (Vaginal Approach). Rectovaginal fistula is an abnormal communication between the rectum and

FIGURE 14-20 Rectovaginal fistula. Examiner's finger puts tension on rectovaginal septum.

vagina (see Figure 14-19). Surgical repair is via the vaginal approach. It includes repair of the perineum, fascia, and muscle-supporting structures between the rectum and vagina, thereby closing the fistula formed between the rectum and the vagina (Figure 14-20). In the presence of a large rectovaginal fistula, as in patients who have had radiation therapy or incurable cancer, a colostomy may be performed (see Chapter 11 for a description of the procedure for colostomy). The surgeon will require an additional pair of sterile

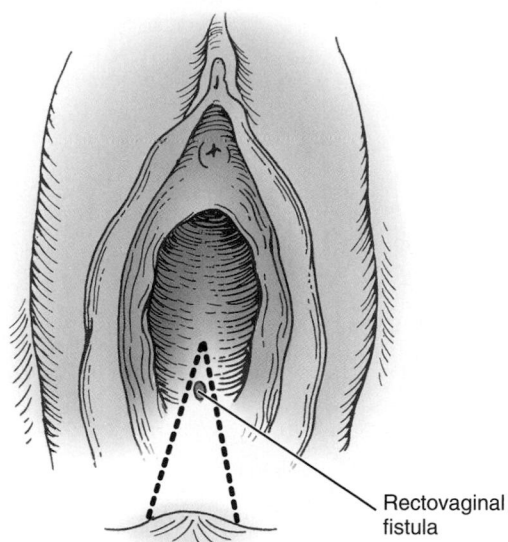

Rectovaginal fistula

FIGURE 14-21 Repair of rectovaginal fistulas of all types is essentially the same as shown here. Portion of scar tissue to be excised is included within dotted lines; repair is as described for complete lacerations of perineum (see Figure 14-18).

gloves if a rectal digital examination is performed during the procedure to prevent cross-contamination.

Procedural Considerations. The basic vaginal instrument tray is required. The patient is placed in the lithotomy position (see Chapter 6 for positioning considerations).

Operative Procedure
1. The surgeon excises the scar tissue and tract between the rectum and vagina (Figure 14-21); edges of fresh tissue are approximated with absorbable sutures (surgeon's preference).
2. The rectum and vaginal walls are mobilized; the rectum is closed with inversion of the mucosa into the rectal canal. Occasionally a myocutaneous flap is used in reconstruction to augment the closure.
3. The vagina is closed transversely or in a sagittal plane different from that of the rectal canal. The vaginal mucosal layer is inverted into the vaginal wall; an indwelling urinary catheter is inserted and a perineal pad applied.

Operations for Urinary Stress Incontinence

Urinary incontinence is the involuntary loss of urine. The three main types of incontinence include stress urinary incontinence (SUI), urge urinary incontinence (UUI), and mixed incontinence (MI), which describes the presence of both types of urinary incontinence simultaneously. Normal micturition depends on a finely coordinated group of voluntary and involuntary movements. As a result of volitional impulses, voiding may be inhibited or stopped by the intrinsic muscles of the bladder neck and proximal urethra and the puborectalis division of the levator ani muscle (see Chapter 15).

Previous pelvic procedures may have resulted in scarring and distortion, with displacement of the bladder neck. Conditions such as uterine prolapse, cystocele, urethrocele, cystourethrocele, or urogenital fistulas after radiation therapy may be associated with stress incontinence.

The type of operation selected depends on the severity of stress incontinence, the extent of the condition causing it, the patient's

ability to use the anatomic mechanism for voluntary inhibition of urination, and any previous procedures. States of stress incontinence are classified in relation to frequency and degree of incontinence, the presence of other diseases, and the function of the pubococcygeal muscle (levator ani). Surgery for SUI entails repair of the fascial supports and the pubococcygeal muscle surrounding the urethra and the bladder neck. This repair is performed through either a vaginal or an abdominal approach. In recent years, retropubic and transobturator suburethral tape has become important in the treatment of stress incontinence (Aschkenazi and Goldberg, 2009). Another available treatment option is the tension-free vaginal tape (TVT) sling (see Chapter 15 for a discussion of this procedure).

The desired outcome of any operation for SUI is to improve the performance of a dislodged or dysfunctional vesical neck, to restore normal urethral length, and to tighten and restore the anterior urethral vesical angle. Operations for SUI can be performed by gynecologists, urologists, and by a new subspecialty of surgeons trained in gynecology and urology known as urogynecologists.

Operative Procedure
Vaginal Approach
1. An indwelling urinary catheter or suprapubic cystostomy catheter is inserted (surgeon's preference). The posterior vaginal wall is retracted, and the surgeon makes an incision through the anterior vaginal wall down to the urethra and bladder.
2. The vaginal wall is dissected from the bladder and urethra; the neck of the bladder is sutured together. The wound is closed as described for anterior vaginal wall repair.

Vesicourethral Suspension. The Marshall-Marchetti-Krantz procedure is fully described in Chapter 15.

Construction of a Vagina

Two basic approaches are used for repairing or overcoming a congenital or surgical defect of the vagina: obtaining a skin graft, which is applied to a mold and placed in the area of vaginal reconstruction; or making a simple opening in the area of vaginal reconstruction and placing a mold to permit spontaneous epithelialization of the area.

Procedural Considerations. For a skin graft, the plastic surgery instrument tray (see Chapter 22) is required, with the addition of a dermatome, marking pen, and nonadherent gauze dressing. For vaginal construction, the basic vaginal instrument tray is required, with the addition of iris scissors, skin hooks, a vaginal mold, Halsted mosquito hemostats, and a ruler.

Operative Procedure
1. The skin graft is taken most commonly from the buttock because it provides a better cosmetic result in young women than the former approaches of harvesting skin from the abdomen or anterior area of the thigh. The donor site is dressed in the routine manner with nonadherent gauze and a pressure dressing.
2. The skin graft is kept in a moist radiopaque gauze sponge until it is ready to be used. Communication of where the graft is on the back table must occur between the scrub persons when there is a change of personnel to prevent the graft from being thrown off the field inadvertently. The graft must be clearly marked on the back table.
3. The surgeon uses sharp dissection to create a vaginal orifice, taking care to prevent damage to the rectum and bladder. A mold is used to apply the donor skin or simply to hold the

FIGURE 14-22 Vaginal reconstruction using split-thickness skin graft.

dissected area open to permit spontaneous epithelialization (Figure 14-22).

Trachelorrhaphy (Cervical Repair)

Trachelorrhaphy is removal of separated or torn surfaces of the anterior and posterior cervical lips and reconstruction of the cervical canal. It is performed to treat deep lacerations of a cervix that is relatively free from infection.

Procedural Considerations. The basic vaginal instrument tray is required, along with an ESU and a conization loop electrode, if desired. An indwelling or straight urinary catheter may be inserted into the bladder, depending on the surgeon's preference. The patient is in the lithotomy position (see Chapter 6 for positioning considerations).

Operative Procedure

1. The labia may be retracted with Allis-Adair tissue forceps or sutures. The surgeon grasps the cervix with a tenaculum.
2. The tissue of the exocervix is denuded with a blade. Using sharp dissection, the surgeon undermines the flaps. Bleeding vessels are clamped and ligated or controlled by a monopolar ESU throughout the procedure. The mucosa is dissected from the cervix.
3. A small distal portion of the cervical canal is coned with a blade or a loop electrode to remove tissue.
4. The denuded and coned areas are covered by transversely suturing the mucosal flaps of the exocervix, using interrupted sutures. Tissue forceps, hemostats, and radiopaque gauze sponges are needed. The sutures are placed in such a manner that the fibromuscular tissue of the cervix is included, thereby eliminating

dead space where a hematoma may form, and providing a complete reconstructed cervical canal.

5. A vaginal pack may be inserted. A perineal pad is applied.

Dilation of the Cervix and Curettage (D&C)

D&C is done for diagnostic purposes for a variety of pelvic conditions, such as abnormal uterine bleeding. D&C is also performed to obtain tissue for diagnosis when carcinoma of the endometrium is suspected, in the study of infertility, or for removal of uterine polyps. A common indication for D&C is incomplete abortion (e.g., miscarriage), or therapeutic abortion. The perioperative nurse should be especially sensitive to the emotional needs of a patient experiencing a miscarriage (Box 14-2).

Procedural Considerations. In a D&C procedure, instruments are introduced through the vagina for the purpose of dilating the cervix. Numerous cervical dilators are available. The patient is in the lithotomy position for this procedure (see Chapter 6 for positioning considerations).

Operative Procedure

1. The surgeon places a Jackson or Auvard weighted speculum in the vagina. A Sims or Deaver retractor is placed anteriorly to expose the cervix. The anterior lip of the cervix is grasped with a tenaculum (Figure 14-23).

2. The direction of the cervical canal and the depth of the uterine cavity are determined by means of a blunt probe or graduated uterine sound.

3. The surgeon dilates the cervix using graduated Hegar or Hanks dilators and/or a Goodell uterine dilator. Lacrimal probes may be needed if severe cervical stenosis is present, such as in patients who are nulligravidas, are postmenopausal, have had scarring

from previous cervical procedures (loop electrosurgical excision procedure [LEEP]), or have undergone radiation therapy in the past.

4. Exploration for pedunculated polyps or myomas may be done with a polyp forceps.

BOX 14-2

Supporting Patients Through Miscarriage or Stillbirth

A diagnosis of pregnancy is often a joyous occasion; however, many women can experience perinatal loss, which is defined as ectopic pregnancy, miscarriage, or fetal death. Miscarriage occurs in approximately 10% to 15% of all pregnancies (e.g., those occurring before 20 weeks of gestation). Stillbirths occur in 1 in 160 pregnancies (e.g., those occurring after 20 weeks of gestation). The primary cause of miscarriage and infant death is birth defects. Perinatal loss may occur with little or no advance warning for the mother, and surgical procedures at this time increase the woman's sense of vulnerability. The perioperative nurse can play a sensitive and supportive role when providing care for patients who present to the OR with miscarriage or cesarean section for stillbirth.

By definition, a miscarriage is a pregnancy loss that occurs before 20 weeks of gestation. In the United States, state laws may stipulate that, in addition, the weight of the fetus is less than 350 g and signs of life are absent. Abortion is the medical term used for both spontaneous and elective pregnancy termination occurring before 20 weeks of gestation. Terms used to identify the diagnosis should also be carefully chosen. Many women find the term abortion harsh and unkind when referring to spontaneous events. Some may feel insulted or misunderstood, believing that abortion refers only to an elective procedure. The term "miscarriage" is more neutral and should be used consistently for early loss. Products of conception are better referred to as "tissue" and the embryo or fetus as "baby," and for infant death, "death" and "died" rather than "lost" or "gone." Also avoid using clinical terminology because this may convey a perceived lack of sincerity and respect.

When discussing perinatal loss with a woman, initiate the conversation by referring to the pregnancy and listen for the patient's use of either the terms "pregnancy" or "baby" when referring to the loss. Such neutrality encourages the woman to express her feelings without being encumbered by what she "should" do and what she "should" feel. Additional suggestions for communicating with parents include the use of phrases and open-ended questions such as:

- "I am sad for you."
- "How are you doing with all of this?"
- "This must be hard for you."
- "What can I do for you?"
- "I am here, and I want to listen"
- "I am sorry"

Avoid the following phrases:

- "Be thankful you have another child."
- "I know how you feel."
- "You have to keep going for her sake."
- "You're young and you can have others."
- "Better for this to happen now, before you knew the baby."
- "There was something wrong with the baby anyway."

Modified from Centers for Disease Control and Prevention (CDC): *National vital statistic report: infant mortality statistics from 2008 period linked birth/infant death data sheet,* May 10, 2012, available at www.cdc.gov/nchs/data/nvsr/nvsr60/nvsr60_05.pdf. Accessed February 23, 2013; March of Dimes: *Loss and grief,* available at www.marchofdimes.com/baby/loss_stillbirth.html. Accessed February 23, 2013; Miles MS: Perinatal loss and grief. In Lowdermilk DL, Perry SE, editors: *Maternity and women's health care,* ed 10, St Louis, 2012, Mosby.

FIGURE 14-23 Dilation of cervix and curettage. Vaginal wall retracted; cervix held by tenaculum; cervix dilated with dilator. Uterine cavity curetted with sharp curettes.

5. Using a sharp curette the surgeon scrapes the interior of the cervical canal to obtain an endocervical tissue specimen. To obtain an endometrial specimen, the surgeon scrapes the endometrial lining of the uterus. For specific identification and the site of specimens, the endocervical specimen is scraped with the curette first, and then a separate specimen is curetted from the uterine endometrium. As with any specimen, a confirmation of its identity is obtained from the surgeon and sent to pathology for diagnosis (see Chapter 2 for a discussion of safe specimen practices).

6. Fragments of endometrium or other dislodged tissues may be removed with warm, moist radiopaque gauze sponges on sponge-holding forceps.

7. The surgeon may take multiple punch biopsies of the suspected cervical lesions with a cervical biopsy forceps to supplement the diagnostic studies.

8. Retractors are withdrawn, the tenaculum is removed from the cervix, hemostasis is evaluated at the site of the tenaculum, and a vaginal pack may be inserted. A perineal pad is applied.

Suction Curettage

Suction curettage is vacuum aspiration of the uterine contents. Aspiration has proved to be a safe and effective method for early termination of pregnancy and for use in missed and incomplete spontaneous abortions. Advantages are less dilation of the cervix, less damage to the uterus, less blood loss, less chance of uterine perforation, and reduced danger of infection. Suction curettage is the treatment of choice for benign gestational trophoblastic neoplasia, more commonly known as hydatidiform mole. Hydatidiform mole is a condition that arises from growth of embryonic tissue containing only paternal genetic origin possibly arising from fertilization by the sperm in a defective egg that has no nucleus or from fertilization of the egg by two sperm. This results in the synthesis of material, which is termed a mole and consists of multiple fluid-filled vesicles resembling a cluster of grapes (Figure 14-24).

Procedural Considerations. Instrumentation required includes the D&C tray, with the addition of one tray of Pratt, Hawkin, or Hank uterine dilators, placenta forceps, urethral catheter, sterile suction cannulae (various sizes), aspirator tubing, a vacuum aspirator unit, and oxytocic drugs. The patient is in the lithotomy position (see Chapter 6 for positioning considerations).

Operative Procedure

1. The surgeon exposes the cervix with an Auvard weighted speculum and an anterior retractor, grasps it with a sharp tenaculum, and draws it toward the introitus.

2. The cervix is dilated enough to be able to insert a 10- to 14-mm curette, depending on the uterus size.

3. The appropriate-size cannula is inserted into the uterus until the sac is encountered. The suction is turned on with immediate disruption and aspiration of the contents. Continued gentle motion of the cannula removes the uterine contents (Figure 14-25). Use of uterine curettes may supplement suction in removing the entire uterine contents but must be done judiciously because it carries the risk of Asherman syndrome (intrauterine adhesions or scarring) from removal of the endometrium.

4. Retractors and tenaculum are removed and a perineal pad is applied.

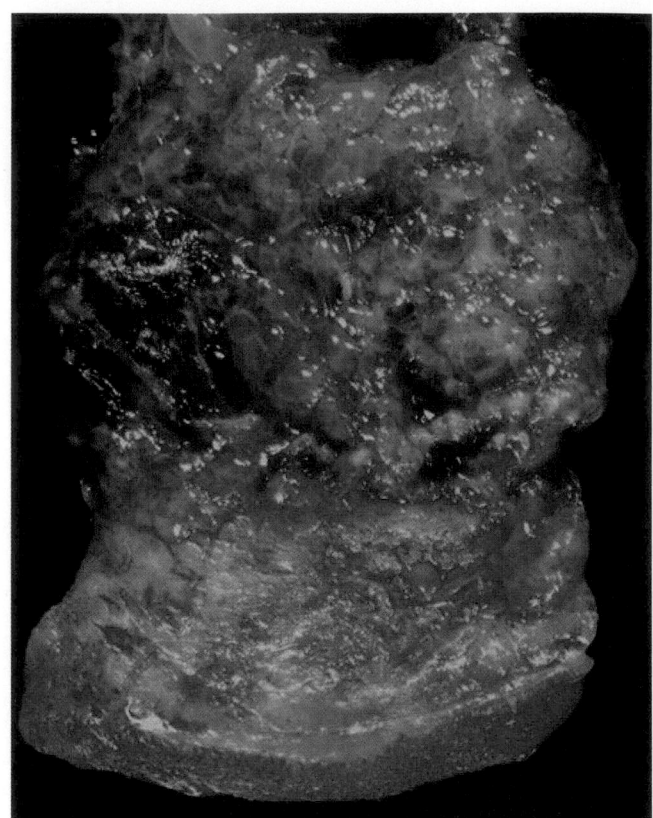

FIGURE 14-24 Complete hydatidiform mole. Enlarged, transparent, and cystically dilated villi fill the uterine cavity. Note vesicles have the appearance of grapelike clusters.

Removal of Pedunculated Cervical Myomas (Cervical Polyps)

Cervical polyps (small pedunculated lesions) stem from the endocervical canal and consist almost entirely of columnar epithelium with or without squamous metaplasia (Figure 14-26). They vary in size and are soft, red, and friable. Bleeding may result from the slightest trauma. Pedunculated lesions are removed from the cervical canal by dissection with a blade or resectoscope. Usually the surgeon performs endometrial and endocervical curettage, and a cytologic smear may be taken because some of these may represent early primary adenocarcinomas.

Procedural Considerations. A D&C tray, the ESU, and a blade electrode or resectoscope are required. The patient is in the lithotomy position (see Chapter 6 for positioning considerations).

Operative Procedure

1. The surgeon grasps the anterior lip of the cervix with a tenaculum. The canal is sounded and dilated either to visualize or to palpate the base of the pedicle.

2. The base of the polyp is dissected out with a blade or monopolar ESU. Bleeding is controlled with a monopolar ESU or manual pressure using a radiopaque gauze sponge. A resectoscope with the use of a monopolar ESU may also be used to dissect the tumor.

3. The tenaculum is removed from the cervix, hemostasis is established, and the retractors are withdrawn.

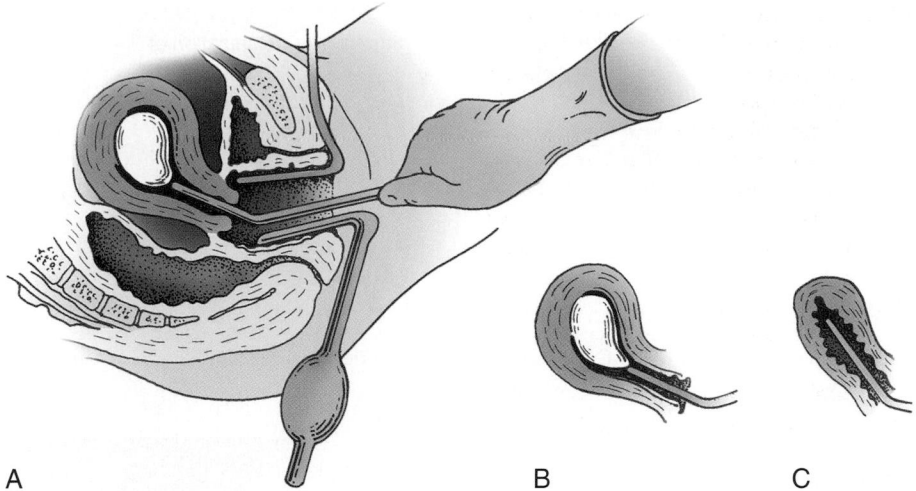

A   B   C

FIGURE 14-25 Suction curettage. **A,** Insertion of cannula. **B,** Gentle suction motion to aspirate contents. **C,** Uterine contents evacuated.

FIGURE 14-26 Cervical polyp. A large polyp protrudes from the external cervical os.

4. A vaginal pack may be inserted for hemostasis if needed. A perineal pad is applied.

Conization Biopsy of the Cervix

Conization biopsy of the cervix is generally performed for the diagnosis or treatment of cervical dysplasia. The procedure may be initiated with colposcopy and punch biopsy, followed by the use of a monopolar ESU, a cone biopsy with either a blade or LEEP. Hemostasis is controlled with a ball electrode and a monopolar ESU.

Procedural Considerations. Instruments required include a D&C tray along with an ESU, a conization electrical loop, and/or a ball-tipped electrode. The patient is in lithotomy position (see Chapter 6 for positioning considerations).

Operative Procedure

1. The surgeon retracts the posterior vaginal wall with a speculum and the anterior vaginal wall with lateral retractors. The outer portions of the cervix are grasped with a tenaculum, and the cervix is drawn toward the introitus. Cystic areas of the cervix

may be treated with a monopolar needle electrode and ESU or laser. An endometrial biopsy may be done (Figure 14-27, *A*). The cervical stroma deep to the site of resection is infiltrated with local anesthetic with epinephrine to provide mechanical and pharmacologic vasoconstriction prior to the procedure. Typically 20 mL of solution is used to provide hemostasis. Bleeding points are coagulated with an ESU or laser.

2. The surgeon uses the electrical loop or a blade (see Figure 14-27, *B* and *C*) to remove the diseased tissue and obtain a histologic specimen for pathologic diagnosis. The surgeon may place a tagging suture at 12 o'clock to determine the position of the specimen for diagnostic purposes. Safe specimen management practices are implemented. The 3-mm ball-tipped electrode and a monopolar ESU may be used for hemostasis.

3. If a wide conization is performed, the cervix rarely requires suturing. Vaginal packing may be used. An indwelling urinary catheter may be inserted. A perineal pad is applied.

Internal Radiation Therapy (Brachytherapy) for Cervical and Endometrial Malignancy

Internal radiation therapy or brachytherapy is used to treat certain cervical and endometrial malignancies, either on its own or in conjunction with external beam radiation treatment (EBRT) and/or chemotherapy. Radiation is either delivered at a low-dose rate (LDR) or at a high-dose rate (HDR) into or near the diseased tissue using several different applicator modes. LDR brachytherapy requires the patient to be admitted to the hospital, whereas HDR brachytherapy is administered on an outpatient basis. For LDR in women who have had a hysterectomy for endometrial cancer, a cylinder containing radioactive material is placed into the vagina (intracavity). If a uterus is still present, as would be the case with primary cervical cancer, a rod (tandem) is placed in the vagina along with small metal holders (ovoids) close to the cervix (tandem and ovoid brachytherapy). Tandem and ovoids are placed in either the OR under general anesthesia or in the interventional radiology department using moderate sedation/analgesia. The radioactive material (LDR) is often loaded into the devices when the patient returns to a shielded hospital room. Patients may remain in the hospital for a couple of days with the radioactive material in place. Cesium has generally replaced radium insertions for treatment of

A

B

C

FIGURE 14-27 A, Endometrial biopsy technique. **B** and **C,** Conization loop used to treat cervical conditions or obtain specimens for diagnostic tests.

malignancy of the cervix and endometrium. Although LDR brachytherapy, typically used with cesium-137 (Cs-137), has been the traditional approach, the use of HDR therapy, used with iridium-192 (Ir-192), is rapidly increasing (Smith and Jhingran, 2012).

Procedural Considerations. The patient is in the lithotomy position. The bladder is drained with an indwelling urinary catheter. The catheter balloon is inflated with a radiopaque medium for radiographic visualization after insertion of the cesium. An indwelling rectal marker is also placed by the surgeon for radiographic visualization. Various types of cesium applicators may be used according to the surgeon's preference and the area of malignancy. The cesium is loaded into the applicators later in the radiation department or in the patient's room under controlled conditions, in which all personnel are monitored by use of a dosimeter.

Interstitial Therapy. Cesium needles are available in various lengths with small diameters for insertion into the tissue surrounding the cervix. They are inserted vaginally with a needle applicator and are used as a supplement to intravaginal or intrauterine sources. To facilitate removal, the needles have wires or threads attached to their distal ends.

Marsupialization of Bartholin Duct Cyst or Abscess

A cyst in a Bartholin gland usually results from retention of glandular secretions caused by blockage in the duct system (Figure 14-28). This causes infection, with resultant scarring of the Bartholin duct. Marsupialization of a Bartholin duct cyst or abscess involves removal or incision of the cyst through the vaginal outlet and drainage of the area. In true marsupialization, the cyst is surgically exteriorized by resecting the anterior wall and suturing the cut edges of the remaining cyst to the adjacent edges of the skin.

Procedural Considerations. The basic vaginal instrument tray is required, with the addition of a 15-gauge needle, syringe and culture tubes (aerobic and anaerobic) to obtain a culture of the cyst if infection is suspected, iodoform or plain gauze packing, and a drain, if desired by the surgeon.

Operative Procedure

1. The labia minora may be sutured to the perineal skin on the lateral side of the thigh to expose the vaginal introitus.
2. A stellate (starlike) incision is then made into the mucosa, which is distended over the cyst.
3. The surgeon dissects the cyst wall. The tissue may be marsupialized, everted with sutures and left open.

FIGURE 14-28 Bartholin abscess.

4. A drain or packing may be inserted, and a perineal pad applied.

Vaginal Hysterectomy

Vaginal hysterectomy is removal of the uterus through an incision made in the vaginal wall and the pelvic cavity. Contraindications to a vaginal approach are a large uterine tumor (either benign or malignant) or pelvic malignancy extending beyond the uterus.

Procedural Considerations. Instrumentation includes the basic vaginal instrument tray. An abdominal gynecologic instrument tray should be available in case laparotomy is indicated. To facilitate dissection and decrease bleeding, the vaginal walls may be infiltrated with a local anesthetic (vasoconstrictors are optional). The patient is in the lithotomy position (see Chapter 6 for positioning considerations).

Operative Procedure

1. The labia minora may be sutured to the medial thigh to expose the vaginal introitus. The surgeon places a weighted vaginal retractor to retract the vaginal wall.
2. A tenaculum or suture ligature is placed on the cervix to permit traction on the cervix.

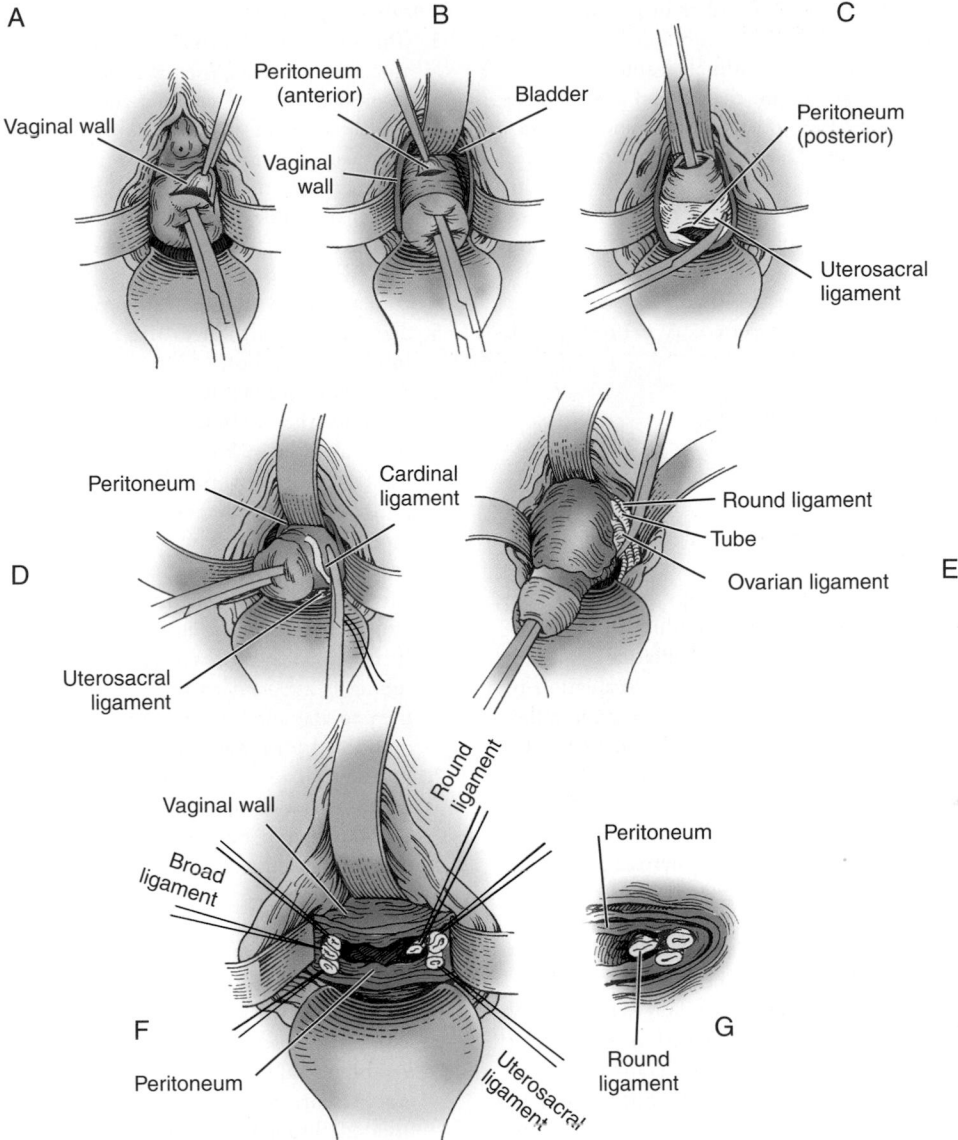

FIGURE 14-29 Vaginal hysterectomy. **A,** Incision of vaginal wall around cervix. Anterior vaginal wall slightly elevated. **B,** Deaver retractor on each side; one Deaver retractor under bladder. Peritoneum opened. **C,** Posterior cul-de-sac opened. Heaney clamp applied to left uterosacral ligament. **D,** Left uterosacral ligament cut and tied. Clamp applied to left cardinal ligament. **E,** Clamp applied to ovarian ligament, round ligament, and fallopian tube. **F,** Uterosacral ligament, broad ligament, and round ligament shown in their respective normal positions. **G,** Peritoneum closed and cardinal ligament, broad ligament, and uterosacral ligament reattached to angle of vagina. Left uterosacral and broad ligaments anchored.

3. The surgeon incises the anterior vaginal wall with a blade through the full thickness of the wall (Figure 14-29, *A*). A circumferential IV saline with epinephrine or vasopressin injection of the submucosa may aid with hemostasis and facilitate with tissue plane dissection. The bladder is freed from the anterior surface of the cervix by sharp and blunt dissection. The bladder is then elevated to expose the peritoneum of the anterior cul-de-sac, which is entered by sharp dissection (see Figure 14-29, *B*).

4. The peritoneum of the posterior cul-de-sac is identified and incised.

5. The surgeon clamps, cuts, ligates, or uses a handheld vessel sealing and dividing device on the uterosacral ligaments (see Figure 14-29, *C* and *D*). If sutures are used the ends of the ligatures are left long and are tagged with a clamp.

6. The uterus is drawn downward, and the bladder is held aside with retractors and moist radiopaque laparotomy pads.

7. The surgeon clamps, cuts, and ligates, or uses a handheld vessel sealing and dividing device on the cardinal ligaments on each side. The uterine arteries are doubly clamped, cut, and ligated or controlled with a handheld vessel sealing and dividing device.

8. The fundus is delivered with the aid of a uterine tenaculum.

9. When the ovaries are preserved, the surgeon clamps and cuts the round ligament or uses a handheld vessel sealing and dividing device bilaterally on the utero-ovarian ligament and the fallopian tube (see Figure 14-29, *E*) and then removes the uterus. These pedicles are ligated if the surgeon uses the clamp and cut technique.

10. The surgeon reapproximates the peritoneum between the rectum and vagina with a continuous suture. Retroperitoneal

obliteration of the cul-de-sac is accomplished by passing sutures from the vaginal wall through the infundibulopelvic ligament and round ligament, through the cardinal ligament, and out the vaginal wall. Sutures are tied on the vaginal aspect of the new vault (see Figure 14-29, *F* and *G*). The round, cardinal, and uterosacral ligaments may be individually approximated for additional support.

11. Any existing cystocele and rectocele and the perineum are repaired. In the presence of prolapse, reconstruction of the pelvic floor may be required.

12. An indwelling urethral catheter is inserted. The vagina may be packed and a drain may be inserted. A perineal pad is applied.

Gynecologic Surgery Using Minimally Invasive Techniques

Hysteroscopy

Hysteroscopy is the endoscopic visualization of the uterine cavity, intracavity, and tubal orifices. Both assessment and operative procedures can be completed during a hysteroscopy procedure. The common indications for hysteroscopy include evaluation of abnormal uterine bleeding (with possible endometrial ablation), location and removal of "lost" intrauterine devices (IUDs), evaluation of infertility, diagnosis and surgical treatment of intrauterine adhesions, verification and excision of submucous leiomyomas or endometrial polyps, resection of uterine septa or submucous leiomyomas, and tubal sterilization. A diagnostic laparoscopy may be done in association with hysteroscopy to assess the patient intra-abdominally. Contraindications for diagnostic or operative hysteroscopy include pregnancy, pelvic infection, cervical malignancy, and, in some instances, heavy bleeding.

A significant potential complication related to hysteroscopy is the intravasation of the fluid used to distend the uterine cavity. Intravasation can lead to hyponatremia. Signs and symptoms of hyponatremia may include bradycardia, hypertension followed by hypotension, nausea, vomiting, headache, visual disturbances, agitation, confusion, and lethargy. The perioperative nurse is responsible for accurately monitoring hysteroscopy fluid intake and output during the procedure. Monitoring may be manual (i.e., calculating the difference between inflow and outflow) or may be automatically calculated on commercially available hysteroscopy pumps, which decrease the chance of human error. If a discrepancy of 1 to 1.5 L or more occurs (less for patients who have compromising medical conditions), the surgeon and anesthesia provider are alerted and consideration is given to terminating the procedure (Kintanar, 2011). At the end of the procedure the hysteroscopy deficit should be communicated to the surgeon, anesthesia provider, and the PACU nurse during handoff report, and documented in the patient's perioperative record. In contrast, intravasation of normotonic solution, although safer, can still lead to congestive heart failure in susceptible individuals.

Procedural Considerations. Instrumentation includes a D&C tray, with the addition of a hysteroscopy tray, polyethylene tubing or pump tubing, fiberoptic light source, the ESU, pressure-infusion pump, and a video camera and monitor. Other instrumentation includes a resectoscope and the instrumentation needed for resection of uterine polyps or submucous leiomyomas, and an endometrial ablation device (if applicable). The patient is in the lithotomy position (see Chapter 6 for positioning considerations).

Operative Procedure

1. The surgeon places an Auvard weighted speculum and an anterior retractor to expose the cervix; the anterior lip of the cervix is grasped with a tenaculum and is drawn toward the introitus.

2. The direction of the cervical canal and the depth of the uterine cavity are determined by means of a graduated uterine sound.

3. The surgeon dilates the endocervical canal with graduated Hegar or Hank uterine dilators to 6, 7, or 8 mm, depending on the size of the hysteroscope or resectoscope (if applicable).

4. The hysteroscope pump tubing is primed using the surgeon's choice of fluid and according to manufacturer's directions.

5. The surgeon introduces the hysteroscope to the level of the internal cervical os.

6. To achieve satisfactory visualization and sustained intrauterine pressure, the uterine cavity is distended with either saline (normal saline solution [NSS]) or 1.5% glycine. Fluids may be under continuous pressure when delivered by means of a pressure-controlled fluid-infusion (hysteroscopic) pump into the irrigating channel of the hysteroscope or (rarely) by direct gravity. The outflow fluid can run freely through the polyethylene tubing connected to the outflow channel of the hysteroscope or drain freely into the under buttocks drainage drape. If an under buttocks drainage drape is used, polyethylene tubing is attached to the bottom of the drainage drape and then to the suction canister, where it can be measured and monitored for a hysteroscopy deficit amount.

7. Exploration of the uterine cavity is begun. A video camera monitor is used to enhance visibility for the operative team. Procedures may be videotaped and pictures taken intraoperatively for record keeping, future reevaluation, and patient teaching.

8. The surgeon may introduce ancillary instruments, such as rigid and flexible biopsy forceps, scissors, grasping forceps, or a tubal occlusive device through the operating channel of the hysteroscope. Insulated coagulation electrodes and an ESU are used with a resectoscope and a "rollerball" electrode.

9. If submucosal leiomyomas or large uterine endometrial polyps are present, a tissue-removing device (MyoSure) may be inserted through the hysteroscope. This device removes submucosal smooth muscle tissue by suctioning and drawing the tissue into the device in order to safely cut and remove it.

10. On completion of the procedure, the hysteroscope and any remaining instruments and retractors are withdrawn. The fluid deficit is reported and recorded. A perineal pad is applied.

Endometrial Ablation

Endometrial ablation is performed to treat abnormal uterine bleeding. The overall goal of endometrial ablation is to create amenorrhea or reduce menstrual bleeding to a normal or tolerable flow for the patient. It may be an alternative to hysterectomy in some patients with chronic menorrhagia. The procedure is performed using either an ESU, thermal energy, or by radiofrequency (RF). Patients who wish to have children in the future are offered other alternative treatments for their abnormal uterine bleeding.

Electrical energy is delivered through an adapted urologic resectoscope using continuous-flow irrigation to either coagulate or resect the endometrium. Endometrial ablation can also be carried out with the use of a resectoscope and an ESU with either a loop or a rollerball electrode attachment. When using the resectoscope, 1.5% glycine is chosen as the distending medium because it is electrolyte-free and compatible with the use of an ESU.

Reported complications associated with endometrial ablation using an ESU include hemorrhage, fluid intravasation, uterine perforation, recurrent bleeding, uterine perforation with injury to bowel and bladder, cervical lacerations, and rupture of a fallopian tube. One of the main disadvantages of using an ESU for endometrial ablation is it must be done in conjunction with a hysteroscopy.

Endometrial ablation using thermal energy can be performed with a uterine balloon catheter. This catheter conforms to the internal uterine contour and contains a heating element. The surgeon performs suction curettage before the therapy to provide maximal balloon contact with the uterine lining. The cervix is dilated to 5 mm, and the balloon catheter is inserted in the uterus until the tip touches the uterine fundus. The surgeon inflates the balloon with sterile D_5W to a pressure of 160 to 180 mm Hg. The solution is heated to a temperature of 188° F (86.6° C) and maintained for 8 to 10 minutes. This procedure may be performed on an ambulatory basis and does not require hysteroscopy (Kintanar, 2011).

Endometrial ablation using RF energy is accomplished using a wandlike device with a retractable triangular mesh end. The surgeon introduces the wand into the uterine cavity, then extends the triangular mesh. The triangular mesh conforms to the uterine cavity and measures its size. The surgeon communicates the uterine cavity measurements to the perioperative nurse, the perioperative nurse confirms these measurements, and inputs them into the RF controller. The surgeon activates the RF wand, where it delivers energy to the uterine cavity for approximately 90 seconds. Once the cycle is completed the triangular mesh is retracted back into the wand and the surgeon removes the wand from the uterine cavity.

A general anesthetic is usually administered, although a paracervical block along with IV conscious sedation/analgesia can be used. Either of these procedures can also be performed in the physician's office using local anesthesia or a paracervical block.

Laparoscopy

Laparoscopy is endoscopic visualization of the peritoneal cavity through the anterior abdominal wall once the establishment of a pneumoperitoneum is accomplished. It is used to investigate and diagnose causes of abdominal and pelvic pain, infertility, and to evaluate pelvic masses. Ancillary procedures such as adhesiolysis, fulguration of endometriotic implants (Figure 14-30), aspiration of cysts or peritoneal fluid for cytologic study, ovarian or tissue biopsy, ovarian cystectomy, oophorectomy, removal of an ectopic pregnancy, tuboplasty, or tubal sterilization may be performed via laparoscopy. Lasers, tissue-sealing devices, or an ESU with either a bipolar and monopolar instrument is often used during laparoscopy.

Procedural Considerations. Laparoscopy requires general anesthesia. Trocar port sites are often infiltrated or injected with local anesthetic prior to trocar insertion into the peritoneal cavity. The perioperative nurse assists with placing the patient in the modified lithotomy position (see Chapter 6 for positioning considerations). The abdomen, perineum, and vagina are prepped and draped for a combined procedure. Specially designed drapes with openings for both abdominal and perineal areas may be used. The bladder is emptied with a straight catheterization or through insertion of an indwelling urinary catheter to prevent injury during trocar port placement.

The surgeon may perform a D&C in conjunction with laparoscopic procedures when indicated. After the cervix is exposed and the position and depth of the uterus are confirmed, the surgeon

FIGURE 14-30 A hemorrhagic area of the right cul-de-sac *(small box)* is seen on magnification to lie adjacent to a clear macule of endometriosis *(large box)* and may contain a gland/stroma complex of endometriosis obscured beneath the hemorrhage. The base of the right uterosacral ligament demonstrates thickening of whitish fibrosis and entrapment of old dark blood between the arrowheads.

introduces a uterine manipulator into the cervix to manipulate the uterus during the laparoscopy for better visibility. Most uterine manipulators have an intrauterine cannula port used for intraoperative chromopertubation. Chromopertubation tests for tubal patency by injecting a diluted mixture of methylene blue or indigo carmine solution through the intrauterine cannula into the cervical canal. If the fallopian tubes are patent, dye can be seen at the tube's fimbriated ends.

The usual instruments for the vaginal portion of the procedure include a D&C tray, with the addition of a uterine manipulator, intrauterine cannula, diluted methylene blue or indigo carmine solution, and a 60-mL syringe with extension tubing for chromopertubation.

An abdominal gynecologic instrument tray should be readily available in the event a laparotomy is indicated.

Operative Procedure

1. The surgeon may inject local anesthetic before making a small vertical percutaneous incision (0.7 to 1.2 cm) at or within the inferior margin of the umbilicus.
2. Elevating the skin with a towel clamp on either side of the umbilicus or grasping below the umbilicus with a radiopaque gauze sponge for traction, the surgeon inserts an insufflation (Veress) needle through the layers of the abdominal wall into the peritoneal cavity. Some surgeons prefer a direct optical access trocar insertion technique or the open laparoscopic Hasson technique to establish the pneumoperitoneum, insufflating through the valve of the trocar sleeve rather than through a Veress needle (see Chapter 11 for a description of these two access approaches).
3. Once the Veress needle is inserted into the peritoneal cavity, a 10-mL syringe partially filled with sterile saline may be attached to the needle and is used for aspiration. If the needle has entered a blood vessel, blood is aspirated. If a loop of intestine or the stomach has been entered, bowel contents or malodorous gas is aspirated. If the needle is free in the peritoneal cavity, nothing is aspirated.
4. The surgeon attaches a plastic or silastic one-way filtration tubing to the Veress needle where it is then connected to a CO_2

gas insufflator. Settings for CO_2 insufflation rate and maximum pneumoperitoneal pressure are confirmed with the surgeon by the perioperative nurse before insufflation begins. Approximately 3 to 4 L of CO_2 is delivered into the peritoneal cavity to achieve pneumoperitoneum. CO_2 is commonly used as the insufflation medium because it is nontoxic, highly soluble in blood, and rapidly absorbed from the peritoneal cavity. The intra-abdominal pressure is usually set between 12 and 15 mm Hg and is closely monitored to prevent overdistention of the abdomen and to ensure free passage of gas into the peritoneal cavity. Veress needles or trocar stopcocks are inspected for leaks as well as to confirm they are in the open position to allow for the free flow of CO_2 into the insufflation tubing. Opening or initial pressures are in the 2- to 8-mm range and slowly rise with insufflation. The abdominal cavity should symmetrically distend with early loss of dullness to palpation over the liver in the right upper quadrant.

5. After insufflation is complete, the Veress needle is withdrawn and replaced with a 5- or 10-mm trocar, covered by a trocar sleeve (port). This is inserted through the abdominal wall and into the peritoneal cavity. The angle of the trocar is approximately 45 degrees toward the concavity of the pelvis. The plastic or silastic one-way filtration tubing is attached to the trocar sleeve and insufflation is resumed. With the trocar sleeve in place, the surgeon withdraws the trocar and introduces the laparoscope.

6. Visualization of the pelvis, lower abdomen, and visceral contents is begun. If the lens of the laparoscope becomes foggy, application of a commercially available defogger solution may control the problem. The laparoscope may also be prewarmed or warmed intraoperatively in a metal scope warmer filled with warm sterile water. Alternatively the surgeon may touch the lens to a loop of intestine to clear it. There are commercial insufflation units that warm the CO_2 either by a separate warming attachment connected to a one-way infiltration tubing or incorporated in the insufflation tubing itself.

7. The anesthesia provider places the patient in Trendelenburg position.

8. The video camera is attached to the laparoscope to aid the surgical teams' visualization, as well as record the procedure for future reference, medical teaching purposes, or patient education. If ancillary instruments such as biopsy forceps, tissue-sealing device, or bipolar forceps are needed, the surgeon inserts a second trocar under direct visualization at the suprapubic region or at the right or left lower lateral oblique region of the abdomen. If needed, a third port is also introduced.

9. The surgeon may test for tubal patency (if applicable) using chromopertubation.

10. After completion of the planned intra-abdominal procedure, the surgeon withdraws the laparoscope, allows the insufflated gas to escape from the trocar port or by suction, and removes any remaining trocar ports. Some surgeons remove the trocar ports under direct vision before removing the laparoscope.

11. The trocar incisions are closed (fascia, if necessary, followed by a subcuticular stitch), and either wound closure strips, small dressings, or skin glue is applied.

12. The surgeon removes the uterine manipulator (if used) and checks the cervix for bleeding. If bleeding is present, pressure may be applied with a radiopaque sponge stick or a suture ligature may be needed.

13. A perineal pad is applied.

FIGURE 14-31 Ruptured ectopic pregnancy with fetus in sac.

Laparoscopic Salpingostomy for Ectopic Tubal Pregnancy

Ectopic pregnancy is defined as any gestation developing outside of the endometrial cavity. Risk factors for developing an ectopic pregnancy include use of IUDs for contraception, pelvic inflammatory disease, tubal ligation, tubal dysfunction (as with endometriosis), in vitro fertilization, smoking, salpingitis, hormonal imbalance, and previous ectopic pregnancy. Although the fallopian tube is the most common site for ectopic pregnancies (occurring in up to 95% of all cases), ectopic pregnancies can also develop on the cervix, on the ovary, or within the peritoneal cavity (Cashion, 2012). Women who experience ectopic pregnancy generally present with abdominal pain, abnormal vaginal bleeding, and a palpable adnexal mass. Diagnosis is confirmed through measurement of human chorionic gonadotropin (hCG) levels and the use of ultrasound to determine the absence of a gestational sac within the endometrial cavity. A serious complication of ectopic pregnancy is tubal rupture and hemorrhage (Figure 14-31). Ultrasound is also useful in identifying free fluid in the peritoneal cavity, which could be blood or cystic fluid. Ruptured ectopic pregnancy is considered a surgical emergency and is associated with severe abdominal pain, tachycardia, and hypotension. The woman with a ruptured ectopic pregnancy may also experience shoulder pain because of irritation of her diaphragm from the hemoperitoneum. Ectopic pregnancy may be treated medically with methotrexate (if unruptured) or surgically through salpingostomy, segmental resection, fimbrial expression, or salpingectomy (Figure 14-32). Methotrexate destroys rapidly dividing cells by blocking folic acid uptake in embryonic cells and is often administered in conjunction with the surgical procedure (Cashion, 2012). Laparoscopic and/or ultrasound-guided application of methotrexate directly into the fallopian tube may also be used. This approach decreases the toxicity of systemic administration of methotrexate (Lobo, 2012).

Procedural Considerations. Procedural considerations for laparoscopic salpingostomy are identical to those for any laparoscopic procedure, with the addition of methotrexate. The surgical team may find that developing a checklist for surgical emergencies such as ruptured ectopic pregnancy assists in efficient care rather than relying on memory alone (Arriaga et al, 2013).

Operative Procedure

1. The operative procedure begins as described in steps 1 through 8 of laparoscopy.

2. Immediate evacuation of blood or fluid is done to enhance visibility and assess the pelvic organs and structures.

FIGURE 14-32 A, Electrodesiccation of the proximal fallopian tube during salpingectomy. **B,** Excision of the fallopian tube.

3. The surgeon mobilizes the distal end of the fallopian tube to perform an adhesiolysis. Grasping forceps are placed on either side of the fallopian tube, and gentle traction is applied.

4. Before making an incision into the tube, coagulation of the serial vessels on both sides of the anticipated incision may be performed. A dilute solution of IV saline and vasopressin may be injected into the mesenteric margin to avoid excessive bleeding (Figure 14-33).

5. A single incision is made with scissors from the mesenteric to the antimesenteric side of the fallopian tube, where the products of conception are exposed.

6. The tissue is removed gently with forceps while constant irrigation (hydrodissection) is maintained with an isotonic solution (Figure 14-34). Vigorous evacuation is avoided so that the highly vascular underlying interstitial layer is not disturbed.

7. Small bleeding vessels can be ligated with a fine, nonreactive suture or with a monopolar ESU. Simple traumatic compression of bleeding margins will also promote hemostasis. Mesosalpingeal vessel ligation may be performed.

8. The tubal incision may be allowed to close by secondary intention or, as in the instance of salpingostomy, the incision may be closed in one or two layers, with 6-0 interrupted sutures.

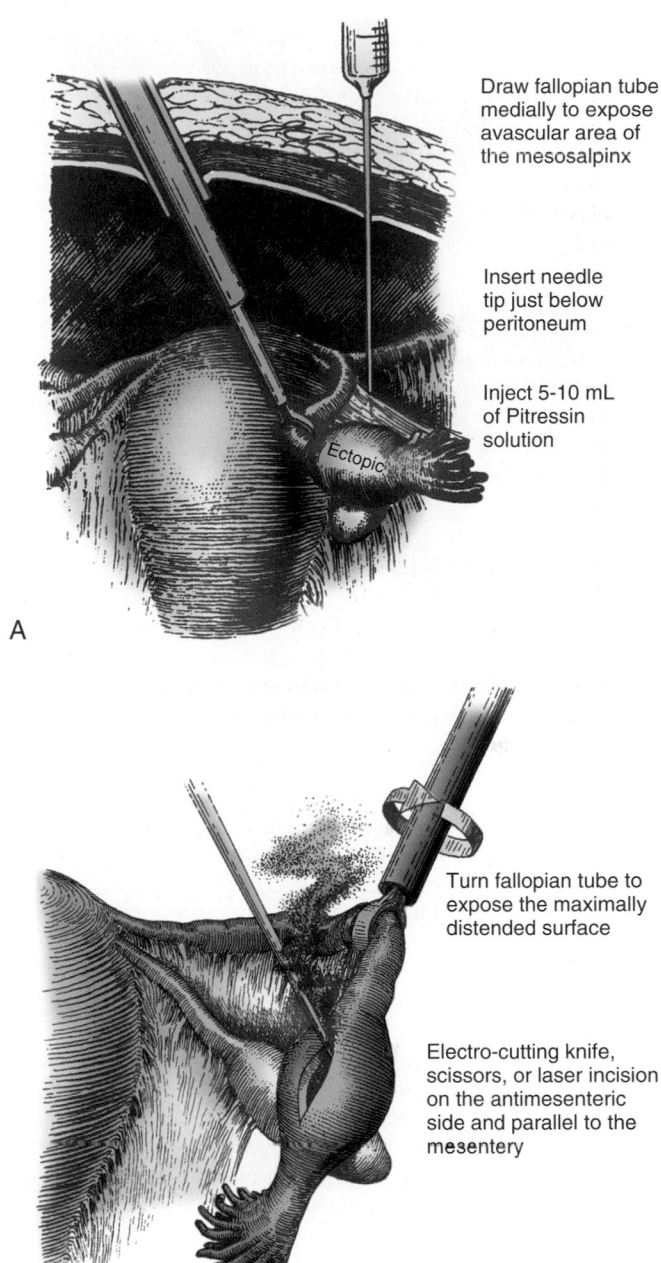

FIGURE 14-33 Salpingostomy. **A,** Injection of vasopressin into mesosalpinx. **B,** Incision made into fallopian tube.

9. The procedure is completed as described in steps 10 through 13 of laparoscopy.

Laparoscopic Ovarian Cystectomy

Ovarian cystectomy is frequently performed via the laparoscopic approach.

Operative Procedure

1. The operative procedure begins as described in steps 1 through 8 of laparoscopy.

2. After successful laparoscopic entry, adhesiolysis is achieved (if applicable).

Insert Aquadissector deep into incision

Fluid under pressure dissects and dislodges ectopic pregnancy and clots

FIGURE 14-34 Hydrodissection (Aquadissector) used to separate ectopic pregnancy from fallopian tube during salpingostomy.

3. On entry, peritoneal washings for cytology are obtained, if indicated. Safe specimen practices are initiated if cytologic washings are obtained.
4. The ovarian cyst is mobilized, and the cortex is grasped with a biopsy instrument.
5. The surgeon incises the cortex to expose the cyst wall with scissors, a monopolar ESU laparoscopic instrument, or the CO_2 laser.
6. The incision is enlarged using scissors, and pressurized hydrodissection is used to separate the cyst from the ovarian stroma.
7. The cyst is dissected, placed in a laparoscopic retrieval bag, and removed intact through a trocar port, or the cyst may be opened, evacuated, thoroughly cleaned by lavage with the hydrodissector, and then removed.
8. If the cyst is opened intraperitoneally, the patient should be placed supine, not in Trendelenburg position, while the fluid is removed and the pelvic cavity is cleaned by lavage. Supine position assists in preventing fluid entry into the upper abdominal cavity.
9. Hemostasis is controlled using a laparoscopic monopolar ESU instrument.
10. The ovary usually does not require suturing; however, if the edges gape widely, the surgeon may loosely approximate them with interrupted 4-0 synthetic absorbable suture.
11. The end of the procedure is completed as described in steps 10 through 13 of laparoscopy.

Laparoscopic-Assisted Vaginal Hysterectomy

Laparoscopic-assisted vaginal hysterectomy (LAVH) offers an alternative to total abdominal hysterectomy (TAH) and vaginal hysterectomy (VH). The patient avoids having a large abdominal incision, extended hospital stay, and long recovery period, which occur with TAH. LAVH is associated with less pain than TAH. Patients who are not candidates for a traditional TAH may be candidates for

LAVH, which allows for morcellation of large benign uterine fibroids that can then be removed through one of the trocar sleeve ports or the vagina.

A morcellation device cores the fibroid or benign enlarged uterus into narrow strips with a circular cutting blade at its tip. A laparoscopic tenaculum inserted through the port of the morcellator is used to control and remove the tissue. The cored narrow strips can be easily evacuated through the port of the morcellator device with each pass of the morcellator. The assistant or surgeon continues to morcellate the uterus until it is small enough to extract through either the vagina or a trocar port. VH does not commonly allow for morcellation of large uterine fibroids.

Although not described here, in laparoscopic-assisted supracervical hysterectomy (LASH), the body of the uterus is removed and the cervix is left intact. In order to remove the benign uterus in a LASH procedure, morcellation is required.

The surgeon uses laparoscopy to visualize the pelvis and can thereby determine whether disease is present. This is not possible with traditional VH. Conditions for LAVH include postmenopausal bleeding, pelvic pain, uterine leiomyomas, and adnexal masses. Patients with postmenopausal bleeding are evaluated for presence of endometrial cancer or atypical endometrial hyperplasia in order to select the appropriate procedure. Contraindications for LAVH may include a history of abdominopelvic surgery, salpingitis or endometriosis, lymphadenectomy, and some types of endometrial cancer or large uterine leiomyomas.

Procedural Considerations. Procedural considerations, accessory instrumentation, and approach are similar to those used in other laparoscopic surgical procedures. The patient is placed in low lithotomy position with attention to positioning interventions to protect the patient from injury (see Chapter 6 for positioning considerations). A two-procedure table setup is used to prevent cross-contamination. One setup is used for the laparoscopic portion of the procedure and the other for the vaginal portion.

Operative Procedure. The operative procedure begins as described in steps 1 through 8 of laparoscopy and may include the following:
1. The broad ligament is dissected with either a blunt or sharp laparoscopic instrument or a laparoscopic monopolar instrument powered by an ESU.
2. Desiccation of the round and infundibulopelvic ligaments is completed using a bipolar coagulation device or with a 5- or 10-mm laparoscopic vessel sealing and dividing device.
3. Continued dissection of the broad ligaments is performed up to the bladder and posterior uterine borders.
4. Dissection continues by freeing the urinary bladder from the lower uterine segment, thus creating a bladder flap.
5. The uterine vessels are sealed bilaterally and divided with a vessel sealing and dividing device or a monopolar ESU laparoscopic instrument using the cutting current. The ESU is used to divide the upper paracervical ligament and devascularize the uterus. The laparoscope and instruments are then removed. The light source is turned off for fire prevention safety. The surgeon, assistant, and scrub person now turn their attention to the vaginal portion of the procedure.
6. The surgeon may inject the vaginal submucosa circumferentially with a diluted sterile IV saline and vasopressin mixture. (See vaginal hysterectomy procedure steps 4 through 12 for the remaining portion of the vaginal procedure.)

7. The surgeon, surgical assistant, and scrub person change their surgical gown and gloves and return to the laparoscopy. The laparoscope is reintroduced to verify hemostasis and to confirm the integrity of the vaginal cuff closure. Irrigation is carried out and any clots are suctioned and removed.

8. The end of the procedure is completed as described in steps 10 through 13 of laparoscopy.

Laparoscopic Robotically Assisted Procedures

Robotic-assisted laparoscopic surgery represents the newest available technology for minimally invasive gynecologic procedures (see Chapter 7, Figure 7-11). It has transformed the way in which surgery is performed. The most common robotic system used in hospitals is the da Vinci surgical system (Intuitive, Inc.) (Walters and Eley, 2011). The system consists of the following three separate components: (1) The *surgeon's console* has a three-dimensional high-definition viewer, hand manipulators, and foot controls. Once docked, the surgeon is seated at the console away from the surgical field and able to manipulate the robotic arms, camera, and magnification of the surgical field. (2) The *vision system* provides a three-dimensional image through an endoscope equipped with stereoscopic cameras and dual optics. There is also a viewing monitor for the assistant and team to visualize the surgical procedure. (3) The *patient cart* has four robotic arms, three of which can be used with robotic 360-degree wristed (i.e., jointed) instruments in 7 degrees of freedom and the other is for holding and stabilizing the endoscope and camera. Robotic technology in gynecologic surgery is used for hysterectomies, pelvic reconstructive surgery, and gynecologic oncology procedures (Gambone, 2010) (Research Highlight). Surgical advantages to robotic-assisted laparoscopic procedures include three-dimensional visualization and magnification of the surgical field, elimination of surgeon hand tremors, ergonomic advantages for the surgeon, and enhanced dexterity with precise and defined microscopic tissue dissection capabilities. Some direct patient advantages compared to traditional open procedures are smaller incisions, reduced blood loss and infection rate, shorter hospital stays, fewer postoperative complications, and less pain (Walters and Eley, 2011; Zender and Thell, 2010). Robotic procedures can also be carried out in extremely obese patients for whom conventional laparoscopy would be ineffective or difficult.

Procedural Considerations. Robotic-assisted laparoscopic procedures are performed under general anesthesia. Procedural considerations applicable to laparoscopic surgery are appropriate for robotic-assisted surgery including both prepping and draping practices. The perioperative nurse and surgical team must be educated and familiar with the specialized equipment used for robotic-assisted surgery to facilitate a smooth and safe experience for the patient. Because steep Trendelenburg position is used intraoperatively, meticulous positioning considerations are used. Face, eye, breast, arm, and hand pads are used to prevent positioning injury. Instrumentation to convert to an open abdominal procedure is always readily available.

Operative Procedure

1. The surgeon places a uterine manipulator (surgeon's preference) into the cervix along with a vaginal balloon occluder. This device is used to manipulate the uterus intraoperatively and to prevent CO_2 from escaping through the vagina during dissection of the uterus and cervix.

RESEARCH HIGHLIGHT

Advantages of Robotic Surgery in Staging of Endometrial Cancer

Minimally invasive surgery (MIS) has long been an integral part of gynecologic surgery. Recent developments in robotic technology offer surgeons certain advantages in performing more advanced gynecologic procedures. Evolutions in MIS instrumentation assist surgeons in overcoming technical and mechanical limitations of traditional laparoscopy.

Using a cohort of 1000 women in a single institution, researchers examined outcomes in an expanding robotic surgical program. The most common indication for surgery within the cohort was women who had endometrial cancer. A total of 337 women undergoing robotic surgery for endometrial cancer staging were compared with the historical data of 131 women who underwent open endometrial staging via laparotomy. Women undergoing robotic surgery for endometrial staging had less blood loss (46.9 vs. 197.6 mL, P < 0.0001), shorter length of hospital stay (1.4 vs. 5.3 days, P < 0.0001), fewer major complications (6.4% vs. 20.6%, P < 0.0001) and higher lymph node counts (15.5 vs. 13.1, P = 0.007). Operative time was longer in the robotic group.

Complication rates between women undergoing robotic and open endometrial cancer staging were also compared. Major complications were higher in open procedures, with wound dehiscence being the most significant. Vaginal cuff dehiscence was higher in robotic procedures.

A subset analysis demonstrated that patients who were morbidly obese (body mass index ≥30 and <40) who underwent robotic surgery for endometrial cancer staging had significant reductions in major complication rates. These findings are consistent with other published studies in obese women undergoing robotic surgery for endometrial cancer staging.

Robotic-assisted MIS effectively surpasses technical obstacles posed by traditional laparoscopy by incorporating 3-D magnified visualization, articulating wristlike instruments, enhancing stability of the operative field and instrumentation, and providing optimal ergonomics for the surgeon. In general, this study reported favorable outcomes using robotic surgery technology for endometrial cancer staging as compared with the laparotomy approach. The major exception was longer operative times in robotic procedures. Future studies are required to explore long-term clinical outcomes, quality of life outcomes, and cost-effectiveness of robotic surgery.

Modified from Paley PJ et al: Surgical outcomes in gynecologic oncology in the era of robotics: analysis of first 1000 cases, *Am J Obstet Gynecol* 204(6):551–559, 2011.

2. A Veress needle is placed and the surgeon establishes an adequate pneumoperitoneum. Alternately, the open Hasson technique (see Chapter 11) may be used.

3. The surgeon incises the skin at or above the umbilicus and inserts a disposable 12-mm trocar port for the camera. Some surgeons place this port either slightly to the right or left of the umbilicus, especially when lymph node dissection is contemplated. The robotic laparoscopic telescope with the attached camera is then introduced into the pelvic cavity. Fire safety practices require that the light source shutter is only opened when the robotic laparoscopic camera is being monitored.

4. Either two or three additional robotic 8-mm trocar ports are created for the robotic instrument arms. A supplementary trocar port (placed on the patient's right or left lateral abdominal area) is created for the assistant to use for any additional instrumentation, removal of specimens, retraction, insertion

and removal of sutures, and for irrigation and suctioning purposes. Once all the trocar ports are placed, the robotic laparoscopic camera is removed and the light source shutter closed for fire prevention safety.

5. The anesthesia provider positions the patient in steep Trendelenburg.

6. The perioperative nurse drives the patient cart up to and between the patient's legs, or to the right or left side of the OR bed (side docking) while observing and maintaining integrity of the sterile field. Patient safety is closely monitored. All team members are attentive when the patient cart is being driven into position and again at the end when the cart is driven away from the patient and parked.

7. Both the surgeon and the surgical assistant attach the robotic camera and instrument arms to their respective trocar ports. The cart is now considered docked.

8. The robotic laparoscopic camera is reintroduced into the abdominal cavity and then, under direct visualization, the robotic instruments are inserted into the pelvic cavity. The monopolar and bipolar cords of the ESU are attached to the robotic instrument scissors and robotic bipolar instrument, respectively.

9. The surgical assistant remains at the sterile field to assist the surgeon and monitor the patient and surgical field throughout the procedure. The surgeon moves to the console to perform the laparoscopic robotic-assisted portion of the procedure.

10. The surgeon begins by bilaterally skeletonizing tissue using the robotic laparoscopic monopolar and bipolar ESU instruments around the infundibulopelvic, round, and broad ligaments as well as the uterine artery pedicles. Once cauterized and desiccated completely, the tissue is divided using the robotic laparoscopic scissor instrument.

11. Additional dissection is performed to divide the cardinal and uterosacral ligament complex bilaterally.

12. Either the scrub person or the surgical assistant provides cephalad pressure on the uterus by means of the uterine manipulator while the surgeon performs a circumferential colpotomy.

13. Once the uterus and cervix are detached, they are delivered into the patient's vagina and positioned to maintain CO_2 pneumoperitoneum by the surgical assistant. If there is suspicion of uterine malignancy, the specimen is removed by the surgical assistant and an occluder inserted into the vagina to maintain CO_2 pneumoperitoneum. If appropriate, pelvic and para-aortic lymph node dissection is now carried out. Specimens can be withdrawn in a retrieval bag through the vagina.

14. The surgeon closes the vaginal cuff using a running absorbable barbed suture.

15. Hemostasis is established and robotic instruments are removed under direct visualization. The robotic laparoscopic camera is then removed along with the trocar ports. The perioperative nurse closes the light shutter for fire safety.

16. The perioperative nurse safely backs the cart away from the patient and parks it away from the surgical field. The cart is now considered undocked.

17. The surgeon returns to the sterile field and, along with the surgical assistant, completes the procedure as in steps 10, 11, and 13 of laparoscopy. The occluder (if used) is removed from the vagina at the end of the procedure.

Laparoendoscopic Single-Site Surgery

The first laparoendoscopic single-site surgery (LESS) for hysterectomy was reported in the early 1990s (Sobolewski et al, 2011).

LESS has recently become a more available option for women undergoing minimally invasive gynecologic surgical procedures. The LESS procedure uses an open Hassan technique, a single-site incision at the umbilicus, and specially designed instruments and endoscopes. Most incisions range from approximately 12 to 25 mm in length; up to four instruments can be inserted and manipulated through a single port at one time.

Most laparoscopic gynecologic surgical procedures such as a LAVH, salpingo-oophorectomy, and laparoscopic tubal ligation (LTL), can be accomplished via the LESS approach. Patient advantages to having a LESS procedure include less postoperative pain; cosmesis; and eliminating the risk for potential injury to the inferior epigastric vessels, as well as the iliohypogastric or the ilioinguinal nerves. These injuries may occur when lateral ports are placed in the traditional laparoscopic surgical approach.

Procedural Considerations. Procedural considerations are the same as with laparoscopic surgery with the addition of one of the many available LESS ports (surgeon's preference), laparoscopic articulating instruments, and a flexible endoscope. As with all laparoscopic procedures, an open abdominal instrument and gynecologic tray is readily available. General anesthesia is administered, a urinary catheter is inserted, and the skin prep and draping are carried out as described in the laparoscopy procedure.

Operative Procedure

1. The surgeon places a uterine manipulator (surgeon's preference) into the cervix, usually along with a vaginal balloon occluder.

2. The surgeon may inject local anesthetic before incising the skin for the open Hasson technique (see Chapter 11).

3. The surgeon inserts the LESS port.

4. A laparoscopic endoscope is placed, followed by the surgeon's choice of laparoscopic instruments.

5. Visualization of the pelvis, lower abdomen, and the visceral contents is begun.

6. The anesthesia provider positions the patient in steep or modified Trendelenburg.

7. The surgical procedure is carried out as described in the similar laparoscopic surgical procedures.

8. The end of the procedure is completed as described in steps 10 through 13 of laparoscopy.

Gynecologic Surgery Using the Abdominal Approach

Total Abdominal Hysterectomy

Total abdominal hysterectomy (TAH) is the removal of the entire uterus, including the corpus and the cervix. TAH may be performed for symptomatic pelvic relaxation or prolapse, chronic pain associated with pelvic congestion, pelvic inflammatory disease, endometriosis, recurrent ovarian cysts, uterine leiomyomas (fibroids), dysfunctional uterine bleeding (DUB) in perimenopausal women, or adenomyosis (Evidence for Practice). TAH procedures are performed with or without bilateral salpingo-oophorectomy (BSO). Approximately 600,000 hysterectomies are performed each year in the United States (Centers for Disease Control and Prevention [CDC], 2012).

Procedural Considerations. The abdominal prep is completed before the vaginal and perineal prep, which includes the cervix. The perioperative nurse uses caution when prepping the vaginal and perineal area to prevent inadvertent splashing of prep solution onto

EVIDENCE FOR PRACTICE

Alternatives to Hysterectomy

When nurses use evidence, they raise their own awareness, give time for thought to the care they provided, and contemplate the evidence that underpins it (Wilkinson, 2013). Hysterectomy is the most common nonpregnancy-related major surgery performed on women in the United States. It is widely accepted as appropriate treatment for cancer and various noncancerous conditions, such as pain, discomfort, uterine bleeding, emotional distress, and related symptoms. Although hysterectomy can alleviate uterine problems, less-invasive treatments are available. Alternatives to hysterectomy recommended by the Agency for Healthcare Research and Quality (AHRQ) are noted in the following table.

Condition	Conservative Surgery	Pharmacologic Therapies		Other Strategies
		Hormonal	Nonhormonal	
Fibroids	Myomectomy	GnRH agonists	NSAIDs	Watchful waiting
	Hysteroscopic or laparoscopic surgery using laser for excision of fibroids			
Endometriosis	Adhesiolysis using laser or an ESU	GnRH agonists	NSAIDs	Watchful waiting
	Laser laparoscopy	Danazol	Analgesics	Biofeedback
	Fulguration of endometriosis sites using an ESU or laser		Opioids for severe pain	
	Nerve blocks	Oral contraceptives		
	Uterosacral nerve ablation			Lifestyle modifications (nutrition/exercise)
Prolapse	Colporrhaphy	Estrogen		Watchful waiting
	Laparoscopic or vaginal suspension techniques			Kegel exercises
				Pessaries
Dysfunctional bleeding	Dilation and curettage	Oral contraceptives		Watchful waiting
	Endometrial ablation			
Chronic pelvic pain	Adhesiolysis	Oral contraceptives	NSAIDs	Watchful waiting
	Uterosacral nerve ablation			Physical therapy
				Nutritional counseling
				Psychologic counseling

ESU, Electrosurgical unit; *GnRH,* gonadotropin-releasing hormone; *NSAIDs,* nonsteroidal antiinflammatory drugs.
Modified from *Common uterine conditions: options for treatment,* AHCPR Pub No. 98-0003, Rockville, MD, December 1997, Agency for Health Care Policy and Research, available at http://archive.ahrq.gov/consumer/uterine1.htm#1. Accessed February 24, 2013.

the already prepped abdomen (AORN, 2013). An indwelling urinary drainage catheter is inserted to provide continual bladder drainage. The patient begins in supine position and is changed intraoperatively to Trendelenburg position. A basic abdominal gynecologic instrument tray and a self-retaining retractor are required. Provisions are made to remove instruments that come into contact with the cervix and vagina from the surgical field, thereby avoiding vaginal contamination of the abdominal incision.

Operative Procedure

1. In an obese patient or for exploration of the upper abdominal cavity, a left rectus (paramedian) or vertical midline incision is usually used. For simple hysterectomy in a woman of normal size, a Pfannenstiel incision is often used. The surgeon opens the abdominal layers and peritoneum as described for laparotomy (see Chapter 11).
2. Once the peritoneal cavity is opened, the anesthesia provider places the patient in Trendelenburg position to provide better visualization of the pelvic organs.
3. A self-retaining retractor is used for exposure and moist radiopaque laparotomy pads are used to pack the intestines into the upper abdomen. The round ligament is grasped with forceps, clamped, cut, and ligated. A handheld vessel sealing and dividing device can be used throughout the procedure where ligaments and vessels are clamped, cut, and ligated. If the surgeon cuts the pedicles, a #10 blade or Metzenbaum

scissors is used; sutures may be tagged with a hemostat for traction. This procedure is done on both sides (Figure 14-35, *A*).
4. Using blunt dissection the surgeon separates the anterior layer of the broad ligament close to the uterus on each side. Bleeding vessels are clamped and ligated. The fallopian tube and the utero-ovarian ligaments are doubly clamped together, incised, and doubly tied with suture ligatures (see Figure 14-35, *B*).
5. The surgeon pulls the uterus forward to expose the posterior sheath of the broad ligament, and incises the ligament with Metzenbaum scissors. Ureters are identified. The uterine vessels and uterosacral ligaments are doubly clamped, divided by sharp dissection at the level of the internal os, and ligated with suture ligatures (see Figure 14-35, *C*).
6. The severed uterine vessels are clamped at the paracervical ligament, cut and suture ligated, or bluntly dissected away from the cervix on each side with the aid of radiopaque gauze sponges on sponge-holding forceps, scissors, and tissue forceps.
7. The bladder is separated from the cervix and upper vagina with sharp and blunt dissection assisted by radiopaque gauze sponges on sponge-holding forceps. The bladder may be retracted with a moist radiopaque laparotomy pad and an angular blade retractor. The vaginal vault is incised close to the cervix with a blade or scissors (see Figure 14-35, *D*).
8. The surgeon grasps the anterior lip of the cervix with an Allis or Kocher clamp. Using scissors, the surgeon dissects the cervix

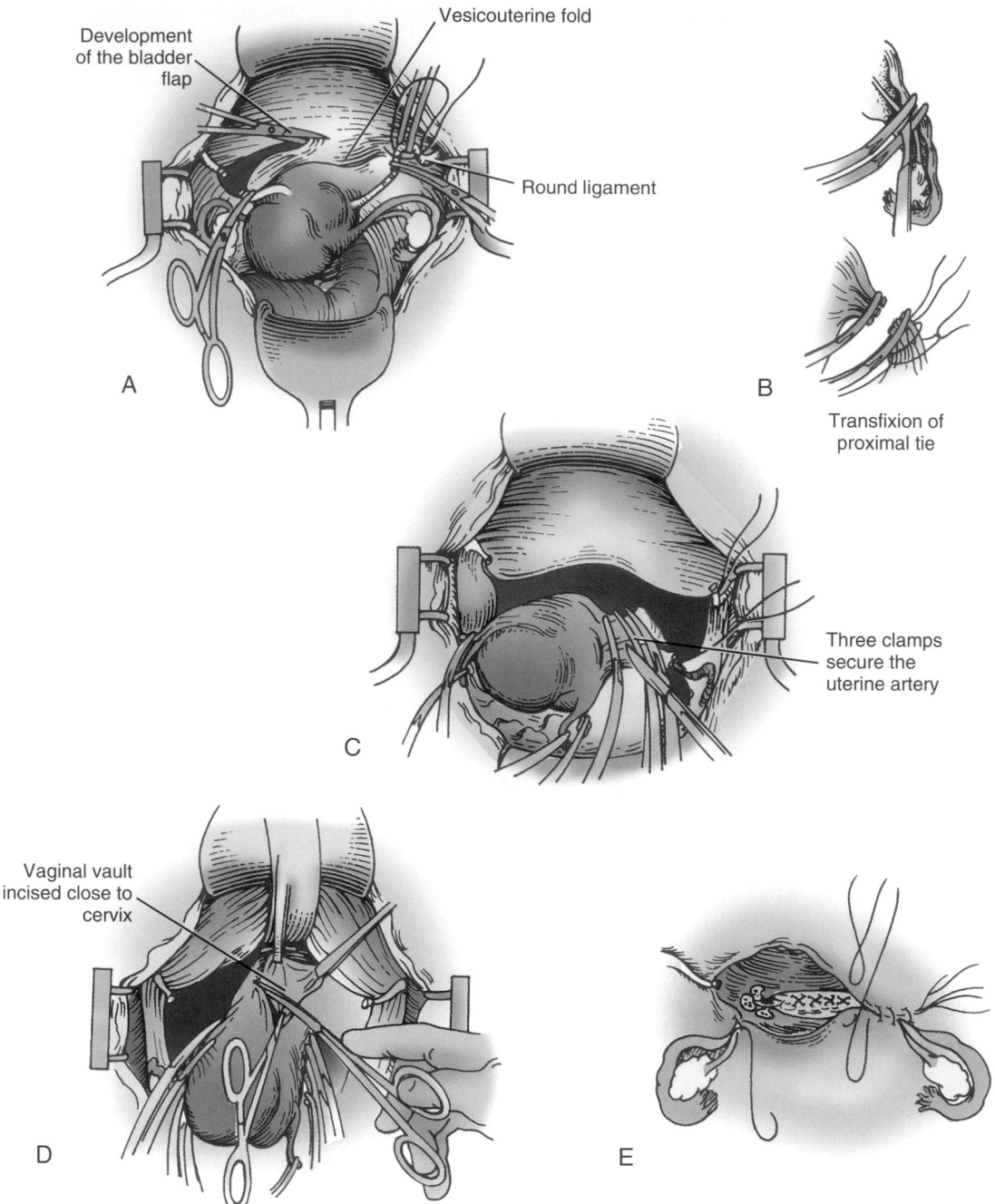

FIGURE 14-35 Abdominal hysterectomy for single fibroid uterus. **A,** Peritoneum retracted with self-retaining retractors, and organs protected with laparotomy packs saturated in warm normal saline solution. Transverse incision made through uterine peritoneum and extended to each side of uterine attachments of round ligaments. Bleeding vessels clamped and ligated. Round ligament grasped, ligated, and cut. **B,** Tube and ovarian ligaments clamped, cut, and sutured. **C,** Uterus pulled forward, posterior sheath of broad ligaments divided, and uterine artery and veins secured by three heavy curved clamps. Pedicle divided, leaving two hemostats on proximal pedicle. **D,** Bladder separated from cervix and upper vagina. Vaginal vault opened and grasped with Allis forceps. Allis forceps placed on anterior lip of cervix, and dissection of cervix carried out to complete its amputation from vagina. **E,** Three connective tissue thickenings anchored to vaginal vault, vaginal mucosa approximated, and vault closed. As shown, peritoneum closed with continuous suture.

and amputates it from the vagina. The uterus is removed. The scrub person places any potentially contaminated instruments used on the cervix and vagina into a discard basin and passes them from the field (including sponge-holding forceps and suction). Bleeding is controlled with hemostats and sutures or a monopolar ESU.

9. The vaginal vault is closed as one layer with interrupted figure-of-eight sutures to ensure the vault of the vagina is closed completely and to prevent any risk for prolapse. Angle sutures anchor all three connective tissue ligaments to the vaginal vault. The pedicles, fallopian tubes, and ovarian ligaments are left free of the vault.

FIGURE 14-36 Classification of uterine leiomyomas.

10. The surgeon may close the peritoneum over the bladder, vaginal vault, and rectum (see Figure 14-35, *E*). The packed radiopaque laparotomy pads are removed, and the omentum is drawn over the bowel.

11. The abdominal wound is closed as described for laparotomy closure (see Chapter 11).

12. An abdominal dressing and perineal pad are applied.

Salpingo-Oophorectomy

Salpingo-oophorectomy is removal of a fallopian tube and all or part of the associated ovary. Unilateral salpingo-oophorectomy may be done to treat chronic salpingo-oophoritis, for ectopic tubal gestation, or for certain disease conditions of the adnexa or large adnexal cysts. Some indications for BSO are malignancy, premalignant states, and as a risk reducing procedure for patients at high risk for malignancy (*BRCA1* or *BRCA2* gene and Lynch syndrome). In most cases this procedure is done laparoscopically unless a large adnexal mass is present.

Procedural Considerations. The basic abdominal gynecologic instrument tray is required.

Operative Procedure

1. The skin is incised, and the abdominal layers are opened, as described for laparotomy (see Chapter 11).

2. The affected tube is grasped with Allis or Babcock forceps. The ureter is first identified and then the infundibulopelvic ligament is clamped with hemostats, cut, and ligated. A laparoscopic vessel sealing and dividing device can be used throughout the procedure where ligaments and vessels are clamped, cut, and or ligated.

3. The mesosalpinx is grasped with hemostats and divided with the suspensory ligament of the ovary.

4. The cornual attachment of the tube is excised with a blade or curved scissors. Bleeding vessels are clamped and ligated.

5. The edges of the broad ligament are peritonealized from the uterine horn to the infundibulopelvic ligament as described for TAH.

6. If both tubes and ovaries are to be removed, steps 2 through 5 are completed on the opposite side.

7. The abdominal wound is closed as described for laparotomy (see Chapter 11).

8. An abdominal dressing is applied.

Abdominal Myomectomy

Uterine fibroids (Figure 14-36) are common benign tumors that arise from the muscular wall of the uterus in 30% to 50% of perimenopausal women in the United States (Katz, 2012). Another term for uterine fibroids is *uterine leiomyomas.* They may also be located in the submucosal area or the subserosal surface of the uterus. On occasion they may become pedunculated and extend into the cervical canal. Rarely a subserosal fibroid may pedunculate and migrate to become a parasitic fibroid attached to the omentum or mesentery. Abdominal myomectomy is removal of leiomyomas, or fibroid tumors, by carefully separating each fibroid from the uterine wall and its blood supply. Myomectomy is usually done in young women who have symptoms indicating the presence of these tumors and who wish to preserve their potential fertility. Fibroids may decrease the chances of conception depending on their location in the uterus (Lobo, 2012).

Uterine fibroids often cause pelvic pain and pressure or may accentuate the severity of bleeding associated with DUB. Fibroids are more common in African American women and become more common during the later reproductive years (Katz, 2012). Myomectomy may be performed as a prophylactic measure with other abdominopelvic surgery. Preoperative preparation may include preoperative patient injections of leuprolide acetate (Lupron), a synthetic version of the naturally occurring gonadotropin-releasing hormone (GnRH) over several months' time, to reduce the volume of the fibroid and decrease its blood supply. This intervention mimics the postmenopausal state for women who receive it because it reduces the amount of estrogen the body synthesizes, thus reducing the size of the fibroid.

Procedural Considerations. The basic abdominal gynecologic instrument tray and an ESU are required. A laser may also be used. The patient is prepped as described for abdominal hysterectomy.

Operative Procedure

1. The procedure begins as in steps 1 and 2 of the TAH.
2. To contract the musculature of the uterine wall, a suitable drug may be injected into the fundus such as a vasopressin and sterile IV 0.9% sodium chloride (NaCl) mixture.
3. The surgeon grasps the fibroid tumor with a towel clip or tenaculum. The broad ligament may be opened with curved hemostats and Metzenbaum scissors to determine the course of the ureter and/or to free the bladder.
4. Each tumor is shelled out of its bed, using blunt and sharp instruments, a monopolar ESU, or the laser. Bleeding vessels are clamped and ligated or an ESU is used.
5. The uterus is reconstructed with interrupted or continuous sutures.
6. The peritoneum is closed over the operative site, and the abdominal wound is closed as described for laparotomy (see Chapter 11).
7. An abdominal dressing and perineal pad are applied.

Cytoreductive Surgery for Ovarian Cancer

Cytoreductive surgery (CSR) is when optimal surgical tumor debulking for ovarian cancer is attempted. Evidence has shown there is an inverse relationship between the amount of tumor left behind at the time of surgery and the patient's overall length of survival rate. The goal of CRS is to leave behind as little tumor as possible; less than 1 cm is adequate to improve survival; no residual gross disease is optimal. Ovarian cancer is the leading cause of gynecologic cancer death in women in the United States. Two thirds of women who present at the time of diagnosis already have intra-abdominal spread with metastatic disease. The death rate for ovarian cancer is high for two main reasons: the disease spreads early and the signs and symptoms of ovarian cancer are vague (Deraco et al, 2011; Fuller, 2011).

Other operative procedures performed during CSR besides a TAH with BSO or supracervical hysterectomy with BSO are omentectomy; rectosigmoid colon resection; mid-transverse colon resection; pelvic lymph node dissection; placement of intraperitoneal chemotherapy catheter; and fulguration of macroscopic tumor on the diaphragm, bladder, pelvic side walls, and liver using either an argon beam coagulator (see Chapter 8 for a discussion of this energy-delivering device) or an ESU.

Procedural Considerations.

The patient is positioned and prepped as described in the LAVH procedure. An indwelling urinary catheter is inserted. Ovarian cancer patients may present with large amounts of ascites and metastatic spread to the omentum, rectosigmoid colon, mid-transverse colon, peritoneum, paracolic gutter, liver, and diaphragm. Instrument requirements are the same as with TAH in addition to long instruments, intestinal staplers, and possibly an argon beam coagulator.

Operative Procedure

1. The skin is incised, and the abdominal layers are opened, as described for laparotomy (see Chapter 11). If ascites is present, a small incision is made into the peritoneum and suction is used to drain the ascites.
2. The surgeon and surgical assistant do a thorough exploration and assessment of the pelvic and abdominal cavity and plan the surgical approach.

3. If omental involvement is visible, an omentectomy will be performed. If no omental involvement is visible, an omental biopsy may be taken. Safe specimen practices are initiated.
4. A TAH with BSO is then performed as described in the TAH and salpingo-oophorectomy procedures.
5. Depending on the extent and involvement of the disease process with other organs, a rectosigmoid resection or other bowel resection (see Chapter 11) may be performed.
6. Fulguration of macroscopic surface tumor sites with an ESU or argon beam coagulator may be performed. Resection of enlarged lymph nodes may also be carried out at this time.
7. An intraperitoneal chemotherapy catheter may be placed into the peritoneal cavity at the end of the procedure. The port for the catheter is inserted and positioned just below the bra line to avoid irritation (Fuller, 2012).
8. The abdominal wound is closed as described in laparotomy (see Chapter 11). Drains may be used.
9. An abdominal dressing and perineal pad are applied.

Radical Hysterectomy (Wertheim)

Radical hysterectomy is en bloc dissection and wide removal of the uterus, tubes, ovaries, entire uterosacral and uterovesical ligaments, and upper vagina; this is often also undertaken with careful removal of all recognizable lymph nodes in the pelvis (Figure 14-37). Complex and extensive dissection of tissue surrounding the ureters, bladder, bowel, and greater vessels of the pelvis is also completed (Tewari and Monk, 2012). There are many variations of radical hysterectomy procedures. The procedure performed depends on the diagnosis and extent of the disease process. Radical hysterectomy is performed for malignancy of the cervix.

Procedural Considerations.

As with any complex surgical procedure, blood loss and urinary output are closely monitored. The patient is prepped and draped as described for TAH. An indwelling urinary catheter is inserted. The basic abdominal gynecologic instrument tray is required, with the addition of long instruments and a self-retaining retractor.

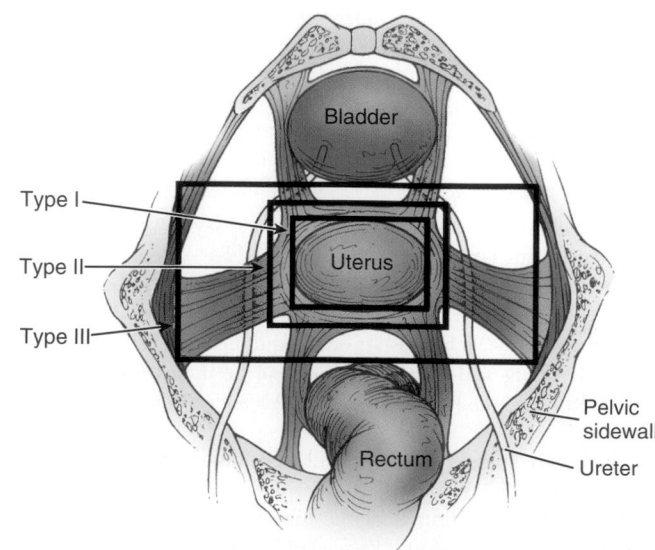

FIGURE 14-37 Different types of hysterectomy: Type I—simple hysterectomy; Type II—modified radical hysterectomy; Type III—radical hysterectomy.

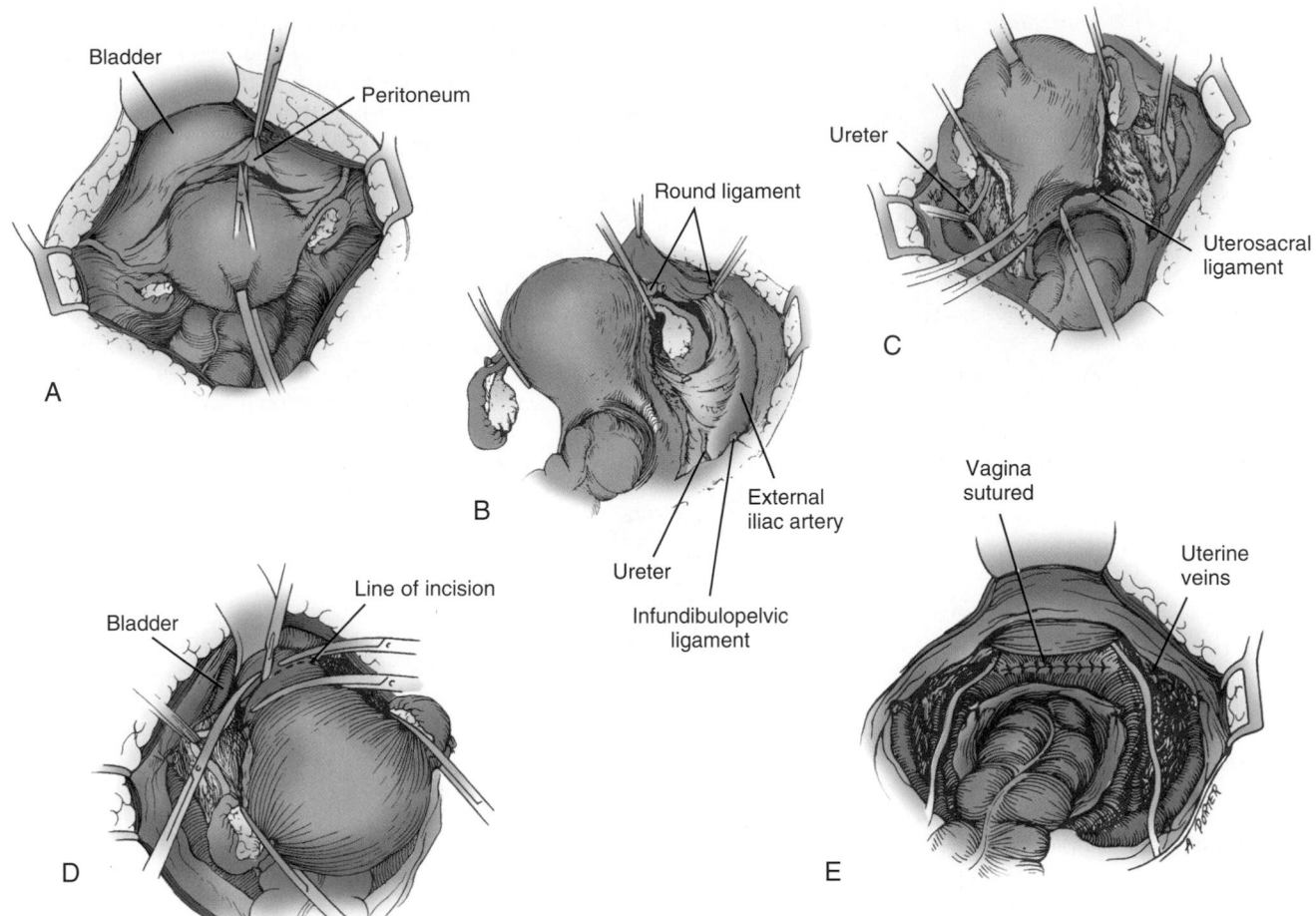

FIGURE 14-38 Wertheim radical hysterectomy. **A,** With upward traction applied on uterus, peritoneum is incised from round ligament to round ligament. **B,** Right round and infundibulopelvic ligaments are ligated and cut, thus exposing right external iliac artery. **C,** Uterus is held upward and forward, exposing cul-de-sac, which is incised as shown by dotted line. **D,** After dissection is completed, vagina is doubly clamped preparatory to transection, after which entire specimen is lifted out en bloc. **E,** Vagina is closed. Peritoneum remains to be reperitonealized.

Operative Procedure

1. The skin is incised, and the abdominal layers are opened, as described for laparotomy (see Chapter 11).

2. The surgeon cuts the peritoneum at its reflection on the anterior surface of the uterus between the round ligaments (Figure 14-38, *A*). Using blunt dissection, the surgeon frees the bladder surface from the cervix and vagina.

3. The right round and infundibulopelvic ligaments are clamped, cut with Metzenbaum scissors, and ligated with sutures or a monopolar ESU to expose the external iliac artery. A handheld vessel sealing and dividing device can be used throughout the procedure where ligaments and vessels need to be clamped, cut, and ligated. The ureter is identified and retracted with a vein retractor (see Figure 14-38, *B*).

4. The lymph and areolar tissues are dissected from the iliac artery, obturator fossa, and ureter with Lahey forceps, small gauze dissectors (also called "Kitners," "peanuts," or "pushers"), and Metzenbaum scissors. A complete lymph node dissection removes tissue from the femoral canal to the bifurcation of the iliac arteries bilaterally. The uterine artery and vein are clamped, cut, and doubly ligated.

5. The surgeon elevates the uterus and opens the cul-de-sac (see Figure 14-38, *C*); the uterosacral and cardinal ligaments are clamped, cut with scissors at some distance from the cervix, and doubly ligated with suture ligatures. Pararectal and paravesical areolar tissues are dissected free to skeletonize the upper vagina, and paraurethral tissues are removed as near to the pelvic walls as possible.

6. If there is an exocervical lesion, the proximal vagina is cross-clamped with Heaney forceps leaving an adequate margin around the cervical lesion (see Figure 14-38, *D*) and divided using a long knife handle and blade. The uterus and surrounding tissues are removed. A monopolar ESU is used to minimize venous oozing from small venules and capillaries. Lowering the head of the OR bed 15 degrees is also helpful in reducing oozing of blood and serum.

7. The surgeon sutures the vagina with an interrupted or running locked stitch, and may insert closed suction drains from above (see Figure 14-38, *E*). The peritoneum may be closed with a continuous running suture.

8. The abdominal wound is closed as described for laparotomy (see Chapter 11). Vaginal packing and drains may be used. A

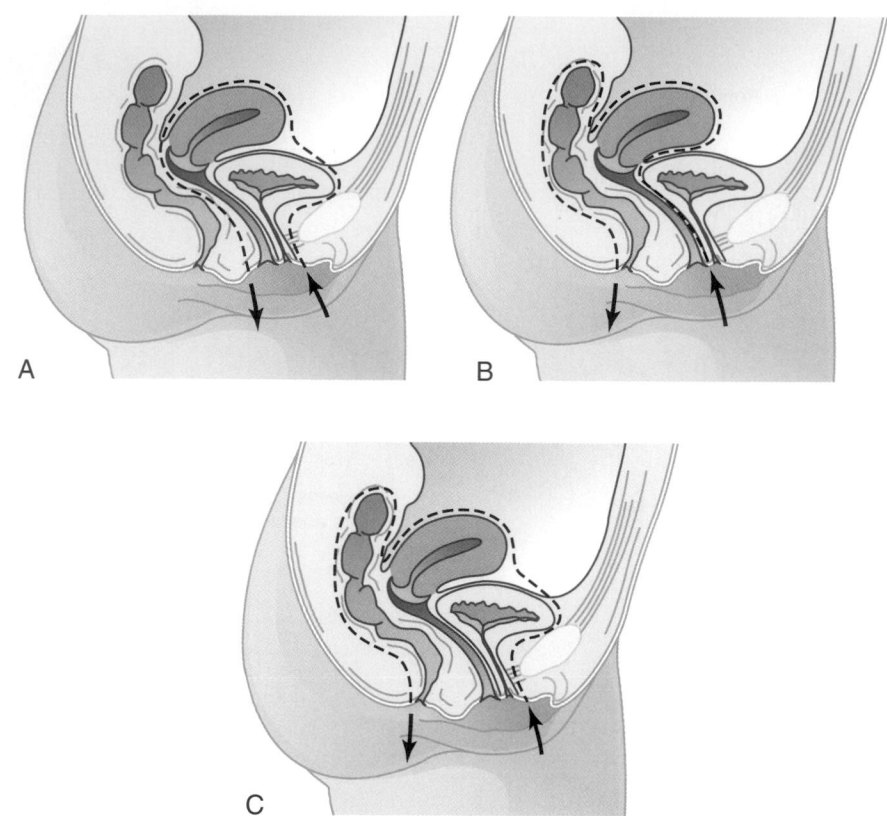

FIGURE 14-39 Organs removed in pelvic exenteration. **A,** Anterior exenteration. **B,** Posterior exenteration. **C,** Total pelvic exenteration.

suprapubic indwelling catheter may be placed to assist in managing postoperative bladder atony and for bladder drainage.

9. An abdominal dressing and perineal pad are applied.

Pelvic Exenteration

Pelvic exenteration is en bloc removal of the rectum, the distal sigmoid colon, the urinary bladder and distal ureters, all pelvic reproductive organs, and lymph nodes. In some patients a perineal phase may also be required to excise all pelvic cancer with a negative margin. In this case, the entire pelvic floor with the accompanying pelvic peritoneum, levator muscles, and perineum may be excised. A partial exenteration, either anterior and or posterior, may be performed, depending on the origin of the carcinoma and the extent of local tissue invasion (Figure 14-39).

Pelvic exenteration is the preferred treatment for advanced or recurrent carcinoma of the cervix after radiation therapy, as long as it can be completely resected with negative margins. Other pelvic carcinomas can be amenable to exenteration (Tewari and Monk, 2012). Exenteration is considered only after a thorough investigation of the patient and disease status to determine if the disease is isolated to the central pelvis, there is a reasonable chance of a cure, and the patient can return to a productive life.

The need to create urinary and bowel diversions is also considered, together with the patient's ability to cope with these diversions postoperatively. Plastic surgery may be required for creation of a neovagina. Psychologic preparation and support of the patient and family by the perioperative nurse and physician are prime requisites.

Procedural Considerations. Utmost care is taken in positioning the patient because of the duration of surgery (see Chapter 6 for positioning considerations). The patient is in supine position with legs abducted in the modified lithotomy position (i.e., lower extremities resting on a well-padded plantar surface rather than on the heel or popliteal area) or slightly elevated in that position to allow access to the perineum without disruptive position changes. Skin prepping includes the abdomen, thighs, perineum, and vaginal vault.

The perioperative team is alert to fluid and blood loss throughout the procedure. Irrigation solutions are accurately measured, and radiopaque laparotomy pads weighed, to more accurately assess blood volume loss, and the anesthesia provider and surgical team must be apprised of the measurements.

When the colon is transected or ureteral drainage is diverted into a segment of the ileum, the gastrointestinal technique (i.e., bowel technique) should be followed as described in Chapter 11.

Separate instrument trays are required for the abdominal and perineal approaches. Extra drapes, gowns, and gloves are readily available.

For the abdominal approach, the basic abdominal gynecologic instrument tray and instruments for abdominoperineal resection (see Chapter 11) are required.

For the perineal approach, the basic vaginal instrument tray is required. To prevent contamination, the anus may be closed with a purse-string suture.

Operative Procedure

1. A long vertical midline incision from the symphysis pubis to the umbilicus is made, and the abdomen is opened as described for laparotomy (see Chapter 11). If a perineal phase is to be performed (in contrast to a supralevator exenteration), a second incision within the perineum encircling the vestibule and anus is also made.

FIGURE 14-40 Pelvic exenteration. **A,** Pelvic viscera in situ as viewed from operating surgeon's vantage point after retractors are placed and small bowel is isolated with moist laparotomy packs. **B,** Empty pelvis after dissection of paravesical and paravaginal tissues and removal of specimen en bloc. **C,** Sagittal view of small bowel above pelvic defect. Perineal packing or drain may be used. **D,** After closure of abdominal wall, colostomy and urostomy stomas are sutured to skin edges.

2. The surgeon explores the peritoneal cavity for metastasis to the liver, the nodes of the celiac axis, the superior mesenteric artery, and the para-aortic tissues.

3. The pelvis is explored, and the peritoneum along the brim of the pelvis is examined for lymph node involvement. Frozen sections may be indicated to be certain that there will be negative margins. The obturator fossa and the region of the uterosacral ligaments are explored. When findings at exploration are negative, retractors are placed and the small bowel is isolated with moist radiopaque laparotomy pads (Figure 14-40).

4. The surgeon frees the sigmoid mesocolon and sections it by means of intestinal clamps and a blade or a stapling device. The proximal end is exteriorized through an opening in the left side of the abdomen; an intestinal clamp is left across the lumen until later, when the permanent colostomy will be secured to the skin (see Chapter 11).

5. The remaining sigmoid mesentery is clamped with Rochester-Péan forceps, cut, and ligated down to and including the superior hemorrhoidal vessels. Long instruments and sutures are used to reach the deep pelvic structures.

6. The distal sigmoid colon is closed with an inverting suture. The sigmoid colon and rectum are freed from the sacrococcygeal area by blunt and sharp dissection.

7. The lateral pelvic peritoneum is cut along the iliac vessels; the ovarian vessels and round ligaments on each side are clamped with Rochester-Péan forceps, cut, and doubly ligated. A hand-held vessel sealing and dividing device can be used throughout the procedure where ligaments and vessels need to be clamped, cut, and ligated.

8. The surgeon incises the peritoneum over the dome of the bladder with a long knife handle and blade or Metzenbaum scissors, and separates the bladder from the symphysis pubis down to the urethra.

9. The ureters are identified and divided 2 to 3 cm below the brim of the pelvis. The proximal end is left open to allow urinary drainage, whereas the distal end is ligated.

10. The external iliac vein is retracted to allow evacuation of the contents of the obturator fossa, leaving the obturator nerve intact. Care must be taken in dissection not to damage the sacral plexus and sciatic nerve. Occasionally some component of the hypogastric (internal iliac) vessels may also be excised.

11. In the perineal phase the surgeon isolates the internal pudendal vessels, ligates them with transfixion sutures, and cuts them. The remaining soft-tissue attachments of the pelvis are clamped and cut. Steps 10 and 11 are then performed on the opposite side.

12. The perineum is incised by an elliptic incision that includes the clitoris and anus. The ischiorectal fat is incised up to the area of the levator muscle.

13. The coccygeal attachment of the rectum is severed. The levator muscles are severed at their lateral attachments by using a long knife handle with a blade; hemostasis is maintained by pressure and traction.

14. The paravesical and paravaginal tissues are resected from the periosteum of the symphysis pubis and superior pubic rami by means of a knife. The specimen is completely freed and removed from the pelvis (Figure 14-41).

15. After residual bleeding vessels are identified and controlled by transfixing ligatures, the surgeon closes the subcutaneous tissue with interrupted sutures. A drain is placed in the wound, and the skin is closed.

16. Further residual bleeding vessels are controlled in the abdomen using a monopolar ESU. On occasion, counted radiopaque laparotomy pads used as packs may be left in the pelvis, to be removed through the perineum after 48 hours. Confirm with the surgeon the number of laparotomy pads left in the surgical site. Follow institutional protocol for documenting counted items such as soft goods that are deliberately left in the surgical site as therapeutic packing (AORN, 2013).

17. The ileal or colonic segment for the conduit is then fashioned, and the ureters are anastomosed to it. The external stoma is placed on the right side of the abdomen.

18. A jejunostomy catheter may occasionally be inserted into the proximal jejunum to aid in postoperative bowel decompression. It is connected to the bowel with a purse-string suture and exteriorized to the skin, where it is sutured in place.

19. A gastrostomy tube may be placed into the stomach in the same manner.

20. Hemostasis is assessed and controlled. The small intestine is carefully repositioned into the pelvis. Packs and retractors are removed.

21. The peritoneum, rectus muscles, and fascial sheaths are closed with interrupted figure-of-eight sutures. The skin is closed with interrupted sutures.

22. The colostomy stoma is prepared by removing the intestinal clamp from the sigmoid colon, opening the colon, and suturing the stoma to the skin edges (see Chapter 11).

23. Dressings are applied to the abdominal wound, drain, and tube sites. Drainage devices are applied to the colostomy and urostomy stomas.

Surgery for Conditions Affecting Fertility

Oophorectomy and Oophorocystectomy

Oophorectomy is removal of an ovary. Oophorocystectomy is removal of an ovarian cyst. Functional cysts constitute the majority of ovarian enlargements, with follicular cysts being the most common. Functional cysts develop in the corpus luteum. Benign cystic teratomas, also known as dermoid cysts, are very common and are composed of ectodermal tissues (sweat glands, hair follicles, and teeth) (Figure 14-42). Other tissues found in dermoid cysts include skin and skin appendages, cartilage, bone, and respiratory tract epithelium (Katz, 2012). Ovarian epithelial tumors, serous cystadenomas, and pseudomucinous cystadenomas are prone to malignant change.

The choice of operation depends on the patient's age and symptoms, findings during physical examination, and direct examination of the adnexa during surgical exploration. If the ovarian tumor is recognized as benign, only the visibly diseased portions of the adnexa are removed. In the presence of dermoid, follicular, and corpus luteum cysts, the cyst is usually enucleated and most of the ovarian parenchyma is preserved. In tubal pregnancy the ectopic pregnancy may be removed from the tube or the entire ectopic fallopian tube may be removed concomitant with, in some instances, the ovary. In most cases, this procedure is done laparoscopically unless there is a large adnexal mass present.

FIGURE 14-41 Total pelvic exenteration specimen: bladder, uterus, cervix, and rectum.

FIGURE 14-42 Gross appearance of a cut-open dermoid cyst. Note the presence of hair-bearing skin.

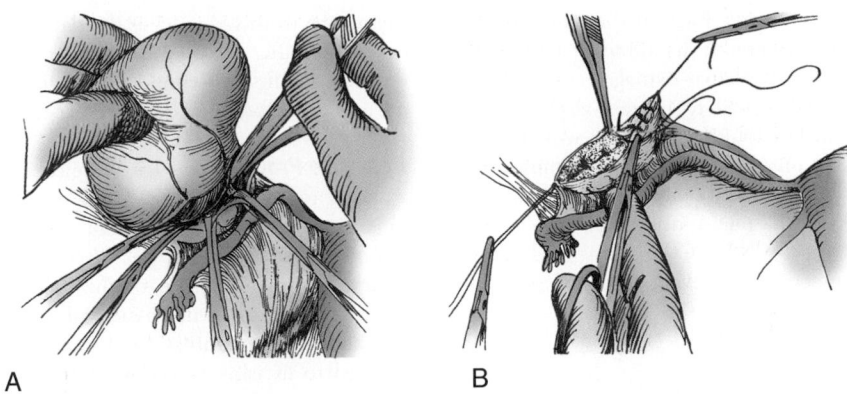

A   B

FIGURE 14-43 Resection of small cyst from ovary. **A,** Incision made around ovary near junction of cyst wall and normal ovarian tissue. Knife handle is convenient instrument for removal of cyst contents. **B,** Wound in ovary closed.

Procedural Considerations. The basic abdominal gynecologic instrument tray is required. An 18-gauge needle and 30- or 60-mL syringe is likely to be needed to aspirate ovarian cyst fluid.

Operative Procedure

1. The skin is incised and the abdominal layers are opened as described for laparotomy (see Chapter 11).
2. After the abdominal cavity is opened, the surgeon has several options:
   a. For removal of a large ovarian cyst, an 18-gauge needle with a 30- or 60-mL syringe attached may be used to aspirate the cyst. Suction is readily available. All normal ovarian tissue is preserved when possible.
   b. For removal of a smaller ovarian cyst, a clamp is placed at the base of the cyst, and the cyst is excised. The wound in the ovary is closed with absorbable suture (Figure 14-43).
   c. For removal of a dermoid cyst, the field is protected with radiopaque laparotomy pads; cystic contents cause irritation if they are spilled into the peritoneal cavity. An incision is made along the base of the cyst between the wall and normal ovarian tissue. The cystic wall is dissected away. The ovary is closed with interrupted or continuous sutures.
   d. For decortication of an enlarged ovary and wedge resection, a large segment of the ovarian cortex opposite the hilum is removed. The cysts are punctured with a needle and collapsed. A wedge of ovarian stroma, extending deep into the hilum, is resected with a #15 blade; the cortex of the ovary is closed with interrupted or continuous sutures.
3. To prevent prolapse of the tube into the cul-de-sac, the tube may be sutured to the pelvic side wall.
4. The abdominal wound is closed as described for laparotomy (see Chapter 11).
5. An abdominal dressing is applied.

Microscopic Reconstructive Surgery of the Fallopian Tube

The obstructed portion of a fallopian tube may be removed and the tube reconstructed to create patency of the remaining portion of the tube, promoting the possibility of fertilization. Reconstructive surgery of the tube, broadly called *tuboplasty,* includes reanastomosis, salpingoneostomy, fimbrioplasty, and lysis of adhesions.

The development of microsurgical techniques has advanced surgical reconstruction of fallopian tubes. Microsurgical techniques are used with mini-laparotomy or laparoscopy, or both. Microsurgical tubal anastomosis permits atraumatic, accurate alignment of fallopian tube segments. The CO_2 laser may be adapted to the operating microscope, or the freehand approach may be used in tubal reconstructive surgery. These procedures may be performed in fertility clinics by fertility specialists.

Procedural Considerations. The patient is in supine position. The surgeon may place a Kahn, Calvin, Rubin, Hui, or Humi cannula or a pediatric Foley catheter into the uterine cavity for intraoperative chromopertubation with diluted methylene blue or indigo carmine solution. Intraoperative chromopertubation can also be achieved by applying a Buxton uterine clamp around the lower segment of the uterus and inserting an Angiocath catheter through the fundus into the cavity. A radiopaque vaginal pack may be inserted to help elevate the uterus.

The basic abdominal gynecologic instrument tray is required, with the addition of iris scissors (one curved and one straight), Adson forceps without teeth, Halsted mosquito hemostats, a tray of Bowman lacrimal probes, Webster needle holders, Frazier suction tip, Kirschner retractor (if desired), and a Buxton uterine clamp (if desired).

Basic microsurgical instruments include microscissors (one curved and one straight), bayonet microscissors, jeweler's forceps, microforceps, fallopian tube forceps, petit-point mosquito hemostats, micro–needle holders (one curved and one straight), ball-tipped nerve hook, and glass or Teflon rods.

Accessory items include micro–needle electrodes for the ESU, electrosurgical pencil, bipolar forceps with cord, irrigator, syringes and blunt needles for irrigation of the tissues, plastic or silastic tubing and connectors, diluted methylene blue or indigo carmine solution, diluted heparinized lactated Ringer's solution, microscope, microscope drape or operative loupes, ESU with monopolar and bipolar capabilities, and a video monitoring system (if desired).

Operative Procedure. Operative procedures for correction of postsurgical tubal occlusion are usually performed under the operating microscope. Other reconstructive procedures vary according to the nature of the pathologic condition of the tube and may be performed under the operating microscope or by use of operative loupes.

In microsurgery, the surgeon ensures no instruments are used in contact with the fallopian tube except those necessary to carry out the surgical technique. Microsurgery for infertility requires the use of specialized and delicate instruments. Each of these instruments is designed to permit gentle, atraumatic handling of tissues and prevent abrasions, lacerations, and vascular damage.

The tissues are continually irrigated to prevent drying of the serosal surfaces. Lactated Ringer's solution alone or with heparin added may be used for this purpose. Meticulous hemostasis is required. Irrigation is also used to identify bleeding vessels. Hemostasis is achieved by an ESU with a micro–needle monopolar electrode or very fine bipolar forceps. When a CO_2 laser is used, smoke from laser vaporization is evacuated to prevent carbon deposits on the tissue.

Tubal Ligation

Tubal ligation is interruption of fallopian tube continuity, resulting in sterilization of the patient. In general, the indication for sterilization depends entirely on the desire of the patient. Certain medical indications and concern for the psychosocial needs of the patient are factors, and occasionally an obstetric indication exists, such as genetic abnormality. However, at least in the United States, sterilization is entirely a voluntary procedure. Thorough presurgical counseling is needed for the patient and her husband or significant other because this procedure is not predictably reversible. Patients may elect to have the procedure performed at an ambulatory surgery center when it is convenient for them.

Tubal ligation may also be performed during or soon after delivery. This timing does not delay the patient discharge time. A precaution to this practice is the danger of hemorrhage, which still exists soon after delivery. With a vaginal delivery, tubal ligation is done on the first or second postpartum day. If a cesarean delivery is done, the tubes may be ligated at that time.

Operative Procedure. Many surgical methods and techniques are available for tubal ligation. Some examples are laparoscopic clips, tubal rings, thermal coagulation, and transcervical tubal occlusion techniques (Newkirk, 2010). The objective of each method is to achieve complete closure of the fallopian tube so conception is prevented. If a segment of each fallopian tube is excised, it is sent for pathologic examination. General surgical considerations are directed to excising a section of each fallopian tube, ligating the severed ends, achieving hemostasis, and incorporating the proximal stump within layers of the mesosalpinx.

Another approach, involving insertion of an expandable spring coil into the fallopian tube to mechanically block it, is accomplished hysteroscopically via the transcervical intrauterine approach. The expandable spring coil device is usually inserted in the surgeon's office. The device is made from titanium, stainless steel, nickel, and Dacron fibers. The device initiates an inflammatory response, with fibrosis of the tubal lumen over a 3-month period (Grochmal et al, 2011).

Transcervical tubal occlusion may also be done by inserting a catheter into each tubal ostium where RF energy is then delivered for 1 minute causing a lesion within the fallopian tube. After the

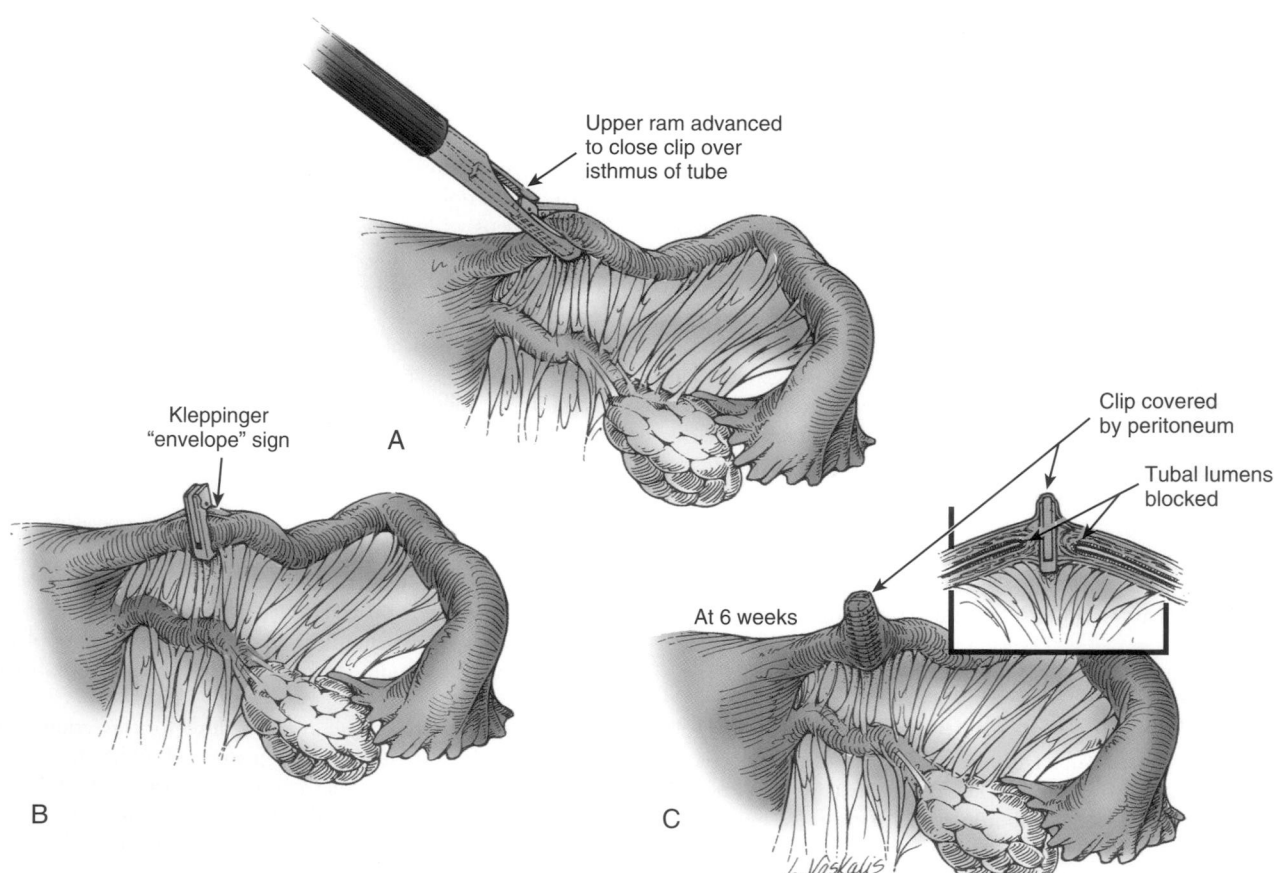

FIGURE 14-44 Spring clip. **A,** Isthmic portion (first 2 to 3 cm of tube) is maneuvered into the open jaws of the clip until it is snug against the hinge. **B,** Closing the clip will create the Kleppinger envelope sign—a fold of tubal peritoneum in the hinge of the clip. **C,** Failure to get the clip completely across the isthmus may result in pregnancy. Some surgeons routinely use two clips close together on each tube.

RF energy is delivered, a 3.5-mm silicone matrix plug is inserted into the lesion portion of the fallopian tube. Both methods of transcervical tubal occlusion require a 3-month follow-up in radiology with a hysterosalpingogram to ensure complete tubal occlusion has occurred (Grochmal et al, 2011).

Laparoscopic Tubal Occlusion

1. The operative procedure begins as described in steps 1 through 8 of laparoscopy.
2. An accessory trocar port is inserted at the suprapubic region for the occluding instrument.
3. Once the tube has been identified and isolated in the grasping forceps sterilization is completed by using a laparoscopic ESU instrument, placement of a spring clip, or silastic band.
   a. Bipolar coagulation occurs when electrical current passes only through the tube from prong to prong. At least 3 cm of the tube is destroyed to prevent spontaneous recanalization. It is recommended the tube be grasped at least 2 to 3 cm away from the uterocornual junction at the time of this procedure. This technique leaves a stump of isthmus to absorb the intra-uterine fluid under pressure and minimize fistula formation, aiding in the future prevention of an ectopic pregnancy.
   b. The *spring clip* occludes the isthmus of the tube by two plastic jaws (Figure 14-44, *A* and *B*). The tube is compressed by a stainless steel spring that presses the jaws together. Spring clip application requires careful surgical technique to ensure the clip is completely across the isthmus of the tube (see Figure 14-44, *C*). Some surgeons apply two spring clips positioned close together on each tube when using this approach.
   c. With a *silastic band* the tube is drawn 1.5 cm into a 0.5-cm-diameter metal cylinder, which destroys approximately 3 cm of the tube (Figure 14-45, *A*). A silastic ring stretched on the outside of the cylinder is released to form an occlusion (see Figure 14-45, *B*). Over time, about 3 cm of the constricted tube undergoes necrosis, and the tubes separate (see Figure 14-45, *C*).
4. Trocar site closure is completed as described for laparoscopy.

Mini-Laparotomy Approach

1. The surgeon creates a 2- to 5-cm transverse incision approximately 6 cm above the pubic hairline. The surgeon may infiltrate the incision with local anesthesia prior to incision or at the end of the procedure.
2. A self-retaining or small handheld retractor is placed through the incision and into the peritoneal cavity. The fallopian tube is grasped with a Babcock clamp and gently pulled up. Spring clips or silastic bands can be applied, or the original Pomeroy method of ligation can be carried out. The Pomeroy technique (Newkirk,

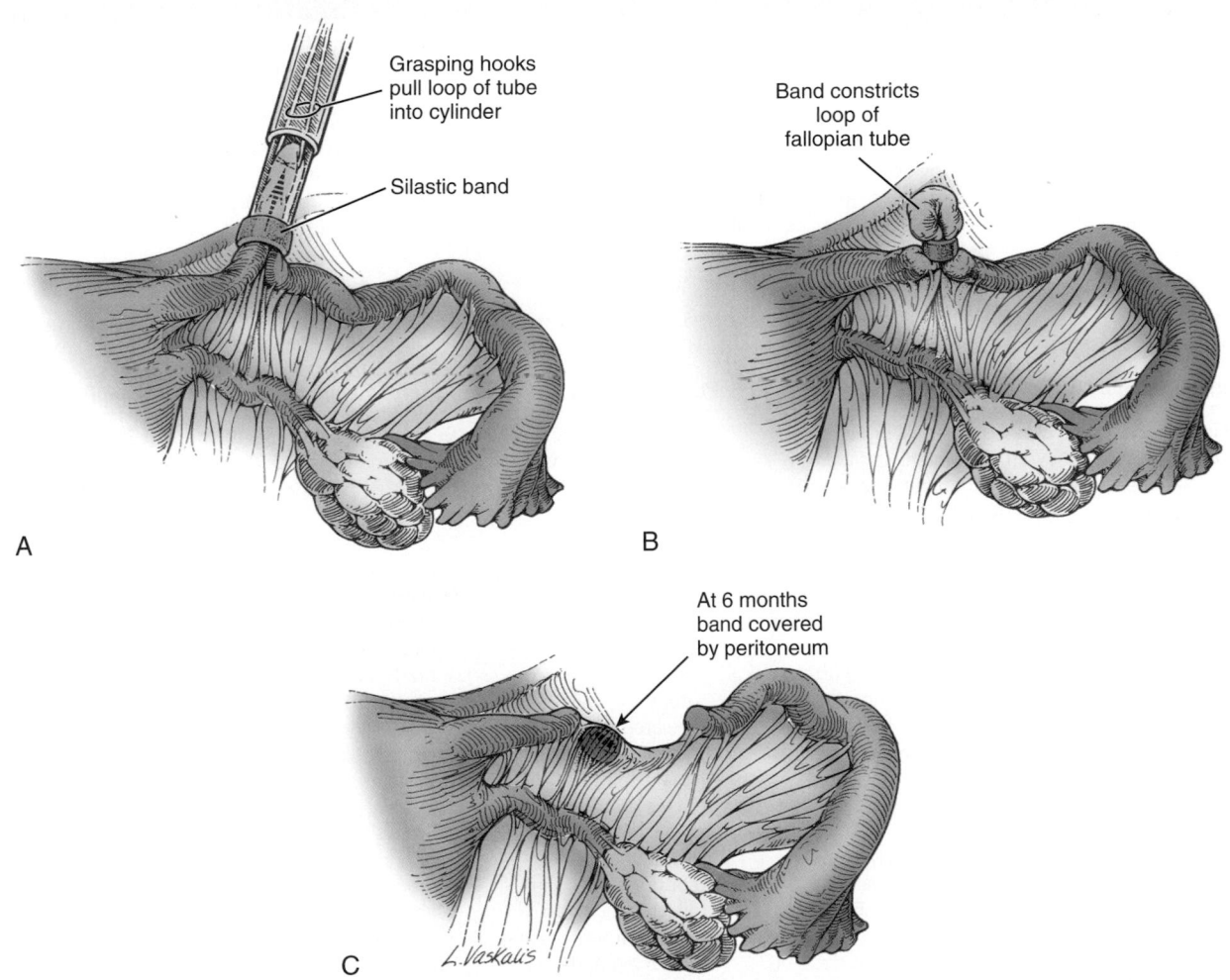

FIGURE 14-45 Silastic band. **A,** About 3 cm of tube is drawn into a 5-mm cylinder over which a silastic band has been stretched. **B,** Releasing the band constricts the knuckle of tube with eventual necrosis. **C,** As with the Pomeroy technique, 6 months later the stumps are about 3 cm apart.

2010) provides a tissue specimen from each tube. Suture material is tied around each tube, and a section of tube is removed. Over time the tubes separate, destroying the passage between the ovary and the uterus.

3. Closure of the incision (fascia, if necessary, followed by a subcuticular running suture) is followed by placement of wound closure strips, small dressings, or skin glue.

Obstetric Surgery

Providing safe, quality nursing care for the perioperative patient is the goal of every surgical team. The interventions necessary to reach this goal intensify with the pregnant woman who presents for surgery. The team is now faced with the challenge of caring for at least two patients, the mother and her child.

Maternal changes in pregnancy increase as gestation progresses and include hormonal fluctuations, mechanical changes to the viscera related to the enlarging uterus, increased metabolic and oxygen demands, and hemodynamic changes. The fetus also has unique metabolic and hemodynamic needs that must be considered. Hazards of performing surgery on the pregnant patient include fetal loss, fetal asphyxia, premature labor, premature rupture of the membranes, and thromboembolic events. These hazards can be increased due to the physiologic changes of pregnancy. These physiologic changes include cardiovascular and hemodynamics, respiratory, GI, coagulation, and renal (Boisseau, 2012; Jones, 2012). Many medications used in the perioperative setting cross into the placental circulation on administration to the mother (Birnbach and Browne, 2009).

Special considerations for the obstetric surgical patient include continuous monitoring of the fetal heart rate, rapid induction for general anesthesia to prevent aspiration, and preparation for the possible use of tocolytics (e.g., medications to decrease uterine activity) to prevent labor (Surgical Pharmacology). Neonatal resuscitative drugs and equipment are readily available when performing surgery on pregnant women in the second trimester and beyond. If the surgical approach allows, the pregnant woman is positioned with a lateral tilt or with a wedge or pillow under her right hip to provide uterine displacement and relieve pressure on the maternal vena cava. This position promotes blood flow to the placenta.

SURGICAL PHARMACOLOGY

Medications Used in Gynecology and Obstetrics

Part of safe perioperative patient care focuses on safe medication practices. Strategies for safe medication administration include standardizing medication labeling both on and off the surgical field, separating sound-alike and look-alike medications, and minimizing interruptions and distractions.

In addition to practicing the "seven rights" (right patient, right medication, right dose, right time, right route, right indication, and right documentation) for the medications he or she administers, the perioperative nurse must be familiar with medications administered to the patient by others (e.g., anesthesia providers, surgeons). Many of the medications used in gynecologic and obstetric surgery are unique to the specialty or have unique uses within the specialty. To be able to constantly modify the patient's plan of care as needed throughout the perioperative period, the perioperative nurse must be familiar with how these medications work, dosage ranges, adverse reactions, and nursing implications.

Oxytocics

Medications that increase motor activity within the uterus by hormonal stimulation, or direct stimulation on the smooth muscles, usually resulting in uterine contractions. Oxytocic medications are used intraoperatively and postoperatively.

Medication/Category	Dosage/Route	Purpose/Action	Adverse Reactions	Nursing Implications
Oxytocin (Pitocin, Syntocinon) *Pharmacotherapeutic:* Uterine smooth muscle stimulant	May be given IV or IM IV: 10–40 units/L of fluid at a rate to control uterine atony IM: 10 units (total dose after delivery)	Control of postpartum bleeding, control uterine atony	Bradycardia, CNS/ brain damage due to rapid propulsion	Monitor BP, pulse, and respirations. Assess for continued bleeding; monitor fundal response to drug.
Methylergonovine maleate (Methergine) *Pharmacotherapeutic:* Ergot alkaloid	May be given PO, IV, or IM PO: Adults 0.2 mg 3 or 4 times a day for up to 7 days IV, IM: Initially 0.2 mg after delivery of anterior shoulder, placenta, or during puerperium; may repeat every 2–4 hr as needed	Prevention/treatment of postpartum, postabortion hemorrhage due to atony Stimulates α-adrenergic, serotonin receptors producing arterial vasoconstriction	Nausea, cramping, vomiting, dizziness, diaphoresis, bradycardia, chest pain, tachycardia, pale, cool, and blotchy skin, facial swelling, increased uterine pain	Monitor BP, pulse every 15 min until stable. Assess for continued bleeding. Monitor fundal response to drug. Assess extremities for color, warmth, movement, and pain.
Dinoprostone (Cervidil, Prepidil, Prostin E2)	Given intracervically Prepidil (endocervical gel): Initially 0.5 mg (2.5 mL); if no cervical or uterine response, may repeat 0.5 mg dose in 6 hr; not to exceed 1.5 mg (7.5 mL) in 24-hr period	To evacuate uterine contents in missed abortion; acts on myometrium causing softening and dilation effect on cervix	Vomiting, nausea, bradycardia, chills/ shivering, diarrhea; may cause hypertonicity with spasm and titanic contraction	Keep gel (Prepidil) refrigerated and bring to room temperature just before use. Use caution when handling to prevent skin contact.

SURGICAL PHARMACOLOGY

Medications Used in Gynecology and Obstetrics—cont'd

Medication/Category	Dosage/Route	Purpose/Action	Adverse Reactions	Nursing Implications
Pharmacotherapeutic: Prostaglandin	Cervidil: (vaginal insert): 10 mg over 12-hr period; remove upon onset of active labor or 12 hr after insertion			Be prepared to treat nausea with antiemetics. Monitor vital signs. Assess for vaginal discharge, cramps, and foul smell.

Tocolytics

Medications that decrease uterine contractility. Most commonly used in the perioperative setting during fetal surgery or in surgical procedures on pregnant females. Tocolytics may also be used in PACU.

Medication/Category	Dosage/Route	Purpose/Action	Adverse Reactions	Nursing Implications
Terbutaline (Brethine, Bricanyl) *Pharmacotherapeutic:* Sympathomimetic (adrenergic antagonist)	May be given PO or IV *Adults:* (maintenance) PO: 2.5-10 mg every 4-6 hr IV: (acute) 2.5-10 mcg/min; may increase gradually every 15-20 min; max 17.5-30 mcg/min	Delays premature labor in pregnancies between 20 and 34 weeks Inhibits uterine contractions	Tremors, anxiety, nervousness, drowsiness, headache, nausea, heartburn, dizziness, flushing and weakness	May decrease serum potassium levels. Assess baseline maternal heart rate and fetal heart rate. Provide emotional support to help ease anxiety.
Magnesium sulfate *Pharmacotherapeutic:* Antacid, anticonvulsive, electrolyte	May be given IV *Adults:* IV: 4-5 g infusion, then 1-2 g/hr continuous infusion; max 40g/24hr	To treat and prevent seizures and eclampsia	Reduced respiratory rate, decreased reflexes, decreased heart rate, hypotension	Assess and monitor renal function. Test patellar reflexes before giving drug to determine baseline. Suppressed patellar reflexes may be sign of impending respiratory arrest. Monitor vital signs. Maintain accurate I&O. Ensure calcium gluconate is available to reverse magnesium sulfate toxicity.

Antimetabolites

Medications that interrupt cell division. Antimetabolite medications may be administered intraoperatively or postoperatively.

Medication/Category	Dosage/Route	Purpose/Action	Adverse Reactions	Nursing Implications
Methotrexate (Rheumatrex, Trexall) *Pharmacotherapeutic:* Antimetabolite	May be given PO, IM, or IV; given IM for ectopic pregnancy IM: 50 mg/m² × 1; may be repeated in 1 week if hCG is rising	Ectopic pregnancies; inhibits DNA, RNA, protein synthesis	Nausea, vomiting, stomatitis, dizziness, blurred vision, photophobia, hepatotoxicity, nephrotoxicity	Encourage patient to maintain scrupulous oral hygiene; be prepared to treat nausea and vomiting. Review good handwashing practices with patient. Discuss need for weekly repeated lab studies to monitor hCG levels.

Miscellaneous Agents

Medication/Category	Dosage/Route	Purpose/Action	Adverse Reactions	Nursing Implications
Mifepristone/ Misoprostol (Medications may be used in conjunction with each other)	Both medications are given PO	Both medications terminate pregnancy		
Mifepristone *Pharmacotherapeutic:* Antiprogestin	*Day 1:* Mifepristone: 600 mg as a single dose	Inhibits activity of endogenous and exogenous progesterone	Diarrhea, abdominal pain, headache, nausea, uterine hemorrhage	Monitor Hgb/Hct. Confirm pregnancy is terminated at 14 days after drug administration. Assess degree of vaginal bleeding.

Continued

SURGICAL PHARMACOLOGY

Medications Used in Gynecology and Obstetrics—cont'd

Medication/Category	Dosage/Route	Purpose/Action	Adverse Reactions	Nursing Implications
Misoprostol (Cytotec) *Pharmacotherapeutic:* Prostaglandin	*Day 3:* Misoprostol: 400 mcg (unless termination of pregnancy has occurred from above medication)	Replaces protective prostaglandins consumed with prostaglandin-inhibiting therapies	Abdominal pain, diarrhea, nausea, vomiting, flatulence, dyspepsia, headache	Give medication immediately following meals. Avoid magnesium containing antacids.
Estradiol cream (Estrace cream) *Pharmacotherapeutic:* Estrogen	Topical cream given intravaginally 0.1 mg/g	Lubricant for vaginal packing for treatment of moderate to severe vasomotor symptoms associated with menopause, hypoestrogenism, and vaginal atrophy	Anorexia, nausea, swelling of breasts, peripheral edema marked by swollen feet and ankles, local irritation, and vaginal discharge	Assess preoperatively for any sensitivity to topical estrogens. Do not use excessive amount of cream. Cream will liquefy from patient's body heat.
Miconazole nitrate cream (Monistat) *Pharmacotherapeutic:* Antifungal	Topical cream given intravaginally Available in 2% and 4% dosage cream	Lubricant for vaginal packing to treat vulvovaginal candidiasis Inhibits synthesis of ergosterol (a vital component of fungal cell formation), damaging fungal cell membrane	Local irritation, vaginal discharge, burning, pruritus, headache, and skin rash	Assess preoperatively for any sensitivity to antifungals, vaginal irritation, burning, and pruritus. Do not use excessive amount of cream. Cream will liquefy from patient's body heat. May interact with latex products.
Sulfathiazole/ sulfacetamide/ sulfabenzamide cream (Triple Sulfa) *Pharmacotherapeutic:* Antiinfective agent	Topical cream given intravaginally Concentration: sulfathiazole 3.42%; sulfacetamide 2.86%; sulfabenzamide 3.7%	Lubricant for vaginal packing, treatment of *Hemophilus* (*Gardnerella*) *Vaginalis* Exerts bacteriostatic action by competitive antagonism of PABA (a component of folic acid synthesis)	Local irritation (erythema), photosensitivity If becomes toxic, can cause Stevens-Johnson syndrome	Assess preoperatively for any sensitivity to sulfa medications or derivatives. Assess skin for rash. Do not use excessive amount of cream. Cream will liquefy from patient's body heat.
Vasopressin (Pitressin, Pressyn) *Pharmacotherapeutic:* Posterior pituitary hormone	Given as a local injection Available in 20 units/mL (is diluted in saline per direction of surgeon)	To help control bleeding; causes vasoconstriction through direct stimulation of smooth muscle; pituitary hormone	Arrhythmia, bradycardia, angina, hypertension, headache, uterine cramping, nausea, vomiting	Potential for confusion related to name; do *not* confuse Pitressin with Pitocin. Monitor vital signs. Verify dilution with surgeon.
Methylene blue (Urolene Blue), methylthioninium chloride *Pharmacotherapeutic:* Antidotes	May be given IV or during chromoperintubation IV: 1% injection 10 mg/mL Chromopertubation diluted in saline per direction of surgeon	To test patency of fallopian tubes or ureters Converts ferrous iron to ferric iron producing methemoglobin	Abdominal pain, dizziness, headache, urine and fecal discoloration, hypertension, N/V, diaphoresis, mental confusion	Warn patient about urine and stool discoloration. Methylene blue stains can be removed with mild bleach solution. Check vitals, and assess for mental confusion.

BP, blood pressure; *CNS* central nervous system; *DNA,* deoxyribonucleic acid; *hCG,* human chorionic gonadotropin; *I&O,* intake and output; *IM,* intramuscular; *IV,* intravenous; *N/V,* nausea or vomiting; *PABA,* para-aminobenzoic acid; *PACU,* postanesthesia care unit; *PO,* by mouth; *RNA,* ribonucleic acid; *VS,* vital signs.
Modified from Hicks RW et al: Implementing AORN recommended practices for medication safety, *AORN J* 96(6):605–622, 2012; Hodgson BB, Kizior RJ: *Saunders nursing drug handbook 2013,* St. Louis, 2013, Saunders; Wiener CP: *Drugs for pregnant and lactating women,* ed 2, Philadelphia, 2009, Saunders; Clinical Pharmacology [database online], Tampa, FL, Gold Standard, Inc., 2013, available at www.clinicalpharmacology.com. Accessed February 24, 2013.

FIGURE 14-46 Principles of Shirodkar operation for treatment of incompetent internal cervical os during pregnancy.

Cervical Cerclage

Incompetence of the cervix is a condition characterized by habitual midtrimester spontaneous abortions. The condition is characterized by a shortening of the length of the cervix (observed on ultrasound) and funneling of the cervix. Surgical intervention is designed to prevent cervical dilation and shortening. This procedure gives better support by means of suture or surgical tape to the cervix. Introduced by Shirodkar in 1951, the cervical cerclage provides a mechanical closure to the cervix. Cerclage is most commonly accomplished via a vaginal approach (Shirodkar and McDonald approaches) or, much less commonly, the abdominal or laparoscopic approach. The Shirodkar technique involves *submucosal* placement of a nonabsorbable heavy purse-string ligature at the level of the internal os to close it (Cashion, 2012). The McDonald cerclage uses a suture to secure and close the cervix by passing suture through four points on the cervix (i.e., 12, 3, 6, and 9 o'clock positions). The vaginal cerclage is generally removed in an office procedure when the woman reaches the thirty-seventh week of gestation (Cashion, 2012; Lewis and Lewis, 2011) or when spontaneous labor begins or the child is delivered by cesarean birth.

Procedural Considerations—Vaginal Approach. A gentle vaginal surgical prep is carried out. The instruments include the basic vaginal instrument tray, with the addition of right and left Deschamps ligature carriers, trocar needles, nonabsorbable sutures for the internal os, and the surgeon's preference for closure of the mucosal incisions.

Operative Procedure—Shirodkar/McDonald

1. Anterior and posterior vaginal retractors are placed, and the cervix is pulled down with smooth ovum or sponge-holding forceps. With smooth tissue forceps and dissecting scissors, the mucosa over the anterior cervix is opened to permit the bladder to be pushed back (Figure 14-46).
2. The surgeon lifts the cervix and incises the posterior vaginal mucosa at the level of the peritoneal reflection. The corners of the anterior and posterior incisions are bilaterally approximated in the area of the lateral mucosa with curved tonsil or Allis forceps.
3. The prepared ligature is placed at the desired level by passage of the material through the approximated tissue and then drawn tight posteriorly to close the cervix; it is then tied. It is not necessary to suture the ligature to the underlying tissues. The suture material used for this ligation is 5-mm Dacron or Mersilene tape. The anterior and posterior mucosal incisions are usually closed with 2-0 absorbable suture to complete the procedure.
4. The McDonald cerclage is performed in a similar manner, using the same instruments, supplies, and preparation. The suture is not buried in the submucosa in the McDonald technique (Figure 14-47).

Procedural Considerations—Abdominal Approach. Transabdominal cerclage is reserved for select women who have a cervix that is so short or damaged that the vaginal approach is not feasible.

FIGURE 14-47 McDonald cerclage.

An abdominal and then vaginal prep are performed. An indwelling urinary catheter may be placed to ensure the urinary bladder remains decompressed. A basic vaginal and an abdominal instrument tray are required. Sutures used for transabdominal cerclage are identical to those used in the vaginal approach.

Operative Procedure—Abdominal Approach

1. The abdomen is opened as described in laparotomy (see Chapter 11) and the viscera retracted. Trendelenburg position may be used to facilitate exposure.
2. The suture material or tape is placed around the uterine isthmus medial to the uterine vessels and fixed to the anterior isthmus, to Mackenrodt ligaments, and to the insertions of the uterosacral ligaments.
3. The abdominal wound is closed as described for laparotomy (see Chapter 11).
4. An abdominal dressing and a perineal pad are applied.

Procedural Considerations—Laparoscopic Approach. The laparoscopic approach may be associated with decreased postoperative pain and morbidity compared with the laparotomy approach. Standard laparoscopic equipment and instruments commonly used in gynecologic procedures are required.

Operative Procedure—Laparoscopic Approach

1. The operative procedure begins as in steps 1 through 8 of laparoscopy.
2. The bladder peritoneum is opened at the level of the uterine isthmus.
3. The surgeon creates a window through the broad ligament medially to the uterine vessels at the level of the internal os.
4. A strip of polypropylene mesh is placed retroperitoneally through the window circumferentially around the isthmus above the cardinal and sacrouterine ligaments.
5. The mesh is anchored with a nonabsorbable suture.
6. The end of the procedure is completed as described in steps 10, 11, and 13 of laparoscopy.

Abdominal Surgery During Pregnancy

The incidence of immediate need for abdominal surgery occurs as frequently among pregnant women as among nonpregnant women of childbearing age. Diagnosis of abdominal problems in the pregnant woman is challenging because of the enlarged uterus and displaced organs. Mild leukocytosis and increased levels of alkaline phosphatase and amylase are normal during pregnancy and may also indicate surgical intraperitoneal processes. Abnormally high or rising laboratory values should be noted. Ultrasound is the safest and most commonly used diagnostic study during pregnancy. MRI also can be used as a diagnostic tool (Jones, 2012; McAteer, 2012). Even though theoretic contraindications exist for the safety of the fetus during radiologic studies, they may be used with minimal to no risk to the fetus. Radiologic studies are often used as an alternative if no other diagnostic tools are adequate (Jones, 2012).

Laparotomy or laparoscopy may be required for conditions such as appendicitis, acute cholelithiasis, ovarian masses, and intestinal obstruction. Appendicitis is the most common nonobstetric surgical condition that complicates pregnancy and occurs in approximately 2 in every 1000 pregnancies (Jones, 2012).

Fetal Surgery

Developments in prenatal diagnosis have progressed to the point where clinicians may consider the fetus to be the patient. Serious congenital anomaly is diagnosable by ultrasonography, alpha-fetoprotein specimen, amniocentesis, chorionic villi sampling, or percutaneous umbilical blood sampling. When an anomaly is identified, a multidisciplinary team reviews the mother's complete medical history and prenatal ultrasonograms. (For more information on fetal surgery, see Chapter 26.)

Cesarean Birth

Cesarean birth, also referred to as *cesarean section* or *C-section,* is delivery of the fetus or fetuses through abdominal (laparotomy) and uterine (hysterotomy) incisions. In general, cesarean birth is used whenever further delay in delivery may seriously compromise the fetus, the mother, or both, or when vaginal delivery cannot be safely accomplished. In recent years cesarean birth has increased due to fetal monitoring, fetal scalp blood sampling for pH determination, and a widespread emphasis on recognition of actual or suspected impairment of fetal well-being if delivery is delayed. Reasons for cesarean birth include failure to progress, malposition and malpresentation, cephalopelvic disproportion, abruptio placentae, toxemia, fetal distress, uterine dysfunction, placenta previa, prolapsed cord, previous pelvic surgery, cervical dystocia, active herpes genitalis, extensive condylomatous disease, and diabetes. Multiple pregnancies also may be an indication for cesarean birth. In certain situations, and after appropriate counseling, elective cesarean delivery may be a medically acceptable option. Cesarean births may be classified as primary (woman's first cesarean), repeat (indicates a previous cesarean birth), elective (a scheduled procedure in either of the previous categories or at maternal request), or emergency (there is an immediate need for intervention). The surgical team may find that developing a checklist for surgical emergencies such as emergency cesarean birth assists in efficient care rather than relying on memory alone (Arriaga et al, 2013).

Cesarean birth is ranked as the most commonly performed major surgical procedure in the United States. In 2010, over a million cesarean sections were performed (HCUPnet, 2011).

Cesarean birth may take place in an OR in the obstetric labor suite or in the main OR. Patients about to undergo cesarean birth need careful assessment and emotional support. Because cesarean birth frequently involves emergency situations, the mother may express grave concern for the infant's well-being. If the mother has participated in childbirth classes, she may believe she has failed in some way. The perioperative nurse remains aware of the psychologic as well as physiologic needs of this patient population. Mothers may choose to remain awake after administration of a regional anesthetic; the mother's birthing partner may be permitted to accompany and support her in the OR and witness the birth (based on hospital policy). The birthing partner will need the perioperative nurse's assistance in preparing for the delivery by washing hands and donning scrub attire or a protective gown. The perioperative nurse reassures and encourages the birthing partner to coach and lend support to the mother during this intensely stressful time. The birthing partner is included in the bonding process that is initiated at birth. The mother, if awake and stable, is shown and encouraged to hold the infant. The perioperative nurse promotes a positive family-centered experience.

If the cesarean birth is performed as an emergency, the family-centered approach may not be feasible. In emergency situations the mother's support person or persons need to be directed to the surgical waiting area, where information will be communicated regarding the condition of the mother and infant. The support person or persons may then accompany the infant as he or she is transferred to the nursery. In an emergency cesarean birth, certain perioperative procedures may be omitted, such as initial surgical counts. When this occurs, institutional protocol for waived counts is initiated.

Procedural Considerations. The patient is supine with elevation of the right side to displace the uterus and prevent vena cava compression. Bony prominences are padded, and the patient positioned in good body alignment with a safety strap above the knees. Antibiotics are administered by the anesthesia provider if not previously given (Research Highlight). The perioperative nurse assists the anesthesia provider with the administration of a regional anesthetic before placing the patient in the supine position. Throughout this process maternal vital signs and fetal heart tones are monitored and recorded per institutional protocol.

If a general anesthetic is used, all preparation, including skin prep, bladder drainage, draping, suction connection, counts, and gowning and gloving of scrubbed personnel, are done before induction. In many hospitals, healthcare providers qualified to deliver newborn care and resuscitation are in attendance for the delivery. A radiant warmer and resuscitative equipment for immediate

---

RESEARCH HIGHLIGHT

Preprocedure Antibiotics Reduce Infection After Cesarean

More than 31% of infants in the United States are delivered by cesarean birth. Surgical-site infection (SSI) rates range from 1.46 to 3.82 per 100 cesarean births, depending on patient risk factors. The 2011 practice guidelines recommend giving prophylactic antibiotics to all women within an hour of cesarean delivery. However, a common practice has been to administer prophylactic antibiotics after the umbilical cord is clamped to avoid masking neonatal sepsis.

An 8-year cohort conducted from 2003 to 2010 in a St. Louis tertiary care hospital implemented five interventions to reduce the risk of postoperative cesarean infection. One implementation was to give the prescribed preoperative prophylactic antibiotic within 1 hour before incision. There were 8668 women who underwent a cesarean birth during the study period. Median age was 26 years (range 12-53 years), 3093 (35.7%) of patients had a body mass index (BMI) of 35 or greater, 2561 (29.5%) were of white race, and 303 (3.5%) had an SSI.

The researchers used time series analysis to determine the effects of the five interventions (after adjusting for secular trends in patient risk factors) on rates of postcesarean SSI. A multivariate analysis showed of the five interventions being studied, the administration of prophylactic antibiotic within 1 hour of incision policy was the only one that was significantly associated with lowering the SSI rate. Implementation of the change in policy resulted in a 48% decrease in SSIs, a reduction of 5.4 SSIs per 100 cesarean deliveries.

Modified from Traytur ND et al: Long-term effect of infection prevention practices and case mix on cesarean surgical site infections, *Obstet Gynecol* 120(2):246–251, 2012.

---

postdelivery care of the infant are available; these infants are considered to be at risk until there is evidence of physiologic stability.

The skin is prepped and draped as for abdominal surgery. The vagina is not prepped. An indwelling urinary catheter is inserted. Instruments include the basic abdominal gynecologic tray, with the addition of Lister bandage scissors, Foerster sponge-holding (ring) forceps, Pennington forceps, cord clamps, a DeLee retractor, delivery forceps, a head extractor (if desired), laboratory tubes for cord blood, a drain (optional), and a bulb syringe.

Operative Procedure

1. The surgeon makes an infraumbilical midline vertical incision or lower transverse Pfannenstiel incision, long enough to allow the infant to be delivered without difficulty. Therefore, the length of the incision varies with the estimated size of the fetus.

2. The abdomen is opened in layers as described in laparotomy (see Chapter 11). The rectus and pyramidalis muscles are separated in the midline by sharp and blunt dissection to expose the underlying transversalis fascia and peritoneum.

3. The peritoneum is elevated with two Crile hemostats about 2 cm apart, then the peritoneum is palpated to rule out the inclusion of bowel, omentum, or bladder. The surgeon opens the peritoneum and enters the abdominal cavity.

4. Bleeding sites within the abdominal incision may be clamped but not ligated until later, unless they obstruct the field of vision. If the patient has a general anesthetic, speed is used to prevent an anesthetized infant. An ESU is used for hemostasis.

5. The surgeon quickly palpates the uterus to determine the size and presenting part of the fetus as well as the direction and degree of rotation of the uterus.

6. The reflection of the peritoneum (visceral) above the upper margin of the bladder and overlying the anterior lower uterine segment is gently separated by sharp and blunt dissection.

7. The developed bladder flap is held downward beneath the symphysis with a bladder retractor such as the DeLee.

8. The uterus is opened with a blade through the lower uterine segment about 2 cm above the bladder flap. Once the uterus is opened the incision can be extended by cutting laterally with a large bandage scissors or by simply spreading the incision by means of lateral pressure applied with each index finger when the lower uterine segment is thin.

9. The presenting membranes are incised. Suction is imperative here, and many surgeons prefer no suction tip (only the large, open end of the suction tubing) during the expulsion and suctioning of amniotic fluid.

10. All retractors are removed. The fetal head is gently elevated manually, by use of obstetric forceps, or with the use of a vacuum apparatus through the incision. Once the fetal head is delivered, the surgical assistant provides transabdominal fundal pressure (Figure 14-48) to aid in the delivery of the shoulders and extremities.

11. As soon as the head is delivered, a bulb syringe or aspirator tip is used to aspirate the exposed nares and mouth to minimize aspiration of amniotic fluid and its contents.

12. Oxytocin (20 units per liter of fluid or as directed by the surgeon) may be administered intravenously by the anesthesia provider as soon as the shoulders are delivered (or after delivery of the infant), so that the uterus contracts. Some surgeons inject 10 units of oxytocin directly into the muscular layer of the uterus either before or after the delivery of the placenta. This use of oxytocin minimizes blood loss.

13. On delivery of the entire infant, the cord is clamped and cut (Figure 14-49), and the infant is given to the member of the

FIGURE 14-48 Fundal pressure applied. Infant's head emerging from hysterotomy.

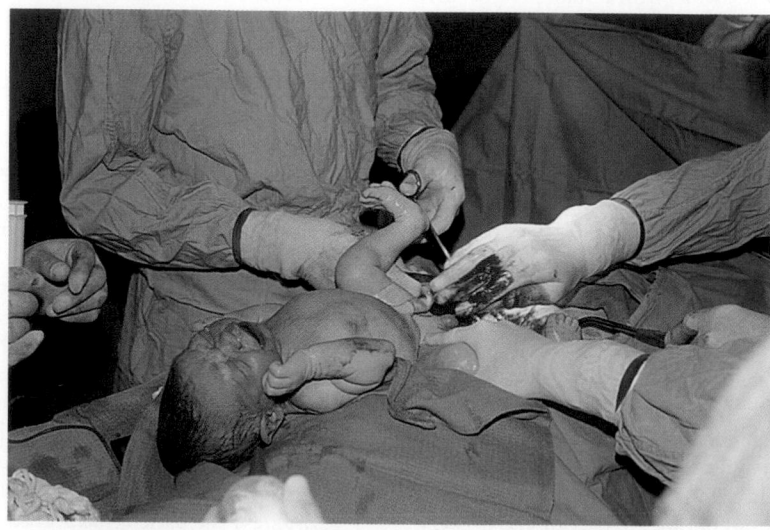

FIGURE 14-49 Cord clamped in preparation for passing infant off field.

team who is responsible for any resuscitation efforts. A sterile gown or sheet is provided to the individual receiving the infant.

14. The edges of the uterine incision are promptly clamped with Péan forceps, ring forceps, Allis clamps, or Pennington clamps.

15. The placenta is delivered and placed in a large receptacle from the back table. Fundal massage or manual removal may be employed to hasten delivery of the placenta and reduce bleeding.

16. One or two separate layers of suture may be used to close the uterine incision. The perioperative nurse and scrub person conduct a count to verify no surgical items have been retained in the uterine cavity.

17. After closure of the uterine incision, hemostasis is established. The cut edges of the visceral peritoneum overlying the uterus and bladder may or may not be approximated. If the surgeon elects to close this layer, it is completed with a continuous running suture.

18. Any blood, blood clots, vernix, and amniotic fluid in the pelvis and peritoneal cavity are removed. The pelvic cavity may be lavaged until clear. The fallopian tubes and ovaries are also inspected. Tubal ligation may be carried out at this point.

19. The peritoneum and each abdominal layer are closed.

20. After the wound is closed, the perioperative nurse massages the patient's fundus and cleans any clots expressed from the vagina.

21. An abdominal dressing and perineal pad are applied.

KEY POINTS

- Surgical procedures on structures of the female reproductive system are performed for diagnostic, therapeutic, or cosmetic purposes.
- A holistic approach with sensitivity to the special needs of women's health and sense of vulnerability is an essential component of perioperative patient care.
- Adult female structures associated with the process of reproduction are the external organs (vulva), the associated ligaments and muscles, the soft tissues and contents of the pelvic cavity, and the bony pelvis.
- The gynecologic patient's history includes a chronologic listing of each pregnancy, length of gestation, type of delivery, complications during pregnancy, duration of labor, and fetal weight; data on menstrual patterns is also collected.
- Lasers are frequently used in gynecologic procedures in conjunction with the colposcope and operating microscope, or the laparoscope.
- Minimally invasive surgery (MIS) and robotic-assisted surgery have specific advantages in approaching and treating gynecologic conditions.
- The incidence of immediate need for abdominal surgery occurs as frequently among pregnant women as among nonpregnant women of childbearing age.
- Cesarean birth is ranked as the most commonly performed major surgical procedure in the United States.

CRITICAL THINKING QUESTION

A 45-year-old patient is scheduled for a laparoscopic robotic-assisted hysterectomy with possible bilateral salpingo-oophorectomy at 7:30 this morning. You are her perioperative nurse. After you have introduced yourself and properly identified her, you start reviewing her medical record for key factors to incorporate in your plan of care. You note she is morbidly obese and has medically controlled hypertension. This morning in preop holding, her BP was 150/86 mm Hg and her fasting blood glucose taken 1 hour ago was 230 mg/dL. She has been fasting for 8 hours and did not take her insulin this morning as she usually does. She did, however, take her blood pressure medication with a sip of water around 5 AM.

What additional perioperative nursing and positioning considerations are you planning for this patient? Will you anticipate monitoring her blood glucose level intraoperatively? If so, how often? Will you add this information to the time-out data you share with the surgical team? When reviewing the patient's medical record, you also note she has had several previous laparoscopic and open abdominal procedures. What additional instrumentation will you have available? What concerns do you have about her metabolic syndrome and the role it will play in her postoperative recovery?

e**volve** *The answers to the Critical Thinking Question can be found at http://evolve.elsevier.com/Rothrock/Alexander.*

REFERENCES

American Cancer Society (ACS): *Cancer facts and figures 2012,* Atlanta, 2012, The Society, available at www.cancer.org/research/cancerfactsfigures/cancerfactsfigures/cancer-facts-figures-2013. Accessed February 23, 2013.

Arriaga AF et al: Simulation-based trial of surgical-crisis checklists, *N Engl J Med* 368:246–253, 2013.

Aschkenazi SO, Goldberg RP: Female sexual function and the pelvic floor, *Expert Rev of Obstet Gynecol* 4(2):165–178, 2009.

Association of periOperative Registered Nurses: *Perioperative standards and recommended practices,* Denver, 2013, The Association.

Berg JA et al: Where are we today: prioritizing women's health services and health policy. A report by the Women's Health Expert Panel of the American Academy of Nursing, *Nurs Outlook* 61(1):5–15, 2013.

Birnbach DJ, Browne I: Anesthesia for obstetrics. In Miller RD, editor: *Miller's anesthesia,* ed 7, Philadelphia, 2009, Churchill Livingstone.

Boisseau L: Care of pregnant patients undergoing nonobstetric surgery, *AORN J* 96(6):636–646, 2012.

Cashion K: Antepartal hemorrhagic disorders. In Lowdermilk DL, Perry SE, editors: *Maternity and women's health care,* ed 10, St Louis, 2012, Mosby.

Cassorla L, Lee JW: Patient positioning and anesthesia. In Miller RD, editor: *Miller's anesthesia,* ed 7, Philadelphia, 2009, Churchill Livingstone.

Centers for Disease Control and Prevention (CDC): *Women's reproductive health: hysterectomy,* Atlanta, 2012, available at www.cdc.gov/ReproductiveHealth/WomensRH/Hysterectomy.htm. Accessed February 23, 2013.

Denholm B: Tucking patient's arms and general positioning, *AORN J* 89(4):755–757, 2009.

Deraco M et al: Advanced cytoreduction as surgical standard of care in hyperthermic intraperitoneal chemotherapy as promising treatment in epithelial ovarian cancer, *Eur J Surg Oncol* 37: 4–9, 2011.

Fuller AF Jr: Surgical management of ovarian carcinoma. In Fischer JE et al, editors: *Fischer's mastery of surgery,* vol 2, ed 6, Philadelphia, 2012, Lippincott Williams & Wilkins.

Gambone JC: Gynecologic procedures. In Hacker NF, editor: *Hacker & Moore's essentials of obstetrics and gynecology,* ed 5, Philadelphia, 2010, Saunders.

Goodman T, Spry C: *Essentials of perioperative nursing,* ed 5, Burlington, MA, 2014, Jones & Bartlett Learning.

Griffin A: The lived spiritual experiences of patients transitioning through major outpatient surgery, *AORN J* 97(2):243–252, 2013.

Grochmal SA et al: Insertion of Essure (hysteroscopically assisted female sterilization). In Pfenninger JL, Fowler GC, editors: *Pfenninger and Fowler's procedures for primary care,* ed 3, Philadelphia, 2011, Mosby.

Healthcare Cost and Utilization Project (HCUPnet): *Patient and hospital characteristics for CCS principle procedure category cesarean section,* 2011, available at www.ahrq.gov//HCUPnet.jsp/. Accessed February 23, 2013.

Healthcare Cost and Utilization Project (HCUPnet): *Statistics for U.S. community hospital stays, principle procedure based on clinical classifications software,* 2009, available at www.ahrq.gov/data/hcup. Accessed February 23, 2013.

Jones HW III: Gynecological surgery. In Townsend CM et al, editors: *Sabiston textbook of surgery*, ed 19, Philadelphia, 2012, Saunders.

Katz VL: Benign gynecologic lesions. In Lentz GM et al, editors: *Comprehensive gynecology*, ed 6, Philadelphia, 2012, Mosby.

Kintanar TA: Endometrial ablation. In Pfenninger JL, Fowler GC, editors: *Pfenninger and Fowler's procedures for primary care*, ed 3, Philadelphia, 2011, Mosby.

Lewis MR, Lewis M: Cervical cerclage. In Pfenninger JL, Fowler GC, editors: *Pfenninger and Fowler's procedures for primary care*, ed 3, Philadelphia, 2011, Mosby.

Lobo R: Ectopic pregnancy. In Lentz GM et al, editors: *Comprehensive gynecology*, ed 6, Philadelphia, 2012, Mosby.

Lowdermilk DL: Structural disorders and neoplasms of the reproductive system. In Lowdermilk DL, Perry SE, editors: *Maternity and women's health care*, ed 10, St. Louis, 2012, Mosby.

McAteer J: Medical-surgical problems in pregnancy. In Lowdermilk DL, Perry SE, editors: *Maternity and women's health care*, ed 10, St. Louis, 2012, Mosby.

Newkirk GR: Permanent female sterilization (tubal ligation). In Pfenninger JL, Fowler GC, editors: *Pfenninger and Fowler's procedures for primary care*, ed 3, Philadelphia, 2010 Mosby.

Shaver J et al: Women's health research agenda for the next decade. A report by the Women's Health Expert Panel of the American Academy of Nursing, *Nurs Outlook* 61(1):16–24, 2013.

Smith JA, Jhingran A: Principles of radiation therapy and chemotherapy in gynecologic cancer: basic principles, uses, and complications. In Lentz GM et al, editors: *Comprehensive gynecology*, ed 6, Philadelphia, 2012, Mosby.

Sobolewski C et al: Laparoendoscopic single site surgery in gynecology, *Obstet Gynecol Clin North Am* 38:741–755, 2011.

Tewari KS, Monk, BJ: Invasive cervical cancer. In Disaia PJ, Creasman WT, editors: *Clinical gynecologic oncology*, 8 ed, Philadelphia, 2012, Saunders.

Walters L, Eley S: Robotic-assisted surgery and the need for standardized pathways and clinical guidelines, *AORN J* 93(4):455–463, 2011.

Wilkinson JE: Reflections on research utilization: meaning, measurement and impact, *Worldviews Evid Based Nurs* 10(1):102, 2013.

World Health Organization (WHO): *Violence against women fact sheet*, 2011, available at www.who.int/mediacentre/factsheets/fs239/en. Accessed February 23, 2013.

Zender J, Thell C: Developing a successful robotic surgery program in a rural hospital, *AORN J* 92(1):72–83, 2010.

CHAPTER 15
Genitourinary Surgery

HELENE KOREY MARLEY

Advances in genitourinary surgery, with the use of robotics, laparoscopic techniques, cryotherapy, brachytherapy, lasers, ultrasonography, lithotripters, innovative diagnostic measures, and minimally invasive surgical approaches, have expanded treatment options. As urologic surgery becomes more complex and far more precise, the perioperative nurse is challenged to maintain up-to-date knowledge, documented competence, and new technical skills. More procedures are performed on an ambulatory or short-stay basis, allowing limited time for patient and family education and discharge planning. The success of surgical intervention and patient outcomes depends greatly on the nurse's ability and knowledge in designing, developing, and implementing an effective perioperative plan of care.

Surgical Anatomy

The normal genitourinary system includes one pair of kidneys, two ureters, the urinary bladder, the urethra, and the prostate gland in the male. Also considered essential to the genitourinary system are the adrenal glands, male reproductive organs, and the female urogynecologic system.

Urine is excreted by the kidneys and conveyed to the bladder through the ureters. Urine is stored in the bladder, which serves as a reservoir until its full capacity (350 to 700 mL) is reached, and is eliminated from the body by way of the urethra. Normal urinary output ranges from 0.5 to 1 mL/kg of body weight per hour for the average adult.

Kidneys

The kidneys are located in the retroperitoneal space along the lateral borders of the psoas muscle, one on each side of the vertebral column at the level of the twelfth thoracic to the third lumbar vertebrae. Usually the right kidney is several centimeters lower than the left because the liver rests superior and anterior to the right kidney (Figure 15-1).

Each kidney is surrounded by a mass of fatty and loose areolar tissue known as *pararenal fat.* A capsule enclosing the renal space is known as the *fascia renalis.* This is composed of *Gerota fascia* (anterior renal fascia) and *Zuckerkandl fascia* (posterior renal fascia). These structures help keep the kidneys in their normal anatomic position. The anterior and posterior relationships of the kidneys are shown in Figure 15-2.

On the medial side of each kidney is a concave area known as the *hilum,* through which the renal artery and vein enter and exit. The renal pelvis, a funnel-shaped structure that lies within the kidney and posterior to the renal vascular pedicle, divides into several branches called *calyces* (Figure 15-3). When surgery is indicated in these structures, a posterior flank approach is preferred. When surgery for removal of a mass is anticipated, a transabdominal or thoracoabdominal incision may be chosen.

The kidneys are highly vascular organs that process approximately one fifth of the body's entire volume of blood at any one time. The blood supply to the kidney is conveyed through the renal artery (a large branch of the aorta) and leaves through the renal vein. On entering the kidney, the renal artery divides into anterior and posterior sections. These undergo further division into interlobular arteries from which smaller afferent branches pass to the glomeruli. Efferent arterioles in the glomeruli then pass to the tubules of the nephron.

The renal lymphatic supply originates beneath the capsule of the kidney and empties into the lumbar lymph nodes at the junction of the renal vascular pedicle and aorta. The nerves of the autonomic (involuntary) nervous system originate from the lumbar sympathetic trunk and from the vagus nerve. Removal of the nerve pathways does not impair renal function. The renal artery and vein with their accompanying nerves and lymphatics are referred to as the *pedicle* of the kidney.

Adrenal Glands

The adrenal glands lie retroperitoneally beneath the diaphragm, capping the medial aspects of the superior pole of each kidney. On the right side the gland is triangular and adjacent to the inferior vena cava; on the left side it is a rounded, crescent-shaped gland posterior to the stomach and pancreas. Each adrenal gland has a medulla, which secretes epinephrine (adrenaline), and a cortex, which secretes steroids and hormones. Secretions from the adrenal cortex are influenced by the activity of the pituitary gland. The adrenal glands are liberally supplied with arterial branches from the inferior phrenic and renal arteries and from the aorta. Venous drainage is accomplished on the right side by the inferior vena cava and on the left by the left renal vein. The lymphatic system accompanies the suprarenal vein and drains into the lumbar lymph nodes.

Ureters

Each ureter is a continuation of the renal pelvis. The ureter extends in a smooth S curve from the renal pelvis to the base of the bladder (Figure 15-4). It is approximately 25 to 30 cm long and 4 to 5 mm in diameter in the adult. This fibromuscular cylindric tube is lined by transitional epithelium (urothelium) and lies on the psoas muscle, passing medially to the sacroiliac joints and laterally to the ischial spines. As urine accumulates in the renal pelvis, slight distention initiates a wave of muscular contractions. This peristaltic activity continues down the ureter, propelling urine into the bladder.

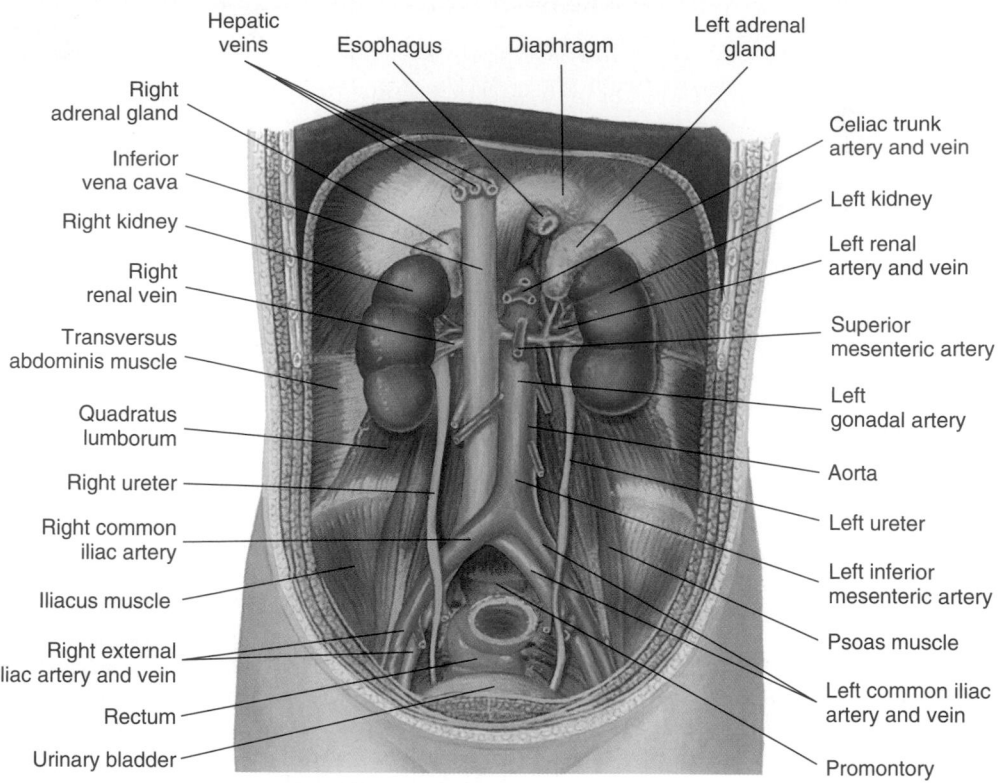

FIGURE 15-1 Location of urinary system organs.

Urinary Bladder

The adult urinary bladder is a hollow, muscular viscus that acts as a reservoir for urine until micturition (voiding) occurs. It has an outer adventitial layer and inner urothelial layer. The trigone, a triangular area, forms the base of the bladder. The three corners of the trigone correspond to the orifices of the ureters and the bladder neck (opening of the urethra) (Figure 15-5). The ureteral orifices, on the proximal trigone at the interureteric ridge, are 2.5 cm apart. The bladder neck (internal sphincter) is formed from converging detrusor muscle fibers of the bladder wall that pass distally to form the smooth musculature of the urethra. Physiologically the bladder fills with urine and expands into the abdominal cavity. The extraperitoneal location is advantageous because a suprapubic (above the pubic arch) incision may be performed without violating the peritoneum and potentially causing intraperitoneal complications.

The main arterial supply of the bladder comprises the superior, middle, and inferior vesical arteries. These vessels are derived from the internal iliac (hypogastric) artery, the obturator and inferior gluteal arteries, and in females the uterine and vaginal arteries. The bladder has a rich venous supply that drains into the internal iliac (hypogastric) vein. The lymphatic system is served by the vesical, external, and internal iliac and common iliac lymph nodes.

The bladder's size, position, and relationship to the bowel, rectum, and reproductive organs varies according to the bladder's distention. In the female the vagina lies dorsal to the base of the bladder and parallel to the urethra (Figure 15-6). In the male the prostate gland is interposed between the bladder neck and the urethra (Figure 15-7). These anatomic relationships influence the symptoms that a patient experiences preoperatively and are important landmarks during pelvic surgery.

The process of bladder evacuation appears to be initiated by nerve cells from the sacral division of the autonomic nervous system. These sacral reflex centers are controlled by higher voluntary centers in the brain. Stimulation of the sacral centers results in contraction of the bladder muscles and relaxation of the bladder outlet sphincters. Muscles inside and adjacent to the urethral wall and from the pelvic floor maintain closure of the sphincters of the bladder, thus enabling continence.

Urethra

The male urethra, normally 20 to 25 cm long, extends from the bladder neck to the tip of the penis and varies in diameter from 7 to 10 mm. It is divided into two portions: the proximal (sphincteric) urethra and the distal (conduit or anterior) urethra, both of which undergo further subdivision. The proximal urethra is commonly referred to as the *posterior urethra,* where it is elevated by the verumontanum, extending from the bladder neck through the prostate and the membranous portion. Within the posterior urethra lie the prostatic and membranous portions (see Figure 15-5). As the urethra exits the prostate and crosses the pelvic (urogenital) diaphragm, it is called the *membranous urethra.* The distal urethra, commonly called the *anterior urethra,* is subdivided into the bulbar, pendulous (penile), and glandular urethras. The bulbar urethra is the area most prone to urethral strictures in the male. The prostatic urethra is approximately 3 cm long and is the widest portion of the urethra. On the floor of the prostatic urethra is the verumontanum, which contains the openings of the ejaculatory ducts. The membranous urethra is the shortest portion, measuring approximately 2.5 cm and extending from the external sphincter to the apex of the prostate. The penile, or pendulous, urethra lies within the

FIGURE 15-2 A, Blood supply of kidneys and relationship of kidneys and ureters to the main arteries and veins and the intraperitoneal organs. **B,** Relationship of the kidneys and ureters to the spinal column.

corpus spongiosum. The urothelium of the urethra is continuous with that of the bladder.

The female urethra is a narrow membranous tube about 3 to 5 cm long and 6 to 8 mm in diameter. Slightly curved, it lies behind and beneath the symphysis pubis, anterior to the vagina. It passes through the internal and external sphincters and the urogenital diaphragm. The periurethral glands of Skene open on the floor of the urethra just inside the meatus. Because the female urethra is so short and in proximity to the anal and vaginal areas, microorganisms find easy access to the bladder and can cause urinary tract infections (UTIs).

Prostate Gland

The prostate gland is a donut-shaped organ composed of fibromuscular and glandular components. It is located at the base of the bladder neck and completely surrounds the urethra. The gland is

FIGURE 15-3 Normal kidney.

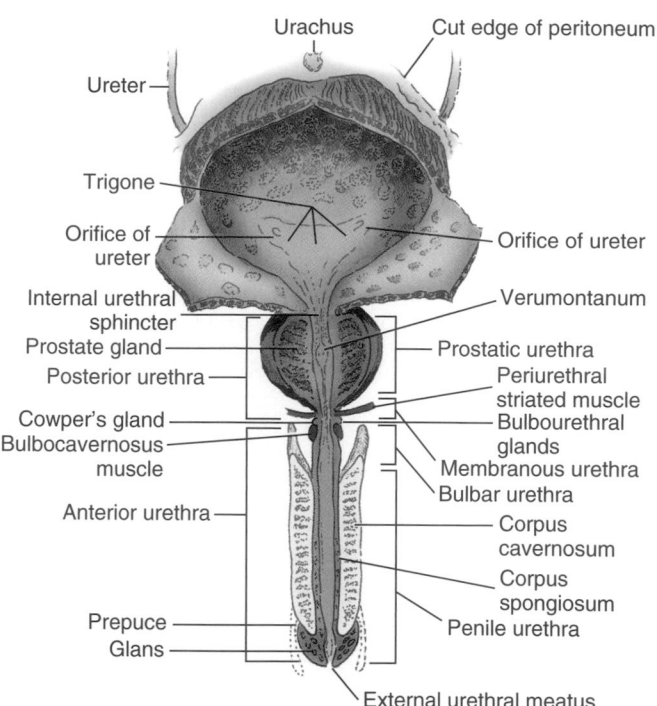

FIGURE 15-5 Anatomy of male urinary bladder, prostate gland, and urethra.

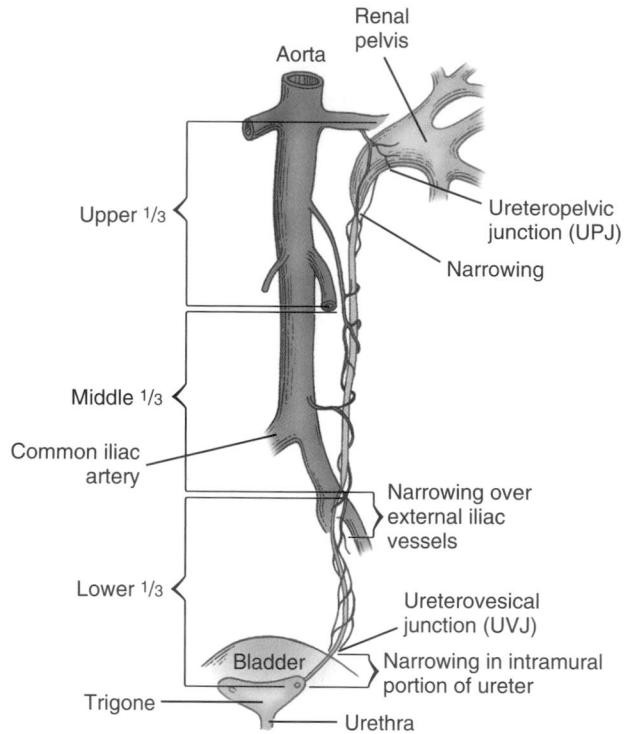

FIGURE 15-4 Anatomy of ureter.

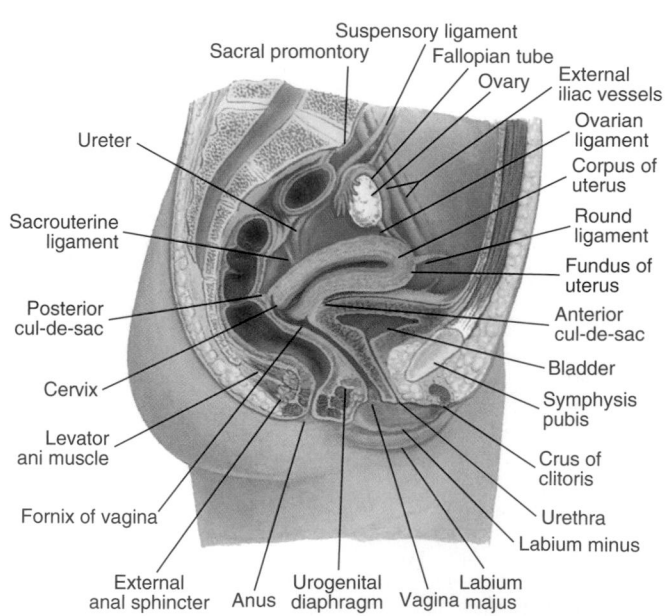

FIGURE 15-6 Female genitourinary and reproductive anatomy.

about 4 cm at the base, is about 2 cm in depth, and normally weighs 20 to 30 g (see Figures 15-5 and 15-7).

The four glandular regions within the prostate have two major zones (the peripheral zone and the central zone) and two minor zones (the transitional zone and the periurethral zone). Many clinicians still refer to prostate lobes as intraurethral lobes (right and left lateral) and extraurethral lobes (posterior and median). The posterior lobe is readily palpable during rectal examination and prone to cancerous degeneration. Benign prostatic hyperplasia (BPH, often

referred to as hypertrophy) generally occurs in the transitional zone (intraurethral lobe).

Behind the prostatic capsule is a fibrous sheath known as the *true prostatic capsule,* which separates the prostate gland and the seminal vesicles from the rectum. This fascia is an important landmark during perineal prostatectomy.

The lobes of the prostate gland secrete highly alkaline fluid that dilutes the testicular secretion as it is excreted from the ejaculatory ducts. These secretions are believed to be essential to the passage of

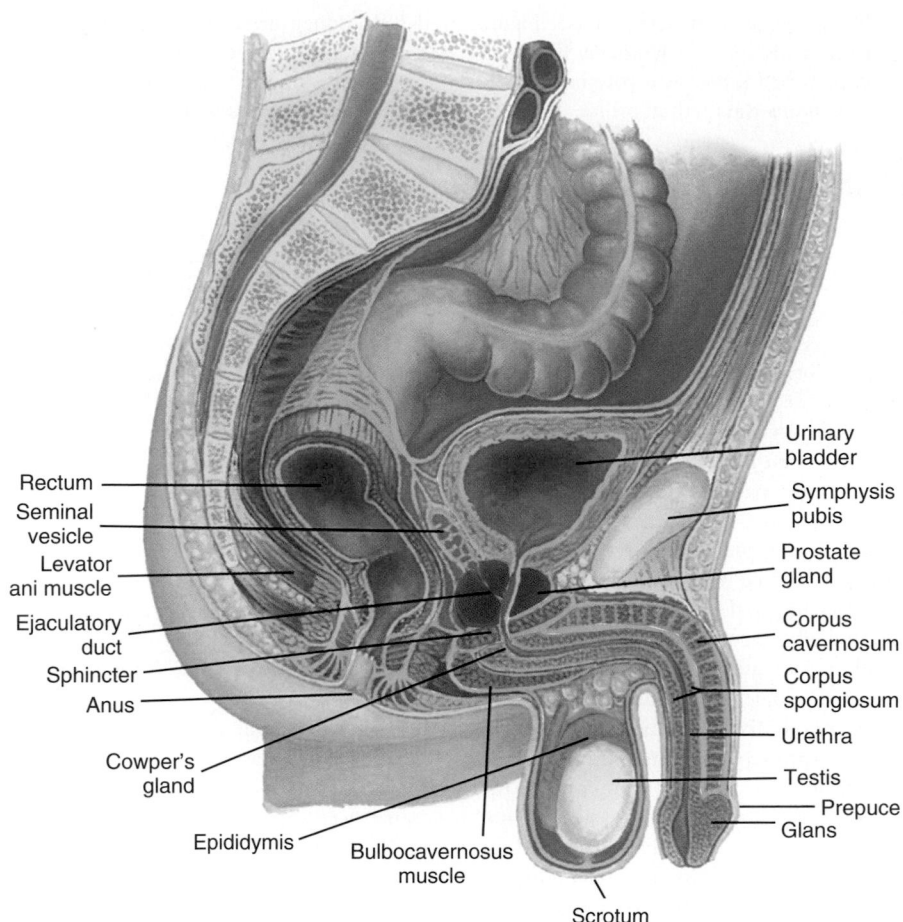

FIGURE 15-7 Male genitourinary and reproductive anatomy.

spermatozoa and helpful in keeping them alive. The arterial supply to the prostate is derived from the pudendal, inferior vesical, and hemorrhoidal arteries.

Male Reproductive Organs

The male reproductive organs include several paired structures: the testes, epididymides, seminal ducts (vasa deferens), seminal vesicles, ejaculatory ducts, and bulbourethral glands. Other organs of the reproductive tract are the penis, prostate gland, and urethra.

The *scrotum* is located behind and below the base of the penis and in front of the anus. Within the scrotum are two cavities, or sacs, that are lined with smooth, glistening tissue—the tunica vaginalis. Normally a small amount of clear fluid is contained in the tunica vaginalis. Each loose sac contains and supports a testis, an epididymis, and some of the spermatic cord. The two sides of the scrotum are separated from each other by a median raphe (septum).

The *testes* manufacture the spermatozoa and also contain specialized Leydig cells that produce the male hormone *testosterone*. Each testis consists of many tubules in which the sperm are formed, surrounded by dense capsules of connective tissue. The tubules coalesce and continue into the adjacent epididymis, where the sperm mature and are stored. At the upper pole of the testis is the appendix testis, a small body that may be pedunculated (stalked) or sessile (flat).

The *epididymis* is a long, convoluted duct located along the posterolateral surface of the testis. It is closely attached to the testicle by fibrous tissue and secretes seminal fluid, which gives the sperm

a liquid medium in which to migrate. The vas deferens (ductus deferens, seminal duct) is a distal continuation of the epididymis as it enters the prostate gland and conveys the sperm to the seminal vesicle.

The *vas deferens* extends from the epididymis into the abdomen and lies within the spermatic cord in the inguinal region. The spermatic cord also contains veins, arteries, lymphatics, nerves, and surrounding connective tissue (cremaster muscle), which give support to the testes. The terminal portion of each vas deferens is called the *ejaculatory duct;* it passes between the lobes of the prostate gland and opens into the posterior urethra.

The *accessory reproductive glands* include the seminal vesicles, prostate gland, and bulbourethral gland. The seminal vesicles unite with the vas deferens on either side, are situated behind the bladder, and produce protein and fructose for the nutrition of the sperm cell. Sperm and prostatic fluid are discharged at the time of ejaculation.

The *Cowper glands* (bulbourethral glands) are located on each side at the juncture of the membranous and bulbar urethras. Each gland, by way of its duct, empties mucous secretions into the urethra.

The *penis* is suspended from the pubic symphysis by the suspensory ligaments. The penis contains three distinct vascular, sponge-like bodies surrounding the urethra: two outer bodies called the *right corpus cavernosum* and *left corpus cavernosum* and an inner body, the *corpus spongiosum urethrae.* These tissues contain a network of vascular channels that fill with blood during erection (see Figure 15-7). At the distal end of the penis the skin is doubly folded to form the prepuce, or foreskin, which serves as a covering for the glans penis. The glans penis contains the urethral orifice.

Perioperative Nursing Considerations

Assessment

Patients entering a hospital or ambulatory surgery unit for genitourinary surgery may exhibit many emotions and reactions, including fear, embarrassment, helplessness, hostility, anger, and grief. To most, a successful surgical outcome is of prime importance. The urology patient population varies from infants with congenital anomalies to elderly people with physiologic impairments. Because many procedures are performed on an ambulatory basis, the nursing staff must prepare to quickly meet patients' specific needs, from preoperative teaching to postoperative home care. The patients' families need to be involved in this preparation process. Patient education begins in the surgeon's office. Communication between the office and perioperative nursing staff allows continuity of care and increases the efficiency and effectiveness of surgical procedures.

In addition to routine admission information, the perioperative nurse will obtain the patient's urologic and cardiac histories. This information includes but is not limited to vital signs, allergies (including latex), the patient's primary problem, history of the present illness, nature of symptoms, and limitations imposed by the disease condition. In some cases patients may be seen who are not having a primary urologic procedure but instead are scheduled for an ancillary urologic procedure (e.g., insertion of ureteral catheters or stents to facilitate positive identification of the ureters and reduce the potential for severing or ligating them during pelvic or abdominal procedures). All data pertinent to the proposed operative procedure should be reviewed. Nursing observation should include the patient's general physical appearance as well as nonverbal behaviors, such as restlessness, which may indicate discomfort or anxiety. Any limitations in mobility or sensory deficits should be noted. Urologic procedures frequently require positions that create unusual stress for the patient, both anatomic and physiologic, such as compression of the vena cava and dependent lung during lateral positioning. Also large amounts of irrigating fluids are frequently used intraoperatively in urologic procedures, which may affect the patient's electrolyte status. Assessment provides the perioperative nurse with data adequate to support preoperative planning, intraoperative implementation, and postoperative evaluation.

The patient may undergo several studies preoperatively, including measurement of levels of serum and urine electrolytes, blood glucose, and blood urea nitrogen (BUN); urinalysis and urine cultures; cardiac enzymes; complete blood count (CBC); prothrombin time (PT) and partial thromboplastin time (PTT); blood chemistry profiles (see the laboratory values in Appendix A); electrocardiogram (ECG); and chest x-ray examination. The nurse reviews the patient's medical history, focusing on medication use (including the use of over-the-counter medications and herbal supplements), any infectious processes, or chronic diseases. Specific genitourinary studies can be found in the patient's medical record. They may encompass all or some of the following: computed tomography (CT) scans, magnetic resonance imaging (MRI), bone and dual energy x-ray absorptiometry (DEXA) scans, positron emission tomography (PET), ProstaScint scans, intravenous (IV) pyelograms or urograms (IVPs or IVUs, respectively), genitourinary flat plate (KUB [kidney, ureter, bladder]), urinary flow studies, fluoroscopic examinations (angiography, cavernosography), prostate-specific antigen (PSA), and ultrasonography. After the nurse reviews the medical record, assessment information is compiled, perioperative nursing diagnoses are identified, and the perioperative plan of care is formulated.

Nursing Diagnosis

Nursing diagnoses related to the care of patients undergoing genitourinary surgery might include the following:
- Anxiety
- Risk for Perioperative Positioning Injury
- Impaired Urinary Elimination
- Risk for Deficient Fluid Volume
- Impaired Gas Exchange
- Sexual Dysfunction

Outcome Identification

Outcomes identified for the selected nursing diagnoses could be stated as follows:
- The patient will verbalize an acceptable anxiety level to the perioperative nurse.
- The patient will be free from injury related to the surgical position.
- The patient will demonstrate or regain a normal pattern of urinary elimination.
- The patient will maintain adequate fluid volume and electrolyte balance.
- The patient will maintain adequate oxygen supply and alveolar ventilation.
- The patient will discuss fears and concerns regarding sexual function.

Planning

Plans of care are the organizing framework for perioperative nursing activities, wherein nursing interventions are clinical processes in a quality health outcome model. Frequently the urology patient presents a complex medical picture. Any alterations in the patient's physical, mental, or emotional status may greatly influence both the surgical and the postoperative course. A review of the patient's record; communication with the patient or family; recognition of specific psychosocial, cultural, ethnic, and spiritual needs of the patient and family; and knowledge gained from other members of the patient care team are all used to formulate the nursing database (see the Sample Plan of Care).

Implementation

The perioperative nurse begins implementation of the patient care plan during the patient interview. Information that is concise and simply presented enhances the final surgical outcome. Meeting the patient's emotional needs is a nursing priority. A calm patient retains more information and is cognitively and emotionally more receptive to perioperative teaching. The nurse provides explanations of what to expect throughout the operative period to allay the patient's fears and nurture confidence in the nursing care provided. Establishment of this relationship is key to assisting patients to minimize the effect of the surgical experience on their coping ability and to be emotionally comfortable. Perioperative nursing care requires not only the collection of pertinent patient data but also the coordination of numerous supplies and equipment to support the smooth implementation of the plan of care.

SAMPLE PLAN OF CARE

Nursing Diagnosis
Anxiety

Outcome
The patient will verbalize an acceptable anxiety level to the perioperative nurse.

Interventions
- Provide an accepting and supportive environment.
- Use touch (as appropriate) to convey caring and support.
- Encourage expression of feelings.
- Promote feelings of self-worth.
- Provide comfort measures (e.g., warm blankets, pillow).
- Facilitate or assist patient in using personally effective coping strategies (e.g., relaxation, deep breathing, music, imagery).
- Maintain patient privacy.
- Encourage participation of patient and family in plan of care.

Nursing Diagnosis
Risk for Perioperative Positioning Injury

Outcome
The patient will be free from injury related to the surgical position.

Interventions
- Maintain proper body alignment.
- Assess range of motion and musculoskeletal, peripheral vascular, and cardiovascular status preoperatively.
- Pad all bony prominences.
- Avoid compression of vulnerable nerves and neurovascular bundles.
- Secure patient to OR bed without friction or pressure.
- Provide support stockings or intermittent pneumatic compression sleeves as indicated.
- Initiate measures to warm patient and maintain normothermia.

Nursing Diagnosis
Impaired Urinary Elimination

Outcome
The patient will demonstrate or regain a normal pattern of urinary elimination.

Interventions
- Include catheter care and measures to facilitate voiding after catheter removal as part of preoperative patient and family education and discharge planning.
- Instruct patient in importance of any postoperative antibiotic or anticholinergic therapy.
- Follow aseptic technique during catheter insertion and connection to drainage device.
- Maintain closed urinary drainage system.
- Note amount, color, and character of urine; report abnormalities.
- Keep drainage tubing and collection device below the level of the patient's bladder.
- Keep urine draining freely; avoid kinks in tubing.
- Check patency of catheter after all position changes.
- Secure drainage tubing to patient to prevent pulling or retraction during transfer.
- Assess bladder for distention.

- Provide patient with information/referral on preventing recurrent urinary tract infection (UTI).

Nursing Diagnosis
Risk for Deficient Fluid Volume

Outcome
The patient will maintain adequate fluid volume and electrolyte balance.

Interventions
- Provide appropriate IV solutions, volumetric pumps, and fluid warmers.
- Monitor patency of all IV lines.
- Record volume of IV and irrigating fluids instilled.
- Monitor electrocardiogram (ECG), vital signs, and cardiopulmonary status as appropriate.
- Monitor blood loss and volume replacement.
- Monitor urinary output, and note color; report output less than 30 mL/hr and changes in color or clarity.
- Collaborate with anesthesia provider in monitoring serum electrolyte status.
- Monitor pH and specific gravity of urine as appropriate.

Nursing Diagnosis
Impaired Gas Exchange

Outcome
The patient will maintain adequate oxygen supply and alveolar ventilation.

Interventions
- Review breathing exercises and use of incentive spirometer with patient preoperatively.
- Position patient to provide maximum lung perfusion; have positioning devices available; check that these are clean and functioning properly.
- Assist anesthesia provider in applying cardiac monitor leads, blood pressure cuff, and pulse oximeter.
- Collaborate with anesthesia provider in monitoring ventilation or perfusion.
- Administer oxygen as required; assist with intubation and maintenance of airway during positioning.
- Assist with collection of arterial blood gases; report results promptly.

Nursing Diagnosis
Sexual Dysfunction

Outcome
The patient will discuss fears and concerns regarding sexual function.

Interventions
- Clarify patient's understanding of risks and benefits of surgical procedure.
- Provide an open, accepting environment for the patient to discuss potentially embarrassing issues.
- Maintain patient privacy and dignity.
- Consider making a referral for patient to discuss options available to achieve sexual function postoperatively.

Patient Safety. The perioperative nurse considers several factors in advocating for the patient during the intraoperative period. Institutions have various protocols and processes in place to support patient safety. A critical safety protocol that the nurse is responsible to follow is to ensure the correct patient, correct procedure, and correct site surgery. Such a protocol includes proper patient identification, proper operative site identification, proper procedure identification, and proper medication identification. All wrong site, wrong procedure, and wrong patient surgery occurrences are considered sentinel events by The Joint Commission (TJC). In addition, the Association of periOperative Registered Nurses (AORN) has established guidelines for patient safety (AORN, 2012a).

To fulfill these requirements, preoperative verification, surgical site marking, and time-out processes must occur for every surgical procedure. What the patient expresses as the intended surgical procedure is compared with what is documented on the operative permit and other items, such as the operating room (OR) schedule. Patient identification is achieved by also asking the patient to state his or her full name and birth date. This information is compared with the patient identification bracelet. Documentation of the processes implemented is completed on the designated institutional form or forms.

The surgical site is marked with a permanent nontoxic marking pen. The patient should be involved in this process. A standard policy needs to be developed within the particular facility as to how marking will be accomplished for urologic, endoscopic, and abdominal procedures, particularly when they involve laterality. This mark should be clearly visible following prepping and draping.

Time-out is a pause in the activity that occurs before the start or incision on all procedures. The entire team stops to verbally confirm the patient's identity, verify the patient's position, state and agree on the procedure and surgical site, and review that all implants and necessary equipment are available and ready (Patient Safety). The nurse documents this process according to hospital policy.

When medications are used intraoperatively, the containers should always be marked with the medication and dose (refer to Chapter 2 for a full discussion of medication safety). The scrub person, who may be a registered nurse or surgical technologist, verifies the medication and dosage verbally when passing the drug in its administration device to the surgeon. Local anesthetics that contain epinephrine should be used with caution in urology. Many urologic interventions involve "end-organs," for example, the scrotum, testicles, and penis. The use of epinephrine in these areas can result in an ischemic situation and should be avoided.

Positioning. Thorough understanding of the urologic OR bed and its functions is essential for optimum patient positioning. The position in which the patient is placed for surgery is determined by the particular operation to be performed. For urologic operative procedures the patient may be placed in the lateral, supine, prone, or lithotomy position. Any of these positions may be exaggerated to give optimum access to the organ involved, particularly in radical surgery of the prostate and bladder. When the patient is supine, his or her arms are placed on padded armboards with the palms up and fingers extended. Armboards are maintained at less than a 90-degree angle to prevent brachial plexus stretch. If there are surgical reasons to tuck the arms at the side, the elbows are padded to protect the ulnar nerve, the palms face inward, and the wrist is maintained in a neutral position (Denholm, 2009). A drape secures the arms. It should be tucked snugly under the patient, not under the mattress. This prevents the arm from shifting downward intraoperatively and

PATIENT SAFETY

Improving Teamwork to Reduce Errors

Publication of the 1999 Institute of Medicine report focused attention on medical errors and the critical importance of patient safety. Reducing errors (such as wrong person, wrong procedure, or wrong site surgery) requires, in part, human solutions, such as improving teamwork and communication in the OR team. Interdisciplinary teamwork is especially important in the so-called high-risk areas in hospitals, such as the OR. Perioperative nurses have long believed that a team approach to patient care reduces errors. Effective teamwork in perioperative patient care consists of knowledge, attitudes, and skills. Developing sustainable efforts to improve teamwork requires thoughtful application. Interventions focused on changing the behavior of team members must first take into account their attitudes. Subsequently, skills and knowledge are assessed, and a training program can be designed to improve teamwork. The benefits of improved teamwork are well exemplified in the time-out process, which aims to enhance effectiveness, increase efficiency, and lower the possibility of error. Preoperative verification processes and the time-out result in fewer errors because these processes are planned by each institution and standardized through use of the Universal Protocol of The Joint Commission. In urology, endoscopic procedures with laterality such as left or right ureteroscopy are marked over the left or right kidney as well as left or right inner aspect of thigh. This is because the surgical site is draped out and all that is visible at the time-out is the perineum and inner thigh. Each member of the OR team knows his or her own responsibilities as well as those of teammates; members look out for each other and note errors before they happen; and members trust one another's judgments and concerns. Teamwork during preoperative verification and the time-out allows proper integration and execution of clinical activities, gives caregivers increased control over their work environment, and provides a safety net against error.

Modified from Caplan RA et al: Practice advisory for the prevention and management of operating room fires; a report by the American Society of Anesthesiologists Task Force on Operating Room Fires, *Anesthesiology* 108:786–801, 2008.

resting against the OR bed rail. Acting as the patient's advocate, the nurse takes considerable care to ensure that the surgical position does not interfere with respiration or circulation. It is essential to avoid displacement of the joints and undue tension on neurovascular bundles or ligaments. A patient positioned laterally (flank position) for renal surgery has the spine extended for greater access to the retroperitoneal space. Padding and stabilized support with gel pads, pillows, sandbags, and straps should be available for precise anatomic positioning and safety (see Chapter 6). When an electrosurgical unit (ESU) is to be used, care must be taken that the patient does not contact metal parts of the OR bed. In some procedures involving stones of the kidneys or ureters, intraoperative fluoroscopy may be required. When fluoroscopy (C-arm) is to be used, the patient must be placed on an OR bed compatible with its use. Whenever possible, the perioperative nurse takes measures to protect the patient from undue radiation exposure to the thyroid and chest areas by using small leaded shields. In urologic procedures it generally is not feasible to shield the reproductive organs during fluoroscopy.

Aseptic Techniques and Safety Measures. Prevention of infection is an important nursing goal in the care of the genitourinary patient. It is, however, seldom possible to confirm freedom from infection intraoperatively or immediately postoperatively. Aseptic techniques must be carefully maintained and monitored. Skin preparation and draping procedures (see Chapter 4) vary, depending on the surgery to be performed and institutional protocols. Special care must be taken when cleansing the perineal area to avoid contamination from the rectum to the urethra. Prepping solutions should be applied with downward strokes and the sponge discarded once it has contacted the inner vaginal or anal areas. Transurethral passage of instruments and catheters requires meticulous technique to prevent retrograde infections of the urinary tract, which account for 32% of all healthcare-associated infections (Scott, 2012).

Visualization of the bladder during transurethral procedures is often enhanced by darkening the room. Provision should be made for proper adjustments to lighting. ESUs and fiberoptic light systems are common adjuncts in urologic surgery. The nurse and scrub person must be familiar with the manufacturer's safety precautions and recommendations during their use.

Use of Irrigating Fluids. When the bladder is entered, sterile distilled irrigating fluid is administered to distend it for effective visualization. Commercially prepared sterile irrigation solutions with appropriate closed administration sets are highly recommended. Such closed systems prevent the inherent risks of cross-contamination. Large volumes of irrigating solutions are frequently used, particularly during more extensive endoscopic procedures. When these solutions are at the room temperature of the OR, they are cold compared with the patient's internal body temperature and can cause hypothermia. Solution-warming units are available commercially and are a useful tool to help decrease this risk. The drawback to these units may be that the warmth delays clotting, thus increasing the risk of blood loss.

Commercially prepared sterile irrigation solutions are available in collapsible bags and rigid plastic containers, both of which have the same advantages: neither depends on air, and each may be hung in series, thus providing continuous irrigation without interruption. Air bubbles, a problem that distorts visibility during the procedure, are eliminated with these systems.

For simple observation cystoscopy, retrograde pyelography, and simple bladder tumor fulgurations, sterile distilled water may be used without complication. However, during transurethral resection of the prostate (TURP), venous sinuses may be opened and varying amounts of irrigant are invariably absorbed into the bloodstream. Studies indicate that the use of distilled water during TURP may result in hemolysis of erythrocytes and possible renal failure. Other important complications include dilutional hyponatremia and cardiac decompensation.

Therefore, a clear, nonelectrolytic, and iso-osmotic solution should be used. The most widely used urologic irrigating fluids are 3% sorbitol, an isomer of mannitol, and 1.5% glycine, an aminoacetic acid solution. In dilute solutions, sorbitol and glycine have many properties that make them particularly useful for irrigation during transurethral prostatectomy. At slightly hypotonic concentrations they do not produce hemolysis. However, if too much intravasation occurs with glycine, an encephalitic state can result from the ammonia produced (Surgical Pharmacology). Because the solutions are nonelectrolytic, they do not cause dispersion of high-frequency current with consequent loss of electrosurgical cutting capacity, as occurs with normal saline.

During ureteropyeloscopy, sterile normal saline is the irrigant of choice unless electrosurgery is to be used. This solution most closely approximates a physiologic solution—an important factor if

perforation and extravasation of fluid into the retroperitoneum occur. If electrosurgery is required, as with a TURP, 3% sorbitol or 1.5% glycine should be used.

Thorough knowledge of the potential hazards encountered intraoperatively during transurethral surgery is extremely important. Although complications are more prevalent in the postoperative stage, close observation during the intraoperative period is essential. Signs and symptoms such as sudden restlessness, apprehension, irritability, confusion, nausea, slow pulse rate, seizures, dysrhythmias, and rising blood pressure may be suggestive of TURP syndrome, a severe hyponatremia caused by systemic absorption of irrigating fluid used during surgery (Han and Partin, 2007). Minimum amounts of fluids should be given and urine output carefully monitored. Irrigation fluid should be under as little pressure as possible and the bladder emptied before it reaches full capacity to prevent intravesical pressure. During ureteropyeloscopy it is frequently necessary to use a pressure bag to ensure adequate visualization of the upper urinary tract. Serum electrolyte values should be obtained, and if a low serum sodium value is reported, hypertonic sodium chloride is administered by means of a slow IV drip, often on a volumetric pump. IV diuretics such as furosemide (Lasix) may be required to prevent possible pulmonary edema associated with the administration of hypertonic saline. If the patient's reaction is severe, surgery may have to be terminated.

Endoscopic and Ancillary Equipment. Cystoscopic and ancillary equipment often varies from one institution to another. Therefore it is valuable to have a reference manual or standard setup cards that illustrate and describe in detail the required instrumentation for each specific procedure.

The basic cystoscopy tray should include instruments and accessory items that are routinely used for all cystoscopy procedures. If ureteral catheterization is planned, catheterizing telescopes or an Albarrán bridge, which can be packaged and sterilized separately, may be easily added to the basic cystoscopy setup. Instruments for transurethral surgery and other special procedures may be wrapped, sterilized, and placed on separate trays so that they are available on request. This concept minimizes handling of the delicate lensed instruments and ultimately reduces costly repairs.

Cystoscopic procedures frequently require additional instrumentation. Instruments of various types and sizes, such as a visual obturator, biopsy forceps, urethral sounds, Phillips filiforms and followers, and Ellik evacuators, are available as prepackaged, sterile, disposable items. The reusable products may also be packaged separately and sterilized.

Ureteral and Urethral Catheters. A variety of ureteral and urethral catheters are designed for specific procedures. Ureteral catheters are manufactured of polyurethane material and are graduated so that the surgeon may determine the exact distance the catheter has been inserted into the ureter (Figure 15-8). Most manufacturers provide sterile disposable catheters wrapped in peel-open packages to allow aseptic handling during ureteral insertion. Some indications for the use of ureteral catheters are to (1) perform retrograde pyelography, (2) identify the ureters during pelvic or intestinal surgery, and (3) bypass partial or complete obstruction that may be present as a result of ureteral tumors, calculi, or strictures. Not uncommonly, it is necessary to insert a ureteral stent in a pregnant female because of hydronephrosis or obstructing calculi.

The most commonly used catheters include the open-ended, whistle tip, cone tip, and olive tip. When a retrograde ureterogram

SURGICAL PHARMACOLOGY

Agents Used in Urologic Surgery

Category	Dose/Route	Purpose/Action	Adverse Reactions	Nursing Implications
Bulking Agents				
Coaptite Macroplastique Botox	Transurethral, periurethral injection 100-300 units	Correct UH, ISD, SUI	Swelling, urinary retention Local tissue infarction/ necrosis, vascular occlusion, embolus	Avoid injection into blood vessels. Do not use bulking agents in presences of acute cystitis, urethritis, or other genitourinary infection.
Irrigants				
Glycine (monocarboxylic amino acid)	1.5%, 3-5 L, intravesical	No hemolysis or dispersion of electrocurrent	Increased ammonia production Encephalitic reaction Biosynthesis of heme Blurred vision CNS disturbances TURP syndrome if absorbed	Contraindicated with clozapine usage. Use with caution in diabetic patients, patients with liver disease; inhibitory neurotransmitter.
Sorbitol (nonelectrolytic, iso-osmotic, hypotonic aminoacetic acid)	3%, 3-5 L, intravesical	Isomer of mannitol, no hemolysis or dispersion of electrocurrent	TURP syndrome if absorbed	Hyperglycemia may occur in patients with diabetes mellitus. Use with caution in patients with renal or cardiac compromise.
Water	Distilled, 3-5 L, intravesical	Irrigant, lyse cancer cells	Hyponatremia, hemolysis of erythrocytes	Avoid with TURP. Intravasation can lead to dilutional hyponatremia, cardiac decompensation, and renal failure.
Normal saline	0.9%, 3-5 L, intravesical	Physiologic irrigant	Hypernatremia	Not for use with electrosurgery. Disperses electrocurrent.
Injectables				
Indigo carmine	40 mg, IV or local	Colorize urine, vessels	Hypertension	Moderately reduces oxygen saturation.
Phenylephrine (Neo-Synephrine)	0.05% (5 mg), SubQ	Vasoconstriction for priapism	Hypertension, reflex bradycardia	May decrease renal blood flow. Contraindicated in patients with hypertension.
Papaverine	30 mg/mL, 2 mL in solution, intercavernosal	Vasodilation, antispasmodic	Dizziness, dysrhythmia, hypotension, flushing, hypothermia	Contraindicated in AV block, pregnancy. Depressed AV or intraventricular conduction, physiologic antagonist.
Vasopressin (Pitressin)	20 units/mL: 2 mL (40 units) in solution, local	Vasoconstriction	Water intoxication, dizziness, headache, pallor	May cause tenesmus, tremors, cramps, abdominal pain, hyponatremia; retards absorption of local anesthetics. Contraindicated in patients with uremia, coronary artery disease, hypertension.
Topical				
Methylene blue	1 mL/100 mL NS, topical	Colorize tissues, vessels	Hypertension, dizziness, headache, anemia, diaphoresis	Do not use in patients with severe renal disease, hemolytic anemia. Destroys erythrocytes; may cause methemoglobinuria.
Other				
B&O suppository (belladonna/opium)	16.2 mg/30 mg, rectal	Prevent/decrease bladder/ureteral spasm	Constipation, decreased sweating	Use with precaution in patients who take MAOIs, agents that affect GI motility, select narcotics. May cause cardiovascular instability, paralytic ileus, respiratory depression, toxin-mediated diarrhea, pseudomembranous enterocolitis.

AV, Atrioventricular; *CNS,* central nervous system; *GI,* gastrointestinal; *ISD,* intrinsic sphincter dysfunction; *IV,* intravenous; *MAOIs,* monoamine oxidase inhibitors; *SubQ,* subcutaneous; *SUI,* stress urinary incontinence; *TURP,* transurethral resection of the prostate; *UH,* urethral hypermobility.

Modified from Daily Med Current Medication Information, available at http://dailymed.nlm.nih.gov/dailymed/about.cfm. Accessed January 8, 2013; Hodgson BB, Kizior RJ: *Saunders nursing drug handbook 2013,* St Louis, 2013, Saunders; NCBI PubChem, available at http://pubchem.ncbi.nlm.nih.gov. Accessed January 8, 2013.

FIGURE 15-8 A, Ureteral catheters. **B,** Adapters.

is indicated, a cone-tipped ureteral catheter may be helpful in occluding the ureteral orifice to accomplish the x-ray study effectively. When a ureteral catheter is left indwelling, a special adapter (see Figure 15-8, *B*) may be connected to the end of the ureteral catheter to facilitate connection to a closed urinary drainage system. A small slit may also be created in the Foley catheter, and the distal end of the ureteral catheter can be slipped into it and taped in place.

Indwelling double-pigtail or double-J stents are available and are passed cystoscopically to reside within the ureter (Figure 15-9). When the guidewire is removed from the core of the stent, a proximal and distal J or "pigtail" forms in the tubing to retain the stents. Many of these stents have a nonabsorbable suture attached to the distal end, which extends through the urethral meatus. A suture may be easily tied to the distal end of those that do not. The surgeon can then remove the stent in the office setting postoperatively without needing to perform a cystoscopy.

Urethral catheters have a multitude of functions as stents, as drainage tubes, and in diagnostic studies in the OR. They are generally divided into two categories—plain and indwelling (retention)—and range in different French (F) sizes, most commonly 10F through 30F. The Foley catheter is the most frequently used retention catheter and is manufactured with a variety of balloon sizes, tip styles, lengths, and eye arrangements.

After transurethral prostatic surgery a three-way Foley catheter with a 30-mL balloon capacity may be left indwelling. This type of catheter is preferred because it facilitates continuous bladder irrigation (CBI), and the large balloon aids in achieving hemostasis in the prostatic bed. The surgeon may apply light traction on the Foley catheter with a leg strap, adhesive catheter anchor, or tape. This traction causes pressure against the bladder neck and aids in hemostasis. The goal is to prevent traumatic catheter removal in men.

A hematuria catheter, a three-way Foley specifically for patients with excessive clot formation, is also available. This catheter is reinforced with a stretch spiral wire within the catheter lining that permits vigorous aspiration without fear of lumen collapse.

Diagnostic studies performed in the cystoscopy suite may require special catheters for specific studies. A Davis or Trattner triple-lumen double-balloon urethrographic catheter or any of a variety of urodynamic catheters may be used to diagnose lesions of the female urethra, such as urethral strictures, diverticula, and fistulas.

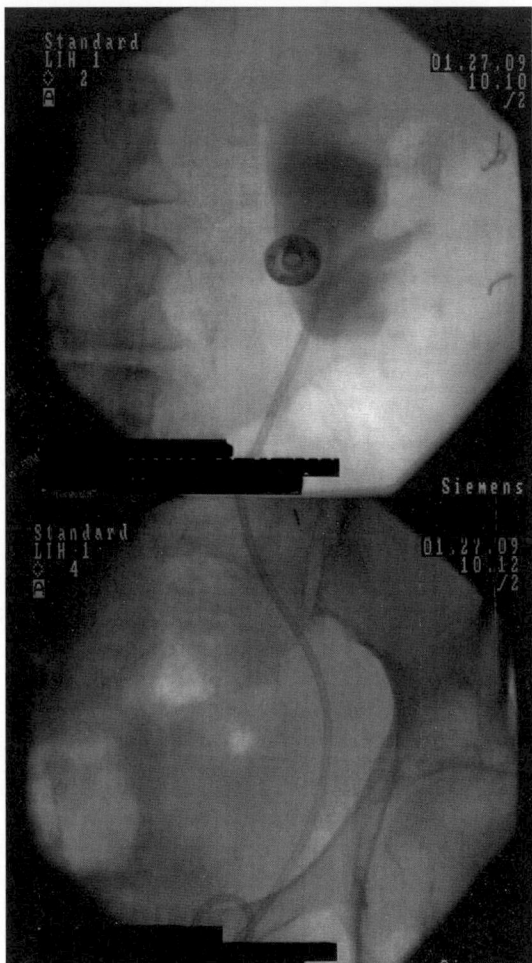

FIGURE 15-9 Double-pigtail stent set.

To accomplish female urethrography, the catheter is inserted through the urethra into the bladder; the two balloons on the catheter are inflated, one in the bladder and one at the external urethral orifice, effectively isolating the urethra. Contrast medium is injected to visualize the entire urethra.

FIGURE 15-10 A, Pezzer (mushroom) catheter. **B,** Malecot (bat-winged) four-winged catheter.

Another type of self-retaining catheter frequently used in the OR is the Pezzer catheter, also known as a *mushroom* catheter (Figure 15-10, *A*). It may be straight or angulated with a large single channel and a preformed tip in the shape of a mushroom. The flexible mushroom tip helps keep the catheter in place. This catheter is used primarily for suprapubic bladder drainage, often for poor-risk patients who have uremia, neurogenic bladder syndrome, or possibly long-standing urinary retention. The catheter is inserted into the bladder through a midline or small transverse abdominal wall incision and secured to the abdomen with suture or tape. The Malecot four-winged catheter, often used as a nephrostomy tube to provide temporary or permanent diversion of urine after kidney surgery and when renal tissue needs to be restored, may also be used for suprapubic drainage (see Figure 15-10, *B*). A Foley catheter of preferred size is frequently chosen for either purpose. Nephrostomy tube replacement is accomplished by introducing the catheter into the surgical tract with a straight catheter guide and securing it in place with a suture or a nephrostomy retention disk that is one size smaller than the nephrostomy tube being used. The flanges of the disk are taped or sutured to the skin. The use of other variations of urethral catheters is described throughout the chapter.

Photography in Urology. The use of photographic and video imaging equipment in urologic surgery serves to document the patient's disease, the progress of a disease process, and long-term follow-up study. It is also an important teaching resource. Video equipment adapts to endoscopic instrumentation and has the capability of projecting an enhanced image on a television monitor, permitting members of the surgical team to observe and learn during the actual surgical procedure. Other visual aids, such as slides and photographs, are used in teaching, as visual references in publication, and as documentation in patient records.

When any form of photography or video imaging is used, the patient's privacy must be ensured and an informed consent should be obtained. Special release forms should also be signed preoperatively by the patient for any videotapes or photographs to be used in teaching or publications.

Evaluation

Before the patient is taken to the postanesthesia care unit (PACU) or observation unit, the perioperative nurse evaluates the patient's general condition. The skin is assessed, and bony prominences, prepped and draped areas, and areas contacted by the attachment of ancillary equipment are observed for signs of pressure, irritation, or other changes from the preoperative status.

Many urology patients are discharged to the PACU with catheters and drains inserted, including urethral, ureteral, suprapubic, and wound drains. A local anesthetic may have been used for either primary analgesia or postoperative pain management (preemptive analgesia); preoperative or intraoperative infiltration of the surgical site blocks sensory input, resulting in postoperative analgesia. A hand-off report to the PACU nurse should include intraoperative position, problems encountered specific to the patient, and the patient's preoperative physical status as well as comprehension and anxiety levels. Documentation of medications administered from the sterile field or by the perioperative nurse intraoperatively should include time of administration, name of medication, dosage, site and route of administration, and the name of the person who performed the application or injection. Drains should be documented as to size and type, insertion site, time and date of insertion, type of collection device, name of the person who performed the insertion, and character of drainage. When several drains are in place, additional labeling on the collection devices is beneficial. Any postoperative observations before or during transport should be recorded. Evaluation should also address whether the patient met the identified outcomes related to specific nursing diagnoses in the perioperative nursing plan of care. Attainment of identified desired outcomes, included in the documentation and report to the PACU, may be phrased as follows:

- The patient verbalized an acceptable anxiety level to the perioperative nurse.
- The patient had no evidence of positional injury; neurovascular status was consistent with preoperative level, and skin integrity was intact.
- The patient maintained patency of the urinary catheter with no signs of blockage or urinary retention. Urinary output remained within normal limits. The patient voids without difficulty after catheter removal.
- The patient had no evidence or signs of fluid volume or electrolyte imbalance; vital signs were stable, arterial blood gases were within normal limits, and urinary output was maintained at acceptable levels.
- The patient maintained adequate gas exchange; lung expansion and O_2 saturation were satisfactory.
- The patient discussed fears and concerns regarding sexual function.

Patient and Family Education and Discharge Planning

Patient and family education and preparation for discharge allow perioperative nurses to plan for the urologic surgery patient's care across a continuum. Information is tailored according to the procedure and the patient's status (Ambulatory Surgery Considerations). Information provided should be presented in language the patient can understand (lay terms) and clarified with the patient by having the patient repeat back in his or her own words the information provided. When possible and with the patient's approval, family members or others who will serve as caregivers should be included in the educational process at the outset. Institutions may find it helpful to inventory the patient education materials available for select surgical procedures. An example of patient education for home care after nephrectomy is presented in Patient and Family Education on page 473.

Discharge instructions should be printed and include community resources and support groups as appropriate for the surgical intervention and the patient's diagnosis. These too should be presented in easily understood terms, reviewed, and confirmed by

AMBULATORY SURGERY CONSIDERATIONS

Cystoscopy, Transrectal Guided Ultrasound of the Prostate

A commonly performed outpatient urologic procedure is a cystoscopy, transrectal ultrasound guided biopsy of the prostate (cysto/TRUS). To minimize complications, patient selection is determined by the healthcare team. Patients classified as physical status 1 or 2, as per the American Society of Anesthesiologists, generally pose no great risk for procedures performed with general, IV moderate sedation and local anesthetics. The majority of cysto/TRUS patients have this procedure performed with IV sedation/local. To decrease pain during and immediately after the procedure, a viscous local anesthetic is injected into the rectum and the urethra after IV sedation is initiated.

Preoperative and postoperative teaching of the patient and his family is essential because the family will be the primary caregiver on discharge. Teaching begins in the surgeon's office. The office staff provides patients with a prescription for antibiotics with instructions to begin the medication 24 hours before the procedure and to continue oral antibiotics postoperatively until the prescription is completed. The office staff also advises the patient to take a cleansing enema 2 to 3 hours before the procedure. Both the antibiotics and the enema decrease the chances of postoperative infection.

Patient and family anxiety levels will be high pending the postoperative diagnosis. The patient may also be anxious because of the nature of the procedure and anesthetic used. The perioperative nurse plays a key role in supporting the patient and his family throughout the ambulatory surgical experience.

Discharge assessment following anesthesia includes:

- Airway patency, respiratory function, and oxygen saturation
- Stable vital signs
- Hypothermia resolved
- Level of consciousness and muscular strength
- Adequate pain control
- Mobility
- Skin color and condition
- Condition of the surgical site
- Intake and output
- Comfort
- Anxiety
- Significant other interaction
- Numeric score if used

Before discharge the nurse instructs the patient to increase his clear liquid intake and monitor urine output. Postoperative burning on urination and blood in the urine as well as blood draining from the rectum are common. Patients are instructed to keep the perineum clean. The nurse ensures that the patient has a prescription for pain medication, clarifies the instructions for dosage and frequency, and instructs the patient to call the surgeon for any temperature higher than 101°F (38°C). The nurse provides all instructions verbally and gives the patient and his family a written copy of the instructions. The patient calls the physician as directed for results of the biopsy.

A postdischarge phone call to the patient is recommended. This allows the nurse to review the patient's postoperative status, provide reassurance if necessary, and reinforce any teaching. The call also provides the patient and his family an opportunity to ask additional questions.

PATIENT AND FAMILY EDUCATION

Home Care Education for the Nephrectomy Patient

Give the patient and the caregiver both verbal and written instructions. Provide them with the name and telephone number of a physician or nurse to call if questions arise. At the end of reviewing home care instructions, have the patient or family member repeat back, in his or her own words, information provided.

General Information
- Review the purpose and explain the type of procedure performed: partial or total nephrectomy.

Wound/Incision Care
- Instruct the patient on caring for the incision and changing the dressing:
  - Wash hands.
  - Inspect the incision for signs of infection.
  - Cleanse the area with an antiseptic agent.
  - If there is no evidence of drainage, leave the site open to the air. Otherwise, cover the incision with sterile gauze squares held in place with tape.
- Teach the patient how to care for the nephrostomy tube, if present.

Special Instructions
- Inform the patient that showering and bathing may be resumed as recommended by the physician.
- Explain how to measure urine output as indicated.

Warning Signs
- Review the signs and symptoms that should be reported to a physician or nurse:
  - Infection: Incision red, warm to touch, painful, with increased or purulent drainage (define)
  - Urinary tract infection: Fever, chills, hematuria ("blood in urine"), flank pain, sudden increase in urinary output

Activity
- Discuss the need to exercise to tolerance and to plan frequent rest periods. Explain that fatigue is common.
- Encourage the patient to discuss allowances and limitations with respect to occupation, recreation, and activities
- Tell the patient to avoid heavy lifting (>10 lb) for at least 6 weeks.
- Advise the patient to avoid contact sports (e.g., wrestling, football) that could endanger the remaining kidney.

Diet
- Inform the patient that a regular diet can be followed unless there are restrictions related to the underlying reason for nephrectomy.
- Encourage the patient to drink 8 to 10 glasses of fluids per day unless restrictions of the underlying disease apply. Half of these should be fruit juices (to maintain electrolyte balance).

Follow-Up Care
- Stress the importance of regular follow-up visits. Make sure the patient has the necessary names and telephone numbers.

Modified from University of Michigan Health System, *Instructions for care following nephrectomy,* 2009, available at http://www.med.umich.edu/1libr/urology/postcare/nephrectomy.htm. Accessed January 11, 2013.

having the patient repeat back in his or her own words the information provided. Any requisite skills that the patient or family will require should be demonstrated, with return demonstrations as time permits. Perioperative nurses may find it helpful to involve institutional resource persons or departments such as the social services department in developing information related to home care services, durable medical equipment, and transfers to aftercare facilities other than home (skilled nursing center, rehabilitation facility, other long-term care facility). Patients and their families need preparation for mastering information and tasks that need to be performed. The goal of such interdisciplinary discharge planning is to provide information for the patient that is comprehensive and easy to use. This is part of perioperative nursing's ethical and professional responsibility to patients; it also meets TJC's requirements of providing consistent patient and family education.

Surgical Interventions

Diagnostic and Endoscopic Procedures

Cystoscopy

Cystoscopy is an endoscopic examination of the lower urinary tract, including visual inspection of the interior of the urethra, the bladder, and the ureteral orifices. In a male patient special attention is given to the examination of the verumontanum (which contains the ejaculatory duct), the bladder neck, and the median and lateral lobes of the prostate. In a female patient the urethra, bladder neck, and bladder are examined.

Cystoscopy is an important diagnostic tool that provides the surgeon with valuable information concerning the patient's urologic condition. Indications for cystoscopy include hematuria, urinary retention, urinary tract infection, cystitis, tumors, fistulas, vesical calculus disease, and urinary incontinence. Urinary incontinence in postmenopausal women may be related to estrogen deprivation.

Procedural Considerations. On arrival to the preoperative area all patients should be greeted by name and identified by their identification bracelet and number. The perioperative nurse should review the chart for operative consent and pertinent laboratory reports; IVPs and any other diagnostic x-ray studies ordered preoperatively should also be available for review. Customarily the patient voids immediately before transport to the OR. The time of urination and the output volume should be documented for ruling out residual urine in the bladder.

After the patient is placed on the cystoscopy bed, correct positioning requires optimum relaxation of muscles of the legs and perineum. Proper positioning is a vital consideration for patient safety and comfort. Allen and Yellofin stirrups are boot-style stirrups that support the foot and calf. These have thick gel padding within the stirrup and provide optimum patient comfort and protection, relieving pressure on the popliteal space. They are especially beneficial for the patient who has limited hip mobility and altered peripheral circulatory status. The nurse should assess the patient's bilateral pedal pulses preoperatively and postoperatively when using any stirrups. Stirrups should be adjusted carefully to avoid undue pressure on the calf. If knee crutches are used, the curve of the yoke suspension should flow outward from the perineum, in the same manner as the patient's legs. Padding the knee crutches reduces pressure on the popliteal areas. If sling stirrups that support only the feet are used, the post should be padded and positioned to prevent pressure on the peroneal nerve. Special pads are designed for use with both of these stirrups.

After the patient is properly positioned, the anesthesia provider may tilt the OR bed so that the patient's head is slightly higher than the buttocks to allow the prep solution to drain into the collecting pan. Pooling of solutions beneath the patient may cause skin reaction and chemical irritation, as well as the potential for burns if an ESU is used. If the cystoscopic procedure requires the use of an ESU, the nurse ensures that the dispersive pad is placed on the patient in direct contact with the skin as close to the operative site as is practical. When placing the ESU pad, the nurse avoids hairy areas, bony prominences, scar tissue, and proximity to prosthetic metal implants or pacemakers.

Next, the nurse or surgeon dons gloves and preps the entire pubic area, including the perineum, with an antimicrobial solution. A disposable drape sheet with a sterile screen material incorporated into it is a standard part of the cystoscopy drape pack. The surgeon and scrub person drape the patient in a manner that ensures aseptic technique is maintained during the urologic procedure. If a general or spinal anesthetic is required, the anesthesia provider administers it before prepping and draping. If a local anesthetic is preferred, the surgeon instills it into the urethra of the male patient after prepping and draping but before instrumentation. For a female patient, the surgeon places a cotton applicator that has been dipped into the anesthetic solution in the urethral meatus. Usually, viscous lidocaine (Xylocaine), 1% or 2%, is used. If the patient is allergic to lidocaine, instillation of 50 to 60 mL of lubricant accompanied by anesthesia-monitored sedation is often adequate to afford the surgeon painless access to the urethra and bladder. The patient should be informed that a sensation of pressure is to be expected.

The basic cystoscopy setup requires a cystoscopy pack, a sterile gown or apron, sterile gloves, a fiberoptic light source, a prep cup and solution, gauze sponges, the cystourethroscope (Figure 15-11), a short bridge and fiberoptic light cord, lateral and foroblique telescopes, a Luer-Lok stopcock, irrigation tubing and sterile water irrigant, and water-soluble lubricant. Additional items that should be sterile and available include a calibrated container to measure residual urine, test tubes with screw tops for urine specimens, an Albarrán bridge and rubber catheter nipples or adapters, a medicine

FIGURE 15-11 Basic instruments for cystoscopy, catheterization, electrosurgery, and retrograde ureteral pyelography (add ureteral catheter of choice). *Left to right,* Bugbee electrodes, single-horn Albarrán deflecting bridge, nipple adapters, stopcock, short double-horn bridge, 23F and 17F foroblique cystourethroscopes and sheaths, 30- and 70-degree telescopes, double-horn Albarrán deflecting bridge, single-horn examining bridge, visual obturator, and fiberoptic cable.

FIGURE 15-12 Flexible cystoscope.

glass for dye, anesthetic solution, disposable 10- and 20-mL syringes, medication labels and a marking pen, a penile clamp (to occlude male urethra after local anesthetic is instilled), contrast material, an ESU and dispersive pad, and a Bugbee electrode.

The flexible cystoscope (Figure 15-12) is used for patients with obstructive symptoms resulting from prostatic hyperplasia and rigid prostatic urethra. In addition, the flexible cystoscope can be used for patients who cannot assume a lithotomy position, such as those with spinal cord injuries or severe arthritis. Flexible cystoscopy may be accomplished with the use of a local anesthetic. It affords the patient a higher degree of comfort, is less traumatic to the urethra, and can be performed in the patient's bed on the nursing unit.

Cleaning, sterilization, disinfection, and maintenance of endoscopic equipment are important procedures in the care of fiberoptic lensed instruments. Ultimately this process reduces costly repairs and ensures the availability of properly functioning instruments. See Chapter 8 for the procedure to correctly process endoscopic equipment.

Endoscopy of the genitourinary tract is considered a class II (clean-contaminated) procedure and, according to the Centers for Disease Control and Prevention (CDC) and the Association for Professionals in Infection Control and Epidemiology (APIC) guidelines, presently requires disinfection rather than sterilization. High-level disinfection with an agent such as activated glutaraldehyde or dialdehyde that can destroy vegetative microorganisms, most fungal spores, tubercle bacilli, and small nonlipid viruses is recommended. In most situations the routine of meticulous cleaning of endoscopic instruments and making sure that all channels are accessed, followed by appropriate high-level disinfection, provides reasonable assurance that the items are safe to use. The level of disinfection is based on the contact time, temperature, and concentration of the active ingredients of the disinfectant, as well as the nature of microbial contamination.

Many institutions are, however, treating endoscopic interventions as sterile procedures because the sterilization of instruments provides the greatest assurance that the risk of infections transmitted by contaminated instruments has been eliminated (see Chapter 4). Some options available include glutaraldehyde solution, hydrogen peroxide solution, an automated peracetic acid unit, an ETO (ethylene oxide, "gas") sterilizer, a hydrogen peroxide and plasma sterilizing unit, and high-vacuum or gravity steam autoclaving for those components that may be sterilized in this manner. The manufacturer's recommendations should always be followed. If soaking is chosen the lid should remain on the soaking container when not in use, and personnel should wear masks when in direct contact with the fumes. It is also imperative that the instrumentation be thoroughly rinsed in sterile distilled water after removal from the soaking solution and before use. Glutaraldehyde residue remaining in the channels or on the lens can result in chemical burns for the patient and the surgeon.

Stone removal, bladder biopsy, and bladder fulguration may be accomplished by using special cystoscopic accessories. This procedure is called a *litholapaxy*. Lowsley forceps, Wappler rigid cup forceps, and flexible foreign body forceps may also be used. Bladder fulguration requires the use of flexible-stem electrodes available in various French sizes and tip configurations such as the ball, cone, dome, and bayonet.

Operative Procedure

1. The surgeon lubricates the cystourethroscope and introduces it into the urethra, withdraws the obturator, and drains the bladder. Residual urine may be measured at this time if the patient voided before the examination. The specimen may be saved for cultures or cytologic studies.
2. The surgeon connects the cystourethroscope to the irrigating system, and inserts and locks the telescope in place. If the patient is awake, telling the patient to try to urinate also helps facilitate passage of the scope. The surgeon controls the rate of flow and volume of fluid by adjusting the stopcock on the scope. If difficulty is encountered during insertion, the visual obturator may be used to introduce the scope under direct vision. This accessory is constructed to smooth the fenestrated edges of the cystourethroscope. It requires the use of the telescope for direct vision and permits irrigation during introduction.
3. For retrograde ureteral catheterization and pyelography, the surgeon passes ureteral catheters through the cystoscope sheath and then through the ureteral orifice and into the ureter via the Albarrán bridge. A radiopaque substance (e.g., nonionic, low-osmolar agents Omnipaque 300 and Optiray 320; or ionic high-osmolar Renografin-60 and Hypaque 50) is injected. Fluoroscopic imaging is used to outline the entire upper urinary collecting system.

Periurethral-Transurethral Injection of Bulking Agents

Coaptite injection is an ambulatory surgery procedure achievable with the patient administered a local anesthetic with or without sedation. Coaptite (calcium hydroxylapatite, Boston Scientific) is a synthetic injectable composed of spherical particles and is prepackaged in a sterile 1-mL syringe containing the coaptite material. Injection needles available are a 14.6-inch, 21-gauge, noncoring needle for transurethral use or for periurethral insertion. Female patients with intrinsic sphincter deficiency (ISD) demonstrated by urodynamic evaluation and male patients (usually after prostatectomy) with incontinence lasting more than 1 year may benefit from this procedure. Other indications for coaptite injection include urethral hypermobility (UH), stress urinary incontinence (SUI) secondary to previous stricture treatment, trauma, or myelodysplasia (Boston Scientific, 2009).

Macroplastique (Uroplasty Inc.) is a bulking product composed of polydimethylsiloxane (a silicone elastomer) particles suspended in a polyvinylpyrrolidone (PVP) carrier gel, and is packaged in a sterile 3-mL syringe containing 2.5 mL of product. Instillation of the bulking agent is achieved by attaching the rigid transurethral needle to the 3-mL syringe containing the agent. The 3-mL syringe is then placed in a manual plunger device and injected. It is designed to treat women with SUI secondary to documented ISD. Macroplastique is permanent implant, nondegradable and nonresorbable and provides a durable effect. Macroplastique is currently approved by the U.S. Food and Drug Administration (FDA) for use in women only (Smith and Wein, 2010).

Botox (onabotulinum toxin A) is FDA approved for neurogenic detrusor overactivity (also called overactive bladder in patients with a neurologic condition) and used off label for idiopathic overactive bladder. Rarely it is also used off label for interstitial cystitis and very rarely for BPH. Doses between 100 and 300 units are used depending on surgeon preference and patient preference. Higher doses are more likely to cause urinary retention or incomplete bladder emptying, requiring intermittent catheterization than lower doses. Patients with neurogenic bladder who already perform intermittent catheterization usually receive higher (300 units) doses, whereas those who do not perform catheterization receive 100 to 200 units. This treatment is covered by insurance for the neurogenic overactive bladder patients (OAB). Repeat injections are generally needed between 12 and 15 months and can be repeated indefinitely (Smith and Wein, 2010).

Procedural Considerations. Coaptite and Macroplastique require no refrigeration. Patient skin testing is not required for either product. Botox is stored in the refrigerator. A urine culture and sensitivity is done approximately 10 days preoperatively. It is optimal to use a video system for the procedure. A basic cystoscopy set is required. The patient is usually positioned in the lithotomy position (Smith and Wein, 2010).

Operative Procedure

1. The surgeon instills urethral anesthetic and may supplement the anesthesia with a perineal block of 1% or 2% lidocaine. Cystoscopic examination is performed before the bulking agent is injected to rule out any associated findings. It is recommended that the irrigation be instilled by use of a pressure bag to minimize extravasation of the material by increasing the intraurethral pressure.
2. The surgeon introduces the injection needle provided by the manufacturer through the cystoscope and places the tip transurethrally, below the urethral mucosa, just distal to the bladder neck. Positioning of the needle tip is accomplished when the surgeon sees the indentation of the urethra by the tip while manipulating the needle.
3. Coaptite and Macroplastique are injected until the urothelium enlarges and meets in the midline, approximating the appearance of lateral lobe enlargement of the prostate. Botox is injected into 10 to 30 locations in the bladder including the trigone.

Transurethral Ureteropyeloscopy

Transurethral ureteropyeloscopy is an endoscopic examination of the ureters and renal pelvis. The use of rigid or flexible ureteroscopes or ureteropyeloscopes provides the opportunity to diagnose filling defects in the ureter and renal pelvis, congenital anomalies (Figure 15-13), hematuria, ureteral obstruction, and damage from trauma. Manipulation, fragmentation, basketing of ureteral and renal calculi, and retrieval of foreign bodies are possible with transurethral ureteropyeloscopy. Extracorporeal shock-wave lithotripsy (ESWL), electrohydraulic lithotripsy (EHL), sonic lithotripsy, or laser lithotripsy may accompany the procedure. It may also be used to manage residual sludge after these treatments.

Ureteral strictures may be treated transurethrally, and biopsies of tumors of the ureter and renal pelvis are performed under direct visualization. Internal ureteral stents may also be inserted for ureteral patency. These range in size from 3F to 8.5F and are available in single-J, double-J, and pigtail configurations.

FIGURE 15-13 Grade 5 bilateral ureteral reflux.

FIGURE 15-14 Flexible ureteropyeloscope and rigid ureteropyeloscope.

Procedural Considerations. The setup is similar to that for a cystoscopy with the addition of a rigid or flexible ureteroscope system (Figure 15-14). A critical factor in this procedure is allowing enough time for careful dilation of the ureter under C-arm fluoroscopy. The flexible ureteroscope has gained popularity because of its inherent tip mobility, which provides a more panoramic view of the entire circumference of the ureter. The perioperative nurse must be prepared to tilt the radiolucent operative bed at head and foot and laterally, as well as raise the bed.

In addition to the standard cystoscopy setup, the following items should be available: a rigid or flexible ureteroscope, ureteral dilators of graduated sizes and styles, size 3F to 5F ureteral stone baskets of various styles, a ureteral grasping forceps, biopsy forceps, snare, scissors, catheters of various styles and sizes, stents, guidewires, balloon dilators, and radiographic contrast material. Patient allergies should be checked before the use of radiographic contrast material.

Operative Procedure

1. The surgeon inserts the ureteropyeloscope and accesses the ureter with a guidewire under fluoroscopic control. The ureter is irrigated as the guidewire is advanced. The scrub person assists by maintaining slight tension on the wire.
2. An additional working guidewire is placed by the surgeon to be used as a safety wire.
3. The surgeon passes the ureteroscope over the working guidewire, biopsies any suspicious lesions, and performs diagnostic pyeloscopy and ureteroscopy. The characteristics of calculi are observed to determine the best treatment approach. Urine may be obtained for cytologic and microbiologic examination. If a calculus is small enough to be delivered through the ureter, the surgeon engages it in a retrieval basket and removes it under visual as well as fluoroscopic control. If, after ureteral dilation, the calculus does not appear to be small enough for delivery, lithotripsy (fragmentation) is performed through the ureteroscope, or ESWL may be performed later. Lithotripsy may be performed with ultrasonic (through a rigid ureteroscope) or electrohydraulic lithotripters or with the tunable pulse-dyed or holmium:yttrium-aluminum-garnet (Ho:YAG) lasers. Appropriate laser precautions must be enforced. Chapter 8 discusses laser safety issues in more depth.
4. The surgeon assesses the ureter for integrity (perforation or laceration) with retrograde pyelography.
5. A ureteral stent is placed over the remaining safety guidewire, and the guidewire is removed.

Surgery of the Penis and the Urethra

Laser Ablation of Condylomata and Penile Carcinoma

Laser ablation of condylomata or penile cancer is the eradication of diseased tissue by means of a laser beam. Laser therapy has been determined to be effective for condylomata and penile cancers that are refractory to other treatments. One of the major advantages of the laser is that heat is distributed evenly to the tissue underlying the lesion. When any laser is being used, precautions appropriate to that system must be initiated (see Chapter 8).

Procedural Considerations. Laser treatment may be performed successfully with local infiltration of an anesthetic. A U-shaped, crater-like lesion of predetermined depth with a 2-mm radius can be created. A power setting ranging from 2 to 20 watts on continuous or super-pulse mode is commonly used. With laser ablation, less edema and necrosis occur, fibrosis is minimized, and rapid healing is facilitated. The argon, CO_2, potassium-titanyl-phosphate (KTP), and neodymium (Nd):YAG lasers are all suitable for this therapeutic application.

Operative Procedure

1. The surgeon moves the beam transversely across the tissue and then in a crosshatch matrix, thereby treating all perimeters of the lesion. Throughout the procedure the surgeon wipes the area with acetic acid (5% vinegar), which results in greater visualization of the diseased tissue and allows therapy to deeper layers.
2. At the end of the procedure the wound is coated with an antibiotic ointment and left uncovered.

FIGURE 15-15 Circumcision.

Circumcision

Circumcision is the excision of the foreskin (prepuce) of the glans penis. Circumcision in adult males is performed for the relief of phimosis, a condition in which the orifice of the prepuce is stenosed or too narrow to permit easy retraction behind the glans. Another condition that may require circumcision is balanoposthitis, an inflamed glans and mucous membrane with purulent discharge. Circumcision may also be performed to prevent recurrent paraphimosis, a condition in which the prepuce cannot be reduced easily from a retracted position. (See Chapter 26 for pediatric considerations during circumcision.)

Procedural Considerations. The perioperative nurse assists in positioning the patient in the supine position. A plastic or minor instrument set and a local anesthetic with IV sedation are sufficient. An ESU should be available.

Operative Procedure

1. The surgeon clamps the prepuce in the dorsal midline and incises it toward the coronal margin (Figure 15-15, *A*), leaving about 5 cm of coronal mucosa intact. If the prepuce is adherent, a probe or hemostat may be used to break up adhesions.
2. A similar procedure is performed ventrally. The two incisions are then joined circumferentially. Alternatively, a superficial circumferential incision is made in the skin with a scalpel at the level of the coronal sulcus and the mucosa at the base of the glans.
3. The surgeon undermines redundant skin between the circumferential incisions and removes it as a complete cuff (see Figure 15-15, *B*).
4. Bleeding vessels are coagulated or clamped with mosquito hemostats and ligated with fine absorbable ligatures.
5. The surgeon approximates the raw edges of the skin incision to a coronal cuff of mucosal prepuce, generally with 4-0 or 5-0 absorbable sutures on atraumatic, plastic cutting, or fine gastrointestinal (GI) needles (see Figure 15-15, *C*).
6. The wound is dressed with petrolatum gauze.

Excision of Urethral Caruncle

A urethral caruncle is a benign lesion or inflammatory prolapse of the external urinary meatus in the female. Excision entails the removal of these papillary or sessile tumors from the urethra.

Procedural Considerations. The perioperative nurse assists with placing the patient in the lithotomy position. A minor or plastic set, an ESU, and a local anesthetic are used. A urethral catheter of an appropriate size may be required if the distal urethral prolapse is severe.

Operative Procedure

1. The surgeon uses a small, fine-tipped Metzenbaum or plastic scissors to expose the tumor and excise it within a wedge of ventral urethral tissue.
2. Figure-of-eight 4-0 absorbable sutures are placed at the edge of the incision to achieve hemostasis.

Urethral Meatotomy

Urethral meatotomy is an incisional enlargement of the external urethral meatus to relieve congenital or acquired stenosis or stricture at the external meatus.

Procedural Considerations. A male patient is placed in the supine position. Female patients are placed in the lithotomy position. Prepping and draping are as described for urethral catheterization. The surgeon administers local anesthesia. A plastic instrument set is required.

Operative Procedure

1. The surgeon places a straight hemostat on the ventral surface of the meatus.
2. An incision is made along the frenulum to enlarge the opening and overcome the stricture.
3. Hemostasis is obtained by clamping the bleeding vessels and ligating them with fine absorbable sutures.
4. The surgeon sutures the mucosal layer to the skin with fine absorbable sutures.
5. A dressing of petrolatum gauze is applied.

Urethral Dilation and Internal Urethrotomy

Urethral dilation and internal urethrotomy are performed to provide relief of distal lower urinary tract obstruction. Urethral strictures or narrowing of the urethra may be caused by a congenital malformation that is usually found at the external urinary meatus. Infection or trauma may also contribute to stricture of the membranous and pendulous urethra. Urethral stricture disease may be treated by periodic and gradual dilation or internal urethrotomy.

Procedural Considerations. The perioperative nurse assists with placing the male patient in the supine position for routine urethral dilation and in the lithotomy position for other procedures. The female patient is placed in the lithotomy position. Prepping and draping are conducted as appropriate to the patient's position and gender. The surgeon administers a local anesthetic either (1) by placing cotton-tipped applicators, which have been dipped into viscous 2% lidocaine (Xylocaine), into the urethral opening or (2) by using a urethral syringe to instill the lidocaine. Female urethral dilation is performed with short, straight metal dilators or with hollow McCarthy dilators. The latter allow a urine specimen to be obtained.

In addition to a cystoscopy setup, required instrumentation includes urethrotomes; the resectoscope working element with sheath, obturator, and cold knives; urethral dilators; Phillips filiforms and followers; Van Buren sounds; and a silicone Foley catheter. Before use, the filiforms and followers should be carefully inspected for damaged or weak points, particularly around the scored-threaded end.

Operative Procedure
Gradual Dilation

1. In a male patient the surgeon lubricates and anesthetizes the urethra with a viscous anesthetic that is instilled into the urethra with a urethral or Uro-Jet syringe. A penile clamp occludes the penile urethra at the coronal sulcus and keeps the anesthetic within the urethra.
2. Phillips filiforms of various tips and sizes are introduced first in an attempt to pass an instrument beyond the urethral stricture. Followers of increasing size are connected to the filiforms and passed through the strictured portion of the urethra, stretching the scarred area (Figure 15-16, *A*).
3. Slow dilation is also achieved with a small catheter or follower left in the urethra. It leads to softening of the stricture over the course of several days.

Internal Urethrotomy

1. The surgeon inserts the assembled visualizing urethrotome into the urethra.

FIGURE 15-16 A, Method of using coudé-tipped bougie for passing stricture. **B,** Variety of urethral sounds (dilators).

2. When necessary, the surgeon feeds a filiform or ureteral catheter into the catheterizing channel to help identify the patent portion of the urethra.

3. The surgeon advances the urethrotome to the desired position, and incises the urethral scar with the blade. The normal urethra is incised 1 cm proximally and distally beyond the stricture to achieve optimum results.

4. A silicone Foley catheter is inserted and left in place for 3 to 5 days after surgery.

Urethroplasty

Urethroplasty is reconstructive surgery of the urethra for strictures, urethral fractures, or narrowed segments of the urethral lumen that are congenital, inflammatory, or traumatic in origin. Urethral grafts are generally required and may include free skin grafts and mobilized vascular flaps. There are many combinations of these procedures, and in all of them some type of temporary urinary diversion may be used, depending on the location and severity of the condition.

Typically the patient complains of obstructive symptoms, frequently associated with a UTI. Techniques used to determine diagnosis include urodynamics (voiding pressures above and below the site of obstruction), urinary flow cytometry, IVU to rule out an upper tract lesion, cystoscopy, and urethrography. The length and density of the diseased urethra are determined to plan the appropriate reconstructive procedure. Any associated UTI must be treated and eradicated before surgical intervention. Definitive repair should not be done for 10 to 12 weeks after use of diagnostic instrumentation to allow the inflammatory reaction to subside.

Procedural Considerations The patient is placed in the exaggerated lithotomy position by the perioperative nurse and one other person. Routine prepping and draping procedures are used with precautions for isolating the anus (e.g., the use of an impervious plastic adherent drape). The setup includes a minor instrument set with fine plastic instruments for dissection and plastic repair. Strictures may be located deep, requiring fiberoptic lighting. An ESU may be required.

Operative Procedure

Johanson Urethroplasty. The Johanson urethroplasty is a two-stage procedure to repair and reconstruct the male urethra for severe urethral stricture disease. Approximately 3 months after completion of the first stage, if the operative site is healing and the patient is voiding adequately, a second-stage procedure is performed. Vascularized flaps of preputial or penile skin may be mobilized to the ventrum by leaving them attached to the outer surface of the prepuce or as an island flap. One modification is the transverse preputial island flap neourethra with glans channel positioning for the meatus. Preputial skin is preferred because of its rich reliable blood supply and non–hair-bearing characteristics.

First Stage

1. The surgeon makes an inverted U incision in the perineum from the inner borders of the ischial tuberosities up to and including the base of the scrotum.

2. A Van Buren sound is passed into the urethra up to the stricture (see Figure 15-16, *B*). The bulbocavernosus muscle is dissected and retracted laterally.

3. The surgeon makes an incision in the urethra over the strictured area and extends it in each direction at least 1 cm beyond the diseased area. The abnormal scar tissue is excised or simply incised, because scrotal skin ultimately increases the lumen.

4. A 28F sound is passed through both the proximal and the distal urethral lumens to rule out further stricture.

5. The surgeon sutures the remaining urethral mucosa to the scrotal skin with 4-0 absorbable sutures.

6. A cystotomy tube to divert the urinary stream may be left indwelling and removed in 5 to 7 days.

Second Stage (Mobilized Vascular Flap)

1. A red rubber catheter is temporarily inserted into the bladder through the proximal urethral stoma.

2. The surgeon incises the penoscrotal skin longitudinally, adjacent to the urethra.

3. A new urethra is constructed by developing the ventral preputial skin that is dissected free and fanned out. The rectangle of skin is rolled into the neourethra and measured.

4. A channel is sharply created on the ventral aspect of the glans, in a plane just above the corpora.

5. The surgeon removes the glans tissue, forming a groove approximately 14F in diameter.

6. Layers of subcutaneous tissue are dissected free from the dorsal penile skin to create an island flap that is spiraled to the ventrum. The surgeon brings the flaps together in the midline and closes with a continuous or interrupted 4-0 absorbable suture.

7. The neourethra is anastomosed proximally to the urethra and carried to the tip of the glans.

8. The dorsal penile flaps are transposed laterally to the midline, and the surgeon excises the excess skin.

9. The surgeon closes with 4-0 absorbable interrupted mattress sutures around the glans and down the penile shaft. A bulky pressure dressing is applied.

10. Suprapubic cystostomy drainage is an option, but a urethral catheter usually suffices.

Horton-Devine Urethroplasty (Urethral Patch Graft). Urethral patch graft is a one-stage operative procedure that incorporates a free skin graft to correct a urethral stricture. Free skin grafts should be at full thickness. Because the free graft must be revascularized, it is important that it have a perfect skin cover of well-vascularized dorsal, preputial, penile skin.

1. The surgeon passes a 17F panendoscope into the posterior urethra, and then passes a 20F urethral dilator into the posterior urethra.

2. A perineal vertical midline incision is made into the urethral lumen. The surgeon reinserts the panendoscope and examines the incision to determine if it crosses the stricture.

3. The defect is measured, and the surgeon makes a circumferential incision on the posterior penile shaft to harvest an oval piece of skin the size of the defect.

4. The epidermal side of the graft is defatted, and 4-0 absorbable sutures are placed at the apex and base.

5. The surgeon sutures the apex into position at the proximal and distal ends of the stricture with the epidermal side toward the urethral lumen.

6. The graft is anastomosed proximally to the urethra with the suture line of the graft next to the corpus. The middle glans dart is fixed to the corpus. The graft is formed into a neourethra over a Silastic stenting catheter.

7. The surgeon reinserts the panendoscope and irrigates the urethra to check for suture-line leaks.

8. A Foley or fenestrated catheter is inserted to serve as a stent.

9. The surgeon approximates and closes the corpus spongiosum over the patched area as a separate layer with interrupted 3-0

absorbable sutures. Subcutaneous 4-0 absorbable sutures are placed.

10. The skin and the graft site are closed with interrupted 4-0 sutures.

11. A suprapubic catheter is inserted to divert urine for healing. Petrolatum gauze is wrapped around the penis and covered with gauze sponges and fluffed dressings. A scrotal support is applied to provide support and pressure.

Penectomy

Penectomy is the partial or total removal of a cancerous penis. The procedure selected depends on the extent of involvement and disease stage. Invasive penile cancer not suited for irradiation because of its size, depth, or location is best dealt with by penectomy. Excision of a 2-cm gross tumor margin is adequate for local management. Partial penectomy may afford a sufficient length for directable and upright urination. At least 3 cm of viable proximal shaft is necessary for consideration of a partial penectomy. If the residual stump is inadequate in length, detachment and mobilization of the suspensory ligaments may be an option in selected patients. A total penectomy is generally required when tumor margins are beyond a 2-cm retrievable length from the penoscrotal junction.

Options are available to limit the extent of the disfiguring surgery used in the past for penile cancer. Chemotherapy agents, often combined with irradiation, are proving effective in shrinking penile carcinomas that would have previously mandated radical penectomy.

Reconstruction is possible after penectomy. Evaluation must take into account sexual, urinary, and cosmetic factors. Extensive or proximally invasive lesions that include the scrotum, perineum, abdominal wall, and pubis necessitate emasculation as well as expanded resection of involved tissues.

Procedural Considerations. The setup necessary is similar to that for any inguinal surgery, with the addition of a medium Penrose drain for use as a tourniquet.

Operative Procedure
Partial Penectomy

1. The lesion is excluded by a towel attached to the planned amputation line. The surgeon applies a penile tourniquet at the base of the penis (Figure 15-17, *A*).

2. After circumferential skin incision, the surgeon divides the cavernous bodies to the urethra with a 2-cm gross margin (see Figure 15-17, *B*).

3. Dorsal vessels are ligated, margins of the tunica albuginea are approximated, and the urethra is dissected proximally and distally (spatulated) to obtain a 1-cm redundant flap (see Figure 15-17, *C*).

4. Without sacrificing the tumor margin, the surgeon divides the urethra. Interrupted sutures are placed on the opposite margins of the tunica albuginea to secure the corpora. The tourniquet is removed, and hemostasis is achieved.

5. After the dorsal urethrotomy, a skin-to-urethra anastomosis is performed. The redundant skin flap is then dorsally approximated (see Figure 15-17, *D*).

6. A small urinary catheter is inserted, and a nonadherent dressing is applied.

Total Penectomy

1. A vertical elliptic incision is made around the penile base (Figure 15-18, *A*).

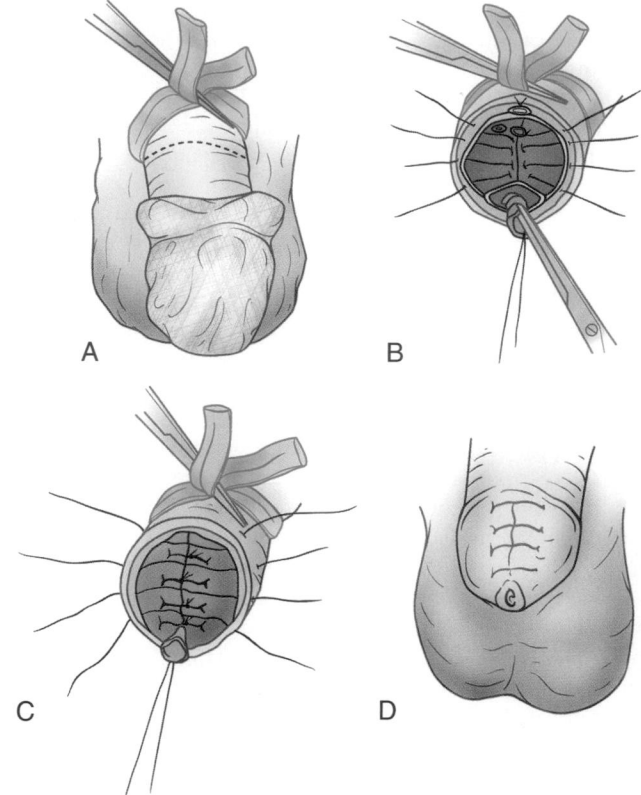

FIGURE 15-17 Partial penectomy.

2. The distal urethra and its ventral traction are divided through an incision in Buck fascia, mobilizing the urethra and aiding its dissection, which extends from the corpora to the bulbar region.

3. The surgeon separates and ligates the corpora (see Figure 15-18, *B*). The suspensory ligaments and dorsal vessels are divided as corporal dissection is carried out.

4. The urethra is transected from the corpora (see Figure 15-18, *C*).

5. An ellipse of skin approximately 1 cm in size is taken from the perineal area. A tunnel is fashioned in the perineal subcutaneous layer of tissue. A traction suture through the tunnel, at the penile base, aids dissection for transposition of the urethra to the perineum (see Figure 15-18, *D*).

6. The surgeon grasps the urethra with forceps and transfers it to the perineum. The urethra is spatulated, and a skin-to-urethra anastomosis is performed through a buttonhole incision in the perineum (see Figure 15-18, *E*).

7. The primary incision is closed horizontally, elevating the scrotum away from the urethral opening (see Figure 15-18, *F*).

8. An indwelling urinary catheter is inserted, and the wound is covered with a nonadherent dressing.

Penile Implant

A penile prosthesis is implanted for treatment of organic sexual impotence. Sexual impotence may be caused by (1) diabetes mellitus, (2) priapism, (3) Peyronie disease, (4) penile trauma, (5) pelvic surgery, (6) neurologic disease (in selected cases), (7) vascular disease, (8) hypertension, and (9) idiopathic impotence. The penile implant serves as a stent to enable vaginal penetration for sexual intercourse. Penile implants are available as malleable one-piece

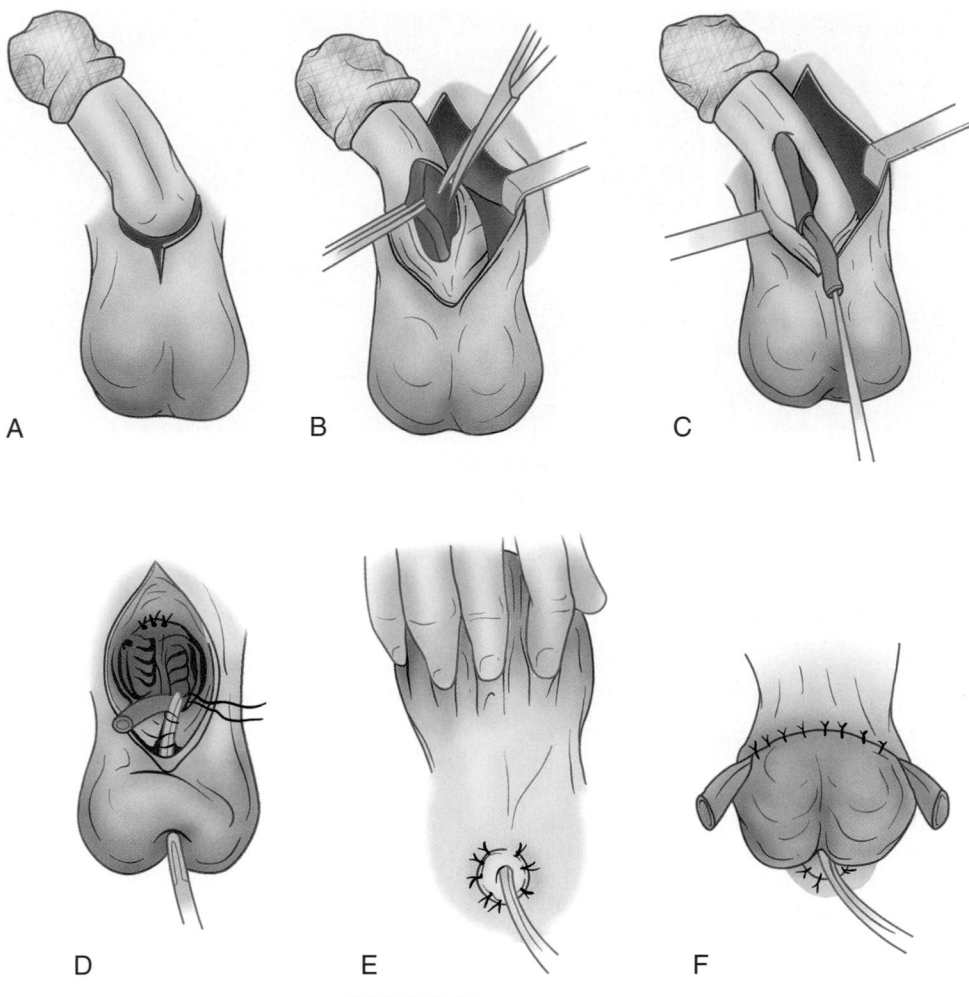

FIGURE 15-18 Total penectomy.

devices, self-contained inflatable devices, and two- and three-piece devices. The procedure described for the inflatable penile implant is for the three-piece device.

Procedural Considerations. The anesthesia provider administers either a spinal or a general anesthetic. The perioperative nurse assists with positioning the patient in either the supine or the lithotomy position, as directed by the surgeon. A 5- to 10-minute skin prep is usually performed before draping is carried out. To prevent urethral injury and potential urinary retention, the surgeon may insert a 14F or 16F Foley catheter to identify the urethra intraoperatively. The ESU may be required. The surgeon may inject a local anesthetic of 0.5% plain bupivacaine (Marcaine) or 1% etidocaine (Duranest) at the beginning of the procedure into the incisional sites. Often a penile block, composed of 0.9% saline (150 mL), 1% plain lidocaine (50 mL), and 30 mg/mL papaverine (2 mL), is instilled intraoperatively before the incision into the corpus cavernosum. This enables the surgeon to evaluate erectile size and provides some postoperative pain management.

The scrub person sets up a separate sterile Mayo stand or small table covered with a plastic drape for the implants. It is recommended that the implants not be in contact with paper or cloth that may shed fiber particles.

The instrument setup includes a minor set with fine instruments, plus Hegar dilators, the penile prosthesis of choice (Figure 15-19), the Furlow inserter, the closing tool, the assembly tool for clamping connectors (Figure 15-20, *A*), and the connectors of choice (see Figure 15-20, *B*). Medications needed in the operative field include 50 mL of 1% lidocaine, 150 mL of injectable 0.9% normal saline, 1 mL of methylene blue (optional by surgeon preference), 2 mL of papaverine, 50 mL of 0.5% bupivacaine or 1% etidocaine, 50,000 units of bacitracin, and 80 mg of kanamycin. Medication safety practices must be implemented for all medications on the sterile field.

A serious risk with a penile implant is infection. Infection rates for first-time implantation are low at 1%, but the rate can rise to as high as 18% with reimplantation procedures. Because of the high risk of infection, models that have been irradiated and embedded with minocycline hydrochloride and rifampin (InhibiZone) are now available (American Medical Systems [AMS], 2009). The sterile team should be double-gloved throughout the procedure. A 5-minute antimicrobial prep of the operative area is critical in reducing skin flora. The anus should be isolated in the perineal approach. Intraoperatively and before insertion of the implant components, a prophylactic antibiotic irrigant of bacitracin and kanamycin in normal saline is used on the implants without rifampin

FIGURE 15-19 A, AMS malleable 650 penile prosthesis. **B,** AMS Ambicor inflatable two-piece penile prosthesis. **C,** AMS tactile inflatable penile prosthesis, three-piece with rifampin (Inhibizone).

FIGURE 15-20 A, *Top to bottom,* Closing tool, Furlow inserter, assembly tool, tubing passer. **B,** Quik-connectors.

and in the insertion sites. Systemic antibiotics may also be required. As with any implant procedure, it is vital to maintain an environment conducive to infection prevention. The perioperative nurse ensures that traffic in and out of the OR is minimized.

It is recommended that the implants with rifampin not be soaked in any solution before implantation because this may cause the antibiotic component to disintegrate. The area to be implanted may be irrigated with antibiotic solution, and the implant itself may be dipped in a sterile solution of 0.9% normal saline to assist with insertion if desired. Prophylactic antibiotic protocols remain the same.

Operative Procedure
Implantation of Noninflatable (Semirigid) Prosthesis

1. The surgeon inserts a 14F or 16F Foley catheter and attaches it to a drainage collection device to be maintained within the sterile field. The amount and color of urine are noted. The catheter is left in place intraoperatively to assist in identifying the urethra.

2. A midline incision is made from the base of the penis into the scrotum for approximately 3 cm. Some surgeons may choose a suprapubic or dorsal penile approach.

3. The surgeon incises the tunica albuginea over the most proximal portion of the corpora in a longitudinal manner, and places stay sutures.

4. The corpora are dilated proximally and distally with 7- to 14-mm Hegar dilators, depending on the diameter of the implant chosen. The corpora are dilated to 1 mm more than the implant size. Care is taken to not perforate the urethra.

5. The surgeon measures the corporal length with a Furlow inserter or sizing instrument.

6. After placement of the closure sutures, the surgeon inserts the prosthesis into the corpora. Proper placement is evident immediately by a change in the configuration of the penis with no buckling of the glans.

7. The surgeon closes the tunica albuginea using the previously placed 2-0 absorbable continuous suture; 3-0 or 4-0 absorbable interrupted sutures are used for skin closure.

8. Petrolatum gauze or 2-inch Kling tube gauze may be used for the dressing.

Implantation of Inflatable Prosthesis

1. The surgeon inserts a 14F or 16F Foley catheter and attaches it to a drainage collection device to be maintained within the sterile field. The amount and color of urine are noted. The catheter is left in place intraoperatively to assist in identifying the urethra.

2. A 3-cm long suprapubic incision is made.

3. The surgeon incises the tunica albuginea of each corpus in the most proximal portion, and places stay sutures.

4. The corpora are dilated distally and proximally with 7- to 14-mm Hegar dilators. Dilation should be 1 mm more than the diameter of the chosen implant. The 700CX implant is 12 mm at its widest point. When this is used, the dilation at the distal end should be 13 mm. The proximal end, however, should be 14 mm to accommodate the input tubing.

5. The surgeon measures the corporal length with the Furlow inserter.

6. Corporal sutures of 2-0 absorbable material are placed along the tunica incision and tagged. Some surgeons prefer to place these sutures last and use the closing tool to prevent puncture of the cylinders.

7. The cylinders are packaged with attached traction sutures of 4-0 braided polyester at the distal end. The surgeon places the suture through the eye of a 2½-inch Keith needle, and slides the needle into the groove of the Furlow inserter.

8. The surgeon guides the Furlow inserter along the corporal tunnel, and pushes the plunger to release the Keith needle, which punctures the glans.

9. The Keith needle is grasped with a heavy hemostat and pulled through the glans, allowing the cylinders to slide to the channel opening. The surgeon removes the Furlow inserter, inserts the cylinder, and guides it to its proper position beneath the glans penis.

10. If necessary, rear tip extenders are added to the proximal end of the cylinder. The proximal end is positioned in the crus.

11. The procedure is repeated on the other side.

12. The surgeon palpates the external inguinal ring and uses blunt dissection to create a path. Dissecting scissors are used to separate the transversalis fascia on the inguinal floor. If the Ambicor implant with self-contained reservoir is being placed, steps 12 through 14 are eliminated.

13. The perivesical space is enlarged to allow palpation of the Cooper ligament. The reservoir is then positioned into the perivesical space.

14. The surgeon fills the reservoir with 65 or 100 mL of saline solution (depending on the reservoir size selected) and pulls it against the floor of Hesselbach triangle.

15. The pump is then placed into the most dependent portion of the scrotum. It is generally positioned on the patient's dominant side. The space is created by blunt dissection lateral to the testicle.

16. The rods and reservoir tubings are connected to the pump with the connectors of choice, using the assembly tool to clamp them in place, and tested for inflation and deflation.

17. The surgeon closes the tunica of the scrotum over the pump with a running stitch of 3-0 absorbable suture.

18. The prosthetic device is left in a partially inflated position to reduce bleeding and promote healing for 24 hours postoperatively (Figures 15-21 and 15-22). (After 24 hours the implants are deflated for the remainder of the "healing phase" so the reservoir pocket heals with the reservoir in "full position" to prevent autoinflation.)

19. The surgeon closes the incision with 4-0 absorbable suture in a running subcuticular stitch, and a dressing is applied.

20. The penis is positioned flush with the lower abdomen for patient comfort. Mesh underpants are useful as a nonadherent support dressing. An ice pack may be applied to reduce swelling.

21. The Foley catheter is left in place during the immediate 24-hour postoperative period and then usually removed.

Deep Dorsal and Emissary Vein Ligation

Undertaken for vascular compromise–related impotence, this procedure entails the ligation or elimination of the penile deep dorsal vein and its tributaries. Care is taken to avoid damage to the arteries and nerves lying alongside the deep dorsal vein. A common cause of erectile dysfunction in patients with organic impotence is vascular compromise. Before surgical intervention is undertaken, a definitive diagnosis of a corporal leak is made through dynamic infusion cavernosometry and cavernosography. Diagnostic results may indicate failure-to-store or failure-to-fill impotence. Patients with vascular compromise in a given anatomic region tend to be compromised elsewhere as well. Many have diabetes or hypertension. Because of this the perioperative nurse must exercise great care in positioning the patient to prevent further damage to the patient's altered tissue perfusion. The cavernous and crural veins are suture-ligated. All circumflex and emissary branches are ligated or coagulated. The suspensory ligament is detached, and the entire deep and accessory dorsal vein is removed.

Revascularization of the Penile Arteries

The relationship of focal arterial occlusive disease to sexual dysfunction has prompted efforts to rectify the resulting impotence. Reconstructive surgery has been attempted in patients who demonstrate correctable vascular disease in the large arteries. The most widely attempted repairs are end-to-end and end-to-side microscopic anastomoses of the distal inferior epigastric artery to the proximal deep dorsal artery near the pubic level, below the rectus muscle and Buck fascia. Paramedian and infrapubic incisions are made, and the arteries are freed and tunneled. This procedure requires both urologic and vascular surgeons.

Surgery of the Scrotum and Testicles

Hydrocelectomy

A hydrocele is an abnormal accumulation of fluid within the scrotum. The fluid is contained within the tunica vaginalis. Excessive secretion or accumulation of hydrocele fluid may be the result of infection or trauma. A hydrocelectomy is the excision of the tunica vaginalis of the testis to remove the enlarged, fluid-filled sac.

Procedural Considerations. The patient is placed in the supine position. Prepping and draping of the patient include routine cleansing of the external genitalia and draping with a fenestrated sheet. A minor instrument set is required, plus a small drain; a 30-mL syringe with a 20-gauge, 2-inch aspirating needle; and a suspensory dressing.

Operative Procedure

1. The surgeon administers a local anesthetic into the cord at the base of the scrotum with 10 to 15 mL of plain 1% lidocaine.

2. An anterolateral incision is made in the stretched skin of the scrotum over the hydrocele mass with a #10 or #15 blade.

3. Bleeding is controlled with Crile hemostats, the ESU, or vessel ligation with 3-0 absorbable ligatures. Stretching the skin of the scrotum compresses the scrotal vessels.

4. An incision is then made between the blood vessels. The fascial layers are incised to expose the tunica vaginalis.

5. The surgeon uses sharp and blunt dissection to free the hydrocele.

6. The sac is opened, and clamps are placed on each side incorporating the tissue adjacent to the tunica vaginalis and the skin.

7. Using Martius clamps, the surgeon everts the incised edges. The tension placed by the Martius clamp compresses the incised edge, controls bleeding, and prevents dissection between the tissue layers.

8. A pouch is created by dissecting between the tunica vaginalis and the dartos layer. Scrotal pressure is released. This pouch will hold the testis after the repair.

9. The surgeon opens the tunica vaginalis and evacuates the fluid contents.

10. The testis is lifted, and the sac is inverted so that it surrounds the testicular attachments and epididymis.

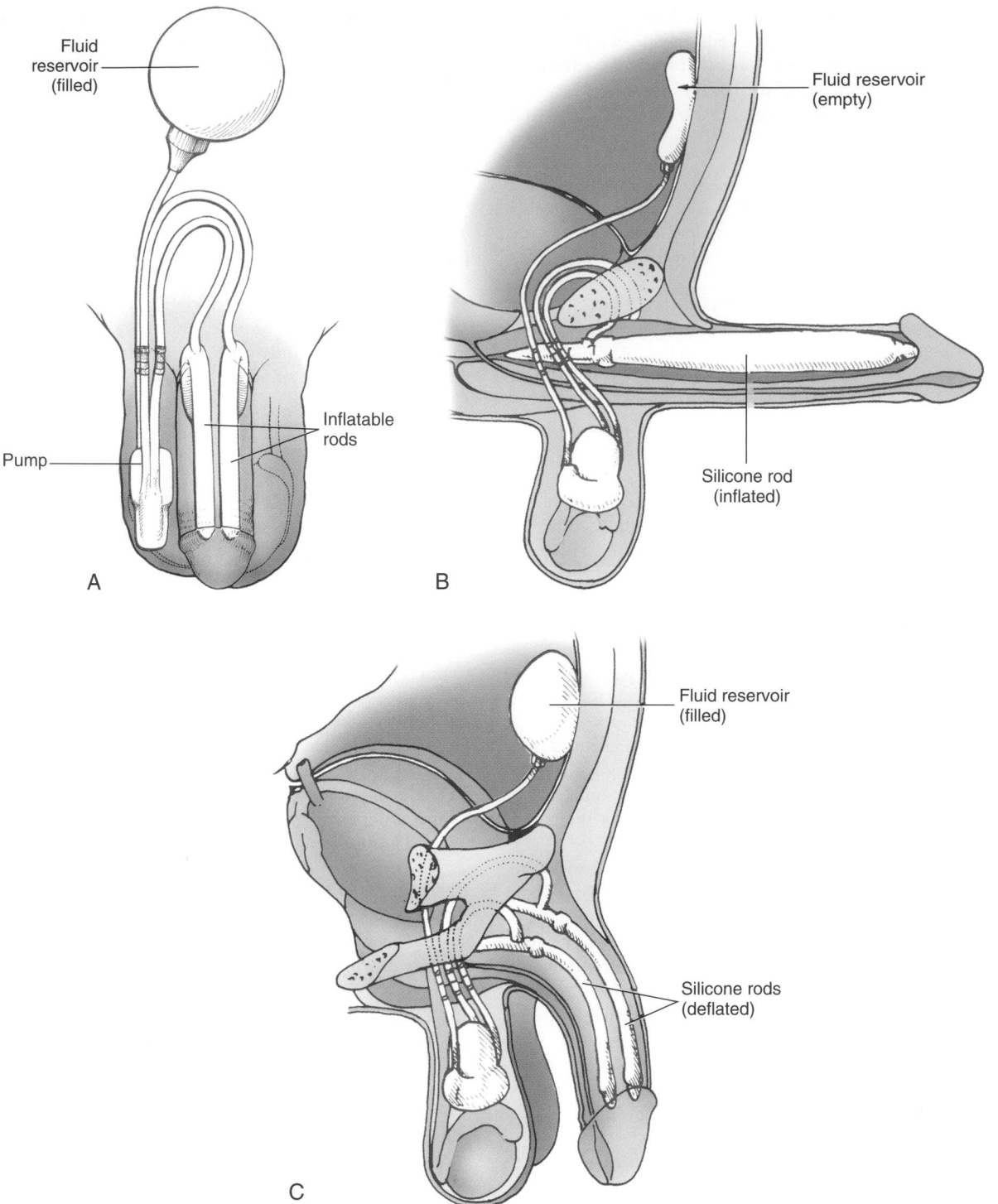

FIGURE 15-21 AMS inflatable 700CX penile prosthesis. **A,** Frontal view. **B,** Sagittal view—penis in erect position. **C,** Sagittal view—penis in flaccid position.

11. Excess tunica vaginalis may be excised. The surgeon sutures the tunica edges along the peritoneal surface with 3-0 absorbable suture in an interrupted fashion to the juncture of the testis. Six to eight sutures are placed around the circumference of the testis (Figure 15-23). Some surgeons elect to sew the sac behind the spermatic cord in an interrupted fashion, and others may choose a continuous radial stitch around the posterior testis and epididymis.

12. The testis is replaced into the scrotum.
13. A drain may be placed into the scrotum and exteriorized through a stab wound in its most dependent portion. The drain is loosely sutured to the external scrotal wall to prevent migration.
14. The surgeon closes the scrotal incision with 3-0 absorbable sutures in a full-thickness continuous manner or in layers with 3-0 and 4-0 continuous absorbable sutures.

FIGURE 15-22 AMS Ambicor inflatable two-piece implant, sagittal view.

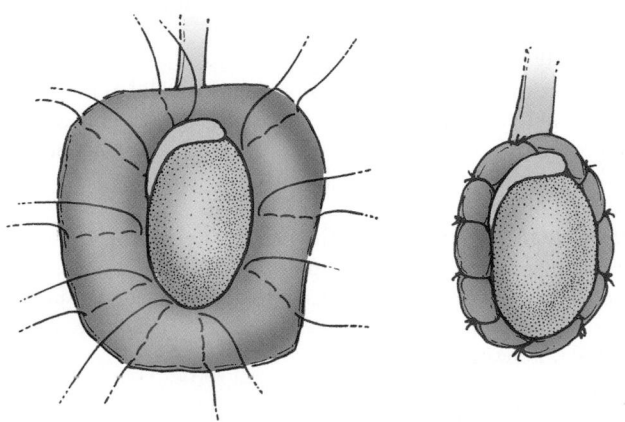

FIGURE 15-23 Hydrocelectomy.

15. A fluff compression dressing contained in a scrotal support or mesh underpants aids in reducing postoperative scrotal edema.

Vasectomy

A vasectomy is the excision of a section of the vas deferens. The operation is usually performed selectively as a permanent method of sterilization. Because of the serious implications of permanent sterilization, particular attention must be paid to acquiring informed consent. Although studies have raised the question of a correlation between prostate cancer and vasectomy, a definitive causal relationship has not been established.

The patient having elective sterilization for birth control is encouraged to return to the office setting for sperm-count analysis. Generally two successive negative counts are sufficient to indicate that sterility has been achieved. Elective vasectomies are frequently performed in the office setting.

Procedural Considerations. The patient usually lies in the supine position. A local anesthetic is used. A minor instrument set and scrotal support are needed.

Operative Procedure

No-Scalpel Approach. The no-scalpel technique was devised in China and has five fundamental principles:

1. Fixation of the vas deferens without entering the scrotal skin
2. Performance under direct vision to prevent damage from blind sharp scrotal penetration
3. Simplified instrumentation
4. Decreased operative time by simplification of the procedure
5. Elimination of an incision or use of a scalpel

The procedure is as follows:

1. The right vas deferens is fixed under the scrotal skin with three fingers.
2. Using a syringe with 1% or 2% plain lidocaine and a small needle, the surgeon raises a small wheal in the median raphe of the scrotum. The needle is advanced along the vas toward the external inguinal ring. Additional lidocaine is injected into the perivasal region.
3. The procedure is repeated on the left side. Pressure is applied to the wheal site to minimize edema.
4. Once adequate anesthesia is accomplished, the right vas is again fixed with three fingers.
5. The surgeon applies a vas ring clamp over the scrotal skin, encircling the vas. Lifting the clamp upward, the skin over the vas is stretched as thin as possible, leaving minimal tissue between the vas and the clamp.
6. The ring clamp is locked in place, and the scrotal skin cephalad to the clamp is stretched with an index finger.
7. The surgeon punctures the skin directly into the vas deferens with the inner prong of the pointed dissecting hemostat. Both prongs of the dissecting hemostat are placed into the puncture site and spread directly on top of the vas.
8. When the surface of the vas is visualized, one prong is used to penetrate the vas itself. The vas is brought out of the wound by twisting the hemostat 180 degrees.
9. The ring clamp is moved to directly encircle the vasal tissue. The vas may then be divided and occluded by intraluminal electrocoagulation, clips, or suture ligation. Fascia should be placed between the severed ends of the vas.
10. The surgeon repeats the procedure on the left side. It is usually possible to place the ring clamp around the left vas through the initial entry site. Sutures are not necessary.
11. After ensuring that there is no bleeding, antibiotic ointment, pressure dressings, and a scrotal support are applied.

Vasovasostomy

Vasovasostomy is the surgical reanastomosis of the vas deferens, generally with the goal of restoring male fertility after vasectomy. Reanastomosis may often alleviate chronic testicular pain, a not infrequent complication after vasectomy. A precise reconnection can be performed with the use of a microscope and a modified two-layer anastomosis. Success rates vary, but in general, patency can be demonstrated by the presence of sperm in the semen within 4 weeks after vasovasostomy (Lipshultz et al, 2007). When there are no longer two viable segments of vas deferens, a similar procedure, the epididymovasostomy, may be performed. This involves anastomosis of a vas deferens to a segment of the epididymis. Postoperative precautions include no lifting or ejaculation for a minimum of

2 weeks. The sperm count and viability of sperm are rechecked at 3- and 15-month intervals. If sperm are not present by 6 months, the operation is considered a failure (Lipshultz et al, 2007).

Procedural Considerations. A minor instrument set is required, with the addition of selected microsurgical instruments and sutures. The procedure is frequently done under monitored anesthesia care with local injection of 0.5% plain bupivacaine (Marcaine) and 1% lidocaine (Xylocaine) in a 50:50 ratio.

Operative Procedure

1. After the vas deferens has been located by external manipulation, the surgeon makes a vertical scrotal incision.
2. The testicle, epididymis, and vas are displaced from the scrotum. The vasectomy site is identified, and the scarred area is excised.
3. The surgeon trims the proximal end of the vas deferens until fluid is expressed. Fluid is collected on a glass slide and examined for the presence of live sperm. Surgery continues even if results for sperm are negative unless an epididymal obstruction exists.
4. The distal end of the vas is resected until a normal lumen is visible.
5. The distal and proximal lumens are then dilated.
6. The surgeon places the two portions of the vas in an approximator clip and inserts a piece of background material underneath to provide contrast and improve visibility. Six stitches of 10-0 nonabsorbable microsuture are placed in the inner layer. The proximal end is sutured through the serosa to the mucosa, and the distal end is sutured through the mucosa to the serosa (Figure 15-24).
7. A second layer of 8 to 10 stitches of 9-0 nonabsorbable suture is placed without penetrating the lumen of the vas.
8. The surgeon closes the incision in two layers with interrupted 3-0 and 4-0 absorbable sutures.
9. Gauze sponges and a scrotal support are placed on the patient to provide a pressure dressing.

Microscopic Epididymal Sperm Aspiration

Microscopic epididymal sperm aspiration (MESA) is a sperm retrieval technique used in men with a reproductive tract blockage (e.g., postvasectomy, congenital absence of the vas deferens). It requires the availability of an in vitro fertilization team so that the aspirated sperm may be immediately processed and used for the selected in vitro technique or frozen for later use. The procedure must be timed according to the partner's cycle of ovulation. Ova are aspirated as an office procedure just before MESA is performed.

MESA should be done using the micropipette technique. The surgeon inserts the tip of a 250- to 350-μm pipette into an epididymal tubule to retrieve sperm cells without contamination by red blood cells. After aspiration the fluid is given to the in vitro fertilization team to process the sperm cells. Processing involves washing debris from the cells, retrieving the most active cells from the sample, and removing any red blood cells, if possible. This is critical because red blood cells significantly interfere with sperm cell function.

After the sperm cells are aspirated, the surgeon closes the epididymal tubule using microscopic technique. If adequate numbers of sperm cells can be obtained from one testis, the other side may be aspirated to add to the sperm bank if this is desirable. It may be necessary to aspirate sperm cells from the rete testis (tubules between the testicles and the epididymal head that carry cells to the head of the epididymis) if sperm cells are not found in tubules closer to the vas deferens.

The sperm cells retrieved may be used for intracytoplasmic injection into the partner's egg (ICSI), the most successful of the in vitro techniques available. This technique is not as dependent on the quality of the sperm as earlier techniques of in vitro fertilization.

Epididymectomy

An epididymectomy is the excision of the epididymis from the testis. Epididymectomy is rarely performed, usually only as a last-choice treatment for degenerative cystic disease, chronic infection, and intractable pain of the epididymis.

Procedural Considerations. The perioperative nurse assists with positioning the patient in the supine position with his legs slightly abducted. The anesthesia provider administers a general, spinal, or regional anesthetic. Setup is as described for hydrocelectomy, plus an ESU, if desired.

Operative Procedure

1. The surgeon makes an anterolateral incision over the testis in the scrotum to expose the tunica vaginalis. The tunica is incised to expose the testis and overlying epididymis.
2. An incision is made along the superior head of the epididymis, which is then sharply dissected from the testis. A portion of the vas deferens may also be excised.
3. Bleeding is controlled with the ESU and absorbable ties.
4. The skin wound is closed with 4-0 absorbable sutures.
5. A small intrascrotal drain may be left in place for 24 to 48 hours.

Spermatocelectomy

Spermatocelectomy is removal of a spermatocele—a lobulated intra-scrotal cystic mass attached to the superior head of the epididymis. Spermatocele is usually caused by an obstruction of the tubular system that conveys the sperm and may be a late complication after vasectomy.

Procedural Considerations. The setup for a spermatocelectomy is as described for a hydrocelectomy, plus a microscope and slides, if desired.

FIGURE 15-24 The two portions of the vas in approximator clip with background material as the proximal end is sutured through the serosa to the mucosa with 10-0 nylon.

Operative Procedure
1. The mass is approached through a scrotal incision as described for hydrocelectomy.
2. The surgeon identifies the structures of the testis and spermatic cord and dissects the cystic structure free.
3. Bleeding is controlled with the ESU.
4. The wound is closed and dressed as described for hydrocelectomy.

Varicocelectomy

A varicocelectomy is the high ligation of the gonadal veins of the testes. Varicocelectomy is done to reduce venous backflow of blood into the venous plexus around the testes and to improve spermatogenesis.

Varicoceles occur more frequently on the left side because the gonadal vein of the left testis unites retroperitoneally with the renal vein at a 90-degree angle and is consequently under greater backpressure. As a result of this unusual backpressure, the pampiniform plexus of the spermatic cord becomes tortuous and engorged, resembling a bag of worms.

Procedural Considerations. The setup for inguinal varicocelectomy is as described for an inguinal hernia repair (see Chapter 13). A microscope may be used to better visualize the vessels involved.

Operative Procedure. The incision may be through a suprainguinal approach or an oblique inguinal approach over the external inguinal ring.
1. The surgeon identifies the structures of the spermatic cord and dissects the vessels free from the vas deferens.
2. The abnormal dilated veins in the inguinal canal are clamped and ligated. The redundant portions are excised. A drain may be placed.
3. The incision is closed in layers.

Testicular Biopsy

A biopsy of the testicle involves a wedge excision of suspicious tissue for diagnostic confirmation. Men experiencing infertility who are azoospermatic or oligospermatic with a normal or minimally elevated level of follicle-stimulating hormone may be evaluated through this means. Biopsy may also be performed to obtain sperm cells for in vitro fertilization techniques.

Procedural Considerations. The perioperative nurse assists with positioning the patient in the supine position, and the anesthesia provider administers a general, regional, or spinal anesthetic. A minor instrument set is used. Special fixatives, such as Bouin or Zenker solution, must be available when pathologic confirmation is required. If retrieval of sperm cells is planned, the perioperative nurse ensures the biopsy specimen is placed in a small amount of saline, kept warm, and taken immediately to the fertility laboratory for aspiration of cells. Formalin destroys the germinal epithelium and should not be used.

Operative Procedure
1. The scrotum is held firmly on its posterior aspect. This causes the skin on the anterior aspect to stretch tightly over the incisional site, forcing the epididymis to remain posterior and allowing the scrotal skin to part without retraction.
2. The surgeon makes a 1- to 2-cm vertical incision, taking care to avoid injury to the epididymis.

3. The incision is continued to the tunica vaginalis. As the tunica is incised, there should be a normal efflux of clear fluid.
4. Absorbable 4-0 stay sutures are placed in the tunica vaginalis. Two more are placed in the tunica albuginea.
5. Using the scalpel in a shaving action, no-touch technique, the surgeon resects a small ellipse of tunica with its tubules. The tissue is placed in the fixative or sent to the histology department as a fresh specimen.
6. The wound is closed in three layers with 3-0 and 4-0 absorbable suture.
7. Gauze sponges and fluffed dressings are placed over and around the scrotum. A scrotal support is applied to provide pressure and support.

Orchiectomy

An orchiectomy is the removal of the testis or testes. Removal of both testes is castration and renders the patient sterile and deficient in the hormone *testosterone,* which is responsible for development of secondary sexual characteristics and potency. This operation, like vasectomy, has legal implications that require attention to acquiring informed consent for surgery. Bilateral orchiectomy is usually performed to control symptomatic metastatic carcinoma of the prostate gland. A unilateral orchiectomy is indicated because of testicular cancer, trauma, or infection. Testicular cancer is the most common solid malignancy affecting males between the ages of 15 and 35. Germ cell tumors account for 95% of testicular tumors. Testicular tumors usually present as a nodule or painless swelling of one testicle. Approximately 30% to 40% of patients complain of a dull ache or heavy sensation in the lower abdomen, perianal area, or scrotum, whereas acute pain is the presenting symptom in 10%. Gynecomastia presents as a symptom due to metastases. Evaluation of the patient includes physical examination, ultrasound, CT, or MRI as well as serum beta-human chorionic gonadotropin (hCG) and alpha fetoprotein (AFP) (Steele et al, 2012). Testicular implants are available for cosmetic purposes. These must be ordered preoperatively based on preoperative measurements for size. This procedure has recently been approached through endoscopic techniques, usually in conjunction with laparoscopic herniorrhaphy.

Procedural Considerations. The perioperative nurse assists with positioning the patient supine, and the anesthesia provider administers a general, spinal, or regional anesthetic. A minor instrument setup is required.

Operative Procedure
Scrotal Approach
1. For benign conditions the incision is made over the anterolateral surface of the midportion of the scrotum.
2. The surgeon carries the skin incision through the subcutaneous and fascial layers through the tunica vaginalis, exposing the testicle.
3. Retractors are placed, and bleeding vessels are clamped and ligated.
4. The spermatic cord is divided into two or three vascular bundles. Each vascular bundle is doubly clamped, cut, and ligated, first with 0 absorbable suture ligature and then with a proximal free 0 absorbable tie.
5. The vas is separately ligated with a 0 absorbable tie. The testis is removed.
6. The procedure is repeated on the opposite side if bilateral excision is planned.

Inguinal Approach

1. For malignant conditions the incision is begun just above the internal ring, extending downward and inward over the inguinal canal to the external inguinal ring.
2. The surgeon exposes the inguinal canal and dissects the spermatic cord free, cross-clamps it, and divides it into vascular bundles at the internal ring.
3. Gentle forward traction is applied to the cord, which is dissected from its bed.
4. The testis is everted into the wound from the scrotum and excised.
5. The procedure is repeated on the opposite side if bilateral excision is planned.
6. Bleeding is controlled with the ESU. A small drain may be placed in the empty hemiscrotum if desired.
7. The surgeon reapproximates the external oblique fascia with 2-0 absorbable interrupted sutures.
8. Subcutaneous tissue, including Scarpa fascia, is closed with 4-0 absorbable sutures.
9. The skin is reapproximated with surgical staples or 4-0 subcuticular sutures.

Radical Lymphadenectomy (Retroperitoneal Lymph Node Dissection)

Radical lymphadenectomy is a bilateral resection of retroperitoneal lymph nodes. Dissection usually includes lymph nodes, channels, and fat around both renal pedicles; the vena cava; and the aorta, including the bifurcation of the aorta. Lymph node dissection is performed for treatment of nonseminomatous testicular tumors or in conjunction with an open prostatectomy for prostate cancer.

Procedural Considerations. The perioperative nurse assists with placing the patient in the supine position. The anesthesia provider administers a general anesthetic. If the dissection is unilateral, the patient is supine with the operative side tilted upward. Long, fine dissection instruments along with basic laparotomy instruments are required.

Although this procedure may be performed laparoscopically, this approach has not yet become the standard of practice because of its technical difficulty.

Operative Procedure

1. The surgeon makes a midline abdominal incision from the xiphoid process to the symphysis pubis.
2. The abdominal contents are explored to determine the degree of gross nodal involvement. The colon is either packed within the abdominal cavity or mobilized and kept moist outside the abdomen.
3. The surgeon opens the posterior peritoneum between the aorta and the vena cava.
4. Using blunt and sharp dissection, the surgeon removes the lymphatic structures and fat en bloc from around both renal pedicles, the vena cava, and the aorta from above the renal hilum to beyond the bifurcation of the iliac vessels on the side of the original testicular neoplasm.
5. The spermatic vessels of the affected side are removed down to and including the stump of the previous orchiectomy.
6. The inferior mesenteric artery may be sacrificed if technically necessary, but the superior mesenteric artery is not disturbed.
7. The ureter on the affected side is skeletonized to remove any perilymphatic tissue.

8. If reperitonealization is desired, the posterior peritoneum is closed with a 2-0 absorbable continuous suture.
9. The surgeon repositions the viscera into the abdominal cavity, and closes the wound in layers, usually without placement of a drain.

Surgery of the Prostate Gland

Glandular hyperplasia of the prostatic urethra usually manifests itself after 50 years of age. Prostatic enlargement may be benign or malignant and may occur in one or more lobes of the prostate but most frequently occurs in the lateral or median lobes. Progressive growth of the hyperplastic gland compresses the remaining normal prostatic tissue, forming what is called a *surgical capsule.* The growth of adenomatous tissue slowly encroaches on the prostatic urethral lumen, causing obstruction of urinary outflow. The surgeon and patient must consider several factors when determining the best route for removal of the prostatic obstruction: the age and medical condition of the patient, the size of the gland and location of the pathologic condition, and the presence of associated medical disease (Patient-Centered Care).

Prostate cancer is the most frequently diagnosed cancer in men and is the second leading cause of cancer death in men (American Cancer Society, 2012). Because of the prevalence of prostate cancer and the similarity of symptoms to BPH, the American Urological Association (AUA) recommends that starting at age 40 the PSA test and digital rectal examination (DRE) be offered to men at average risk (Evidence for Practice).

A blood sample is drawn to determine the PSA level, followed by a DRE. The blood is often drawn first because manipulation of the gland has been known to alter the efficacy of the PSA test. The PSA test is considered a valuable tool for early detection of carcinoma of the prostate, but if used alone, it will miss 20% to 30% of all prostate cancers. If the test value is elevated, the patient is at risk for carcinoma of the prostate; a PSA value greater than 10 ng/mL is highly suggestive of prostatic carcinoma. Clinical evaluation and an elevated PSA usually indicate the need for a transrectal ultrasound needle biopsy to confirm the diagnosis. When the results of the biopsy are positive for malignancy, additional diagnostic studies are indicated including measurement of free and total serum PSA II levels, bone scans, and CT and MRI scans of the pelvis (Ignatavicius, 2013).

The most commonly used system to grade prostate cancer is the Gleason score. To calculate the Gleason score, the pathologist evaluates the prostatic tissue to determine which type of cell is the most common and which type is the second most common and gives each of the two cell types a score from 1 to 5. The two scores are combined to determine the total score. Higher numbers are an indication of more abnormal, aggressive cancer cells. Men with a Gleason score of 2 to 4 are generally cured by surgery; scores from 5 to 6 indicate mildly aggressive cancer cells; a score of 7 indicates the cancer is moderately aggressive. Scores between 8 and 10 indicate highly aggressive tumors and are associated with a poor prognosis after surgery (Epstein, 2007). Additional prostate cancer staging tools are the tumor, node, metastasis (TNM) system and the AUA system (Box 15-1).

If the prostate gland is cancerous, a radical retropubic or radical perineal prostatectomy, in conjunction with open or laparoscopic pelvic lymph node dissection, is usually performed. TURP may also be used in men who cannot have a radical prostatectomy, or to relieve symptoms caused by prostate cancer before other treatments begin. Select patients with well-differentiated or moderately differentiated lesions may be candidates for transperineal, ultrasonically guided implantation of radium seeds (brachytherapy) or cryoablation of the prostate (cryotherapy). Newer therapies for prostate cancer are being developed (Research Highlights on page 491). Many patients desire to retain sexual function. The surgeon may attempt to save the neurovascular bundles in what is termed a nerve-sparing approach. The site and size of the prostatic lesion, however, often determine if this can be achieved successfully and without undue risk to the patient.

Surgery for prostate enlargement may be preceded with a biopsy procedure. Depending on the results of the biopsy, a variety of procedures are available to address the benign or malignant condition.

Prostatic Core Needle Biopsy

Needle biopsy of the prostate is indicated for patients in whom prostatic cancer is clinically suspected. It may be accomplished transrectally with a needle designed for this purpose or transperineally.

Procedural Considerations. Needle biopsy of the prostate has the risk of both intraoperative and postoperative bleeding. A cystoscopic examination may accompany a needle biopsy. Most needle

---

PATIENT-CENTERED CARE

The trend in health care is shifting from traditional disease-centered models to a focus on patient-centered care. The Agency for Healthcare Research and Quality (AHRQ) notes that in a patient-centered model, patients become active participants in their own care and receive services designed to focus on their individual needs and preferences, in addition to advice and counsel from health professionals.

One method that can be useful to engage the patient is a symptom severity questionnaire. An example of a patient-centered care questionnaire is the American Urological Association (AUA) severity index for ranking benign prostatic hyperplasia (BPH) symptoms. Because BPH is rarely life threatening but can have a considerable effect on a patient's quality of life, treatments are more preference-driven than for conditions such as cancer, so patients must be involved more fully in treatment decisions.

Each of the seven questions included asks the patient to rank a particular symptom on a scale of 0 to 5, with 5 being the most severe. The symptoms are incomplete emptying, frequency, intermittency, urgency, weak urinary stream, hesitancy, and nocturia. On completion of the test, the numbers are added up in order to determine the overall severity of BPH-related symptoms. Based on these totals, the patient's symptoms are classified as mild, moderate, or severe.

According to a survey of more than 500 urologists, 99% were aware of and used the AUA symptom severity index, and 21% of those had altered their diagnosis and management strategies because of it. Measures of symptoms and BPH-specific health status provide the most detailed and sensitive measures of treatment effectiveness from the patient's perspective, according to AHRQ-funded researchers.

The AUA severity index is described below:
1. Over the past month or so, how often have you had a sensation of not emptying your bladder completely after you finished urinating?
2. Over the past month or so, how often have you had to urinate again less than 2 hours after you finished urinating?
3. Over the past month or so, how often have you found you stopped and started again several times when you urinated?
4. Over the past month or so, how often have you found it difficult to postpone urination?
5. Over the past month or so, how often have you had a weak urinary stream?
6. Over the past month or so, how often have you had to push or strain to begin urination?
7. Over the last month, how many times did you usually get up to urinate from the time you went to bed at night until the time you got up in the morning?

For questions 1-6, there is a choice of six possible answers: never; less than one time in five; less than half the time; about half the time; more than half the time; almost always. Question 7 has six possible answers, ranging from 0 to 5 or more.

Modified from Agency for Healthcare Research and Quality: Expanding patient-centered care to empower patients and assist providers, *Research in Action* Issue 5, Publication No. 02-0024, Rockville, MD, available at www.ahrq.gov/qual/ptcareria.htm. Accessed January 13, 2013; Rickert J: Patient-centered care: What it means and how to get there, *Health Affairs Blog*, January 24, 2012, available at http://healthaffairs.org/blog/2012/01/24/patient-centered-care-what-it-means-and-how-to-get-there/. Accessed January 13, 2013.

EVIDENCE FOR PRACTICE

Diagnosing and Managing Prostate Cancer

Early detection is important in diagnosing and managing prostate cancer. Information relating to a patient's profile in initiating the algorithm (see page 490) includes the following:

Risk Factors
1. *Age:* After 50 years old, the risk increases rapidly; about 64% of all prostate cancer cases are diagnosed in men ages 65 and older. Although the lifetime risk for prostate cancer is 3%, prostate cancer is the most common noncutaneous cancer in men in the United States, and the second leading cause of male cancer mortality.
2. *Race:* African American men and Jamaican men of African descent have the highest prostate cancer incidence rates in the world.

3. *Diet:* High dietary fat is associated with a greater risk for developing cancer.
4. *Family history:* Risk is increased for men who have first-degree relatives with prostate cancer.

Candidates for Early Detection
1. Men 40 years old or older with a life expectancy of 10 years or longer.

Diagnostic Measures Used in Combination for Early Detection
1. DRE
2. Serum PSA
3. Biopsy if indicated (three of four men undergoing biopsy will not have cancer)

Continued

EVIDENCE FOR PRACTICE

Diagnosing and Managing Prostate Cancer—cont'd

Screening for Prostate Cancer: Clinical Summary of U.S. Preventive Services Task Force (USPSTF) Recommendation

Population	Men Younger than Age 75 Years	Men Age 75 Years or Older
Recommendation	No recommendation Grade: I (Insufficient Evidence)	Do not screen Grade: D
Risk assessment	Prostate cancer is more common in older men, African Americans, and men with a family history of prostate cancer. The same uncertainties about the effects of screening that apply to other men also apply to these higher-risk men.	
Screening tests	The prostate-specific antigen (PSA) test is more sensitive than the digital rectal examination (DRE). The conventional PSA test cut-point of 4.0 g/L misses some early cancer. However, lowering the cut-point would increase the rate of false-positive results. Variations of PSA screening have not yet been demonstrated to improve health outcomes.	
Screening intervals	If PSA screening reduces mortality, screening every 4 years may be as beneficial as annual screening.	
Interventions	Management strategies for localized prostate cancer include watchful waiting, active surveillance, surgery, and radiation therapy. There is no consensus regarding optimal treatment.	
Balance of harms and benefits	• The harms of screening include the discomfort of prostate biopsy and the psychological harm of false-positive test results. • Harms of treatment include erectile dysfunction, urinary incontinence, bowel dysfunction, and death. A proportion of those treated, and possibly harmed, would never have developed cancer symptoms during their lifetime.	
	For men younger than age 75 years, evidence is inadequate to determine whether screening improves health outcomes. Therefore, the balance of harms and benefits cannot be determined.	For men age 75 years or older and for those whose life expectancy is 10 years or fewer, the incremental benefit from treatment of prostate cancer detected by screening is small to none. Therefore, harms outweigh benefits.
Suggestions for practice	Clinicians should discuss the potential benefits and known harms of PSA screening with their patients younger than age 75 years. Men in this age group should be informed of the gaps in the evidence, and their personal preferences should guide the decision of whether to order the test.	
Other relevant USPSTF recommendations	A list of USPSTF recommendations on cancer screening can be found at www.preventiveservices.ahrq.gov.	

Prostatitis, benign prostatic hyperplasia, and prostate cancer can all be associated with elevated serum PSA levels. Other factors that are known to cause elevations in PSA levels include urethral or prostatic trauma and infection.

Modified from U.S. Preventive Services Task Force: *Screening for prostate cancer: clinical summary of U.S. Preventive Services Task Force recommendation,* August 2008, available at www.uspreventiveservicestaskforce.org/uspstf08/prostate/prostatesum.htm. Accessed October 10, 2012.

biopsies are performed in the surgeon's office or ultrasound department.

The most significant potential complication of a biopsy is systemic infection. This risk can be decreased with antibiotic administration before and after the procedure and bowel cleansing before the examination. The patient is given antibiotic therapy 24 hours before the procedure and is advised to use a sodium phosphate enema 2 to 3 hours before the test is performed. Before the examination, an antiseptic solution mixed with a viscous local anesthetic often is instilled into the rectum and allowed to coat the tissues for 5 to 15 minutes. The surgeon may also inject local anesthetic into the prostate and seminal vesicles transrectally with a 22-gauge,

22-cm injection needle through the needle guide on the transducer.

Operative Procedure

Transrectal, Ultrasonically Guided Biopsy. Transrectal, ultrasonically guided biopsy is commonly performed in the surgeon's office using a high-frequency transrectal ultrasound transducer to assess the prostate gland. The technique allows the surgeon to assess the size, volume, and shape of the prostate and the likelihood of the presence of a malignancy. Biopsy specimens of suspicious areas or lesions may be obtained with a needle passed across the rectal wall, with the aid of ultrasound guidance. The needle penetrates the

---

BOX 15-1

American Urological Association Prostate Cancer Stages

Stage A: Clinically Unsuspected Disease
A1   Focal carcinoma, well differentiated
A2   Diffuse carcinoma, usually poorly differentiated

Stage B: Tumor Confined to Prostate Gland
B1   Small, discrete nodule of one lobe of the gland
B2   Large or multiple nodules or areas of involvement

Stage C: Tumor Localized to Periprostatic Area
C1   Tumor outside prostate capsule, estimated weight ≤70 g, seminal vesicles uninvolved
C2   Tumor outside prostate capsule, estimated weight >70 g, seminal vesicles involved

Stage D: Metastatic Prostate Cancer
D1   Pelvic lymph node metastases or ureteral obstruction causing hydronephrosis, or both
D2   Bone, soft tissue, organ, or distant lymph node metastases

Modified from Nelson WG et al: Prostate cancer. In Abeloff MD et al, editors: *Abeloff's clinical oncology,* ed 4, Philadelphia, 2008, Churchill Livingstone.

RESEARCH HIGHLIGHT ▌▌

The Use of Metformin as an Adjuvant Treatment for Prostate Cancer

Current clinical trials use the medication metformin in prostate cancer patients prior to radical prostatectomy. Metformin is a relatively safe drug used for blood sugar control in type 2 diabetic patients. It has been noted in recent years that metformin might have a variety of anticancerous effects not only in prostate cancer but also several different types of cancer.

The latest clinical trials have suggested the possibility of better postoperative outcomes following radical prostatectomy surgery. Studies suggest its role in chemoprevention, while being well tolerated by the patient. Metformin data show promising effects not only in reducing insulin resistance but also inhibiting metabolic parameters causing a decrease in prostate-specific antigen (PSA) results prior to surgery.

Clinical trials are still being directed toward using neoadjuvant metformin for interruption in the cancer metabolic pathway.

Modified from Joshua M et al: A phase II study of neoadjuvant metformin in prostatic carcinoma, *J Cancer Res* 72:8, 2012.

RESEARCH HIGHLIGHT ▌▌

Prostate Cancer Research

Prostate cancer research continues to be an area of great growth and interest. Investigators are looking at prostate cancer genomics for markers of indolent versus aggressive disease. Researchers are hopeful that understanding the genetics of an individual's prostate cancer will allow a more individualized approach to treatment and will assist with treatment decisions.

Advanced stages of prostate cancer are generally treated successfully for some period of time with androgen deprivation therapy. When disease progresses despite this therapy it is termed castrate-resistant prostate cancer. Investigators are studying novel treatment agents, primarily immunotherapies, to address this patient population. Sipuleucel-T is an autologous dendritic cell therapeutic vaccine designed to augment the patient's own immune response to the cancer. Phase III studies have shown a 4-month improvement in survival in patients randomized to the vaccine.

Modified from Wiklund F: Prostate cancer genomics: can we distinguish between indolent and fatal disease using genetic markers? *Genome Med* 2:45, 2010, available at http://genomemedicine.com/content/2/7/45. Accessed September 30, 2012.

---

seen in cross section. To evaluate the prostate in the sagittal planes, the surgeon rotates the probe clockwise or counterclockwise (Figure 15-25). A series of 12 biopsy specimens is generally taken with a disposable "core biopsy" needle. These are taken from the right and left medial and lateral apices, the right and left midline, and the right and left medial and lateral bases. Lesions as small as 2 to 3 mm are visible with this procedure.

Transperineal Biopsy. The perioperative nurse assists with placing the patient in the lithotomy or lateral position. The procedure may be performed with the patient receiving a general, regional, or local anesthetic. The surgeon performs a rectal examination to identify the induration. The needle is inserted through the perineal skin and guided ahead until the tip is against the lesion. The biopsy specimen is taken in the same fashion as described for the transrectal approach. Some surgeons may incise the site with the #11 or #15 scalpel and place a 4-0 absorbable closing suture.

The surgeon may also use the transperineal approach to perform template biopsies with ultrasound guidance, using the brachytherapy (seed implant) template. The perioperative nurse assists with placing the patient in the lithotomy position, and secures his scrotum toward the abdomen with a transparent adhesive dressing. The surgeon positions the brachytherapy grid, template fixation device, and probe with cradle adjacent to the patient's perineum. Using the ultrasonic transrectal transducer the surgeon measures the prostate and calculates its total volume. Biopsies are then obtained transperineally through the template grid.

Transurethral Resection of the Prostate Gland

In TURP, the surgeon passes a resectoscope into the bladder through the urethra and resects successive pieces of tissue from around the bladder neck and the lobes of the prostate gland, leaving the capsule intact. The resectoscope has a stabilized cutting loop that is used to resect tissue and coagulate blood vessels by means of electric current. The electric current that powers the electrode is supplied by a high-frequency ESU. The current settings are specified by the surgeon, who activates the cutting or coagulating current with a foot pedal during the course of the procedure.

rectal mucosa with a core biopsy system. Color-flow imaging may also be used to help identify areas that are likely invaded with prostatic carcinoma or have acute and chronic inflammation. Highly vascular areas carry a greater probability of harboring a carcinoma. A full bladder helps delineate the base of the prostate.

The surgeon visualizes the prostate in three dimensions, allowing more accurate localization of abnormalities and extent of disease. For the axial view, the transrectal transducer is placed deeply into the rectum, just proximal to the seminal vesicles, to about 10 cm above the anal verge. Here the vas deferens may be distinguished. The transducer is slowly withdrawn to the level of the base of the gland, enabling visualization of the inner gland. Seminal vesicles are

FIGURE 15-25 Schematic drawing of zonal anatomy of the prostate (*nonshaded area* is peripheral zone). **A,** Coronal view. **B,** Axial view. **C,** Sagittal image showing prostate *(P)*, seminal vesicles *(S)*, and rectum *(R)*. **D,** Transverse image of seminal vesicles *(S)*.

TURP is one surgical method of treating benign obstructive enlargement of the prostate gland. Several factors influence the surgical approach: size of the gland and location of the pathologic condition, age and condition of the patient, and presence of associated diseases.

Procedural Considerations. The instrument setup for TURP is as described for cystoscopy with additional necessary instruments. The four principal types of resectoscopes are McCarthy, Nesbit, Iglesias, and Baumrucker. Adult resectoscopes range in size from 24F to 28F and have the following components: foroblique telescope, operating element, cutting loops, and postresectoscope sheaths and obturators. A TURP requires a resectoscope (multiple working elements); a foroblique telescope as well as a backup telescope; stabilized or unstabilized cutting loops; a postresectoscope sheath with its corresponding articulated obturator; a high-frequency cord; a short bridge; a Toomey syringe or the Ellik or Urovac evacuator; van Buren sounds; a 22F or 24F, 30-mL, three-way Foley catheter; a disposable urologic drape with rectal sheath; and a system for continuous bladder irrigation and urinary drainage. Supplementary instruments include a resectoscope adapter and a lateral telescope.

The continuous-flow resectoscope (CFR) has unique components that include an outlet stopcock to which a suction tube is attached, an inflow tube on the inner sheath, and outflow holes on the outer sheath. These features enable the surgeon to resect tissue without interruption to empty the bladder, as must be done with the standard resectoscope. In addition to the CFR, which replaces the standard resectoscope, the setup includes thick-walled Silastic suction tubing and a continuous-flow pump. The continuous-flow

technique decreases intravesical pressure on the bladder during the procedure, provides a clearer field of vision because of the constant inflow and outflow of irrigant, reduces the operating time because the resection process need not be interrupted to evacuate the bladder, and provides a "still" bladder for the resection of bladder tumors.

A continuous flow of isotonic and nonelectrolytic irrigating fluid is necessary to ensure transmission of electric current and clear visualization throughout surgery. Irrigating solution such as 3% sorbitol or 1.5% glycine, 3 to 5 L, may be connected in tandem to provide a constant flow. Warming units, available for these solutions, help eliminate the hypothermia often experienced when large amounts of cold irrigants are used. On the other hand, when solutions are warm, the patient may show a tendency to bleed more. The perioperative nurse must remain alert as to the status of the irrigation solution and replace it as required.

During transurethral prostatic surgery, the return of irrigation fluid must be monitored because intravasation and absorption of fluid into open prostatic venous sinuses or bladder perforation may occur. The perioperative nurse should be aware of the early signs and symptoms and measures used to remedy these complications (Young et al, 2009). The patient usually experiences significant respiratory changes and abdominal discomfort. Continued extravasation and absorption can lead to hypovolemia and hyponatremia. Other important observations are rigidity and swelling of the lower abdomen, coupled with changes in sensorium. If extravasation of irrigating fluid is evident, the surgical procedure is discontinued and a cystogram is obtained immediately to determine if bladder perforation has occurred. Insertion of a Foley catheter is generally all that

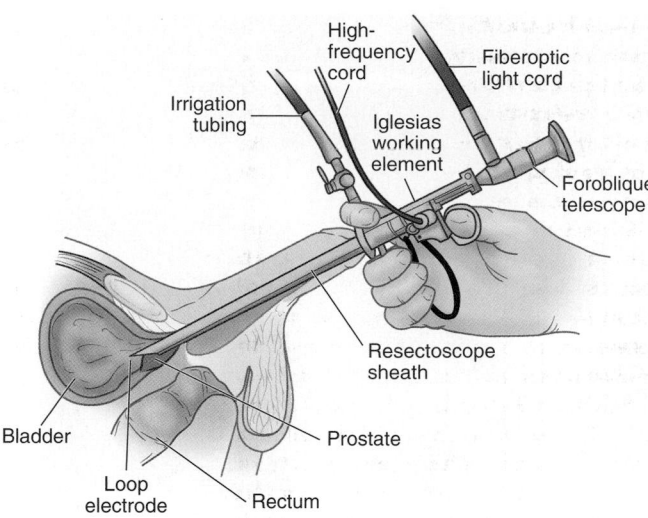

FIGURE 15-26 Sectional view illustrating removal of portion of hypertrophied middle lobe of prostate gland with Iglesias resectoscope.

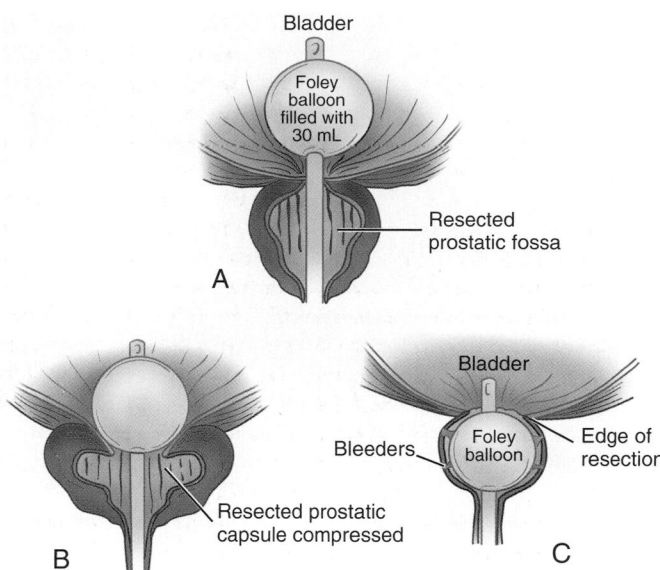

FIGURE 15-27 **A** and **B,** Proper position for Foley catheter with inflated balloon beyond prostatic capsule. **C,** Improper position.

is necessary to control the situation. In the rare instance of a major perforation, surgical closure may be accomplished through a cystotomy incision.

Operative Procedure

1. The surgeon dilates the urethra with sounds sized from 20F to 30F.
2. Cystourethroscopy is performed to assess the degree of prostatic obstruction and to inspect the bladder. Some surgeons perform this diagnostic procedure several days before surgery, whereas others perform the examination in the OR immediately before surgery.
3. The surgeon passes a well-lubricated postresectoscope sheath with its fitted Timberlake obturator into the urethra.
4. The Timberlake obturator is removed, and the working element (resectoscope), assembled with the foroblique telescope and cutting loop, is inserted through the sheath.
5. The irrigation tubing, light cord, and high-frequency cord are appropriately connected, and the surgeon opens the stopcock to allow the irrigation fluid to fill the bladder.
6. With the bladder distended, the surgeon inspects the prostatic urethra and bladder trigone.
7. After determining the location of the ureteral orifice, the surgeon begins electrodissection, alternating cutting and coagulating currents as required (Figure 15-26).
8. The bladder is drained, washing out prostatic tissue and small blood clots. At times the surgeon may use the Ellik evacuator to remove resected prostatic tissue. The Ellik is used by removing the working element of the resectoscope, fitting the nozzle of the evacuator onto the resectoscope sheath, and removing the bladder contents by manual pulsatile pressure. The scrub person ensures an Ellik or Urovac evacuator or a Toomey syringe is readily available for manual irrigation. Fluid may be drawn from the irrigant directly into the resectoscope sheath through the already attached tubing.
9. When the resection is completed, the surgeon inspects the prostatic fossa to ensure that all bleeding points have been coagulated.

10. The resectoscope is then removed, and a Foley catheter (22F or 24F, two-way or three-way, 30-mL balloon) is inserted into the bladder for urinary drainage. The balloon is inflated (Figure 15-27, *A*), pulled gently in traction against the bladder neck, and secured, to help control venous bleeding (see Figure 15-27, *B*). The Foley balloon must not be inflated within the prostatic fossa (see Figure 15-27, *C*), where it may cause excessive bleeding from the resected prostatic capsule. If desired, continuous irrigation with gravity drainage is initiated, with normal saline as the bladder irrigant instead of sorbitol or glycine. A 3- to 4-L urinary drainage system is suggested to avoid frequent emptying of the drainage bag.

Transurethral Incision of the Prostate

Transurethral incision of the prostate (TUIP) is a procedure in which the prostate is incised at the 5 and 7 o'clock positions to provide relief of obstruction, with results similar to those provided by a complete transurethral resection but with a lower incidence of bladder neck contracture and retrograde ejaculation. The shorter operative time inherent with the procedure minimizes fluid absorption and may decrease postoperative pulmonary and cardiovascular complications. The procedure may be performed with cold or hot knives as well as the standard resectoscope, or laser fiber (TULIP). This procedure is appropriate for sexually active patients with moderate to small obstructive prostates without a significant middle-lobe component. One major disadvantage is the potential for missing occult prostatic cancer. Despite this, some clinicians view this as an underused, feasible form of treatment.

Transurethral Incision of the Ejaculatory Ducts

Transurethral incision of the ejaculatory ducts is performed for the relief of obstructed ejaculatory ducts, a common condition in men with chronic prostatitis and prostatic calculi. Symptoms closely mimic prostatodynia and include aching in the perineal and genital areas with no lasting or significant improvement from conservative therapy (antibiotics and analgesics). The resectoscope loop is guided

FIGURE 15-28 A, Dilated seminal vesicle (ejaculatory duct) with resectoscope loop approaching. **B,** Resectoscope loop entering dilated seminal vesicle (ejaculatory duct).

with transrectal ultrasound imaging to the dilated ejaculatory ducts, and the obstructed ducts are resected (Figure 15-28). Calculi may be fragmented if necessary and removed. A catheter generally is not needed.

Photoselective Vaporization of the Prostate

The KTP laser is now used to treat BPH or prostatic enlargement. *Green-light photoselective vaporization of the prostate (PVP)* is a new minimally invasive approach performed on an outpatient basis. The approach is the same as with other endoscopic techniques. A non-contact laser fiber is used to heat the prostate tissue and rapidly vaporize it to a penetration depth of 0.8 mm with minimal to no blood loss. Vaporization occurs from within the tissues, where the collagen matrix eventually bursts as a result of the vapor buildup. The laser is operated in a continuous wave mode and induces a coagulation zone of only 1 to 2 mm in thickness. This prevents the excessive sloughing of necrotic tissue. The patient may not always need a Foley catheter following the procedure.

Interstitial Laser Coagulation of the Prostate

Interstitial laser coagulation (ILC) with the Indigo laser is a minimally invasive procedure for treatment of urinary outflow obstruction secondary to BPH. It is indicated for men older than 50 years with a median or lateral prostatic lobe volume of 20 to 85 mL. Designed for those men who wish to minimize the risk for incontinence and impotence found with conventional TURP, this procedure is now performed in the office setting about 80% of the time.

The procedure is contraindicated for the treatment of prostate cancer and for those patients who had previous brachytherapy with radioactive seeds. However, some physicians may elect to perform ILC before brachytherapy (or cryotherapy) in the hopes of minimizing, if not relieving, the postoperative voiding symptoms associated with these more definitive treatments.

Procedural Considerations. The patient is placed in the lithotomy position and prepped as for cystoscopy. An optional local anesthetic with oral or monitored IV sedation is generally adequate. Oral sedation is used more commonly with the office-based procedure; if the surgery takes place in the hospital or ambulatory center, monitored IV sedation may be used. An ultrasound machine with

FIGURE 15-29 Indigo Optima laser unit with diffuser-tip fiber.

transrectal capability is often used to measure the size of the prostate gland and determine the appropriate number of laser applications (sticks). Some surgeons choose to measure by cystoscopy alone.

The setup includes a 17F or 23F panendoscope and 30-degree fiberoptic lens, ultrasound and transrectal transducer, and the Indigo laser machine with laser fiber (Figure 15-29). The fiber has graduated black depth markings used to guide placement into the prostate gland. The laser machine automatically times each "stick" for 2 minutes, 30 seconds. The perioperative nurse ensures that all laser safety precautions are observed (see Chapter 8).

Operative Procedure

1. The surgeon inserts the transrectal transducer and measures the prostatic volume. (This may have been performed as an office procedure preoperatively.) Local anesthetic may be injected

through the transducer guide pin with an 8-inch spinal needle or with the 8-inch collagen injection needle if ultrasound is not used.

2. Cystoscopy is performed, and the prostatic urethra is evaluated.

3. The surgeon introduces the laser fiber through the panendoscope and passes it into the lateral lobe of the prostate gland through the urethral wall to the desired depth.

4. This is repeated one to three times on each side, depending on the measured prostatic volume.

5. A TUIP may be performed using the bare-tip fiber.

6. A 16F or 18F urethral catheter is inserted and connected to straight drainage. A 16F suprapubic Foley catheter may also be used and attached to irrigation or drainage.

Transurethral Microwave Therapy (TUMT)/Transurethral Needle Ablation (TUNA)

TUMT is a minimally invasive method of applying heat to the prostate gland for the relief of the symptoms associated with BPH and bladder-outlet obstruction. TUMT maintains temperatures in the urethra, sphincter, and rectum at a level that is physiologically safe while heating the tissue deep within the transitional zone of the prostate. A water-cooled catheter is combined with microwave radiation to the lobes of the prostate. This treatment is an office-based procedure.

Transurethral needle ablation (TUNA) is also a minimally invasive office procedure for the treatment of BPH of the median and lateral lobes. This technique delivers radiofrequency (RF) energy through two electrodes that are embedded in a special urethral catheter. Specific target areas of the prostate are thermally ablated by the RF energy and combined inductive heating of water molecules, leaving the urethra and the remainder of the prostate intact.

Simple Retropubic Prostatectomy

Simple retropubic prostatectomy is the enucleation of hypertrophic prostatic tissue through an incision in the anterior prostatic capsule by an extravesical approach. The retropubic approach offers excellent exposure of the prostate bed and vesical neck and readily controllable intraoperative and postoperative bleeding.

A preoperative bowel prep and antibiotic therapy are the standards of care for all open prostatectomies.

Procedural Considerations. The perioperative nurse assists with positioning the patient in a slight Trendelenburg position with the pelvis elevated and the legs slightly abducted. Although the draping procedure must conform to individual OR policies, the following procedure is suggested for draping the patient:

1. The first towel, with a cuff, is placed under the scrotum.

2. The next three towels are placed around the lower abdominal incision site, followed by a sterile laparotomy sheet.

3. A fifth towel, folded in half, is placed over the penis and scrotum below the retropubic incision site and secured with two nonperforating towel clamps.

The instrument setup includes a basic laparotomy set and bladder and prostatic instruments (Figures 15-30 and 15-31). The following supplies should be readily available: Jackson-Pratt drains; water-soluble lubricant; Toomey and Asepto syringes; urinary drainage system; 20F, 5-mL Foley catheter; 22F or 24F, 30-mL Foley catheter; 10- and 30-mL syringes; and a self-retaining retractor such as the adjustable Omni-Tract surgical UO400 urology retractor system (Figure 15-32).

FIGURE 15-30 Curved and straight Lowsley tractors in open position.

FIGURE 15-31 A, Urethral suture guides. **B,** Roth grip-tip urethral suture guide.

Operative Procedure

1. The surgeon inserts a 20F or 22F Foley catheter with 30-mL balloon into the urethra and through the bladder neck and inflates it. This is clamped and maintained within the sterile field. Frequently a three-way catheter is used for continuous bladder irrigation.

2. Through a Pfannenstiel or low vertical midline incision, the surgeon incises the anterior rectus sheath along with portions of the internal and external oblique muscles.

3. The rectus abdominis muscles are retracted laterally to expose the space of Retzius.

4. After placement of traction sutures, the anterior portion of the prostatic capsule is incised transversely (Figure 15-33, *A*).

FIGURE 15-32 Adjustable Omni-Tract surgical UO400 urology retractor system.

5. The prostatic adenoma may be dissected or finger-enucleated from the surgical capsule (see Figure 15-33, *B*).
6. The surgeon places hemostatic sutures at the 5 and 7 o'clock positions, encompassing the vesical neck and prostatic capsule, to ligate the primary blood supply to the prostate. Other bleeding points within the capsule may be suture-ligated with 2-0 absorbable sutures.
7. The prostatic capsule incision is closed with either a continuous or an interrupted 0 absorbable suture (see Figure 15-33, *C*).
8. A drain is placed in the space of Retzius and exteriorized through the fascia and skin via a separate stab incision.
9. The abdominal incision is then closed in layers, and the wound is dressed.
10. If continuous bladder irrigation is to be used, normal saline solution irrigation is initiated through a 3-L closed irrigation system.

Suprapubic Prostatectomy

Suprapubic prostatectomy is the removal, through a transvesical approach, of periurethral glandular tissue obstructing the outlet of the urinary tract. A low midline, or Pfannenstiel, incision may be used. One advantage of the suprapubic approach is that it allows access for surgical correction of any existing bladder condition such as vesical calculi or vesical diverticula. Control of bleeding is a major consideration in any prostatectomy and is one disadvantage of the suprapubic approach. Because the prostate is located beneath the symphysis pubis, ligation of bleeding capsular vessels is difficult. However, control of hemorrhage and replacement of blood loss, coupled with skilled perioperative nursing care and early mobilization of the patient, have greatly minimized complications.

Procedural Considerations. Spinal, epidural, or general anesthesia may be selected for patients having a suprapubic prostatectomy,

A

B

C

FIGURE 15-33 Retropubic prostatectomy.

depending on their medical condition. The patient is placed in a slight Trendelenburg position with the umbilicus elevated and the legs slightly abducted. Draping and instrumentation are as described for retropubic prostatectomy.

Operative Procedure

1. The surgeon inserts a 20F or 22F Foley catheter with 30-mL balloon into the urethra and through the bladder neck and inflates it. This is clamped and maintained within the sterile field. This maneuver facilitates identification of the bladder.
2. A transverse or midline lower abdominal incision is made through the skin and the two layers of superficial fascia (Figure 15-34, *A*).
3. The external and internal oblique muscles are cut along the lines of the original incision.
4. The surgeon clamps, electrocoagulates, or ligates any bleeding vessels.
5. The rectus muscles are separated in the midline and retracted laterally.
6. After the placement of traction sutures, the surgeon opens the bladder at the dome with a scalpel. Liquid contents are aspirated, and the bladder incision is enlarged.

FIGURE 15-34 Suprapubic prostatectomy.

7. The bladder is visually and manually explored for calculi, a tumor, or diverticula.

8. The surgeon manually enucleates the adenomatous tissue using the tip of the index finger inserted through the vesical neck into the prostatic urethra (see Figure 15-34, *B*). If difficulty is experienced with the enucleation, the surgical assistant may place a finger into the rectum to elevate the prostate gland. Aseptic technique is maintained during enucleation with the use of a sterile second glove on the hand used in the rectum.

9. After enucleation is completed, attention is directed to maintaining good hemostasis by suture ligation of the vesical neck at the 5 and 7 o'clock positions. Other significant bleeding points may also be ligated.

10. A suprapubic catheter is placed into the bladder lumen through a small stab incision.

11. A 22F or 24F, two-way or three-way Foley catheter with a 30-mL balloon is inserted into the urethra in place of the original one, and the balloon is inflated to a size that prevents the catheter from falling or being pulled into the prostatic fossa (see Figure 15-34, *C*).

12. The surgeon closes the cystotomy incision with interrupted 2-0 absorbable sutures.

13. A drain is left along the cystotomy incision, exteriorized through a separate stab wound, and secured to the skin with a silk suture.

14. The muscles, fascia, and subcutaneous tissues are closed in layers, and a dressing is applied.

15. To reduce clot formation and maintain catheter patency, normal saline irrigation solution may be connected to the Foley catheter to provide continuous irrigation to the bladder. Continuous irrigation may be initiated during closure.

Simple Perineal Prostatectomy

Simple perineal prostatectomy is the removal of the prostate gland through a perineal approach. A perineal approach is most suitable when open prostatic biopsy is desired and, after receipt of pathologic confirmation, radical excision is to follow. Other advantages include preservation of the bladder neck, improved urethrovesical anastomosis, and easier control of bleeding. Some surgical disadvantages are (1) inability to perform biopsy of the iliac and obturator nodes for determining extension of disease and (2) possible formation of urethrorectal fistulas.

Procedural Considerations. The patient is placed in an exaggerated lithotomy position with the legs above the level of the pelvis. The perioperative nurse places a bolster beneath the sacrum to allow the perineum to be as parallel to the OR bed as possible, with the buttocks extending several inches over the bed edge. Stirrups should be well padded to protect the popliteal fossa. Intermittent pneumatic compression devices are recommended to assist peripheral vascular flow. The patient is often placed in a steep Trendelenburg position. Well-padded shoulder braces, placed over the acromial processes in a manner to prevent stretch or pressure injury, may be required to prevent the patient from sliding upward on the bed. Routine skin preparation is carried out and includes an interior rectal prep. Special draping is as follows:

1. A towel folded in half is placed over the pubic area.
2. Two towels with a cuff are placed on either side of the perineum.
3. Two legging drapes, with points down, are placed over the legs.
4. One impervious drape is placed over the anus.
5. A large sheet fully opened with a large cuff is placed across from one stirrup to the other and secured by towel clamps.
6. A laparotomy sheet follows, with the short end to the floor.

The instrument setup is as described for suprapubic prostatectomy, omitting abdominal self-retaining retractors and adding straight and curved Lowsley tractors, Roux retractors, Jackson retractors with short and long blades, Doyen vaginal retractors, Young retractor, perineal prostatic retractors, Sauerbruch retractors, and a narrow and wide self-retaining perineal retractor, such as the Thompson retractor or the Omni-Tract surgical UO100 pelvic retractor system.

Operative Procedure

1. A curved Lowsley tractor is placed through the urethra into the bladder and held back by the surgical assistant, causing the prostate to be pushed down toward the perineum.
2. An inverted U-shaped incision is made from one ischial tuberosity to another, curving just anteriorly to the anus (Figure 15-35, *A*).
3. Three Martius or Allis clamps are secured to the posterior edge of the incision and retracted downward, over the anal drape.

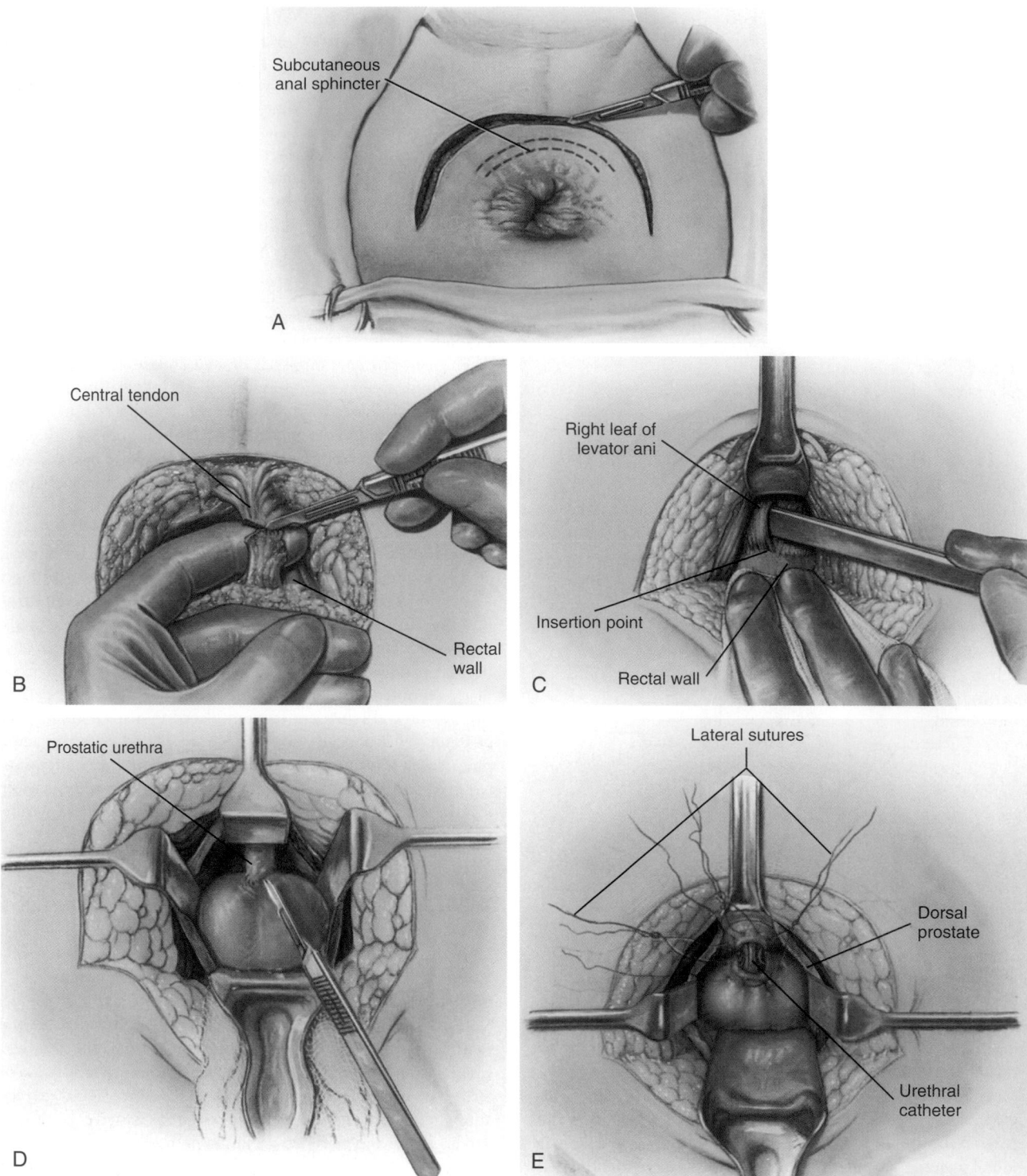

FIGURE 15-35 Simple perineal prostatectomy.

4. The surgeon clamps any subcutaneous bleeders with straight mosquito hemostats and electrocoagulates or ties them with 3-0 absorbable ligatures.
5. The central tendon is isolated, clamped, and cut distally to the external anal sphincter (see Figure 15-35, *B*).
6. The rectourethral muscle is incised and pushed downward from the central tendon.

7. The levator ani muscle is exposed and retracted laterally (see Figure 15-35, *C*).
8. The prostate gland is exposed. The surgeon may send biopsies of the prostate for pathologic confirmation. If the results are negative, the prostatic adenoma is removed. If the frozen section reveals malignancy, a radical prostatectomy may be done at this time.

9. If simple enucleation is to be performed, the prostatic capsule is incised and the Lowsley tractor is removed (see Figure 15-35, *D*).

10. The urethra is divided, and the Young prostatic retractor is inserted.

11. The blades are opened, drawing the prostate down, and the adenoma is manually enucleated from the surgical capsule.

12. A 22F Foley catheter with a 30-mL balloon is inserted through the urethra into the bladder.

13. Bleeding is controlled at the 5 and 7 o'clock positions.

14. The capsulotomy incision is repaired with a continuous 2-0 absorbable suture (see Figure 15-35, *E*).

15. A drain is left in place at the level of the capsulotomy incision.

16. The surgeon reapproximates the subcutaneous tissue with 3-0 absorbable suture.

17. The skin incision is reapproximated with 4-0 absorbable subcutaneous sutures.

18. The wound is dressed according to the surgeon's preference and taped or held with a supportive device, such as mesh underpants.

Transrectal Seed Implantation (Interstitial Radiotherapy with Brachytherapy)

Brachytherapy of the prostate gland is a procedure that requires a collaborative, multidisciplinary approach to patient care. The radiation oncologist and medical physicist, in addition to the surgeon, are vital to an optimum outcome from the initial planning stage throughout the postoperative surveillance. Preplanning is required to determine the size of the prostate, dose of each seed, the spacing necessary between each seed, and the number of seeds required. A template plan is developed preoperatively by using the ultrasound and the probe-anchoring equipment to measure and map the appropriate seed sites within the prostate. This may be accomplished in the surgeon's office, radiology department, or oncology clinic. The implant plan is finalized at the time of surgery.

The facility that offers this treatment must be licensed for "Group 6" with the radioactive materials licensing department of their respective state. If seed implantation is indicated as an adjunct to radiation therapy, it should be performed 3 to 4 weeks after the radiation treatment.

During percutaneous implantation of iodine-125 or palladium-103 seeds, the patient is positioned in the lithotomy position. The surgeon visualizes the prostate with transrectal ultrasonic imaging, and locates the midportion of the prostate on a transverse image. This location becomes an index for positioning the axial ultrasound plane at the base of the prostate. Approximately 2 to 3 hours should be allowed from start to completion. The procedure is amenable to outpatient management using a regional or general anesthetic.

Iodine seeds are commercially available in titanium-encased rods called magazines that absorb the electrons. The rods have to be secured by the attending radiologist, who brings them to the procedure and monitors their handling. They cannot go to central processing unless a radiologist or radiology technician accompanies through the process, so the perioperative nurse ensures that the recommended practices for immediate use sterilization are followed (Association of periOperative Registered Nurses [AORN], 2012b). These seeds may also be obtained embedded in an absorbable suture that allows them to remain positioned appropriately in relation to themselves and their location within the prostate and minimizes the risk of seed migration. Palladium seeds, which are not presently available prethreaded, are plated onto a graphite pellet. The pellets are loaded into titanium tubes with a lead marker. The half-life of iodine-125 (60 days) is longer than that of palladium-103 (17 days) and allows the therapy to be delivered over the duration of tumor cell replication, altering the ability of the tumor cells to multiply. Compared to iodine-125, palladium-103 affords a larger dose of radiation in a shorter time interval to more rapidly growing tumors.

Procedural Considerations. Percutaneous implantation of radioactive seeds allows the delivery of significantly higher doses of radiotherapy to the prostate than provided by external beam therapy. The radius of penetration around each seed is only 5 mm, thus sparing adjacent organs. The typical radiation dose that can be delivered by external beam may be 6500 centigrays (cGy), whereas the dose that can be delivered with implantation of seeds alone is in the range of 12,000 to 16,000 cGy. Some patients may receive hormone therapy to shrink the prostate gland for 3 months before implantation, and some will undergo radiation therapy before implantation. Patients with stage A or stage B prostate cancer are appropriate candidates, and selection is not influenced by a rise in the PSA level, biopsy specimens indicative of further involvement, or age. Ideal patients for brachytherapy treatment as monotherapy are those with low-risk parameters (PSA ≤10, Gleason score 6 or less, low-volume disease on biopsy).

Possible complications include the risk of intraoperative seed displacement into the bladder; implantation too close to the urethra, resulting in postoperative urethral stricture or prolonged dysuria; and implantation into the perineum if the needles are withdrawn too quickly. There is also the chance of migration of seeds, placed just outside the periphery of the gland and in the periprostatic plexus, to the lung. The nurse instructs the patient to avoid extended contact with children and pregnant females and to keep a 15-foot distance from this population group for 6 to 8 weeks. The patient must strain his urine, and any seeds expelled should be retrieved and returned to the oncologist. Body wastes are not considered hazardous, however.

Bleeding from the percutaneous sites is minimal, but postoperative ecchymosis of the perineum is to be expected. Other postoperative complications that may occur in the first 12 months include acute cystitis, prostatitis, and urinary retention. Late complications may include chronic prostatitis with cystitis, urethral stricture with contracture, stress with urge or total incontinence, proctitis, and impotence. Some patients may require post-treatment TURP, bladder-neck incision, suprapubic catheter insertion, or urethral dilation to alleviate the aforementioned conditions. Much less commonly, rectovesical or rectoprostatic fistula can occur, requiring interventions such as laparotomy, colostomy, and urinary diversion. Patients are generally able to void 24 to 48 hours after implantation. The perioperative nurse positions the patient in the lithotomy position with assistance. The scrotum must be secured cephalad to allow a clear operating field. The surgeon places a traction stitch through the lateral edges of the scrotum and anchors it to the groin region.

With an experienced team, seeding is done with real-time ultrasound imaging. Throughout the procedure, random room checks with a Geiger counter are performed to determine radiation levels. All personnel, surgical equipment, and trash (including disposable drapes) are scanned before leaving the room at the end of the procedure.

Operative Procedure. Before seeding is begun, the surgeon positions the ultrasound transducer so that the posterior margin of the prostate is parallel to the axis of the ultrasound transducer. The direction of seed insertion and the transverse images of the prostate must have a similar appearance to those on the preoperative volume study. The volume study and implant worksheet are used for continual verification of coordinates. The surgeon attaches a stabilizer bar to the OR bed. This secures the "stepping unit," which allows a 5-mm incremental forward-and-backward motion of the probe. The sled that holds the transducer is attached to the stepping unit. The probe must be securely anchored so that the position of the prostate relative to the needles used to implant the seeds remains unaltered throughout the procedure. For the needles to be positioned appropriately, the template with labeled grid is attached to the transrectal transducer so that the needles placed through the probe grid match the grid locations on the plan. The grid is labeled alphabetically *Aa, Bb, Cc,* and so on, with the center of the prostate corresponding to *D* on the grid. The plan is designed to avoid the urethra, bladder neck, and rectum to prevent urethrorectal fistula formation, irradiation of the bladder, and scarring at the bladder neck level.

1. At the beginning of the procedure the surgeon inserts a urethral catheter, drains the bladder, and then refills it with 150 mL of sterile water. The bladder then provides an "acoustic void" to better visualize the prostate. If fluoroscopy is used, contrast medium can be instilled into the bladder to delineate the position of the bladder neck.

2. The surgeon removes the urethral catheter during implantation of seeds to avoid placement of seeds close to the urethra. The catheter causes the tissue surrounding the urethra to be compressed, and if attempts are made to implant seeds into this compressed tissue, penetration of the catheter and urethra may occur. The catheter also causes an acoustic shadow that prevents visualization of the anterior prostate gland.

3. The scrub person covers the ultrasound probe with a sterile probe cover filled with 15 mL of sterile water to remove the artifact. Alternatively, a gel-filled probe cover can be placed on the end of the ultrasound probe. Filling with too much fluid will change the configuration of the prostate and alter the anatomic presentation. The transducer will be aimed with the tip upward at a 10- to 20-degree angle (Figure 15-36). The posterior wall of the prostate must be far enough away from the probe so that the posterior row of seeds is placed just inside the posterior capsule. Seeds are implanted by means of loaded

needles placed into the prostate according to the template plan, with the midline seeds placed slightly off center to avoid the urethra. Alternatively, individual seeds can be placed through the hollow needles with a Mick applicator that uses a long plunger.

4. Stabilization of the prostate may be achieved with stabilization needles placed laterally to the center into the right and left lobes and then removed once the anterior seeds are in place. Another method is to use a Foley catheter as a retractor for implantation of the periphery and until implantation near the urethra occurs. The best method may be to overcompensate for the rotation of the prostate by angling or turning the needle slightly opposite to the direction desired.

5. The most anterior seeds are placed first so that imaging of the anterior portion of the gland is not obscured by the ultrasonic shadows created by seeds placed posteriorly. If strands are used, hydrocortisone (Anusol-HC) is used to seal the bevel before implantation. Strands should be cut cleanly with electrosurgery to seal the ends and avoid frayed ends, which may be split further when the stylet is inserted into the needle, adversely affecting seed placement.

6. Contrary to normal needle insertion with the bevel up, these needles are placed into the prostate with the solid, or back, side up. Every effort is extended to avoid implanting seeds into the bladder or too close to the urethra, which causes significant postoperative irritative symptoms.

7. When placing the anterior needles, passage of the needle may be prevented by the inferior arch of the pubic bone. The needle tip is visualized as a bright echo, and the angle may be altered to compensate for the bone. Alternatively, the placement of the anterior seeds may be postponed until the end when the template may be dropped down, the probe positioned parallel to the pubic arch, and the needles inserted past the anterior portion into the prostate. Rarely, the template may need to be removed from the ultrasound probe at the conclusion of the procedure to allow "freehand" placement of anterior needles.

8. The needle is inserted beyond the desired site and then retracted. The first seed determines where the balance will lie because the seeds fall into a plane that follows the first seed in a specific needle. The target volume is greater than the actual volume of the prostate so the capsular edge of the prostate and just beyond are also subjected to seed penetration (Figure 15-37). These peripherally placed seeds have a higher energy and may have a greater tendency for migration if the tissue is not dense enough to hold the seed in place.

9. The distribution of seeds is generally 80% peripheral and 20% central.

10. The surgeon performs a cystoscopy at the end of the treatment so that seeds protruding into the urethra or left in the bladder may be removed.

11. A Foley catheter is placed and left for 24 to 48 hours.

Transrectal Cryosurgical Ablation of the Prostate Gland

Cryoablation of the prostate is a feasible, minimally invasive option for patients with localized or locally advanced prostate cancer. This method of treating the prostate gland can be used either as primary therapy or as a salvage procedure for local recurrence of prostate adenocarcinoma after previous external radiation therapy, brachytherapy, or even previous cryoablation. Cryoablation causes cell death through crystallization within the intercellular and extracellular spaces that exert mechanical shear forces on the cell

FIGURE 15-36 Transducer on stepping unit and slide, angled upward to "get under" the pubic bone.

FIGURE 15-37 Fluoroscopic view of completed seed implant.

membranes, osmotic changes, and cellular hypoxia. Complications related to the procedure include urinary incontinence, urethral slough, rectourethral fistula, UTI, and post-cryoablation erectile dysfunction (Langenhuijsen et al, 2009).

Procedural Considerations. The perioperative nurse assists with positioning the patient in a dorsal lithotomy position with the legs raised high enough to allow placement of a stabilizer bar that is affixed directly to the operating table. The ultrasound probe can then be placed on a sled with the use of brachytherapy. Because of the positioning required for the procedure and the length of the procedure (i.e., average 2 hours), the patient is at increased risk for developing deep vein thrombosis (DVT). The perioperative nurse initiates DVT precautions (e.g., elastic stockings, intermittent pneumatic compression device sleeves) as part of the plan of care. Patients treated with cryosurgery are generally admitted to the hospital after the procedure and discharged the following morning, unless bleeding, fever, or anesthetic complications prevent their discharge.

Operative Procedure

1. The surgeon performs a cystoscopy to assess the external sphincter, prosthetic urethra, bladder neck, and location of the ureteric orifices on the bladder trigone.
2. At the conclusion of the cystoscopy the surgeon fills the bladder with sterile irrigant to facilitate percutaneous insertion of a suprapubic cystotomy tube.
3. A guidewire is then introduced into the bladder on removal of the cystoscope, to facilitate later passage of the urethral warming device.
4. The surgeon tacks the scrotum away from the perineum with suture.
5. The transrectal ultrasound probe is then affixed to the table and inserted for visualization of the prostate gland. Volume and length measurements of the prostate are made at this time.
6. The perioperative nurse attaches the needles to the cryosurgery machine to allow circulation of the argon and helium gases through the device tubing. Before insertion of the needles into the perineum, the perioperative nurse and scrub person test the needles in the saline to ensure production of an ice ball.

7. After all needles are in place, the surgeon advances the urethral warming device over the guidewire previously placed in the urethra. This warming catheter remains for the duration of the procedure, and is often left in place for up to 1 hour following the cryoablation treatment. The use of the urethral warming catheter is crucial to the safety of this procedure, and cryoablation of the prostate should not be done without its use.
8. Using ultrasound guidance in the transverse and longitudinal planes, the surgeon inserts the cryosurgery treatment needles and thermocouple needles for temperature monitoring. The needles are positioned according to a template that allows for uniform freezing of the prostate gland. Alternatively, needle placement can be tailored by the surgeon to allow for focal cryoablation as clinically indicated. The needle probes are placed at least 1 cm from the location of the urethra, to minimize risk of damage to this structure and to the urinary sphincter.
9. Freezing is initiated in the anterior portion of the prostate (upper needles), and progress of the ice ball is monitored with ultrasound as the ice front progresses to the posterior aspect and apex of the prostate gland.
10. After all tissue has been frozen using a double-freeze technique, the surgeon removes the cryoprobes. Active warming of the prostate can be achieved with circulation of helium through the hollow needles, and this also facilitates removal of the needles at the conclusion of the procedure.
11. If the urethral warming catheter is to remain in place, the patient is transferred to the recovery room with the urethral warmer and circulating machine, which can be transported on an IV pole. One hour following the procedure, the warming catheter is removed and replaced with a Foley catheter, which is usually removed the morning after surgery.
12. The suprapubic catheter allows for urinary drainage for the first 1 to 2 weeks. The tube can then be clamped for a voiding trial after prostate swelling has subsided enough to allow micturition to occur.

Nerve-Sparing Radical Retropubic Prostatectomy with Pelvic Lymphadenectomy

Radical prostatectomy is the treatment preferred for patients with organ-confined carcinoma of the prostate. This procedure involves removal of the entire gland, its capsule, and the seminal vesicles. Important anatomic structures that affect erectile function are within the surgical field. Whenever possible, the surgeon attempts to spare the posterolateral neurovascular bundles, supplying the corpora cavernosa, to preserve potency. Those with tumors confined in the prostatic capsule are the best candidates for nerve-sparing procedures. In the presence of more advanced tumor extension, the surgeon attempts to spare one of the bundles, allowing the chance for potency.

Procedural Considerations. Patient preparation and basic surgical instrumentation are as for the simple retropubic approach. Additional supplies include long-tipped, right-angled clamps; urethral suture guides; a Bookwalter or Wishbone (UO400) self-retaining retractor; long Martius clamps; straight and right-angled clip appliers and clips; and right-angled scissors.

Operative Procedure

1. The surgeon creates a vertical midline lower abdominal extraperitoneal incision.

2. A bilateral pelvic lymphadenectomy is performed, removing the external iliac, obturator, and hypogastric nodes en bloc. Lymphadenectomy is done primarily for tumor staging.

3. The surgeon exposes the puboprostatic ligaments, and incises the endopelvic fascia on each side of the gland to the puboprostatic ligaments (Figure 15-38, *A*). Right-angled scissors are used to divide the puboprostatic ligaments. The dorsal vein complex is easily subject to injury, and excessive venous bleeding may occur during this phase of the procedure. The scrub person and the perioperative nurse need to be alert to this potential complication.

4. A plane is developed between the lateral prostatic border and the levator ani muscles with sharp and blunt dissection. Once visualized, the muscle is dissected laterally to the urogenital diaphragm.

5. The surgeon ligates and divides the collateral veins originating from the levator ani muscle and running laterally to the puboprostatic ligaments to free the apex of the prostate.

6. The dorsal venous complex, supplying the penis, is carefully retracted medially. Once a plane is developed, the venous complex is separated from the urethra with a long-tipped, right-angled clamp. The venous complex is ligated with 0 or 2-0 absorbable ligatures. Some surgeons opt to use a stapler designed for this purpose. The complex is then transected with a #15 scalpel. Backbleeding, from the vessels onto the anterior surface of the prostate, is suture-ligated.

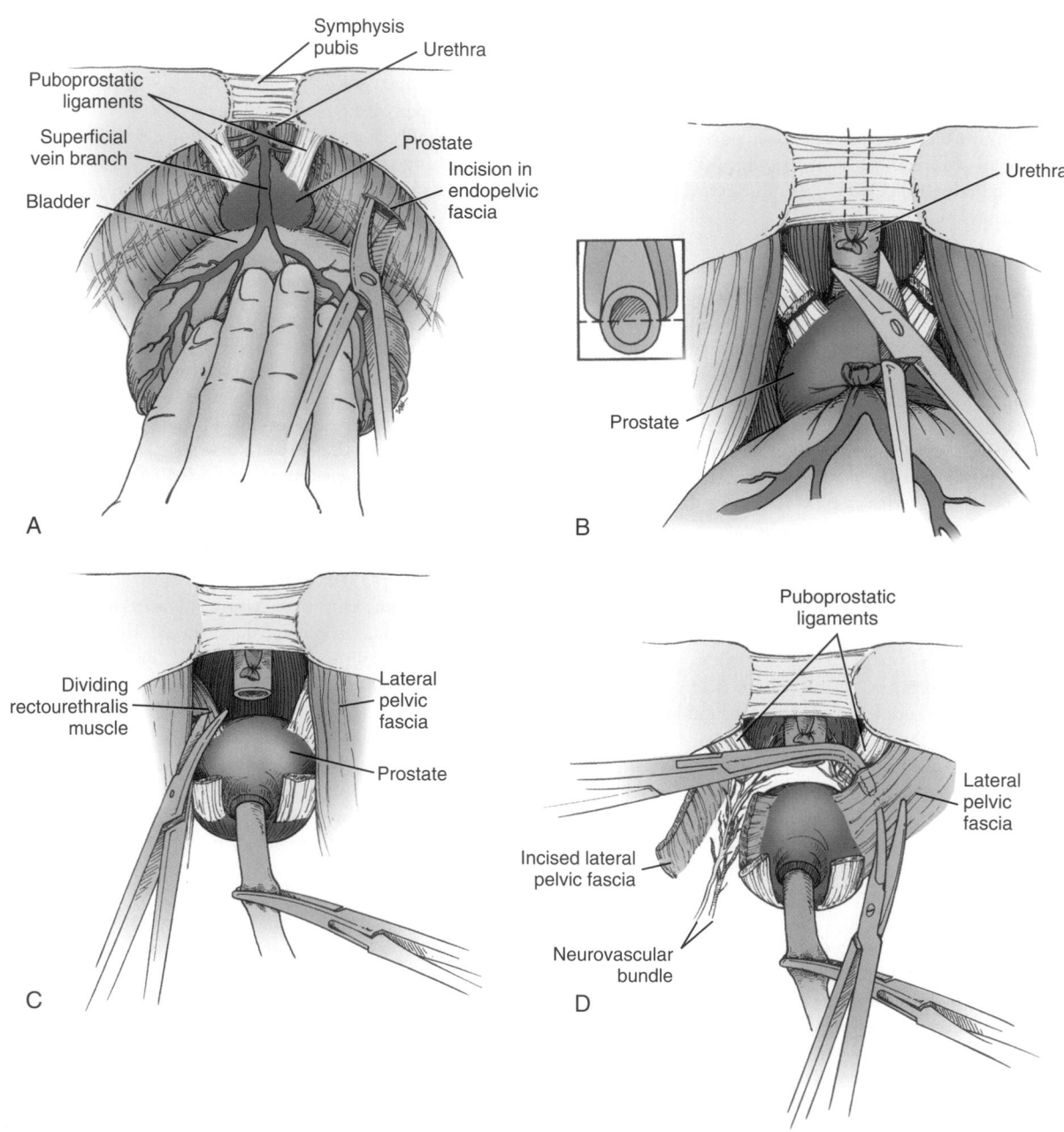

FIGURE 15-38 Radical retropubic prostatectomy.

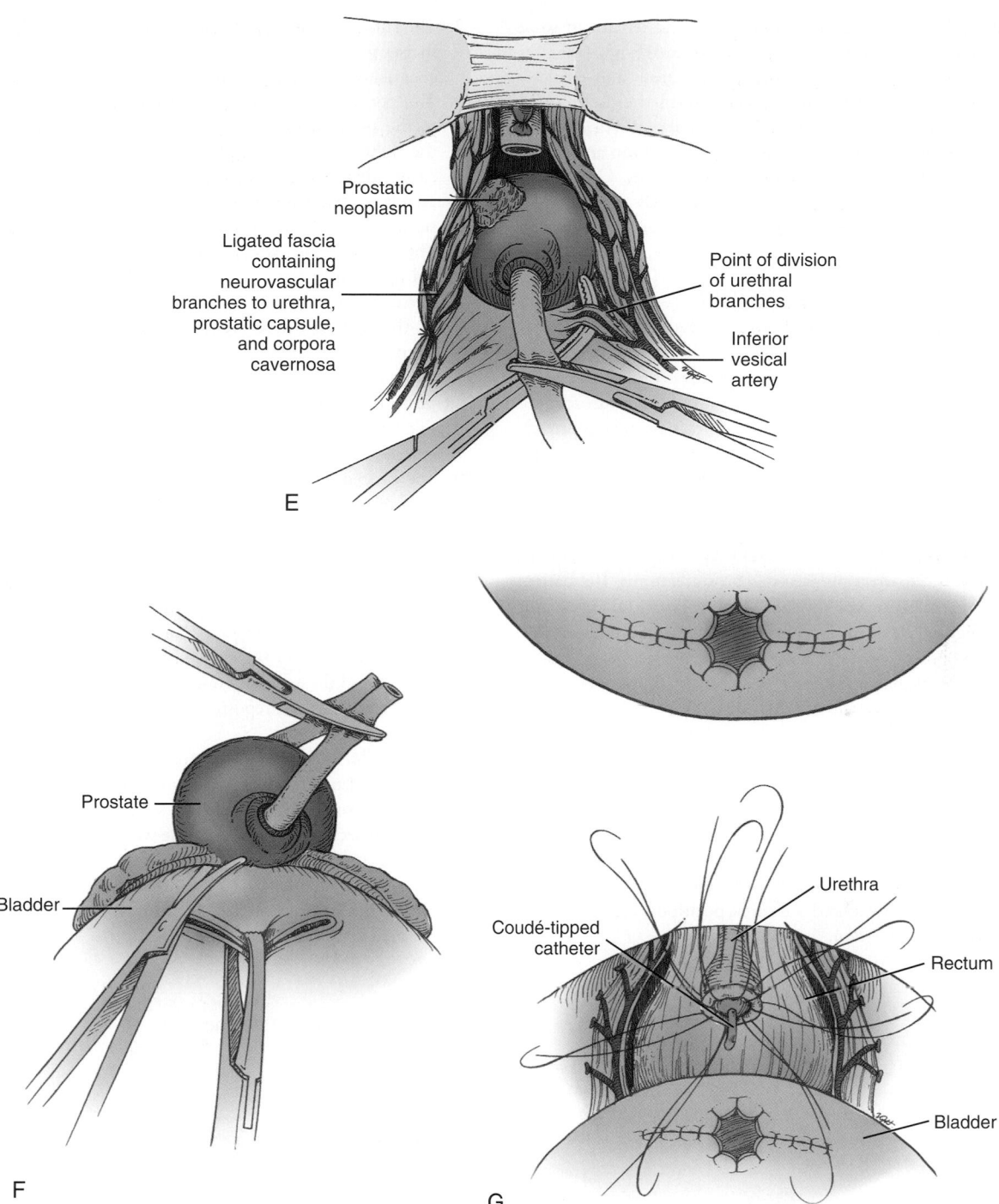

FIGURE 15-38, cont'd Radical retropubic prostatectomy.

7. The surgeon uses a right-angled clamp to mobilize the urethra from the rectourethralis muscle between the two neurovascular bundles, avoiding damage to them.

8. A Penrose drain or vessel loop is passed around the urethra. The surgeon elevates and divides the urethra with a long-handled scissors or scalpel (see Figure 15-38, *B*). The catheter is clamped proximally and pulled upward through the urethral incision, where it is cut and held cephalad.

9. The posterior urethra is transected (see Figure 15-38, *B*).

10. The surgeon dissects the rectourethralis fibers free from and medial to the neurovascular bundles (see Figure 15-38, *C* and *D*).

11. Next the surgeon enucleates the prostate, divides the bladder neck, and clip-ligates the seminal vesicles (see Figure 15-38, *E* and *F*).

12. Once bleeding is controlled, the urethral suture guide is inserted in place of the Foley and six 2-0 absorbable sutures on a ⅝-inch curved needle are placed inside to outside on the

distal urethral segment. These are tagged and left uncut to be anastomosed to the bladder neck (see Figure 15-38, *G*).

13. The surgeon trims and everts the bladder neck and creates a rosebud stoma. The sutures are placed from the urethra to a corresponding position on the bladder neck. When all are placed, they are brought together in single fashion and tied.

14. Closure is as for simple retropubic prostatectomy. Continuous postoperative irrigation is rarely used. A 22F, 30-mL Foley catheter is inserted and placed to gentle traction, and dressings are applied.

Radical (Total) Perineal Prostatectomy

Patient preparation and instrumentation are the same as for simple perineal prostatectomy. The radical approach is accompanied by laparoscopic or low abdominal lymph node dissection, if not previously performed as a separate procedure. Currently, laparoscopy is performed more frequently than the standard incisional approach. Supplies needed for laparoscopy include standard laparoscopic instrumentation, three 10-mm trocars, one 5-mm trocar, an insufflation needle, a video camera unit, and CO_2 insufflation supplies.

Procedural Considerations. Two operative setups are necessary. Most commonly, laparoscopy precedes prostatectomy. The patient is in the supine position for the laparoscopy, with the area of the umbilicus slightly elevated. Intermittent pneumatic compression devices and preoperative Foley catheterization are necessary. Instruments should be available in the OR to convert to an open procedure if necessary. Lymph nodes may be sent for frozen section, primarily for tumor staging.

Operative Procedure
Laparoscopic Lymph Node Dissection

1. The surgeon inserts the Veress needle and insufflates the abdomen.

2. Trocars are placed as follows: 10-mm trocars at the 12 o'clock (umbilicus), 3 o'clock, and 9 o'clock positions; a 5-mm trocar at the 6 o'clock position.

3. The surgeon grasps the peritoneum over the vas deferens, and incises it with scissors. The vas is identified, clipped or electrocoagulated, and divided.

4. The peritoneal dissection is continued laterally and cephalad to the sigmoid colon on the left and the ascending colon on the right.

5. After identification of the spermatic cord structures, iliac vessels, ureters, and psoas muscle, the surgeon extends the incision to the pubic ramus.

6. The Cloquet node is identified and freed from under the external iliac vein.

7. Dissection continues until the obturator nerve is isolated.

8. At the level of the bifurcation of the common iliac vein, the large lymph channel is located and removed. Endo Clips or scissors-coagulation may be used. Clips offer a lower risk of postoperative lymphocele.

9. In a similar fashion the tissue overlying the external iliac artery is removed.

10. The procedure is repeated on the opposite side.

11. Hemostasis is achieved and the trocars are removed. Each trocar is removed under direct observation with the laparoscope, to allow for identification of inner abdominal wall bleeding sites.

12. After evacuation of the CO_2 from the abdomen, the fascia layers are closed at the 12, 3, and 9 o'clock positions.

13. The surgeon closes the skin with 4-0 absorbable subcuticular sutures and dresses the wound.

14. The patient is then repositioned and prepared for radical perineal prostatectomy.

Radical Perineal Prostatectomy. Surgical approach is as for simple perineal prostatectomy (Figure 15-39).

1. The surgeon incises a layer of subcutaneous fascia and uses blunt dissection to create a space within the ischial rectal fossa (Figure 15-40, *A*).

2. The central tendon is incised, permitting dissection to be carried out beneath the triangle formed by the superficial external anal sphincter (see Figure 15-40, *B*).

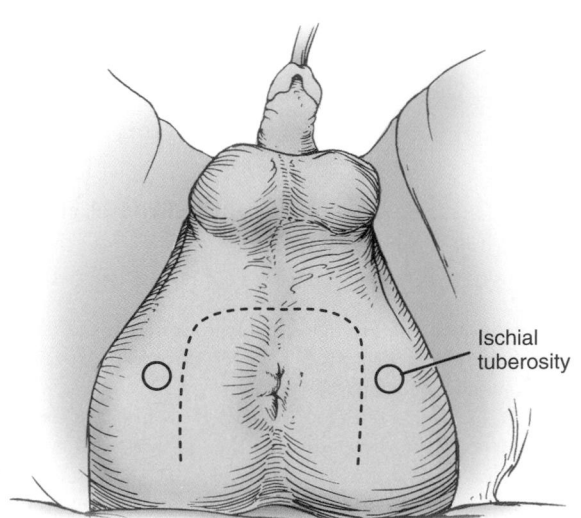

Ischial tuberosity

FIGURE 15-39 Radical perineal prostatectomy, draping and incision.

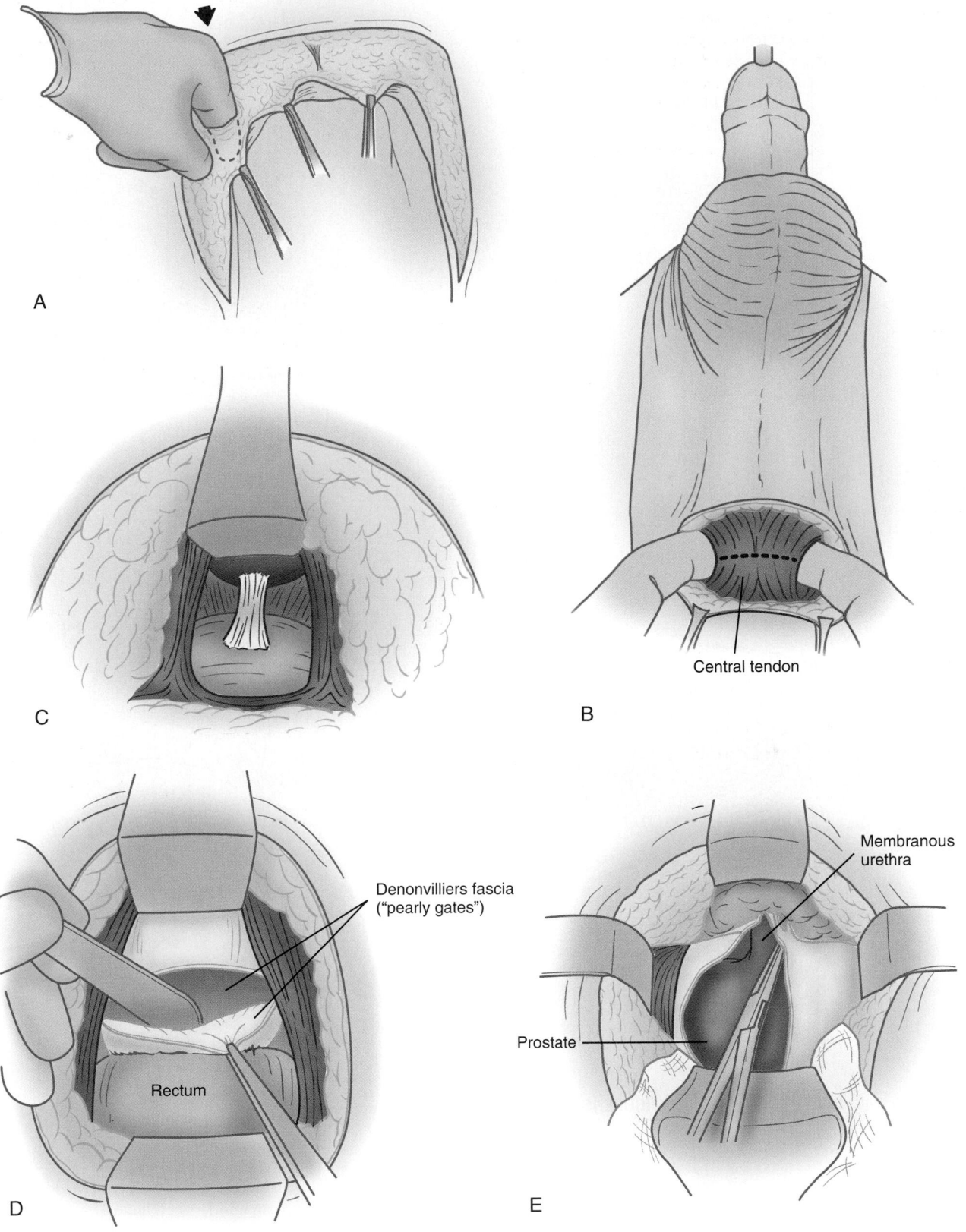

FIGURE 15-40 Radical perineal prostatectomy.

A

B

Central tendon

C

D

Denonvilliers fascia
("pearly gates")

Rectum

E

Membranous
urethra

Prostate

Continued

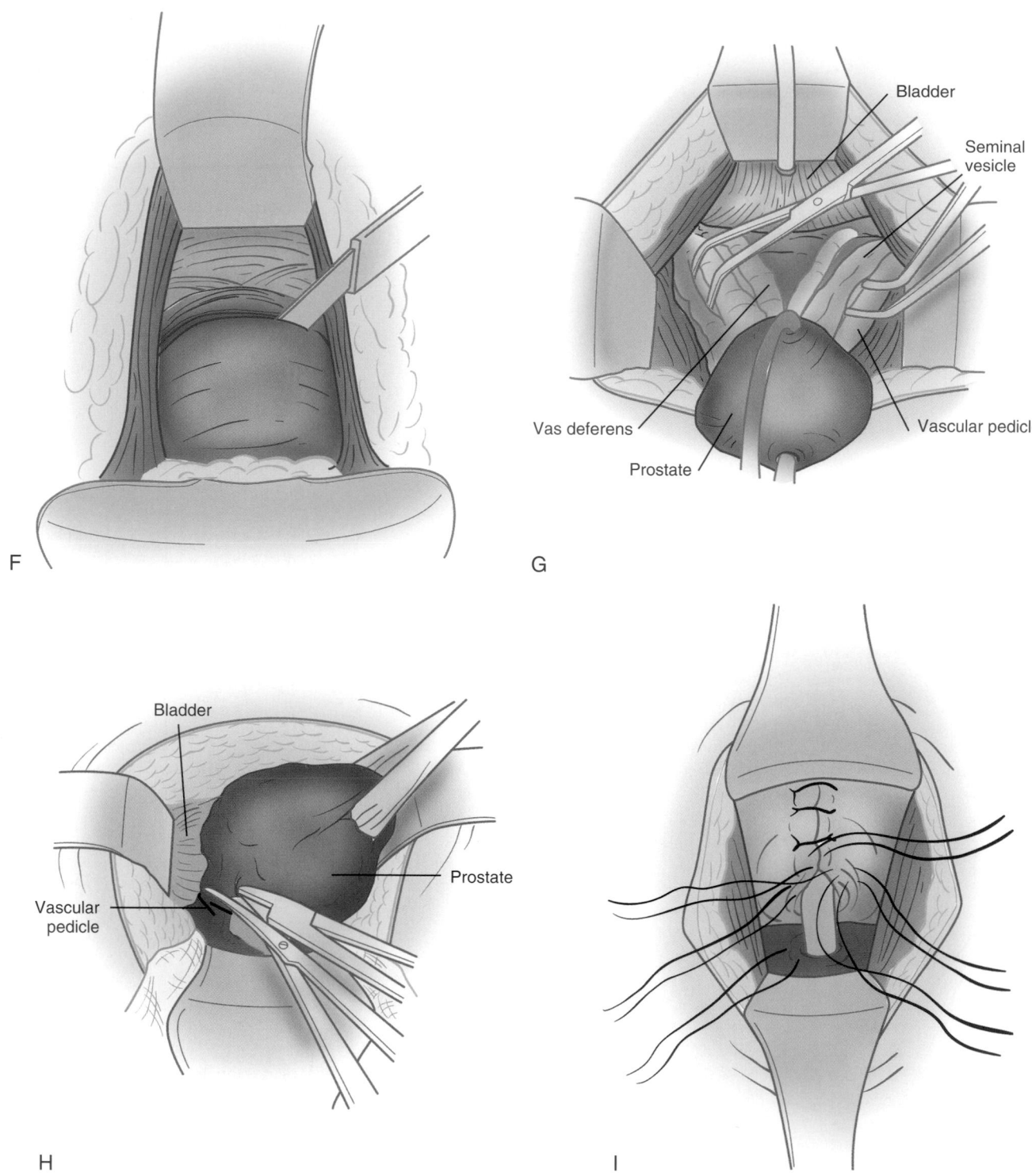

FIGURE 15-40, cont'd Radical perineal prostatectomy.

3. The assistant retracts the sphincter to provide visualization of the rectourethralis (see Figure 15-40, *C*).
4. The true prostatic capsule is exposed by incision of the overlying fascia (see Figure 15-40, *D*).
5. After dissection of the periprostatic fascia unilaterally, the surgeon passes a right-angled clamp around the membranous urethra and incises it (see Figure 15-40, *E*).

6. Using a knife the surgeon severs the posterior bladder neck and retracts the bladder superiorly (see Figure 15-40, *F*).
7. Blunt dissection is used to develop a plane between the anterior bladder and the posterior prostate and seminal vesicles (see Figure 15-40, *G*).
8. The surgeon identifies the vascular pedicles at the 5 and 7 o'clock positions, and incises and divides them (see Figure 15-40, *H*).

9. Before closure of the bladder neck, the surgeon may place vest sutures of 0 or 2-0 absorbable material in a mattress fashion in the open bladder neck at the 2 and 10 o'clock positions and left long for later lateral perineal placement (see Figure 15-40, *I*).

10. Once the reanastomosis is accomplished, the vest sutures are crossed, passed through the perineal body laterally and parallel to the urethra (anterior to the incision), and secured either just beneath the skin or to the skin with suture buttons.

11. After placement of the Foley catheter, the surgeon reanastomoses the urethra to the bladder neck with four to six 2-0 absorbable sutures placed at the 2, 4, 8, and 10 o'clock positions. Some surgeons opt to place sutures at the 6 and 12 o'clock positions as well.

12. A drain is placed anteriorly to the rectal surface and exteriorized through the incision line or through a separate stab wound.

13. The wound is closed as described in the simple procedure.

Laparoscopic Radical Prostatectomy

Laparoscopic radical prostatectomy (LRP) is a minimally invasive approach that may be offered to some patients in centers where practitioners are skilled in the technique. Patient selection is the same as that for radical retropubic or perineal prostatectomy. Those patients who have undergone androgen deprivation, radiation, or perineal surgery may not be good candidates for the procedure, however. Advantages to an LRP over an open procedure are decreased intraoperative blood loss (attributable to the tamponade effect of the pneumoperitoneum on the venous sinuses, and improved access to and visualization of vascular structures), shorter hospital stays, and decreased postoperative pain. The return to continence and sexual potency is reported to be comparable with other approaches. Some practitioners suggest that retaining sexual potency is more likely because the neurovascular bundles may be visualized under magnification and therefore are more readily preserved (Gonzalgo, 2008). Because of the high cost of the numerous disposable items needed, many institutions may opt to not offer this approach to their patients.

Procedural Considerations. Generally no bowel prep is performed preoperatively. IV administration of a third-generation cephalosporin and 2500 units of low-molecular-weight subcutaneous heparin on the morning of surgery is standard treatment.

With the assistance of at least one additional person, the perioperative nurse positions the patient in low lithotomy position with his arms at his sides. The abdomen, entire perineal area, and the upper and inner thigh region are prepped. This entire area is draped open, and separate leggings are used. The anesthesia provider places the patient in the Trendelenburg position. The perioperative nurse positions the video monitor between the patient's legs. A Foley catheter is inserted into the urethra and attached to drainage. After the procedure, heparin is given once daily for 2 weeks postoperatively. The drain and Foley catheter are generally removed on the third postoperative day, and the patient is discharged.

Operative Procedure

1. The surgeon inserts the Veress needle and insufflates the abdomen. Once an internal pressure of 15 mm Hg of CO_2 is achieved, the needle is removed and replaced with a 10-mm trocar.

2. The laparoscope is used to inspect the interior of the abdominal wall. A second incision is then created at McBurney point, a 10-mm trocar is inserted, and the CO_2 line is moved and reattached to this port to prevent fogging of the lens.

3. Three small incisions are made for 5-mm trocar placement: one inferolateral to McBurney point, one in the left iliac fossa, and the third midline between the umbilicus and pubis.

4. If a lymph node dissection is to be performed, this is accomplished first as described in laparoscopic lymph node dissection.

5. The surgeon incises the peritoneal reflection to expose the vas deferens and seminal vesicles. The vasal artery is coagulated, and the vas is transected bilaterally. The seminal vesicles are transected bilaterally and well mobilized.

6. Denonvilliers fascia is incised longitudinally close to the ampulla of the vas and seminal vesicles and placed on mild traction. Once the prerectal fat is visible, the surgeon begins inferior blunt dissection to the posterior surface of the prostate. Dissection is carried to the rectourethralis muscle.

7. The bladder is filled through the Foley catheter with approximately 120 mL of sterile saline to pull it posteriorly and help identify the bladder contours.

8. An incision is made medial to the medial umbilical ligament for the initiation of bladder dissection. This is carried to the vas and up the abdominal wall anteriorly and caudally until contact is made with the pubic ramus.

9. The urachus is divided in the midline and dissected to the level of the symphysis pubis, across the space of Retzius. A bipolar or monopolar dissector is often used for this purpose.

10. After the bladder is freed anteriorly and laterally, the surgeon manually empties it with a suction or syringe device.

11. The surgeon coagulates and incises the dorsal vein. The fascia of Zuckerkandl (fat) covering the prostate is resected or pushed laterally cephalad. The periprostatic space is entered, and the endopelvic fascia is incised on its line of reflection.

12. The puboprostatic ligaments are incised to allow dissection of the dorsal venous complex. This is accomplished with a curved monopolar or bipolar scissors. The vessels surrounding the dorsal venous complex are electrocoagulated with bipolar forceps and then ligated with 2-0 absorbable ligature passed from one side to the other.

13. Using sharp and blunt dissection, the surgeon develops a plane between the bladder neck and prostate. The anterior wall of the urethra is incised, and the Foley catheter is deflated and pulled into the operative field. The lateral and posterior urethral walls are then incised.

14. The posterior bladder neck is finally incised and the retrovesical space entered. The prostatic pedicles are bilaterally electrocoagulated with bipolar forceps.

15. A lateral incision is made to expose and preserve the neurovascular bundles on each side. They are dissected free of the prostatic base to the entrance of the pelvic floor and posterolateral to the urethra.

16. The surgeon transects the dorsal vein complex and retracts it anteriorly to expose the anterior urethral wall. A knife is used to cut across the anterior urethra, and a urethral suture guide is pushed through the urethrotomy into the pelvis. The posterior wall is then transected.

17. The prostate is retracted superiorly and the remaining attachments freed.

18. The surgeon creates the urethrovesical anastomosis with interrupted 3-0 absorbable sutures using two needle holders. Once

all sutures are placed and tied, the Foley is reinserted and the bladder filled to check the patency of the anastomosis.

19. A specimen collection bag is passed through the second port at McBurney point and opened. The prostate is placed in the sac, the sac is closed, and the string is cut. The port is removed and the string to the sac is placed on the abdomen outside the port, a mosquito clamp is attached to the end, and the port is reinserted.

20. Abdominal pressure is lowered to 5 mm Hg, and peritoneal incisions are left open. A drain is placed in the pelvis through the lower left port and sutured to the skin. The abdominal muscles are split, and the specimen is extracted after removal of the trocar. All trocars are then removed and the incisions closed in a routine manner.

Robotic-Assisted Laparoscopic Radical Prostatectomy

Robotic-assisted surgery uses robotic equipment to imitate the surgeon's movements, allowing for operative access through five small portal incisions rather than large incisions, which results in shorter recovery times. The robotic system enhances the surgeon's range of motion and precision and allows surgeons to preserve nerves crucial to urinary continence and erectile function. Benefits of robotic-assisted prostatectomy are similar to benefits of laparoscopic surgery. Patients have only five or six small incisions, a shorter hospital stay, decreased blood loss, and a shorter time before the catheter is removed. Men who have undergone the procedure also have decreased incidence of postoperative urinary incontinence and improved sexual function compared with patients who undergo open prostatectomy (Gonzalgo, 2008).

The robotic surgical system consists of a surgeon console, a cart with interactive robotic arms, jointed instruments that mimic the dexterity of the human hand and wrist, and a high-resolution three-dimensional endoscope and image processing equipment. The system provides a three-dimensional stereoscopic display as the surgeon uses the master arms to make surgical movements that are translated into real-time movements of the instrument tips (see Figure 7-11).

The role of the perioperative nurse during robotic laparoscopic radical prostatectomy procedures begins with competency in the OR. Because use of this technology requires special skills, nurses should become familiar and proficient with all aspects of the procedure.

Procedural Considerations. Before the patient's arrival to the OR the perioperative nurse and scrub person collaborate to ensure all the necessary instrumentation and equipment are available for the procedure. Depending on the robotic system used, a standard laparoscopic setup is used with the addition of the robotic instrumentation and equipment, including the control station, the surgeon's console that provides the interface to the robot, and the robotic arms.

Patients undergoing robotic prostatectomy receive a general anesthetic. The perioperative nurse assists with positioning the patient in the supine position with his legs in Allen stirrups. Once the procedure begins, the anesthesia provider places the patient in the Trendelenburg position to displace the viscera from the pelvis into the upper abdomen to improve visualization. Once the patient is positioned and draped, the patient instrument cart is docked, and instruments are inserted into the patient; even if the patient's condition deteriorates and something needs to be done that involves moving the patient, the patient cannot be moved until the

instruments are removed or it could cause serious damage to the internal organs (Uffort and Jensen, 2011). Surgeons may use a transperitoneal or extraperitoneal approach to the prostatectomy. The transperitoneal approach is described in the next section.

Operative Procedure

1. The surgeon inserts a 22F Foley catheter and maintains it within the sterile field.

2. Pneumoperitoneum is established using either a Veress needle placed at the base of the umbilicus or an open trocar placement with a Hasson technique, depending on the surgeon's preference.

3. The surgeon inserts the 0-degree endoscope through the 12-mm cannula and places the remaining ports as described under direct vision: two ports are inserted on each side of the pararectus and two additional ports are placed two to three fingerbreadths medial to the patient's right and left anterior superior iliac spine.

4. The sterile team docks the robot, and the perioperative nurse transfers the cart with the robotic arms to the field and assists the scrub person with draping. The scrub person assists with connecting the robotic manipulators and other system components.

5. The surgeon moves to the console and the assistant remains in the sterile field to operate the clip applicator and suction devices.

6. From the remote location at the console, the surgeon incises the peritoneum over the vas deferens and divides them.

7. The seminal vesicles are dissected and the surgeon incises Denonvilliers fascia.

8. Using blunt dissection, the surgeon develops a plane between Denonvilliers fascia and the rectum. The surgeon identifies the endopelvic fascia, dissects it, and makes a bilateral incision.

9. The Foley catheter is removed and the assistant replaces it with a metal sound. Using a figure-of-eight 2-0 polyglactin suture, the surgeon suture-ligates the deep dorsal venous complex. The sound ensures that the urethra is not incorporated into the ligature (Figure 15-41).

FIGURE 15-41 Intraoperative view demonstrating passage of a suture incorporating the deep dorsal vein complex during robotic-assisted laparoscopic radical prostatectomy.

FIGURE 15-42 Intraoperative view demonstrating the use of a running continuous suture for the vesicourethral anastomosis.

10. Using ultrasonic shears or the monopolar ESU, the surgeon incises the anterior and posterior bladder neck. Endo Clips are placed along the lateral pedicles as necessary for hemostasis.
11. Dissection continues along the lateral surface of the prostate and the neurovascular bundles are identified.
12. The surgeon divides the dorsal vein and divides the urethra distal to the apex of the prostate.
13. The gland is freed and placed in an entrapment bag.
14. Using a running or interrupted 2-0 polyglactin suture, the surgeon performs the urethrovesical anastomosis (Figure 15-42). The assistant fills the bladder with 100 to 150 mL of irrigant to test the anastomosis. Any visible leaks are repaired with additional suture.
15. A closed-suction drain is placed in the prevesical space.
16. The assistant extends the incision at the umbilical port site and removes the specimen.
17. The surgeon closes the port incisions.

Surgery of the Bladder

Operations on the urinary bladder may be performed through an open abdominal incision or a transurethral route. Diagnostic procedures are often undertaken via the transurethral route. Bladder tumors, diverticula, congenital defects, or trauma may necessitate an open abdominal approach. A thorough diagnostic workup and endoscopic examination help to determine the appropriate surgical approach to be used. Radical procedures, such as total cystectomy, are performed for the treatment of invasive carcinoma of the bladder and require permanent urinary diversion.

For most open-bladder surgery the patient is placed in the supine position with a bolster under the pelvis. The Trendelenburg position may be desired because this position tilts the head down and allows the viscera to fall cephalad. This allows excellent exposure of the pelvic organs, including the bladder. The patient is draped as described for routine suprapubic prostatectomy, using a disposable impermeable drape that is placed immediately below the bladder incision. A catheter may be inserted into the urethra and the bladder distended with sterile saline at the start of surgery for easy identification. An ESU is required. The instrument setup for open-bladder operations requires a basic laparotomy set, plus

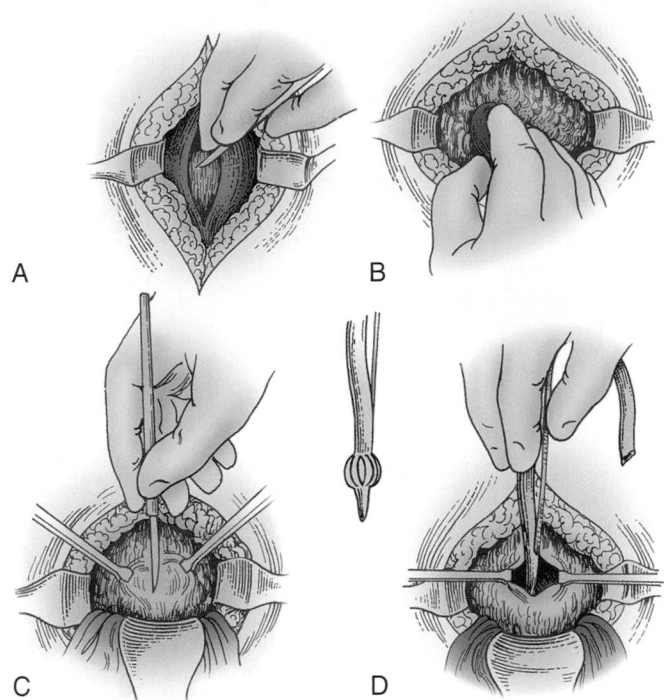

A   B

C   D

FIGURE 15-43 Suprapubic cystostomy.

Mason-Judd bladder retractors, long and short thyroid traction forceps, retropubic needle holders (or other long needle holders), one trocar, vessel loops, a catheter stylet, a closed-wound suction system, and assorted Foley, Pezzer, and Malecot catheters.

Suprapubic Cystostomy

Cystotomy is an opening made into the urinary bladder through a low abdominal incision. When a drainage tube is inserted into the bladder through an abdominal incision, the procedure is a cystostomy.

Procedural Considerations. The patient is in the supine position. Anesthesia may be general, spinal, or local with sedation. A basic laparotomy set is generally sufficient for the procedure. Foley catheters ranging from 22F to 30F should be available, as well as Malecot suprapubic catheters and a drainage bag. Frequently a flexible cystoscopy is incorporated as part of the procedure.

Operative Procedure

1. After making a vertical or Pfannenstiel incision the surgeon divides the rectus fascia along the midline (Figure 15-43, *A*).
2. The bladder is distended with saline solution that is instilled with an Asepto syringe through a catheter.
3. The surgeon uses sharp and blunt dissection to dissect free the dome of the bladder (see Figure 15-43, *B*).
4. Using a pair of Martius forceps, the surgeon grasps the walls of the bladder on either side of the midline (see Figure 15-43, *C*).
5. Two traction sutures may be placed through the bladder wall and held with straight hemostats.
6. The surgeon incises the bladder downward with a scalpel. Bleeding vessels in the bladder wall are clamped and ligated.
7. The bladder contents are aspirated with a suction device.

FIGURE 15-44 Laser fulguration.

FIGURE 15-45 Resectoscope with bridge.

uncovered during this short resection procedure, water absorption with hemolysis and systemic complications such as hyponatremia do not occur. In addition, cancer cells released during the procedure tend to absorb water, causing them to rupture and lyse rather than remain viable and capable of implanting themselves into the raw surface of the bladder created by the surgery. When the procedure is completed, the surgeon passes a large catheter, usually a 24F, into the bladder and connects it to drainage.

Transurethral Laser Ablation of Bladder Tumors

The Nd:YAG or Ho:YAG laser may be used to destroy small recurrent bladder tumors and to coagulate the tumor bed of larger bladder tumors resected with an electrosurgical loop. A powerful, highly focused beam of light in the near-infrared range is transmitted to the tumor site through a flexible glass fiber. This laser fiber is passed through the catheter channel of a cystoscope, and the fiber is directed by a deflecting laser bridge (Figure 15-45). The advantages of a laser in the eradication of bladder tumors are as follows: (1) bleeding is minimized, (2) only sedation is required, (3) the operating time is shortened, (4) there is minimal damage to healthy tissue, and (5) postoperative drainage of the bladder by a urethral catheter is not needed.

Alternatives to Surgery for Superficial Bladder Cancer

Patients with various types of cancer may be treated in the urology office setting with various therapeutic modalities including the instillation of chemotherapeutic solutions. These measures may be initiated instead of surgery or as an adjunct to surgery. Instillations are aimed at eradicating existing disease, reducing tumor recurrence and progression, and improving overall patient survival (Steinberg, 2011).

Patients with bladder cancer that has been staged as Ta, carcinoma in situ (CIS), and T1 may be treated with intravesical, antineoplastic chemotherapy agents such as *thiotepa* (Thioplax), *mitomycin C* (Mutamycin), *doxorubicin* (Adriamycin), and *etoglucid* (Epodyl). Chemotherapy has become the treatment of choice for low-risk patients.

Immunotherapy with *bacille Calmette-Guérin (BCG)* (TheraCys or Tice) is used to treat patients considered to have high-risk tumors. BCG, through an unknown mechanism, strengthens the body's immune reaction to cancer and is considered the most effective therapy for recurrent and residual bladder cancer.

Combination chemotherapy and immunotherapy have become standard treatment for patients with metastatic transitional cell carcinoma. BCG has been combined with *mitomycin C* and with *interferon alfa-2b*. The latter combination has been highly effective, rescuing approximately 60% of those who failed with BCG alone (Steinberg, 2011).

Trocar Cystostomy

Trocar cystostomy consists of draining the bladder by puncture with a needle or trocar and inserting a catheter.

8. The bladder opening may be extended if the bladder is to be explored for diverticula or calculi.
9. The surgeon inserts a large-size Malecot or Pezzer catheter into the bladder (see Figure 15-43, *D*).
10. The incision is closed snugly about the catheter with absorbable sutures to render the closure watertight around the cystostomy tube.
11. The muscle, fascia, and subcutaneous tissue are closed with absorbable suture.
12. The surgeon closes the skin with staples or suture.
13. The cystostomy tube is secured to the skin with a 0 or 2-0 nonabsorbable suture to prevent it from being inadvertently dislodged from the bladder. A drain such as a Jackson-Pratt may be left in the prevesical space.
14. The wound is dressed, and the cystostomy tube is connected to a straight urinary drainage system.

Transurethral Resection of Bladder Tumors

Bladder lesions may be removed using a standard resectoscope, working element, loop, and a foroblique telescope, which is passed through the urethra into the bladder. A 24F cystoscope sheath with a catheterizing bridge and biopsy forceps may be used to remove bladder tumors located at the very top or dome of the bladder (Figure 15-44). Transitional cell carcinoma of the bladder is one of the most difficult lesions to track because it can occur wherever there is transitional cell lining of the urinary tract. Bladder cancer has a tendency to recur in other areas of the bladder, even after complete resection of the original lesion.

Usually the surgeon removes not only the bladder lesion but also a portion of the bladder muscle underlying the lesion so that the pathologist can determine if any tumor has invaded the muscle. Random biopsy specimens of the normal bladder lining are also taken to ascertain if microscopic transitional cell carcinoma in situ is present. Lesions that deeply invade the muscle must be treated with an open surgical procedure, such as a partial cystectomy or total cystectomy.

The resection technique, setup, and preparation of the patient are virtually the same as those for TURP. The anesthesia provider administers a general, spinal, or regional anesthetic. A retrograde pyelogram may be done to check for lesions in the upper urinary tract.

Sterile water is recommended as an irrigating solution in transurethral resection of bladder tumors. Because few vessels are

Procedural Considerations. A minor instrument set along with a metal probe and grooved director, an Anthony suction tube and tubing, and trocar catheters or a prepackaged cystostomy kit is required. A local anesthetic may be used.

Operative Procedure

1. The surgeon nicks the skin at the site of the puncture with a scalpel and inserts the trocar into the bladder.
2. The trocar obturator is withdrawn, the bladder is drained through the trocar by suction, and a catheter is passed through the trocar cannula into the bladder.
3. The surgeon removes the cannula and sutures the catheter to the wound edges. The wound is dressed.

Suprapubic Cystolithotomy

Suprapubic cystolithotomy is the removal of calculi from the bladder. Obstructions, such as prostatic enlargement or foreign bodies, are common causes of bladder calculi and may be corrected at the time of surgery. In the past, special transurethral instruments such as the lithotrite were commonly used to crush vesical calculi manually. Bladder stones are often eradicated via the electrohydraulic lithotripter, which fragments the stone within the bladder by using an electric current to initiate shock waves (Figure 15-46, *A*), or by ultrasonic lithotripsy.

During ultrasonic lithotripsy ultrasound waves are transmitted through a hollow metal probe, which creates vibration at the tip. When applied to the surface of a calculus, the vibrating tip drills and fragments the calculus. This mechanical disintegration is continued until the stone is reduced to small fragments that are evacuated by suction through the hollow center of the probe (see Figure 15-46, *B*). The Ho:YAG laser may also be used for fragmentation of bladder calculi.

Procedural Considerations. Instruments for open-bladder operations along with Millin T-shaped stone forceps, Millin capsule forceps, and Lewkowitz lithotomy forceps are required.

Operative Procedure. The surgical approach is similar to that described for suprapubic cystotomy. When the bladder is opened, calculi are identified and extracted. If indicated, bladder outlet obstruction is repaired.

Repair of Vesical Fistulas

Vesical fistulas occurring between the bladder and the intestines or vagina may be repaired surgically. *Vesicointestinal fistulas* may be caused by ulcerative colitis, diverticulitis, or neoplasms of the colon or rectum. *Vesicovaginal fistulas* may be a complication of radiotherapy for cervical cancer, endoscopic procedures involving surgery of the trigone or vesical neck, obstetric injuries, and hysterectomies.

Procedural Considerations. The instrument setup is as described for open-bladder operations. Intestinal instruments (see Chapter 11) are necessary for vesicointestinal fistulas. For vesicovaginal fistulas, vaginal preparation and a colporrhaphy set (see Chapter 14) with colostomy or ileostomy instruments are used.

Vesicointestinal fistulas are more common than vesicovaginal fistulas. Of the intestinal fistulas, the sigmoid colon is most often involved (Figure 15-47). A colostomy proximal to the fistula may be performed to protect the repaired segment of bowel. The communicating area of bladder and bowel is totally resected. Generally, an end-to-end bowel resection is performed after excision of the involved intestinal segment. The bladder is then repaired in three layers.

FIGURE 15-46 A, Electrohydraulic lithotripter. **B,** Ultrasonic lithotripter.

FIGURE 15-47 Vesicoenteric fistulogram (cystogram) showing contrast material in bladder *(B),* sigmoid colon *(S),* and rectum *(R).*

If the fistula is at the dome of the bladder, the approach will be transperitoneal, transvesical, or a combination of the two. If the fistula is in the trigone of the bladder, a vaginal approach may be used. A suprapubic tube is usually left in the bladder.

Operative Procedure
Vesicovaginal Fistula Repair—Vaginal Approach

1. Before placing the patient in the hyperflexed lithotomy or Kraske position (jackknife), the surgeon inserts a suprapubic catheter, clamps it, and connects it to closed drainage. If the intended position is Kraske, separate draping material and instrumentation are set up for the suprapubic catheter insertion with the patient supine. The catheter is secured, and the patient is turned for the procedure.

2. The area is draped with a lithotomy or laparotomy sheet as indicated per the patient's position.

3. The surgeon sutures the labia to the outer groin or inner thigh for retraction and visualization.

4. A weighted vaginal retractor is placed posteriorly, and the defect is examined. A relaxing vaginal incision may be necessary at the 5 or 7 o'clock position.

5. The surgeon inserts a 4F ureteral catheter through the fistula, and dilates the tract to admit an 8F balloon catheter. The balloon is inflated, and the catheter is used as a retractor.

6. The area is infiltrated with vasopressin (Pitressin) solution.

7. The surgeon incises the vaginal mucosa and perivesical fascia around the defect outside of the scarred tissue.

8. Two planes are developed—one between the mucosa and fascia and one between the fascia and the bladder wall—with fine scissors, forceps, and gauze (Kittner) dissectors.

9. The bladder wall is freed from the vaginal wall.

10. The vesical defect is grasped with Martius clamps, the scarred edges are everted, and the defect is closed vertically with interrupted 3-0 absorbable sutures after removal of the catheter previously placed. In some instances, a labial pedicle or full-thickness flap (Martius flap) may be placed between the vesical closure and the vaginal closure (Figure 15-48). This prevents suture-line stress and overlay and removes the need for a relaxing incision. Larger fistulas that do not adequately reapproximate may necessitate a vascularized muscle flap to reinforce closure.

11. The surgeon approximates the perivesical fascia and vaginal mucosa separately with transverse interrupted 3-0 absorbable sutures. A one-sided ellipse of vaginal mucosa may be excised to offset the closure.

12. Alternatively, an inverted-U incision may provide more exposure than other incisions and result in a posterior flap that completely covers the site of the defect.

13. The surgeon unclamps the suprapubic catheter, removes the labial stitches, and loosely packs the vagina.

Vesicovaginal Fistula Repair—Transperitoneal (Transvesical) Approach

1. The patient is placed in the low lithotomy and moderate Trendelenburg position. Both the perineum and the abdomen are prepped and draped appropriately. A laparoscopy pack works well for this approach.

2. The surgeon inserts ureteral catheters and places a 16F Foley catheter in the bladder and clamps it.

3. Tight gauze packing is placed into the vagina.

4. The surgeon makes a vertical midline or Pfannenstiel incision.

5. The peritoneum is incised and bluntly dissected from the dome of the bladder.

6. The small bowel is packed cephalad.

7. Stay sutures of 2-0 absorbable material are placed in the bladder dome, and the bladder is opened.

8. The surgeon divides the bladder wall and overlying peritoneum down to the fistula. Stay sutures are placed periodically to serve as retractors for bladder elevation.

9. The peritoneum is incised transversely at the level of the fistula, forming a pedicle flap.

10. The vagina and bladder are separated widely on each side of the fistula. An assistant places upward pressure on the packing to facilitate dissection.

11. As the fistula is exposed, the surgeon excises it until it is completely removed. A probe may be used to localize it, if small, or an 8F balloon catheter may be inserted and used for traction during dissection.

12. The bladder and vagina are freed from each other until there is enough mobility for separate closures.

13. The surgeon closes the vagina, without tension, with inverting 2-0 or 3-0 interrupted sutures in two layers.

FIGURE 15-48 Creation of Martius flap.

14. The peritoneal flap is swung into the defect and sutured in place for reperitonealization. A long, attached peritoneal or free peritoneal pedicle flap may be needed for reperitonealization. Alternatively, the omentum may be manipulated from behind the right side of the colon for an omental graft. A vascularized muscle flap may be placed for fistulas resulting from radiation necrosis.

15. A 22F Malecot catheter and a wound drain are inserted and pulled through separate stab wounds in the abdomen.

16. The ureteral catheters are removed, and the bladder mucosa and submucosa are closed in separate layers with 2-0 or 3-0 absorbable suture in a running fashion.

17. The muscularis and adventitia are externally approximated with interrupted 3-0 sutures.

18. The wound is closed in layers.

19. Dressings are applied, the Foley is unclamped, the packing is removed, and the vagina is loosely repacked.

Vesicosigmoid Fistula Repair—Abdominal Approach

1. With the patient in the Trendelenburg position, a 20F or 22F, 5-mL Foley catheter is inserted and the bladder filled with 100 mL of sterile water. After the patient is prepped and draped as described for laparotomy, a midline, or paramedian, and transperitoneal incisions are made.

2. The surgeon explores the abdomen.

3. The descending colon and sigmoid colon are mobilized by incising along the fascia fusion line of Toldt.

4. The involved loop of colon is identified. If a walled-off inflammatory mass is found, a transverse colostomy may be performed and a two-stage intervention considered.

5. Using blunt dissection, the surgeon separates the fistulous tract.

6. A probe is inserted to determine the extent of involvement.

7. The defects in the bladder and bowel are debrided to obtain healthy tissue. Large inflammatory masses require a colon resection.

8. The surgeon closes the bladder in two layers with a 3-0 absorbable submucosal running stitch and a 2-0 absorbable interrupted muscularis and adventitial stitch.

9. The edges of the bowel defect are trimmed to reach normal tissue, and stay sutures are placed on each side.

10. The cavity is pulled transversely, and the mucosa and submucosa are closed in one pass with a Connell stitch of 3-0 chromic catgut.

11. The surgeon approximates and closes the muscularis and serosa in one pass with 4-0 silk Lembert sutures.

12. The abdomen is irrigated with 2000 mL of sterile saline with an attempt to reach all areas.

13. A sump-style drain is placed intraperitoneally, and a Penrose or small Jackson-Pratt drain is placed suprapubically, exiting through separate stab wounds.

14. The surgeon closes the abdomen in layers in the conventional manner. If a colostomy was performed, it is opened for fecal diversion and the appropriate appliance applied.

15. Gauze and bulky absorbable dressings are applied and secured; Montgomery straps may be used.

Vesicourethral (Marshall-Marchetti-Krantz) Suspension

A Marshall-Marchetti-Krantz suspension is performed for the correction of stress incontinence caused by an abnormal urethrovesical angle. The intent of the Marshall-Marchetti-Krantz operation is to bring the bladder and urethra into the pelvis by suturing paraurethral vaginal tissue to the back of the symphysis pubis. A modification of this technique is the Burch procedure. The approach mimics the Marshall-Marchetti-Krantz until placement of the buttressing sutures. Instead of attempting difficult periosteal sutures, the surgeon places nonabsorbable size 0 sutures into the Cooper ligament from each side of the bladder neck. The Burch procedure is technically easier, and long-term results are fairly equivalent.

A large percentage of patients with stress incontinence are obese and have diabetes. It is important to evaluate for these conditions and prepare for proper patient management (i.e., positioning concerns relating to peripheral vascular circulation and pressure points, skin breakdown, risk for infection, wound healing).

Procedural Considerations. The patient is usually placed in a moderate Trendelenburg position, frog-legged, with supports under each knee to allow for intraoperative vaginal manipulation. Abdominal and vaginal preps are required. A Foley catheter is inserted at the beginning of surgery. Both the surgeon and assistant double-glove for vaginal manipulation. Basic laparotomy and abdominal hysterectomy instruments (see Chapter 14), if needed, are used. Postoperatively, the patient commonly has a vaginal pack, a urethral catheter with or without a suprapubic catheter, and possibly a wound drain.

Operative Procedure

1. The surgeon makes a suprapubic transverse incision and exposes the prevesical space of Retzius.

2. The bladder retractor is positioned with small, moist laparotomy packs in place.

3. Using blunt dissection, the surgeon frees the bladder and urethra from the posterior surface of the rectus muscle and symphysis pubis.

4. The assistant places two fingers into the vagina, lifting the urethra upward against the symphysis pubis to facilitate ease of repair of the periurethral musculofascial structures.

5. A heavy, nonabsorbable atraumatic suture on a Heaney needle holder is placed through the supporting fascia of the vaginal wall on each side of the urethra. The suture is passed through the symphysis pubis, providing support to the urethra and bladder neck. Generally, a row of three heavy, nonabsorbable sutures is placed on each side of the urethra, the most proximal located just at the vesical neck.

6. The surgeon closes the wound in layers.

7. The vagina may be packed with 2-inch packing, which is removed after 24 to 36 hours.

Tension-Free Vaginal Tape Sling

A tension-free vaginal tape (TVT) sling is indicated for women diagnosed with urethral hypermobility, intrinsic sphincter deficiency, and pure stress incontinence caused by pelvic floor relaxation. It will not correct urge incontinence, although it may be used in women with combination stress and urge incontinence. This patient will need to have her urge incontinence controlled in another manner. It appears to be a viable option for the overweight and older female and for women who have had previous corrective measures that failed. It is not recommended for younger women who are pregnant or intend to become pregnant. Other contraindications include patients with intrinsic bleeding problems or who are receiving anticoagulant therapy. Risks include bladder perforation, perforation of pelvic viscera adherent to the pubis, retropubic

FIGURE 15-49 A, Uretex self-anchoring urethral support system. **B,** Pelvitex polypropylene mesh.

hemorrhage and hematoma formation, infection, and urinary retention.

The tape is composed of polypropylene mesh (Figure 15-49) encased in a plastic sleeve that has a center slit and is secured to a large, curved trocar needle at each end. A T-shaped introducer is attached to these needles for passage of the sling material. The mesh is passed through the pelvic tissue and positioned under the urethra, creating a supportive sling. Unlike other corrective procedures for incontinence, no screws, anchors, or internal sutures are required.

Procedural Considerations. The procedure may be performed using a local anesthetic with monitored sedation. After the sedation is administered, the perioperative nurse places the patient in the lithotomy position.

Operative Procedure

1. A 16F or 18F Foley catheter is inserted to drain the bladder.
2. The surgeon injects local anesthetic through the skin and into the muscle and fascia lateral to the midline and just above the symphysis pubis, bilaterally. Vasopressin (Pitressin) is commonly added to the anesthetic to help control bleeding.
3. Additional local anesthetic is injected suburethrally into the anterior vaginal mucosa to the retropubic space, bilaterally.
4. The surgeon performs a cystoscopy to confirm integrity of the bladder wall, urethral patency and length, and location of the ureters.
5. Two incisions, 0.5 to 1 cm in length, are made in the abdominal skin over each injection site.
6. The surgeon places a weighted speculum in the vagina, and grasps the anterior vaginal mucosa with two Allis clamps.
7. Using a #10 or #15 scalpel the surgeon makes a 1.5-cm incision into the anterior vaginal mucosa, 1 cm to the right of the external meatus.
8. Blunt Metzenbaum scissors are used to dissect suburethrally and periurethrally to the level of the endopelvic fascia.
9. The surgeon inserts a rigid stylet into the Foley catheter, and inserts the catheter into the bladder.
10. The bladder neck and urethra are deflected away to allow passage of the first needle by holding the Foley with its stylet against the inner ipsilateral thigh. An Allis clamp or hemostat may be placed in the center of the sling material to prevent twisting of the mesh or its sleeve.
11. After attaching the introducer, the first needle is passed 1 cm lateral to the urethra with the curve of the needle in the palm of the surgeon's hand. The needle penetrates the urogenital diaphragm behind the symphysis pubis.

12. Two fingers of the other hand are placed over the skin incision, the needle is pushed through the retropubic space, and the introducer is removed. The needle is guided up to partially protrude through the abdominal wall.
13. Before the trocar needle is extracted and removed, the surgeon removes the Foley and performs a cystoscopy. When bladder integrity has been confirmed, the first needle may be brought out through the abdominal wall and cut from the sling material, and a hemostat is attached to the mesh and sleeve.
14. The procedure is then repeated on the other side with the Foley directed toward the ipsilateral inner thigh during insertion and passage of the needle.
15. Once the tape is in place, the surgeon positions an 8F Hegar dilator between the tape and the urethra for tension testing. The patient is asked to cough, and the tape is adjusted until there is no leak or only a few drops of fluid are lost during coughing. The plastic sleeves are then removed by pulling them up through the abdominal incisions. The excess mesh that protrudes is cut at the skin surface.
16. The surgeon closes the vaginal mucosa with a running stitch of 2-0 chromic suture. Wound closure strips or skin sutures are used to close the abdominal incisions.
17. A perineal pad may be placed to absorb any vaginal bleeding. Abdominal dressings are applied at the surgeon's discretion. Vaginal packing and a postoperative Foley catheter are usually not necessary.

Transvaginal Sling with Bone Anchor

Indications and contraindications for this procedure are the same as those for the TVT sling procedure. The patient with severe osteoporosis may not be a good candidate for this technique because the bone anchors may not integrate into the pubic bone properly.

Risks with this technique include bladder perforation, inadequate fixation of the bone anchor (this generally requires abandoning the method and using a different type of sling approach), urinary retention, pain, osteitis pubis or osteomyelitis of the pubic bone, and recurrent incontinence.

Procedural Considerations. The procedure may be performed using a local anesthetic with monitored sedation. After the sedation is administered, the perioperative nurse places the patient in the lithotomy position. A formal incision may not be necessary for this procedure.

Operative Procedure

1. Before the procedure the scrub person loads a bone screw with preloaded #1 polypropylene suture onto the bone drill. A plastic cover fits over the screw, protecting the patient during insertion.
2. A Foley catheter is inserted, the bladder drained, and the catheter clamped.
3. The surgeon places Allis clamps on the mucosa and pulls gently upward to expose the anterior vaginal wall.
4. Tension is put on the polypropylene stitch that protrudes through the handle of the bone drill. The surgeon inserts the drill into the vagina in a line parallel to the plane of the symphysis pubis, and holds the drill head against the pubic bone (Figure 15-50).
5. Insertion is complete when the polypropylene stitch stops rotating. Fixation of the screw is tested with a gentle downward tug on the suture. The bone screws should lie lateral to

FIGURE 15-50 A, Bone anchor on bone drill with #1 polypropylene. **B,** Bone drill ready; polypropylene extends out handle *(arrow).* **C,** Bone drill in place.

FIGURE 15-51 Fascia lata graft being placed for suburethral sling procedure.

the symphysis pubis in the posterior mid-third of the pubic bone.

6. The Foley is opened and drained. If the urine is bloody a cystoscopy is performed. Some surgeons choose to routinely perform cystoscopy after each screw insertion to evaluate bladder patency.
7. A right-angle clamp is used to follow the tunnel of the polypropylene suture upward. A small puncture is created in the urethropelvic ligament to allow passage of the sling material into the retropubic space. The sling material may be cadaveric fascia or polypropylene mesh.
8. The surgeon creates a 2-cm tunnel between the midurethra and bladder neck, behind the vaginal wall.
9. The sling material is perforated with a Keith needle, and the polypropylene suture is passed through the eye of the needle. The suture is then transferred to the sling material. This is done twice on each end of the material.
10. The material is passed through the tunnel (Figure 15-51).
11. Following cystoscopy, steps 4 through 6 are repeated on the contralateral vaginal wall. The polypropylene sutures are tied individually so that the material lies close to the pubic bone.

12. The vagina is sutured on each side with a single stitch of absorbable 2-0 suture.
13. A vaginal pack soaked in antibiotic or estrogen cream is inserted. The Foley catheter is drained and attached to a closed drainage system.

Implantation of InterStim Sacral Nerve Stimulator (Neuromodulator)

The InterStim system is indicated for the treatment of urinary urge incontinence, urinary retention, and significant urgency-frequency in patients who have failed or could not tolerate other measures (Gross et al, 2010). The procedure is performed in two stages. During the first stage a lead is implanted and connected to an external stimulator. The patient is discharged and undergoes a trial period that lasts from 2 to 4 weeks to determine if the device will be effective. During this trial period the patient maintains a diary to track symptoms and postvoid residuals. If the trial is successful, the patient will return for the subcutaneous implantation of a pulse generator.

Some precautions must be taken by the patient who has had this device implanted. MRI studies are not recommended. Caution should be taken and the device turned off if the ESU will be used during any future surgery the patient might undergo. Female patients should be instructed to carry their purses on the opposite side of the implant.

Procedural Considerations. The perioperative nurse assists with positioning the patient in the prone position with a 30-degree flexion at the hips. Pillows may be placed under the patient's abdomen to support the lumbar area and decrease lordosis. Pillows are also placed under the ankles to elevate the feet and prevent pressure on the toes.

C-arm fluoroscopy is used to visualize sacral landmarks and verify lead position intraoperatively. Although general anesthesia may be used, monitored sedation with a local anesthetic is preferable so that the patient may verbally respond to nerve stimuli during the procedure. It is suggested that no IV muscle relaxants be administered because this will affect the physiologic response to the stimulator. If electrocoagulation is needed, a bipolar system should be used, because unipolar current could travel into the sacral foramen. The patient is typically discharged from the hospital on the same day.

The nurse preps the patient's sacral area, buttocks, and perineum and applies the test stimulation ground pad to the patient's heel. An alternative to this placement is the calf or skin below the rib cage or iliac crest. The pad is approximately 5 to 8 cm in size. The pad is attached by a test stimulation cable to the external stimulator. The patient is draped to expose the entire buttock area so that responses to nerve stimulation may be assessed. The feet and lower legs are also exposed to allow visualization of muscle response.

The surgeon locates and marks the sacral outline, S3 foramen, posterior iliac spine, coccygeal tip, and midline. To locate these landmarks, the surgeon palpates the upper border of the greater sciatic notch. The S3 sacral foramen is approximately one finger-breadth from the midline, whereas the S2 and S4 foramina are one fingerbreadth above and below S3. The sacral crest corresponds to S4, and the S3 foramen is 9 cm above the coccygeal tip and 2 cm from the midline.

Operative Procedure

1. The surgeon inserts the needle into the S3 foramen. The external stimulator is activated to confirm correct placement of the needle. A bellows response (flattening of the perineum) and flexion of the great toe indicate the needle is in the S3 foramen.
2. The guidewire is inserted into the foramen needle.
3. A 5-mm stab wound is created for the lead introducer.
4. The surgeon slides the lead introducer, consisting of dilator and sheath, over the guidewire and advances it into the foramen. The depth marker on the directional guide is aligned with the top of the dilator.
5. The dilator is then removed, and the sheath remains in place.
6. The surgeon inserts the tined lead, with its stylet (Figure 15-52), and passes it through the sheath until the second white

FIGURE 15-52 InterStim tined lead.

marker is aligned with the back of the sheath. The four electrodes on the lead are now exposed and visible on fluoroscopy.

7. Nerve responses are again assessed at this time by connecting the mini-J hook on the patient cable to the uninsulated section of the foramen needle. The electrodes are numbered zero to three, and the connector contacts on the needle correspond to these numbers. Beginning at the distal tip of the needle, all four electrodes are tested. The lead is repositioned according to the verbalized and visualized responses of the patient. The foramen producing the best results is chosen.
8. After the electrodes are in optimal position, the lead body proximal to the sheath is held in place and the sheath is slowly backed out of the wound. This is often accomplished under fluoroscopy.
9. As the sheath is withdrawn, the tines on the lead open, anchoring it in place.
10. The surgeon creates a tunnel for the subcutaneous neurostimulator generator pocket by means of the same incision. Placement is in the upper buttock below the beltline.
11. A pocket is created with the bipolar ESU. The pocket depth should not be greater than 4 cm to avoid interference with programming and shifting of the neurostimulator. The ideal pocket is 3 to 5 cm below the superior iliac crest and lateral to the outer sacral edge.
12. The surgeon uses the tunneling tool with its metal tip and plastic tube to develop the tunnel from the lead to the intended pocket. Once tunneling is achieved the metal tip is removed and the tool is withdrawn, leaving the plastic tubing in place. The proximal lead end is then fed through the tubing to the pocket, and the tubing is removed. The protective boot is placed over the end of the lead. Leads may be placed bilaterally at the surgeon's discretion.
13. The percutaneous extension is then tunneled from the eventual generator site to the opposite posterior iliac side, and exits the skin. This is then attached to the external device.
14. The incisions at all wound sites are closed. The wounds are dressed with small gauze and an occlusive dressing.

If the patient has a good response (50% or greater decrease in symptoms), then the area of generator site is extended in a second stage and the generator is connected to the lead (Figures 15-53 and 15-54). The percutaneous extension is pulled out through the other side and taken away from the field.

Male Perineal Sling

The male perineal sling is designed to improve male incontinence by increasing outlet resistance. Using cadaveric dermis, fascia lata, or pericardium, the surgeon places a triangular sling under the bulbous urethra and anchors it with six screws that are placed into the inner portion of the descending ramus just below the symphysis pubis. Other treatments for incontinence, including the use of botulinum A toxin, are being investigated.

Bladder Augmentation

Augmentation enterocystoplasty is a procedure performed to surgically enlarge the bladder capacity. A wide range of conditions that were previously treated with urinary diversion may now be successfully managed with this technique. Indications include reflex incontinence unresponsive to medical management, detrusor hyperactivity with compromised bladder function, chronically contracted bladder resulting from radiation or repeated infections, and neuropathic bladder combined with recurrent urinary tract infections or

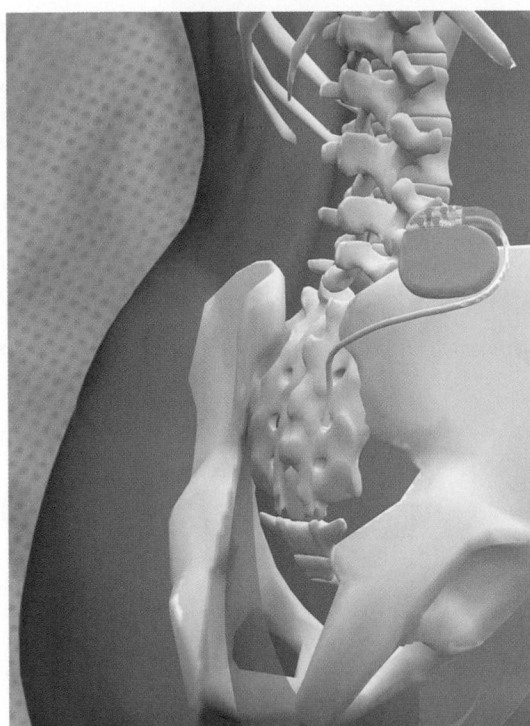

FIGURE 15-53 Graphic placement of InterStim.

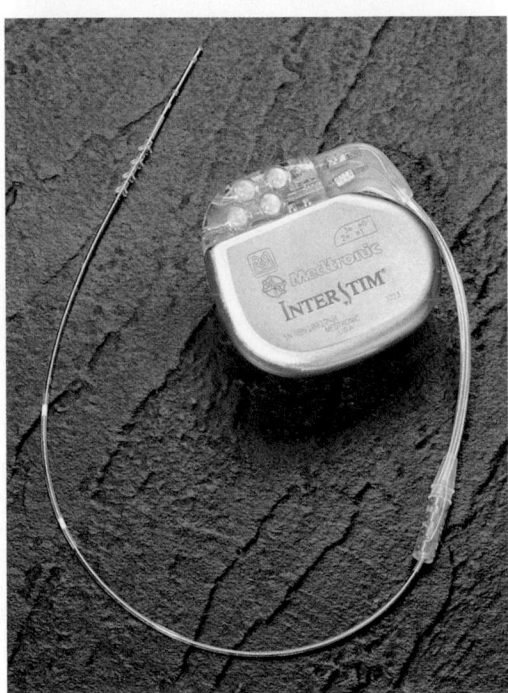

FIGURE 15-54 InterStim implant.

compromised renal function. A segment of bowel is used to augment the bladder. The bowel is re-formed into a semispheric shape to decrease peristaltic contractions and anastomosed to the opened bladder dome. The result is a low-pressure reservoir that provides improved bladder capacity and urinary compliance. Almost all segments of bowel as well as the stomach have been used for bladder

augmentation. Selection depends on anatomic factors, functional characteristics, and the surgeon's preference. In some cases, ureteral reimplantation or associated bladder-outlet procedures are incorporated in a one-stage procedure.

Postoperatively, intermittent catheterization and bladder irrigations may be necessary. The patient must be able and willing to learn and perform these procedures and must be accepting of this alteration in lifestyle.

Procedural Considerations. The nurse assists with positioning the patient in the supine position after the anesthesia provider administers a general or regional anesthetic. The female patient may be in a frog-leg or lithotomy position, particularly if access to the perineum is necessary. The entire abdomen and genitalia are prepped and draped. The surgeon inserts a Foley catheter after the patient has been prepped and draped so that the bladder can be filled to capacity for visualization during the procedure. Basic laparotomy and intestinal instruments are required.

Operative Procedure

1. The surgeon makes a supraumbilical to symphysis midline abdominal incision.
2. The peritoneal cavity is exposed using a Bookwalter or similar retractor.
3. The surgeon examines the intestines and stomach, and chooses the appropriate segment for reconstruction (Figure 15-55, *A*).
4. A sagittal bladder incision is made from 2 cm cephalad to the bladder neck anteriorly across the anterior bladder wall, the peritonealized dome surface, and the posterior bladder wall to 2 cm above the posterior interureteric ridge. This causes the bladder to be bivalved in a clam-shaped design.
5. The surgeon places bilateral traction sutures along the bladder incision.
6. The length of the incision is measured to correlate with the corresponding segment of bowel or stomach. Average length required is 25 cm.
7. The surgeon mobilizes the segment of bowel and closes the mesentery cephalad so that the segment is on the retroperitoneum. The segment is left attached to its mesentery to maintain blood supply (see Figure 15-55, *B*).
8. The isolated segment is opened, trimmed, and detubularized. The surgeon then folds it double and sutures it to form a cup patch (see Figure 15-55, *C*).
9. Anastomosis is accomplished with a running, intermittent locking, absorbable suture, beginning at the posterior apex and running up each side.
10. With one third of the attachment complete, the surgeon places sutures at the anterior apex and runs them bilaterally to meet cephalad (see Figure 15-55, *D*).
11. The surgeon fills the bladder to check the integrity of the anastomosis.
12. Abdominal closure is performed, and dressings are applied. The Foley catheter will remain for 7 to 14 days. Some surgeons may choose to place a suprapubic catheter instead of a Foley.

Implantation of Prosthetic Urethral Sphincter

Implantation of a prosthetic urethral sphincter is usually done as a last measure for patients with stress incontinence when other modalities have failed. Problems with the device have included foreign-body reaction, persistent urethral pressure causing urethral erosion, and fluid hydraulic failure. The artificial sphincter unit has

FIGURE 15-55 Ileocystoplasty for bladder augmentation.

an abdominally placed, pressure-regulated reservoir that maintains a constant predetermined pressure on the periurethral cuff. Because of the connection between the reservoir and cuff, any increase in intra-abdominal pressure transmits more fluid into the cuff. This connection allows for a compensatory increase in urethral resistance during coughing or straining.

The scrotal or labial pump shifts the fluid into the cuff to the reservoir to allow bladder emptying. The fluid reenters the cuff through a resistor in about 60 to 120 seconds. The locking button in the AMS 800 artificial sphincter unit traps fluid in the reservoir to allow activation of the cuff. The sphincter is available in a single-cuff and double-cuff model.

Procedural Considerations. Standard laparotomy and lithotomy setups are required, as well as the sphincter components, contrast material diluted according to the manufacturer's recommendations, and an antibiotic solution. The patient is placed in a modified lithotomy position.

Stricture disease is more commonly found in the male population, and the most common cuff placement is around the bulbous urethra. Bladder neck placement of the cuff is generally reserved only for females.

Operative Procedure
Bulbous Urethral Cuff

1. Perineal and transverse suprapubic incisions are made.
2. The surgeon mobilizes the bulbous urethra through a midline perineal incision (Figure 15-56, *A*).
3. A 2-cm space is created beneath the bulbocavernosus muscle and around the bulbous urethra.
4. The surgeon places the cuff, tab end first, around the bulbous urethra (see Figure 15-56, *B*).
5. The reservoir is placed beneath the rectus muscle through the suprapubic incision (see Figure 15-56, *C*).
6. The surgeon attaches the pump to the tubing passer, introduces it through the suprapubic incision, and transfers it to the

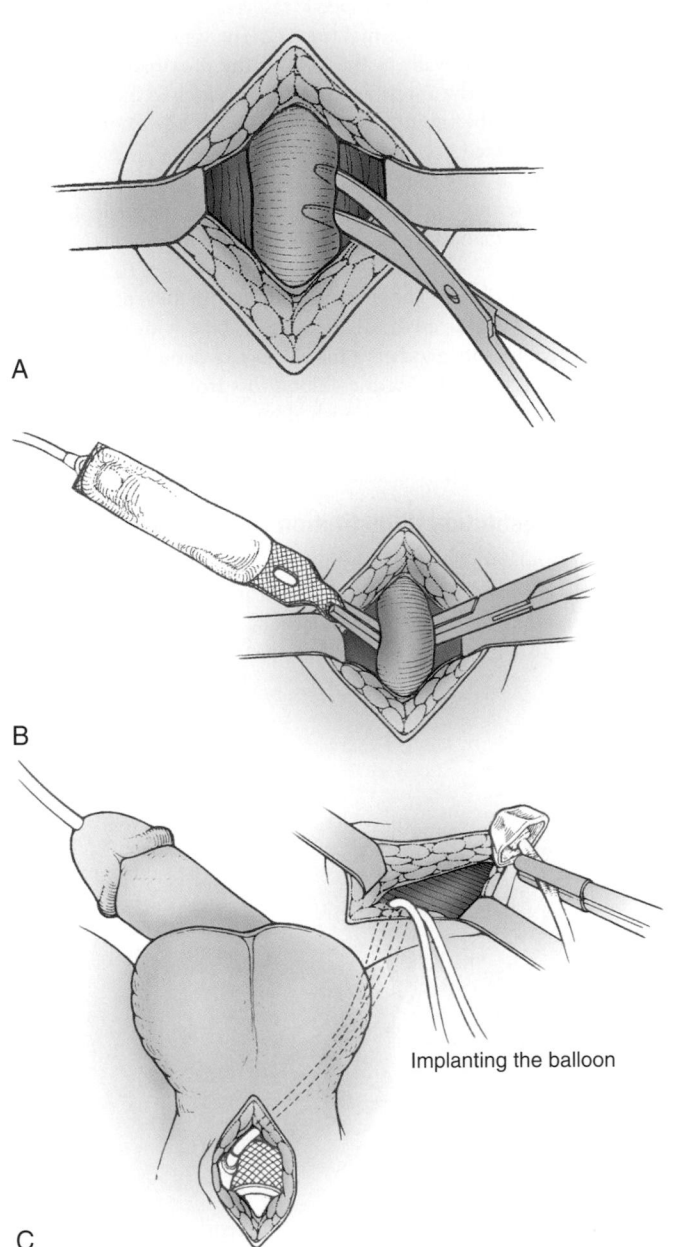

A

B

Implanting the balloon

C

FIGURE 15-56 Implantation of artificial urinary sphincter.

A

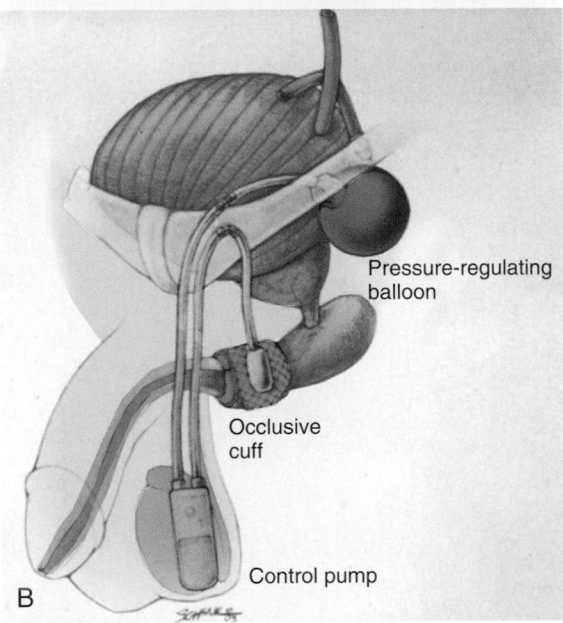

Pressure-regulating balloon

Occlusive cuff

Control pump

B

FIGURE 15-57 A, AMS 800 single-cuff artificial urinary sphincter. **B,** Final placement of artificial urinary sphincter.

scrotum through a subcutaneous tunnel created between the two incisions. The reservoir, cuff, and pump are connected and filled with contrast material or injectable saline to the appropriate volume (Figure 15-57).

7. The wound is closed and dressed with gauze sponges. A urethral catheter is usually not inserted.

Radical Cystectomy with Pelvic Lymphadenectomy

Cystectomy is the total excision of the urinary bladder and adjacent structures along with pelvic lymph nodes. Cystectomy is a surgical consideration when a vesical malignancy has invaded the muscular wall of the bladder or when frequent recurrences of widespread papillary tumors do not respond to endoscopic or chemotherapeutic management. The patient should be medically able to withstand surgery with the expectation of reasonable longevity. Total cystectomy necessitates permanent urinary diversion into an ileal or colonic conduit. In a male patient, the prostate gland, seminal vesicles, and distal ureters are removed with the bladder and its peritoneal surface. In a female patient, the bladder, urethra, distal ureters, uterus, cervix, and proximal third of the vagina are removed.

Procedural Considerations. The perioperative nurse places the patient in the supine position. Instruments are as described for major abdominal procedures. For a male patient, if the prostate and seminal vesicles are to be removed, prostatectomy instruments should be added. For a female patient, vaginal and abdominal hysterectomy as well as plastic surgery instruments should be added (see Chapters 14 and 22).

Operative Procedure. A midline incision from the epigastrium to the symphysis pubis, curving to the left of the umbilicus, is generally used.

1. The surgeon enters the peritoneal cavity above the umbilicus. The entire urachal remnant is clamped, divided, and ligated with heavy silk ligatures (Figure 15-58, *A*). It will be removed en bloc with the bladder.

2. The bladder dome is lifted at its peritoneal surface, and dissection proceeds laterally on either side with ligation of the major vesical arteries to the level of the vas deferens or round ligament (see Figure 15-58, *B*).

3. The surgeon divides the vas deferens and cuts the urethra at the level of the pelvic diaphragm.

4. The ureters are identified and traced to the bladder. Care is taken to preserve the adventitial tissue (see Figure 15-58, *C*).

5. Abdominal exploration and pelvic lymphadenectomy with frozen sections are performed to rule out metastatic disease.

6. In the male patient the bladder is then retracted to expose the endopelvic fascia and puboprostatic ligaments. The prostate, dorsal venous complex, and seminal vesicles are dissected free, as described for a radical retropubic prostatectomy (see Figure 15-58, *D*). These will be removed in continuity with the bladder.

7. In the female patient the broad ligament is bilaterally incised posterior to the fallopian tube and ovary to the level of the posterior vagina to be removed en bloc with the bladder (see Figure 15-58, *E*). The endopelvic fascia is incised at the bladder neck to expose the proximal urethra. The vagina is then incised along the lateral walls to the level of the proximal urethra and bladder neck. The anterior vaginal wall is incised in a U fashion to circumscribe the urethra (see Figure 15-58, *F*). The vagina is reconstructed.

8. The surgical specimen consists of the bladder, distal ureters, prostate, seminal vesicles, and distal vas in the male and the uterus, fallopian tubes, and ovaries in the female and is removed en bloc.

9. The surgeon ligates the urethra with absorbable suture. If urethrectomy is indicated, this is done en bloc with the bladder.

10. Radiopaque soft goods are placed in the denuded pelvis, and pressure is applied to reduce blood loss from oozing.

11. Urinary diversion is accomplished by means of an isolated ileal or colonic conduit, an orthotopic diversion, or a continent urinary diversion.

Bladder Substitution (Substitution Cystoplasty)

The ideal candidate for a bladder replacement after cystectomy for carcinoma is a patient with a normal urethra; a proximally located, well-differentiated bladder tumor; absence of carcinoma in situ; and proof, in the male patient, that the prostatic urethra is free

FIGURE 15-58 Radical cystectomy.

E   F

FIGURE 15-58, cont'd Radical cystectomy.

of disease. High-dose radiation offers appreciable risks for postoperative complications and is contraindicated with enterourethral anastomosis. A discussion of techniques to create a neobladder follows.

Right Colocystoplasty. Depending on the extent of involvement, the right side of the colon may be used to replace the bladder, the bladder and prostatic urethra, or the bladder and prostate with a direct enteric-to-proximal bulbar urethral anastomosis. This procedure has become more functionally effective with the use of intermittent self-catheterization and selective implantation of a prosthetic urinary sphincter.

Ileocecal Bladder Substitution. The ileum has been used as a reservoir to restore urinary continuity because it possesses a low intraluminal pressure. However, the short mesentery does not always permit the bowel to reach the urethra and results are not consistently successful. There have been significant incidences of recurrent carcinoma, renal damage, incontinence, strictures, fistula, hypokalemia, anemia, suture-line breakdown, and stone formation after the procedure. Although most patients attain daytime urinary control, a small percentage still have problems with enuresis. Deterioration of the upper urinary tract as a result of infection and obstruction has historically been a significant risk with this procedure, and therefore ileocecal substitution is met with mixed reactions and recommendations.

Sigmoidocystoplasty. Because of the sigmoid colon's ease of construction, bladder proximity, decreased obstruction from mucus, and large capacity, it has been more appealing as a tissue source to many surgeons in their attempt to create a new bladder. More efficient emptying with a larger reservoir capacity seems to occur with a sigmoid replacement. Results yield higher intraluminal pressures, more effective urinary flow rates, and less nocturnal incontinence than with ileal segments.

Ileoascending Bladder Substitution. In an effort to improve the intestinal reservoir's capacity and antirefluxing effectiveness, the use of the ascending colon as a continent reservoir was introduced. This technique has several anatomic advantages over other methods of bladder replacement. The segment used can include the hepatic flexure and proximal transverse colon. A large-capacity reservoir is obtained, and colonic incision or tailoring is not required to achieve an appropriate shape. It easily reaches any site within the pelvis and can be anastomosed directly to the urethra without tension.

Orthotopic Ileocolic Neobladder (Le Bag). The Le Bag continent diversion technique uses the right colon and ileum as an orthotopic bladder replacement. Bladder substitution relies on meticulous dissection of the prostatic apex with preservation of the urinary sphincter and neurovascular bundles, as well as a watertight urethral anastomosis. Most patients have achieved a high degree of daytime continence and a minimum of nocturnal enuresis. Short-term complications encountered include bleeding, infection, urinary extravasation, bladder perforation, urethral stricture, fistula formation, urinoma, and small-bowel obstruction. Long-term problems include chronic constipation or diarrhea, compromised enterohepatic circulation, vitamin B_{12} deficiency, and urinary incontinence in a small percentage of patients.

Considerations influencing patient selection include age, general health, and fitness for extensive, complicated surgery. Contraindications include previous radiation therapy, bowel disease (diverticulosis, Crohn disease, colitis), and other major medical problems. Preoperative urethral biopsy specimens are frequently taken to rule out tumor or cellular atypia in the urethra, which would prevent this particular intervention.

Procedural Considerations. The patient is placed in the supine position. Intermittent pneumatic compression devices are applied before the induction of anesthesia. A cystectomy and prostatectomy or hysterectomy are performed. Major deep intestinal, bladder, and prostate or hysterectomy instruments, as well as a large self-retaining retractor, are needed.

Operative Procedure

1. After cystoprostatectomy, the right side of the colon is reflected medially along the mesentery to the hepatic flexure. The distal ileum that is to be used in the neobladder is inspected.

2. The surgeon divides the small bowel, positions it in an S shape, and places stay sutures of 2-0 or 3-0 absorbable material.

3. The posterior walls are sewn from inside to outside with running 3-0 absorbable suture.

4. A seromuscular wedge of the dependent cecum is excised, and the mucosa is everted with 4-0 absorbable sutures to form a bladder neck.

5. The left ureter is brought retroperitoneally under the sigmoid mesentery, a submucosal tunnel is created, and the ureters are reimplanted through the colonic wall. Anastomosis is done from the interior of the pouch.

6. The surgeon places anchor sutures of 3-0 or 4-0 silk at the outer entry point. The wall of the colon is anchored to the psoas muscle with 3-0 or 4-0 silk to prevent migration of the neobladder.

7. Ureteral stents are placed and exteriorized through the colonic segment and a separate abdominal stab wound, along with a catheter, to serve as a suprapubic tube.

8. Sutures of 2-0 absorbable material are placed around the urethral stump and tagged.

9. The surgeon inserts a Foley catheter into the urethra in a retrograde manner, and the urethra is anastomosed to the neobladder at the point of the new bladder neck.

10. The neobladder is closed in an intestinal fashion or with a GI stapler in a side-to-side anastomosis. Wound drains are placed, the bladder filled to test for leaks, and the wound closed.

Cutaneous Urinary Diversions

Ileal Conduit. The ileal conduit is the classic method by which the urine flow is diverted to an isolated loop of bowel. One end of the isolated loop is exteriorized through the skin so that the urine can be collected in a drainage bag, which is intermittently emptied. The surgeon consults with the enterostomal therapist preoperatively to determine the stoma site. The selected site, usually in the right lower quadrant of the abdomen, above the beltline, is marked with a fine needle dipped in methylene blue to prevent erasure during skin preparation. The goal is to create a round, protruding stoma without wrinkles in the skin, to prevent urine leakage under the collecting device. The candidate for ileal diversion must have a retrievable ureter at least 1 cm in diameter with a thick, well-vascularized wall. The patient must be able to care for the appliance. Conditions amenable to diversion include neurogenic bladder, interstitial cystitis, and bladder carcinoma. Cystectomy may be performed before or after this procedure, depending on the patient's diagnosis. In cases that do not involve bladder cancer, the surgeon may choose to leave the bladder in situ rather than subject a debilitated patient to further surgery. In certain cases of extensive bladder carcinoma, the surgeon may elect to treat the patient with radiation in an attempt to decrease the size of the tumor and neutralize the regional lymph nodes before performing cystectomy.

Procedural Considerations. The perioperative nurse assists with positioning the patient in the supine position. Abdominal and GI instruments are required. A cystectomy, prostatectomy, or hysterectomy may also be done at the time of the surgery. Endostapling devices, with absorbable staples, should be available.

Operative Procedure

1. The bladder is decompressed with a catheter.
2. The surgeon enters the abdomen through a midline abdominal incision and places a self-retaining abdominal retractor to exclude the viscera from the region of dissection.

3. The ureters are identified and severed approximately 2.5 cm from the bladder.

4. The surgeon creates a retroperitoneal tunnel so that the left ureter lies close to the right ureter.

5. The distal ileum and mesentery are inspected to identify the bowel's blood supply.

6. A drain is passed through the mesentery, midway between the two main arterial arcades adjacent to the ileum at the proximal and distal ends of the selected segment. This segment usually makes up 15 to 20 cm of the terminal ileum, a few centimeters from the ileocecal valve. The ileocecal artery is preserved to maintain adequate circulation to the isolated ileal segment.

7. The surgeon incises the peritoneum over the proposed line of division of the mesentery.

8. Intestinal clamps are placed across the ileum, and the bowel is divided flush with the clamps.

9. Using GI technique (also referred to as bowel technique; see Chapter 11), the surgeon closes the proximal end of the isolated ileal segment first with a layer of absorbable sutures and then with a second layer of interrupted 2-0 nonabsorbable sutures.

10. The proximal and distal segments of ileum are reanastomosed end-to-end in two layers.

11. The surgeon closes the mesenteric incision with interrupted nonabsorbable sutures.

12. The closed proximal end of the conduit segment is fixed to the posterior peritoneum.

13. The ureters are implanted in the ileal segment, using fine instruments and 4-0 absorbable ureteral sutures on atraumatic needles.

14. The surgeon separates the peritoneum and muscle of the abdominal wall lateral to the original incision with blunt dissection.

15. The abdominal opening for the stoma is made, and the distal opening of the ileal conduit is then drawn through a fenestration in the muscle, fascia, and skin.

16. The ileum is fixed to the fascia with 2-0 sutures. A rosebud stoma is constructed as the ileum is sutured to the skin using subcuticular stitches (Figure 15-59).

17. Ureteral stents are usually left in the stoma, and a urinary collecting pouch is placed over the rosebud stoma to collect urine.

18. The surgeon inserts closed-suction wound drains and closes the abdominal incision. The skin is reapproximated.

Continent Urinary Diversions

The Kock pouch, the right colocystoplasty, and the Camey version of the ileocystoplasty have been modified for anastomosis to a urethral stump or the prostatic capsule, resulting in effective continent bladder replacement. All continent urinary diversions create an easily catheterized stoma and a nonrefluxing ureteral anastomosis. Different parts of the bowel and the stomach have been used as continent reservoirs. The choice of the antireflux mechanism depends on the implantation site. The stoma does not require an appliance; therefore, the site may be placed below the beltline or bikini line, permitting it to be catheterized when the patient is sitting. It may be anastomosed to the proximal urethra, thus forming an orthotopic bladder.

Ileal Reservoir (Kock Pouch)

Procedural Considerations. A continent reservoir formed into a U configuration is constructed from a section of ileum proximal

FIGURE 15-59 Rosebud suture technique for stoma.

to the ileocecal valve. The legs of the U are sewn together at the antimesenteric border. The intestine is opened adjacent to the antimesenteric border, and the back wall of the pouch is reinforced with absorbable suture.

Continence is achieved by the valve mechanism with the nipple valve attached to the skin. Nipple valves are created proximally and distally by intussusception of the bowel into the reservoir cavity. Once the nipples are fixed to the sidewall of the reservoir with absorbable suture or polyglycolic staples, the anterior wall is closed. The ureters are anastomosed to the afferent limb of the pouch, preventing reflux. The efferent limb is drawn through the stoma site and anchored to the abdominal wall fascia.

Operative Procedure

1. The mesentery is divided and suture-ligated or staple-ligated along the avascular plane between the superior mesenteric artery and the ileocolic artery.
2. The surgeon divides the bowel, and four segments are measured and marked with silk suture tags. These segments will serve as the efferent conduit, the pouch, and the afferent limb.
3. A portion of the proximal ileum is resected and discarded along with a wedge of mesentery. Suction is passed down the lumen to clear any fecal material or mucus.
4. The surgeon closes the proximal end of the bowel with suture or staples.
5. The segment to be used is spread out in a U shape. The sides are sewn together with 3-0 absorbable suture in a running stitch or connected using a GI endostapler.
6. The surgeon uses the ESU to incise the bowel laterally to the suture in the two loops. The medial edges are oversewn with 3-0 or 4-0 silk.
7. The mesentery is cleared on the limb segments, and the lumens are intussuscepted into the open pouch.
8. Synthetic mesh is used to serve as a strut to prevent peristomal herniation and to fix the base of the efferent nipple to the

abdominal wall, facilitating catheterization. The thoracoabdominal (TA) or similar endostapler is used to form each nipple and to attach the nipples to the back wall of the pouch.

9. An 8F stenting catheter is placed inside the nipple of the efferent conduit to prevent the formation of a collar that is too tight.
10. The surgeon secures the limbs with 3-0 or 4-0 silk suture.
11. The pouch is closed with sutures or the endostapler.
12. The ureters are anastomosed, as described in the "Ileal Conduit" discussion, to the afferent limb.
13. A small stoma site is prepared, as described in the "Ileal Conduit" discussion. A catheter of choice is placed in the stoma for postoperative care. Stents may be placed in the ureters for the immediate postoperative period. This necessitates initial placement of an ileostomy appliance until all systems are functioning.
14. A drain is placed, which exits through a separate stab wound.
15. The surgeon closes the wound. Retention sutures may be used. Bulky absorbent dressings are applied; Montgomery straps may be used.

Indiana Pouch

Procedural Considerations. The Indiana pouch technique is a modification of the original ileocecal diversion. The surgeon constructs a continent reservoir from the right side of the colon, which may include the ileum and cecum, the ileocecal valve, and ascending colon. Surgery proceeds as for any diversionary procedure. The ileocecal valve is reinforced with nonabsorbable suture. Two rows of nonabsorbable suture are used to then imbricate the ileal segment, which serves as a limb that can be catheterized once it is exteriorized to the skin level as a stoma. The cecal segment is detubularized by incising along the taenia and anastomosing the distal edge horizontally to the proximal portion. Intussusception of the ileocecal valve into the cecum and narrowing of the ileal segment attached to the skin allow for continence.

Operative Procedure

1. The large bowel is split down the antimesenteric border for approximately three quarters of its length.
2. The U-shaped defect is closed.
3. The surgeon sutures the terminal ileum along its length over a small Robinson catheter in an intestinal fashion.
4. The pouch is filled with 400 mL of saline, and a larger catheter is placed to determine ability to be catheterized.
5. The ureters are tunneled into the cecum through its taenia and then tacked to the outer bowel wall. The cecum is secured to the pelvic wall. Ureteral stents may be placed.
6. The pouch is secured to the abdominal wall.
7. The surgeon prepares the stomal site as described in the "Ileal Conduit" discussion.
8. A 22F Malecot drain is placed in the reservoir to drain the cecostomy, exiting through a separate stab wound.

Surgery of the Ureters and Kidneys

Stones, infections, and tumors are the most common causes of urinary tract obstruction, necessitating surgery to prevent renal obstruction and subsequent renal failure. Obstruction may also result from congenital malformations or previous operations on the urinary tract (Figure 15-60).

The ureter has three areas of narrowing where calculi may become lodged and pose a potential problem with pain and obstruction: (1) the ureteropelvic junction (UPJ), (2) the crossing of the ureter

FIGURE 15-60 Some common causes of urinary tract obstruction. *UPJ,* Ureteropelvic junction.

Labels in figure: Hydronephrosis; UPJ obstruction; Retroperipheral scar tissue; Compressing extrinsic tumor; Aberrant vessel; Calculus; Intrinsic tumor; Calculus; Chronic infection; Aperistaltic distal segment

over the external iliac vessels, and (3) the ureterovesical junction (UVJ). Urine may sometimes cause calculi to be washed down the ureter to produce severe ureteral colic. The majority of renal calculi are spontaneously passed into the bladder. However, if they become lodged in the ureter, surgical intervention may be indicated.

Although the causes of many kidney stones are obscure, certain conditions, such as obstruction, stasis, and imbalance of metabolism, predispose to their formation. Stones consist of various elements: calcium oxalate, calcium phosphate, magnesium ammonium phosphate, uric acid, calcium carbonate, and cystine. An increase in the concentration of any of these compounds can cause tiny crystals to form; as these clump together, they begin to form a stone. Stones removed during surgery are subjected to chemical analysis and should be submitted in a dry jar. Fixative agents such as formalin should not be used.

Stones in the renal pelvis may fall into the UPJ and obstruct the flow of urine. However, stones less than 3 cm in diameter may also pass down the ureter and lodge at a more distal location. A stone may remain in a renal calyx and continue to enlarge, eventually filling the entire renal collecting system (staghorn calculus). Diverticula may form and harbor stones that can be difficult to reach and treat. Hydroureteronephrosis, infection, and destruction of renal parenchyma frequently result from unrelieved obstruction.

Hypothermia may be used as an adjunct to renal stone surgery as a means of prolonging the safe period of renal ischemia. Several methods enable renal cooling: ice slush or cold saline solution, surface cooling coils, perfusion of cold solutions through the renal artery, or a variation of these basic techniques, such as perfusion of the renal pelvis with saline that has been cooled by a coil immersed in ice slush.

A refrigeration unit "slush machine" that produces sterile slush provides a cost-effective, time-saving alternative to the other methods of slush preparation. Commercially synthesized ultrafiltrate of sterile plasma in liter bottles is also available for use as the slush. Alternatively, a rigid plastic container of 1000 mL of normal saline or lactated Ringer's solution may be placed on its side in a freezer several hours before surgery. To prevent the solution from solidifying, the container should be rotated one-half turn every 20 to 30 minutes. Sterile slush may then be poured directly into a sterile basin as required.

The surgical approach in renal surgery depends on the patient's condition, the amount of exposure needed, and the surgical procedure to be performed. There are three principal surgical approaches to the kidney. The simple *flank,* or *transabdominal,* incision is most frequently used and may include removal of the eleventh or twelfth rib. The incision begins at the posterior axillary line and parallels the course of the twelfth rib. It extends forward and slightly downward between the iliac crest and the thorax. For the *lumbar* incision, the patient may be initially positioned supine and then rotated to lateral and slightly forward over protective bolsters with the operative side up. This effectively places the flank in an oblique position, causing the abdominal viscera to fall away from the operative incision, and affords an excellent approach to the renal pedicle. Alternatively, the patient may be placed prone with bolsters under the affected side to provide elevation. The *thoracoabdominal* exposure is used primarily for large upper-pole renal neoplasms. The tenth and eleventh ribs are usually removed, and the chest cavity is opened, collapsing the lung. The leaves of the diaphragm are separated to expose the kidney.

Ureteral Surgery

Ureterostomy (ureterotomy) is opening the ureter for continued drainage from it into another body part. Cutaneous ureterostomy is diversion of the flow of urine from the kidney, through the ureter, away from the bladder, and onto the skin of the lower abdomen. A suitable urinary collecting device is then placed over the ureteral stoma.

Ureterectomy is complete removal of the ureter. This procedure is generally used in collecting system tumors and includes nephrectomy and the excision of a cuff of bladder.

Ureteroureterostomy is segmental resection of a diseased portion of the ureter and reconstruction in continuity of the two normal segments.

Ureteroenterostomy is diversion of the ureter into a segment of the ileum (ureteroileostomy, or more commonly, ileal urinary conduit) or into the sigmoid colon (ureterosigmoidostomy). Ureteroneocystostomy (ureterovesical anastomosis) is division of the distal ureter from the bladder and reimplantation of the ureter into the bladder with a submucosal tunnel.

Reconstructive operations may be indicated because of a pathologic condition of the bladder or lower ureter that interferes with normal drainage. Conditions requiring urinary diversion or reconstruction of the urinary tract include malignancy, cystitis, stricture, trauma, and congenital ureterovesical reflux. Invasive vesical malignancy requiring surgical removal of the bladder necessitates urinary diversion.

Ureterocutaneous transplant, ureterosigmoid anastomosis, and ileal conduit are urinary diversionary procedures performed when the bladder is no longer functioning as a proper urine reservoir. Etiologic factors causing irreparable vesical dysfunction are chronic inflammation, interstitial cystitis, neurogenic bladder, exstrophy, trauma, tumor, and infiltrative disease (amyloidosis). Ureterolithotomy is incision into the ureter and removal of an obstructing calculus.

Procedural Considerations. The site of the incision and position of the patient depend on the nature of the proposed surgery. The patient may be placed in the supine position for abdominal surgery, in the modified Trendelenburg position for low abdominal or pelvic surgery, or in the lateral position for high- or midureteral obstructing calculi. The perioperative nurse ensures that the patient's arms are supinated when on armboards; in lateral position the upper arm is placed on an overbed armboard such as the Allen lateral arm support and the lower arm is supinated on a padded armboard. The kidney rest should lie just under the dependent iliac crest.

Instruments include a nephrectomy set, plus plastic instrumentation for pyeloplasty. Additional instruments may be required, depending on the type of operation and the surgical approach used.

Operative Procedure
Ureteral Reimplantation

1. The surgeon exposes the ureter through an incision determined by the location of the pathologic condition. A ureteral catheter, passed retrograde, may be used to facilitate identification and isolation of the ureter.
2. The ureter is dissected free with long forceps and scissors, picked up with fine traction sutures, freed from the surrounding tissues, and severed at the desired level.
3. The surgeon ligates the distal end of the ureter and transfers the proximal stoma to the site of anastomosis. The anastomosis is accomplished with fine dissection instruments and fine atraumatic sutures.
4. A soft splinting stent is usually left in place until healing has taken place and free drainage is ensured. The wound is closed in layers and dressings applied.

Ureterocutaneous Transplant (Anastomosis). The surgical approach is the same as that for a low ureterolithotomy.
1. The ureter is divided as far distally as possible.
2. The surgeon passes the severed ureter retroperitoneally through the lower abdominal wall and sutures it to the skin with an absorbable everting suture of 4-0 on an atraumatic needle to form a stoma. The ureter is handled gently with plastic instruments, fixation forceps, and iris scissors.
3. A small Silastic stenting catheter is passed up into the ureter and left in place for 48 to 72 hours, as ureteral edema subsides. The patient requires a urine-collecting device after surgery.

Ureterosigmoid Anastomosis
1. The surgeon enters the peritoneal cavity through a lower left paramedian incision.
2. The major portion of the large bowel is protected with moist laparotomy packs.
3. Deep retractors are placed, and the surgeon uses long forceps and scissors to incise the posterior peritoneum.
4. The ureters are identified, divided close to the bladder, mobilized, and brought through the posterior peritoneal incision to

lie near the sigmoid. Traction sutures and smooth tissue forceps are used to handle the ureters.
5. The sigmoid colon is mobilized to prevent tension on the ureteroenteric anastomosis.
6. Using 3-0 nonabsorbable suture material, the surgeon sutures the sigmoid colon to the pelvic peritoneum at a point where the ureter falls easily on the bowel.
7. Using a scalpel with a #15 blade, the surgeon makes an incision into the taenia of the sigmoid down to the mucosal layer. The edges of the taenia are undermined to create two parallel flaps.
8. The ureter is laid on the bowel mucosa, and a small slit is made through the mucosa into the lumen of the colon.
9. With fixation forceps and iris scissors, the surgeon bevels the ureter to lie flat in the tunica incision.
10. The distal ureter is anchored to the bowel mucosa with 4-0 absorbable ureteral sutures on atraumatic needles. The other ureter is anastomosed in the same manner in a position slightly above the first.
11. The tunicae are then loosely reapproximated over the ureter with 4-0 absorbable sutures, creating an antireflux anastomosis.
12. The surgeon closes the posterior peritoneum with absorbable sutures. Drains are exteriorized retroperitoneally. The incision is closed and dressings applied.

Ureterolithotomy
Procedural Considerations A KUB x-ray examination should be done immediately before surgery to determine the exact location of the stone. The surgeon may also schedule a cystoscopic examination preoperatively and may attempt to remove the stone endoscopically. The location of the stone determines the surgical approach. A stone high in the ureter requires a flank incision with possible removal of the twelfth rib; a more distal ureteral stone requires a lower abdominal incision.

Operative Procedure
1. After exposure of the ureter, the stone may be kept stationary with Babcock clamps or vessel loops applied above and below it.
2. With a #15 blade, the surgeon makes an incision in the ureter directly over the stone, which may be easily removed with Randall stone forceps.
3. A 10F catheter is passed proximally up and distally down the ureter while irrigating with saline to check for ureteral patency and to dislodge any remaining stone fragments.
4. The surgeon closes the ureter with 4-0 or 5-0 absorbable sutures. All stones should be placed in dry receptacles and sent to the chemistry laboratory for analysis.

Kidney Surgery

See Box 15-2 for terms pertaining to kidney surgery.

Procedural Considerations. Patient preparation and instrument setup are as described for ureteral surgery.

Operative Procedure
Pyelotomy and Pyelostomy
1. The surgeon incises the pelvis of the kidney with a small scalpel blade. Fine traction sutures may be placed at the edges of the incision for gentle retraction while the pelvis and calyces are explored.
2. In pyelostomy, a small Malecot or Foley catheter is placed through the incision into the renal pelvis. Pyelotomy is used only

BOX 15-2

Terms Pertaining to Kidney Surgery

Nephrostomy: Creation of an opening into the kidney to maintain temporary or permanent urinary drainage. A nephrostomy is used to correct an obstruction of the urinary tract and to conserve and permit physiologic functioning of renal tissue. It is also used to provide permanent urinary drainage when a ureter is obstructed or for temporary urinary drainage immediately after a plastic repair on the kidney.

Nephrotomy: Incision into the kidney, usually over a collecting system containing a calculus.

Pyelolithotomy: Removal of a calculus through an opening in the renal pelvis.

Pyelostomy: Making an opening in the renal pelvis for temporarily or permanently diverting the flow of urine.

Pyelotomy: Incision into the renal pelvis used as an access to stones in the renal pelvis or collecting system.

FIGURE 15-61 Kuntz laser working element.

for very short periods of renal drainage because tubes tend to be dislodged easily from the renal pelvis.

Percutaneous Nephrolithotomy. Percutaneous nephrolithotomy facilitates the removal or disintegration of renal stones using a rigid or flexible nephroscope (Figure 15-61) passed through a percutaneous nephrostomy tract. Accessory instrumentation, such as the ultrasound wand, electrohydraulic lithotripter probe, laser fiber, stone basket, and stone grasper, is passed through the lumen of the nephroscope.

Ideally the patient is in good health and not obese and the calculus is 1 cm or less in diameter, free-floating, radiopaque, and solitary. However, there is a high population of obese patients who undergo percutaneous nephrolithotomy. Advances in technology complemented by the experience gained by the uroradiology team have allowed patients with more complex problems to be managed in this manner. Patients who have undergone previous renal surgery, have stone recurrence, or have an established nephrostomy tract may also benefit from this procedure.

Creation of the nephrostomy tract and removal of the stone can be accomplished by three different methods. Proper placement of the nephrostomy wire can decrease the operating time significantly. In the *one-step procedure,* creation of the nephrostomy tract, tract dilation, and stone removal are completed in a single session. This method is generally preferred unless there are contraindications. In the *immediate two-step procedure,* the radiologist places the nephrostomy tube under radiographic guidance and the surgeon removes the stone later the same day or the next morning. The second step is usually done in the OR with the patient administered a general anesthetic. In the *delayed two-step procedure,* the nephrostomy tract is established after the patient has been administered a local anesthetic. The patient is discharged the following day with a 22F or 24F nephrostomy tube connected to drainage. The patient is readmitted to the hospital 5 to 7 days later for the percutaneous removal of the stone after the patient has been administered a general anesthetic.

Of basic concern during the operative phase are the patient's position and body temperature, the potential for sudden and rapid blood loss, the type of anesthesia, medications required during surgery, and catheter management during and after the procedure.

The patient's position, which may be prone or up to 30 degrees prone-oblique, and the draping procedure depend on whether the surgery is performed in the radiology department or the OR and the type of x-ray equipment that will be used.

Endopyelotomy. Endopyelotomy is currently considered the first-line therapy for primary and secondary UPJ obstruction in adults and secondary UPJ obstruction in children.

Procedural Considerations. Acucise endopyelotomy is the simultaneous dilation and incision of a ureteral stricture under fluoroscopic guidance. Only basic cystoscopic equipment and C-arm fluoroscopy are needed for this procedure. The Acucise balloon catheter will pass through a standard 25F cystoscope sheath.

Operative Procedure

1. The surgeon places an open-ended ureteral catheter into the distal ureter, and a retrograde pyelogram is performed to define the area of stenosis. A guidewire is then advanced into the renal collection system.
2. The Acucise catheter is placed over the guidewire and passed through the cystoscope. The Acucise catheter should be rotated under direct cystoscopic vision so the cutting wire is in correct lateral orientation.
3. The surgeon advances the cutting balloon catheter over the super stiff guidewire until the UPJ stenosis is visualized. At the UPJ and in the proximal and midureter, the cutting wire is positioned laterally.
4. After visualizing the wire in the lateral position, the surgeon gently inflates the balloon with dilute contrast media to ensure correct positioning across the UPJ.
5. After ensuring proper grounding of the patient, the cutting wire is activated at 75 to 100 watts (pure cut) for 5 seconds, and simultaneously dilute contrast is again instilled into the dilating balloon under continuous, fluoroscopic guidance. As the balloon inflates, the stricture is incised.
6. The incision is completed and a retrograde pyelogram is performed through the Acusise catheter to confirm extravasation at the incision site.

The surgeon removes the internal stent at 6 weeks postoperatively using a flexible cystoscope in males or a rigid cystoscope in females. Patients typically return 12 weeks following stent removal for postoperative IV pyelogram or differential renal scan with furosemide washout to confirm efficacy of the endopyelotomy.

Extracorporeal Shock-Wave Lithotripsy (ESWL). ESWL units use water-filled cushions adjacent to the kidney area. An x-ray image intensifier with two monitors is used to visualize the kidney stone at the focal point of the shock wave. After every 100 shocks, fluoroscopy is used to locate remaining stone particles. Adjustments are made, and the patient is repositioned before further treatments. ESWL is often used with percutaneous nephrolithotomy and transurethral ureteropyeloscopy if the patient does not pass the gravel.

Stones that are treated with ESWL are fragmented by the energy focused on the stone with the lithotripter. The shock waves are administered from 30 minutes to 2 hours. Shock waves reverberate inside the stone, causing fragmentation with ultimate complete or partial destruction of the calculus. The amount of destruction depends on the number and energy of the shock waves delivered and the stone's hardness. This technique is effective because shock waves can be transmitted and focused through tissue without loss of energy. A loud, reverberating, popping sound occurs each time a wave pulse is activated. It is advisable that earplugs be worn.

The requirement for anesthesia is determined by the power of the shock wave, the area of shock-wave entry at the skin level, and the size of the shock-wave focal point. The summation of shock waves used during the procedure can cause pain at the skin level. Typically a general, spinal, or local anesthetic is used with the older lithotripters. Modern versions allow for lithotripsy with only IV sedation, oral sedation, or a transcutaneous electrical nerve stimulation (TENS) unit.

The use of a stent before ESWL depends on the patient and the character of the stone or stones. The patient should have a negative urine culture before stent placement. Studies show that complication rates decrease if a stent is used with a stone larger than 1.5 cm. A stent placed before ESWL tends to decrease the need for ancillary interventions, reduces overall complications, and assists in proper positioning for ESWL by delineating the ureteral anatomy and the precise stone location. On the other hand, those patients who tend to readily form stones may demonstrate calcification of the ureteral stent in a relatively short time. Without a stent the risk of silent renal obstruction resulting in loss of kidney function, obstruction of the ureter, nephritis, and sepsis is increased.

Complications related to ESWL are attributable to the cavitation effects of treatment and are proportional to the number of shocks. The ability of the kidney's tubular cells to survive shock waves is related to the number of shock waves to which the kidney is exposed and not to the energy level. Gross hematuria is seen almost universally, resolves in 12 to 48 hours, and is believed to be attributable to parenchymal edema that spontaneously heals within 1 week. Subcapsular or perirenal hematoma caused by perinephric fluid collections may occur and appears to be higher in the hypertensive patient. Subcapsular hematoma may resolve in 6 weeks or may take up to 6 months, whereas perirenal hematoma is relieved usually in a matter of days. Impairment of renal function may be seen in patients with solitary kidneys. Iliac artery and vein thromboses have been reported with lithotripsy for ureteral stones. The majority of lithotripsy patients demonstrate little or no long-term morbidity.

Laser Lithotripsy. Laser lithotripsy has become an exciting alternative to ESWL and electrohydraulic lithotripsy (EHL). The Ho:YAG, tunable pulse-dyed (coumarin), Er:YAG (erbium:yttrium-aluminum-garnet), the tunable Alexandrite (a chromium-doped mineral), or the Q-switched Nd:YAG laser systems have the ability to disintegrate stones without damaging soft tissue. The technique may be used during a ureteropyeloscopy or nephroscopy or to manage ureteral stones instead of performing a ureterolithotomy. When the laser probe is discharged in direct contact with the calculus, plasma (ionized gas) coats the stone's surface. This plasma expands with repeated firings, creating a shock wave that fractures the stone. Normal saline is used for continuous irrigation throughout the procedure. It is not necessary to immobilize the calculus. Everyone in the room must wear laser goggles, and all laser precautions apply (see Chapter 8).

Dismembered Pyeloplasty. *Pyeloplasty* is revision or plastic reconstruction of the renal pelvis. Pyeloplasty is performed to create a better anatomic relationship between the renal pelvis and the proximal ureter and to allow proper urinary drainage from the kidney to the bladder. A temporary nephrostomy is often included to protect the plastic reconstruction of the UPJ. Tissue healing usually occurs in 10 to 12 days, and the nephrostomy tube is removed once ureteral patency is demonstrated. *Ureteroplasty* is reconstruction of the ureter distal to the UPJ. A *dismembered pyeloplasty* is the combined correction of the redundant renal pelvis and resection of a stenotic portion of the UPJ.

Procedural Considerations. The instrument setup is as described for nephrectomy, plus fine plastic and vascular instrumentation and Randall stone forceps. A ureteral stent and red rubber catheters also are used. The perioperative nurse assists with positioning the patient in the lateral position.

Operative Procedure

Open Approach

1. The surgeon exposes the kidney and upper ureter through a supracostal flank incision.

2. Gerota fascia is entered, and the renal pelvis and ureter are freed while the kidney is rotated medially.

3. The surgeon frees the ureter and stabilizes it with a vessel loop below the level of the UPJ.

4. A 4-0 stay suture is placed in the tip of the ureter, and the ureter is incised, trimmed, and shaped to the desired contour with fine forceps and scissors.

5. Anchoring sutures of 4-0 material are placed for traction during reconstruction of the renal pelvis. A diamond-shaped incision is made into the renal pelvis, and the tissue is removed. The Y-V-plasty technique may be followed. It converts a Y-shaped surgical incision of the renal pelvis into a V by drawing the apex of the arms of the Y to the foot of the Y with absorbable sutures.

6. Sutures are placed at each end of the refashioned renal pelvis, passed to the ureteral stoma, and tagged. The pelvis is irrigated free of clots. The sutures are run in a continuous manner, creating the anastomosis.

7. A Silastic tubing may be used to stent the repaired pelvis until adequate healing has occurred. A nephrostomy tube is also placed within the pelvis to divert urine safely while the edema in the area of the repair resolves.

8. The surgeon closes Gerota fascia over the repair.

9. A drain is placed where the pelvis was reconstructed, and the surgical incision is closed in layers.

Laparoscopic Approach. UPJ obstruction has joined the rank of surgeries that may be treated laparoscopically. Generally a standard transperitoneal approach is used. The patient may be placed supine with a lateral tilt or in lateral decubitus and the bed rotated to access the ports.

After placement of four trocars as in laparoscopic nephrectomy, the surgeon frees the proximal ureters and renal pelvis. The obstruction at the UPJ is excised, and a spatulated anastomosis is performed using running or interrupted sutures. A ureteral stent is usually left in place.

Decreased postoperative pain and shorter hospitalization make this approach appealing. A higher degree of skill is required for this technique, however, making it an option that has not become standard treatment as yet.

Nephroureterectomy—Open Approach.
Nephroureterectomy is removal of a kidney and its entire ureter. This procedure is indicated for hydroureteronephrosis of such a degree that reconstructive repair is impossible. It is also used for collecting system tumors of the kidney and ureter.

Procedural Considerations. Open nephroureterectomy requires an extension of the incision anteriorly with the patient positioned semilaterally and fully prepped and draped for the surgeon to access the flank and lower abdomen. Only one instrument set is required, but a second skin-prep setup and set of sterile drapes may be necessary. An alternative to open nephroureterectomy is laparoscopic nephroureterectomy.

Operative Procedure

1. The surgeon exposes the kidney and upper ureter and performs a nephrectomy as described in the following procedure. The kidney may be placed in a plastic bag to prevent possible spillage of tumor cells.
2. The ureter is mobilized as far distally as possible. The OR bed is adjusted so that surgery on the lower ureter may proceed. The lower ureter and bladder are identified and mobilized.
3. The ureter and a small cuff of the bladder are removed in continuity, and the bladder is repaired with a single layer of 2-0 absorbable interrupted sutures. The ureter and cuff of bladder are pulled superiorly, and the intact kidney and ureter are removed.
4. An 18F or 20F Foley catheter is left in the bladder, and a drain is placed behind the bladder. The incision is closed in layers.

Nephrectomy—Open Approach.
Nephrectomy is the surgical removal of a kidney. It is performed as a means of definitive therapy for many renal problems, such as congenital UPJ obstruction with severe hydronephrosis, renal tumor, renal trauma, calculus disease with infection, cortical abscess, pyelonephrosis, and renovascular hypertension.

In routine renal surgery the patient is placed in the lateral position with the dependent iliac crest over the kidney rest. The operative flank is uppermost, with the patient's back brought to the edge of the OR bed. The upper arm is supported on an overhead arm support, and the lower arm is supinated on a padded armboard. It may be flexed slightly at the elbow and angled cephalad to promote better access to the flank. The patient's legs are positioned by placing a pillow between them and flexing the lower leg at the knee. The upper leg remains extended. The kidney rest is then raised, and when the desired bed flexion is achieved, 3-inch adhesive tape is used to stabilize the patient throughout surgery. Routine skin preparation and draping procedures are carried out.

Procedural Considerations. The nephrectomy setup includes a routine laparotomy setup; kidney instruments (Figure 15-62); a variety of red rubber, Malecot, or Pezzer catheters; a wound drainage system; and vessel loops. In certain nephrectomies the chest or the GI tract may be opened. If the chest is opened, appropriate instruments and postoperative chest drains are needed. Rib resection requires the addition of a Finochietto rib retractor, a large Matson costal periosteotome, an Alexander costal periosteotome, right and left Doyen rib raspatories, a Bethune rib cutter, a double-action duckbill rongeur, a Bailey rib approximator, and a Langenbeck periosteal elevator. When the GI tract is opened, GI technique is used for the anastomosis.

Operative Procedure

1. The incision is carried through the skin, fat, and fascia. Bleeding vessels are clamped and ligated.
2. The surgeon exposes and incises the external oblique, internal oblique, and transversalis muscles in the direction of the initial skin incision.
3. If necessary, a rib or ribs (eleventh and/or twelfth) may be resected to provide better access to the kidney. The surgeon strips the periosteum with an Alexander costal periosteotome and Doyen rib raspatory. A scalpel and heavy scissors are used to cut through the lumbocostal ligaments. The rib is grasped with an Ochsner clamp and cut with rib shears, removing the portion necessary to expose the kidney. Gerota fascia is identified and incised with Metzenbaum scissors.
4. The surgeon extends the incision and uses blunt and sharp dissection to expose the kidney and perirenal fat. The scrub person should save all perirenal fat that is removed during surgery, placing it in a small basin of normal saline for possible use as a bolster to stop bleeding.
5. The ureter is identified, separated from its adjacent structures, doubly clamped, divided, and ligated with absorbable 0 suture.
6. The kidney pedicle containing the major blood vessels is isolated and doubly clamped; each vessel is triply ligated with heavy nonabsorbable ties. Each vessel is then severed, leaving two ligatures on the pedicle, and the kidney is removed (Figure 15-63).
7. The renal fossa is explored for bleeding, and necessary hemostasis is achieved. The fossa is then irrigated with normal saline, and the irrigant is removed by suction.
8. The surgeon closes the fascia and muscle in layers with interrupted absorbable sutures. Retention sutures may be used in obese or chronically ill patients in whom wound healing may be delayed.
9. The skin edges are approximated with sutures or skin staples, and the dressing is applied.

Laparoscopic Nephrectomy.
The approach for laparoscopic nephrectomy may be transabdominal (transperitoneal), extraperitoneal (retroperitoneal), or intraperitoneal. Transabdominal is the most common approach. Indications for laparoscopy are generally for benign disease, although more radical surgeries have been accomplished in this manner. A full mechanical antibiotic bowel prep is prescribed. Although surgery time may be longer than typical for an open procedure, postoperative recovery time, analgesia requirements, and total hospital stay are lessened. The procedure always includes cystoscopy with placement of a renal balloon catheter, a ureteral catheter, and a Foley urethral catheter under C-arm fluoroscopy. Indigo carmine may be injected into the skin overlying the renal pelvis.

The patient is initially placed on a beanbag in the supine position. A standard laparoscopy instrument and equipment setup that includes three 5-mm trocars, an insufflation needle, and two 10- to 12-mm trocars is used. Cystoscopic and ureteroscopic supplies are needed, as well as a 0.035-gauge Bentson guidewire, an occlusion balloon catheter, a 0.035-gauge Amplatz stiff guidewire, a 16F Foley catheter and drainage bag, indigo carmine, an irrigator-aspirator, a 1-L bag of saline, a 1-L pressure bag (to pressurize the irrigant to 250 mm Hg), a #12 or #11 knife blade, 10-mm clip appliers, the entrapment sack, and tissue morcellator. An open setup should always be available in the event laparoscopy is unsuccessful.

Procedural Considerations. The patient is prepped and draped as for laparotomy. Use of a draping pack with four large adherent

FIGURE 15-62 A, Kidney clamps. *Top to bottom,* Satinsky (vena cava) forceps; Herrick kidney forceps; Mayo-Guyon kidney forceps. **B,** Randall stone forceps tips. *Top to bottom,* ¼ curved, ½ curved, ¾ curved, full curved. **C,** Gil-Vernet retractors, front view. **D,** *Top to bottom,* Love nerve retractors: straight, front view; 90-degree angle, side view. **E,** *Top to bottom,* Little retractors, medium: front view, side view.

drape sheets, instead of a standard laparotomy sheet, affords better access for the port sites.

The patient may be placed in lateral decubitus position on a deflated beanbag positioner at the outset or turned after endoscopic intervention. Ensuring that the patient is adequately secured to the OR bed is critical. Before prepping the patient, the bed is tilted laterally to afford a central abdominal access. The patient is prepped and draped, and access of the first three ports is achieved. Before the surgeon inserts the remaining trocars, the anesthesia provider returns the bed to its normal configuration so that the patient is again in lateral decubitus position. The kidney rest is then elevated, and the operation continues.

Some surgeons begin the procedure with the patient supine. The patient's contralateral arm is padded with thick foam from the shoulder to the fingertips. The patient is prepped and draped for thoracoabdominal surgery. Extra draping materials are used when the patient is repositioned.

Operative Procedure

1. The surgeon accesses the peritoneal cavity through a 1-cm transverse, subumbilical stab-wound incision. After elevation of the anterior abdominal wall with towel clips, the Veress needle is inserted with the stopcock valve control in the closed position.

2. After the Veress needle is in place, sterile saline is dropped into the lumen of the needle and the valve of the needle is opened. If the saline enters freely (a successful test), the abdominal cavity is inflated with CO_2 until a pressure of 15 to 20 mm Hg is obtained. If saline does not enter freely, it indicates improper placement of the needle.

3. The surgeon nicks the rectus fascia with the knife blade, and replaces the Veress needle with the 10-mm trocar. Towel clips are again used on each side of the incision to stabilize the abdominal wall during insertion.

4. The 10-mm laparoscope is inserted.

5. A second incision is made immediately below the costal margin in the midclavicular line, and a 10- to 12-mm trocar is inserted.

6. The surgeon inserts the first of three 5-mm trocars through a small incision 2 cm below the umbilicus in the midclavicular line.

7. The last two 5-mm trocars are placed, one in the anterior axillary line level with the umbilicus and one subcostal in the anterior axillary line. All trocars are then withdrawn until 2 to

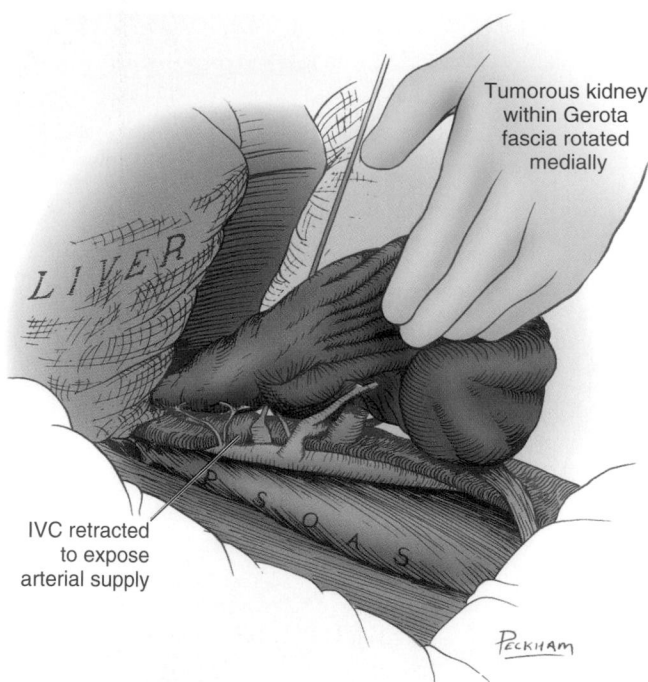

FIGURE 15-63 Nephrectomy. *IVC,* Inferior vena cava.

FIGURE 15-64 Interior view of exposing right kidney laparoscopically.

3 cm of each sheath protrudes into the abdomen. The surgeon may use polypropylene suture to secure the side arm ports to the patient's skin. Each trocar site is laparoscopically inspected after trocar insertion to identify any bleeding or perforation. On occasion it may be necessary to extend the incision for trocar insertion.

8. The ascending or descending colon is completely mobilized with electrosurgical scissors and deflected medially. The retroperitoneum is opened.
9. Using gentle motion on the ureteral catheter, the surgeon identifies and dissects the ureter. A Babcock forceps is clamped around the dissected ureter for retraction.
10. The ureter is dissected until the lower pole of the kidney is visualized (Figure 15-64). Any veins encountered are clipped twice proximally and twice distally. The kidney is cleared of surrounding tissue and freed laterally and superiorly. Gerota fascia is entered to free the adrenal gland and exclude it from the dissection.
11. The renal artery and vein are identified and cleared to create a 360-degree window around each vessel. The clip applier is inserted through the 10- to 12-mm port. Two clips are placed on the specimen side, and three clips are placed on the stump side of both the artery and the vein, which are then sharply incised.
12. Two pairs of clips are placed proximally and distally on the ureter, which is sharply incised. The specimen end is grasped, and the kidney is moved into the upper abdominal quadrant.
13. The surgeon introduces the entrapment sac through the 10- to 12-mm port. The bottom of the sac is pulled into the abdomen with graspers until the neck of the sac clears the end of the port and is then unfurled.
14. The sac is opened, and the ureteral stump with attached kidney is placed inside. The drawstrings are pulled tight, closing the mouth of the sac.

15. The anesthesia provider returns the patient to the supine position by tilting the OR bed, and the sac strings are extracted through the umbilical port. Under laparoscopic observation, the surgeon removes the port, and the neck of the sac is brought to lie on the abdominal surface. The tissue morcellator is inserted into the sac, and the kidney is morcellated under suction in a clockwise fashion.
16. The surgeon removes the instrumentation from the abdominal cavity, observing each trocar site, during and after removal, to ensure that hemostasis has been achieved. Fascial layers at the 12-mm trocar sites are closed with 2-0 or 3-0 absorbable suture in a figure-of-eight pattern.
17. Using a 4-0 absorbable suture, the surgeon performs a subcuticular closure of all port sites.

Heminephrectomy. Heminephrectomy is removal of a portion of the kidney. It is usually indicated for conditions involving the lower or upper pole of the kidney, such as calculus disease, or trauma limited to one pole of a kidney. In rare instances in which a patient has only one kidney, such surgery may be used for renal neoplasms to avoid the need for dialysis and subsequent renal transplantation.

Procedural Considerations. The setup is as described for nephrectomy with the addition of vascular and bulldog clamps.

Operative Procedure

1. The surgeon mobilizes the kidney and its pedicle as described for nephrectomy. The main vessels may be temporarily occluded for only 20 to 30 minutes, after which progressive renal damage may occur. Local hypothermia may be indicated to prolong ischemic operating time.
2. The renal capsule is incised and stripped back.
3. A wedge of kidney tissue containing the diseased or damaged cortex is excised. The surgeon clamps the interlobar fat or arcuate and interlobular arteries with Hopkins clamps and suture-ligates them with 4-0 absorbable suture on urologic needles.
4. The surgeon reapproximates the open collecting system with a continuous 4-0 suture.
5. Perirenal fat is placed in the area in which tissue was excised, and the renal parenchyma is reapproximated with horizontal mattress sutures.
6. If possible, the renal capsule is reapproximated with a continuous 2-0 suture.

Laparoscopic Partial Nephrectomy. Laparoscopic partial nephrectomy is usually indicated for the removal of a tumor, leaving more kidney than a heminephrectomy (Caceres et al, 2009).

Procedural Considerations. The setup is as described for laparoscopic nephrectomy.

Operative Procedure

1. Steps 1 to 8 of the laparoscopic nephrectomy procedure are repeated.
2. The surgeon locates the tumor and then clears the fat around it. The surgeon tries to keep the fat directly above the tumor in tact so the pathologists can confirm no advancement into the fat.
3. A 0.5- to 1-cm margin around the tumor is marked with the ESU. Some surgeons may use laparoscopic ultrasound to see the depth of the tumor.
4. The anesthesia provider administers IV mannitol and the surgeon clamps the hilum to prevent blood loss. Clamp time needs to be minimized to 30 minutes or else icing of the kidney is needed.
5. A scissors is used to sharply excise the tumor. If the collecting system of the kidney is entered, this needs to be closed separately. It can be checked for watertight closure with IV indigo carmine. Surgical bolsters and Floseal are generally used for hemostasis.
6. After the sutures are placed, the surgeon removes the hilar clamp and monitors for bleeding. A closed wound drain system may be placed.
7. The surgeon removes the instrumentation from the abdominal cavity, observing each trocar site, during and after removal, to ensure that hemostasis has been achieved. Fascial layers at the 12-mm trocar sites are closed with 2-0 or 3-0 absorbable suture in a figure-of-eight pattern.
8. Using a 4-0 absorbable suture, the surgeon performs a subcuticular closure of all port sites.

Radical Nephrectomy. Radical nephrectomy is excision of the kidney, perirenal fat, adrenal gland, Gerota capsule (fascia), and contiguous periaortic lymph nodes. This procedure is performed for parenchymal renal neoplasms. In the open approach, a lumbar, transthoracic, or transabdominal approach to the kidney is used, depending on the size and location of the lesion. The transthoracic or transabdominal approach is preferred because the blood vessels of the kidney can be more easily reached and ligated before the tumor is mobilized, decreasing the possibility of tumor embolization into the bloodstream. For the laparoscopic approach a retroperitoneal or transperitoneal approach may be used.

Procedural Considerations. The setups are as described for open nephrectomy and laparoscopic nephrectomy.

Operative Procedure. In general the procedure is as described for nephrectomy with two exceptions: (1) the renal pedicle is ligated before the kidney is mobilized, and (2) Gerota capsule is not incised but is removed en bloc with the kidney. Involved lymph nodes surrounding the renal pedicle are excised. A chest tube is inserted if the transthoracic approach is used.

Kidney Transplant

Kidney transplant entails transplantation of a living-related or cadaveric donor kidney into the recipient's iliac fossa (Figure 15-65). It is performed in an effort to restore renal function and thus maintain life in a patient who has end-stage renal disease.

Transplant from a Living Donor. The kidney donor must be in good health. ABO (blood typing) and histocompatibility (human leukocyte antigen [HLA] tissue typing) along with a negative white

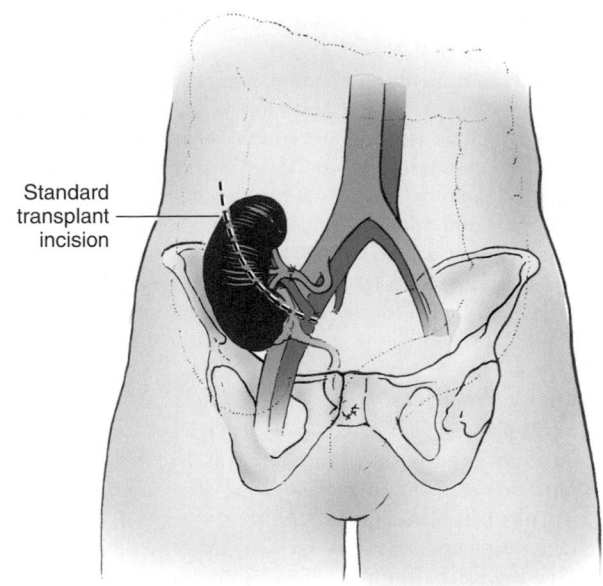

Standard transplant incision

FIGURE 15-65 Transplanted kidney in recipient's iliac fossa.

cell (lymphocyte) crossmatch determine donor-recipient compatibility. It is not necessary to match the Rh factor. After the donor has been chosen, a complete workup that includes history, physical examination, chest x-ray examination, ECG, CBC, BUN and creatinine values, blood chemistry profiles, coagulation studies, viral titers, and serologic testing is performed. Renal function is assessed by monitoring three creatinine clearances, urinalysis, and blood and urine cultures if hospitalized 72 hours or longer, followed by IVP and excretory urography. A flush aortogram assesses the vascular anatomy, and renal angiography pinpoints the kidney of choice while ruling out the presence of renal lesions. A kidney with a single renal artery is preferred, but kidneys with double and triple arteries may be used if necessary. If there is a family history of diabetes, a 5-hour glucose tolerance test is also performed (United Network for Organ Sharing [UNOS], 2012).

The ideal living donor is an identical twin, although a family member, friend, or altruistic donor may donate an organ. The living donor and the kidney recipient arrive in the preoperative registration area the morning of surgery. The patients are then brought to the preop holding area to be prepared for surgery (Mucksavage et al, 2011).

Procedural Considerations. Two adjacent ORs are prepared for the procedures; surgery on the donor and surgery on the recipient proceed simultaneously.

Usually the left kidney is chosen for removal because the left renal vein is longer than the right renal vein. Two IV lines and a Foley catheter are required. The patient is placed on a beanbag positioning device and moved into a modified flank position with the torso in a 30-degree lateral decubitus position with the right side down following endotracheal intubation. The lower arm is positioned extended outward on a well-padded armboard at a right angle to the torso; the upper arm is positioned on an elevated lateral armboard. The hips are rolled slightly posteriorly to allow exposure of the lower abdominal midline. Three pillows are placed between the patient's legs, and the ankles and feet are appropriately padded. An axillary roll is also placed and the radial pulse is confirmed in the right wrist. The bed is flexed to 30 degrees, and the upper portion is angled downward to approximately 140 degrees. The skin is prepped from midchest to pubis and draped to expose the flank area (Mucksavage et al, 2011).

Required instruments and equipment are identical to those for a nephrectomy plus an IV pole and supplies for the sterile perfusion table. These include electrolyte solution (placed in an iced basin until needed), cystoscopy tubing, a large kidney basin with iced saline solution, an olive tip, a 30-mL syringe, Gerald forceps, tenotomy scissors, a smooth Christmas tree tip, mosquitos, and Kelly hemostats (Mucksavage et al, 2011).

An electrolyte solution of histidine-tryptophan-ketoglutarate (HTK) or UW (University of Wisconsin) solution that contains 10,000 units of heparin is used to flush the harvested kidney (Mucksavage et al, 2011).

Operative Procedure
Open Approach

1. The donor nephrectomy procedure is as described for nephrectomy; however, the ureter and renal vein and artery require meticulous dissection.
2. Maximum length of the ureter is achieved by dividing it at or below the pelvic rim if possible. To preserve adequate ureteral vascularization, the surgeon is cautious not to skeletonize the ureter.
3. Particular care is taken to remove the maximum length of the renal vein and artery. Obtaining the maximum length of the left renal vein sometimes requires partial occlusion of the inferior vena cava with a Satinsky clamp and dissection of a portion of the inferior vena cava. This is done after the ureter has been freed.
4. Repair of the inferior vena cava is made with a continuous 4-0 or 5-0 vascular suture.
5. Five minutes before the surgeon clamps the renal vessels, 5000 units of heparin sodium and 12.5 g of mannitol are systemically administered to the patient to prevent intravascular clotting and maximize diuresis.
6. Furosemide, mannitol, and IV fluids are administered to the donor to maintain adequate urinary output from the donor's remaining kidney.
7. Gentle handling of the kidney is essential. Team members must prevent undue traction on the vascular pedicle, which may induce vasospasm and reduce perfusion of the kidney.
8. To reduce warm ischemia time the surgeon double-clamps the vein and the artery, excises the kidney, and immediately places it in iced saline solution on a sterile back table, where the kidney is flushed with the designated electrolyte solution. Warm ischemia time (from the clamping of renal vessels to a point at which the kidney is perfused with cold electrolyte solution) should be kept to a minimum to prevent acute tubular necrosis and to maintain maximum renal function after transplantation.
9. Gerald forceps are used to expose the renal artery to permit insertion of an olive tip or smooth Christmas tree cannula. The cold electrolyte solution passes through the IV tubing and the needle catheter, flushing any remaining donor's blood from the kidney. This also decreases the kidney's metabolic rate by lowering its temperature. Flushing time is usually 2 to 5 minutes.
10. After flushing the surgeon may trim the vessels of adventitia to facilitate the vascular anastomosis to the recipient's iliac vessels.
11. The kidney, in iced saline solution and HTK or UW solution, is covered with sterile drapes and taken by the surgeon to the room in which the recipient's iliac vessels have been exposed.
12. Wound closure for the donor is as described for nephrectomy.

Hand-Assisted Laparoscopic (HAL) Approach. The HAL approach allows surgeons direct hand contact with the operative field, maximizing tactile feedback and minimizing surgical injury to the patient. HAL differs from standard laparoscopy because surgeons are also able to introduce their hand into the operative field.

Procedural Considerations. A gel-port hand-port and three or four trocars are used. Generally, the hand-port and a 5-mm trocar are the working ports; a 10-mm trocar is used for the laparoscope, and an additional 5-mm trocar may be used if extra retraction is needed. Instruments required include the following: two 5-mm atraumatic graspers, 5-mm curved dissecting scissors, a coagulating hook, a bipolar grasper, two needle holders, a clip applier, a vascular stapler, and an atraumatic retrieval bag without a system for opening and closing it and a minimal opening of 15 cm. In addition, the standard open setup needs to be ready with open vascular instrumentation, a smooth Christmas tree adapter, sterile cystoscopy tubing, and sterile iced saline for ex vivo perfusion.

Operative Procedure

1. The surgeon creates a supraumbilical incision for the hand-port. After the hand-port is placed, a 10-mm trocar is placed through the hand-port to introduce pneumoperitoneum. A camera is introduced through the trocar to directly visualize the placement of the 5-mm working port, approximately two fingerbreadths cephalad to the hand-port. The 10-mm camera port is placed three fingerbreadths inferior to the xiphoid. An additional 5-mm trocar may be placed in the flank at the convex border of the kidney if extra retraction is necessary.
2. A bipolar ESU is used to incise the left lateral peritoneal reflection.
3. The descending colon is reflected medially from the beginning of the splenic flexure down to the level of the sigmoid colon, incising the phrenocolic ligaments completely. Care is taken to ensure no bowel injury or mesenteric defect occurs.
4. The surgeon divides the lienorenal and splenocolic ligaments at the inferior border of the spleen, allowing the spleen to be retracted superiorly and to mobilize the splenic flexure medially.
5. Gerota fascia is exposed by mobilizing the descending colon medially.
6. The plane is developed between Gerota fascia and the mesentery, adjacent to the lower pole of the kidney.
7. The plane medial to the gonadal vein and the ureter is developed and the structures are dissected off the psoas muscle, taking care not to devascularize the ureter.
8. The surgeon continues to dissect the medial aspect of the upper pole of the kidney, which is mobilized until the upper pole is completely free.
9. The left renal vein is then freed from its adventitial attachments and the adrenal and lumbar veins are identified, doubly clipped on both sides, and divided between clips.
10. After elevating the kidney, the surgeon performs additional dissection, usually posteriorly to the renal vein to identify and isolate the renal artery and after dividing the fibro-fatty and lymphatic tissue around the vessels.
11. The renal artery is dissected out, taking care to ensure there is space to pass the endovascular gastrointestinal anastomosis (GIA) stapler around the artery and vein.
12. The entire kidney is then freed of all its adventitial attachments.
13. The anesthesia provider administers 40 mg of furosemide (Lasix) and 12.5 mg of mannitol and 3000 units of heparin via the patient's IV.

14. Next the gonadal vein is double-clipped and divided and the ureter is triple-clipped and divided at the level of the iliac vessels.

15. After 3 minutes of systemic heparinization, the renal artery and vein are transected individually and sequentially with the endovascular GIA stapler.

16. The kidney is placed in the large basin with iced saline and flushed on the back table with 1 L of cold HTK or UW solution.

17. After the kidney is flushed, as described in the open donor nephrectomy, the kidney basin is covered with a drape and taken to the recipient OR.

18. The surgeon irrigates the peritoneum and achieves hemostasis. A drain may be inserted into the peritoneal space for a short time postoperatively.

19. The wounds are sutured and dressings applied (Mucksavage et al, 2011).

Transplant from a Cadaveric Donor. The ideal cadaveric donor is young, free from infection and cancer, normotensive until a short time before death, and under hospital observation several hours before death. Permission to harvest the donor kidney must be obtained from the family and the medical examiner after brain death has been unequivocally established. Awareness of existing state legislation in this complex area is advisable.

The donor is completely evaluated. The medical history is reviewed for any possible contraindications, such as chronic disease, ongoing systemic infection, IV drug abuse, malignancy, heart or lung disease, trauma to the donor organ, and the presence of human immunodeficiency virus (HIV). Laboratory studies include blood typing, urinalysis, urine and blood cultures, BUN, serum creatinine, CBC, hepatitis B antigen evaluation, Venereal Disease Research Laboratory (VDRL) for the presence of venereal disease, and p24 antigen capture assay for the presence of HIV antigen. Evaluation of arterial blood gases, electrolyte values, and liver enzymes is also necessary. Because of improvements in medical therapy, the only absolute contraindications to organ donation are HIV and metastasis.

Preoperative management of the cadaver donor is vital to the success of the transplant. Organ perfusion, oxygenation, and hydration must be maintained. Arterial blood gas evaluation determines ventilatory support, and dopamine may be administered if fluids alone are not able to maintain an adequate systolic blood pressure. Urine output is monitored, and antibiotics may be administered to combat and prevent infection.

Procedural Considerations. After brain death has been established, the donor is taken to the OR with respiratory and cardiac function maintained mechanically. The donor is placed in the supine position and is prepared for a laparotomy. Anticoagulant and α-adrenergic receptor-blocking agents are administered systemically during the procedure. Adequate renal perfusion and function are maintained with IV fluids and diuretics.

Instruments and equipment are the same as those for nephrectomy, with the addition of Metzenbaum scissors, suture scissors, vascular forceps, DeBakey forceps, Dean hemostatic forceps, mosquito hemostats, DeBakey clamps, angled clip appliers with medium and large clips, bulldog clamps, vascular clamps, Deaver retractors, Harrington splanchnic retractors, vascular needle holders, a sternal saw or Lebsche knife and mallet, umbilical tapes, electrolyte solution (lactated Ringer's, Sachs, or Collins), cold packing in an iced basin until needed, an IV pole, IV extension tubes, a kidney basin with cold (4° C [39.2° F]) IV saline solution, a three-way stopcock, an 18-gauge needle catheter, a centimeter ruler, the perfusion machine or kidney transplantation equipment, and ice.

Operative Procedure

1. The surgeon makes a midline incision from the xiphoid process to the symphysis pubis with bilateral supraumbilical transverse extensions through the skin, subcutaneous layer, fascia, and muscle.

2. Hemostasis is obtained with clamps, ties, suture ligatures, and the ESU.

3. The kidney, renal vessels, and ureter are carefully dissected with Metzenbaum scissors, DeBakey forceps, and Dean hemostatic forceps.

4. The anesthesia provider administers 15,000 units of heparin sodium intravenously 5 to 10 minutes before the renal vessels are clamped.

5. The usual method of resection is en bloc resection (harvesting of donor kidneys) (Figure 15-66), which involves the removal of sections of the inferior vena cava and aorta with both kidneys in continuity.

6. The surgeon makes an incision along the route of the small bowel mesentery up to the esophageal hiatus.

7. The entire GI tract, spleen, and inferior portion of the pancreas are mobilized by dividing the celiac axis and the superior mesenteric artery, exposing the entire retroperitoneal region.

8. Using vascular clamps, the surgeon clamps and divides the inferior vena cava and aorta below the renal vessels.

9. Lumbar tributaries are secured with metal clips and are divided.

10. The kidneys and ureters are freed from their surrounding soft tissues.

11. The ureters are divided distally at the pelvic brim.

12. The surgeon clamps and divides the suprarenal aorta and inferior vena cava at the level of the diaphragm, close to the bifurcation.

13. The vessels and kidney are severed and the aorta and vena cava ligated.

14. After removal of the kidneys, immediate perfusion with cold (4° C [29.2° F]) UW or electrolyte solution is carried out. The kidneys are placed in a container of cold saline solution and surrounded by saline slush in an insulated carrier or placed on a hypothermic pulsatile perfusion machine for transport. While kidney perfusion is begun, the abdominal lymph nodes and spleen are removed for use in tissue typing.

15. The incision is closed with interrupted sutures, and artificial life-support systems are terminated. The perioperative nurse cares for the patient's body, preserving privacy, and dignity at the patient's death.

Transplant Recipient. Each potential recipient is judged individually in regard to kidney transplantation. Most people younger than 55 years are acceptable; older patients are less tolerant of postoperative complications. Contraindications for renal transplantation include: (1) systemic disease that precludes major surgery, (2) oxalosis (a metabolic disorder), (3) a positive HLA cytotoxic antibody screen, (4) untreatable cardiovascular disease, (5) active cancer, and (6) noncompliance (Ibrahim and Kasiske, 2008). If required, a patient may need to undergo bilateral nephrectomy before renal transplantation for uncontrollable hypertension, for kidney infections, or for reflux when there is a significant history of infections. Occasionally a large polycystic kidney may need to be removed to create a space for the new kidney. Splenectomy may be performed

FIGURE 15-66 En bloc resection.

at this time to improve leukopenia and enhance the effects of myelosuppressive and immunosuppressive drugs.

The transplant recipient requires optimal nutritional support and adequate dialysis. All potential sources of infection must be treated. Most commonly these include teeth, bladder, nasal sinuses, and skin. The patient may need a short course of hemodialysis to control fluid overload or electrolyte imbalances. A repeat cytotoxic crossmatch with fresh serum specimens should follow hemodialysis. Preoperative antibiotics are commonly administered. Other important diagnostic tools for preoperative evaluation are chest x-ray examination, abdominal ultrasonography, voiding cystourethrography, liver function studies, hematologic assays, and serum values for screening hepatitis, HIV, and viral diseases.

Procedural Considerations. The perioperative nurse positions the patient in the supine position. A Foley catheter is inserted into the bladder by sterile technique. Approximately 100 mL of antibiotic mixed in an IV bag of 0.9% normal saline is instilled into the bladder through cystoscopy tubing. The bladder is filled and drained four times. The fifth instillation of 100 mL is left in the bladder and the cystoscopy tubing is clamped until the time of the ureteral anastomosis. The patient is prepped from nipples to groin and draped.

Operative Procedure

1. The surgeon makes a curved right lower quadrant incision through the skin, subcutaneous layer, fascia, and muscle.
2. Bleeding is controlled with clamps, ties, and an ESU.
3. The inferior epigastric vessels are divided between suture ligatures.
4. Retroperitoneal dissection is performed by mobilizing the peritoneum superiorly and medially.
5. A self-retaining Bookwalter retractor is placed once exposure is attained.
6. Using Metzenbaum scissors and DeBakey forceps, the surgeon dissects along the entire length of the hypogastric artery and the external and common iliac arteries to the bifurcation of the aorta, continuing down the internal iliac artery.
7. The internal iliac artery is ligated distally and divided, with proximal control maintained by a vascular clamp.
8. The iliac vein may be dissected free by ligating and dividing the internal iliac venous branches with 3-0 nonabsorbable sutures or ligating clips. More commonly, only the hypogastric artery and that portion of iliac vein to be anastomosed are dissected free.
9. The donor kidney is brought into the operative field in a large basin of iced saline and HTK or UW solution.
10. The surgeon uses mosquito hemostats, 4-inch DeBakey forceps, and curved and straight fine scissors to make the necessary alterations on the donor kidney vessels to facilitate the anastomoses.
11. A Lambert Kay clamp is placed on the internal iliac vein.
12. A #11 blade is used to make a 1-cm incision in the iliac vein between the clamps.
13. The vessel is rinsed with heparin sodium solution (10 units/mL) in a 30-mL syringe with an olive tip.
14. Angled Potts scissors are used to extend the incision to accommodate the donor renal vein.
15. The surgeon performs the anastomosis of the donor kidney renal vein to the side of the recipient's iliac vein with 15-0 double-armed vascular sutures.
16. In like manner the renal artery is anastomosed end-to-end with the proximal portion of the internal iliac artery using 15-0 vascular sutures.
17. Before placing the final sutures, the vessels are irrigated proximally and distally with heparin sodium solution with a 30-mL syringe with an olive tip.
18. The Lambert Kay clamps are removed from the venous vessels, and the anastomosis is checked for leakage.

19. The clamp on the internal iliac artery is then released, and the anastomosis is checked.
20. Meticulous inspection is made of the hilum and surface of the kidney for bleeding and infarction.
21. The anesthesia provider administers diuretics intravenously as needed.
22. Attention is then directed to the ureter and bladder.
23. Two Gerald forceps are used to grasp the anterior bladder wall.
24. Using a scalpel with a #10 knife blade, the surgeon makes a 4-cm anterior incision.
25. The ureter is passed through the bladder wall and tunneled suburothelially for 2 to 2.5 cm.
26. The surgeon sutures the spatulated end of the ureter into the bladder urothelium with four to six 15-0 atraumatic absorbable sutures, creating a ureteroneocystostomy.
27. A 6F ureteral stent is passed through the ureteroneocystostomy, up to the renal pelvis, and out through the urethra with the Foley catheter. This stenting catheter will remain in place for 36 to 48 hours to ensure ureteral patency during a period in which ureteral edema may occur.
28. Retractors are removed, and the bladder is closed with 5-0 atraumatic absorbable suture.
29. The renal anastomoses are again checked for bleeding.
30. The cystoscopy tubing is disconnected from the Foley catheter and a urometer is attached to the Foley catheter to monitor postoperative urine output.
31. Closed wound suction drains are inserted into the wound, exteriorized through the skin laterally, and secured with 2-0 nonabsorbable suture on a cutting needle.
32. Muscle and fascial layers are closed with a single layer of 0 nonabsorbable sutures on a large atraumatic needle.
33. The subcutaneous layer is closed with 3-0 absorbable sutures on an atraumatic needle.
34. Skin closure is accomplished with skin staples, and dressings are applied.

Adrenalectomy

Adrenalectomy is partial or total excision of one or both adrenal glands. It may be performed for several reasons: hypersecretion of adrenal hormones; neoplasms of the adrenal gland; or for secondary treatment of neoplasms elsewhere in the body that depend on adrenal hormonal secretions, such as carcinoma of the prostate and breast; and pheochromocytoma.

Care of the patient with pheochromocytoma carries with it particular concerns for the perioperative nurse. These patients are subject to extreme elevations in blood pressure, often accompanied by tachycardia, and hypovolemic states that can induce vascular collapse. If an adrenal tumor is being excised, early ligation of the adrenal vein is crucial in avoiding a sudden blood pressure elevation from the manipulation of the gland. After tumor removal there will be a rapid drop in blood pressure that can be minimized by maintenance of blood volume and administration of norepinephrine. With bilateral adrenalectomy, cortisone replacement is instituted.

Procedural Considerations. Adrenalectomy may be approached as a laparoscopic or an open procedure. The laparoscopic approach is generally associated with less morbidity and shorter hospital stays. For unilateral adrenalectomy the patient may be placed in the lateral or supine position, depending on the intended approach. If both glands are to be removed the supine or prone position is selected. The prone position is especially useful for a known disorder, such as aldosteronism, localized benign lesions, and solitary adenomas of Cushing disease, and for debilitated patients with an advanced neoplasm.

The setup for a lateral approach is like that described for nephrectomy, including rib resection instruments, vascular instruments, and vessel clips and appliers. The setup for an abdominal approach is like that described for laparotomy, including vascular instruments, extralong scissors, tissue forceps, Rochester-Péan forceps, Mixter forceps, and needle holders. Penrose tubing is needed for retraction. Vessel clips and appliers also may be needed, as well as various sizes of nonabsorbable braided sutures.

The setup for the posterior approach is like that described for the lateral approach. The patient is placed prone in a 35-degree jackknife position with the kidney rest under the inferior margin of the anterior rib cage. Both arms should be carefully extended cephalad with adequate support under each shoulder.

Operative Procedure
Laparoscopic Approach

1. The surgeon makes a 1.5-cm incision at the tip of the twelfth rib. The thoracolumbar fascia is entered by blunt dissection, and the 12-mm balloon dissector is placed behind Gerota fascia and along the anterior axillary line. The balloon is inflated with 800 mL of saline, and the laparoscope is used to confirm balloon placement.
2. The operating balloon trocar is then placed in this position.
3. The surgeon inserts two 10-mm trocars on each side of the initial trocar, along the costal margin, in the anterior and posterior axillary line.
4. The fourth trocar is placed along the posterior costal margin.
5. Dissection begins near the renal hilum, incising into Gerota fascia.
6. The surgeon identifies, clips, and divides the adrenal arteries.
7. The anterior, lateral aspect of the gland is freed from the upper pole of the kidney.
8. The adrenal vein is clipped and divided.
9. The surgeon mobilizes the posterior, superior, and anterior surfaces of the adrenal gland. A fan retractor is used to retract the pancreas and spleen, or pancreas and liver, depending on which side the gland is being excised.
10. The adrenal branches of the inferior phrenic vessels and any accessory vessels are clipped and divided. The gland is removed through the original port using a retrieval sac. Hemostasis is achieved. The trocars are then sequentially removed, the incisions closed, and dressings applied.

Lateral Approach—Open

1. A flank, thoracolumbar, or transthoracic incision is performed as described for nephrectomy.
2. The rib underlying the chosen approach is resected or deflected for optimum exposure of the upper pole of the kidney.
3. The surgeon enters between the eleventh and twelfth ribs in a flank approach, the tenth and eleventh ribs in a thoracolumbar approach, and the ninth and tenth ribs in a transthoracic approach.
4. Using scissors, the surgeon makes an opening through the transverse fascia.
5. The pleura and diaphragm are protected with moist laparotomy packs, and Gerota fascia is incised to expose the kidney and adrenal gland.

6. The surgeon identifies the gland and dissects it free from the upper pole of the kidney with scissors and Babcock forceps.

7. The blood supply of the gland is identified, clamped or clipped, and divided. Bleeding vessels are ligated.

8. To release the gland the left adrenal vein, a branch of the left renal vein, is separated by clamping and cutting. The right adrenal vein, a tributary of the vena cava, is also divided. Fine vascular sutures may be required to repair inadvertent injury to the vena cava.

9. When hemostasis has been ensured, the surgeon closes the wound in sequential layers: muscle, fascia, subcutaneous tissue, and skin. Dressings are then applied.

Abdominal Approach

1. The surgeon incises the abdominal wall with an upper abdominal incision, and the peritoneal cavity is opened and explored.

2. Hemostasis is established.

3. The abdominal wound is retracted, and the surrounding organs are protected with moist laparotomy packs.

4. The surgeon opens the retroperitoneal area near the diaphragm on the left side, exposing the renal fascia.

5. The renal fascia is opened to reveal the left kidney and adrenal gland.

6. Using blunt and sharp dissection, the surgeon frees the adrenal gland from the kidney, clamps all bleeding vessels, and ligates them with 3-0 nonabsorbable sutures.

7. After all bleeding is controlled, the surgeon replaces the kidney in the renal fascia, and closes it with interrupted 0 absorbable sutures.

8. The peritoneum is closed over the left kidney and renal fascia.

9. The abdominal retractors are rearranged to provide access to the peritoneum over the right kidney and adrenal gland. Care must be taken to prevent trauma to the liver.

10. The surgeon repeats the procedure on the right side, taking care to clamp and ligate the short adrenal vein.

11. The abdomen is inspected for bleeding vessels, which are clamped and ligated.

12. The wound is closed and dressings applied.

Posterior Approach

1. The surgeon makes an incision over the eleventh or twelfth rib.

2. The periosteum is elevated, avoiding the nerves and vessels on the inferior margin.

3. The diaphragm and pleura are displaced superiorly, the appropriate rib is resected and hemostasis is achieved.

4. Gerota fascia is incised, and through sharp and blunt dissection the surgeon exposes the posterior aspect of the upper pole of the kidney.

5. The surgeon mobilizes the upper pole and places a padded retractor to deflect the kidney downward for the approach to the adrenal gland.

6. The suprarenal fat is meticulously dissected.

7. Vessel clips are used for control of smaller vessels.

8. Dissection continues superiorly, laterally, and inferiorly while the integrity of the hilum of the adrenal gland is maintained.

9. Using right-angled clamps, the surgeon frees, divides and ligates the adrenal vein and artery.

10. Babcock clamps are used for manipulation and removal of the adrenal gland.

11. Bleeding is controlled, and the wound is inspected for injury to renal structures.

12. The surgeon closes Gerota fascia with interrupted absorbable sutures.

13. The wound is closed and dressings applied.

Key Points

- A variety of surgical techniques and approaches in the field of urologic surgery offer patients many options for treating benign and malignant conditions.

- Urologic procedures on men are more prevalent due to the prevalence of benign and malignant prostatic conditions. Benign prostatic hyperplasia (BPH) is one of the most common diseases of aging men, ranking in the top 10 most commonly diagnosed conditions in men older than age 50. Prostate cancer is the most frequently diagnosed cancer in men and is the second leading cause of cancer death in men.

- Key factors to consider in planning patient care include positioning and attention to fluid and electrolyte balance. Many procedures require lithotomy positioning, which has a high potential for patient injury. The use of various solutions to aid in visualization and electrocautery during transurethral resection of the prostate (TURP) procedures may contribute to hyponatremia.

Critical Thinking Question

You are assigned as the perioperative nurse for a 58-year-old man who will undergo a robotic radical prostatectomy. The patient states he has a history of hypertension and inguinal hernia repair but denies any other history. However, while positioning the patient you note that he has bilateral incisional scars consistent with hip arthroplasty. His range of motion is severely inhibited in both joints. What risk factors must you take into consideration concerning positioning? How can traditional lithotomy positioning place the patient into further danger? What alternative position(s) would be safer for the patient?

@volve *The answers to the Critical Thinking Question can be found at http://evolve.elsevier.com/Rothrock/Alexander.*

REFERENCES

American Cancer Society: *Cancer facts and figures 2012*, Atlanta, 2012, American Cancer Society.

American Medical Systems (AMS): *Erectile dysfunction*, 2009, available at www.americanmedicalsystems.com/prof_erectile_restoration_product_objectname_prof_male_700_inflatable.html. Accessed January 7, 2013.

Association of periOperative Registered Nurses (AORN): *Creating a patient safety culture guideline. In Perioperative standards and recommended practices*, Denver, 2012a, The Association.

Association of periOperative Registered Nurses (AORN): Recommended practices for sterilization in the perioperative practice setting. In *Perioperative standards and recommended practices*, Denver, 2012b, The Association.

Boston Scientific: *Coaptite injectible implant*, 2009, available at www.bostonscientific.com/templatedata/imports/collateral/Gynecology/broc_coaptite_02_us_all_ug.pdf. Accessed December 29, 2012.

Caceres F et al: Laparoscopic partial nephrectomy, *Actas Urol Españ (English Edition)* 35(8): 487–493, 2009.

Denholm B: Tucking patient's arms and general positioning, *AORN J* 89(4):755–757, 2009.

Epstein JL: Pathology of prostatic neoplasia. In Wein AJ et al, editors: *Campbell-Walsh urology*, ed 9, Philadelphia, 2007, Saunders.

Gonzalgo ML: Minimally invasive surgical approaches and management of prostate cancer, *Urol Clin North Am* 35:489–504, 2008.

Gross C et al: Sacral neuromodulation for nonobstructive urinary retention: a meta-analysis, *Female Pelvic Med Reconstr Surg* 16(4):249–253, 2010.

Han M, Partin AW: Retropubic and suprapubic open prostatectomy. In Wein AJ et al, editors: *Campbell-Walsh urology*, ed 9, Philadelphia, 2007, Saunders.

Ibrahim HN, Kasiske BL: Donor and recipient issues. In Brenner BM, Levine SA, editors: *Brenner & Rector's the kidney*, ed 8, Philadelphia, 2008, Saunders.

Ignatavicius DD: Care of male patients with reproductive problems. In Ignatavicius DD, Workman ML, editors: *Medical-surgical nursing: patient-centered collaborative care*, ed 7, St Louis, 2013, Saunders.

Langenhuijsen JF et al: Cryosurgery for prostate cancer: an update on clinical results of modern cryotechnology, *Eur Urol* 55:76–86, 2009.

Lipshultz LI et al: Surgical management of male infertility. In Wein AJ et al, editors: *Campbell-Walsh urology*, ed 9, Philadelphia, 2007, Saunders.

Mucksavage P et al: Laparoscopic transperitoneal nephrectomy for renal cancer: The University of California, Irvine, technique, *J Endourol* 25(2):195–200, 2011.

Scott RD: *The direct medical costs of healthcare-associated infections in U.S. hospitals and the benefits of prevention*, October 2012, Centers for Disease Control and Prevention, available at www.cdc.gov/ncidod/dhqp/hai.html. Accessed January 7, 2013.

Smith AL, Wein A: Recent advances in management of bladder overactivity, *F1000 Med Rep*, 11(2):9, 2010.

Steele G et al: *Clinical manifestations, diagnosis, and staging of testicular germ cell tumors*, 2012, available at UpToDatewww.uptodate.com/contents/clinical-manifestations-diagnosis-and-staging-of-testicular-germ-cell-tumors#H1. Accessed: December 29, 2012.

Steinberg GD: Response to Lammers and Witjes article: new developments in intravesical therapy for non-muscle-invasive bladder cancer, *Expert Rev Anticancer Ther* 11(9):1331–1332, 2011.

Uffort EE, Jensen JC: Side docking the robot for robotic laparoscopic radical prostatectomy, *JSLS* 15(2):200–202, 2011.

United Network for Organ Sharing (UNOS): *A guide to calculating and interpreting the kidney donor profile index (KDPI)*, 2012, available at http://optn.transplant.hrsa.gov/ContentDocuments/Guide_to_Calculating_Interpreting_KDPI.pdf 2012. Accessed January 11, 2013.

Young E et al: Perioperative fluid management, *AORN J* 89:167–178, 2009.

CHAPTER 16

Thyroid and Parathyroid Surgery

MARIA MARINELLI

Manifestations of thyroid glandular diseases include goiter, benign and malignant nodules, hyperthyroidism, hypothyroidism, and inflammatory conditions. Goiters have been described since 2700 BCE, before the thyroid gland was even identified. During the Italian Renaissance, around 1500, Leonardo da Vinci depicted two glands located on either side of the larynx. In 1543 Vesalius labeled the tissue "laryngeal glands." However, Thomas Wharton, in a 1656 publication titled *Adenograpahia,* is credited with replacing the term as the "thyroid gland," with a Greek origin word *(thyreoeides),* meaning "shield shaped." The first documented thyroid surgery occurred in the twelfth century, described by Roger Frugardi. High mortality rates of 40% were the norm until medical advances in anesthesia, antisepsis, and hemostasis were developed during the 1800s. Two notable thyroid surgeons, C.A. Theodore Billroth (1829-1894) and Emil Theodor Kocher (1841-1917), revolutionized the treatment of thyroid diseases. Kocher received the Nobel Prize in 1909 for his advances in thyroid surgery, performing more than 2000 surgeries, with a 4.5% death rate. He captured the title "Father of Thyroid Surgery" for his high rate of surgical achievement in the field of thyroid surgical procedures (Hunter and Jobe, 2010).

Today surgeons continue to perform surgical procedures on the thyroid gland for various underlying causes. Surgery ranges from lobectomy and isthmectomy for papillary microcarcinomas (lesions smaller than 1 cm) to near-total and total thyroidectomies for symptomatic multinodular goiters. Technologic advances have added new approaches to thyroid and parathyroid surgery, such as minimally invasive surgery (MIS) techniques. Emergence of endocrine surgery as a surgical subspecialty that requires advanced postgraduate training has evolved due to the complexity in management of surgical disorders of thyroid, parathyroid, adrenal glands, and neuroendocrine pancreas tumors (Wang, 2011).

Surgical Anatomy

Thyroid Gland

The thyroid gland (Figure 16-1) is a highly vascular organ that lies in the anterior portion of the neck, deep to the paired strap muscles, resting on the midline of the trachea. It is attached to the cricoid and trachea by the ligament of Berry. The inferior border of the thyroid varies and may be located above or below the sternal notch. It consists of right and left lobes united by a middle portion, the isthmus, and it weighs approximately 20 g (Figure 16-2). The isthmus is situated near the base of the neck, between the second and fourth tracheal rings, and the lobes lie beside the larynx, trachea, and esophagus. The pyramidal lobe, a long, thin projection of thyroid tissue protruding cephalad from the isthmus, is found in

about 30% of patients at surgery; it is the vestige of the embryonic thyroglossal duct and migrates from the foramen cecum at the base of the tongue.

Blood supply to the thyroid is from the superior thyroid artery, which originates from the external carotid artery, and from the inferior thyroid artery, which originates from the thyrocervical trunk of the subclavian artery. The points at which these two arteries enter the thyroid gland are referred to as "poles" of the thyroid and are important anatomic landmarks during surgery. The thyroid gland is drained by three pairs of veins (superior, middle, and inferior thyroid veins). Occasionally a single thyroid artery (thyroidea ima) may arise directly from the arch of the aorta or the innominate artery and rise in front of the trachea to enter the midline of the gland inferiorly.

The recurrent laryngeal nerve, a branch of the vagus nerve, innervates the intrinsic muscles of the larynx. The right recurrent laryngeal nerve loops under the subclavian artery and ascends in an oblique direction lateral to the tracheoesophageal groove. The recurrent laryngeal nerve contains both motor and sensory fibers. The motor component innervates the abductor muscles of the true vocal cords. The sensory component supplies sensation to the larynx below the vocal cords. During surgery, care is taken to identify and protect this nerve. Immediate hoarseness occurs if the nerve is divided on one side. If the recurrent nerve is injured bilaterally, acute paralysis of both vocal cords may obstruct the airway and require emergency tracheotomy. Injury to the external branch of

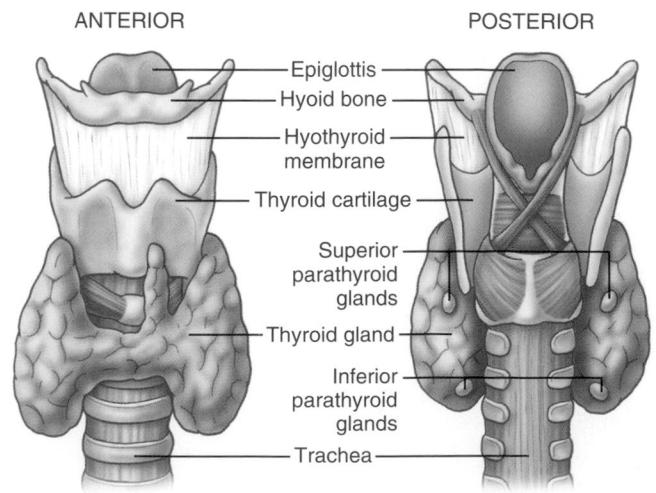

FIGURE 16-1 The thyroid gland.

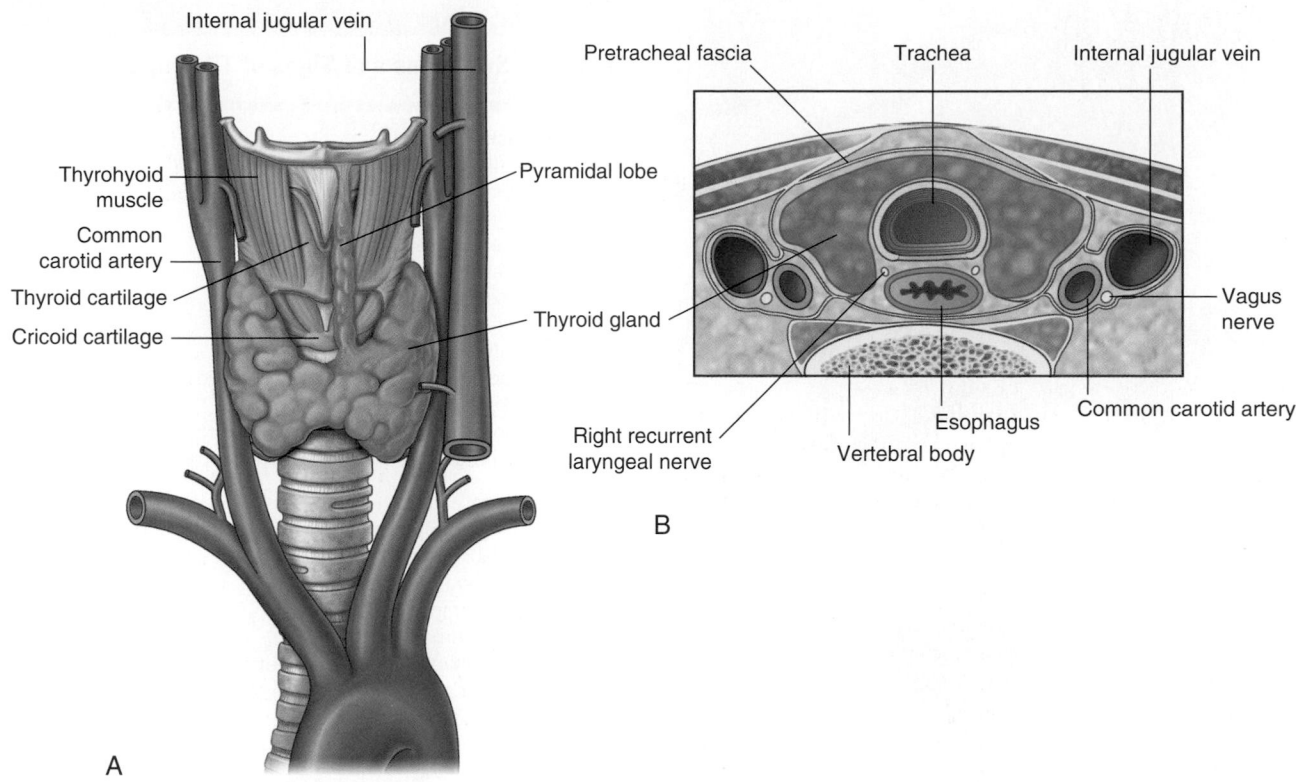

Internal jugular vein

Thyrohyoid muscle

Common carotid artery

Thyroid cartilage

Cricoid cartilage

Pyramidal lobe

Thyroid gland

A

Pretracheal fascia   Trachea   Internal jugular vein

Vagus nerve

Common carotid artery

Right recurrent laryngeal nerve   Vertebral body   Esophagus

B

FIGURE 16-2 Thyroid in relation to surrounding structures.

the superior laryngeal nerve, which innervates the cricothyroid muscle, results in difficulty shouting or singing high notes.

The thyroid gland produces three hormones: thyroxine (T_4) and triiodothyronine (T_3) (together known as the *thyroid hormones*) and calcitonin. T_3 and T_4 cannot be synthesized without iodine and regulate energy metabolism and growth and development. Calcitonin inhibits calcium resorption from bone and increases calcium storage in the bone. In addition, calcitonin increases renal excretion of calcium and phosphorus and decreases serum calcium levels. When elevations in serum calcitonin are found in the patient's blood work, medullary thyroid cancer is suspected. When there is a family history of thyroid cancer, family members are encouraged to seek genetic testing for medullary thyroid carcinoma (Lewis et al, 2011). Thyroid-stimulating hormone (TSH) is synthesized by the anterior pituitary, and stimulates the production and release of thyroid hormones and the uptake of iodine.

Parathyroid Gland

The parathyroid glands are small ovoid masses, usually four in number, situated behind the thyroid lobes. Normal parathyroid glands are generally small, lobular, and yellow, but their color may vary from yellow to mahogany. They are usually found in pairs and are about the size of a lentil bean. It can be challenging to differentiate the gland from a lobule of fat, a thyroid nodule, or lymph node. Thyroid adenomas generally, although not always, tend to be larger, asymmetric, and more red-brown than normal parathyroids (Figure 16-3). The upper pair of glands lies in proximity to the posterior portion of the superior pole of the thyroid; the lower pair usually (about 60% of the time) lies near the posterior lateral aspect of the lower pole of the thyroid. Ectopic parathyroid glands, more

common in the inferior parathyroid glands, may be found in the superior mediastinum, especially within the thymus and as low as the pericardium. To allow for interdisciplinary communication between pathologists, radiologists, surgeons, endocrinologists, and anesthesiologists, a classification system is used to determine the most commonly located positions for enlarged parathyroid glands (Harris et al, 2012). Each parathyroid gland measures approximately $3 \times 3 \times 3$ mm and generally weighs less than 50 mg; the upper glands are generally smaller than the lower ones. Both the upper and lower parathyroid glands receive their blood supply from the inferior thyroid artery (Figure 16-4). Because the blood supply to the superior parathyroid stems from that of the supply to the inferior parathyroid, disrupting supply to the inferior parathyroid compromises the supply to the upper parathyroid.

The parathyroid glands secrete parathyroid hormone (PTH), an antagonist to calcitonin. Both PTH and calcitonin work together to maintain calcium homeostasis (Figure 16-5) by increasing calcium removal from storage in bone and increasing absorption of calcium by the intestines. A recent study (Kim, 2012) concludes that an insufficient number of parathyroid glands is the cause of hypocalcemia after total thyroidectomy and node dissection. Therefore, preserving at least one parathyroid gland after a routine thyroidectomy may prevent permanent hypocalcemia.

Perioperative Nursing Considerations

Assessment

Appropriate pharmacologic measures used in treatment of hyperthyroidism include antithyroid drugs, iodine, and β-adrenergic

BOX 16-1

Common Symptoms and Signs of Thyroid Dysfunction

Hypothyroidism

- Fatigue, lethargy, weakness
- Weight gain, puffy face
- Cold intolerance, decreased sweating
- Dry, sparse, coarse hair; dry skin
- Anemia, pallor
- Hoarse voice, decreased hearing
- Poor concentration, depression
- Muscle stiffness and pain
- Generalized interstitial edema, inelastic cold skin
- Bradycardia, cardiac hypertrophy
- Constipation, decreased libido
- Menstrual irregularity (especially heavy menses; infertility)

Hyperthyroidism

- Vision changes: myopathy, ophthalmopathy, and exophthalmos
- Emotional lability, restlessness
- Irritability, mood changes
- Exercise intolerance, fatigue
- Dependent edema
- Weight loss, thirst, increased appetite
- Heat intolerance and flushing
- Hyperactivity, especially children
- Bounding, rapid pulse
- Increased sweating
- Insomnia, exhaustion
- Muscle weakness, tremor
- Dyspnea on mild exertion
- Frequent bowel movements
- Menstrual irregularity (oligomenorrhea; infertility)
- More common in elderly: tachycardia and atrial tachydysrhythmias, palpitations, cardiomegaly

Modified from Lewis S et al: *Medical-surgical nursing*, ed 8, St Louis, 2011, Mosby.

FIGURE 16-3 A, A right upper parathyroid adenoma in situ. The thyroid gland is retracted to the midline. The recurrent laryngeal nerve enters the operative field inferiorly and tracks superiorly in the tracheoesophageal groove. The carotid sheath lies lateral to the nerve. The adenoma is the lobular mahogany mass located at the superior pole of the thyroid. **B,** Parathyroid adenoma after removal.

blockers. Medications are considered useful in treating symptoms during the thyrotoxic states and in returning the thyroid hormone levels and metabolism to a normal state. Radiation therapy or surgery is ultimately necessary because the medication regimen is not considered a "cure." Preoperatively the patient with hyperthyroidism most likely has had appropriate drug therapy that has returned thyroid hormone levels and metabolic state to normal (Lewis et al, 2011). Perioperative nurses assess for any symptoms that relate to accelerated metabolism (Box 16-1). The patient's baseline vital signs are noted for an abnormally elevated resting pulse rate, elevated systolic blood pressure, and cardiac symptoms, such as palpitations or atrial fibrillation. Studies show that patients with overactive thyroid conditions have an increased risk of various heart problems, particularly atrial fibrillation, that may lead to premature death (Burman and Rodoni, 2012). The perioperative nurse should determine whether anticoagulant and thyroid medications are being taken by the patient. The patient's cardiac and respiratory rates, muscle strength, elimination patterns, history of weight loss, heat intolerance, and emotional status are reviewed. The patient, especially a young one, may be anxious about the disease state and the success of surgery, and may express concerns about neck surgery and its cosmetic results. Patients who are concerned about body image should have the opportunity to discuss these issues with the

perioperative nurse. Vocalists may be especially concerned about whether surgery will adversely affect their voice. The anesthesia provider may choose to use an endotracheal tube with a smaller diameter than usual in order to minimize any trauma to the vocal cords. Skin integrity should be determined; patients with hyperthyroidism may have finely textured skin and edema in the lower extremities, placing them at higher risk for skin breakdown. The most typical complications specific to thyroid surgery, although infrequent, are hypoparathyroidism and injury to the recurrent laryngeal nerve. Preoperative assessment of the patient's voice tone and quality should therefore be noted.

Large thyroid nodules may cause tracheal shift and present a challenge to the anesthesia provider for intubation and airway management. The size of thyroid enlargement should be noted preoperatively and steps taken to prepare the operating room (OR) in anticipation of a difficult intubation. The "difficult airway" anesthesia cart should be in the room along with, preferably, two anesthesia providers and the circulating nurse standing by to assist with induction. The anesthesia provider will not extubate a patient who has been difficult to intubate until the anesthestic gases have dissipated and level of consciousness is such that the patient can protect his or her own airway and maintain oxygen saturation with spontaneous breathing. If there is concern about postoperative edema and ensuing airway obstruction from a difficult induction, the anesthesia

FIGURE 16-4 Posterior view of thyroid and parathyroids. Note relation to carotid sheath and esophagus. Note pathway of recurrent laryngeal nerves.

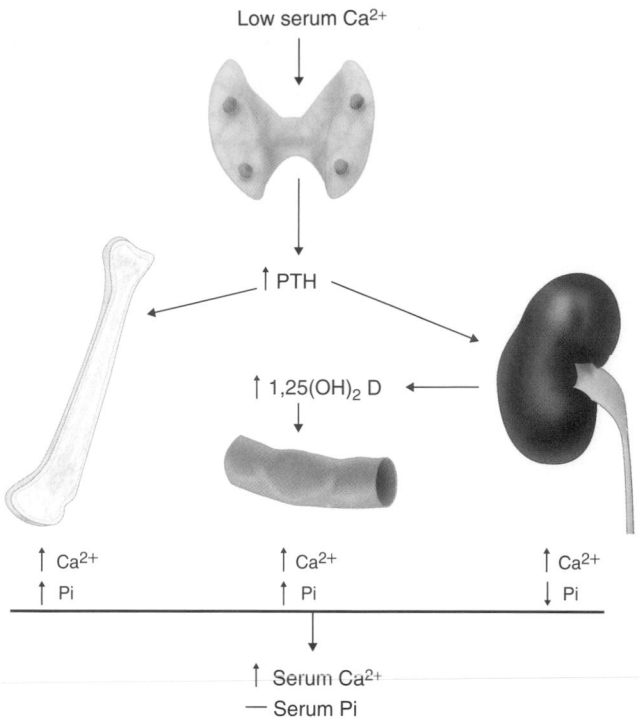

Low serum Ca²⁺

↑ PTH

↑ 1,25(OH)₂ D

| ↑ Ca²⁺ | ↑ Ca²⁺ | ↑ Ca²⁺ |
| ↑ Pi | ↑ Pi | ↓ Pi |

↑ Serum Ca²⁺
— Serum Pi

FIGURE 16-5 Homeostatic response to a fall in serum calcium (Ca^{2+}). *Pi,* Inorganic phosphate; *PTH,* parathyroid hormone; *1,25(OH)₂D,* biologically active form of vitamin D.

provider may administer steroids intraoperatively and choose to leave the tube in postoperatively.

Grossly enlarged thyroids are also more difficult to excise, and intraoperative bleeding is more common and profuse. Finger dissection may be unavoidable and small vessels that retract and contract may rupture during emergence or postoperatively, leading to hemorrhage. Hemorrhage may cause tracheal compression and airway compromise. Generally, patients who have larger glands excised will require a drain for postoperative wound drainage (Byrne, 2013). They must be closely monitored during emergence from anesthesia and postoperatively; excessive swelling at the operative site, with or without poor air exchange, must be treated as a potentially life-threatening emergency. The instrument table should be kept sterile until the patient is extubated and has left the OR. A tracheotomy tray with tubes should be readily available should an emergency tracheotomy be necessary.

In addition to clinical signs and symptoms, results of diagnostic tests should be reviewed (Evidence for Practice). Tests performed most commonly before thyroid surgery include measurements of TSH, T_3, and T_4 levels; radioisotope or ultrasonic scans; and an electrocardiogram (ECG).

Thyroid Assessment. In addition to palpation of the thyroid gland for size, contour, consistency, lymph nodes, fixation, tenderness, and bruits, ultrasound is often the first diagnostic test performed (Lewis et al, 2011). Computed tomography (CT) and magnetic resonance imaging (MRI) scans are used to assess a thyroid with suspected malignancy for encroachment of the tumor outside the thyroid capsule into the adjacent tissue of the neck. Scans are the most effective means to evaluate local invasion of surrounding tissue.

EVIDENCE FOR PRACTICE

Screening for Thyroid Dysfunction

A number of symptoms and signs are well-established manifestations of thyroid dysfunction (see Box 16-1). A thorough history and physical are required. A history of being exposed to neck or whole-body radiation or being raised in iodine-poor areas may lead to thyroid cancer. A rapidly expanding neck mass, new onset of hoarseness, neck or ear pain, or cough are symptoms of concern. Patients with a fixed, immobile mass and/or hoarseness, dysphagia, or respiratory symptoms require computed tomography or magnetic resonance imaging as part of evaluation. These symptoms may be indicative of metastasis (Loevner and Mukherji, 2008). Although calcifications were formerly considered a benign finding, some thyroid cancers demonstrate eggshell calcifications.

The American Association of Clinical Endocrinologists (AACE, 2012) practice guidelines for the diagnostic evaluation of hyperthyroidism and hypothyroidism recommend TSH assay as the single best screening test. Hyperthyroidism results in a lower-than-normal TSH level (suppressed TSH secretion). To diagnose hyperthyroidism accurately, TSH assay sensitivity, the lowest reliably measured TSH concentration, must be 0.02 milli-international unit/L or less.

An elevated serum TSH concentration is present in both overt and mild (subclinical) hypothyroidism. In the latter, the free thyroid hormone (fT_3 and fT_4) levels are, by definition, normal.

Hypothyroidism results from undersecretion of thyroid hormone. In the United States, hypothyroidism affects nearly 11 million people each year. The most common cause of primary hypothyroidism is chronic autoimmune thyroiditis (Hashimoto disease). The most valuable laboratory test is measurement of TSH and free T_4 levels. Clinical hypothyroidism is treated with levothyroxine (L-thyroxine) replacement therapy. The AACE supports treating subclinical hypothyroidism if TSH levels are greater than 10 microunits/mL or if TSH levels are between 5 and 10 microunits/mL in conjunction with goiter or positive antibodies or both. Antithyroid peroxidase antibody (TPOAb) measurements are also considered when evaluating patients with subclinical hypothyroidism.

Serum TSH measurement is the single most reliable test to diagnose all common forms of hypothyroidism and hyperthyroidism, with high sensitivity (98%) and specificity (92%). Periodic TSH measurements are done after 6 months and then at 12-month intervals, or more frequently if the patient's symptoms indicate.

fT₃, Free triiodothyronine; *fT₄,* free thyroxine; *TSH,* thyroid-stimulating hormone.
Modified from American Association of Clinical Endocrinologists: Clinical practice guidelines for hypothyroidism in adults, *Endocr Pract* 18(6):e1–e45, 2012; Loevner LA, Mukherji SK: *Thyroid and parathyroid glands: imaging, treatment, and beyond,* Philadelphia, 2008, Saunders.

Ultrasound and autopsy studies show more than 50% of healthy adults have thyroid nodules, yet only 3% to 5% are found to be palpable. Although most nodules are benign, 7% to 29% are cancerous. There are an estimated 60,000 new cases of thyroid cancer each year, with a 3:1 female-to-male ratio (ACS, 2013). The surveillance program of the National Cancer Institute estimates the prevalence of thyroid cancer is less than 1% of the population (Harris et al, 2012). The lifetime risk of developing thyroid cancer is 1 in 97 (Howlader et al, 2013). From 2005 to 2009, the median age at diagnosis for cancer of the thyroid was 50 years. Approximately 1.8% were diagnosed younger than age 20; 15.5% between ages 20 and 34; 20.4% between ages 35 and 44; 24% between 45 and 54, 19% between 55 and 64; 11% between 65 and 74; 5.9% between

75 and 84; and 1.4% at 85 years and older. Thyroid cancer is poised to become one of the most common cancer diagnoses in living cancer patients (Grebe, 2009).

Preoperative Testing

Thyroid Isotope Scan (Thyroid Scintigraphy). A thyroid nodule, the most common endocrine problem in the United States, is any abnormal growth of thyroid cells. Most nodules are discovered during routine physical examination, because they rarely are symptomatic. Imaging of the normal thyroid with radionuclide agents shows normal size, shape, position, and function of the thyroid, with no areas of decreased or increased uptake. Nodules that are *hot* demonstrate increased uptake of radionuclide agent; this may indicate benign adenoma or localized toxic goiter. *Cold nodules* are hypofunctioning or nonfunctioning and may indicate cyst, nonfunctioning adenoma or goiter, lymphoma, localized area of thyroiditis, or carcinoma. Two commonly used agents in thyroid imaging are radioactive iodine and technetium 99m-pertechnetate ($^{99m}TcO_4^-$).

Ultrasonic Scan. Ultrasonic scans are the treatment of choice to evaluate thyroid nodules and are useful to determine the size and number of nodules within the thyroid as well as to monitor size progression during follow-up. Involvement of the vessels in the neck or mediastinum, although rare, can occur. It is critical that the surgeon and operative team know this before surgery. Radiologic evaluation frequently dictates the extent of the surgery. Several new ultrasonic techniques have been applied to the thyroid. Three-dimensional (3D) ultrasound has proven to be more accurate. Tissue harmonic imaging (THI) uses the first harmonic of the transmitted frequency for image formation and results in images with less "noise." These techniques improve image clarity but do not improve lesion characterization.

Ultrasonography also helps facilitate accurate needle placement and sampling of the target nodule during fine-needle aspiration (FNA).

Fine-Needle Aspiration. When a tissue sample for pathologic examination is required, FNA of a palpable nodule is considered one of the most effective methods for identifying malignancy. FNA has high accuracy and low risk, and is cost-effective. A suspicious nodule usually implies a follicular neoplasm, which can be benign or malignant, and requires removal and evaluation by the histology department. The procedure is usually performed under ultrasound guidance, but may be performed in the surgeon's office. Several samples are usually taken from various parts of the nodule, and are rated on a 1 to 6 scale ranging from benign to clearly malignant. When metastatic disease is found on preoperative imaging, an altered operative and disease management plan will be established for the patient. FNA is not suggested for diagnosing parathyroid carcinoma because of the potential for seeding or spreading of the malignant parathyroid cells (Harris et al, 2012). Patient preparation for FNA should include the following information:

- You will be lying down for the procedure and may expect coldness on your neck from the prepping solution.
- Local anesthesia may or may not be used.
- Once the prick of the needle is felt, no talking, swallowing, or moving is allowed.

FNA may be an emotionally stressful procedure for the patient. Vials of ammonia should be kept in the room in case the patient feels faint. Lowering the head (using Trendelenburg position or sitting with the head down) is also important to treat vasovagal syncope. Postprocedure education should include (1) the necessity of refraining from using aspirin or aspirin-containing medications or nonsteroidal antiinflammatory drugs (NSAIDs) for the next 24 hours, and (2) the expectation of seeing a half-dollar–size bruise at the FNA site (Patient-Centered Care). There are no restrictions on food or activity.

Preoperative Patient Education. Preoperative patient education for partial or total thyroidectomy includes an explanation of perioperative events, discussion of the incision site and type of dressing to be used, and explanation of any drains, if anticipated. Pain assessment and pain management therapy are reviewed. Patients are advised that there are various ways of protecting their eyesight during surgery, and if ointment is used, they can expect temporary blurred vision when they first open their eyes. If intermittent pneumatic compression devices are to be used for deep vein thrombosis (DVT) prophylaxis, their use and sensation is explained. The patient is encouraged to flex and extend the neck slowly early in the postoperative period. As mentioned, a baseline description of vocal cord function is noted preoperatively. (For further discussion of patient education, see Patient and Family Education and Discharge Planning on page 547.)

Parathyroid Assessment. Elevation of serum PTH level in association with hypercalcemia is diagnostic of hyperparathyroidism in most cases. Normal PTH levels are between 15 and 65 pg/mL; also diagnostic is a serum calcium level greater than 1 mg/dL above normal (8.5 to 10 mg/dL) and a bone density T-score of less than −2.5 at any site (Yeh et al, 2012). Causes of primary hyperparathyroidism are single adenoma (80% to 85%), four-gland hyperplasia (10% to 15%), and rarely parathyroid carcinoma (less than 1%).

PATIENT-CENTERED CARE

Patient-centered care emphasizes recognition of the patient, the patient's family, or other designee as full partners in care delivery. When perioperative nurses provide patient education, either verbally or through written materials, they should not only be tailored to the patient's individual situation but also be easily understood. Here are some suggestions for patient-centered communication when providing patient education:

- Be concise. ("You had a fine-needle aspiration of your thyroid gland today.")
- Focus on need to know information. ("Here are some important things to know.")
- Use words of one or two syllables.
- Avoid use of medical terms; use words laymen would use. ("An 'aspiration' means getting a small piece out through a needle.")
- Speak or write material in the first person. ("You will have a bruise about the size of a half dollar.")
- Do not use fancy fonts or bold fonts; use bold only for items that are of critical importance. ("Call 911 if you have a hard time swallowing.")
- Ask the patient to "teach-back" the material to you rather than ask if the patient understood you. ("Please tell me in your own words what you can eat or drink this afternoon.")
- Be sure the patient can state the name of the surgical procedure. ("What is the name of the operation you had today?")
- Treat patients, their family or designee with courtesy and respect. ("What else can I help you with?")

FIGURE 16-6 A, Early three-dimensional sestamibi image shows uptake in mass *(asterisk),* in salivary glands *(arrowheads),* and in thyroid gland *(arrow).* **B,** Late three-dimensional sestamibi image shows retention of radiotracer in the adenoma *(asterisk),* with absence of radiotracer in the thyroid gland. Salivary glands normally retain radiotracer on late images.

Nuclear Medicine. Preoperative localization studies with a parathyroid sestamibi scan (Figure 16-6) or high-resolution ultrasonography can identify parathyroid adenomas with high sensitivity (70% to 80%). Sensitivity decreases significantly for hyperplasia (less than 50%).

Improvements in anatomic detail may be achieved by using the single-photon emission computed tomography/CT (SPECT/ CT). This system uses software that depicts 6 to 16 slices of tissue and produces 3D images that help differentiate the parathyroid tissue from lymphadenopathy and thyroid pathologies (Harris et al, 2012).

Four-Dimensional CT. This uses a multiphase multidetector CT that provides rapid volumetric acquisition and in-plane spatial resolution of 1 mm or better, which provides a roadmap for the operating surgeon. There is more precise visualization of the parathyroid glands, and detailed anatomic information provided with this CT scan (Harris et al, 2012).

Hyperparathyroidism causes an increase in the level of serum calcium and a decrease in the level of serum phosphate. Nursing diagnoses and plans of care are based on these imbalances and the severity of associated symptoms. Some patients are asymptomatic, whereas others have symptoms that manifest themselves as disturbances in the central nervous system or cardiovascular, renal, gastrointestinal, or musculoskeletal system (Box 16-2).

Assessment includes determining whether the patient is apathetic or emotionally irritable; whether there is muscle weakness and atrophy, back or joint pain, nausea, vomiting, constipation, peptic ulcer disease, or cardiac dysrhythmia; and whether there is renal damage, stones, or disease. If any of these are present, the plan of care is adjusted. Otherwise, perioperative patient education and nursing management of the patient undergoing parathyroidectomy are essentially the same as those for thyroidectomy. In the early postoperative period for both thyroidectomy and parathyroidectomy, the patient is closely observed for any signs of hypocalcemia. The serum calcium level reaches its lowest level in 48 to 72 hours after surgery and returns to normal within the following 2 to 3 days. Symptoms include numbness and tingling of extremities and around the lips. Hyperactive tendon reflexes and a positive Chvostek sign (tapping on the facial nerve elicits contraction of facial muscles) can be demonstrated on physical examination. Tetany may develop and is exhibited by carpopedal spasms, tonic-clonic convulsions, and laryngeal stridor, which can be fatal.

BOX 16-2

Parathyroid Dysfunction

Hyperparathyroidism
Definition
Overactivity of one or more of the parathyroid glands; excessive secretion of parathyroid hormone causes an increase in the level of calcium (hypercalcemia)

Signs and Symptoms
- Polyuria, polydipsia, kidney stones
- Abdominal pain, constipation, nausea, anorexia
- Fractures of ribs, spine
- Joint or back pain
- Depression, paranoia, mood swings
- Muscle weakness and atrophy

Complications
- Cardiac dysrhythmias, cardiac failure
- Gastric ulcer
- Pathologic fractures
- Renal disorders: kidney stones, urinary tract infections, renal failure
- Pancreatitis
- Stupor/coma

Hypoparathyroidism
Definition
Deficiency of parathyroid hormone, necessary to maintain normal levels of serum calcium; may occur as a result of radiation therapy for head and neck cancer or as a postoperative complication from thyroid or parathyroid surgery; symptoms are related to reduced calcium levels (hypocalcemia)

Signs and Symptoms
- Personality disturbances: anxiety, depression, irritability
- Tetany: muscle cramps, spasms (hands, face, feet); paresthesias: numbness and tingling (around mouth, lips, and tongue)
- Dry, scaly skin; brittle nails; thin, patchy hair
- Weak tooth enamel/dental caries
- Cataracts

Complications
- Cardiac dysrhythmias
- Seizures
- Psychoses
- Cardiac arrest

Modified from Copstead LE, Banasik J: *Pathophysiology*, ed 4, St Louis, 2010, Saunders.

Nursing Diagnosis

Nursing diagnoses related to the care of patients undergoing thyroid and parathyroid surgery might include the following:
- Impaired Swallowing related to mechanical obstruction (enlarged thyroid preoperatively; edema or hematoma postoperatively)
- Risk for Imbalanced Body Temperature related to altered metabolic rate and surgical environment
- Disturbed Body Image related to surgical scar in prominent location
- Ineffective Airway Clearance related to obstruction (enlarged thyroid preoperatively; edema or hematoma postoperatively) or bilateral recurrent laryngeal nerve injury
- Impaired Gas Exchange related to postoperative bleeding or swelling or inability to move secretions

Outcome Identification

Outcomes identified for the selected nursing diagnoses may be stated as follows:

- The patient will maintain normal swallowing.
- The patient will maintain normal body temperature.
- The patient will verbalize decreased disturbance in feelings related to body image.
- The patient will maintain a patent airway.
- The patient will maintain effective gas exchange.

Planning

The perioperative nurse and surgical technologist should know the OR team members who will participate in the procedure as well as the roles each team member will assume (Haynes et al, 2009). Careful planning, assessment, and tailoring the plan of care to the surgery and specific patient needs reduce inherent risks. The perioperative nurse should consider a patient who is not at optimal weight at high risk for pressure ulcer development and plan on padding pressure areas to prevent skin and tissue damage. Intraoperatively, warm saline should be provided for irrigation and a forced-air warming device used. Patients with hypothyroidism are at increased risk of becoming hypothermic (Hegarty et al, 2009).

A rapidly progressive and potentially fatal complication for patients with hyperthyroidism is thyroid storm (thyrotoxic crisis) (Copstead and Banasik, 2010). The perioperative staff must recognize and differentiate between uncomplicated thyrotoxicosis and thyroid storm (Box 16-3) and be prepared to act quickly. Thyroid storm can occur in patients whose hyperthyroidism has been partially controlled or has been left untreated. Thyrotoxic crisis can be precipitated by a stressful event, such as surgery. By planning a quiet, calm atmosphere and helping the patient relax, the perioperative nurse can reduce the risk of thyroid storm. Collaborating with the surgical and anesthesia team, the perioperative nurse plans for appropriate interventions to assist in reducing body temperature and heart rate, provides oxygen and intravenous solutions, and administers medications as prescribed in the event thyrotoxic crisis occurs (Surgical Pharmacology).

A Sample Plan of Care for a patient undergoing thyroid and parathyroid surgery is on pages 546 to 547.

Implementation

Positioning. Proper patient positioning on the OR bed is crucial for optimal exposure of the thyroid gland. The patient is positioned supine. Some surgeons prefer a beach chair position or a wedge under the back. Hyperextension of the neck is required for maximal exposure. A headrest provides proper support, keeps the head straight, and prevents aggravation of prior neck problems. Alternatively, a shoulder roll may be used. The arms are tucked at the side, the elbows are padded to protect the ulnar nerve, the palms faced inward, and the wrist is maintained in a neutral position (Denholm, 2009). A drape secures the arms. It should be tucked snugly, but not tightly, under the patient, not under the mattress. This prevents the arm from shifting downward intraoperatively and resting against the OR bed rail. All pressure points should be padded, especially for patients not at optimal weight. Should the patient be too large to tuck the arms safely at the sides, arm sleds or side extensions for the OR bed may be used to accommodate the arms. Reduction of venous congestion can be accomplished by a 30-degree reverse-Trendelenburg tilt of the OR bed.

Skin Preparation. The operative area (chin and anterior neck region, lateral surfaces of the neck from the earlobes down to the

---

BOX 16-3
Thyroid Storm

Mortality/Morbidity

Thyroid storm is a fulminating state that is fatal if untreated, with death rates of 20% to 30%. It is an acute manifestation of hyperthyroidism.

Physical Symptoms

Thyroid storm may be difficult to differentiate from signs of uncomplicated thyrotoxicosis. It is an accentuation of the same signs. Onset is heralded by high-grade fever, mental obtundation, and decompensation of one or more organ systems as a result of severe hypermetabolism.

Guidelines are presented in the following table comparing symptoms of uncomplicated thyrotoxicosis and thyroid storm:

Uncomplicated Thyrotoxicosis	Thyroid Storm
Heat intolerance, diaphoresis	Hyperpyrexia, temperature in excess of 106°F (41.1 C), dehydration
Sinus tachycardia, heart rate 100-140 beats/min	Heart rate faster than 140 beats/min, hypotension, atrial dysrhythmias, congestive heart failure
Diarrhea, increased appetite with weight loss	Nausea, vomiting, severe diarrhea, abdominal pain, hepatocellular dysfunction with jaundice
Anxiety, restlessness	Confusion, agitation, delirium, frank psychosis, seizures, stupor, or coma

Causes

Causes of rapid rise in thyroid hormone levels:

- Thyroid or parathyroid surgery
- Radioiodine therapy, iodinated contrast dye
- Withdrawal of antithyroid drug therapy
- Vigorous thyroid palpation
- Thyroid hormone medication

Other common precipitating factors:

- Infection
- Emotional stress
- Tooth extraction
- Diabetic ketoacidosis
- Hypoglycemia
- Trauma
- Bowel infarction
- Parturition
- Pregnancy toxemia
- Pulmonary embolism
- Cerebrovascular accident
- Gestational trophoblastic disease

---

outer aspects of the shoulder, and upper anterior chest region to the nipples) is prepped with an antimicrobial solution. Appropriate precautions are taken to prevent pooling of solution under the neck or in the axillary area. When using an alcohol-based prep solution around the head and neck, there is an increased risk for a surgical fire. Follow the manufacturer's directions for the prep solution carefully; the patient's skin should be totally dry and all fumes from the prep solution should be dissipated prior to draping. Bed sheets or towels that become soaked with a flammable prep solution should be removed from the OR. After the skin prep, the patient is draped with sterile towels and a fenestrated sheet. A sterile towel, lap sponge, or self-adherent tape strips may be placed on each side of

SURGICAL PHARMACOLOGY

Thyroid Storm

Preoperative Prophylactic Care for Thyroid Storm
Use potassium iodide (KI) preoperatively in thyrotoxicosis to decrease thyroid blood flow.

Emergency Care During Thyroid Storm
- Maintain a patent airway and adequate ventilation.
- Administer supplemental oxygen.
- Establish vascular access for fluid resuscitation or medication administration.
- Monitor intake and output.
- Give antithyroid drugs as prescribed: propylthiouracil (PTU, Propyl-Thyracil), 300-900 mg/day; methimazole (MMI) (Tapazole), up to 60 mg/day.
- Administer sodium iodide solution, 2 g/day IV as prescribed.
- Initiate continuous cardiac monitoring.
- Prepare the patient for insertion of a central venous pressure line.
- Give propranolol (Inderal, Detensol), 1-3 mg IV as prescribed; administer slowly, over 3 minutes.
- Esmolol (Brevibloc), 500 mcg/kg IV followed by 50-200 mcg/kg, minimum maintenance dose, is useful in patients at risk for complications from beta-blockade and cardiovascular collapse.
- Guanethidine or reserpine is substituted for propranolol in patients with congestive heart failure (CHF), cardiac failure, bronchospasm, or history of asthma (do not use for patients who are in cardiovascular shock or collapse).
- One hour after administration of PTU or MMI, hormone release can be inhibited by large doses of iodine, which reduce thyroidal iodine uptake. Lugol solution, 30 gtt/day orally in 4 divided doses, or a saturated solution of potassium iodide, 5 gtt orally or via an NG tube q6hr, can be used.
- Ipodate sodium, 0.5-3 g/day PO, can be administered instead of iodine.
- Patients unable to take PTU or MMI also can be treated with lithium 300 mg PO q6hr in conjunction with iodine. Adjust lithium dose to maintain levels at about 1 mEq/L.
- Plasmapheresis, plasma exchange, peritoneal dialysis exchange transfusion, and charcoal plasma perfusion are other techniques to remove excess circulating hormone for patients who do not respond to the initial line of management.
- Monitor vital signs every 30 minutes or more frequently as patient's condition dictates.
- Provide comfort measures.
- Control hyperthermia with application of ice packs and a cooling blanket.
- Give nonsalicylate antipyretics such as acetaminophen (normally 650 mg PO q4hr).
- Aggressive fluid and electrolyte therapy, 3-5 L/day, is needed for dehydration and hypotension.
- Provide multivitamins, especially vitamin B_1, to prevent Wernicke encephalopathy.
- Glucocorticoids reduce iodine uptake and must be used with caution because they have significant adverse effects.
- Dexamethasone (Decadron, Dexone), 2 mg IV q6hr, or hydrocortisone (Cortef, Solu-Cortef), 100 mg IV q8hr, may be given.
- Control hypertension with agents such as guanethidine (Ismelin), 1-2 mg/kg/day orally, or reserpine, 2.5-5 mg IM q4-6hr.
- Treat heart failure if present.
- Educate patient and family about symptoms of thyroid storm and that they should call 911 for these symptoms.

IM, Intramuscular; *IV,* intravenous; *NG,* nasogastric; *PO,* orally.
Modified from Copstead LE, Banasik J: *Pathophysiology,* ed 4, St Louis, 2010, Saunders; Crawford A, Harris H: Thyroid imbalances: dealing with disorderly conduct, *Nursing 2012* 42(11):45–50, 2012; Czako P, Meyers A: *Thyrotoxic storm following thyroidectomy,* available at emedicine.medscape.com/article850924. Accessed May 27, 2013; Simmons S: Detecting thyroid disease, *Nursing 2010* 40(7):22–29, 2010.

SAMPLE PLAN OF CARE

Nursing Diagnosis
Impaired Swallowing related to mechanical obstruction (enlarged thyroid preoperatively; edema postoperatively)

Outcome
The patient will maintain normal swallowing.

Interventions
- Keep suction line and suction catheter connected and ready until patient is discharged from OR.
- Monitor for and report difficulty swallowing during emergence from anesthesia or transport to PACU.
- Gently suction oropharyngeal secretions as required.
- Keep vein open postoperatively until patient can swallow without difficulty.

Nursing Diagnosis
Risk for Imbalanced Body Temperature related to altered metabolic rate

Outcome
Patient's body temperature will be maintained within normal range.

Interventions
- Monitor patient's temperature; report abnormalities.
- Provide light covers if temperature is elevated or patient states that he or she is too warm.
- Use forced-air warming device intraoperatively as needed to maintain temperature.
- Use fluid warmer for intravenous fluids as needed to maintain body temperature.
- Change linens preoperatively and postoperatively if wet from perspiration.
- Avoid using plasticized drapes.

Nursing Diagnosis
Disturbed Body Image related to surgical scar

SAMPLE PLAN OF CARE—cont'd

Outcome

The patient will verbalize decreased disturbance in feelings related to body image.

Interventions

- Describe incision location in natural fold of skin.
- Explain that techniques used for surgical closure minimize scarring.
- Instruct patient in postoperative turning measures that decrease strain on suture line.
- Suggest that jewelry, scarves, and certain necklines can be used to cover scar until normal fading occurs.
- Advise patient to refrain from prolonged exposure to direct sunlight or tanning salons while incision is healing.

Nursing Diagnosis

Ineffective Airway Clearance related to obstruction secondary to enlarged thyroid (preoperatively), edema (postoperatively), or laryngeal nerve injury

Outcome

The patient's airway will remain patent.

Interventions

- Position patient so that enlarged gland does not obstruct airway. Head of transport vehicle may need to be elevated preoperatively. Postoperatively the head of the bed may need elevation to 30 to 45 degrees to ease air exchange and minimize edema.
- Assist anesthesia provider during induction and extubation. Have oxygen and suction available.
- Monitor respiratory rate and signs of respiratory distress (stridor, wheezing, dyspnea, labored respirations).

- If distress occurs because of recurrent laryngeal nerve injury, a tracheotomy may be required. Have oxygen, suctioning equipment, and a tracheotomy tray available.
- Observe neck dressing and back of neck for signs of edema or bleeding (postoperatively). Hemorrhage at the incision site or respiratory distress from tracheal compression may require urgent reintubation for airway protection and a return to the OR for wound reexploration.

Nursing Diagnosis

Impaired Gas Exchange related to postoperative bleeding or swelling, bilateral recurrent laryngeal nerve surgical injury, or inability to move secretions

Outcome

The patient's gas exchange will remain effective.

Interventions

- Monitor respiratory status and results of pulse oximetry.
- If patient is extubated in OR, be prepared to assist anesthesia provider; closely observe for respiratory stridor or respiratory obstruction (recurrent laryngeal nerve malfunction). Tracheotomy may be required; oxygen, suctioning equipment, and a tracheotomy tray should be available. A trach tube with a high-volume, low-pressure cuff is often indicated postoperatively for patients with head and neck cancer.
- Assess and document color of nailbeds.
- Monitor surgical site for swelling and bleeding.
- Suction patient's secretions as needed.
- Monitor patency of surgical drain and amount/nature of drainage in collection device, as applicable.
- Instruct patient in coughing and deep breathing: supporting the neck; place both hands behind the neck when coughing to reduce strain on the suture line (postoperative).

PACU, Postanesthesia care unit.

---

the neck to prevent blood from pooling under the neck during surgery. Self-adherent tape strips or drapes also promote maintenance of the integrity of the sterile field and reduce the risk of intraoperative fire hazard by sealing off the operative site from anesthetic vapors that may have leaked and become trapped under the drapes. If lap sponges are used on each side of the neck during the draping of the patient, they should be noted on the count sheet to avoid confusion when accounting for all items used throughout the procedure. After draping is complete, a time-out is taken. All personnel stop and listen attentively during the time-out. The following must be verified: correct patient, correct site, and correct procedure to be performed; special patient considerations and supplies may also be included. In addition, all antibiotics given to the patient should be verbalized; include the dose, time, and amount given. The time-out is documented. The surgeon then marks the incision site with a marking pen or the pressure of a full-length fine silk tie to help ensure a wound line that blends with the patient's neck creases and skin lines.

Evaluation

Evaluation of intraoperative interventions determines the effectiveness of the plan of care. The hand-off report to postanesthesia care unit (PACU) or ambulatory recovery unit includes the surgical procedure, type of anesthesia used, local anesthetics administered, location of drain (if any), dressing used, condition of skin

postoperatively, and any other information specific to the patient's postoperative care. Documentation, using facility protocol, reflects achievement of patient outcomes related to planned interventions; these should also be included in the hand-off nursing report to PACU personnel. Outcomes identified for the selected nursing diagnoses may be stated as follows:

- The patient will maintain normal swallowing.
- The patient will maintain normal body temperature.
- The patient will verbalize decreased disturbance in feelings related to body image.
- The patient will maintain a patent airway; there was no edema or hematoma at the surgical site or signs of respiratory distress.
- The patient will maintain adequate gas exchange; O_2 saturation remain normal. The patient will be extubated without incident.

Patient and Family Education and Discharge Planning

Patient education and discharge planning include any family members, significant others, or even friends who will help the patient at home (Patient and Family Education). Written discharge instructions are provided and orally reviewed, with clarification of information and correction of misperceptions. The name and telephone number of the physician or nurse to call with questions is provided, as is information regarding a follow-up office appointment, if available. General information, such as the name of the thyroid or parathyroid procedure and any changes that will occur

PATIENT AND FAMILY EDUCATION

Home Care After a Thyroidectomy

- Give both patient and caregiver *verbal* and *written* instructions. Provide the name and telephone number of a physician or nurse to call if questions or problems arise. Have patient and/or caregiver verbally repeat instructions in his/her own words. Allow time for questions.
- Advise patient to sit up slowly and allow his/her legs to dangle for 1 to 2 minutes before getting up. The caregiver should accompany the patient on the first walk at home.
- Explain and discuss with patient the surgical procedure performed. The patient should be able to state the name of the surgical procedure performed.
- Wound/incision care
  - Teach patient to keep the surgical site clean and dry.
  - Review methods to conceal surgical site without affecting healing. Suggest loosely buttoned collars, high-neck blouses, jewelry, or scarves.
  - Explain that paper strip(s) over wound will peel off in 7 to 10 days; when ends curl, it may be removed.
  - Advise patient that incisions approximated with surgical glue may have glue peeled off at a prescribed postoperative day.
  - Inform patient that lotion may soften healing scar and improve its appearance (if approved by physician).
- Warning signs: review signs and symptoms that should be reported to physician or nurse.
  - *General:* respiratory distress, bleeding
  - *Wound infection:* redness, warmth, swelling, persistent drainage from site, unrelieved tenderness
  - *Total thyroidectomy:* signs and symptoms of hypothyroidism: intolerance to cold; decreased body temperature; dry, rough, or scaly skin; puffy face, hands, and feet; periorbital edema; decreased blood pressure; bradycardia; nonspecific fatigue, weakness; decreased exercise tolerance; weight gain; constipation; anorexia; delayed deep tendon reflexes; muscle aches and joint stiffness; speech changes (slowed, slurred, monotonous); somnolence, lethargy; impaired memory, inattentiveness, slow cognition; loss of initiative; paranoia, depression, agitation; decreased libido; female: decreased or missed menstrual cycles; abdominal distention
  - *Parathyroid damage:* signs of hypocalcemia: numbness, tingling, twitching, spasm, tetany
- Medication management
  - Review medication reconciliation form.
  - Explain purpose, dosage, schedule, and route of administration of any prescribed drugs, as well as side effects to report to physician or nurse.
  - Provide list of all medications patient is to take (including those that are not newly prescribed; this is part of discharge medication reconciliation and safety).
  - Discuss importance of not taking over-the-counter medications without first checking with physician or nurse.
  - If patient had total thyroidectomy, explain importance of taking thyroid replacement medication regularly.
- Activity
  - If patient has parathyroid damage, explain need for calcium supplements.
  - Encourage patient to discuss allowances and limitations with respect to occupation, recreation, and activities.
  - Teach prescribed head and neck exercises: flexion, lateral movement, hyperextension.
  - Teach importance of balance between activity and rest.
  - Discuss need to maintain well-balanced diet.

Follow-Up Care

- Stress importance of regular follow-up visits to monitor thyroid levels: thyroid-stimulating hormone (TSH), thyroxine (T_4). Make sure patient has necessary names and telephone numbers.

Modified from Lewis S et al: *Medical-surgical nursing*, ed 8, St Louis, 2011, Mosby; Workman LM: Care of patients with problems of the thyroid and parathyroid glands. In Ignatavicius DD, Workman ML, editors: *Medical-surgical nursing: patient-centered collaborative care*, ed 7, St Louis, 2013, Saunders.

as a result of the surgery, is explained. Signs and symptoms to report include those of hypocalcemia. The patient should report any numbness or tingling around the lips or extremities, twitching, or spasms. Explore the patient's concerns, anxieties, thoughts, and feelings. The advent of thyroidectomies and parathyroidectomies performed in ambulatory surgery centers has introduced a new set of needs and challenges for the patient, family, and perioperative staff (Ambulatory Surgery Considerations).

Surgical Interventions

Unilateral Thyroid Lobectomy, Subtotal Lobectomy, Bilateral Subtotal Lobectomy, Near-Total Thyroidectomy, and Total Thyroidectomy

Unilateral thyroid lobectomy or *hemithyroidectomy* is the removal of one thyroid lobe with excision of the isthmus. The isthmus is completely removed to prevent postoperative hypertrophy in response to the lobectomy with subsequent airway impingement. *Subtotal lobectomy* is a lobectomy that spares the posterior capsule and a portion of adjacent thyroid tissue. *Bilateral subtotal thyroidectomy* is

removal of both lobes of the thyroid in the fashion stated for subtotal thyroidectomy. *Near-total thyroidectomy* is a total lobectomy with contralateral subtotal thyroidectomy. *Total thyroidectomy* is the removal of both lobes of the thyroid and all thyroid tissue present. For patients with cancer of the thyroid, total or near-total thyroidectomy is the desired treatment. Following surgery, the thyroid cancer patient may be treated with radioactive ablation therapy for residual or metastatic disease and thyroid hormone suppression therapy. The patient is then monitored by physical examination, laboratory studies (serum thyroid function and thyroglobulin levels), and radioactive scans.

The purpose of the surgical intervention relates to the patient's medical diagnosis. *Goiter* refers to any enlargement of the thyroid gland and includes both benign and malignant nodules; the enlargement is visible over the anterior neck (Wilson and Giddens, 2009). *Benign adenomas* are encased in a fibrous capsule, distinct from surrounding thyroid tissue. *Malignancies* occur most commonly in patients younger than 20 or older than 60 years. Excising the lymph nodes with suspected or known cancer of the thyroid remains a standard therapy. Radiologic studies aid in the understanding of nodal metastasis and determining which levels of the neck to dissect.

AMBULATORY SURGERY CONSIDERATIONS

Patient Teaching, Preparation, and Screening: An Emphasis on Health Literacy

Thorough patient teaching and preparation with written instructions are critical for ambulatory surgery patients and their families. Limited health literacy has been related to problems comprehending discharge information. Nurses require strong critical thinking, clinical reasoning, and assessment skills to screen patients for problems that may preclude discharge to home. Safe and successful ambulatory surgery depends, in part, on recognizing which patients can be sent home and which patients should be admitted.

Nurses verify that patients have arranged for someone to drive them home and for a caregiver (family/friend) to assist during the first 24 hours at home. Surgery cannot be done on an ambulatory basis if these arrangements have not been made.

Patients are thoroughly and carefully screened as to eligibility for ambulatory thyroidectomy or parathyroidectomy. Ambulatory surgery is contraindicated in patients with grossly enlarged thyroids or comorbid medical conditions, such as cardiac disease, uncontrolled hypertension, brittle diabetes, and sleep apnea. Patients who had a difficult intubation or who bled excessively during surgery should be excluded from discharge on the same day as surgery.

Nurses also ascertain the patient's ability to understand and cooperate with discharge instructions. Part of health literacy is ensuring that the patient can process and understand health information.

The patient is sent home with prescriptions for pain management, calcium supplements, thyroid hormone (if indicated), and other medications specific to preexisting conditions. All medications should be reviewed (discharge reconciliation) and a list provided. Lower health literacy and a high number of medications may result in less understanding of medication regimens (Marnanova et al, 2011).

Patients must meet discharge criteria from ambulatory surgery: be fully awake, alert, and oriented and able to void, swallow, and drink fluids without nausea or vomiting.

Deep breathing, early mobility at home, and hydration are emphasized.

Patients are cautioned not to drive or drink alcohol for at least 24 hours.

Patients and families are under physical and emotional stress and often will find the environment and information received overwhelming (McCarthy et al, 2012). Standardized printed discharge instructions from the surgeon, specific to the surgery performed, with space available to customize information for the patient, provide a valuable tool and reference resource for the patient and family/caregiver to use at home. This too is part of health literacy among ambulatory surgery patients.

Nurses verify that the patient and caregiver understand the symptoms indicating a significant problem that needs immediate attention, as well as actions to take and people to contact in case of an emergency. These include signs and symptoms of dyspnea, hemorrhage, thyroid storm, and hypocalcemia. Speak in plain language when describing signs and symptoms. Validate that the patient has no language barriers to understanding discharge instructions (Karliner et al, 2012). Ask the patient to repeat these instructions in their own words.

The patient should be instructed to call the physician's office for a follow-up visit if this has not been arranged.

Modified from Karliner LS et al: Language barriers and understanding of hospital discharge instructions, *Med Care* 50(4):283–289, 2012; Marnanova M et al: Health literacy and medication understanding among hospitalized adults, *J Hospl Med* 6(9):488–493, 2011; McCarthy DM et al: What did the doctor say? Health literacy and recall of medical instructions, *Med Care* 50(4):277–282, 2012.

Contralateral metastasis is generally associated with large tumors. Young patients tend to respond favorably to treatment and have a better prognosis than older patients. Recent studies show that elderly patients are at a greater risk for postoperative complications with twice the risk of postoperative complications in patients ages 65 to 79 and five times the risk in patients ages 80 and older (Grogan, 2012).

Graves' disease, the most common cause of hyperthyroidism, is associated with diffuse, bilateral enlargement of the thyroid gland. Surgery is reserved for those patients who fail medical therapy (antithyroid drugs and radioactive iodine) or have a contraindication to medical therapy. *Hashimoto's thyroiditis* is believed to be an autoimmune disease in which nontender enlargement of the gland occurs. Surgery is performed to relieve compressive symptoms. *Nontoxic nodular goiter* involves production of insufficient hormones and is noninflammatory; in such cases thyroid tissue proliferates in an apparent attempt to produce the minimal hormonal requirement. Surgery may be indicated to relieve tracheal or esophageal obstruction or to rule out a malignant nodule of the thyroid. *Total thyroidectomy* may be done for malignant tumors (Box 16-4). An intraoperative frozen section may be indicated to confirm the diagnosis. If the diagnosis is not definitive by frozen section, a hemithyroidectomy may be the treatment of choice. If the permanent histologic report is benign, the patient's unaffected thyroid lobe is preserved. If, however, the pathologic analysis demonstrates that the thyroid mass is malignant, a total thyroidectomy is often recommended.

Minimally invasive approaches to thyroid surgery arose in the late 1990s and early twenty-first century for treatment of small thyroid nodules. These include minimally invasive open thyroidectomy (MIT) and minimally invasive video-assisted thyroidectomy (MIVAT). Minimally invasive thyroid surgery is performed for both partial and total thyroidectomies. Although it remains more expensive than open procedures, robotic-assisted transaxillary methods for thyroidectomies are becoming more common (Hunter and Jobe, 2010). Researchers continue to conduct studies on natural orifice transendoscopic surgery (NOTES); in the future, skin incisions may become obsolete for some surgeries (Research Highlight on page 550). Of interest also is the relationship of various factors on patient outcomes in thyroid surgery (Research Highlight on page 551).

Minimally invasive thyroidectomies reduce postoperative pain, decrease hospital length of stays, and improve cosmetic results. Minimizing dissection and resultant dead space eliminates the need for external drains in most cases. Smaller incisions, minimal use of surgical drains, and prophylactic calcium supplementation have enabled thyroid surgery to be performed safely with better surgical and cosmetic outcomes (Yu et al, 2012).

MIVAT is generally reserved for thyroid nodules within specific size limits as well as for low-stage papillary thyroid carcinomas. As MIVAT has evolved and surgeons have become more proficient

BOX 16-4

Malignant Thyroid Nodules

Papillary Carcinoma
- Most common form (>70%)
- Poorly encapsulated
- Calcifications present—uncommon in other carcinomas

Follicular Carcinoma
- Second most common form (10%)
- Well differentiated
- Associated with iodine deficiency

Hürthle Cell Tumor
- Derived from follicular epithelium
- Accounts for 3% of thyroid malignancies
- Associated with regional nodal metastasis

Medullary Carcinoma
- Undifferentiated tumor
- Accounts for 5% of thyroid malignancies
- Higher death rate than differentiated

Anaplastic Carcinoma
- More common in females and elderly
- Highly aggressive
- Rapidly fatal; death usually occurs within 1 year of diagnosis

Uncommon Carcinomas
- Primary lymphoma
- Metastatic thyroid tumors

Modified from Hunter JG, Jobe BA: *Schwartz's principles of surgery*, ed 9, New York, 2010, McGraw-Hill.

RESEARCH HIGHLIGHT

Using Robotics in Thyroid and Neck Dissection Surgeries

A variety of studies have been reviewed for using robotics in thyroid surgical procedures. Several recent studies that have a great potential for advancing thyroid surgery are presented here.

Lee and Chung (2012) reviewed 23 reports, which included three multicentered trials, and concluded that robotic thyroidectomies and robotic modified neck dissection (MRND) using a gasless transaxillary approach (TAA) yielded identical or superior levels of safety when compared with conventional open or endoscopic surgery for thyroid carcinomas. Furthermore, these reports noted additional benefits including reduction in pain, lower morbidity rates, improved swallowing function, and superior cosmetic results.

Kang and colleagues (2011) reported on 1000 cases using the gasless robotic TAA and determined that the technique is a safe surgical alternative for select patients who have low-risk thyroid cancer. They also concluded that future instrumentation and robotic developments will gradually enable TAA surgery to be performed on advanced thyroid cancer patients. In addition, suitable operator experience advances both the safety and reliability of these TAA procedures (see Research Highlight on page 551).

Richmon and colleagues (2011) reported on the transoral robotic-assisted approach for thyroidectomy (TORS). Using human cadavers his group performed minimally invasive surgery by modifying the transoral approach, placing the camera in the midline oral vestibule. This technique allowed an excellent view of the central neck area, and enabled the surgeons to perform successful surgeries in the central compartment of the neck.

Modified from Kang S et al: Prospects of robotic thyroidectomy using a gasless, transaxillary approach for the management of thyroid carcinoma, *Surg Laparosc Endosc Percutan Tech* 21(4):223–229, 2011; Lee J, Chung WY: Prospects of robotic thyroidectomy using a gasless, transaxillary approach for the management of thyroid carcinoma, *Curr Opin Oncol* 24(1):7–15, 2012; Richmon J et al: Transoral robotic assisted thyroidectomy with central neck dissection: preclinical cadaver feasibility study and proposed surgical technique, *J Robot Surg* 5(4):279–282, 2011.

with the technique, the only absolute contraindications for its use are thyroid malignancies beyond low-stage papillary carcinoma and preoperative evidence of lymph node metastasis. Relative contraindications include prior conventional thyroidectomy, nodules with a diameter larger than 35 mm and volume greater than 30 mL, and a history of thyroiditis.

Procedural Considerations

The patient is positioned supine. A drape pack with fenestrated sheet is required along with a basic instrument set and thyroid instruments. An electrosurgical unit (ESU), an exhaust system for surgical smoke (AORN, 2013), gauze dissectors, and a small drain (optional) are commonly used. A headlight for the surgeon and assistant may be required. A nerve monitor may be used during surgery to protect the recurrent laryngeal nerves. The patient is prepped from the chin to the upper chest, using fire safety precautions. Surgeons may also use the harmonic scalpel or tissue fusion device. The heated blade of the harmonic scalpel retains its heat longer than an ESU blade. Appropriate precautions must therefore be used to avoid inadvertent burning of adjacent tissue. Thyroidectomies are done through a small incision, and visualization is critical for successful extraction. Bleeding can obscure the view and hinder the progress of the surgery. Therefore, surgeons may use hemostatic agents intraoperatively to maintain hemostasis.

Operative Procedure—Open Thyroidectomy

Figure 16-7 provides an overview of safe thyroidectomy principles.

1. A transverse incision (slightly curved and symmetric) is made parallel to the normal skin line crease of the neck, through the skin and first layers of the cervical fascia and platysma muscle, about 2 cm above the sternoclavicular junction.
2. An upper skin flap is undermined to the level of the thyroid notch of the thyroid cartilage; double skin hooks or Allis clamps are placed on the dermis and retracted anteriorly and superiorly to facilitate dissection. A lower flap is then undermined to the sternoclavicular joint. A knife, fine curved scissors, tissue forceps, and gauze sponges are used to undermine the flaps. Bleeding vessels are clamped with hemostats and ligated with fine nonabsorbable sutures. Lateral retraction with a vein retractor or army-navy retractor helps identify the plane for dissection.
3. Flaps are held away from the wound with stay sutures inserted through the cervical fascia and platysma muscle or by a self-retaining retractor.
4. The fascia in the midline is incised between the strap (sternohyoid and sternothyroid) muscles with a knife. Care must be taken to preserve the anterior jugular veins. The fascia may be lifted on either side with forceps during the dissection to help define the plane of dissection and protect the jugular vessels. The sternocleidomastoid muscle may be retracted with a loop

RESEARCH HIGHLIGHT ||

Influence of Experience on Surgeon Performance in Thyroidectomy

Though complication rates can vary greatly during a surgeon's career, the potential for decline in performance among very experienced surgeons remains unclear. Some have suggested that human factors such as fatigue, circadian rhythms, scheduling, or staffing may contribute to an increase in patient safety problems for surgical procedures performed later in the workday or workweek (Sessler et al, 2011). This has been shown to not be true. Other research has examined surgeons' years of experience or compliance with published guidelines, such as evidence-based practice guidelines, as risk factors for surgical site infection (Hubner et al, 2011). That research concluded that no correlation existed between surgeons' individual adjusted risks for surgical site infections (SSIs) and their adherence to guidelines or their years of experience.

In this multicenter study (Duclos et al, 2012), researchers examined the association between surgeons' experience and postoperative complications in thyroid surgery. The study population was composed of 3574 thyroidectomy patients, surgery performed by 28 different surgeons, at five different hospitals over the course of a 1-year period.

Of significance, these researchers discovered that patients were at higher risk of complications when operated on by inexperienced surgeons and those in practice for 20 years or more. Surgeons between 35 and 50 years of age had better outcomes than their younger or older colleagues. When surgery was performed by surgeons in practice for 20 years or more, the probability of complications increased considerably.

The researchers concluded that surgeons' performance varies over the course of their careers, and optimum performance cannot be achieved or maintained passively by accumulating experience. Clearly this research suggests that factors contributing to poor performance in experienced surgeons should be studied further with larger populations of surgeons, in various settings, and in other surgical specialties to corroborate a link between experience and performance.

Modified from Duclos A et al: Influence of experience on performance of individual surgeons in thyroid surgery: Prospective cross sectional multicentre study, *BMJ*, published online Jan 11, 2012; Hubner M et al: Surgical site infections in colon surgery: the patient, the procedure, the hospital, and the surgeon, *Arch Surg* 146:1240–1245, 2011; Sessler DI et al: Operation timing and 30-day mortality after elective general surgery, *Anesth Analg* 113:1423–1428, 2011.

retractor. Ordinarily it is not necessary to divide the strap muscles. However, if additional exposure is required, such as with a very large gland, they may be divided between clamps using Mastin muscle clamps, Kocher clamps, or hemostats and a knife. The divided muscles are retracted from the operative site to expose the target lobe.

5. The inferior and middle thyroid veins are ligated with fine nonabsorbable sutures or hemoclips, and divided with Metzenbaum scissors.

6. The lobe is first rotated medially, and loose areolar tissue is then divided posteriorly and medially toward the tracheoesophageal sulcus with hemostats and Metzenbaum scissors. Small gauze sponges are used for blunt dissection. Bleeding is controlled with hemostats, hemoclips, and ligatures, as well as with the ESU; a bipolar ESU may also be used. The recurrent laryngeal nerve, which enters the larynx immediately posterior to the

FIGURE 16-7 Safe thyroid principles emphasize the following: division of all branch vessels on the capsule of the thyroid with fine mosquito hemostats to prevent injury to the superior laryngeal nerve while detaching the superior thyroid artery and to prevent injury to the parathyroid glands while detaching the inferior thyroid artery; mobilization of parathyroid glands *(arrows)* by medial-to-lateral dissection to preserve their vascular pedicle; constant awareness of the location of the recurrent laryngeal nerve *(A)*, especially near its penetration into the larynx.

cricothyroid articulation, is identified and carefully preserved. Electrocoagulation should not be used in the vicinity of the recurrent or superior laryngeal nerves because the spread of current could damage these nerves. Nerve integrity monitoring systems (NIMSs) are a helpful adjunct in identifying and preserving the recurrent laryngeal nerves, but are not a substitute to visualization. The monitoring device is located in the endotracheal tube inserted by the anesthesia provider during anesthesia induction. Vigorous suction and dissection may cause injury to the nerve and parathyroid glands. Bilateral injury to each external branch of the superior laryngeal nerve (EBSLN) results in paralysis of the cricothyroid muscles, and makes it impossible to produce high-pitched sounds. Although surgeons must maintain visual identification of the recurrent laryngeal nerve, a randomized controlled study revealed a significant improvement in identifying the nerve, and a decreased risk of early phonation changes following a thyroidectomy when the NIMS monitoring device was used (Barczynski et al, 2012). The scrub person should prepare a radiopaque 4 × 8-inch sponge on the end of a forceps for the surgeon or assistant to use in gently blotting the area.

7. The thyroid lobe is pulled downward, a Lahey goiter or polar retractor inserted as necessary, and the avascular tissue between the trachea and upper pole of the thyroid dissected by means of Metzenbaum scissors.

8. The superior thyroid artery is defined by blunt dissection with a peanut sponge on a clamp; it is then isolated with a right-angle clamp. The artery is ligated with nonabsorbable suture or clamped with hemoclips, and divided. Care is taken here to avoid injury to the superior laryngeal nerve. The upper parathyroid gland is often identified at this time.

9. The inferior thyroid artery is identified and preserved. The inferior parathyroid is likewise identified. Only branches of the inferior thyroid artery that do not supply the parathyroid glands are ligated, using fine forceps, sutures, and scissors. The thyroid lobe is then dissected away from the recurrent laryngeal nerve with Metzenbaum scissors and hemostats. Bleeding vessels are clamped with hemostats or hemoclips, and ligated with fine nonabsorbable sutures.

10. The lobe is elevated with Babcock clamps and freed from the trachea with fine scissors, forceps, knife, and hemostats, or with cautious electrodissection. The fibrous bands attached to the trachea and cricoid cartilage are divided.

11. The isthmus of the gland is elevated with fine forceps and divided between hemostats with scissors, removing the lobe and isthmus. The cut edge of the remaining thyroid may be oversewn to maintain hemostasis. If a pyramidal lobe is present, it is removed, along with the lobe to which it is attached, to its termination in the neck, which may reach the hyoid bone. If it is necessary to transect the hyoid bone, a small bone cutter is used.

12. The cut surface of the opposite lobe requires careful hemostasis. Interrupted sutures may be used for this purpose as well as for reapproximation to the pretracheal fascia.

13. The excised thyroid is examined for inadvertent parathyroid inclusion. If a parathyroid is present, it is removed and reimplanted.

14. The strap muscles, if severed, are reapproximated with fine interrupted absorbable or nonabsorbable sutures. If necessary, a drain is inserted into the thyroid bed and exteriorized through the midline. Some surgeons prefer to drain the wound laterally through the sternocleidomastoid muscle and the lateral aspect of the incision, believing that this produces better healing and cosmetic results. A hemostatic agent may be placed in the lateral gutter to facilitate hemostasis.

15. The edges of the platysma muscle are reapproximated. The skin edges are then reapproximated with subcuticular fine absorbable sutures.

16. Wound closure tapes or surgical glue is applied to the wound edges, and gauze dressings, if required, are placed on the wound with minimal tape.

Complications of thyroidectomy include hemorrhage, seroma formation, pneumothorax when extended thyroid dissection is done, and injury to the recurrent laryngeal or superior laryngeal nerves.

Substernal or Intrathoracic Thyroidectomy

Extensions of goiters enlarging into the substernal and intrathoracic regions may occur. If they cause tracheal and esophageal obstruction, they are usually excised surgically. Longer instruments are sometimes required. Splitting the sternum is rarely necessary because access to the substernal part of the gland is usually satisfactory through the standard thyroid incision.

Minimally Invasive Thyroidectomy

Minimally Invasive Open Thyroidectomy

The length of the incision is the major difference between minimally invasive and traditional thyroidectomy. Because of its smaller size, the site of the incision is critical for optimum access and visualization. After the incision is made, the remaining procedure is the same as that for conventional thyroidectomy (Hunter and Jobe, 2010).

Minimally Invasive Video-Assisted Thyroidectomy (MIVAT)

Procedural Considerations. The possibility of conversion to open thyroidectomy should be included on the operative consent form. Instruments and supplies for a possible open procedure are readied. Surgical skin preparation is done as in an open procedure in the event conversion is necessary. A set of long Miccoli instruments is added to the standard thyroid or neck dissection setup. A 30-degree endoscope and harmonic scalpel with scissors are used to ligate and divide vessels. Fire safety precautions are implemented for illuminated light cords, endoscopes, light sources, and cable connections.

Intraoperative Procedure

1. The patient is positioned and draped as for thyroidectomy. A horizontal incision of 3 cm or less is marked and then carefully made between the sternal notch and cricoid cartilage, usually less than 2 cm inferior to the cricoid (Figure 16-8).

FIGURE 16-8 A, Minimally invasive video-assisted thyroidectomy (MIVAT) incision location. **B,** MIVAT incision length.

2. Subcutaneous tissue is electrodissected and the raphe of strap muscle is then separated superiorly and inferiorly for about 3 cm. The anterior jugular veins are preserved.

3. Blunt dissection is used to separate the strap muscle from the thyroid.

4. The middle thyroid vein is clipped and divided.

5. Miccoli retractors are used to retract the strap muscles and soft tissue, exposing the superior lobe and vascular bundle.

6. The endoscope is introduced to visualize the upper pole. Three persons are needed: the surgeon, an assistant for retraction, and an endoscopist.

7. Miccoli spatula-shaped and aspirator dissectors are used to dissect the superior pole and vascular bundle (Figure 16-9). Care is taken to identify and preserve the external branch of the superior laryngeal nerve.

8. The thyroid lobe is then retracted medially and its lateral and posterior attachments are dissected. The recurrent laryngeal nerve and parathyroids are protected and preserved (Figure 16-10).

9. After sufficient mobilization of the lobe, the remainder of the procedure is accomplished under direct visualization. The isthmus is transected to complete the lobectomy.

10. The same procedure is repeated on the other side for complete thyroidectomy.

11. Hemostasis is achieved, the wound is irrigated, strap muscles are reapproximated, and the skin is closed (Figure 16-11).

Postoperatively, analgesics, antiemetics, and prophylactic antibiotics are administered in the PACU. Preoperative thyroid hormone supplementation is continued. For inpatients, ionized calcium and albumin levels are checked in the PACU and then every 6 to 8 hours. Hypocalcemia is a serum calcium level less than 8 mg/dL. If patients are discharged the same day as surgery, prophylactic calcium supplements will be prescribed for several weeks. Ambulatory patients are provided with contact information and told to notify their surgeon immediately if they experience signs of hypocalcemia. Early signs include perioral numbness or paresthesia and a positive Chvostek sign.

Thyroglossal Duct Cystectomy

Thyroglossal duct cysts (TDCs) are the most common congenital cyst found in the neck. These cysts are the second most common

FIGURE 16-9 Video-assisted dissection of the right superior pole.

FIGURE 16-10 Identification of the recurrent laryngeal nerve during video-assisted right thyroid lobectomy. A parathyroid gland is also identified.

FIGURE 16-11 A, Surgical scar at 2 weeks. **B,** Surgical scar at 6 weeks.

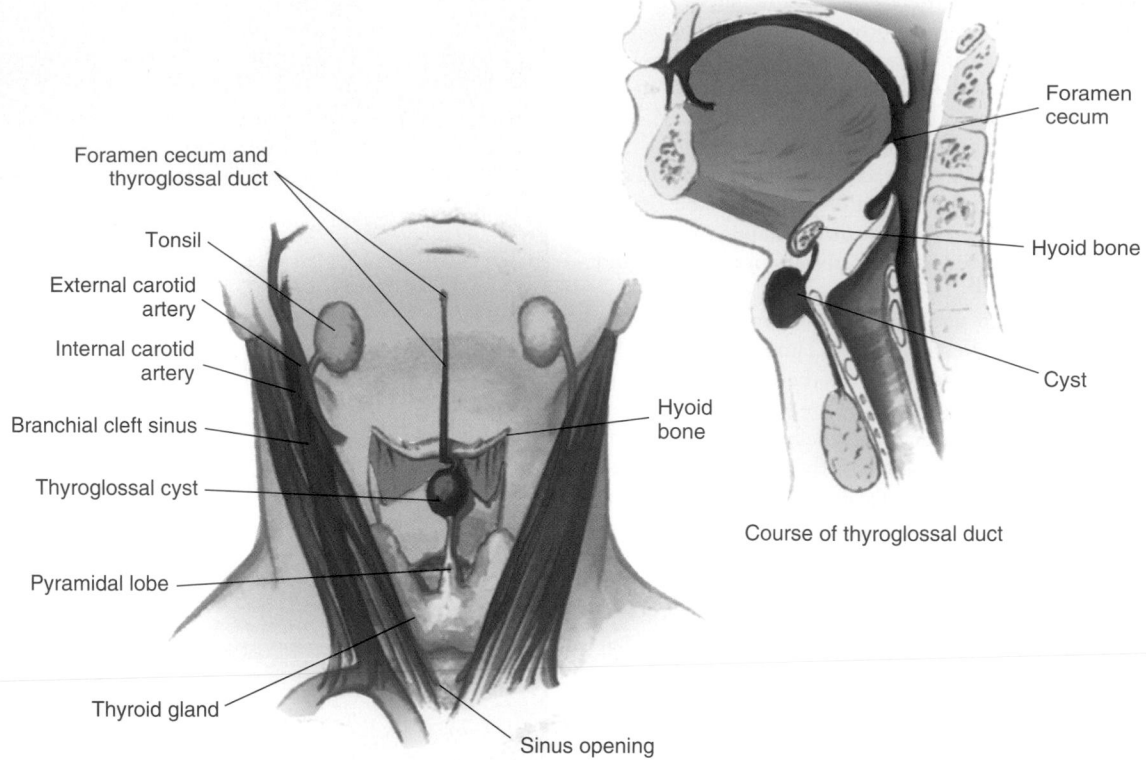

FIGURE 16-12 Thyroglossal cyst showing both anterior and lateral views.

type of pediatric neck mass. Although this cyst may be found in patients of any age, most are noted during childhood; 50% usually are seen before 20 years of age and about 70% by 30 years of age. The thyroglossal duct is an embryonic structure arising from the descent of the thyroid gland into the anterior portion of the neck. Usually the cyst presents as an asymptomatic midline swelling and is painless. Occasionally the cyst may become infected due to its proximity to the oral cavity. When present in an adult, it exists as a pretracheal cystic pouch attached to the hyoid bone, with or without a sinus tract to the base of the tongue at the foramen cecum (Figure 16-12). Thyroglossal duct cystectomy, often referred to as the Sistrunk procedure, requires complete excision of the cyst in continuity with its tract, the central portion of the hyoid bone, and the tissue above the hyoid bone extending to the base of the tongue to avoid recurrent cystic formation and to prevent infection. Only 1% of TDCs are malignant on histology; the prognosis for treating this malignancy is very good (Abuabara et al, 2010).

Procedural Considerations

The perioperative nursing assessment should be appropriate to the patient's age because the patient is frequently a child or teenager. Reassurance and age-appropriate information about the procedure are given. The patient is positioned supine, with the neck supported in extension. Bone instruments are needed in addition to the basic instrument set.

Operative Procedure

1. After the head is extended and the chin elevated, a transverse incision is made between the hyoid bone and thyroid cartilage through the subcutaneous tissue.

2. The platysma muscle is incised and flaps raised as described for thyroidectomy.
3. The strap (sternohyoid and sternothyroid) muscles are separated in the midline.
4. Sharp and blunt dissection is used to mobilize the cyst and duct, up to the attachment to the hyoid bone. The hyoid bone is transected twice, removing the center section with bone-cutting forceps. The segment of bone and the cyst are freed from adjacent structures.
5. The duct is traced superiorly through or near the hyoid up to the musculature of the tongue and removed completely. Methylene blue dye injection is used occasionally to visualize the whole tract.
6. The cyst is removed and the strap muscles closed with interrupted fine nonabsorbable sutures. A drain may be placed. The skin is then closed with subcuticular fine absorbable sutures and dressings are applied.

Neck Dissection

Neck dissection after a total thyroidectomy in a patient with carcinoma remains controversial because there is a high correlation of recurrence of cancer with little effect on long-term survival despite neck dissection. Lateral neck dissection is reserved for patients who have clinically proven metastatic disease or gross metastasis along the jugular vein; tumor histologic type is considered as well. Central compartment dissection is reserved for those who have clinically apparent or suspicious nodes first noted during the primary surgery.

Patients are closely monitored postoperatively with ultrasound and thyroglobulin to screen for recurrence. Adjuvant radioactive iodine ablation is used for high-risk thyroid cancer patients, including those with residual disease in the thyroid bed, large tumors, multifocal disease, nodal metastasis, vascular and extrathyroidal invasion, and cancer with an aggressive history as well as younger patients with distant metastasis (Loevner and Mukherji, 2008). Surgery is the treatment of choice for resectable recurrent thyroid carcinoma. The overall 10-year survival rate is 90%.

Parathyroidectomy

Parathyroidectomy is excision of one or more parathyroid glands. Normal or atrophic glands are generally not removed. The presence of adenomas (hypersecreting neoplasms), hyperplasia, or carcinoma requires surgical excision. For carcinomas, resection of the ipsilateral thyroid lobe and lymph nodes is essential, although metastasis may still occur by way of the bloodstream. Any residual parathyroid cancer may secrete PTH, causing hypercalcemia and its attendant problems.

Previously, the gold standard for parathyroidectomy was bilateral neck exploration with biopsy of all four glands to confirm the presence of adenoma or hyperplasia. New technologies, however, offer less invasive surgical options that pinpoint the affected gland and obviate the need to biopsy, and potentially damage, healthy parathyroid glands. The four-gland exploration for single-gland involvement is being replaced by radio-guided, minimally invasive ambulatory procedures using intraoperative PTH levels and/or the gamma probe. Patients with a negative sestamibi scan are excluded from minimally invasive parathyroidectomy protocols although intraoperative PTH levels are still helpful in identifying multiple adenomas (Loevner and Mukherji, 2008). Often the diagnosis of an adenoma can be made by gross inspection of the glands by the surgeon, but such diagnoses must be confirmed histologically by the pathologist.

Minimally invasive techniques cannot be used for hyperplasia. Hyperplasia requires removal of three and one-half glands through a bilateral neck exploration. A portion of a gland must remain to prevent hypocalcemia and its complications.

Procedural Considerations

During bilateral neck exploration multiple biopsies may be performed to determine the presence or absence of parathyroid tissue. Numerous specimen containers should be available (Patient Safety). When parathyroidectomy using a minimally invasive approach with intraoperative PTH assays is planned, the perioperative nurse verifies that a pathologist is alerted and ready to analyze blood samples and tissue specimens. If the surgeon is performing a focused parathyroidectomy (as described under Minimally Invasive, Focused Parathyroid Surgery), several blood tubes are required to measure PTH levels intraoperatively. The circulating nurse notes excision time and collaborates with the anesthesia provider to anticipate and handle post-excision blood samples. Mediastinotomy instruments should be available (see Chapter 23). The patient is positioned, prepped, and draped as described for thyroidectomy. Hemoclips should be available.

Operative Procedure—Open Approach

In the classic open approach, with the thyroid gland visible, bilateral neck exploration of the "normal" locations of the four parathyroid glands is conducted. Meticulous hemostasis by means of mosquito hemostats and fine ligatures is a prerequisite to location and identification of these small glands.

The thyroid gland is gently rotated anteriorly to provide access to the posterior thyroid sulcus, where the parathyroid glands are

almost always found. Identification of the parathyroid vascular pedicle, as it leaves either the superior thyroid artery or the inferior thyroid artery, is a means of locating both the inferior and superior glands. Metzenbaum scissors, mosquito hemostats, hemoclips, and gauze dissector sponges are used during dissection.

Attention then turns to the posterolateral surface of the thyroid lobe or just beneath the lower thyroid pole, where the inferior parathyroid glands are frequently found. Finding the vascular pedicle from the inferior thyroid artery may aid in identification (see Figure 16-4). Occasionally the lower pair is found in the thymic capsule or tissue, in which case a portion of the thymus is resected. A mediastinotomy is indicated for a small percentage of patients. Thoracoscopy (see Chapter 23) is also a successful, minimally invasive technique that may be used to remove parathyroid tumors that are deep in the mediastinum.

If one of the parathyroid glands shows evidence of disease, an effort is made to find other glands on the same side to ensure that they are disease-free. When found, biopsy is performed, and the area is marked with a hemoclip. The surgeon resects the diseased gland by clamping the vascular pedicle with mosquito hemostats, dividing with small scissors or a knife, and ligating with a fine nonabsorbable suture or hemoclip. The amount of parathyroid tissue that should be removed remains controversial and relates to whether single or multiple glands are involved. As noted, a portion of a gland must remain to prevent hypocalcemia and its complications.

A current alternative for multiple gland involvement is to excise all four glands and to transplant a portion of one in an accessible site, such as the neck or forearm, for later removal if hypercalcemia recurs. The amount of remaining parathyroid tissue can then be adjusted to regulate PTH to the desired level. This eliminates reexploration and potential injury to the recurrent laryngeal nerves. The parathyroid is morsellized and divided into several segments. An incision is made in the forearm or neck, and four separate grooves with purse-string sutures are made in the muscle. Some parathyroid tissue is placed and secured in each groove. The sites are then marked with one, two, three, and four hemoclips, respectively. If PTH levels remain high, the sites can be easily identified by the clips and more parathyroid tissue excised.

The neck region is then explored for aberrant parathyroid tissue, which is also resected. The remainder of the procedure is as described for the thyroid gland.

Minimally Invasive, Focused Parathyroid Surgery

Although a variety of minimally invasive techniques have evolved, a widely used procedure is the focused minimally invasive open approach (focused parathyroidectomy [FP]), in which imaging has identified a single parathyroid lesion. A localization study with sestamibi scan or ultrasound is used to identify the offending adenoma and to determine an optimum incision site.

PTH-Guided Parathyroidectomy.
A relatively new approach is the intraoperative intact, rapid assessment PTH approach. Given that blood samples must be drawn before, during, and after the procedure to measure PTH levels, an arterial line is inserted and a baseline PTH measurement is obtained preoperatively.

A 2-cm incision is made in the neck based on the localization studies. Once the suspect parathyroid gland is exposed, a pre-excision blood sample is taken. As a result of manipulation, the pre-excision blood level may test higher than the baseline level. The pre-excision level becomes the marker for measuring the post-excision drop in PTH level.

The excised gland is placed in sterile saline and kept on the instrument table until the pathologist confirms a sufficient drop in PTH blood levels. A drop of 50% or more is considered verification that the parathyroid adenoma was excised. Blood levels are also drawn at 5, 10, and 20 minutes post excision. When the adenoma is excised, a dramatic drop in PTH level is frequently achieved by the 10-minute post-excision PTH sample. If the 10-minute drop is significant, the surgeon may opt not to have the pathologist run a 20-minute post-excision blood sample. If the hormone level fails to drop sufficiently, the ipsilateral parathyroid is explored as the next most likely adenoma. False positives have been reported in patients who have slow metabolic rates, are renal insufficient, or have large adenomas (3 g or greater) (Loevner and Mukherji, 2008).

Any normal parathyroid that was excised and placed in saline is then morcellized with a #15 blade to increase surface area and then reimplanted. After the fascia is reapproximated, a clamp or scissors is used to create a groove in the strap muscle. A purse-string stitch of fine nonabsorbable suture is placed around the groove. The morcellized parathyroid tissue is placed inside the groove and the purse-string tightened and tied. Parathyroid tissue responds well to reimplantation.

Sestamibi-Guided Parathyroidectomy.
Another minimally invasive technique is the sestamibi-guided, or radio-guided, parathyroidectomy. Minimally invasive parathyroidectomy (MIP) is considered the treatment of choice for hyperparathyroidism (HPT) when a singular adenoma is present (Richards et al, 2012). Technetium-99m sestamibi is the imaging method of choice for localization of the parathyroid for patients with primary hyperparathyroidism. Sestamibi is administered preoperatively and a gamma probe used intraoperatively to pinpoint the adenoma. MIP is usually an ambulatory surgery procedure that has a 95% success rate using sestamibi imaging techniques. A higher success rate is also noted when an experienced endocrine surgeon consults in the radiology study interpretation (Richards et al, 2012).

KEY POINTS

- The thyroid gland is situated in the ventral aspect of the neck and is composed of right and left lobes anterolateral to the trachea and connected by an isthmus.
- Hyperthyroidism occurs when tissues are exposed to high levels of circulating thyroid hormone.
- Diagnosis and management of this clinical syndrome are based on the patient history, clinical presentation, and blood work results, including T_3, T_4, and thyroid-stimulating hormone (TSH).
- Radioiodine uptake and thyroid scans may be performed along with ultrasound.
- Treatment for hyperthyroidism includes antithyroid medication, radioiodine, and surgery.
- Hypothyroidism is a deficiency in thyroid hormone. It may be overt or subclinical. It is a common chronic condition and more common in women than men.
- Thyroid storm is an acute manifestation of hyperthyroidism.
- Patients with thyroid disease need frequent follow-up and sound nursing education.
- The four parathyroid glands are small and located behind the thyroid gland. They monitor and control calcium by secreting parathyroid hormone (PTH) to closely control serum calcium levels.
- In hyperparathyroidism, calcium builds up, potentially leading to atherosclerosis, hypertension, increased risk for atrial fibrillation, palpitations, osteopenia, osteoporosis, and formation of kidney stones.
- Head and neck irradiation in childhood and long-term lithium therapy are associated with a higher prevalence of primary hyperparathyroidism.
- A serum calcium level greater than 13.5 mg/dL can produce life-threatening cardiac dysrhythmias.
- Parathyroidectomy may be completed on an ambulatory surgery basis.

CRITICAL THINKING QUESTION

Your patient, Ms. J., is a 30-year-old who has just undergone a thyroidectomy in OR #6. The surgeon has left the OR and you are the circulating nurse in the room. It is lunchtime, and a new perioperative nurse (J.R.) comes into the room to give lunch relief to the surgical technologist (A.S.), who is cleaning up her instruments and preparing to take them to the decontamination area. J.R. says that she will take the instruments to the decontamination area, and that A.S. needs to go to lunch now; she has many lunch reliefs to do today. The hospital policy requires that the scrub person remain in the room until the patient has been transferred to the PACU, but J.R. is unaware of this policy. As a novice perioperative nurse, she is concerned with the tasks of preparing for the next surgery. You are finishing the documentation at the computer station, and turn around to see the anesthesia provider is having difficulty with the patient's airway. He has just extubated the patient, and his assistant has left the OR. You are alone in the room with this patient in distress. What would your priority nursing actions be at this time? What needs to be established for patient safety? What is the most probable cause for the patient's respiratory distress, and what actions will you need to perform to provide this patient with a positive patient outcome?

℮volve *The answers to the Critical Thinking Question can be found at http://evolve.elsevier.com/Rothrock/Alexander.*

REFERENCES

Abuabara A et al: Thyroglossal duct cyst, *Rev Sul-Bras Odontol* 7(2):244–246, 2010.

American Cancer Society (ACS): *Cancer facts and figures 2013*. Atlanta, Ga: American Cancer Society, 2013. Available at http://www.cancer.gov/cancertopics/pdq/treatment/thyroid/HealthProfessional/page1. Accessed May 23, 2013.

Association of PeriOperative Registered Nurses: *Perioperative standards and recommended practices*, Denver, 2013, The Association.

Barczynski M et al: Randomized control trial of visualization versus neuromonitoring of the external branch of the superior laryngeal nerve during thyroidectomy, *World J Surg* 36(6):1340–1347, 2012.

Burman KD, Rodondi N: Thyroid condition linked to heart problems, *Arch Intern Med*, April 23, 2012, available at http://newshealth.com/2012/04/23/thyroid-condition-linked-to-heart-problems-study. Accessed August 22, 2013.

Byrne MD: Little gland, big problems, *OR Nurse* 7(1):22–29, 2013.

Copstead LE, Banasik J: *Pathophysiology*, ed 4, St Louis, 2010, Saunders.

Denholm B: Tucking patient's arms and general positioning, *AORN J* 89(4):755–757, 2009.

Grebe SKG: Diagnosis and management of thyroid carcinoma: a focus on serum thyroglobulin, *Expert Rev Endocrinol Metab* 4(1):25–43, 2009.

Grogan R: Thyroid surgery riskier for older patients, *J Clin Endocrinol Metab*, March, 2012.

Harris R et al: Modern approach to surgical intervention of the thyroid and parathyroid glands, *Semin Ultrasound CT MRI* 33(2):115–122, 2012.

Haynes AB et al: A surgical safety checklist to reduce morbidity and mortality in a global population, *N Engl J Med* 360(5):491–499, 2009.

Hegarty J et al: Nurses' knowledge of inadvertent hypothermia, *AORN J* 89(4):710–713, 2009.

Howlader N et al: *SEER cancer statistics review, 1975-2009 (Vintage 2009 Populations)*, available at http://seer.cancer.gov/csr/1975_2010/results_merged/sect_26_thyroid.pdf. Accessed May 23, 2013.

Hunter JG, Jobe BA: *Schwartz's principles of surgery*, ed 9, New York, McGraw-Hill, 2010.

Kim YS: Impact of preserving the parathyroid glands on hypocalcemia after total thyroidectomy with neck dissection, *J Korean Surg Soc* 83(2):75–82, 2012.

Lewis S et al: *Medical-surgical nursing*, ed 8, St Louis, 2011, Mosby.

Loevner LA, Mukherji SK: *Thyroid and parathyroid glands: imaging, treatment, and beyond*, Philadelphia, 2008, Saunders.

National Cancer Institute: *Based on Nov 2011 SEER data submission*, available at http://seer.cancer.gpv/csr/1975_2009_pops09. Accessed September 2, 2012.

Richards M et al: Technetium-99m sestamibi imaging: are the results dependent on the reviewer? *J Surg Res* 177(1):97–101, 2012.

Wang T: Endocrine surgery, *Am J Surg* 202:369–371, 2011.

Wilson SF, Giddens JF: *Health assessment for nursing practice*, ed 4, St Louis, 2009, Mosby.

Yeh MW et al: Surgery for primary hyperparathyroidism, *Ann Surg* 255(6):1179–1183, 2012.

Yu JJ et al: Minimally invasive video-assisted thyroidectomy for the early-stage differential thyroid carcinoma, *J Transl Med* 10(Suppl 1):S13, 2012.

Most surgical procedures of the breast are performed to establish a definitive diagnosis or to treat breast cancer. Changing hormone levels from puberty throughout the remainder of life affect breast tissue in its physical and microscopic characteristics. In association with these changes, numerous aberrations and tumors can occur.

The occurrence of breast changes, benign or malignant, are some of the most emotionally upsetting health problems confronting women. Besides skin cancer, breast cancer is the most common cancer in American women. The most significant risk factors for developing breast cancer are being a woman and growing older (Breast Cancer.org 2012). Estimates are that one in eight women in the United States will develop breast cancer during her life. If the cancer is detected early, there is a 98.5% 5-year survival rate (Surveillance Epidemiology and End Results, 2013). Breast cancer risk doubles if a woman's mother, sister, or daughter had breast cancer. Early menarche (before 12 years of age) and a late natural menopause (after 50 years of age) are associated with a slightly increased risk for developing breast cancer. Further, a woman who has cancer in one breast is at increased risk for cancer in the other breast (American Cancer Society [ACS], 2012). Heightened public awareness, an increased number of women practicing self-examination, early detection of breast masses by mammography, and reduced use of hormone replacement therapy following the results of a large study called the Women's Health Initiative have started to slow the annual increase in breast cancer mortality.

Surgical Anatomy

The breasts are bilateral mammary glands that lie on the pectoralis major fascia of the anterior chest wall. They are surrounded by a layer of fat and are encased in an envelope of skin. The breasts extend from the second to the sixth ribs and horizontally from the lateral edge of the sternum to the anterior axillary line. The largest part of the mammary gland rests on the connective tissue of the pectoralis major muscle and laterally on the serratus anterior (upper outer quadrant of the breast), with a normal globular contour occurring as a result of fascia support (Cooper ligaments) (Figure 17-1). An elongation of mammary tissue normally extends laterally on the pectoralis major toward the axilla and is known as the *tail of Spence* (Figure 17-2).

Each breast is made up of 12 to 20 glandular lobes separated by connective tissue. Each lobe drains by a single lactiferous duct that opens on the nipple. The nipple, located at about the fourth intercostal space, forms a conical projection into which the ducts open independently of each other on the surface. A pigmented circular area called the *areola* surrounds the nipple. Smooth muscle fibers of the areola contract to allow for nipple projection.

Three major arterial systems (Figure 17-3) supply the mammary glands with blood. The major supply of blood comes from the perforating branches of the internal mammary arteries, derived from the internal thoracic artery. The breast is additionally supplied by the lateral thoracic and thoracoacromial arteries as well as posterior intercostal arteries. Veins that mainly drain the breasts are the axillary along with the subclavian, intercostals, and internal thoracic veins.

Lymph drainage generally follows the course of the vessels. Greater than 75% of lymph drainage, chiefly from the lateral quadrants, drains to the axillary lymph nodes. The remainder of lymph drains to either the parasternal nodes, the opposite breast (medial quadrants), or the inferior phrenic nodes' lower quadrants (Figure 17-4). The internal thoracic nodes are few, but are responsible for most lymph drainage from the inner half of the breast. Thus the lymph system can also be a channel for the spread of malignant disease from the breast to associated areas of the chest wall or to the axilla.

The breast's sensory nerve supply is primarily threefold: the anterior cutaneous branches of the upper intercostal nerves, the third and fourth branches of the cervical plexus, and the lateral cutaneous branches of the intercostal nerves (Hunt et al, 2010).

The mammary glands are affected by three types of physiologic changes: (1) those related to growth and development, (2) those related to the menstrual cycle, and (3) those related to pregnancy and lactation. The mammary glands are present at birth in males and females. Hormonal stimulation, however, produces the development and function of these glands in females. Estrogen promotes growth of the ductal structures, whereas progesterone promotes lobular development. Occasionally developmental errors of the breast occur. Additional nipples or extra mammary tissue in the axilla or over the upper abdomen may be present. Absence of one or both nipples may also occur and may be associated with absence of the underlying pectoral muscle and chest wall.

Benign Lesions of the Breast

Fibrocystic change in the breast is an all-encompassing term used to describe many different breast changes. Examples of benign lesions that are generally considered when fibrocystic changes are discussed are multiple lesions of fibrous disease, intraductal papilloma, cysts, and solid masses such as fibroadenoma (Table 17-1). These changes affect almost all women at some time in their lives. Frequently pain is present, which calls attention to the problem. Pain, fluctuations in size, and multiple lesions are common features that help differentiate these generally benign lesions from cancer.

Nipple discharge is more commonly associated with benign lesions than with cancer. A postmenopausal woman who has some duct ectasia or who has borne children can manually produce nipple discharge. The most common cause of serous or serosanguineous

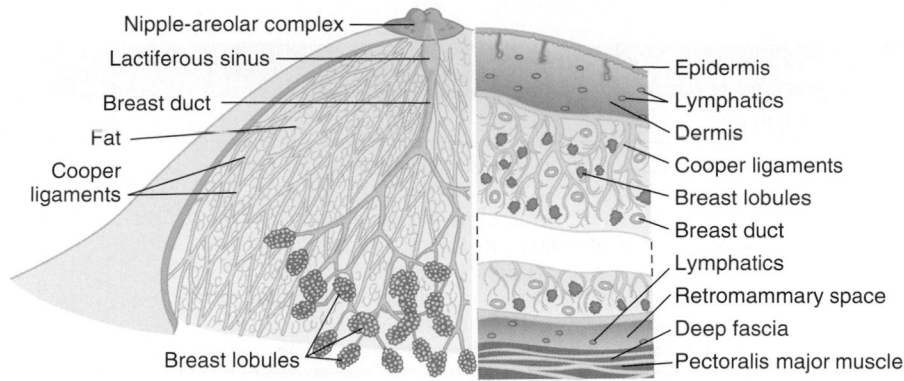

FIGURE 17-1 Normal mature resting breast.

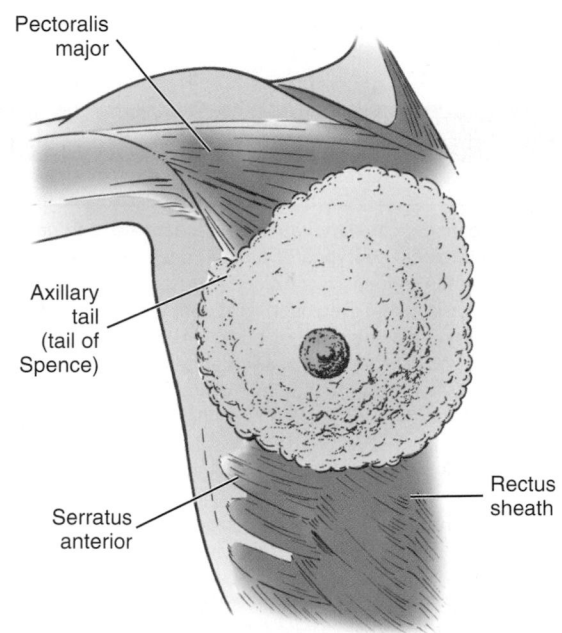

FIGURE 17-2 Normal distribution of mammary tissue of adult female.

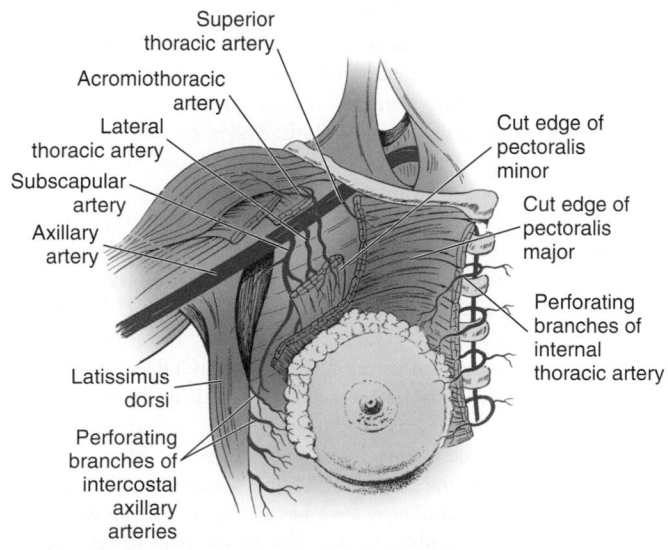

FIGURE 17-3 Normal arterial blood supply of the breast.

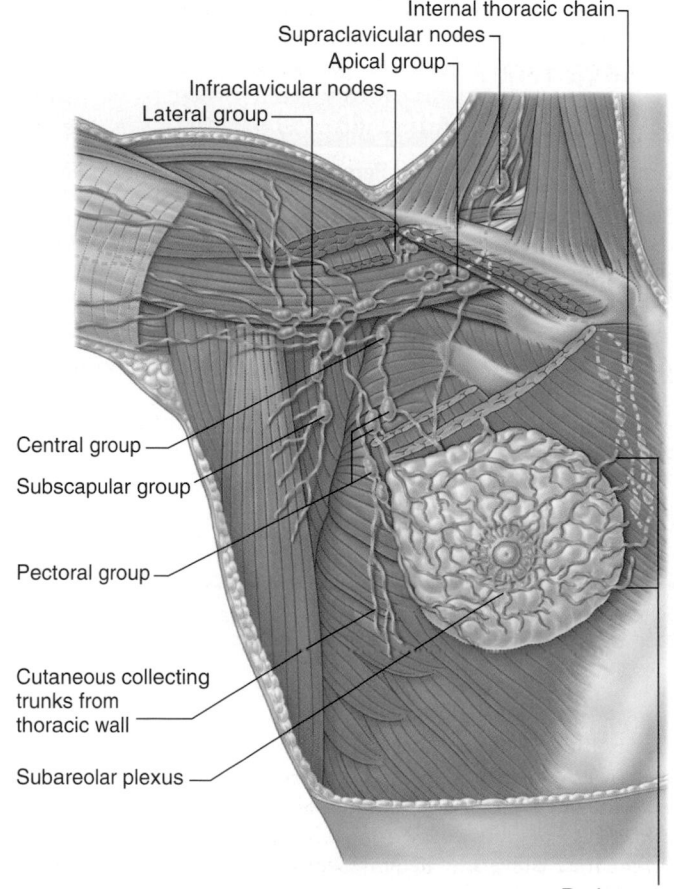

FIGURE 17-4 Axillary lymph node groups.

nipple discharge is a benign intraductal papilloma, along with medications such as tricyclines and antidepressants. Discharge is usually significant only if it is spontaneous and persistent. The discharge may be clear or bloody (Townsend et al, 2012). Chronic unilateral nipple discharge, especially if bloody, should prompt an investigation for occult carcinoma.

Breast Cancer in Men

Breast cancer in men is rare; less than 1% of breast carcinomas arise in men. The average age at diagnosis is approximately 68 years. Risk

TABLE 17-1

Typical Presentation of Benign Breast Disorders

Breast Disorder	Description	Incidence
Fibroadenoma	Most common benign lesion; solid mass of connective tissue that is unattached to surrounding tissue	Teenage years into 30s
Fibrocystic breast disease (FBD)	*First stage:* Characterized by premenstrual bilateral fullness and tenderness *Second stage:* Presence of bilateral, multicentric nodules *Third stage:* Presence of microscopic and macroscopic cysts	Late teens and 20s
Ductal ectasia	Hard, irregular mass or masses with nipple discharge, enlarged axillary nodes, redness, and edema; difficult to distinguish from cancer	Women approaching menopause
Intraductal papilloma	Mass in duct that results in nipple discharge: mass is usually not palpable	Women 40-55 years of age

Modified from American Cancer Society: *Noncancerous breast conditions,* 2012, Atlanta, Author; Ignatavicius DD, Workman ML: *Medical-surgical nursing: patient-centered collaborative care,* ed 7, St Louis, 2013, Saunders; Imaginis: *Non-cancerous breast conditions 2011,* available at www.imaginis.com/breast-health-non-cancerous/benign-breast-conditions. Accessed January 27, 2013.

TABLE 17-2

Types of Invasive Breast Cancer

Breast Cancer Type	Percent of Breast Cancers	Specific Features
Ductal carcinoma in situ (DCIS)	85-90	Can appear as microcalcifications, can vary widely in appearance, and can have features of other histologic subtypes of breast cancer. If untreated, 60%-100% of cases advance to invasive carcinoma.
Lobular carcinoma in situ (LCIS)	10	A marker for future breast cancer risk. Begins in milk (lobules) glands of breast, may become invasive, grows as single file of malignant cells around ducts and lobules and presents most often as a poorly defined mass.
Medullary carcinoma	5	Forms distinct boundary between tumor tissue and normal tissue, well circumscribed, frequent phenotype of *BRCA1* hereditary breast cancer, contains lymphocytes.
Tubular	2	Infrequently metastasizes to lymph nodes, slow growing, long-term survival approaches 100%.
Inflammatory carcinoma	1-5	Rapidly growing, often with metastasis present at diagnosis, first manifestations are breast skin edema and redness and warmth with dimples or ridges. It can be confused with mastitis. More common in African American women.

Modified from Breast Cancer.org: *IDC type: tubular carcinoma of the breast 2012,* available at www.breastcancer.org/symptoms/types/tubular. Accessed January 27, 2013; Townsend CM et al: *Sabiston textbook of surgery: the biological basis of modern surgical practice,* ed 19, Philadelphia, 2012, Saunders.

factors include increased age, radiation exposure, estrogen treatment, Klinefelter syndrome, heavy alcohol intake, obesity, female relatives with a breast cancer diagnosis, and families in which breast cancer susceptibility gene 2 *(BRCA2)* mutation has been identified (Ohio State University Medical Center, 2013). The most common type of tumor is infiltrating ductal carcinoma. Paget disease of the nipple, inflammatory carcinoma, and intraductal cancer have also been reported in men. Symptoms include breast lumps, nipple inversion, nipple discharge, pain or pulling feelings and skin or nipple changes such as dimpling, puckering, redness, or scaling. Staging of male breast cancer is identical to staging for female breast cancer. Treatment may include surgery, radiation therapy, chemotherapy, and hormone therapy. Before hormone therapy begins, a hormone receptor test is done to determine if estrogen and progesterone receptors are present. Adjuvant therapy of radiation, chemotherapy, or hormone treatment can be given after to destroy cancer cells that cannot be detected. According to a large study of male breast cancer, male patients have more advanced disease at diagnosis, lower 5-year survival rates, and shorter median overall survival rate than women (Healthday, 2013).

Breast Cancer in Women

Breast cancer affects primarily women. Until it can be prevented, early detection is the best hope for cure. It has, in the past, been recommended that all women should practice monthly self-examination to detect palpable lesions, and they should immediately report any changes or masses to a physician. However, the efficacy of breast self-examination (BSE) in decreasing cancer mortality is being questioned. Allen and colleagues (2010) suggest patients with breast cancer risk factors such as gene mutation, family history, obstetric and gynecologic history, demographics, and environmental risk factors should be taught BSE. The U.S. Preventive Services Task Force (USPSTF) does not recommend BSE (Centers for Disease Control and Prevention [CDC], 2012). The most common form of breast cancer at present is infiltrating ductal carcinoma (Table 17-2).

The cause of breast cancer remains unknown. Many factors, including environmental, dietary (National Cancer Institute [NCI], 2011), and familial influences have been suggested as contributors to its development (Table 17-3). The belief that breast cancer spreads by direct extension from its initial site in the breast to

TABLE 17-3

Risk Factors for Breast Cancer

Factors	Comments
High Increased Risk (Relative Risk >4)	
Female gender	99% of all breast cancers occur in women.
Age >50 years	Greatest risk for women occurs during ages 50-69 years.
Genetic factors	Inherited mutations of *BRCA1* and/or *BRCA2* increase risk.
History of previous breast cancer	Risk for developing cancer in opposite breast is five times greater than average population at risk.
Breast density	Dense breasts contain more glandular and connective tissue, which increases the risk for developing breast cancer.
Moderate Increased Risk (Relative Risk 2.1-4)	
Family history	One first-degree relative with breast cancer moderately increases risk.
Biopsy confirmed atypical hyperplasia	The overactive growth of cells increases risk.
Ionizing radiation	Women who received frequent low-level radiation exposure to thorax have increased risk, especially if exposure occurred during periods of rapid breast formation.
High postmenopausal bone density	High estrogen levels over time both strengthen bone and increase breast cancer risk.
Low Increased Risk (Relative Risk 1.1-2)	
Reproductive history (nulliparity or first child born after age 30)	Childless women have an increased risk, as do women who bear their first child near or after age 30.
Menstrual history (early menstruation or late menopause or both)	Risk for breast cancer rises as interval between menarche and menopause increases. Women who undergo bilateral oophorectomy before age 35 have only 40% of risk for breast cancer compared with women who undergo natural menopause.
Oral contraceptives	There is a slight increase in breast cancer risk in women taking oral contraceptives.
Hormone replacement therapy (HRT)	Use of estrogen and progesterone increases risk; routine use of hormone therapy for osteoporosis and heart disease is no longer recommended.
Obesity	Postmenopausal obesity (especially increased abdominal fat), increased body mass, insulin resistance, and hyperglycemia have been reported to be associated with increased risk for breast cancer.
Alcohol	Risk is dose dependent; consumption of 3 to 14 drinks per week is associated with a slight increase in risk; risk increases with increased consumption.
High socioeconomic status	Breast cancer incidence is greater in women of higher education and socioeconomic background. This relationship is possibly related to lifestyle differences, such as age at first birth.
Jewish heritage	Women of Jewish Ashkenazi heritage have higher incidences of *BRCA1* and *BRCA2* genetic mutations.

Modified from American Cancer Society: *Breast cancer facts and figures 2010-2011*, Atlanta, 2012, Author; Ignatavicius DD, Workman ML: *Medical-surgical nursing: patient-centered collaborative care*, ed 7, St Louis, 2013, Saunders.

adjacent lymph nodes may not always be correct. Breast cancer may be a systemic condition at the time of diagnosis. Distant metastases may have already occurred without adjacent lymph node involvement at the time of palpable detection. This could explain why radical breast surgery of the past, which involved removal of the affected breast and all axillary and thoracic lymph nodes, did not greatly lower mortality. Survival from breast cancer is best when detected early, reducing axillary lymph node involvement and improving long-term survival. Tumor size can usually be correlated with involvement of lymph nodes. The larger a tumor is, the more likely it is that lymph nodes are involved.

Less radical surgery is the treatment of choice today. Most small noninvasive and invasive breast cancers are treated by breast conservation therapy (BCT). Surgical excision of the tumor, the use of radiation therapy alone, or a combination of surgery, chemotherapy, and radiation therapy are treatment recommendations. The use of adjuvant chemotherapy is particularly recommended for premenopausal women with axillary node metastasis. Studies show that similar therapy can benefit node-negative breast cancer patients. New studies and new therapeutic options are continually being developed and tested.

Clinical use of accelerated partial breast irradiation (APBI) is a current treatment. In APBI the radiation is focused on the area of greatest risk for tumor recurrence, the lumpectomy site, instead of whole breast irradiation (WBI). Such focused radiation treatment therapies reduce the traditional 6-week radiation treatment plan to 1 week to 3 weeks (ACS, 2012). Although external beam radiation therapy of the whole breast after lumpectomy has been the standard of care for treating early stage breast cancer, APBI is being used increasingly as an alternative treatment option for carefully selected patients.

Brachytherapy, also known as internal radiation, is another delivery method of radiation. Radioactive seeds are placed precisely into the adjoining cancerous breast tissue. There are two kinds of brachytherapy: interstitial and intracavitary. In interstitial brachytherapy, many small, hollow catheters are inserted into the breast around the lumpectomy area and are left in place for several days. Radioactive pellets are inserted into the catheters for short periods each day and then removed. It is not as common today as intracavitary brachytherapy, which is a form of APBI that involves placing a source of radiation into the lumpectomy site for a short period and removing it. It is usually administered twice a day for 5 days on an outpatient basis (ACS, 2012). Clinicians are likely to prefer the newer intra-cavitary brachytherapy technique for APBI because this method is less invasive and less technically demanding than interstitial techniques.

Minimally invasive cryoablation technology to freeze and destroy solid breast tumors is another option for treatment of a breast tumor. Another breast surgery alternative is focused ultrasound (FUS) with magnetic resonance guidance (MRgFUS), which allows for imaging and tissue temperature monitoring while controlling the FUS beam direction during ablation of breast lesions (Tempany et al, 2011).

Screening Technologies

Imaging methodologies, such as mammography and ultrasonography (US), have helped detect breast masses too small for clinical detection. A recent study supports the need to identify and track breast cancer screening disparities in the United States (Research Highlight). The American Cancer Society (ACS) recommends clinical breast exams by a physician every 3 years for women ages 20 to 39 years, with annual clinical breast exams and mammograms for women 40 and older (Table 17-4). Women who are at high risk should have magnetic resonance imaging (MRI) and a mammogram every year. High-risk women include those who have a known breast cancer susceptibility gene 1 *(BRCA1)* or breast cancer susceptibility gene 2 *(BRCA2)* mutation, those who have a first-degree relative with a *BRCA1* or *BRCA2* gene mutation, and those who have a history of breast cancer, ductal carcinoma in situ (DCIS), lobular carcinoma in situ (LCIS), atypical ductal hyperplasia, or atypical lobular hyperplasia (ACS, 2012). The USPSTF advises women ages 50 years and older to have a screening mammogram every 2 years (CDC, 2012). Many professional organizations such as the American Medical Association, American College of Surgeons, American College of Obstetricians and Gynecologists, and the American College of Radiology advocate mammography to begin at age 40.

The most common screening mechanism for asymptomatic women is mammography (Figure 17-5). In mammography the entire breast is visualized as x-ray beams are directed in several planes through it. Mammograms detect abnormal-appearing densities, irregular or spiculated margins, microcalcifications, and clusters of calcium deposits that are clinically nonpalpable. Screening mammography is the most helpful in early detection because it can discover cancer several years before physical symptoms such as a lump develop. Often previous mammograms are used for comparison. The accuracy of mammography depends on careful x-ray technique and breast size, structure, and density. Radiation dosage varies with individuals and techniques. As a result of improved radiologic techniques, radiation exposure in a mammogram is very low. The benefits of this screening mechanism far outweigh the minute risks

---

RESEARCH HIGHLIGHT

Cancer Screening in the United States

The percentage of U.S. citizens screened for cancer remains below national targets with noteworthy differences among racial and ethnic populations, according to a federal study examining cancer screening disparities among Asian and Hispanic groups. Based on responses to the 2010 National Health Interview Survey (NHIS), 72.4% of women overall followed the screening recommendation of the U.S. Preventive Services Task Force (USPSTF) for breast cancer, significantly less than the *Healthy People 2020* target of 81.1%. Cervical and colorectal cancer screenings were also below target. Screening rates for all three cancers were considerably lower among Asians compared with other groups. Hispanics were less likely to be screened for cervical and colorectal cancer compared with non-Hispanics. Significantly, lower breast, cervical, and colorectal cancer screening exists in people without any usual source of healthcare or health insurance. Age, race, ethnicity, education, length of residence in the United States, and financial resources for healthcare were variables explored in this study. Education level was associated positively with screening. This study supports the need to identify and track cancer screening disparities, providing guidance for development of programs to increase use of screening tests in order to meet *Healthy People 2020* targets and decrease cancer mortality and morbidity.

Modified from Centers for Disease Control and Prevention: *Study finds racial and ethnic disparities in U.S cancer screening rates,* 2012, available at www.cdc.gov/media/releases/2012/p0126_cancer_screening.html. Accessed January 27, 2013; *Healthy People 2020,* available at www.cdc.gov/nchs/healthy_people/hp2020.htm. Accessed June 15, 2013.

TABLE 17-4

American Cancer Society Breast Cancer Screening Guidelines for Asymptomatic Women*

Age	Screening Activity
20-39 yr	Breast self-examination (BSE) optional Clinical breast examination (CBE) every 3 yr
40 yr and older	BSE optional CBE annually prior to mammogram Annual mammogram

*Asymptomatic women identified to be at higher risk need to have individualized screening plans that may differ from these guidelines.
Modified from American Cancer Society: *Breast cancer facts and figures 2011-2012,* Atlanta, 2012, Author, available at www.cancer.org/research/cancerfactsfigures/breastcancerfactsfigures/breast-cancer-facts-and-figures-2011-2012. Accessed January 27, 2013.

FIGURE 17-5 Mammographic features of malignancy. **A,** A stellate mass. The combination of a density, surrounding spicules, and distortion of the breast architecture strongly suggests a malignancy in this mammogram. **B,** Clustered microcalcifications. Fine, irregular, and branching forms suggest malignancy in this mammogram. Fine calcifications, less than 0.5 mm in size, are more often associated with cancer than are larger, coarse calcifications.

FIGURE 17-6 Mammogram section. Craniocaudal view of breast. Arrow indicates breast lesion localized by wire before surgical excision.

BOX 17-1

BI-RADS Assessment Scores

Category 0: The screening mammogram indicates additional screening is necessary. Prior mammograms, if available, are used for comparison. Additional imaging may include spot compression, magnification, special mammographic views, or ultrasound.
Category 1: The results are negative.
Category 2: The findings are benign.
Category 3: The findings are probably benign. Short-term follow-up is advised.
Category 4: The findings are suspicious. Biopsy is considered.
Category 5: The findings are highly suggestive of malignancy. Preliminary biopsy is needed; surgical treatment likely required.
Category 6: Known biopsy-proven malignancy. This category may be used for a second opinion before excisional biopsy, radiation therapy, chemotherapy, or mastectomy or for following tumor response during chemotherapy.

BI-RADS, Breast Imaging Reporting and Data System.
Modified from Townsend CM et al: *Sabiston textbook of surgery: the biological basis of modern surgical practice,* ed 19, Philadelphia, 2012, Saunders.

of radiation exposure. Advances in computer-assisted detection allow the computer to analyze the mammogram, placing asterisks and triangles on small potential problem areas, which a radiologist then reviews. In some instances, such as when a lesion previously detected in a mammogram is too small to palpate, mammograms are repeated immediately before surgery. The lesion is localized by the insertion of a needle or a wire within a needle (often referred to as "needle" or "wire" localization) (Figure 17-6). If screening mammography reveals a suspicious area, the patient is asked to return for diagnostic mammography.

Digital mammography, also known as full-field digital mammogram (FDDM), is similar to a standard mammogram in that an x-ray is used to take images of the breast. The mammograms are recorded and viewed on a computer where the image size, brightness, or contrast in certain areas of the film can be adjusted and seen more plainly. Digital images can be sent electronically to other sites for viewing and consulting with breast specialists. Radiologists also can use software to interpret digital mammograms. Digital screening mammograms are more accurate than film screening mammograms, with a 70% detection rate compared with 55% for film screens. Women most likely to benefit from digital screening are those younger than 50 with dense breast tissue and who are premenopausal or perimenopausal (ACS, 2012). When a palpable mass or other abnormality is identified on screening mammography, additional diagnostic mammographic views are obtained, and the radiologist assigns a Breast Imaging Reporting and Data System (BI-RADS) score (Box 17-1). US may then be ordered.

US differentiates between solid and cystic lesions. A cyst is a fluid-filled sac and is considered a benign finding. A solid mass may suggest malignancy and requires further evaluation. As a screening methodology alone, its sensitivity and specificity are less definitive than mammography. US can be useful with dense or dysplastic breasts and in pregnant or lactating women. Women 30 to 39 years of age benefit most from US, which has a sensitivity of 95.7% compared with 60.9% for mammography and discovers more cancerous lesions than mammography (Lehman et al, 2012).

MRI is used as an adjunct to mammography in the detection of breast lesions. MRI uses a strong magnet to produce a complete image of the breast. There is no radiation. Breast MRI can image dense breast tissue, which shows poorly with conventional mammography. The ACS recommends that MRI be used for women at high risk. Such women include those who have known breast cancer–associated *BRCA1* or *BRCA2* gene mutations, have a first-degree relative with a *BRCA1* or *BRCA2* gene mutation, have a

lifetime risk of breast cancer of 20% to 25% or greater according to risk assessment tools, and had radiation therapy to the chest between 10 and 30 years of age. MRI also better determines definite size of the cancer and is useful in women with breast augmentation.

Molecular breast imaging (MBI) refers to a number of modalities that use a radiopharmaceutical agent in scanning, including breast-specific gamma imaging (BSGI) and positron emission mammography (PEM). It involves injection of a short-lived radiotracer, which is absorbed by breast tissue and preferentially so by breast tumors. MBI is especially useful in detecting breast cancer in women with dense breasts, those who present with a palpable abnormality not found on mammogram or US, and those who cannot tolerate MRI or who have metallic implants (Kaplan, 2011).

Deoxyribonucleic acid (DNA)–based genetic testing for *BRCA1* and *BRCA2* is recommended for women with family histories that suggest risk for these gene mutations. These mutations lead to the development of hereditary breast and/or ovarian cancer in affected women. Individuals with a harmful *BRCA* mutation have a lifelong chance of up to 80% risk of developing breast cancer and are more likely to be diagnosed before menopause (Breast Cancer.org., 2012). To test for *BRCA1* and *BRCA2*, a blood DNA sample is needed for full-length gene sequencing. A genomic profiling tool for breast cancer, approved in the United States, is specifically for estrogen-receptor–positive, node-negative breast cancer. One of the test results is a recurrence score, which correlates the chance of a specific tumor returning in the next 10 years. Genetic counseling is suggested before and after the workup (Townsend et al, 2012).

Diagnostic Techniques

Once a mass is identified, the physician has multiple techniques to establish a diagnosis. During a fine-needle aspiration biopsy (FNAB) the physician or radiologist anesthetizes a small area of the breast with lidocaine. FNAB is mainly used for differentiation of solid from cystic masses but may also be performed when a new, dominant, unexplained mass is found in the breast. A 22- or 25-gauge needle attached to a 20-mL syringe is inserted into the mass, and a small amount of the contents is aspirated, then prepared on a slide for cytologic examination. Cyst fluid is usually cloudy and dark green or amber. If the mass is solid, the needle is repetitively inserted into the mass while steady negative pressure is applied to the syringe; suction is released and the needle is withdrawn. The slides are then fixed and submitted to pathology. Cytologic evaluation does not reveal if the cancer is invasive or noninvasive, so most physicians advise a core needle biopsy for histologic diagnosis before a surgical procedure (Townsend et al, 2012).

A core needle biopsy is similar to a FNAB but a larger needle is used because actual breast tissue is removed rather than a sampling of cells. Core needle biopsy is preferred over excisional biopsy because it is minimally invasive and less expensive (Townsend et al, 2012). The types of core biopsies are US-guided core biopsy and stereotactic core biopsy. US-guided core biopsy does not require surgery. A large biopsy needle is placed into the breast tissue and the US aids in confirming the proper needle placement for biopsy. US can also distinguish many benign lesions such as fluid-filled cysts. Tissue samples are then obtained through the needle. In stereotactic core biopsy, a large biopsy needle is inserted into the breast tissue; computerized mammographic pictures facilitate needle placement using digital imaging so the precise location of breast tissue is biopsied. Tissue samples are then withdrawn through the needle (Cleveland Clinic, 2009).

Surgical Treatment Options

Surgical treatment ranges from minimally invasive breast biopsy, BCT, wide excision of the tumor mass, or modified radical mastectomy involving the breast and axillary lymph nodes. In some cases, salpingo-oophorectomy is considered (Domchek et al, 2010). BCT surgeries are alternately called segmental mastectomy, lumpectomy, partial mastectomy, wide local excision, and tylectomy (Hunt et al, 2010). The goal of surgery is removal of the cancerous mass with a margin of normal tissue and a good cosmetic result. When a specimen of breast tissue is sent to the laboratory, it is inked to mark the relationship between the tumor and the surgical margins of the excision. The pathologist evaluates these margins on all sides of the tumor for malignant cells. If a margin is positive it indicates that malignant cells may remain in the breast. Additional surgery is usually required until the margins contain only normal tissue (Stephan, 2009).

The choice of procedure depends on the size and site of the mass, the characteristics of the cells, the stage of the disease, and the patient's choice. A breast cancer diagnosis is usually staged to measure the extent of the disease and to classify patients for possible treatment modalities (Figure 17-7 and Table 17-5). The TNM (T = tumor; N = node; M = metastasis) classification has been adopted as a mechanism to clinically stage this disease. Staging results are used in designing a specific treatment plan. Radiation therapy, chemotherapy, or hormonal therapy may be used with surgery or as alternative treatment methods. An intravenous (IV) access port may be surgically placed for later infusion of chemotherapeutic medications, fluids, or nutrition as well as to withdraw blood and laboratory specimens (Ambulatory Surgery Considerations).

Excised tumors or core needle biopsies are evaluated for their estrogen-binding and progesterone-binding abilities. Techniques have been developed to assess the ability of breast cancer to bind with estrogen and progesterone. This positive binding capability identifies the patient with a hormone-dependent tumor (Figure 17-8). It is estimated that about two thirds of all breast cancers are positive for estrogen binding, a majority of which are also positive

TABLE 17-5	
Staging of Breast Cancer	
Stage 0	Carcinoma in situ LCIS—abnormal cells in lining of a lobule DCIS—intraductal carcinoma; abnormal cells that are in lining of a duct
Stage I	Tumor <2 cm with no axillary lymph node involvement
Stage IIa	Cancer cells found in axillary lymph nodes, or tumor is <2 cm with metastasis to axillary lymph nodes, or tumor >2 cm but not >5 cm with no metastasis to axillary lymph nodes
Stage IIb	Tumor >2 cm but not >5 cm with positive axillary lymph nodes or tumor >5 cm with negative axillary lymph node involvement
Stage IIIa	Tumor ≤5 cm with metastasis to axillary lymph nodes that are attached to each other or to other structures or has spread to lymph nodes behind the breast bone; or tumor ≥5 cm with spread to axillary lymph nodes that are alone or attached to each other or to other structures or has spread to lymph nodes behind the breast bone
Stage IIIb	Tumor of any size that has grown into the chest wall or skin of the breast causing swelling of the breast or nodules in breast skin and may have spread to axillary lymph nodes that are attached to each other and to other structures and may have spread to lymph nodes behind the breast bone
Stage IIIc	Tumor of any size that has spread either to the lymph nodes behind the breast bone and axillary lymph nodes or to the lymph nodes above or below the collarbone
Stage IV	Distant organs

DCIS, Ductal carcinoma in situ; *LCIS,* lobular carcinoma in situ.
Modified from Breastcancer.org: *Stages of breast cancer,* available at: www.breastcancer.org/symptoms/diagnosis/staging.jsp. Accessed January 27, 2013; National Cancer Institute at the National Institutes of Health: *Breast cancer treatment (PDQ),* available at www.cancer.gov/cancertopics/pdq/treatment/breast/Patient/page2. Accessed January 27, 2013.

for progesterone binding. The presence of these receptor sites is favorable to hormone manipulation, with the goal of preventing breast cancer cells from receiving estrogen stimulation. In these patients, who also have negative axillary nodes, it is decidedly preferable to obtain a genomic profile of the primary cancer to find out the risk for recurrence (Townsend et al, 2012). Use of selective estrogen receptor modulators (SERMs) and estrogen receptor down-regulators (ERDs), in addition to surgery and chemotherapy, increase disease-free survival in premenopausal women with positive binding for estrogen. Postmenopausal women benefit from aromatase inhibitors (AIs). They appear to work better than estrogen receptor modulators on certain breast cancers, with fewer side effects.

Some of the most promising data reported for advanced breast cancer involves human epidermal growth factor receptor 2 (HER-2), a cellular proto-oncogene coding for a transmembrane receptor. Agents such as trastuzumab (Herceptin), to target HER-2 were first approved for treatment of metastatic HER-2–positive breast cancer in 1998. In 2012, pertuzumab was approved for use in combination with trastuzumab and with the chemotherapy agent docetaxel (Baselga et al, 2012). It is indicated for use in patients with metastatic HER-2–positive breast cancer who have not received previous

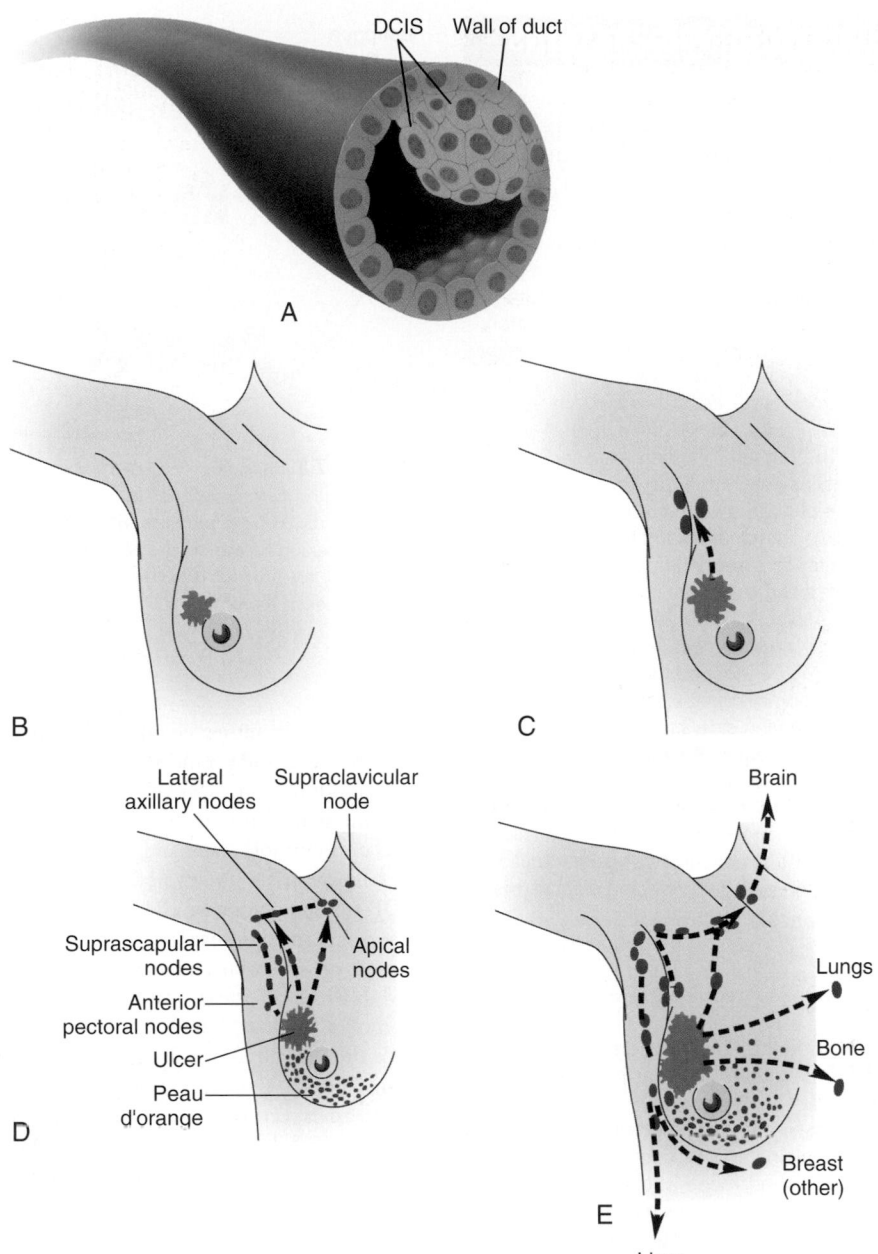

FIGURE 17-7 Anatomic staging of breast cancer. **A,** Stage 0 is carcinoma in situ. Lobular carcinoma in situ (LCIS) is defined as abnormal cells that are in the lining of a lobule. LCIS seldom becomes invasive cancer. However, having LCIS in one breast increases the risk of cancer for both breasts. Ductal carcinoma in situ (DCIS) is defined as abnormal cells that are in the lining of a duct. DCIS is also called intraductal carcinoma. The abnormal cells have not spread outside the duct. They have not invaded the nearby breast tissue. DCIS sometimes becomes invasive cancer if not treated. **B,** Stage I: tumor <2 cm with no axillary lymph node involvement. **C,** Stage IIa: cancer cells found in axillary lymph nodes, or tumor ≤2 cm with metastasis to axillary lymph nodes, or tumor >2 cm but not >5 cm with no metastasis to axillary lymph nodes. Stage IIb: tumor >2 cm but not >5 cm with positive axillary lymph node involvement, or tumor >5 cm with negative axillary lymph node involvement. **D,** Stage IIIa: tumor ≤5 cm with metastasis to axillary lymph nodes that are attached to each other or to other structures, or has spread to lymph nodes behind breast bone; or tumor >5 cm and has spread to axillary lymph nodes that are alone or attached to each other or to other structures, or has spread to lymph nodes behind the breast bone. Stage IIIb: tumor of any size that has grown into the chest wall or skin of the breast, causing swelling of the breast or nodules in breast skin; may have spread to axillary lymph nodes that are attached to each other and to other structures and may have spread to lymph nodes behind the breast bone. Inflammatory breast cancer: breast is red, swollen (at least stage IIIb). Stage IIIc: tumor of any size that has spread either to the lymph nodes behind the breast bone and axillary lymph nodes or to the lymph nodes above or below the collarbone. **E,** Stage IV: distant metastatic cancer.

AMBULATORY SURGERY CONSIDERATIONS

Port Insertion

A breast cancer patient who needs further medical treatment may opt to have an implanted venous access port placed under the skin in the chest, abdomen, or upper arm. This access port is used for frequent or continuous infusions of chemotherapeutic agents, solutions, other medications, pain management medication, or blood products as well as for procurement of blood samples. Consequently the patient's veins do not need to be repeatedly accessed. Port insertion is commonly done in an ambulatory surgery setting by a surgeon or in the interventional radiology department by a radiologist. The port has a soft, pliable plastic catheter that is threaded into a large central vein such as the subclavian, internal jugular vein, or a vein in the upper or lower arm under x-ray guidance. The catheter is then attached to the port chamber (a metal or plastic base with a rubber dome), which is placed under the skin. The patient is instructed to refrain from consuming solid foods or full liquids for at least 6 hours before the procedure. Clear liquids may taken 2 hours before the procedure. Regular medications may be taken the morning of the insertion unless instructed otherwise. Aspirin, clopidogrel (Plavix), or warfarin should be discontinued prior to surgery. Ask the physician when these medications need to be stopped; usually they can be resumed the next day. Medication allergies are noted. The protocol for correct person, procedure, and side/site is observed. After the procedure the patient will be observed for approximately 1 hour before discharge. Discharge instructions are as follows:

- Give both the patient and the caregiver verbal and written instructions and the telephone numbers of the physician and nurse so that questions or concerns can be addressed.
- Review the purpose of the port insertion and discuss how long it will stay in place.
- Discuss protecting the skin over the port and keeping the incision clean and dry.
- Avoid any strenuous activities involving the chest and arms for at least 10 days.
- If fever, chills, swelling, redness, bleeding, discharge, shortness of breath, or chest pain develops, seek prompt medical attention.
- No blood pressure measurement or blood draws are to be done from the arm containing an arm port.
- The port needs to be flushed monthly to keep it patent. Demonstrate this technique and have the patient repeat critical steps for port flushing. Flushing may also be performed by an oncology nurse or home care nurse.
- Explain that removal of the port will be an ambulatory procedure when it is no longer needed medically.
- Magnetic resonance imaging with magnetic strength of 3 or lower is permitted. Metal detectors will not harm the port. Have your port identification card with you.

Modified from Banerjee I, Mehta D: *Use of port-A-cath in chemotherapy*, available at http://lookingforcure.org/index.php?option=com_content&view=article&id=103:use-of-port-a-cath&catid=42:chemotherapy&Itemid=55. Accessed January 27, 2013; Liang E: *Portocath insertion-patient information guide*, available at www.sir.net.au/portacath_pi.html. Accessed January 27, 2013; Teichgräber UK et al: Central venous port systems as an integral part of chemotherapy, *Dtsch Arztebl Int* 108(9):147–154, 2011, published online March 4, 2011, available at www.ncbi.nlm.nih.gov/pmc/articles/PMC3063378. Accessed January 27, 2013.

FIGURE 17-8 Physiology of estrogen and the estrogen receptor, shown schematically. Estrogen binds to estrogen receptors, translocates to the nucleus of the cell, and interacts with cellular deoxyribonucleic acid (DNA). This interaction results in the transcription of estrogen-responsive genes, such as the receptor for progesterone. In addition, other genes are induced by the estrogen receptors that influence cell growth and differentiation.

treatment with either chemotherapy or HER-2–targeted therapy. Research and understanding of the immune system, development of methods to evaluate aspects of the immune response, and ongoing development of monoclonal antibodies continue to transform the field of immunotherapy and breast cancer treatment (Modi, 2011).

Clinical trials are exploring the clinical effectiveness of poly ADP-ribose polymerase (PARP) enzyme inhibitors (Surgical Pharmacology) in triple-negative breast cancer (TNBC) patients. These tumors are estrogen and progesterone hormone receptor negative and HER-2/neu negative. TNBC is found in younger women, women of African American or Hispanic descent, and individuals with *BRCA1* mutations. It also is associated with a worse prognosis than other breast cancer subtypes (Winer, 2011).

Breast cancer patients are increasingly seeking and using complementary and alternative medicine (CAM) and integrative therapies to enhance their surgical and medical treatment. (See Chapter 30 for a full discussion of integrative therapies.) Besides using products such as green tea, botanicals, vitamins E and C, and flaxseed, breast cancer patients are incorporating massage therapy and meditation and enlisting the help of dietitians and nutritionists as they battle breast cancer (NCI, 2012).

Perioperative Nursing Considerations

Assessment

Patients undergoing breast surgery will likely be extremely apprehensive about the possibilities of having a malignancy, losing a body part, facing a negative reaction from her spouse and family, and experiencing a negative change in self-image. For this reason patients may have nurse navigators guide them through the maze of breast cancer treatment options and requirements (Research Highlight). During a preoperative interview the perioperative nurse continues to assess the patient's level of anxiety and possible causes, such as the possibility of a cancer diagnosis. Identification of fears and concerns helps in planning appropriate nursing interventions. The patient should identify the breast (and, if possible, the quadrant

SURGICAL PHARMACOLOGY

Drugs Used in Breast Cancer

Medication Category	Dosage/Route	Purpose/Action	Adverse Reactions	Nursing Implications

Anastrozole
Functional class:
  Antineoplastic
Chemical class:
  Aromatase inhibitor
	1 mg daily by mouth	Advanced breast cancer not responsive to other treatment in estrogen receptor–positive patients (usually postmenopausal), patients with advanced disease on tamoxifen, adjunct treatment in early breast cancer. Highly selective nonsteroidal aromatase inhibitor, lowers serum estradiol concentrations	Hot flushes, headaches, lightheadedness, nausea, vomiting, rash, leukopenia, chest pain, hypertension, edema, angina, myocardial infarction, cerebral infarct	Stevens-Johnson syndrome; take calcium and vitamin D for bone loss/fracture; increase in size of tumor and increased bone pain may occur and will subside rapidly.

Exemestane
Functional class:
  Antineoplastic
Chemical class:
  Aromatase inhibitor
	25 mg by mouth after meals; may need 50 mg/day if taken with a potent CYP3A4 inducer	Advanced breast cancer not responsive to other therapies. Lowers serum estradiol concentrations	Headache, depression, insomnia, anxiety, fatigue, hot flushes, nausea, lymphopenia, dyspnea	Assess blood pressure for hypertension and bone mineral density; use reliable contraception; do not breastfeed.

Fulvestrant
Functional class:
  Antineoplastic
Chemical class:
  Estrogen receptor antagonist
	500 mg on days 1, 15, 29, and monthly thereafter as an IM injection	Advanced breast cancer in estrogen receptor–positive patients	Headache, nausea, vomiting, rash	Encourage nutritious diet with iron and vitamins; store in refrigerator; report vaginal bleeding immediately; increase in size of tumor; use contraception.

Letrozole *Functional class:* Antineoplastic, nonsteroidal aromatase inhibitor	2.5 mg daily by mouth	Early advanced or metastatic breast cancer in postmenopausal women	Headache, lethargy, nausea, vomiting, anorexia, rash, pruritus, myocardial infarction (MI), cerebrovascular accident (CVA), endometrial carcinoma, vaginal bleeding, second malignancies	Regular assessment of hepatic function studies; may administer with bisphosphonates to increase bone density; nutritious diet with iron and vitamins; report vaginal bleeding.
Poly ADP-ribose polymerase (PARPs) inhibitors *Functional class:* Antineoplastic	Varies; 200 mg bid	Treat triple-negative breast cancer patients. Causes the *BRCA* genes to function improperly because of the mutation	Fatigue, somnolence, mood alteration	Report anything that may be considered a side effect; very little reported.

Raloxifene
Functional class:
  Bone reabsorption inhibitor
Chemical class:
  Hormone modifier, selective estrogen receptor modulator
	60 mg daily by mouth	Breast cancer prevention, treatment of osteoporosis in postmenopausal women, breast cancer prophylaxis. Reduces resorption of bone and decreases bone turnover; mediated through estrogen receptor binding	Nausea, hot flushes, leg cramps, CVA, pulmonary embolism (PE), insomnia, peripheral edema, fever, weight gain	Regular hepatic studies done during therapy; bone density baseline obtained; administer vitamin D, calcium supplement; weigh weekly and report 5-lb weight gain; avoid staying in one position for long periods.

Tamoxifen
Functional class:
  Antineoplastic
Chemical class:
  Antiestrogen hormone
	Breast cancer: 20 to 40 mg daily by mouth for 5 years
	High-risk breast cancer and DCIS: 20 mg daily by mouth for 5 years
		Prevention of breast cancer following surgery or radiation; advanced breast cancer not responsive to other therapies in estrogen-positive patients. Inhibits cell division by binding to cytoplasmic estrogen receptors	Hot flushes, headache, lightheadedness, nausea, vomiting, rash, stroke, uterine malignancy, thrombocytopenia, PE, uterine malignancy, leukopenia	Do not break, crush, or chew tablets; obtain complete blood count (CBC) with differential and platelets regularly; encourage nutritious diet; increase fluids; routine eye exams.

bid, Twice daily; *DCIS,* ductal carcinoma in situ.

Modified from Skidmore-Roth L: *2013 Mosby's nursing drug reference,* ed 26, St Louis, 2013, Mosby; Winer EP: *State-of-the-art treatment for triple negative breast cancer,* CME/CE, February 22, 2011, available at www.medscape.org/viewarticle/737322_transcript. Accessed January 27, 2013.

RESEARCH HIGHLIGHT ||

Patient Navigation in Breast Cancer

Breast cancer is a strategic field for patient navigation because of known survival benefits of early detection through clinical breast examination, mammography, and early intervention. Navigation is important in breast cancer care because of acknowledged racial gaps in breast cancer screening and care across the disease spectrum. African American women frequently present with late stage breast cancer due to not obtaining recommended screening tests and not reporting clinical symptoms. Reviews of U.S. cancer studies yield strong evidence that white patients receive more assertive treatment for breast cancer than African American patients, resulting in higher morbidity among non-white populations. African American women missed more treatment appointments during breast cancer treatment. Missed appointments correlates with shorter survival rates.

This study reviewed published research over a 9-year period evaluating the usefulness of breast cancer navigators across all aspects of the disease process. Consolidated Standards of Reporting Trials (CONSORT) guidelines were followed to make certain correct and critical research was reviewed. After applying inclusion criteria, there were 12 data-based articles evaluating patient navigators' effectiveness in breast cancer. Most studies (66%) included predominantly samples of non-white women. Efficacy criteria indicated a positive trend toward adherence to breast cancer screening, follow-up of diagnostic abnormalities, initiation of breast cancer treatment, and stability or improvement in quality of life with patient navigation in breast cancer.

There were several limitations to this review of navigational research. It did not address the potential navigational needs of women with more advanced breast cancer. Also the extent of the navigation protocol was not well defined in any study. Some navigators were not nurses.

Nursing needs input into navigation training, evaluation, and development of care protocols to ensure that patients are provided accurate, streamlined, and evidence-based care.

Modified from Robinson-White S et al: Patient navigation in breast cancer, *Cancer Nurs* 33(2):127–139, 2010.

of the breast) where the mass is located and participate in surgical site marking. The perioperative nurse may reinforce the patient's understanding of the proposed surgical procedure, verify that the patient can correctly state its name, and correct misunderstandings (as appropriate). Identifying the patient's support systems and coping mechanisms helps manage anxiety and enhances the discharge planning process. If the patient has lost a relative or close friend to breast cancer, her coping mechanisms may be affected because of memories of that loss.

Nursing Diagnosis

Based on the nursing assessment, the perioperative nurse uses nursing diagnoses to develop a plan of care. Nursing diagnoses related to the care of patients undergoing breast surgery might include the following:

- Anxiety related to fear of cancer, the surgical intervention, or biopsy results
- Disturbed Body Image related to loss of body part
- Risk for Injury related to use of electrosurgery
- Deficient Knowledge related to unfamiliarity with perioperative routines

Outcome Identification

Outcomes are derived from nursing diagnoses. They direct the perioperative nurse in selecting nursing interventions that will prevent, or intervene in, the actual or high-risk areas identified in the nursing diagnoses. Outcomes identified for the selected nursing diagnoses could be stated as follows:

- The patient will verbalize a level of anxiety that is personally acceptable.
- The patient will discuss feelings regarding body image changes resulting from the surgical procedure.
- The patient will experience no untoward injury from electrosurgery.
- The patient will verbalize an understanding of perioperative procedures.

Planning

Using nursing diagnoses and desired outcomes, the perioperative nurse can individualize a plan of care for each patient and allow for communication with other colleagues on the patient care team. The plan of care for a patient undergoing breast surgery can include nursing interventions that allow the patient freedom to express concerns, have specific questions answered, and discuss breast reconstruction options, as appropriate. The Sample Plan of Care shows such an example. As part of planning patient care, priorities are established and a method of ensuring continuity of care ensured.

Implementation

Before surgery the perioperative nurse should procure the necessary supplies, instruments, and equipment for the planned operation. The patient's operative site is marked by the surgeon outside of the operating room (OR) before any medications are given. Mammogram films or other imaging studies should be available in the OR for the surgeon's review; their presence may be confirmed during the preoperative briefing and/or time-out. The facility protocol for identifying the correct surgical site should be followed. Often this consists of a checklist that is initiated during the time-out and includes verbal communication among surgical team members, review of the medical record and informed consent, confirmation of imaging studies, and direct observation of the marked surgical site. IV antibiotics, started within 1 hour before the incision is made, may be administered (Patient Safety). For breast surgery, the site and side must be verbally verified with each member of the surgical team during the time-out. A breast biopsy, performed after the patient has received a local anesthetic, will require adjunct sedation and monitoring equipment (e.g., electrocardiogram [ECG], pulse oximeter, blood pressure apparatus). Patient allergies should be reviewed to avoid allergic or toxic reactions to local anesthetics, antibiotics, or pain medications. For a mastectomy, extra soft goods and instrumentation are often needed. An electrosurgical unit (ESU) or a surgical laser is used to provide both hemostasis and tissue dissection. Safe practices when using devices that generate surgical smoke require the use of a smoke evacuation system and accessories in both open and laparoscopic procedures (Association of periOperative Registered Nurses [AORN], 2013). (See Chapter 8 for a full discussion of the ESU and surgical smoke evacuation.) The incision site may be drained postoperatively with a closed wound suction device. Ensuring availability of supplies before the procedure allows the nurse to maintain a comforting presence while supporting, monitoring, and caring for the surgical patient.

After transfer to the OR bed, the patient is placed supine with the operative side near the edge of the bed. The arm on the involved

SAMPLE PLAN OF CARE

Nursing Diagnosis
Anxiety related to fear of cancer, the surgical intervention, or obtaining biopsy results

Outcome
The patient will verbalize a level of anxiety that is personally acceptable.

Interventions
- Encourage questions and allow time for verbalization of fear, distress, and anxiety. Use active listening and reflective questions.
- Review the surgeon's explanation of the planned procedure and the reason for it (as appropriate).
- Assess verbal and nonverbal signs of anxiety.
- Provide emotional support and comfort measures (warm blankets, touch as appropriate).
- Maintain quiet, calm environment.
- Demonstrate warmth and acceptance of the patient's anxiety.
- Determine the patient's personally effective coping techniques (or recommend some), such as relaxation, rhythmic breathing, or guided imagery. Support the patient in using these.
- Record patient's reactions.

Nursing Diagnosis
Disturbed Body Image related to loss of body part

Outcome
The patient will discuss feelings regarding body image changes resulting from the surgical procedure.

Interventions
- Allow patient to discuss concerns about her sexual attractiveness, loss of confidence, or perceived loss of femininity.
- Promote an environment of support, respect, and comfort.
- Discuss available resources and options (external prosthesis, alternatives in garments and dress, reconstructive surgery, as appropriate). Make referrals to nurse on discharge unit or community agency as indicated.
- Maintain patient's privacy.
- Encourage a visit by a Reach to Recovery volunteer (as applicable).

Nursing Diagnosis
Risk for Injury related to use of electrosurgery

Outcome
The patient will experience no untoward injury from electrosurgery.

Interventions
- Position dispersive pad as close to operative site as possible.
- Note any metal implants patient may have and do not place dispersive pad over these sites.
- Select a site that is clean and dry, with good muscle mass; note and document the condition of the skin at the selected site.
- Protect dispersive pad from fluids and contact with metal objects.
- Ensure that all prep solutions have dried before activating the unit.
- Activate electrosurgical unit after dispersive pad and active electrode are connected.
- Set power setting as low as possible to achieve desired effect. Document power settings used.
- Use holster for active electrode on the sterile field.
- Provide supplies to remove excess char buildup from active electrode (as applicable).
- Check dispersive pad contact and all connections after changes in position or requests to increase power.
- Evaluate and document the condition of the skin on removal of the dispersive pad.

Nursing Diagnosis
Deficient Knowledge related to unfamiliarity with perioperative routines

Outcome
The patient will verbalize understanding of perioperative procedures.

Interventions
- Assess the patient's experience with previous surgical procedures.
- Review surgical team use of correct site surgery verification protocols.
- Explain that skin will be cleansed with antiseptic solution at the surgical site and that solution may feel cold.
- Provide clear and concise explanations of all nursing interventions.
- Explain roles of the healthcare team members present in the OR.
- Encourage questions.
- Describe types of dressings and equipment that may be used postoperatively. If lymph node dissection is performed, describe use of incisional closed wound drainage systems.
- Teach back. Ask the patient to explain in her own words what type of surgery will be performed.

---

side, with the palms up and fingers extended, is carefully placed on a padded armboard at no greater than 90 degrees to prevent brachial plexus stretch. If there are surgical reasons to tuck the arms at the side, pad the elbows to protect the ulnar nerve, turn the palms inward, and maintain the wrist in a neutral position (AORN, 2013). Depending on the location of the lesion and the planned surgery, a small pad can be placed under the operative side to facilitate exposure of the incision area. Positioning the OR bed in slight Fowler position with a lateral tilt away from the surgeon can also facilitate exposure. The anesthesia provider or the circulating nurse places a forced-air warming device on the patient away from the surgical site (Evidence for Practice).

Skin preparation ("prep") depends on the location of the lesion and the surgery intended. Antimicrobial skin prep solutions vary according to surgeon preference. For a breast biopsy, the area prepped is usually the affected breast and the immediate surrounding skin. For a mastectomy, the area prepped can extend from above the clavicle to the umbilicus and from the opposite nipple to the bed line of the operative side, including the axilla, and possibly the upper arm on the operative side (Hueske, 2008) (Figure 17-9). Some surgeons caution against vigorous scrubbing of the surgical site to prevent possible seeding of cancer cells from the main mass. Appropriate precautions to prevent pooling of solution under the patient and to reduce the risk of surgical fire are taken during skin prep procedures.

Surgical draping exposes the affected breast and the preoperative site mark. For mastectomy, the arm on the operative side is draped free, using a stockinette and drapes that allow free movement of the arm to facilitate access to the axilla. A final time-out check is performed before the incision is made.

PATIENT SAFETY

Reducing Surgical Site Infections After Breast Cancer Surgery

The Centers for Disease Control and Prevention (CDC) wound classification system considers breast surgery as "clean." The surgical site infection (SSI) rate for clean surgical procedures is projected to be less than 1.5%. Nonetheless, this retrospective study explored perioperative reasons that could be connected with a higher probability of a patient developing an SSI after breast cancer surgery. Researchers reviewed medical records of patients with breast cancer who had mastectomies and breast conserving surgery (BCS) between January 2005 and August 2007 at a university associated cancer referral center in Bogota, Colombia. No surgical procedures in which contaminated "dirty" wounds existed or patients whose final pathology reports ruled out cancer were included. All patients received antibiotics within 45 minutes of incision. Preoperative and intraoperative recommendations from the CDC with regard to preventing SSI were practiced. The breast surgeries were performed by one breast surgeon and residents.

Signs and symptoms of infection and postoperative wound care were taught to the patients before discharge. Patients' wounds were evaluated postoperatively in the clinic by nurses. Preoperative data collected included age, comorbidities, American Society of Anesthesiologists (ASA) physical status classification score, history of breast cancer surgery, and neoadjuvant treatment. Intraoperative information gathered was surgical procedure, length of surgery, and estimated blood loss. Postsurgical data included whether the patient was hospitalized or an ambulatory surgery patient, signs and symptoms of SSI, along with the date of diagnosis and manner of treatment. Other data included histologic diagnosis, removed tissue weight, and number of lymph nodes removed, as applicable.

In the 199 studied patients, the SSI rate was 19.1% (38 cases). Patients who underwent radical breast surgery had a 29.4% SSI rate and those who had BCS had a 3.8% SSI.

The findings of this study remind the perioperative team that SSI after breast cancer surgery is higher than the expected clean classification. Basic, evidence-based nursing and surgical team practices to prevent the spread of transmissible infections should be implemented (see Chapter 4 for a thorough discussion of essential elements of sterile technique), such as the following:

- Wear clean, facility laundered scrub attire and head covers that cover all hair.
- Apply surgical masks when in the presence of sterile supplies or a person scrubbing in preparation for a surgical procedure.
- Select and apply surgical gowns and drapes that are safe, efficacious, and cost-effective.
- Use sterile technique appropriately; perform surgical hand antisepsis for the prescribed amount of time. Don a surgical gown and double-glove (use closed gloving for self and closed assisted gloving for other team members if you are the scrub person) to set up sterile supplies.
- If you are the circulating nurse, strictly adhere to skin preparation protocols for the breast and other tissue areas that are part of the planned surgery.

Modified from Angarita FA et al: Perioperative variables associated with surgical site infection in breast cancer surgery, *J Hosp Infect* 79(4):328–332, 2011; Recommended practices for sterile technique. In AORN: *Perioperative standards and recommended practices*, 2013.

EVIDENCE FOR PRACTICE

Unintended Perioperative Hypothermia

Hypothermia, a core body temperature less than 97°F (36°C), is a common occurrence in surgical patients. A slight drop in perioperative normothermia can be associated with considerable morbidity and mortality. ORs are typically kept below 73°F (23°C); this is the temperature required to maintain normothermia for all but the quickest surgical procedures. Room temperature is the single most critical factor influencing actual heat loss. Up to 20% of patients experience unintended perioperative hypothermia (UPH). Anesthetized patients cannot move to a warmer environment or take other actions to warm themselves. Anesthesia also alters thermoregulatory mechanisms.

More than 10 years of research illustrate the adverse effects of mild hypothermia in perioperative patients. These include a threefold increase in the incidence of morbid cardiac outcomes, increases in surgical blood loss, a 20% increase in allogeneic transfusion, and a tripling of surgical site infections (SSIs). The Surgical Care Improvement Project (SCIP) has focused institutional efforts to decrease hypothermic complications during and after surgery. Although oral temperature measurement is supported by strong evidence as the method best approaching core temperature, its use is not practical in OR settings. For surgical patients the same modality of temperature measurement should be used throughout the perianesthesia period for comparison purposes. Heat loss from patient radiation (thermal) and convection are the two most significant sources in the operative environment. Anesthetics have a serious effect on thermoregulatory body mechanisms. General anesthesia inhibits cold-induced vasoconstriction, which promotes patient hypothermia. Epidural and spinal anesthesia each decreases the shivering and vasoconstriction thresholds. A regionally anesthetized patient thinks herself to be warm when she is actually being cooled. Sedatives and analgesics may impair thermoregulatory control even further.

SSI is the most serious complication from hypothermia associated with administration of anesthetics. Wound infections are likely the most significant cause of morbidity, greater than all other anesthetic complications combined. Myocardial ischemia, prolongation of medication effects, increased surgical bleeding, shivering, breaks in skin integrity, increased length of stay, and patient dissatisfaction with care are other untoward processes associated with hypothermia. Actions to maintain normothermia include determining patient temperature on admission, assessing for signs and symptoms of hypothermia, implementing passive thermal warming measures, maintaining room temperature at or above 75°F (24°C), instituting active warming for patients who are hypothermic, prewarming the patient for 30 minutes, performing frequent intraoperative temperature monitoring, limiting skin exposure, warming intravenous fluids, and reassessing temperature on arrival and discharge to the postanesthesia care unit (PACU). Monitoring body temperature and avoiding perioperative hypothermia through active and passive warming measures are important in preventing complications.

Modified from Hart SR et al: Unintended perioperative hypothermia, *Oshsner J* 11:259–270, 2011.

FIGURE 17-9 Diagram of skin surgical preparation.

During implementation of the plan of care, the perioperative nurse continues to collect data, continually reassesses the patient's needs and the needs of the surgical team, initiates nursing interventions, and documents all care delivered. Formats for documenting perioperative patient care vary from institution to institution. However, documentation of patient problems and nursing interventions addressing these problems is essential. For the patient undergoing breast surgery, consideration should be given to documenting the patient's level of anxiety, the surgical position and accessory positioning devices used, the time-out, the location of the ESU dispersive pad, unit settings and identification number, results of perioperative monitoring, medications administered by the perioperative nurse or from the sterile field, specimens collected, and any closed wound drainage systems inserted into the surgical wound.

Evaluation

Evaluation of the patient before discharge from the OR includes both general observation parameters important for every surgical patient and specific evaluation of the goals of the plan of care. The patient's skin at dependent pressure sites, skin prep sites, and the dispersive pad placement site are assessed and any change in skin integrity documented. The hand-off report to the nurse in the postanesthesia care unit (PACU) includes any unusual events or patient problems during surgery, the incorporation of any closed wound drainage systems in the wound, and achievement of identified patient outcomes. These outcomes, based on the nursing diagnoses selected, should be part of documentation as well as the nursing report. Outcomes identified for the selected nursing diagnoses could be stated as follows:

- The patient will verbalize an acceptable level of anxiety; she communicated her specific anxieties, her facial expression and body structures were relaxed, and her vital signs remained within her normal range.
- The patient will discuss feelings regarding possible body image changes resulting from the surgical procedure; her preferred coping strategies were reviewed and supported during the procedure.
- The patient will experience no untoward injury from electrosurgery; there were no skin changes at the site of the dispersive pad.

- The patient will verbalize an understanding of perioperative procedures; she cooperated with requests and was provided with ongoing explanations.

Patient and Family Education and Discharge Planning

Discharge planning should begin as soon as the patient is informed of the necessity for surgery or when the nurse first meets the patient. According to the extent of the anticipated surgery, information about appropriate exercises to enhance recovery, prosthetic devices, reconstruction options, and available community support groups should be explained to the patient. The perioperative nurse provides or reinforces information based on the patient's desire for information, readiness to learn, and anxiety level.

The patient is often discharged within hours of or the day after surgery. The patient and other caregivers need to be instructed regarding aseptic wound care, care for the closed wound drainage system (if present), and pain management. Possible signs of complications should be included, along with instructions regarding when and how to notify the physician. Postoperative exercises need to be taught to the patient to facilitate her return to normal activities. Nursing home care or a visiting nurse may be necessary and should be coordinated with the physician and the patient. A follow-up telephone call to the patient can help the nurse assess the patient's ability to cope with her diagnosis and surgery. The Patient and Family Education box on page 572 provides sample discharge information for the patient undergoing breast surgery.

Late and long-term effects of breast cancer treatments should be reviewed with the patient. Fatigue, insomnia, loss of appetite, fear of recurrence, anxiety, depression, and "chemobrain" are common symptoms seen in cancer survivors (Research Highlight). These signs and symptoms should be reported to the physician and nurse so intervention can be initiated (Barclay, 2009).

Surgical Interventions

Biopsy of Breast Tissue

The diagnosis of breast lesions using a minimally invasive procedure, as discussed in diagnostic techniques, is preferred. In an *incisional biopsy*, a portion of the mass is surgically excised using a curved incision line. The tissue is sent for pathologic examination. In an *excisional biopsy*, the entire tumor mass is excised along with a small margin of normal tissue from adjacent tissue for examination as with incisional biopsy.

Procedural Considerations

Biopsy is usually performed after the patient has been administered a local anesthetic, a local anesthetic with IV moderate sedation/analgesia, a laryngeal mask airway (LMA), or a general anesthetic with intubation depending on the patient's condition and medical history. The short delay between biopsy and further treatment has not been shown to adversely affect survival. However, when an extensive surgical procedure is anticipated in conjunction with the biopsy or when multiple lesions are to be excised and the amount of local anesthetic would exceed the maximum safe dose, general anesthesia is induced. A minor instrument set is used for biopsy; the ESU is often requested. Separate instruments are used for each biopsy site when there are multiple lesions. Perioperative staff should be sensitive to the fact that the patient may be alert during the procedure and use caution with oral pathology reports called over a speaker phone. Pathology reports, especially if the report

PATIENT AND FAMILY EDUCATION

Discharge Instructions and Home Care for Breast Surgery Patients

Give both the patient and the caregiver *verbal* and *written* instructions. Provide them with the name and telephone number of a physician or nurse to call if questions arise. Use visual aids to assist in instruction.

General Information

- Review explanation of the disease, the surgical procedure performed, and adjuvant therapy to be carried out.
- Explain that if the axillary nodes were removed, the affected arm may swell and is less able to fight infection. Discuss measures to prevent lymphedema:
  - Exercise arm daily (provide specific exercises).
  - Report loss of shoulder or joint mobility.
  - When healing is complete, begin strengthening and stretching exercises.

Wound/Incision Care (Select Applicable Education Based on Surgical Procedure Performed)

- Encourage the patient to look at her incisions so she can see what is normal. Teach her how to care for the skin at the site of surgery.
  - Advise her that there may be a dry gauze dressing over the incision site and the drain site.
  - Provide information regarding dressing changes, amount of fluid leakage at closed wound drainage system site that is normal, when to change soiled drain-site dressing (including emptying and measuring drain reservoir), and what to report to a physician or nurse.
  - Discuss numbness in the area of surgery and typical sensations (heaviness, tingling, and "pins and needles"). These are likely to resolve by 1 year after surgery.
- For modified radical mastectomy:
  - Teach the patient to change the dressing, assess the appearance of her incision and closed wound drainage system site, milk or strip clots through the drainage tubing to maintain patency, empty the drainage container, and record the amount and character of drainage.
  - Caution her not to abduct the affected arm or elbow above the shoulder until closed wound drainage systems are removed.
  - Instruct her to report any redness or drainage around the closed wound drainage system.
  - Instruct her to avoid use of deodorants or antiperspirants until stitches and drains have been removed from the axilla and the wound has healed. If no closed wound drainage system is present, she may shower.
  - Caution her not to allow injections, placing of intravenous lines, drawing of blood, or taking of blood pressure in her affected arm if axillary dissection was done.
  - Instruct her to avoid wearing constricting clothing or jewelry on her affected arm and to carry her handbag on the unaffected arm if axillary dissection was done.
  - Discuss types of temporary and permanent prostheses available; assist with referral as needed.
  - Advise her not to use an external prosthesis or bra pad until swelling has subsided and incisional healing is complete. Tell her to check with a physician or nurse before getting fitted for a breast prosthesis. This usually occurs about 6 weeks after surgery as long as wounds are healing and any postoperative edema has resolved.
  - Discuss types of reconstruction available (as appropriate).
  - Stress importance of continuing breast self-examination and mammography of her unaffected breast.

Warning Signs

- Review signs and symptoms that should be reported to a physician or nurse:
  - Swelling of arm
  - Drainage from incision, excessive drainage or blood in drainage unit, difficulty keeping container flat
  - Infection: redness, purulent drainage, pain, incision warm to touch

Medications

- Explain purpose, dosage, schedule, and route of administration of any prescribed medications, as well as side effects to report to a physician or nurse. Have her repeat these back or review them with you (medication reconciliation). If she is taking an opioid analgesic, initiate a bowel protocol (including a laxative and stool softener) to prevent constipation.
- Discuss alternative methods of postoperative pain management: visualization, guided imagery, meditation, relaxation, biofeedback, music, and other personally effective techniques.

Activity

- Encourage discussion of allowances and limitations with respect to occupation, recreational sports, or activities.
- Encourage resumption of self-care activities (feeding, combing hair) and activities of daily living as tolerated.
- Explain that sexual activity may be resumed when desired. The partner should use a position that does not place pressure on her chest wall.
- Discuss the need to continue postmastectomy exercises to regain full range of motion (as applicable).

Follow-Up Care

- Stress the importance of regular follow-up visits. Make sure she has the necessary names and telephone numbers.
- Prepare her for adjuvant therapies: hormone therapy, chemotherapy, and radiation therapy.

Psychosocial Care

- Encourage verbalization about feelings and fears regarding diagnosis, adjunctive therapy, actual and perceived changes in body image and sexuality.
- Encourage patient and family to seek individual or group counseling to reduce emotional stress and help with effective coping.

Referrals

- Provide referrals to the breast care navigator (if available) (see Research Highlight: Patient Navigation in Breast Cancer); if not, refer to a home health service and social services as indicated.
- Assist the patient to obtain referral services to breast cancer survivorship programs and contact support groups, such as the American Cancer Society's Reach to Recovery program, to cope with alterations in body image and other concerns.
- Encourage follow-up care with the patient's primary care provider for ongoing healthcare needs.
- Remind the patient to continue breast self-examination and to have an annual mammogram as prescribed.
- If chemotherapy or radiation therapy is prescribed post discharge, ensure that the patient and family have specific instructions about appointments, anticipated side effects, and self-management at home.
- Provide reliable printed and online resources for patient and family education. (Note: This chapter has many reliable online references for patient and family information/education.)

Modified from Canobbio MM: *Mosby's handbook of patient teaching*, ed 3, St Louis, 2006, Mosby; Mosby's nursing: *Evidence-based nursing: monographs breast cancer*, 2012, available at www.nursingconsult.com/nursing/evidence-based-nursing/monograph?monograph_id=198261. Accessed January 27, 2013 (subscription required); UCSF Medical Center: *Mastectomy: instructions after surgery*, available at www.ucsfhealth.org/education/mastectomy_instructions_after_surgery/index.html. Accessed January 27, 2013.

confirms malignancy, should be discussed when the patient is fully awake and has a support system available.

Operative Procedure—Open Breast Biopsy

1. An incision in the direction of the skin lines (curvilinear) or along the border of the areola is made over the tumor mass. The circumareolar incision gives the best cosmetic result. If the lesion is located in an extremely lateral or medial site, a radial incision may be used.
2. Gentle traction is applied to the mass with holding forceps. If the lesion is small, the entire mass and an edge of normal tissue are removed by sharp dissection. If a large lesion is present, a small incisional biopsy of the main mass is done. The specimen should not be placed into a formalin solution if a frozen section or further studies are to be done on the tissue to determine cancer treatment for the patient. Formalin immersion prevents frozen-section examination. For diagnostic biopsies, the surgeon orients the specimen and the pathologist should ink all margins. This assists the surgeon in reexcision if the pathologist finds positive margins on the specimen. The tissue can be examined by frozen section to determine immediate diagnosis if desired. If a 48-hour permanent section is required for definitive

diagnosis, the patient is scheduled at a later time for any further surgery that may be necessary.

3. If the lesion is benign, hemostasis is ensured and subcutaneous breast tissue approximated with absorbable suture. A cosmetic subcuticular skin closure is used when possible.

Operative Procedure—Open Breast Biopsy with Needle (Wire) Localization

In some instances, such as when a lesion previously detected on mammogram is too small to palpate or the lesion is not amenable to stereotactic core biopsy, needle (wire)-localization breast biopsy (NLBB) may be done. Mammograms are repeated immediately before surgery. The lesion is localized by the insertion of a needle or a wire within a needle. The wire is placed within the suspected area, and the distal end is left on the outside of the skin. The needle may be left in place or removed after insertion of the wire (see Figure 17-6). The needle or wire is then protected by a cup taped over the wire for protection during transport and the patient sent to the OR for surgical biopsy. Care is taken during transfer to the OR bed and gown removal not to dislodge or bump the wire. Similar care is taken during positioning, prepping, and draping. Images are sent to the OR with the wire entry visible on the film, or should be available on the computer system in the suite.

1. The skin incision is placed precisely over the expected location of the mammographically determined lesion to minimize tunneling through the breast tissue.
2. Dissection is carried out using the wire as a guide.
3. Tissue around the wire is removed en bloc with the wire and sent for specimen mammography in the radiology department. Radiography can also be done intraoperatively.
4. The patient is kept on the OR bed with the sterile field maintained until confirmation that the lesion has been excised. It is then sent from radiology or the OR to the pathology department.
5. Needles and portions of needle/wire must be counted.

Incision and Drainage for Abscess

Incision of an inflamed and suppurative area of the breast is performed to drain an abscess. Breast abscesses occur most frequently during the first 4 weeks of breastfeeding. Staphylococcal or streptococcal organisms enter the breast through abraded or lacerated nipple surfaces or through the lactiferous ducts. Chronic abscesses are rare. Drainage is required when the breast abscess is apparent. Biopsies may be done for additional diagnosis along with cultures for appropriate antibiotics.

Procedural Considerations

Breast abscess is very painful and may require surgery with the patient administered a general anesthetic. Instruments are the same as those for a biopsy.

Operative Procedure

1. Generally a radial incision extending outward from the nipple or a circumareolar incision is preferred. A short incision into the thoracomammary fold may be used for deep breast abscesses in the lower or outer quadrant.
2. After skin incision the wound is deepened until pus is encountered.
3. A curved hemostat is directed into the cavity to determine the extent of the abscess. Specimens for aerobic and anaerobic organisms are usually taken for culture.

4. Loculations are broken up by exploring the cavity with the index finger.

5. The opening is enlarged to ensure adequate drainage, the cavity is irrigated with warm saline solution with or without antibiotics, and bleeding vessels are ligated with absorbable sutures or coagulated.

6. The wound is drained or loosely packed with medicated gauze. Healing occurs by second intention.

Breast-Conserving Surgery

Lumpectomy, also known as partial mastectomy or wide local excision, is a procedure that is breast conserving. It is removal of a tumor mass with a margin of 1 to 1.5 mm of normal tissue. The Margin-Probe system, which emits an electric field and senses the returning signal from tissue under evaluation, may be used to examine specimen margins (Box 17-2). Tumors exhibit greater vascularization, a different polarization of cell membranes, and other anatomic differences over healthy tissue, resulting in a different electromagnetic "signature." The probe is used to detect the characteristic signature of cancer, helping surgeons verify they obtained clean margins in the tumor specimen.

Surgical clips may be left in the operative site to assist the radiation oncologist. Breast-conserving surgery (BCS), with subsequent radiation therapy, is often the treatment of choice for small tumors. It is not an option for patients who have two or more cancer sites in separate quadrants of the breast; persistent positive margins after reasonable surgical attempt; diffuse, malignant-appearing microcalcifications; or for patients who have undergone previous radiation to the affected breast. BCS, combined with sentinel node or axillary node dissection (Figure 17-10) and irradiation in stage I and stage II breast cancers, yields long-term survival equivalent to mastectomy and axillary staging. If one or more axillary nodes are involved, chemotherapy is recommended.

Procedural Considerations

In patients with large breasts, increased bleeding may occur, requiring the ESU, a smoke evacuation system, and additional hemostatic clamps.

Operative Procedure

The procedure is as described for excisional biopsy.

BOX 17-2

MarginProbe System

In investigational studies, the MarginProbe system was able to intraoperatively identify positive margins that required reexcision in patients with DCIS. There was a decrease in the need for reexcision (13% with the MarginProbe system) versus 37% in control groups. In patients with DCIS and invasive carcinoma, the decrease in reexcision rates was 17% versus 33%. The device led to overall decreases in reexcision rates compared with the standard procedure of lumpectomy without appreciably increasing the total amount of tissue removed. Failure to achieve appropriate margins has key consequences for the patient such as returning for additional surgery, delay administration of adjuvant therapies, psychologic and physical stress, and potential for an inferior cosmetic result from breast conserving surgery.

In an international multicenter study, patients were randomized in the OR after lumpectomy to either the device or a control group. When the device was used in patients with DCIS alone, the reexcision rate declined by 50% and when used with patients who had invasive cancer and DCIS, the results were the same. Further studies are needed to investigate device application in histologic subgroups.

DCIS, Ductal carcinoma in situ.
Modified from Boolbol SK: *Novel device reduces re-excision after lumpectomy,* Breast Cancer Symposium, Medscape Medical News, reported September 11, 2012, available at www.medscape.com/viewarticle/770744. Accessed January 27, 2013.

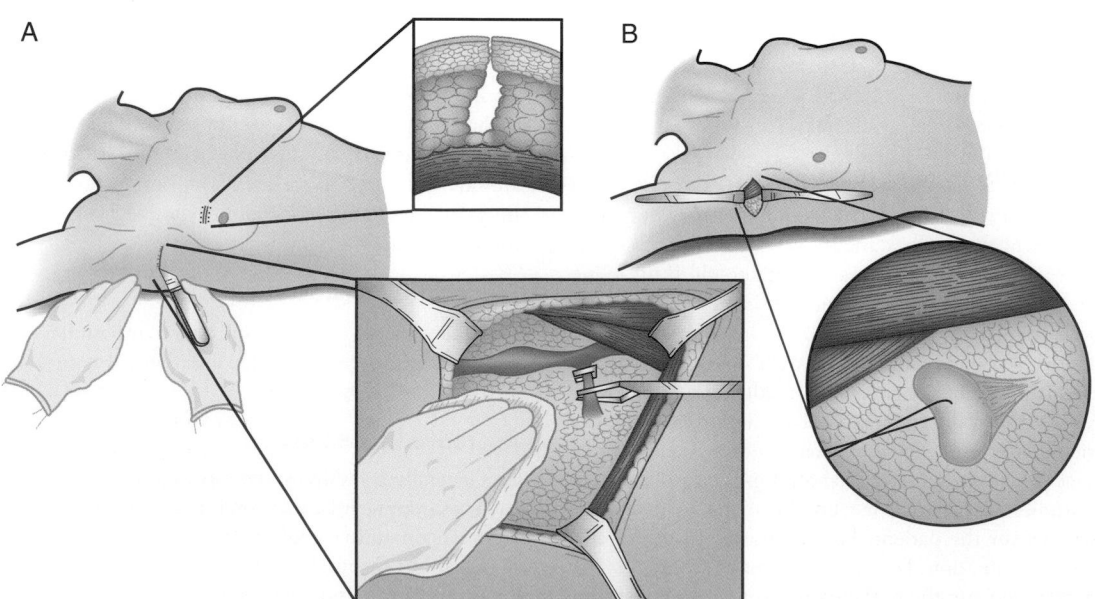

FIGURE 17-10 Breast-conserving surgery. **A,** Incisions are placed directly over the mass to be removed. A transverse incision in the low axillary region is used for sentinel node biopsy or axillary dissection. *Inset,* Excision cavity of breast conserving surgery. **B,** In sentinel node biopsy, a similar transverse incision is made that may be located by percutaneous mapping with the gamma probe if radiolabeled colloid is used. The sentinel node is located by its staining with dye, radioactivity, or both, and dissected free as a single specimen.

Sentinel Lymph Node Biopsy

Identification and microscopic examination of the sentinel lymph nodes (SLNs), the first lymph nodes along the lymphatic channel from the primary tumor site, helps determine the need for additional or more extensive surgeries and treatments of early stage invasive breast cancer for patients thought to have low to moderate risk for involvement of lymph nodes. It is believed that if the cancer cells have traveled through the lymph nodes, the cells will lodge in the first nodes. The sentinel node is not located in the same site in every patient. If sentinel nodes are negative, no other nodes in the lymph node channel are likely to be involved. Evidence of a positive node may require an axillary lymph node dissection (ALND) and adjunct therapy (Kass et al, 2007). ALND may not be recommended for patients with positive SLNs who will be treated with subsequent adjuvant systemic therapies and whole-breast radiotherapy (Giuliano et al, 2011). It doesn't apply to patients with palpable nodal disease, those who have received preoperative chemotherapy, and those who have undergone mastectomies or who do not receive postoperative radiotherapy or partial-breast radiotherapy. Complications of SLN biopsy include risk of allergic reactions to the blue dye, isotope usage, rare instances of sensory or motor nerve damage, and pain.

Procedural Considerations

The procedure for SLN biopsy is similar to that for breast biopsy. Sentinel node identification is accomplished by injection of either isosulfan blue dye, methylene blue dye, or a radiocolloid (technetium 99 [^{99m}Tc]), a gamma-emitting material. Isosulfan blue is contraindicated in patients with known hypersensitivity to the dye; careful patient monitoring and observation are mandatory, and a crash cart should be available in the instance of severe anaphylactic reaction. The procedure is coordinated with staff of the nuclear medicine department and requires use of a sterile handheld detector if technetium is used. In addition to a minor instrument set, if isosulfan blue is used, a 5-mL syringe, a 25-gauge needle, an alcohol wipe, and the dye are required. For technetium, the gamma-tracer probe, counter, and sterile sleeve for the probe are required. Multiple specimen containers should be on hand along with pathology request forms. The surgeon may request that each specimen be numbered on the specimen container and the pathology request form. Safe practices for handling surgical specimens are implemented. A number of studies have shown that using a combination of isosulfan blue dye and technetium results in the lowest false-negative results (Townsend et al, 2012). SLN biopsy is replacing levels I and II axillary lymph node dissection as the standard procedure for staging an axillary lymph node–negative patient (Patient-Centered Care).

Operative Procedure—Using Isosulfan Blue Dye or Methylene Blue Dye

1. Dye is injected around or near the tumor, or dye may be injected into the area of the breast mass that has been exposed as part of a breast biopsy (Townsend et al, 2012).
2. This may be followed by a lymphatic massage (Townsend et al, 2012).
3. The sentinel nodes stained with the blue dye are identified and excised.
4. The nodes are sent fresh to the pathology department for examination.
5. Based on the results, the surgeon may or may not proceed with further axillary lymph node dissection or the planned surgery, or he or she may elect breast conservation (see Figure 17-10).

Operative Procedure—Using Technetium

1. The tumor or previous biopsy site is injected with a small amount of radioactive tracer 20 minutes to 8 hours before the surgery. It can also be injected after anesthesia is induced and the time-out completed.
2. This is followed by massage.
3. A handheld detector is passed over the top of the patient's chest to identify the area of the sentinel node by a positive reading. The probe may also be used with the addition of a sterile sleeve during excisional biopsy. Isosulfan blue dye may be used in conjunction with technetium during a procedure to enhance visibility of nodes.
4. The surgeon marks the skin with a marking pen to indicate the reactive area.
5. The area is prepped, and the surgeon proceeds with the planned procedure for excisional biopsy of the sentinel lymph node.

Axillary Lymph Node Dissection

Axillary lymph node dissection (ALND) (Figure 17-11) is removal of axillary nodes through an incision in the axilla after determining that the sentinel node is malignant. Removal and examination of the axillary nodes allow staging (see Figure 17-7) of the disease. Adjunct treatment can be more accurately planned when the pathologic stage is determined.

Procedural Considerations

The patient is placed supine on the OR bed with the operative side near the bed edge. The arm on the operative side is extended to less than 90 degrees on an armboard. The skin is prepped and draped as previously described.

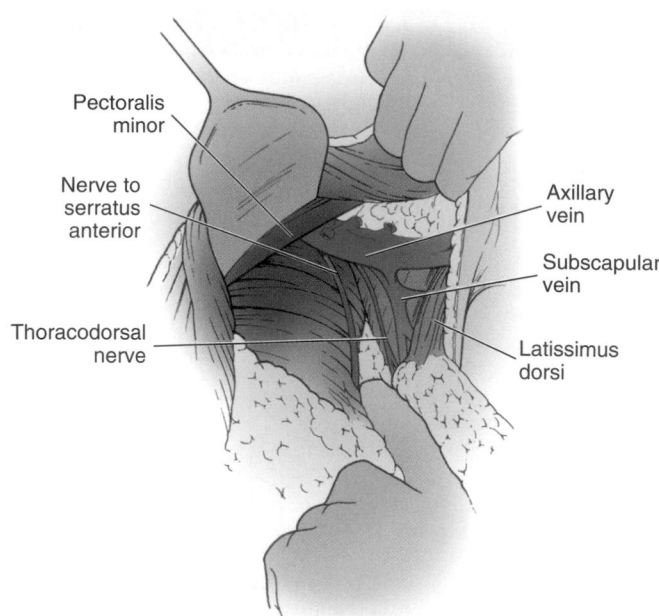

FIGURE 17-11 Axillary dissection.

Operative Procedure

1. An incision is made slightly posterior and parallel to the upper lateral border of the pectoralis major muscle or transversely across the axilla, below the hair line.
2. The fascia is incised over the pectoralis muscle and the pectoralis minor muscle is exposed. Major blood and lymphatic vessels are clamped and ligated. Use of the ESU is avoided around the axillary vessels and nerves to reduce the risk of inadvertent injury and subsequent impaired muscle function.
3. The tissue over the axillary vein is incised.
4. Lymph nodes between the pectoralis major and pectoralis minor muscles are removed. Care is taken not to injure the medial and lateral nerves of the pectoralis major muscle.
5. Axillary fat and lymph nodes are freed from the chest wall and axillary vein carefully so it is not skeletonized, because this increases risk for lymphedema (Tsangaris, 2011). The long thoracic nerve is identified along the chest wall near the axillary vein, and the thoracodorsal nerve posteriorly is dissected free from the specimen.
6. The fat and nodes are removed.
7. A closed wound drainage system is usually placed through a separate stab incision for lymphatic drainage, and the wound is closed (Tsangaris, 2011).

Subcutaneous Mastectomy

Subcutaneous mastectomy is removal of all breast tissue with the overlying skin and nipple left intact. This is also called nipple-sparing surgery (NSM) (Tsangaris, 2011). This procedure is recommended for patients who have central tumors of noninvasive origin, chronic cystic mastitis, hyperplasic duct changes, multiple fibroadenomas, or who have undergone several previous biopsies. This technique may also be used in women undergoing risk-reducing mastectomy and offered to patients with smaller tumors far from the nipple with favorable pathologic features (Rusby, 2010). Breast reconstruction may be undertaken at the time of mastectomy or at a later date (if desired by the patient).

FIGURE 17-12 Simple mastectomy. **A,** Skin incisions are generally transverse and surround the central breast and nipple-areolar complex. **B,** Skin flaps are raised sharply to separate the gland from the overlying skin and then the gland from the underlying muscle. Simple mastectomy divides the breast from the axillary contents and stops at the clavipectoral fascia.

Procedural Considerations

The patient is positioned as for a biopsy. If reconstruction is to be undertaken, appropriate equipment and supplies (see Chapter 22) are also required.

Operative Procedure

1. An incision is usually begun in the inframammary crease and may be made on the medial or lateral aspect of the breast. Some surgeons initially remove and preserve the nipple areola complex by using lateral extensions of wide circumareolar incisions.
2. Blunt dissection is performed to elevate the breast from the pectoral fascia.
3. The breast tissue is separated from the skin, attempting to remain in a plane between the subcutaneous tissue and the breast. Dissection is carried out toward the axilla. With care, 90% or more of the breast tissue, including the tail of Spence, can be removed. Some lymph nodes in the axillary area also may be removed. Bleeding vessels are clamped and ligated.
4. To assess the nipple areolar complex (NAC) base for tumor on permanent histologic evaluation, the NAC is inverted through the incision and a thin slice of tissue is removed from the base to establish a true margin. This ensures viability of the NAC while obtaining an adequate tissue sample (Tsangaris, 2011).
5. A closed wound suction catheter typically is inserted. The wound is closed, and a light pressure dressing applied.

Simple Mastectomy

Simple mastectomy is removal of the entire involved breast without lymph node dissection (Figure 17-12). A simple mastectomy is performed to remove extensive benign disease, if malignancy is believed to be confined only to the breast tissue, or as a palliative measure to remove an ulcerated advanced malignancy.

Procedural Considerations

The patient is positioned as for a biopsy.

Operative Procedure

1. Through a transverse elliptic incision (see Figure 17-12, *A*), using a knife, curved scissors, and the ESU, the skin edges are freed from the fascia. Bleeding vessels are clamped with hemostats and ligated with sutures or electrocoagulated.
2. The skin edges of the wound can be protected with warm, moist laparotomy pads; the breast tissue is grasped with Allis forceps and is dissected free from the underlying pectoral fascia with curved scissors, a knife, or an ESU.

3. The tumor and all breast tissue are removed. The axillary fat pad is not entered unless the procedure is being performed in conjunction with sentinel lymph node biopsy (SLNB) (Kass, 2007). Bleeding vessels are clamped and ligated or electrocoagulated.

4. A closed wound drainage catheter is inserted and anchored to the skin with a fine suture. The wound is closed with fine sutures or staples; a dressing is applied.

Modified Radical Mastectomy

Modified radical mastectomy is performed after a tissue biopsy with a positive diagnosis of malignancy and removes the involved breast and all or partial axillary contents (Figure 17-13). This surgery is only considered after careful discussion among patient, family, and surgeon. A modified radical mastectomy is done to remove the involved area with the hope of decreasing the spread of the malignancy. This surgery's elliptic incision encompasses the nipple-areolar complex, a biopsy scar if an open biopsy has been performed, and excess skin of the breast. The underlying pectoral muscles are not removed. Patients who meet criteria for mastectomies may be considered for immediate reconstruction (see Chapter 22). The type of reconstruction should be based on the patient's cosmetic and physiologic needs (Tsangaris, 2011).

Procedural Considerations

The patient is placed supine on the OR bed with the operative side near the bed edge. The arm on the operative side is extended to less than 90 degrees on a padded armboard. The skin is prepped and draped as previously described. Tissue removed during surgery will be submitted for microscopic analysis to further classify it (type, tumor size, grade, invasion, lymphocytic response, clean margin size). Additional analyses such as hormone receptor status (estrogen and progesterone positive or negative) and HER-2/neu expression may also be performed. This information assists the oncologist in planning subsequent adjuvant therapies (Ignatavicius and Workman, 2013).

Operative Procedure

1. An oblique elliptic incision with lateral extension toward the axilla is made through the subcutaneous tissue (see Figure 17-13, A). The bleeding points are controlled with hemostats and ligatures or electrocoagulation.

2. The skin is undercut in all directions to the limits of the dissection with a #3 knife handle with a #10 blade, curved scissors, or the ESU. Knife blades need to be changed frequently to ensure precise dissection.

3. The margins of the skin flaps are covered with warm, moist laparotomy pads and then retracted. The fascia and breast are resected from the pectoralis major muscle (see Figure 17-13, B), starting near the clavicle and extending down to the midportion of the sternum. The pectoralis muscle is left intact.

4. The intercostal arteries and veins are clamped and ligated.

5. The axillary flap is retracted for dissection of the axilla. Careful attention is directed to preventing injury to the axillary vein and to the medial and lateral nerves of the pectoralis major muscle.

6. The fascia is dissected from the lateral edge of the pectoralis muscle (see Figure 17-13, C). Vessel ligation is performed in the axilla and adjacent to the sternum. The fascia is then dissected from the serratus anterior muscle. The thoracic and thoracodorsal nerves are preserved (see Figure 17-13, D).

7. The breast and axillary fascia are freed from the latissimus dorsi muscle and suspensory ligaments (see Figure 17-13, E). The specimen is then passed off the field.

8. The surgical area is inspected for bleeding sites, which are ligated and electrocoagulated. The wound is irrigated with normal saline. Closed wound suction catheters are inserted into the wound through stab wounds and secured to the skin with a nonabsorbable suture on a cutting needle (see Figure 17-13, F).

9. A few absorbable sutures may be used in the subcutaneous tissue to approximate the skin edges. The incision is closed with suture material of choice, staples, or a running subcuticular stitch.

10. Wound closure tapes, antibiotic ointment, and Adaptic may be applied.

11. The dressing can be a simple gauze dressing or a bulky absorbent dressing held in place by a surgical bra or ACE bandage.

KEY POINTS

- Each breast has 15 to 20 lobes; each lobe has many smaller lobules, which end in dozens of tiny bulbs that can produce milk. These are all linked by ducts, which in turn lead to the nipple in the center of the areola.
- There are many benign breast conditions such as breast tumors and solitary lumps, fibrocystic changes, nipple problems and discharge, and infections or inflammation.
- Fibroadenomas in the breast are composed of both glandular and connective tissue. They usually occur in women between 20 and 30 years of age and are benign breast tumors.
- A woman has about a 1 in 8 chance of being diagnosed with breast cancer at some time during her life (13% chance).
- Breast cancer in men is rare—less than 1% of all breast cancers occur in men.
- Although the strongest risk factor for breast cancer is age, other risk factors include a personal or family history of breast cancer, having dense breasts, beginning to menstruate before age 12, starting menopause after age 55, having a first full-term pregnancy after age 30, never having been pregnant, obesity after menopause, alcohol use, and inherited changes in certain genes.
- *BRCA1* and *BRCA2* are genes that belong to a class of genes known as tumor suppressors. Mutation of these genes has been linked to both hereditary breast and ovarian cancers.
- After breast cancer has been diagnosed, tests are conducted to determine if cancer cells have spread within the breast or to other parts of the body.
- A biopsy is performed to determine the type of breast cancer, hormone receptor (estrogen, progesterone, or both) and HER-2 presence. This aids in developing treatment plans.
- Lumpectomy is a surgical procedure that involves removing a suspected malignant tumor or lump, and a small margin of surrounding tissue, from the breast.
- Simple or total mastectomy involves removing the entire breast tissue but not the muscle tissue under the breast. This mastectomy can be combined with a sentinel lymph node biopsy (SLNB) (see page 579).
- In a traditional mastectomy the surgeon removes an ellipse of skin that includes the skin of the nipple/areolar complex.
- In a nipple-sparing mastectomy, an incision is made around the nipple but the areola is left intact.
- The first node that the fluid passes through in a group of lymph nodes is called the sentinel lymph node.

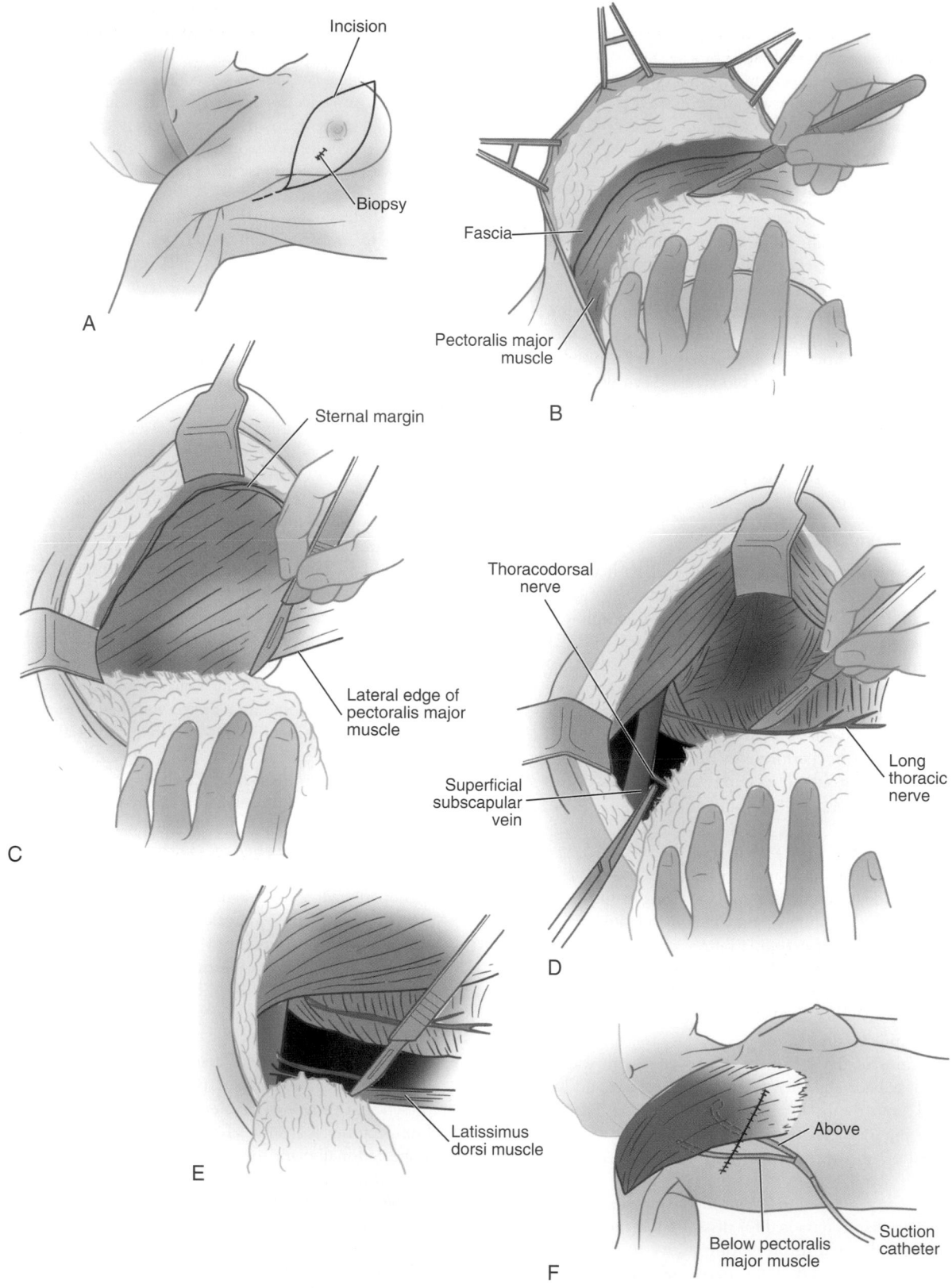

FIGURE 17-13 Modified radical mastectomy. **A,** Lines of incision. **B,** Resection of breast from lateral edge of pectoralis major muscle. **C,** Dissection of breast from lateral edge of pectoralis major muscle. **D,** Thoracodorsal and long thoracic nerves identified. **E,** Resection from latissimus dorsi muscle. **F,** Incision is closed, and closed wound drainage systems are placed.

- SLNB is done by removing one to five sentinel lymph nodes from an underarm. The nodes are then examined by a pathologist to determine if they are positive for cancer cells.
- Following breast cancer surgery, patients should have a physical exam and a review of symptoms every 3 to 6 months for the first 2 to 3 years, then every 6 months until year 5, and annually thereafter. They should continue to have annual mammograms of the other breast.

CRITICAL THINKING QUESTION

Your patient, M.J., 48 years old, is undergoing a left breast lumpectomy with sentinel lymph node dissection. She weighs 73 kg. After you interview the patient and review her chart for all pertinent information and required permits, you notice that the surgeon did not order an antibiotic. Is an antibiotic required for this breast surgery procedure? If so, what antibiotic might be ordered? What is the common dose? Because breast surgery is often classified as a "clean" procedure, why might an antibiotic be ordered?

Ꮎvolve *The answers to the Critical Thinking Question can be found at http://evolve.elsevier.com/Rothrock/Alexander.*

REFERENCES

Allen TL et al: The breast self-examination controversy, what providers and patients should know, *J Nur Pract* 6:444–451, 2010.

American Cancer Society: *Detailed guide, breast cancer*, 2012, available at www.cancer.org/cancer/breastcancer/detailedguide/index. Accessed January 27, 2013.

Association of periOperative registered nurses: Recommended practices for a safe environment of care. In *Perioperative standards and recommended practices*, Denver, 2013, The Association.

Barclay L: Cancer survivorship care: an expert interview with Miriam E. Sleven, RN, MS, OCN, *Medscape* May 04, 2009, available at www.medscape.com/viewarticle/702286. Accessed January 27, 2013.

Baselga J et al: Pertuzumab plus trastuzumab plus docetaxel for metastatic breast cancer, *N Engl J Med* 366:109–119, 2012.

Breast Cancer.org, 2012, available at www.breastcancer.org/symptoms. Accessed January 27, 2013.

Centers for Disease Control and Prevention: *Study finds racial and ethnic disparities in U.S. cancer screening rates*, 2012, available at www.cdc.gov/media/releases/2012/p0126_cancer_screening.html. Accessed January 27, 2013.

Cleveland Clinic: *Understanding benign breast disease*, 2009, available at http://my.clevelandclinic.org/disorders/breast_disease/. Accessed January 27, 2013.

Domchek SM et al: Association of risk reducing surgery in BRCA1 or BRCA2 mutation carriers with cancer risk and mortality, *JAMA* 304(9):967–975, 2010.

Giuliano AE et al: Axillary dissection vs. no axillary dissection in women with invasive breast cancer and sentinel node metastasis: a randomized clinical trial, *JAMA* 305(6):569–575, 2011.

Healthday: *Men's breast cancer often more deadly, study suggests*, at healthday.com/Article.asp?Aid=664452 5/4/13. Accessed June 15, 2013.

Hueske RD: *Mosby's PDQ for surgical technology: necessary facts at hand*, St Louis, 2008, Mosby.

Hunt KK et al: The breast. In Brunicardi FC et al, editors: *Schwartz's principles of surgery*, ed 9, New York, 2010, McGraw-Hill.

Ignatavicius DD, Workman ML: *Medical-surgical nursing: patient-centered collaborative care*, ed 7, St Louis, 2013, Saunders.

Kaplan DA: *Beyond the mammogram: molecular breast imaging emerges*, Diagnostic imaging, 2011, available at www.diagnosticimaging.com/articles/beyond-mammogram-molecular-breast.imaging. Accessed January 27, 2013.

Kass RP et al: Breast procedures. In Souba WW et al, editors: *ACS surgery: principles & practice*, ed 6, Canada, 2007, Decker Publishing.

Lehman CD et al: Accuracy and value of breast ultrasound for primary imaging evaluation of symptomatic women 30-39 years of age, *Am J Roentgenol* 199:1169–1177, 2012.

Modi S: *Case challenges: improving clinical outcomes in patients with HER2-positive breast cancer*, May 2011, available at www.medscape.org/viewarticle/742366. Accessed January 27, 2013.

National Cancer Institute: *What you need to know about breast cancer*, 2011, available at www.cancer.gov/cancertopics/wyntk/breast. Accessed January 27, 2013.

National Cancer Institute: *Thinking about complementary and alternative medicine: a guide for people with cancer*, 2012, available at www.cancer.gov/cancertopics/cam/thinking-about-CAM. Accessed January 27, 2013.

Ohio State University Medical Center: *About breast cancer in men*, available at http://medicalcenter.osu.edu/patientcare/healthcare_services/breast_health/about_breast_cancer_men/Pages/index.aspx. Accessed January 27, 2013.

Rusby JE: Nipple-sparing mastectomy, *Br J Surg* 97(3):305–316, 2010.

Stephan P: *How surgical margins affect breast cancer treatment decisions*, 2009, available at www.breastcancer.about.com/od/diagnosis/tp/surgical_margins.htm. Accessed January 27, 2013.

Surveillance Epidemiology and End Results: Available at seer.cancer.gov/statfacts/html/breast.html. Accessed January 27, 2013.

Tempany CMC et al: Focused ultrasound surgery in oncology: overview and principles, *Radiology* 259(1):39–56, 2011.

Townsend CM et al: *Sabiston textbook of surgery: the biological basis of modern surgical practice*, ed 19, Philadelphia, 2012, Saunders.

Tsangaris TN: Breast cancer: surgical therapy. In Cameron JL, Cameron AM, editors: *Current surgical therapy*, ed 10, Philadelphia, 2011, Saunders.

Winer EP: *State-of-the-art treatment for triple negative breast cancer*, CME/CE, February 22, 2011, available at www.medscape.org/viewarticle/737322_transcript, Accessed January 27, 2013.

CHAPTER 18

Ophthalmic Surgery

EILEEN MIELCAREK

Eyesight is not essential to life, but quality of vision enables us to have a higher quality of life. Much of what we learn throughout our lifetime and how we understand and navigate our world is through our vision. In 2012 Bausch + Lomb surveyed more than 11,000 people in 11 countries to gauge eye care habits and perceptions. Their survey, the Barometer of Global Eye Health, revealed that respondents said they would rather lose a limb, lose 10 years of their life, or receive a 50% cut in income rather than lose 50% of their vision (Bausch + Lomb, 2012). Early detection of eye disease through regular eye examinations can provide the most effective treatment when needed and ultimately preserve vision.

There is a disconnect between Americans' fear of losing their vision and not taking the necessary steps to preserve and enhance their eyesight. The previously mentioned survey revealed that more than two thirds of respondents did not have a recent eye examination—the most basic step necessary to preserve eyesight. In addition, 7 in 10 consumers said they were somewhat or very knowledgeable about their eye healthcare, yet 97% of eye doctors say the public does not sufficiently understand proper eye healthcare. Part of the disconnect could be attributed to the fact that sick or diseased eyes often look normal and certain diseases exhibit no warning signs (Bausch + Lomb, 2012).

The ocular surgical interventions discussed in this chapter are delicate, are microscopic, and demand careful planning and execution by both the surgeon and the perioperative staff. As technology advances in eye care, surgical interventions become more detailed and require advanced instrumentation as well as more planning and participation. Emerging technology requires a partnership with high-tech computers and precise instrumentation. The perioperative nurse must keep abreast of changes in technology, procedural techniques, safety issues, efficiency, communication, and patient education resources to provide optimal care to ophthalmic surgery patients.

Surgical Anatomy

The eyes are one of the more complex organs of the human body. Vision begins with a focal point of light, which travels through the cornea, lens, and vitreous fluid, and lands on the retina to be sent to and interpreted by the brain. Clear vision requires all of the following: healthy, functioning eye structures; adequate light; intact neurovascular communication with the brain; and the brain's effective interpretation of the images relayed. The following cycle, if completed in the full sequence, leads to accurate visual images.

1. Light rays emanate from an object in the field of vision and transmit to the eye. These light rays pass through the clear cornea, which accounts for approximately 65% of the refractive power of the eye.

2. Iris muscles control the size of the pupil to allow the appropriate amount of light into the eyes.

3. The rays pass through the crystalline lens, which changes shape to accommodate the refraction and focus between distant and near images. The lens accounts for 35% of the refractive power of the eye.

4. The rays travel through the clear vitreous fluid and land directly on the macula, the central part of the retina and the area of highest sensitivity for details. The nerve endings of the retina pass the images as nerve impulses through the optic nerve to the brain, where the occipital area interprets the images (Figure 18-1).

The American Academy of Ophthalmology (AAO) recommends that healthy adults receive an eye examination every 2 years, even if vision is normal and unchanged. Children should receive a baseline eye examination by an ophthalmologist prior to starting school, even if no signs of impairment or complications are presented. Diabetic individuals of any age should see an ophthalmologist every year because they are at higher risk for eye diseases (AAO, 2012).

Refractive Apparatus

As light rays pass through the eye, there are opportunities for the light not to land directly on the macula. Refractive errors occur when images do not focus and fall directly on the retina, but these can be corrected with eyeglasses or contact lenses. Myopia (e.g., nearsightedness) occurs when the focal point of the light rays is behind the retina. Hyperopia (e.g., farsightedness) occurs when the light rays focus in front of the retina. Astigmatism occurs when the cornea is cylindrically shaped instead of spherical, and the light rays diverge as they reach the retina. Presbyopia is the natural aging of the eye in which the lens cannot change shape and accommodate for the focusing needed to see close objects. Myopia, hyperopia, and astigmatism are considered lower-order aberrations that account for the majority of refractive errors. Higher-order aberrations are complex microscopic irregularities presented on the surface of the cornea, lens, and retina that can affect the quality of visual acuity.

Eyeglasses that minimize images are prescribed to refocus light rays in myopic patients; eyeglasses that magnify images are prescribed for hyperopic patients; and magnifying bifocals or reading glasses are prescribed for presbyopic patients, usually after age 40. Presbyopia occurs in everyone older than age 45, even if they have perfect distance vision. The unit of measure in refraction is called a diopter. The more diopters required to correct vision, the worse unaided vision one has (Figure 18-2).

Cornea

The cornea is the transparent, avascular window through which light passes to the retina; it joins the white sclera at a transitional zone called the limbus. The cornea is composed of five layers: the

FIGURE 18-1 Anatomy of the eye. Horizontal section through left globe.

epithelium, Bowman's membrane, the stroma, Descemet's membrane, and the endothelium. The epithelium consists of constantly renewing cell layers with many nerve endings, accounting for the cornea's great sensitivity to foreign bodies and abrasions. Bowman's membrane is connective tissue thickening that forms a barrier to trauma and infection under the epithelium. If damaged, Bowman's membrane does not regenerate and a permanent scar is formed. The stroma accounts for 90% of the corneal thickness and is composed of precisely layered fibers. If this layering is disrupted (for example, by edema), the corneal clarity decreases. Descemet membrane is a thin layer between the endothelial layer of the cornea and the stroma. The corneal endothelium is a single layer of hexagonal cells that acts as a fluid pump to keep the cornea clear by maintaining the proper level of stromal dehydration for clarity. Because corneal endothelial cells do not regenerate, damage to this layer may cause persistent corneal edema and loss of transparency (Figure 18-3).

The *sclera* is the opaque "white" part of the strong external layer, and is made up of collagenous fibers loosely connected with fascia. The sclera receives the attachments of the extraocular muscle tendons, and is pierced by the ciliary arteries and nerves posteriorly by the optic nerve. The sclera provides the eye with form and shape and encompasses the entire side and back of the eye.

Conjunctiva

The conjunctiva is a thin, transparent mucous membrane divided into a palpebral portion (lining the inside of the eyelids) and a bulbar portion (lining the surface of the globe). The junction

FIGURE 18-2 A, Emmetropia (perfect vision). **B,** Myopia (nearsightedness). **C,** Hyperopia (farsightedness). **D,** Astigmatism can present with hyperopia or myopia.

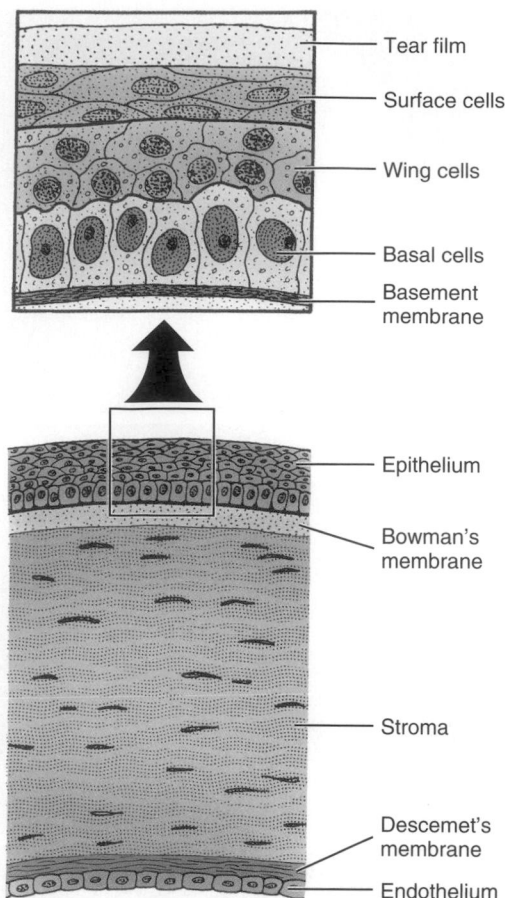

FIGURE 18-3 Five layers of cornea. *Inset,* Layers of epithelium.

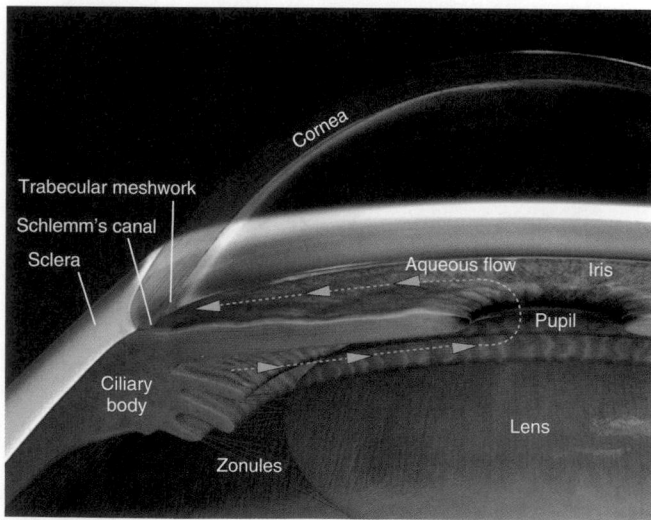

FIGURE 18-4 Anterior chamber, ciliary body, and aqueous circulation.

between the palpebral and bulbar conjunctivae forms a forniceal sac (Figure 18-4).

Crystalline Lens

The biconvex lens is suspended behind the iris and connected to the ciliary body by delicate collagenous strings called *zonules.* The lens changes shape and focus (accommodation) by either relaxation or tightening of the zonular fibers. Over time (particularly after age 40), the lens and lens zonules becomes progressively less elastic, resulting in *presbyopia.* This loss of accommodative power is typically corrected by reading glasses or bifocals.

Vitreous Humor

The vitreous body is a transparent, gelatinous mass composed of 99% water and 1% collagen and hyaluronic acid. It fills the posterior four fifths of the eyeball and is adherent to the retina at the vitreous base. The vitreous supports the shape of the eye internally and gives the eye its shape.

Retina

The retina is an extension and modification of the brain designed to perceive light and relay visual signals through the optic nerve back to the occipital brain. The central portion of the retina is called the macula and is responsible for central detailed vision (20/20), while the peripheral retina is responsible for spatial orientation, night vision, and peripheral vision. The visual sensory nerve endings of the retina pass the images as nerve impulses through nerve fibers of the optic nerve to the brain, where the occipital area interprets the images.

Supporting Structures

Nerve and Blood Supply

The optic nerve (second cranial nerve) extends between the posterior eyeball and the optic chiasm. This cranial nerve carries visual impulses as well as the sensations of pain, touch, and temperature from the eye and its surrounding structures to the brain, where it can be interpreted. The ophthalmic artery, the main arterial supply to the orbit and globe, is a branch of the internal carotid artery. It divides into branches supplying the globe, muscles, and eyelids. The central retinal artery and central retinal vein travel through the optic nerve and provide a separate blood supply for the retina.

Lacrimal Apparatus

The lacrimal gland produces aqueous tears and secretes them through a series of ducts onto the anterior ocular surface, thereby keeping the cornea moist and washing away any debris. The tears then flow inward to the puncta, from which they are conducted by the canaliculi to the lacrimal sac and finally pass into the nasolacrimal duct. The lacrimal apparatus effectively functions like a sink, with a faucet (main and accessory lacrimal glands) and drain (lacrimal puncta, canaliculi, sac, and nasolacrimal duct) (Figure 18-5).

Eyelid

Eyelids provide protection to the eye from debris and foreign bodies, as well as provide continuous tear moisture to the cornea (blinking). The anterior eyelid layers contain the eyelid skin, ocular adnexa (eyelashes and associated glands), and subcutaneous tissue, lymphatics, and muscles. The tarsus is a plate of dense fibrous tissue that forms the main scaffolding of the eyelids. Within the tarsus are the meibomian glands, which secrete the oily component (sebum) of the tear film. The orifices of these sebaceous glands are found at the eyelid margin just posterior to the eyelashes.

The palpebral fissure refers to the space between the margins of the two eyelids. When the eye is closed, the fissure becomes a mere slit and the cornea is completely covered by the upper eyelid. The upper eyelid is more mobile and larger than the lower. The eyelids

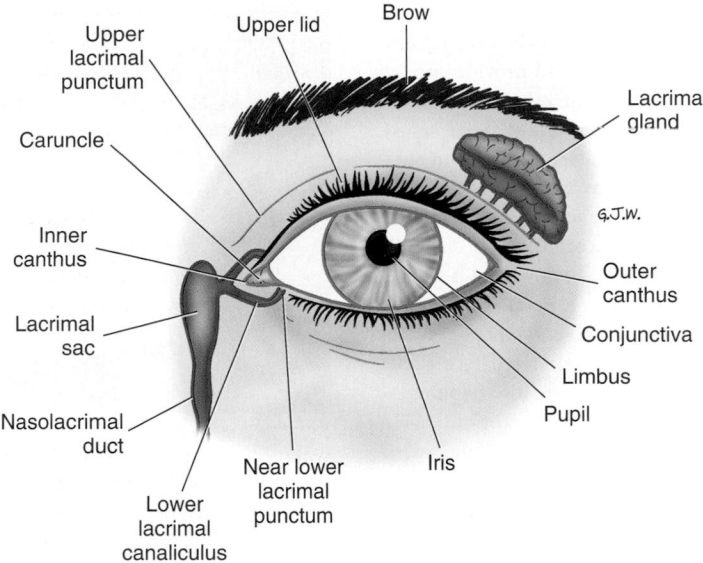

FIGURE 18-5 Lacrimal apparatus.

are closed by the orbicularis oculi muscle, and the upper lid is opened by the levator muscle.

Tears

Tears are essential for keeping the cornea lubricated to maintain clarity and optical performance. Tears have three layers; the mucous layer that sits closest to the cornea, the aqueous water layer, and the oily lipid layer. Aqueous tears are created by the lacrimal glands located within the upper temporal eyelid, mucous layer by conjunctival cells, and oily layer by meibomian glands in the eyelid. The cornea does not have blood vessels or blood flow, so tears provide antibodies and nutrition to the cornea, as well as flush out irritations and debris.

Muscles

Seven separate eye muscles control the movement of the eyeball. The muscles work in yoked pairs, with ocular movements generated by an increase in the tone of one set of muscles and a decrease in the tone of the antagonistic muscles. Named according to their relative position on the eyeball, the extraocular muscles of the eyeball include the four recti (the *superior rectus, inferior rectus, medial rectus,* and *lateral rectus*) and two oblique muscles (the *superior oblique* and *inferior oblique*). Except for the inferior oblique muscle, these muscles originate from the back of the orbit. The extraocular muscles are supplied by cranial nerves III (oculomotor, supplying the superior, inferior, and medial recti), IV (trochlear, supplying the superior oblique), and VI (abducens, supplying the lateral rectus) (Figure 18-6).

Perioperative Nursing Considerations

Assessment

Patients undergoing eye surgery range from premature infants with retinopathy of prematurity or congenital conditions to elderly patients whose conditions result from the aging process. These patients need assessment of both their vision and general health status. A preoperative visit to the eye clinic or surgeon's office

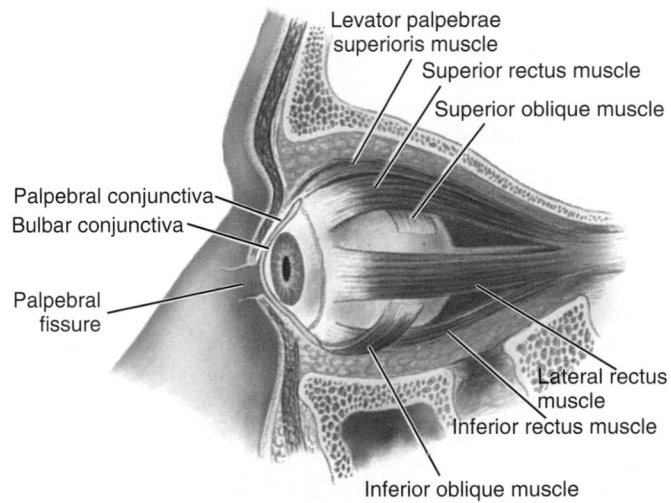

FIGURE 18-6 Orbit and muscles. Medial rectus is located on nasal side of globe.

typically completes the diagnostic testing and physical examination pertinent to the presenting eye condition subsequently requiring surgery. Communication with the physician's office staff to coordinate patient preparation and teaching and to collate preoperative test results increases the efficiency and effectiveness of preoperative procedures. Perioperative nurses contact patients preoperatively by phone to provide needed information concerning the day of surgery and to obtain initial preoperative assessment information.

The perioperative nursing staff must be prepared to meet the specific needs of each patient and family, collaborate and communicate effectively for continuity of patient care, and prepare the patient for home care. On admission, a staff member should fully orient the patient to the physical surroundings. Constant description and reinforcement are important to visually impaired patients. Approaching the patient from the unaffected side increases the patient's independence and decreases the possibility of startling the patient.

The assessment is designed to collect and disseminate pertinent information and must be carried out in a comprehensive, yet efficient, manner. A standard set of parameters should provide enough information to facilitate appropriate care in the event of an emergency. Physiologic information (e.g., height, weight, vital signs), psychosocial factors (e.g., support systems, fears, anxiety), and environmental, education, and self-care needs are assessed. The general health history includes completing a comprehensive list of current medication therapy (often the patient is asked to bring currently prescribed medications to the appointment). The medical history is very important in cueing the nurse to evaluate for ocular manifestations of systemic disease. For example, the patient may present for retinal surgery as a consequence of retinopathy related to diabetes mellitus. Additional discharge planning factors are also explored.

Data may be collected from family or significant others or directly from physicians or their office staff. Throughout the assessment process the nurse encourages the patient toward self-actualization and assuming an active role in his or her healthcare needs. All information should be documented so that it is readily available to others.

An ocular history, which includes the patient's primary problem, history of the present condition, symptoms, and visual limitations, is collected from the patient's initial visit to the eye care provider's office, and the nurse confirms these findings. Some common forms of ocular examination are shown in Figure 18-7.

An external examination of the eye, including lids, lashes, conjunctivae, and lacrimal apparatus, should have been performed to detect any deviations from normal. The corneal reflex should have been tested and the cornea inspected for superficial irregularities. Pupil size and contour, as well as pupillary reaction, both direct and consensual, should be noted. Shallow anterior chamber depth alerts staff members to the potential for high pressures resulting from angle closure with dilation of the pupil.

The function of the extraocular muscles should have been determined. Movement should be synchronous, and visual lines should meet on a fixed object. Documentation of this examination must be descriptive, accurate, and concise. It is of value later in assessing the outcome of the procedure. The following observations are also important:

- General appearance of the eye (edema, asymmetry, redness, condition of conjunctiva, sclera, and skin around eyes)
- Symptoms of irritation (itching, burning)
- Position of eyelids (opened and closed), condition of upper and lower lid surfaces, eyelid spasm
- Visual acuity, pupillary dilation (note if pupils are equal, round, reactive to light, and accommodative), visual fields
- Extraocular muscle movement
- Drainage from eye
- Current and significant past medical problems (eye disease, diabetes, cardiovascular disease, hypertension, allergies)
- Current medication history, including anticoagulants, analgesics, herbs, and nutritional supplements
- General: vital signs; restlessness, discomfort, anxiety; limitations in mobility; presence of prosthesis

After the assessment information has been compiled, nursing diagnoses are identified and the plan of care for the entire perioperative period is developed.

Nursing Diagnosis

Nursing diagnoses related to the care of patients undergoing ophthalmic surgery might include the following:

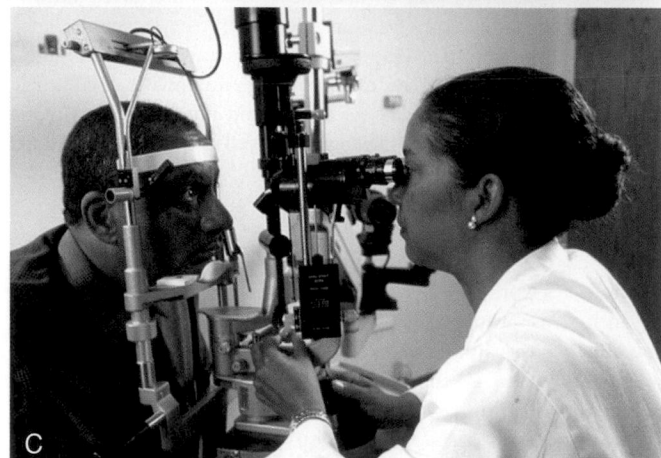

FIGURE 18-7 A, The optical coherence tomography (OCT) machine takes cross section images of the retina, cornea, and anterior segment. It is used to diagnose glaucoma, retina issues, and cornea abnormalities. The femtosecond laser machine has a live OCT incorporated for real-time viewing. **B,** After the eyes are dilated, an indirect ophthalmoscope provides the eye care professional with a wider view of the retina. **C,** A slit lamp, with its high magnification, allows the eye care professional to examine the front of the eye.

- Deficient Knowledge or Readiness for Enhanced Knowledge related to diagnosis, surgical intervention, and home care management
- Anxiety related to vision loss, surgical intervention, awake status during surgical intervention, fear of the unknown and surgical outcome

- Acute and/or Chronic Pain related to increased intraocular pressure and surgical intervention
- Risk for Infection related to surgical interventions

Outcome Identification

Outcomes identified for the selected nursing diagnoses could be stated as follows:

- The patient, family, or significant others will verbalize knowledge of the diagnosis, planned surgical intervention, medication management, and requirements for home care maintenance before discharge.
- The patient will verbalize an acceptable level of anxiety and use personally effective coping mechanisms.
- The patient will remain comfortable during surgical intervention as determined by response on a verbal pain scale.
- The patient will be free from signs and symptoms of postoperative infection.

Planning

Plans of care are the framework for organizing activities in the perioperative period. Although ophthalmic surgery is often perceived as minor because of the small incision site and relatively short surgery period, the perioperative nurse must be fully prepared for potential complications or emergencies. Patients who are admitted for ophthalmic surgery often have complex medical histories. After a review of the patient's record, supplemented by a patient or family interview or collaboration with colleagues, the data collected are incorporated into an individualized perioperative plan of care. A Sample Plan of Care for a patient undergoing ophthalmic surgery can be found on page 586.

Implementation

Managing and Monitoring Patient Safety Needs. A key aspect of the perioperative nurse's role is patient safety. Because many ophthalmic procedures are performed with local anesthesia, the circulating nurse or an additional perioperative nurse must be prepared to monitor the patient and provide supportive care. Reassurance is especially important for patients who are awake because they can usually see and hear the surgery progressing. Ophthalmic patients, like other surgical patients, have increased sensitivity to noise and activities within the operating room (OR). The OR should be kept quiet and peaceful to decrease anxiety and increase cooperation, thereby reducing the need for deep sedation.

Both the scrub person, who may be a registered nurse or surgical technologist, and the perioperative nurse, must also manage additional patient safety needs. Foreign substances must not be introduced intraocularly. Lint-free drapes should be used to create the sterile field. Gloved hands should not touch the portion of an instrument used in an intraocular wound, and debris should be cleansed from instruments with cellulose sponges.

Members of the perioperative team have several important responsibilities in the preparation of the room and the equipment. Technologic advances in ophthalmic surgery require that perioperative nurses be familiar with equipment and check each piece carefully before the patient arrives in the OR. Organization and grouping of the outlet cords must be checked to ensure clear walking areas. The availability of specially ordered intraocular lens implants or prostheses needs to be checked to prevent delay or cancellation of the procedure. Scrupulous attention to aseptic technique is essential in preventing endophthalmitis (infection within the eye) and possible blindness. Safety-focused

communication within the perioperative nursing team includes the following:

- *Identification:* The perioperative nurse asks the patient to state his or her name and compares the name on the wristband with the name on the chart and surgical schedule while verbally confirming it with the patient or a family member. The use of two identifiers, such as birth date or medical record number, is recommended.
- *Verifications:* The patient or family member should also state which eye is the operative site and which procedure is being performed. The nurse reviews the surgical consent, surgeon's preoperative orders, and OR schedule to determine if the correct operative eye has been prepared (including verification of operative eye using the word "right" or "left" [abbreviations are not accepted], marking of operative site, and dilation, if appropriate) and other procedures have been carried out according to facility policies on correct-site surgery. Such a policy may require that before the administration of eyedrops or medication, the nurse asks the awake patient which eye is the operative site. If there is any discrepancy among the patient's response, the informed consent, the physician's orders, ophthalmic history, and exam, the discrepancy is corrected during the preoperative verification process. Immediately before the incision, this information, along with any implants or special needs, is reconfirmed during the time-out (Patient Safety).

Preventing Infection. As in any practice of nursing the number one way to prevent infection within ophthalmic surgery is hand washing. The Association of periOperative Registered Nurses (AORN) recommends hands should be washed on entering the perioperative setting, before and after every patient contact, before putting on or after removing gloves or other personal protective equipment, any time there has been contact with blood or other potentially infectious materials, before and after eating, before and after using the restroom, before leaving the healthcare facility, and when hands are visibly soiled (AORN, 2013).

To prevent endophthalmitis, patients receive an antibiotic prior to surgery, and the physician may also use a topical antibiotic such as vancomycin given intracamerally, for gram-positive coverage which is responsible for more than 90% of endophthalmitis (Shorstein, 2013) (Evidence for Practice). Symptoms of endophthalmitis are noticed 48 to 72 hours following surgery (Jeng, 2012). Toxic anterior segment syndrome (TASS) is a sterile postoperative inflammatory reaction caused by a noninfectious substance that enters the anterior segment, resulting in toxic damage to intraocular tissues. The process typically starts as early as 4 hours following the procedure and up to 48 hours after cataract surgery. A recent study showed that TASS presented in cases nearly 2.5 years after the surgery and were more likely to occur in more difficult surgery cases (Krader, 2012). TASS is limited to the anterior segment of the eye, is always Gram stain and culture negative, and usually improves with steroid treatment. The primary differential diagnosis is infectious endophthalmitis. Review of the literature indicates that possible causes of TASS include intraocular solutions with inappropriate chemical composition or concentration, pH, osmolarity, preservative, denatured ophthalmic viscosurgical devices, enzymatic detergents, bacterial endotoxin, oxidized metal deposits and residues, and factors related to intraocular lenses such as residues from polishing or sterilizing compounds. An outbreak of TASS is an environmental and toxic control issue that requires complete analysis of all medications and fluids used during

SAMPLE PLAN OF CARE

Nursing Diagnosis
Deficient Knowledge or **Readiness for Enhanced Knowledge** related to diagnosis, surgical intervention, and home care management

Outcome
The patient, family, or significant others will verbalize knowledge of the diagnosis, planned surgical intervention, medication management, and requirements for home care maintenance before discharge.

Interventions
• Determine knowledge level.
• Identify barriers to communication.
• Assess readiness to learn.
• Identify psychosocial status.
• Assess coping mechanisms.
• Implement measures to provide psychologic support.
• Elicit perception of surgery.
• Encourage patient participation in decision-making and planning for postoperative care.
• Reinforce physician's explanations and clarify any misconceptions.
• Provide instructions based on age and identified needs.
• Include family members in preoperative teaching.
• Evaluate response to instructions.
• Evaluate environment for home care.
• Identify expectations of home care.

Nursing Diagnosis
Anxiety related to vision loss, surgical intervention, awake status during surgical intervention, and fear of the unknown and surgical outcome

Outcome
The patient will verbalize an acceptable level of anxiety and use personally effective coping mechanisms.

Interventions
• Allow the patient time to verbalize concerns.
• Help the patient identify sources of anxiety.
• Assist the patient to identify personal strengths and external resources; reinforce personally effective coping mechanisms.
• Observe for increased anxiety demonstrated through behavior (e.g., hand tremor, shakiness, restlessness, facial tension, voice quivering, increased perspiration).
• Provide information and answer questions honestly.
• Use touch (as appropriate) to communicate reassurance.
• Control environmental stimuli in the OR.

Nursing Diagnosis
Acute Pain and/or Chronic Pain related to increased intraocular pressure and/or surgical intervention

Outcome
The patient will remain comfortable during surgical intervention as determined by response on a verbal pain scale.

Interventions
• Identify cultural and value components related to pain.
• Instruct patient to verbalize pain during procedure performed using local anesthetic or sedation; use a validated pain rating scale.
• Observe for physical signs of pain, such as facial grimacing, groaning, muscle tightening, or changes in vital signs.
• Alert surgeon to any patient reports of significant pain from the injection or signs of toxicity (e.g., tinnitus, tingling around the mouth) if using local anesthesia.
• Ensure patient understands what is happening during the procedure (e.g., stinging or pressure from local anesthetic injection) and how long it will last.
• Monitor the presence of, or an increase in eye pain, pain around orbit, blurred vision, reddened eye, abdominal pain, nausea, vomiting, neurologic changes, and changes in visual fields; initiate appropriate action.
• Implement measures to provide psychologic support.
• Implement pain guidelines; administer medications as prescribed.
• Instruct the patient to refrain from excessive exertion, such as crying, coughing, straining, lifting, bending, rubbing the eyes, and blowing the nose postoperatively.
• Discuss other methods to promote patient comfort, such as music, guided imagery, relaxation techniques.

Nursing Diagnosis
Risk for Infection related to surgical intervention

Outcome
The patient will be free from signs and symptoms of surgical site infection.

Interventions
• Document any preexisting infection, if patient is immunocompromised, or other conditions that compromise resistance to infection.
• Maintain an aseptic perioperative environment.
• Adhere to good handwashing practices.
• Minimize length of invasive procedure by planning care.
• Initiate traffic control.
• Maintain continual surveillance.
• Determine and record the wound classification.
• Instruct the patient and family in self-care, including postoperative antibiotic therapy if prescribed.
• Teach the patient and family to wash hands before instilling any ophthalmic medications.
• Instruct the patient and family to watch for signs and symptoms of infection including redness, pain, swelling, drainage, and changes in visual acuity postoperatively and to report these problems promptly to the physician.

---

surgery, as well as complete review of OR and sterilization protocols.

Safety Measures in Administering Medications. Medications used in the perioperative period are extremely important to the procedure's outcome and the patient's safety. Drugs for diagnosing and treating eye disorders are potent; one error could result in total, irreversible blindness.

The patient's medical and ocular histories determine the selection of an appropriate ophthalmic agent. The perioperative nurse should be knowledgeable about the specific medication ordered, including purpose, strength, action, duration, adverse reactions,

PATIENT SAFETY

Using an Ophthalmic-Specific Checklist

More than 70% of the serious adverse events reported to The Joint Commission (TJC) are related to communication breakdowns during the entire perioperative period (ECRI, 2009). Using checklists to ensure critical information is shared among team members is one strategy to promote a safe environment of care and enhance communication. An example of a comprehensive ophthalmic-specific checklist is provided below. The checklist was developed by a task force comprised of members from the American Academy of Ophthalmology (AAO), the American Society of Ophthalmic Registered Nurses (ASORN), and other key ophthalmic societies and divides surgical care into three main phases: before anesthesia sign-in, time-out before incision, and the postoperative sign-out before transferring the patient to the recovery area.

Before Anesthesia Sign-In
☐ Patient has confirmed:
  • Allergies
  • Consent
  • Identity
  • Procedure
  • Site
☐ Site marked
☐ History and physical reviewed
☐ Presurgical assessment complete
☐ Anesthesia safety check done

Does patient have difficult airway/ aspiration risk?
☐ Not applicable
☐ No
☐ Yes: equipment/assistance available

Before Incision Time-Out
☐ All team members have introduced themselves by name and role
☐ Surgeon, anesthesia provider and nurse orally confirm:
  • Patient
  • Site
  • Procedure
☐ Surgeon and nurse orally confirm:
  • Antibiotic
  • Devices
  • Dyes
  • Gas
  • Implant style and power
  • Mitomycin-C/antineoplastics
  • Tissue

Anticipated Critical Events
☐ Surgeon reviews:
  • Critical or suspected steps
    ☐ None anticipated
    ☐ Reviewed
  • Operative duration
☐ Anesthesia provider reviews any patient-specific concerns
☐ Nursing team reviews:
  • Sterility (including indicator results)
  • Equipment issues
  • Concerns

Before Leaving Or Sign-Out
☐ Nurse orally confirms with team the name of procedure recorded:
  • Instrument, sponge, sharps count correct:
    ☐ Not applicable
    ☐ Yes
  • Specimen labeled (including patient name):
    ☐ Not applicable
    ☐ Yes
☐ Nurse orally confirms with team whether there are any equipment issues to be addressed
☐ Surgeon, anesthesia provider, and nurse discuss key concerns for recovery and management of this patient reviewed

Patient Label
Date of Surgery: _____

Signature/Time   Signature/Time   Signature/Time

Modified from ECRI Healthcare Risk Control Executive Summary: Risk and quality management strategies 17, Supplement A, September 2009, available at www.ecri.org/Forms/Documents/Communication.pdf. Accessed March 28, 2013; AAO, OMIC, ASCRS, ASORN, OOSS Task Force: Sample ophthalmic, June 26, 2012, available at www.asorn.org/resources/safe_surgical_checklist. Accessed March 28, 2013.

route of administration, and contraindications. This information should be included in the patient's initial assessment. For example, mydriatic and cycloplegic eyedrops may be contraindicated in narrow-angle glaucoma.

The nurse checks the medication label for name, strength, and expiration date during preparation and before administration. This precaution is especially important because many ophthalmic drugs are distributed in single-dose units that closely resemble each other. The patient must be positively identified, and the site of the administration must be clearly translated from the physician's orders. Handwashing between patients when administering eyedrops is imperative, and Standard Precautions should be followed. The nurse ensures that intraocular solutions are separated from those not used intraocularly.

All solutions on and off the sterile field must be clearly labeled. To meet The Joint Commission's (TJC) *2013 National Patient Safety Goals,* medications in a procedural setting must have labels that include drug name, strength/concentration, and amount. Medication errors are the most common medical errors (TJC, 2013). Staff members may be more likely to label medications when preprinted labels are provided. Preprinted labels and sterile waterproof pens and labels are commercially available to avoid smearing from liquids.

Instillation of Eyedrops. Most medications prescribed for the eye are administered in the form of eyedrops. Perioperative nurses should have a firm grasp of instilling eyedrops, and confirm that patients know how to properly instill drops for their postoperative care. Certain diseases such as arthritis can impede a patient's ability

EVIDENCE FOR PRACTICE

Decreasing Postoperative Endophthalmitis with Intracameral Antibiotics

Postoperative endophthalmitis, defined as an inflammatory condition of the aqueous and/or vitreous humor, is a very serious complication that can occur after any ocular surgery that disrupts the integrity of the globe. In the United States, reports of postoperative endophthalmitis after cataract surgery have ranged from 0.40 to 2.65 per 1000 cases (Shorstein, 2013).

Postoperative endophthalmitis is generally the result of the perioperative introduction of bacteria to the patient's eye either from the patient's skin, lashes, or conjunctiva, or from contaminated instruments. Patients usually present between 1 and 6 weeks after surgery with symptoms of moderate to severe eye pain, decreased vision, photophobia, conjunctival hyperemia, discharge, chemosis (conjunctival edema), ocular and periocular inflammation, and hypopyon (pus in the anterior chamber) Endophthalmitis can result in decreased or permanent loss of vision.

Eye with endophthalmitis, illustrating a hypopyon.

The practice of using antibiotic prophylaxis to prevent endophthalmitis after cataract surgery is well established in the medical community; however, there is no consensus on the most appropriate agent or route to use. In European studies the use of intracameral cefuroxime was found to be effective in preventing endophthalmitis. An advantage of using the intracameral route is that the dose achieved in the anterior chamber is much higher than that achieved with topical administration.

Shorstein and partners (2013) undertook a study to determine postcataract surgery endophthalmitis in relation to practices for administering antibiotic prophylaxis using intracameral injections of cefuroxime, moxifloxacin, or vancomycin. Their ecologic time-trend study evaluated 16,264 cataract surgeries between 2007 and 2011. In 2007 patients received postoperative antibiotic eyedrops, but no intracameral injection. Patients undergoing surgery in 2008 and 2009 received postoperative antibiotic eyedrops and intracameral cefuroxime (unless contraindicated). A departmental policy requiring intracameral injection was implemented in 2010. In 2010 and 2011 all patients received intracameral injections of cefuroxime, moxifloxacin, or vancomycin and postoperative antibiotic eyedrops. Cefuroxime was the primary medication used for injection; moxifloxacin or vancomycin was used for patients with medication allergies.

Endophthalmitis cases were identified via electronic record using diagnosis codes for a 12-month period after each cataract surgical procedure. Cases meeting the criteria for endophthalmitis were then manually reviewed by the study author. Incidence rates were calculated for each of the time periods identified using the number of cases of postoperative endophthalmitis as the numerator and the total number of cases performed as the denominator.

Nineteen cases of endophthalmitis occurred in 16,264 cataract surgeries. The rates during the three time periods were as follows: 3.13 infection rate per 1000 cases in 2007; 1.43 infection rate per 1000 cases in 2008-2009; and 0.14 infection rate per 1000 cases in 2010-2011. The infection rate declined 22-fold with the use of intracameral injection.

The authors concluded that an increase in the use of intracameral injection coincided with a large decline in the risk for endophthalmitis. There was a slight advantage to combining topical antibiotics with intracameral injection, and this warrants further study.

Modified from Clark WL et al: *Postoperative endophthalmitis,* 2013, available at http://emedicine.medscape.com/article/1201260-overview. Accessed March 19, 2013; Durand ML: Endophthalmitis. In Mandell GL et al, editors: *Mandell, Douglas, and Bennett's principles and practice of infectious diseases,* ed 7, Philadelphia, 2010, Churchill Livingstone; Egan DJ et al: *Endophthalmitis,* 2011, available at http://emedicine.medscape.com/article/799431-overview. Accessed March 19, 2013; Shorstein NH et al: Decreased postoperative endophthalmitis rate after institution of intracameral antibiotics in a Northern California eye department, *J Cataract Refract Surg* 39:8–14, 2013.

to instill his or her own eyedrops. The perioperative nurse should confirm that a caretaker is able to instill drops on behalf of the patient before being discharged.

Before administering eyedrops, the perioperative nurse should perform hand hygiene. The patient may be supine or sitting, with the head tilted back slightly. The nurse instructs the patient to look upward and then gently pulls the lower eyelid open to expose the lower conjunctival sac (Figure 18-8). The prescribed number of drops is then administered without touching the tip of the dropper to the eye or the nurse's fingers. The natural blinking distributes the drug evenly onto the eye surface.

To minimize systemic absorption of certain eyedrops, such as atropine, or maximize the absorption of the drop within the eye, the nurse may instruct the patient to immediately keep the eyelid

closed and gently press on the nasolacrimal duct for 1 minute to prevent absorption into the circulatory system. When a toxic drug is instilled, the nurse uses a tissue or clean cotton ball to dry the inner corners of the patient's eyelids after each drop to minimize systemic absorption of the drug. When multiple eyedrop prescriptions are required, each drop of medicine should be allowed to fully absorb within the eye before proceeding to the next drop. The nurse should wait at least 1 minute between the application of multiple medicines. The nurse instructs the patient to keep the eyelids closed to maximize absorption.

The nurse provides education about the expected effect of each medication so the patient is able to evaluate its effectiveness, detect signs and symptoms of adverse reactions, and know when to notify the perioperative personnel concerning problems. The patient should also be well-informed of the special considerations associated with specific medications so that appropriate safety precautions can be taken.

Ophthalmic Pharmacology. Numerous medications are used during ophthalmic surgery (Surgical Pharmacology)

Anesthesia

Local Anesthesia. The three types of ocular blocks are sub-tenon (parabulbar), peribulbar, and retrobulbar. The typical anesthetic agents used in the blocks are 2% lidocaine, 0.75% bupivacaine, and hyaluronidase (enzyme). The total volume that

Text continued on p. 594

FIGURE 18-8 An eye care professional applies eyedrops to dilate a patient's pupils. Positioning of the patient may require applying eyedrops from the left (**A**) or right side (**B**).

SURGICAL PHARMACOLOGY

Medications for Ophthalmic Surgery

Medication/Category	Dosage/Route	Purpose/Action	Adverse Reactions	Nursing Implications
Mydriatics (Dilation)				
Phenylephrine (Neo-Synephrine, Mydfrin)	Topical: 2.5%, 10%; rarely used 0.5% Dosage per surgeon's order	Dilates pupil but permits focusing; causes vasoconstriction of conjunctiva and anterior vessels; used for objective examination of retina, testing of refraction, easier removal of lens; used alone or with a cycloplegic	Corneal micro-deposits noted in almost all patients treated for more than 6 months (can lead to blurry vision) Hypertension, nausea, fever, narrow-angle glaucoma, interacts with tricyclic antidepressants	Standard red cap. Use preoperatively. Check for effect on cardiac and lung conditions; can stimulate sympathetic receptors. Lasts 4-6 hr.
Cycloplegics (Dilation)				
Tropicamide (Mydriacyl)	Topical: 0.25%, 0.5%, 1% Dosage per surgeon's order	Dilates pupil by paralyzing iris sphincter and accommodation muscles; anticholinergic, used for examination of fundus, refraction, uveitis, and relief of pain from ciliary spasm	Interacts with tricyclic antidepressants, cardiovascular effects in higher doses Use may cause delusions	Standard red cap. Use preoperatively. May precipitate attack of narrow-angle glaucoma. Lasts 4-6 hr.
Atropine	Topical: 0.5%, 1% Dosage per surgeon's order	Anticholinergic; dilates pupil; potent	Mydriasis, blurred vision, photophobia, decreased visual acuity, tearing, dry eyes or dry conjunctiva, eye irritation, crusting of eyelid	Standard red cap. Used preoperatively. Patient may be sensitive to light. May use slight pressure on lacrimal punctum to prevent systematic absorption. Lasts 7-14 days.

Continued

SURGICAL PHARMACOLOGY—cont'd

Medications for Ophthalmic Surgery

Medication/Category	Dosage/Route	Purpose/Action	Adverse Reactions	Nursing Implications
Cyclopentolate (Cyclogyl)	Topical: 0.5%, 1%, 2% Dosage per surgeon's order	Anticholinergic; dilates pupil; inhibits focusing	Extremely narrow anterior chamber angles Use with caution in Down syndrome patients Not used younger than 1 year of age Tachycardia Hypertension	Standard red cap. Used preoperatively. Duration up to 24 hr.
Epinephrine PF mixture	Intracameral or topical: (1:1000)/0.3 mL Dosage per surgeon's order	Dilates pupil; added to bottles of balanced salt solution (BSS) for irrigation to maintain pupil dilation; constricts blood vessels to prevent bleeding		Red cap. Syringes should be well marked to measure 0.3 mL. Comes in 1-amp vial.
Combination Dilation Eyedrops				
Hydroxyamphetamine (Paredrine, Paremyd), tropicamide (Mydriacyl)	Topical: Hydroxyamphetamine 1%; tropicamide 0.25%. Dosage per surgeon's order	Combination of parasympathetic antagonist and sympathetic agonist; simplifies process of dilation	Tachycardia Hypertension Contraindicated for closed-angle glaucoma	Red cap. Onset 15 min. Duration 45-60 min. Combination medication helps with high-volume surgical centers.
Intracameral Injections				
Epi-Shugarcaine	9 mL BSS Plus 3 mL 4% lidocaine/4 mL epinephrine 1:1000 PF (bisulfate free)	Used to dilate pupil; helps maintain dilation intraoperatively; used for floppy iris syndrome and patients with small pupils	Inflammation or foreign body sensation Contraindicated if allergic to any of the ingredients	Caution: Must be precisely mixed by perioperative nurse according to surgeon's order. Different strengths and mixtures possible. Use blunt-tip 25- to 30-gauge cannula, 2-mL syringe.
Miotics (Parasympathetic Constriction)				
Carbachol (Miostat)	Intracameral: 0.01% in 1.5-mL vial Dosage per surgeon's order	Potent cholinergic; constricts pupil; used intracamerally during anterior segment surgery	Ciliary or accommodative spasm, blurred vision, reduced night vision, diaphoresis, increased salivation, urinary frequency, nausea, diarrhea, bronchial asthma Use with caution with Parkinson disease	Green packaging. Use blunt-tip anterior chamber needle. Used intraoperatively.
Acetylcholine chloride (Miochol-E)	Intracameral: 1% 1:100 solution in 2-mL dual-chamber univial Dosage per surgeon's order	Cholinergic; rapidly constricts pupil by activating parasympathetic; used intraocularly during anterior segment surgery to constrict a dilated pupil	Iris spasm that may be painful, flushing of face, corneal edema, decompensation, allergies to any ingredients	Onset 15-30 sec. Comes from medication dispensing system. Preset vials with green lettering.
Pilocarpine hydrochloride	Topical: 1%, 4% Dosage per surgeon's order	Cholinergic; constricts pupil; used topically for lowering intraocular pressure in glaucoma	Acute uveitis, headaches, decreased night vision	Green top. Used preoperatively and postoperatively. Lasts 4-6 hr.

SURGICAL PHARMACOLOGY—cont'd

Medications for Ophthalmic Surgery

Medication/Category	Dosage/Route	Purpose/Action	Adverse Reactions	Nursing Implications
Topical Anesthetics				
Tetracaine hydrochloride (Pontocaine)	Topical: 0.5% Dosage per surgeon's order	Anesthetic and pain reliever	Can compromise cornea epithelium Category C pregnancy and lactation	Red cap bottle. Used preoperatively and postoperatively. Onset 5-20 sec. Duration of action 10-20 min. If pain persists contact surgeon.
Proparacaine hydrochloride (Ophthaine)	Topical: 0.5% Dosage per surgeon's order	Anesthetic and pain reliever	Known hypersensitivity to any component of the solution Softening and erosion of corneal epithelium have been reported	White cap bottles. Used preoperatively. Onset 5-20 sec. Duration of action 10-20 min. If pain persists contact surgeon.
Lidocaine hydrochloride gel (Akten)	Topical: 3.5% Most often used 10 min before surgery Dosage per surgeon's order	Anesthetic and pain reliever	Known hypersensitivity to any component of the solution	Used preoperatively. Apply to the surface of the eyeball under the upper and lower lids. Can desensitize corneal nerves and may lead to neurotrophic corneal ulcers and melting.
Injectable Anesthetics				
Lidocaine (Xylocaine), lidocaine MPF	1%, 2%, 4% Dosage per surgeon's order	Anesthetic and pain reliever; local skin injection retrobulbar and peribulbar	Known hypersensitivity to any component of the solution Cardiac and CNS watch	Preoperatively and intraoperatively. Onset 4-6 min. Duration of action 40-60 min, 120 min with epinephrine. MPF solution is preservative free.
Bupivacaine (Marcaine, Sensorcaine), bupivicane MPF, hyaluronidase (Hydase) (enzyme)	0.25%, 0.50%, 0.75%; hyaluronidase: 1 mL Dosage per surgeon's order	Anesthetic and pain reliever; local skin injection facial nerve block; hyaluronidase is occasionally added to bupivacaine to enhance diffusion of the anesthetic	Watch in dosage for hepatic or renal disease	Preoperatively and intraoperatively. Onset 5-11 min. Duration of action 8-12 hr with epinephrine. Often used in 0.75% combination with lidocaine for blocks. MPF solution is preservative free.
Mepivacaine (Carbocaine)	1%, 2% Dosage per surgeon's order	Local anesthetic and pain reliever; injection: block	Long acting, can affect cardiac and CNS	Onset 3-5 min. Duration of action 120 min, greater with epinephrine.
Viscoelastics/Adherents				
Sodium hyaluronate chondroitin sulfate (Healon, GV5, Amvisc, Provisc, Viscoat, Duovisc)	Intracameral: Prepared syringes; dose labeled on syringe to surgeon's order	Coats and protects corneal endothelium, intraocular structure and tissue; helps increase volume to push structures away such as filling capsular bag	Increased IOP, punctate keratitis, cystoid macular edema, postcapsular opacity No known contraindications if used according to manufacturer's instructions	Some brands require refrigeration. Allow 30 min to warm to room temperature. Check manufacturer's inserts for single-use syringe. GV 5 requires surgeon certification.

Continued

SURGICAL PHARMACOLOGY—cont'd

Medications for Ophthalmic Surgery

Medication/Category	Dosage/Route	Purpose/Action	Adverse Reactions	Nursing Implications
Irrigants				
BSS (Endosol)	Topical and intracamerally	Used to keep cornea moist during surgery; also used as internal irrigant into anterior or posterior segments	Corneal edema has occurred Use with caution with diabetic patients during vitrectomy	Solution most used in eye surgery. Used preoperatively and intraoperatively. Preservative free; do not use for more than one patient.
BSS enriched with bicarbonate, dextrose, and glutathione (BSS Plus, Endosol Extra)	Intracameral; not for injection or IV infusion	Used as internal irrigant into anterior or posterior segment; provides better metabolic support for ocular tissues during long procedures	When corneal endothelium is abnormal irrigation, trauma can cause bullous keratopathy	Used intraoperatively. Need to reconstitute immediately before use by addition of part 1 to part 2 with transfer device. Never use part 1 or part 2 alone; may result in damage to the eye.
Steroid Antiinflammatory Agents				
Betamethasone sodium phosphate and betamethasone acetate suspension (Celestone)	Injection: Comes in single-use local infiltration	Injected and used to treat severe allergic and inflammatory conditions in ocular conditions; also used with blocks	Foreign body sensation	Stored in medication dispensing system. Used preoperatively and intraoperatively.
Dexamethasone (Decadron)	Injection: 4 mg/mL Injected into conjunctiva	Adrenocortical; injected subconjunctivally postoperatively for inflammation prophylaxis and used to treat severe allergic and inflammatory conditions	Fungus infection, increased IOP	Stored in medication dispensing system. Used intraoperatively.
Prednisolone (Pred Forte, Econopred, Inflamase)	Topical drops suspension: 1% Dosage per surgeon's order	For reducing inflammation and severe allergic conditions	Elevated IOP and cataract formation	Pink cap. Shake bottle before use. Preoperatively and postoperatively.
Fluromethalone (FML, Flarex)	Topical eyedrops, suspension, or ointment: 0.1%, 0.25% Dosage per surgeon's order	For reducing inflammation and severe allergic conditions	Elevated IOP and subcapsular cataract formation	Pink cap. Shake bottle before applying to cornea postoperatively. Use ointment form for longer-lasting dose.
NSAIDs				
Nepafanec (Nevanac), flurbiprofen (Ocufen), ketorolac (Acular), diclofenac (Voltaren), bromofenac (Xibrom)	Topical eyedrops: 2-4 times daily	Topical treatment of inflammation	Adverse effect is corneal melting	Gray cap. Used preoperatively and postoperatively.
Antiinfectives				
Aminoglycosides: gentamicin (Genoptice, Gentake), besifloxacin (Besivance, Moxeza), tobramycin (AKtobe, Tobrex), norfloxacin (Chibroxin) ophthalmic	Topical drops: 2-4 times daily Dosage per surgeon's order and manufacturer's instructions	Topical treatment of bacterial superficial ocular infections	Allergic reaction to ingredients, itching, redness	Brown or tan cap. Used preoperatively and postoperatively.
Quinolones: gatifloxacin (Zymaxid), ofloxacin (Ocuflox), ciprofloxacin (Ciloxan), levofloxacin (Iquix, Qioxin), moxifloxacin (Vigamox) ophthalmic	Topical drops: 2-4 times daily Dosage per surgeon's order and manufacturer's instructions	Topical treatment of superficial bacterial ocular infections at time of surgery	Allergic reaction to ingredients, itching, redness	Brown or tan cap. Used preoperatively and postoperatively.

SURGICAL PHARMACOLOGY—cont'd

Medications for Ophthalmic Surgery

Medication/Category	Dosage/Route	Purpose/Action	Adverse Reactions	Nursing Implications
Injectable Antiinfectives				
Cefazolin (Ancef, Kefzol)	1 g mixed with 4.8 mL sterile water. Use 0.5 mL for subconjunctival injections Dosage per surgeon's order	Prophylactically injected subconjunctivally/ intracamerally for endophthalmitis	Hypersensitivity to any component	Perioperative nurse mixes medicine. Careful calculation and validation that dosage is correct. Stability and sterility must be maintained. Syringes must measure low concentrations, no air bubbles left in syringe. 6-24 hour expiration.
Vancomycin	1 g mixed with 20 mL sterile water Dosage per surgeon's order	Prophylactic for eye infections	Hypersensitivity to any component	Perioperative nurse reconstitutes drug according to manufacturer's instructions. Careful calculation and validation of dosage. Syringes must measure low concentrations, no air bubbles left in syringe.
Tobramycin	Dosage per surgeon's order	Intravitreal injections for active endophthalmitis	• Lid itching • Hypersensitivity to any component	Careful calculation and validation that dosage is correct. Syringes must measure low concentrations, no air bubbles left in syringe.
Miscellaneous				
Cocaine	Topical: 1%-4%	Used on cornea to loosen epithelium before debridement and on nasal packing to reduce congestion of mucosa; topically used for packing for dacryocystorhinostomy	• Damage or soften corneal epithelium • Sloughing of tissue with too much vasoconstriction	Never injected. Must be kept with controlled substances.
Hyperosmotic agent, mannitol (Osmitrol)	IV dosage per surgeon's order	IV osmotic diuretic to reduce intraocular pressure	• Use with caution in renal disease, dehydration, diuresis	Administered by anesthesia provider in IV bottle.
Trypan (VisionBlue)	Intracameral: 0.6%	For capsule staining and identification in complex cataract	Can stain IOL implant up to 1 wk if not irrigated out of the eye	Precaution: Confirm label for ophthalmic use. Follow manufacturer's instructions.
Tissue plasminogen activator (TPA) (Activase)	6.25 to 25 mcg per 0.1 mL Loaded into syringe after defrosted	Used to treat fibrin formation in postvitrectomy patients; lysis of clots on retina	Bleeding	Drug is stored in frozen single-dose aliquots. Must be defrosted at least 30 min to reach room temperature. See Chapter 7.
Corneal fibrin glue (Tisseal, Evicel, Artiss)	Corneal glue IV 500 mg or 125 mg to 500 mg orally q6hr			
Acetazolamide sodium (Diamox)		Carbonic anhydrase inhibitor; IOP lowering by suppressing the secretion of aqueous humor	Swelling of lens, myopia, gastrointestinal intolerance, drowsiness, lethargy, depression, renal sulfa hypersensitivity	Orange packaging. Administered by anesthesia provider through IV. Communicate about sulfa allergies and report to surgeon if there is a reaction. Receive order from surgeon to discontinue use.

Continued

SURGICAL PHARMACOLOGY—cont'd

Medications for Ophthalmic Surgery

Medication/Category	Dosage/Route	Purpose/Action	Adverse Reactions	Nursing Implications
Antimetabolite				
Mitomycin (MMC), fluorouracil (5-FU)	Topical: 0.2 to 0.4 mg/mL for 90 sec or longer per surgeon's orders	Antimetabolite used topically to inhibit scar formation in glaucoma-filtering procedures and pterygium excision	• Known reaction to any components • MMC is toxic and potentially hazardous; avoid exposure to unintended tissue	Chemotherapeutic drug. Handle and discard in compliance with OSHA and facility policies for safe use of antineoplastics. Oncology department and pharmacy have instructions that must be followed.

BSS, Balanced salt solution; *CNS,* central nervous system; *IOL,* intraocular lens; *IOP,* intraocular pressure; *MPF,* Methylparaben Free; *NSAIDs,* nonsteroidal antiinflammatory drugs; *OSHA,* Occupational Safety and Health Administration; *PF,* preservative free.
Modified from Bartlett J: *Ophthalmic drug fact sheet,* St Louis, 2011, Wolters Kluwer Health; Gyang KO: *Ocular drugs handbook: an easy reference guide to eye medications,* Bloomington, IN, 2008, AuthorHouse.

may be mixed is generally 10 mL; however, usual volume given is much less and depends on technique chosen by the surgeon. The ocular blocks are performed by the surgeon because of the proximity to major nerve endings and muscles.

Ocular Blocks. The *retrobulbar block* has the highest risk of all the ocular blocks. This block uses a 3-L syringe armed with a retrobulbar needle. This needle's tip is specially designed not to lacerate blood vessels. The surgeon places the needle inferior to the globe, outer one third of the orbital rim. After the needle is past the equator, it is then directed toward the orbital apex while the patient is looking upward and inward. This block is given retro, or behind the eye (muscle cone). The advantages of this widely used block are the relatively small volume of solution required, excellent anesthesia, and loss of voluntary eye muscle control. The risks of this block include perforation of the globe, hemorrhage, damage to the optic nerve, and injection of the muscle; a major risk is brainstem anesthesia (Figure 18-9).

The *peribulbar block* carries a moderate risk and is given outside of the muscle cone. The surgeon begins with the needle in the inferior lateral orbital rim. It is then directed under and away from the globe. The peribulbar block uses a larger volume of local anesthetic and diffuses into the retro space. The advantages of this block include increased safety because there is less chance of hitting the optic nerve or causing brainstem anesthesia. Risks associated with this block are perforation (smaller risk than the retrobulbar block), hemorrhage, unpredictable akinesia, conjunctival chemosis, and extended lead time for effects to set up (Figure 18-10).

A *subtenon block* is administered after the skin preparation. The surgeon makes a small inferior nasal incision with a dissection past the equator of the globe using blunt scissors. The injection is given inferior nasal to the globe using a blunt cannula. The advantages of this block include increased safety because the surgeon is unlikely to perforate the globe, relatively quick onset, and smaller volumes than the peribulbar block. The disadvantages of the subtenon block are chemosis, inconsistent akinesia, and the time for the block to take effect.

Topical Anesthesia. The most common ophthalmic anesthetic agents are proparacaine and tetracaine. These topical anesthetics are useful to check intraocular pressure and temporarily relieve pain for

FIGURE 18-9 Retrobulbar block.

diagnostic purposes. Topical anesthetic is given in the OR prior to the facial prep. Each medication is applied in the superior and inferior conjunctival fornices with the patient in supine position. The cornea becomes numb with first drop, but the conjunctiva is more difficult to numb and may require another application. The process is finished with the application of lidocaine gel to the upper

FIGURE 18-10 Peribulbar block.

FIGURE 18-11 Draped patient. The scrub person keeps the cornea moist with saline solution during eye surgery.

and lower conjunctival surface. Advantages of topical anesthesia include no risk of perforation or retrobulbar hemorrhage and quick onset. The disadvantages include no akinesia and no block of the seventh nerve to prevent the patient from squeezing the eye.

Positioning. Positioning the patient for ophthalmic surgery generally requires additional devices for stabilizing the head, protecting bony prominences, and providing appropriate alignment to prevent peripheral neurovascular injury. The ophthalmology stretcher, which is a combination transport device and OR bed, is often used as the surgical bed for convenience and comfort. This special bed, with a tapered head end, allows for closer access to the patient's face and eliminates several transfers for the patient. The perioperative nurse positions the patient with a foam donut or headrest under the head and a firm pillow under the knees. The nurse tucks the patient's arms at the side, pads the elbows to protect the ulnar nerve, faces the palms inward, and maintains the wrists in a neutral position; a drape secures the arms (Denholm, 2009). The drape should be tucked snugly under the patient, not under the mattress. This prevents the arm from shifting downward intraoperatively and resting against the OR bed rail.

If patients are to be sedated, the nurse asks if they are comfortable and offers reassurance that there are ways to increase comfort. Some elderly patients prefer not to discuss their discomfort for fear of being bothersome, so it is important to pay attention to their body language and cues.

Intraocular surgery is usually carried out with the use of a microscope. A special wrist rest may be used to stabilize the surgeon's hands and may include perforated tubing or bar to provide oxygen under the drapes. The nurse should attach the tube to the bed and secure it approximately 2.5 cm below the patient's lateral canthus before draping. The wrist rest may be placed unilaterally or may encircle the head. A strip of tape may be placed over the patient's forehead (avoiding the eyebrows) and secured to the operative bed to provide head stabilization.

Prepping. The operative site is prepped under aseptic conditions, usually after the anesthetic is administered. A sterile prep tray commonly contains sterile normal saline solution, irrigation bulb, basins, gauze sponges, cotton-tipped applicators, towels, and antimicrobial skin disinfectant.

Some surgeons order one or two drops of 5% povidone-iodine solution administered to the eye surface before the prep of the face and eyelids to decrease the number of surface microbes. Unless the patient has been administered a general anesthetic, a topical anesthetic drop is placed to minimize the stinging sensation. Povidone-iodine may be contraindicated in patients with allergic reactions to *topical* iodine. For these patients a mixture of baby shampoo and balanced salt solution (BSS) can be used as the agent for the facial prep instead of iodine.

The nurse cleans the patient's lid margins by inverting the lids and cleaning with cotton-tipped applicators moistened with antimicrobial skin disinfectant, taking care to prevent the solution from entering the patient's ears. The eye may be then irrigated with normal saline solution using an irrigating bulb. When toxic chemicals or small particles of foreign matter must be removed, the eye surface and conjunctival sac are thoroughly flushed with tepid sterile normal saline solution using an irrigation bulb or an Asepto syringe. The nurse dries the prep area so the drape will adhere. The surgical prep must be completed at least 3 minutes before the procedure begins so the solution has adequate time to dry.

Draping. Special concerns for eye surgery draping include repelling water, eliminating lint and fiber particles, and providing adequate air exchange for patients receiving local anesthetics. A cardboard bridge that adheres to the sides of the patient's face may be used to support the drape above the patient's mouth and nose. The surgeon may request that the nurse place a Mayo stand above the patient before the draping process to provide a platform to decrease the weight of the drapes and surgical handpieces/tubing on the patient. The use of a one-piece disposable drape, with a self-adherent, fenestrated plastic section for the eye, eliminates the need to lift the patient's head during draping and facilitates drape removal at the end of the procedure. The eyelids may be separated when applying the self-adherent plastic eye drape to keep the eyelashes out of the operative eye. A fluid drainage bag with wicking strip may also be adhered to the plastic eye drape.

In an alternative method, the surgeon may drape the head with a half-sheet and two towels, use a large sheet or U-drape or split sheet to cover the patient and OR bed, and place a fenestrated plastic eye drape over the operative site (Figure 18-11).

Instrumentation. Additional instruments, depending on the type of procedure, can be added to the basic instrument set. Special surface finishes are used to reduce light reflection. Instruments are designed with round handles for smoother motion and rotation under the microscope. The instruments are to be placed on the Mayo stand; the order of their use can also be listed on the surgeon's preference card or computerized pick list.

A variety of ophthalmic forceps are designed for specific use with different tissues of the eye. Fixation forceps, used to hold tissue firmly in place or provide traction before incision, have an angled tooth that overlaps for secure fixation. Suturing forceps, used to pick up wound edges for dissection or suturing, are single-toothed forceps with the tooth at a right angle to the shank of the forceps. Tying forceps have a flat platform for holding suture as it is tied.

Care and Handling. To maintain the quality and precision of all ophthalmic instruments, including microsurgical instruments, strict criteria for care and handling must be followed. Storage cases protect instrument tips and cutting surfaces. The instruments should be inspected under magnification when purchased and before and after each use, observing for burrs on tips, nicks on cutting surfaces, and alignment of jaws. The scrub person should clean eye instruments used during the procedure with nonfibrous sponges to avoid damaging delicate instrument tips. Personnel handling instruments should know the name and purpose of each instrument. Tissue can be damaged by the use of an inappropriate instrument, and instruments can be damaged by inappropriate use. After use, the instruments should be cleaned, thoroughly dried, and terminally sterilized before storage in protective containers.

It is recommended that microsurgical instruments undergo ultrasonic cleaning with distilled water and an appropriate enzymatic cleansing agent. They can be individually handheld or immersed together in the ultrasonic cleaner as long as they are not touching each other. Instruments should be rinsed with distilled water and thoroughly dried. A hot air blower (never a towel) should be used for drying instruments. Instrument lubricant should not be used on an irrigating cannula because residue can be introduced into the eye and cause damage.

In addition to basic care and handling, a routine preventive maintenance program should be established for sharpening, realigning, and adjusting the precision eye instruments. Keeping an instrument in good repair is much less expensive than buying a new one. Disposable instruments offer accessibility and quality assurance; for example, forceps are properly aligned for each use because they have not been used on other procedures. Benefits for the institution include elimination of costs related to repairs. Knives are available that have safety features of retractable blades to be in compliance with the Needlestick Safety and Prevention Act, requiring implementation of safer medical devices to minimize occupational exposure to bloodborne pathogens from accidental sharps injuries, which remains a serious problem.

Range of Equipment Used. A wide range of equipment is used in ophthalmic surgery. The perioperative team's knowledge of proper functioning and troubleshooting should be confirmed through inservice education and training specific to new equipment. For safety, all items must be used according to the manufacturer's directions and tested for proper performance before the patient enters the OR. Although the products and manufacturers may vary, the following are some of the typical pieces of equipment and accessories used in ophthalmic surgeries:

- *Phacoemulsification machines (phaco):* These machines produce ultrasound frequency vibrations, which in a fluid medium emulsify and break up the cataract. Irrigation and aspiration (I/A) handpieces are used. The phaco tips and handpieces can be chosen with different diameters and straight or curved tips.

Ultra-chopper tips are available for torsional handpieces. With these advanced ultra-chopper tips the scrub person must be aware of the high speed in which they function; the slightest wrong movement may shatter the cataract. Bipolar electrosurgical unit (ESU) and anterior vitrectomy handpieces may also be attached when needed. The surgeon controls the foot pedal and chooses one of the following modes by depressing the pedal to a certain position: irrigation alone; irrigation and aspiration; and irrigation, aspiration, and phacoemulsification combined. Some machines also have an anterior vitrector. As the surgeon manipulates the handpiece and operates the foot pedal to emulsify the lens nucleus, the perioperative nurse monitors the function of the instrument and operates the console controls to change settings such as irrigation bottle height. The irrigation used with this machine is BSS. Modern tubing attached to the handpiece has low compliance and helps reduce the intraoperative fluid surge that may occur after an occlusion blockage suddenly releases. It is important to ensure that all parts of the phaco machine are functioning properly prior to the procedure. Improperly used phaco units can cause corneal burns.

- *Posterior vitrectomy machines:* Functions on these machines may include vitrectomy with cutter handpieces for removal of vitreous; extrusion for gentle aspiration near sensitive retina and macula; oil infusion; bipolar electrosurgery or diathermy; and motorized cutting with electric scissors attachment. Foot pedal or manual control can set eye pressure and cut and suction rates.

- *Cryotherapy machine:* The cryotherapy machine is generally used to cause an inflammatory reaction in the retinal tissue that seals a break or tear. The unit uses nitrous oxide as the freezing agent. Adequate pressure settings are needed for acceptable levels of freeze. External and intraocular handpieces are available.

- *Lasers:* Lasers are used for various applications in eye procedures, whether for clearing an opacified posterior capsule after cataract surgery, for reshaping or creating a flap of the cornea, or for direct use inside the eye during posterior vitrectomy. Settings must be confirmed with the surgeon. Everyone in the OR when the laser is in use must wear appropriate protective eyewear according to the laser's wavelength. Warning signs are posted on doors, and windows are covered to avoid scatter outside the room.

- *ESU units:* Bipolar or monopolar ESU may be used. The return electrode monitor placement must follow manufacturer's guidelines. Fire precautions must be observed, especially in the presence of oxygen.

- *Operating microscope:* Most ophthalmic procedures are performed using a surgical microscope. Proper care and maintenance of the operating microscope are essential to ensure optimal functioning and durability of this sophisticated, expensive piece of equipment. It is the perioperative nurse's responsibility to adjust the microscope's oculars (eyepieces) prior to surgery to obtain the clearest view of the operating field. The perioperative nurse must be familiar with how to adjust pupillary distance (e.g., the distance between pupils of the user's eyes) and diopter settings on the oculars for operator vision correction to work without eyeglasses comfortably. The angle of the ocular should also be adjusted for appropriate viewing and personal comfort without scrunching or stretching. Users who have significant astigmatism should wear their eyeglasses and set the oculars at zero because uncorrected astigmatisms cannot be entered into the microscope's ocular setting. If there is an uncorrected refractive error, the minus (myopia) or plus (hyperopia) error should

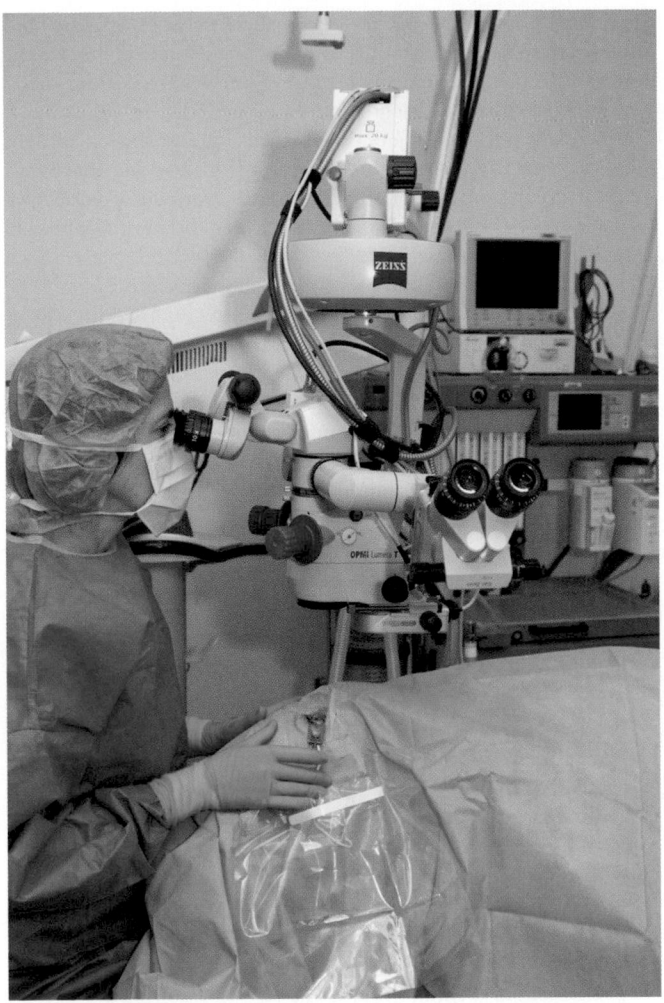

FIGURE 18-12 When the patient is in position, the perioperative nurse sets the microscope into focus. Head is positioned properly for surgery.

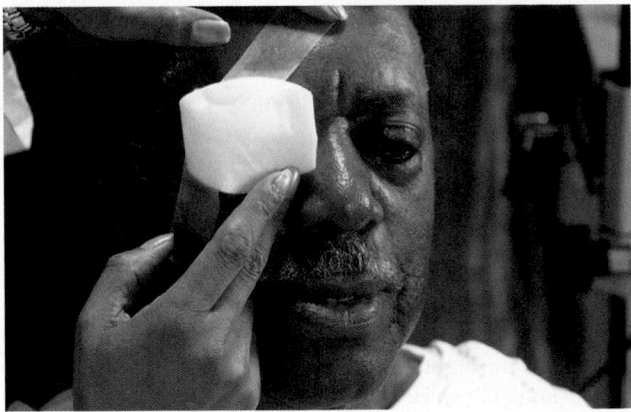

FIGURE 18-13 Application of a protective eyepatch.

be entered on the ocular dial, each hash mark indicting a diopter of correction. Users should be aware of their own refractive errors because they can cause decreased visual acuity during surgery. For safety, the microscope should be tested and adjusted for proper performance before the patient enters the room. The centering buttons on the microscope for the vertical plane and horizontal planes should be set before the procedure begins by pushing each button once. The microscope spotlight should be in gross focus, obtained by manually raising or lowering the microscope head or the OR bed height. Some microscopes used for other applications such as plastic surgery may use light sources that are so bright they damage the retina. The nurse must ensure that the microscope used in ophthalmic surgery is specifically intended for and safe for eye surgery. Other responsibilities for the circulating nurse include full command of how the scope needs to be focused and all the movements of the arms of the scope. Microscopes are adjusted for right eye and left eye procedures (Figure 18-12).

Ophthalmic Sutures. Sutures used in ophthalmic surgery are very fine and range in size from 4-0 to 10-0. Handling and arming these sutures can be a challenge for the scrub person with uncorrected presbyopia. Fine eye sutures produce minimum reaction and

discomfort for the patient. They should be handled as little as possible to avoid weakening and fraying. Ophthalmic needles also are very delicate and must be handled with extreme care and inspected for evidence of burrs before use.

Ophthalmic Dressings. At the completion of the operation, the operative eye area is cleansed with saline sponges. After plastic procedures on the lids or lacrimal ducts, antibiotic ophthalmic ointment may be thinly spread over the skin and eyelashes to prevent adhesion of the bandage.

The initial dressing is a sterile eye pad secured with nonallergenic tape (Figure 18-13). After intraocular operations, when external pressure on the eyes might be harmful, the initial dressing is covered with a protecting, perforated aluminum plate or plastic eye shield. Postcataract dressings range from traditional eye pads to collagen corneal shields rehydrated in an antiinfective-antiinflammatory solution to no dressing at all. A pressure bandage, consisting of a folded eyepatch covered with a second single-layer eyepatch, may be used when a compression effect is desired.

Application of Corneal Shields. Contact lenses, applied directly onto the cornea, are used by patients to correct refractive errors instead of eyeglasses. It is important for the perioperative nurse to confirm the patient has removed all contact lenses prior to surgery and understand they must abstain from contact lens use until the ophthalmologist permits. Collagen corneal shields look like contact lenses and are used postoperatively to distribute postoperative medication and protect the eye after surgery.

Perioperative nurses should be able to apply corneal shields to the patient's eye with comfort. The nurse applies a glove to the dominant hand and places the corneal shield on the index finger. Using the nondominant hand, the upper eyelid is gently lifted while pulling down the lower lid with the middle finger of the dominant hand. The nurse instructs the patient to slightly look up and then gently places the corneal shield on the cornea and instructs the patient to blink the shield into place. The corneal shield may naturally fall out of the eye during the postoperative period, usually within 4 to 12 hours. The nurse discusses this with the patient and reinforces that it is a normal process and the shield should be reapplied.

Evaluation

The nurse evaluates the patient's general condition before transport to the postanesthesia care unit (PACU) or observation unit. The general appearance of the skin is assessed, with areas around the face and bony prominences noted for redness or other changes from the preoperative condition.

A hand-off report to the receiving nurse in the PACU or observation area includes postoperative positioning requirements, potential problems specific to the patient, and preoperative anxiety level and use of coping mechanisms.

Evaluation should address whether the patient met the desired perioperative nursing outcomes; the patient's responses may be documented as outcome statements. The following examples are based on the nursing diagnoses identified in the plan of care:

- The patient, family, or significant others verbalized knowledge regarding the diagnosis, planned intervention, medication management, and requirements for home care maintenance.
- The patient verbalized an acceptable level of anxiety and used effective coping mechanisms.
- The patient remained comfortable during the intervention as determined by pain scale response.
- The patient will remain free from signs and symptoms of surgical site infection.

Patient and Family Education and Discharge Planning

Patient education is one of the nurse's greatest contributions. Some facilities have programs with group teaching for patients; in other settings, education is provided individually. Depending on the setting, the nursing role in patient education may include review of preoperative expectations, individual patient needs, surgeon's instructions, procedure, intraocular lens (IOL) choices (if applicable), and overview of the surgery experience.

Implementation of the plan of care actually begins during the patient interview. Planning to meet the patient's educational needs should play an equal role with meeting other needs. Verbal review and reinforcement of information initially provided in the physician's office ensures consistency in teaching. Written material and audiovisual media (closed circuit television, DVDs, tablet computers, photos, and patient information websites) may be used to enhance patient education programs but do not eliminate the need for direct interchange with patients and feedback from them.

Family members or friends should be included to add support and increase understanding of the planned surgery. The loss of sight produces the same staged coping behaviors of grieving that move the individual from denial to acceptance. Thorough preoperative preparation of the patient and in most cases the family, who will assist with care at home in the postoperative period, plays a vital role in the successful outcome of the surgical procedure. The National Quality Forum (NQF) describes truly high-quality care as also culturally competent care. Provision of culturally appropriate care can increase efficiency and improve patient satisfaction besides improving outcomes (NQF, 2012). General guidelines for patient and family education for the patient undergoing ophthalmic surgery include the following:

- Purpose and desired results of preoperative eyedrops and sedation
- Explanation of what to expect from the anesthetic
- Activities and routines of the intraoperative period
- What to expect immediately after surgery, including pain and visual acuity
- Designated driver after procedures
- Verbal and written instructions for use of eyedrops and other medications
- Any limitations on activities (bending, lifting, eye rubbing, special positioning)
- Wound care, protective sunglasses
- Signs and symptoms of complications
- Follow-up postoperative phone calls from the ambulatory surgery center, as applicable
- Who to call with questions or concerns
- Follow-up appointments

The Patient and Family Education box has additional examples of instructions specific to cataract surgery.

PATIENT AND FAMILY EDUCATION

Discharge Instructions and Home Care After Cataract Surgery

- Give both the patient and the caregiver verbal and written instruction. Provide them with the name and telephone number of the surgeon or nurse to call if questions arise. Stress handwashing for patient and caregiver.
- Advise the patient to avoid squeezing the eyelids shut or touching the eyes postoperatively.
- Encourage the patient to wear eyeglasses during the day to avoid rubbing the eye and provide protection from environmental hazards.
- Review the signs and symptoms that should be reported to the surgeon or nurse such as sudden onset of eye pain or pressure, photophobia, sudden decrease in vision, sudden and severe headaches, excessive redness or watering of eyes, swelling, nausea, or vomiting. Discuss the need to wear an eye shield while sleeping the first week postoperatively. Tape may be used to hold the shield in place. The patient should avoid sleeping on the stomach or operated side for the first week after surgery.
- Discuss that vision may not be clear for the first few days postoperatively.
- Instruct that sunglasses must be worn at all times while outside after cataract surgery to avoid ultraviolet light damage and reduce glare and photophobia.

- Reinforce that if the patient is receiving a standard intraocular lens (IOL) implant he or she will still need to wear eyeglasses; however, the prescription may not be as strong. Approximately 3 to 6 weeks after surgery, the new prescription will be given with proper healing and the surgeon's advice. Vision may feel unbalanced until the new prescription is ordered and the trained optician delivers new eyeglasses.
- Discuss that if an advanced technology multifocal IOL is implanted, it may take time for the visual acuity to adjust completely (up to 3 months), especially until after the second eye is operated on.
- Remind the patient not to use eyedrops from previous surgeries because this may promote infections. An eyedrop checklist should be given to the patient to keep track of the eyedrop schedule. Review the proper instillation of eyedrops with patient and caregiver. (Note: If the surgery on the second eye was just performed, the patient may still be taking drops for the first eye. Review the specific drops for each eye and provide a checklist for each eye. Instruct the patient to follow the surgeon's directions for tapering drops for the first eye.)
- Instruct the patient not to use handkerchiefs to wipe the eyes if eyedrops spill over; instead use disposable single-use tissues.

PATIENT AND FAMILY EDUCATION

Discharge Instructions and Home Care After Cataract Surgery—cont'd

- Advise the patient to avoid constipation by drinking plenty of water and eating a diet high in fiber.
- Explain the need to avoid strenuous exercise for 2 to 3 weeks. Check with the physician before resuming heavy occupational or recreational activities. Note that sexual relations can usually resume after 1 week.
- Discuss limiting the amount of computer and close reading during the first few days after surgery because this may dry out the eyes and prevent the new IOL from stabilizing.

- Review that pets, although lovable, carry dander and germs that can irritate the surgery site. Discuss precautions with the patient and caregiver such as not sleeping in the same bed as the pets and to be conscious of contacting pet saliva.
- Stress the importance of regular follow-up care with the physician.

Modified from Canobbio MM: Mosby's handbook of patient teaching, St. Louis, 2006, Mosby; Goldblum K et al: *The surgical patient journey: from the office to discharge to home—pre-op office care, pre-op medical clearance, intraoperative, discharge and home,* Presentation at American Society of Ophthalmic Registered Nurses (ASORN) annual meeting, Chicago, 2012.

Surgical Interventions

Surgery of the Lens

Cataract Extraction

Cataract surgery is the leading diagnosis for ambulatory surgery visits, with more than 3 million lens extractions performed yearly in the United States (Ambulatory Surgery Considerations). It is estimated that more than 24 million Americans older than age 40 have a cataract, and this number is expected to increase as the baby-boomer population ages over the next 20 years (National Eye Institute [NEI], 2012a).

Normally, light passing through a clear lens projects a sharp image onto the retina. The lens is made of mostly water and protein and over time some of the protein may clump together, leading to clouding of the lens (cataract). Ultraviolet light has been linked to the acceleration of cataract development. The vision gradually gets worse as the lens changes from clear to a yellow or brown (Figure 18-14). The cataract eventually makes it difficult to differentiate certain colors and difficult to read or perform routine activities. Other symptoms include blurred vision, difficulty using current

AMBULATORY SURGERY CONSIDERATIONS

Caring for Patients Undergoing Day Surgery in Ambulatory Surgery Centers

Most eye surgeries are performed on an outpatient basis or in stand-alone ambulatory surgery centers, which limits the personal interaction with nurses compared with inpatient surgeries. Efficiency, increased flow, and work management concerns also reduce the time for perioperative nurses to bond with and care for the surgery patient. The patients still desire and require a hands-on approach to their eye care, so finding an appropriate balance between comforting care and efficiency to meet the surgery centers's bottom line can be challenging.

Perioperative nurses often observe anxious behavior in surgery patients, yet little acknowledgment or intervention is taken to document or respond to the anxiety. A patient-centered care approach to nursing may be lost to efficiency and a mechanistic approach to patient care. The psychologic and psychosocial aspects of outpatient surgery nursing will continue to emerge as the field of healthcare changes.

The five simple steps to help alleviate anxiety for day surgery patients are information provision, personal control, self-efficacy, therapeutic care of self, and environmental considerations. Implementing these practices into the care of surgery patients helps bridge the gap between efficiency and patient-centered care.

1. *Information provision:* Anesthesia and pain as well as unexpected wait times are common causes of presurgery anxiety. Dispelling common misconceptions of eye anesthetics and a formal delivery of information may dispel anxiety. The nurse should avoid using terms like "quick and simple procedure" because it may create anxiety postoperatively if patients feel they are not healing fast enough.

2. *Personal control:* Unfamiliar hospital environments, strange staff members, decreased cognition with medications, and externally enforced strict schedules can diminish a patient's real or perceived sense of control. Targeted communication and minor decision-making questions may increase the sense of control over situations and thus provide a sense of control over the patient's body and healthcare.

3. *Self-efficacy:* Resiliency and the ability to cope with stressful situations has a positive influence on recovery. A planned and detailed program of at-home care can increase feelings of confidence and self-efficacy for the patient.

4. *Therapeutic use of self:* Social support from the nurses and relatives can ease pre- and postoperative anxiety. Enhance optimism by openly discussing fears and offering encouraging statements like "reliable effective medications." Realistic optimism can be used to negate unrealistic negative fears by opening up channels of honest dialogue.

5. *Environmental considerations:* The surgery center can be a busy, noisy, bright, and bustling center of activity, which can create anxiety for patients who may need to consciously reduce fears by listening to music, talking with friends, or spending quiet time to themselves before surgery. Proximity to other surgery patients can increase or exaggerate fears and anxiety. Describing the sounds and sites around them and stating aspects of safe and effective equipment, policies, and procedures may reduce anxiety. Using touch (if welcomed by the patient) or reducing the sterile appearance of the environment can limit the negative effect of the surroundings.

Modified from Mitchell M: A patient centered approach to day surgery nursing, *Nurs Stand* 24:44:40–46, 2010.

FIGURE 18-14 A hypermature age-related corticonuclear cataract with a brunescent (brown) nucleus.

eyeglasses, having poor night vision, noticing glare from headlights or lamps, perceiving that sunlight is too bright, and double vision. In addition to age-related cataracts, the following other types of cataracts exist:

- *Congenital*—Children may be born with cataracts or develop them throughout their youth.
- *Traumatic*—After eye injury or electric shock, cataracts may develop even years later.
- *Secondary*—After eye surgery for other conditions, cataracts may develop, or they may be associated with other health problems such as diabetes, steroid use, smoking, and prolonged exposure to sunlight.

Cataract removal is warranted when they interfere with everyday activities such as driving, reading, and watching television. The presence of a cataract may also create difficulties for the ophthalmologist to assess vitreous and retina issues. Potential complications, though rare, are discussed as part of informed consent prior to surgery. In a patient with vision in only one eye, the risks and benefits of surgery must be carefully evaluated. The potential problems include vision-threatening infections, bleeding, inflammation, loss of vision, double vision, and high or low eye pressure.

Certain medications and diseases may prevent the pupil from properly dilating or may cause unexpected iris contractions during surgery. Intraoperative floppy iris syndrome (IFIS) may cause complications during cataract surgery, but those complications are partially reduced when proper precautions are taken in at-risk patients. Patients who are under long-term treatment for glaucoma therapy, who use alpha-blockers such as tamsulosin (Flomax), or who have diabetes are more prone to IFIS.

Patients who had had previous refractive surgery such as laser-assisted in situ keratomileusis (LASIK) or photorefractive keratectomy (PRK) have a compromised cornea and postoperative refractions are less predictable. Optiwave refractive analysis (ORA) can be used intraoperatively to analyze the reflected wave of light exiting the eye and give the surgeon an accurate measure of the eye's focusing capabilities and better predict the postcataract results for visual acuity. The ORA measurement is completed after the cataract nucleus has been removed but before the IOL has been inserted.

Patients expect to see well without glasses as early as the day after surgery. It is important to manage the postoperative visual expectations of patients so they understand proper healing times and fluctuations. If patients are scheduled for surgery in both eyes a few

weeks apart, they may experience some imbalances because one eye has postoperative refraction and the other eye has preoperative vision. This imbalance is not an indication of the final visual acuity outcome of cataract surgery. The stronger the presurgery eyeglass prescription the more likely imbalances may occur and the more the perioperative nurse must communicate the imbalances so the patients are prepared and avoid premature disappointment. Patients with cataracts in both eyes generally have their procedures performed at separate times, usually 4 to 8 weeks apart.

Months or years after cataract surgery, residual epithelial cells may grow back on the capsular bag causing opacification of the posterior capsule and a haze in the vision. The YAG laser may then be indicated for capsulotomy, creating a hole in the center of the capsule to allow light to pass through and restore clear vision.

There are two separate stages of cataract surgery; the removal of the cataractous lens with the extracapsular cataract excision (ECCE) phaco method, or the intracapsular cataract extraction (ICCE) method and the insertion of an artificial IOL to restore visual acuity. The femtosecond laser is a newer technology that some surgeons use to perform capsulorrhexis prior to the ECCE or ICCE procedure (Figure 18-15) (Research Highlight). All perioperative personnel using specialized ophthalmic instruments and equipment must have thorough knowledge of the operation as well as problems that may be encountered and actions to correct them.

In the ECCE procedure the anterior portion of the capsule is opened in a controlled manner using a 25-gauge needle or a capsule forceps. Phaco uses high-frequency ultrasonic energy to break the hardened lens material into fragments that can then be aspirated from the eye with saline. The surgeon removes only the lens nucleus from the eye, leaving the posterior capsule behind to hold the IOL implant. The ICCE method of cataract removal consists of removing the entire lens within its capsule with a cryoprobe and is rarely performed except in the event of a dislocated lens. If an ICCE is scheduled, alpha-chymotrypsin (Catarase, Chymar), an enzyme that acts to weaken the zonules of the lens is used, and a cataract cryoprobe needs to be available.

Intraocular Lens. Extraction of the cataractous lens removes one of the major refractive components of the eye. Four options for replacing this lost refractive power are: (1) IOL implantation, (2) astigmatism IOL implantation, (3) advanced technology bifocal (multifocal) IOL implantation, or (4) aphakia (no implant), which requires the use of thick eyeglasses postoperatively. IOLs offer many advantages to patients, including reduced dependence on eyeglasses and reduced thickness of any eyeglass correction needed.

The invention and adoption of the IOL since the late 1990s has allowed cataract surgery to become a procedure of choice with increased visual freedom rather than a last resort option with limited vision recovery. The redefinition of aging in the baby-boomer generation has spurred research for improved performance of IOLs. Active adults understand cataract surgery has also become refractive surgery and can significantly reduce their dependence on eyeglasses and contact lenses. The expectations of vision after cataract surgery have increased and patients are demanding more and requiring better outcomes. The perioperative nurse holds a crucial job in the ophthalmic surgical team to provide detailed, educated, and accurate assistance to help achieve the patient's heightened expectation of results.

IOLs are made of silicone or acrylic resin and are available in various diopter powers. The necessary diopter power customized for each patient is determined by measuring the curvature of the

FIGURE 18-15 A, The femtosecond laser is used in cataract surgery to perform the capsulorrhexis. The room is nonsterile and adjacent to the OR. **B,** The patient is positioned under the femtosecond laser with a speculum in place and docking cone in position for the surgeon.

Modified from Slade S: *Laser refractive cataract surgery,* Pennsylvania, 2012, Bryn Mawr Communications; Roberts TV et al: Surgical outcomes and safety of femtosecond laser cataract surgery: a prospective study of 1500 consecutive cases, *Ophthalmology* 20:227–233, 2013; Roberts TV et al: Femtosecond laser cataract surgery: technology and clinical practice, *Clin Exper Ophthalmol* 41(2):180-186, 2013.

RESEARCH HIGHLIGHT

Femtosecond Lasers and Cataract Surgery

References to cataract surgery date back as early as the 6th century BC, when a curved needle was inserted into the eye to detach the lens and let it sink to the bottom of the eye. During the 20th century, innovation developed the intraocular lens (IOL) to reduce thick postoperative eyeglasses, phacoemulsification techniques to improve IOL placement, and the advanced technology multifocal IOL to decrease dependence on eyeglasses. The next advancement for cataract surgery is the use of the femtosecond (FS) laser.

LASIK surgery created a desire in patients for better visual acuity without glasses, as well as an acceptance to pay out of pocket to improve their vision, and ultimately a higher expectation of vision after cataract surgery. Femtosecond lasers improve precision, reproducibility, and change the concept of cataract surgery from a surgery for older people to laser refractive cataract surgery that can enhance one's lifestyle.

FS refers to the speed of the optical pulse of the laser: one quadrillionth of a second (10^{-15}). This short pulse duration allows less tissue damage during surgery as well as more precisely focused ablation in the cornea or anterior chamber. The laser can be set to different depths to reach different levels within the anterior chamber, all without generating heat during the ablation process. The use of the FS laser during cataract surgery can create more accurate initial incisions, yielding more predictable and standardized results. These findings are significant because a fraction of a millimeter in eye surgery can alter the desired postsurgery results.

Roberts and colleagues undertook a single-center, prospective, consecutive cohort study to evaluate the rate of complications in a series of procedures using the FS laser for cataract surgery. All procedures were in two stages, the first stage taking place using the FS to create the anterior capsulotomy, nuclear fragmentation, and primary and side-port corneal incisions. The second stage took place in the OR using phacoemulsification techniques with insertion of an IOL.

Study participants were divided into two groups; group one was composed of the first 200 patients in series and the second group was the remaining 1300 cases. All study participants were similar in demographic characteristics (e.g., age, axial length, keratometric diopters).

Complications included anterior radial and posterior capsule tears, posterior lens dislocation, suction breaks, manual corneal incisions, papillary constriction, and anterior capsule tags. The incidence of majority complications in group two was statistically lower compared with the initial group.

The authors note that their complication rate was comparable to rates found in the literature for manual cataract surgery, and that continuing surgeon experience, modification of techniques, and improved technology will determine the effect of FS lasers on the quality of cataract surgery and patient outcomes.

patient's cornea (keratometry) and the axial length (length from cornea to retina). A complex mathematic formula is then used to calculate the correct lens power needed for the desired results. This work is performed in the surgeon's office, and the desired IOL orders are transmitted to the hospital a week before surgery date.

The standard IOL implant reimbursed by insurance can reduce the prescription for hyperopia or myopia, but does not correct for astigmatism or presbyopia. After cataract surgery the patient's distance prescription can be significantly reduced, but he or she will most likely need to wear some form of bifocal glasses for most activities.

Advanced technology multifocal IOLs are becoming more accepted by physicians and patients. Nationwide 17% of all IOL implants are advanced technology bifocal implants (Slade, 2012); however, some surgeons insert advanced technology IOLs in nearly 40% of their patients, with these numbers expected to go up. When the advanced technology multifocal IOL option is chosen, the patient's expectations of visual acuity after surgery are heightened. The astigmatism and multifocal IOLs require an extra out-of-pocket expense for the patients, furthering their higher expectations on performance and visual acuity.

Toric IOLs are designed to reduce hyperopia or myopia as well as astigmatism so as to reduce a patient's dependence of eyeglasses for distance as much as possible. Toric IOLs have different optical power and focal length in two orientations perpendicular to each other. The patient will still need eyeglasses for close reading and computer work, but will gain freedom from eyeglasses for activities such as driving and watching television. Advanced technology bifocal or accommodating IOLs are the most advanced IOL and give the patient the most freedom from eyeglasses because they correct for distance as well as reading. Patients have reported excellent visual acuity results with the bifocal IOLs. Advanced technology IOLs also require more preparation, precision, and detailed work on the surgeon's behalf, which requires extra attention by the attending perioperative nurse.

Over the past years numerous microsurgical techniques have been developed for IOL insertion through a smaller self-sealing incision, and most recently through a clear corneal incision. With the advent of the smaller 2.8-mm or less incision diameter, IOLs have evolved to become foldable. The scrub person is required to understand the importance of proper folding techniques. IOLs that are folded incorrectly into the injector can be inserted upside down or backward, negatively affecting postsurgical refractions. The more the surgeon has to manipulate the incorrectly folded IOL, the higher the risk of inflammation. Astigmatism and multifocal IOLs require more precise attention while folding into the injector because they have a smaller room for error and require more precise insertion by the surgeon. IOL manufacturers have started supplying IOLs in a preloaded injector to reduce the instance of misloading (Figure 18-16).

Perioperative nursing personnel must be familiar with specific institutional policies pertaining to IOLs and their use. The AAO developed recommendations to minimize the occurrence of preventable errors such as wrong IOL implant, damaged IOL implantation, or upside down IOL loading and implantation. The recommendations emphasize the importance of heightened communication and verifications of preoperative calculations of lens style and power ordered, and documentation as a written order. It is recommended that the surgeon have some form of written documentation regarding the case specifics and IOL specifications (white board or copy of operative plan taped to microscope) available to view when scrubbed, gowned, and seated at the surgical microscope (Ronge, 2013).

Posterior chamber lenses (PCLs) can be implanted only when the cataract was removed by ECCE. Placement behind the iris in the bag or in the sulcus is the most physiologic position for an artificial lens (posterior chamber lens) and is the most common method. Anterior chamber lenses (ACLs), placed in front of the iris, are used in the absence of capsular support, including after vitreous loss or ICCE and for secondary lens implantation (when the cataract was previously removed without lens replacement).

FIGURE 18-16 The intraocular lens (IOL) is folded into the injector by the scrub person, handed to the surgeon, and the surgeon places the folded IOL into the capsular bag. In some instances the haptics need to be adjusted with a Sinskey hook to line up the refraction.

Procedural Considerations. Preoperative dilating drops, both sympathetic agonists (phenylephrine) and parasympathetic antagonists (tropicamide, cyclopentolate, atropine, homatropine), are instilled at prescribed intervals in the preoperative area. The nurse administers a drop of topical preservative-free tetracaine 0.5% numbing agent into the operative eye before the patient enters the OR. The patient is instructed to keep this eye closed to prevent the cornea from drying. As the patient is being positioned on the OR bed, the nurse administers another drop of tetracaine. During the procedure an intraocular anesthetic solution is usually injected, and can be combined with intracameral epinephrine, lidocaine, and BSS (Epi-Shugarcaine) to help with poorly dilating pupils.

An armrest is positioned on the operative side, and the patient's head and the microscope are adjusted. The patient is instructed to look at the light of the microscope and told where to fixate. If the patient cannot open the eye, a facial nerve block should be considered. If the patient cannot fixate on the light at all, the surgeon may administer a retrobulbar block.

Instrumentation varies with the surgeon's preference but usually includes:

- Phaco handpiece and tip
- Irrigation/aspiration handpiece and tips
- BSS

- Phaco blades (based on surgeon preference)
- Capsule forceps
- Lens manipulators
- Hydrodissection cannula
- Pupil expander: iris retractor or Malyugin ring
- IOL forceps
- Lens positioner hook
- IOL and IOL injector

The nurse also ensures the following are available for unexpected procedures:

- Anterior vitrectomy handpiece
- Beehler forceps to dilate the pupil
- Sutures: 10-0 nylon or 10-0 Vicryl (polyglactin)
- Secondary IOL

Machine settings are specific for each brand of phaco machine and are not interchangeable. Power and vacuum settings, irrigation bottle height, and foot pedal positions are examples of settings that must be adjusted for each machine and for each surgeon. Perioperative nurses should continually consult the instruction manuals for the machines and review the necessary settings to avoid complications or delays. Overall, through teamwork and adequate training and monitoring for competency, the surgical team can optimize technology for safety and efficiency in cataract surgery regardless of the equipment used.

Pressures in the anterior and posterior chambers are generally equal. After the surgeon makes the incision into the anterior chamber, aqueous fluid leaks out. Pressure in the anterior chamber falls below that in the posterior chamber, and vitreous from the back of the eye tries to push forward and could carry other structures with it. To minimize the risk from these pressure gradients, the surgeon injects thick viscoelastics early in the procedure, which do not leak.

The surgeon may choose to make the incision on two different points of the eye. An incision near the limbus, where the cornea meets the sclera, should not have an effect on the postsurgical refraction, where an incision point in clear cornea can purposefully adjust the postsurgical astigmatic refraction.

Operative Procedure

1. The surgeon places an eyelid speculum after draping.
2. A 1-mm stab incision (paracentesis, tiny incision in cornea opposite the main incision) is made at 5 o'clock in the left eye or at 11 o'clock in the right eye into the anterior chamber.
3. Intercameral anesthesia may be inserted: 1 mL of unpreserved lidocaine is slowly injected into the anterior chamber through a 30-gauge cannula using a tuberculin syringe.
4. The surgeon injects viscoelastic material into the anterior chamber to deepen the chamber and widen the pupil.
5. The temporal or superior corneal incision is made with a keratome (diamond gem or single-use blade). Some surgeons may use a caliper to mark the incision width, and may use a second knife to make a vertical cut before the horizontal pass with the keratome (Figure 18-17, A).
6. BSS is continuously sprayed onto the eye to keep the cornea moistened and reduce the risk of dryness during surgery.
7. A capsulotomy and capsulorrhexis are performed with a capsulorrhexis forceps or other surgeon preferred instrument. This step of tearing the capsule in a controlled manner is critical in creating a round, stable opening into the capsular bag (e.g., the saclike structure remaining within the eye after the phaco

FIGURE 18-17 Clear cornea cataract extraction. **A,** A 2.6-mm or smaller incision is made into the cornea. **B,** Manual capsulorrhexis is performed on anterior capsule of lens. **C,** Nucleus of lens is loosened by hydrodissection. **D,** Nucleus of lens is "cracked" into four quadrants and removed with phacoemulsification. **E,** Irrigation and aspiration (I/A) handpiece is used to strip the remaining cortex from the capsule. **F,** Intraocular lens (IOL) is folded. **G,** IOL is placed into the capsular bag.

process) (see Figure 18-17, *B*). The IOL is placed within this structure).

8. Using a 30-gauge cannula and BSS solution, the surgeon performs hydrodissection (and sometimes hydrodelineation) to separate the center/nucleus from the capsule and maneuver the lens within the capsule (see Figure 18-17, *C*).
9. The surgeon uses a phaco tip to sculpt the nucleus with ultrasound vibration.
10. A second supporting instrument is inserted through the left-handed paracentesis incision to help rotate and divide the cataractous nucleus into quadrants (see Figure 18-17, *D*).
11. Cataractous nucleus removal usually proceeds in two phases: nuclear sculpting, wherein the nucleus is cracked or sculpted into smaller fragments, and quadrantic emulsification of those fragments. If the cataract is too hard to emulsify, the surgeon can express the nucleus the lens manually. This is known as non-phaco ECCE.
12. After removing the lens nucleus, the surgeon places an I/A tip into the eye and uses it to remove the remaining cortical material (see Figure 18-17, *E*). This combination of irrigation and aspiration is intended to maintain equilibrium within the eye. Removing the cortex minimizes postoperative inflammation.
13. The surgeon may polish the posterior capsule or aspirate anterior lens epithelial cells with a burred instrument.
14. The surgeon injects viscoelastic material to inflate the anterior chamber and capsular bag.
15. A posterior chamber IOL is carefully folded into the injector by the scrub person (following manufacturer's loading guidelines), passed to the surgeon, and placed into the eye by unfolding the

capsular bag (see Figure 18-17, *F* and *G*). The IOL is centrally positioned with a Sinskey hook or the I/A tip. The surgeon may need to widen the corneal incision before placing the IOL.

16. The surgeon uses the I/A tip to remove any remaining viscoelastic material to let the eye pressures stabilize. Leaking of the wound may be controlled or prevented by hydrating the wound edges. Occasionally a 10-0 nylon suture is necessary for diabetic, elderly, or extremely active patients or dense cataract removals.

17. Topical antibiotics or combination antibiotic-corticosteroid ointment or drops are placed on the eye. A shield is applied to prevent dust and debris from entering the surgery site and to prevent the patient from touching the eye.

Anterior Segment Vitrectomy

The main indications for vitrectomy in the anterior segment are as follows:

- Vitreous loss during cataract extraction
- Opacities in the anterior segment
- Complications associated with vitreous in the anterior chamber
- Miscellaneous causes, such as hyphema, pupillary membranes, and residual soft lens material

Procedural Considerations. The procedure varies according to the surgeon's preference. A pathologic condition in the anterior segment can be approached through a limbal incision, as in lens extraction with vitreous loss, or through an open sky approach, after trephine incision for penetrating keratoplasty. Most phaco equipment has a vitrector that can be quickly attached if needed.

Operative Procedure
Anterior Vitrectomy for Vitreous Loss During Cataract Extraction

1. The surgeon introduces the vitreous cutter into the eye through the cataract wound. Saline infusion may be through the handpiece or a separate cannula with infusion line.
2. The cutter is placed in the middle of the pupil, posterior to the iris, and enough vitreous is removed to ensure that no vitreous remains in the anterior chamber and that the iris has fallen back into its normal position.
3. The pupil is constricted with acetylcholine chloride intraocular solution. The anterior chamber may be re-formed with BSS.
4. The procedure is completed as for a lens extraction.

Anterior Vitrectomy for Anterior Segment Opacities, Hyphema, Pupillary Membranes, and Residual Soft Lens Material

1. Appropriate fixation sutures or a lid speculum is placed.
2. The surgeon makes an incision at the limbus either through clear cornea or under a conjunctival flap. One to three incisions are made, depending on the vitreous cutter chosen and the technique.
3. If a multifunction probe is not used, the surgeon places an infusion cannula into one incision and the vitreous cutter into another incision. A third incision may be used for an accessory instrument. The vitreous, blood, or other material is removed.
4. The surgeon closes the incisions and patches the eye.

Surgery of the Retina

Vitreoretinal Surgery

Vitreous fluid fills about two thirds of the eye, helps keep the round shape of the eyeball, and is originally attached to the retina. The vitreous slowly liquefies, atrophies, and shrinks as we age. The vitreous then can become stringy, and shadows can be cast onto the retina, causing "floaters" ("cobwebs" or specks that float in the field of vision). They may look like spots, threadlike strands, or squiggly lines. Floaters are more noticeable when looking at bright objects, such as a white piece of paper. Floaters are more common in patients who have diabetes, have undergone cataract surgery, or are nearsighted. Over time the floaters usually settle below the line of sight but do not completely disappear. Floaters in and of themselves generally do not require treatment. However, if a patient experiences a sudden increase in the number of floaters, retinal examination is warranted to rule out a retinal tear, break, or hole (NEI, 2012b).

The retina, the light-sensitive layer of tissue lining the eye, sends visual signals via the optic nerve to the brain. Attached to the retina are millions of fine fibers intertwined with the vitreous. The shrinking vitreous in an aging eye causes the fine fibers to pull on the retinal surface. When the fibers break the vitreous separates and shrinks from the retina, causing traction on the retina. Normally the vitreous detaches from the retina (a posterior vitreous detachment). However, sometimes the vitreous can create traction on the retina and pull a piece of the retina with it, creating a retinal tear. Fluid can then leak under the retina into the subretinal space, leading to a retinal detachment; symptomatic breaks (manifested as new floating objects or flashing lights) are likely to progress to a retinal detachment (Patient and Family Education).

Posterior vitreous detachments (PVDs) are usually not sight threatening and, like floaters, typically do not require treatment. Patients at risk for the development of PVD are those who are

---

PATIENT AND FAMILY EDUCATION

Discharge Instructions and Home Care After Retina Surgery

- The patient's main issues at home postoperatively are pain management, positioning, using postop drops, and coping with visual impairment.
- For small-incision vitrectomy, pain control is generally not a problem. Patients are generally comfortable and using acetaminophen and a cold compress to increase comfort.
- With more extensive vitrectomy or scleral buckle surgery, additional pain management is needed. Scleral buckle patients generally need a long-acting periocular anesthetic to help with the first 6 to 8 hours. After that, prescription doses of nonsteroidal antiinflammatory medications or narcotics are helpful. Ice compresses help considerably as well as postoperative cycloplegic drops by preventing ciliary spasm.
- Positioning after retinal detachment repair, or macular hole repair is important. Perioperative nurses can help by starting the positioning during the most crucial first few hours. The nurse should review with the patient how to position him- or herself and provide tips for doing so comfortably.
- Proper usage of drops can be a challenge for some patients, especially those with considerable lid and conjunctival swelling from surgery. Demonstrating tips for instilling the drops is helpful.
- Many retinal patients, even those with an excellent visual prognosis, have to cope with temporary visual impairment. Many patients have gas in the vitreous, leaving the operated eye severely limited visually. Educating the patient and ensuring adequate assistance at home is key.

nearsighted and more than 50 years of age, although the condition is very common after age 80. Again, it may not be noticeable but will simply be annoying because of an increase in floaters. A small but sudden increase in new floaters is a symptom of vitreous detachment. Flashes of light in side vision may also occur (NEI, 2012b).

Occasionally some of the vitreous fibers pull so hard on the retina that it causes a retinal detachment (RD)—the sensory retina (neural layer) is separated from the underlying retinal pigment epithelium layer. A sudden increase in floaters or flashing lights (a result of traction on the retina) is a cardinal symptom of RD and an indication for evaluation by a retina specialist as soon as possible. The dilated eye examination is the only way to diagnose the exact cause of the vision problem; potentially, permanent loss of vision can occur without timely treatment (NEI, 2012c).

An additional symptom of retinal detachment is the appearance of a "curtain" in the field of vision, from above, below, or the side. Retinal detachment generally occurs because of retinal tears or holes associated with injury, degeneration, or vitreous contraction. Other much less common causes include inflammation, retinal vascular problems, or even tumors of the retina and choroid. Patients who have previously had cataract surgery are at higher risk for retinal detachment. Males are more likely to develop RD than females, and the condition is more common in people older than 40 years (NEI, 2012c). Other risk factors include history of nearsightedness or retinal detachment in the other eye, family history of RD, presence of lattice degeneration (thinning of the retina in nearsighted people), and occurrence of an eye injury.

Other retinal diseases can produce changes that require vitreoretinal surgery. These generally include conditions that impair the ability of light to reach the retina (i.e., obstruction of the visual axis), or cause traction on the retina, produce fluid accumulation (i.e., exudation), leading to swelling within or under the retina. Occasionally surgery is performed for diagnostic reasons, to deliver medication in a targeted fashion, or to relieve intractable inflammation.

Microvascular disease is related to the eye's vulnerability as a result of its dense network of capillary vessels. Diabetes leads to retinal changes (diabetic retinopathy). The presence of diabetes for more than 15 years significantly increases the likelihood of developing some form of retinopathy, typically bilaterally. However, the severity may be different between eyes. Retinopathy is classified in either of the following ways:

- *Background, or nonproliferative:* In this form of retinopathy disease is confined to the retinal surface. Retinal capillary walls develop microaneurysms (bulges) that can lead to leakage and the development of exudates within the retina. Hemorrhages occur within the retina and are reabsorbed. Capillary membrane changes result in blocked capillaries and thereby retinal ischemia. Eventually deterioration progresses to the next stage.
- *Proliferative:* Neovascularization, or the formation of new retinal blood vessels, can develop within the retina in an attempt to relieve ischemic anoxia secondary to microvascular damage caused by diabetes. These new vessels are fragile and can rupture spontaneously, causing bleeding, and they are very permeable, causing leakage. Hemorrhage into the retina or vitreous can consequently ensue, leading to severe visual loss (Figure 18-18).

Neovascularization can develop into scar tissue that can produce traction, which may distort or even detach the retina. In retinal detachment, pigment or blood cells are freed in the vitreous, causing flashes and floaters. Fluid from the vitreous cavity can seep through the retinal tears into the subretinal space and progressively detach

FIGURE 18-18 **A,** Proliferative retinopathy, an advanced form of diabetic retinopathy, occurs when abnormal new blood vessels and scar tissue form on the surface of the retina. **B,** Fundus photo showing scatter laser surgery for diabetic retinopathy.

the retina. The part of the retina that has separated from its nutritional source becomes damaged and relatively nonfunctional. On occasion inflammatory or scar tissue can develop on the retinal surface, leading to an epiretinal membrane that can distort vision. As the inflammatory or scar tissue, which is firmly attached to the retina, contracts, the retina can wrinkle or "pucker." When the wrinkle is over the area of the macula, the central vision becomes blurred and distorted.

In the same manner, as the shrinking vitreous pulls the retina, peripherally causing tears and detachment, vitreous traction centrally can produce problems. When the macula is affected, it is more serious because of the effect on central vision, and is called a macular hole. Both macular pucker and macular hole have the same symptoms—distorted, blurred vision (NEI, 2012d). Additionally, a macular hole may present with distortion of straight lines and difficulty reading. Vision ranges from 20/25 to 20/400 (the latter for untreated macular hole). Fifty percent of very early macular holes close on their own.

Various types of retinal detachment are as follows:
- *Rhegmatogenous:* This is the most common type. Fluid exudate from a tear or break in the retina leaks under the retina, separating it from the retinal pigment epithelium (RPE).
- *Tractional:* This form of retinal detachment is often secondary to diabetic retinopathy, especially if untreated. The retina also

separates from the RPE, but it is attributable to the contraction of scar tissue on the retina's surface.

- *Exudative or serous:* In inflammatory retinal disease or trauma, fluid exudate leaks under the retina. In this type, however, there are no breaks or tears in the retina.

Location of the pathology on the retina affects visual symptoms. Macular pucker, for example (also called epiretinal membrane, pre-retinal membrane, retina wrinkle, or internal limiting membrane disease), generally affects the macula, located in the center of the retina. The macula normally provides sharp, central vision needed for reading, driving, and fine detail work, and when puckered can cause blurred, distorted central vision.

Various modalities for surgical treatment include laser treatments, scleral buckling, vitrectomy, and retinopexy. In addition to any of these therapies, freeze treatment (cryopexy) may be performed in the surgeon's office for small holes and tears to help "weld" and reattach the retina (NEI, 2012d).

Laser Treatment in Diabetic Retinopathy

Laser energy is used to apply burns to peripheral retinal tissue to help neovascularization regress. The pathophysiologic mechanism for regression of neovascularization is not completely understood, but is thought to occur as a result of the reduced retinal oxygen requirement as a result of the scarred retinal tissue. This method of eliminating abnormal vascularization is called panretinal photocoagulation (PRP). Again, in principle, early diagnosis and control of blood glucose levels are paramount, because laser treatment does indeed partially destroy the retina in order to help arrest neovascularization. Thus, surgeons use the laser before excess damage occurs, electrocoagulating minute hypoxic areas to prevent the new vessels from forming (Phillips, 2012). Laser treatments may begin in an office setting or later within the OR in conjunction with surgeries. The laser may be applied through the slit lamp, with the indirect ophthalmoscope, or directly during vitrectomy surgery using an intraocular endolaser probe (see Figure 18-18).

Vitrectomy

Vitrectomy is narrowly defined as removal of all or part of the vitreous gel (body). In the broader clinical sense of the term, vitrectomy surgery can also include the excision and removal of fibrotic membranes, removal of epiretinal membranes, and electrocoagulation of bleeding vessels. In its normal state the vitreous gel of the eye is transparent. In certain disease states, bleeding from damaged or newly formed vessels may cause the vitreous to become opaque, which may severely decrease vision. In addition to the patient's inability to see, the surgeon is unable to visualize the retina and therefore treat the underlying pathologic condition before permanent damage can occur. In these cases vitrectomy surgery is indicated to restore the patient's vision and to allow the surgeon to institute treatment if indicated.

Formation of membranes may block the visual axis and cause decreased vision. Contraction of these membranes may produce traction-type or rhegmatogenous retinal detachment. In these cases vitrectomy surgery is indicated to relieve the underlying pathologic processes leading to decreased vision.

Posterior Segment Vitrectomy. A pathologic condition in the posterior segment is usually approached through the pars plana, which is tissue that is anterior to the anterior attachment of the retina, typically located 3 to 4 mm from the limbus (corneoscleral junction). Because the pars plana has no retinal tissue, entry at this site

poses little risk for retinal detachment. The main indications for posterior segment vitrectomy through the pars plana are as follows:

- Long-standing vitreous opacities
- Advanced diabetic eye disease
- Severe intraocular trauma
- Retained foreign bodies
- Proliferative vitreoretinopathy
- Retinal detachment from giant tears
- Endophthalmitis
- Diagnostic vitreous biopsy

Essentially, vitrectomy vacuums any pooled blood to enhance clarity. Complications of vitrectomy include retinal detachment, retinal tears, cataract, and infection. Of course, the risk of no treatment can be total loss of vision.

Procedural Considerations. Vitrectomy of the posterior segment is a microsurgical procedure requiring a viewing system (e.g., operating microscope with an X-Y coupling, zoom lens, and fine focus), contact lens system or noncontact wide-angle viewing system (e.g., Biom), an illumination system, a cutting-suction-infusion system, and accessory instruments (Figure 18-19).

The surgeon can hold the contact lens in place by hand or can suture it for stabilization. Another option to a sew-on lens is the use of a noncontact panoramic wide-angle viewing system. This system allows a wide, noncontact view of the macula and is mounted to the microscope and swings out of the way for extraocular phases of the vitrectomy. Other advantages are that it provides a good view under air, eliminates the time needed to sew on a lens, and does not require an assistant to hold the lens. The eye may be rotated freely to view the extreme periphery. The image is inverted by a manual knob, foot pedal, or hand control.

The infusion system consists of a 500-mL bottle of buffered BSS (such as BSS Plus or Endosol Extra), a standard IV administration set, and an infusion needle or sleeve. The level of intraocular pressure can be varied by elevating or lowering the infusion bottle in relation to the patient's eye and by adjusting the digital readout of the nitrogen gas–forced infusion.

The suction and cutting systems vary in sophistication and technology. All cutters engage tissue into a port and then cut it by the shearing action between the edges of a moving and a nonmoving part. Guillotine cutters have a linear back-and-forth action, whereas reciprocating or oscillating cutters rotate in a clockwise-counterclockwise fashion. Suction is operated with a pump controlled by a foot switch to maintain the level of aspiration. The cutter may be part of a single-use multifunction handpiece.

An endolaser or indirect laser delivery system is usually available for photocoagulation. Illumination for vitrectomy is *external,* using the operating microscope for anterior segment vitrectomy; and *internal,* using a fiberoptic light pipe (endoilluminator) for posterior segment vitrectomy. A special light pipe (cannonball) that illuminates a wider area is needed if a wide-angle viewing system is used on the microscope.

Replacement of the vitreous with air is facilitated with a special air-exchange unit that may be incorporated into the multifunction vitrectomy machine. Other substances for intraocular tamponade are liquid perfluorocarbons, silicone oil, perfluoropropane gas (C_3F_8), and sulfur hexafluoride gas (SF_6).

Several accessory instruments may be used for pars plana vitrectomy, depending on the extent of the procedure. Microhooks, picks, and subretinal forceps and scissors are used for dissection, peeling, and removing membranes (Figure 18-20). These instruments can be manually operated with a thumb control or run with compressed

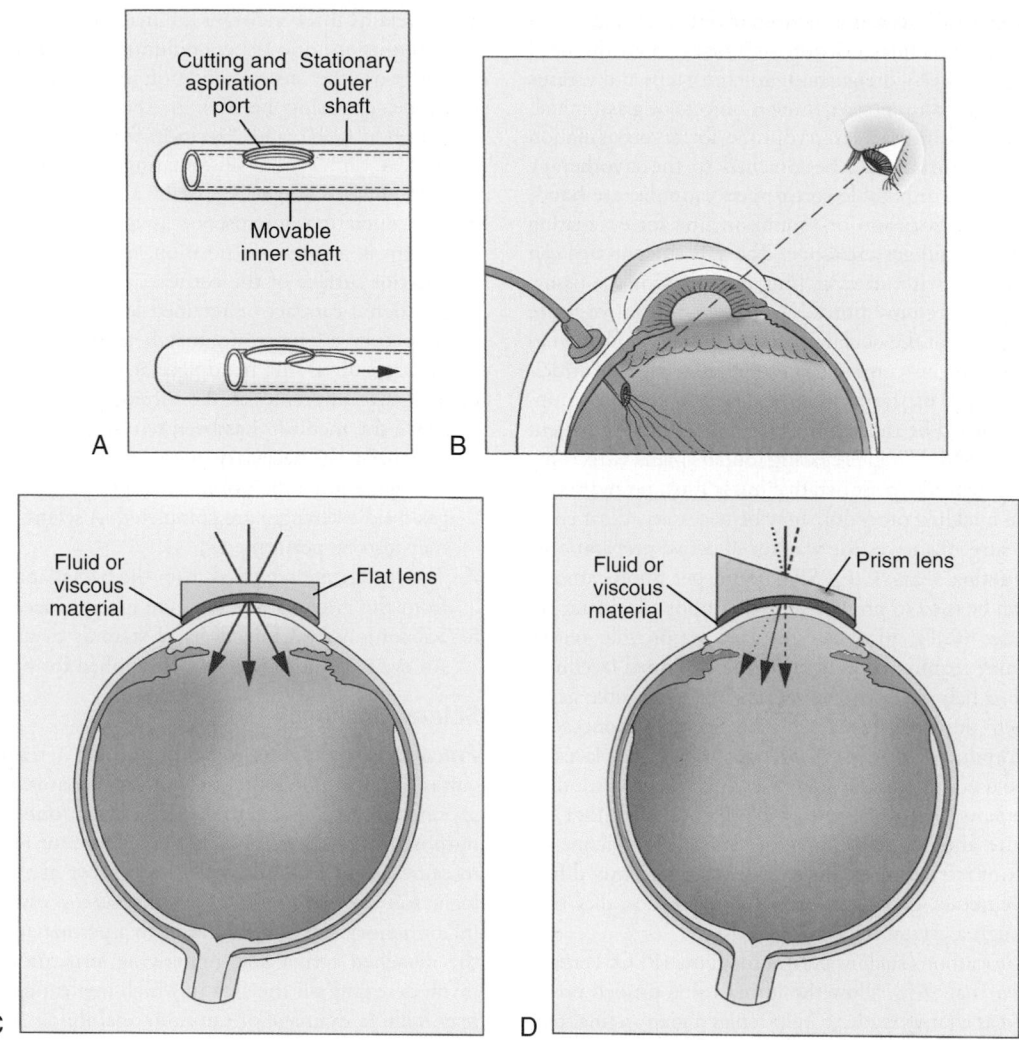

FIGURE 18-19 Essential components for vitrectomy. **A,** Vitrector probe with its cutting/aspirating port close to the tip of the intraocular portion of the handpiece. **B,** Infusion cannula, placed in pars plana, is viewed for correct position. **C,** Flat contact lens, resting on cushion of fluid or viscoelastic material on the cornea, is used for viewing posterior half of the vitreous cavity and retina. **D,** Prism contact lens used for viewing anterior structures in the vitreous cavity.

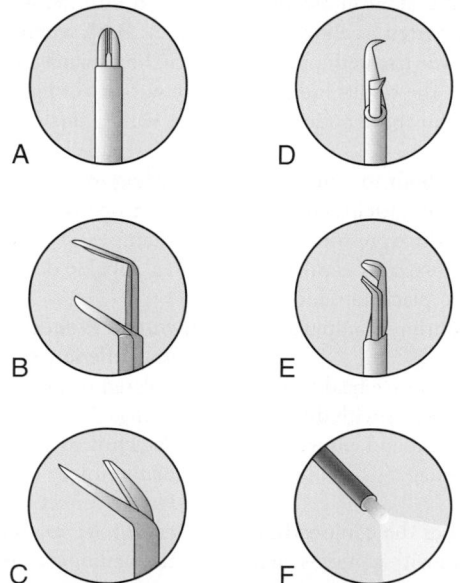

FIGURE 18-20 Tips of microinstruments used in vitrectomy procedures. **A** and **B,** Peeling forceps. **C,** Horizontal scissors. **D,** Vertical scissors. **E,** Membrane peeler and cutter (MPC). **F,** Lighted pick.

air from the automated vitrectomy console. Even smaller 23- and 25-gauge trocars allow for finer instrumentation without the need for suturing the trocar sites. Foreign-body microforceps and various magnetic devices are used to retrieve foreign objects of glass, metal, or other substances. An intraocular cryoprobe for cryocoagulation directly on the retina surface can be attached to the cryotherapy device. Flute needles or disposable soft-tipped cannulae are hand-held or attached to an extrusion or aspiration line for evacuating pools of blood or for fluid-gas exchange. The soft silicone tips can come close to the retina without scratching or damaging the tissue.

To prepare for a vitrectomy procedure, the perioperative nurse must know the location of the ocular problem, the surgeon's plan to address the problem, the instrumentation to be used, and the anticipated extent and length of the procedure. Instrument and equipment functioning should be thoroughly checked before the patient is transferred into the OR. When preparing for pars plana vitrectomy in the posterior segment, the perioperative nurse must be aware that a combined scleral buckling procedure may be necessary. Clear communication with surgeons paves the way for effective preparations.

In the case of retinal tears, C_3F_8, SF_6, liquid per fluorocarbons, and silicone oil can be used to provide retinal tamponade. Intraocular expansible gases (C_3F_8, SF_6) can be used to provide retinal tamponade, but may require the patient to be positioned facedown for several weeks to help reattach the retina. The expansible gas is slowly absorbed by the body (over a period up to 3 months) as aqueous humor produced by the ciliary body slowly displaces it. Silicone oil can be used for complicated cases and when positioning is difficult for patients. The disadvantage of silicone oil is that the patient will require another procedure to remove the silicone oil because the index of refraction of silicone oil is significantly different than that of vitreous, giving patients the impression that they are "looking through a crystal ball."

Liquid perfluorocarbons such as perfluorooctane (PFO; Perfluoron), being heavier than BSS, allow the retina to be pushed posteriorly and are used as a tamponade to help repair a giant retinal tear. The liquid is then removed from the posterior segment. Silicone oil is a highly viscous oil with a high surface tension that mechanically limits fibrovascular proliferation. The oil may be left in place, but it is recommended that it be removed within 1 year if the retina is reattached and stable. Silicone oil may cause increased intraocular pressure and secondary glaucoma. The NEI supported a nationwide clinical trial comparing treatment of proliferative vitreoretinopathy with silicone oil or long-acting intraocular gas. The results indicate that either treatment is effective and surgeons thus have options in treating such cases (NEI, 2012d).

Vitrectomy procedures vary from less than 1 hour to more than 3 hours (Figure 18-21). When a long procedure is anticipated, care must be taken to protect the patient's skin and reduce pressure areas. A foam mattress pad, heel and elbow protectors, and elasticized stockings may be used. A wrist support may be placed around the patient's head to support the surgeon's wrist during manipulation of the intraocular instruments.

Because of the amount of fluid used in the operative field during this procedure the perioperative nurse carefully assists with draping to allow for removal of infusion fluid from the field and ensures the electric foot pedals are protected from fluid damage.

Operative Procedure

1. The surgeon places a lid speculum and incises the conjunctiva.
2. The surgeon sutures the infusion line in place with a purse-string suture (for 20-gauge surgeries) and checks it for proper placement.

3. Generally, three incisions are made through the pars plana: one for infusion, one for endoillumination, and one for a vitreous cutter or other instrumentation (e.g., pick, forceps, scissors, laser probe, extrusion needle). In the right eye these incisions are placed at 8, 10, and 2 o'clock; for the left eye, this corresponds to 2, 4, and 10. An illuminating chandelier can also be placed for bimanual surgery, typically at the 6 o'clock position.
4. The operating microscope is aligned. A wide-angle viewing system is swung into position, or a fundus lens is fixed on the anterior surface of the cornea.
5. If a dense cataract or retained lens material blocks the view of the retina, a lensectomy may be performed with a Fragmatome or other ultrasonic handpiece at this time.
6. The surgeon removes the vitreous under direct visualization. Once the medium has been removed and the retinal condition visualized, the necessary injections or treatments (endolaser photocoagulation, repair of macular pucker, insertion of silicone oil, gas-fluid exchange) are completed. A scleral buckling procedure may also be performed.
7. The trocars are removed from the pars plana incisions. Cultures from the vitreous washings are taken if necessary.
8. Subconjunctival injections of steroids or antibiotics are given. An eye pad and shield may be applied for protection of the eye.

Scleral Buckling

Procedural Considerations. In treating retinal detachment, the aim is to return the retina to its normal anatomic position. For this specific procedure, repair is done from outside the globe. The purpose of the scleral buckling procedure for retinal detachment is to cause an intrusion or push into the eye at the site of the pathologic source. Treatment by diathermy or cryotherapy causes an inflammatory reaction that leads to a permanent adhesion between the detached retina and underlying structures. The surgery also involves sealing off the area in which the tear or hole is located and may include drainage of the subretinal fluid.

The procedure may be performed using general anesthesia or monitored anesthesia care (MAC) with local blocks. The scleral buckling may be done using episcleral (working outside of the sclera) technique or by scleral dissection (making a partial-thickness incision into the sclera and creating flaps to expose the underlying tissue). Both techniques may include drainage of subretinal fluid, encircling bands, diathermy, light coagulation, or cryotherapy. Cryosurgery or light coagulation may be used alone or in combination with a buckling procedure. A detailed drawing of the retina may be made before surgery and is displayed in the operating suite according to surgeon preference. On the basis of this drawing, the surgeon opens the conjunctiva to a previously determined extent, for example, 90 degrees for a simple horseshoe tear or 360 degrees for an aphakic detachment.

Operative Procedure (Figure 18-22)

1. The inferior, superior, lateral, and medial rectus muscles are isolated using 0 silk ties as traction sutures.
2. Using the indirect ophthalmoscope, the surgeon locates the detachment and tear and marks the site with nonpenetrating diathermy by indentation or with a methylene blue marking pen.
3. Under direct visualization the surgeon applies the retinal cryoprobe to the external surface of the globe in the area of the pathologic condition and treats the area. An ice ball is seen to form in the proper areas until the entire lesion has been treated.

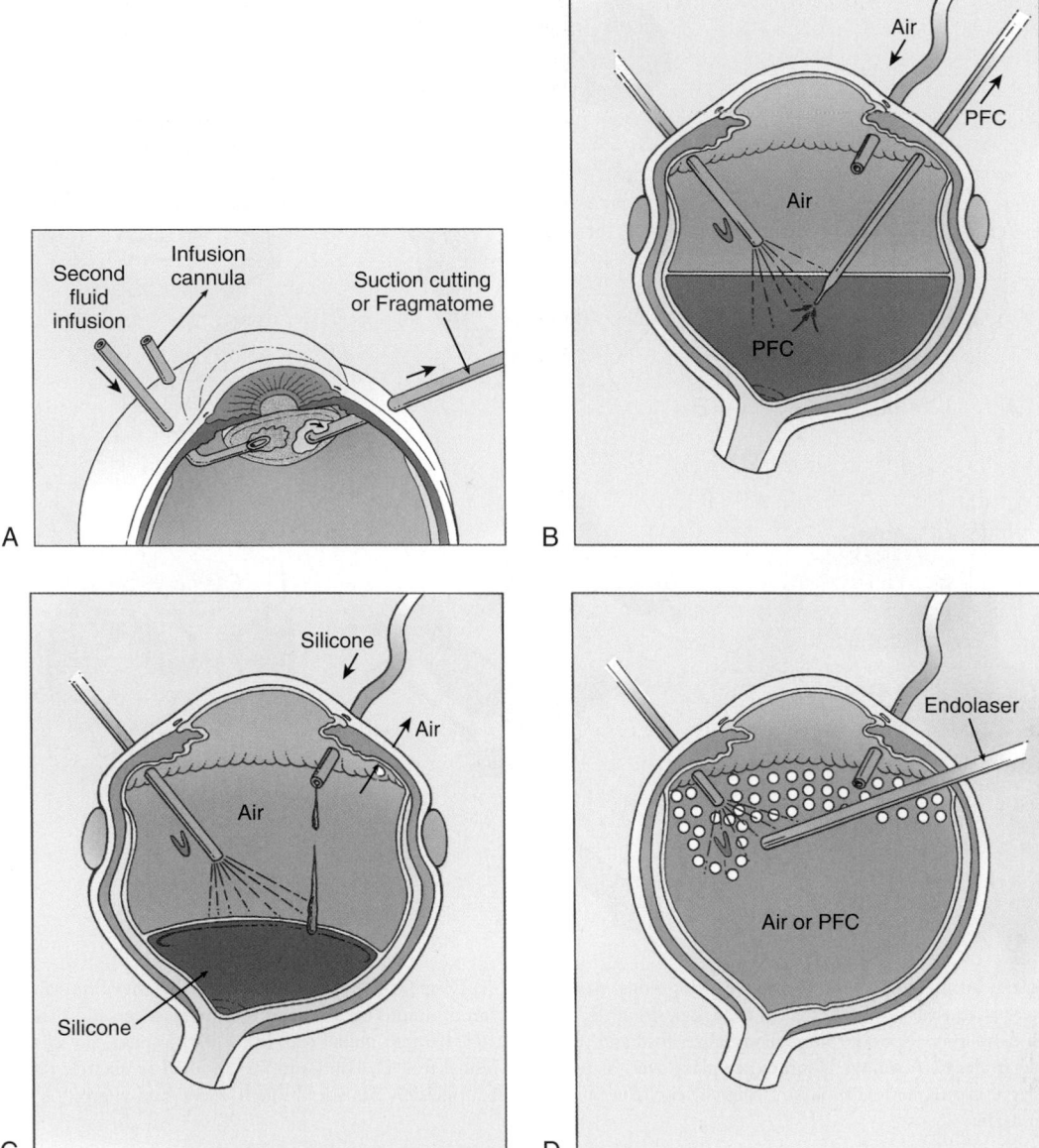

FIGURE 18-21 Procedures done with vitrectomy. **A,** Pars plana lensectomy performed with a second infusion line. **B,** Air/perfluorocarbon (PFC) exchange. The PFC has been placed in the vitreous cavity for removal of subretinal fluid and anatomic reattachment of the retina. Air under positive pressure is then placed through the infusion cannula as the PFC is simultaneously extruded through the tapered needle. **C,** Silicone/air exchange. Silicone is inserted through the infusion cannula as a temporary intraocular tamponade. Silicone is heavier than air and fills the globe from the bottom up, and the air escapes through the sclerotomy site. In silicone/fluid exchange, the silicone floats on the fluid and the fluid is removed with an extrusion needle. **D,** Endolaser photocoagulation is performed after the retina is returned to its normal position.

4. The buckling component of the procedure secures silicone bands, sponges, plates, or tires to the sclera. The surgeon places nonabsorbable sutures (4-0 or 5-0) into the sclera surrounding the lesion and ties them over the silicone sponge, causing the outer shell of the eye to be pushed toward the elevated retina.

5. If an encircling band is to be used, the surgeon places mattress sutures into the sclera in four quadrants. A silicone band is passed 360 degrees around the eye under the sutures and the rectus muscles. The sutures are tied, and a self-holding Watzke sleeve is applied to the band to maintain a predetermined circumference. This causes a 360-degree constriction of the outer coats into the eye.

6. If drainage of subretinal fluid is desired, the surgeon chooses an area under direct visualization in which a significant fluid level exists under the retina, and places a diathermy mark on the sclera. The sclera is split to the choroid, and a small amount of diathermy is applied to the choroid bed. A 27-gauge ½-inch needle is then used to puncture the choroid into the subretinal space to permit fluid drainage.

FIGURE 18-22 Scleral buckling operation for treatment of retinal detachment. **A,** Diagram of retina showing detachment of retina of temporal half of left eye, with retinal tear at equator of globe at 1:30 o'clock position. **B,** Examination of fundus by means of ophthalmoscope and handheld lens and depression of sclera with diathermy electrode. Surgeon visualizes field and places electrode beneath retinal tear; burn mark is made on sclera at site of retinal tear with diathermy electrode. **C,** A sponge is sutured in place over treated site of retinal tear. **D,** Band and tire are used to encircle the eye. **E,** Placement of Watzke silicone sleeve is one method to secure edges of encircling band. **F,** Small incision is made through sclera, and choroid is finely incised to allow subretinal fluid to drain.

7. Air or replacement fluids may be introduced into the eye after draining the subretinal fluid. This is usually done through the pars plana under direct visualization.

8. The surgeon removes the traction sutures from around the muscles and closes the conjunctiva with 7-0 absorbable suture. A subconjunctival injection of an antibiotic, steroid, or both may be given, and an eye pad is applied.

Retinopexy

In pneumatic retinopexy an intraocular injection of an air bubble or therapeutic gases provides pressure against retinal breaks, allowing the detached retina breaks to approximate the pigment epithelium. Retinopexy may be used in combination with scleral buckling and posterior vitrectomy; it may be performed as part of an ambulatory procedure for treatment of certain retinal detachments, using laser photocoagulation with injection of the gas bubble followed by specific postoperative positioning. The gases are drawn through a Millipore 0.22-μm filter and may be mixed with filtered air so that the concentration may be varied. The gas bubble is a ratio mixture of gas and air. The higher the concentration of gas to air, the longer the bubble remains in the eye before being "absorbed." Patient positioning after retinopexy is often facedown for several days to weeks but may include tilting the head to one side or the other as well. The head position is determined by the location of the retinal tear or hole. For example, if the retinal tear or hole is located superior temporal in the right eye, the patient would be instructed to tilt the head down and to the left, so the bubble will float upward and to the right where the tear or hole is located. The larger the tear or hole, the longer the bubble needs to be in contact with the area to be reattached (Figure 18-23).

SF_6 is a colorless, odorless, and nontoxic gas. It increases 2.5 times in volume within 48 hours after injection by drawing other gases, specifically nitrogen and oxygen, from the surrounding tissues. SF_6 bubbles remain for at least 10 days.

FIGURE 18-23 Pneumatic retinopexy. **A,** Gas bubble is injected through the pars plana. **B** and **C,** The bubble closes and supports the retinal break. After a 7- to 10-day healing period and when the retina is returned to normal position, laser surgery or cryotherapy can be performed to seal the break.

C_3F_8 is a colorless, odorless, and nontoxic gas. It quadruples its volume within 48 hours after injection. A 1-mm bubble can remain up to 30 to 50 days.

Because SF_6 and C_3F_8 are expansible gases, certain precautions are required. Patients are given a wristband to wear that states what kind of gas bubble is in their eye and when it was instilled. If they require surgery, they need to alert the anesthesia provider of the presence of the gas bubble. The intent of instilling a gas bubble is to sustain its size and hold the retina in place. SF_6 and C_3F_8 are inert, very insoluble in water, and poorly diffusible. Because nitrous oxide (N_2O) is 117 times more diffusible than SF_6, it rapidly enters the gas bubble. With continued administration of N_2O, the injected gas bubble can increase to three times its original size. Intraocular pressure (IOP) can increase from 14 to 30 mm Hg; 18 minutes after discontinuation of N_2O, IOP decreases along with the smaller bubble size. Such quick and wide variations in bubble size can negatively affect the surgical outcome. Therefore, N_2O should be discontinued at least 20 minutes before an intravitreal gas injection to ensure stable bubble size and IOP. Some anesthesia providers avoid using N_2O for any case in which intravitreal gas injection is anticipated. Patients are instructed to avoid air travel until the gas bubble is completely resolved or decreased to a level of 5% of the vitreous volume. Cabin pressurization in air travel will cause severe enlargement of the gas bubble with an increase in IOP and eye pain. Car or train travel to high elevations should also be avoided unless the change in altitude is done gradually. N_2O should be avoided so long as there is gas in the eye. The exposure to N_2O could reexpand the bubble, increase IOP, and thereby occlude the retinal artery with loss of vision.

Overall, a great majority of patients with retinal detachment can be successfully treated. This is a great advance considering some of the same conditions were inoperable 40 years ago. Visual outcomes, however, are not always predictable, and additional treatment may be necessary. A successful anatomic result of retinal reattachment unfortunately does not always correlate with improvement in visual function. It may take up to several months to evaluate the final visual result. Occasionally even with the best efforts and multiple attempts at repair, treatment may fail; sight may not be able to be restored. This discussion is part of informed consent. Repairing a detachment before the macula detaches provides the best visual results.

Surgery for Glaucoma

Glaucoma is a group of diseases that include optic neuropathy and associated visual field loss for which elevated IOP is one of the primary risk factors. Glaucoma is caused from a buildup of fluid in the eye, which causes pressure on the optic nerve. This pressure gradually begins to damage a person's peripheral vision with little warning signs, and if left untreated may cause permanent blindness (Figure 18-24). Generally once the loss of peripheral vision occurs from glaucoma it cannot be restored (Patient-Centered Care).

Glaucoma can be treated with pressure-reducing drops and medications, with laser treatments such as Argon laser trabeculectomy (ALT) or selective laser trabeculectomy (SLT) or with surgery. Research continues to look for alternate treatment (Research Highlight).

Iridectomy

Peripheral iridectomy is removal of a section of iris tissue (Figure 18-25). Peripheral iridectomy is usually performed as part of a trabeculectomy procedure or when laser iridotomy is not feasible because of cloudy cornea or uveitis. Peripheral iridectomy is used to treat acute, subacute, or chronic angle-closure glaucoma when extensive peripheral anterior synechiae have not formed. This procedure is performed to reestablish communication between the posterior and anterior chambers, thus relieving pupillary block and permitting the iris root to drop away from the trabecular meshwork to reestablish the outflow of aqueous fluid through Schlemm's canal.

Operative Procedure
1. The speculum is introduced.
2. A small beveled incision is made at the superior limbus, or a perpendicular incision is made in the clear cornea.
3. The surgeon grasps the peripheral iris with forceps, pulls it through the incision, and excises it with a scissors.
4. The iris is repositioned by gently stroking the cornea with a blunt spatula or muscle hook. The iris can also be repositioned by irrigating with BBS.
5. A clear corneal incision is closed with 10-0 nonabsorbable suture, and a limbal incision is closed with an absorbable suture. Intracameral antibiotics may be injected, and an eye pad is applied.

A   Normal vision

B   Cataract

C   Glaucoma

D   Diabetic Retinopathy

FIGURE 18-24 Comparative views with **(A)** normal vision, **(B)** a scene as it might be viewed by a person with cataract, **(C)** a scene as it might be viewed by a person with glaucoma, and **(D)** a scene as it might be viewed by a person with diabetic retinopathy.

PATIENT-CENTERED CARE

Patient-centered care recognizes the obligation to understand and meet patients' expectations, and partnerships between nurses and patients are a cornerstone of patient-centered care. It is especially important to fulfill that obligation in providing care to ophthalmology patients who may be experiencing challenges with visual acuity. Providing patient-centered care is further challenged by the ambulatory nature of most ophthalmic procedures. Nursing theorist Jean Watson states, "Clinical care and health care practices are grounded in human communication, human interactions and relationships. At the same time, approaches to system solutions are often disconnected from relationships and caring."

In the scenario that follows the nurse practices patient-centered care by considering the effect of communication and relationships on the outcomes of his care.

Mr. B. is an energetic 76-year-old African American male with glaucoma in both eyes and a dense cataract in the left eye. Glaucoma has left him blind in the right eye, with some peripheral loss in the left eye. Mr. B. has been married for 45 years and goes to church every Sunday with his wife. She is the main caregiver and holds his hand when they walk to minimize bumping into objects from his decreased visual acuity. He is active in his community and accompanies his wife to her different volunteer activities.

In providing patient-centered communication for Mr. B., the nurse notes, "I see on your consent for today's surgery that you are having a trabeculectomy on the left eye combined with cataract removal and implementation of a lens. Can you tell me in your own words what that means?" She then listens carefully to determine that Mr. B. understands the procedure. An indication that Mr. B. understands might include his response of:

"The doctor tells me that the pressure in my good eye is too high, like a basketball that has too much air in it. She wants to make a release valve so that fluids can drain and stop the high pressure. The doctor also said I have a cataract and she will remove that and put a new lens in at the same time. I might have to keep taking my pressure drops, but I may have to take them less often if the surgery works."

The nurse considers Mr. B.'s preexisting blindness in the right eye and the fact that his left eye will be patched postoperatively, so he will be fully blind during the initial postoperative recovery room visit. He will need constant assistance in navigating the room. Mr. B. will be prone to bumping into objects and falls, so the staff should take all precautions necessary.

Prior to discharge, Mr. B.'s patch will be removed. The perioperative nurse should work with his wife to orient him to the room and those around him. Even with the patch removed the patient's visual acuity will be greatly diminished the first 24 hours and he will continue to require constant care. Mr. B. should have light perception and can count fingers and see blurry images until further healing occurs. The nurse partners with the patient and his wife to ensure they both understand to continue the eyedrop regimen and make sure labels can be seen by the patient. They may need to use a magnifying glass or write larger letters on forms and medicine bottles. The nurse reinforces that Mr. B. will be required to wear the shield while sleeping, so he will not be able to navigate by himself. The nurse may also explore community assistance as part of patient-centered care to assist Mr. B. and his wife through the initial recovery period and challenges associated with partial blindness.

Modified from Frampton SB, Guastello S: Patient-centered care: more than the sum of its parts, Planetree's patient-centered hospital designation program, *AJN* 110:9, 50–53, 2010; Watson J, Frampton SB: Human interaction and relationship-centered caring. In Frampton SB, Charmel PA, editors: *Putting patients first: best practices in patient-centered care*, San Francisco, 2008, Jossey-Bass.

Implantable Telescope FDA Approved to Improve Visual Acuity in Late-Stage Macular Degeneration Patients

Advanced macular degeneration (AMD) is a progressive eye disease that once moderate to severe progressions have occurred there are minimal surgical interventions for the reparation of visual acuity. In the United States more than 60,000 people have central vision loss from the advanced stage of macular degeneration. Although most patients with AMD do not go completely blind, the disease has a devastating effect on quality of life and independence.

A telescope can be monocularly implanted in the capsular bag to magnify the incoming images. AMD causes vision loss in the central field of view. By magnifying incoming images the picture is expanded and displaced to the healthier peripheral retina, where it can then be interpreted by the brain. With the incoming light and visual stimulus projecting on to the healthy parts of the retina, patients can see and recognize objects they would otherwise not be able to see with their natural lens.

The implementation of the telescope is similar to cataract surgery because it is placed in the capsular bag after the lens has been removed. There is increased risk to the cornea because the telescope cannot be folded like an intraocular lens (IOL) and requires a larger 12-mm incision site. Corneal edema and reduced endothelial cell counts postoperatively are risks of the surgery. In the Hudson (2008) study, cell loss mostly occurred within the 3 months after implementations and generally stabilized after 6 to 12 months. Endothelial cell loss was significantly less in the surgeon's fourth case and beyond compared with the first cases, suggesting a learning curve for the surgeon and nurses.

Patients with the implantable telescope saw clinically significant improvement in best correctable visual acuity (BCVA) compared with the control group. The surgery group saw an average of 3 lines of improvement in visual acuity compared to 0.5 line in the control group. After 2 years of follow-up 7.5% of the control group lost 3 lines or more of acuity due to AMD progression, whereas only 0.6% of the telescope group lost visual acuity. The results show that the implantable telescope can provide substantial benefits to the patient with end-stage macular degeneration.

Modified from *Centra Sight Treatment for Advanced Macular Degeneration*, available at www.centrasight.com. Accessed March 17, 2013; Hudson H et al: Implantable telescope for end-stage age related macular degeneration: long term visual acuity and safety outcomes, *Am J Ophthalmol* 146:664–673, 2008.

FIGURE 18-25 Peripheral iridectomy.

Trabeculectomy (Filtration Surgery)

Trabeculectomy is a filtering procedure accomplished by incising a conjunctival flap and a scleral flap, creating a fistula, performing an iridectomy, and creating the filtering bleb. Trabeculectomy is often combined with cataract removal (phacoemulsification) and insertion of an IOL (Figure 18-26).

Procedural Considerations. Adjunctive medical therapy to decrease postoperative fibrosis includes application of an antimetabolite-soaked sponge (5-fluorouracil [5-FU] or mitomycin C) placed under the conjunctival flap. Multiple sponges are used to create diffuse blebs. Because 5-FU and mitomycin C are antimetabolites, nursing precautions for handling hazardous waste must be carried out. The perioperative nurse must wear gloves while drawing up the antimetabolite from the vial to transfer to the operative field. All items used with the medication should be disposed as hazardous waste. Instruments that contact antimetabolites should be washed separately.

Operative Procedure

1. Incisions are made into the conjunctiva and Tenon capsule, dissection is done, and a conjunctival Tenon capsule flap is created. Hemostasis is obtained with bipolar coagulation.
2. If antimetabolite is to be used, the surgeon applies it for 90 seconds to the sclera using multiple sponges before making any incision into the sclera. A small piece of sponge is saturated in the antimetabolite (5-FU or mitomycin C) and placed between the conjunctival Tenon capsule flap and the sclera. The sponge is left in place for 3 to 5 minutes, then the site is irrigated vigorously with copious amounts of BSS.
3. The surgeon creates a square or triangular partial-thickness scleral flap (300 μm).
4. The scleral flap is retracted, and the surgeon makes an incision into and through the limbus into the anterior chamber with the tip of the blade. The limbal incision is extended to a rectangular flap of deep limbal tissue, which is then excised to create the fistula.
5. An iridectomy is performed.
6. The surgeon replaces the scleral flap and closes it with interrupted 10-0 nonabsorbable sutures. The conjunctival Tenon capsule flap is closed with a running suture, and the conjunctiva is closed.
7. BSS is injected through a cannula into the anterior chamber to deepen the anterior chamber and elevate the conjunctival bleb.
8. An eye pad and shield are applied.

Glaucoma Drainage Devices

Several types of drainage devices have been implanted into the posterior subconjunctival space with varying success when filtering procedures have been unsuccessful. These include the Molteno implant, Krupin valve, Ahmed device, Baerveldt device, and Schocket implant. Complications have been reduced through modifications in design and technique (Figure 18-27).

Procedural Considerations. The glaucoma drainage device (GDD) and the pericardium or donor patch may be soaked in an antibiotic solution. The drainage device and graft are documented as implants per facility procedure.

FIGURE 18-26 Trabeculectomy. **A,** Sponge soaked in antimetabolite is placed on sclera and (**B**) held in place for 90 seconds. **C,** Area is thoroughly irrigated. **D,** Scleral flap is formed. **E,** Incision is made into anterior chamber. **F and G,** Fistula is created by removing a flap of limbal tissue.

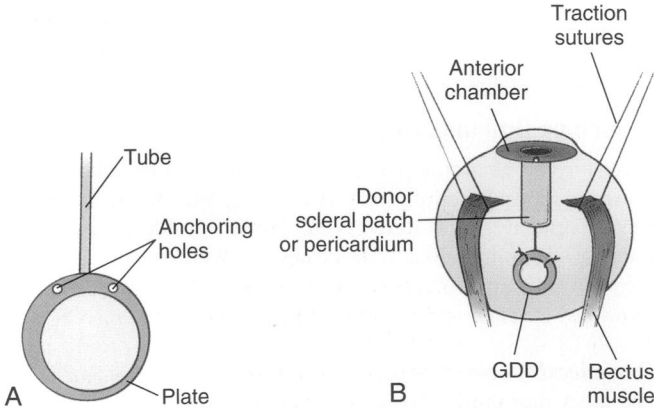

FIGURE 18-27 Glaucoma drainage devices (GDDs). **A,** Components of GDD. **B,** GDD in place. Tip of drainage tube in anterior chamber. Donor scleral patch or pericardium covering tube from plate to edge of cornea.

Operative Procedure

1. The surgeon incises the conjunctiva and exposes the sclera.
2. Two rectus muscles are isolated using silk ties as traction sutures.
3. The surgeon takes measurements for placement of the plate of the device. The plate is then sutured to the sclera.
4. After the patency of the device is checked, the surgeon inserts an occluding suture into the drainage tube.
5. With a needle, a tunnel is created into the anterior chamber for the tube and paracentesis tract.
6. The tube is trimmed and inserted into the anterior chamber. The surgeon sutures the tube to the sclera with 9-0 nonabsorbable suture.
7. The tube is covered with patch graft of donor sclera or pericardium.
8. The occluding suture is passed through the Tenon capsule and the conjunctiva into the inferior cul-de-sac, secured with absorbable suture, and trimmed.

9. The surgeon removes the traction sutures from around the rectus muscles, and closes the conjunctiva with a continuous 7-0 absorbable suture.

10. Antiinfective agents are injected subconjunctivally. The eye is dressed with an eye pad and shield.

Canaloplasty

Canaloplasty is a surgical procedure performed when a small microcatheter is inserted into the eye around the trabecular meshwork. A viscoelastic is injected into the catheter to dilate it; this enlarges the main drainage channel (Schlemm's canal). After the channel is enlarged the catheter is removed and a suture is placed within the channel. The suture is tightened to make sure the channel stays open. Opening the channel allows aqueous to flow out of the eye, thereby reducing the intraocular pressure. The microscope is tilted at a 45-degree angle to enhance visualization (make sure that the microscope is designed to be tilted at this angle) (Dansby-Kelly, 2010).

During this procedure a microscope and bipolar ESU must be used. The instruments include an anterior segment tray, curved Stevens iris scissors, #15 blades, and lamellar or crescent blades. Medications to be used during this procedure are anesthetic eye-drops or injections (per surgeon's or anesthesia provider's preference), BSS, viscoelastic, antibiotic and steroid injection, antibiotic eye ointment, and cycloplegic drops. The surgeon makes a small limbal incision into the anterior chamber, injects a viscoelastic, and passes a small catheter around the trabecular meshwork around Schlemm's canal. Ophthalmic ointment is applied followed by a patch and shield.

Surgery of the Conjunctiva

The conjunctiva is a transparent and elastic membrane that lines the inner surface of the eyelids and covers the sclera. Lacerations caused by injury as well as deficits resulting from excision of tumors, cysts, nevi, or pterygia can usually be repaired by simple undermining and suturing.

Pterygium Excision

A pterygium is a fleshy, triangular encroachment of conjunctiva onto the peripheral area of the cornea. Pterygia occurrence has been linked to increased exposure to ultraviolet light, so it is important to wear polarized sunglasses while outside during the day. Because pterygia tend to recur, surgery is delayed until vision is affected by encroachment on the visual axis, high astigmatism, or irritation.

Operative Procedure. Pterygia surgery can be done under topical, peribulbar, or less commonly retrobulbar anesthesia. A pterygium can also be excised totally and the limbus treated with an eye cautery or bipolar ESU. The sclera is typically covered using a conjunctival autograft or amniotic membrane graft, or less commonly the sclera is left bare (Figure 18-28).

Surgery may be combined with application of the chemotherapeutic agent mitomycin C (typically 0.02 mg/mL) for recurrent cases. In addition, a diamond burr drill may be used to smooth the corneal and limbal surfaces after the removal of tissue. More recently, surgeons have adopted the use of fibrin tissue adhesive in place of sutures for conjunctival grafts or amniotic membranes.

Excisional Biopsy

Any suspect lesion of the conjunctiva can be removed by a simple elliptic excision and sent for pathologic examination. The

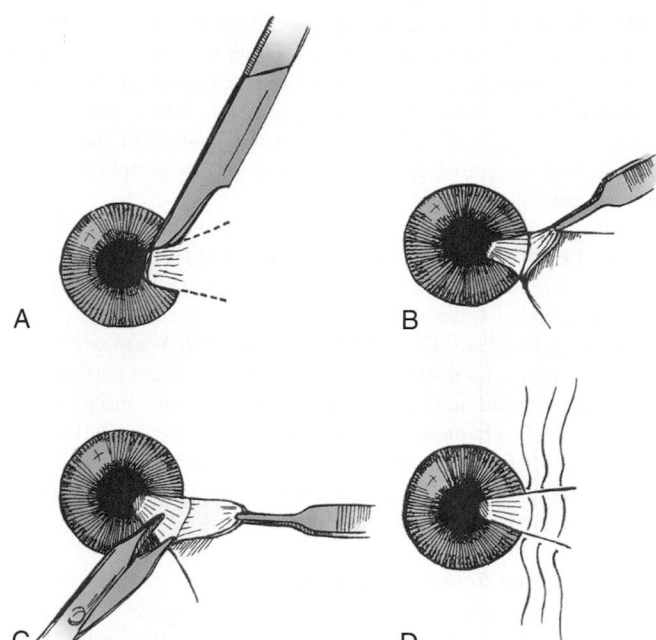

FIGURE 18-28 McReynolds technique for pterygium excision. **A,** Cornea around head of pterygium is incised. **B,** Pterygium flap is dissected upward, leaving clear cornea. **C,** Lower margin of pterygium is dissected, and whole pterygium is freed from sclera. **D,** Sutures are placed for closure of conjunctiva.

conjunctiva may or may not be closed, depending on the surgeon's particular technique.

Surgery of the Cornea

Surgery of the cornea is indicated for a variety of conditions in which cosmetic, therapeutic, restorative, or refractive outcomes are desired.

Repair of Lacerations

Corneal lacerations may be closed with direct appositional suturing with 10-0 suture viewed through an operating microscope or with a tissue adhesive, such as cyanoacrylate monomers. The sterile tissue adhesive is applied to well-dried tissue that has been properly oriented anatomically. It polymerizes and seals the wound on contact with the tissue. Culture specimens are usually obtained at the time of surgery. Antibiotics are injected subconjunctivally before the dressing is applied.

Refractive Corneal Procedures

Keratorefractive procedures are corneal procedures designed to correct myopia, hyperopia, and astigmatism. These procedures require reshaping the cornea to change the refractive power of the eye to reduce or eliminate the need for eyeglasses and contact lenses. The types of corneal refractive surgeries include PRK, LASIK, and custom wavefront guided LASIK. Whereas most refractive procedures are truly surgical, few are performed in traditional hospital or outpatient surgical facilities. However, refractive surgery has been performed for so many years that these same patients who are aging will present themselves for cataract surgery. It is recommended that the perioperative nurse be familiar with this branch of eye surgery.

LASIK Surgery. With the LASIK procedure the curvature of the corneal stroma is reshaped using an excimer laser to ablate certain areas. For nearsighted patients the central curvature of the cornea is flattened by removing stromal tissue from the center of the cornea. For farsighted patients the central curvature of the cornea is steepened by removing stromal tissue from the periphery of the cornea, leaving the center untreated.

Advances in LASIK have allowed surgeons to improve the overall results of LASIK surgery. Wavefront guided LASIK surgery corrects for the lower order aberrations (refractions) as well as the patient's individual higher order aberrations. Custom guided LASIK (Intralase), a U.S. Food and Drug Administration (FDA)–approved femtosecond laser, is used to create the corneal flap. It can perform the cutting more accurately, quicker, and without using a mechanically moving metal keratome. This technology is more precise because the laser reads the patient's eye and uses these findings for calculations. During this precise process, stable eye positioning is paramount for the best results.

Photorefractive Keratectomy (PRK). PRK is a surface ablation technique that involves manual scraping to remove the corneal epithelium and to shape the surface of the cornea with the cool light of the excimer laser. Surface ablation avoids the complications of flap formation in LASIK and provides excellent visual results. A major drawback, however, is delayed visual rehabilitation and pain from the regrowth of corneal epithelium, though it can be controlled with topical and oral therapy. PRK is performed if a patient has thin corneas, previous corneal scarring, or other corneal diseases.

LASEK Surgery. Laser epithelial keratomileusis (LASEK) is similar to PRK because the procedure is performed on the surface of the cornea. After numbing the eye with topical anesthetic drops, the surgeon loosens the epithelium with a diluted alcohol solution and mechanically pushes it aside. A laser is then used to treat the corneal surface, similar to PRK and LASIK procedures. The epithelial flap is then returned to its original position, and a bandage contact lens is placed for the duration of the healing process, which may take several days.

Corneal Transplantation (Keratoplasty)

A corneal transplantation (keratoplasty) is performed when the patient's cornea is thickened or opacified by disease and degeneration. The transparency of the cornea may be impaired as a result of scars, infection (bacterial, fungal, or viral), thermal or chemical burns, corneal dystrophies, edema after intraocular surgery, or keratoconus (abnormal steepening). Corneal transplantation, in which corneal tissue from one human eye is grafted to another, is done to improve vision when the retina and optic nerve are functioning properly; it was first performed in 1905. Because the cornea is tissue that lacks blood vessels, it can be transplanted with less rejection and at a 90% success rate. Corneal transplant is one of the most frequently performed human transplant procedures, with more than 1 million performed since 1961 (Eye Bank Association of America [EBAA], 2011). Lamellar grafts can be used to treat a pathology that is not of full thickness. One type of lamellar surgery, called deep anterior lamellar keratoplasty, is commonly used for patients who have keratoconus or partial-thickness corneal scars. If successful, the corneal stroma and epithelium are able to be replaced while keeping the host endothelium, which decreases the risk of transplant rejection and improves graft stability. Due to the technical difficulty of this procedure, it is common to convert to a full-thickness penetrating procedure. A new technique used for posterior corneal pathology is Descemet stripping endothelial keratoplasty (DSEK). This is used for patients who have Fuchs dystrophy, corneal edema due to intraocular surgery, or failed corneal transplants. It consists of replacing the endothelium without transplanting the entire cornea. It offers improved corneal clarity with less astigmatism, shorter healing times, and less chance of wound dehiscence and rejection. Deep lamellar endothelial keratoplasty (DLEK) is an emerging and evolving technique. It consists of replacing the endothelium without transplanting the full cornea to restore vision. This technique offers the potential for highly predictable corneal power for extended periods without the astigmatism that often occurs with penetrating keratoplasty. The transplanted endothelium is inserted into the host through a small incision, greatly reducing the risk of infection.

Phototherapeutic keratectomy (PTK) procedures use excimer laser ablation to remove superficial corneal lesions and smooth the corneal surface. PTK can be used for conditions that would require corneal transplant and may delay or replace the occurrence of penetrating keratoplasty in some cases.

Procurement of Corneas. Education on eye donation and transplantation is important for all surgical staff so that they understand that ocular tissue is a donated gift. Corneas and scleral grafts are not the same as other implants pulled off the shelf prior to surgery; they are gifts that were given by families as they were grieving the loss of their loved ones and should be treated as such (Drury, 2012).

The eye bank may be a central community agency or may be owned and operated by a hospital. Eye banks help coordinate the procurement of eyes from recently deceased persons under the EBAA guidelines. People of any age can be eye donors, and poor eyesight or cataracts do not influence eye viability (EBAA, 2011). The donor's family, medical, and social histories are reviewed. It is not necessary to perform antigen matching as with other tissue or organ transplants, but blood serum tests for human immunodeficiency virus (HIV) and hepatitis B and C virus are performed on the donor. The procurement team removes donor eyes within 6 hours of death in accordance with legal regulations. Tissue, such as a cornea, must be recovered, processed, and transplanted in controlled surgical environments. If the donor eye is unsuitable for the cornea to be transplanted, the eye can be used for research or education.

Many individuals have signed donor cards or eye-donor designation on their drivers' licenses. A special consent form is required and should be signed by the authorized next of kin and by a hospital representative designated by institutional policy. Federal regulations require hospitals to report all deaths and imminent deaths to organ procurement organizations. With the collaboration of hospitals, organ procurement organizations, and eye and tissue banks, the family of every potential donor is informed about the option to donate organs or tissues.

The enucleations may be done in the hospital morgue or emergency department under aseptic conditions. The procured cornea is placed in Optisol GS sterile buffered tissue culture medium within 12 hours of death and transplanted within 3 to 7 days. Optisol GS sterile buffered tissue culture medium contains polypeptides, dextran, and antibiotics (gentamicin and streptomycin) and can preserve a donor cornea for 14 days under refrigeration. It is best if corneal transplantation is performed in 2 or 3 days because the cornea may become boggy from constant exposure to the tissue culture solution.

Donor Tissue Procurement

Procedural Considerations. Postmortem preparation includes elevating the donor's head with a pillow to minimize edema in the face or near the eye. The eyes are irrigated and lightly taped closed to avoid pressure on the eye. A small ice pack may be applied to the forehead or over the eyes if the donor is not in a refrigerated morgue within 1 hour of death.

For the procurement procedure, the eyes are washed and irrigated in the routine manner of preparation for eye surgery. The sterile field, drapes, and instruments are essentially the same as those for an enucleation on a living patient (see pages 622-624).

Operative Procedure

1. Eye specimen jars are labeled for right and left eyes.
2. The speculum is inserted, and after routine enucleation the donated eye is placed with the cornea up and secured in a metal eye cage or on gauze in the sterile specimen jar.
3. The eye sockets are packed with cotton, and the lids are closed.
4. Specimen jars are sealed with tape and labeled with the donor's name or identification number, time of death, time of enucleation, and date. The jars are placed on crushed ice in an insulated carrier and transported to the eye bank. The entire cornea with a scleral rim is placed in Optisol GS before transplant.

Corneal Transplant

Procedural Considerations. For the transplant procedure the nurse positions and preps the patient in the same fashion as a cataract procedure. Corneal transplant is typically done under local or general anesthesia. For local anesthesia, most surgeons use a retrobulbar or peribulbar block in addition to a facial block. It is very important to have adequate akinesia and anesthesia so the patient cannot squeeze the eyelids after removal of the host corneal button. It is also important for the anesthesia provider to keep the patient comfortable during this crucial step in transplantation. Any posterior pressure during this time can lead to suprachoroidal hemorrhage or expulsion of the intraocular contents. For this reason, many surgeons give mannitol to lower intraocular pressure prior to the surgery (see Surgical Pharmacology).

Operative Procedures

Penetrating Keratoplasty (Figure 18-29)

1. After insertion of a wire lid speculum, the surgeon may place a Flieringa ring or bridle sutures to support the structure of the eye. If a ring is used, the surgeon secures it in place with four 5-0 Dacron sutures.
2. A corneoscleral button that has been refrigerated and stored in Optisol GS is removed from its container.
3. The surgeon places the donor corneoscleral button on a sterile Teflon block with the epithelial (outside) surface down. Using the corneal trephine as a punch, the surgeon presses out the button. A drop of Optisol GS may be used to cover the donor button until it is implanted.
4. Using a handheld trephine or a disposable suction trephine, the surgeon excises a corneoscleral button from the recipient's cornea. The diameter of the cornea removed from the recipient's eye is usually 0.25 mm smaller than the graft taken from the donor's eye.
5. Peripheral iridectomies or iridotomies may be performed at this time at the surgeon's discretion, or a cataract extraction with IOL implantation may also be performed if the lens is opaque.
6. The surgeon places the graft into the opening of the recipient's eye and anchors it in place with four single-armed sutures placed

FIGURE 18-29 Corneal transplantation. **A,** Eye of patient who will undergo corneal transplantation. Flieringa fixation ring is sutured in place with 5-0 nonabsorbable sutures. **B,** Corneal trephine is placed on recipient cornea, and partial penetration is made approximately three quarters through stroma. **C,** Anterior chamber is entered through groove, and the remainder of button is excised with right and left corneal microscissors. **D,** Corneal button is removed. **E,** Donor cornea graft is sutured in place with four sutures. **F,** Donor cornea graft is sutured in place with interrupted or continuous 10-0 nonabsorbable suture (**G** and **H**).

at the four cardinal meridians, viewed through an operating microscope. Some surgeons pre-place sutures in the graft. The surgeon sutures the graft to the host with either continuous or interrupted 10-0 nonabsorbable sutures.

7. Air or sodium hyaluronate may be injected into the anterior chamber of the recipient's eye to keep the iris from adhering to the suture line. Mydriatic or miotic solutions are used at the surgeon's discretion.
8. A subconjunctival injection of antibiotic solution or a topical application of antibiotic drops may be used at the completion of the procedure. Antibiotic ointment is applied, followed by an eye pad and a protective shield.

Lamellar Keratoplasty

1. The surgeon inserts the eye speculum, then places the superior rectus and inferior rectus bridle sutures (if needed).
2. The perioperative nurse presents the donor eye from the eye bank to the sterile field; the scrub person washes it in BSS.
3. If the lamellar graft has not already been cut by the eye bank, the surgeon will make a groove to the desired depth in the cornea using a trephine. The lamellar graft is completed using either a keratome or sharp dissection with a blade, and the graft is placed in Optisol solution or BSS.
4. The recipient cornea is trephined to the appropriate depth. The surgeon can then perform a lamellar resection, removing the anterior part of the cornea. If a deep anterior lamellar keratoplasty is being performed, the surgeon may insert a needle or

cannula into the deep corneal stroma after placing the groove. Air is then injected to find a plane for dissection between the corneal stroma and the inner layer of the cornea called Descemet membrane. This is called the "big bubble technique."

5. The surgeon sutures the donor tissue in place with an interrupted or continuous 10-0 nonabsorbable suture.
6. A mydriatic agent and subconjunctival or topical antibiotics may be used.
7. An eyepatch is applied.

Descemet Stripping Endothelial Keratoplasty

1. The surgeon inserts a lid speculum and uses a trephine to mark the corneal epithelium for the size of endothelial graft that will be placed. Multiple paracentesis incisions are made, and a viscoelastic agent is injected to maintain a formed anterior chamber. A temporal corneal incision is made.
2. Using a reverse Sinskey hook the surgeon scores and strips the Descemet membrane. Venting incisions may be placed full thickness through the remaining host cornea using a sharp point blade. Aspiration is then used to remove the viscoelastic from the anterior chamber, and an anterior chamber maintainer is typically placed to facilitate graft placement.
3. Attention is directed to the donor corneal button. The button may be cut by the eye bank, or may need to be cut to the appropriate thickness using a microkeratome and artificial anterior chamber system.
4. The endothelial graft can be inserted into the anterior chamber by several different methods. Many graft inserters are available that attach to the irrigation on a phaco unit. Other common methods of insertion include the use of a Busin glide or folding, using forceps.
5. After the graft is in the anterior chamber, a 10-0 nonabsorbable suture is placed at the wound and the graft is unfolded so the endothelial surface is facing down. When the graft is in good position, a cannula is used to inject an air bubble under the graft, displacing it up against the corneal stroma and increasing the intraocular pressure so the graft will adhere to the posterior cornea. The air is typically left in position for 30 minutes to 1 hour after which part of it is released in order to prevent pupillary block. Some surgeons may perform an iridectomy and leave a full air bubble in the eye. The surgeon may remove the air in the OR or at a slit lamp.
6. Antibiotic and mydriatic drops are then placed on the eye and the eye may be patched.

Surgery of the Lacrimal Gland and Apparatus

Surgery of the lacrimal gland is usually performed for treatment or diagnosis of tumors of the lacrimal fossa or to correct epiphora, which is abnormal overflow of tears related to a congenital or acquired obstruction of the lacrimal drainage system.

Surgery of the Lacrimal Fossa

Surgery of the lacrimal fossa is performed for biopsy of any structure in the lacrimal fossa.

Operative Procedure. The lacrimal fossa, which is in the upper temporal quadrant of the orbit, may be approached directly through the lid or through the conjunctiva by everting the upper lid. The lacrimal gland is divided into a palpebral and an orbital part by the orbital septum. Surgery on the palpebral portion may produce a dry eye.

Nasolacrimal Duct Procedures

Operative Procedure
Simple Probing

1. Using a punctual dilator, the surgeon widens the tear duct opening along the medial aspect of the upper and lower eyelids.
2. A lacrimal probe (sizes vary from 00 to 4) is passed through the punctum, canaliculus, lacrimal sac, and nasolacrimal duct into the nasal cavity (under the middle meatus)
3. Adequacy of the duct opening is confirmed via metal-on-metal contact with the probe within the nasal cavity or via irrigation of fluorescein-tinged saline through the tear duct, aspirated in the nose.

Probing with Intubation.
After opening the duct as described in the previous procedure, the surgeon may place a Silastic tube or stent in one or both canaliculi to reduce the chance of postoperative obstruction.

The surgeon threads the polyglactin leader on the stent through a stylet inserted into the punctum and retrieves it from the nasal cavity in the nose with a hook. Bicanalicular stents may use a pliable metal rod attached to the Silastic tube.

Dacryocystorhinostomy

Dacryocystitis (Figure 18-30) is an infection in the lacrimal sac, which may result in a localized cellulitis. Chronic or recurrent dacryocystitis in adults may necessitate probing or dacryocystorhinostomy (DCR) because of resistant obstruction of the nasolacrimal duct related to infection-associated scarring, dacryolith (calculus in the duct), or trauma. Another indication for a DCR may be intolerable epiphora (tearing) resulting from tear duct laceration following medial orbital wall fracture. DCR is the establishment of a new tear passageway for drainage directly into the nasal cavity. The minimally invasive approach to DCR surgery includes the use of a transconjunctival incision, lasers, and endoscopic techniques. This approach to DCR is generally associated with less pain and low risk of infection.

Procedural Considerations. The nasal cavity is anesthetized topically with cocaine just before surgery. The surgery is performed after the patient has been administered a local or general anesthetic (Figure 18-31).

FIGURE 18-30 Chronic infection of lacrimal sac (dacryocystitis) causes swelling of inner lower corner of eye socket.

FIGURE 18-32 Transconjunctival approach. Clamp everts eyelid during surgery for chalazion. Viscous contents of chalazion will be removed with curette.

FIGURE 18-31 Dacryocystorhinostomy. **A,** Skin incision for dacryocystorhinostomy or dacryocystectomy. **B,** Lacrimal sac and lacrimal bone exposed. Opening made in lacrimal bone and lacrimal crest. **C,** Posterior flap of wall of sac sutured to posterior flap of nasal mucosa. **D,** Anterior flap of wall of sac sutured to anterior flap of nasal mucosa (drawing is somewhat distorted for visualization of relative positions). **E,** Canaliculi are intubated with Silastic tubes. **F,** Tubes are secured to lateral nasal wall and allowed to slide back into nose.

Operative Procedure

1. An external incision is made in the medial canthal area or inside the nose when an internal approach is used.
2. Blunt dissection is carried through the orbicularis down to the nasal bone. The orbicularis is separated from the bone with a Freer elevator. The lacrimal fossa sac is exposed.
3. The surgeon uses a hemostat to press an opening through the lacrimal bone. If this is unsuccessful, the anterior lacrimal crest is perforated with a power burr or mallet and chisel. The opening is enlarged to a 10-mm circle with a Kerrison rongeur, and hemostasis is obtained with bone wax if necessary.
4. The inferior punctum is dilated, and a probe is passed into the lacrimal sac.
5. The lacrimal sac and nasal mucosa are incised with H flaps. The surgeon sutures the posterior nasal mucous membrane flap to the posterior lacrimal sac flap with 4-0 absorbable suture.
6. The surgeon passes the first end of the wire stylet of a Silastic lacrimal duct intubation set through the upper canaliculus, through the opening, and out through the nose (under the inferior meatus). The procedure is repeated for the lower canaliculus.
7. The anterior nasal mucous membrane flap is sutured to the anterior lacrimal sac flap with 4-0 absorbable suture to create a bridge over the Silastic tubing. The tubing remains in place until the sutures become absorbed, thereby acting as a stent around which epithelial union between the lacrimal and nasal mucosa can occur.
8. The orbicularis is closed with 6-0 absorbable suture. Skin margins are approximated and closed with nonabsorbable 6-0 suture. Antibiotic ointment is applied to the incision.
9. The surgeon cuts the wire stylets off the Silastic tubing, and ties the ends of the tubing together. The tubing is sutured to the lateral nasal wall with 6-0 nonabsorbable suture. The tubing is cut so that it retracts into the nostril. An absorbent sponge may be taped under the nostrils.

Surgery of the Eyelids

Oculoplastic procedures performed on the eyelids include treatment of chalazion, entropion, ectropion, dermatochalasis, and ptosis; biopsy and excision of eyelid tumors; and repair and reconstruction of eyelid trauma or postbiopsy damage.

Removal of Chalazion

Obstruction of the meibomian gland due to secretions may lead to a chalazion, manifesting as a variably firm bump in the eyelid. Although chalazia can become infected, this is not primarily an infectious process. If persistent, incision and drainage of the chronic chalazion may be warranted (Figure 18-32).

Procedural Considerations. Incision of chalazion is often performed in an office setting, but pediatric and very anxious patients may require intravenous sedation. Local anesthesia, with 1:100,000 epinephrine in the local anesthetic, is usually used. The majority of chalazia are surgically approached from the conjunctival side of the tarsal plate, but cutaneous incisions or repair of friable cutaneous tissue may be required.

Operative Procedure (Transconjunctival Approach)

1. The surgeon everts the affected lid to expose the chalazion and applies a chalazion clamp.
2. A vertical incision is made on the inner lid surface with a sharp blade; the small lesion is curetted, or the chalazion wall is excised, in part or in toto.
3. Hemostasis is achieved through use of the bipolar ESU.
4. The wound is left open for drainage. Cutaneous sutures are placed when needed. Pressure eyepatching may be performed.

FIGURE 18-33 Wies procedure for entropion. Placement of an everting mattress suture across a transverse blepharotomy.

Repair of Entropion

Entropion occurs when the eyelid margin inverts. It may cause significant corneal irritation, attributable to rubbing of inturned eyelashes against the ocular surface. The most common type is *involutional entropion,* in which laxity and degeneration of fascial attachments between the pretarsal muscle and the tarsus permit the pretarsal muscle to override the lid margin during contraction. *Cicatricial entropion* is attributable to contraction of either the upper or the lower tarsus and its conjunctiva, causing inturned lashes (trichiasis) to abrade the cornea. Commonly used surgical techniques for entropion repair include lateral tightening of a lax eyelid via either a tarsal strip procedure or a pentagonal wedge resection, and suture eversion (via either a Wies or a Quickert suture technique).

Procedural Considerations. The causes of entropion vary, as do corrective procedures, depending on the pathologic process. Local topical and infiltrative anesthetic is typically used, and antiinfective ointment is applied postoperatively.

Operative Procedures

Blepharoplasty of Lower Lid for Involutional Entropion

1. The surgeon injects local anesthetic into the lower lid through the conjunctiva using an angled needle.
2. The skin is marked, and an incision is made in the lateral canthus.
3. The orbicularis is dissected off the orbital septum.
4. The skin excision is extended across the lower lid.
5. The orbital septum is incised to expose fat pockets, which can be excised.
6. The surgeon removes extra fat, and hemostasis is achieved.
7. After incising the lateral canthus, the surgeon pulls the lower lid laterally and shortens (tightens) it to correct entropion.
8. The tarsus is reattached to the lateral canthal tendon, and the lower lid fascia is reattached to the orbicularis.
9. The excess skin is pulled up, marked, and excised.
10. The skin incisions are closed.

Wies Procedure for Cicatricial Entropion (Figure 18-33)

1. A marking pen is used to draw a parallel line 4 mm below the lower lid margin; the local anesthetic is then injected.
2. The surgeon places a double-armed 4-0 nonabsorbable retraction suture through the conjunctiva and lower lid 4 mm from the lateral canthus and 4 mm from the medial canthus.
3. A lid plate retractor is placed behind the lower lid as it is pulled up with the traction suture. The surgeon uses a #15 blade to make the skin incision on the marked line.
4. The lid plate retractor is placed in front of the lid, and the lower lid is everted using the traction suture. The conjunctiva is incised with the #15 blade.
5. A full-thickness blepharotomy is extended laterally and medially with scissors.
6. The surgeon passes one end of the double-armed 4-0 suture through the conjunctiva and lower lid tendons and between the orbicularis and tarsus on the medial aspect of the lower lid. This process is repeated approximately 4 mm laterally with the other end of the 4-0 suture.
7. Six mattress sutures are placed and tied to evert the lower lid.
8. Excess skin is excised, and the skin incision is closed with 7-0 nonabsorbable suture.

Repair of Ectropion

Ectropion (sagging and eversion of the lower lid), usually bilateral, is common in older adults. Ectropion may be caused by the relaxation of the orbicular muscle and canthal tendons. Symptoms include tearing, conjunctival infection, irritation, and inadequate corneal protection leading to injury to the cornea. Surgery is indicated when facial paralysis is permanent or when scarring follows lacerations, lesions, or penetrating injuries and the cornea becomes exposed, resulting in ulceration and photophobia.

Procedural Considerations. The causes of ectropion vary, and corrective procedures also vary depending on the pathologic process. Local anesthetic is typically used, and antiinfective ointment and

FIGURE 18-34 Lateral canthal sling procedure for ectropion. **A,** A cantholysis of the lower arm of the lateral canthal tendon is performed. **B,** Horizontal laxity of the lid is relieved by stretching the lid temporally until it fits tightly against the globe. A tarsal lateral canthal tendon strip is isolated. **C,** Using a cotton applicator, tissue is cleaned from the periosteum of the lateral rim of the orbit. **D,** The tarsal tendon strip is sutured to the periosteum along the inner surface of the lateral wall of the orbit.

ice compresses are applied postoperatively. The Müller muscle conjunctival resection (MMCR) can be done with an internal approach by starting the incision from the inside lower eyelid.

Operative Procedure
Lateral Canthal Sling Procedure (Figure 18-34)
1. One method of correction for ectropion is the lateral canthal sling procedure, which repositions and tightens the lower lid in a horizontal direction.
2. The lateral canthus is incised, and a strip of tarsus and lateral canthal tendon is isolated.
3. The surgeon sutures the tarsus/tendon to the periosteum along the inner surface of the lateral wall of the orbit, thereby tightening the lid and correcting the ectropion.

Plastic Repair for Dermatochalasis

Dermatochalasis is a condition of drooping skin and herniated fat of the upper and lower lids that causes the skin of the upper eyelids to hang down over the palpebral fissure, sometimes obscuring vision. It may occur in older adults who have lost normal elasticity in the skin of their upper lids or in individuals who have persistent angioneurotic edema with stretching of the skin of the eyelids. If ptosis is present, it accentuates the condition. Dermatochalasis is

corrected with blepharoplasty of the redundant skin of the upper or lower eyelids (refer to Chapter 22 for procedural considerations and the operative procedure).

Surgery for Unilateral or Bilateral Ptosis

Ptosis is true drooping of the upper lid and may be congenital or acquired. In congenital ptosis there usually is developmental weakness of the levator muscle. The condition may be unilateral or bilateral. The child often compensates by raising the eyebrow or tilting the chin upward. Acquired ptosis can be neurogenic, myogenic, or involutional, which is manifested by a gradual stretching or dehiscence of the levator aponeurosis. The eyelid crease may be high or absent. Ptosis can affect the visual field and the cosmetic appearance of the eye (Figure 18-35).

Procedural Considerations. The objective of ptosis surgery is to achieve a good cosmetic result, expand the superior visual field, and restore function with elevation of the lid. Many surgical procedures have been devised, directed at the levator aponeurosis, frontalis muscle, or the levator-Müller muscle complex. These muscles are the elevating forces of the upper lids. Local anesthesia may be preferred in cooperative individuals so that intraoperative adjustments can be made. Frontalis suspension uses fascia lata or synthetic

FIGURE 18-35 Ptosis surgery before (A) and after (B).

materials to attach the tarsus to the frontalis, bypassing the ineffective levator muscle. Harvesting fascia lata requires an additional incision in the leg.

Operative Procedure

Levator Aponeurosis Repair (Figure 18-36)

1. The surgeon marks the existing or potential eyelid crease. With the skin of the upper lid held taut, the skin incision is made.
2. An incision is made through the orbicularis. The surgeon dissects the orbicularis off the orbital septum and the levator aponeurosis anterior to the tarsus.
3. The aponeurosis is incised across the tarsus and dissected off the orbicularis. The levator is reattached to the tarsus with interrupted 6-0 suture.
4. If the patient is awake, he or she is asked to look forward and the sutures are adjusted as needed.
5. The pretarsal orbicularis is sutured to the aponeurosis to reconstruct the lid crease.
6. The surgeon closes the skin incision with a running 6-0 nonabsorbable suture.

Frontalis Suspension (Figure 18-37)

1. The upper lid is marked, one incision is made in the lid crease, and two incisions are made above the eyebrow.
2. The surgeon places a lid plate behind the upper lid, exposes the tarsus, and secures the suspension material (fascia graft or a synthetic implant) to the tarsus with nonabsorbable sutures.

3. Using a Wright needle, the surgeon passes the suspension material away from the globe deeply into the orbital septum and out through one eyebrow incision.
4. The remaining end of the suspension material is passed in the same manner.
5. The surgeon sutures the pretarsal orbicularis to the tarsus to form the lid crease.
6. The lid incision is closed with a running 6-0 nonabsorbable suture.
7. The surgeon passes the long end of the suspension material under the skin between the brow incisions to complete the loop, and sutures the ends of the material together.
8. The brow incisions are closed with interrupted 6-0 nonabsorbable suture.

Excisional Biopsy

Excisional biopsy is removal of lesions for diagnostic examination. Basal cell carcinomas account for 95% of neoplastic lesions of the lid; the treatment of choice is excision with frozen-section analysis or Mohs technique.

Operative Procedure. Through-and-through excision of skin, muscle, tarsus, and conjunctiva is followed by careful structural closure of anatomic spaces. Depending on the type, extent, and location of the lesion, rotation flaps or free grafts may be necessary.

Plastic Repair for Traumatic Injuries

Lacerations of the lids, including damage to the inferior canaliculus, are repaired surgically. Paramount for success is the careful approximation of the borders of the lid margin and the ends of a torn canaliculus.

Operative Procedure. Lacerations of the lid margin are closed with a 6-0 silk suture to align the gray line of the lid that lies between the lash follicles and the orifices of the meibomian glands. Once this anatomic line has been approximated, all other sutures are placed, maintaining the approximation. If the canaliculus has been lacerated, the lacrimal drainage system is intubated with a silicone tube and the canaliculus and lid are reconstructed around the tube.

Surgery of the Globe and Orbit

Surgery of the globe (eyeball) and orbit is usually performed because of trauma. Rupture of the eyeball may be direct at the site of injury or, more frequently, indirect from an increase in intraocular pressure that causes the wall of the eyeball to tear at weaker points, such as the limbus. When the intraocular contents have become so deranged that useful function is prohibited or the blind eye becomes painful, removal of the eye contents (evisceration procedure) or of the entire eyeball (enucleation) is indicated. If either procedure is required, an inert globe or a coralline hydroxyapatite (coral) implant may be inserted as a space filler and to aid in the movement of a prosthesis (artificial eye). Fractures of the orbit are discussed in Chapter 22.

Enucleation

Enucleation is removal of the entire eyeball, with the severing of its muscular attachments and optic nerve. This life-altering procedure is indicated for a blind, painful eye; intraocular tumors; and as a last resort after trauma. Usually a round implant is inserted into the socket to replace the globe and provide support for a prosthetic eye. Sphere implants may be coralline (hydroxyapatite) or synthetic

FIGURE 18-36 Levator aponeurosis repair for ptosis. **A,** Eyelid crease is marked. **B,** Skin incision is made, and the orbicularis and orbital septum are divided while dissection proceeds toward the orbital rim. **C,** The anterior surface of the tarsus is exposed, and the aponeurosis is separated from the Müller muscle. **D,** The aponeurosis is reattached to the tarsus with partial-thickness permanent sutures. Lid contour and position are adjusted. **E,** The eyelid crease is created by suturing the pretarsal orbicularis muscle to the aponeurosis, and the skin is closed.

FIGURE 18-37 Frontalis suspension for ptosis. One method used to suspend the eyelid from the brow.

FIGURE 18-38 Patients who have an enucleation can have excellent cosmetic results when fitted with an ocular prosthesis designed by a board certified ocularist.

though glass and silicone implants are still commonly used. Hydroxyapatite, a lightweight coral-like material, may be used as the foundation for a prosthetic eye because its porous structure encourages fibrovascular ingrowth. The hydroxyapatite implant is wrapped in human donor sclera or Silastic sheeting before insertion into the orbital space. New porous polyethylene implants have the advantage of allowing the rectus muscles to be sutured directly to the implant, thus eliminating the wrapping and expense of donor sclera. Suturing rectus muscles to the orbital implant enables improved postoperative movement of the ocular prosthesis (Figure 18-38).

The patient typically consults with an ocularist 4 to 6 weeks after enucleation or evisceration surgery for a prosthetic eye. A temporary prosthesis may be inserted while a custom-made prosthesis is fabricated. The prosthesis fitting process takes about 7 hours to complete. A mold of the socket is made using a type of wax, and the prosthesis is fabricated and painted to match the seeing eye. After insertion of the prosthesis the patient follows up 1 month after to ensure proper fitting, and then once per year to evaluate its size and to resurface (polish) the prosthesis to maintain the health of surrounding socket tissue. An appointment is warranted if the prosthesis becomes uncomfortable, feels rough to the touch, or changes in appearance, such as the lids appearing droopy or the eye turning in, out, up, or down. The nurse should stress the importance of protecting the visually viable eye with protective glasses anytime damage could occur, such as participating in sports, yard work, or housework.

Operative Procedure

1. The surgeon places a speculum retractor into the palpebral fissure.
2. The conjunctiva is divided around the cornea with sharp and blunt dissection.
3. The medial, lateral, inferior, and superior rectus muscles are divided, leaving a stump of medial rectus muscle. If a coralline hydroxyapatite implant with donor sclera is used, the four rectus muscles and two oblique muscles are identified and secured with 6-0 suture (to be used to reattach muscles to cut-out areas in

donor sclera) before the muscles are disinserted. The two oblique muscles are similarly detached, but are often not subsequently secured to the orbital implant.
4. Using blunt-pointed curved scissors, retractors, hemostats, and forceps, the surgeon separates the globe from the Tenon capsule. The eye is rotated laterally by grasping the stump of the medial rectus muscle.
5. A large curved hemostat is passed behind the globe, and the optic nerve is clamped for 60 seconds. The hemostat is removed, the enucleation scissors are passed posteriorly, and the optic nerve is transected. The oblique muscles are severed as the eye is lifted out of the socket by the stump of the medial rectus muscle.
6. Hemostasis is provided with either pressure via a sterile test tube or packing with saline-soaked sponges.
7. The muscle cone is filled with an implant, and the rectus muscles may then be sutured to the surface. Tenon capsule and the conjunctiva are carefully closed over the implant in separate layers.
8. A plastic socket conformer is placed into the cul-de-sac.
9. A pressure dressing with eye pads is applied.

Evisceration

Evisceration is removal of the contents of the eye, leaving the sclera and the attached muscles intact.

Operative Procedure

1. A sharp-pointed knife is inserted through the limbus anterior to the iris. The conjunctiva is not separated from the sclera as it is for enucleation.
2. The surgeon removes the contents of the eye (iris, vitreous, lens).
3. The choroid adhering to the sclera is removed with curettes.
4. Bleeding is controlled with delicate hemostatic forceps, ESU, and sutures.
5. A plastic or coral implant is placed within the empty shell.
6. Using nonabsorbable 4-0 or 5-0 suture, the surgeon approximates the conjunctival and scleral edges.
7. A pressure dressing is applied.

Exenteration

Exenteration is removal of the entire orbital contents, including the periosteum, for certain malignancies of the globe or orbit. The procedure may also include removal of the external structures of the eyelids.

Procedural Considerations. General anesthesia is usually administered.

Operative Procedure

1. Depending on circumstances, exenteration of the eye may include the removal of the lids. An incision is made down to the orbital rim, through the periosteum, and around the entire orbit.
2. The surgeon frees the periosteum from the orbital walls and apex of the orbit with periosteal elevators.
3. The optic nerve is clamped, and the entire contents of the orbit are removed en bloc.
4. Hemostasis is obtained using the ESU and bone wax.
5. A skin graft or temporal muscle implant may be used to fill the orbital cavity or iodoform gauze is used to fill the cavity.
6. A pressure dressing is applied. The cavity is allowed to granulate.

KEY POINTS

- Surgery on the eyes requires precision and detailed preoperative planning. A millimeter in eye surgery can mean the difference between a successful surgery and one with undesired results. The eyes work together binocularly, so surgery on one eye may expose decreased vision or issues in the second eye.
- Cataract surgery is the most performed outpatient surgery in the United States and with advancements in technology can restore and even improve a patient's vision to reduce the need for eyeglasses.
- Glaucoma surgeries do not restore vision, but rather prevent further damage from the progressing disease. Patients with glaucoma may have limited peripheral vision that requires the nurse, forms and papers, and medication bottles to be in their central field of vision to view.
- Retina issues are a serious threat to vision and retina surgeries are more often emergency in nature. A combination of injections and surgery may be needed to repair damage. Retina surgery may be needed after an initial unrelated eye surgery so detailed histories and review of medications and postoperative care are needed.
- The cornea accounts for two thirds of the refraction and is the first layer of the eye in the visual system. Damage from foreign objects or accidents are more likely to occur on the cornea.

CRITICAL THINKING QUESTION

You are assigned to the ophthalmology OR for the day and have seven cataract procedures scheduled for your room. The first three patients were on schedule but the fourth patient did not show up or call the surgery center to cancel, so the supervisor has moved the fifth and remaining patients up in time to fill the gap. The fifth patient is checked in and ready for surgery and the surgeon was made aware of the changes. What factors must you consider and prepare for the remaining surgeries to avoid complications or delays?

©volve *The answer to the Critical Thinking Question can be found at http://evolve.elsevier.com/Rothrock/Alexander.*

REFERENCES

American Academy of Ophthalmology: *Living eye smart*, available at http://geteyesmart2-px.ez/c/.com/eyesmart/living/index.cfm. Accessed December 1, 2012.

Association of periOperative Registered Nurses (AORN): Recommended practices for hand hygiene in the perioperative setting. In *Perioperative standards and recommended practice*, Denver, 2013, The Association.

Bausch + Lomb: *Barometer of global eye health study*, 2012, available at www.bausch.com/en/Our-Company/Recent-News/Fact-Sheet. Accessed March 14, 2013.

Dansby-Kelly A: *Ophthalmic procedures in the operating room and ambulatory surgery center*, ed 3, San Francisco, 2010, American Society of Ophthalmic Registered Nurses.

Denholm B: Tucking patient's arms and general positioning, *AORN J* 89(4):755–757, 2009.

Drury D: *Executive director, Transplant Services Center, UT Southwestern Medical Center, personal correspondence with the author*, November 26, 2012.

Eye Bank Association of America (EBAA): *Frequently asked questions: corneal transplant*, 2011, available at www.restoresight.org/about-us/frequently-asked-questions. Accessed March 16, 2013.

Jeng B: Perioperative strategies to reduce postoperative infection, *Ocul Surg News Prevent Periop Infect* (Supplement):3–7, 2012.

Krader C: Difficult surgery a factor for TASS, *Ophthalmol Times* 37(21):48, 2012.

National Eye Institute (NEI, 2012a): *NEI health information: facts about cataracts*, available at www.nei.nih.gov/health/cataract/cataract_facts.asp. Accessed December 1, 2012.

National Eye Institute (NEI, 2012b): *NEI health information: facts about floaters*, available at www.nei.nih.gov/health/floaters/index.asp. Accessed December 1, 2012.

National Eye Institute (NEI, 2012c): *NEI health information: facts about retinal detachment*, available at www.nei.nih.gov/health/retinaldetach/index.asp. Accessed December 1, 2012.

National Eye Institute (NEI, 2012d): *NEI health information: facts about macular pucker*, available at www.nei.nih.gov/health/pucker/index.asp. Accessed December 1, 2012.

National Quality Forum (NQF): *NQF endorses healthcare disparities and cultural competency measures*, 2012, available at www.qualityforum.org/News_And_Resources/Press_Releases/2012/NQF_Endorses_Healthcare_Disparities_and_Cultural_Competency_Measures.aspx. Accessed March 15, 2013.

Phillips N: *Berry & Kohn's operating room technique*, ed 12, St Louis, 2012, Mosby.

Ronge LJ: Human error during cataract surgery: right patient, wrong lens, *Eye Net Magazine*, available at www.aao.org/publications/eyenet/200603/feature.cfm. Accessed April 8, 2013.

Shorstein NH et al: Decreased postoperative endophthalmitis rate after institution of intracameral antibiotics in a Northern California eye department, *J Cataract Refract Surg* 39:8–14, 2013.

Slade S: *Laser refractive cataract surgery: science, medicine, and industry*, Bryn Mawr, PA, 2012, BMC Bryn Mawr Communications.

The Joint Commission (TJC): *2013 Patient safety goals*, available at www.jointcommission.org/assets/1/6/2013_HAP_NPSG_final_10-23.pdf. Accessed March 14, 2013.

CHAPTER 19

Otorhinolaryngologic Surgery

TROY J. DEROSE

Otorhinolaryngology is the study and science of the human ear *(oto),* nose *(rhino),* and throat *(laryngo).* It is a specialty that continues to evolve as a result of cutting-edge technology; high-powered surgical microscopes; narrower, flexible endoscopes; computer imaging; wound care improvements; and navigation systems that communicate with radiologic imaging. Such advances yield significant gains in improving the health and surgical outcomes of patients with physical ailments of the head and neck. This chapter comprehensively and respectively reviews perioperative care of patients undergoing surgical procedures to the ear, nose, head, and neck.

Surgical Anatomy

External, Middle, and Inner Ear

The ear is a sensory organ that identifies, localizes, and interprets sound as well as maintains equilibrium. Hearing is the sense by which sounds are appreciated. Referred to as the "watchdog of the senses," hearing is the last sense to disappear when one falls asleep and the first to return when one awakens. The physical nature of sound results from the compression and rarefaction of pressure waves and moving molecules, but the sensations humans actually experience are the product of complex mechanical, electrical, and psychologic interactions in the ear and central nervous system. Three anatomic segments—the external ear, middle ear, and inner ear—work together to provide hearing and balance (Figure 19-1).

The *external ear* includes the auricle (or pinna) and external auditory canal, and is composed of cartilage covered with skin. The auricles are fixed in position and lie close to the head; they concentrate incoming sound waves and conduct them into the external auditory canal. Both ears provide stereophonic hearing that gives us very specific sound localization capabilities. Without binaural hearing, determining where sounds emanate can be difficult; this is a common problem for patients with unilateral or asymmetric hearing loss.

The external auditory canal, an S-shaped pathway leading to the middle ear, is approximately 2.5 cm in length in adults and shelters the tympanic membrane. Its skeleton of bone and cartilage is covered with very thin, sensitive skin. The canal lining is protected and lubricated with cerumen, a waxy substance secreted by sebaceous glands in the distal third of the canal. Cerumen helps to trap foreign material and has a mildly acidic pH that reduces bacterial levels in the outer ear.

Located at the end of the external auditory canal is the *tympanic membrane* (eardrum) (Figure 19-2). It is a thin structure with three distinct layers: an outer squamous epithelial layer in continuity with

the skin of the external ear canal, a fibrous middle layer for strength and support, and a medial mucous membrane layer that is continuous with the lining of the middle ear.

The *middle ear* is filled with air, which flows from the nasopharynx through the eustachian tube. It is divided into three areas: the epitympanum (upper), mesotympanum (middle), and hypotympanum (lower). Posteriorly, the epitympanic portion of the middle ear communicates with the mastoid air cells of the temporal bone via the mastoid antrum. The mucous membrane of the middle ear is continuous with that of the pharynx and the mastoid cells, making it possible for infection to travel to the middle ear (otitis media) and mastoid cells (mastoiditis). The eustachian tube serves to aerate the air-filled spaces of the temporal bone and to equalize pressure in the middle ear with atmospheric pressure. It is normally closed at rest and actively opens during yawning, sneezing, or swallowing. A chain of three small articulated bones (ossicles) extends across the middle ear cavity and conducts vibrations (airborne sound waves) from the tympanic membrane across the middle ear into the oval window and the fluid-filled inner ear (Figure 19-3).

The *malleus* (hammer) consists of a head, neck, handle, and short process. The handle and short process are attached to the undersurface of the eardrum, and the head articulates with the body of the incus in the upper segment of the middle ear called the epitympanum or "attic." The *incus* (anvil) consists of a body and long and short processes (see Figure 19-2). The distal end of the long process of the incus is called the lenticular process and articulates with the capitulum (head) of the stapes, which is the third, innermost bone. The *stapes* (stirrup) consists of a head, neck, anterior and posterior crura, and a mobile footplate that is secured to the oval window by an annular ligament. The movable joints between these ossicles contribute to a lever system that amplifies the received sound and transmits and converts vibrations from ambient air to the fluid of the inner ear.

The inner ear is protected from loud noise by the *tensor tympani* muscle, which draws the drum inward to increase tension and restricts its ability to vibrate, and the *stapedius* muscle, which contracts and tightens the stapes in the oval window to reduce the intensity of vibrations passing through the ossicles into the inner ear. The middle ear and mastoid are supplied with blood from the branches of the internal and external carotid artery systems.

The *inner ear* is a membranous, curved cavity located in the petrous portion of the temporal bone; it contains hair cell receptors that provide us with both hearing and balance. The inner ear consists of a bony labyrinth filled with a watery fluid (perilymph) that surrounds and bathes a membranous labyrinth filled with another fluid with distinct electrolyte characteristics, called the endolymph. The bony labyrinth includes the cochlea and the vestibular labyrinth.

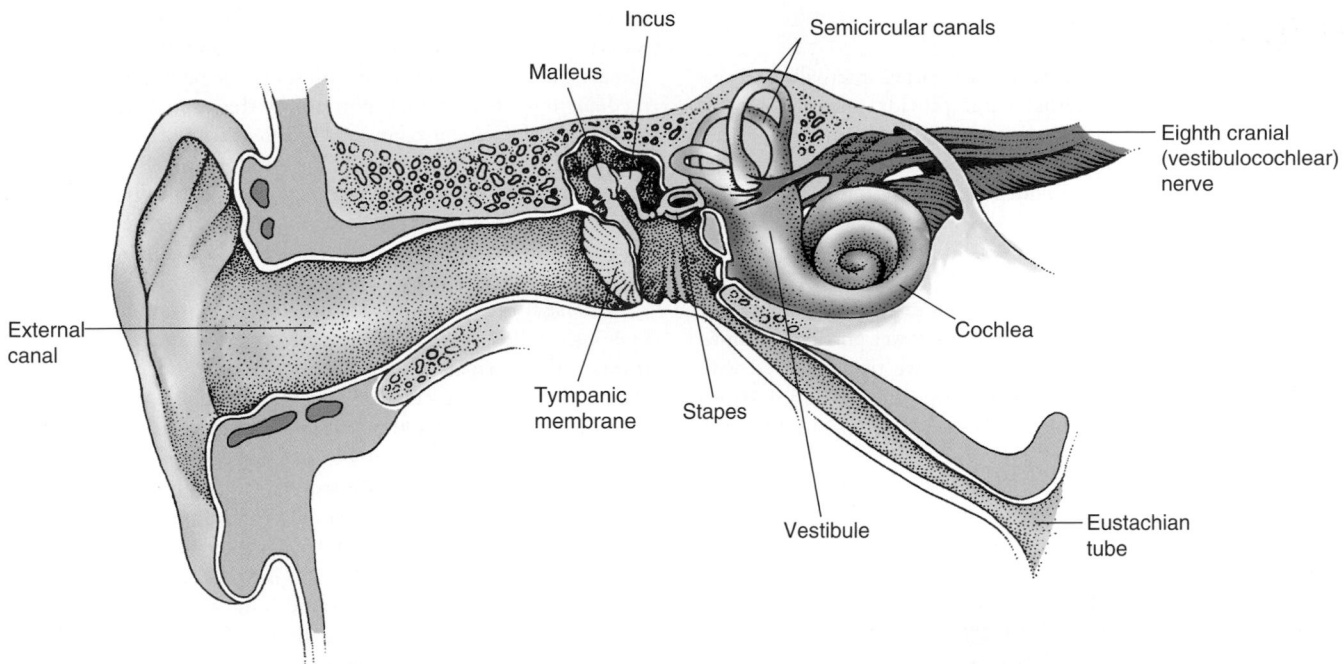

FIGURE 19-1 Anatomic structures of the external ear, middle ear, and inner ear.

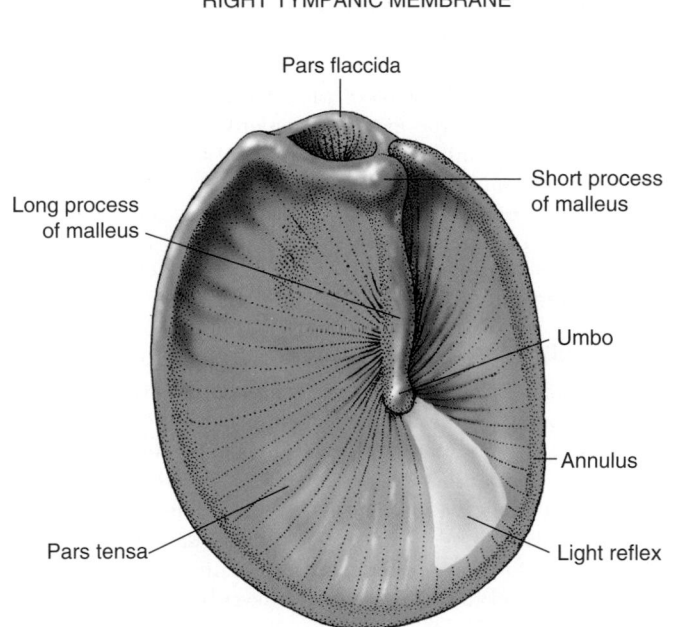

FIGURE 19-2 Structural landmarks of the tympanic membrane.

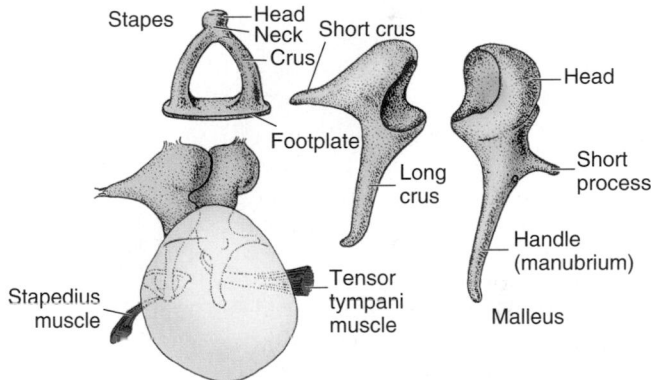

FIGURE 19-3 Articulated ossicles of the right middle ear.

The *cochlea* resembles a snail shell. It is divided into three compartments: the scala vestibuli, which is associated with the oval window; the scala tympani, which is associated with the round window; and the cochlear duct. The scala vestibuli and scala tympani are filled with perilymph, whereas the cochlear duct contains endolymph. On the basilar membrane of the cochlea lies the organ of Corti—the neural end organ for hearing. Its neuroepithelium projects thousands of hair cells that are set into motion by vibrations passing through the ossicles and oval window to the perilymph. The hair cells convert the mechanical energy of wave movement from

vibration in the perilymph into electrochemical impulses. The *vestibular labyrinth* is composed of the utricle, the saccule, and three semicircular canals, referred to as the *lateral, superior,* and *posterior canals.* They are positioned at right angles to one another and are responsible for detecting angular acceleration that can be elicited with any head or body movement. Each canal contains a sense organ (crista) that responds to fluid movement in the endolymph, which triggers impulses in the vestibular branch of the acoustic nerve. Cristae are stimulated by angular accelerations and movements, such as head turning. The maculae of the utricle and saccule of the vestibular labyrinth are gravity oriented. Linear accelerations are detected by the utricle and saccule; they both have a mat of sensory cells *(otoconia)* imbedded in a gelatinous material covered with calcium deposits. The weight of these otoconia constantly orients us to the direction of gravity. Their inertia gives information about linear accelerations. The combined signals from the cristae of the semicircular canals and the sensory cells of the utricle and saccule provide a sense of balance and orientation in space. The internal auditory branches of the basilar artery supply the inner ear.

Nasal Anatomy

The nose is covered with skin and is supported internally by bone and cartilage. The two external nares provide openings for the passage of air through the nasal cavity. These openings contain internal hairs for the filtration of coarse particles that are sometimes carried by air. The nose is divided into the prominent external portion and the internal portion known as the *nasal cavity* (Figure 19-4). The chief purpose of the nose is to prepare air for use in the lungs.

The nasal bones and the frontal process of the maxilla form the upper portion of the external nose, and the lower portion is formed by a group of nasal cartilages and connective tissue covered with skin (Figure 19-5). The nostrils and the tip of the nose are shaped by the major alar cartilages. The nares are separated by the *columella,*

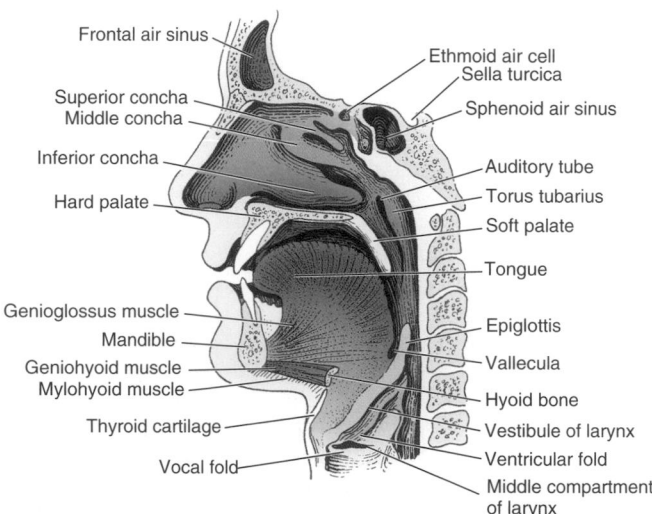

FIGURE 19-4 Sagittal section of the face and neck.

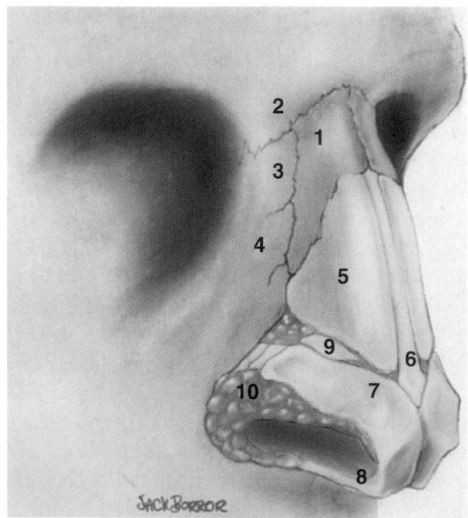

FIGURE 19-5 Nasal bony framework. *1,* Nasal bone; *2,* frontal bone; *3,* lacrimal bone; *4,* maxillary bone; *5,* upper lateral cartilage; *6,* nasal septum; *7,* lower lateral cartilage, lateral crus; *8,* lower lateral cartilage, medial crus; *9,* sesamoid cartilage; *10,* fibrofatty tissue.

which is formed by the lower margin of the septal cartilage, the medial parts of the major alar cartilages, and the anterior nasal spine, all of which are covered with skin. The nasal cavity is divided medially into right and left portions by the *nasal septum.*

The *nasal septum* is composed of three structures: the nasal cartilage, the perpendicular plate of the ethmoid bone, and the vomer bone. The septum is covered by mucoperichondrium on either side that contains blood vessels and mucus-secreting cells. The rich blood supply warms and moistens the air, and the sticky mucus traps dust, pollen, and other small particles.

The nasal cavity communicates with the outside by its external openings, called the *nares.* The nares open into the nasopharynx through the choanae. The nasal cavity is also associated with each ear, sharing the torus tubarius (opening of the eustachian tube in the nasopharynx) with the paranasal sinuses (frontal, maxillary, ethmoidal, sphenoidal) through their respective orifices (meatus). The nasal cavity also communicates with the conjunctivae through the nasolacrimal duct. The nasal cavity is separated from the lingual cavity by the hard palate and soft palate (see Figure 19-4) and from the cranial cavity by the ethmoids. It is held together by periosteal covering over bone and by perichondrium, which extends over the cartilages. The turbinate bones of the nasal structure are arranged one above the other, separated by grooves that are composed of pseudostratified columnar ciliated respiratory epithelium. The turbinates act to increase the turbulence of airflow to humidify and regulate the temperature of air that is naturally inspired. This area is commonly referred to as the *sphenoethmoidal recess* and contains bony shelves known as the the *superior, middle,* and *inferior meatus* or *turbinates* (Figure 19-6).

The nasal sinuses serve as air spaces and communicate with the nasal cavity through the meatus. Anteriorly, on each side of the skull, the frontal sinus, the anterior ethmoidal sinus, and the maxillary sinus (antrum of Highmore) drain into the middle meatus; the posterior ethmoid and the sphenoid sinuses drain into the spheno-ethmoidal recess (see Figure 19-6).

Throat Anatomy

Oral Cavity

The *oral cavity* is composed of the mouth and salivary glands. The mouth is formed by the cheeks, the hard palate, the mandible, and the tongue. It extends from the lips to the junction of the hard and soft palates. The portion of the mouth outside the teeth is the buccal cavity, and that on the inner side of the teeth is the lingual cavity. The hard palate forms the upper boundary of the oral cavity. The hard palate is formed by the maxilla and palatine bones. The mandible and floor of the mouth form the lower boundary of the oral cavity (Figure 19-7).

The *salivary glands* consist of three paired glands: the sublingual, the submandibular, and the parotid. They communicate with the mouth and produce saliva, which serves to moisten the mouth and initiate digestion of carbohydrates. The minor salivary glands exist in the submucosa of the cheeks, tongue, palates, and floor of the mouth, pharynx, lips, and paranasal sinuses.

The *sublingual gland* lies on the undersurface of the tongue beneath the mucous membrane on the floor of the mouth and the side of the tongue, on the inner surface of the mandible. The many tiny ducts of each gland separately enter the oral cavity on the sublingual fold.

The *submandibular gland* lies partly above and partly below the posterior half of the base of the mandible and on the mylohyoid

Anterior cranial fossa
Crista galli
Ethmoid air cell
Middle meatus
Maxillary sinus
Inferior meatus
Hard palate

Frontal air sinus
Orbit
Middle concha
Septum
Inferior concha

FIGURE 19-6 Vertical section through the nose. Plane of the section passes slightly obliquely through the left first molar tooth and behind the second right premolar tooth. The posterior wall of right frontal sinus is removed.

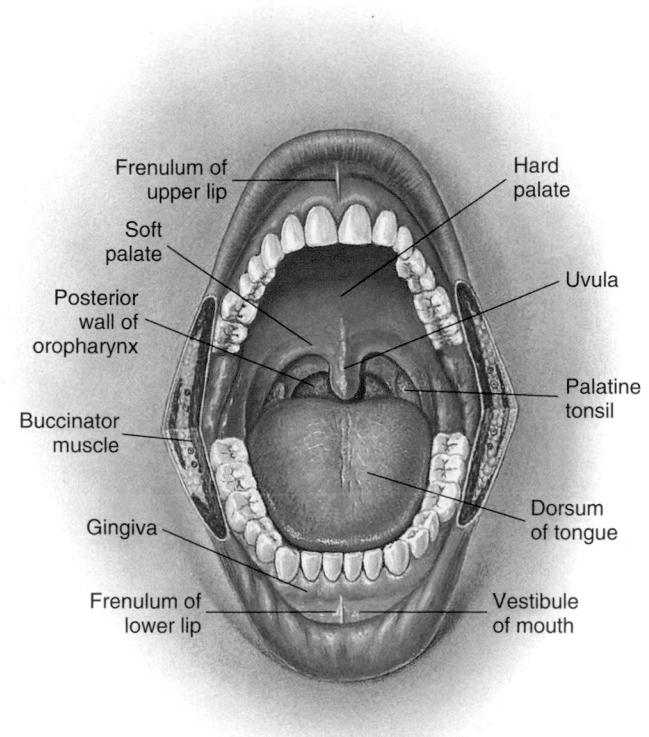

Frenulum of upper lip
Soft palate
Posterior wall of oropharynx
Buccinator muscle
Gingiva
Frenulum of lower lip

Hard palate
Uvula
Palatine tonsil
Dorsum of tongue
Vestibule of mouth

FIGURE 19-7 Anatomic structures of the oral cavity.

and hyoglossus muscles. Its duct (Wharton duct) runs superficially beneath the mucosa of the floor of the mouth and enters the oral cavity behind the central incisors.

The *parotid gland,* the largest of the salivary glands, lies below the zygomatic arch in front of the mastoid process and behind the ramus of the mandible; it is divided into a superficial portion and a deep portion. The parotid duct (Stensen duct) pierces the buccal pad of fat and the buccinator muscle, finally opening into the oral cavity opposite the crown of the upper second molar tooth.

Pharynx

The pharynx extends from the posterior portion of the nose to the esophagus and larynx and serves as a channel for both the digestive and respiratory systems (Figure 19-8). It is composed of muscular and fibrous layers with a mucous membrane lining. It is approximately 13 cm long and lies anterior to the cervical vertebrae and posterior to the nasal and oral cavities. The pharynx is associated above with the sphenoid sinus and the basilar part of the occipital bone, and it joins the esophagus below. Seven cavities communicate with the pharynx: the two nasal cavities, the two tympanic cavities, the mouth, the larynx, and the esophagus. The pharynx comprises three groups of constrictor muscles. Each muscle fits within the one below, and each inserts posteriorly in the median line with its mate from the opposite side. The constrictor muscles provide constriction of the pharynx for swallowing. Between the origins of the constrictor muscle groups are the so-called *intervals,* through which ligaments, nerves, and arteries pass. The pharynx is divided anatomically into three sections: the nasopharynx, the oropharynx, and the hypopharynx.

Nasopharynx. The nasopharynx lies posterior to the nasal cavity and extends over the soft palate. It communicates with the oropharynx through the pharyngeal isthmus, which is closed by muscular action during swallowing. Infection can spread from the nasopharynx to the middle ear through the eustachian tube.

Oropharynx. The oropharynx lies posterior to the oral cavity and extends from the palate to the level of the hyoid bone. The tonsils are situated on each side of the oropharynx, lodged in a tonsillar fossa that is attached to folds of membrane-containing muscle. The palatine tonsils (a pair of oval structures) are the only lymphatic organs covered with stratified squamous epithelium. The lateral surface of each tonsil is usually covered with a fibrous capsule. The anterior and posterior tonsillar pillars join to form a triangular fossa, with the posterior lateral aspects of the tongue at its base. The lingual tonsils are lodged in each fossa. The adenoids, or pharyngeal tonsils, are suspended from the roof of the nasopharynx and consist of an accumulation of lymphoid tissue.

Hypopharynx. The hypopharynx extends from the hyoid bone and empties into the esophagus posteriorly and the larynx anteriorly.

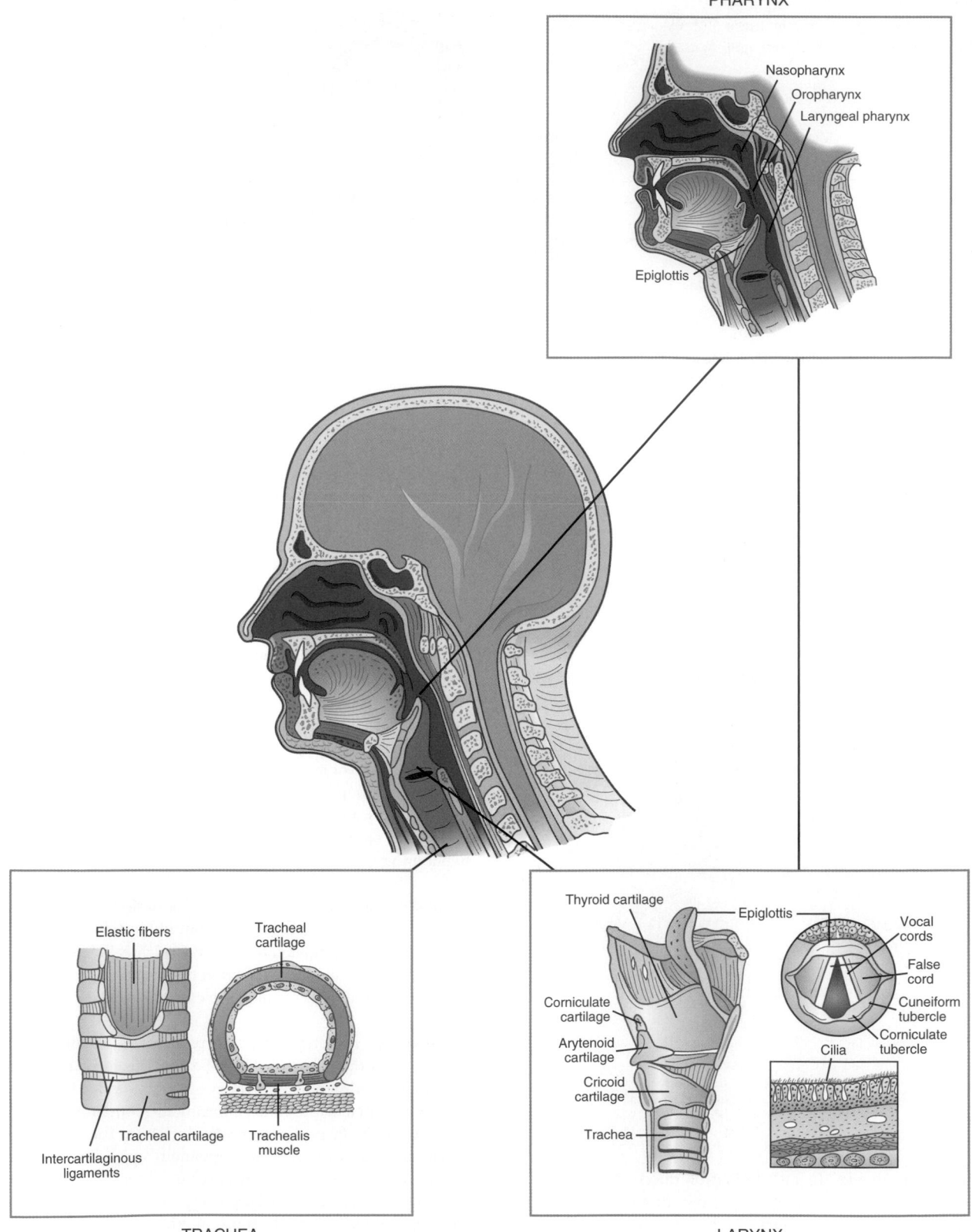

PHARYNX

Nasopharynx
Oropharynx
Laryngeal pharynx

Epiglottis

Elastic fibers
Tracheal cartilage

Intercartilaginous ligaments
Tracheal cartilage
Trachealis muscle

TRACHEA

Thyroid cartilage
Epiglottis
Vocal cords
False cord
Corniculate cartilage
Cuneiform tubercle
Arytenoid cartilage
Corniculate tubercle
Cricoid cartilage
Cilia
Trachea

LARYNX

FIGURE 19-8 Structures of the upper airway.

The piriform sinuses are bound medially by the arytenoepiglottic fold and laterally by the thyroid cartilage and hypothyroid membrane. The fossae are involved in speech.

Larynx and Associated Structures

Larynx. The larynx is a cartilaginous box that lies midline in front of the fourth, fifth, and sixth cervical vertebrae between the trachea and the root of the tongue, at the upper front part of the neck. The location of the larynx between the gastrointestinal (GI) and respiratory systems is strategic in protecting the airway during swallowing and breathing. The larynx has three main functions: as a passageway for respiration, as a valve to prevent aspiration, and as a vibratory source for vocalization.

The larynx can be divided into three portions: *supraglottis* (or upper portion above the true vocal cords), *glottis* (level of the true vocal cords), and *subglottis* (below the true vocal cords). The upper portion of the larynx is continuous with the pharynx above and includes the epiglottis, vallecula, and the laryngeal cartilages. Its lower portion joins the trachea. The skeletal structure provides for patency of the enclosed airway. The complex muscle action and arrangement of tissues within the larynx provide for closure of the lumen, to protect against trauma and entrance of foreign bodies, and for speech.

Laryngeal Cartilages. The skeletal framework of the larynx consists of cartilages and membranes. Of the nine separate cartilages, three are single and six are arranged in pairs. The main cartilages of the larynx include the thyroid, the cricoid, the epiglottis, two arytenoid, two corniculate, and two cuneiform. The thyroid cartilage, or Adam's apple, forms the anterior portion of the voice box. The cricoid cartilage is a complete cartilaginous ring that resembles a signet ring; it rests beneath the thyroid cartilage and supports the airway (see Figure 19-8). The epiglottis is a slightly curled, leaf-shaped, elastic, fibrous membrane that is attached in the midline to the upper border of the thyroid cartilage. The epiglottis helps protect the larynx during swallowing. Contraction of the cricothyroid muscle pulls the thyroid cartilage and the cricoid cartilage to tighten the vocal cords and close the glottis. The arytenoid cartilages, which rest above the signet-ring portion of the cricoid cartilage, support the posterior portion of the true vocal cords.

Laryngeal Ligaments. The extrinsic ligaments of the larynx are those connecting: (1) the thyroid cartilage and epiglottis with the hyoid bone, and (2) the cricoid cartilage with the trachea. The intrinsic ligaments of the larynx are those connecting several cartilages of the organ to each other. They are considered the elastic membrane of the larynx.

The mucous lining of the larynx blends with fibrous tissue to form two folds on each side of the larynx. The upper set is known as the *false vocal cords.* The lower set is called the *true vocal cords* because they are concerned primarily with the speaking voice and protection of the lower respiratory channels against the invasion of food and foreign bodies. The region of the larynx at the true vocal cord level is called the *glottis,* a triangular space between the vocal cords. During swallowing, the rising action of the muscular larynx, the closure of the glottis, and the doorlike action of the epiglottis all serve to guide food and fluid into the esophagus.

Laryngeal Muscles. The laryngeal muscles perform two distinct functions: the extrinsic muscles (Figure 19-9) regulate the degree of tension on the vocal cords, and the intrinsic muscles open and close the glottis. The spoken voice also depends on the sphincter action of the soft palate, tongue, and lips. The muscle action of the larynx permits the glottis to close either voluntarily or involuntarily by reflex action. The closure of the inlet by this mechanism protects the respiratory passages. The closure of the glottis and the action of the vocal cords are precisely coordinated to produce the voice.

Trachea. The trachea is a cartilaginous tube about 15 cm in length and 2 to 2.5 cm in diameter. It begins in the neck and extends from

FIGURE 19-9 Extrinsic muscles of the larynx.

the lower part of the larynx, on a level with the sixth cervical vertebra, to the upper border of the fifth thoracic vertebra. It descends anteriorly to the esophagus, enters the superior mediastinum, and divides into right and left main bronchi. The trachea is composed of a series of C-shaped rings of hyaline cartilage. The posterior surface of the trachea is flattened rather than round because the cartilaginous rings are incomplete. The carina is a ridge on the inside of the bifurcation of the trachea. It is a landmark during bronchoscopy and separates the upper end of the right main branches from the upper end of the left main branches of the bronchi. Branches from the arch of the aorta—the brachiocephalic (innominate) and left common carotid arteries—are in close relation to the trachea. The cervical portion of the trachea is related anteriorly to the sternohyoid and sternothyroid muscles and to the isthmus of the thyroid gland.

Musculature of the Neck

A layer of deep cervical fascia surrounds the neck like a collar and is attached to the trapezius and sternocleidomastoid muscles. The sternocleidomastoid muscle extends from the upper part of the sternum and medial third of the clavicle to the mastoid process. The trapezius muscle extends from the scapula, the lateral third of the clavicle, and the vertebrae to the occipital prominence. The relationship of these muscles to each other and to the adjacent bone creates triangles used as anatomic landmarks.

The pretracheal fascia of the neck lies deep in the strap muscles (sternothyroid, sternohyoid, thyrohyoid, and omohyoid) and partially encloses the thyroid gland, trachea, and larynx. The pretracheal fascia is pierced by the thyroid vessels. It fuses with the front of the carotid sheath on the deep surface of the sternocleidomastoid muscle. The carotid sheath consists of a network of areolar tissue surrounding the carotid arteries and vagus nerve.

Laterally the carotid sheath is fused with the fascia on the deep surface of the sternocleidomastoid muscle; anteriorly it is fused with the middle cervical fascia along the lateral border of the sternothyroid muscle. Lying between the floor and roof of this triangular formation of muscles are the lymph glands and the accessory nerve. Arteries and nerves traverse and pierce this triangle.

Proximal Structures

Cranial Nerves

The trigeminal (fifth cranial) nerve supplies sensory innervation to the face, oral cavity, nose, nasal cavity, and maxillary sinuses. It provides motor innervation to the muscles of mastication.

The right and left facial (seventh cranial) nerves are responsible for all the movements of the facial muscles. Both nerves have a very complex and tortuous course from the brainstem to the motor endplates of the facial musculature. The facial nerve enters the internal auditory meatus along with the eighth (vestibulocochlear) cranial nerve and travels through the internal auditory canal, passing through the labyrinthine portion of the temporal bone to the geniculate ganglion, where it turns sharply and passes superior to the oval window. It then turns inferiorly through the mastoid and exits through the stylomastoid foramen. There are three primary branches of the facial nerve in the temporal bone: the greater superficial petrosal nerve controls lacrimation, the stapedial branch controls the stapedius muscle, and the chorda tympani nerve carries the taste sensation to the anterior two thirds of the tongue.

The vestibulocochlear (eighth cranial) nerve connects the inner ear to the brain through its brainstem nuclei and ascending neural

FIGURE 19-10 Advanced cancer of the mouth with metastasis to the neck.

pathways. The recurrent laryngeal branch of the vagus (tenth cranial) nerve is the important motor nerve of the intrinsic muscles of the pharynx and larynx.

Lymphatic System

The lymphatic system serves both immunologic and circulatory functions. Interstitial fluid, which may contain bacteria, viruses, or tumor cells, is returned to the blood circulation through the lymphatic channels. As the lymph nodes trap the foreign matter, the nodes may become enlarged, infected, or the focus of metastatic cancer (Figure 19-10).

The nasal cavity, the paranasal sinuses, and the pharynx drain into the retropharyngeal nodes. The mouth, lips, and external nose are drained by the submandibular nodes. The lymphatics of the tip and lateral aspects of the tongue drain to the submental nodes, and the posterior tongue lymphatics drain to the cervical nodes.

The lymphatic drainage of the neck can be divided into superficial and deep nodes (Figure 19-11). Lymph nodes of the neck can be further classified into subzones. Level Ia nodes are submental nodes; level Ib nodes are submandibular nodes. Level IIa nodes are upper jugular nodes anterior to cranial nerve IX. Level IIb nodes are upper jugular nodes posterior to cranial nerve IX. Level III nodes are middle jugular nodes. Level IV nodes are lower jugular nodes. Level Va nodes are posterior triangle nodes of the spinal accessory group, and level Vb nodes are posterior triangle nodes of the transverse cervical artery and supraclavicular group. Level VI nodes are anterior tracheal nodes. Level VII nodes are superior mediastinum nodes.

Perioperative Nursing Considerations

Assessment

Assessment is a systematic and intentional process of collecting and interpreting data concerning a patient's health history and status

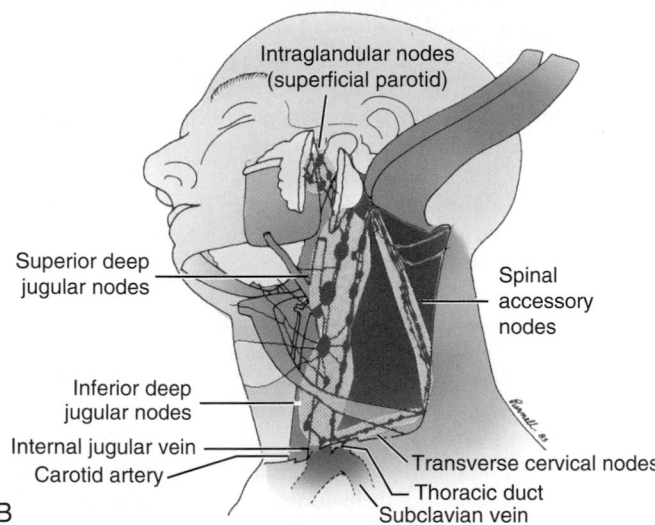

FIGURE 19-11 Lymphatic drainage of neck. **A,** Superficial cervical and facial nodal drainage patterns. **B,** Deep cervical lymphatic drainage patterns. Note that the sternocleidomastoid muscle is reflected.

	TABLE 19-1	

Types of Hearing Loss

Classification	Definition	Causes
Conductive	Loss of hearing acuity resulting from failure to conduct sound from external ear to middle ear	Blockage of external canal with cerumen or foreign bodies Edema Trauma Infection Tympanic perforation Otosclerosis, ossicular chain fixation
Sensorineural	Loss of hearing acuity resulting from failure to conduct sound to inner ear (cochlea or acoustic nerve)	Ototoxic medications Exposure to loud noise Trauma Meniere disease Tumor Presbycusis Infectious disease (measles, mumps, meningitis)
Mixed	Loss of hearing acuity resulting from combination of conductive and sensorineural factors	Develops secondary to either conductive or sensorineural loss (e.g., patient with presbycusis and impacted cerumen)

---

with diagnoses related to the head and neck. Familiarity with otorhinolaryngologic conditions is essential for effective patient assessment. Information obtained helps develop nursing diagnoses, which direct nursing plans, interventions, and evaluation. A nursing preoperative assessment is usually obtained either in person during scheduled preoperative evaluation or by telephone before the day of surgery. The perioperative nurse should review this assessment as well as the physician's evaluation to prepare for patient care in the operating room (OR). The assessment should include a review of the following:

- *Communication status.* Approximately 17% (36 million) of American adults report some degree of hearing loss severe enough to cause problems with communication and about 2 to 3 of every 1000 children in the United States are born deaf or hard-of-hearing (National Institute on Deafness and Other Communication Disorders [NIDCD], 2010). Hearing loss may be classified as conductive, sensorineural, or mixed (Table 19-1). Nurses must determine the best way to communicate with the patient who is hard-of-hearing (Evidence for Practice). Patients who are unable to speak because of vocal cord dysfunction must be provided an alternate means of communication (e.g., pen and paper, erasable board). Nurses must assess for adaptive responses—lip reading, sign language, written communication—and the effect of the patient's communication status on daily life (e.g., inability to hear traffic, alarms, or telephone; inability of voice to be heard because of hoarseness; voice volume issues; reluctance to communicate).

- *Respiratory status.* Observe and note the quality and character of respirations; observe and note the quality and character of the voice—hoarseness, "hot potato" voice (e.g., voice that lacks resonance, sounds muffled, and evidences a distortion of vowels, as if the speaker has a hot potato in his/her mouth), or hyponasal speech; note inspiratory stridor, expiratory stridor, hemoptysis, or dyspnea.

- *Physical status.* Observe problems in range of motion in all four extremities; note joint replacements, back or neck stiffness or pain, or trismus. Assess facial symmetry, landmarks, color, position, and presence of deformities, lesions, and nodules; note presence or absence of rhinorrhea or otorrhea. Note any cranial nerve involvement (e.g., inability to look downward, nystagmus, facial asymmetry, and facial paresis).

- *Presence of a mass.* Note the length of time the mass has been evident; note if the size of the mass decreased after antibiotic therapy; note a fixed mass versus a mobile mass.

- *Nutritional status.* Note any weight loss, including length of time weight loss occurred. Patients with diagnosed and undiagnosed neoplasms may be nutritionally depleted from dysphagia, tumor, chemotherapy, or radiation therapy.

- *Emotional status and anxiety level.* Observe for restlessness, poor eye contact, facial tension, or increased perspiration.

Strategies for Communicating with a Hearing-Impaired Patient

Hearing deficits in patients must be considered when performing assessment, planning and implementing interventions, and providing education. Preexisting and postoperative hearing deficits can present a communication challenge for patients, their families, and perioperative nurses. Recommended strategies for communicating with a hearing-impaired patient include the following:

- Position yourself directly in front of the patient. Most people who have hearing loss rely heavily on seeing the speaker's face (best distance is about 3 feet).
- Ensure that the room is well lighted, making sure the light is shining at the speaker and not in the patient's eyes.
- Get the patient's attention before beginning to speak.
- Ask the patient what you need to do so that he or she can best understand you.
- If one ear is better than the other, move closer to the less-affected side.
- Speak clearly and slowly using a good elocutionary style (do not exaggerate mouth movements).
- Do not shout. Shouting raises the frequency of sound and makes understanding more difficult.
- Try not to mumble or lower the sound intensity of words at the end of sentences.
- Decrease background noise as much as possible; turn off medical equipment alarms if possible when attempting communication with the patient.
- Do not chew gum and speak at the same time.
- Keep hands and other objects away from your mouth and the speaker's mouth when talking to the patient.
- When family members are present, speak directly to the patient. Do not refer to the patient in the third person.
- Minimize distractions.
- Rephrase rather than repeat—the patient may not have understood a particular word or phrase.
- Have the patient repeat back, in his or her own words, your statements to assess understanding.
- Use appropriate hand motions.
- Be patient and relax. By working together you can help maximize effective communication.
- Write messages on paper if the patient is able to read.

Modified from Bierschbach JL: Care of patients with ear and hearing problems. In Ignatavicius DD, Workman ML, editors: *Medical-surgical nursing: patient-centered collaborative care,* ed 7, St Louis, 2013, Saunders; Medwetsky L: Hearing loss. In Duthie EJ et al, editors, *Practice of geriatrics,* ed 4, Philadelphia, 2007, Saunders.

- *Pain.* Observe location and character of odynophagia, sore throat, facial pain, or otalgia. Note preoperative medications and the time they were administered. Begin education for pain management before discharge.
- *Allergies.* Note allergic reactions to medications, foods, or latex.
- *Medication history.* Note medications taken by the patient for the presenting condition and any other diagnosed medical condition. Medications should include prescription medications; over-the-counter medications; vitamins; herbals; nutraceuticals; ototoxic drugs, including salicylates, aminoglycosides, furosemide, streptomycin, quinine, and ethacrynic acid; or any chemotherapy. Ensure key participants in the patient's care are aware of the medication history (Ambulatory Surgery Considerations).
- *Past responses to anesthesia.* Local anesthetics are often used either as the sole means of anesthesia for minor procedures or as an adjunct to procedures performed using monitored anesthesia care or general anesthesia. The patient's account of previous dental experiences with local anesthetics can provide a clue as to how the patient will respond to local anesthetic agents. Cardiac status should be noted because many surgeons use epinephrine as an additive to the local anesthetic to achieve vasoconstriction and minimize blood loss. The epinephrine effect may contribute to cardiac dysrhythmias and an increased potential for cardiac arrest.
- *Patient's knowledge and understanding of the surgical procedure.* Note questions and provide answers, or ask surgeon to clarify information for the patient (Patient-Centered Care). Review equipment and care (e.g., suctioning, packing, drains) that will be part of the postoperative regimen and possible communication deficits related to the procedure (e.g., inability to speak after laryngeal procedures, decreased hearing after otologic procedures).
- *Patient's support system.* Note family members' names and their location during the surgical procedure, and explain that a nurse will communicate with them during the procedure regarding the patient (as applicable).

In addition to standard office diagnostic procedures performed by the surgeon, several other tests may be performed before the patient arrives in the OR. Study results of most significance to the perioperative team that should be available in the OR are listed under laboratory data in Appendix A. Radiology studies are described as follows.

Medication Reconciliation

Medication reconciliation is defined by The Joint Commission (TJC) as the comparison of medications a patient should be using (and is actually using) to the new medications that are ordered for the patient, and resolves any discrepancies. Medication reconciliation is an important element of National Patient Safety Goal 3, Improve the Safety of Using Medication (TJC, 2013).

Reconciliation of medication information can prevent prescribing errors, such as duplicate prescriptions, incompatible medications, and overprescribing. The patient entering the perioperative setting may be at risk for medication errors because of decreased

communication with the patient's primary care physician or other treating specialists. Otorhinolaryngologic patients may also have communication challenges (auditory or vocal) that increase the risk of error in obtaining an accurate medication history. In ambulatory surgery, perioperative nurses typically review the patient's medication history in the preoperative period and then review medications again in the postoperative or discharge phase. Nurses can positively affect patient safety and reduce the risk for prescribing errors by following medication safety practices, using medication reconciliation processes, and implementing these risk-reduction strategies:

AMBULATORY SURGERY CONSIDERATIONS

Medication Reconciliation—cont'd

- Collect a current home medication list (including dose and frequency along with allergies, drug intolerance information, and immunization history) for each patient on admission.
- Validate the home medication list with the patient whenever possible; a family member, significant other, or surrogate decision maker may be involved. This involvement should occur at all interfaces of care, and on admission to and discharge from the facility.
- Have the home medication list available for the physician whenever writing orders; place the reconciling form in a consistent highly visible location within the patient chart.
- Assign primary responsibility for collecting the home list to someone with sufficient expertise, within a context of shared accountability.
- Assign responsibility for comparing admission orders with the home medication list; identifying discrepancies, interactions, and so on; and reconciling variances to someone with sufficient expertise.
- Reconcile medications within specified timeframes (within 24 hours of admission; shorter timeframes for high-risk drugs, potentially serious dosage variances, and/or upcoming administration times).
- On discharge from the ambulatory surgery setting, in addition to communicating the updated medication list to the next

provider of care during the hand-off report, provide the patient with the complete list of medications that he or she will be taking after discharge, as well as instructions on how and how long to continue taking newly prescribed medications. Encourage the patient to carry the list and share it with any care providers, including primary care and specialist physicians, nurses, pharmacists, and other caregivers.
- Adopt a standardized form to use for collecting the home medication list and for reconciling the variances (includes both electronic and paper-based forms).
- Develop clear policies and procedures for each step in the reconciliation process.
- Provide access to drug information and pharmacist advice at each step in the reconciliation process.
- Provide orientation and ongoing education on procedures for reconciling medications to all healthcare providers.
- Provide feedback and ongoing monitoring.
- When the patient is unable to actively or fully participate in the medication reconciliation process and has requested assistance from another person(s) (e.g., family member, significant other, surrogate decision maker), involve the authorized person(s) in the medication reconciliation process.

Modified from The Joint Commission (TJC): *Hospital national patient safety goals,* 2013, available at www.jointcommission.org/assets/1/18/NPSG_Chapter_Jan2013_HAP.pdf. Accessed March 23, 2013; Brown S: Overcoming the pitfalls of medication reconciliation, *Nurs Manage* 43(1):15–72, 2012.

PATIENT-CENTERED CARE

Ensuring that the process of informed consent is respected for patients is a mandate of The Joint Commission (TJC) and an important facet of patient-centered care. Otorhinolaryngology patients may be at more risk for communication errors due to hearing or phonation. Paulson (2010) notes, "The idea of informed consent is often associated with the piece of paper signed before a procedure rather than the continuum of communication that happens during the course of the medical care of patients." Responsibility for explaining the surgical procedure, risks, benefits, and possible complications lies with the surgeon, but nurses can play an important role in ensuring the patient is fully cognizant of the implications of surgery and advocating for additional communication with the physician if necessary. Some talking points and questions nurses can use to assess a patient's understanding of the informed consent process include:

- Tell me what health problem you're being treated for today.
- Can you describe in your own words what the physician will be doing to you?
- Tell me where on your body you will have surgery.
- Can you tell me in your own words what you expect to happen as a result of this surgery?
- Tell me what you think the risks are for this operation.
- What do you know about different ways to treat your problem?

TJC also suggests that healthcare workers can support the informed consent process through the following actions:

- Arrange for language services to help with treatment of patients whose preferred language is not English or who are deaf.
- Make sure that appropriate auxiliary aids and services are available during treatment of patients who have sensory impairments (e.g., hearing aids, speech generating devices, alphabet boards, speaking valves, interpreters for the deaf, etc.).
- Provide augmentative and alternative communication (AAC) resources to help in treating patients with communication impairments (e.g., alphabet boards, picture boards, teletype for the deaf).
- Note the use of communication assistance in the medical record, and communicate needed aids and services to staff.
- Use informed consent materials that meet health literacy needs. Materials should be written at a fifth grade or lower reading level. Consider revising written materials to address the health literacy needs of all patients. Use readability tests, divide complex information into bullet points, and modify document font, layout, and design to improve readability.

Modified from Paulson E: A new look at informed consent: recent guidelines prompt patient-centered approach, *ENT Today,* August 2010, available at www.enttoday.org/details/article/806315/A_New_Look_at__Informed_Consent_Recent_guidelines_prompt_patient-centered_approach.html. Accessed March 24, 2013; Patek A et al: Improving patient-provider communication: a call to action, *J Nurs Adm* 39(9):372–376, 2009; The Joint Commission: *Advancing effective communication, cultural competence, and patient- and family-centered care: a roadmap for hospitals,* Oakbrook Terrace, IL, The Joint Commission, 2010, available at www.jointcommission.org/assets/1/6/aroadmapforhospitalsfinalversion727.pdf. Accessed March 24, 2013.

Computed Tomography (CT). CT scans are radiographic studies that visualize structures by producing serial sections, many times clinically referred to as "cuts," through planes of the head and neck. CT imaging provides visualization of bone, soft tissue, and adjacent intracranial and extracranial pathologic conditions. Intravenous (IV) injection of iodine contrast agents produces visual enhancement of some anatomic structures and pathologic tissues, including highly vascularized tumors. CT is the study of choice to assess intratemporal bone pathologic conditions and to evaluate the paranasal sinuses and adjacent structures. It is also used in the assessment of the oral cavity and neck.

Magnetic Resonance Imaging (MRI). MRI is an imaging modality using powerful magnetic and radiofrequency waves to reproduce cross-sectional images of the human body without exposing the patient to ionizing radiation. On an MRI scan, fat and fluid produce high-intensity signals, which appear as bright areas, whereas bone and air emit weak signals and appear as darkened areas. MRI is often used with CT imaging in a complementary fashion when evaluating lesions in and around bone for a variety of head and neck conditions, including tumors in the oral cavity, external auditory canal, middle ear, and mastoid.

Audiogram. Patients scheduled for otologic surgery may have undergone evaluation of their hearing through audiograms to determine whether they have normal hearing, conductive hearing loss, or sensorineural hearing loss (see Table 19-1). Two types of audiometric testing—pure tone and speech audiometry—are performed on patients with suspected hearing loss.

Nursing Diagnosis

Nursing diagnoses related to the care of patients undergoing otorhinolaryngologic surgery might include the following:
- Anxiety
- Acute Pain
- Risk for Ineffective Breathing Pattern
- Risk for Bleeding
- Disturbed Body Image
- Impaired Verbal Communication

Outcome Identification

Outcomes identified for the selected nursing diagnoses could be stated as follows:
- The patient will be able to identify factors that cause anxiety and verbalize an ability to cope.
- The patient will communicate adequate pain control and display absence of physiologic indicators of pain (e.g., tachypnea, tachycardia, pallor, hypertension).
- The patient will demonstrate effective breathing patterns.
- The patient will maintain a hematocrit level of 30 mg/dL or greater or a hemoglobin level of 12 to 14 mg/dL.
- The patient will experience a sense of self-worth and self-respect.
- The patient will establish an effective communication method with staff and family.

Planning

The development of a plan of care is based on the preoperative assessment, nursing diagnoses, expected outcomes, and the surgery being performed. Patients undergoing otolaryngologic procedures may have special communication needs that must be considered in planning effective care. The perioperative nurse should determine

the best way to communicate with patients who have hearing deficits or impaired vocalization. Information given to the patient should be reinforced as needed throughout the perioperative experience. The OR environment must be quiet and free of any loud noise. Intraoperative noises, such as those from suction, electrosurgical units (ESUs), and other equipment, should be explained to the locally anesthetized patient before they are generated. This will help avoid startling the patient and adversely affecting the success of the surgery. Patients receiving local anesthetics need to remain still during the procedure, so providing for comfort measures becomes especially important. The room temperature should be regulated at a comfortable setting, and the patient should be adequately covered to maintain normal body temperature.

Preparation of the OR includes checking the availability and functional capacity of suction, the surgeon's headlight and light source, and the ESU. It is essential that the x-ray view box is in working order and appropriately located so that scans may be easily viewed by the surgeon during the procedure. In endoscopic cases the navigation tower and monitor should be rolled to the head of the table and tested to ensure proper functioning of the light source for the camera wands and suction. If the surgeon plans on videorecording the case, assurance that the video recorder is adequately working is needed before the start of the case.

A Sample Plan of Care for a patient undergoing otorhinolaryngologic surgery is shown on pages 637-638.

Implementation

The nurse ensures the following interventions are instituted for the patient:
1. Use the institutional verification process immediately before surgery to identify the correct surgical site. This should include verifying the operative side and site with the patient or family and confirmation through review of the medical record, informed consent, diagnostic test reports, and other members of the surgical team during the time-out.
2. Verify that the patient has maintained nothing-per-mouth (NPO) status as directed and that requested laboratory studies are on the medical record.
3. Provide calm, careful, and comforting nursing measures to reduce the patient's anxiety. Allow the patient time to comply with requests, and explain the sequence of perioperative events.
4. Allow patients who wear hearing aids to wear them to the OR. Carefully remove the hearing aids at the time of or after anesthesia induction, or leave them in place if local anesthesia is used. Prescription eyewear should be brought into the holding area because hearing-impaired patients may require them to assist in lip reading when instructions and procedures are explained. If the patient has impaired vocalization, the nurse should ensure that the patient's preferred method of communication (e.g., pen and paper, artificial larynx) is available. Disposition of any assistive devices brought into the OR must be documented on the record.
5. Protect patients with impaired communication from injury. The perioperative nurse must control the environment because excess stimulation interferes with the patient's ability to hear, vocalize, and comply with instructions and explanations.
6. Carefully review instructions for patients receiving local anesthetics. Remind the patient of the need to remain immobile during the procedure and report any adverse symptoms related to the anesthetic. Symptoms of adverse drug reactions include skin changes, such as rash or itching; restlessness; unexplained

SAMPLE PLAN OF CARE

Nursing Diagnosis
Anxiety

Outcome
The patient will be able to identify factors that cause anxiety and verbalize an ability to cope.

Interventions
- Assess the patient's level of anxiety (alertness, ability to comprehend, ability to perform activities of daily living [ADLs]).
- Maintain a calm and safe environment.
- Assist the patient in identifying possible sources of stress.
- Allow the patient to ventilate and ask questions. Assess the patient for desire for preoperative visit by people with altered communication methods.
- Following the protocol in place, inform the patient and family what to expect on the day of surgery and describe the environment of care (preoperative area, OR, postanesthesia care unit).
- Introduce members of the surgical staff. Explain activities performed by the nursing staff in simple language the patient can understand.
- Assure the patient that he or she will be informed before any procedure is done.
- Provide time for the patient and family to express fears and concerns. Provide factual, accurate information.
- Note expressions of distress and anxiety.
- Prevent unnecessary body exposure during transfer and positioning.
- Control external stimuli and noise levels.

Nursing Diagnosis
Acute Pain

Outcome
The patient will communicate adequate pain control and display absence of physiologic indicators of pain (e.g., tachypnea, tachycardia, pallor, and hypertension).

Interventions
- Review with the patient normal coping mechanisms that are personally effective; support and encourage these during surgical intervention. As appropriate, consider nonpharmacologic measures such as guided imagery, music, and relaxation exercises.
- Describe the anticipated sequence of perioperative events.
- Explain that some initial discomfort (e.g., pinprick followed by slight burning and then numbness) may be felt during the administration of local anesthetic.
- Inform the patient before the injection of local anesthetic; provide support and reassurance; evaluate patient response.
- Observe for, document, and report any changes in the patient's vital signs (blood pressure, heart rate and rhythm, respiratory rate, oxygen saturation), skin condition, and mental status.
- Be aware of the maximum recommended dosage of local anesthetics and be alert for signs of allergic reactions or toxic responses.
- Ask the patient whether he or she is experiencing any pain; communicate the presence of pain sensation to the surgeon.
- Administer sedation or analgesics as ordered by the surgeon. Describe the purpose and expected response to the medication administered. Document medications administered.
- Verify with the patient that the desired response has been achieved.

Nursing Diagnosis
Risk for Ineffective Breathing Pattern

Outcome
The patient will demonstrate effective breathing patterns.

Interventions
- Assess respiratory status and breathing pattern. Monitor respiratory rate, rhythm, and depth and oxygen saturation (pulse oximetry). Maintain oxygen saturation at greater than 90%. Report any variances from normal.
- Note any restlessness, apprehension, agitation, lethargy, or repeated swallowing. Use a penlight to examine the throat for bleeding if nasal, oral cavity, or laryngologic procedures were performed. Notify the surgeon if bleeding is present.
- Have emergency medications and airway equipment available.
- Elevate the head of the bed (to decrease edema, which can interfere with breathing).
- Increase humidification with a bedside humidifier or a humidified facemask.
- Encourage the patient and family to increase frequency of oral hygiene.

Nursing Diagnosis
Risk for Bleeding

Outcome
The patient will maintain a hematocrit of 30 mg/dL or greater or a hemoglobin of 12 to 14 mg/dL.

Interventions
- Assist with the insertion of intravenous (IV) lines and fluid replacement therapy. Keep IV lines patent.
- Provide blood or blood products for fluid replacement; assist in replacement therapy and patient monitoring.
- Estimate blood loss on soft goods and drapes; communicate to anesthesia provider and surgeon.
- Record the amount of irrigation used.
- Document the contents of the suction canisters.
- Monitor and document hourly urine output (as applicable); communicate results of measurements.
- Observe for signs of shock (e.g., hypotension, abnormal electrocardiogram [ECG]); report signs, and initiate corrective nursing actions.
- Observe for signs of excess blood loss (e.g., rapid, weak pulse; rapid respirations; cool, moist skin; early, slight rise in blood pressure); report signs, and initiate corrective nursing actions.
- Collaborate with the collection and interpretation of intraoperative blood analyses.

Nursing Diagnosis
Disturbed Body Image

Outcome
The patient will experience a sense of self-worth and self-respect.

Interventions
- Acknowledge normalcy of emotional response to actual or perceived change in body structure or function. Experiencing stages of grief over loss of a body part or function is normal and typically involves a period of denial, the length of which is variable.
- Encourage the patient to verbalize feelings and self-perceived changes related to health status and surgical procedure.
- Involve the family or significant others in initial communication with patient.
- Encourage the patient to ask questions.
- Discuss referrals for support groups.

Continued

SAMPLE PLAN OF CARE—cont'd

Nursing Diagnosis
Impaired Verbal Communication

Outcome
The patient will establish an effective communication method with staff and family.

Interventions
- Plan in advance to obtain necessary assistive devices or interpreters.
- Inform the entire healthcare team of the patient's communication challenges and any interpretive services to be used.

- Agree on a method of communication preoperatively to be used postoperatively. Suggestions include the following:
  - Writing with a pen or pencil and paper, or using an erasable slate
  - Hand signals or signs, body expressions
  - Picture board
- Consult with the surgeon regarding requirements for voice rest.
- Place IV lines in the nondominant hand.
- Adapt written materials (e.g., consent forms, discharge instructions) as necessary; include visual information such as symbols, pictures, or diagrams to help understanding.

---

anxiety or fearfulness; diaphoresis; and complaints of blurred vision, tinnitus, dizziness, nausea, palpitations or acute changes in heart rate, disturbed respiration, pallor or flushing, and syncope. Emergency drugs, suction apparatus, and resuscitation equipment, including a defibrillator should be readily available.

7. Remain with the patient throughout the induction phase of anesthesia.
8. Perform any hair removal by clipping. Protect the patient's eyes during skin preparation.
9. Promote normothermia through the use of thermal warming blankets, forced–air warming units, and warm IV and irrigating solutions.
10. Use graduated compression stockings and intermittent pneumatic compression devices to decrease the risk of deep vein thrombosis (DVT) and pulmonary embolism (PE) during long surgical procedures.
11. Document the serial number and lot numbers of any implanted materials according to institutional policy.
12. Initiate and document laser safety precautions if the laser is used (see Chapter 8).

Preoperative Room Preparation. Before the patient enters the OR, the nurse and scrub person (who may be a surgical technologist or a registered nurse) gather the equipment and supplies for the scheduled procedure. A well-organized surgical environment can significantly reduce anesthesia time and enable the perioperative nurse to spend more time attending to the patient's preoperative and intraoperative needs. Planning includes identifying equipment, instrumentation, furniture, and positioning accessories necessary to perform the surgery—the operating microscope, video system, monopolar and bipolar ESUs, suction, nerve integrity monitors, specialty instrument sets, prosthetic devices, drill and irrigation accessories, and the laser. A dedicated otorhinolaryngologic specialty storage cart centrally houses assorted prostheses, drill burrs and accessories, and dressing and packing materials, which contributes efficient intraoperative care.

Positioning. The supine position with modifications is used during otorhinolaryngologic procedures. The perioperative nurse gathers the supplies necessary to ensure the patient's comfort in a supine position. These usually include a foam headrest or a pillow for under the knees and warm blankets. The nurse pads the patient's extremities at pressure points and at major nerves. A pillow should be placed under the thighs, and the legs should be slightly angled to decrease pressure on the patient's back. Gel or foam heel pads are

placed under the heels to prevent pressure ulcers. This positioning should be carried out before the patient is anesthetized to ensure comfort. Arms are placed on padded armboards or wrapped with gel pad wraps with the palms up and fingers extended. Armboards are maintained at less than a 90-degree angle to prevent brachial plexus stretch. If there are surgical reasons to tuck the arms at the side, the elbows are padded to protect the ulnar nerve, the palms face inward, and the wrist is maintained in a neutral position (Denholm, 2009). A drape secures the arms. It should be tucked snuggly under the patient, not under the mattress. This prevents the arm from shifting downward intraoperatively and resting against the OR bed rail. Placing IV lines in an arm that is to be tucked at the side should be avoided, but when this is not avoidable, patency of those lines must be ensured.

Otologic Surgical Positioning. Microscopes are used for most otologic procedures. Based on the design of the microscope and the OR bed used, the patient may be placed on the bed in the reverse position—with the head at the foot of the bed—to facilitate proper placement of the microscope mounted on a floor stand and to allow adequate space for the surgeon and assistant to be positioned on sitting stools near the surgical site.

The patient is placed supine with the operative side as close to the edge of the OR bed as possible, with the head turned and the operative ear upward. This positioning gives the surgeon access in viewing all areas of the middle ear and mastoid. One or more safety or restraining belts are used to secure the patient on the OR bed to ensure safety when turning or rotating the bed. During some procedures, such as mastoidectomy, the patient's head may be secured in position by placing tape across the head and attaching it to the frame of the OR bed. For other procedures, such as myringotomy, the patient's head may be immobilized and supported on a foam headrest. A donut-shaped foam head support helps immobilize the head and permits easy adjustment of the angle while the operating microscope is being used.

To protect the nonoperative ear, the perioperative nurse should ensure that it is in the center of the donut hole and that the headrest does not cause any pressure on the ear. The dependent arm on the nonoperative side must also be well padded and properly positioned to minimize pressure injury; the patient's body weight could cause injury when the OR bed is rotated laterally to optimize surgical access. Special consideration must be given when the patient's head is positioned for surgery, especially when general anesthetics are used. Extremes in neck extension and head torsion can cause injury to the brachial plexus or cervical spine. Other options to assist in patient positioning are determined by the otologic procedure to be performed and by the surgeon's preference. They may include ophthalmic headrests with a crescent-shaped pad, a padded horseshoe-shaped headrest, or a headrest with skull pins such as the Mayfield, which is used in certain neurologic procedures.

Positioning of the surgeon is equally important to the success of the surgery. The surgeon's chair should be positioned at a height and distance that allow comfortable access to the operative site. The use of hydraulic or electric chairs enables the surgeon to adjust the position to meet these needs.

Rhinologic Surgical Positioning. A standard headrest may be used to maintain the head in normal position but is not necessary. The entire bed is turned 180 degrees to allow the right-handed surgeon to work from the patient's right side, and the right arm is tucked in at the patient's side. Pad the elbows to protect the ulnar nerve; place the palms facing inward and the wrist in a neutral position. Depending on the procedure, the left arm may be maintained by the anesthesia provider and usually has the IV line placed in it for easier access. The anesthesia provider will be at the patient's head. Positioning the bed in the reverse Trendelenburg position greater than 45 degrees uses gravity to help minimize intraoperative bleeding. The scrub person may stand at the patient's head or near the patient's waist next to the surgeon's right arm (Figure 19-12). The Mayo stand can be positioned at the head and to the side of the bed; however, it is most commonly positioned over the patient's chest, depending on where the scrub person is standing. If indicated for the procedure, the perioperative nurse assists with setting up the navigation towers and video monitor equipment at this time.

Oral Cavity/Pharyngeal/Laryngeal/Neck Surgical Positioning. The nurse assists with placing the patient in the supine position. A shoulder roll may be used for hyperextension of the neck. The headrest should allow easy movement of the head from side to side yet maintain support. The patient's arms are often tucked at the sides as described earlier in this section to allow access of the surgical team to the operative site. If a microscope or video equipment is used, the OR bed may be turned to accommodate this equipment.

Robotic-Assisted Surgery Positioning. Positioning for robotic-assisted surgery is similar to positioning used for other otorhinolaryngologic procedures. After the patient is anesthetized, protective eye shields are placed over the patient's eyes. An instrument

FIGURE 19-12 Nasal procedure with the scrub person on the right side of the surgeon.

clamping arm is fastened to the side of the bed and attached to a Davis mouth gag that has been carefully placed into the patient's mouth. The robotic equipment is then positioned over top of the patient's mouth or head.

Anesthesia. Both the use of general anesthesia and the infiltration of a local anesthetic agent (local anesthesia) have advantages during otorhinolaryngologic surgery. General anesthesia provides airway control and allows the patient to remain still throughout the procedure, thereby making surgery technically easier to perform, but requires particular attention to extremes in head positioning, possible air emboli, the control of bleeding, and, for otologic procedures, the effects of nitrous oxide in the middle ear. All anesthetics create an oxygen-rich atmosphere, and the perioperative team must consider the patient's safety in this environment (Patient Safety).

Local anesthesia is used alone or as an adjunct to many procedures. Safe administration of medication is essential for achieving optimal outcomes. Lidocaine is frequently combined with epinephrine. A concentration of 1:200,000 provides maximum vasoconstriction, but some surgeons prefer a concentration of 1:100,000. Cocaine 4% topical solution is the second medication that is used commonly for rhinologic procedures. It is a good vasoconstrictor with the added benefit of anesthetic properties. Some surgeons use a nasal decongestant instead of cocaine for nasal vasoconstriction. These decongestants do not produce some of the cardiac effects seen with cocaine. Because nasal and sinus surgeries are performed in such a confined space, vasoconstriction becomes crucial for appropriate visualization of the surgical field. Hypertension can increase bleeding despite the use of vasoconstrictive agents and may need to be managed medically by the anesthesia provider intraoperatively if the field becomes compromised and surgery is impaired (Surgical Pharmacology).

For rhinologic procedures, before the patient arrives in the OR the nurse prepares a separate prep table, which includes a labeled container of the vasoconstrictor solution, x-ray–detectable cottonoid patties (usually ½ × 3 inches with attached strings), bayonet forceps, and a small nasal speculum. The surgeon soaks the cottonoid patties with the vasoconstrictor solution and usually packs the nose with the patties before prepping and draping, to allow time for the vasoconstrictive properties to take effect. The patties are left in place. Some surgeons also inject local anesthetic at this time, but others may wait to inject at the time of surgery. Maximum vasoconstriction occurs in approximately 10 to 12 minutes after epinephrine is administered. If a local anesthetic is to be injected next, the prep table should also include a 10-mL Luer-Lok syringe, appropriate-size needle (usually 25 gauge, 1½ inches), and labeled lidocaine (0.5% to 2%, according to surgeon's preference). Additional syringes, needles, and labeled local anesthetic solution should be available on the sterile field for additional administration intraoperatively. Additional labeled cocaine solution and cottonoid patties should be available on the sterile field as well. The nurse and scrub person ensure that the cottonoid patties are counted before and at the end of the procedure. (If a pattie is placed extremely posterior along the nasal floor, it can slide past the palate and be swallowed or aspirated by the patient.)

Topical agents used in laryngeal surgery include epinephrine, phenylephrine hydrochloride, or cocaine. These agents may be applied on a cottonoid pattie or sprayed directly onto the vocal cords. Lidocaine 4% (Xylocaine) may be instilled into the trachea

Text continued on p. 643

PATIENT SAFETY

Managing the Risk of Fire in Oxygen-Rich Environments

Three elements must be present for fire to occur: heat source, fuel, and oxygen. All elements are present in the OR. According to the ECRI institute, surgical fires occur 550 to 650 times a year. In these fires, 44% involve the patient's head, neck, and upper chest (ECRI, 2009).

Patients undergoing otorhinolaryngologic procedures are at greater risk for fire injury because of the proximity of the surgical field to high concentrations of oxygen. Devices used in this specialty (e.g., lasers, fiberoptic light cables, electrosurgical unit [ESU], high-speed surgical drills and burrs) further contribute to risk by providing a heat source and fuel.

The tenets of fire safety are discussed in length in Chapter 2. Specific recommendations that perioperative nurses caring for otorhinolaryngologic patients must consider include:

- Awareness of risk factors. Oxygen vents into the atmosphere from facemasks, nasal cannulae, and uncuffed endotracheal tubes, accumulating under surgical drapes. This creates an oxygen-enriched atmosphere within the proximity of the surgical site for otorhinolaryngologic procedures.
- Discussion of risk. The perioperative nurse and scrub person should collaborate prior to procedures to plan for risk and ensure that sterile saline is available on the surgical field, a holster is used for the active ESU electrode, and that the volume of music, conversation, and ambient room noise are reasonable so that the audio from the ESU or laser can be heard. A careful review of the facility protocol for handling fire in the OR, to include verification of the location of fire pull alarms, extinguishers, and evacuation routes is essential and should not be minimized.
- Implementation of specific safety protocols for the use of the laser and the ESU in the airway includes:
  - A laser-resistant endotracheal tube should be used, and the tube should be chosen to be resistant to the laser used for

the procedure (e.g., CO_2, Nd:YAG, etc.) The cuff of the laser tube should be filled with saline and colored with an indicator dye such as methylene blue. Before activating the laser, the surgeon should inform the anesthesia provider so that the oxygen concentration delivered to the patient can be safely reduced. Additionally, the surgeon should wait a few minutes before activating the laser to allow the oxygen concentration to diminish.
- Cuffed endotracheal tubes should be used whenever possible for airway procedures. Before activating the ESU inside the airway, the surgeon should give the anesthesia provider adequate notice that the ignition source is about to be activated. The anesthesia provider should reduce the oxygen concentration to the minimum required to prevent hypoxia, and the surgeon should wait a few minutes before using the ESU to allow the oxygen concentration to diminish.
- Scavenging with the wound suction may be used to reduce the oxygen concentration in the operative field.
- Soft goods (cottonoid patties, and cottonoid strings) should be moistened when used in oxygen-rich environments to reduce the ignition potential from sources such as the laser or ESU.
- If an uncuffed endotracheal tube must be used, moistened soft goods should be used around the field to minimize leakage and reduce potential heat buildup.
- Immediate halt to the procedure when early warning signs of a fire are noticed. For fire in the airway or breathing circuit, the endotracheal tube should be removed and all flammable and burning materials should be removed from the airway. Delivery of all airway gases should stop, and saline should be poured into the patient's airway to extinguish any residual embers and cool the tissues.

Modified from Association of periOperative Registered Nurses: Recommended practices for a safe environment of care: *AORN Perioperative standards and recommended practices,* Denver, 2013, The Association; ECRI: New clinical guide to surgical fire prevention, *Health Devices* 38(10):314–332, 2009; Everson CR: Fire prevention in the perioperative setting: perioperative fires can occur everywhere, *Periop Nurs Clin* 3:333–343, 2008; Richter GT, Willging JP: Suction cautery and electrosurgical risks in otolaryngology, *Int J Pediatr Otorhinolaryngol* 72:1013–1021, 2008.

SURGICAL PHARMACOLOGY

Medications Commonly Used in Otorhinolaryngologic Surgery

Category	Dosage/Route	Purpose/Action	Adverse Reactions	Nursing Implications
Local Anesthetics				
Lidocaine, 0.5% or 1%	Local injection	Blocks pain and temperature fibers; used as medium to dilute epinephrine Local anesthetic	Cardiovascular, hypotension, confusion, dizziness, headache, somnolence, tremor, injection site pain, cardiac arrest, cardiac dysrhythmias, seizure	Contraindicated in hypersensitivity to amide locals. Use with caution in CHF, bradycardia, hypovolemia, liver disease, renal impairment.
Tetracaine (Pontocaine)	Topical: 0.25%-0.5% by nebulization or direct application	Blocks pain, suppresses gag reflex; local anesthetic	Pain, redness, irritation on initial contact	Solution must be refrigerated. Frequently given by way of an atomizer. Remind patient not to eat, drink, or chew gum for at least 1 hour after procedure or until cleared by physician; return of gag reflex should be determined before discharge from PACU.

SURGICAL PHARMACOLOGY

Medications Commonly Used in Otorhinolaryngologic Surgery—cont'd

Category	Dosage/Route	Purpose/Action	Adverse Reactions	Nursing Implications
Benzocaine/ tetracaine/ butamben (Cetacaine)	Topical: Available in gel, liquid, and spray	Blocks pain, suppresses gag reflex; local anesthetic	Dry mouth, dizziness	Spray is given by way of metered applicator; 1- to 2-sec spray is approximately 200 mg/sec. Should not be used over prolonged periods. Remind patient not to eat, drink, or chew gum for at least 1 hour after procedure or until cleared by physician; return of gag reflex should be determined before discharge from PACU.
Benzocaine	Topical: Available in 20% gel and 20% spray	Blocks pain, suppresses gag reflex, local/topical anesthetic	Dry mouth, dizziness	Spray delivers 180-200 mg/sec when container is full, 60-80 mg/sec when inverted. Remind patient not to eat, drink, or chew gum for at least 1 hour after procedure or until cleared by physician; return of gag reflex should be determined before discharge from PACU.
Lidocaine hydrochloride	Available as 4% solution, 2% viscous solution	Local anesthetic	High doses may cause cardiac dysrhythmias, minor burning and stinging of mouth and throat on initial contact	Provide patient with emesis basin to expectorate any secretions. Patient may be instructed to gargle or swish with viscous solution to numb oral cavity in preparation for introducing Abraham cannula with 4% solution.
Cocaine hydrochloride	4% topical swab; packing instilled into cavity or spray; may be applied directly to vocal cords or other laryngeal structures on pledgets to promote vasoconstriction	Local anesthetic (also used as vasoconstrictor)	CNS depression, CNS stimulation, anxiety, tachydysrhythmia, seizures; may interact with cannabis, promethazine (Phenergan), and St. John's wort	Contraindicated in hypersensitivity to cocaine products. Use with caution in acutely ill patients or children, on severely traumatized mucosa, or when sepsis is present in area of intended application.
Vasoconstrictors				
Oxymetazoline hydrochloride (Afrin Nasal Spray, Neo-Synephrine 12 Hr, Nasacon)	Nasal spray: 0.05%	Nasal decongestant used for vasoconstriction	Headache, insomnia, nervousness, nasal congestion, rebound congestion, dry nasal mucosa, nasal stinging/ burning, sneezing, cardiac dysrhythmias, hypertension, tachydysrhythmia	Contraindicated in patients hypersensitive to oxymetazoline or other adrenergic agents, narrow-angle glaucoma. Use with caution in patients with cardiovascular disease, concurrent MAOI or tricyclic depressant therapy, diabetes, hypertension, prostatic enlargement, thyroid disease.
Epinephrine	1:100,000 to 1:200,000	Used for local anesthetic; vasopressor, topical antihemorrhagic	Palpitations, tachydysrhythmia, paleness and sweating, nausea and vomiting, asthenia, dizziness, headache, tremor, pain in eye, anxiety, apprehension, nervousness, dyspnea, cardiac dysrhythmias, hypertensive crisis, pulmonary edema	Should not be used in patients with hypersensitivity to epinephrine products, narrow-angle glaucoma (ophthalmic form) within 2 weeks of MAOI (inhalational form). Proceed with caution in presence of cerebrovascular insufficiency, diabetes, geriatrics, heart disease, coronary insufficiency, hypertension, thyroid disease, pregnancy.

Continued

SURGICAL PHARMACOLOGY

Medications Commonly Used in Otorhinolaryngologic Surgery—cont'd

Category	Dosage/Route	Purpose/Action	Adverse Reactions	Nursing Implications
Topical Antibiotics				
Mupirocin (Nasal Bactroban)	Topical: 2%	Antibacterial and lubricant for nasal packing, applied topically to skin incisions	Dermatologic, nasal stinging and burning, disorder of taste, headache	Do not use with patients hypersensitive to mupirocin products. Prolonged use may result in overgrowth of nonsusceptible organisms including fungi; not intended for open wounds or mucous membranes. Good for intranasal MRSA.
Bacitracin	Topical ointment: 500 units/g	Antibacterial, topical antibiotic	Swelling, contact dermatitis, pruritus	Apply with sterile tip applicator or cotton swab.
Ciprodex	Ciprofloxacin: 3 mg/mL Dexamethasone: 1 mg/mL (0.3%; dexamethasone 0.1%) 10 drops into the affected ear once a day for 7 days	Fluoroquinolone derivative; interferes with DNA gyrase with steroid combination		Has been shown in randomized clinical trials to be more effective at resolving acute OE than neomycin/polymyxin/ hydrocortisone.
Ciprofloxin otic	Otic solution (Floxin Otic): 0.3% 10 drops into the affected ear once a day for 7 days	Fluoroquinolone derivative; interferes with DNA gyrase	Taste perversion, pruritus, site irritation; dizziness, earache, and vertigo in ~1% of patients studied	Commonly reported side effects include pruritus and bitter taste if used with a perforated tympanic membrane.
Topical Antifungals				
Vosol	3 or 4 drops q6hr until ears are dry and free of infection	A solution containing acetic acid (2%) in a propylene glycol vehicle containing propylene glycol diacetate (3%), benzethonium chloride (0.02%), and sodium acetate (0.015%)	Stinging on administration of an acutely inflamed ear from an external auditory infection	Contraindicated for the inner ear; ruptured TM.
Chloramphenicol powder 0.5%: reconstitute 25 mg/vial	2 or 3 drops 3 or 4 times per day for 7 days via powder insufflator	Dichloroacetic acid derivative	Prolonged use: Headache, contact sensitivity, pruritus	Effective against yeast and bacteria, for chronic wet ears/ mastoid cavity; commonly used in combination powder with tolnaftate and sodium sulfacetamide powder.
Boric acid powder: reconstitute 7.5 g/15.375 g	1 or 2 drops 4 to 6 times per day for 7 days via powder insufflator	Weak acid; boron often used as an antiseptic	Repeated skin contact of damaged skin with boric acid can cause nausea, vomiting, diarrhea, loss of appetite, weakness, confusion, abnormalities in menstruation and hair loss	Avoid in children; toxicity and death reported with prolonged use. Avoid during pregnancy.
Tolnaftate topical powder (1%)	A typical dosage is 3 or 4 drops into affected ear 4 times daily for 7 days via powder insufflator	A synthetic topical thiocarbamate antifungal agent	It is unknown if tolnaftate is absorbed through the epidermis or if detectable systemic concentrations of tolnaftate are achieved in the blood.	Effective in the treatment of fungal OE; commonly used in combination powder with chloramphenicol and sodium sulfacetamide powder.
Sulfanilamide powder	A typical dosage is 3 or 4 drops into affected ear four times daily for 7 days via powder insufflator	Sulfonamides inhibit bacterial dihydropteroate synthase by competing with p-aminobenzoic acid (PABA). This action interferes with the conversion of PABA into folic acid, an essential component of bacterial development.	Pruritus; limited data available	Effective in the treatment of fungal OE; commonly used in combination powder with chloramphenicol and tolnaftate powder.

SURGICAL PHARMACOLOGY

Medications Commonly Used in Otorhinolaryngologic Surgery—cont'd

Category	Dosage/Route	Purpose/Action	Adverse Reactions	Nursing Implications
Steroids				
Triamcinolone acetonide (Aristocort, Kenalog)	Topical	Used topically to lubricate packs or expand packing	Hypertension, atrophic condition of skin	Use with caution in patients with hypertension, hypothyroidism, pregnancy. Do not use with hypersensitivity to triamcinolone acetonide; local, viral, fungal, or bacterial infections.
Cortisporin otic suspension (neomycin and polymyxin B sulfates/hydrocortisone)	Topical	Used after otologic surgery as an antiinflammatory/antibiotic agent	Itching, pain, stinging, burning, ototoxicity	When administering to patient, do the following: Tilt patient's head in opposite direction of affected ear. Instill prescribed number of drops toward ear canal, not directly onto eardrum. (Tip: To promote correct placement of drops in children pull auricle down and posterior; in adults pull auricle up and posterior.)

CHF, Congestive heart failure; *CNS,* central nervous system; *DNA,* deoxyribonucleic acid; *MAOI,* monoamine oxidase inhibitor; *MRSA,* methicillin-resistant *Staphylococcus aureus; OE,* otitis externa; *PACU,* postanesthesia care unit; *TM,* tympanic membrane.
Modified from Skidmore-Roth L: *Mosby's drug guide for nurses with 2014 update,* ed 10, St Louis, 2013, Mosby; Hodgson BB, Kizior RJ: *Saunders nursing drug handbook 2013,* St Louis, 2013, Saunders; Chow AW: Infections of the oral cavity, neck, and head. In Mandell GL et al, editors: *Principles and practice of infectious diseases,* ed 7, Philadelphia, 2009, Churchill Livingstone.

to decrease the cough reflex when it becomes an obstacle to a thorough physical assessment.

Local anesthesia combined with sedation or monitored anesthesia care is often used for surgery in the premeatal region and for stapedectomy and uncomplicated middle ear procedures of less than 2 hours' duration, some rhinologic procedures, and some excisional neck procedures. Sedation should render the patient calm, comfortable, cooperative, and able to understand and communicate. Patients should not be overmedicated to the point of demonstrating obtunded reflexes or being out of touch with their surroundings. Documentation should follow institutional policy for recording intraoperative medications administered (Association of periOperative Registered Nurses [AORN], 2013a).

Preparation of the Operative Site. If hair removal is absolutely necessary, clipping is preferred because shaving may injure the skin and increase the risk of infection. Postauricular and endaural incisions extending upward from the meatus require hair to be about 1 to 2 cm away from the proposed incision site so that hair will not be in the operative field. Long scalp hair is easily managed and kept out of the way with tape or lubricant. It is good practice to pull the top layer of hair out of the way and only clip under the hair, to help maximize normal hair aesthetics postoperatively. Plastic adhesive drapes can be applied circumferentially around the proposed incision site, or a clear sterile drape laid over the entire surgical area. Parotid surgery may require hair removal from just below the temple to a line even with or slightly behind the pinna of the ear. Head and neck surgeries may require removal of hair on the chest to the nipple area on both sides. Thorough drying of the surgical area after the prep has been applied is critical for proper adhesion of the drapes to the skin so sterility is maintained throughout the operative procedure.

A povidone-iodine solution is generally used (unless the patient is allergic to iodine) to prep the surgical site for otologic and head and neck procedures. Povidone-iodine 10% solution is generally considered safe for the middle ear space and has not been found to be ototoxic in animal studies; however, in the presence of a tympanic membrane perforation, swabbing of the ear canal skin is preferred to instillation or pooling in the ear canal to prevent large volumes of prep solution from entering the middle ear space. All other surgical prep solutions, such as chlorhexidine and alcohol, are considered ototoxic and should be strictly limited to the outer ear and surrounding skin. Head and neck procedures may involve extensive skin preparation and usually include the entire area from the chin to the nipples; it may also include a donor skin graft site if a defect or large flap coverage is anticipated. Some surgeons prefer the patient's face to be included in the prep, depending on the type of surgery anticipated and the site of the lesion. If a flap may be raised to reconstruct a defect, saline should be available to remove the discoloration from the skin to allow the surgeon to check for flap viability.

Prepping the nose and face may be done for rhinologic and laryngeal or oral cavity procedures, depending on the surgical procedure and institutional policy. These areas are considered "dirty" and not possible to prep as effectively as other surgical sites, such as an abdomen. The surgical field is maintained in sterile fashion, and these procedures usually have a "clean contaminated" wound classification (see Chapter 4).

Facial Nerve Monitoring. Audible facial nerve monitors are used intraoperatively during procedures in which the facial nerve is at risk. The purpose of this monitoring technique is to assist in the early identification of the nerve, to increase the possibility of its preservation by minimizing trauma, and to assess its integrity after

FIGURE 19-13 Nerve integrity monitor system for intraoperative facial nerve monitoring.

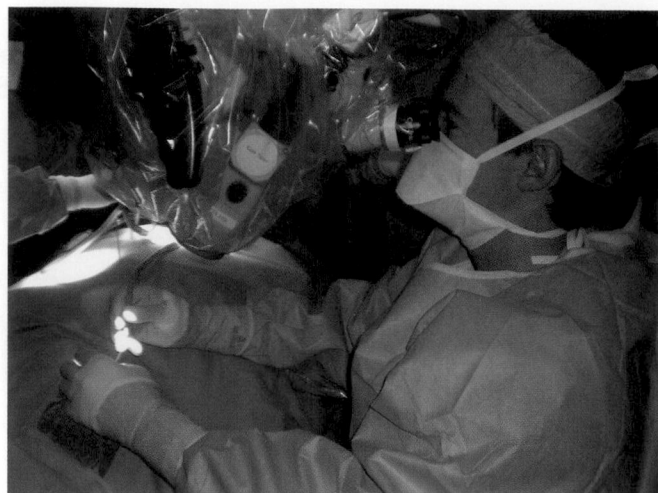

FIGURE 19-14 Surgeon in correct seated position for otologic surgery.

dissection (Seubert et al, 2009). Electrodes are placed into the facial muscles before the patient is draped. Consultation and communication with the anesthesia provider are essential because the use of muscle relaxants and long-term paralyzing agents must be avoided. In the setting of a tympanic membrane perforation, lidocaine should not be allowed to spill into the middle ear space when injecting the ear canal, as temporary facial paralysis can ensue from topical anesthesia of a dehiscent facial nerve in the tympanic segment. Facial nerve monitoring is commonly used during acoustic neuroma and mastoid surgery (Figure 19-13).

Draping. Barrier draping minimizes the risk of postoperative infection. Draping technique is based on the surgeon's preference and the procedure to be performed.

Otologic Procedure Draping. Draping may be minimal for procedures such as myringotomy. For major otologic procedures, plastic adhesive drapes are applied around the ear to keep the patient's hair out of the surgical field. A sterile, plastic aperture drape is placed over the surgical site with the ear exposed through the opening. The surgeon may elect to expose a portion of the face on the affected side to observe facial movement.

Three or four towels are draped over the aperture drape around the ear and may be secured with nonpenetrating towel clips. A fenestrated drape is unfolded over the patient, with the opening centered over the operative site. An alternative method is the use of a split sheet with the split end secured at the base of the ear and the open flaps wrapped around the patient's head. Disposable drapes with adhesive backing may be used to secure the sheet to the patient.

During mastoid surgery and for resections of acoustic tumors, fluid-collection pouches may be attached to the drape. These pouches will catch fluid runoff when drilling and irrigation are planned. The operating microscope is draped to extend the sterile field (Figure 19-14).

Special consideration must be given to the selection of draping material used during ear surgery and to the technique for removing powder from surgical gloves. Powder and lint cling to gloves and can be transferred to instruments and introduced into the ear. They act as a foreign body in the wound, causing the formation of granulomas in the middle and inner ear, and may contribute to irreversible hearing loss. Therefore, gloves worn by the surgical team should be rinsed to remove powder and lint. Lint-free drapes should be used.

Rhinologic Procedure Draping. Draping is done for most rhinologic cases. A small sheet with a towel on top of it is placed under the patient's head, and the towel is secured around the hairline with a nonpenetrating towel clip. A split sheet is then placed around the head. It is good practice to place a towel over the endotracheal (ET) tube if one is in place; this helps prevent the adhesive portion of the split sheet from sticking to the ET tube and inadvertently pulling on the tube after the procedure is completed and drapes are removed. Except during certain endoscopic procedures, the patient's eyes should be covered with moist gauze or towels if the patient is awake or taped closed if the patient has received a general anesthetic, protecting the eyes from nasal drainage or injury from instruments.

Oral Cavity, Pharyngeal, Laryngologic, and Neck Procedure Draping. Draping of the patient for a laryngeal procedure for a benign lesion (intraoral approach) is minimal, with the primary focus being protection of the patient's eyes and face. This may be accomplished by: (1) placing ointment in the patient's eyes; (2) taping the eyelids closed with a nonabrasive, nonirritating tape; (3) applying moist padding over the tape (if use of a laser is anticipated); and (4) placing self-adhering eye pads over the moistened pads. A head drape may be placed over the patient's face to expose only the lips and chin.

Draping for neck procedures often varies according to surgeon preference and is similar to the draping procedures described for rhinologic surgery. After the surgeon marks the incision site, the site is cleansed with antiseptic prep. Sterile towels are squared off around the field, then secured in place with either towel clips or staples. A "scrunched" towel may be set underneath the lobule of each ear onto the OR table to collect any drainage. A split sheet is then applied. Additional drapes may be needed if skin grafts or flaps are used for reconstructive procedures.

Surgical Microscope. A surgical microscope is often used to provide illumination and magnification for complex procedures to the ear, laryngeal surgery, or reconstructive free flap procedures following neck surgery. Several kinds of surgical microscopes with different attachments are available for otologic and laryngologic surgery. The microscope may be floor or ceiling mounted. Optimal light is provided by a xenon or halogen light source. Numerous types of monocular and binocular heads are available for the microscope. These heads may be fixed in a straight or angled plane, or they may be designed to be adjustable in an inclinable plane. For operations through an ear speculum, the microscope provides direct light and permits the surgeon to select a magnification of ×6, ×10,

×16, ×25, or ×40. A common eyepiece magnification for an otologic microscope is ×12.5, and the usual objective (lens) is 250- or 300-mm focal length (f). A 400-mm lens is used for laryngeal surgery. The total magnification is determined by multiplying the magnification of the eyepiece times that of the microscope body times that of the objective. The type of head and objective selected is based on the surgeon's preference. Microscopes equipped with a variable distance feature allow the surgeon to adjust the focal length from 200 to 400 mm without changing the lens objective. Video equipment may be attached to the microscope, which allows other team members to follow the procedure and to anticipate the necessary instrumentation. Before lenses are placed into the microscope they should be checked to ensure that they are free from lint, dust, fingerprints, and soil. The surgeon adjusts the microscope before it is draped for surgery and manipulates it during the procedure. The microscope is draped with a sterile cover for otologic surgery, but is often left undraped for laryngeal procedures. It is necessary to keep the drape material away from the light source fan of the microscope. Doing so allows cool air to continue to circulate and avoids overheating of the fan, which could prematurely burn out the lamp and cause a fire. When micromanipulators are secured to transmit laser energy to tissue through the operating microscope, special microscope laser drapes must be used. These drapes have an opening in the plastic at the base of the micromanipulator covering the objective, allowing laser energy to pass through the opening of the drape without burning the drape.

Care should be taken when removing the drapes from the microscope to avoid discarding the eyepieces with the drapes or dropping them on the floor. Eyepieces have been lost or damaged in this manner, necessitating costly repair or replacement.

When the microscope is not in use it should be kept in a locked, upright position and stored in an area that is away from traffic, free from dust, and properly ventilated. Ideally a set of eyepieces should be left in the scope to prevent the inside of the scope from becoming dusty. The microscope may also be covered with either a protective cover or a plastic bag.

Equipment and Instrumentation. Equipment that may be used in otorhinolaryngologic surgery includes an ESU (both monopolar and bipolar), a forced–air warming unit or other device to maintain normothermia, and headlights. Lasers assist in vaporization of scar tissue, granulomas, and cholesteatomas without damaging surrounding tissue and may be used for select otolaryngologic procedures. Lasers used in this specialty include the carbon dioxide (CO_2), potassium titanyl phosphate (KTP), erbium:yttrium-aluminum-garnet (Er:YAG), and neodymium:yttrium-aluminum-garnet (Nd:YAG) lasers. Lasers can be secured to the operating microscope and laser energy delivered to the tissue by means of a micromanipulator. Laser energy is delivered directly to tissue by fiberoptic probes, which can be navigated around obstructing structures.

Advances in robotic-assisted surgery are creating a synergistic complement to endolaryngeal and head and neck surgery. Transoral robotic surgery (TORS) has been used for laryngectomy, sleep apnea procedures, thyroidectomy, and some skull base procedures (Oliveira et al, 2012). Robotic surgery is described in detail in Chapter 8.

For complex reconstructive procedures in the neck, a handheld Doppler unit (to determine the viability of blood vessels) or an electromyographic nerve monitor (to determine the location and quality of nerves) may be used.

Specimen cups, labels, and a marking pen should be available on the sterile field because often several specimens are obtained. Institutional procedure for correct patient and specimen identification should be followed (AORN, 2013b).

The basic principles of care, handling, and sterilization of instruments are discussed in Chapter 4. The instrumentation used in otorhinolaryngologic surgery is quite specific and is discussed with each surgical intervention. Head and neck instrumentation combines general surgical instruments and procedure-specific instruments. Many procedures use delicate microinstruments that should be handled individually and should not be allowed to physically contact each other. Fine tympanoplasty and stapedectomy instrumentation should be kept in special storage and sterilization trays. These trays help separate instruments, aid in quick identification, protect the instruments from damage, and facilitate handling during surgery. Instruments used in the path of the operating microscope may have an ebony glare-reducing finish. Handles of assorted knives and dissectors may be flat, hexagonal, or round for better gripping or handling during surgery. The shaft of these instruments may be straight, angled, or bayonet shaped.

Powered Equipment. A power sagittal saw is used for complex neck procedures. A power drill and assorted rotating burrs are essential for middle ear surgery and some sinus procedures. Many drills are commercially available that are pneumatically or electrically driven. Pneumatic drills must have high torque (power) and more than 20,000 revolutions per minute (rpm) (speed). Some surgeons believe electrically powered drills offer equal torque but better control of the drill tip.

A selection of burrs including assorted sizes of round cutting burrs and diamond polishing burrs should be available. A diamond burr cuts slowly and grinds the bone away rather then tearing into it; it is commonly used around vital structures. Cutting burrs assist in quickly removing bone from areas not close to vital structures. The grooves or teeth of burrs must be clean of bone dust. Bone-cutting burrs tend to clog more easily than coarse-toothed burrs. A sterile wire brush may be used to keep burrs clean intraoperatively. Bone dust must be prevented from settling in areas such as those in stapedectomy, tympanoplasty, endolymphatic sac, or fenestration surgery. A sterile field continuously flooded with irrigation solution helps to lessen clogging of the burr and washes away bone dust.

Evaluation

Perioperative nursing care should be evaluated at the completion of the procedure before the patient is transported to the postanesthesia care unit (PACU) or ambulatory recovery area. If the patient has received a local anesthetic, the nurse will have had the opportunity to evaluate care on an ongoing basis, communicating with the patient throughout the procedure.

At the conclusion of the procedure, the nurse assesses the patient for any breathing difficulty. Patients who have undergone nasal surgery may have packing, which can inhibit breathing; however, the patient should be able to breathe normally through the mouth. Patients who have undergone oral cavity or laryngeal surgery are at risk for airway edema. The head of the PACU bed should be elevated before transport to the unit for all otorhinolaryngologic patients. Because of the proximity of the facial nerve to many structures within the anatomic field for otorhinolaryngologic procedures, the nurse must evaluate the patient's facial nerve function. This evaluation requires the patient's cooperation in smiling, closing the eye, and wrinkling the nose on the operative side. If facial palsy is observed and does not resolve within 2 hours of the procedure, it may be caused by surgical trauma. The nurse assesses skin integrity at positional pressure sites and the ESU dispersive electrode site documents the findings. The amount of drainage present on any dressings is also noted.

During evaluation, the perioperative nurse determines if the patient met the outcomes in the plan of care. Some outcomes can be reached during the preoperative and intraoperative phases of care; they are evaluated before the patient's discharge from the OR. Others require ongoing monitoring and measurement in the postoperative phase. A complete hand-off report allows the PACU or intensive care unit (ICU) nurse to detect significant changes in the patient's condition at an early stage. Special considerations should also be included, such as the necessity for flexion of the neck to avoid disruption of the suture line of the trachea in a patient who has undergone tracheal resection. Repeated swallowing should be noted because this may indicate posterior nasal or oral cavity bleeding. Part of the hand-off report to the PACU or nursing unit should include the outcomes of care provided:

- The patient identified factors that caused anxiety and verbalized effective coping; frequent explanations were provided, which assisted in coping with an unknown environment.
- The patient communicated adequate pain management using a pain scale and demonstrated effective coping with the physical and psychologic effects of pain. Vital signs remained stable; there were no electrocardiogram (ECG) or central nervous system (CNS) changes.
- The patient demonstrated effective breathing patterns. Respiratory rate and depth were within normal limits, and the respiratory pattern appeared effective with no cyanosis or other signs of hypoxia.
- Intraoperative bleeding was kept at a minimum during the case, keeping the patient safe from a dangerous amount of surgical blood loss.

- The patient verbalized understanding of anticipated postoperative alteration in the senses of hearing or smell and taste.
- The patient verbalized feelings regarding disturbances in body image, interacted positively with perioperative staff, maintained eye contact, and identified personally effective coping strategies.
- The patient is able to communicate effectively (ongoing) and use an alternative method (specify) of communication.

Patient and Family Education and Discharge Planning

Patient and family education is an important component of the age-appropriate and culturally sensitive care provided by perioperative nurses. Visual teaching aids, teaching brochures, and written discharge instructions provide the patient with knowledge of the surgery and what to expect during the postoperative period. Preoperative patient education includes preparing the patient for alterations in body image and function, if applicable to the planned procedure. Alternate methods of communication must be discussed before disruption of oral or laryngeal function, or hearing. The presence of edema, drains, or dressings; changes in mobility; side effects of surgery or anesthesia; possible complications of surgery; and the pertinent signs and symptoms of these complications must be discussed. The OR environment and presence of equipment should be described to the patient preoperatively to keep anxiety at a minimum. Specific instructions based on the type of surgery performed must be reviewed with the patient, focusing on important areas, such as management of pain and discomfort, restriction of activity levels, and observation for signs of infection. Printed information should be reviewed with the patient, and the patient should repeat back the key points that are essential to a successful recovery. By the time of discharge, patients and family members should have a thorough knowledge and understanding of what to expect during the postoperative recuperation period (Patient and Family Education).

PATIENT AND FAMILY EDUCATION

Patient Education for Otorhinolaryngologic Surgery

The following information is applicable to all otorhinolaryngologic procedures. Instructions unique to specific procedures are also included. Teaching is best accomplished using a variety of methods (e.g., conversation, printed materials, written instructions) and should include evaluation of the patient's understanding of the material, such as by having the patient or caregiver "teach back" the concepts previously discussed.

Preprocedural Teaching—All Procedures
- Review the physician's explanation of the procedure and its purpose; encourage the patient to ask questions and to discuss any fears or anxieties. Discuss the need for informed consent for surgery and anesthesia.
- Tell the patient that nothing-per-mouth (NPO) status must be maintained as directed by the anesthesia provider.
- Describe the OR environment and sequence of events that occur, explaining what the patient will see, feel, and hear during the perioperative experience.
- Provide information about what to expect if a local anesthetic is used (e.g., some discomfort may occur during the initial administration of a local anesthetic; if epinephrine is used with the local agent, the resulting weak, quivering feeling and increased heart rate are effects of the epinephrine and disappear after a few minutes).

- Remind the patient undergoing a local procedure that there will be pressure at some point but not pain. Encourage the patient to inform the perioperative nurse and surgeon if any discomfort is felt during the procedure. Discuss a mechanism to communicate when unable to speak. A gesture as simple as raising the hand nearest to the nurse monitoring the patient may be appropriate.
- Inform the patient that the skin will be cleansed with bactericidal soap or antiseptic solutions to remove bacteria.

Otologic/Laryngologic Procedures
- Review the use of an erasable board, paper and pencil, flash cards, or other communication board if applicable to the surgery performed.
- Encourage questions and verbalization of fears and anxieties regarding possible loss of voice or hearing.

Review of Postprocedural Care—All Procedures
- Explain that the patient will be in high Fowler position to lessen edema, improve coughing and deep breathing, and provide comfort. Advise patients to use pillows or a wedge to elevate the head by 30 degrees for the first 24 hours after discharge. Note that some patients use a recliner chair at home for comfort.
- Discuss the importance of frequent deep breathing and coughing.

PATIENT AND FAMILY EDUCATION

Patient Education for Otorhinolaryngologic Surgery—cont'd

- Explain the presence of any dressings and drainage tubes.
- Review pain management, encouraging the patient to use mild analgesics when possible.
- Remind the patient to limit the Valsalva maneuver (e.g., coughing, straining at stool) to prevent tissue damage or bleeding.
- Inform the patient that some bruising and swelling can be expected after many procedures, but will gradually subside.
- Note that some numbness may be noted postoperatively but gradually disappears.
- Heavy lifting or strenuous activity should be avoided until directed by the surgeon.

Rhinologic Procedures

- Inform the patient that if a nasal pack is inserted, there may be some difficulty in swallowing. When the patient attempts to swallow, a sucking action occurs in the throat because the packing does not allow air passage through the nose, thereby creating a partial vacuum.
- Review the procedure for changing the mustache dressing (or drip pad) that is in place postoperatively to absorb any drainage.
- This is usually a folded 2 × 2-inch gauze pad placed under the nose and secured by tape. Blood-tinged secretions in the nasopharynx are normal in the first few hours after the procedure.
- Advise the patient that forceful nose blowing must be avoided for a time to prevent movement of the rearranged nasal structures.
- If necessary to clear nasal passages, the patient should sniff gently.
- Review the importance of humidification. As directed by the surgeon, patients may use a humidifier at home to reduce nasal dryness.
- Note that the sense of smell is diminished for a time after surgery but gradually returns.

Otologic Procedures

- Avoid rapidly moving the head, bouncing, or bending over for 3 weeks.
- Exercise caution when coughing or blowing the nose; open both the nose and mouth if sneezing is unavoidable.
- Avoid drinking through a straw.

Oral Cavity/Laryngologic Procedures

- Rinse the mouth as directed by the surgeon; avoid contact with agents that may inflame the mouth, such as mouthwashes that contain alcohol.
- Perform oral hygiene after each meal or as often as needed.
- Use a soft toothbrush, sponge brush, or gauze for oral care.
- Use and apply topical analgesics and anesthetics as ordered by the physician.
- Observe voice rest as directed by the surgeon.
- Use humidification to decrease dryness and increase comfort.

Home Care—All Procedures

Give both the patient and the caregiver *verbal* and *written* instructions. Provide them with the name and telephone number of a physician or nurse to call if questions arise. Use visual aids to assist in instruction.

- General information
  - Review any explanation about the procedure and any specific follow-up care.
  - Review the signs and symptoms that should be reported to the surgeon or nurse:
    - Infection of the incision: redness, drainage, pain, warm to touch
    - Fever
    - Dyspnea without exertion
    - Difficulty swallowing
    - Bleeding or discharge of clear fluid from the ear or nose
    - Vertigo—lasting more than 24 to 48 hours after surgery
- Activity
  - Remind the patient to plan frequent rest periods.
  - Assist the patient to begin self-care as soon as possible.
  - Review any restricted activities such as driving, swimming or diving, and air travel.
- Follow-up care
  - Stress the importance of regular follow-up visits. Make sure the patient has the necessary names and telephone numbers to contact the surgeon.

Modified from Bierschbach JL: Care of patients with ear and hearing problems. In Ignatavicius DD, Workman ML, editors: *Medical-surgical nursing: patient-centered collaborative care,* ed 7, Philadelphia, 2013, Saunders; Christensen BL: Care of the patient with a respiratory disorder. In Christensen BL, Kockrow EO, editors: *Adult health nursing,* ed 6, St Louis, 2010, Mosby; Rebar CR: Care of patients with oral cavity problems. In Ignatavicius DD, Workman ML, editors: *Medical-surgical nursing: patient-centered collaborative care,* ed 7, St Louis, 2013, Saunders.

Surgical Interventions

Otologic Procedures

The majority of otologic procedures are performed either through the ear canal or from behind the ear. Incisions through the ear canal include endaural and transcanal approaches. The postauricular approach is made through an incision from behind the ear (Figure 19-15).

Endaural Approach

The endaural incision is made in two steps, using a #15 blade on a knife handle. The first incision starts at the superior meatal wall about 1 cm in from the outer edge of the meatus and extends down the posterior meatal wall to the edge of the conchal cartilage. The second incision on the superior meatal wall extends upward to a

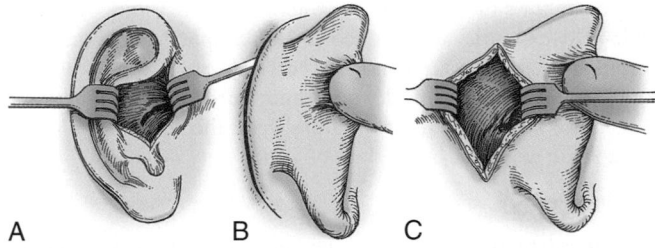

FIGURE 19-15 Surgical incisions. **A,** Endaural. **B,** Postauricular. **C,** Postauricular incision retracted.

point halfway between the meatus and upper edge of the auricle. This approach offers direct access to the external auditory meatus and tympanic membrane and may be used for meatoplasty, canalplasty, selected tympanic membrane perforations, and stapes surgery.

FIGURE 19-16 A, In purulent otitis media, pus under pressure pushes eardrum outward, resulting in bulging tympanic membrane. **B,** Radial myringotomy incision.

Transcanal Approach

The transcanal approach is used for those procedures that are limited to the mesotympanum, hypotympanum, and tympanic membrane. The incision entails a superiorly based tympanomeatal flap through the ear canal and involves making a semilunar canal skin incision anywhere from 2 to 10 mm lateral to the tympanic membrane. For exposure, the skin, fibrous annulus, and tympanic membrane are elevated as a unit. Posterior tympanomeatal flaps may be used in stapedectomy, labyrinthectomy, myringoplasty, tumor biopsy, ossiculoplasty, and removal of glomus tympanicum tumors. Congenital cholesteatomas are best approached by superior tympanomeatal flaps, whereas perforations of the tympanic membrane may be accessed through an inferior tympanomeatal flap (Chole and Suddath, 2010).

Postauricular Approach

The postauricular incision is made 2 to 5 mm behind the ear as the surgeon follows the curve of the posterior auricular fold, providing wide-field exposure and a versatile and adaptable incision. It is commonly used for tympanoplasty procedures; it is also used to expose the mastoid process for a mastoidectomy, endolymphatic sac procedure, labyrinthectomy, or translabyrinthectomy resection of an acoustic neuroma.

Myringotomy

A standard myringotomy is an incision in the pars tensa of the tympanic membrane. Myringotomy is often accompanied by the aspiration of fluid under pressure in the tympanum, and the subsequent placement of small, hollow, pressure equalization tubes (PETs) (also known as *tympanostomy* or *myringotomy tubes*). It is indicated for acute otitis media (AOM) in the presence of an exudate that has not responded to antibiotic therapy. AOM occurs in 84% to 93% of all children. Otitis media with effusion (OME) occurs in 80% of children younger than age 10 years. The majority

of children with AOM have spontaneous resolution. Hearing loss is the main concern when fluid is present in the middle ear (OME) (Thrasher, 2011). If left untreated, hearing loss can affect language development. If the fluid persists more than 8 to 12 weeks and is accompanied by hearing loss, removal of the fluid and placement of ventilating tubes in the eardrum are necessary.

Otitis media, although more common in the pediatric population, is also seen in adults. Tympanic fibrosis is common in adults and is a result of repeated infections that occurred in childhood. Acute otitis media is a collection of infected pus in the middle ear. The patient may have severe pain and bulging of the tympanic membrane (Figure 19-16). Failure to respond to oral antibiotics and analgesics or other complications, such as facial nerve paralysis, may require a myringotomy. By release of the pus or fluid, hearing is restored and the infection can be controlled. The procedure may be performed for chronic serous otitis media in which the presence of fluid in the middle ear produces a hearing loss. Frequently tubes are inserted into the tympanic membrane (Figure 19-17) to allow ventilation of the middle ear. Myringotomy tubes may be used for the treatment of colds and fluid in the ear on a short-term basis (a few months), on an intermediate basis (6 to 18 months), and in long-term treatment (years) for chronic situations. Tubes may also be placed in patients undergoing hyperbaric therapy to prevent ear pain and tympanic rupture while in the hyperbaric chamber. Care must be taken to avoid getting water in the ears while the tubes are in place. Myringotomy is usually performed on an ambulatory surgery basis. A recent alternative to tube placement is CO_2 laser–assisted myringotomy, in which the laser energy is used to create a precise hole in the tympanic membrane. This remains open for 4 to 6 weeks. Laser-assisted myringotomy is done using a topical anesthetic and may be performed in the physician's office.

Procedural Considerations. Myringotomy with tube placement is considered a clean procedure. In adult patients the procedure may

A

B

C

FIGURE 19-17 A, Tube (placed on end of alligator forceps) being inserted into tympanic membrane. **B,** Tube in place. **C,** Several types of plastic tubes that may be inserted into tympanic membrane. Purpose of the tubes is to aerate the middle ear and reduce middle ear infections.

be performed using a topical anesthetic. Pediatric patients generally require general anesthesia. The surgeon may wear gown and gloves or gloves only, depending on the policy related to Standard Precautions at the institution in which the procedure is performed. Myringotomy procedures require a sharp knife for making incisions into the tympanic membrane. Sterile, disposable, single-use blades are supplied with integrated handles or as single blades that may be secured into reusable handles. Myringotomy blades are spear-, lancet-, and sickle-shaped and are a matter of the surgeon's preference. The instrument setup includes a myringotomy knife and disposable blade, assorted sizes of aural specula, ear curettes, suction tip and tubing, a delicate Hartmann forceps, metal aural applicators, a curved needle, a culture tube (if cultures are to be taken),

and myringotomy tubes (as applicable). Several types of disposable myringotomy tubes are available for implantation, depending on the length of time the surgeon wishes the tube to remain in place (see Figure 19-17). Once the tube falls out, the tympanic membrane incision usually heals.

Operative Procedure

1. With the head and microscope in position, the surgeon inserts the aural speculum into the ear canal. The external canal is cleaned of excess cerumen using a wire loop curette. With a sharp myringotomy knife, the surgeon makes a small, curved or radial incision in the anterior inferior quadrant of the pars tensa (see Figure 19-2).
2. A culture may be taken to determine the type of organism present. Pus and fluid are suctioned from the middle ear.
3. A tube may be inserted into the incision with alligator forceps or a tube inserter. Care should be taken to consult the manufacturer's directions for handling the tube.
4. Antibiotic drops (e.g., ofloxacin 0.3% otic) may be instilled after positioning the tube.
5. A cotton ball may be placed in the external canal at the end of the procedure.

Tympanoplasty

Tympanoplasty is the surgical repair of the tympanic membrane and the tympanum and the reconstruction of the ossicular chain. It is indicated for conductive hearing losses caused by perforation of the tympanic membrane as a result of trauma or infection, for ossicular discontinuity, for chronic or recurrent otitis media, for progressive hearing loss, and for the inability to safely bathe or participate in water activities as a result of perforation of the tympanic membrane with or without hearing loss.

Perforation of the tympanic membrane is the most common ear injury necessitating surgical intervention. Perforations may result from (1) direct injury (e.g., cotton applicators, pencil), (2) blow to the ear, and (3) injury from temporal bone fractures. Early diagnosis is the key to proper management.

Conductive hearing loss is caused by an obstruction in the external canal or middle ear, which impedes the passage of sound waves to the inner ear. It may be attributable to disease of the middle ear or tympanic membrane. Occasionally the tympanic membrane does not heal after myringotomy.

Ossicular discontinuity may result from chronic otitis media, trauma, or cholesteatoma—a skin cyst that erodes bone. Various methods and materials are used in constructing a closed, air-contained middle ear cavity and restoring a sound-pressure transforming action. Among these materials are high-density polyethylene, silicone, hydroxyapatite, and titanium prostheses.

Procedural Considerations. The ear is prepped and draped as previously described. An endaural or postauricular approach may be used. Both approaches provide similar functional results. The procedure most often is performed after the patient has been administered a general anesthetic.

Operative Procedure

1. The following three approaches may be used when performing a tympanoplasty:
   a. When an *endaural approach* is used, a Lempert speculum is introduced into the external meatus of the ear canal, and the microscope is appropriately positioned. The surgeon

injects lidocaine with epinephrine postauricularly and into the external meatus and external auditory canal. The end-aural incision is made as detailed previously and then the tympanomeatal incision is made using a sharp, round knife.

b. When a *postauricular approach* is used, the surgeon injects lidocaine with epinephrine postauricularly. An ear speculum is introduced, and the microscope is appropriately positioned. Additional lidocaine is injected into the external auditory canal. The microscope head is moved from directly over the patient's ear. The surgeon incises the skin behind the fold of the ear with a #15 blade. Bleeding vessels are coagulated. An incision is then made into the periosteum down to the bone, and the periosteum is elevated from behind the incision with a Lempert elevator.

c. During the *transcanal approach,* the surgeon injects the four quadrants of the fibrocartilaginous canal with a 1% or 2% lidocaine solution with 1:100,000 epinephrine. An endaural speculum gently compresses the tissue edema resulting from the injection and assists in the placement of a speculum within the confines of the bony canal. A 30-gauge needle is used to inject the skin of the bony canal. Various canal incisions can be made, all of which accomplish the same goal of lifting the posterior ear canal skin and the tympanic membrane in continuity. Once the incisions have been made, the skin is elevated to the tympanic annulus, subcutaneous tissue at the tympanomastoid suture is dissected, and bleeding is controlled before the middle ear is reached.

2. At this point the surgeon or the assistant harvests a section of temporalis fascia for the graft material used in the repair of the tympanic membrane. Lidocaine with epinephrine may be injected under the fascia to separate it from the temporalis muscle. The surgeon uses a narrow Shambaugh elevator or duckbill elevator to separate the fascia and excises the amount needed using small, sharp scissors or a knife blade. The fascia is trimmed of excess tissue with small, sharp scissors and set aside to dry on a Teflon cutting block that is standard in most otologic instrument trays. Some surgeons prefer to thin the fascia by using a House Gelfoam press before placing the graft on the cutting block.

3. The canal skin may be elevated from the canal with a duckbill elevator, curved needle, gimmick, or similar microinstrument, or it may be removed (lateral/overlay tympanoplasty), depending on the size and location of the tympanic membrane perforation.

4. The surgeon uses a sickle knife, curved needle, 45- or 90-degree pick, or cup forceps to remove all the epithelium from the drum surrounding the perforation edges of the tympanic membrane in preparation for receiving the graft. This is referred to as "freshening the edges" and is a critical step in promoting reepithelialization of the graft.

5. If an edge of the perforation or tympanic membrane cannot be visualized because of the bony canal, the surgeon uses a microcurette or drill to remove the overhang of bone.

6. The middle ear is explored with a pick or similar instrument, and any epithelium is removed with an alligator, or cup, forceps. The surgeon inspects each ossicle to ensure that it is intact and mobile.

7. If the malleus or incus is diseased or eroded, it may be removed and replaced with a partial ossicular replacement prosthesis (PORP). Ossicles that are removed may be reshaped with the aid of a drill and small burr and replaced. If all ossicles are diseased or eroded, they may be removed and replaced with a total ossicular replacement prosthesis (TORP). This step is accomplished with microinstrumentation, such as Bellucci scissors, cup forceps, malleus nipper, incudostapedial joint knife, sickle knife, picks, and a curved needle.

8. The surgeon prepares the graft for insertion. The edges are trimmed with a #15 blade or sharp scissors to fit the shape of the ear canal and the size of the perforation. The surgical site is suctioned with a microsuction device. Hemostasis may be achieved by applying very small, epinephrine-soaked Gelfoam balls with an alligator forceps.

9. Different tissues—such as temporalis fascia or loose connective tissue, tragus perichondrium, and vein grafts—have been used for a tympanoplasty procedure. The most common tissue used is temporalis fascia. Most surgeons prefer to use autograft tissue, although homograft tympanic membranes have also been used. The risk of transmission of infectious disease has reduced homograft use. For easier manipulation, the graft may be dipped in water or saline before its insertion with alligator forceps. A gimmick, sickle knife, pick, curved needle, or similar microinstrument is used to position the graft into place. Small pieces of absorbable gelatin sponge may be packed below the graft in the middle ear space to ensure support and position. The graft and tympanomeatal flap are then laid back into place and Gelfoam packing is used to secure the flap, remnant tympanic membrane, and graft in the proper position. This outer ear canal packing is left in place for 1 to 2 weeks postoperatively and removed in the surgeon's office.

10. The external ear canal is then packed with bioresorbable packing; moistened, absorbable, gelatin sponge pledgets; or antibiotic ointment.

11. The incision is closed with suture of the surgeon's preference.

12. A pressure dressing consisting of fluffed gauze placed around the ear and an elastic gauze wrapped around the affected ear and the head may be applied for the first 24 hours to reduce swelling. Commercially prepared postauricular incision dressings are available.

Mastoidectomy

Mastoidectomy is the removal of diseased bone of the mastoid process and mastoid space. Before the introduction of antibiotic therapy, mastoidectomy was commonly performed for infection. Although occasionally still performed to eradicate infection, it is more frequently used to treat cholesteatoma. Cholesteatoma is the result of accumulation of squamous epithelium and its products in the middle ear and mastoid. It occasionally forms a cystlike mass. As it expands it is destructive to the middle ear and mastoid. As a result, the diseased bone (ossicles and mastoid bone) must be removed to prevent recurrence of the cholesteatoma.

There are three types of mastoidectomy. A *simple mastoidectomy* is removal of the diseased bone of the mastoid with preservation of the ossicles, eardrum, and canal wall. This procedure is performed to eradicate chronic infections unresponsive to antibiotics or to remove cholesteatoma. A *modified radical mastoidectomy* is removal of the diseased bone of the mastoid along with some of the ossicles and the canal wall. The eardrum and some of the ossicles remain, leaving a mechanism for the patient to hear. A canal-wall-up mastoidectomy is similar to the modified mastoidectomy without removing the posterior ear canal wall. The benefit of a canal-wall-up mastoidectomy is that the patient's ear canal will appear and function normally. Canal-wall-down mastoid cavities require maintenance with debridement of aculeate debris at least yearly.

A *radical mastoidectomy* is removal of the canal wall along with the ossicles and tympanic membrane. It is rarely performed except for unresectable disease. With either the modified radical or the radical mastoidectomy, a meatoplasty is performed to enlarge the ear canal opening. This facilitates cleaning the mastoid bowl that has been created.

Procedural Considerations. The surgical team preps and drapes the patient as for a tympanoplasty. An endaural or postauricular incision may be used, but most surgeons believe that the postauricular incision offers better exposure to all areas of the mastoid and middle ear. A drill is used to remove diseased bone and tissue. Facial nerve monitoring is used to alert the surgeon to the proximity of the nerve within the surgical field.

Operative Procedure

1. Steps 1 to 6 from the tympanoplasty procedure are performed.
2. The surgeon uses a drill with a large cutting burr to drill the mastoid bone under direct vision. As the mastoid cavity is created, the scrub person should be able to anticipate changes needed in burr size. Once the vital structures have been identified, diseased bone is removed by use of diamond burrs of the appropriate size. The surgeon may interrupt drilling to explore areas of the mastoid with a pick, curved needle or annulus elevator, or with other microinstruments to identify surrounding structures.
3. On completion of the mastoidectomy, the surgeon focuses on the middle ear. Diseased ossicles are removed, middle ear mucosa is inspected and removed if necessary, and all evidence of cholesteatoma is removed. Depending on the extent of the disease and the reliability that the patient will be available for follow-up care, the surgeon then reconstructs the ossicular chain or prepares the cavity created by a radical mastoidectomy. Some surgeons do not reconstruct at the time of mastoidectomy but reconstruct as a second-stage operation, which serves the added purpose of reexploring the middle ear and mastoid for residual or recurrent cholesteatoma.
4. The surgeon may pack the mastoid cavity and middle ear with an absorbable gelatin sponge or other bioresorbable material. The external auditory canal may be packed with bioresorbable material, an absorbable gelatin sponge, or antibiotic ointment.
5. The incision is closed and dressing applied in similar fashion to that used for postauricular tympanoplasty (as detailed previously).

Stapedotomy

Stapedotomy is removal of the stapes superstructure and creation of a fenestra (opening) in the fixed stapes footplate for treatment of otosclerosis and placement of a prosthesis to restore ossicular continuity and alleviate conductive hearing loss. Otosclerosis is the formation of abnormal bone around the stapes footplate, resulting in immobility of the footplate. Sound waves cannot be transmitted adequately through the oval window and round window to be changed into electrochemical impulses in the cochlea.

There are two types of procedures for replacing the immobile stapes. In *stapedotomy* the footplate of the stapes is not removed; only the superstructure is removed. A hole is made in the stapes footplate, and the prosthesis is secured laterally to the long process

of the incus and positioned medially over the hole created in the footplate. A CO_2 laser may also be used for stapedotomy—to create (drill) a hole in the footplate of the stapes for insertion of a prosthesis or to vaporize the stapedial tendon. Ideally, laser energy should be completely absorbed by the footplate and should not heat the perilymph or damage the inner ear (House and Cunningham, 2010). The laser stapedotomy offers improved postoperative hearing results while reducing postoperative dizziness and sensorineural hearing loss. An older procedure that is still used today, however, not as frequently as in years past, is the *stapedectomy*. In stapedectomy the entire stapes (superstructure and footplate) is removed, a graft is placed over the oval window, and a prosthesis is attached laterally to the long process of the incus and positioned medially on the graft over the oval window. Both of these procedures may be performed using monitored anesthesia care (MAC) or local anesthesia for adults, enabling the surgeon to test hearing before the conclusion of the surgery. Certain patient populations, such as children, patients with anxiety, and non–English-speaking patients, may find it difficult to remain immobile during the procedure, and general anesthesia is recommended in these populations to facilitate surgery and patient comfort.

Procedural Considerations. Various materials are used as the prosthesis for the stapes; the most common are stainless steel, titanium, platinum, nitinol, and Teflon. The most common types are either bucket-handle or piston prostheses (Figure 19-18). Both are secured to the incus and extend to the stapes footplate to reconstitute the ossicular chain. The use of stainless steel materials may present a risk for prosthesis displacement and subsequent sensorineural hearing loss if the patient undergoes MRI studies in the future.

Robinson
stainless steel piston

Shea
Teflon piston

Fisch-McGee
stainless steel piston

Teflon wire piston

FIGURE 19-18 Stapedectomy prostheses. *Top left,* Prostheses used after the footplate has been removed. *Top right and bottom,* Footplate had been "drilled" to accept a prefabricated piston precisely.

The prosthesis of choice is determined by the surgeon's experience and preference. The scrub person must be aware of each step in the procedure and hand the instruments to the surgeon expediently. Because the oval window is left uncovered, some perilymph may leak from the inner ear into the middle ear. This leak subjects the patient to the possible complication of a sensorineural hearing loss postoperatively.

Microsuction tips (18- to 26-gauge) are used in this procedure because large suction tips may suction perilymph from the oval window, resulting in permanent hearing loss as well as promoting bleeding in the middle ear. After the incision and reflection of the flap, footplate hooks are used because the tips on picks are too large and long and may cause damage rather than assist in the procedure.

Operative Procedure—Stapedotomy

1. The surgeon or the assistant may harvest a temporalis fascia, fat, perichondrium, or vein graft at the start of the procedure to cover the oval window. Depending on the surgeon's graft preference, the ear, hand, or a portion of the abdomen may be prepped for the graft. Most surgeons use temporalis fascia or postauricular subcutaneous tissue because it is within the surgical field and easily accessible.

2. The ear speculum is introduced, and the microscope is appropriately positioned. The surgeon cleans any cerumen or debris from the ear canal and may gently wash the canal with physiologic irrigating solution.

3. The surgeon injects lidocaine with epinephrine into the ear canal.

4. An ear speculum is inserted, the tympanomeatal flap is created, and the tympanic membrane is reflected forward, exposing the middle ear.

5. If visualization of the ossicles is inadequate because of the overhang of bone, the surgeon may use microcurettes or a drill to remove enough bone to allow proper visualization. Attempts to save the chorda tympani nerve are made because it controls taste from the anterior two thirds of the tongue. If this nerve obstructs the view of the stapes, it may on rare occasion be divided for exposure, and at the conclusion of the procedure the neural ends are reapproximated.

6. The surgeon may measure the distance from the incus to the stapes footplate at this time or after the removal of the stapes. It is accomplished with a depth gauge and done to ensure the proper fit of the prosthesis.

7. The incudostapedial joint is disarticulated to allow fracture and subsequent removal of the stapes, usually accomplished through the use of a joint knife or right-angled hook.

8. Both crura of the stapes are treated with a laser or fractured laterally, usually with a footplate pick or curved needle, and the superstructure is removed with alligator forceps. The surgeon may take this opportunity to ensure hemostasis, using tiny sponges soaked in epinephrine and applying suction with a microsuction tip. The laser helps coagulate middle ear vessels, thus improving hemostasis.

9. An opening is created in the footplate with a laser or a sharp footplate pick. If the footplate is extremely thick, a microdrill may be used. If a stapedectomy is to be carried out, each half of the footplate is removed using a Hough hoe, footplate pick, or footplate hook.

10. The oval window is inspected to ensure that it is long enough, and then a measuring stick is used to approximate the correct size prosthesis required for reconstruction.

11. Holding the prosthesis with alligator forceps, the scrub person passes it to the surgeon. The prosthesis is introduced into the middle ear with the shaft resting against the oval window graft.

12. The wire is positioned over the long process of the incus using picks, Hough hoes, or footplate hooks. Once it is in proper position, the surgeon crimps the wire onto the long process of the incus to ensure its attachment.

13. The surgeon may test the patient's hearing by softly whispering to the patient (if the procedure is performed with the patient administered a local anesthetic) or by touching the malleus with a pick and observing for mobility of the malleus, incus, and stapes prosthesis (if performed with the patient administered a general anesthetic).

14. Tiny pieces of the previously harvested graft tissue are then placed around the base of the prosthesis to ensure its stability. Alligator forceps, picks, a gimmick, and similar instruments may be used for this step.

15. The tympanomeatal flap is returned to its original location. The external ear canal may be packed with an antibiotic gel or ointment or a moistened, compressed gelatin sponge.

16. Cotton is placed in the concha of the ear, and an adhesive bandage or small dressing is usually applied to the graft site.

Ossicular Chain Reconstruction

Ossicular reconstruction may be required for long-standing recurrent ear infections. It is commonly performed for the replacement of the incus portion of the ossicular chain. There are many surgical techniques for ossicular reconstruction.

Natural and synthetic prosthetic materials are available for ossicular reconstruction or replacement. The autologous ossicle (incus or head of malleus) taken from the patient's ear is often used, particularly in children who do not have a cholesteatoma. A synthetic PORP or TORP is indicated for reconstitution of the ossicular chain.

Alloplastic materials for partial and total ossicular reconstruction prostheses are available. Hydroxyapatite is used in many prostheses because its mineral content is very similar to that of bone and it is well tolerated by the middle ear, thereby decreasing extrusion rates. Because it is brittle, it is often combined with other materials to allow it to be more easily trimmed for a precise fit in the middle ear. Titanium is another material used frequently in middle ear prostheses. Titanium is ideal for ossicular reconstruction because of its properties of being rigid and lightweight. Regardless of the type of prosthesis used, the surgeon must sculpt or trim it to bridge the ossicular gap by simulating the ossicular configuration and preserving the lever mechanism of the middle ear.

Procedural Considerations. PORP refers to an ossiculoplasty with a strut from the head of the stapes to the tympanic membrane (or graft) or manubrium. TORP refers to a strut extending from the footplate to the tympanic membrane (or graft) or manubrium. The patient is prepped and draped as for stapedotomy or tympanoplasty.

Operative Procedure. The procedure steps are similar to those for stapedotomy, except that the stapes footplate is not removed or opened.

Labyrinthectomy

Labyrinthectomy is a procedure that eliminates the vestibular and auditory function of the labyrinth to relieve severe vertigo. The procedure is usually performed when the disease is unilateral, a shunt or decompression procedure has been ineffective, and the affected ear has severe or total loss of hearing. Because the inner ear is removed, the patient may be very dizzy for several days until the brainstem begins to compensate for the destroyed labyrinth. The operation also leaves the ear with no residual hearing.

Procedural Considerations. The procedure is most commonly performed via the transmastoid approach. The patient is prepped and draped as described for the tympanoplasty or mastoidectomy procedure.

Operative Procedure

1. The surgeon creates a postauricular incision and performs a simple mastoidectomy.
2. The vertical segment of the facial nerve is identified, and the incus is disarticulated and removed.
3. The horizontal, posterior, and superior semicircular canals are drilled and removed. The neuroepithelium is completely removed from the ampullae of the three semicircular canals. The vestibule is exposed and the neuroepithelium from the utricle and saccule is removed.
4. The incision is closed in layers. An external pressure dressing of elastic gauze is applied.

Transmastoid, Translabyrinthine Approach

Procedural Considerations. The patient is prepped and draped as described for mastoidectomy. Neurologic intensive care is required for the first 24 hours. Preoperatively, ointments protect the eye and the eyelid is taped closed, or an adhesive bubble is placed over the eye to trap moisture. This protection is continued into the postoperative period unless a tarsorrhaphy (suturing the eyelid closed) is performed intraoperatively.

Operative Procedure

1. Steps 1 to 7 from the mastoidectomy procedure are performed.
2. After completing the mastoidectomy, the surgeon continues the dissection using cutting and diamond burrs until the internal auditory canal and the posterior fossa bone are removed.
3. The bone immediately over the facial nerve is removed by the use of nerve excavators and picks.
4. Using a facial nerve knife, neurectomy knife, sickle knife, neurectomy scissors, or micropick, the surgeon incises the facial nerve sheath. The majority of surgeons do not incise the epineurium of the facial nerve, and decompression only is felt to be equally efficacious and less traumatic to the nerve itself.
5. Hemostasis is achieved by the use of moistened, absorbable gelatin sponge; cottonoids; oxidized cellulose; bipolar ESU; or a combination of these.
6. The incision is closed and a pressure dressing of elastic gauze applied.

Middle Cranial Fossa Approach

Procedural Considerations. The patient's hair is clipped almost to the midline on the affected side. Povidone-iodine solution generally is used for the prep, which includes the portion of the head that has been clipped, the affected side of the face, and the neck. The surgeon injects lidocaine with or without epinephrine subcutaneously above the ear to assist in hemostasis. The patient's eye on the affected side is protected as previously described.

Operative Procedure

1. The surgeon incises the temporalis muscle and elevates it with a Lempert, Shambaugh, or similar type of elevator.
2. Hemostasis is achieved by clamping and tying vessels or by electrocoagulation.
3. The surgeon drills a square of bone from the temporal bone to expose the middle cranial fossa dura. (The bone is saved for replacement at the end of the procedure.)
4. A self-retaining retractor with a blade for retraction of the middle fossa (e.g., Fisch middle fossa retractor, House-Urban retractor) is inserted.
5. The microscope is positioned appropriately, and the surgeon elevates the dura from the floor of the middle fossa with a Freer elevator, a gimmick, or similar instruments.
6. Once hemostasis is achieved and the blade is inserted over the dura to expose the middle fossa, drilling may proceed.
7. When the bone becomes quite thin, the surgeon may remove the remaining bone with excavators to avoid damaging the nerve sheath.
8. The facial nerve sheath can be incised with a facial nerve knife, neurectomy knife, neurectomy scissors, or microknife.
9. The retractor is removed when hemostasis is achieved, and the bone flap is replaced.
10. The temporalis muscle is approximated and sutured, the incision closed, and a pressure dressing applied.

Removal of Acoustic Neuroma (Vestibular Schwannoma)

Acoustic neuromas arise from the Schwann cells of the vestibular portion of the eighth cranial (acoustic) nerve and are therefore more appropriately termed *vestibular schwannomas*. These tumors are benign but may grow to a size that produces symptoms of cerebellar and brainstem origin. Bilateral vestibular schwannomas are a common finding in patients with neurofibromatosis type 2 (NF2) (Briggs, 2010).

Most patients experience unilateral tinnitus and hearing loss—the main symptoms of a possible acoustic neuroma. However, depending on the rate and direction of tumor growth, signs and symptoms may include hearing loss, tinnitus, vertigo, headaches, double vision, diplopia, decreased corneal reflex, decreased blink reflex, impaired taste, reduced lacrimation, facial paralysis, diminished gag reflex, vocal cord paralysis, atrophy or fasciculation of the tongue, weakness of the sternocleidomastoid and trapezius muscles, disturbance in balance and gait, hydrocephalus, lethargy, confusion, drowsiness, and coma.

Several surgery centers have developed great expertise in acoustic neuroma surgery, which requires the combined team of a neurologist and a neurosurgeon.

Procedural Considerations. The translabyrinthine approach for the removal of an acoustic tumor reduces mortality and morbidity and offers a good chance of saving the facial nerve if the tumor has not directly invaded it. The patient should be informed about the presence of a Foley catheter, arterial line, temperature probe, clipped hair, and graft-site incision. The patient's hair is clipped to the midline of the affected side. Some patients prefer to have the entire head clipped to facilitate wearing a wig. This option should be presented preoperatively to enable the patient to make a decision before surgery. The surgical team preps and drapes the patient as described for labyrinthectomy. The surgeon injects lidocaine (with or without epinephrine) subcutaneously behind the ear. A facial nerve monitor is routinely used in the excision of cerebellopontine angle tumors. An intermittent pneumatic compression device is used intraoperatively and for the first 24 to 48 hours postoperatively or until the patient is ambulatory to decrease the risk of DVT and PE.

Operative Procedure

1. The surgeon makes a postauricular incision slightly longer and more posterior than the incision for mastoidectomy and elevates the periosteum from the mastoid bone with a Lempert, Shambaugh, or similar type of elevator.
2. Self-retaining retractors are inserted, and the cortical mastoidectomy is begun with a large cutting burr.
3. The microscope is positioned, and the attic is opened to visualize the ossicles. The sigmoid sinus, middle fossa dura, and superior petrosal sinus are left in place with a thin covering of bone. The semicircular canals are exposed. The incus is removed with alligator forceps or cup forceps and suction.
4. The surgeon excises the semicircular canals with the drill. The utricle and saccule are removed, and the aqueduct of the vestibule is drilled out to expose the internal auditory canal 270 degrees circumferentially.
5. Using nerve excavators, Fisch dissectors, or picks, the surgeon removes the remainder of bone from the dura of the internal meatus, posterior fossa, middle fossa, and petrosal angle. The wedge of bone between the facial and superior vestibular nerves (Bill's bar) is removed.
6. The dura is opened with microscissors or a dura knife. The surgeon dissects the tumor with a gimmick, Freer microelevator, microinstrument, and bipolar forceps (with or without suction). Hemostasis is achieved with a moistened, absorbable gelatin sponge; cottonoid patties; oxidized cellulose; or the bipolar ESU.
7. The tumor is removed by the use of pituitary cup forceps, long alligator forceps, and similar instruments.
8. Graft material (e.g., fat, fascia, or muscle) is obtained to pack the mastoid cavity created from the drilling. The packing is performed meticulously to avoid a cerebrospinal fluid leak.
9. The wound is closed and a thick pressure dressing applied.

Assistive Hearing Devices

A variety of assistive devices are available to patients with hearing loss, including phone amplifiers, closed captioning broadcasts, Telecommunication Device for the Deaf (TDD), and electronic devices, such as hearing aids. Technology has evolved tremendously in the field of otology, enabling surgeons to use surgically implantable devices in the treatment of hearing loss. These devices have greatly benefited the recipients, allowing some to distinguish sounds for the first time. Research continues in this field to develop applications for conditions previously considered untreatable and to refine and improve existing technology.

Cochlear Implantation. Technologic advances have given the deaf patient new hope in the area of cochlear implantation. The device is implanted in the cochlea, with the receiver resting in the mastoid (Figure 19-19). As the device receives sound through the receiver, it emits electrical impulses through the transmitter into the cochlea and along the acoustic nerve. These impulses are interpreted as sound in the auditory area of the brain, which is in the temporoparietal area of the cerebral cortex. The patient must be taught to interpret these sounds, which requires extensive training. Adult candidates for cochlear implantation generally possess the following characteristics: (1) severe or profound hearing loss with pure-tone

FIGURE 19-19 Cochlear implant system. Sound is transformed into an electrical signal in a speech processor. The signal is transmitted from an external to internal induction coil, which is connected to an electrode implanted near the cochlear nerve.

average of 70-dB hearing loss, (2) use of appropriately fitting hearing aids or a trial with amplification, (3) aided scores on open-set sentence tests of less than 50%, (4) no evidence of central auditory lesions or lack of an auditory nerve, and (5) no evidence of contraindications for surgery in general. Pediatric candidates (1) are 12 months through 17 years of age, (2) have profound sensorineural hearing loss, (3) experience minimal benefit from hearing aids, (4) have no evidence of central auditory lesions or lack of an auditory nerve, and (5) have no evidence of contraindications to surgery (Wackym and Runge-Samuelson, 2010). Appropriate auditory training and psychologic counseling are needed after appropriate selection of candidates.

Operative Procedure

1. A *modified postauricular incision is used.* The posterior flap, including the temporalis muscle, is elevated, exposing the underlying bone. The site of the internal receiver is identified, and with a special drill a circular depression in the squamous portion of the temporal bone is made to house the receiver.
2. A mastoidectomy is performed with preservation of the bony ear canal and opening of the facial recess.
3. The surgeon secures the internal receiver in the depressed area in the temporal bone, and introduces the intracochlear electrode through the facial recess via a cochleostomy into the cochlea. It is secured in place with a piece of temporalis fascia.
4. The wound is closed. The patient is observed for 2 to 4 weeks until the wound is completely healed. Then the external signal processor is fitted and programmed. This allows transmission of an electrical signal, picked up at an ear-level microphone and processed in a microprocessor worn on the body.

Osseointegrated Bone-Anchored Hearing Implants

Conventional hearing aids transmit sound using air conduction and bone conduction. Traditional bone-conduction hearing aids are

FIGURE 19-20 Bone-anchored hearing aid (BAHA) components. **A,** External processor; **B,** abutment and fixture.

FIGURE 19-21 Cross section showing fixture and abutment.

external and secured to the head with a spring device. Their design may make them uncomfortable and obtrusive, causing headaches and skin abrasions. The quality of sound is inferior, and they are associated with high battery consumption. Air-conduction devices use an earmold that fits into the ear canal. These devices may be contraindicated for patients with physical abnormalities that prevent the insertion of the earmold into the canal and for those who have chronic eczema, ear drainage, or inflammation in the ear canal. Osseointegrated bone-anchored hearing implants are designed for patients with moderate to severe conductive and sensorineural hearing loss (unilateral or bilateral). Ideally, implantable hearing devices should improve sound quality, provide comfort, improve appearance, and reduce the risk of chronic ear infections. Surgical implantation of hearing devices may be performed on an ambulatory basis using local or general anesthetics. The device is usually implanted in the ear with the best cochlear function.

Osseointegrated bone-anchored hearing implants (BAHA, by Cochlear Corp. and Ponto by Oticon Medical) eliminate many of the disadvantages associated with traditional external bone-conduction hearing aids. The implant is designed for patients 5 years of age and older with moderate to severe conductive hearing loss (unilateral or bilateral) caused by congenital malformations but who maintain good cochlear function (down to 45-dB hearing loss) and for patients with otitis media, cholesteatoma, otosclerosis, microtia, and canal atresia who are unable to benefit from conventional amplification. The device is approved and also used in patients with single-sided deafness, most commonly from sudden profound hearing loss or after surgical excision of an acoustic neuroma. The BAHA/Ponto system consists of a conventional microphone and amplifier, a specially designed transducer, and a coupling device to attach the device to the skin-penetrating and bone-anchored implant (Figure 19-20). The area behind the ear is prepped and draped, and the implant site is marked. It is important to ensure that the hearing aid does not touch the pinna, which may cause acoustic feedback. A semicircular incision is made around the proposed fixture site. A titanium fixture is permanently implanted (tapped) into the mastoid bone, and a permanent skin penetration is made with a titanium snap coupler (Figures 19-21 and 19-22). A sound processor is fitted and adjusted to the patient's hearing loss 8 to 12 weeks after the implantation, depending on the age of the patient and ensuring the osseointegration process has taken place (Lustig and Santina, 2010) (Figure 19-23). When the BAHA/Ponto

FIGURE 19-22 Bone-anchored hearing aid (BAHA) abutment.

system is placed in young children, the sound processor is fitted in 3 to 6 months to ensure adequate osseointegration.

Rhinologic (Nasal) Procedures

Rhinologic surgery is performed to correct structural issues of the nose and to treat sinusitis and other conditions; it is also used as an adjunctive procedure to treat other disorders (e.g., pituitary neoplasms). Procedures that involve both internal and external nasal reconstruction can be done with local anesthetics, usually supplemented with IV sedation and analgesia. If the patient is particularly apprehensive or anxious, a general anesthetic may be more appropriate.

Treatment of Epistaxis

Patients with nasal bleeding usually control the problem themselves with direct pressure application. When their efforts fail, they seek help from their physician or an emergency department (ED). When more conservative measures (which involve vasoconstrictive agents

FIGURE 19-23 Patient with an implanted bone-anchored hearing aid. The implant is positioned to avoid contact with the pinna, which could cause acoustic feedback if the device were driven at maximum output.

FIGURE 19-24 Posterior nasal packing with syringe for balloon inflation.

and nasal packing) taken in the ED fail, surgical intervention becomes necessary.

When epistaxis occurs, the first step of treatment is to spray oxymetazoline nasal spray in both nares and apply direct pressure to the patient's nose. An initial hold of 15 minutes is recommended. Thereafter, inspection of the anterior nose and posterior oral pharynx should be performed to determine if the site of bleeding is anteriorly based in the nose or posteriorly located deep in the nasal cavity. Evidence of a posterior bleed is usually demonstrated by a trickling flow of blood from the nasopharynx running down along the posterior pharyngeal wall during an oral inspection. Blood may also appear on the tongue and the patient may complain of swallowing blood. Anterior epistaxis characteristically trickles down the front of the face onto the upper lip. Anterior septum bleeds (in patients without coagulopathy), identified appropriately and timely, can often be easily controlled with silver nitrate sticks. If oxymetazoline spray and direct pressure fail to arrest the bleed, packing with nasal tampons or posterior packs should be considered. Various gelatin packing is available for selective patients. Brisk bleeding usually requires a nasal tampon or endoscopic surgical control, whereas slower oozing may be appropriately treated with oxymetazoline spray, direct pressure, and gelatin packing with close monitoring and follow-up.

The length of the pack should be based on the suspicion of where the bleed originates. Longer packing (8- or 10-cm packing) is considered when bleeds are more posterior in the nasopharynx. More anterior bleeds can be packed with 4.5-cm packing. Packing should be generously coated with antibiotic ointment and inserted in a horizontal angle following the floor of the nose. The packing is then sprayed with saline or oxymetazoline spray, and expands. The patient should receive broad-spectrum antibiotics, such as oral third-generation cephalosporins, and instructed to follow up in 2 to 3 days for removal of packing.

Balloon nasal packing has an exterior balloon along the tube length as well as an anchoring balloon on the end (Figure 19-24). The anchoring balloon is first inflated, and then the pressure balloons are inflated to compress bleeding vessels. If commercial

balloon sinus packing is not available, a Foley catheter may be used. A clamp can be placed on the Foley to prevent sliding back into the nasopharynx. Close attention to the ala must be observed to prevent alar necrosis. If this fails to stop the oozing and other hemostatic agents, such as gelatin-based packing, silver nitrate sticks, or oxidized cellulose, fail to halt the bleed, an endoscopic approach to control the epistaxis is warranted. The endoscopy is performed in the OR with the use of general anesthesia or conscious sedation. Occasionally ligation of the ethmoid, or internal maxillary artery, is necessary and should be considered for persistent bleeds. Embolization of the internal maxillary arteries may be considered as well. Endoscopic ligation of the sphenopalatine artery has been recently described and found to be useful in controlling persistent bleeds.

The setup for endoscopic control of epistaxis is the same as that for all nasal case prepping and draping. Using an endoscope, the surgeon focuses attention on the Kiesselbach plexus in the anterior nasal cavity and on the sphenopalatine artery because these are common sites of persistent bleeds. Suction ESU should be used to control any visual bleeding and to clear the nasal passages of clot or oozing. Other surgical options include transmaxillary artery ligation, internal maxillary artery ligation, anteroposterior ethmoid ligation, transnasal endoscopic sphenopalatine artery ligation, and submucosal supraperichondrial septoplasty and in extremely rare cases, ligation of the external carotid artery.

Nasoseptoplasty or Submucous Resection of the Septum

A nasoseptoplasty is straightening of either the cartilaginous or the osseous portions of the septum that lie between the flaps of the mucous membrane and the perichondrium. When the nasal septum is deformed, fractured, or injured, normal respiratory and nasal function may be impaired, interfering with airflow and sinus drainage. Deviations of the septum involving cartilage, bony parts (spurs), or both may block the meatus and compress the middle turbinate on that side, thereby resulting in an obstruction of the sinus opening. Septal deviations tend to produce sinus disease and nasal polyps.

The objective of the procedure is to establish an adequate partition between the left and right nasal cavities, thereby providing a clear airway through both the internal and external cavities of the nose.

Procedural Considerations. The procedure may be performed using local anesthesia, MAC, or general anesthesia. Regardless of

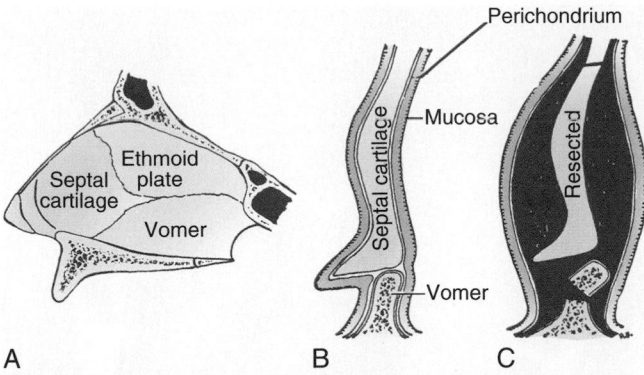

FIGURE 19-25 A, Primary components of septum. Incision line is for Killian-type submucous resection. **B,** Septum with deviated cartilage and spur at junction of vomer and septal cartilage. **C,** Resection of obstructive parts after careful elevation of the mucoperichondrium and mucoperiosteum.

FIGURE 19-26 Reduction of nasal fracture. **A,** A Boies elevator is placed along the lateral wall of the nose to a point below the nasofrontal angle. The distance to the ala is marked with the thumb. **B,** The elevator is then placed under the depressed nasal bone, lifting it into position; the opposite thumb carefully exerts downward pressure on the elevated contralateral bone.

the method chosen, the surgeon uses topical and injected anesthetics to aid in hemostasis. In most cases the surgeon wears a headlight to improve visualization of the intranasal structures.

Operative Procedure

1. The surgeon opens the nostril with a nasal speculum and incises through the mucoperichondrium of the septum with a #15 blade. Using a Freer elevator, the tissues are separated and elevated.
2. Deviated cartilage and bony, thickened structures are trimmed or removed with a septum punch and a nasal cutting forceps.
3. The surgeon trims the bony septal spurs with a punch forceps or chisel, gouge, and mallet. Suction is used to expose the field. Bleeding is controlled by insertion of additional cottonoids soaked with a topical hemostatic agent or by using an ESU.
4. The perpendicular plate of the ethmoid as well as the vomer may be removed by means of a suitable septum-cutting forceps (Figure 19-25).
5. The incision is sutured with 4-0 absorbable atraumatic suture on a small, straight needle.
6. Plastic or Silastic nasal splints may be inserted to prevent adhesions and septal hematoma. Some surgeons use mattress sutures to provide a patent airway while maintaining support for the septum.
7. A mustache dressing (i.e., a piece of 2 × 2–inch gauze folded and placed below the nose and secured with tape across the face or bridge of the nose) is applied. A small ice bag (e.g., a surgical glove filled with ice) may be applied to the nose.

Closed Reduction of Nasal Fracture

The nose is the structure most susceptible to trauma because it is seated midface. The paired nasal bones are thin and project like a tent on the frontal process of the maxilla. If the trauma is caused by a direct frontal blow, usually both nasal bones are fractured, displaced outward, and depressed into the ethmoid sinus, and the septal cartilages become displaced. Noncontrast CT scans of the sinuses may be performed with protocols compatible with endoscopic navigation systems to have an accurate sense of extension of deviation or possible injury to surrounding sinuses and structures.

Procedural Considerations. Simple nasal fractures often can be managed with topical and local anesthesia. However, as with most nasal procedures, if the patient is significantly anxious, general anesthesia may be necessary. Topical and local anesthetics are used with a general anesthetic to provide vasoconstriction and enhance visualization for the procedure. The surgical team preps and positions the patient for nasal surgery.

Operative Procedure

1. The surgeon packs the nose with cottonoid patties saturated with 4% cocaine. The local anesthetic is injected as previously described. When epinephrine is used, 10 minutes is the optimum time to wait for the effects of the hemostatic agent. This period of time will vary with other agents.
2. A Boies elevator is inserted into the nostril, and the nasal bones are elevated and molded into place by external manipulation (Figure 19-26).
3. Nasal packing or a Denver splint may be used to stabilize the reduction because sometimes the bony fragments tend to return to a depressed status.

Sinus Surgery

Sinusitis can be either recurrent acute, or chronic. It is caused by bacteria and fungi and may be associated with anatomic abnormalities of the nose, such as a deviated septum or poor drainage pathways from the sinuses. Medical management of acute bacterial sinusitis involves a course of appropriate antibiotic therapy for 10 days to 2 weeks. If a patient does not respond to medical treatment for acute bacterial sinusitis or if sinus complaints persist, surgical drainage of the sinuses is indicated. Traditionally open surgical treatments involved destructive procedures such as Caldwell-Luc, external ethmoidectomy and sphenoidectomy, and frontal sinus obliteration. Sinus procedures can be performed intranasally with or without the aid of endoscopes and video or through an open approach determined by which sinus cavity is involved. These

FIGURE 19-27 Endoscopic suites demonstrating navigation systems and monitors.

FIGURE 19-28 Computed tomography (CT) scan of maxillary and ethmoid sinuses. Note septal deviation to the left, maxillary sinus ostia, turbinates, and ocular muscles.

procedures have been replaced by modern endoscopic sinus surgery. Noninvasive fungal sinusitis is treated by endoscopic removal. Invasive fungal sinusitis is frequently fatal and requires aggressive endoscopic debridement with a prolonged course of antifungals.

Functional Endoscopic Sinus Surgery (FESS). FESS provides a more functional approach to treat sinus disease. Procedures performed endoscopically decrease trauma to normal structures, reduce morbidity, and shorten the healing process for the patient. Endoscopic procedures offer an advantage over open procedures because of direct visualization of the tissue and anatomic structures. Dedicated endoscopic sinus and skull base suites present a popular option for FESS because of the ease of setup, use of multiple monitors, and rooms that free up floor space (Figure 19-27).

FESS involves the endoscopic resection of inflammatory and anatomic defects of the sinuses while preserving natural function in a surgical procedure that is minimally invasive. Because of the anatomic relationship to the brain and orbit, this procedure has many risks, which should be incorporated into the informed consent process. It is considered to be a technically demanding surgery, and techniques vary significantly. Most surgeons prefer the endoscope to be attached to a video monitor, but some prefer to look directly through the eyepiece. The operative instruments are introduced into the nose alongside the endoscope.

If there is obstruction of outflow (e.g., allergy, septal deflection, spurs) between the mucosa and the sinus, mucociliary clearance is inhibited and secretions are retained in the sinus. This predisposes the patient to sinus infections and mucocele. The following sections are discussed with the understanding that they are more commonly performed endoscopically but may be done with an open approach as necessary. The purpose of FESS is to ensure adequate drainage of the sinuses by resecting tissue and creating increased aeration of the sinuses.

Procedural Considerations. FESS can be performed after induction of general anesthesia or MAC, depending on the surgeon's and patient's preference. The setup for FESS is the same as the setup for any nasal surgery in terms of prepping, draping, and positioning. The instruments required are the basic nasal set, video equipment including monitor, and light source with the appropriate

light cord adapted to the type of endoscope used. The endoscopes used in sinus surgery are much like endoscopes used in other procedures. They are 4 to 5 mm in diameter and have different directions of view: 0, 30, 70, 90, or 120 degrees. Lenses are chosen based on the sinus to be operated on. Often if work is to be done in several sinus cavities, the surgeon may change lenses intraoperatively to obtain the optimal view in each cavity.

In addition to endoscopes, other instruments that may be used in FESS include endoscopic suction tips and suction elevators, biopsy forceps, forceps for retracting and cutting or excising tissue, and scissors. Patients undergo preoperative CT studies to determine the specific areas affected by the sinusitis. These CT scans should be available in the OR and will be referenced by the surgeon during the surgery (Figure 19-28).

The video equipment is located at the head of the bed. The surgeon operates from the right side of the patient, the scrub person stands at the right of the surgeon, and the surgical assistant usually stands across from the surgeon on the opposite side of the table. More commonly the surgeon, the assistant, and the scrub person stand during the procedure. The rest of the surgical team can view the procedure on the video monitor.

Image-guided navigational systems are especially useful in revision sinus surgery, in which the familiar anatomy of the sinuses has been altered by previous surgery and the typical landmarks of the sinuses are now changed. From a safety standpoint and to reduce the risk of a revision surgery, many surgeons will not attempt a revision sinus procedure without having a navigational system available.

Several navigational systems are available, and many of these systems have applications for different types of surgeries, so the initial expense of the machine itself can be defrayed if it is shared with different surgical specialties, such as neurosurgery. Also technical components to facilitating this type of sinus surgery must be

FIGURE 19-29 Entellus procedure kit.

FIGURE 19-30 Entellus express device with light fiber.

mastered by the perioperative nursing staff, who must develop competence in system setup, transfer of the CT scan data into the system, and perform maintenance procedures.

To avoid possible injury, the scrub person should pass instruments in the closed position and never over the patient's face. They should be passed smoothly and carefully so that the surgeon's eyes do not leave the endoscope or video monitor, limiting distractions. Some surgeons will request a suction-irrigation device that provides visualization of the sinus recesses by allowing simultaneous suction and irrigation of the operative field. Antifog solutions and endoscopic scrubbing devices are also used to improve visibility during the procedure.

Another consideration that is crucial to a successful outcome in FESS is to maintain the integrity of the patient's orbit. The patient's eyes must be visible to the surgeon at all times to avoid injury to the orbit or to immediately recognize injury if it occurs. The surgeon monitors for movement of the eyeball or appearance of an intraorbital hematoma.

Encroachment of the orbit can be recognized if yellow tissue is seen, because orbital fat is yellow. This finding should be communicated immediately to the surgeon. Another good technique is for the scrub person to place all tissue removed by the surgeon into a small labeled container of normal saline or lactated Ringer's solution on the surgical field. If any of the tissue floats, the surgeon should be notified immediately.

Balloon Sinuplasty. Balloon sinuplasty (Figures 19-29 and 19-30) is an alternative surgical technique to FESS by which the paranasal sinus ostia are dilated open with a balloon catheter inserted over a guidewire or Lusk probe via direct visualization (video endoscopy) and then inflated into the ostia creating a patent ostium (Research Highlight). This procedure can only be performed on the frontal, maxillary, and sphenoid air cells. The ethmoid sinuses still need to be addressed by the endoscopic approach.

Nasal Polypectomy. Nasal polyps are benign, grapelike clusters of mucous membrane and connective tissue lining the nose or sinuses. When the polyps become large, they obstruct the free passage of air, make breathing difficult, and cause a change in speech quality (Figure 19-31). Endoscopic nasal polypectomies are often performed with other sinus procedures that also require removal of diseased tissue. Because of the aggressive nature of polyps, microdebriders are particularly helpful in these cases. They can greatly shorten surgical time by their mechanism of morcellating the polyp and removing it by immediate suctioning while controlling bleeding, as opposed to each polyp being manually extracted with an instrument in small pieces. Cases involving inverting papilloma often recur and frequently require repeat polypectomies as symptoms recur.

Procedural Considerations. Nasal polypectomy setup is as for any intranasal procedure, with the addition of endoscopic equipment. Additional instruments may include a nasal polyp snare if a microdebrider is not used. Packing is typically not needed or used.

Operative Procedure
1. The surgeon applies topical anesthetic and administers the local anesthetic.
2. The lens of the endoscope is treated with antifog solution before the endoscope is introduced into the nose.
3. The surgeon enlarges the natural ostium of the maxillary sinus with a Lusk probe to provide physiologic drainage through the middle meatus. This creates a maxillary antrostomy and allows a larger drainage pathway into the ostiomeatal complex.
4. The diseased tissue is visualized through the endoscope, and the surgeon uses straight or angled true-cuts to remove it.
5. If an anterior ethmoidectomy is indicated, the surgeon inserts the endoscope into the ostiomeatal complex and performs the ethmoidectomy by taking small bites of the honeycombed bones with straight true-cuts and removing them manually or with suction. This reduces the many-celled ethmoid labyrinth into one large cavity to ensure adequate drainage and aeration.
6. A sphenoidotomy is created by biting an opening into one or both of the sphenoidal sinuses with a straight true-cut. It is usually performed only if sphenoid sinus disease is present on

RESEARCH HIGHLIGHT

Balloon Sinuplasty Versus Functional Endoscopic Sinus Surgery (FESS)

Rhinosinusitis is generally the end result of a blocked osteomeatal complex and disturbed mucociliary transport. Surgical options for treating rhinosinusitis focus on opening the sinus ostia to improve aeration and mucosal function. In FESS techniques, instruments are used to remove bone to and physically alter structures, aerate, and create a larger meatus. Balloon sinuplasty involves the passage of a balloon catheter over a guidewire to the stenosed area. The balloon is inflated and dilates the passage, allowing the surgeon to open narrowed ostia without removing bone or tissue. Long-term studies of balloon sinuplasty have demonstrated the safety and efficacy of the procedure (Weiss et al, 2008).

Two studies published in 2012 sought to determine if there were any advantages of balloon sinuplasty over FESS in treating chronic rhinosinusitis. Achar and colleagues conducted an open, randomized controlled pilot study with 24 adult participants using the sinonasal outcome test questionnaire and saccharine clearance time (SCT) to determine outcomes and effectiveness of one technique over the other. The questionnaire and SCT tests were administered preoperatively, and at 6 months after surgery. Study participants ranged in age from 29 to 64 years and were equally divided into a FESS group and a balloon sinuplasty group. Analysis of the outcome data between the two groups showed that the balloon sinuplasty group had a greater improvement of subjective symptoms per the questionnaire and that SCT improved as well. The balloon sinuplasty group also had a shorter recovery time of 2.2 days versus 5 days for the FESS group.

Thottam and colleagues studied 31 pediatric patients using a two-group retrospective cohort blinded chart review methodology. The mean age of their participants was 9.3 years. Within the participant group, 16 were treated with FESS and 15 were treated with balloon sinuplasty. All procedures resulted in symptom improvement; 92.6% of the participants undergoing sinuplasty had reduction of symptoms at the 2- to 4-week postoperative mark versus 64.3% who underwent FESS. The balloon sinuplasty group also had significant improvement in congestion and cessation of antibiotic use over the FESS group.

Both studies have demonstrated the effectiveness of balloon sinuplasty as a viable treatment option for rhinosinusitis and indicated some advantages to the sinuplasty procedure over FESS. Ongoing studies with larger study groups are needed to determine sustainability of these early results.

Modified from Weiss RL et al: Long-term outcome analysis of balloon catheter sinusotomy: two-year follow-up, *Otolaryngol Head Neck Surg* 139:S38–S46, 2008; Achar P et al: Endoscopic dilatation sinus surgery (FEDS) versus functional endoscopic sinus surgery (FESS) for treatment of chronic rhinosinusitis: a pilot study, *Acta Otorhinolaryngol Ital* 32:314–319, 2012; Thottam PJL et al: Functional endoscopic sinus surgery (FESS) alone versus balloon catheter sinuplasty (BCS) and ethmoidectomy: a comparative outcome analysis in pediatric chronic rhinosinusitis, *Int J Pediatr Otorhinolaryngol* 76(9):1355–1360, 2012.

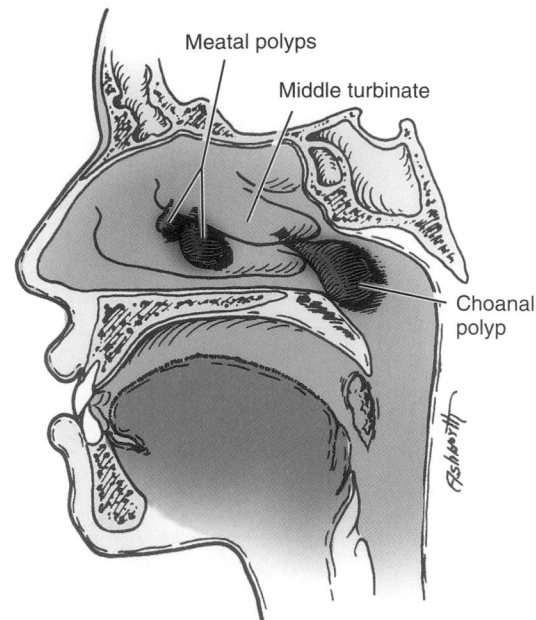

FIGURE 19-31 Nasal polyps. A choanal polyp is usually single and originates in the maxillary sinus; however, most polyps are found in the middle meatus.

9. Absorbable gelatin film or packing may be placed into the patient's middle meatus to maintain patency and reduce stenosis. If used, it is rolled into a cylindric splint and set in place with bayonet forceps. Some surgeons use nonabsorbable packing. An antibiotic ointment may be applied to the splint first, according to the surgeon's preference. The gel splints dissolve gradually, or they may be removed with irrigation.

10. A mustache dressing is applied.

Caldwell-Luc with Antrostomy. The purpose of an antrostomy is to establish a large opening into the wall of the inferior meatus, which ensures adequate gravity drainage and aeration. This large opening allows removal of the diseased tissues in the sinuses under direct vision. The Caldwell-Luc approach is also used to access the maxillary artery in cases of extreme epistaxis. The procedure requires an incision into the canine fossa of the upper jaw and exposure of the antrum for removal of bony diseased portions of the antral wall and contents of the sinus (Figure 19-32).

Endoscopic Transnasal Repair of Cerebrospinal Fluid Leak. Cerebrospinal fluid (CSF) leaks are usually created by surgery or trauma. Although rare, spontaneous CSF leaks do occur. CSF leaks are associated with morbidity such as general malaise and headache. More importantly, a leak can lead to meningitis and fast deterioration of a patient. CSF leaks occur when the bony cranial vault and its underlying dura are breached. Such leaks may be broadly categorized as traumatic or nontraumatic in origin. Traumatic causes can be further subclassified into surgical and nonsurgical, with surgical causes divided into planned or unplanned (Prosser et al, 2011). Patients usually complain of clear rhinorrhea with a salty taste from the nose, worse when either leaning forward or lying flat. Headache may accompany the rhinorrhea because of low spinal column pressures. Diagnosis is confirmed by sending the nasal fluid to the laboratory to test for β_2-transferrin, a protein specifically found in CSF.

CT. Sphenoidotomies are often done with ethmoidectomies because once the ethmoid labyrinth is removed, the surgeon has excellent access through a lateralized middle turbinate exposing the sphenoidal sinuses.

7. The surgeon may perform a frontal sinusotomy by opening the frontal recess anterior to ethmoid air cells. If more severe disease is present, a frontal sinus drill-out may be indicated.

8. Because no incisions are made, no sutures are required. Epistaxis should be controlled endoscopically until it becomes a slow ooze.

FIGURE 19-32 Caldwell-Luc operation.

FIGURE 19-33 Carcinoma of the dorsal tongue.

A CT cisternogram assists with diagnosing the leak and often helps locate the site of dehiscence. Prepping and draping of the patient are performed in the same sterile fashion as for an endoscopic transsphenoidal approach to resection of pituitary mass, including prepping one lateral thigh and abdomen for potential graft use. All steps are followed as in a transsphenoidal resection of mass while paying close attention to the location of the carotids on the navigation system. When the leak is found, a decision on what type of closure to use is made by the otolaryngology/neurosurgical team.

Oral Cavity/Laryngologic/Pharyngologic/Neck Procedures

Surgery of the Oral Cavity and Pharynx

The oral cavity is susceptible to both benign and malignant lesions, in part because of environmental risk factors. Oral malignancies can be linked to specific carcinogens, the most important being tobacco usage (without and in combination with heavy alcohol consumption). It is estimated by the American Cancer Society (ACS) that in 2013 about 36,000 people will be diagnosed with oral cavity or oropharyngeal cancer and 6850 will die from these cancers. Incidence rates are more than twice as high in men as in women and are greatest in men who are older than 50 years. The recent rise in human papillomavirus (HPV)–linked cancer has risen dramatically over the past decades. HPV DNA is now found in about two out of three oropharyngeal cancers. The rising rate of HPV-related cancers is thought to be due to changes in sexual practices, particularly to an increase in oral sex (ACS, 2013).

Benign or malignant lesions of the tongue, floor of the mouth, alveolar ridge, buccal mucosa, or tonsillar area are excised depending on extensiveness of disease, involvement of surrounding vessels and nerves, and candidacy for surgery (Figures 19-33 and 19-34). Benign or small malignant tumors of the oral cavity may be excised without a neck dissection, though in the presence of diagnosed or highly suspicious metastatic disease, a selective neck dissection may be performed in an effort to control a cancerous growth in the upper jugular lymphatic chain of the neck.

Prior to treatment of carcinoma of the floor of the mouth with involvement of the mandible, a CT scan or MRI of the face and neck should be obtained to evaluate extension of the disease. A

FIGURE 19-34 Carcinoma of the right tonsil.

portion of the tongue is resected and may require a combined operation with reconstructive surgeons. A tracheostomy, percutaneous endoscopic gastric tube, neck dissection, and composite resection of both the mandible and the tongue with free flap reconstruction may be considered for extensive disease. When the primary intraoral

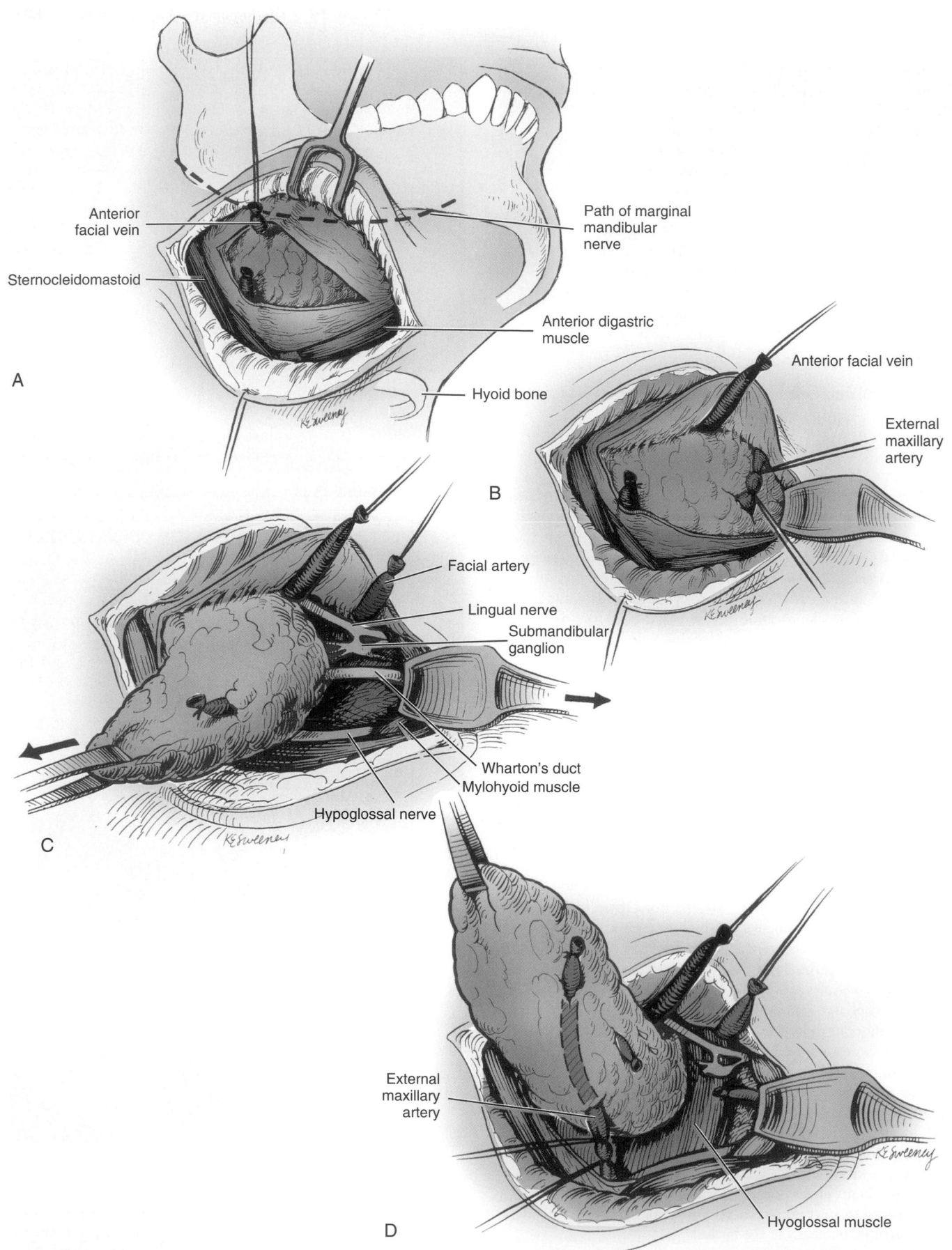

FIGURE 19-35 Excision of submandibular gland. **A,** Submandibular incision made in a natural skin crease 3 to 4 cm inferior to the mandible. The marginal mandibular nerve generally lies just superficial to the anterior facial vein. **B,** The external maxillary artery is identified on the submandibular gland. **C,** The mylohyoid muscle is retracted anteriorly and submandibular gland posteriorly. This exposes the lingual nerve, submandibular ganglion, and Wharton's duct. **D,** The hypoglossal nerve, running between the hypoglossal and mylohyoid muscles. The external maxillary artery must be divided a second time.

lesion is confined to the tongue, a neck dissection and a hemiglossectomy are performed without resection of the mandible. In the presence of a lesion of the tonsil or an extensive lesion of the base of the tongue with pharyngeal wall involvement, resection of the mass may require removal of portions of the base of the tongue, pharyngeal wall, and soft palate to secure an adequate margin of normal tissue around the lesion. In recent years nonsurgical management with chemoradiotherapy has advanced for select oropharyngeal tumors. A free flap may be considered to fill a soft tissue defect if one is created from surgical resection. Psychologic preparation of the patient is extremely important because these procedures may be done for a minor lesion in the oral cavity or may be the first stage of much more extensive surgery in the head and neck area. A supportive and accepting family is important to the patient because of the possibility of disfigurement after surgery.

Procedural Considerations. The patient is positioned supine with the shoulders elevated. Generally, endotracheal anesthesia is used, and a pharyngeal pack of moist gauze may be inserted in the mouth. Instruments and supplies vary, depending on the surgical intervention.

Operative Procedure. Although the procedure may be scheduled as a local excision, frequently lesions of the oral cavity require more extensive excision. The setup should be designed to include the instruments for a neck dissection, or they should be readily available. For some tumors of the oral cavity, a tracheostomy is performed to ensure a patent airway after surgery. A laser may be used to excise locally confined lesions of the oral cavity.

Salivary Gland Surgery

Disorders of the salivary glands typically fall into one of three categories: inflammatory, obstructive, and neoplastic. Inflammatory conditions, such as bacterial or viral infections, can lead to salivary gland abscesses and ductal stone formation. Obstructive conditions can be a secondary consequence of inflammatory processes. Masses of the salivary glands may be benign or malignant, and 70% of them occur in the parotid gland. Three quarters of these parotid masses are benign (Elluru, 2010). Perioperative nurses will facilitate surgical care for patients experiencing any of these conditions.

Excision of the Submandibular Gland. Excision of the submandibular gland is performed to remove mixed tumors and calculi associated with extensive chronic inflammation. An incision is made below and parallel to the mandible and extending to beneath the chin to remove the gland and tumor.

Procedural Considerations. The team positions the patient supine, with the affected side up. The instruments include a minor neck dissection setup. A set of lacrimal probes should also be added to the instrument setup if exploration of the submandibular (Wharton) duct is necessary during surgery. The perioperative nurse must ensure that no local anesthetic is delivered to the sterile field if identification of major nerves is anticipated. A nerve stimulator and bipolar ESU may be requested.

Operative Procedure

1. The surgeon makes a small skin incision below and parallel to the mandible, extending forward to beneath the chin (Figure 19-35, *A*). The platysma is incised with scissors; the skin flaps and undersurface of the platysma and cervical fascia covering the gland are undermined with fine hooks, tissue forceps, and Metzenbaum scissors (see Figure 19-35, *B*).

2. The mandibular branch of the facial nerve is retracted with a small loop retractor or nerve hook.

3. The submandibular gland is elevated from the mylohyoid muscle (see Figure 19-35, *C*). The edge of the muscle is retracted anteriorly to expose the lingual veins and nerve and the hypoglossal nerve, which is identified and preserved.

4. The gland is freed by blunt dissection, and the submandibular duct is clamped, ligated, and divided with care to prevent injury to the lingual nerve.

5. The facial artery is clamped, ligated, and divided. The submandibular gland is removed (see Figure 19-35, *D*).

6. The wound is closed with interrupted absorbable sutures. The skin edges are approximated with nonabsorbable sutures. A drain is inserted into the submandibular bed and secured to the skin. Dressings are applied.

Parotidectomy. Parotidectomy may be performed to treat recurrent parotitis, but it is more commonly performed as part of the management of parotid gland tumors. In parotidectomy for tumor removal, the tumor and a portion of or the entire parotid gland are removed through a curved incision in the upper neck, in front of the earlobe, or through a Y-type incision on both sides of the ear and below the angle of the mandible. Even when a mass in the parotid gland is benign, the closeness of the facial nerve makes removing the entire mass surgically challenging (Figure 19-36). The facial nerve exits the stylomastoid foramen, enters the substance of the salivary gland, and then bifurcates into the temporofacial and cervicofacial branches, variably communicating with the gland. These branches then further divide into the temporal, zygomatic, buccal, and marginal mandibular and cervical branches near the edge of the parotid. The gland is divided artificially into a *superficial* and a *deep* lobe according to its relationship to the facial nerve. The possibility of damaging the facial nerve (resulting in facial nerve

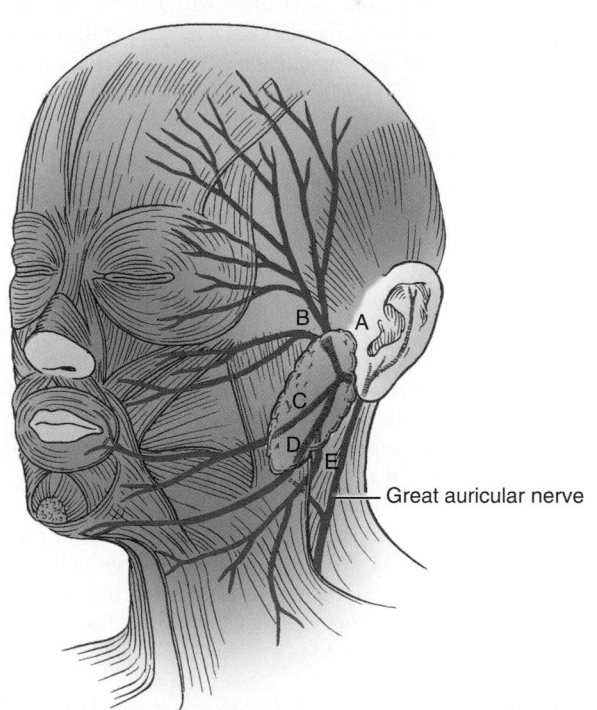

FIGURE 19-36 Branches of facial nerve. *A,* Temporal; *B,* zygomatic; *C,* buccal; *D,* mandibular; *E,* cervical.

weakness or paralysis) during the dissection of the gland should be considered carefully by all patients contemplating parotidectomy. Therefore, the surgeon must understand that the most definitive way of avoiding damage to the facial nerve is to identify it early in the procedure. In addition, the patient should understand that a more radical procedure might be required if a malignant tumor is discovered to involve adjacent structures.

Procedural Considerations. The patient is positioned supine with the entire affected side of the face up. The entire side of the face, the mouth, the outer canthus of the eye, the ear, and the forehead are prepped and left exposed.

The instrument setup is a neck dissection set. A nerve stimulator or nerve integrity monitor should be available. A set of lacrimal probes should be included in the setup if exploration of the ductal system of the parotid is necessary during the course of surgery. Bipolar ESU may also be required.

Operative Procedure

1. The incision (Figure 19-37) may extend from the posterior angle of the zygoma downward in front of the tragus of the ear and behind the lobule of the ear backward; the incision continues over the mastoid process and then downward and forward on the neck parallel to and below the body of the mandible (a chin incision also may be used). Bleeding vessels are controlled by hemostats and fine ligatures or with an ESU.

2. Using fine-toothed tissue forceps and scissors, the surgeon elevates the skin flaps as described for thyroidectomy (see Chapter 16) and retracts the flap with silk sutures fastened to clamps.

3. The surgeon exposes and retracts the upper portion of the ster-nocleidomastoid muscle. The auricular nerve is identified, and the lower part of the parotid gland is elevated with curved hemostats.

4. The superficial temporal artery and vein and external jugular vein are identified by means of blunt dissection. The surgeon dissects the parotid tissue from the cartilage of the ear and the tympanic plate of the temporal bone. The temporal, zygomatic, mandibular, and cervical branches of the facial nerve are identified and preserved.

5. The surgeon removes the diseased portion of the parotid gland, which can be superficial or deep.

   a. The *superficial portion* of the parotid gland containing the tumor is removed. In some cases the entire superficial portion is removed, followed by ligation and division of the parotid duct (Figure 19-38).

   b. When the *deep portion* of the parotid gland must be removed, the facial nerve is gently retracted upward and outward and then the parotid tissue is removed from beneath the nerve. Kocher retractors are used to retract the mandible. The external carotid artery is identified. In many cases the internal maxillary and superficial temporal arteries are clamped, ligated, and divided.

6. The surgeon closes the wound in layers with absorbable suture. If a tissue defect is observed or anticipated overlying the resected portion of the parotid gland, abdominal fat may be harvested. A small drain is inserted, the skin is closed with fine nonabsorbable suture, and a pressure dressing may be applied depending on the surgeon's preference.

Uvulopalatopharyngoplasty. Uvulopalatopharyngoplasty (UPPP) is performed primarily to relieve obstructive sleep apnea (OSA) and snoring (Figure 19-39). UPPP is not a substitution for the use of

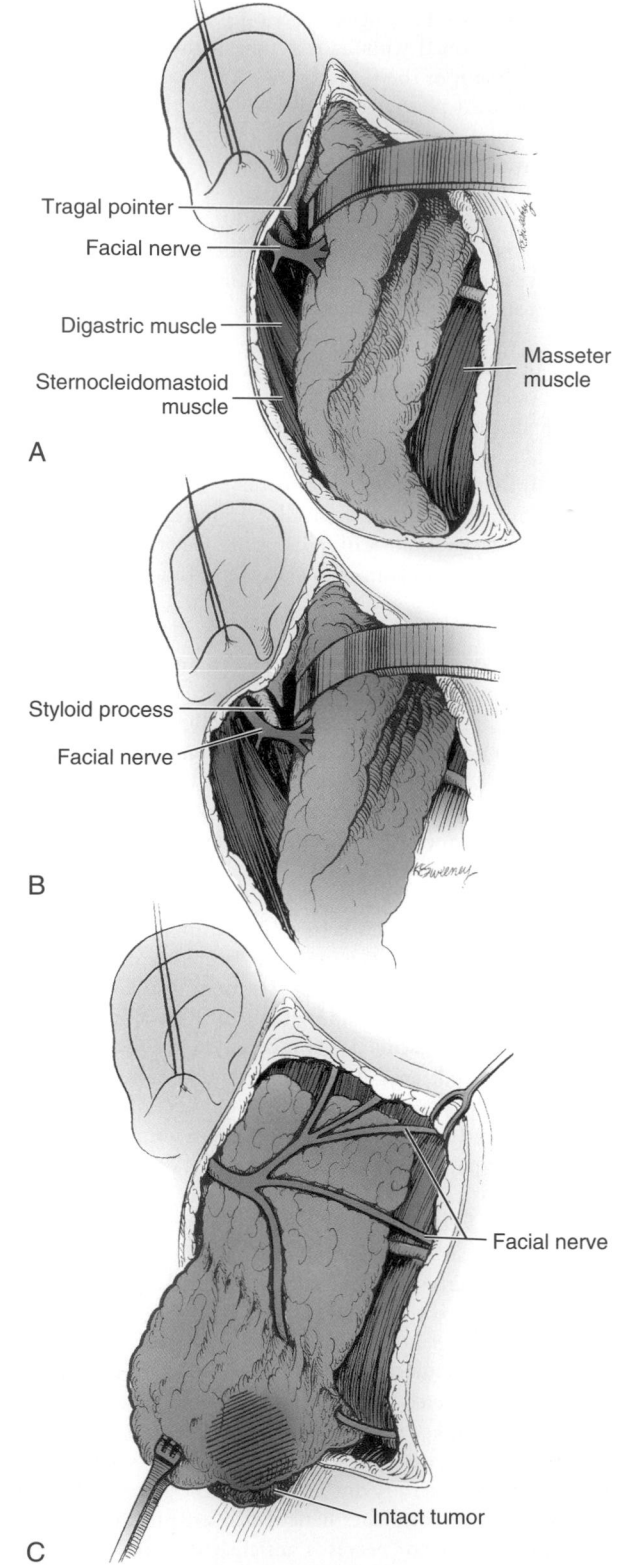

A

B

C

FIGURE 19-37 Operative technique for parotidectomy. **A,** Blunt dissection of parotid gland from the external auditory canal cartilage exposes the tragal pointer. The facial nerve lies approximately 1 cm deep and slightly antero-inferior to the pointer and 6 to 8 mm deep to the tympanomastoid suture line. **B,** Facial nerve exits stylomastoid foramen to run anteriorly between the styloid process and attachment of digastric muscle to the digastric ridge. **C,** Nearly completed process with tumor within intact superficial parotidectomy specimen.

FIGURE 19-38 Surgical removal of superficial parotid mass.

Patient predisposed to OSA

Apneic episode

FIGURE 19-39 Sleep apnea syndrome is a condition in which airflow is temporarily obstructed during sleep. Airflow obstruction occurs when the tongue and the soft palate fall backward and partially or completely obstruct the pharynx. The obstruction may last from 10 seconds to as long as 2 minutes. During the apneic period the patient experiences severe hypoxemia (decreased PaO_2), hypercapnia (increased $PaCO_2$), and acidosis. These changes interrupt sleep and cause the patient to partially awaken. When the patient begins to awaken, the tone of the muscles of the upper airway increases. The tongue and soft palate move forward, and the airway opens. Apnea and arousals occur repeatedly during the night, separated by several normal breaths. The cause of sleep apnea is not definitely known. However, three factors appear to be involved: (1) shape of the upper airway, (2) neural control of the respiratory muscles, and (3) hormonal balance. *OSA,* Obstructive sleep apnea.

continuous positive airway pressure (CPAP), though the procedure may be considered when conventional use of CPAP fails. Two or more of the following indications are reason to perform the operation:

• An O_2 saturation that drops below 80%
• Apnea index worse than 20
• Significant daytime sleepiness

• Heroic snoring, producing social or marital problems
• Cardiac dysrhythmias, other than tachycardia or bradycardia, during sleep

Procedural Considerations. On occasion, tracheostomy may be performed with UPPP because of postoperative edema with subsequent risk of airway obstruction. The tracheostomy tube is removed and the incision is closed when the danger of postoperative edema and bleeding has passed. Because some of these patients are obese (causing the tissue of the pharynx to sag during sleep), preoperative planning should include obtaining an assortment of tracheostomy tubes, including extra-long tubes, before the start of the procedure. Care must be taken in positioning the obese patient to ensure proper body alignment. Emergency tracheotomy or bronchoscopy should be anticipated in the event of airway obstruction after anesthesia induction. The surgeon may choose to administer a local anesthetic with the anesthesia provider monitoring the patient. The ease of intubation should have already been determined by this time, choosing the safest method of intubation (i.e., fiberoptic intubation, video laryngoscope). Once the method of intubation has been established and an airway is secured, a general anesthetic may be delivered. The team positions the patient supine with a shoulder roll to hyperextend the neck. If the tonsils are present, a tonsillectomy is performed along with the UPPP. When inspecting the incision in the postoperative period, care should be taken not to disturb it with a tongue blade, if one is used to provide access for inspection. The patient must not use a straw for fluid intake because it might disturb the suture line. Gentle oral cavity rinsing is recommended several times daily to decrease the chance of postoperative infection and to increase patient comfort.

Operative Procedure

1. The surgeon inserts a McIvor mouth gag.
2. The surgeon may outline the tissue to be resected using an ESU blade. The incision may be completed with the ESU or with a #3 knife handle with a #15 blade or a #7 knife handle with a #12 blade. The incision is made in the soft palate and anteriorly to the tonsillar pillar (if the patient has not previously undergone a tonsillectomy) or posteriorly to the tonsillar pillars (if the patient has undergone a tonsillectomy) (Figure 19-40).
3. Larger blood vessels may be clamped until the tissue is removed, or a suction coagulator or hand-controlled ESU handpiece may be used to obtain hemostasis as the tissue is excised.
4. After the tissue is removed and hemostasis is achieved, the surgeon uses absorbable sutures to approximate the edges of the mucosa. Depending on the surgeon's preference, 2-0 and 3-0 absorbable suture should be available. Needle holders should be long enough to allow the surgeon ease in delivering the atraumatic needle to the edges of the mucosa.
5. The surgeon irrigates the oral cavity and inspects the incision before the patient is transferred from the OR.

Tonsillectomy. A tonsillectomy (and occasionally an adenoidectomy) is indicated primarily for either relief of pharyngeal obstruction or for recurrent pharyngitis or tonsillitis. The child with a surgical tonsil must have documented recurrent throat infections (seven in 1 year, five in 2 years, or three in 3 years) (Baugh et al, 2011). Indications for adult tonsillectomy include chronic infection, airway obstruction secondary to hypertrophy, and suspected neoplasms.

Pharyngeal obstruction is revealed by a history of sleep disordered breathing. Mouth breathing, snoring, pauses in breathing, restless sleep, waking at night, and enuresis may be related to

FIGURE 19-40 Technique of palatopharyngoplasty as advocated by Simmons and associates.

obstruction. Daytime somnolence and an inability to concentrate may also be indicators of poor sleep quality. Tonsil size is graded on a scale of one to four, with one being contained within the tonsillar fossa, and four with the tonsils touching each other in the middle of the pharynx. Adenoids are not able to be visualized through the mouth, but symptoms of adenoid enlargement can include mouth breathing, nasal congestion, rhinorrhea, and hyponasal speech. Flexible nasolaryngoscopy and lateral neck radiography can aid in diagnosis of nasopharyngeal obstruction.

An additional reason for tonsillectomy would be a marked difference in size. Lymphoma on rare occasion may present in this fashion. Unusually enlarged tonsils in an immunosuppressed transplant recipient may also be indicative of post-transplant lymphoproliferative disorder.

Other indications include dysphagia from obstructing tonsils, halitosis from tonsilloliths, recurrent adenoiditis contributing to sinusitis, or otitis media.

Cold knife and snare technique with or without the ESU, and the harmonic ultrasound scalpel and bipolar radiofrequency ablation techniques may all be used for tonsillectomy. Both the harmonic ultrasonic scalpel and the bipolar radiofrequency wand cut and coagulate at the same time, resulting in very little blood loss. Hemostasis is achieved by the production of a protein plug in the end of the cut vessel from the ultrasonic or plasma energy of the devices. The harmonic scalpel generates operative site temperatures of 158° to 176°F (70° to 80°C), and the radiofrequency wand produces a slightly lower temperature of 140°F (60°C) (Told, 2010).

Cold knife and snare is the oldest and most widely recognized method of tonsil removal. Bleeding must be controlled by other means such as electrocautery, vasoactive topical agents, packing, or placement of absorbable sutures.

The harmonic scalpel technique uses an ultrasonic generator that passes energy to a special titanium rod that vibrates at 55,000 times per second (Hz) for controlled vaporization of tissue. The ultrasonic energy also generates enough heat (158° to 176°F [70° to 80°C]) through the disposable scalpel tip to form protein plugs in the severed ends of blood vessels. The vapor that is generated from cell destruction helps undermine the tissue layers as well (Told, 2010).

The bipolar radiofrequency technique can be used for both tonsillectomy and adenoidectomy. It produces tissue vaporization by passing a bipolar radiofrequency current through normal saline resulting in the production of a plasma field of sodium ions. This plasma field is able to vaporize tissue at low temperatures (140°F [60°C]) and coagulate blood in any severed vessels (Told, 2010). The wand in this unit contains both suction and bipolar ESU and is twice the diameter of the harmonic scalpel.

FIGURE 19-41 Patient positioned for tonsillectomy with Davis mouth gag in place.

Procedural Considerations. The patient is positioned supine with the head hyperextended using a dropped headrest or a shoulder roll. The head must be secured on a donut-style headrest or on head pads. An oral endotracheal tube with a preformed bend, such as the Ring, Adair, Elwin (RAE), is used to facilitate visualization of the surgical field (Figure 19-41). The neck is extended by placing a small roll under the shoulders. Typical draping includes a head drape and an impervious sheet over the patient; no prep is used. A tonsil instrumentation set is used. A harmonic scalpel setup and radiofrequency ablation unit are required for their respective procedures.

Operative Procedure
Cold Knife and Snare Technique

1. The surgeon inserts a mouth gag retractor with a size-appropriate tongue blade, taking care to keep the tongue in midline position with the endotracheal tube protected by the blade.
2. The posterior and lateral walls of the pharynx are carefully inspected and palpated to detect abnormally positioned vessels.
3. The tip of a 12 French red rubber catheter is advanced through one of the nares, into the nasopharynx and out through the mouth. The catheter is gently stretched, and the two ends are clamped snugly with a Kelly clamp near the upper lip to retract the soft palate forward.
4. Next, the surgeon places a throat pack in the posterior pharynx, ensuring it is easily retrievable at the end of the procedure.
5. A tonsillar tenaculum is placed at the midpoint of the tonsil to apply medial traction on the tonsil, thereby tenting the tonsil into the tonsillar fossae and oral cavity.
6. Using a curved tonsil knife, the surgeon makes an incision down to the palatoglossus muscle along the posterolateral aspect of the muscle in the plane of the muscle fibers and follows with blunt dissection starting from the superior portion of the tonsillar bed and working downward toward the lower one third or inferior portion of the tonsillar bed.
7. A snare is applied over the tonsil, tightened, and then closed to bluntly dissect the tonsil from the tonsillar bed. The ESU is used along with sutures and packing to control bleeding.
8. At this point the mouth gag is released for a brief period, then reopened. The nasopharynx and oropharynx are reinspected to ensure that there is no further bleeding from vessels that may have been compressed by the opened mouth gag.
9. The oropharynx may be irrigated with 50 to 60 mL of normal saline solution to evaluate for additional signs of bleeding. The endotracheal tube cuff should be inflated, or the anesthesia provider should maintain positive pressure inflation during the irrigation to prevent inadvertent passage of the irrigation into the trachea.
10. The red rubber catheter is removed. The mouth gag retractor is carefully removed from the oral cavity to prevent inadvertent extubation of the patient.
11. Dentition, temporomandibular joint mobility, and perioral skin are reinspected for inadvertent surgical complications.

Harmonic Scalpel Technique

1. Steps 1 to 5 from the cold knife and snare technique are performed.
2. The surgeon uses the blunt, curved back portion of the tip with extremely light downward pressure to dissect the tonsil from the bed, moving inferiorly or superiorly, depending on how easily the tonsil releases.
3. After the tonsil is completely released from the bed, the surgeon reapplies the tenaculum to facilitate removal of the tonsil from the palatopharyngeus muscle of the posterior pillar.
4. The surgeon controls any residual bleeding by placing the flat portion of the dissection tip against the bleeding site and gently tamponading the bleeding. Small amounts of capillary bleeding also can be controlled by lightly moving the activated tip over the bleeding site until the bleeding stops or a light char appears.
5. The tonsillar beds are painted with sucralfate liquid, and the self-retaining retractor is released to check for residual bleeding. The posterior throat pack is removed and the posterior pharynx is then thoroughly suctioned, if necessary.

Radiofrequency Tonsillectomy

1. Steps 1 to 5 from the cold knife and snare technique are performed.
2. The surgeon uses the tip of the wand to carefully dissect the anterior portion of the tonsil away from the surrounding muscle.
3. The surgeon controls any residual bleeding with the ESU portion of the device.
4. The tonsillar beds are painted with sucralfate liquid, and the self-retaining retractor is released to check for residual bleeding. The posterior throat pack is removed, and the posterior pharynx is then thoroughly suctioned, if necessary.

Adenoidectomy. Children with polysomnogram-proven sleep disorder breathing and hypertrophic adenoids should have their adenoids assessed as a complete workup. Obstructive upper airways from hypertrophic adenoids can be easily evaluated using flexible nasopharyngoscopy by an otolaryngologist. Surgical removal of hypertrophic adenoids to relieve upper airway obstruction is often performed to create a patent nasal airway. Adenoidectomy by curette, ablation, radiofrequency, and powered microdebriders has been described in the pediatric otolaryngology literature. Hemostasis is achieved depending on the method chosen, by electrocautery, radiofrequency, or direct pressure (using angled mirrors or endoscopic visualization).

Laryngeal Surgery

Laryngeal surgery may be performed for diagnostic reasons or as a means of treatment for benign as well as malignant conditions (Figure 19-42). This type of surgery involves both endoscopic and traditional "open" approaches and always has the potential to alter the patient's ability to communicate verbally in the postoperative period. As is the case with oral cavity malignancies, cancerous lesions within the laryngeal structures are often attributed to environmental factors, such as tobacco and alcohol use. Benign conditions, such as vocal cord polyps and nodules, are often treated with laryngeal surgery (Figure 19-43).

Endoscopic Procedures

Laryngoscopy. Laryngoscopy is direct visual examination of the interior of the larynx by means of a rigid, lighted speculum known as a *laryngoscope* to obtain a specimen of tissue or secretions

FIGURE 19-42 Large granular tumor on the true cord.

FIGURE 19-43 Bilateral vocal cord polyps.

for pathologic examination. Vocal cord visualization also may be accomplished in the office setting with a flexible fiberoptic nasopharyngolaryngoscope.

Procedural Considerations. Most rigid laryngoscopies are performed with the patient receiving a general anesthetic. If the patient is unable to tolerate general anesthesia, a local or topical anesthetic of lidocaine, tetracaine, cocaine, or benzocaine-tetracaine is administered. The patient should be sufficiently relaxed by reassurance and by pharmacologic preparation if the procedure is performed using local anesthesia. Sedatives may be administered before surgery. Immediate preoperative assessment should include the presence of any dental appliances and loose teeth and the condition of dental work. Any stiffness or immobility of the neck or shoulders should be evaluated. Respiratory problems such as asthma must receive careful attention. The patient should be cautioned about not eating or drinking after surgery until the gag reflex has returned and swallowing occurs without difficulty. The nurse or scrub person prepares a local anesthesia setup for the surgeon. An operative laryngoscope instrument set with laryngoscopes, light carriers, biopsy forceps, and telescopes is used.

If the surgeon wishes to perform a suspension laryngoscopy, a self-retaining laryngoscope holder is added to the instrument table, as well as microlaryngeal instruments, which include scissors, cup forceps, and alligator forceps. A special platform may be mounted onto the OR bed, or a Mayo stand may be placed above the patient's chest and over the OR bed to provide a place for the laryngoscope holder to rest. The surgeon normally uses the operating microscope with a 400-mm lens during suspension laryngoscopy. The team positions the patient supine to facilitate visualization of the vocal cords. A shoulder roll should be available if slight hyperextension of the neck is necessary to assist in visualization of the larynx. Laryngoscopy instrumentation should remain set up in the room until the patient is transferred because the equipment may be needed if the patient experiences laryngospasm postoperatively and requires intubation.

Operative Procedure

1. The anesthesia provider places moist gauze pads or tape over the patient's eyes to protect them from the instrumentation and to prevent injury and irritation from secretions during the procedure. The head may also be wrapped in a sterile towel. A sterile drape may be used to cover the patient. A tooth guard or moistened soft goods are placed to protect the patient's teeth.

2. The surgeon introduces the spatula end of the laryngoscope into the right side of the patient's mouth and directs it toward the midline; then the dorsum of the tongue is elevated so that the epiglottis is exposed.

3. The surgeon tips the patient's head backward, then lifts it upward as the laryngoscope is advanced into the larynx.

4. The larynx is examined, a biopsy is taken, secretions are aspirated, and bleeding is controlled.

Microlaryngoscopy. Microlaryngoscopy facilitates improved diagnosis and allows the surgeon to view with relative ease areas that previously were inaccessible or difficult to visualize. It may also be used for minor surgery of the larynx, especially for the removal of polyps or nodules on the vocal cords. (Intralaryngeal surgery using the laryngoscope is often referred to as *phonosurgery.*) Instrumentation may vary according to surgeon preference.

Procedural Considerations. If the procedure is done to remove polyps or nodules from the vocal cords, the patient must be cautioned to observe complete voice rest postoperatively. The patient should be provided with a pencil and paper or erasable slate to aid in communication. The patient's restriction on speaking should be noted on the nursing plan of care and on the front of the chart.

The basic instrument setup for laryngoscopy is used. Microlaryngeal instruments and a self-retaining laryngoscope holder are added to the setup. The microlaryngeal instruments are 22 cm long to allow use with the microscope, and are long enough to keep the surgeon's hands out of the visual field. The patient's head is adjusted to allow visualization of the larynx. The surgeon usually adjusts the microscope. The microscope lens should have a 400-mm focal length. Focal length is the distance from the lens to the operative area and is the point at which the field can be clearly viewed through the microscope. Beyond this point the field becomes blurry. The 400-mm lens gives the surgeon a 40-cm focal length, or working distance.

Carbon Dioxide Laser Surgery of the Larynx. Surgeons often use the CO_2 laser to treat lesions of the larynx and vocal cords. This laser is efficient and has a high power output. The beam destroys tissue at a precise point with minimal destruction of the surrounding tissue. It is especially useful in surgeries such as removal of webs in the larynx, vocal cord papillomas, and carcinoma in situ of the larynx, as well as benign endobronchial lesions.

Procedural Considerations. The basic setup for laryngoscopy and microlaryngoscopy is used. All instrumentation used for laser laryngoscopy should be ebonized. A general anesthetic is usually administered. The operating microscope with a 400-mm lens is used, with the laser micromanipulator attached to the microscope head. The beam should also be tested for proper working order before use on the patient. Extreme care should be used when handling this delicate piece of equipment. A smoke evacuator should be used to remove the laser plume—a smokelike steam rising from the impact site; high-filtration laser masks should be worn by personnel. Where minimal plume is generated, central wall suction with an in-line filter may be used for plume evacuation (AORN, 2013c). All other laser precautions apply (see Chapter 8).

Adjunctive Procedures. Although the following procedures do not technically involve the larynx, they are often performed by otorhinolaryngologists in conjunction with laryngeal surgery and are of particular use in the diagnostic arena.

Bronchoscopy. The trachea, bronchi, and lungs are visualized directly with a rigid or flexible bronchoscope that has a fiberoptic lighting system. A rigid scope gives a larger viewing area, whereas a flexible scope is easily inserted into the patient and manipulated.

(Bronchoscopy is fully described in Chapter 23.) The Nd:YAG laser may be used for lesions of the trachea or bronchi, depending on the type of lesion. Most diagnostic bronchoscopies are performed using topical anesthetics and moderate sedation, requiring careful patient monitoring by the perioperative nurse.

Esophagoscopy. Esophagoscopy is the direct visualization of the esophagus and the inner stomach organ. This procedure is used to observe the area for extension of tumor, to remove tissue and secretions for study, or to evaluate for second primary tumor sites.

Procedural Considerations. Esophagoscopy facilitates the diagnosis of esophageal carcinoma, diverticula, hiatal hernia, stricture, benign stenosis, and varices. Patients with suspected obstruction, symptoms of bleeding, or regurgitation may require endoscopy. The Nd:YAG laser may be used to treat some of these lesions. Esophagoscopy may also be used for therapeutic manipulations, such as removal of a foreign body or insertion of an esophageal bougie to treat esophageal stenosis. A set of rigid esophagoscopes, light carriers, biopsy forceps, and bougies is used.

Operative Procedure

1. The scrub person inserts the fiberoptic light carrier into the esophagoscope and attaches the fiberoptic light cord. A thin layer of lubricant is applied to the scope. The surgeon passes the scope into the mouth. The tongue, epiglottis, laryngeal inlet, and cricopharyngeal lumen are identified. If necessary, a person holding the patient's head may be required to tip the head backward while extending the neck anteriorly. Usually the esophagoscope is passed to the right side of the tongue, and the patient's head is turned slightly to the left.

2. When the scope has passed the inferior constrictor muscles, the patient's head is moved in various directions so that all areas of the esophageal wall may be examined.

3. Specimens of secretions from the esophageal lumen may be obtained with an aspirating tube and suctioning apparatus. In some cases saline may be injected through the esophagoscope's aspirating channel and the fluid withdrawn immediately for histologic study. A tissue biopsy may be taken. After biopsy the area is assessed for bleeding and the esophagoscope is then removed.

Triple Endoscopy (Panendoscopy). When laryngoscopy, bronchoscopy, and esophagoscopy are performed in a single session on a patient, the procedure is termed *triple endoscopy* or *panendoscopy.* The order in which the procedures are performed depends on the surgeon's preference. The purpose of triple endoscopy is usually diagnostic. While inspecting for a malignancy, the surgeon views the structures, takes specimens for biopsy, and possibly makes smears or washings of the suspect areas. For any of the aforementioned endoscopic procedures, all equipment or instrumentation should be set up and be in working order (i.e., light carriers in place; light cables connected and working). Instrumentation to be used through the various scopes (i.e., suction tips, telescopes, and biopsy forceps) should be checked for appropriate length. Specimens taken during endoscopic procedures should be labeled and removed from the back table as soon as possible. In some instances it may be helpful to indicate on the label that the specimens are microscopic.

Transoral Robotic Surgery (TORS). TORS provides a mechanism to approach tumors of the upper aerodigestive tract through a natural body orifice—the mouth. In otolaryngology this technique has been applied to malignant tumors of the oral cavity, most often, and now is even used as a primary and salvage approach to oral cancers of the tongue, tonsils, and pharynx. Other uses for

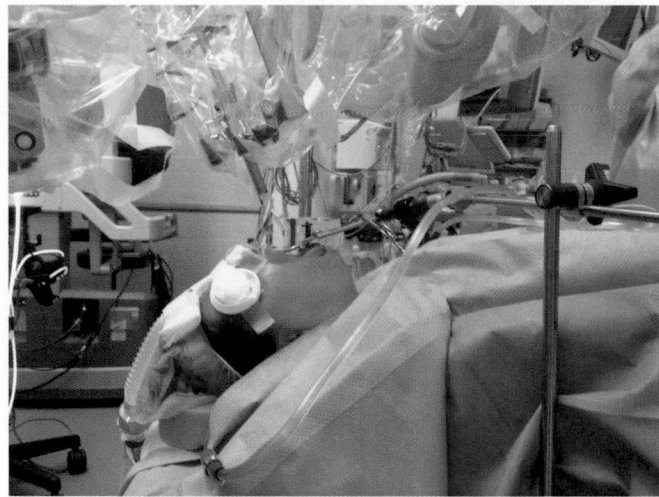

FIGURE 19-44 Base of tongue robotic resection for hypertrophic lingual tonsils.

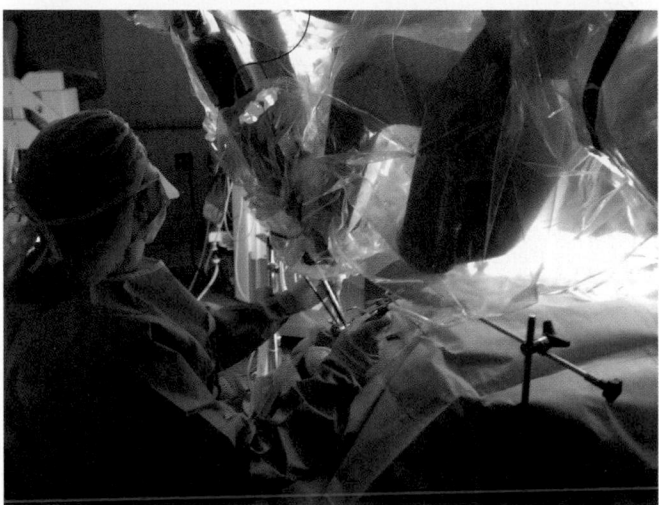

FIGURE 19-45 Bedside assistant in robotic resection of hypertrophic lingual tonsils.

robotic-assisted surgery within otorhinolaryngology include transaxillary endoscopic thyroidectomy, laryngotracheal reconstruction, removal of hypertrophic lingual tonsils, and debulking of the tongue base for obstructive sleep apnea (Figures 19-44 and 19-45).

Iseli (2009) mentions that robotic surgery has low morbidity and acceptable functional outcomes, but also mentions that T4 and late stage cancers were associated with poorer functional outcomes and were at greater risk of enterogastric feeding and poor swallow outcomes. Moore and colleagues (2012) concluded that with appropriate adjuvant therapy, TORS achieves excellent functional results for patients with oropharyngeal squamous cell carcinoma, and oncologic outcomes are equivalent or superior to results of other surgical and nonsurgical treatments (Research Highlight).

Advances in robotic-assisted technology have allowed manufacturers to construct manipulators that mimic and, in some cases, improve the motion of the human shoulder and wrist (Hillel et al, 2008). Additional information about the mechanics of robotic-assisted surgery is available in Chapter 8.

Transoral Robotic Surgery in the Treatment of Oropharyngeal Cancer

The American Cancer Society projects that about 36,000 people will get oral cavity or oropharyngeal cancer, and an estimated 6850 people will die of these cancers in 2013. Traditional approaches to surgical treatment of these cancers have included wide resections (e.g., mandibulotomy, neck dissections) or when possible transoral resections.

Transoral robotic surgery (TORS) offers an alternative to a wide resection and may be suitable for some patients. This study used a prospective review to determine the effect of TORS on long-term functional (e.g., airway and swallowing) and oncologic outcomes (e.g., disease control, recurrence, and survival) on squamous cell carcinoma of the tonsil or base of tongue.

Investigators studied 66 patients who had a minimum of 2-year follow-up after TORS for ororpharyngeal squamous cell carcinoma. TORS was performed in conjunction with neck dissection, with most patients undergoing a unilateral dissection on the same day as the TORS procedure. Depending on the final pathology reports, some patients also underwent adjuvant radiation therapy.

A review of the functional outcomes of surgery determined that 98.5% of patients were tracheostomy free and 95.5% were able to meet their nutritional needs without a gastrostomy tube. Oncologic outcomes measured noted that 95.5% of the patients were still alive at follow-up, and 92.4% had no evidence of recurrence.

The investigators note that TORS offers organ preservation and maximizes function. The return of swallowing function is a distinct advantage of the TORS approach. Other advantages include effective tumor and lymph node staging in a single setting, tissue and neurovascular supply preservation, and decreased morbidity.

Modified from Moore EJ et al: Long-term functional and oncologic results of transoral robotic surgery for oropharyngeal squamous cell carcinoma, *Mayo Clin Proc* 87(3):219–225, 2012; American Cancer Society: *Oral cavity and oropharyngeal cancer*, 2013, available at www.cancer.org/cancer/oralcavityandoropharyngealcancer/detailedguide/oral-cavity-and-oropharyngeal-cancer-key-statistics. Accessed March 23, 2013.

Open Neck and Laryngeal Procedures

Tracheostomy. Tracheostomy is the opening of the trachea and the insertion of a cannula through a midline incision in the neck, below the cricoid cartilage. A tracheostomy may be permanent or temporary. It is used as an emergency procedure to treat upper respiratory tract obstruction, which can be caused by bilateral vocal cord paralysis, swelling of the neck or airway caused by trauma, allergic reactions, or neoplasms. It is also used as a prophylactic measure in the presence of chronic lung disease, in extensive neck resections when massive upper airway edema is anticipated, or if radiation-induced edema is expected during the treatment of cancers involving the tongue and neck. Tracheostomy is also considered the gold standard for treating sleep apnea in which obstruction may occur. Tracheostomy may be performed to permit easy and frequent pulmonary toileting on patients having a difficult time managing and expectorating their own secretions. Additionally, tracheostomy should be performed on patients experiencing prolonged intubation to avoid overgrowth of granulation tissue and subsequent subglottic stenosis.

The nurse carefully evaluates the patient's psychologic status because of the altered body image, which may be temporary or permanent depending on the disease entity involved. Tracheostomy care should be explained carefully and thoroughly so that the patient will understand why self-care should be performed frequently. Reinforcement should be given regarding the ability to communicate with others by means of a pencil and paper or message board. As recovery progresses and secretions diminish, the patient can be shown how to occlude the opening of the tube for brief periods to be able to speak a few words. The patient also must be taught the mastery of tracheostomy self-care. If a tracheostomy tube with a disposable inner cannula is inserted, the nursing staff must ensure that the patient has replacement cannulae in the event occlusion or blockage occurs in the immediate postoperative period.

Procedural Considerations. Before tracheostomy tubes are inserted, the cuffs should be tested for air leaks by inflating and then deflating the balloon. Cuffed tracheostomy tubes are used on patients at risk for aspiration, patients receiving positive-pressure ventilation, or patients who have undergone skull base surgeries involving open communication of the sinuses into the intracranium, where it is desirable to avoid pneumocephalus. The patient is placed in a supine position, with the shoulders raised by a small rolled sheet to slightly hyperextend the neck and head. Using a skin marker, the surgeon marks a midline incision site halfway between the sternal notch and the cricoid cartilage, between the second and third tracheal rings. The neck is prepped and sterile drapes are applied. A soft suction catheter should be available on the sterile field for suctioning after the tube is inserted. An additional tracheostomy tube of the same size and the obturator should be kept with the patient at all times, in the event the tube becomes dislodged or plugged with secretions. This practice expedites changing the tracheostomy tube with minimal potential for complications to the patient.

Operative Procedure

1. The surgeon injects lidocaine with epinephrine into the subcutaneous tissue across the tracheotomy site previously marked with a surgical marker.
2. A horizontal incision is made with a #10, #15, or #11 blade. Soft tissues and muscle are divided, using blunt hemostats and sharp dissection through the platysma and the overlying strap muscles. The thyroid gland is identified; attention is directed to the isthmus with the intention of transecting this area of the gland. Occasionally the isthmus can be retracted from the surgical site without transection (Figure 19-46).
3. The plane between the isthmus and the trachea is separated by the surgeon with a blunt hemostat, exposing the thyroid gland so the surgical assistant can carefully transect it with the ESU blade. This exposes the underlying tracheal rings—usually the second and third. In some cases two curved clamps may be inserted through this incision across the isthmus, and then the isthmus is transected.
4. The transected ends of the isthmus are oversewn or suture-ligated with absorbable sutures.
5. After identifying the trachea, the surgeon makes a horizontal incision with a #11 blade through the second and third tracheal rings. The incision is extended and the tracheostomy tube is inserted.
6. Two 2-0 silk sutures are then sewn into the trachea for future use during the first tracheostomy change. In two motions, one silk suture is inserted into the trachea, and then retrieved with the needle driver through the horizontal incision. This is then repeated with another silk suture through the bottom half of the horizontal incision.
7. Air knots are tied into each of the sutures and secured with tape onto the chest so they are ready for easy retrieval for retraction

A   B   C   D

FIGURE 19-46 Operative technique for elective tracheostomy. **A,** Retractor exposing trachea by drawing the isthmus of the thyroid upward. **B,** Alternative method to that shown in **(A).** Isthmus of thyroid is divided to expose the trachea. **C,** Two tracheal rings are cut, and upper ring is partially resected. Tracheal hook pulls trachea from depth of wound nearer surface. **D,** Insertion of tube.

during the first tracheostomy change, about 5 to 7 days later. By tradition, one air knot is placed in the upper stay suture and two air knots are placed in the lower stay suture to allow for easy identification and proper retraction at the time of tracheostomy tube change or in the event of tracheostomy tube dislodgement. The air knots are cut and removed once the first tracheostomy change takes place.

Laryngofissure. Laryngofissure is an opening of the larynx for exploratory, excisional, or reconstructive procedures that cannot be accomplished endoscopically.

Procedural Considerations. A laryngofissure may be performed when access to the intrinsic larynx is necessary. The thyroid cartilages are split in the midline, and the true vocal cords and false vocal cords are incised at the midline anteriorly. A neck dissection instrument set is required, plus an oscillating power saw. A tracheotomy is performed as the first step of the procedure and the tracheostomy tube is left in place postoperatively to ensure a patent airway.

Operative Procedure

1. The surgeon makes a transverse incision through the skin and first layer of the cervical fascia and platysma muscles, approximately 2 cm above the sternoclavicular junction or in the normal skin crease. The upper skin flap is undermined to the level of the cricoid cartilage, and the lower flap is undermined to the sternoclavicular joint.
2. Bleeding vessels are clamped with mosquito hemostats, and ligated. The strap muscles are elevated and incised in the midline.
3. The surgeon cuts the thyroid cartilages with an oscillating saw, and visualizes the true vocal cords through an incision into the cricothyroid membrane. The true vocal cords are divided in the midline (anterior commissure), and the interior of the larynx is exposed.

Partial Laryngectomy. Partial laryngectomy is removal of a portion of the larynx. It is performed to remove superficial neoplasms that are confined to one vocal cord or to remove a tumor extending up into the ventricle or the anterior commissure or a short distance below the cord. A cancer confined to the intrinsic larynx is generally a low-grade malignancy and tends to remain localized for long periods. The patient should be prepared for an altered voice quality postoperatively as well as for the possibility of total laryngectomy if the tumor proves too extensive for partial resection. Types of partial laryngectomies include a vertical hemilaryngectomy, supraglottic laryngectomy, and supracricoid laryngectomy. With surgical excision of the tumor along with

postoperative administration of chemotherapy concurrently with external beam radiation therapy, it is possible to preserve some laryngeal function. The goal of partial laryngectomy is to avoid removing the entire larynx and to preserve the patient's natural swallowing ability. A successful partial laryngectomy should leave the patient with the ability to phonate, though usually with a more hoarse voice. The otolaryngologist must carefully stage the laryngeal cancer via a panendoscopy with biopsy and determine the overall candidacy of the patient who may receive a partial laryngectomy. If tumor extension does not warrant a partial laryngectomy, a total laryngectomy must be performed. Steps and procedural considerations for a total laryngectomy are described next.

Total Laryngectomy. Total laryngectomy is the complete removal of the cartilaginous larynx, the hyoid bone, and the strap muscles connected to the larynx and possible removal of the preepiglottic space with the lesion. A wide-field laryngectomy is done when there is a loss of mobility of the cords and to treat cancer of the extrinsic larynx and hypopharynx (Figure 19-47). Malignant tumors of the extrinsic larynx are more anaplastic and tend to metastasize. When laryngeal carcinoma involves more than the true cords, a prophylactic (preventive) modified, or selective, neck dissection is done to remove the lymphatics. Depending on the extent and severity of disease in the neck, a radical neck dissection may be warranted though rarely routinely performed.

Laryngectomy presents many psychologic problems. The loss of voice that follows total laryngectomy is traumatic for the patient and family. The patient may be taught to talk by using either an esophageal voice or an artificial larynx. The esophageal voice is produced by the air contained in the esophagus rather than by that in the trachea. Speech requires a sounding air column. With instruction and practice, the patient is able to control the swallowing of air into the esophagus and the reintroduction of this air into the mouth with phonation. The sounding air column is then transformed into speech by means of the lips, tongue, and teeth. A tracheoesophageal fistula facilitates insertion of a tracheoesophageal prosthesis or valve for the purpose of speech. This fistula may be created during the initial surgical procedure (primary tracheoesophageal puncture [TEP]) or at a later date when healing has occurred. Because the stump of the trachea is exteriorized to the skin of the neck to form a permanent stoma, all the patient's breathing is done directly into the trachea and no longer through the nose and mouth. The nose no longer moistens this air. Drying and crusting of the tracheal secretions occur. Humidification may be provided with a humidified tracheostomy collar or a humidified moisture exchange system later during the healing process (Patient and Family Education). The patient will be anxious to know about postoperative voice quality, which depends on the specific procedure performed.

Procedural Considerations. The team positions the patient supine with the neck extended and shoulders elevated by a shoulder roll or folded sheet. A general anesthetic is administered. Airway considerations are paramount when approaching a patient with

FIGURE 19-47 Wide-field defect following removal of the larynx.

laryngeal cancer. An awake tracheostomy may be performed initially to control the airway, and occasionally patients have previously placed tracheostomy tubes. If the tracheostomy is performed initially or is preexisting, the use of a cuffed, wire-reinforced, flexible endotracheal tube will ensure effective delivery of the anesthetic and give the surgical team flexibility as the larynx and trachea are manipulated during the surgical procedure. An effective suction apparatus is essential. The proposed operative site, including the anterior neck region, the lateral surfaces of the neck down to the outer aspects of the shoulders, and the upper anterior chest region, is prepped and draped in the usual manner. The instrument setup is a neck dissection set.

Operative Procedure

1. The surgeon makes a midline incision from the suprasternal notch to just above the hyoid bone. Skin flaps are undermined on each side. The sternothyroid, sternohyoid, and omohyoid muscles (strap muscles) on each side are divided by means of curved hemostats and a knife.

2. The suprahyoid muscles are severed from the portion of the hyoid to be divided. The hyoid bone is skeletonized with care to preserve the hypoglossal nerves. Bleeding vessels are clamped and ligated.

3. The surgeon exposes and ligates the superior laryngeal nerve and vessels on each side with long, curved fine hemostats and fine ligatures.

4. Next, the isthmus of the thyroid gland is divided between hemostats. Each portion of the thyroid gland is dissected from the trachea with Metzenbaum scissors and fine tissue forceps. The superior pole of the thyroid is retracted. The superior thyroid vessels are freed from the larynx by sharp dissection. Sometimes one or both lobes of the thyroid gland are included in the resection for oncologic purposes.

5. The surgeon rotates the larynx. The inferior pharyngeal constrictor muscle is severed from its attachment to the thyroid cartilage on each side.

6. The endotracheal tube is removed. The trachea is transected with care to keep an adequate margin from the tumor. The upper resected portion of the trachea and the cricoid cartilage are held upward with Lahey forceps. A balloon-cuffed, wire-reinforced endotracheal tube is inserted into the distal portion of the trachea.

PATIENT AND FAMILY EDUCATION

Teaching Laryngectomy Care

Below are suggested steps for the nurse who is teaching a patient to care for a laryngectomy stoma. Information needs to be modified according to the type of tube or stent the patient has in place.

1. Remove, inspect, and clean your laryngectomy tube twice daily and as needed for secretions.
   • Be sure to remove and clean inner cannula to maintain patency.
2. While your tube is out, look at your stoma for breakdown and crusting. Wipe any crust away from the stoma to prevent aspiration (inhalation of foreign material).
   • Use half-strength hydrogen peroxide and a cotton-tipped applicator to clean your stoma.
   • Wipe with normal saline after using the hydrogen peroxide.
3. Administer saline every 4 hours and as needed (this is to help you cough).

   • Place a few drops of saline into your stoma to initiate coughing. If you are unable to cough and clear the saline instillation, you must immediately provide suction.
4. Suction your tube as needed so you breathe easily.
5. Use humidification. Humidification is extremely important to help with secretion management. You should wear humidification at night and while in your room.
   • If you wear a heat and moisture exchange (HME) cassette, change the cassette daily or if it gets very wet from your secretions. If you can't tolerate HME or if you need supplemental oxygen, remove HME and use humidified oxygen via a tracheostomy collar.
   • If you are not fitted for HME (i.e., you have a Bivona vent or a laryngectomy tube), provide humidification via a tracheostomy collar at 28% as frequently as possible.

PATIENT AND FAMILY EDUCATION

Teaching Laryngectomy Care—cont'd

Proxy Lary tube.

Proxy Lary with heat and moisture exchange (HME).

Bivona tracheostoma vent.

Shiley laryngectomy tube.

Modified from Rozencwaig H, Shumway B: *Best practice teaching tool for laryngectomy care, patient education, 2013,* Thomas Jefferson University Hospital, Department of Otolaryngology, Philadelphia.

FIGURE 19-48 Removal of the larynx en bloc.

7. The surgeon frees the larynx from the cervical esophagus and attachments by sharp and blunt dissection. A moist pack is placed around the endotracheal tube to help prevent leakage of blood into the trachea.

8. The pharynx is entered. In most cancers of the intrinsic larynx, the pharynx is entered above the epiglottis. The surgeon extends the mucous membrane incision along either side of the epiglottis; the remaining portion of the pharynx and cervical esophagus is dissected well away from the tumor by means of fine-toothed tissue forceps, Metzenbaum scissors, knife, and fine hemostats. The specimen is removed en bloc (Figure 19-48).

9. The surgeon inserts a nasal feeding tube through one naris into the esophagus; closure of the hypopharyngeal and esophageal defect is begun with continuous inverting fine 3-0 absorbable suture. The nasal tube is guided down past the pharyngeal suture line.

10. The pharyngeal suture line is reinforced with running horizontal or vertical mattress Vicryl sutures; the suprahyoid muscles are approximated to the cut edges of the inferior constrictor muscles.

11. The surgeon uses a knife and heavy scissors to increase the diameter of the tracheal stoma. The two portions of the thyroid behind the tracheal opening are approximated with interrupted nonabsorbable sutures, thereby obliterating dead space posterior to the upper portion of the trachea.

12. Using a blade, the surgeon makes a small puncture wound through the neck, lateral to the incision, using the tips of a hemostat inserted on the inner wound bed as a guide.

13. The hemostat is then stabbed into the puncture wound, grasping the distal drain tubing and pulling it through until the fluted portion of the drain is visible in the wound bed. The drain is trimmed and measured to fit into the wound.

14. The drain is secured to the skin just lateral to where the puncture wound was made, and an air knot is tied using square knots.

15. The surgeon closes the edges of the deep cervical fascia and the platysma separately.

16. Next, the surgeon inserts a laryngectomy tube into the tracheal stoma. A pressure dressing may be applied to the wound and

neck, although some surgeons prefer leaving the wound without dressings to observe the skin flaps.

Radical Neck Dissection. In a radical neck dissection, the tumor, all soft tissue from the inferior aspect of the mandible to the midline of the neck to the clavicle end posterior to the trapezius muscle, and lymph nodes are removed en bloc from the affected side of the neck. This procedure is done to remove the tumor and metastatic cervical nodes present in malignant lesions as well as all nonvital structures of the neck. Metastasis occurs through the lymphatic channels by way of the bloodstream. Diseases of the oral cavity, lips, and thyroid gland may spread slowly to the neck. Radical neck surgery is done in the presence of cervical node metastasis from a cancer of the head and neck that has a reasonable chance of being controlled. Sentinel node biopsy may also be performed in conjunction with a neck dissection.

A prophylactic neck dissection implies an elective neck dissection when there is no clinical evidence of metastatic cancer in the cervical lymph nodes.

Procedural Considerations. The team positions the patient supine. General endotracheal anesthesia is induced before the patient is positioned for surgery. A shoulder roll may be placed to slightly hyperextend the neck, with the head slightly turned to the contralateral side. The head of the bed may be slightly elevated to reduce venous bleeding.

During the procedure the anesthesia provider works behind a sterile barrier at the patient's unaffected side. The preoperative skin prep is extensive, including the neck, lower face, and upper chest. The patient's neck is draped so as to leave a wide operative field. On occasion, local muscle flaps are harvested to cover and protect the carotid artery (as when a patient has received extensive previous radiation therapy). If this is the case, the thigh area is also prepped and draped with sterile towels in readiness for obtaining a dermal graft before closure of the neck wound. It is usually more convenient to use the thigh on the same side as the neck dissection. Patient and family education includes tracheostomy care (if applicable), pain management, care of the surgical incision, reportable signs and symptoms, healthful behaviors, and review of physical therapy exercises.

Operative Procedure

1. The surgeon may use one of several different incisions, including the Y-shaped, H-shaped, or trifurcate incision (Figure 19-49), all of which aim for complete lymphadenectomy while preserving good, viable skin flaps.

2. The upper curved incision is made through the skin and platysma with a knife, tissue forceps, and fine hemostats; ligatures are used for bleeding vessels. A monopolar ESU may be used to control skin edge bleeding.

3. The upper flap is retracted, then the vertical portion of the incision is made, and the skin flaps are retracted anteriorly and posteriorly with retractors. The anterior margin of the trapezius muscle is exposed by means of curved scissors. The flaps are retracted to expose the entire lateral aspect of the neck. Branches of the jugular veins are clamped, ligated, and divided.

4. The surgeon clamps the sternal and clavicular attachments of the sternocleidomastoid muscle with curved Péan forceps and then divides them with a knife. The superficial layer of deep fascia is incised. The omohyoid muscle is severed between clamps just above its scapular attachment.

5. Using sharp and blunt dissection, the surgeon opens the carotid sheath. The internal jugular vein is isolated by blunt dissection and then doubly clamped, doubly ligated with medium silk,

FIGURE 19-49 Dissection incisions. **A,** Latyshevsky and Freund. **B,** Freund. **C,** Crile. **D,** Martin. **E,** Babcock and Conley. **F,** McFee. **G,** Incision used for unilateral supraomohyoid neck dissection. **H,** Incision used for bilateral supraomohyoid neck dissection.

and divided with Metzenbaum scissors. A transfixion suture is placed on the lower end of the vein.

6. Next, the common carotid artery and vagus nerve are identified and protected. The fatty areolar tissue and fascia are dissected and removed using Metzenbaum scissors and fine tissue forceps.

Branches of the thyrocervical artery are clamped, divided, and ligated.

7. The surgeon dissects the tissues and fascia of the posterior triangle, beginning at the anterior margin of the trapezius muscle and continuing near the brachial plexus and the levator

scapulae and scalene muscles. During the dissection branches of the cervical and suprascapular arteries are clamped, ligated, and divided.

8. The anterior portion of the block dissection is completed. The omohyoid muscle is severed at its attachment to the hyoid bone. Bleeding is controlled. All hemostats are removed, and the operative site may be covered with warm, moist laparotomy packs.

9. The surgeon severs and retracts the sternocleidomastoid muscle. The submental space is dissected free of fatty areolar tissue and lymph nodes, from above downward.

10. The deep fascia on the lower edge of the mandible is incised; the facial vessels are divided and ligated.

11. The submandibular triangle is entered. The submandibular duct is divided and ligated. The submandibular glands with surrounding fatty areolar tissue and lymph nodes are dissected toward the digastric muscle. The facial branch of the external carotid artery is divided. Portions of the digastric and stylohyoid muscles are severed from their attachments to the hyoid bone and on the mastoid. The upper end of the internal jugular vein is elevated and divided. The surgical specimen is removed.

12. The entire field is examined for bleeding, then irrigated with warm saline solution. If necessary, a skin graft may be placed to cover the bifurcation of the carotid artery, extending down approximately 4 inches, and sutured with 4-0 absorbable suture on a very small cutting needle.

13. Closed-wound suction drains are placed into the wound.

14. The surgeon approximates the flaps with interrupted fine non-absorbable sutures or with skin staples. A bulky pressure dressing may be applied to the neck, depending on the surgeon's preference.

Modified Radical Neck Dissection. Modified radical neck dissection (Figure 19-50) includes the en bloc removal of all node-bearing tissue in the anterior and posterior cervical triangles, the tail of the parotid gland, and cervical sensory nerves with sparing of the following structures: the sternocleidomastoid muscle, internal jugular vein, and eleventh cranial nerve. Depending on the extent of the cervical neck disease diagnosed by physical examination along with supportive imaging exams, a modified radical neck dissection is procedurally idealized first by the surgeon unless late-stage malignancy requires a more extensive neck dissection, such as a radical. The goal of a modified neck dissection is to preserve as much of the normal anatomic structures of the neck as possible and remove only diseased neck content, tumor-invaded structures, and lymph nodes. Performing an appropriate neck dissection results in minimal morbidity to the patient, provides invaluable data to accurately stage the patient, and guides the need for further therapy.

Procedural Considerations. This modified type of neck dissection facilitates removal of a tumor and lymph nodes suspected of metastases and allows the patient a minimal defect and minimally impaired shoulder function. With radical and modified neck dissection, the surgeon and medical and radiation oncologists may decide on a course of postoperative radiation therapy or chemotherapy. The decision depends on the type and location of tumor, stage of disease, and patient's condition. Patients undergoing neck dissection are usually admitted overnight for observation of swelling, bleeding, or hematoma. A neck bleed is an airway emergency and needs immediate attention.

Reconstructive Procedures. Depending on the surgical defect, head and neck surgical procedures to remove malignant tumors may also involve reconstructive procedures. The wound may be closed

FIGURE 19-50 Right modified neck dissection with retraction of the right sternocleidomastoid muscle exposing cranial nerves and jugular vein.

primarily, or local flaps and split-thickness skin grafts (as for facial and intraoral defects) or full-thickness skin grafts (as for nasal and facial defects) may be used. Split-thickness skin grafts and full-thickness skin grafts are ideal for small surgical defects.

Surgical flaps for the head and neck are chosen to fill surgical defects by their ability to survive in poorly vascularized areas. The surgeon chooses the surgical flap option (e.g., regional rotational, pedicled, or free microvascular) that provides the best aesthetic result for the patient based on location of the surgical defect, size of the defect, and vascular condition and whether bone, such as the fibula, is needed to be harvested due to invasive disease.

Regional flaps, classified as either myocutaneous or fasciocutaneous, are typically rotated locally to fill large defects in the head and neck. Pectoralis major flaps raised on the long axis of the pectoral branch of the thoracoacromial artery are known for reliability, versatility, and strength (Figure 19-51). A deltopectoral flap is usually used to fill cutaneous defects of the head and neck and is a pedicled flap based on the second and third perforating branches of the internal mammary artery. The lattisimus dorsi flap is a pedicled flap or a free tissue transfer flap receiving its blood supply from the thoracodorsal artery, which arises from the subscapular axis, which can be used to fill large defects of the head and neck.

Free or microvascular flaps represent another reconstructive option for otorhinolaryngologic surgery. Perioperative nurses must incorporate the factors of increased surgical and anesthesia time (approximately 8 to 12 hours), positioning needs, and advanced equipment needs when planning care for the patient undergoing a

FIGURE 19-51 Right pectoralis flap with two chest drains and one right neck drain.

FIGURE 19-52 Harvest of radial forearm osteocutaneous flap for repair of the mandible.

FIGURE 19-53 Anterolateral thigh free flap.

and fascia. It is important to note that all patients receive a preoperative Allen test.

The anterolateral thigh free flap (Figure 19-53) is most often supplied by perforating vessels arising from the descending branch of the lateral circumflex artery. Its potential bulkiness is deemed advantageous and can be harvested as a subcutaneous, fasciocutaneous, myocutaneous, or adipofascial flap, increasing its versatility. Fibula free flaps are commonly used in otolaryngology when tumor, osteonecrosis, or infection erodes or invades the mandible and reconstruction requires bone harvest.

KEY POINTS

- The specialty of otorhinolaryngology focuses on disorders of the ear, nose, and throat.
- Patients undergoing otorhinolaryngologic surgery are considered a communication-vulnerable population due to possible deficits in hearing and phonation.
- Maintenance of the patient's airway is critical in many otorhinolaryngologic procedures.
- Perioperative nurses must be familiar with otorhinolaryngologic anatomy and a variety of surgical procedures and techniques to provide effective care to this patient population.
- Technology continues to evolve in this specialty, with new indications and experience with robotic-assisted surgery and other advancements in endoscopic techniques.

CRITICAL THINKING QUESTION

Mr. L. is a 46-year-old who underwent a parotidectomy and is recovering in the step-down unit of the PACU. He is being prepared for discharge. His wife contacts the nurse because Mr. L. is complaining of increased pain, has facial swelling, is having trouble closing his eye on the operative side, and has some mild drooping around his mouth. He is pale, rates his pain at 8 on a 10-point scale, and has a pulse rate of 110. His blood pressure is 150/90 and his respiratory rate is 20 and shallow. The PACU nurse calls the surgeon and alerts the perioperative nurse of Mr. L.'s status. What should the perioperative nurse anticipate as next steps for Mr. L.?

free flap procedure. When the tissue is removed for the free flap, veins and arteries are microscopically connected, nerve grafts may be used, and bone must be connected with the use of plates and screws. The Doppler unit is also used intraoperatively and postoperatively to detect occlusions or spasms of the vessels.

The free temporoparietal fascial (TPF) flap is the most commonly used free fascial flap. The TPF flap offers the advantages of thin, nonbulky, supple, and highly vascularized tissue with a size of up to 14 × 17 cm. Other advantages include an inconspicuous donor site scar, the option for simultaneous donor and recipient site dissections, and the capacity for inclusion of bone from the outer table of the calvarium. Disadvantages include a long and tedious dissection and post-harvest alopecia (Mankani and Pribaz, 2010).

The radial forearm flap, based off the radial artery and accompanying paired venae comitantes, is the most commonly used free flap for oropharyngeal and osteocutaneous reconstruction, such as the reconstruction of defects of the floor of the mouth with or without partial or total tongue involvement (Figure 19-52). If needed, radial bone may be harvested along with the skin paddle

evolve *The answer to the Critical Thinking Question can be found at http://evolve.elsevier.com/Rothrock/Alexander.*

REFERENCES

American Cancer Society (ACS): *Oral cavity and oral pharyngeal cancer*, 2013, available at www.cancer.org/acs/groups/cid/documents/webcontent/003128 -pdf.pdf. Accessed March 22, 2013.

Association of periOperative Registered Nurses (AORN): Recommended practices for perioperative health care information management, *Perioperative standards and recommended practices*, Denver, 2013a, The Association.

Association of periOperative Registered Nurses (AORN): Recommended practices for the care and handling of specimens in the perioperative environment, *Perioperative standards and recommended practices*, Denver, 2013b, The Association.

Association of periOperative Registered Nurses (AORN): Recommended practices for laser safety in practice settings, *Perioperative standards and recommended practices*, Denver, 2013c, The Association.

Baugh RF et al: Clinical practice guidelines: tonsillectomy in children, *Otolaryngol Head Neck Surg* 144(1 Suppl):S1–S30, 2011.

Briggs R: Central neural auditory prosthesis. In Flint PW et al, editors: *Cummings otolaryngology: head and neck surgery*, ed 5, Philadelphia, 2010, Mosby.

Chole RA, Suddath HH: Chronic otitis media, mastoiditis and petrositis. In Flint PW et al, editors: *Cummings otolaryngology: head and neck surgery*, ed 5, Philadelphia, 2010, Mosby.

Denholm B: Tucking patients' arms and general positioning, *AORN J* 89(4):755–757, 2009.

Elluru RG: Physiology of the salivary glands. In Flint PW et al, editors: *Cummings otolaryngology: head and neck surgery*, ed 5, Philadelphia, 2010, Mosby.

Hillel AT et al: Applications of robotics in laryngeal surgery, *Otolaryngol Clin North Am* 41(4):781–791, 2008.

House JW, Cunningham CD: Otosclerosis. In Flint PW et al, editors: *Cummings otolaryngology: head and neck surgery*, ed 5, Philadelphia, 2010, Mosby.

Iseli TA: Functional outcomes after transoral robotic surgery for head and neck cancer, *Otolaryngol Head Neck Surg* 141(2):166–171, 2009.

Lustig LR, Santina CC: Implantable hearing aids. In Flint PW et al, editors: *Cummings otolaryngology: head and neck surgery*, ed 5, Philadelphia, 2010, Mosby.

Mankani MH, Pribaz J: Free flap donor sites. In Weinzweig J, editor: *Plastic surgery secrets plus*, ed 2, St Louis, 2010, Mosby.

Moore E et al: Long-term functional and oncologic results of transoral robotic surgery for oropharyngeal squamous cell carcinoma, *Mayo Clin Proc* 87(3):219–224, 2012.

National Institute on Deafness and Other Communication Disorders (NIDCD): *Quick statistics* 2010, available at www.nidcd.nih.gov/health/statistics/ quick.htm. Accessed March 21, 2013.

Oliveira CM et al: Robotic surgery in otolaryngology and head and neck surgery: a review, *Minim Invasive Surg*, Article ID 286563, 2012.

Prosser JD et al: Traumatic cerebral spinal fluid leaks, *Otolaryngol Clin North Am* 44(4):857–873, 2011.

Seubert CN et al: Neurologic monitoring. In Miller RD, editor: *Miller's anesthesia*, ed 7, Philadelphia, 2009, Churchill Livingstone.

Thrasher RD: *Middle ear, otitis media with effusion*, August 2011, available at http://emedicine.medscape.com/article/858990-overview. Accessed December 1, 2012.

Told TN: Tonsillectomy and adenoidectomy. In Pfenninger JL, Fowler GC, editors: *Pfenninger and Fowler's procedures for primary care*, ed 3, St Louis, 2010, Mosby.

Wackym PA, Runge-Samuelson CL: Cochlear implantation: patient evaluation and device selection. In Flint PW et al, editors: *Cummings otolaryngology: head and neck surgery*, ed 5, Philadelphia, 2010, Mosby.

CHAPTER **20**
Orthopedic Surgery

BARBARA BOWEN

The word *orthopédie* is derived from the Greek *orthos,* meaning "straight," and *paideia,* meaning "rearing of children." It was first used by Nicholas Andry in 1741 in the title for a book addressing the prevention and correction of skeletal deformities in children. Orthopedic surgery has been defined by the American Academy of Orthopaedic Surgeons' Board of Orthopaedic Surgery as "a broad based medical and surgical specialty dedicated to the prevention, diagnosis, and treatment of diseases and injuries of the musculoskeletal system" (American Board of Orthopaedic Surgeons [ABOS], 2012).

Orthopedic surgery is an ever-changing field that is a challenge for the perioperative nurse. Technologic advances in the multitude of systems and hardware used have resulted in improved treatment of orthopedic disorders. In addition to understanding anatomic and physiologic responses, the perioperative nurse should have a general understanding of the concepts and purposes of these systems to provide the most safe and efficient care. Knowledge of the principles of bone fixation and healing and the relationship of bone and soft tissues provide a strong basis to ensure continued understanding of the care required for the orthopedic patient.

Surgical Anatomy

Anatomic Structures

The 206 bones of the body form the appendicular or axial framework that supports soft tissues, provides storage areas and reservoirs for minerals, and serves as a site for formation of blood cells (Figure 20-1). The skeletal system is composed of varied elements, including bone, muscle, and associated structures.

Bone remains in a constant state of formation and resorption, preventing development of excessive thickness or thinness. These processes are related to individual metabolism and absorption of calcium, vitamin D, and phosphorus. Levels of minerals affect disease processes, causing bone changes. A layer of connective tissue called *periosteum* covers all bone. Bone formation at the cellular level is initiated by the osteoblasts. Osteocytes, which make up 90% of all cells in the adult skeleton, are responsible for maintaining bone. Osteoclasts resorb bone (Miller, 2012).

Muscles are masses of tissue that cover bones and provide movement to the skeletal system. Muscles interact with nerves, minerals, skin, and other connective tissue to contract and extend. Individual muscles are short or long and vary in diameter, depending on their position on a specific bone.

Ligaments, tendons, and cartilage also form the skeletal structures. Ligaments are bands of dense connective tissue that hold bone to bone. They provide stability to a joint by encircling or holding ends of bone in place. Tendons are tough, long strands of fibers that form the ends of muscles. They transmit forces to bone or cartilage without being damaged. Cartilage is a layer of elastic, resilient supporting tissue found at the ends of the bones. It forms a cap over the bone end to protect and support the bone during weight-bearing activities and provides a smooth gliding surface for joint movement. Cartilage is aneural (without nerves), alymphatic (without lymph tissue), avascular (without blood vessels), and high in water content. The lack of vascularity and loss of water from cartilage during a lifetime are causes of resulting degenerative disease, such as arthritis. Weight bearing and joint movements keep cartilage from becoming thin or damaged and help prevent degenerative conditions.

Joints are articulations where bones are joined to one another or where two surfaces of bones unite. Joints are classified by the type of material between them or according to movement. Material between joints is fibrous, cartilaginous, or synovial. The type of movement is synarthrotic (immovable), amphiarthrotic (slightly movable), or diarthrotic (freely movable). Synarthrotic joints are connected by fibrous tissue or ligaments (e.g., the suture type of joints holding the bones of the skull; connections between two bones, such as the radius and ulna). Amphiarthrotic joints are connected by cartilage. Joints of this type include the symphysis pubis, intervertebral joints, and manubriosternal joint. The majority of joints are diarthrotic; these are the only joints with one or more ranges of motion. These joints are lined with a synovial membrane and are called *synovial joints*. Examples include the knee, cervical vertebrae 1 and 2 (C1 and C2), the radius articulating on the wrist bones, the hip, and the shoulder.

The two types of bone tissue are *cortical* and *cancellous*. Cortical bone is the hard bone forming the outer shell—the main supporting tissue. Cancellous bone is soft and spongy—located at the iliac crest, tibia, sternum, and ends of long bones. It contains the red bone marrow for hematopoiesis.

Bones are divided according to their shape: long, short, flat, irregular, and round (Figure 20-2). Long bones are present in the limbs and consist of a shaft and two ends; the ends generally flare out, are covered with articular cartilage, and provide a surface for articulation and musculotendinous attachment. Short bones, such as the carpals and tarsals (in the wrist and midfoot areas, respectively), are present where the structure is strong but limited movement is required. Flat bones are the scapula, the sternum, and the pelvic girdle. Irregular bones are found in the skull and vertebral column. Round bones, or sesamoid bones (resembling a sesame seed), are found within tendons. The patella is a large sesamoid bone; however, most are small, such as the two found on the head of the first metatarsal, which form the "ball" of the foot.

Long bones consist of a shaft (diaphysis) and two ends (epiphyses). The shaft is composed of compact bone. The epiphyses flare

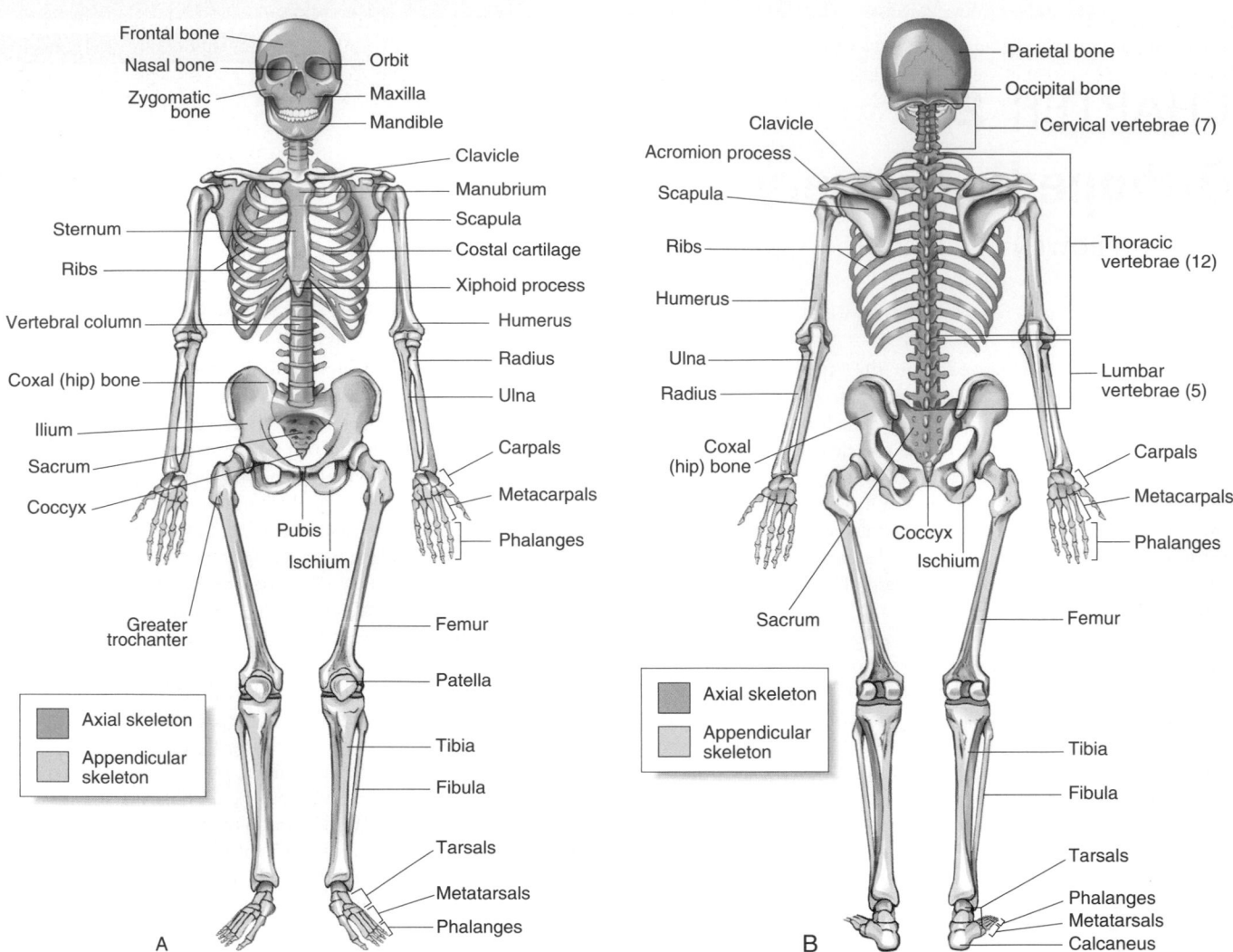

FIGURE 20-1 A, Anterior view of the skeleton. **B,** Posterior view of the skeleton.

out and consist of cancellous bone. They are covered by cartilage, which provides a cushion and offers protection during weight bearing and movement. Until skeletal maturity, a line of cartilage called the *epiphyseal plate* separates the epiphysis from the diaphysis. Fractures in this region by children can be devastating because they often lead to malformation and permanent limb shortening.

Trabeculae are located within cancellous bone and consist of an interconnecting network of bone oriented along the lines of stress. These structures are important for weight bearing, providing strength to withstand stress placed on the bone. The periosteum is a thin, outer covering of bone containing nutrient arteries for nourishment of bone cells. Disruption of these periosteal vessels after bone trauma can influence the ability of bone to heal. The haversian system consists of thousands of microscopic units found in the cortical bone. These units of matrix cells, canals, and conduits allow flow of nutrients and facilitate calcium absorption.

Vertebrae

Vertebrae form the longitudinal axis of the skeleton. The vertebral bodies are connected by several cartilaginous joints, which enable the vertebrae to flex, extend, or rotate while being held together. Intervertebral disks and ligaments connect the bodies of adjacent

vertebrae. The ligamenta flava bind the laminae of adjacent vertebrae together. Other ligaments connect the spinous processes and vertebral bodies.

Seven cervical vertebrae form the skeletal framework of the neck. Twelve thoracic vertebrae support the thoracic region, and five lumbar vertebrae support the small of the back. Below the lumbar vertebrae lie the sacrum and coccyx. Each of these bones is composed of fused vertebrae—five for the sacrum and four for the coccyx.

The vertebral column is curved. After birth there is a continuous posterior convexity. As development occurs, secondary posterior concavities develop in the cervical and lumbar regions, resulting in improved balance.

Each area of the vertebral column has specific bony structures. General features include a body (except the first two cervical vertebrae) on the anterior part. The posterior portion of the vertebrae consists of a neural arch formed by pedicles and laminae and the spinous and transverse processes.

Shoulder and Upper Extremity

The clavicle, which is a long, doubly curved bone, serves as a prop for the shoulder and holds it away from the chest wall. The clavicle rests almost horizontally at the upper and anterior part of the thorax, above the first rib. It articulates medially with the manubrium of the sternum and laterally with the acromion of the scapula; it is tethered to the underlying coracoid process of the scapula by the coracoclavicular ligaments.

The scapula (shoulder blade) is a flat, triangular bone that forms the posterior part of the shoulder girdle, lying superior and posterior to the upper chest. The glenoid cavity on the lateral side of the scapula provides a socket for the humerus (the bone of the upper arm). The acromion process articulates with the clavicle medially. The scapula is attached to the thorax by muscles.

The shoulder (pectoral) girdle consists of the glenohumeral, sternoclavicular, and acromioclavicular (AC) joints (Figure 20-3). The glenohumeral joint has a multidirectional range of motion, whereas the latter two joints have limited motion. The AC joint, located at the top of the shoulder, is the articulation between the outer end of the clavicle and a flattened articular facet situated on the inner border of the acromion. The muscles immediately surrounding the shoulder joint are the supraspinatus, infraspinatus, teres minor, and subscapularis; together they are referred to as the *rotator cuff*. These muscles stabilize the shoulder joint, whereas the powerful deltoid, pectoralis major, teres major, and latissimus dorsi muscles move the entire arm. Shoulder girdle strength and stability are maintained by the soft tissue integrity—not the bony structures. A pathologic condition in this area can be the result of bone, soft tissue, or combined injury.

The humerus is the longest and largest bone of the upper extremity. It is composed of a shaft and two ends. The proximal end, or head, has two projections—the greater and lesser tuberosities (Figure 20-4). The circumference of the articular surface of the humerus is constricted and is termed the *anatomic neck*. The anatomic neck marks the attachment to the capsule of the shoulder joint. The constriction below the tuberosities is called the *surgical neck* and is the site of most fractures.

The greater tuberosity is situated at the lateral aspect of the humeral head. Its upper surface has three impressions where the supraspinous, infraspinous, and teres minor tendons insert. The lesser tuberosity is situated in the anterior neck and has an impression for the insertion of the tendon of the subscapular muscle. The attachment sites for the rotator cuff, the tuberosities, are separated

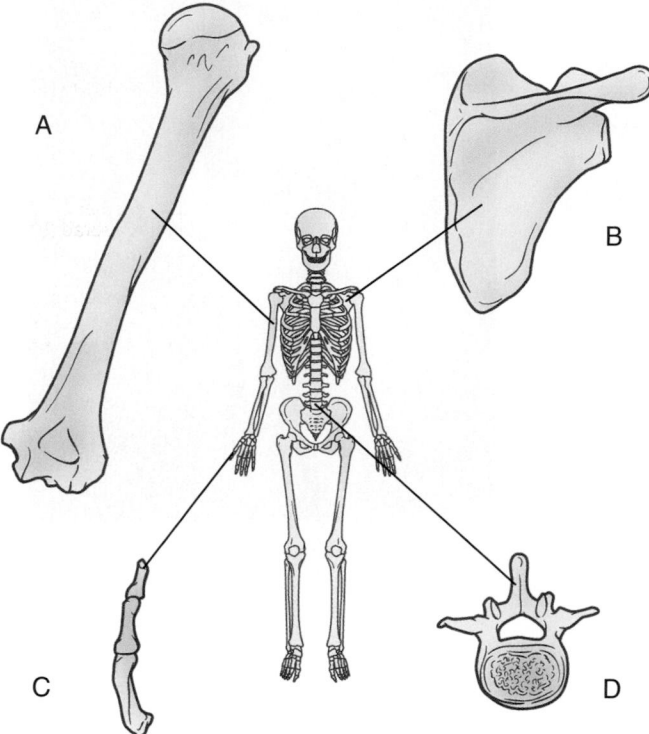

FIGURE 20-2 Types of bones, as examples. **A,** Long bones (humerus). **B,** Flat bones (scapula). **C,** Short bones (phalanx). **D,** Irregular bones (vertebra).

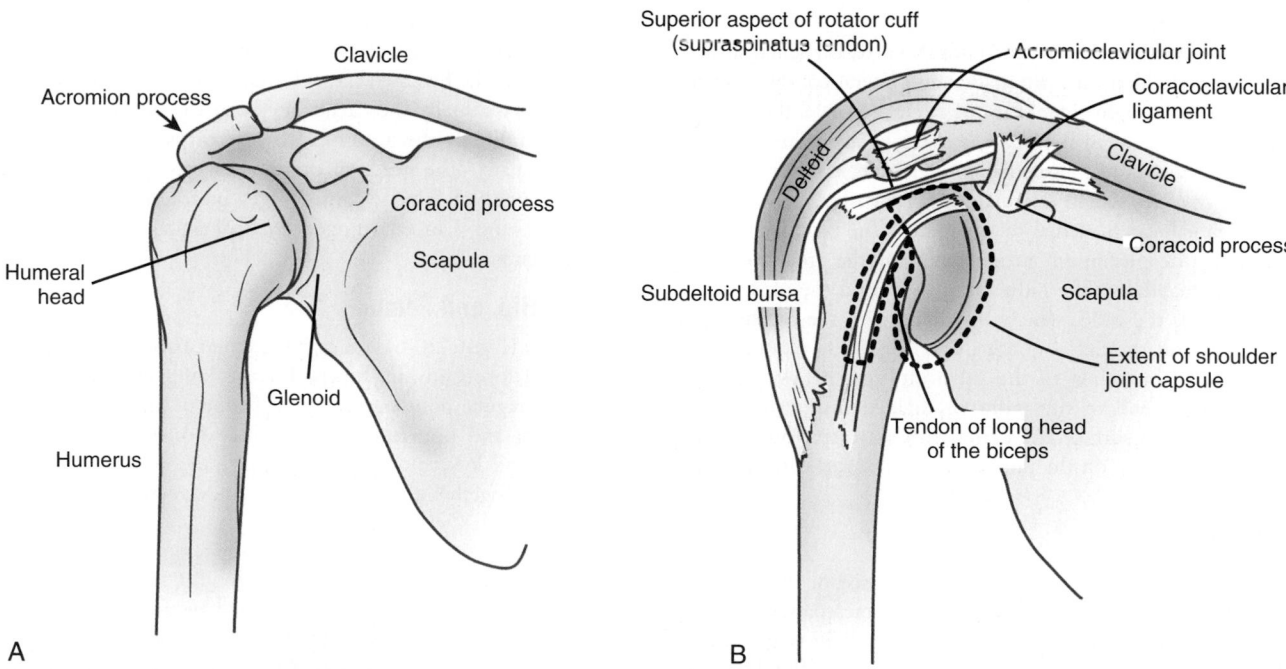

FIGURE 20-3 Shoulder. **A,** Joint showing anterior view. **B,** Girdle showing articulations.

FIGURE 20-4 Bones of the arm, anterior view, showing the humerus, radius, and ulna.

from each other by a deep groove (bicipital groove), in which lies the tendon of the long head of the biceps muscle of the arm. The tendon of the pectoralis major inserts on the lateral margin of the bicipital groove, and the latissimus dorsi and teres major insert on the medial margin.

The distal humerus flattens and ends in a broad articular surface. The surface is divided into the medial and lateral condyles, which are separated by a slight ridge. On the lateral condyle, the rounded articular surface is called the *capitulum,* which articulates with the head of the radius. On the medial condyle, the articular surface is termed the *trochlea,* which articulates with the ulna.

The ulna is located medial to the radius. The proximal portion of the ulna, the olecranon, articulates with the trochlea of the humerus at the elbow. The radius rotates around the ulna. At the proximal end is the head, which articulates with the capitulum of the humerus and the radial notch of the ulna. The tendon of the biceps muscle is attached to the tuberosity just below the radial head. The distal end of the radius is divided into two articular surfaces. The distal surface articulates with the carpal bones of the wrist, and the surface on the medial side articulates with the distal end of the ulna.

Wrist and Hand

The skeletal bones of the wrist and hand consist of three distinct parts: (1) the carpals, or wrist bones; (2) the metacarpals, or bones of the palm; and (3) the phalanges, or bones of the digits (Figure 20-5).

The eight carpal bones are arranged in two rows. The distal row, proceeding from the radial to the ulnar side, includes the trapezium,

trapezoid, capitate, and hamate; the proximal row consists of the scaphoid (also called the *navicular*), lunate, triquetrum, and pisiform. Functionally, the scaphoid links the rows as it stabilizes and coordinates the movement of the proximal and distal rows. Each carpal bone consists of several smooth articular surfaces for contact with the adjacent bones, as well as rough surfaces for the attachment of ligaments. The five metacarpal bones (long bones) are situated in the palm. Proximally they articulate with the distal row of carpal bones, and distally the head of each metacarpal articulates with its proper phalanx. The heads of the metacarpals form the knuckles. The phalanges, or fingers, consist of 14 bones in each hand—2 in the thumb and 3 in each finger. Each phalanx consists of a shaft and two ends.

Pelvis, Hip, and Femur

The pelvis (Figure 20-6) is a stable circular base that supports the trunk and forms an attachment for the lower extremities. It is a massive, irregular bone created by the fusion of three separate bones. The largest and uppermost of the three bones is the ilium, the strongest and lowermost is the ischium, and the anterior-most is the pubis. Together these are termed the *os coxae,* or innominate bone.

The acetabular portion of the innominate bone and the proximal end of the femur (Figure 20-7) form the hip, which is a ball-and-socket joint. The hip joint is surrounded by a capsule, ligaments, and muscles that provide stability. The iliofemoral ligament connects the ilium with the femur anteriorly and superiorly, and the ischiofemoral and pubofemoral ligaments attach the ischium and pubis

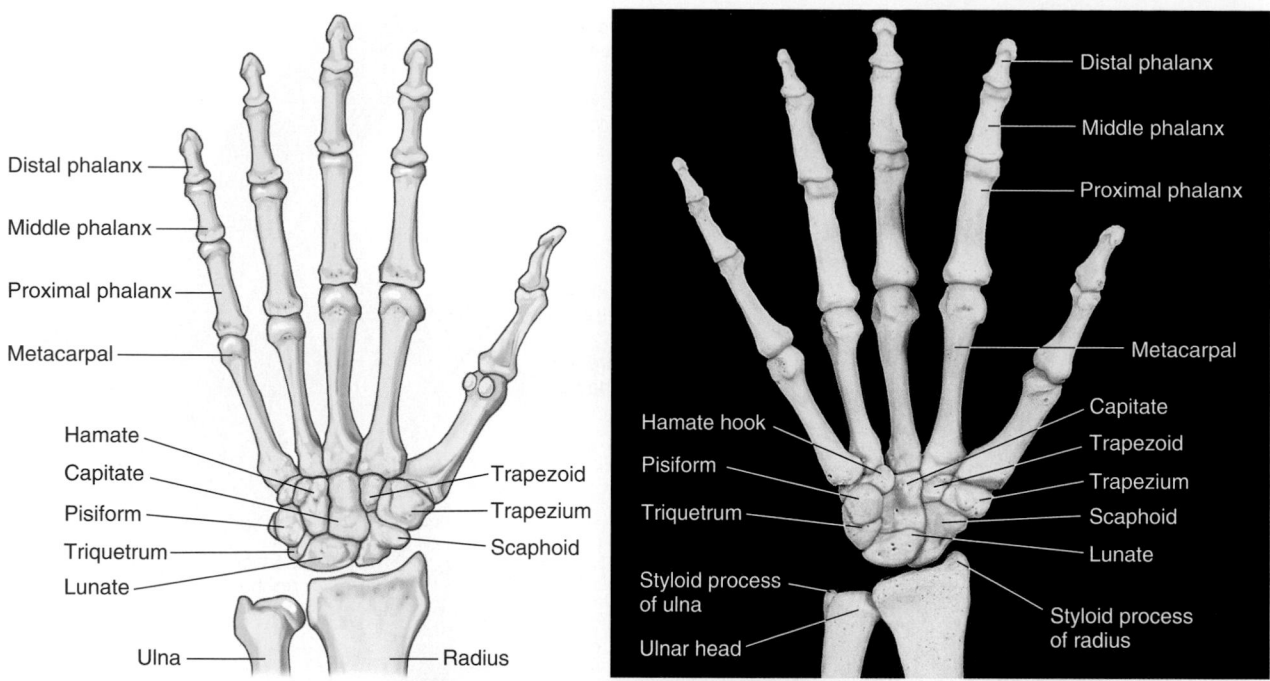

FIGURE 20-5 Bones of the wrist and hand, palmar view.

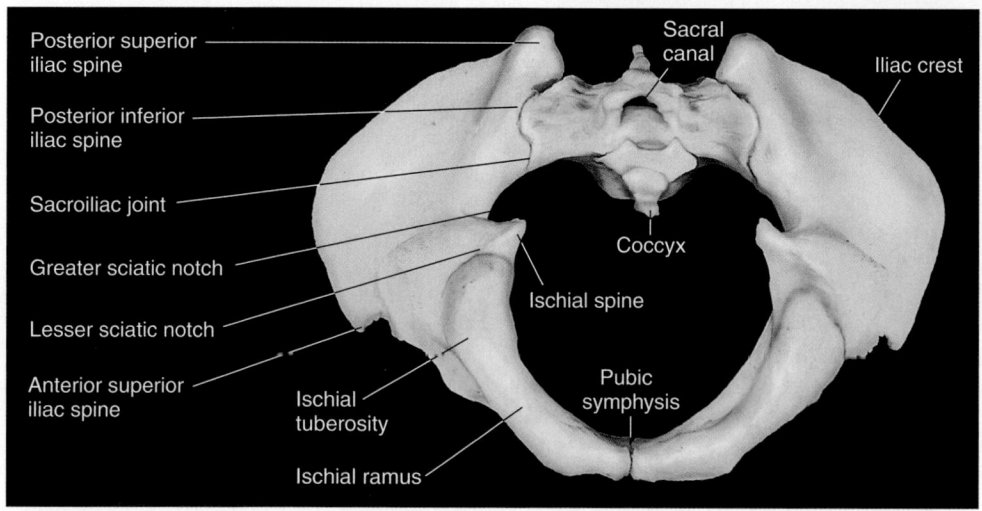

FIGURE 20-6 Pelvis, superior view.

to the femur, respectively. The acetabulum is a deep, round cavity that articulates with the head of the femur. The proximal end of the femur consists of the femoral head and neck, the upper portion of the shaft, and the greater and lesser trochanters (Figure 20-8).

The greater trochanter is a broad process that protrudes from the outer, upper portion of the shaft and projects upward from the junction of the superior border of the neck with the outer surface of the shaft. It serves as a point of insertion for the abductor and short rotator muscles of the hip.

The lesser trochanter is a conical process projecting from the posterior and inferior portion of the base of the neck of the femur at its junction with the shaft. It serves as a point of insertion for the iliopsoas muscle. The lower end of the femur terminates in the two condyles. Anteriorly, the condyles are separated from one another

by a smooth depression, called the *intercondylar,* or *patellar, groove,* forming an articulating surface for the patella. Posteriorly, they project slightly, and the space between them forms the intercondylar fossa—a supporting structure for neurovascular structures.

The upper or condylar end of the tibia presents an articular surface corresponding with those of the femoral condyles. The articular surface of the two tibial condyles forms two facets, which are deepened by the semilunar cartilage into fossae for the femoral condyles.

Knee, Tibia, and Fibula

The knee joint (Figure 20-9) consists of two articulations. One articulation is between each condyle of the femur and the tibial plateau; the other is between the patella and the femur. These areas

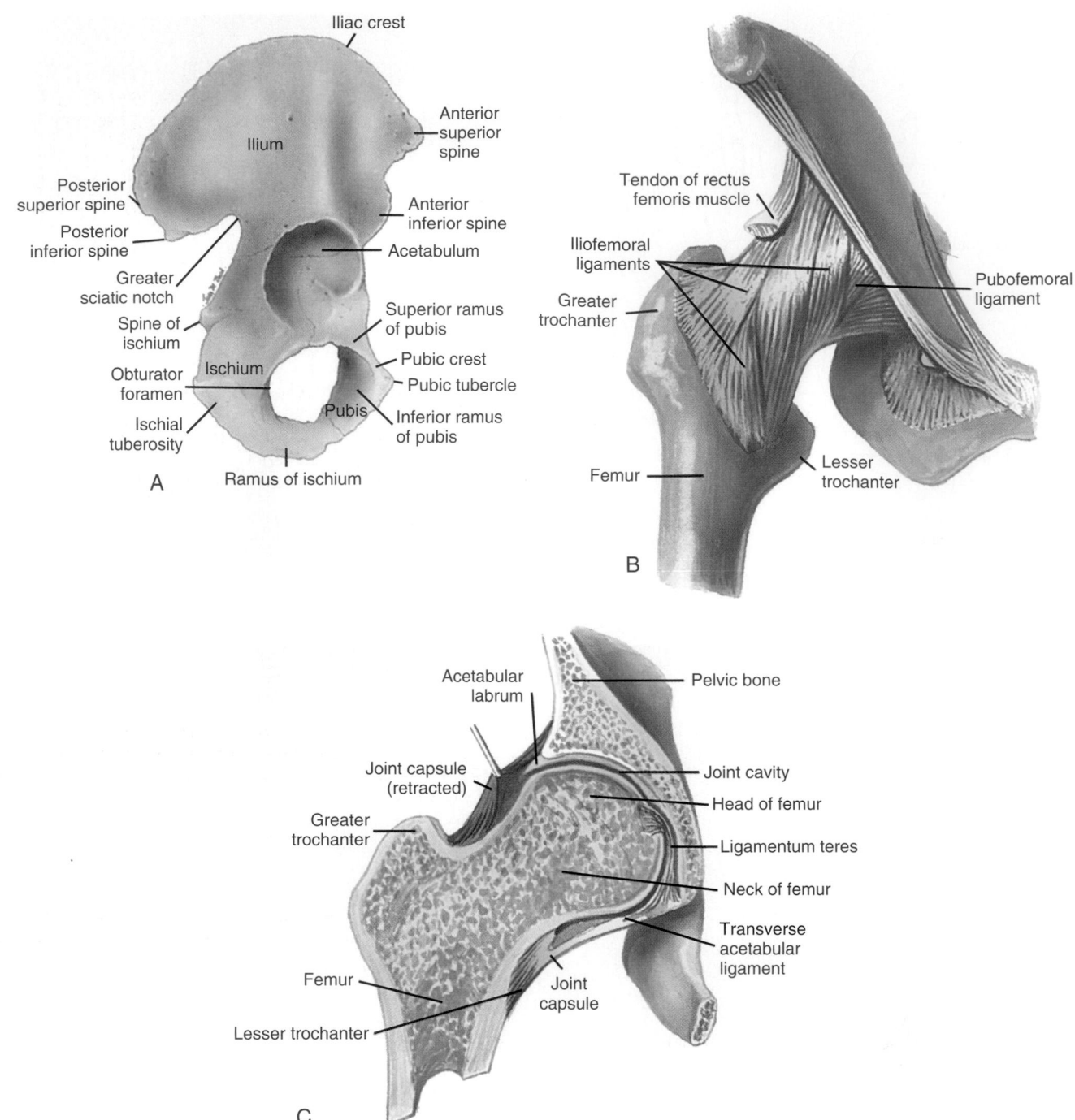

FIGURE 20-7 Hip joint. **A,** Coxal bone disarticulated from the skeleton. **B,** Ligamentous structure. **C,** Bone structure.

are subject to degenerative changes, often requiring reconstructive surgery. The bones of the knee joint are connected by extra-articular and intra-articular structures. The extra-articular attachments consist of the joint capsule, multiple muscular attachments, and two collateral ligaments. The intra-articular ligaments consist of the two cruciate ligaments and the attachments of the menisci.

The patella, or kneecap, is anterior to the knee joint in the intercondylar groove, or trochlea, of the distal femur. It is a sesamoid bone contained within the quadriceps tendon. The anterior surface of the patella is united with the patellar tendon as the

tendon originates and inserts above and below the knee joint. The posterior surface of the patella articulates with the femur.

The capsule of the knee joint is attached proximally to the femoral condyles, and it is attached distally to the condyles of the tibia and to the upper end of the fibula. The capsule is reinforced anteriorly by the patellar and quadriceps tendon, on the sides by the medial and lateral collateral ligaments, and posteriorly by the popliteus and gastrocnemius muscles.

The cruciate ligaments (Figure 20-10), consisting of two fibrous bands, extend from the intercondylar fossa of the femur to

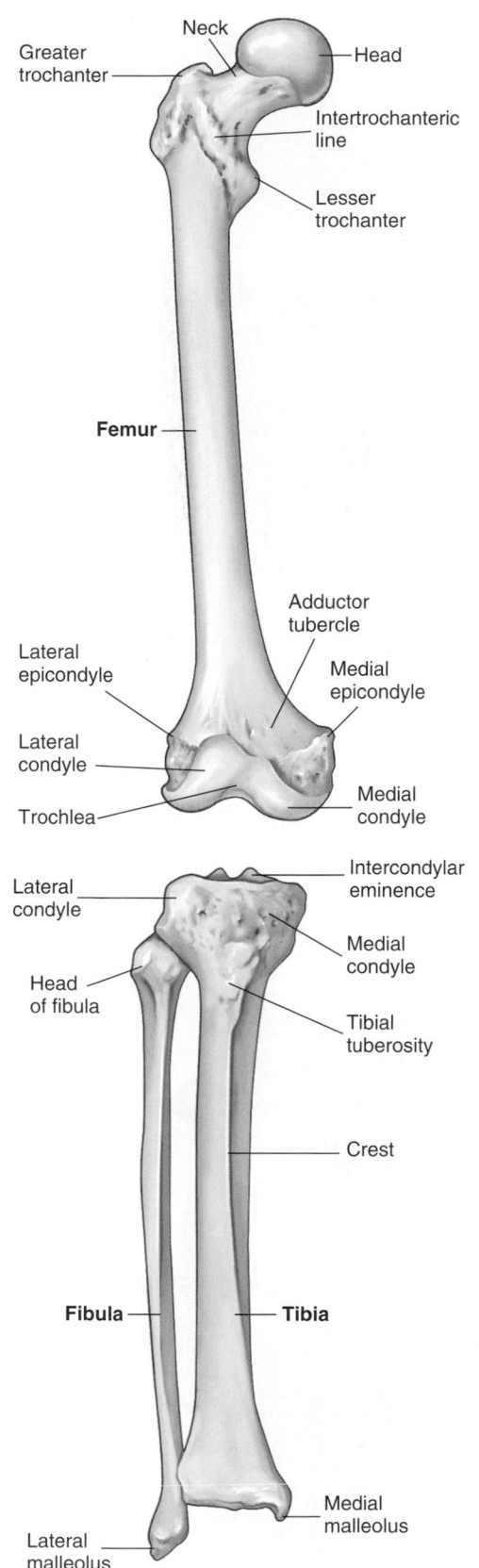

FIGURE 20-8 Bones of the upper *(top)* and lower leg *(bottom)*.

FIGURE 20-9 Bones of the knee showing the tibia and fibula. **A,** Anterior aspect. **B,** Posterior aspect.

attachments anterior and posterior on the intercondylar surface of the tibia.

The menisci are interposed between the condyles of the femur and those of the tibia (see Figure 20-10). Each meniscus is attached to the joint capsule. The ends of the cartilage are attached to the tibia in the middle of its upper articular surface. These structures are almost totally avascular, and degenerative changes are usually permanent.

Synovial membrane lines the capsule of the joint and covers the infrapatellar fat pad, parts of the cruciate ligaments, and portions of the bone. The portion of the knee joint cavity that extends upward in front of the femur is called the *suprapatellar pouch,* or *bursa* (Figure 20-11).

The tibia is the larger and stronger of the lower leg bones. The fibula is smaller and located more laterally, articulating at the proximal end with the lateral condyle of the tibia. The proximal end of

FIGURE 20-10 Bony structures of the knee joint.

FIGURE 20-11 Superficial aspect of the knee joint.

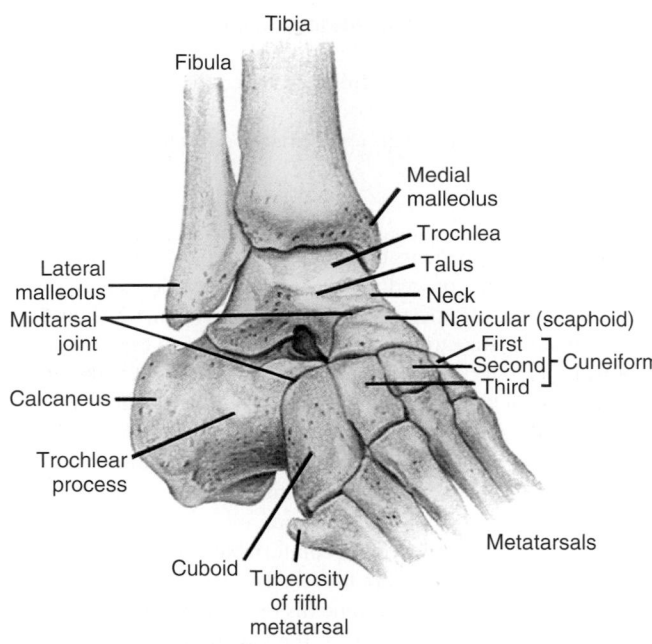

FIGURE 20-12 Anatomy of the ankle.

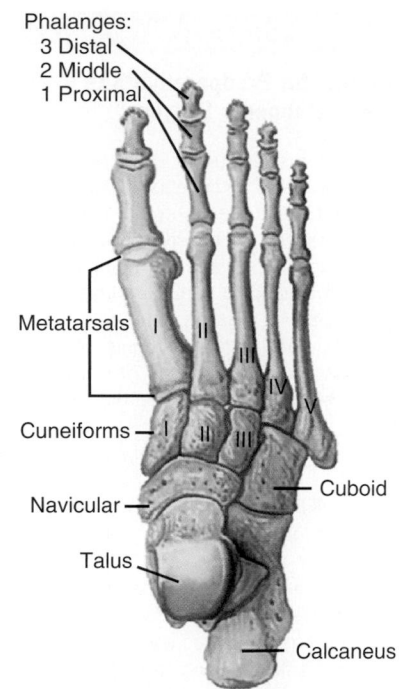

FIGURE 20-13 Bones of the foot viewed from above.

the tibia articulates with the femur to form the knee joint. Distally the tibia articulates with the fibula and with the talus, forming the ankle joint.

Ankle and Foot

The ankle is a hinge joint, formed by the distal end of the tibia and fibula and the proximal end of the talus. The tibia (medial and posterior malleoli) and fibula (lateral malleolus) form a mortise (notch) for the reception of the upper surface of the talus and its facets. The talus is an irregular bone consisting of a body, neck, and head. The bones are connected by ligaments that spread out from the malleoli to attach to the talus, calcaneus, and navicular bones (Figure 20-12). A thin capsule surrounds the joint.

The bony framework of the foot (Figure 20-13) comprises 7 tarsal bones, 5 metatarsal bones, and 14 phalanges. The calcaneus forms the heel and gives support to the talus. The cuboid bone articulates proximally and posteriorly with the calcaneus and distally with the fourth and fifth metatarsals and the third cuneiform bones.

The navicular bone articulates with the cuneiform bones, which lie side by side just anterior to it. The metatarsal bones articulate proximally with the tarsal bones and distally with the bases of the first phalanges of the corresponding toes. There are two phalanges for the great toe and three for each of the other toes.

Perioperative Nursing Considerations

Assessment

Assessment of the orthopedic patient is dynamic, beginning with initial patient consultation. The history and physical are done in the usual fashion. Preoperatively, the nurse takes special care to document any functional losses that are caused by the disability. The social situation of the patient should also be documented both in the physician's office and again in the hospital chart, because this may affect discharge planning. Familiarity with orthopedic procedures and anticipated patient outcomes improves the ability to

gather appropriate information and complete the nursing process. Obtaining patient-specific information from the physician also enhances the perioperative nursing assessment. The signed operative consent provides information to confirm the scheduled procedure or procedures and verify the operative site and side as discussed by Guido (2010) and per The Joint Commission's (TJC) Universal Protocol for correct site surgery (TJC, 2012). The consent is usually obtained before admission to the surgery suite and should be reviewed for accuracy and completeness.

Additional measures that should be undertaken to verify the correct operative side and site include marking the surgical site and having the patient verify the site with the surgeon during the marking process; using a verification checklist (which includes documents such as the medical record, x-ray films, imaging studies); using verbal verification by the patient of his or her identity, surgical site/side, and planned surgical procedure; confirming this information during the time-out by each member of the surgical team; and monitoring safe site protocol compliance with these procedures (Evidence for Practice).

The perioperative nurse reviews the patient record, noting relevant aspects of the history and physical examination; the nature of the problem and its onset; and results of radiographic studies, laboratory data, and other findings. The nursing history is reviewed to determine physical, psychosocial, cultural, spiritual, and other needs. The nurse assesses the patient's range of motion, neurovascular status, and general condition. The patient's understanding of the surgical procedure and postoperative rehabilitation is determined, and patient education is begun.

Assessment information helps the nurse determine specific needs related to surgical positioning, skin preparation, equipment, instrumentation, and supplies. Environmental safety is also considered, including room temperature, traffic flow, lighting, and personnel attire.

Universal Protocol for Preoperative Site Verification as Indicated for Orthopedic Surgery

The Joint Commission's Universal Protocol for correct patient, procedure, and surgical side and site as well as the AORN Position Statement on correct site surgery both emphasize verification and marking of the surgical site (or invasive procedure site), especially when it involves laterality, levels, or multiples. As part of this process, protocols are used to verify the correct patient, correct procedure, correct patient position, and availability of necessary equipment, implants, imaging studies/equipment, or other special requirements. These protocols are part of the preoperative verification process as well as the time-out before the start of the surgical procedure.

For surgery a recommended protocol may involve these additional steps:

- Preoperative skin marking of the procedure site is present.
- Preoperative films or images are present in the OR or procedure room.
- A time-out, including patient identity (using two unique identifiers); procedure to be performed; correct patient position; correct procedure side, level, or site; and presence of necessary implants, imaging, equipment, or other special requirements.
- Provisions for delaying the procedure if there are any discrepancies by any members of the surgical team. If there are discrepancies, the procedure will not proceed until the institution's reconciliation procedure is initiated and the results of the reconciliation documented.
- Use of opaque instruments to mark the specific bony landmarks when intraoperative imaging is necessary. X-rays are taken and compared with the preoperative films or images by the surgeon performing the procedure.

Modified from The Joint Commission: Universal protocol, available at www.jointcommission.org/assets/1/18/UP_Poster1.PDF. Accessed January 5, 2013.

The nurse communicates information with other members of the perioperative team. The information collected helps the perioperative nurse plan and coordinate activities, facilitate a smooth transition, and reduce operative time.

Nursing Diagnosis

Nursing diagnoses related to the care of patients undergoing orthopedic surgery might include the following:
- Anxiety
- Risk for Peripheral Neurovascular Dysfunction
- Risk for Perioperative Positioning Injury
- Impaired Gas Exchange
- Risk for Infection
- Risk for Imbalanced Body Temperature

Outcome Identification

Outcomes identified for the selected nursing diagnoses could be stated as follows:
- The patient will verbalize concerns and apprehension related to surgery and recovery.
- The patient will be free from peripheral neurovascular dysfunction.
- The patient will be free from perioperative positioning injury.

- The patient will maintain adequate ventilation and oxygen exchange.
- The patient will be free from postoperative surgical site infection.
- The patient will maintain appropriate body temperature intraoperatively.

Planning

The care of surgical patients undergoing any type of surgery requires planning for routine procedures that are always followed, as well as anticipating the unexpected. The perioperative nurse should be consistent and systematic in the planning process to expedite actual steps required to facilitate the surgical procedure. Care of the orthopedic patient presents unique challenges because of the psychosocial, physical, and technical aspects of patient care. Planning includes attention to environmental factors, positioning, transfusion supplies, equipment, and instrument needs, in addition to practices that will prevent complications.

The optimal environment is comfortable for the patient and surgical team. The patient should feel relaxed and secure enough to allow the surgical team to become his or her advocates during the procedure. Physical preparation of the environment changes with individual patients. At the time the procedure is posted in the operating room (OR), traffic flow is considered to determine room location. The temperature is selected for the procedure with consideration given to the age and general health of the patient, attire worn by the operative personnel (body exhaust suits), or use of polymethylmethacrylate (PMMA) (bone cement). The patient's temperature should be monitored for all but very brief surgical procedures, such as those lasting less than 30 minutes. To maintain normothermia, the perioperative nurse might consider using warming blankets preoperatively to prewarm the patient in the holding area, warming the ambient room temperature, warming intravenous (IV) fluids, warming the skin surface with a forced-air warming device intraoperatively, and using warm cotton blankets at the end of the surgical procedure.

Equipment and instrumentation needed for the procedure are planned before the patient's arrival in the OR; orthopedic procedures may vary significantly because of the patient's physical condition or age. It may be necessary to communicate with the manufacturer's representative to facilitate obtaining items needed for the procedure. It is common for healthcare industry representatives to bring requisite orthopedic instruments to the OR or to act as a product resource regarding new equipment. However, industry representatives must comply with all institutional policies and Association of periOperative Registered Nurses (AORN) standards defining requirements and procedures and restrictions that govern their presence in the OR (AORN, 2006).

The nurse reviews the procedural information to plan positioning and protective measures. Aseptic technique is essential in the perioperative environment and should be considered a priority when caring for the orthopedic patient. Osteomyelitis is an infection of the bone that can remain unrecognized for a long time and requires expensive, intensive treatment. Osteomyelitis can lead to severe bone loss and possible loss of a limb. Preventive measures, including administration of antibiotics within 60 minutes of the initial incision, have been demonstrated to be efficacious in preventing surgical site infection.

OR equipment such as defibrillators and resuscitative equipment must always be available, functional, and familiar to staff. This includes supplies needed for emergency treatment of a patient's condition, such as malignant hyperthermia or unanticipated blood loss. All medications and solutions along with their containers should be labeled both on and off the surgical field. Equipment alarms should be activated with appropriate settings and should be sufficiently audible. Orthopedic procedures may also require a change in the plan of care in the event of a fracture, damage to vascular integrity, or changes in the patient's condition, requiring an understanding of methods and equipment needed to manage these situations.

The nursing process requires continual reassessment and modifications. An effective plan entails communication, creating a culture that supports patient safety, creation of an optimal environment, and effective use of human and physical resources (AORN, 2013a). A Sample Plan of Care for a patient undergoing orthopedic surgery follows.

Implementation

Implementing care for the orthopedic surgical patient requires an understanding of anatomic, physiologic, psychologic, cultural, spiritual, and technical patient needs. Orthopedic surgical procedures demand special equipment, instruments, and psychomotor skills that differ from those required by other specialties. Implementation includes an understanding of the procedures, patient needs, perioperative practices, and perioperative nursing interventions to protect the patient while delivering care.

The nurse should provide explanations to the patient about the intraoperative phase, including the anticipated sequence of events, personnel, environment, required positioning, and procedures such as administration of a regional anesthetic and application of a tourniquet. The patient may be alert during the procedure; therefore, noise from power equipment and activities that will occur should

SAMPLE PLAN OF CARE

Nursing Diagnosis
Anxiety

Outcome
The patient will verbalize concerns and apprehension related to surgery and recovery.

Interventions
- Encourage verbalization of feelings, expression of fear, and questions about procedure, anticipated outcome, postoperative rehabilitation, pain management, and home care/self-care requirements.
- Explain anticipated routine activities (diagnostic studies, OR environment, preoperative holding area, postanesthesia care unit [PACU]), and encourage questions.
- Encourage patient and family participation in decision-making activities related to discharge planning.
- Demonstrate respect, and attend to patient's individual needs and those of the family or significant others.
- Remain with patient; ensure other personnel are introduced.
- Provide comfort and care, for example, through the use of warm blankets, touch, hand holding.
- Discuss any other concerns with the patient and family, and initiate appropriate referrals.

Nursing Diagnosis
Risk for Peripheral Neurovascular Dysfunction

Outcome
The patient will be free from peripheral neurovascular dysfunction.

Interventions
- Complete and document a preoperative neurovascular assessment including skin color and temperature, pulses, motor strength and movement, and sensation; reassess and document at procedure conclusion.
- Position patient with proper body alignment, considering range of motion or any limitations in mobility.
- Protect vulnerable neurovascular structures and prevent pressure injury by properly padding bony prominences and pressure points.
  - For the brachial plexus, pad the elbow, avoid excessive abduction, and secure arm gently on locked armboard.
  - For the radial nerve, pad the wrist and secure it gently on an armboard or at the patient's side.
  - For the medial or ulnar nerves, pad and tuck the arm carefully at the patient's side or on an armboard.

- For the peroneal nerve, place a pillow at the knee (but not under it) and support the lower extremities; ensure that restraining straps are not tight and do not compress the knee.
  - For the tibial nerve, keep equipment off the lower extremities.
- Apply pneumatic tourniquet correctly, observing, verifying, and documenting pressure settings and tourniquet inflation time.
- Provide padding (air mattress or gel pads) when long surgical times are expected or patients are predisposed to peripheral vascular compromise.
- Anticipate patient's and surgical team's needs to minimize surgical time.

Nursing Diagnosis
Risk for Perioperative Positioning Injury

Outcome
The patient will be free from perioperative positioning injury.

Interventions
- Assess range of motion; identify joints at risk for injury caused by immobilization, pain, trauma, or arthritic or other disease processes.
- Position arthritic joints carefully to prevent strain.
- Observe and document condition of patient's skin before transfer to the OR bed and again at conclusion of procedure.
- Use proper lifting and transfer techniques when transferring the patient to and from the OR bed to prevent shearing forces on skin.
- Keep sheets on OR bed dry and wrinkle-free.
- Ensure that personnel with knowledge of the patient's condition and equipment are available to supervise and assist with transfer of the patient.
- Use proper restraint devices to protect patients from falls or movement of the extremities.
- Avoid extending or flexing extremities beyond range of motion when there is resistance.
- Protect skin in dependent areas from pooling of solutions.
- Use positioning devices, such as pillows, to maintain position; use a small head pillow under the head if head and neck are normally bent slightly forward.
- Pad all dependent pressure sites; provide extra padding for patients with decreased circulation.
- Protect vulnerable neurovascular areas from compression.

Nursing Diagnosis
Impaired Gas Exchange

Continued

SAMPLE PLAN OF CARE—cont'd

Outcome

The patient will maintain adequate ventilation and oxygen exchange.

Interventions

- Review preoperative evaluation of the patient's pulmonary status.
- Assist anesthesia provider in airway management.
- Ensure full chest excursion when positioning, particularly in the lateral and prone positions.
- Collaborate with anesthesia provider in monitoring vital signs, oxygen saturation, ventilation, cardiac rhythm, and blood loss.
- Complete a vascular assessment (pulse, sensation, movement, temperature, and color check) preoperatively, and compare with postoperative status.

Nursing Diagnosis
Risk for Infection

Outcome

The patient will be free from postoperative surgical site infection.

Interventions

- Confirm that the patient has complied with preoperative skin cleansing (as appropriate).
- Implement strict aseptic practices for preparing the patient's skin, draping the patient and equipment, opening supplies and equipment for the procedure, removing hair (as necessary), and controlling traffic patterns in the OR.
- Prepare for pulsatile lavage or irrigation (as needed).

- Initiate antibiotic therapy preoperatively and/or intraoperatively per physician's orders; check for medication allergies before antibiotic administration.
- Implement procedure-specific activities, such as using body exhaust systems and pulsatile lavage.
- Anticipate equipment needs, and check equipment function; implement safety precautions when using equipment.
- Sterilize instruments according to policy and procedure and the manufacturer's guidelines.
- Handle implants according to manufacturer's recommendations.

Nursing Diagnosis
Risk for Imbalanced Body Temperature

Outcome

The patient will maintain normothermia intraoperatively.

Interventions

- Obtain and document baseline preoperative temperature.
- Initiate preoperative warming with either warmed blankets or forced hot air warming device.
- Maintain temperature in the OR between 68° and 73° F (20° to 23° C) if possible.
- Monitor patient temperature throughout the procedure.
- Use warming devices and warming blankets during the procedure.
- Warm fluids as necessary.
- Minimize patient exposure to room air.
- Place warm blankets on patient immediately after surgery.

---

be explained. Immobilization devices, such as splints, casts, braces, and drains, also should be explained.

Positioning and Positioning Aids. The orthopedic patient requires proper positioning on the OR bed or specialty bed to provide adequate exposure of the operative area, maintain body alignment, minimize strain or pressure on nerves and muscles, allow for optimal respiratory and circulatory function, and provide adequate stabilization of the body. Selection of position depends on several factors, including the type of procedure, the location of the injury or lesion, and the preference of the surgeon. Guidelines for placing the patient in the supine or recumbent position are followed (see Chapter 6), with modifications to facilitate the specific orthopedic procedure.

Procedures performed in lateral, prone, or modified positions require positioning aids and devices to support these positions. Patients undergoing surgical procedures risk neuromuscular and skin injury. The nurse's preoperative assessment should be thorough to plan the position, taking into consideration the prevention of neurovascular compromise, the potential for impaired chest excursion, and the danger of falls. The safety strap does not always provide adequate security, and other methods of securing the patient on the OR bed may need to be implemented. The surgeon is responsible for selecting the position and ensuring that adequate exposure can be obtained. The perioperative staff must understand the meaning of terms such as *flexion, extension, abduction,* and *adduction* when positioning the patient. The staff must also be thoroughly familiar with the function of the orthopedic surgical bed and its various attachments (e.g., the leg attachment for arthroscopy, the three-point positioner for lateral position, and positioning devices for shoulder procedures).

Many orthopedic operations require a device for holding the extremities. Various holders are available for both upper and lower extremities. Positioners used intraoperatively can be sterilized for the procedure, resulting in the ability to reposition as needed throughout the procedure. These types of positioners include the shoulder positioner (Figure 20-14), Alvarado foot holder (Figure 20-15), and ankle distractor (Figure 20-16). Many other orthopedic positioning devices are also available.

The lateral position is sometimes used for a total hip arthroplasty. Padded anterior and posterior supports may be positioned at the umbilicus and lumbar regions, respectively, to hold the patient in the lateral position. A vacuum beanbag positioning device can also achieve the lateral position. Pressure points on the lateral area of the skull, ear, axilla, hip, knee, and ankle should be adequately padded. The patient's feet are placed in the neutral position to prevent excessive plantar flexion or dorsiflexion. A conscientious effort should be made by the surgical team to avoid leaning on the patient during the procedure.

The patient is positioned prone for surgery on the posterior aspect of the body, including the spine; posterior portion of the shoulder, arms, and legs; and Achilles tendon; and for posterior iliac bone graft harvesting. This position presents a challenge for the anesthesia provider to monitor and manage the airway because of the potential for impaired chest excursion and gas exchange. The patient's extremities need to be moved through a normal range of motion when transferring and positioning into the prone position. Vascular integrity is always assessed before the patient is moved into position and reassessed after the patient is positioned; the nurse should note the quality of pulses, extremity warmth, and capillary refill.

FIGURE 20-14 Shoulder positioner allows distraction of the joint for visualization.

FIGURE 20-16 Ankle distractor, noninvasive, for distraction of the joint and visualization.

FIGURE 20-15 Alvarado foot holder used during total joint procedures to position the extremity for exposure.

FIGURE 20-17 Andrews bed used for prone positioning.

The prone position is often attained with the use of adjunctive frames, such as the Wilson, Hastings, Canadian, Relton-Hall, Cloward saddle, or Andrews, or with the Andrews bed (Figure 20-17). Each frame has qualities that meet the patient or physician's needs. The Hastings and Andrews frames and the Andrews bed maintain the patient in a modified knee-chest position. The frames require assembly and are labor-intensive when positioning; some can be used only with certain beds. The Andrews bed is similar to

the Andrews frame but has the attachments built in and is used exclusively for this position.

On an OR fracture bed (Figure 20-18), generally used for femoral neck and shaft fixation, the team places the patient in supine or lateral position to allow exposure of the surgical site while maintaining alignment. The patient's legs are positioned on outriggers, allowing access by the image intensifier to obtain multiple radiographic views. Applying or releasing traction can be done to reduce the fracture or aid in intramedullary surgical techniques. Like all positioning devices, the fracture bed must be set up by experienced personnel and padded adequately. There are several moving parts that can cause injury if not operated properly.

If the patient is positioned supine, special attention must be paid to the arms. Arms are placed on padded armboards with the palms up and fingers extended. Armboards are maintained at less than a 90-degree angle to prevent brachial plexus stretch. If there are surgical reasons to tuck the arms at the side, the elbows are padded to

FIGURE 20-18 Patient positioned on the orthopedic fracture bed for femoral neck, femoral shaft, or tibial fixation, with image intensifier in position.

protect the ulnar nerve, the palms face inward, and the wrist is maintained in a neutral position (Denholm, 2009). A drape secures the arms. It should be tucked snuggly under the patient, not under the mattress. This prevents the arm from shifting downward intraoperatively and resting against the OR bed rail.

Surgical Prep. A primary concern in orthopedic surgery is the prevention of infection. The orthopedic surgical prep must be meticulously carried out using aseptic technique. Physicians often instruct patients to complete a scrub prep with an antimicrobial agent before arrival for surgery. The surgical prep for the orthopedic patient may include preoperative removal of hair from the surgical site. Surgical shave preps contribute to the possibility of infection caused by abrasion and cutting of the skin. If hair removal from the incisional site is ordered, it should occur immediately before surgery, using clippers or a depilatory (AORN, 2013b). Trauma patients require precautions during the skin prep to prevent further injury caused by solution contact with membranes or injury to the bone and soft tissue from movement.

Skin preparation is performed to remove microorganisms from the operative site. The site should be prepped with a broad-spectrum antimicrobial agent. The prep proceeds from the incision site to the periphery. Pooling of the prep solution beneath the patient or tourniquet must be avoided. Prep solutions should be allowed to dry before draping; this is a fire safety precaution and may be included in the time-out. The groin and anal areas should be isolated when the surgical site is on the upper third of the leg.

Devices such as leg stirrups may help support an extremity to complete a circumferential prep. When multiple extremities or other areas, such as a bone graft site, are prepped, cross-contamination of previously prepped areas must be prevented. Knowledge of aseptic technique and the ability to organize the activity are important in proper preparation of the surgical site.

Draping. Applying sterile drapes is the final step in preparing the patient for the operation. The surgeon and scrub person, who may be a registered nurse or surgical technologist, cover the patient's extremities with a cloth or water-impervious stockinette—a cylindric drape that is rolled up the arm or leg. Impervious sheets are essential when large amounts of fluid are used, such as during arthroscopy and wound irrigation. Prefabricated disposable drapes with fenestrations for the upper and lower extremities are available.

Antimicrobial incise drapes can be used to isolate the surrounding area from the incisional site. Many of these drapes contain iodophor-impregnated adhesive, which slowly releases iodine during the procedure, inhibiting proliferation of organisms from the patient's skin. They are contraindicated for patients with an allergy to iodophors. An alcohol skin wipe may be done before placement of the antimicrobial incise drape.

Equipment and Supplies. Orthopedic ORs require a variety of special equipment and accessories in addition to routine OR equipment. Nitrogen-powered, battery-powered, and electrically powered equipment, video systems, pneumatic tourniquets, laminar airflow systems, x-ray equipment, lasers, and special orthopedic tables are included in the operative armamentarium. Manufacturers' pamphlets with illustrations and directions on equipment use and sterilization should be readily available for reference.

Radiographic Intervention. Radiographic intervention is widely used in orthopedic surgery. Many procedures require portable x-ray or fluoroscopy machines. Fluoroscopy, also known as *image intensification* or *C-arm,* allows the team to view the progression of the procedure, confirming fracture reduction or intramedullary reaming of the humerus, femur, or tibia. An x-ray technician operates radiographic equipment. An understanding of equipment placement, function, and safety precautions is necessary. The perioperative nurse is responsible for communicating with the radiology personnel concerning the procedure, aseptic technique, and traffic flow in the OR. X-ray cassettes brought onto the sterile field are draped with a sterile plastic cover. Lead aprons and thyroid shields are to be worn by all personnel in proximity to the x-ray equipment, and personnel should be monitored for exposure to radiation. Measures should be taken to protect patients from direct and indirect radiation exposure, and these should be documented on the perioperative nursing record.

Pneumatic Tourniquets. Pneumatic tourniquets are frequently used for procedures involving the extremities. A tourniquet is a fabric-covered cylindric bladder inflated by compressed gas or ambient air. It applies circumferential pressure on arterial and venous circulation, which results in a relatively bloodless surgical field; this promotes visualization of structures during the procedure. Limb exsanguination is achieved by elevating the limb or by wrapping it, distally to proximally, with an ACE or Esmarch rubber bandage before tourniquet inflation. The majority of tourniquets used today are run by a microprocessor for regulation of pressure and time setting, providing both auditory and visual feedback for the user.

Tourniquet safety should be a priority; the surgical team should understand recommended parameters and precautions. Safety guidelines for the use of tourniquets include preventive measures and evaluation (AORN, 2013c). Preoperative assessment of the patient includes determining contraindications for use, including compartment syndrome, McArdle disease (e.g., glycogen storage disease), hypertension, or other vascular problems. If the tourniquet must be used for patients with these conditions, specific guidelines must be observed.

Before applying the tourniquet cuff, the nurse checks all components of the tourniquet equipment for proper functioning. Inflation pressures are established based on the systolic blood pressure, age of the patient, and circumference of the extremity. Duration of tourniquet inflation should be kept to a minimum. It is recommended in the average, healthy 50-year-old person to apply continuous tourniquet pressure less than 1 hour on the upper extremity and less than 2 hours on the thigh. Tourniquet pressure should not exceed the recommended maximum cuff pressure limits of 300 to 350 mm Hg for the thigh and 250 to 300 mm Hg for the arm and the lower leg. Kleinert and colleagues (2012) note the interval between inflation and deflation should be 5 minutes for every 30 minutes of tourniquet ischemia to minimize effects on muscle and nerves.

The tourniquet should be placed on the extremity without compression on bony structures and superficial neurovascular structures. The person placing the cuff should ensure it is positioned as high as possible without pinching skinfolds. Soft padding or stockinette is wrapped around the extremity and kept free of wrinkles and gatherings beneath the cuff. Cuffs should overlap a minimum of 3 inches and a maximum of 6 inches; excess overlap can pinch skinfolds. A tourniquet cuff that is too short can loosen after inflation. Care must be taken to ensure that the line from the air supply to the cuff is not kinked.

Tourniquet equipment should be checked periodically and serviced when problems arise. Injury from tourniquets may result from inadequate precautions, faulty preparation, or use of inaccurate equipment. The gauges and other related equipment should be checked with commercially available test equipment. Patient evaluation requires assessment of the extremity (skin color, temperature, pulses, movement, sensation) after removal of the tourniquet. Abnormal findings need to be reported to the surgeon and documented (Patient Safety).

New technology has provided a bloodless field. Hemaclear is a sterile one-step application of a tourniquet cuff and the associated pressure. The cuff is applied over the hand or foot using sterile technique and then rolled upward to the desired height. The rubber band within the fabric provides the tourniquet effect and produces the bloodless field. Hemaclear is a disposable, single-use item.

Traction. The surgeon uses traction preoperatively, intraoperatively, or postoperatively for prevention or reduction of muscle spasm, immobilization of a joint or body part, reduction of a fracture or dislocation, and treatment of a joint disorder. Traction alignment must be constant.

Various traction techniques can be used, including manual, skin, and skeletal (Figure 20-19). In manual traction the hands provide the forces pulling on the bone being realigned. Skin traction uses strips of tape, digital straps, moleskin, or an elastic bandage applied directly to the skin. Common forms of skin traction are Buck extension and Russell traction. Skeletal traction applies forces directly to the bone, using pins. Manual and skin traction can be applied in the emergency department or patient room, whereas skeletal traction is applied preoperatively in the emergency department or in the OR.

Skeletal traction is often used in conjunction with the OR fracture bed, using the traction attachment to aid in reduction of a long bone fracture. Postoperatively the patient may be confined to bed with balanced skeletal traction using a Thomas splint (Figure 20-20) and a Pearson attachment. Some cervical spine fractures or injuries may require Crutchfield or Gardner-Wells tongs or a cervical halo inserted directly into the skull to stabilize the vertebrae and reduce spinal cord damage or further injury. Application of skeletal traction requires the use of sterile supplies, including a traction bow, pins, and drill.

PATIENT SAFETY

Safe Tourniquet Use

Recommended practices from AORN help the perioperative nurse effectively manage cases that involve tourniquets. Patient safety is the primary concern when using tourniquets intraoperatively. All OR personnel responsible for the tourniquet should be familiar with current standards. The primary purpose of the tourniquet is to occlude blood flow to the extremity, providing a bloodless surgical site. Competency associated with the use of tourniquets should be demonstrated by the OR staff. All tourniquets should be maintained according to manufacturers' guidelines including cleaning, sterilizing, and testing. Disposable tourniquets are available for single use. The integrity and function of the base unit should be tested before each use. Personnel should be familiar with the application of the tourniquet, recommended pressures, maximum times for inflation for extremities, and contraindications for tourniquet use. OR personnel must be aware of the risks of exceeding the time limits and should inform the surgeon at regular intervals of the tourniquet inflation time. The nurse is responsible to assess and document patient outcomes at the end of the procedure.

Modified from Association of periOperative Registered Nurses (AORN): Recommended practices for the use of the pneumatic tourniquet in the perioperative practice setting. *Perioperative standards and recommended practices,* Denver, 2013, The Association.

  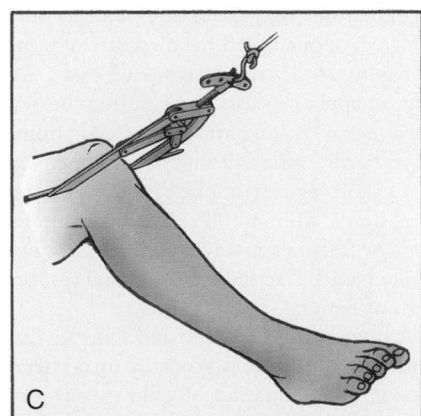

FIGURE 20-19 Traction techniques. **A,** Manual. **B,** Skin. **C,** Skeletal.

FIGURE 20-20 Thomas splint balanced suspension.

The perioperative nurse ensures the patient's postoperative bed is prepared with the correct traction frames. Nursing care of the patient in traction should include ensuring that the traction is continuous and skin tapes or skeletal pins are secured. Neurovascular status should be checked routinely, including skin color, pulse, temperature, and sensation. Changes from baseline or normal value must be reported.

Postoperative Immobilization. Postoperative immobilization may require use of a cast, splint, or other supplies designed for the specific anatomic part. A cast is a common method of immobilizing a fractured bone during healing (Patient and Family Education). The forces of distraction, rotation, and malalignment can be overcome with the application of a cast. Closed reduction with a cast may be an option, thus minimizing the disadvantages and complications of open reduction, such as infection and tissue damage.

The surgeon uses plaster or synthetic materials such as fiberglass for casting. Plaster is less expensive, with a greater weight-to-strength ratio (it requires a greater weight of plaster to produce the same strength of fiberglass). Plaster casts may be burdensome if the casts are too heavy. They are routinely used as the primary cast after surgical procedures and are replaced later with a lighter fiberglass cast to promote patient mobility.

Casting material sets up and hardens rapidly once activated with water, and such a property necessitates that it be prepared with all necessary materials. Soft padding or stockinette should be applied to the patient's extremity before the cast is applied to protect the skin from thermal injury while the plaster sets, as well as to protect the skin from undue abrasion and pressure. The plaster must be prepared, applied, and handled carefully and safely.

Figure 20-21 shows types of casts. After wrist fractures the surgeon applies a short arm cast from below the elbow to the metacarpal heads. A long arm cast extends from the axilla to the metacarpal heads, immobilizing forearm or elbow fractures. The surgeon uses a short leg cast, applied from the tibial tuberosity to the metatarsal heads, to immobilize the ankle and foot. The long leg cast is used for fractures involving the femur, tibia, or fibula or for complicated ankle fractures. The femoral cast brace is used in the treatment of femoral shaft fractures.

A snug-fitting thigh cast and short leg cast are hinged at the knee joint. The cast brace is generally used after 4 to 6 weeks of skeletal traction after initiation of callus formation at the fracture site. A cylinder cast incorporates the leg from the groin to the ankle and is applied when complete knee immobilization is required. This is

PATIENT AND FAMILY EDUCATION
Casts

Explanation of the Cast
The cast is only one of several devices used to promote the healing of broken bones. Surgeons also use traction and pins, or a combination of these three devices, to help heal broken bones. The cast has the advantage of being less expensive, requiring little care on the patient's part, and allowing the patient mobility. The cast also encloses and immobilizes the broken bone and injured soft tissues to prevent movement that could cause further injury and to keep the bone in place for proper healing. The cast may be made of plaster or of a synthetic material, such as fiberglass. Although the plaster cast is heavy, the surgeon can mold a plaster cast more easily for a close fit over severe injuries. The synthetic cast is lightweight and easier to move around.

Cast Care
- Keep a plaster cast dry; cover it or wrap it in a plastic bag when bathing or going out in the rain or snow.
- Check with the surgeon about immersing a fiberglass (or other synthetic) cast in water. The surgeon may permit immersion if there are no surgical wounds under the cast.
- Maintain good skin care around the cast. However, do not:
  - Insert objects, such as a coat hanger, under the cast.
  - Put any creams, lotions, or powder inside the cast.

Things to Watch for and Report to Your Surgeon or Nurse
The skin under the cast will feel warm at first because of the reaction that occurs during the setting process. However, warm areas on the cast later may indicate infection; notify the surgeon or nurse at once.

Watch for increased pain or soreness under the cast, particularly around a bony prominence such as the wrist or ankle not relieved by repositioning the body. Check the skin color and temperature periodically. When the tip of a finger or the big toe that extends from the cast is squeezed until it is white, the pink color should return within 4 to 6 seconds. If skin color does not return within 4 to 6 seconds or if the skin is red, blue, white, or otherwise discolored, notify the physician. If fingers or toes are cool, cover them. If they do not warm up in 20 minutes, call the physician. Call the physician immediately if any of these other symptoms occur:
- An increase in swelling and pain. Some swelling is common at first. The surgeon may have advised to elevate the cast after it was applied. The cast should feel snug for the first 48 hours. If it continues to feel too snug and causes pain and swelling, call the surgeon.
- A tingling or burning sensation.
- An inability to move muscles around the cast.
- A foul odor detected around the edges of the cast.
- Any drainage that may show through the cast.
- Any cracks or breaks in the cast.
- Marked loosening of the cast, allowing the parts inside the cast to move fairly easily.

Modified from Canobbio MM: *Mosby's handbook of patient teaching*, ed 3, St Louis, 2006, Mosby; Eiff MP, Hatch RL: *Fracture management for primary care*, ed 3, Philadelphia, 2011, Saunders.

often required after surgery involving soft tissue reconstruction around the knee.

The hip spica cast is used when complete leg immobilization is desired. The patient's trunk, affected side, and unaffected side may all be incorporated into the cast. Spinal immobilization is accomplished with a body jacket.

FIGURE 20-21 Types of casts. **A,** Short arm cast. **B,** Long arm cast. **C,** Plaster body jacket cast. **D,** One and one-half hip spica cast.

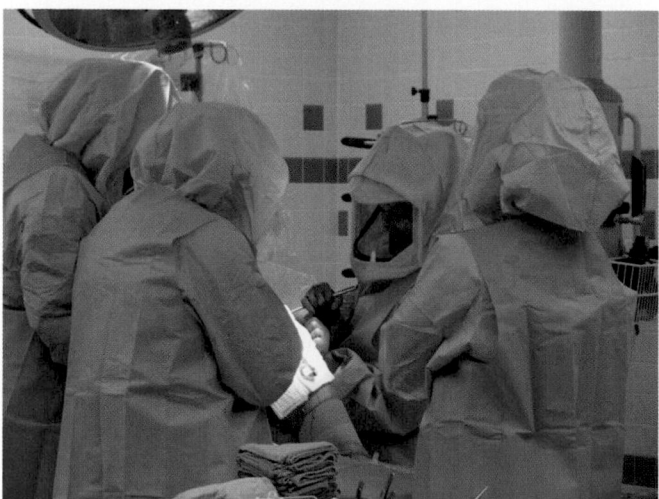

FIGURE 20-22 Body exhaust system used in arthroplasty.

Splints may also be used for postoperative immobilization but are not circumferential and allow for swelling and closer observation of the surgical site.

Another immobilization device is the abduction pillow, used after total joint replacement. This prevents the patient's leg from adducting, or rotating internally, and the hip from flexing, which could cause dislocation of the hip. Further discussion of this and other devices is included with the description of various surgical interventions.

Lasers. Laser application has been increasing in the field of orthopedics. Its use mandates safety precautions, certification, patient consent, and protective attire (see Chapter 8 for a full discussion of lasers and laser safety). Laser types include carbon dioxide, holmium:yttrium-aluminum-garnet (Ho:YAG), neodymium:YAG (Nd:YAG), potassium titanyl phosphate (KTP), erbium:YAG (Er:YAG), and excimer. Laser technique differs for use on bone, muscle, tendon, and cartilage. Lasers have been used successfully for osteotomy, revision arthroplasty (removal of PMMA), nerve and tendon repair, arthroscopy, and diskectomy.

Airflow Control. Airflow control in the orthopedic OR is critical to prevent introduction of microorganisms. Surgical site infections may result from airborne bacteria or transient bacteria from the patient or surgical team (AORN, 2013d). Laminar airflow is a system designed to provide highly filtered air and continuous air exchange for reducing airborne bacteria. Body exhaust suits are also used as a defense against airborne bacteria (Figure 20-22). Aseptic practices, sterile technique, and conscientious behaviors in ORs using conventional airflow can be used to maintain low rates of surgical site infections.

Postoperative Management. The nurse begins planning the patient's postoperative management during the preoperative period. Special equipment may include continuous passive motion (CPM) machines, pain management devices and techniques, compression devices, and blood salvage. CPM machines stimulate the healing effect on articular tissues, including cartilage, tendon, and ligaments, without interfering with healing incisions over the moving joint. The benefits of CPM include inhibition of adhesion formation and joint stiffness, decreased pain and swelling, early functional range of motion, and decreased effects of immobilization. The device is applied early in the postoperative period.

Pain management may include insertion of an epidural catheter, use of a patient-controlled analgesia (PCA) pump, or local administration of pain medication through a pain pump. The advantages of using these techniques include rapid pain relief, increased patient satisfaction, and, often, less use of medication than with traditional intramuscular analgesics. These techniques can be used independently or in combination. In using the PCA pump, a predetermined IV dose of the prescribed pain medication is administered. It allows continuous infusion of analgesic as well as bolus administration when the patient feels it is necessary.

Management of fluid and electrolyte balance may include use of intraoperative autologous transfusion or postoperative blood salvage. A potential problem with salvage of large amounts of blood is depletion of clotting factors; therefore, coagulation problems should be identified. Postoperative blood salvage is accomplished with a closed-drainage system. It requires a complete understanding of the system for safe use.

Instruments and Accessory Items. Orthopedic surgical procedures require an extensive inventory of instruments and implants and specific instruments to implant and apply hardware. Revision surgery requires that the perioperative staff be prepared with the appropriate tools and extractors needed to remove an old implant and an understanding of equipment use. Preoperative planning is essential for orthopedic surgery.

Implant Inventories. Implant inventories include plates and screws, intramedullary nails and rods, total joint implants, and a host of accessory items. Surgeon preference, patient population, and equipment cost are considered when selecting stock items. The surgical team must ensure these items are stocked in a timely fashion to prepare for consecutive implant use.

Inventory should be organized by manufacturer, type of implants (e.g., total hip, knee), and comparative sizes. Some may be provided on a loaner or consignment basis. Staff must be familiar with the varied types and refer to the manufacturer's information pertaining to each implant. Practices should ensure that the correct implant is opened on the operative field to prevent unnecessary expense or error in placement. Confirmation of the implant by the surgeon, scrub person, and perioperative nurse is essential before opening the implant onto the field.

Many different alloys are used in manufacturing implants. However, all devices implanted in a patient must be of the same metallic composition to prevent galvanic corrosion; internal fixation implants used during an orthopedic procedure should be of the same metal. Screws, for example, should be of the same composition as the metal plate affixed to the bone. Alloys used most frequently include stainless steel, cobalt-chromium, and titanium-vanadium-aluminum.

Internal fixation devices should never be reused. Resulting imperfections, such as abrasions or scratches, increase the potential for corrosion and weakening of the implant. Bending implants to conform to the contour of the bone should be avoided whenever possible to prevent loss of strength. When bending is necessary, the proper bending press should be used. Once an implant is bent, it should not be reshaped or straightened; doing so may weaken the implant.

Orthopedic equipment and implants require special care, storage, and handling. When possible, implants should be individually wrapped and processed. Today's implants, excluding some plates and screws, are packaged separately by the manufacturer. During sterilization, implants should not be placed in a position in which knocking or bumping might occur. Appropriate sterilizing cases and trays should be used, and implants should be sterilized according to the manufacturer's instructions. An internal fixation device that has become damaged as a result of improper storage or handling must be discarded.

The perioperative nurse assigned to orthopedic patients should have a working knowledge of the general types and sizes of implants that might be selected. Templates of radiographs are often made preoperatively, providing a general idea of the size of the implants needed.

The U.S. Food and Drug Administration (FDA) requires strict guidelines in properly documenting and tracking implant devices. Documentation should include, but not be limited to, the patient's permanent record, the operative record, and an implant registry maintained by the OR. Many manufacturers now include mailers to return information to the company for data collection. Information to be recorded includes the lot and serial numbers and the manufacturer, size, type, and anatomic position of the implants used.

Orthopedic Instrumentation. Orthopedic instrumentation varies from very small to large instruments. Some procedures require multiple instrument containers (sets). Organization of instrument sets for multiple uses prevents the need for duplication and requires thoughtful consideration of anatomic and physiologic needs. When preparing for a procedure, the perioperative nurse should open the minimum number of instruments yet be prepared for unexpected or untoward events. Careful planning and preparation of instrumentation ensure efficient use of time and equipment.

Instruments that do not function properly (as a result of dullness, poor adjustment, lack of lubrication, damage, improper fit, or incomplete cleaning) are primary sources of complaints and problems in the OR. Instrument maintenance is vital to ensure availability for the procedure and ease in completion of the procedure. Instruments should be used for the intended purpose during the procedure. Movable parts should be lubricated after each cleaning and checked for cracks or damage after each use. The perioperative nurse is responsible for instrument maintenance and familiarity with sterilization and packaging procedures.

The following basic bone instrument sets should be available in the orthopedic OR. Soft tissue instrument sets appropriate for the size of the anatomic site are used for procedures not requiring bone instruments or in addition to the sets. Additional instruments and special equipment are mentioned with the discussion of various surgical interventions.

- *Hip set:* Total hip arthroplasty or fractures of the neck and proximal femur
- *Total knee set:* Total knee arthroplasty or supracondylar and distal femoral fractures
- *Shoulder set:* Shoulder arthroplasty and other shoulder procedures
- *Large bone set:* Bone work on the large bones, including hip, knee, upper arm, and elbow
- *Extremity or small bone set:* Bone work on the hand or foot
- *Fusion or bone graft instruments:* Additional instruments necessary for an autograft

Powered Surgical Instruments. Powered surgical instruments used in the OR have eliminated the need for many hand-operated tools, thereby reducing operative time and improving technical results. They are available as air-driven, battery-driven, or electrically driven equipment. Fingertip control provides the surgeon speed and power. Variable-speed saws, drills, and reamers offer wide flexibility. Power equipment has a safety control that prevents inadvertent activation; this should be engaged when passing the instrument to the surgeon or assistant. The perioperative nurse and scrub person should monitor the sterile field to make certain that powered instruments are not rested on the patient when they are not in use.

It is important to follow the manufacturer's recommended cleaning, sterilizing, and lubricating instructions. With proper care, powered surgical instruments have a long life span and many uses.

Suture Material. Suture material requires increased tensile strength and minimal degradability for the select type of tissue. Tendons and ligaments are fibrous, avascular tissues, resulting in a slower healing process than that occurring in tissues rich in blood supply. Absorbable suture may be used for sewing tendon or ligaments to bone. Nonabsorbable sutures, including polyester and surgical steel, are also used. For various ligament replacement grafts, a harvested tendon may be customized with multiple strands of suture material, increasing tensile strength and length of time until fibrous union occurs.

Polymethylmethacrylate. PMMA (bone cement) is an acrylic, cement-like substance composed of a liquid methyl methacrylate monomer and a powder methyl methacrylate-styrene copolymer. The powder component is 10% barium sulfate, U.S. Pharmacopoeia (USP), which provides radiopacity to the finished product. The liquid monomer is highly flammable, and the OR should be properly ventilated. Caution should be exercised during mixing of the two components to prevent excessive exposure of OR personnel to the vapors of the monomer. This exposure can cause irritation of the respiratory tract and eyes. Personnel in a room where methyl methacrylate is being mixed should not wear soft contact lenses. Many special hoods and mixing devices are available to minimize staff exposure to the fumes. Additionally, the use of antibiotic-impregnated PMMA bone cement has been shown to decrease the infection rates in total joint arthroplasty (Srivastav et al, 2009).

Adverse patient reactions with PMMA include transitory hypotension, cardiac arrest, cerebrovascular accident, pulmonary and fat embolus, thrombophlebitis, and hypersensitivity reaction. Cardiac arrest and death, although uncommon, have resulted after insertion of bone cement. Adverse reactions have been attributed to a combination of factors, including a rise in intramedullary canal pressure causing embolic phenomena, a possible chemical and blood reaction causing sudden hypotension, and certain preexisting patient conditions. More research is needed to discover the exact cause of adverse reactions. Patient care should include collaborating with the anesthesia provider before insertion of PMMA and then monitoring for side effects after insertion.

Medications. Antibiotics, hemostatics, and antibacterial agents are used commonly. Antibiotics are delivered both intravenously and locally in irrigation solutions. Common antibiotics used in irrigation include polymyxin and bacitracin. Irrigation may also be delivered using pulsatile lavage, with antibiotics added to the solution. Hemostatic agents may include bone wax, gelatin foam, thrombin, microfibrillar collagen, and parecoxib sodium (Surgical Pharmacology). Parecoxib sodium is a liquid, sprayable hemostatic agent consisting of collagen, thrombin, the patient's own platelets, and fibrinogen. Antibacterial ointments are preimpregnated in gauze dressings from the manufacturer or are applied before the application of the dressing. Other medications used during orthopedic procedures include steroids, local anesthetics, antifibrinolytics, and normal saline. Local anesthetics are often injected near the end of the surgical procedure to minimize postoperative pain.

Protective Measures. Orthopedic procedures require caution as a result of the use of fluids for irrigation or bloody procedures. Personnel protective measures include handling items (blades, sharp instruments, bone) cautiously to prevent inadvertent punctures or cuts and wearing protective masks, eyewear, or a face shield as well as protective attire, including gowns and boots. Sharp bone edges are a hazard and can puncture gloves and skin. Double-gloving or protective gloves should be used to protect the patient and personnel.

Bone Banking. The American Association of Tissue Banks (AATB) accredits and periodically inspects bone-banking programs to ensure that specific standards are followed in the retrieval, processing, storage, and distribution of bone allografts (AATB, 2011). Allografts are frozen until use. Vacuum-sealed freezers are monitored with an alarm. When requested for a procedure, the bone allograft is delivered to the field, slightly thawed, cultured, and washed with an antibiotic solution. Banked bone is available in many shapes of cortical and cancellous tissue.

Records are maintained on both donors and recipients. Donor records provide the donor identification, medical history (with circumstances of death if applicable), laboratory results, and graft description. Recipient records include recipient identification, surgeon and organization implanting the graft, surgical procedure, culture results, and any adverse reactions. Like other implants, the recipient's operative record should include the name of the bone bank from which the allograft was received, type of allograft, tissue number, and expiration date if applicable.

Evaluation

Evaluation is an ongoing process throughout the procedure. The perioperative nurse evaluates the patient, considering the nursing diagnosis and achievement of identified outcomes. This part of the nursing process provides feedback regarding the effectiveness of the plan, its implementation, and alterations needed for improving patient care. Was the patient protected from peripheral neurovascular injury? Was the patient free from perioperative positioning injury? Was adequate oxygenation maintained? Does the patient have more questions pertaining to recovery and rehabilitation? The answers will dictate whether there is a need to maintain or modify

---

SURGICAL PHARMACOLOGY

Medications Commonly Used in Orthopedic Surgery

Medication/Category	Dosage/Route	Purpose/Action	Adverse Reactions	Nursing Implications
Bupivacaine hydrochloride injection 0.5%	Injection via local infiltration, peripheral nerve block, and caudal and lumbar epidural blocks; 5-mL dose of 0.25% or 0.5% (12.5 to 25 mg); maximum dose 400 mg/day	Local anesthetic for pain management during surgery	Weak or shallow breathing; fast heart rate, gasping, feeling unusually hot; slow heart rate, weak pulse; feeling restless or anxious, ringing in the ears, metallic taste, speech problems, numbness or tingling around the mouth, tremors, feeling lightheaded	Monitor vital signs. Patients should be informed in advance that they may experience temporary loss of sensation and motor activity.
Bone wax	Topical application: 2.5 g	Sterile mixture of beeswax and isopropyl palmitate, a wax-softening agent, used to help control bleeding from bone surfaces	Delayed healing, increased infection and inflammation	Look for signs and symptoms of the adverse reactions postoperatively.
Topical thrombin	5000 to 20,000 international units applied topically on the bleeding area	Used to reduce bleeding and absorb blood	Incision site complications, increased bleeding times	Must be reconstituted prior to use.

Modified from Hodgson BB, Kizior RJ: *Saunders nursing drug handbook 2013*, St Louis, 2013, Saunders; Lukens bone wax, package insert. Available at www.angioedupro.com/Sharpoint-LOOK/dfu/062608_BoneWax_901%20902%20FINAL.pdf. Accessed January 4, 2013.

the plan. The evaluation information is shared with the nurse caring for this patient postoperatively to provide continuity of care.

The following sample outcome statements apply to evaluating care of the orthopedic patient when using the nursing diagnoses identified earlier in this chapter:

- The patient verbalized fears and feelings and indicated that anxiety and apprehension were lessened.
- The patient was free from peripheral neurovascular dysfunction on discharge to the PACU as evidenced by presence of pulses, warmth of the extremity, good capillary refill, and intact movement and sensation.
- The patient was free from injury related to perioperative positioning as evidenced by maintenance of skin integrity and absence of reddened areas.
- The patient maintained adequate ventilation and perfusion as evidenced by blood gases, arterial saturation, and vital signs within normal limits.
- The patient was free from surgical site infection as evidenced by temperature within normal limits and a clean and dry incision site.

Patient and Family Education and Discharge

Discharge planning and patient education should be initiated when the healthcare provider evaluates the patient for surgery. It should continue when the patient comes into contact with the healthcare system and should involve a multidisciplinary approach. A method of planning the overall care from preadmission to discharge is to place a patient on a clinical guideline or care path based on "best practice"—a multidisciplinary case management tool. Best practices define the expected processes of care. Essentially they are strategies of care developed with the intent of encouraging physicians and other healthcare providers who care for the same surgical patient population to agree to a specific sequence of common interventions. Included with the clinical guideline on the patient's medical record is a set of orders that mirrors the guideline and allows the physician to make minor changes to the protocol. Receiving feedback from all disciplines involved in the patient's care and discharge planning is beneficial in reducing variance and improving efficiency, outcomes, and costs.

For the patient undergoing orthopedic surgery, patient and family education and discharge planning in the following areas are essential: wound care and dressing changes, pain control, wound assessment, physical and occupational therapy, personal care, housekeeping, mobility, nutrition, prescriptions other than pain medication, extended anticoagulant therapy, application and removal of orthopedic appliances, and follow-up with a physician. Information concerning these content areas should be described, discussed, and reinforced with written instructions. Perioperative nurses should ensure that the patient and family understand the instructions, have the opportunity to demonstrate a requisite skill if that is part of home care and convalescence, and have time to ask questions and address concerns (Patient-Centered Care). A sample of written educational material that might be provided to the orthopedic surgical patient with a cast is presented in the Patient and Family Education box on page 694.

Surgical Interventions

Allografts and Autografts

Bone grafting using allografts or autografts may be used: (1) to fill cavities after removal of large amounts of bone that might result in

Preoperative patient education is an important part of the perioperative experience for patients undergoing total joint surgery. Using clear and simple language and avoiding the use of medical jargon while providing patient education can foster understanding and help decrease unnecessary anxiety for patients and their families.

A nurse discussing pain management with a patient might say, "Today I will be the nurse taking care of you during your hip replacement. During the preoperative class, preventing pain following surgery was addressed. One of the ways to help with pain after the surgery is by putting a plastic tube into the hip area. Once you are awake, you will notice this tube is connected to a ball. This plastic tube puts pain medication directly and automatically into the hip joint after surgery. You do not have to do anything. Additional pain medication is ordered for you as well. The nurses will check on you to make sure you are pain free and comfortable following your surgery. It's important for you to let us know if you need additional pain medication."

As a follow-up to the information provided the nurse should ask the patient to "teach-back" the information using his or her own words to describe the protocol for postoperative pain management.

instability, (2) to fill bony defects, and (3) to promote union of fractures at the time of open reduction. The type of graft used depends on the location of the fracture or defect, the condition of the bone, and the amount of bone loss as a result of injury. Bone grafts may be used for procedures involving revision of joints if there is significant bone loss caused by resorption or mechanical destruction after removal of bone cement.

The bone graft may be the patient's own bone (autogenous in origin and referred to as *autograft*) or bone obtained from a tissue bank (homogeneous in origin and referred to as *allograft*). Autografts are often harvested from the iliac crest, where there is cortical and cancellous bone. Various harvesting techniques are used. Struts of cortical bone from the iliac crest can be fashioned to the desired shape and used in areas needing structural strength. The amount of cancellous bone is plentiful. It is used to promote bone growth in areas of defect. Local bone graft material may be taken from the site of injury. Allografts are used when bone is not available from the patient because of the lack of sufficient quantity or because a secondary procedure is undesirable for the patient.

Procedural Considerations

Cancellous grafts may be taken from the ilium, olecranon, or distal radius; cortical grafts may be taken from the tibia, fibula, iliac crest, or ribs. When the recipient site of an autogenous graft is diseased, instruments used for the recipient site must be separated from donor graft site instruments. The operating team must change their gowns and gloves to take the bone graft and again follow the procedure to prevent cross-contamination. The patient is positioned to allow exposure to the surgical site. A sandbag may be placed beneath the area for easier access.

The instrumentation for taking a bone graft includes soft tissue instruments and a bone graft set. Grafts may be harvested with hand instruments, power tools such as an oscillating saw, or high-speed tools such as the Midas Rex. Power tools may be necessary if a uniformly shaped graft is needed to fill a defect. Because hemostasis is sometimes difficult to achieve as a result of the vascular nature of bone, wound drains may be desirable.

Operative Procedure

Harvest of Bone Graft. A cancellous bone graft consists of spongy bone usually taken from the anterior or posterior crest of the ilium. A cortical bone graft, consisting of hard, dense bone, is removed from the crest of the ilium or the tibia. The location of the crest of the ilium is subcutaneous, allowing exposure without difficulty.

1. The surgeon makes an incision along the border of the iliac crest, and strips, elevates, and retracts the muscles on the outer table of the ilium.
2. Strips of the iliac crest can be removed with an osteotome or oscillating saw.
3. A cortical window may also be made in the outer table, and the surgeon may use curettes or gouges to remove cancellous bone chips.
4. A drain may be inserted. The surgeon closes the wound in layers and applies a pressure dressing.

Electrical Stimulation

The healing process in bone involves several stages (Figure 20-23). When a bone is damaged such as during a surgical procedure or fracture, bleeding occurs. The amount of extravasated blood depends on the vascularity of the fracture site. The blood exudate infiltrates the surrounding area, where a clot is formed. Fibroblasts invade the hematoma and form a fibrin meshwork.

As osteoblasts invade the fibrin meshwork, blood vessels develop to build collagen. After several days, calcium deposits may form in the granulation tissue. These deposits eventually form new bone, known as *callus*. Within the callus, cartilage cells develop a temporary semirigid tissue that helps stabilize the bone fragments. The callus is immature bone that is remodeled by new connective tissue cells (osteoblasts) of the periosteum and the inner membrane of the bone cavity. Through this process, mature bone is formed, excess callus is resorbed, and trabecular bone is placed.

After several months, depending on the age and physical condition of the individual, the bone becomes firmly united, although the ossification process is not yet completed. Complete union of the fractured bone or joint is determined by means of clinical and radiologic examination.

Healing of bone is classified by degree. *Delayed union* signifies that healing has not occurred within the average time. The average time depends on many factors, and delayed unions must not be considered nonunion until the healing process has ceased without bony union. *Malunion* signifies that the fracture has united with deformity sufficient to cause impairment of the function or a significant angulation of the extremity. *Nonunion* signifies that the process of healing has ended without producing bony union; in this case, electrical stimulation may be used.

Electrical stimulation is artificially applied electrical current that induces or influences the formation of new bone. Various types of stimulators (Figure 20-24) are available for treatment of nonunion, including invasive (implantable), semi-invasive (percutaneous), and noninvasive (capacitance coupling). The bone stimulator of choice depends on the patient, pathologic condition, and the physician's comfort with the device.

The bone-growth stimulator is used in patients with high risk of nonunion. It can be used to provide electrical stimulation for treatment of nonunion, delayed union, congenital pseudarthrosis, and bone defects. It may be used with or without internal fixation devices, external fixation devices, or bone grafting. Patients who have undergone previous surgery, who have sustained significant tissue loss, or in whom bone grafting is contraindicated are candidates. Electrical stimulation requires long periods of immobilization of the site. This prolonged immobilization may impede rehabilitation.

Procedural Considerations

Instructions for implanting and components selected vary according to the type. The position of the patient depends on the implant site.

In addition to the implant of the surgeon's choice and the implant-specific instrumentation, a soft tissue set is used. Curettes, osteotomes, or bone rasps are used for bony debridement and to scarify the donor bed. Power drills with drill bits may be necessary to create access through the bone for the electrical leads.

Operative Procedure

1. The surgeon exposes the site and debrides it as necessary.
2. A bone slot is fashioned, spanning the nonunion site.
3. The surgeon makes a second incision about 8 to 10 cm from the first one and dissects the tissue. Before the generator is implanted, hemostasis must be achieved. The use of electrosurgical equipment may interfere with function of the bone-growth stimulator.
4. Using blunt or sharp dissection, the surgeon creates a subcutaneous channel for the cathode.
5. The surgeon guides the long cathode lead through the channel.

FIGURE 20-23 Bone-healing process. **A,** Hematoma formation. **B,** Fibrin network formation. **C,** Invasion of osteoblasts. **D,** Callus formation. **E,** Remodeling.

FIGURE 20-24 Bone-growth stimulator used after procedures to induce bone formation.

6. The generator is carefully implanted near the skin surface. The generator should be inserted into soft tissue, not against bone or metal fixation devices; it should not create a bulge beneath the skin.

7. The surgeon places the electrical coils in the prepared bone slot in equal lengths above and below the fracture site.

8. Cancellous bone grafts are placed between the coils if large bony defects are being treated.

9. Routine closure of the subcutaneous and skin tissue is carried out. After union has occurred (5 to 6 months), the surgeon removes the generator, usually under local anesthesia.

Fractures and Dislocations

A fracture is a break in the continuity of a bone. The care of fractured bones or dislocation of a joint is complicated when there is trauma to the soft tissues, including muscles, nerves, ligaments, and blood vessels. Bone diseases, which can increase the risk of a fracture, can be metabolic, infectious, or degenerative. Metabolic diseases are disorders of bone remodeling. The most common are osteoporosis, osteomalacia, and Paget disease, all of which may result in bone fractures. The most common infectious process is osteomyelitis. Degenerative musculoskeletal conditions are associated with aging. Osteoarthritis is the most common degenerative change.

Osteoporosis is one of the most common and serious of bone diseases and is responsible for more than 2 million fractures a year. Osteoporosis-related fractures most commonly occur in the hip, spine, and wrist, but any bone can be affected. About one in two women and one in four men older than age 50 will break a bone due to osteoporosis (National Osteoporosis Foundation [NOF], 2013).

Osteoporosis is characterized by excessive loss of calcified matrix, bone mineral, and collagenous fibers, causing a reduction of total bone mass. Decreasing levels of estrogen and testosterone in the older adult result in reduced new bone growth and maintenance of existing bone. Inadequate intake of calcium or vitamin D; lack of weight-bearing activities, exercise, and physical activity; smoking; and caffeine intake are other contributing factors. Osteoporotic bone is porous, brittle, and fragile, fracturing easily under stress. This results in susceptibility to spontaneous fractures and pathologic curvature of the spine.

Osteomalacia is a metabolic bone disease characterized by inadequate mineralization of bone as a result of vitamin D deficiency, which leads to a reduced absorption of calcium and phosphorus. Risk factors for development of osteomalacia include malabsorption problems, vitamin D and calcium deficiencies, chronic renal failure, and inadequate exposure to sunlight. Medical treatment includes dietary supplements and exposure to sunlight.

Paget disease is a disorder affecting older adults. It is characterized by proliferation of osteoclasts and compensatory increased osteoblastic activity, resulting in rapid, disorganized bone remodeling. The bones are weak and poorly constructed.

Types of Fractures

Fractures are classified into two main groups: closed fractures and open or compound fractures. *Closed fractures* are those in which there is no communication between the bone fragments and the skin surface. *Incomplete closed fractures* are those in which the whole thickness of the bone is not broken but is bent or buckled, such as in greenstick fractures, which commonly occur in prepubertal children. *Open fractures* exist when the break in the bone communicates with a wound in the skin. These fractures are usually considered contaminated, requiring measures to control potential infection.

The many varieties of fracture architecture (Figure 20-25) include: (1) transverse fracture, in which the fracture line runs at a right angle to the longitudinal axis of the bone; (2) longitudinal and spiral fractures, which runs along the length of the bone; (3) oblique fracture in which bone is twisted apart (similar except that oblique is shorter than spiral); (4) comminuted fracture, in which the bone fragments splinter into more than two pieces; (5) compression fracture, in which one fragment is driven into the other end and is relatively fixed in that position; and (6) pathologic fracture, in which a bone fractures easily because it is weakened by disease. A fracture in the shaft of a long bone is described as being in the proximal, middle, or distal third or at the junction of one of these two divisions. A fracture of one of the bony prominences of the end of a long bone is described as a fracture of that prominence by name. Examples include a fracture of the olecranon, medial malleolus, or lateral condyle of the femur.

An epiphyseal separation occurs when a fracture passes through or lies within the growth plate of a bone. When this occurs in a child with immature bone, impediment to limb length and growth may occur. These injuries require immediate and expert treatment.

An avulsion fracture results in a ligamentous attachment remaining intact on a separated bone fragment. This may occur after joint dislocation or rotational injury, such as the femoral condyle separating from the tibial plateau. A dislocation (luxation) is a complete displacement of one articular surface from another. This injury can disrupt neurovascular structures, requiring immediate attention. A subluxation is a partial dislocation, often indicated by ligamentous instability.

Principles of Fracture Treatment

The purpose of fracture treatment is to reestablish the length, shape, and alignment of the fractured bones or joints and restore anatomic function. Acute fracture treatment is necessary to alleviate neurovascular compromise. The surgical team should consider the following principles when providing care for the patient: (1) the patient's extremity or fracture site must be handled gently; (2) initial general medical treatment must be provided; (3) equipment and personnel must be readily available to treat impending or existing shock and to control hemorrhage; (4) aseptic technique must be maintained; (5) positioning must allow adequate circulatory and respiratory function with adequate exposure; and (6) patient comfort must be considered.

The primary goal in treatment of an upper extremity fracture is to preserve mobility and restore range of motion, enabling the individual to perform skilled and delicate work. In fractures of a lower extremity, the objectives of surgery are to restore alignment and length and provide stability of the extremity for weight bearing.

In the presence of open fractures involving soft tissues, several associated conditions may arise, including: (1) secondary hemorrhage, (2) infection, (3) severe damage to soft tissues, (4) damage to blood vessels and nerves, and (5) Volkmann contracture (ischemic paralysis).

Basic Treatment Techniques

Closed Reduction. The surgeon may treat fractures with closed reduction—manipulating the fragments into position without incising the skin. When possible this is the treatment of choice because it decreases the opportunity for infection, improves results (including bone union of the fracture), and minimizes the recovery period. Significant bone comminution, periosteal damage, or soft tissue entrapped within the fracture site may result in complications.

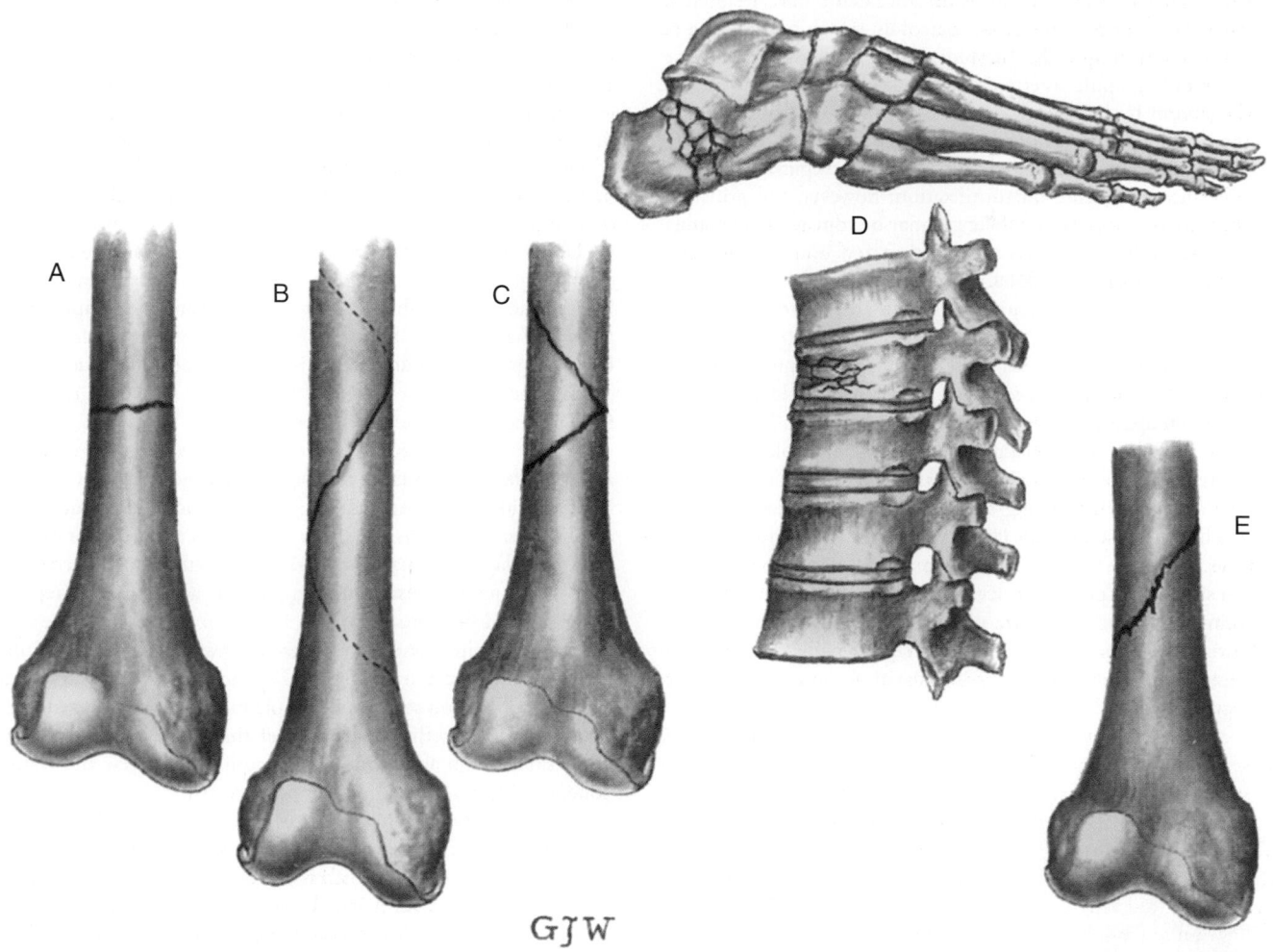

GJW

FIGURE 20-25 Fracture types, which may be open or closed. **A,** Transverse. **B,** Longitudinal or spiral. **C,** Comminuted. **D,** Compression. **E,** Oblique.

Procedural Considerations. The choice of anesthesia depends on the site of fracture and the patient's condition. A closed reduction can be performed with: (1) infiltration of local anesthetic agent into the fracture site (hematoma block), (2) IV regional anesthesia (Bier block), (3) regional or spinal nerve block, or (4) general anesthesia. Closed reduction may take place before an open procedure to reduce the fracture site. Skeletal traction may also be applied to the fracture site, requiring a surgical skin prep and application of drapes. The perioperative nurse consults with the surgeon to determine the appropriate casting or brace materials and makes certain they are readily available to prevent loss of fracture reduction. Instrumentation and supplies should be available in the event it is necessary to open the fracture site and apply fixation.

Operative Procedure

1. The surgeon uses manual traction to manipulate the fragments into alignment.
2. Reduction is confirmed using radiography (x-ray or fluoroscopy).
3. After reducing the fracture the surgeon immobilizes it with casting material or bracing techniques.

External Fixation. External fixation of fractures provides rigid fixation and reduction with the ability to manage severe soft tissue wounds. Because of the increased chance of infection in patients with an open fracture, external fixation is often the preferred treatment. Advantages of external fixation include the absence of casting material, fracture stabilization at a distance from the injury site, ability to perform subsequent procedures such as skin grafts or vascularized grafts, minimal joint interference, early mobilization, and the ability to use internal fixation or other skeleton-fixation devices at the same time or sequentially.

Indications for external fixation include: (1) severe open fractures, (2) highly comminuted closed fractures, (3) arthrodesis, (4) infected joints, (5) infected nonunion, (6) fracture stabilization to protect arterial or nerve anastomoses, (7) major alignment and length deficits, (8) congenital deformities, and (9) static contractures. External fixation provides a bridge between fracture reduction and insertion of an internal fixator such as an intramedullary nail, allowing time for vascular recovery. Internal fixation can take place at a later date.

Many improvements have been made in the design and articulations of external fixation devices. The fixators can be applied to most anatomic sites. The available external fixators vary greatly in design; however, all contain three main components: (1) bone-anchoring devices (threaded pins, Kirschner wires), (2) longitudinal supporting devices (threaded or smooth rods), and (3) connecting elements (clamps and partial or full rings). Improvements have resulted in the use of lightweight and stronger materials, which are radiopaque, for use as connecting rods. The radiopaque feature prevents postoperative radiographic interference when viewing the fracture site for progress in healing.

The Ilizarov device uses principles of tension-stress and distraction to correct bone defects and limb-length discrepancies. It is not routinely used for acute fracture fixation; however, the principles and technique are similar. Limb length may be adjusted with gradual bone distraction of bone ends, stimulating new bone formation.

Procedural Considerations. External fixators are applied using sterile technique after the patient has been administered a general or regional anesthetic. Radiographic imaging ensures fracture reduction after closed manipulation; it also ensures proper pin placement. Because the incision site is small to allow introduction of pins, a soft tissue set appropriate to the site will be necessary. Many different external fixators are available for use. Some examples are shown in Figures 20-26 and 20-27. Irrigation and debridement at the fracture site and surrounding soft tissue may be necessary if soft tissue is damaged, so pulsatile lavage with 3000 mL of normal saline solution should be available. The surgeon will use a power drill at the pin sites, and a periosteal elevator if necessary for blunt or sharp dissection. An appropriate-size pin cutter should also be available to shorten the pins if the need arises. The dressing consists of an antibacterial ointment, antibiotic-impregnated gauze, or nonadherent gauze with gauze overwrap.

Operative Procedure
1. The fracture is reduced manually.
2. The surgeon incises the skin.
3. Using a periosteal elevator, the surgeon dissects the periosteum from the bone if necessary.
4. The surgeon predrills the cortex, using a drill sheath to protect surrounding soft tissue.
5. Hand drilling or low-speed power drilling is used to insert the half pins above and below the fracture.
6. Universal joints are slipped over the pins and joined with a connecting rod.
7. The surgeon tightens the frame using the appropriate wrenches.
8. Radiography or fluoroscopy is used to confirm reduction and alignment.
9. Dressings are applied to the pin sites.

Internal Fixation. Internal fixation is often the treatment of choice for correction of fractures of long bones or those in the hip region. Application of compression plates and screws and insertion of pins, intramedullary rods, nails, or wiring are methods of internal fixation. Fractures of most anatomic parts in adults can be repaired using internal fixation.

Many principles and techniques apply when using internal fixation. Types of screws (Figure 20-28) include cortical, cancellous, lag, pre-tapped, and self-tapping. Cortical bone screws have threads that are closer together and narrower than other types of threads. These threads run along the entire length of the screw and transfix bone, gaining purchase (grab) of bone cortex.

Cancellous bone screws feature threads that are broader and farther apart than those of cortical screws. Cancellous screws are used in cancellous bone, which is less dense than cortical bone; the bone accumulates within the threads to provide the purchase for fixation. Like cortical screws, cancellous screws can traverse fracture sites and hold plates onto bone. The screw threads do not completely traverse the bone through the opposite cortex. Cancellous screws are commonly used when fractures occur at the condylar ends of the shaft.

Plating of a fracture may occur with or without dynamic compression (Figure 20-29). Dynamic compression uses screw and plate configurations to apply forces through the fracture site. Semitubular plates are less rigid and do not have the ability to produce dynamic compression. This type of plate is used in the forearm and fibula, where weight bearing, which could break the plate, is not a factor.

FIGURE 20-26 AO/ASIF pelvic external fixator, double frame using tube-to-tube clamps.

FIGURE 20-27 Dynawrist dynamic wrist external fixator.

FIGURE 20-28 Types of screws used for fixation with or without plating systems.

Closed Reduction with Percutaneous Pinning. The surgeon may reduce fractures using closed reduction methods of manipulation and traction combined with percutaneous insertion of pins, intramedullary nails, or rods. Pins can be placed percutaneously (Figure 20-30) to fix fractures involving the digits, wrist, elbow, and foot. A rod or nail is placed percutaneously (Figure 20-31) in a large bone such as the humerus or femur. Closed reduction is, however, a misnomer because small openings in the soft tissue and bone are made to facilitate introduction of the devices. These incisions are considerably smaller than those created when repairing the fracture using open reduction. The advantages of closed reduction over open reduction and internal fixation are: (1) a lower incidence of infection and (2) absence of additional soft tissue or vascular damage.

Open Reduction and Internal Fixation (ORIF). Open reduction and internal fixation provides exposure of the fracture site and uses pins, wire, screws, a plate and screw combination, rods, or nails to correct the fracture (Figure 20-32). Surgeons use ORIF when they are unable to reduce a fracture by closed methods and skeletal traction is not indicated. The advantage is that anatomic alignment of the fracture can usually be obtained and verified through direct observation. Fractures that are comminuted or difficult to reduce

can be more effectively treated using this technique. The incidence of infection and nonunion, however, is increased when the wound is opened.

The procedure varies for each anatomic site, using the principles for specific fixation devices. Several procedures described in the text identify steps for completion of open reduction and internal fixation. Reference examples include the following:

- *Pin fixation:* Application of a unilateral frame
- *Wire fixation:* Reduction of patellar fracture, tension banding of the olecranon
- *Screw fixation:* Correction of scaphoid fractures
- *Plate and screw fixation:* Repair of a comminuted distal humeral fracture
- *Rod or nail fixation:* Correction of fractures of the shaft of the humerus, femoral shaft, or tibial shaft

Surgery of the Shoulder

Correction of Acromioclavicular Joint Separation

Acromioclavicular joint separation (Figure 20-33), a common occupational and athletic injury, results from a force applied downward, most commonly from a fall, directly to the top of the shoulder. The ligamentous support of the distal clavicle in the form of the coracoclavicular, coracoacromial, and acromioclavicular ligaments is disrupted. The result is either a posterior or a superior displacement of the lateral end of the clavicle.

The purpose of surgery in an acutely injured patient is to reestablish the proper relationship between the clavicle and the acromion, thereby reducing long-term shoulder pain and increasing function. This is accomplished by replacing the coracoclavicular ligaments with heavy suture or Mersilene tape or by inserting a screw through the clavicle and into the coracoid process. It may also be necessary to stabilize the acromioclavicular joint by placing a smooth Steinmann pin across the acromion and into the clavicle. Sometimes the distal end of the clavicle is also resected. If resection of the clavicle is the only treatment required, this may be completed

FIGURE 20-29 Plating a closed forearm fracture using dynamic compression showing final position of the screw insertion.

FIGURE 20-30 Percutaneous pinning of a supracondylar fracture. **A,** Severely displaced supracondylar fracture. **B** and **C,** Treated by closed reduction and percutaneous pinning.

arthroscopically. Shoulder arthroscopy is detailed in the Arthroscopy of the Shoulder section of Arthroscopy, p. 758.

Procedural Considerations. The perioperative nurse assists in placing the patient in the supine or semi-sitting position with a sandbag or folded sheet under the affected shoulder. The patient's shoulder is positioned slightly off the OR bed (Figure 20-34) to allow full range of motion, or if mobility of the arm is unnecessary, a shoulder positioner is used. The head is turned to the opposite side, taking care not to overstretch the nerves of the brachial plexus. The scrub person assists with draping the patient's arm with a stockinette to the midhumeral level.

A soft tissue set and bone instrumentation specific for the shoulder are required. Depending on the technique used, bone screws

FIGURE 20-31 Rod placement for femoral fracture.

and their instrumentation, freecutting needles, bone-anchoring devices, and power instruments may be necessary.

Operative Procedure
Coracoclavicular Suture Fixation
1. A curved incision is made to expose the acromioclavicular joint, the distal end of the clavicle, and the coracoid process.
2. The surgeon exposes the acromioclavicular joint and removes any loose fragments or debris.
3. Mattress sutures are placed in the ruptured coracoclavicular ligaments but not tied.
4. The surgeon places drill holes in the clavicle above the coracoid in the anteroposterior (AP) plane.
5. A #5 nonabsorbable suture is placed beneath the base of the coracoid and superiorly through the two holes in the clavicle. With the joint reduced, the sutures are tied.
6. If instability is still a concern, the surgeon places small Kirschner wires across the acromioclavicular joint, through the lateral border of the acromion. The ends of the wires are bent 90 degrees at the lateral border to prevent proximal migration.
7. The surgeon ties the sutures previously placed in the coracoclavicular ligaments.
8. The acromioclavicular joint capsule and the origins of the deltoid and trapezius muscles are repaired.
9. A sling-and-swathe bandage is then applied to the extremity.

Correction of Sternoclavicular Dislocation

Traumatic dislocation of the sternoclavicular joint usually occurs from an indirect blow on the anterior shoulder while the arm is abducted. The clavicle most frequently is displaced anteriorly, but posterior or retrosternal dislocations can occur. Posterior dislocation can be more severe because injury to the trachea, esophagus, thoracic duct, and large vessels of the mediastinum is possible. Except in severe cases, dislocation of the sternoclavicular joint is treated nonoperatively with manual traction and immobilization bandages.

Clavicular Fracture

Fractures of the clavicle are some of the most common bony injuries. These injuries rarely require surgical intervention. The majority of clavicular fractures are the result of an indirect or direct blow on the clavicle or shoulder. The most common site of clavicular

FIGURE 20-32 Types of internal fixation for fracture repair. **A,** Plate and screws for transverse or short oblique fracture. **B,** Transfixion screws for long oblique or spiral fractures. **C,** Transfixion screws for long butterfly fragment. **D,** Fixation for short butterfly fragment. **E,** Medullary fixation.

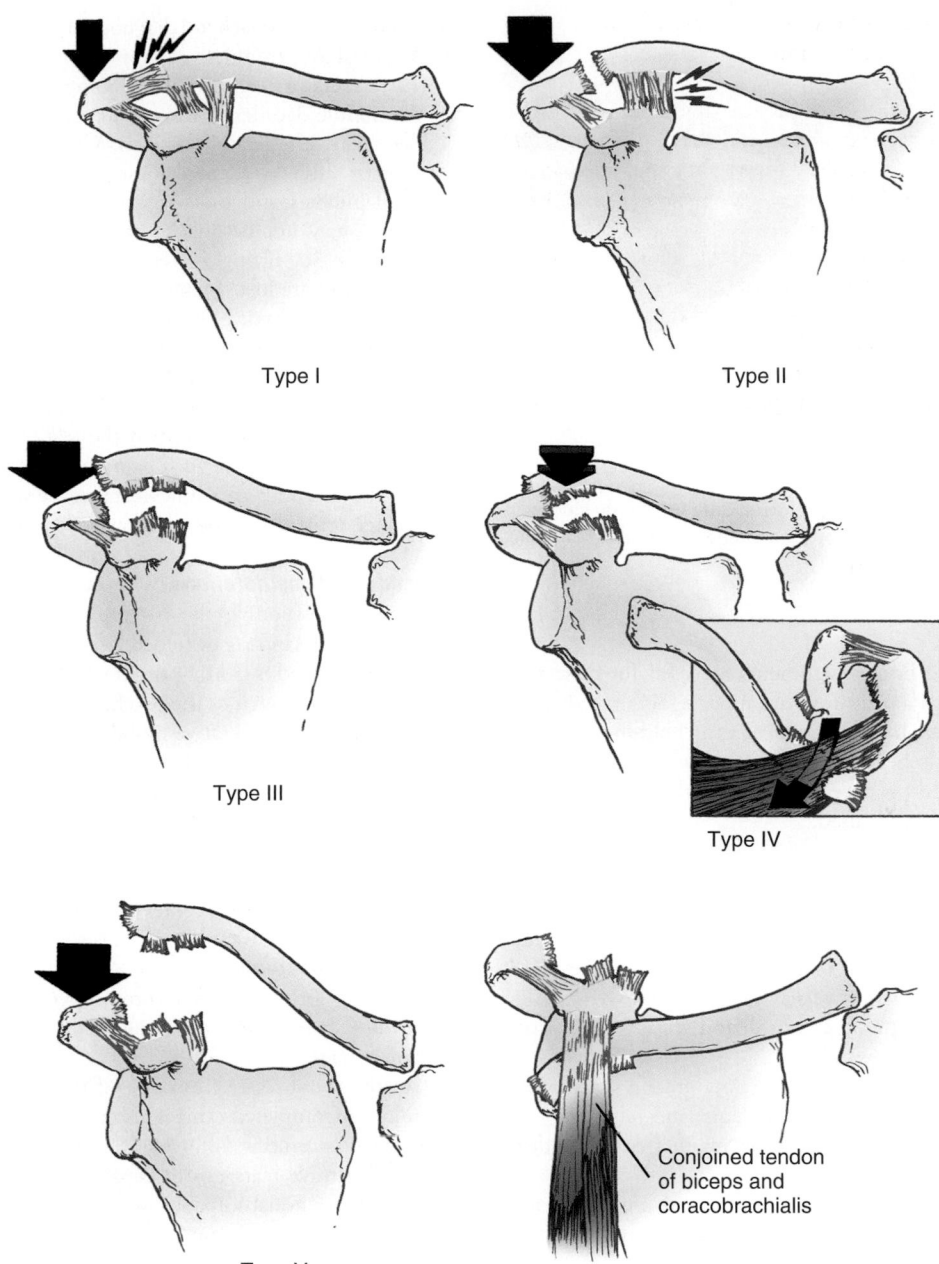

Type I

Type II

Type III

Type IV

Type V

Type VI

Conjoined tendon
of biceps and
coracobrachialis

FIGURE 20-33 Classification of acromioclavicular injuries. *Type I,* Neither acromioclavicular nor coracoclavicular ligaments are disrupted. *Type II,* Acromioclavicular ligament is disrupted, and coracoclavicular ligament is intact. *Type III,* Both ligaments are disrupted. *Type IV,* Ligaments are disrupted, and distal end of clavicle is displaced posteriorly into or through trapezius muscle. *Type V,* Ligaments and muscle attachments are disrupted, and clavicle and acromion are widely separated. *Type VI,* Ligaments are disrupted, and distal clavicle is dislocated inferior to coracoid process and posterior to biceps and coracobrachialis tendons.

fractures is the middle-third portion of the bone, mainly at the middle- and outer-third junction.

Clavicular fractures are usually treated by immobilization in a figure-of-eight splint. The chances of nonunion are greatly increased when open reduction is used for a clavicular fracture. The outcome may result in a bony prominence, which may be disturbing to the patient; the overriding fragments are resorbed with time.

Clavicular fractures may require open reduction and internal fixation after nonunion, neurovascular compromise that cannot be resolved with reduction, distal clavicular fracture with torn coracoclavicular ligaments in the adult, or persistent wide separation of the fragments with soft tissue entrapment. Surgery is necessary when the fracture is displaced enough to cause underlying damage to the vessels and brachial plexus. Open reduction is accomplished with a tubular plate and screws or intramedullary pin fixation.

Procedural Considerations. The perioperative nurse assists with positioning the patient in the supine or semi-sitting position with a sandbag or folded sheet under the affected shoulder. The patient's head is turned to the opposite side, and care is taken to not stretch the nerves of the brachial plexus. The scrub person assists the surgeon with draping the entire extremity after it is prepped. Soft

FIGURE 20-34 Positioning for a surgical procedure on the shoulder with the patient in a semi-sitting position and support beneath the affected shoulder.

tissue instruments and bone instruments are used for dissection. Bone-reduction forceps and clamps are used to obtain reduction, and Kirschner wires may be used to temporarily hold the reduction. Permanent reduction is held with either Steinmann pins or plate and screws. A power drill is necessary to apply these. In the case of a nonunion, bone grafting is used.

Operative Procedure

1. The surgeon makes a 2.5-cm incision over the fracture site. The incision may need to be extended for comminuted fractures.
2. Dissection is carried down to the clavicle, taking care not to strip periosteum or disrupt vessels or nerves.
3. The surgeon exposes the fracture site and reduces the fracture with bone-holding forceps.
4. If pinning the clavicle is to be done, a Steinmann pin is passed into the medial fragment medullary canal and removed.
5. The pin is then passed in the same manner into the distal fragment.
6. The surgeon reduces the fracture again, and uses a threaded Steinmann pin across the fracture site through both fragments to transfix it.
7. If plating the clavicle is to be done, a small semitubular plate is used with at least two screw holes on each side of the fracture site.
8. The surgeon strips a small portion of the periosteum from the clavicle so that a plate can be applied to the anterior surface.
9. Extreme care must be taken when drilling screw holes to avoid damage to the subclavian vein and thoracic contents.
10. After closure, an immobilization sling is applied.

Correction of Rotator Cuff Tear

Most rotator cuff tears occur through the insertion of the tendinous fibers of the supraspinatus muscle that attaches onto the greater tuberosity of the proximal humerus. In severe tears the remaining tendons of the cuff, the subscapularis, infraspinatus, and teres minor, may also be involved. Supraspinatus syndrome, also known as *impingement syndrome,* can involve multiple pathologic conditions, such as calcium deposits, bicipital tendinitis, subacromial bursitis, tenosynovitis, and other nonarticular lesions along with a

cuff tear. The approach to diagnosis and treatment is similar for both partial and complete rotator cuff tears.

Partial rotator cuff tears and impingement usually affect people in the middle decades of life or later and are often attributable to a long-term degenerative process. Complete tears of the rotator cuff occur after accidental injury of younger patients, such as baseball pitchers and football quarterbacks. Patients with rotator cuff tears may not be able to initiate abduction of the shoulder because the stabilizing forces of the ruptured tendons on the humeral head are lost. Many rotator cuff tears can be treated conservatively with physical therapy and nonsteroidal antiinflammatory drugs (NSAIDs).

A variety of procedures may be performed for these conditions when conservative treatment is unsuccessful. Methods of repair depend on the size and shape of the tear. The common goal is to restore joint stability, alleviate pain, and allow the patient to return to normal activities. In some instances a significant reduction in pre-injury activity may be permanent.

Procedural Considerations. The perioperative nurse assists the surgeon in positioning the patient in the supine or semi-sitting position with a sandbag or folded towel under the affected shoulder. The patient's head is gently turned to the opposite side, taking care to avoid undue stretch to the brachial plexus. A shoulder positioner can be used if intraoperative mobility of the arm is not a factor. In addition to a bone set and a soft tissue set, shoulder instruments are required. The remaining equipment needs depend on the severity of the tear. Minor tears may require no more than heavy nonabsorbable suture. Major tears require a power drill and burr and possibly a microsagittal saw. Fixation may be gained with bone-anchoring devices. Free needles will be necessary if these are used.

Operative Procedure

1. The surgeon makes an anterosuperior deltoid incision and divides the coracoacromial ligament at the acromial attachment.
2. A subacromioplasty (resection of the undersurface of the acromion) is completed. This is also primary treatment for impingement syndrome.
3. Small, simple tears can be repaired by suturing the torn edges with heavy nonabsorbable sutures.
4. Massive tears may require attaching the torn edges to the greater tuberosity using bone-anchoring devices.
5. If the defect cannot be bridged, the surgeon may transpose a flap from the subscapularis tendon and suture it to the supraspinatus and infraspinatus muscles.
6. If impingement is involved or solely the cause of a rotator pathologic condition, other measures involving the same approach are taken.
7. The surgeon excises any calcium deposits encased in the tendon to alleviate mechanical obstruction or performs an acromioplasty.
8. After closure, a sling is applied.

Patients with small tears may begin motion on the third to fourth postoperative day. Larger tears may require immobilization for 2 to 8 weeks.

Correction of Recurrent Anterior Dislocation of the Shoulder

The anterior fibers of the shoulder capsule become stretched and weakened as a result of frequent dislocations of the shoulder joint.

More than 150 operations or modifications have been devised to treat recurrent anterior dislocation. The goals are to: (1) prevent recurrence, (2) prevent surgical complications, (3) prevent creation of arthritic changes, (4) maintain joint motion, and (5) correct the problem. The surgeon selects the procedure appropriate for the patient's condition that will satisfy the conditions necessary to correct the problem. A stapling procedure was once common treatment of recurrent dislocation, but it has been replaced by other accepted procedures.

Procedural Considerations. The surgeon and perioperative nurse place the patient in the supine or semi-sitting position with a sandbag or folded sheet under the shoulder. The patient's arm is draped free so that the extremity can be manipulated. The surgeon makes an anterior curved incision or a longitudinal incision in the anterior axillary fold over the shoulder joint, depending on the location of the tear and procedure planned. A soft tissue set and a bone set are required, as well as a set of instruments specific to shoulder surgery, power drill and burr, bone-anchoring devices, and free needles.

Operative Procedure

Bankart Procedure. For the Bankart procedure (Figure 20-35), the scapula is not elevated with a sandbag or folded sheet. The surgeon reattaches the attenuated anterior capsule to the rim of the glenoid fossa with heavy sutures. The glenoid fossa rim is decorticated with a curette to provide a raw surface to which the capsule is attached. Special instruments designed for the Bankart procedure, such as the curved awl and humeral head retractor, facilitate the surgery, although the capsule may be attached with bone anchors, obviating the use of the awl. If the coracoid process is to be removed to obtain better operative exposure, a drill, bone screws, and washer should be available for reattachment. Postoperatively the extremity is immobilized in a sling or shoulder immobilizer. Shoulder motion is begun 3 days postoperatively, and the patient may return to contact sports or heavy labor after approximately 6 months.

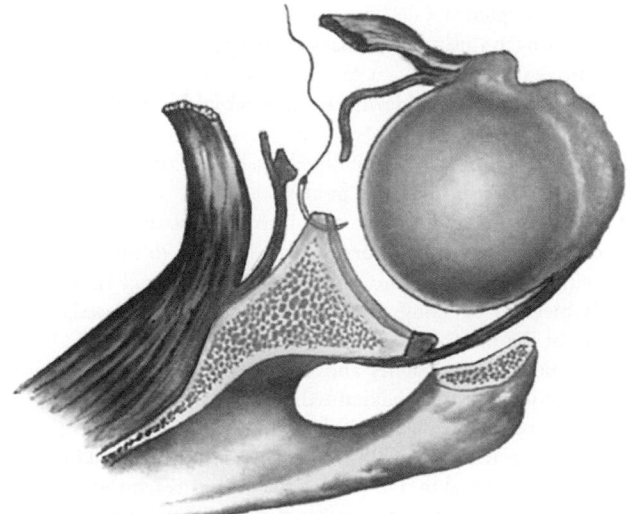

FIGURE 20-35 Bankart procedure for restoration of shoulder stability. Holes are made in the rim of the glenoid, and the free lateral margin of the capsule is sutured to the rim of the glenoid. The medial margin of the capsule is sutured to the lateral surface.

Putti-Platt Procedure. The steps of the Putti-Platt procedure are similar to those of the Bankart procedure in that the joint capsule is sutured to the glenoid rim. In addition, the Putti-Platt procedure requires the lateral advancement of the subscapularis. This produces a barrier against dislocation of the shoulder. This procedure is rarely useful when the anterior capsular mechanism is of poor quality.

The surgeon divides the subscapularis tendon 2.5 cm medially to its insertion. The glenoid and humeral head are inspected using palpation to assess osteochondral changes. The lateral portion of the subscapularis is sutured to the anterior glenoid rim. The medial portion of the subscapularis is sutured to the rotator cuff at the greater tuberosity. The layers of the shoulder joint are imbricated (overlapped), a technique used often in soft tissue reconstruction. The incision is closed, and a shoulder immobilizer is applied. The immobilizer is worn for approximately 3 weeks. External rotation of the arm should be avoided immediately after the repair.

Bristow Procedure. In the Bristow procedure the coracoid process, along with the attached muscles, is detached and inserted onto the neck of the glenoid cavity, where it is attached with a screw through the subscapularis muscle. This stabilizes the anterior joint capsule and prevents recurrent dislocation. A Bristow procedure is considered an appropriate alternative when the anterior capsular mechanism is of poor quality. Disadvantages of this procedure are: (1) internal rotation contracture, (2) inattention to labrum or capsule disorders, (3) potential for injury to the musculocutaneous nerve, (4) reduction of internal rotation power by shortening of the subscapularis muscle, (5) possible limitation of external rotation, (6) possible penetration of the screw into the articular surface of the glenoid, and (7) later development of early joint disease of the shoulder.

Correction of Humeral Head Fracture

Comminuted fractures of the humeral head (Figure 20-36) with displacement may require open reduction and internal fixation with screws or pins or closed reduction with a humeral nail or rod. However, if the fracture is badly comminuted, a prosthetic replacement is indicated. Traumatic or degenerative arthritic shoulder joints may be so painful or dysfunctional that a total shoulder joint replacement is necessary.

Extensive rehabilitation for the shoulder is required. Surgery should be performed as soon as possible because delay can allow time for increasing scar formation, contracture of the muscles, and increasing osteoporosis of the bone fragments. The shoulder is the most difficult joint in the body to rehabilitate because it has: (1) the greatest range of motion, (2) a second space beneath the acromion that must be mobilized, and (3) many muscles that enter into complex movements.

Surgery of the Humerus, Radius, and Ulna

Fractures of the Humeral Shaft

Closed manipulation and immobilization usually reduce a fractured humerus as well as minimize the risk of nonunion and infection. When closed reduction is impossible or when nonunion of the fracture has occurred, surgery is indicated. The fracture is reduced and held with intramedullary fixation, a compression plate, a lag screw, or a rigid locking nail, with distal and proximal bone screws that transfix the rod within the canal. This last device can control rotation of the fracture fragments and prevent distraction at the

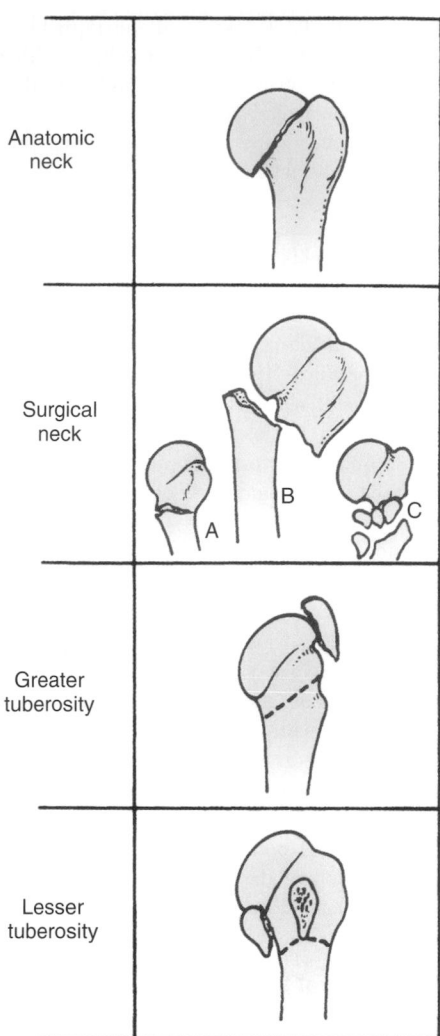

Anatomic
neck

Surgical
neck

A   B   C

Greater
tuberosity

Lesser
tuberosity

FIGURE 20-36 Fractures and fracture-dislocations relate to the pattern of displacement. Fractures can occur in two, three, or four parts.

fracture site (Figure 20-37). Multiple flexible nails may be used if more rigid nails are not available. A bone graft may be used, depending on both the extent of the fracture and the length of time since injury. Compression plating of shaft fractures is usually reserved for supracondylar involvement or when other treatment has failed.

Procedural Considerations. Fluoroscopy and permanent radiographs are required to ensure proper alignment, reduction, and placement of implants. The perioperative nurse arranges for intraoperative radiology support and a radiolucent OR bed before the patient's arrival in the OR suite. The surgeon and nurse position the patient supine with the body near the edge of the bed to facilitate moving the arm. The extremity is prepped and draped from the middle of the chest to below the elbow.

A soft tissue set and a large bone set are required. In addition, the intramedullary fixation device of choice and the required instruments for its insertion are needed. PMMA may be used in the case of pathologic fractures. Instruments that are required for harvesting bone graft might be needed as well. A traction tray may be used to gain reduction. A power drill is necessary if screws are used to lock the device. Sterile x-ray cassette covers are needed for permanent intraoperative films.

Operative Procedure
Medullary Fixation: Antegrade Technique

1. Proper length and alignment of the fracture must be attained with traction. Nail length should ensure proximal burying to avoid subacromial impingement and be 1 to 2 cm proximal to the olecranon fossa. The surgeon makes a skin incision from the lateral point of the acromion over the tip of the greater tuberosity. The fascia is incised, and the greater tuberosity is palpated.

2. Using a small awl, the surgeon enters the greater tuberosity and confirms placement with fluoroscopy in both AP and lateral views.

3. The surgeon removes the awl and inserts a ball-nosed reamer guidewire, advancing it down the medullary canal (periodically verified with fluoroscopy). Confirmation is made with each step to ensure that the wires, reamers, or implant has not fractured through the cortex along the shaft.

4. The guidewire is advanced to within 1 to 2 cm of the olecranon fossa, avoiding distraction or shortening.

5. If Enders nails are used, each one is advanced in the same fashion as the guidewire.

6. Nail length can be determined by using a second guidewire of the same length held against what remains extended from the humerus. The difference between the length protruding and the length remaining on the second rod is the approximate length requirement of the humeral nail. Another method uses a nail-length gauge that is held directly against the upper arm, viewed with fluoroscopy, and read directly on the gauge.

7. Enders nails may be held directly against the arm and viewed with fluoroscopy to determine proper length. If Enders nails are used, the surgeon drives two or three nails down the shaft, across the fracture site, and into the distal fragment. Fluoroscopy is used to confirm proper placement and reduction.

8. If intramedullary nailing is to be accomplished, the surgeon may use a cannulated reamer over the guidewire to ream the humerus. Reaming of the canal is completed in 0.5-mm increments. The humerus becomes smaller in diameter. Reaming is gentle to ensure that protrusion through the bone does not occur. The bone is reamed 0.5 to 1 mm larger than the selected nail diameter.

9. The surgeon uses a medullary exchange tube to maintain fracture reduction.

10. The ball-tipped guidewire is replaced with a non–ball-tipped guidewire.

11. The medullary nail is assembled for impaction with the appropriate outrigger and drill guides.

12. The surgeon guides the nail into the proximal end of the humerus, and uses the humeral nail driver to impact the nail within the canal. Care must be taken to avoid splitting the humerus or creating a supracondylar fracture by wedging the tip of the nail.

13. As the nail approaches and crosses the fracture site, manual reduction must be maintained.

14. The scrub person attaches the proximal drill guide to the nail impactor with the nail coupled; the surgeon makes a stab wound in the skin and pushes the nail to reach the bone.

15. An 8-mm drill sleeve is inserted through the drill guide, followed by a 2.7-mm drill guide into the first guide.

16. The surgeon scores the cortex with the 2.7-mm trocar, and transfixing of the hole is completed with a 2.7-mm drill from the lateral to distal areas of the cortex.

FIGURE 20-37 Placement of the humeral rigid locking nail with distal and proximal screws. **A,** After incision and exposure, a femoral awl is used to make an entry portal. **B,** Guidewire is advanced into the center of the epicondylar region. **C,** After reaming, the nail is advanced over the fracture site and seated. **D,** Proximal and distal locking takes place after the correct screw placement is determined.

17. The humeral screw-depth gauge is inserted and read directly to determine the appropriate screw size.
18. A 4-mm fully threaded humeral screw is inserted to the selected length. The surgeon confirms the screw position by inserting a guidewire down the end of the nail, where it is impeded by the transfixing screw.
19. Fluoroscopy is used to target the distal humeral locking screw.
20. The surgeon creates a second percutaneous access from the anterior to posterior cortex of the bone to the bone surface of the humerus.
21. With the freehand technique, the cortex of the bone is scored followed by insertion of the 8-mm handheld drill sleeve and the 2.7-mm drill bit.
22. The selected size of humeral screw is gauged and inserted. Placement is confirmed with fluoroscopy, and the impactor assembly is removed from the nail.
23. Full-view radiographs are obtained in both dimensions, and the wound is irrigated and closed.

NOTE: Many variations of approach and technique are used, depending on the complexity of the fracture and any associated injury. Often the fracture site may have to be opened if it is comminuted or will not reduce properly through closed techniques. The radial nerve or other neurovascular structures may become entrapped or traumatized, requiring exploration and repair.

Although this type of antegrade fixation, using locked rods, is preferred for this type of fracture, it is not the only method. Often a retrograde technique is used, with the patient in the prone or lateral decubitus position. The retrograde technique, used more commonly in the care of femoral shaft fractures, is described on page 720.

Distal Humeral Fractures (Supracondylar, Epicondylar, and Intercondylar)

Distal humeral fractures are classified into several types, depending on location and the presence or absence of articular involvement (Figure 20-38). Supracondylar fractures of the humerus do not involve the articular surface and can generally be treated with closed reduction and casting. Transcondylar fractures may or may not have articular involvement, and this will dictate treatment. Intercondylar fractures involve both condyles with a comminution of injury, are intra-articular, and present the greatest challenge for the surgical team. Fractures of the articular components—the capitulum and the trochlea—are usually the result of a fall on an outstretched arm. The force drives the radial head to shear off the capitulum, producing an intra-articular fragment. The lateral or medial condyles and epicondyles are also subject to fracture by various mechanisms.

Patients may present with a single isolated fracture or any combination, as previously mentioned. Neurovascular and other soft tissue trauma is considered in selecting the type of reduction and fixation. Screws, pins, a variety of different plates, and dynamic compression technique can be used for internal fixation. Certain fixation techniques of the distal portion of the humerus may require an osteotomy of the olecranon (proximal ulna) to properly align and affix hardware (Figure 20-39). The general goals of treating these injuries are to: (1) maintain neurovascular integrity, (2) restore normal joint articulation, (3) preserve motion of the joint, and (4) correct other soft tissue injuries.

Procedural Considerations. Regional anesthesia can be used for procedures on the distal end of the humerus. Bone graft harvesting may require use of general anesthesia. The patient may be prone with the elbow flexed over a small table, supine with the arm over the chest, supine with the arm on a hand table, or in the lateral position. A tourniquet is placed before the surgical prep and inflated during surgery as needed.

A soft tissue set, a large bone set, and a bone graft set are needed, in addition to a compression set, bone-holding clamps, reconstruction plates, and smooth Kirschner wires. A power drill and Kirschner wire driver are needed to apply the hardware.

Operative Procedure
ORIF Comminuted Distal Humeral Fracture (Figure 20-40)
1. The surgeon makes an incision over the distal humeral fracture site.
2. The fracture is exposed and reduced using bone-reduction clamps and temporary small, smooth Kirschner wires, driving them across the fracture site with the power drill.
3. A cancellous bone screw is placed using drill and tap to transfix from one condyle to the other. The surgeon is careful not to violate the joint surface with the threads of the screw.
4. If the reduction is maintained, the surgeon removes the Kirschner wires.
5. A one-third tubular or reconstruction plate is contoured to the shape of the distal humeral fracture and applied to bridge the fracture fragments.
6. Throughout the entire procedure, the articular surface is periodically inspected to ensure integrity. The plates are held in place by hand while the patient's elbow is moved through its range of motion. The plates should not encroach on the olecranon or coronoid fossa (distal end of the ulna) because this limits flexion and extension of the arm.
7. The bone is drilled and tapped from one cortex to the other with the appropriate drill and tap. The screw is inserted and seated

FIGURE 20-38 Classification of distal humeral fractures. **A,** Supracondylar. **B,** Transcondylar. **C,** Lateral condyle with trochlea. **D,** Medial condyle. **E,** Intercondylar with comminution.

FIGURE 20-39 Osteotomy of the olecranon with placement of a lag screw and tension band wire fixation.

FIGURE 20-40 Repair of the comminuted distal humeral fracture with 3.5-mm reconstruction plates.

FIGURE 20-41 Tension band technique used for repair of the olecranon.

to the bone surface on the plate. This is done for all subsequent screws, observing the fracture site and articular surface.

8. Interfragmentary screws may be used in addition to the cortical screws spanning the condyles. If osteotomy of the olecranon was previously done for exposure, it is reattached using the tension band technique with a cancellous bone screw and heavy-gauge (18 or 20 gauge) wire (Figure 20-41).

9. The surgeon irrigates the wound, places a drain (as needed), and closes the incision. A long arm posterior splint is applied.

Olecranon Fracture

If the olecranon fracture fragment is small, it may be excised and the triceps tendon reattached to the ulnar shaft. This does not result in loss of stability of the elbow joint. However, larger fragments must be reduced and held with internal fixation. Osteotomy of the olecranon is often done electively for surgical exposure (see previous section) and repaired in the same fashion as for a traumatic fracture.

Procedural Considerations. The patient is placed in the prone position with the arm on an armboard or hand table. A soft tissue

FIGURE 20-42 Operative procedure: tension banding with stainless steel wire passed through drill holes; figure-of-eight adds stability to the fracture.

set, a bone set, AO/ASIF instrumentation (AO/ASIF is the abbreviation for Swiss Association of Osteosynthesis/Association for the Study of Internal Fixation), heavy stainless steel wire (16 and 18 gauge in long lengths), a wire tightener, Kirschner wires, bone-reduction clamps, a power drill, and Kirschner wire driver are needed.

Operative Procedure
Tension Banding (Figure 20-42)
1. The surgeon makes an incision over the olecranon and exposes the fracture.
2. A drill hole is made in the distal fragment, traversing the bone.
3. Stainless steel wire is passed through the drilled holes, crossed over, and pulled toward the tip of the olecranon.
4. After using the drill and tap, the surgeon uses a cancellous bone screw to attach the proximal fragment to the distal, stopping short of totally seating the screw.
5. The surgeon pulls the wire and loops it around the exposed shaft of the screw while reduction is maintained manually or by using a reduction clamp. The wire can be tightened using the wire tightener. Two smooth Steinmann pins, bent over the exposed portion to hook the loop of wire, can substitute for the cancellous screws.
6. The remaining screw is threaded into the bone; the fracture site is observed for opposition.
7. The wound is irrigated and closed. Drains are generally not necessary. A long arm posterior splint is placed.
   NOTE: Using this technique requires early active motion of the arm. Compression of the fracture site is achieved by moving the elbow through its range of motion and applying force by the hardware.

Transposition of the Ulnar Nerve

Transposition of the ulnar nerve involves freeing the nerve from a groove at the back of the medial epicondyle of the humerus and bringing it to the front of the condyle. The ulnar nerve is frequently

divided or damaged after fracture or wounds to the elbow caused by trauma. Dislocation of the elbow may also cause ulnar nerve damage. Late traumatic neuritis may occur after an old injury, resulting in stretching of the ulnar nerve. The hand appears atrophied, and sensory loss is extensive. In severe cases, a claw hand deformity develops.

Procedural Considerations. The perioperative nurse assists with positioning the patient supine with the extremity slightly flexed on a hand table or over the chest. A tourniquet is applied to the upper arm, and the entire arm (fingers to tourniquet) is prepped and draped. A soft tissue set is required. Bone instruments may be required.

Operative Procedure
1. The surgeon makes an incision on the lateral aspect of the elbow near the epicondyle.
2. The fascia and the flexor carpi ulnaris muscle are divided.
3. The surgeon frees the ulnar nerve and dissects the medial intermuscular septum.
4. The nerve is then drawn anteriorly and placed deep into the brachialis flexor muscle origin.
5. The wound is irrigated and closed. A drain is not necessary. A short arm posterior splint is applied to the elbow postoperatively.

Excision of the Head of the Radius

Fractures of the radial head can be displaced or nondisplaced, segmental, or comminuted. Complications can arise when treatment is delayed, causing limitation of motion, pain, and post-traumatic arthritis. A congruous radial head is essential for proper rotation of the forearm at the elbow. Consequently, in an adult it is necessary to excise the radial head if a severely comminuted fracture with angulation interferes with rotation. The radial head should never be excised in children. The outcome for the patient undergoing radial head excision may result in some permanent loss of pronation and supination of the forearm. Noncomminuted fractures that are easily reduced can be treated using closed reduction and casting.

Procedural Considerations. The patient is supine with the arm over the chest or on a hand table. A tourniquet is applied. A soft tissue set, a small bone set, and an oscillating microsaw with blades are needed.

Operative Procedure
1. The surgeon makes an incision on the shaft of the radius from 5 cm distal to the radial head, extending proximally over the lateral humeral condyle.
2. Dissection is continued between the extensor carpi ulnaris and extensor digitorum muscles onto the joint capsule.
3. With the head and neck of the radius exposed through the joint capsule, the surgeon irrigates the joint to clear bone debris and blood clots.
4. The surgeon excises the radial head just proximal to the radial tuberosity, and removes all the periosteum to limit new bone formation. The remaining annular ligament is also excised. The fragments of the radial head should be saved and readily available so that they may be reassembled to ensure that all fragments have been retrieved.
5. The wound is closed, and a long arm posterior splint is applied with the elbow at 90 degrees.

Correction of Fractures of the Proximal Third of the Ulna with Radial Head Dislocation (Monteggia)

The Monteggia type of fracture presents with a proximal ulnar fracture and dislocation of the radial head. The fracture is rarely treated with open reduction in children. The open technique is often used to treat adults. A direct blow to the ulnar aspect or a fall while the arm is hyperextended produces this type of injury. If the open reduction approach is chosen, closed reduction of the radial dislocation is attempted and often is successful. At times the annular ligament may prevent reduction of the radial head dislocation, and open reduction becomes necessary. Deforming forces of the forearm vary, depending on the location of the fracture in relation to the insertion of muscles. These forces are often encountered when treating forearm injuries. The dynamic compression technique uses compression plates that are stockier and stronger than the semitubular plates mentioned earlier for distal humeral fractures. They are used to plate shaft fractures, where stress forces on the shaft are greater and stronger plates are required.

Procedural Considerations. The patient is placed in the supine position with or without a hand table. A tourniquet is applied and inflated as needed. A soft tissue set and a large bone set are required, as well as bone-reduction clamps and bone-grasping forceps, AO/ASIF instrumentation, plates and screws, and a power drill.

Operative Procedure

Fixation with Dynamic Compression Plate (Figure 20-43)

1. The surgeon performs a closed reduction to reduce the radial head dislocation.
2. An incision is made; the ulnar fracture site is dissected.
3. The surgeon strips the periosteum and reapproximates the fragments using bone-reduction and bone-grasping forceps.
4. The bone is assessed for placement of a small- or large-fragment dynamic compression plate (DCP), with at least three screw holes proximal and three distal to the fracture site.
5. A concentric (neutral) hole is drilled into the ulna (through one of the screw holes on the plate) to the opposite cortex.
6. After the hole is gauged, the selected size of screw is inserted, with purchase of the opposite cortex ensured. The surgeon inserts a second screw on the opposite fragment in the neutral position.
7. On either side of the fracture site, an eccentric (loading) hole is drilled in the same fashion to the opposite cortex. The hole is gauged and tapped, and the screw is inserted.
8. The selected screw is entered eccentrically into the plate. As the screw seeks the center of the screw hole while riding the bevel of the screw hole, it compresses the fracture site. The surgeon tightens this screw completely, and slightly loosens the other screws.
9. The fracture site is now visualized radiographically as the action of the screw in the plate compresses the fracture site.
10. The remaining bone screws are inserted following the same procedure.
11. The wound is irrigated and closed; a drain may or may not be inserted.
12. A long arm posterior splint is placed with the arm in 110 to 120 degrees of flexion.

Correction of Colles Fracture with External Fixation

Colles fracture is a dorsally angulated fracture of the distal end of the radius. Most of these fractures can be managed successfully with

FIGURE 20-43 Fixation with dynamic compression plate. **A,** Gliding hole with drill bit. **B,** Fracture is reduced, drill sleeve is inserted, the fracture is drawn together, a hole is drilled, and a screw is inserted in the neutral position to correct the fracture. **C** and **D,** One screw is inserted in load position (eccentric) into the other fragment; as the screw is tightened, axial compression is generated. **E,** Lag screw inserted across the fracture site. **F,** Remaining screws inserted in the neutral position.

closed reduction and immobilization, but external fixation is especially useful in the case of a comminuted intra-articular fracture. Internal fixation is indicated when the distal end of the radius is severely comminuted and displaced. In these cases, Kirschner wires are used for internal fixation.

Procedural Considerations. The patient is in the supine position with the arm extended on a hand table and may require traction by means of finger traps. A soft tissue set and a small bone set are required, along with a power drill, small elevator, and the external fixation device of choice. Fluoroscopy is necessary.

Operative Procedure

1. Small incisions are made, and the surgeon places two pins through the second metacarpal—one at the base and the other

distal-ward a distance equal to the span between the openings in the fixator.
2. Two pins are placed in the radius 8 cm from the styloid.
3. The surgeon confirms pin placement radiographically in both the AP and lateral views.
4. A frame is constructed to incorporate all four pins.
5. Reduction of the fracture is obtained, and the surgeon secures the frame.
6. Postreduction films are obtained to check alignment and pin position.

Surgery of the Hand

Hand surgery has become highly specialized. The perioperative nurse encounters numerous procedures for treating bone, soft tissue, or both. Many of the techniques and principles used to treat large bone defects are used in the treatment of hand injuries. Hand procedures range from carpal tunnel release to complex digit reimplantation.

Tourniquets and regional anesthetics are often used for hand surgery. The OR team usually sits down at a hand table but may move to areas such as the iliac crest for bone grafting. The instruments for hand surgery are common to orthopedics but on a smaller scale. Many instruments and reconstruction systems have been developed primarily for hand surgery. Air- or battery-powered drills and saws are frequently used. The surgery often requires the use of eye loupes (glasses for magnification) or a microscope.

Carpal Tunnel Release

Carpal tunnel syndrome results from entrapment of the median nerve on the volar surface of the wrist; it is caused by thickened synovium, trauma, or aberrant muscles. Carpal tunnel syndrome is frequently seen in patients with rheumatoid synovitis or malaligned Colles fracture and is associated with obesity, Raynaud disease, pregnancy, and occupational injuries. The symptoms are pain, numbness, tingling of the fingers, and weakness of the intrinsic thumb muscles. These symptoms are usually reversible after the flexor retinaculum is incised so that the compressed median nerve is relieved. Carpal tunnel release may be completed endoscopically or by open incision.

Procedural Considerations. The patient is placed in the supine position with the arm extended on a hand table. A tourniquet is applied to the forearm or upper arm. A hand set is required. The endoscopic approach requires use of specialized equipment.

Operative Procedure—Open Approach
1. The surgeon makes a curvilinear, longitudinal volar incision from the proximal side of the palm, paralleling the thenar crease and extending to the crease of the wrist across the wrist joint.
2. The deep transverse carpal ligament is divided, taking care to avoid damage to the median nerve.
3. At this point the release is completed.
4. If indicated, the surgeon performs a tenosynovectomy.
5. The wound is closed, and a compression dressing and volar splint are applied.

Excision of Ganglions

A ganglion is a cystic lesion arising from a joint capsule or tendon sheath and containing glassy, clear fluid. Ganglions are most common on the dorsum of the wrist, palm of the hand, and dorsolateral aspect of the foot. Ganglions appear as firm masses that vary in size. They may resolve spontaneously but occasionally require excision because of discomfort or for cosmetic reasons.

Procedural Considerations. The perioperative nurse assists with positioning the patient supine with the arm extended on a hand table, and applies the tourniquet as directed by the surgeon. A hand set is required.

Operative Procedure
1. The surgeon makes a transverse incision over the ganglion.
2. The ganglion is excised with a rim of normal joint capsule or tendon sheath at its base.
3. The wound is irrigated and closed, and a pressure dressing is applied. A plaster splint may also be applied to immobilize the affected joint.

Correction of Carpal Fractures

Most fractures of the carpal bones are treated by closed reduction and immobilization. However, it is occasionally necessary to operate on a fracture because of acute instability, delayed union, or nonunion. The scaphoid is the most commonly fractured carpal bone. Internal fixation is accomplished with Kirschner wires, small compression screws, or mini fragment compression plates and screws. A bone graft from the distal end of the radius or olecranon may be taken.

For displaced or unstable scaphoid fractures, the Herbert bone screw (Figure 20-44) has several advantages: (1) strong internal fixation, (2) compression at the fracture site with reversed threads at each end of the screw, and (3) reduced time required for external immobilization.

Procedural Considerations. The patient is supine with the arm extended on a hand table. A tourniquet is applied and fluoroscopy should be available. A soft tissue set and a small bone or hand set are required in addition to the Herbert screw set. If a mini fragment compression set is used, a power drill and smooth Kirschner wires will also be needed. A bone graft set should also be available.

Operative Procedure (Figure 20-45)
1. The surgeon makes a longitudinal skin incision over the palmar surface of the wrist.
2. The superficial palmar branch of the radial artery is ligated and divided.

FIGURE 20-44 Herbert bone screw placement.

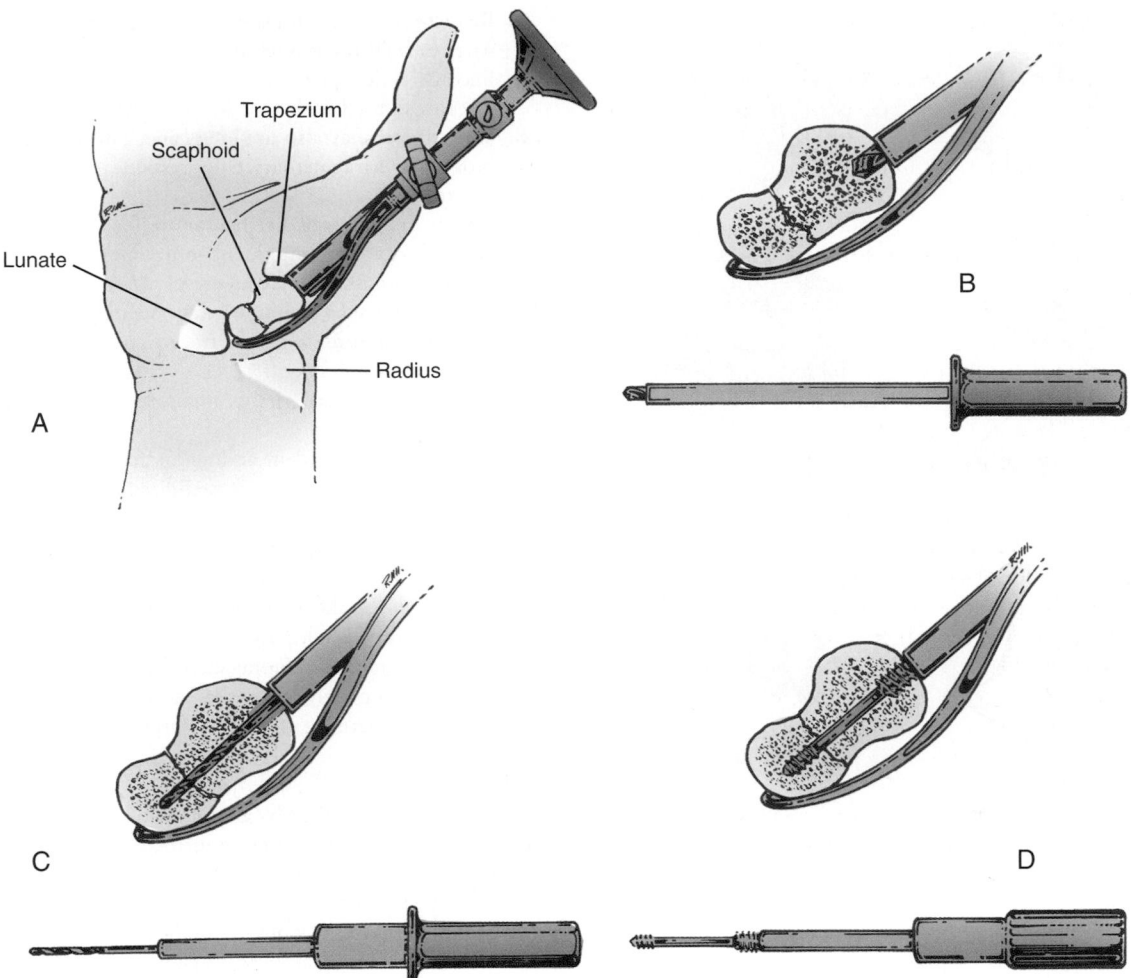

FIGURE 20-45 Repair of the scaphoid. **A,** Fracture site is exposed. **B,** Alignment guide reduces the fracture and guides all subsequent instrumentation. **C,** The screw hole is drilled by hand, and the tap is inserted. **D,** The Herbert bone screw is inserted through the drill guide.

3. The surgeon incises the flexor carpi radialis tendon sheath and retracts it to expose the capsule of the wrist.
4. The capsule is entered, and the scaphoid fracture is identified and inspected to determine the need for bone grafting.
5. The surgeon manipulates the fracture to reduce it and inserts small Kirschner wires to temporarily hold the reduction.
6. The scaphoid fracture is reduced and held with the Herbert jig.
7. A short drill bit and then a long drill bit are inserted to create a channel for the screw.
8. The surgeon inserts the Herbert screw and turns it until it is seated within the scaphoid.
9. Bone graft is placed around the fracture site if needed. (The loss of significant bone can often be corrected by fashioning a strut of bone from graft.)
10. The wound is irrigated and closed.
11. A splint is applied with a thumb spica or long arm cast incorporating the thumb.

Surgery of the Hip and Lower Extremity

Fractures of the Acetabulum

Fractures of the acetabulum usually result from high-energy injuries such as motor vehicle accidents and falls with a landing on the extended extremities. The fracture is directly related to the force transmitted to the femoral head through the greater trochanter or lower leg. Management of these fractures can often present the surgical team with a complex and challenging task. Indications for internal fixation of acetabular fractures include: (1) greater than 2 mm of displacement, (2) presence of intra-articular loose bodies, (3) inability to reduce under closed methods, (4) unstable fractures of the posterior acetabular wall, and (5) open fractures. Internal fixation is usually delayed 3 to 10 days to allow time for the patient to be evaluated and clinically stabilized. Until internal fixation is undertaken, the fracture is reduced by means of closed methods and the patient is maintained in skeletal traction. General anesthesia may be required for closed reduction and placement of skeletal traction when the acetabular fracture is severely displaced or dislocated. The fractures are divided into five basic groups: (1) fractures of the posterior wall, (2) posterior column, or (3) anterior wall; (4) anterior column; and (5) transverse fractures (Figure 20-46). Internal fixation is accomplished with reconstruction plates and screws, total hip replacement with bone grafting (see Total Hip Arthroplasty, p. 734), or fusion if the fracture cannot be reduced.

Procedural Considerations. The surgical approach depends on the type and area of the fracture and the surgeon's preference. The

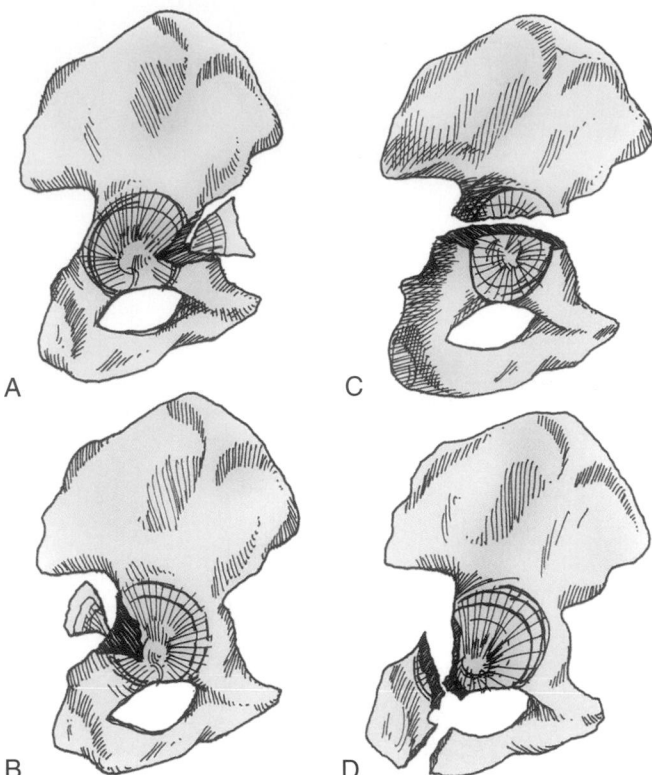

FIGURE 20-46 Acetabular fractures. **A,** Anterior wall. **B,** Posterior wall. **C,** Transverse. **D,** Posterior column.

perioperative nurse assists in placing the patient on a fracture or standard OR bed in the lateral or supine position. A general anesthetic is usually administered, but the procedure can be performed solely with a regional block or concurrent epidural infusion. Procedures of this magnitude can be lengthy and involve considerable blood loss. Appropriate measures should be taken to avoid complications from these factors. The room should remain warm, the patient protected from pressure injury, and red blood cell salvaging techniques used.

A soft tissue set, large bone and acetabular instruments, pelvic reduction clamps, reconstruction plates and screws (both 3.5 and 4.5 mm), plate-bending irons, and a femoral distractor are necessary. A total hip set should be available. Also needed are Kirschner wires and Steinmann pins, large-fragment bone screws, pulsatile lavage supplies, and power drill and reamer. Fluoroscopy may be used for this procedure.

Operative Procedure
Posterolateral Approach
1. The surgeon makes a lateral incision over the acetabular fracture site.
2. The joint is opened and the femur dislocated from the acetabulum.
3. The surgeon uses self-retaining or handheld hip retractors to maintain exposure of the acetabulum.
4. Femoral distraction or osteotomy of the trochanter may be used to improve visualization and access to the fracture.
5. The surgeon reduces the fracture using bone clamps, forceps, and a ball spike.

6. Reduction is accomplished in gradual steps using Kirschner wires to hold the fragments temporarily in place.
7. Reconstruction plates are fitted and contoured to the fracture site and secured with screws.
8. The surgeon may also use long cancellous lag screw fixation to provide interfragmentary compression, particularly in column fractures.
9. A bone graft may be needed for additional fixation. A femoral head allograft technique is sometimes used, in which the allograft is mushroomed to create a new acetabulum.
10. The surgeon uses pulsatile lavage to irrigate the wound with antibiotic solution to ensure the articular surfaces are free from loose bodies.
11. The wound is closed, drains are inserted, and pressure dressings are applied.

The leg is maintained in abduction and external rotation with traction. Once the fracture is stabilized, traction is no longer necessary.

NOTE: If there is associated traumatic dislocation of the hip with the acetabular fracture, the dislocation should be treated promptly. The dislocation should be reduced as soon as possible and skeletal traction inserted if needed to maintain reduction. Acetabular fractures often accompany femoral shaft fractures, which also need to be treated concurrently with the surgeon's desired method (see Femoral Shaft Fractures: Internal Fixation, p. 720).

Hip Fractures

Hip fractures are classified by anatomic location and can be categorized as femoral neck fractures, intertrochanteric fractures, and subtrochanteric fractures (Figure 20-47), and these can each be subclassified. Fracture-dislocations also have a classification system and treatment protocol. Fractures of the greater or lesser trochanters alone are less common and can usually be treated nonoperatively.

Femoral neck fractures and intertrochanteric fractures commonly require open reduction and internal fixation. Neck fractures are more common in women because of several factors, including osteoporosis. Most elderly patients require a comprehensive preoperative medical evaluation to define and treat anesthetic risks. However, efforts should be made to correct the fracture as soon as possible to avoid complications related to immobility, skin pressure, pulmonary congestion, and thrombophlebitis. Avascular necrosis and degenerative changes can occur as a result of diminished blood supply to the femoral head, resulting in irreversible changes. Buck traction may be placed preoperatively to reduce discomfort from muscle spasm caused by overriding of fracture fragments.

Manipulation, reduction, and internal fixation of these fractures are greatly facilitated by use of the OR fracture bed, which also permits adequate radiographic examination to determine placement of the internal fixation.

Intertrochanteric Fractures. Intertrochanteric fractures occur most frequently in older patients. The fractures usually unite without difficulty. However, because the lower extremity is externally rotated at the fracture site, internal fixation is necessary to prevent malunion. Internal fixation allows patients to be mobilized earlier, thereby decreasing mortality and morbidity.

Procedural Considerations. The patient is placed in the supine position on the OR fracture bed, and the surgeon reduces the fracture by manipulating the extremity and then confirming with fluoroscopy. Various internal fixation devices, including Ambi, Free-Lock, dynamic hip screw (DHS), and medullary fixation, may be

FIGURE 20-47 Proximal femur fractures. **A,** Midcervical. **B,** Comminuted subtrochanteric. **C,** Intertrochanteric.

FIGURE 20-48 Intertrochanteric fracture repair with compression plate. **A,** Guide pin is inserted. **B,** Depth of guide is measured. **C,** Lag screw channel is reamed. **D,** Tube/plate is applied, and lag screw is inserted.

used. Success of the procedure is determined by bone quality, fragment configuration, adequate reduction, implant design, and implant-insertion technique. Intraoperative blood loss is minimized because the hip joint is not opened.

A soft tissue set and a large bone set are required in addition to the compression hip screw instrumentation and implants, bone-reduction and plate-holding clamps, and a power drill and reamer.

Operative Procedure
Free-Lock Compression Plate and Lag Screw (Figure 20-48)
1. The surgeon reduces the fracture as previously described.
2. Reduction is checked in both the AP and lateral views with fluoroscopy.
3. The surgeon makes an incision from the greater trochanter distally to accommodate the length of the implant.

4. The dissection is completed through the fascia lata, and the vastus lateralis is exposed.

5. The reduction is visually confirmed and the surgeon inserts the guide pin after determining the angle plate to be used. A 135-degree angle plate is commonly used.

6. The pin should be centralized in the femoral head approximately 1 cm short of the femoral articular surface. Care must be taken to not enter the joint space because this might result in arthritic changes. Further penetration of the pin through the acetabulum and into the pelvis can damage large vessels or bowel. A second pin can be used to control rotation in high neck or unstable fractures.

7. The surgeon uses a conical cannulated drill bit over the guide pin to open the lateral cortex.

8. The depth gauge is placed over the guide pin. The size of the required lag screw is determined from the guide.

9. A double-barrel reamer is adjusted to correspond to the depth of the guide pin. The cortex is reamed over the guide pin to create a channel for the lag screw and barrel of the compression plate.

10. The lag screw channel is tapped to the full distance of reaming to allow proper seating of the lag screw, particularly in young patients with firm bone. Reaming depth of osteoporotic bone is reduced 5 mm, and the tap depth is reduced approximately 1 to 2 cm to allow sufficient screw purchase.

11. The surgeon may confirm the plate angle with a trial. Once confirmed, the nurse opens the implants (plate and lag screw) to the back table.

12. The scrub person assembles the plate, lag screw, and insertion wrench with the centering sleeve. A screw stabilizer is passed through the center of the insertion wrench and threaded into the lag screw.

13. The surgeon places the entire assembly over the guide pin, and advances the lag screw to the desired depth with periodic verification with fluoroscopy. Penetration of the lag screw through the femoral articular surface must be avoided.

14. The insertion wrench is disassembled, and the barrel of the compression plate is placed over the lag screw. The barrel of the plate should fully cover the lag screw. The plate is seated on the lateral femoral shaft.

15. The surgeon secures the plate to the shaft of the femur with plate-holding forceps. The guide pin is removed. At this point, traction can be released to allow compression of the fracture site.

16. Screw holes are made using the drill guide and a 3.5-mm drill bit. The length is determined, and cortical screws are inserted through the screw hole on the plate with sufficient purchase on the opposite cortex of the shaft. The top screw hole on the plate can accept a 6.5-mm cancellous screw, which can be angled for better purchase in comminuted fractures.

17. Traction is released if not done previously. The surgeon inserts a compression screw into the barrel of the screw and threads it into the back of the lag screw, compressing the fracture site. The compression screw exerts a powerful force. The amount of compression applied should correlate with the quality of the bone.

18. The wound is irrigated and closed. Two closed suction drains may be inserted during closure.

Weight bearing may begin as early as the first postoperative day, depending on reduction and quality of bone.

NOTE: Many of the same techniques and principles of long bone fracture fixation are used in treating various types of hip fractures.

The different screw types, dynamic compression, and lag screw effect are described throughout the chapter.

Femoral Neck Fractures: Internal Fixation

Anatomic reduction is necessary before internal fixation of femoral neck fractures because of the high incidence of associated complications, such as nonunion and avascular necrosis of the femoral head. The degree of displacement, tamponade pressure from intracapsular bleeding, and delays in reduction and fixation can affect the blood supply to the femoral head. These factors contribute to death of the femoral head and failed fixation. Growing children may sustain fractures through the epiphyseal growth plate (slipped capital femoral epiphysis). These injuries are treated by reduction and internal fixation of the femoral head, similar to the procedures used in the adult. The Garden and AO nomenclatures are the most popular classifications for grading the fractures. Pins of various designs, such as Knowles and Hagie pins, and universal cannulated screws (Figure 20-49) are used for fixation (Figure 20-50). In cases of severe comminution or avascular necrosis of the femoral head, the patient may require a prosthetic replacement (see Total Joint Arthroplasty, p. 734).

Procedural Considerations. The perioperative nurse assists with positioning the patient on the OR fracture bed, and a general or regional anesthetic (spinal or epidural) is administered. Slight traction and external rotation are adjusted on the affected side. A soft tissue set and a large bone set are required, as well as the fixation device of choice with instrumentation, Kirschner wires, Cobra retractors, a power drill, and fluoroscopy.

Operative Procedure
Cannulated Screw Fixation for Nondisplaced Femoral Neck Fractures

1. The surgeon makes a 5-cm lateral incision over the greater trochanter and exposes the fracture.

2. The dissection is carried through the subcutaneous and fascial layers; the vastus lateralis is detached anteriorly and retracted, exposing the femoral neck.

3. Two guide pins are driven into the middle of the femoral head, one anterior and one posterior, within 5 mm of subchondral bone; a third pin is placed adjacent to the medial cortex at a 135-degree angle. The surgeon is careful to not violate the articular surface.

4. The guide pins are measured for correct screw length, and the cannulated screws are inserted over the guide pin without applying compression until all are seated.

5. Compression of the anterior screws is completed first and the posterior screws last to avoid collapse of the posterior aspect of the neck.

6. Traction is released, and the fracture site is visualized with fluoroscopy while the hip is rotated through a full range of motion.

7. Radiographs are taken to verify the position of the screws; the wound is irrigated and closed.

NOTE: Screw protrusion into the joint space can be disastrous to the articular surface. Radiopaque dye can be injected to rule out communication with the joint.

Femoral Head Prosthetic Replacement: Unipolar and Bipolar Implants

With the development of current cement fixation techniques and the evolution of the modular bipolar and monopolar design, the

FIGURE 20-49 Cannulated screw system.

FIGURE 20-50 Internal fixation with cannulated screws (AO technique). **A,** Guidewire parallel to anteversion wire. **B,** Guidewire placed over positioning wire through diamond-patterned positioning holes. **C,** Guidewire placed through each outer triangle of holes. **D,** Cannulated tap passed over guidewire to tap near cortex. **E,** Large cannulated screw inserted over guidewire. **F,** Remaining screws inserted in same manner.

use of fixed endoprostheses such as the Austin-Moore and Thompson designs declined. During the early 1980s the bipolar system in conjunction with a cemented femoral stem became popular. Bipolar endoprostheses (Figure 20-51) were introduced to reduce the shear stresses affecting the acetabular surface, decreasing the motion and

friction between the prosthetic head and the acetabulum that is seen with conventional (unipolar) endoprostheses. A femoral head prosthesis is snapped into a rotating polyethylene-lined cup that, when inserted, moves as one unit. Friction occurs between the ball and plastic instead of between the head and the acetabulum. This was

FIGURE 20-51 Modular bipolar endoprostheses.

a revolutionary design in the mechanics of hip motion and stresses. Current data, however, have some surgeons and engineers reevaluating the use of bipolar prostheses. It is believed that bipolar motion subsides after fibrous growth has taken place, allowing for only unipolar motion. There have also been reports of bone resorption and subsequent prosthetic loosening in cases in which bipolar prostheses were used. Researchers are evaluating evidence of metallic head wear of the polyethylene cup, creating microscopic debris with a subsequent chemical lysis of bone. Thus there has been resurgence in the use of unipolar heads for femoral head replacement.

Trends in healthcare toward cost reduction precipitated the development of the *diagnosis-related group (DRG) prosthesis*. The modular design was retained, allowing for different combinations of head size, neck length, and stem size. Instead of being bipolar, the head is solid, or unipolar, and the stem is the result of a less costly manufacturing process. The most cost-effective prosthesis is still the original Austin-Moore design, which may be selected for those patients whose life expectancy is short and who have a minimal level of activity. If major deficiencies in the acetabular side of the joint are present, a total joint arthroplasty may be performed. In deciding between the hemiarthroplasty and total hip reconstruction, the patient's medical condition, age, and level of activity must be considered.

Current biomaterials, methods of fixation (cemented versus uncemented), prosthetic life, and modular components allow conversion of a hemiarthroplasty (reconstruction of one side of the joint) to a total hip arthroplasty, provided that the femoral component is adequately fixed. Depending on the patient's condition, the acetabulum may eventually require arthroplasty as a result of degenerative changes. Improved technology and surgical technique have increased the life span of implanted components. The portion of the implant that articulates within the acetabulum can be removed and replaced with a smaller femoral head. The acetabulum is then prepared for prosthetic implantation by various means of fixation. The ability to convert from hemiarthroplasty to total arthroplasty reduces the amount of surgery required.

Procedural Considerations. The patient is placed in the lateral position after the administration of a general or regional anesthetic. The perioperative nurse preps the patient from the umbilicus down to and including the foot. Instrumentation for total hip replacement should be available but not opened until inspection of the resected joint is completed to determine if a total arthroplasty is required.

The soft tissue and the large bone sets are required, as well as the endoprosthesis instruments, trials, and implants. A power reciprocating or sagittal saw may be necessary. Templates or a calipers is used to measure the size of the femoral head. Bone cement and the supplies for preparing and inserting it also should be available.

Operative Procedure
Modular Austin-Moore Endoprosthesis. Both posterior and anterior approaches can be made to the hip to place an endoprosthesis. The posterior approach is quicker and generally involves less blood loss, but detractors suggest that there is a higher dislocation rate and a greater chance of infection because of the proximity of the incision to the anus. Although both approaches are widely used, the posterior approach is described as follows:

1. The surgeon makes a linear incision from 5 cm below the posteroinferior iliac spine toward the posterior aspect of the greater trochanter and distally along the posterior aspect of the proximal femur for 7 mm.
2. The capsule is entered, and the femoral head is removed and gauged with the template. Fragments that may be loose in the acetabulum or attached to the ligamentum teres are removed.
3. The surgeon inserts a trial cup into the acetabulum, and applies axial compression while checking clearance of the extremity's lateral motion.
4. The femoral neck is fashioned to achieve an accurate prosthetic fit.
5. Using a punch, the surgeon opens the medullary canal from the femoral neck. The intramedullary canal is reamed and rasped to accommodate the prosthesis.
6. Once the canal is prepared, the surgeon inserts the prosthesis of choice with or without bone cement.
7. A unipolar or bipolar assembly is snapped onto the neck of the femoral stem. The height of the head determines the neck length and is selected after trial reduction.
8. The hip is reduced, and closure is accomplished in layers over suction drains.

Femoral Shaft Fractures: Internal Fixation

Fractures involving the femoral shaft are very common in today's orthopedic OR. Prolonged immobility, with its attendant complications, and disability can result if femoral shaft fractures are not managed appropriately. The femur is the largest principal load-bearing bone in the body. Fractures of the femoral shaft can be surgically treated with several available techniques. Considerations for treatment are type and location of fracture (location on shaft), the number of segments involved, the degree of comminution (Figure 20-52), and the activity level of the patient. Femoral shaft fractures are often associated with ipsilateral (same-side) trochanteric or condylar fractures. Pathologic fractures often occur in this region.

Possible treatment methods for femoral shaft fractures are closed reduction, skeletal traction, and femoral cast bracing. External fixation has limited utility when fractures associated with surgical site infection or neurovascular compromise are treated, but it may serve

FIGURE 20-52 Femoral shaft fractures. **A,** Transverse. **B,** Oblique. **C,** Spiral. **D,** Comminuted. **E,** Longitudinal split. **F,** Complete bone loss.

temporarily until internal fixation can be performed. Although plates and screws are used for femoral shaft fractures, their use has been widely disputed because of complications such as bent or broken plates, refractures, and deep surgical site infections. Intramedullary (IM) fixation devices have become the preferred method of treatment. IM nails and rods increase the load sharing of the bone, making the implant less likely to fracture. Bone healing requires a load across the fracture site to promote osteosynthesis and prevent refracture. The open or closed method of intramedullary nailing can be used with locked and nonlocked nails. Closed methods of intramedullary fixation often minimize exposure of the surgical site and decrease surgical time, resulting in less opportunity for infection.

Intramedullary nail and rod designs vary: (1) flexible nails such as the Rusch or Enders type, (2) standard rods such as the Sampson and AO rods, and (3) interlocking nails (see Fractures of the Humeral Shaft, p. 707) such as the Grosse-Kempf and Russell-Taylor varieties. Closed reduction and intramedullary nailing with or without locking screws have become the method against which other methods are measured. Incidences of scarring, blood loss, and infection are all favorable. Fracture hematoma remains intact at the fracture site, which is important in bone healing, and the rate of bone union is increased.

Procedural Considerations. General or epidural anesthetics are used. The patient is placed on the OR fracture bed in the supine position, traction applied, and the fracture manually reduced and confirmed with fluoroscopy. If the fracture is profoundly unstable, the surgeon must take care during manipulation to prevent neurovascular complications. For open IM fixation, extra retractors and bone instruments may be required. For a percutaneous reduction, a soft tissue set and a large bone set are required in addition to the IM nail implants and associated instruments, a power reamer and drill, and long guidewires for reamers. This procedure requires the use of fluoroscopy. A skeletal traction tray with Steinmann pins may be necessary.

Operative Procedure
Russell-Taylor Rod With or Without Locking Screws

1. The surgeon makes an incision over the tip of the greater trochanter and continues it proximally and medially for 6 to 8 cm. The fascia of the gluteus is incised, and the piriformis fossa is palpated.
2. With a threaded guide pin followed by cannulated reamers or by use of an awl, the surgeon identifies the trochanteric fossa and penetrates the cortex. A 3.2-mm guide rod is inserted to the level of the fracture. A curved guide pin is available for more severely displaced fractures.
3. Under fluoroscopy, the surgeon advances the guidewire across the fracture site and into the distal fragment until the ball tip of the guidewire reaches the level of the epiphyseal scar. A second guidewire is held against the portion of the guidewire extending out of the proximal femur, and the length is measured. That measurement is subtracted from 90 mm (total guidewire length) to determine the length of the intramedullary nail required.
4. The cannulated reamers are placed sequentially over the guidewire. The entire femur is reamed at 0.5-mm increments. The entire shaft, and especially the fracture site, should be visualized with fluoroscopy as the reamers pass.
5. The final reamer size should be verified with the reamer gauge. The femur is reamed 1 mm over the selected nail diameter. Inserting a nail in an inadequately reamed femur or inserting a nail that is too large can cause severe bone splitting and comminution.
6. The proximal screw guide/slap hammer is assembled onto the nail. The nail is oriented to match the curve of the femur.
7. Using the handle of the inserter, the rotation of the nail is controlled and the nail is driven into the femur. The nail is fully seated when the proximal screw guide is flush with the greater trochanter. The surgeon disengages the inserter from the slap hammer.
8. Using the power drill and correct drill sleeves, the surgeon drills a 4.8-mm hole through both cortices and measures the depth directly off the bit.
9. Through the appropriate drill sleeve, a 6.4-mm self-tapping locking screw is inserted and the drill sleeve is removed.
10. By fluoroscopy, the distal screw holes are confirmed as perfect circles on the screen. The distal targeting device is mounted on the nail, followed by the left or right adapter block. The adapter block is adjusted until the calibration reads the length of the nail. The crosshairs are aligned in the adapter to the holes in the distal nail, with confirmation by fluoroscopy.
11. The surgeon makes an incision through the adapter block over the distal femur to the lateral cortex. Following the same steps

as those for placing the proximal screw, one or two distal locking screws are inserted. There are various freehand techniques for inserting distal locking screws.

Surgery of the Lower Leg (Distal Femur, Tibia, and Fibula)

Many procedures on the lower leg use the same principles of fracture fixation already mentioned. Meticulous detail is required to ensure proper alignment and optimal surgical results for the patient. As in the hip, fractures around the knee require secure fixation to allow bone healing, preserve motion, and provide joint mobility as early as possible. Fracture treatment for the various described injuries is based on location and the pattern of fracture. Methods of fixation for the distal end of the femur and proximal end of the tibia include pins, wire, compression plates, intramedullary nails, supracondylar plates, and cannulated screws. Multiple-trauma patients with one or a combination of fractures may require more than one method of fixation. Open reduction and internal fixation must ensure anatomic restoration of the joint surface and rigid fixation, and allow early motion of the knee joint.

Most operations on the knee are performed with the patient in the supine position and the leg prepped and draped from the groin to the middle of the calf or including the entire foot. It is occasionally necessary for the surgeon to operate with the foot of the OR bed dropped and the patient's knee flexed to 90 degrees. Consequently, it is important for the nurse to position the patient so that the knee is at a break in the bed; if it is necessary, the lower leg can then be flexed at the knee during the operation. A tourniquet is often used.

Femoral Condyle and Tibial Plateau Fractures

The joint surfaces are often involved with fractures of the distal end of the femur and proximal end of the tibia. Anatomic alignment of the articular surfaces is necessary to provide joint stability and decrease the chance of post-traumatic arthritis. Nonunion is the most common complication in supracondylar fractures, leading to failure of surgery. As with humeral head and hip fractures, it is important that the articular surfaces are reposed as close as possible to avoid future degenerative changes. Unfortunately these often cannot be avoided, and patients with this type of injury often face future joint arthroplasty and replacement (see Total Joint Arthroplasty, p. 733).

Distal femoral fractures result in varying degrees of comminution. Condylar fractures can be unicondylar or bicondylar, with separation of both condyles (Figure 20-53). Type A fractures are extra-articular. Type B are single condyle fractures in the sagittal or coronal planes, whereas type C fractures are T and Y configurations. Type C fractures have varying degrees of shaft and condylar comminution, presenting the greatest treatment challenge.

Simple, nondisplaced distal femoral fractures can be treated with closed reduction and immobilization by casting if anatomic reduction is achieved. Nondisplaced extra-articular fractures can be treated with a hinged cast brace. Comminuted fractures in this region can also be treated in this manner if shortening and angulation are minimal. Traction can be used initially to augment this type of treatment. Distal femoral fractures are treated with open reduction if distal tibial traction and manipulation attempts fail. Flexible nails, locking intramedullary nails, blade plates, condylar compression screws, and condylar buttress plates are accepted methods of treating condylar fractures. Attention must be given to the attachment of the cruciate ligaments, which originate in the condylar

notch and may require fixation of a partial or full disruption as a result of the injury to the knee (see Arthroscopic Anterior Cruciate Ligament Repair, p. 756).

Tibial plateau fractures historically have been attributed to bumper or fender injuries, but a variety of falls or other traumas frequently are the cause. Compression force of the distal end of the femur on the tibia produces the various types of plateau fractures. Commonly this occurs from abduction of the tibia while the foot is planted, driving the lateral femoral condyle into the lateral tibial plateau. There are several classification systems based on fracture and dislocation patterns. The general theme of these fracture classifications and examples of their treatment can be summarized by the following types (Figure 20-54): (1) pure cleavage, unicondylar fracture, (2) cleavage fracture combined with local depression, (3) pure central depression, (4) medial condylar wedge with depression or comminution, (5) bicondylar but with continuity of diaphysis and metaphysis, and (6) comminution with dissociation of metaphysis from diaphysis. Fractures of the tibial plateau are often associated with dislocation, which may spontaneously reduce at the time of trauma.

Special attention must be given to the possibility of neurovascular insult, which must be addressed immediately. Elevation and fixation of the depressed fracture are the focus for treatment of plateau fractures. As with distal femoral fractures, the articular surfaces and cruciate insertion require reapproximation and fixation. Repair to the menisci and ligaments should occur simultaneously to prevent knee instability.

Blade plates, buttress plates, and cannulated screws are all methods by which fractures of the tibial plateau are fixed. Severe fractures are treated using multiple buttress plates and screws (Figure 20-55). Bone graft from the iliac crest and fibular head autograft are often used when there is a significant amount of bone lost to comminution with proximal tibial fractures.

Supracondylar Fractures of the Femur

Fractures of the distal femur in the multiple-trauma patient are treated early to promote rapid ambulation, which decreases complications caused by immobility. In an effort to deliver quick fracture reduction and stabilization, many orthopedic trauma systems have been developed. Often these are the same systems used in daily orthopedic procedures with modifications to expedite implantation and fixation. Some of the intramedullary devices do not require reaming.

Procedural Considerations. Initial stabilization of the patient may immediately precede the nailing procedure. Often other team members are attending to treatment of other systems. The perioperative nurse is challenged to control traffic, coordinate team efforts, and protect the patient from increased risk of infection by the inadvertent contamination of instruments and implants. The patient is placed in the supine position after induction of general or regional anesthesia. If possible, the patient is positioned on the OR fracture bed; if not, a radiolucent OR bed is used. A pneumatic tourniquet may be applied as high up on the femur as possible, taking care to protect the genitals during placement. The nail can be inserted using the closed or open technique.

The soft tissue set and large bone set are required, as well as the intramedullary supracondylar nail implant (Figure 20-56) and the instruments necessary for its insertion. A power drill, guidewires, intramedullary rod set, and fluoroscopy also are needed. In addition, Steinmann pins, Kirschner wires, bone-reduction clamps, and

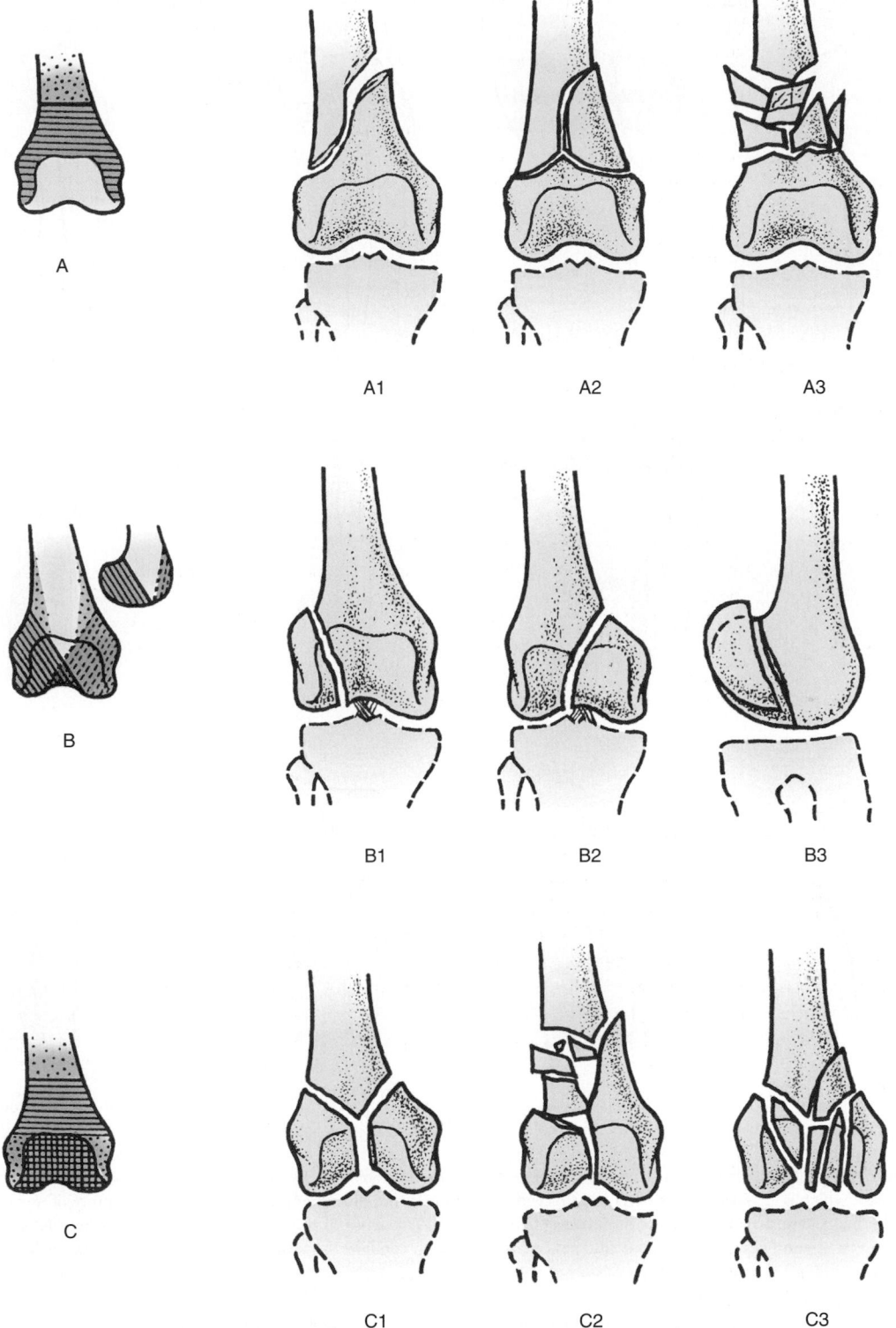

FIGURE 20-53 Classification of fractures of distal femur.

A. Type I

B. Type II

C. Type III

D. Type IV

E. Type V

F. Type VI

FIGURE 20-54 Classification of fractures of the tibial plateau. **A,** *Type I:* Pure cleavage fracture. **B,** *Type II:* Cleavage combined with depression. Reduction requires elevation of fragments with bone grafting of resultant hole in metaphysis. Wedge is lagged on lateral aspect of cortex protected with buttress plate. **C,** *Type III:* Pure central depression. There is no lateral wedge. Depression may also be anterior or posterior or involve whole plateau. After elevation of depression and bone grafting, lateral aspect of cortex is best protected with buttress plate. **D,** *Type IV:* Medial condyle either is split off as wedge or may be crumbled and depressed, which is characteristic of older patients with osteoporosis (not illustrated). **E,** *Type V:* Note continuity of metaphysis and diaphysis. In internal fixation both sides must be protected with buttress plates. **F,** *Type VI:* Essence of this fracture is fracture line that dissociates metaphysis from diaphysis. Fracture pattern of condyles is variable, and all types can occur. If both condyles are involved, proximal tibia should be buttressed on both sides.

a bone graft set should be available. Occasionally a primary total knee arthroplasty is performed, and the appropriate instruments should be available should that possibility exist.

Operative Procedure
Intercondylar Fracture of the Femur, T Type (AIM Supracondylar Intramedullary Nail).
1. The surgeon makes a standard midline skin incision with parapatellar arthrotomy. Depending on the degree of intra-articular extension, the incision may be as small as 2.5 cm or involve lateral eversion of the patella to gain visualization of the entire joint.
2. Articular fractures should be anatomically reduced and secured with 6.5- or 8-mm cannulated screws placed in the anterior and posterior aspects of the condyles to allow adequate space for the placement of the nail.
3. Using an awl, the surgeon makes an entry hole into the femoral canal just anterior to the femoral insertion of the posterior cruciate ligament. Care is taken to ensure anatomic alignment of the condyles to avoid varus or valgus femoral alignment.

FIGURE 20-55 Severe fractures are treated by use of multiple buttress plates and screws.

FIGURE 20-56 Supracondylar nail.

4. The hole is enlarged with the nonadjustable step reamer to accept the largest diameter of the chosen nail. Further reaming of the canal is necessary only in the case of nonunion, when the canal is reamed 0.5 to 1 mm larger than the size of the selected nail.
5. The selected nail is attached to the screw-targeting jig, which is then locked into place by the jig adapter. Before the nail is inserted, the alignment of the jig and nail holes is carefully checked by manually inserting the sheath and trocar through the selected holes.
6. The surgeon places the nail in the prepared canal and advances it retrograde either by hand or with gentle blows of a mallet on the jig adapter. The nail should be countersunk approximately 3 to 5 mm below the articular surface.
7. The screws may then be placed using the targeting jig and sheath and trocar assembly. The surgeon makes a small lateral incision and advances the sheath and trocar to the femoral cortex. A 5.3-mm drill bit is advanced through the medial cortex, and the length is measured from the calibrated drill bit or by use of a depth gauge. The appropriate 6.5-mm cortical screw is inserted, and the process is repeated for placement of the second screw.
8. Proximal locking of the nail is then performed in a similar fashion, taking care to use the appropriate holes in the targeting jig for the length of nail inserted. The 3.8-mm drill bit and 4.5-mm self-tapping screws are used to fill these holes after femoral rotation and alignment are confirmed with fluoroscopy.
9. The jig adapter and screw-targeting jig are removed, and an end cap is placed into the distal end of the nail. The surgeon irrigates the wounds and closes them in layers. A compression dressing is applied.

Range-of-motion and muscle-strengthening exercises are begun on the first postoperative day. Care is taken to protect against varus and valgus stresses. The patient is discouraged from bearing weight on the extremity until there is radiographic evidence of healing.

Supracondylar Fracture (Compression Plate)

1. The lateral area of the distal end of the femur is exposed above and below the knee joint.
2. The surgeon reduces the fracture site and inserts multiple Kirschner wires for fixation.
3. A calibrated Steinmann pin is placed transversely across the condyles parallel to the joint line. The pin must stop 8 to 10 mm short of the medial cortex.
4. The length of the lag screw is gauged when it is read directly on the calibrated Steinmann pin, and adjustable double reamers are used to ream to this depth.
5. A lag screw is inserted across the condyles, followed by the compression screw.
6. The surgeon secures the plate to the femoral shaft with cortical bone screws and confirms the repair by fluoroscopy.
7. The incision site is irrigated and closed. A knee immobilizer is placed.

Medial and Lateral Y-Type Tibial Plateau Fractures

1. The surgeon makes a long anterolateral incision, starting 2.5 cm above the superolateral aspect of the patella and tendon and proceeding distally around the patella to the anterior aspect of the tibia just below the tibial tuberosity. The distal end of the tibial shaft should be exposed.
2. The level of the prepatellar bursa is identified. The surgeon uses blunt dissection beneath the skin and retracts the proximal end of the tibia to expose it from midline medially to midline laterally.
3. Using a tibial bone plug, the surgeon detaches the patellar tendon and exposes both the medial and lateral articular surfaces. The articular surface is reconstructed using temporary Kirschner wires. A contoured T-plate is attached to the medial aspect of the tibia using cancellous screws in the proximal portion and cortical screws in the distal portion. A smaller T-plate is inserted on the lateral side and secured in the same manner. The Kirschner wires are removed. Care should be taken

to ensure that the screws do not interfere with each other as they traverse from opposite sides of the tibia.

4. The surgeon reattaches the patellar tendon using a 6.5-mm cancellous screw through the bone plug.

5. The wound is closed and immobilized at 30 degrees with a posterior splint.

Patellectomy and Reduction of Fractures of the Patella

Patellectomy was a frequently performed procedure until the early 1970s. It is possible to excise a portion of the patella (for comminuted fracture) or the entire patella (for painful degenerative arthritis) without significantly affecting ordinary activities. However, patellectomy has been shown to significantly reduce power of extension as the joint extends, which is the most important function of the knee. Other complications associated with patellectomy are: (1) slow return of quadriceps mechanism strength, (2) quadriceps muscle atrophy, and (3) loss of knee protection from the patella. Removal of the entire patella may result in relative lengthening of the knee extensor mechanism, which necessitates overlapping of the quadriceps tendon at the time of operation to prevent a lag in knee extension. Patellectomy should be performed only when comminution is extensive and reconstruction of the articular surface of the patella is not possible.

If the fracture consists of two large fragments that can be anatomically reduced, fixation is accomplished with a tension band, a circumferential loop technique, or bone screws. Tension band wiring produces compression forces across the fracture site and results in earlier union and immediate mobility of the knee.

Procedural Considerations. The patient is supine. The tourniquet is applied, and the leg is prepped and draped. A soft tissue set and a bone set are required, along with a power drill and bits, bone-reduction clamps, 18-gauge wire, heavy needle holders, and a wire tightener.

Operative Procedure

1. The surgeon makes a transverse curved incision over the patella.

2. Using sharp and blunt dissection the surgeon exposes the surface of the patella, the quadriceps, and the patellar tendons.

3. The joint is irrigated, and the fracture is reduced with bone-reduction clamps.

4. One length of wire is passed around the insertion of the patellar tendon and then around the quadriceps tendon. A second wire is passed more superficially through the bone fragments.

5. The fracture is overcorrected, and the wire is tightened with the wire tightener. In flexing the knee or contracting the quadriceps, the condyles press against the patellar fragments, producing compression at the fracture site.

Correction of Recurrent Dislocation of the Patella

Recurrent dislocation of the patella can be the result of violent initial dislocation or more commonly from underlying anatomic abnormalities. The underlying condition causes an abnormal excursion of the extensor mechanism over the femoral condyles. Dynamic forces, such as the vastus lateralis, and static forces, such as those arising from the shape of the patella, tend to displace the patella laterally. Dislocations occur when there are extreme displacing forces combined with internal rotation of the femur and flexion of the knee. If untreated, patellar dislocations will deteriorate the knee

by causing abnormal patellofemoral articulation, chondromalacia, and meniscal tears.

Conservative treatment aimed at quadriceps strengthening may be indicated in some patients. Numerous procedures have been designed to realign the knee extensor mechanism. All the procedures include incising the lateral quadriceps tendon and shifting the insertion of the patellar tendon medially or distally to the original insertion of the tibia.

Procedural Considerations. The patient is positioned supine. The tourniquet is applied, and the leg is prepped and draped. A soft tissue set and a bone set are required, along with a large-fragment screw set, a power drill, a microsagittal saw, and osteotomes.

Operative Procedure
Patellar Realignment (Elmslie-Trillat)

1. The surgeon makes a lateral parapatellar incision beginning proximally to the patellar pole, laterally around the patella, and extending to 2 cm distally and just laterally to the tibial tuberosity.

2. A skin flap is developed and retracted medially to expose the capsule. A medial arthrotomy is completed, the joint is inspected, and any pathologic condition present is repaired.

3. The lateral retinaculum is released from the vastus lateralis proximally and the patellar tendon distally.

4. Using a ½-inch osteotome, the surgeon scores the tibial tuberosity medially and laterally, just below the fat pad and under the patella.

5. The surgeon continues the osteotomy using a microsagittal saw distally for 4 to 6 cm, and leaves the periosteum hinged at the distal-most part of the osteotomy.

6. The entire segment, with patellar tendon attached, is displaced medially and manually held in place while moving the knee through a range of motion. Tracking of the patella on the femoral groove is completed by systematically moving the knee medially in increments.

7. A cancellous bone bed is prepared at the point of reattachment of the tibial tuberosity.

8. The surgeon displaces the tuberosity medially and places a 6.5-mm cancellous bone screw.

9. The wound is irrigated and closed, and a long leg cylinder cast is applied. The cast is bivalved immediately.

Repair of Collateral or Cruciate Ligament Tears

The stability of the knee depends on the integrity of the cruciate and collateral ligaments. If any of these supporting structures is damaged, an unstable knee is likely unless properly repaired. Injuries to these supporting structures are usually not isolated. More frequently, several of the ligaments are injured at the same time. For example, the injury commonly referred to as the "terrible triad" includes a torn anterior cruciate ligament (ACL), torn medial meniscus, and torn medial collateral ligament.

The knee demonstrates grave disability with major ligamentous disruption. The *collateral ligaments* reinforce the knee capsule medially and laterally. They resist varus and valgus stresses on the knee. The *cruciate ligaments* control anteroposterior stability. Along with the ligaments, the muscle groups stabilize the joint and control movement. Because muscle strength is the first line of defense for the knee, damage is repaired to protect the ligaments. For optimum function of the joint, damaged structures should be reconstructed as close as possible to the original anatomic structures. If the knee is left untreated, osteoarthritis will develop.

Injury to a single cruciate ligament may not significantly compromise knee function. When the injury is combined with other injuries, surgery may be warranted. Surgeons may use various types of ligament grafts to replace or augment the cruciate ligaments. Autografts, allografts, and artificial substitutes are available. Ligament substitutes act as a scaffold, stent, or augmentation of the torn cruciate ligaments. Scaffolds support the soft tissue initially to allow ingrowth of the host tissue. Stents protect the joint from excessive stress while the permanent ligament substitute is healing. Augmentation, as by the patient's own iliotibial band, protects the graft initially after repair of a partial tear. Synthetic ligaments, which are less popular, include carbon-fiber grafts, polyglycolic acid material, Dacron, polyester, and polytetrafluoroethylene.

All synthetic grafts are subject to mechanical failure from weakening with fragmentation and synovitis. These are recommended for salvage procedures only when conventional reconstruction has failed and when other autogenous tissue is unavailable for substitution. Biologic materials from animals, such as bovine xenografts, are also available for ligament substitution, although they are subject to increased risk of infection, synovitis, and rejection. Homogeneous allografts are the substitute of choice for knee reconstruction when no autogenous graft is available from the patient. Disadvantages of homogeneous allografts include long-term weakening, possible rejection, and the possibility of infectious disease transfer.

Autogenous tissues are currently the substitute of choice, with the middle third of the patellar tendon and a block of patella being the most reliable. To minimize necrosis and maintain graft strength, the fat pad with its blood supply may be preserved along with the patellar tendon. Using this graft and other soft tissue autografts, the cruciate-deficient knee can be reconstructed arthroscopically. A combination of a torn ACL, medial meniscus, and medial collateral ligament in the past often indicated the need for an open procedure (arthrotomy). With developing technology, many of these procedures can now be done arthroscopically. When reconstructing the cruciate ligament, the surgeon must have the graft biomechanically correct to maintain proper function. Many devices and systems are used to provide placement assistance and gauge appropriate graft tension. These devices are used either separately or in some combination. Though the variations are many, the principles are the same.

Procedural Considerations. The patient is positioned supine with a tourniquet applied to the upper area of the thigh. The perioperative nurse preps the patient from the upper area of the thigh down to and including the foot. Soft tissue instruments, arthroscopy instruments, ACL reconstruction instruments, Steinmann pins, reconstruction guides (Figure 20-57), and a tension isometer are required. A power drill, microsagittal saw, and burrs are essential. The fixation device of choice should also be available. Meniscal repair instruments should be in the room.

Operative Procedure

Anterior Cruciate Repair. The surgeon performs an examination under anesthesia (EUA) immediately after induction of anesthesia, when the ligaments are completely lax, to evaluate the severity of the injury.

1. The surgeon makes a straight midline or slightly medial incision across the knee.

FIGURE 20-57 Reconstruction guide used for ligament repair.

2. Meniscus tears in the vascular zone (peripheral) are repaired with arthroscopic meniscal repair instruments or cutting needles with a heavy absorbable suture to repair the meniscofemoral and meniscotibial ligaments. If the meniscus is not repairable, the surgeon will perform a partial meniscectomy.

3. Using a power saw and osteotome, the surgeon harvests patellar and tibial bone plugs from the middle third of the patellar tendon.

4. A notchplasty is then performed, debriding and smoothing the lateral intercondylar wall with a burr and curette.

5. The surgeon uses the ligament guide to develop the femoral and tibial osseous tunnels and passes guidewires from the lateral area of the femoral condyle and tibial tubercle into the intercondylar notch at isometric points near the anatomic attachment site of the ACL.

6. The pins are then overdrilled with cannulated drills as close to the size of the patellar tendon graft as possible. The tunnels are smoothed with a curette.

7. Sutures are placed through drill holes at both ends of the graft to pass the graft through the tunnels.

8. The surgeon passes the graft through the femoral and tibial osseous tunnels and fixes it at both ends with interference screws, staples, or polyethylene buttons.

9. The medial collateral ligament and posterior oblique ligament are then individually repaired at their insertion sites with bone screws and spiked washers.

10. Additional extra-articular repair is done if necessary.

11. The surgeon closes the wound over intra-articular and subcutaneous drains, and a locking knee brace or knee immobilizer is applied.

Popliteal (Baker) Cyst Excision

Baker cysts occur in joints, frequently affecting the popliteal fossa. Baker cysts are often painful and can become very large, especially when associated with rheumatoid arthritis. Cysts in the popliteal fossa occur without a precipitating cause in children; in adults they often indicate an intra-articular disease process, such as rheumatoid arthritis, or a torn meniscus.

Procedural Considerations. In contrast to many other operative procedures on the knee, the patient is placed in the prone position. A soft tissue set and a bone set are required.

Operative Procedure

1. The surgeon makes an oblique incision in the popliteal area over the mass and divides the fascia to expose the mass.
2. Using blunt dissection, the surgeon frees the cyst and clamps it at the base of its attachment to the joint capsule.
3. The cyst is divided, and the pedicle is inverted and closed.
4. After the mass has been removed, the surgeon irrigates and closes the wound.

   Postoperatively, the knee may be immobilized in extension with a posterior splint.

Correction of Fractures of the Tibial Shaft

The location of the tibia results in frequent exposure to injury. Open fractures are more common in the tibia than in other major bones because one third of its surface is subcutaneous. Tibial shaft fractures are difficult to treat. The blood supply to the tibia is more precarious than that of other long bones because of its lack of enclosure by heavy muscle. The presence of hinge joints at the knee and ankle allows no adjustment for rotational deformity after fracture, so special care is required to correct for rotation during reduction and fixation. Rotational deformities are often seen. Delayed union, nonunion, and infection are fairly common complications. Closed reduction and casting provide excellent healing without significant complications, but this treatment can require casting for 6 months or more. Surgical reduction and internal fixation generally allows for earlier weight bearing and a shortened period of casting; however, the rate of complications is higher.

In general, torsional fractures seem to heal better and are more amenable to treatment than transverse fractures. It is theorized that twisting injuries cause less damage to endosteal vessels than that caused by transverse fractures, in which periosteum and endosteal vessels are torn circumferentially. The important prognostic indicators for tibial fractures are as follows: (1) the amount of initial displacement, (2) the degree of comminution, (3) the presence or absence of infection, and (4) the severity of soft tissue injury, excluding infection. As a rule, high-energy fractures, such as those caused by motor vehicle accidents or crushing injury, have a much worse prognosis than low-energy fractures, such as those caused by falls on ice or skiing accidents.

Because intramedullary tibial nailings do not cause a significant increase in infections, external fixation of open tibial shaft fractures is less commonly performed. However, in the presence of gross contamination, severe soft tissue and vascular injury, bone infection, and delayed treatment, external fixation is the treatment of choice. The Ilizarov external fixation device is indicated when bone loss is significant and limb lengthening is required. Plate and screw fixation is another method in which tibial shaft fractures can be treated, although infection and nonunion of tibial shaft fractures are twice as likely with this method. Plate and screw fixation is indicated when intra-articular fragments of the knee and ankle are associated with the injury. Closed intramedullary nailing is the treatment of choice in tibial shaft fractures because infection is less likely to occur and the periosteal blood supply is preserved. Static locking nails (locking both proximal and distal ends of the nail) are indicated for fractures with comminution, bone loss, and lengthening osteotomies. Dynamic locking nails (locking the end closest to the fracture site) are indicated for proximal or distal tibial fractures, nonunions, and malunions. Locking tibial nails include the Russell-Taylor and the Grosse-Kempf tibial nail.

The key to successful treatment of open tibial fractures, as in all open fractures, is meticulous and systematic debridement of all foreign matter and devitalized tissue. The surgeon is careful to minimize devascularization when reducing and fixing the fracture. Systemic antibiotics and those delivered by pulsatile lavage help reduce the chance of infection.

Procedural Considerations. The patient is usually administered a general or regional anesthetic while still on the hospital bed or the transport vehicle and then transferred to the OR fracture bed. The perioperative nurse assists with positioning the patient supine with the affected hip flexed approximately 45 degrees and the knee at 90 degrees. This positioning provides a horizontal orientation of the tibia. Using a calcaneal traction pin or table foot holder, traction is applied and rotational alignment obtained. After rotational alignment is obtained, a tourniquet is applied and the leg is prepped and draped. Some surgeons prefer to use a standard OR bed, breaking it at the knee. This obviates the need to insert the calcaneal traction pin and allows for easier maneuvering of the tibia during insertion of the locking screws.

A soft tissue set and a large bone set are required, in addition to the intramedullary nail and insertion instruments of choice. A power drill and reamer-driver are needed to use the necessary intramedullary reamers. Fluoroscopy is needed as well. If open plating is being considered, the plates of choice and the large-fragment screws need to be available as well as bone-reduction clamps.

Operative Procedure

Closed or Open Tibial Intramedullary Nailing (Figure 20-58)

1. If the open technique is required, the fracture site is exposed, reduced, and irrigated as necessary. Focus is then turned toward the nailing procedure.
2. The surgeon makes a 5-cm incision medial to the patellar tendon to just below the tibial tuberosity.
3. Using a curved awl, the surgeon opens the medullary canal just proximal to the tibial tuberosity.
4. A guide rod (3.2 mm) is inserted into the shaft of the tibia down to the fracture site. The proximal fragment is reduced distally and the guide rod advanced into the distal fragment. Rod types include the straight guide rod for simple fractures, a curved guide rod for displaced fractures, and a cutting tip for an obstructed canal.
5. The length of the required nail is determined by the guide rod method (see Operative Procedure under Femoral Shaft Fractures: Internal Fixation, p. 720) or by using the nail-length gauge and confirming with fluoroscopy.
6. With cannulated reamers over the guide rods, the surgeon reams the entire tibia 1 mm larger than the nail to be inserted. Inserting a nail too large for the canal can have a detrimental effect.
7. The driver, proximal drill, guide, and hexagonal bolt are assembled onto the tibial nail.
8. The surgeon inserts the nail over the guide rod and, with a mallet, drives it down the proximal fragment to enter the distal fragment, crossing the fracture site. The nail is not fully seated.
9. The guide rod is removed to prevent incarceration, and the surgeon completes the seating of the nail. The proximal tip of the nail should be flush with the tibial entry site.

FIGURE 20-58 Tibial intramedullary nailing. **A,** Attachment of nail to proximal drill guide. **B,** Driving nail over guide rod. **C,** Final seating of nail with its tip flush with tibial entry portal. **D,** For proximal interlocking, cortex is dimpled. **E,** Depth measurements are made. **F,** Locking screw length is confirmed. **G,** Self-tapping screw is inserted through drill sleeve.

10. Proximal locking is accomplished with the corresponding drill and tap through the proximal drill guide for 5-mm cortical bone screws.
11. Using the distal targeting device or a freehand technique, the surgeon inserts the distal screws. The 5-mm cortical bone screws are inserted, traversing the tibia through the tibial nail.
12. The surgeon irrigates the wounds. If bone graft is to be used, the surgeon places it around the fracture site and then closes the wound. Dressings are applied, and a cast or splint for immobilization may be applied.

Dynamization, or removal of either the proximal or the distal screws, may take place after 3 months for fractures that are stable but lack callus. Dynamization produces compressive forces at the fracture, thereby promoting osteogenesis.

Tibial Dynamic Compression Plating

1. The surgeon makes a longitudinal incision large enough to accommodate the selected plate lateral to the tibial crest and exposes the fracture site.
2. The periosteum is stripped only enough for application of the plate. Circumferential stripping can diminish blood supply.
3. The surgeon reduces the fracture, places a plate across the fracture site, and secures the plate with bone-holding and plate-holding forceps. The plate may have to be contoured with a handheld or plate-bending press.
4. Using the neutral drill guide, the surgeon drills a 3.2-mm bicortical hole into the plate screw hole close to the fracture site, gauges it, and taps to 4.5 mm. The first bone screw is inserted, ensuring purchase of the screw on the opposite cortex.
5. Using the load drill guide (eccentric), the surgeon drills a second hole next to the fracture line in the opposite fragment. Drill and tap are accomplished as in the previous step. As the screw enters the bone, it will seek the center of the screw hole (the screw is eccentric, and the screw hole is beveled). The fracture site is brought under compression as the screw seats into the hole.
6. The wounds are irrigated. If bone graft is to be used, the surgeon places it around the fracture site and then closes the wound. Dressings are applied, and a cast or splint for immobilization may be applied.

Surgery of the Ankle and Foot

Correction of Ankle Fractures

Ankle fractures include fractures of the medial malleolus (tibia), lateral malleolus (fibula), and posterior malleolus (posterior aspect of the articular surface of the distal end of the tibia). They may or may not be associated with ligamentous injury. Ankle fractures can be classified in anatomic lines as unimalleolar, bimalleolar, and trimalleolar. Because medial malleolar and posterior malleolar fractures involve the distal weight-bearing articular surface of the tibia, open reduction and anatomic alignment are necessary. Fixation of the lateral malleolus is also important because it forms the ankle mortise—the socket formed by the distal tibia and fibula into which the body of the talus fits.

Anatomic reduction prevents the occurrence of degenerative joint disease. Displaced fractures are treated with pins, malleolar or bone screws, or plates and screws (Figure 20-59). Bimalleolar fractures can be treated with closed reduction and casting, but approximately 10% of these eventually develop a nonunion. The lateral malleolus (distal end of the fibula) is important for lateral and rotational stability of the joint. Open reduction and internal fixation using Steinmann pins or screws placed obliquely into the tibia

FIGURE 20-59 Plate-screw placement for lateral malleolar fragment repair using one-third tubular plate.

is a common technique. Lateral malleolar fractures can be fixed with the cancellous lag technique—overdrilling the first fragment and allowing compression of the fragments. Fracture of the lateral malleolus can also be treated with a Rush rod, inserted through the fragment and into the fibular canal. Compared with the other varieties of fractures, trimalleolar fractures require surgery more frequently. The posterior lip of the articulating surface of the tibia is usually involved and needs to be anatomically reduced to minimize degenerative changes. Cannulated screws can provide efficient reduction of a posterior fragment.

Procedural Considerations. The patient is in the supine position. The affected leg is prepped and draped after application of a pneumatic tourniquet. If the lateral ankle is involved, a padded sandbag is placed beneath the hip to internally rotate it. A soft tissue set; a small bone set; a small-fragment set with plates, screws, and pins; a power drill; and bone-reduction clamps are required.

Operative Procedure
ORIF Trimalleolar Fracture

1. The surgeon makes medial and lateral incisions across the ankle.
2. The posterior malleolar fracture is exposed and reduced with bone-holding clamps and manipulation.
3. The surgeon inserts two Kirschner wires above the anterior tibial lip to temporarily reduce the fracture. The wires are directed anteriorly to posteriorly, to engage both fragments.
4. A drill hole is made anteriorly to posteriorly through both fragments. After measuring with a depth gauge, a malleolar, small cancellous, or other preferred screw is inserted through the fracture. The wires are removed.
5. The surgeon manipulates the lateral malleolar fracture into reduction.
6. If the fracture is oblique and not comminuted, the surgeon reduces it with one or two lag screws placed anteriorly to posteriorly. If the fracture is transverse, the surgeon inserts a long screw or medullary pin across the fracture line into the canal of the proximal fragment. A small semitubular or one-third tubular plate is applied if the fracture occurs above the syndesmosis.

7. Once the posterior and lateral malleolar fractures have been fixed, the medial malleolar fracture is finally reduced using bone clamps.

8. The reduction is held with two Kirschner wires while a hole is drilled through the medial malleolus into the metaphysis of the tibia.

9. Using a depth gauge, the surgeon determines the screw length. The malleolar screw is inserted across the fracture site and the Kirschner wires are removed.

10. If rotational stability is needed, the surgeon may add an additional smaller screw or compression wiring.

11. Intraoperative radiographs are taken in AP, lateral, and mortise views.

12. The wounds are irrigated and closed, and a short or long leg cast or splint is applied.

Triple Arthrodesis

The talocalcaneal (subtalar), talonavicular, and calcaneocuboid joints must be fused in patients with pronounced inversion or eversion deformities of the foot. Such deformities occur in clubfoot, poliomyelitis, and rheumatoid arthritis. Occasionally this operation is necessary for patients who have pain resulting from degenerative or traumatic arthritis, such as that occurring after intra-articular fractures of the calcaneus. Triple arthrodesis limits motion of the foot and ankle to plantar flexion and dorsiflexion.

Procedural Considerations. The perioperative nurse assists with positioning the patient in the supine position and preps the patient from the midcalf down to and including the foot. The perioperative nurse should consult with the surgeon before the procedure to determine if bone grafting is anticipated so the patient's iliac crest area can be prepped.

A soft tissue set; a small bone set; a power saw, drill, or rasp; a bone graft set; and the AO compression plates and screws or bone staples to hold the fusion are required. Kirschner wires can be used to provide temporary fixation. A small lamina spreader is helpful in providing exposure.

Operative Procedure

1. An anterior or anterolateral approach is used.
2. The surgeon exposes the subtalar and calcaneocuboid joints and the lateral portion of the talonavicular joint.
3. The surgeon incises the capsules of the talonavicular, calcaneocuboid, and subtalar joints circumferentially to obtain as much mobility as possible. If this release allows the foot to be placed into a normal position, removal of large bony wedges is not required.
4. Using an osteotome, power saw, or power rasp, the surgeon removes the articular surfaces of the calcaneocuboid joint, the subtalar joint, and the talonavicular joint. The small lamina spreader is used to expose these surfaces. Care is taken to save all bone removed for later use in the fusion.
5. The removed bone is cut into small pieces to be used for bone grafting. If the quantity is insufficient, the surgeon will harvest additional bone from the anterior ilium. Most of the bone is placed around the talonavicular joint and in the depth of the sinus tarsi.
6. Smooth Steinmann pins, staples, or screws are used for internal fixation.
7. The wound is closed over a suction drain. A short leg cast or splint is applied.

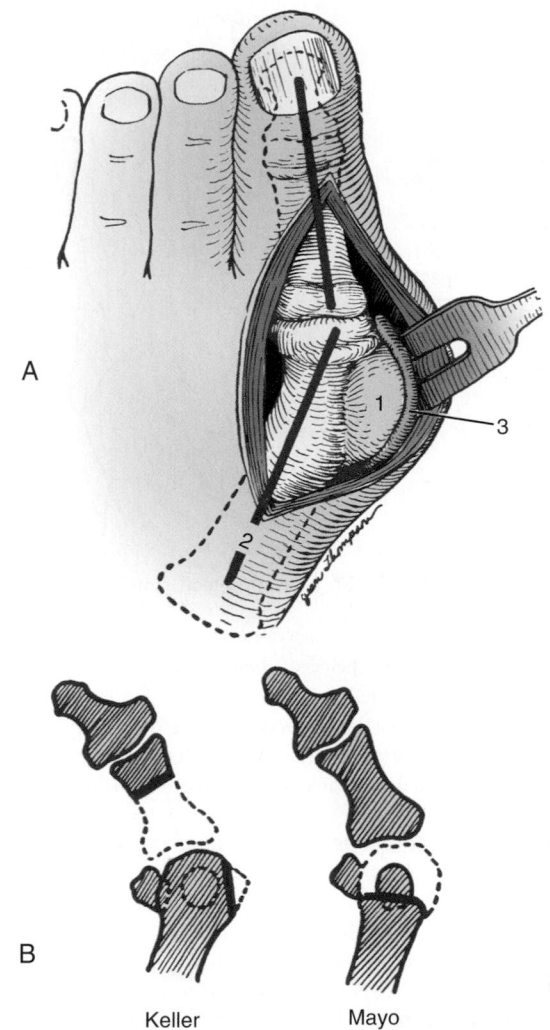

FIGURE 20-60 Bunionectomy. **A,** Bunion. *(1),* Exostosis of metatarsal head; *(2),* hallux valgus deformity; *(3),* overlying bursa. **B,** Operations for hallux valgus.

Bunionectomy

A bunion (hallux valgus) is a soft tissue or bony mass at the medial side of the first metatarsal head. It is associated with a valgus deformity of the great toe (Figure 20-60). A bunion is caused by a basic structural defect of the foot, which predisposes to the development of this deformity. Ill-fitting shoes accentuate the situation and speed the development of bunions. Bunions are more common in women because of shoe styles, including high heels and pointed toes. Other factors that may contribute to this deformity are heredity, flat feet, foot pronation, longer first toe, muscle imbalance, and inflammatory disturbances of the feet.

Symptoms include pain on the dorsomedial aspect of the first metatarsal head or directly over the medial exostosis, swelling of the big toe, painful plantar callus, and plantar keratosis. Discomfort to the entire foot occurs as the forefoot becomes more fatigued and symptomatic, with pain radiating to the leg and knee.

Hallux valgus is treated with a variety of surgical procedures (Figure 20-61). All these procedures remove the exostosis and attempt to realign the great toe by removal of bone, transfer of

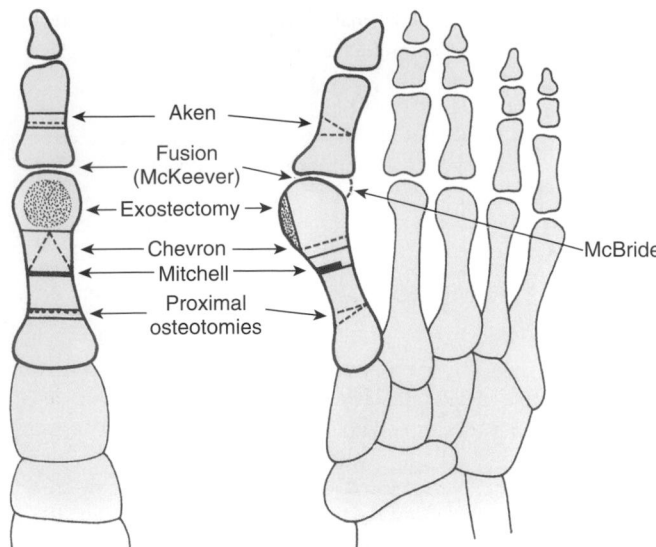

FIGURE 20-61 Types of bunionectomies.

tendons, osteotomy of the first metatarsal shaft, or appropriate imbrication of soft tissue.

The goals of surgery are correction of the deformity (cosmesis), resection of the abnormal bony components (reconstruction), and restoration of normal or near-normal range of motion (function).

Procedural Considerations. The anesthesia provider administers a general or regional anesthetic, and a tourniquet is applied. The foot and leg are prepped and then draped using a sterile stockinette.

A soft tissue set, a small bone set, Kirschner wires, a power wire driver, and a microsagittal saw are required.

Operative Procedure
Keller Procedure

1. The surgeon makes a midline, straight, medial incision beginning at the neck of the proximal phalanx and extended proximally.
2. Using blunt and sharp dissection, the surgeon exposes the joint capsule. A flap incision is made to expose the underlying hypertrophic bone found at the dorsomedial aspect of the first metatarsal head.
3. All soft tissue attachments are removed from the base of the proximal phalanx.
4. The surgeon uses a power-oscillating saw to resect the proximal third of the proximal phalanx.
5. Proper alignment of the toe is maintained as one or two 0.062-inch Kirschner wires are placed in the center of the medullary canal of the phalanx and then driven into the metatarsal head, neck, and shaft.
6. The surgeon irrigates and closes the wound. A bandage is applied to maintain the toe in the correct position.
7. Postoperative convalescence requires a minimum of 6 weeks.

Correction of Hammer Toe Deformity

The term *hammer toe* is most often used to describe an abnormal flexion posture of the proximal interphalangeal joint of one of the four lesser toes. This deformity causes painful calluses to develop on the dorsal joints of the four lesser toes because the cocked-up digits rub against the shoes. Incising the long extensor tendon to

the toes and fusing the proximal interphalangeal joint treat the deformities. A smooth Kirschner wire is frequently used to stabilize the fusion and position the toe properly during the postoperative period.

Procedural Considerations. The patient is positioned supine. An ankle tourniquet is applied. The foot is prepped and draped. A soft tissue set, a small bone set, Kirschner wires, and a power wire driver are required.

Operative Procedure

1. The surgeon makes an elliptic incision over the proximal interphalangeal joint measuring 5 to 6 mm wide with a 2- or 3-mm lateral extension on either side.
2. The capsular tissue of the distal third of the proximal phalanx and proximal interphalangeal joint is entered to expose the defect completely.
3. Using a small rongeur or microsaw, the surgeon resects the distal third portion of the proximal phalanx. After the capital fragment is excised, the surgeon debrides the remaining portion of the distal proximal phalanx with a rongeur or rasp.
4. Digital alignment can be maintained with small Kirschner wires.
5. The surgeon irrigates and closes the wounds. A sterile dressing and orthopedic shoe are applied for postoperative recovery.

Correction of Metatarsal Fractures

Metatarsal fractures occur in various sites. These fractures have a reduced healing potential because metatarsals consist mainly of cortical bone, which lacks vascularity. Treatment is determined by the extent of the fracture—the greater the displacement, the greater the need for reduction. In general, transverse and short, oblique, midshaft fractures of the metatarsals are internally fixed because of their instability and displacement. Pins, wires, screws, and plates are used for internal fixation of metatarsal fractures. The simplest method is Kirschner wire fixation.

Procedural Considerations. The patient is placed in the supine position, a tourniquet is applied, and the foot is prepped and draped. A soft tissue set, a small bone set, Kirschner wires, and a power wire driver are required.

Operative Procedure

1. The surgeon makes a small incision over the fracture and identifies and retracts the distal fragment.
2. A smooth Kirschner wire is driven distally, exiting the skin.
3. The surgeon uses a wire driver to drive the wire proximally into the canal of the proximal fragment.
4. If the fracture is more complex or comminuted, the surgeon may cross two Kirschner wires through the fracture to transfix the fracture site.
5. The incision is closed, and a postoperative shoe is applied.

Metatarsal Head Resection

Patients with rheumatoid arthritis frequently have dorsally dislocated toes and prominent and painful metatarsal heads on the plantar surfaces of their feet. Excision of all the metatarsal heads commonly relieves the pain and corrects an associated bunion deformity.

Procedural Considerations. The patient is placed in the supine position, a tourniquet is applied, and the foot is prepped and draped. A soft tissue set, a small bone set, Kirschner wires, a power wire driver, and a power microsagittal saw are required.

Operative Procedure
Clayton Technique

1. A transverse plantar incision is made, and tissue is dissected to the metatarsal heads.
2. Using a microsagittal saw the surgeon removes the metatarsal heads and half the proximal phalanges.
3. The surgeon transects the extensor tendons; they are not repaired.
4. The skin is closed, and a dressing and postoperative shoe are applied.

Pelvic Fractures and Disruption

Patients with multiple trauma often present with multiple fractures that can be life-threatening. Complications of pelvic fractures include injury to not only major vessels and nerves but also major visceral organs, such as the intestines, bladder, and urethra. Factors influencing mortality include associated visceral injury, hemorrhage, and head injury.

Pelvic fracture classification is divided into three main groups (Table 20-1). *Type A fractures* are stable, without ring involvement (A1) or minimally displaced fractures of the ring (A2). *Type B fractures* are rotationally unstable and vertically stable and are also subclassified: B1 is an open book fracture, B2 has ipsilateral compression, and B3 has contralateral compression. *Type C fractures* are both rotationally and vertically unstable: C1 is unilateral, C2 is bilateral, and C3 is associated with the acetabulum. Radiographic films, computed tomography (CT) scan, and magnetic resonance imaging (MRI) all prove useful in determining the type and appropriate treatment for pelvic trauma.

Treatment is based on classification and may include closed manipulation and reduction or internal and external fixation. Internal and external fixation can be used concurrently in the treatment of some pelvic fractures.

Type A fractures are stable and can be treated nonoperatively. Type B1 fractures may be treated with external fixation or anterior plate fixation. Type C fractures usually require open procedures to fix the fractures with plates and screws, and reduction of sacral disruptions with transiliac rods or screws. Type C fractures may be treated with external fixation when the patient is hemodynamically unstable and a quicker, simpler procedure is prudent.

External fixation is the most widely recommended treatment for type B fractures of the pelvis. A technique similar to that of external fixation of extremity fractures is done in the OR with anesthesia and sterile conditions. If external fixation is to be used, the earlier it is attempted the greater the chance of success.

Procedural Considerations

This procedure is often done during other emergent and trauma resuscitative efforts. The patient's entire pelvic area is prepped and draped. Pin placement is performed to complete the reduction. A soft tissue set is needed in addition to the external fixator of choice and the instruments for its insertion, including a power drill.

Operative Procedure
AO External Fixation

1. The surgeon reduces the pelvic disruption manually and confirms it radiographically. It may be impossible to completely reduce the disruption without skeletal traction using a distal femoral pin.
2. Kirschner wires are inserted percutaneously to determine the position of the pin placement, taking into consideration the inward and downward crest slope.
3. The surgeon places parallel rows of pins into the anterior iliac crest area by drilling the outer cortex and placing 5-mm half-pins medially and distally. The pins should enter cancellous bone between the outer and inner tables of ilium.
4. Three universal frames are placed over the pins as close to the skin as possible for maximum rigidity.
5. Optimal reduction of the fracture is visualized using radiography. The surgeon applies the crossbar, and compression and distraction maneuvers are used to maintain the reduction.
6. The surgeon removes the crossbar and applies the connecting rods with couplers.
7. After the couplers are in place, the surgeon reattaches the crossbar and tightens the joints of the frame.
8. The pin sites of tented skin are released. The wounds are dressed with iodine ointment and gauze.
9. The frames are left in place generally for 8 to 12 weeks.

Total Joint Arthroplasty

Arthroplasty of the joints is performed to restore motion of the joint and function to the muscles and ligaments. It is indicated in individuals with a painful, disabling arthritic joint that is no longer responsive to conservative therapy. In the past, the procedure was reserved for those with a less active lifestyle, and surgeons treated patients with reconstructive procedures such as arthrodesis or osteotomy because of the unknown life expectancy of the materials used in the manufacturing of the prostheses. Technologic advances in the prostheses used today allow the younger patient, or the very active older person, to undergo joint replacement. Many total hip and knee replacements are done each year. Improvements in implant design, materials, and fixation techniques are ongoing, as is research on enhancing soft and hard tissue healing.

The classic combination of metal on polyethylene is the mainstay of joint implants. Metals used in hip and knee implants include *cobalt-chromium* (weight-bearing femoral head) and *titanium* (stems of hips and tibial components). The acetabulum and tibial articulating surfaces continue to be substituted with *ultra-high-molecular-weight polyethylene* (UHMWPE), which provides superior wear characteristics. Other designs have emerged in total hip arthroplasty, including metal on metal and the use of ceramic femoral heads.

At one time it was thought that bone cement was the weak link in the longevity of a joint implant because of a relatively high rate of loosening of cement-fixed implants, especially in younger, more

---

TABLE 20-1

Classification of Pelvic Injuries

Type A	Stable
	A1—Fractures of pelvis not involving ring
	A2—Stable, minimally displaced fractures of ring
Type B	Rotationally unstable, vertically stable
	B1—Open book
	B2—Lateral compression: ipsilateral
	B3—Lateral compression: contralateral (bucket handle)
Type C	Rotationally and vertically unstable
	C1—Unilateral
	C2—Bilateral
	C3—Associated with an acetabular fracture

active patients. In response to this belief, alternative methods of fixation have been developed. One method involves the application of a precoat of PMMA to the femoral stem to enhance bonding of the prosthesis to the cement mantle. Another method involves the attachment of a porous metal surface to parts of the femoral stem and the entire outer surface of the acetabular component. Most of the porous surfaces are composed of multiple layers sintered in place, creating interconnecting, open pores among the various particles. This allows for the ingrowth of bone to occur, ultimately anchoring the prosthesis in place. "Porous coating" was an attempt to eradicate what was termed *cement disease*—a lysis of bone around the prosthesis causing early loosening. It is now believed that this condition is caused by "wear debris"—particulate matter being shed from metal-to-polyethylene interfaces—and not necessarily from the effects of PMMA.

Bone cement, or PMMA, has received considerable attention in the search for optimal bone-to-implant fixation. Cement seems to exhibit various degrees of porosity depending on mixing methods and cement pressurization within the canal. Bone cement must prevent motion at the implant interface. Porosity can lead to fatigue and fracture, which ultimately can lead to implant loosening. Local tissue effects of PMMA may include: (1) tissue protein coagulation caused by polymerization, (2) bone necrosis caused by occlusion of nutrient metaphyseal arteries, and (3) cytotoxic and lipotoxic effects of nonpolymerized monomer.

Despite the high rate of success of total joint implantation over the years, there are numerous potential complications. They are generally divided into medical complications, mechanical complications, and infections. Medical complications include, but are not limited to, cardiac dysrhythmias, myocardial infarction, hemorrhage (Research Highlight), and pulmonary emboli. Mechanical complications are implant breakage, loosening, and wear. Infection in the patient with a total joint implant is a catastrophic complication that usually requires additional surgery and prolonged hospitalization.

Most surgeons recommend the routine use of antibiotics in primary and revision joint arthroplasty. Antibiotic coverage is initiated preoperatively, continued during lengthy procedures, and administered for 24 to 48 hours postoperatively. The Surgical Care Improvement Project (SCIP) measures have been instituted by the TJC in order to prevent surgical site infections (TJC, 2012). Pulsatile lavage systems with antibiotic irrigation are used to keep tissues moist, remove debris, and dilute bacteria that may be present. Multimodal pain management has led to decreased complications and length of hospital stay (Research Highlight).

Total Hip Arthroplasty

Total hip arthroplasty is a common orthopedic procedure performed on patients with hip pain caused by degenerative joint disease, rheumatoid arthritis, or avascular necrosis. A total hip replacement can be cemented, noncemented, or hybrid. Hybrids involve cementing one component, usually the femoral stem, and then inserting a metal-backed, porous-coated acetabular component in a press-fit state. Hybrid arthroplasty is a controversial procedure for two reasons. The first relates to research that demonstrates that wear debris is increased with the larger metal-to-polyethylene interface present in the metal-backed, porous-coated acetabular component. The second relates to cost. The metal-backed, porous-coated acetabular component is significantly more expensive than the all-polyethylene component. Consequently, patient selection is very important in determining which type of component is best.

The primary function of the femoral component is the replacement of the femoral head and femoral neck after resection. The femoral head should ultimately sit where it reproduces the center of rotation of the hip. The neck length is variable and is built into several different heights of femoral heads that are eventually seated onto the Morse taper of the femoral stem. The version (implant rotation within the canal) is very important; too much anteversion or retroversion leaves the hip prone to dislocation. The normal position of the proximal femur is in 10 to 15 degrees of anteversion.

Femoral stems can be collarless or have collars that sit down on the resected femur. Collars produce forces on the bone and may be desired in cases of osteoporotic bone, where bone genesis may be diminished because of the disease process.

Acetabular cups have also presented challenges in trying to maintain fixation within the socket. When cement techniques of the 1970s were used, femoral loosening plateaued about 5 years after surgery. Wear properties of the UHMWPE are also a concern. For this and other reasons associated with component failure, the idea of modularity was developed. Modular components, such as a polyethylene cup that snaps into a metal acetabular shell, greatly decrease the amount of surgery needed in the case of some revisions. In the case of excessive cup wear or a short femoral neck, surgery

---

RESEARCH HIGHLIGHT ▐▐

Preventing Blood Loss with Tranexamic Acid

Tranexamic acid (TA) use in total joint surgery has been successful in minimizing blood loss. Surgery and venous stasis result in the activation of the fibrinolytic system and the release of tissue plasminogen activator. TA inhibits fibrinolysis by blocking the lysine-binding sites of the plasminogen. Studies have found by administering TA prior to incision, there was a significant decrease in postoperative bleeding. Reductions in postoperative drainage and blood transfusions were noted.

Modified from Sepah YJ et al: *Use of tranexamic acid is a cost effective method in preventing blood loss during and after total knee replacement*, available at www.josr-online.com/content. Accessed June 1, 2012; Singh J et al: Effects of tranexamic acid on blood loss during total hip arthroplasty, *J Orthop Surg* 18(3):282–286, 2010.

RESEARCH HIGHLIGHT ▐▐

Postoperative Pain Management

Patients undergoing a total joint arthroplasty in the past have experienced differing amounts of pain postoperatively. Recent studies have shown multimodal pain management beginning preoperatively is key to successfully limiting patient pain following surgery. Preoperative medications can include antiinflammatories, neuromodulators, and oral narcotics given preemptively. Intraoperative injections are the second line of defense for pain management. These could include a combination of local anesthetics, ketorolac, and corticosteroids. Local anesthetic can also be delivered directly to the surgical site via a continuous pain pump. Postoperative pain management with patient-controlled analgesia pumps, femoral blocks, and oral medication supplemented with injections were used. Decreased narcotic consumption, decreased length of stay, and improved patient pain scores were found when using a multimodal approach to pain management.

Modified from Post ZD et al: A prospective evaluation of two different pain management protocols for total hip arthroplasty, *J Arthroplasty* 25:410–415, 2010; Mullaji A et al: Efficacy of periarticular injection of bupivacaine, fentanyl, and methylprednisone in total knee arthroplasty: a prospective, randomized trial, *J Arthroplasty* 25:851–857, 2010.

is minimized with the ability to exchange the modular components without removing the implants fixed to the bone.

Acetabular cups come with a textured back for cement fixation and may have standoff pegs to allow an appropriate cement mantle. Noncemented cups usually are porous coated and may have screw holes to aid in anchoring the less-than-stable cup. The presence of screw holes in an acetabular component is another controversial issue. Some believe that more wear debris is created with micromotion between the screw head and the cup as well as between the uneven surface of the screw and the polyethylene liner.

Prostheses are available for every patient's needs. Modular hip systems allow the orthopedic surgeon to choose from an array of interchangeable components that have been developed. Various femoral head sizes (22, 26, 28, and 32 mm) are available to maintain proper center of rotation. Acetabular cups may be snap fit, low profile, or deep profile, which adds additional thickness to the medial wall, where bone loss may be significant.

With modular systems, unipolar or bipolar cups are also an option when the acetabular articular surface is relatively normal. The unipolar and bipolar cups with appropriate head sizes are designed to fit on various modular system stems.

Custom prostheses or revision and extra-long stems are available when bone loss is significant. These implants are used in cases of revision when fixation is needed farther down the femoral canal or in oncologic cases in which tumor and corresponding bone have been resected.

Young, active individuals with strong, healthy bones are ideal candidates for noncemented total hip replacement arthroplasties. Elderly patients with osteoporosis and poor-quality bone are usually candidates for cemented components because their bones may lack the compressive strength to support weight-bearing forces.

Several different surgical techniques have been developed for total hip arthroplasty. Surgical techniques have improved over the years focusing on minimizing soft tissue insult.

Hip Reconstruction (Cemented). Numerous implants are available for total hip implantation. Many of the implants can be used for the same surgical indications, and one implant may not function any better than another, provided that all other conditions and techniques are the same. The instruments required to implant any one device cannot be used for another. During the preoperative verification process and time-out, the perioperative nurse and scrub person collaborate to ensure that all the instrumentation is available.

PMMA adheres to the polyethylene and metal but not to the bone. It fills the cavity and interstices of the bone and forms a mechanical bond. PMMA is manufactured as a liquid monomer and a powder, and is mixed under sterile conditions by the scrub person in the OR at the time of implantation. It usually takes 10 to 12 minutes to harden. Because of the potentially harmful effects of PMMA fumes to the nasal epithelium, an exhaust system should be used during the mixing process.

Procedural Considerations. The patient is positioned in the lateral decubitus position and secured in place with anterior and posterior bolsters. This position is essential to ensure correct anatomic placement of the acetabular cup. The perioperative nurse verifies that the patient's bony prominences are adequately padded. The skin prep is completed from the level of the umbilicus down to and including the foot; then the patient is draped. The radiographs are overlaid with the implant templates.

A soft tissue set and a large bone set are required. In addition, the total hip implants and corresponding instrumentation, acetabular reamers, hip retractor set, power reamer driver and saw, and

pulse lavage with a 3-L bag of normal saline solution are needed. If PMMA is used, femoral canal suction wicks, a cement restrictor and its inserter, and PMMA including its mixing supplies will be needed. If a trochanteric osteotomy is performed, the equipment of choice for its reattachment will be required.

Revision of total hip arthroplasties requires the same instrumentation as for cemented total hip reconstruction in addition to cement removal instrumentation, fluoroscopy, and the revision implants and their corresponding instrumentation.

Operative Procedure
Cemented Modular Hip System, Posterior Approach

1. The surgeon makes an incision 2.5 cm distal and lateral to the anterosuperior iliac spine and curves the incision distally and posteriorly over the lateral aspect of the greater trochanter and lateral surface of the femoral shaft to 5 cm distal to the base of the trochanter.

2. The surgeon divides the tensor fasciae latae over the greater trochanter, and carries this distally to the extent of the incision. Dissection is carried proximally between the interval of the gluteus medius and the tensor fasciae latae muscles.

3. The anterior fibers of the gluteus medius tendon are tagged and detached from the trochanter. The surgeon incises the capsule longitudinally along the anterosuperior surface of the femoral neck. In the distal part of the incision, the origin of the vastus lateralis may be either reflected distally or split longitudinally to expose the base of the trochanter and proximal part of the femoral shaft.

4. After completing the capsulotomy, the surgeon dislocates the hip. Adduction and external rotation present the femoral head anteriorly into the surgical site.

5. The surgeon places the femoral osteotomy guide over the lateral femur to identify the point on the femoral neck where the osteotomy should be made. Some femoral osteotomy guides also gauge the neck length required. The surgeon marks the level and uses an oscillating or a reciprocating saw to complete the femoral osteotomy.

6. The femur is retracted to expose the acetabulum, allow completion of the capsulotomy, and expose the bony rim of the entire acetabulum.

7. The surgeon inspects the acetabulum, removes any osteophytes, and reams the articular cartilage with bone-conserving reamers in a circumferential manner. The smallest reamer is progressed in a graduated method 1 or 2 mm at a time until the cartilage is reamed down to expose osteochondral bone. A hemispheric shape and bleeding bone should result.

8. Remaining soft tissue is curetted from the floor of the acetabulum, and cystic areas are filled with cancellous bone from the femoral canal and packed with a bone tamp. Any other bone grafting of major bony defects is accomplished using the fixation method of choice (bone screws).

9. Several 6-mm holes are drilled into the floor of the acetabulum, aimed into the ilium, ischium, and pubis. Holes are undercut using curettes. These prepared holes act as anchoring areas for the bone cement.

10. Trial acetabular components are placed on the positioning device and positioned in the socket. The surgeon assesses the cup for size, position within the socket, and the relationship of the component compared with the bony margins of the acetabulum.

11. The prepared acetabular socket is lavaged, dried with wicks, and filled with cement that has been injected and pressurized with an injection gun. The surgeon positions the acetabular

shell component and holds it motionless until the cement polymerizes. Extruded cement is trimmed from around the edge of the component. A polyethylene insert is later snapped into the shell.

12. A radiopaque soft good is placed in the acetabulum to protect the component from bone debris and subsequent cement as attention is turned to the femur.

13. Dropping the patient's foot toward the floor and internally rotating and pushing the leg proximally expose the proximal femur. The surgeon accesses the femoral canal using a box osteotome or trochanteric reamer followed by the T-handle canal reamer.

14. Beginning with the smallest broach, the surgeon alternately impacts and extracts the proximal femoral canal. Progressively larger broaches are used to crush and remove cancellous bone until cortical bone is reached. A broach that is not advancing should not be used because this could result in shattering the femur.

15. With the final broach seated to the desired depth in the canal, the neck is prepared with a calcar reamer. The broach remains while the surgeon places the femoral trial component along with the various-size head, neck, and offset trial components.

16. The trial component is removed, and the canal is lavaged and brushed to accommodate the PMMA.

17. A cement restrictor is inserted into the femoral canal. The femoral components are passed and assembled on the back table.

18. The cement is injected and pressurized within the femoral canal.

19. The femoral component, with the proximal and distal centralizers, is inserted into the canal with or without the femoral head.

20. The surgeon positions the appropriate size of femoral head onto the stem, and reduction is carried out. The joint is taken through a range of motion to check for positioning, stability, and the limit to which dislocation occurs.

21. Depending on the surgeon and the surgical approach, the greater trochanter may or may not have been removed for exposure of the hip joint. If removed, it is reattached with 18-gauge wire or a cable grip system.

22. The surgeon closes the wound in layers over suction drains. The skin is closed with staples, and a sterile dressing is applied to provide compression to the wound.

23. An abduction pillow or splint is placed between the patient's legs postoperatively if stability of the joint is of concern.

Hip Reconstruction (Noncemented). Fixation with a noncemented prosthesis is initially accomplished by a tight fit and intimate contact of the implants within bone of substantial strength. As with all prosthetic designs, it is essential to fill the medullary canal and wedge the prosthesis in as tightly as possible to provide temporary press-fit fixation. These prostheses closely follow normal anatomic shape. Only the instrumentation corresponding to the implant should be used. Precise machining of the femoral canal must be ensured. Acetabular components are usually press-fitted, but many systems provide holes for screw fixation if stability of the prosthesis is in doubt. Sufficient time is then allowed for the cancellous bone to heal by growing into the porous portions of the prosthesis.

The healing process requires the same amount of time as a long bone cortical fracture (approximately 3 months). The patient must

be cautious after the procedure and protect the operative hip from excessive compression, rotation, and shear stresses.

Procedural Considerations. The position and incision are the same as those used for the cemented total hip replacement. The radiographs and implant templates are placed on the view box.

Operative Procedure
Noncemented Anatomic Medullary Locking (AML) Hip System (Figure 20-62)

1. After the incision is made, the surgeon enters the capsule and dislocates the femoral head.

2. A pilot hole is established in the trochanteric fossa as an intramedullary reference point.

3. The surgeon uses progressively sized fully fluted rigid reamers to ream the intramedullary canal.

4. A femoral neck osteotomy is achieved by positioning an osteotomy template along the axis of the femur and cutting at the level of the collar.

5. The surgeon clears the soft tissue from the acetabulum and reams it with hemispheric reamers.

6. Trial acetabular sizers are placed to determine the correct position and size of the prosthetic component.

7. The surgeon uses a hollow osteotome in the femoral canal to connect the pilot hole to the osteotomy site.

8. Femoral broaches are then inserted to enlarge the intramedullary space for trial insertion.

9. The surgeon may use a power calcar planer placed over the trunnion of the broach to contour the femoral neck.

10. A trial head and neck component is positioned onto the fitted broach, and a trial reduction is carried out.

11. If trial reduction is satisfactory, the surgeon removes all the trial components.

12. The appropriate size of acetabular component is inserted into the acetabulum, and a polyethylene insert is locked into place.

13. The femoral component is placed into the canal, and the modular head is seated on the trunnion.

14. Reduction of the hip is followed by standard closure with drains.

15. Abduction of the hip is maintained postoperatively with a foam abduction pillow if necessary.

Minimally Invasive Total Hip Arthroplasty. Minimally invasive total hip arthroplasty (MITHA) has resulted in minimized scarring, reduced patient morbidity, a shortened hospitalization period, and an accelerated rehabilitation process (Dorr et al, 2010). MITHA can be performed with a single or double incision. For a single incision, the patient is placed in a lateral position; the patient is supine for a double-incision procedure. With double-incision MITHA, the acetabular and femoral components are inserted through two small incisions, one anterolateral and one posterolateral, each approximately 5 cm long. The technique spares the muscles and tendons around the hip.

Procedural Considerations. As with any joint replacement, templates of the x-rays preoperatively are recommended. A regular OR bed with x-ray capability is used. The perioperative nurse should alert the radiology department that fluoroscopy will be used. Equipment should be arranged carefully (Figure 20-63). The patient is positioned supine with a small bolster placed under the pelvis on the operative side. The patient's entire leg, from above the waist to the ankle, is then prepped and draped in the usual fashion. The time-out includes confirmation of the correct patient, site, side, procedure, position, and implants.

FIGURE 20-62 Noncemented hip reconstruction. **A,** After the incision, the Charnley retractor is placed, the tensor fasciae latae is incised, and the gluteus medius is detached. **B,** An anterior capsulotomy is completed. **C,** The hip is flexed, adducted, and externally rotated to dislocate from the acetabulum. **D,** The femoral neck is cut by use of an oscillating saw blade. **E,** The rim of the acetabulum is debrided of labrum, redundant capsule, and marginal osteophytes. **F,** The acetabulum is reamed; after reaming, the appropriate drill guide is inserted into the acetabulum.

Continued

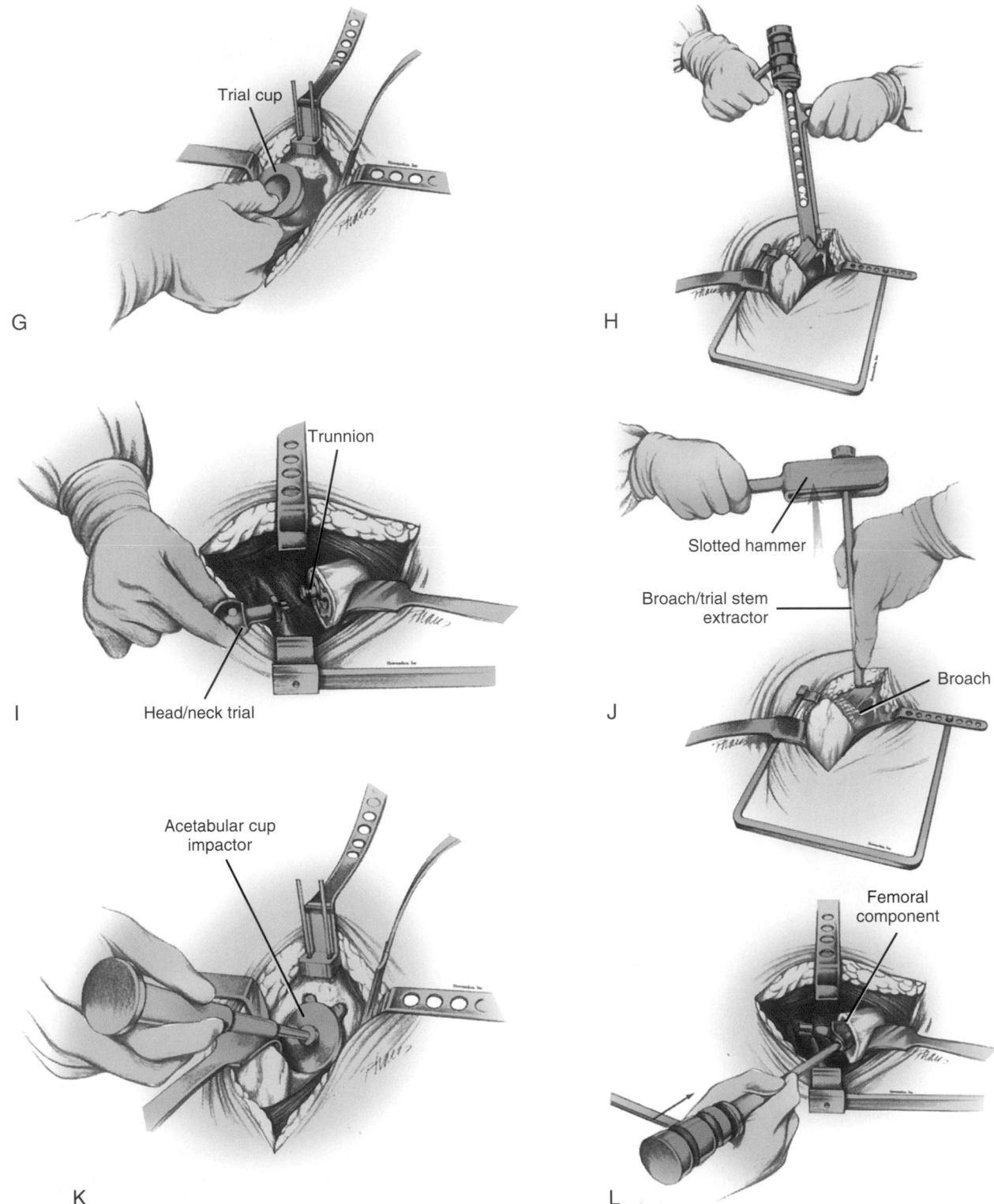

FIGURE 20-62, cont'd **G,** After drilling the holes for the acetabular fixation pegs, the trial acetabular cup is inserted. **H,** The proximal wedge of cancellous bone is removed, and the appropriate size of femoral broach is introduced down the axis of the femoral canal. **I,** The trial head is placed on the broach trunnion of trial reduction. **J,** With the slotted hammer the femoral broach is extracted; the trial acetabular cup is removed. **K,** Acetabular fixation pegs are seated, the acetabular cup is introduced, and the component is seated. **L,** The femoral canal is irrigated with pulsatile lavage and dried with suction and soft goods; the femoral canal is plugged and filled with methylmethacrylate; the femoral component is inserted.

M   N

FIGURE 20-62, cont'd M, The femoral head component is placed on the trunnion. **N,** The femoral head is impacted, the femur is reduced, and the wound is irrigated before closure.

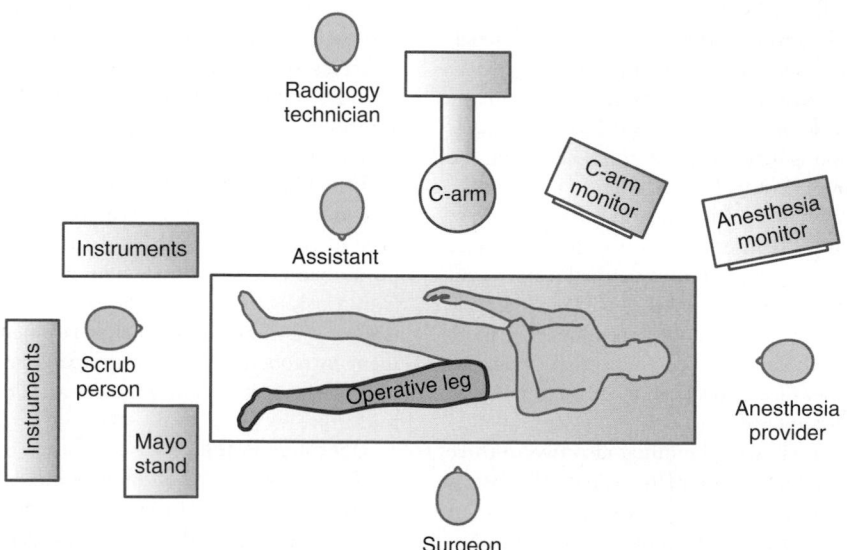

FIGURE 20-63 Illustration of room setup, including positioning of C-arm and monitor, for minimally invasive total hip arthroplasty (MITHA).

Operative Procedure (VerSys Hip System)

1. The C-arm is used to define the femoral neck. The surgeon makes the anterior incision directly over the femoral neck from the base of the femoral head. The lateral femoral cutaneous nerve is identified and located, and then carefully retracted along with the sartorius using an Army Navy retractor. A second retractor is used for the tensor fasciae latae laterally. This exposes the lateral border of the rectus femoris.

2. The surgeon uses an electrosurgical unit (ESU) for hemostasis of the lateral femoral vessels. The Army Navy retractors are extended deeper as the rectus femoris is dissected with a #10 blade on a long handle. An extended blade ESU pencil may also be used.

3. The surgeon incises the femoral capsule and fat pad. A Cobb elevator is used to move the tissue medially underneath the rectus muscles and laterally off the femoral neck, allowing exposure of the capsule over the femoral neck.

4. Two curved lighted retractors are placed outside the capsule around the femoral neck, perpendicular to it. If additional leverage is needed, retractor handle extenders may be attached and used. The femoral capsule is incised in line with the femoral neck lateral to the midline to facilitate future placement of the head of the femoral prosthesis. Sutures can be used to retract the capsule so that the femoral head and neck are clearly visible.

5. Fluoroscopy may then be used to verify osteotomy position. Using the oscillating saw, the surgeon places a high femoral neck cut and uses a straight, 4-cm osteotome to complete it. A second cut is then made, and a threaded Steinmann pin is inserted to remove the small wafer of bone. This allows enough room for the surgeon to make the final femoral neck cut.

6. The surgeon uses fluoroscopy to check the angle and length of resection. It is important for the surgical team to help keep the leg in neutral position, especially during these cuts. The femoral

head is then removed while the surgical assistant applies gentle traction on the leg.

7. Three lighted anterior retractors are placed: one superiorly in the line of the incision, over the acetabulum, and the second and third at 90-degree angles to the first. Once the acetabulum is exposed, sharp and blunt dissection is used to remove remaining tissue and synovium.

8. Reaming starts with the acetabular reamer that is close to the template size. C-arm visualization is used during the reaming. After reaming is completed to the acceptable size, the trial components are placed to determine fit. C-arm images are used to confirm location and size. The positioning bolster is removed at this time. The appropriate-size cup and liner are then chosen. The acetabular component is then seated using the offset shell inserter, retractors are removed, and the cup is impacted into place. Multiple images are taken to check the placement and position of the cup while impacting. The inserter is then removed. If screws are used, a drill, screws, drill guide, depth gauge, and flexible screwdriver will be required. Once the cup and screws are in place, their position is again checked with fluoroscopy. The liner is inserted.

9. The second incision is found by direct palpation. The nonoperative leg is adducted. The operative leg is fully adducted, externally rotated, and flexed over the nonoperative leg. Location is verified by fluoroscopy. A stab wound is made in the posterior lateral buttock and extended to 1.5 to 3 cm as needed. Sharp dissection is used to spread the tissue along the coaxial pathway to the piriformis fossa.

10. Downward pressure is applied to the operative knee to elevate the trochanter. The surgeon inserts the tissue protector and reams the femoral canal beginning with the lateral reamers. All reamers should be inserted in the locked position. After the lateral reaming is complete, intramedullary reamers are used. The surgeon uses fluoroscopy at regular intervals throughout the reaming process to ensure centralization in the canal. The tissue protector is then removed.

11. The surgeon rasps the canal, with the initial rasp two to three times smaller than the template size of the canal. The rasp is tapped into place until fully seated; its position is verified with fluoroscopy. The canal is rasped until proper sizing and positioning are obtained. The C-arm is used to check the final depth, fill, and positioning of the rasp with the apex of the calcar.

12. Trial reduction is done with the final rasp in place. The provisional head is placed on the rasp, and the hip is reduced by providing longitudinal traction and internal rotation. The surgeon moves the hip through a full range of motion. Fluoroscopy may be used to check the levels of the lesser trochanters for possible leg length discrepancies. Once trial reduction is complete, the rasp is removed by way of a posterior exit and the head through the anterior incision.

13. Two lighted anterior retractors are placed in the posterior incision to keep the tissue away from the stem as it is placed in the femoral canal. Once the implant is through the skin and properly rotated, the implant driver is attached. Gentle traction is placed on the leg in neutral abduction. Once the femoral component is within the capsule of the hip, the patient's operative leg is repositioned; it is fully adducted, externally rotated, and flexed over the nonoperative leg. The stem is impacted until it is fully seated. Fluoroscopy is used to ensure proper seating and alignment.

14. The surgeon pulls the neck of the femur through the wound and places the trial head. Traction is placed on the hip, and the hip is then turned into internal rotation. Range-of-motion and leg length assessment is then done.

15. After the final trial reduction is performed, the surgeon dislocates the hip to put the final head in place. Hip dislocation is done using a dull bone hook and external rotation of the hip. Two sutures are placed in the capsule: one medially and the other laterally. This is done before the head is reduced to prevent the capsule from invaginating posteriorly. The prosthetic head can then be seated and impacted. Gentle traction and internal rotation are used to reduce the hip. A final range-of-motion and leg length assessment is performed.

16. The surgeon irrigates the incisions with antibiotic irrigation. A local anesthetic such as bupivacaine (Marcaine) may be infiltrated into the incision, the two previously placed sutures tied, and additional sutures placed to fully close the capsule. A drain may be placed.

Anterolateral Approach for Total Hip Arthroplasty. Bertin and Rottinger (2004) originally described an anterolateral modified Watson-Jones approach to preserve hip abductor function. This approach, between the hip abductor and the tensor fasciae latae, preserves the abductor muscles (Shigemura et al, 2012). It also provides additional inferior surgical field rather than a direct lateral approach and is better in preserving the soft tissue than a direct lateral approach.

Procedural Considerations. The patient is supine on the OR bed, and a hip bolster is placed under the sacrum with the inferior edge of the bump at the ischial tuberosity. A contralateral post is positioned at the opposite side of the torso. Both legs are draped with stockinettes within the sterile field. This surgical approach facilitates accurate component placement and leg length measurement intraoperatively. This approach also provides good visualization of the acetabulum with the aid of specific angled Hohmann retractors.

Operative Procedure

1. The surgeon makes an oblique incision between the anterosuperior iliac spine and the grater trochanter (or through a straight incision made at the anterior border of the trochanter). Visualization of the acetabulum is made with the angled Hohmann retractors. An osteotomy of the femoral neck is made, and a corkscrew facilitates the removal of the femoral head.

2. The Hohmann retractors are repositioned and the surgeon prepares the acetabulum for reaming by removing remaining cartilage with Kocher clamp and knife. The acetabular reaming begins and progresses as the surgeon assesses for cup size and position within the socket. The prepared socket is then lavaged with antibiotic irrigation and the component is placed along the insert.

3. Hyperextension of the hip provides better access to the proximal femur and is accomplished by placing the operative leg under the nonoperative leg, held in place by the second assistant. Using an ESU and a bone hook, the surgeon releases the posterior capsule. Two double-footed retractors are placed over the greater trochanter between the bone and the abductor muscle. A small metal curette is used as a canal finder followed by a canal reamer.

4. The surgeon begins with zero femoral broach, impacting down the canal, followed by sequentially larger broaches until cortical bone is reached. With the final broach seated at the desired

depth, the surgeon places the trial femoral and neck components. The hip is reduced with traction and internal rotation, and the legs are straightened and leg lengths measured. Trial reduction with adjustment of the leg lengths is easily accomplished in the supine position.

5. Once sizes are determined, the patient's leg is again positioned under the nonoperative leg and the Hohmann retractors replaced. The surgeon removes the trial components and lavages the femoral canal with antibiotic irrigation. The femoral component is inserted along with the trial femoral head; leg lengths are again measured. After the final size is determined, femoral head is impacted. The hip is reduced and a final range of motion is performed to check for stability in extension, adduction, and internal rotation.

6. The wound is lavaged and—with a simple juxtaposition of the interval between the vastus lateralis, gluteus medius, and iliotibial muscle—closed.

7. Superficial layers are then closed according to surgeon preference. Dressings are placed.

Total Knee Arthroplasty

Total knee arthroplasty is a surgical procedure designed to replace the worn surfaces of the knee joint. Patients complain of knee pain and instability. Degenerative rheumatoid or traumatic arthritis can result in severe destruction of the entire knee joint, or only the medial or lateral compartments of the knee joint can deteriorate as a result of extreme varus or valgus deformity. Arthroplasty of the knee has been successful in relieving these symptoms. Success depends on patient selection, component design, surgical technique, and rehabilitation.

The challenge of finding the optimal knee implant is in reproducing the complicated range of motion of the knee. Motion of the knee occurs in three planes: flexion and extension, abduction and adduction, and rotation. Designs of total knees should allow preservation of the normal ligaments whenever possible while providing soft tissue balance when necessary to maintain stability.

Total knee implants may be classified into three different categories, according to the portions of the knee to be replaced. *Unicompartmental* implants are used to replace just one opposing articular surface (medial or lateral) of the femur and tibia. *Bicompartmental* designs, mentioned only to demonstrate the progression of total knee design, replaced both the medial and lateral surfaces of the femur and tibia. Most of the total knee replacements completed today are *tricompartmental* implants, which replace not only the opposing femorotibial joint but also the patellofemoral joint.

The tricompartmental knees are further divided into three categories (Figure 20-64). *Unconstrained* prostheses have very little constraint built in between the femoral and tibial components and depend on the integrity of soft tissues to provide stability of the reconstructed joint. Where there is significant deformity and the need for soft tissue release, the surgeon may decide to use a *semiconstrained* prosthesis, which lends itself to more inherent stability necessitated by ligamentous deficiency. *Fully constrained* prostheses are linked together with pure hinges, rotating hinges, and nonhinged designs. They are used in the presence of considerable bone loss, instability, deformity, and revision surgery where bone loss has been significant. Fully constrained prostheses do not provide a normal range of motion, and such a lack of motion leads to excessive wear, implant loosening, and breakage.

Methods of fixation of total knee implants include both cemented and noncemented techniques. The noncemented variety

FIGURE 20-64 Knee arthroplasty implants. **A,** Unconstrained hinge. **B,** Semiconstrained hinge. **C,** Fully constrained hinge.

encompasses both porous bony ingrowth and press-fit designs. The choice of implant and method of fixation depend on the predisposition of the bone, the patient's age and activity level, and the surgeon's comfort with a particular technique. Previous designs did not retain the posterior cruciate ligament, which led to increased joint instability. Newer designs allow the posterior cruciate to be retained. Some surgeons believe that the retention of the posterior cruciate ligament dictates the need for absolute ligament balancing beyond what may be possible in the reconstructed knee.

In the interest of more cost-effective use of medical resources, new designs have been developed for the less-active patient with a shorter expected life span. The femoral component design is a symmetric design that can be used on either the left or the right knee. The tibial component is composed entirely of UHMWPE, thereby lowering manufacturing costs. Both components are placed with the use of PMMA.

Procedural Considerations. The perioperative nurse assists with positioning the patient supine. A tourniquet is applied to the upper thigh. The surgical prep is completed. A soft tissue set and a large bone set; the total knee instruments, trials, and implants of choice; a power drill and saw; PMMA and cement supplies; and a pulse lavage are required.

Operative Procedure
NexGen Total Knee Arthroplasty (Figure 20-65)

1. With the knee flexed, the surgeon makes a straight midline incision from 3 to 4 inches above the patella, ending at the patellar tubercle.
2. The capsule is entered medially. After making a median parapatellar incision, the surgeon places Kocher clamps on both lateral and medial sides of the capsule, and reflects the patella laterally to expose the entire tibiofemoral joint.
3. Hypertrophic synovium, a portion of the infrapatellar fat pad, is excised using a toothed forceps and knife or the ESU, and

FIGURE 20-65 Total knee implant, instrumentation, and procedure. **A,** After exposure of the intercondylar notch, the femoral sizer is placed at the distal end of the femur. **B,** After the femoral canal is reamed, the femoral intramedullary alignment guide is inserted and passed up the medullary canal. **C,** Correct rotational alignment is maintained; the anterior femoral cutting guide is attached to the femoral intramedullary alignment guide. **D,** The femoral cutting guide is mounted in place. **E,** The femur is resected. **F,** Femoral cuts are completed.

FIGURE 20-65, cont'd Total knee implant, instrumentation, and procedure. **G,** The tibial alignment guide is placed and secured; the tibia is resected. **H,** The tibia is sized. **I,** The tibia is reamed. **J,** The tibia is impacted. **K,** The tibial trial is inserted.

Continued

FIGURE 20-65, cont'd Total knee implant, instrumentation, and procedure. **L,** The patella is measured. **M,** The patella is sized. **N,** The patella is drilled.

then the osteophytes are removed using a rongeur. This allows easy access to the medial, lateral, and intercondylar spaces and facilitates soft tissue releases, should the need arise.

4. The knee is flexed to 90 degrees, and Hohmann retractors are placed deep to the collateral ligaments and anterior to the posterior capsule as well as laterally to the patella to protect these structures during resection of the proximal tibia. A Richardson retractor is placed medially to protect the medial collateral ligament (MCL).

5. The surgeon positions the distal cutting alignment guide extramedullary and parallel to the proximal tibial spine. Proper rotational alignment is established by positioning the appropriate malleoli wings parallel to the transmalleolar axis. The alignment rod is proximally placed just slightly lateral to the tibial tubercle.

6. The osteotomy saw is then used to resect the proximal portion of the tibia. The distal cutting guide is removed. Alignment is

checked with a Gerber guide (spacer block with the alignment rod) by placing the guide on the tibia. This checks the tibial cut for valgus alignment. The tibia is then sized with templates.

7. Before proceeding further, the surgeon ensures that the extremity can be moved into normal mediolateral (ML) alignment in extension. If not, additional soft tissue balancing is performed until the normal mechanical axis is obtained.

8. The AP cutting guide is then used to size the femur. The guide yoke is attached to the AP block, and the yoke is slipped under the muscle anteriorly on the periosteum. The middle nail is hammered into place, while pressing down on the guide yoke. Then by pulling up on the yoke, the valgus alignment is achieved such that it is square with the tibial cut. The block is then nailed into place with two pins.

9. With the AP femoral guide in place, the surgeon positions right-angle retractors to protect the MCL and lateral collateral

ligament (LCL). The anterior and posterior portions of the femur are resected. The tibial and femoral cuts are checked for balance and size at the same time with a tibial block.

10. After the flexion balance is determined, the distal femoral cutting block is set. The tensor, placed in flexion, is then slowly moved into extension. Tension is placed on the extension gap by dialing between 30 to 40 pounds of pressure on the tensor. The amount of pressure dialed on the tensor is based on the patient's size and tightness of the ligaments. The distal cutting jig is then placed in the tensor. After the jig is secured, the surgeon drills two pin holes and removes the tensor. The distal cutting guide is then placed in the exact two pin holes made by the distal cutting jig. The knee is then flexed, and the distal portion of the femur is resected.

11. The surgeon uses the appropriate spacer block to ensure equal tension in flexion and extension.

12. The knee is placed in flexion; the femoral notch and chamfer guide is centered between the epicondyles and impacted until fully seated. Three anterior fixation pins secure the guide to the femur. The surgeon drills two $\frac{1}{4}$-inch holes into the distal end of the femur, and cuts the anterior and posterior chamfers with the oscillating saw. The box osteotome is used to make the notch cut from the proximal end of the finishing guide. A power saw is used to resect the posterior femoral condyle remnants to ensure adequate flexion clearance. The femoral trial is then positioned.

13. The tibial size is reassessed using the tibial templates. The selected tibial template is then positioned rotationally and drilled, and the appropriate-size centering punch is used to cut through the subchondral bone. The tibial trial is then placed.

14. The surgeon measures the patella and places two towel clips onto the distal and proximal portions of the patella tendon, and then performs the appropriate amount of resection. The patellar template is placed over the resected surface, and the cruciate channels are created using the patellar drill through the slots in the template.

15. A trial reduction is performed. If this reduction proves satisfactory with regard to alignment and ligament laxity, the surgeon removes the trial components, irrigates with a pulsatile lavage, and places the permanent components. These can be inserted without bone cement, with bone cement, or with a combination of both.

16. Drains are placed in the joint depending on the surgeon's preference. The joint is closed and a compression dressing is applied to the leg. The tourniquet can be released before closure or after the dressing has been applied.

Postoperative care consists of rapid mobilization and strengthening, with a target discharge of 2 to 3 days postoperatively.

Stryker Navigation Total Knee Arthroplasty

Procedural Considerations (Figure 20-66). During the surgical approach the company representative will initialize (set up) the Smart Tools instrumentation with the scrub person. Healthcare industry representatives can provide valuable technical support to the perioperative team. Integration of surgical instrumentation and computers results in the ability to build a customized digital map of the patient's anatomy and navigate the surgical instruments according to this map. Successfully executed steps are marked with a blue checkmark and are graphically visualized. Proper setup is achieved when all Smart Tools are shown inside the camera's working space. Advantages to using a navigation system include the increased

FIGURE 20-66 Stryker navigation tracking equipment.

ability to verify the accuracy of cuts in less visible areas, decreased blood loss, and improved feedback to the surgeon about the patient's soft tissue balance.

A tourniquet, foot holder, and ESU are required. Antibiotics and heparin usually are ordered.

Operative Procedure

1. The capsule is entered medially. After making a median parapatellar incision, the surgeon places Kocher clamps on both lateral and medial sides of the capsule, and reflects the patella laterally to expose the entire tibiofemoral joint.

2. The surgeon begins to raise the medial flap using the ESU at the anterior tibia.

3. With a finger to retract medially, the surgeon places the tibial anchoring pin (self-tapping screws) at the distal aspect of the exposure. Drilling is then undertaken from the anterior to posterior tibial cortex using a 3.2-mm drill bit parallel to the joint line and rotated approximately 30 degrees medially.

4. Using a depth gauge, the surgeon rounds off to the size larger than measured (pins are available in 5-mm increments).

5. The scrub person places the pin on a T-handle for the surgeon to manually screw in the anchoring pin.

6. For the femoral anchoring pin, the surgeon next drills from the anterior to posterior femoral cortex, measures with a depth gauge, rounds up to the next larger size, and inserts the pin with a T-handle.

7. The blue tracker (B = bottom) is attached to the tibial pin and the green tracker to the femoral pin. Trackers should be placed so they are facing the camera attached to the navigation system.

8. The femoral head is registered. The hip is placed at 0 to 20 degrees of flexion and then at 45 degrees of flexion. As the leg is rotated, the LED locations yield a set of data points relative to the size of the femoral head.

9. The distal femur is then registered. The medial and lateral condyles, the center of the knee, and the AP axis of the knee are digitalized to identify the articulating surfaces.

10. The proximal tibia is then registered. The center of the tibia, AP axis, and medial and lateral tibial plateaus are traced in a similar fashion to the femur, which identifies the slope of the tibia.

11. The knee is moved through range of motion from full extension to full flexion. This kinematic datum is calculated and then recorded. Once data are recorded, the trackers are removed.

12. The surgeon excises any hypertrophic synovium and a portion of the infrapatellar fat pad using a toothed forceps and knife or ESU; the osteophytes are removed with a rongeur. This allows easy access to the medial, lateral, and intercondylar spaces and facilitates soft tissue releases, should the need arise.

13. The knee is flexed to 90 degrees, and Hohmann retractors are placed to the MCL and immediately anterior to the posterior capsule as well as laterally to the patella to protect these structures. A Richardson retractor is placed medially to protect the MCL. The surgeon uses a Kocher clamp and knife to resect the medial and lateral menisci as well as remnants of the ACL and posterior cruciate ligament (PCL).

14. The surgeon places the navigated tibial cutting guide on the proximal tibia. A cutting guide is attached to the horseshoe device and then the blue tracker to the tibial anchoring pin and the green tracker to the femoral anchoring pin. With two pins, the guide is anchored. The position is confirmed with the navigation system, and the trackers and horseshoe device are then removed.

15. The surgeon uses a 5.5-mm round burr to open the tibial surface and then drive the keel punch slightly anteriorly. The guide and pins are then removed.

16. The horseshoe device is placed with the opening posterior on the distal femur with two pins. The distal femoral cutting guide is attached to the device, and the blue tracker is attached to the blue anchoring pins. Finally, the green tracker is attached to the femoral anchoring pins.

17. The surgeon manipulates the cutting guide to the distal femur. The first pin is driven into the guide and adjusted, and then the second and third pins are placed. The horseshoe and pins are removed. The saw is flushed with the cutting guide, the green top is attached, and the blue Gurba guide is set on the tibial surface to check the cuts.

18. The femoral 4-in-1 cutting guide is placed, and the pin is placed and cut with the saw. The LCL and MCL are protected with a finger or right-angled retractors and the pins removed.

19. The Booth retractor is then placed over the tibia. After the notch guide and pin are placed, the surgeon cuts the tibia to an appropriate depth, using a saw as well as chamfer cuts. The pins and guide are then removed.

20. Next, the patella is measured; then two towel clips are placed onto the distal and proximal portions of the patellar tendon, and the appropriate resection is performed. The surgeon places the patellar template over the resected surface, and creates the cruciate channels using the patellar drill through the slots in the template.

21. Trial components are placed, trackers attached, and the knee moved through a full range of motion. The trials and anchoring pins are then removed.

22. PMMA is prepared. Bone surfaces are irrigated with a pulsatile lavage, and the permanent components are placed. These can be inserted without bone cement, with bone cement, or a combination of both.

23. Drains are placed in the joint depending on the surgeon's preference. The joint is closed in the usual fashion, and a compression dressing is applied to the leg. The tourniquet can be released before closure or after the dressing has been applied.

Postoperative care consists of rapid mobilization and strengthening, with a target discharge of 2 to 3 days postoperatively.

Total Knee Revision Arthroplasty

Revision arthroplasty may be indicated if the patient's original knee replacement wears out or loosens, or fails as a result of repeated dislocation, infection, or trauma. Total joint revision can be a very demanding and complicated procedure. Attention to detail, anticipation, and preparation are essential. Important patient information includes the preoperative x-rays, bone scan, laboratory results (including aspiration results), and physical findings.

Procedural Considerations. The perioperative nurse assists with placing the patient in supine position with a footrest for the affected leg. An OR bed with x-ray capability is used. Following the induction of anesthesia the surgeon performs an EUA. Although one of the most difficult aspects of revision surgery is that there is no clear-cut sequence of events, it is best, if possible, to approach revision surgery using the same logical sequence for each procedure. This allows all members of the surgical team to anticipate the steps in the procedure and the needs of the patient. In the case of revision arthroplasty for infection, antibiotics are held, usually at the surgeon's request, to allow for one final attempt to recover an organism. Tissue and fluid cultures are obtained when the initial incision is made through the capsule and into the joint space. Once the cultures are obtained, antibiotics are given.

Instrumentation includes a basic knee set, primary total knee instrumentation, and trials (in case only one portion of the prosthesis is revised); revision instrumentation to extract the components and cement; instrumentation and trials for the revision components; cementing system and extra cement (usually double the amount of cement used in a primary total knee arthroplasty); and power equipment including saw, reamer, and burrs.

Operative Procedure. The previous skin incision is usually used. This maintains adequate blood flow to the skin. The skin is marked to reapproximate the skin edges after surgery. A tourniquet cuff is applied after determining that there are no contraindications based on the patient's medical and surgical history.

1. Using a #10 blade, the surgeon incises through the scar from the original surgery.

2. With heavy-toothed forceps and blade, the surgeon undermines skin on each side of the incision; this allows the skin to be more easily closed at the end of the procedure.

3. After exposing the capsule, the surgeon uses a clean #10 blade to make a medial parapatellar incision into the joint. A Kocher is placed on the medial side of the capsule, and a towel clip is placed laterally, immediate to the patella, to aid with eversion.

4. Both tissue and fluid cultures are taken. Antibiotics are then administered by the anesthesia provider.

5. Using heavy-toothed forceps or a Kocher, the surgeon performs a synovectomy with a knife or the ESU. A clean dissection is needed to allow visualization of the bone-prosthesis interface and to remove any synovitis caused by poly debris or metallosis (metallosis is a nonsuppurative osteomyelitis that occurs around metal implants as a result of corrosion or hypersensitivity reaction).

6. The surgeon uses a periosteal elevator to peel away the medial ligament, which was stripped during the original surgery.

7. The knee is dislocated with posterior placement of a Hohmann retractor immediately behind the tibia. A second Hohmann

retractor is placed laterally to the patella and LCL. Medially, a Richardson retractor provides protection of the MCL.

8. If possible, the surgeon removes the poly tibia insert to allow better visualization and an increased work space.

9. Using an osteotomy saw with a small blade, the surgeon removes the tibial plate at the bone-prosthesis interface. If the saw is unable to complete the cuts, $\frac{1}{4}$- or $\frac{1}{2}$-inch curved osteotomes may be used to gain access to the posterior lateral corner. Cement is then removed from the canal using a Kocher clamp, $\frac{1}{4}$-inch straight osteotome, chisels, mallet, and curettes. If the cement is deep, a heavy-toothed alligator forceps may be required.

10. After the tibia and cement are removed, the surgeon recuts the tibia surface using an osteotomy saw and alignment guide. Sometimes the tibia is completely revised before the next step. If so, the tibial template, pins, mallet, and punch will be needed.

11. With the patella everted, a Booth retractor is placed under the femur. Using a $\frac{1}{2}$-inch curved osteotome and mallet, the surgeon removes the femoral component. A $\frac{1}{4}$-inch curved osteotome may be required if there are metal pegs at the distal end on the femoral component or at the posterior edge of the prosthesis. Once both sides of the prosthesis are loosened, it should fall off. If not, a femoral distractor will be used.

12. Any remaining cement is removed using osteotomes, chisels, or the saw. Any cement in the canal will be removed with a Kocher clamp or alligator forceps.

13. Next, the posterior capsule is addressed. With the leg in extension, the surgeon places a lamina spreader between the femur and tibia. Using curettes and a rongeur, the scar on the posterior capsule is removed to improve postoperative range of motion.

14. After the capsule is released, attention is turned to rebuilding the femur. This is done by using a series of guides and trial components.

15. Augmentation of both tibia and femur components can be done using either metal augments or bone grafting. Balance between the femur and tibia is obtained first in flexion and then in extension.

16. The last component to be revised is the patella. Two towel clips are placed, distal and proximal on either side of the patella, and the button is removed, using a large-blade osteotomy saw. All poly buttons can be readily removed by this method. However, a metal-backed patella requires the additional use of a $\frac{1}{4}$-inch osteotome. Any remaining cement is removed from holes with a curette or 6-mm burr on a drill. The patella will be recut using a large-blade osteotomy saw.

17. The guide is placed on the patella, and the drill is used for new holes. The trial button is placed, the patella inverted, and the knee placed through a range of motion.

18. All components are removed, and the knee is irrigated with antibiotic solution using pulsatile lavage. The bone edges are dried with suction and clean soft goods. This is done while the cement is being mixed.

19. Components can be cemented all at once or in stages, depending on the surgeon's preference.

20. The femur is usually cemented first. The Booth retractor is placed under the femur, and cement is put on the posterior phalanges of the femoral component and then on the distal edges of the bone. The component is placed on the end of the femur and impacted with an impactor and mallet. The cement is removed using glue knives anteriorly, laterally, and medially. Posterior glue is removed using curettes. The Booth retractor is then removed.

21. Hohmann retractors are placed posteriorly and laterally; a Richardson retractor can be placed medially if necessary. The surgeon applies cement on the tibia surface and on the tip of the tibial stem. The tibial component is then placed and impacted. Remaining cement is removed using glue knives or bayonet forceps. The retractors are removed, and the knee is relocated.

22. Cement is applied to the patella in the predrilled holes as well as on the patella button itself. The button is placed on the patella and held with a patella clamp. Remaining cement is again removed using a glue knife or bayonets.

23. Drains are used at the discretion of the surgeon, and the wound is closed.

Total Shoulder Arthroplasty

Indications for the prosthetic replacement of the shoulder joint include physically induced or accidental injury or degenerative arthritis. The procedure may be a hemiarthroplasty with reconstruction of the humeral side or a total arthroplasty with replacement of the humeral head and glenoid (Figure 20-67).

Procedural Considerations. The patient is placed in a 30-degree semi-sitting position with the arm draped free on a padded armboard and the shoulder hanging slightly off the OR bed to allow movement through the entire range of motion. The perioperative nurse confirms that the patient's head is supported to avoid neck extension. A pad is placed beneath the scapula.

A soft tissue set and a large bone set; shoulder instruments; PMMA and cement supplies; the implants with associated instrumentation and trials; a power drill, reamer, and saw; and a pulsatile lavage system are needed.

Operative Procedure
Neer Total Shoulder Arthroplasty (Figure 20-68)

1. The surgeon makes a 16-cm incision from the midacromion distally along the deltopectoral groove.

2. The cephalic vein is identified, and the surgeon opens and retracts the deltopectoral groove.

3. The deltoid attachment may be removed if the patient is large or muscular, which may affect rehabilitation.

4. The long head of the biceps is identified as the landmark between the tuberosities and rotator interval.

5. The surgeon elevates the subscapularis from the underlying capsule and divides it 2 cm medially to the bicipital groove, and places a stay suture.

6. The subscapularis is retracted medially with the lesser tuberosity, thereby exposing the joint and associated structures.

7. The capsule is exposed by elevation. The surgeon uses an elevator placed beneath the capsule to protect the axillary nerve. The long head of the biceps is left undisturbed and free in its groove so that it will continue to function as a depressor of the head after surgery.

8. After external rotation the fractured humeral head is removed. The incision site is irrigated to remove blood and clots from the joint.

9. The surgeon examines the proximal humeral shaft to select the appropriately sized stem, available in various lengths and diameters.

FIGURE 20-67 Total shoulder arthroplasty. **A,** The patient is positioned, and a deltopectoral incision is made to release the capsule. **B,** The humeral head is removed with a reciprocating saw. **C,** After exposure of the glenoid, a fenestration for the glenoid component is made. **D,** The glenoid bow is curetted.

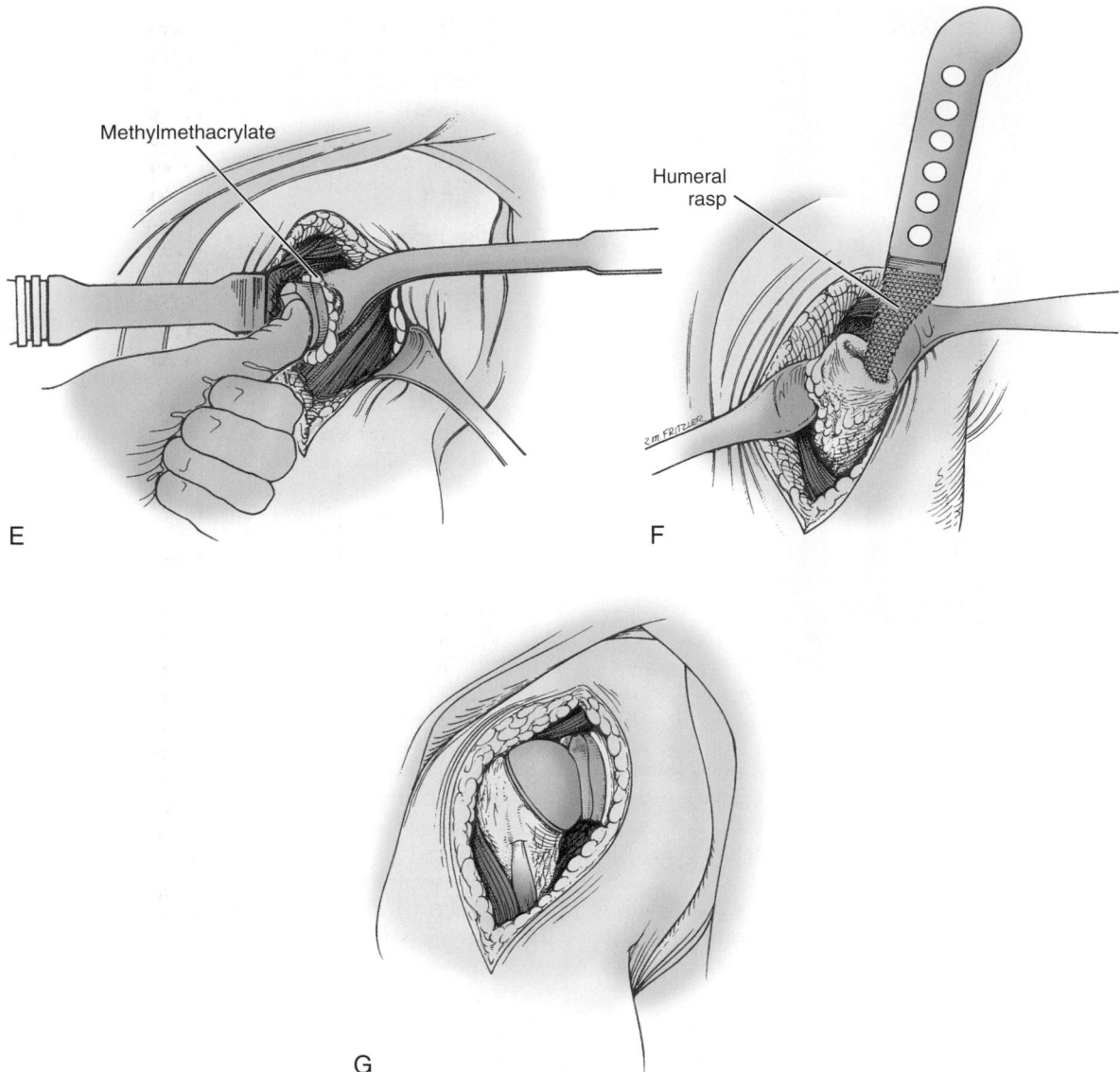

Methylmethacrylate

E

Humeral rasp

F

G

FIGURE 20-67, cont'd Total shoulder arthroplasty. **E,** Cancellous bone is evacuated and cement impressed. **F,** The humeral shaft is rasped. **G,** The humeral component is inserted.

10. Marginal osteophytes are trimmed.
11. The glenoid is inspected for integrity and sized for a prosthesis if it is to be replaced.
12. A central hole for a prosthesis fit is made into the glenoid with a high-speed burr and curette.
13. Stem diameter and length are estimated to check the prosthesis for fit. The largest stem diameter possible is used.
14. With the shaft held forward and upward, the surgeon locates the intramedullary canal with a long curette. A $\frac{1}{4}$-, $\frac{3}{8}$-, or $\frac{1}{2}$-inch drill bit is selected to correspond to the diameter of the canal; depending on the prosthesis stem length, the surgeon drills down the medullary canal 5 or 6 inches. Final preparation of the shaft is accomplished with the appropriately sized tapered reamer.
15. A heavy-gauge nonabsorbable suture is passed through holes that have been drilled on the tuberosities. The surgeon checks the length of the rotator cuff by pulling the tuberosities distal to the collar of the prosthesis.

16. Neck length and stability of the joint are determined before final impaction of the prosthesis.
17. A check for 35- to 40-degree retroversion is done by palpating the epicondyles at the elbow.
18. The implant is seated on the calcar with a driver and mallet, with its articular surface protected with a moist sponge. Just before final seating, further trimming of high spots with an osteotome or high-speed burr may be required. PMMA is used except in young patients, in whom a firm press-fit can be achieved.
19. Wires or sutures are passed through the holes in the neck of the prosthesis, reducing the tuberosities beneath the collar, and are secured. If wires are used they are buried in drill holes in the bone.
20. The surgeon reduces the shoulder. The interval of the rotator cuff is closed and the biceps tendon reattached if previously detached.
21. The joint is irrigated as each compartment and layer is closed.

FIGURE 20-68 Neer shoulder prosthesis.

22. A closed-drainage system is inserted between the rotator cuff and deltoid, avoiding contact of the drainage tubes with the axillary artery. Routine closure is accomplished.
23. Dressings are placed between the body and the arm. A shoulder immobilizer is applied.

Passive range-of-motion machines may be used for patients prone to adhesion or contracture. Pendulum and gentle exercise are permitted at 10 days.

Total Elbow Arthroplasty

Although not as prevalent as arthroplasty of the shoulder, knee, or hip, total elbow replacement (Figure 20-69) is indicated for patients with traumatic lesions or excessive bone loss from rheumatoid or degenerative arthritis, resulting in elbow instability and pain or bilateral elbow ankylosis. The design of implants and methods of fixation for postoperative stability have presented challenges that have been overcome in arthroplasty of other joints but remain a challenge in elbow arthroplasty. Postoperative stability of the elbow implant depends largely on the soft tissues surrounding the joint. There are devices that provide more constraint for the patient with significant soft tissue laxity or loss of bone stock. The Coonrad-Morrey, Tri-Axial, and Pritchard-Walker are just a few of the total elbow prostheses available.

The prosthesis may be used with or without PMMA, depending on the quality of the diseased bone and the design of the implant. If PMMA is not used, bone grafting with local bone that has been resected may be used to help seat the ulnar component snugly and achieve adequate bony contact against the porous coating of the metal ulnar component. After elbow arthroplasty, patients with degenerative arthritis generally have better results than those with injury.

Procedural Considerations. The perioperative nurse assists with positioning the patient in the supine or semi-Fowler position with

the arm over the chest. A tourniquet is applied and can be inflated if needed. The arm is prepped from shoulder to fingers and draped. A soft tissue set and a small bone set; the total elbow implants and instruments; a power saw, drill, and burr; an awl; heavy-gauge wire; and a wire tightener are needed. PMMA and cement supplies as well as a pulsatile lavage system are required if the prosthesis is placed with the use of PMMA.

Operative Procedure

1. The limb is exsanguinated, and the tourniquet is inflated to the desired pressure.
2. The surgeon makes a midline posterior incision, protecting the ulnar nerve.
3. The triceps mechanism is elevated in continuity with the periosteum, and the elbow joint is explored.
4. The surgeon explores the distal end of the humerus, proximal end of the ulna, and radial head while preserving the collateral ligaments.
5. The midportion of the trochlea is removed to allow access to the distal end of the humerus; the medullary canal is opened with a high-speed burr, and the canal is entered with a twist hand reamer.
6. The distal end of the humerus is notched with the appropriate cutting guide.
7. A high-speed burr is used to drill through subchondral bone to allow access to the medullary canal of the ulna and serially ream the canal.
8. After the humerus and ulna have been prepared for insertion of the trial prosthesis, the surgeon evaluates the elbow for flexion and extension. Bony adjustments are made where necessary.
9. The surgeon irrigates with pulsatile antibiotic lavage to clean the canals of all bone fragments.
10. The canal is dried before implant insertion, and the preparation is checked before the cement is mixed to ensure that the correct size of component is available.
11. The surgeon inserts the cement into the canals followed by the prosthesis. Flexion and extension of the elbow are avoided until the cement has hardened.
12. Any bone graft that may be required is secured with wire or pins.
13. The tourniquet is deflated, and hemostasis is achieved.
14. The triceps mechanism is repaired. The incision site is irrigated and closed. A drain may be inserted.
15. A long arm posterior splint is applied with the elbow at 90 degrees.

Total Ankle Joint Arthroplasty

Indications for total ankle arthroplasty include: (1) failed arthrodesis, (2) bilateral ankle arthritis when arthrodesis has already been performed on one ankle, (3) after talectomy because of avascular necrosis, and (4) revision of a previous arthroplasty. Total ankle joint arthroplasty is reserved for older or more sedentary patients, as long-term results tend be extremely poor. Ankle arthrodesis should be considered first in joint reconstruction. Total ankle replacement prostheses are made of high-density polyethylene and metal components.

Procedural Considerations. The patient is positioned supine and the tourniquet cuff is applied. The leg is prepped and draped. A soft tissue set, a small bone set, the total ankle joint replacement

FIGURE 20-69 Total elbow arthroplasty. **A,** The arm is draped free, and the incision is made. **B,** The tip of the olecranon is excised with an oscillating saw. **C,** The canal is identified with a burr, and the canal is opened with a twist reamer. **D,** The capitellum is measured and cut. **E,** The medullary canal is cleaned and dried, and bone cement is inserted. **F,** The ulnar prosthesis is inserted, followed by cementing and inserting of the humeral components.

instrumentation set and implants, a power drill and saw, a pulsatile lavage system, and PMMA cement and supplies are necessary.

Operative Procedure (Figure 20-70)

1. The surgeon makes an anterior incision over the ankle joint.
2. Using blunt and sharp dissection the surgeon exposes the tibiotalar joint and talus dome.
3. Once the center of the talus is identified and marked, a sizing template is used to mark the tibia.
4. A defect that is 1-inch wide by ⅜-inch deep is made using the air drill. Anchoring holes can be made in the tibia. The template is positioned in the defect while the foot is distracted.
5. The talus is marked, and using a reciprocating saw the surgeon makes a groove that is ½-inch deep by 3/16-inch wide to accommodate the talar component.
6. A trial fit is carried out to ensure that the talar unit is in the center of the talus and that the tibial unit is parallel to the plane of the floor, both centered over the dome of the talus.

7. Once trial reduction is complete, the talar and tibial components are cemented into place.
8. The ankle joint is irrigated and closed, a drain inserted, and a posterior splint applied.

Metacarpal Arthroplasty

Metacarpal joint replacement is most often performed in patients who have pain or a disabling deformity associated with rheumatoid or degenerative arthritis of the metacarpophalangeal or interphalangeal joints. The results of rheumatoid reconstructive surgery are generally good, and pain can be eliminated and joint alignment and joint stability restored in the majority of patients. The greatest problems after surgery are weakness of grasp and pinch, and progression of the disease in adjacent joints.

Procedural Considerations. The patient is positioned supine with the arm extended on a hand table. A tourniquet is applied, and the entire extremity is prepped and draped. A hand set,

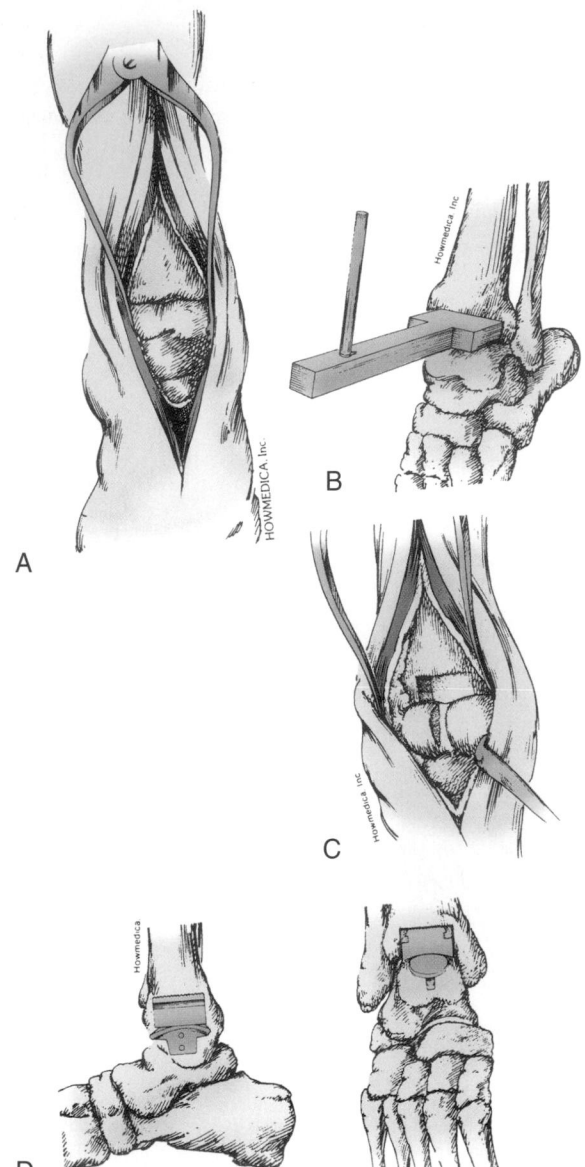

FIGURE 20-70 Total ankle arthroplasty. **A,** An anterior incision is made, and the tibiotalar joint and talus dome are exposed. **B,** The sizing template is used to mark the tibia. **C,** An air drill is used to create a defect, and anchoring holes are prepared. **D,** Trial reduction is completed, and the talar and tibial components are cemented into place.

instrumentation for implants, and implants are required, as well as a high-speed burr.

Operative Procedure

1. Incisions are made on the dorsum of the appropriate fingers.
2. The surgeon excises the proximal and distal portions of the joints and reams the intramedullary canals.
3. Sizers are used to facilitate a correct fit of the prosthesis.
4. Once the appropriately sized implant is determined, the surgeon positions it into the canal (Figures 20-71 and 20-72) and makes tendon and ligament repairs as indicated to improve stability.
5. The joint is irrigated and closed, and a bulky dressing is applied.
6. A short arm posterior splint is applied for immobilization.

FIGURE 20-71 Metacarpophalangeal implant.

FIGURE 20-72 Silastic implant for finger joint.

Metatarsal Arthroplasty

Silastic implantation is indicated in the treatment of deformities associated with rheumatoid arthritis, hallux valgus, hallux rigidus, and a painful or unstable joint.

Procedural Considerations. The patient is positioned supine. A tourniquet cuff is applied, and the entire extremity is prepped and draped. A small bone set is required, as well as the implant instruments and implants, a power wire driver, and the microsagittal saw.

Operative Procedure

1. The incisions are made over the appropriate joints.
2. The surgeon resects the proximal phalanx and removes exostosis from the metatarsal head.
3. The medullary canal is reamed, and trial implants are fitted.
4. The surgeon determines the appropriate sized metatarsal implant and seats it.
5. The wound is irrigated and closed.
6. A bulky compression dressing and orthopedic shoe are applied for early ambulation.

Arthroscopy

Progress and development of arthroscopy and arthroscopic procedures have changed the approach, diagnosis, and treatment of many joint ailments. Arthroscopic techniques require skill and accomplishment in identifying three-dimensional relationships. The advantages of arthroscopic surgery surpass the disadvantages. Among the advantages are: (1) decreased recovery and rehabilitation time; (2) smaller incisions; (3) less inflammatory response; (4) less postoperative pain, scarring, and extensor disruption; (5) reduced complications; (6) reduced hospital stay and cost; and (7) easier, more rapid surgical procedures (Ambulatory Surgery Considerations).

Disadvantages usually relate to the size and delicacy of the instruments. Maneuverability within a joint may be difficult and produce scuffing and scoring of the articular surfaces.

Improvements in scope and camera systems, sharper scope optics, and miniaturization have made operative arthroscopy a logical extension of diagnostic arthroscopy. Surgical arthroscopy has also been aided with the development of numerous second puncture instruments and devices to repair and excise defects. There are a multitude of motorized shaving and abrader systems. Irrigation systems provide regulated distention of the knee joint by infusing normal saline or lactated Ringer's solution. These systems may

AMBULATORY SURGERY CONSIDERATIONS

Arthroscopic Surgery

Ambulatory surgery has long been part of orthopedic surgery. Recent advances in minimally invasive surgery and postoperative pain management have led to even more orthopedic procedures being performed in an ambulatory setting.

The most important factor in ambulatory surgery is patient selection. Surgical, anesthesia, and nursing departments should work together to define the criteria to identify suitable candidates for ambulatory surgery. Red flags should identify any patient with potential problems that indicate inability to tolerate the surgical procedure as an outpatient.

Preoperative assessment can determine which patients are the best candidates for ambulatory surgery. Careful review of health history, social history, and potential limitations postoperatively is vital in the initial assessment. Special attention to mobility both preoperatively and postoperatively is key for the orthopedic ambulatory surgery patient. Patients who will experience significant limited mobility postoperatively, live alone with no help available postoperatively, and have multiple medical comorbidities are not ideal candidates for orthopedic ambulatory surgery. Patient education is initiated during the preoperative assessment. Gait-training, pain management, postoperative instructions, and transportation should be addressed preoperatively as well as arrangements for any special equipment necessary for postoperative recovery. Attention to postoperative details before surgery will prevent delays with patient discharge postoperatively.

The anesthesia evaluation is done during preadmission testing during which the anesthesia provider will develop a plan of care best suited for the patient and the anticipated surgery. Patient comorbidities, length of procedure, and positioning during the procedure as well as the surgery itself are taken into consideration when establishing a plan of care.

Knee Arthroscopy

Knee arthroscopy is a common orthopedic ambulatory surgery procedure. New technology and approaches in surgery allow additional procedures to be done through the arthroscope. Once the patient has been identified as a candidate for ambulatory surgery, preoperative planning for preadmission testing, anesthesia evaluation, and patient education begin. The popular choice of anesthesia is one of two types based on patient history. Choices include regional or general anesthesia. Most providers prefer regional anesthesia for knee arthroscopy because of the decreased complication rates postoperatively. On the day of surgery the history and physical are again reviewed with the patient. The surgical site is marked according to standards established by The Joint Commission and facility policy. The patient is taken to the OR, anesthetized, prepared, and positioned for surgery. With regional anesthesia, those patients who would like to remain alert during the procedure can do so, watch the surgery on the monitor, and even converse with the surgeon about the findings. Once the surgery is over, a local anesthetic is injected into the joint to minimize pain. The length of the postoperative period depends on the regional anesthetic and the dose used. Patients will regain sensation and motion from trunk down to toes. Strength should be taken into consideration when gait-training is initiated. Patients may be discharged once discharge criteria are met, physician orders are reviewed with the patient, written discharge instructions and prescriptions are given to the patient, and the responsible adult escort is present. Phone numbers for any emergency should be listed on both physician and hospital discharge sheets.

function by gravity flow or are mechanized with built-in microprocessors to monitor joint pressures and adjust accordingly. Lasers and ESUs can be used in tandem with arthroscopic equipment. Integrated video systems can record and store still and video images on film, tape, or digitally for education and documentation.

Arthroscopy is commonly performed on the knee, shoulder, and wrist. It is used less often in the elbow, hip, and ankle. Many corrective procedures that previously required an arthrotomy or other open procedure can be completed with the assistance of the arthroscope.

Arthroscopic equipment has certain requirements for care and handling. Fiberoptics, lenses, and cameras are heat sensitive, requiring consideration for sterilization. Temperatures and moisture generated by steam autoclaves can damage materials used in video equipment or deteriorate the sealant, making the moisture accessible to the lens. Alternatives to steam sterilization for this equipment are ethylene oxide, cold sterilization, and high-level disinfection (see Chapter 4 for a discussion of sterilization methods).

Scopes, lenses, and fiberoptic cords should be handled carefully, and cords should never be kinked or twisted. Gradual deterioration and fiber breakage occur in mishandled cables, and light cannot be transmitted. When stored, the cords should be loosely coiled or hung.

Two types of arthroscopy may be performed. *Diagnostic arthroscopy* is for patients whose diagnosis cannot be determined by history or physical examination or whose CT or MRI findings are insufficient to warrant surgical exploration. Diagnostic arthroscopy may be performed before an anticipated arthrotomy, and surgical treatment may be modified on the basis of the findings of the arthroscopic examination. *Operative arthroscopy* is for patients presenting with an intra-articular abnormality or ligamentous injury.

Arthroscopy of the Knee

The knee is the joint in which arthroscopy lends itself to the greatest number of diagnostic and surgical procedures. Arthroscopic surgery of the knee is indicated for diagnostic viewing, synovial biopsies, removal of loose bodies, resection of plicae, shaving of the patella, synovectomy, partial meniscectomy, meniscus repair, and ACL reconstruction. Anesthesia for knee arthroscopy may be general, spinal, or local. Tourniquet cuffs are often placed on the thigh but are inflated only if bleeding obscures the view. If there are no contraindications, an epinephrine solution may be injected at the portal sites or diluted into the distention fluid.

Procedural Considerations. The perioperative nurse assists with positioning the patient in the supine position on a standard OR bed. The surgeon may perform an EUA before the patient is placed in position for the arthroscopy. The foot end of the bed may be flexed 90 degrees (Figure 20-73). A lateral post can be attached to the bed at the level of the midthigh. This post can provide a method of countertraction to open the medial side of the joint, providing better visualization of structures. After the leg is prepped the entire extremity is draped to allow complete range of motion and manipulation of the knee joint. The procedure requires specialized equipment for fluid collection and personnel protection.

Instruments and equipment needed for an arthroscopy depend on whether the procedure is diagnostic or operative. Diagnostic arthroscopy instruments include arthroscopy instrumentation; arthroscopes of 30 and 70 degrees; video with camera, light source, and peripheral equipment (Figure 20-74); an arthroscopy pump and tubing (Figure 20-75); inflow and egress cannulae

FIGURE 20-73 Positioning for a knee arthroscopy to enhance visualization.

FIGURE 20-74 Arthroscopy tower with video monitor, light source, camera, and shaver system.

FIGURE 20-75 Arthroscopy pump.

FIGURE 20-76 Cannulae.

(Figure 20-76); 3-L bags of normal saline or lactated Ringer's solution; and a spinal needle. Operative arthroscopy instruments depend on the procedure planned. Arthroscopic powered shavers and abraders (Figure 20-77) are almost universally used. Instruments specific for ACL reconstruction or meniscal repair will be needed if those procedures are planned.

Operative Procedure
Diagnostic Arthroscopy

1. The surgeon marks the anteromedial and anterolateral joint lines and portal positions with a skin marker.

2. The skin areas for portal placement are infiltrated with 1% lidocaine with 1:200,000 epinephrine. If the knee has an effusion, the surgeon aspirates it with a 16-gauge needle on a 60-mL syringe, followed by injection of a small amount of distending fluid.

3. After creating a small stab incision with a #11 blade, the surgeon inserts the irrigation cannula and trocar into the lateral suprapatellar pouch near the superior pole of the patella. Lactated Ringer's or normal saline solution is connected to the cannula, and the joint is distended using gravity or a pressure-sensitive arthroscopy pump.

4. An additional stab incision is then made anterolaterally or anteromedially 2 to 3 mm above the tibial plateau or patellar

tendon at the joint line. A sharp trocar and sheath are inserted through the stab wound and just through the capsule.

5. A blunt trocar is used to pass the sheath into the knee joint. The surgeon removes the trocar and inserts a 30-degree scope into the sheath. The light source and video camera are connected to the scope.

A

B

FIGURE 20-77 Arthroscopic shaver (**A**), with console (**B**).

6. The inflow may remain in the suprapatellar area, and the egress tubing is connected to the arthroscope, or the position may be reversed.

7. A spinal needle can be introduced under direct vision to determine the best angle for an opposite portal for insertion of probes and operative instruments. The cruciates and menisci are probed to determine integrity and tears.

8. The scope is moved to the opposite portal to allow a complete examination to be performed.

9. The joint is irrigated periodically and at the end of the procedure to maintain good visualization and clear the joint of blood and tissue fragments.

10. The surgeon closes the portals with nylon or undyed polyglactin suture and $\frac{1}{2}$-inch wound closure strips.

11. Bupivacaine (Marcaine) 0.25%, 30 mL, with epinephrine 1:200,000 may be injected intra-articularly to minimize bleeding and postoperative pain.

12. Gauze dressing, soft padding, and 4- and 6-inch elastic bandages are applied.

Operative Arthroscopy. Operative arthroscopy includes procedures for resection of synovial plica, patellar debridement, excision of meniscal tears, partial or total meniscectomy, lateral retinacular release, removal of loose bodies, abrasion or drilling of osteochondral defects, synovectomy, treatment of osteochondritis dissecans, meniscal repairs, and ACL reconstruction.

Arthroscopic Resection and Repair of Meniscal Tear. Menisci are important structures in the knee joint that distribute load across the joint and provide capsular stability. A tear in the meniscus is the most common knee injury requiring arthroscopic surgery (Figure 20-78). Although both menisci can sustain tears, the medial meniscus is injured much more frequently than the lateral one.

Treatment of meniscus tears is aimed at preserving the structures. Some minor tears heal with immobilization, but some persist and cause symptoms. In these more severe cases surgical intervention is necessary. A partial or complete meniscectomy may be necessary to alleviate troublesome symptoms such as locking, pain, and swelling (Figure 20-79). Partial meniscectomy is preferred, leaving a peripheral rim to share load bearing and stabilize the knee. Complete meniscectomy removes all of this load-bearing protection and reduces knee stability. The goal is to leave an intact, balanced rim.

Arthroscopic meniscal repair is widely accepted as the standard of care. Arthroscopy provides better exposure than an arthrotomy

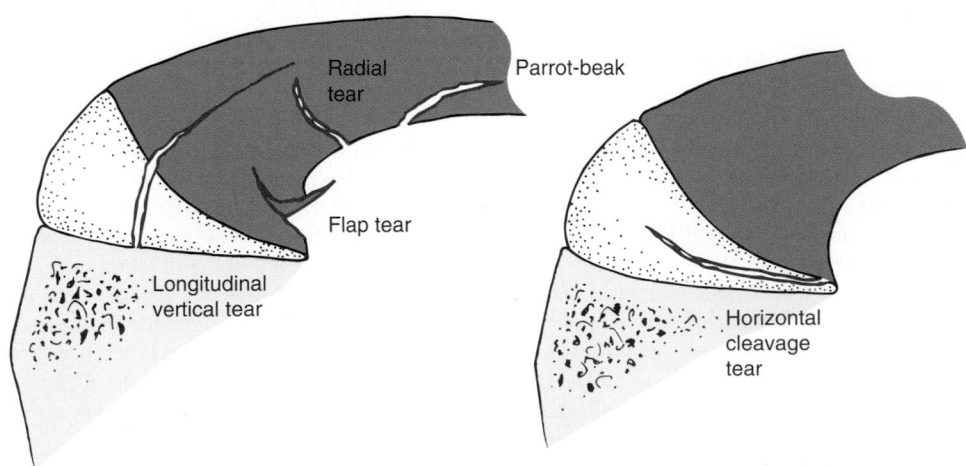

FIGURE 20-78 Types of meniscal tears.

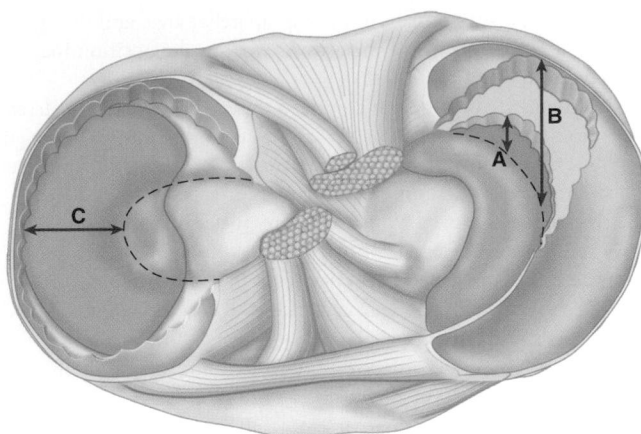

FIGURE 20-79 Types of meniscal excision. **A,** Partial menisectomy. **B,** Subtotal menisectomy. **C,** Total menisectomy.

does and enables the surgeon to approach the meniscus from the inner margin, where most tears begin. Suture repair is appropriate for meniscal tears occurring in the vascular zone (outer 10% to 25%) that heal predictably with repair and immobilization.

Operative Procedure
1. Steps 1 through 9 of the diagnostic arthroscopy procedure are performed.
2. Working and scope portals are determined. The lateral bucket handle tear is identified, displaced, and reduced with a probe.
3. The surgeon cuts the attachment of the anterior horn of the meniscus with a hook knife and clamps it with a grasper.
4. An accessory portal is determined with a spinal needle.
5. The surgeon maintains traction and twisting motions on the meniscal horn to present a better edge to divide the remainder of the tear. Various scissors or push knives can be used to complete resection.
6. The motorized shaver is used to trim any frayed edges of the meniscus.
7. Limited debridement of chronic tears is completed to clean the edges.
8. When the medial meniscus is to be sutured, the surgeon places a cannula next to the inner edge of the tear. Two long meniscal-stitching needles with synthetic absorbable suture are inserted into the cannula, through the meniscus, across the tear, and through the capsule.
9. The surgeon palpates the needle tips beneath the skin, and makes a small incision to pull the suture out of the joint.
10. The sutures are tied over the capsule. Positioning the cannula enables either horizontal or vertical sutures to be placed.
11. After completing partial menisectomy or suture repair, the surgeon irrigates the joint.
12. The incisions are closed, and the knee is lightly dressed and wrapped with soft rolled padding and elastic bandages.

Arthroscopic Anterior Cruciate Ligament Repair. The ACL is an important stabilizing structure of the knee and is the most frequently torn ligament. Injury is usually a result of simultaneous anterior and rotational stresses. Candidates for ACL reconstruction are active individuals with instability that is sufficient to interfere with their activities and that has failed to respond to bracing, rehabilitation, exercises, and other nonoperative treatment methods. The selected treatment method depends on the classification and

FIGURE 20-80 Example of a bone tunnel plug.

severity of the tear, the experience and preference of the surgeon, and a history of a previous failed repair.

ACL reconstruction may be intra-articular, extra-articular, or a combination of both. Arthroscopic repair causes less patellar pain and decreased disturbance of extensor mechanisms and therefore is becoming the treatment of choice if there is no other significant capsular instability or gross disruption of the knee joint.

ACL repair most often involves replacement of the ligament with a substitute. Substitutes include autografts, allografts, and synthetic ligaments. Autografts are the method of choice, with a free central-third patellar tendon graft attached to patellar and tibial bone blocks used most often. The semitendinosus tendon and iliotibial band are sometimes used instead. Autografts may be used alone or augmented, although synthetic augmentation devices have fallen out of favor because of the development of chronic synovitis.

Procedural Considerations. Instrumentation for an ACL repair includes all instruments required for an operative arthroscopy. In addition, an ACL reconstruction guide system, fixation device of choice (bone screws, staples, spiked washers, or interference screws), bone tunnel plugs (Figure 20-80), a power drill, and microsagittal saw are needed. If the surgeon believes that isometric placement of the graft is important, a tension isometer will be needed, as well as a system for finding that intra-articular position.

Operative Procedure: Reconstruction of the ACL with Patellar Tendon Graft
1. The surgeon performs an EUA immediately after anesthesia induction to further evaluate the stability of the knee.
2. A diagnostic arthroscopy is then carried out through the standard anteromedial and anterolateral portals.
3. Any meniscal tears or other intra-articular injuries are treated before attending to the ligament.
4. The surgeon debrides any remaining ACL tissue with a full-radius resector.
5. A notchplasty is then performed, widening the intercondylar notch with a 4.5-mm arthroplasty burr, rasp, osteotome, and curettes. Notchplasty aids in arthroscopic visualization and protects the graft from abrasion and amputation.
6. After preparation of the intercondylar area, the surgeon makes a small incision on the distal lateral aspect of the femur and extends the incision to the flare of the lateral femoral aspect of the condyle. A femoral aiming device is positioned, and a guide pin is inserted from the femoral site into the posterosuperior region of the intercondylar notch at an isometric point (Figure 20-81). Another small incision is made anteriorly, below the knee and medial to the tibial tubercle.
7. The tibial aiming device is positioned, and the surgeon inserts a guide pin from the anterior tibial incision into the intercondylar notch, anterior and medial to the center of the tibial anatomic attachment site of the ACL.
8. The pins are then replaced with a heavy suture passing through the femoral and tibial pin sites.
9. Isometric placement of the guide pins is checked with a tensioning device that is attached to the heavy suture. The knee is

FIGURE 20-81 Femoral aiming device positioned for anterior cruciate ligament reconstruction.

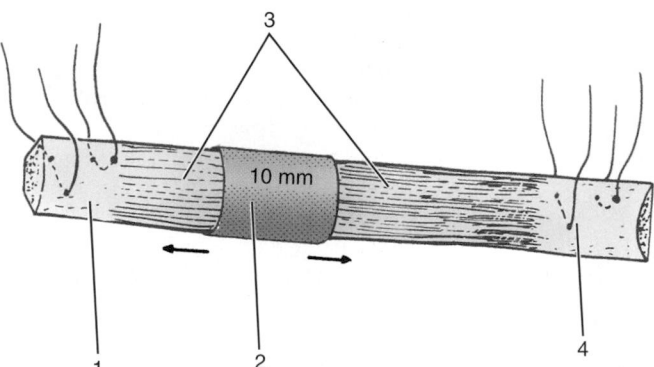

FIGURE 20-82 Sizing tubes are used to determine the minimum diameter of tunnel necessary for passage of the graft.

FIGURE 20-83 Three drill holes are placed into each bone block of the patellar graft, and a heavy suture is placed into each drill hole.

FIGURE 20-84 A patellar tendon graft is affixed by tying of sutures over bone buttons at the tibial and femoral drill holes.

moved through a range of motion to determine correct isometric measurement.

10. Once isometric positioning is determined, the surgeon makes a longitudinal skin incision to the midline near the patellar tendon.

11. The central third portion of the patellar tendon with tibial and patellar bone plugs is harvested with a mini-saw and osteotome. The graft is sized to the appropriate width, usually 10 to 12 mm, using sizing tubes (Figure 20-82).

12. Heavy nonabsorbable suture is placed through drill holes made at each end of the graft in the bone plugs (Figure 20-83).

13. The guide pins are then reinserted and overdrilled with cannulae that are close in width to the prepared graft. Overdrilling establishes the tunnels so that they are in the center of the previous insertion sites of the ACL.

14. The surgeon smoothes the femoral and tibial osseous tunnels with curettes, a rasp, or an abrader. If the tunnels are made before the graft is harvested, they are temporarily occluded with bone tunnel plugs to minimize fluid extravasation.

15. Both ends of the graft are fixed with a barbed staple, bone screw with washer, interference screw, or ligament button (Figure 20-84).

16. The incisions and joint are irrigated and closed.

17. A hinged knee brace may be applied over the dressing. The brace allows 10 to 90 degrees of motion.

Arthroscopic Posterior Cruciate Ligament Repair. Surgical procedures for tears of the PCL are considered if significant disabling instability has occurred. Patients usually return to adequate function without operative treatment. The arthroscopic procedure for repair of the PCL is similar to the technique used to repair the ACL, except that isometric placement is posterior within the joint and the femoral attachment is proximal to the medial epicondyle.

Arthroscopy of the Shoulder

Shoulder arthroscopy is a useful diagnostic and therapeutic tool in the management of shoulder disorders. It is particularly beneficial in evaluating and managing patients with chronic shoulder problems. Arthroscopy provides extensive visualization of the intra-articular aspect of the shoulder joint and is performed for removal of loose bodies; lysis of adhesions; synovial biopsy; synovectomy; bursectomy; stabilization of dislocations; correction of glenoid labrum, biceps tendon, and rotator cuff tears; and relief of impingement syndrome.

Procedural Considerations. The patient is either in the lateral position or in a sitting position using a "beach chair" positioner. The lateral position is maintained using a vacuum beanbag positioning device or lateral rolls with a kidney rest. Three-inch adhesive tape is secured across the patient's hips. Proper padding of the uninvolved axilla and lower extremity is important to prevent soft tissue or neurovascular problems. The affected extremity is placed in a shoulder suspension system, and Buck traction or a Velcro immobilizer is applied to the forearm to achieve adequate distraction to the glenohumeral joint. The extremity is abducted 40 to 60 degrees and forward-flexed 10 to 20 degrees, with 5- to 15-pound weights placed on the pulley system. Weight may be added to further distract the glenohumeral joint, taking care not to overstretch the axillary artery.

The shoulder is prepped and draped free, permitting full range of motion during the procedure.

The operative instruments and arthroscope commonly used for the knee may also be used in the shoulder, plus an 18-gauge needle, switching sticks, and a Wissinger rod. A variety of fixation devices (screws and tacks) can be used to repair bony defects and tears of the labrum.

Operative Procedure (Figure 20-85)

1. An 18-gauge spinal needle is inserted through the posterior soft spot and directed anteriorly toward the coracoid process, where the surgeon's index finger has been positioned.

FIGURE 20-85 Shoulder arthroscopy. **A,** The spinal needle is inserted for dilation of the joint if indicated. **B,** An incision is made over the glenohumeral joint. **C,** The arthroscope sleeve and sharp trocar are inserted. **D,** The arthroscope is inserted and attached to the inflow and outflow tubing, video camera, and light source. **E,** Operative instruments are placed through the portal.

2. The glenohumeral joint is distended with normal saline or lactated Ringer's solution. This facilitates entry of the arthroscope.

3. The surgeon injects bupivacaine (Marcaine) 0.25%, 2 to 3 mL, with epinephrine 1:200,000 along the needle track to minimize bleeding.

4. With the needle removed, the surgeon makes a stab incision with a #11 blade over the needle site.

5. The arthroscope sleeve and sharp trocar are then introduced through the posterior joint capsule.

6. After the capsule has been penetrated, the surgeon replaces the sharp trocar with a blunt obturator to enter the joint.

7. The arthroscope is inserted and attached to inflow and outflow tubing, the video camera, and the light source.

8. Operative instruments are placed through an anterior portal that is established laterally to the coracoid process by using a Wissinger rod. A third portal can be established near the anterior portal or supraspinous fossa portal. Switching sticks are used to change portals.

9. The surgeon moves the arm and rotates it as needed to visualize various structures in and around the joint.

10. Glenoid tears can be repaired with the insertion of an absorbable fixation tack.

11. At the conclusion of the procedure, the joint is irrigated. The surgeon may inject a long-acting local anesthetic into the joint and subacromial space through the portal to minimize postoperative discomfort.

12. The puncture wounds are closed and dressed with a sterile 4 × 4 gauze pad. The patient's arm is placed in a sling for recovery.

Arthroscopy of the Elbow

The elbow joint is accessible to arthroscopic examination, although it requires more attention to detail than the knee because instruments must be placed through deeper muscle layers and close to important neurovascular structures.

Arthroscopy of the elbow, both diagnostic and operative, has become fairly routine. Indications for its use include extraction of loose bodies, evaluation or debridement of osteochondritis dissecans of the capitulum and radial head, partial synovectomy in rheumatoid disease, debridement and lysis of adhesions of post-traumatic or degenerative processes at or near the elbow, diagnosis of a chronically painful elbow when the diagnosis is obscure, and evaluation of fractures of the capitulum, radial head, or olecranon.

Procedural Considerations. General anesthesia is preferred to local anesthesia because it affords complete comfort to the patient and provides total muscle relaxation.

The perioperative nurse assists with placing the patient in either the supine or the prone position. In the supine position the forearm is flexed on an armboard or placed in a prefabricated wrist gauntlet connected to an overhead pulley device and tied off at the end of the OR bed. This provides excellent access to both the medial and lateral aspects of the elbow, allows the forearm to be freely pronated and supinated, and places the important neurovascular structures in the antecubital fossa at maximum relaxation.

A tourniquet is routinely used for hemostasis. The entire arm, including the hand, is prepped and draped.

The three portals most commonly used for diagnostic and operative arthroscopy of the elbow are the anterolateral, anteromedial, and posterolateral.

Operative arthroscopy instruments commonly used for the knee may also be used in the elbow. However, smaller-diameter scopes and instruments may be desired instead.

Operative Procedure

1. The surgeon outlines the bony anatomic landmarks with a sterile marking pen before beginning the procedure. Lateral structures to be marked and identified are the radial head and the lateral epicondyle. The medial epicondyle is also marked.

2. An 18-gauge needle is inserted anteriorly to the radial head from the lateral side, and the joint is distended.

3. After distending the joint with approximately 15 to 30 mL of lactated Ringer's or normal saline solution, the surgeon makes a stab wound incision with a #11 blade, and inserts the sharp trocar with cannula through the joint capsule.

4. The sharp trocar is replaced with the blunt obturator to provide safe entry of the cannula into the joint.

5. The surgeon replaces the blunt obturator with the scope and attaches it to the video and light source.

6. A second portal and third portal are established anteromedially and posterolaterally for triangulation. With the patient's elbow flexed to 90 degrees and adequate distention maintained at the time of insertion of the instruments, the surgeon displaces the neurovascular structures anteriorly. This provides a greater area above the medial and lateral humeral epicondyles in which to insert the various instruments.

7. Outflow and inflow are controlled by alternating the valve on the scope or using a separate 18-gauge needle with drainage tubing.

8. After diagnostic and operative procedures have been completed, the joint is irrigated, the puncture sites are sutured, and a compression dressing is applied with soft rolled padding and elastic bandages.

Arthroscopy of the Ankle

The talocalcaneal articulations are complex and play an important role in the movements of inversion and eversion of the foot. The subtalar joints function as a single unit, but anatomically they are divided into anterior and posterior joints. The surgeon and perioperative nurse must be familiar with the extra-articular anatomy of the ankle to prevent neural or vascular damage.

Indications for ankle arthroscopy include osteochondral fragments or loose bodies, persistent ankle pain after trauma and despite adequate conservative treatment, biopsy, post-traumatic arthritis of the ankle joint, unstable ankle before lateral ligamentous reconstruction, and osteochondritis dissecans of the talus.

Procedural Considerations. General anesthesia is preferable because manipulation and distraction of the joint to obtain adequate arthroscopic viewing require muscle relaxation. The position of the patient is based on the surgeon's preference. The patient may be supine with the knee flexed approximately 70 degrees or supine with a sandbag under the buttock of the operative side. Ankle and thigh holders may be used; when better posterior visualization is necessary, a distractor may be used to increase the space between the tibia and talus. A tourniquet is placed around the upper thigh but is not used unless excessive bleeding, uncontrolled by irrigation, is encountered. Routine skin prepping and draping are done. Miniaturized instruments and needle scopes for the ankle are used.

Operative Procedure

1. Using a sterile marking pen, the surgeon outlines important extra-articular anatomic structures on the skin.

2. The surgeon examines the ankle joint, using the anterolateral portal. The anteromedial joint line is palpated, and an 18-gauge, 1½-inch needle is inserted into the joint.
3. Sterile plastic extension tubing is attached to the needle, and a 50-mL plastic Luer-Lok syringe filled with normal saline is connected to the tubing to distend the joint. Approximately 15 to 20 mL is needed.
4. After intra-articular injection is confirmed by the ease with which the saline can be injected and by palpation of the joint as it is distended, the surgeon makes a small incision with a #11 blade over the site of the anterolateral portal.
5. A hemostat is then inserted and used to dissect to the capsule.
6. The surgeon places the sheath of the arthroscope and sharp trocar into the incision, angles them approximately 30 to 45 degrees laterally, and inserts them with a sharp plunge as joint distention is maintained. Entrance into the joint is felt as the sleeve and trocar "pop" through the capsule and is confirmed by the rush of saline on removal of the trocar from the sheath.
7. The arthroscope is inserted into the sheath, the needle is removed, and the plastic tubing and syringe are attached to the stopcock on the arthroscope sleeve. The video camera and light source are connected to the scope. Joint distention must be maintained.
8. Triangulation through other portals is easily done by first inserting the 18-gauge needle for localization while viewing with the arthroscope. Posterior viewing is done in the same fashion except that the patient is usually placed in the prone position and instruments are inserted through the posterior portals.
9. After the procedure is completed the surgeon irrigates the joint, closes the wounds with wound closure strips or a single suture, and covers the wound with a dressing and short leg compression elastic wrap.

Surgery of the Spine

Treatment of Back Pain

Back pain is a natural result of degenerative and arthritic change, punctuated by protrusion or rupture of a disk. It gradually progresses but may also disappear gradually. With aging, a degenerative disk-space narrowing or facet arthropathy begins to appear radiologically. The lower lumbar spine carries the burden of the body's weight, holds a person upright, and returns the body to the vertical position from sitting, lying, or a bent-over position. Degenerative changes, ruptured disk, and facet arthropathy develop at the lowest two limb segments, where the greatest weight, torsion, and shearing stress occur. This degeneration sometimes extends into the upper and middle spine.

Cervical-spine degenerative disk narrowing also develops most often at the two lowest cervical spaces, which are also the levels of greatest stress resulting from movement of the head and neck. Sometimes lumbar or cervical degenerative changes develop early from excessive repetitive movements or injury.

Epidural steroid injections, electrodes, stimulators, braces, or traction may be used to treat back pain. A natural recovery may result after 6 or 7 days of intense pain, subsiding between 6 weeks and 4 months. Motor and sensory deficits usually disappear with resolution of pain. The ability to recover without surgery depends on fragment size and compression on the nerve root. Neural compression remains the major indication for disk excision.

Spinal fusion is a consideration, usually for patients with demonstrable post-traumatic, postsurgical, rheumatoid, infectious, or neoplastic instability.

Procedural Considerations. After assessment the patient-specific plan of care is implemented. Radiographs are obtained. The perioperative nurse assesses the patient's bilateral pulses and range of motion in all of the extremities. Elastic wraps or intermittent pneumatic compression devices may be placed. The patient is positioned prone to eliminate lordosis, reduce venous congestion, and keep the abdomen free with chest rolls or special frames after inducing general anesthesia. Depending on the extent of the procedure, blood availability may be required. The skin is prepped and the area draped. A spinal laminectomy set is used, in addition to a spinal retractor of choice and a bipolar ESU. Hemostatic adjuncts such as gelatin foam, oxidized cellulose strips, thrombin, and bone wax should be available.

Operative Procedure
Laminectomy

1. The surgeon makes a midline incision over the affected disc and carries it sharply down to the supraspinous ligament.
2. The supraspinous ligament is incised, and the muscles are dissected subperiosteally from the spines and laminae of the vertebrae. These are retracted with a self-retaining retractor.
3. The surgeon denudes the laminae and ligamentum flavum with a curette.
4. A small part of the inferior margin of the lamina is removed with a rongeur.
5. The ligamentum flavum is grasped and incised where it fuses with the interspinous ligament, and this flap is then sharply removed to expose the dura.
6. The dura is then retracted medially, and the nerve root is identified.
7. Once identified, the nerve root is retracted medially so that the underlying posterior longitudinal ligament can be exposed.
8. The surgeon incises the posterior longitudinal ligament over the intervertebral space in a cruciate fashion, and enters the disk space with a pituitary grasping forceps.
9. The disk material is systematically removed, taking care not to exceed the distance to the anterior annulus. A complete search for additional fragments of nucleus pulposus, both inside and outside the disk space, is then carried out.
10. Residual bleeding is controlled with bipolar coagulation.
11. The surgeon closes the wound with absorbable sutures in the supraspinous ligament and subcutaneous tissue. Various nonabsorbable sutures or staples are used for skin closure.

Minimally Invasive Spine Surgery

Advances in technology have made minimally invasive spinal surgery (MISS) available to certain patients. Candidates for MISS are carefully selected by the surgeon. Conditions that may be amenable to MISS include disk herniation, spinal stenosis, and kyphosis. The need to convert from MISS to the traditional incision must be discussed with the patient before the surgery, and the perioperative nurse and scrub person must prepare for that possibility. The microdiskectomy procedure, used to treat disk herniation, is described below.

Procedural Considerations. The perioperative nurse and scrub person ensure that all equipment is available and assembled before the patient's arrival into the OR. Equipment needed includes the C-arm, microscope, and radiolucent spinal table. After the administration of a general anesthetic, the patient is positioned prone on the radiolucent spinal table. Care is taken to ensure proper padding

FIGURE 20-86 Wanding maneuver is used to change the position of the tubular retractor and reach different areas of the spine.

FIGURE 20-87 Pedicle screw placement using the MaXcess retractor and SpheRx fixation system by NuVasive, Inc.

of bony prominences and proper positioning of extremities. The skin is prepped and draped. Instrumentation for MISS includes the tubular microdiskectomy set and the tubular retractor. A high-speed drill and hemostatic agents such as gelatin foam, thrombin, and bone wax should be available. The perioperative nurse places intermittent pneumatic compression devices on the patient.

Operative Procedure

1. The surgeon inserts an 18-gauge spinal needle in the back at the level of the disk herniation and confirms the correct level with the C-arm.
2. The surgeon makes a 1- to 1.5-cm incision at the previously identified level.
3. A Cobb elevator and sequentially sized dilators are used to serially dilate the soft tissues, preserving the integrity of the muscles and ligaments.
4. The surgeon inserts a tubular retractor and connects the flex arm directly to the spinal table.
5. The tubular retractor is used as a viewing portal to visualize and operate on the spine (Figure 20-86).
6. The surgeon confirms the level again with x-ray and moves the draped microscope into position.
7. Using the long electrode on the ESU, the surgeon dissects the tissue.
8. A high-powered burr and/or assorted sizes of Kerrison punches are used to remove part of the caudal lamina.
9. After identifying the nerve roots, the surgeon enters the disk space and removes the extruded disk material with pituitary grasping forceps.

10. Gelatin foam and cotton pledgets are used to control bleeding along with the bipolar ESU.
11. The surgeon irrigates and closes the wound.

Pedicle Fixation of the Spine

Pedicle screw fixation (Figure 20-87) is a method of surgical fixation of the spinal column. Screw fixation was initially used in an attempt to avoid postoperative external immobilization and prolonged bed rest. Pedicle screw fixation has been used most often in degenerative processes, particularly iatrogenic instability after decompression, degenerative and isthmic spondylolisthesis, and diskogenic disease. It is also indicated for tumor, trauma, degenerative spinal disorders, postoperative hypermobility, and infection.

Three basic approaches for fixation have been described as the procedure has evolved. Each has improved on the first, based on anatomic placement of the screw. Positioning and placement of the screw within the spine are established after direct visualization of the pedicle.

Procedural Considerations. After the administration of a general anesthetic, the patient is positioned prone. The skin is prepped, and drapes are applied. A spinal laminectomy set is used in addition to the instrumentation and implants of choice, a spinal retractor, power equipment such as a high-speed motorized hand tool, and hemostatic adjuncts such as gelatin foam, thrombin, and bone wax. A bone graft set is needed to harvest graft from the iliac crest.

Operative Procedure

1. The surgeon makes a standard midline incision. The surgeon follows the steps as described in the laminectomy procedure to expose the spine.
2. The areas of the pedicles to be fixated are located using external landmarks.
3. The surgeon removes the posterior cortical wall at the entrance site using a high-speed burr.
4. A Penfield dissector is used to identify the entrance hole through the pedicle.
5. The surgeon inserts a gearshift probe to identify the path into the vertebral body.

6. The hole is tapped (5.5-mm tap) and widened.

7. The surgeon places the screw(s). Guidelines for screw sizes are 7 mm for S1, L5, and L4; 6.25 mm for L3 and L2; and 5.5 mm for L1 and T12.

8. A posterolateral graft is performed, using graft strips from the iliac crest.

9. The surgeon contours the plate or rod to approximate the patient's physiologic lordosis. The longitudinal device is locked onto the screws in the appropriate position.

10. A screw-plate system may require oblique and transverse washers between the screw head and plate to provide a flush fit at the screw-plate interface.

11. The foramina are checked for patency before closure. The excess portion of the screw is cut close to the upper locking device.

12. A suction drain is placed; the wound is closed in layers.

Treatment of Scoliosis

Scoliosis is a three-dimensional deformity (Figure 20-88) with lateral deviation of the spinal column from the midline; it may include rotation or deformity of the vertebrae. Types are congenital, juvenile, adolescent, and adult. School screening programs provide quick and simple detection. For effective treatment of scoliosis, early detection is critical.

Scoliosis can be idiopathic or congenital and may result from muscular or neurologic diseases or unequal leg lengths. Numerous posterior and anterior segmental spinal instrumentation systems are available for treating idiopathic scoliosis. As a consequence, fixation strategies are more complex than they were with Harrington instrumentation. The newer systems provide better sagittal control and more stable fixation, allowing quicker mobilization of the patient. On thin patients, however, the bulk of these implants may be a problem.

Posterior Spinal Fusion with Harrington Rods. Posterior spinal fusion is most frequently performed in adolescence, when the laterally deviated curve is still flexible. Harrington rods are internal splints that help maintain the spine as straight as possible until the vertebral body fusion has become solid. Distraction rods are placed on the concave side of the curve, and compression rods are placed on the convex side. On the convex side of the curve, three to eight hooks are inserted in the transverse processes of the vertebrae and pulled together with a threaded rod. In this way the scoliotic deformity can be corrected as much as the flexibility of the spine allows.

FIGURE 20-88 Scoliotic deformity.

The posterior elements of the vertebrae are denuded of soft tissue, and the bone graft is added. Blood loss can be expected, and an accurate record of the loss must be maintained. After surgery the patient is placed in an immobilizing jacket.

Some disadvantages of the Harrington rod system over other systems are that there is only end-point fixation, rod breakage is increased, fixation is less, sagittal plane curves are difficult to manage, distraction for correction is not always desired, and the patient is required to wear a postoperative cast or brace. Other systems have evolved from the Harrington rods that are used for correction of some scoliotic deformities. It remains a feasible treatment of idiopathic scoliosis.

Procedural Considerations. The patient is placed in the prone position on a spinal table or a spinal frame to facilitate respiration. Before the procedure begins, an x-ray cassette is placed under the patient so that a radiograph for accurate identification of the vertebrae to be fused can be taken during the operation. A single straight longitudinal incision is made down the midline of the back. Because of the amount of bleeding, the skin and subcutaneous tissues are often infiltrated with a vasoconstricting solution, such as epinephrine.

Basic spinal instrumentation and bone graft instruments are required, plus the Harrington rod instrumentation. A large pin cutter, designed to cut large pins but provided with a small end so that it will fit in the wound, should be available.

Operative Procedure

1. The appropriate hooks are selected and inserted. The surgeon inserts a Harrington distraction rod of appropriate length through the two proximal self-adjusting hooks, which have been placed under the laminae.

2. A rod clamp is clamped onto the Harrington rod just below the hook, and a single regular spreader is used to obtain the first inch of distraction.

3. The Bobechko spreader is used to span over the first hook, closest to the smooth part of the rod, to apply distraction force on the most proximal hook.

4. The surgeon inserts two C-locking rings around the first ratchet immediately below the hook to prevent dislodgement of the hooks. The excessive length of protruding rod above the most proximal hook is removed with a rod cutter. The compression is tightened.

Luque Segmental Spinal Rod Procedure. The Luque segmental method uses smooth L-shaped stainless-steel rods, usually $\frac{3}{16}$ or $\frac{1}{4}$ inch in diameter, with sublaminar wires placed at every level possible. It is more secure and longer than the Harrington rod system and was the first system to use multiple-point fixation. Luque instrumentation applies corrective forces to the spinal segments at each level, thereby spreading the corrective forces throughout the length of the deformity. Two Luque rods are wired to both sides of the spine. The rods are contoured to achieve no more than 10 degrees of increased correction beyond that exhibited on preoperative x-ray study.

Procedural Considerations. The patient is placed in the prone position as described for the Harrington rod procedure. Patient care is provided (see Laminectomy, p. 760). A straight midline incision is made in the back. Because of the amount of bleeding, the skin and subcutaneous tissues are often infiltrated with a vasoconstricting solution, such as epinephrine. Basic spinal instrumentation is required. In addition, Luque rods and instrumentation, a wire tightener and cutter, and bone graft instruments are needed.

Operative Procedure

1. The ligamentum flavum is detached, exposing the neural canal.
2. The surgeon passes doubled stainless steel suture wire under the lamina. The wire loop is cut later to form two wires at each level.
3. Total bilateral facetectomies are made, forming posterolateral troughs for subsequent bone grafts.
4. Wedge osteotomies may be necessary in severe immobile curves to avoid stretching the spinal cord during correction.
5. The wire loop is cut, resulting in two separate wires at each level.
6. The surgeon secures the L bend to the base of the spinous process to prevent rod migration.
7. Initial placement of the convex rod is made, followed by initial placement of the concave rod.
8. Transverse wiring is done to add increased stability to the system.
9. Stabilization of the lumbosacral joint is corrected by bending the rods distally to form sacral bars.

Cotrel-Dubousset System Procedure. The Cotrel-Dubousset system (Figure 20-89) provides three-dimensional correction of spinal deformities without sublaminar wiring and neurologic risks. This instrumentation permits distraction, compression, and derotation. The scoliotic curve is corrected by derotation and, at the same time, restores the normal sagittal contours. In addition to correction of scoliosis, the Cotrel-Dubousset system can be applied to correct kyphosis or lordosis and to stabilize and rebuild the spine after tumor resection or after injury. No external support is necessary. The Cotrel-Dubousset system has no ratchets or notches. It consists of metallic rods with diamond crosscut patterns on which hooks and screws can be positioned in any position, level, or degree of rotation. The rod is held in the open hooks with blockers. The rods are then interlocked with devices for transverse traction. The Cotrel-Dubousset system was the forerunner to the systems used today, such as the Texas Scottish Rite Hospital (TSRH) system and the Isola system.

Procedural Considerations. The patient is placed in the prone position after induction of general anesthesia. Patient assessment and precautions for the prone position are initiated. Basic spinal instrumentation is required in addition to the Cotrel-Dubousset system and instrumentation as well as the instruments used for harvesting the bone graft.

Operative Procedure

1. Closed hooks are inserted at both ends of the surgical site, and open hooks are inserted at various levels between the closed hooks.
2. Decortication and facet excision are done at the remaining interposed vertebral levels for rod placement.
3. Bone graft is placed in the areas that will be under the rod.
4. The surgeon bends the appropriate concave rod to shape for sagittal-plane correction and manipulates it into the end hooks.
5. Stabilization along the length is achieved with blockers that anchor the rod into the open hooks.
6. The spine is then derotated using the rod holders. The frontal-plane scoliosis curve becomes the sagittal-plane kyphosis.
7. Hooks are reseated for secure fixation.
8. To correct kyphosis, the surgeon bends the convex rod to shape and seats it.
9. Once the rods are placed, the surgeon applies the device for transverse traction (DTT), usually near the ends of the rods, to complete the stabilization.
10. Remaining bone graft is then applied to the fusion area.

Texas Scottish Rite Hospital Crosslink System. The TSRH crosslink system (Figure 20-90) is a multicomponent stainless steel implant used to lock spinal rods together rigidly. Locking the rods increases construction stiffness and prevents rod migration. The system was originally designed for the Luque segmental system to prevent migration between the rods and wires before complete fusion occurred. By rigidly crosslinking the rods, loss of scoliotic correction was reduced. This system can also be used with the Harrington and Cotrel-Dubousset systems. Crosslinks are indicated when the rigidity of a spinal system alone is not sufficient to generate fusion in a reasonable amount of time.

Procedural Considerations. The patient is administered a general anesthetic and positioned prone. The skin is prepped, and drapes are applied. A spinal laminectomy set is used. Spinal instrumentation and implants, a spinal retractor, and power equipment such as a high-speed handheld tool are necessary. Hemostatic adjuncts such as gelatin foam, thrombin, oxidized cellulose, and bone wax should be available.

Operative Procedure

1. Eyebolts are placed on the spinal rods before the rods are implanted.
2. The surgeon secures the rods with hooks or wires, depending on the system used.

FIGURE 20-89 Cotrel-Dubousset system, representing rotation of rods.

FIGURE 20-90 Texas Scottish Rite Hospital (TSRH) crosslink system.

3. After the rods are positioned, cross plates of varying widths accommodating different rod-to-rod distances are bolted in place between the rods and nuts.

Anterior Spinal Fusion with Isola Instrumentation. Isola instrumentation involves screw fixation into each vertebral body, complete disk excision and grafting, and segmental connection of the vertebral bodies. A semirigid rod connects the segments. The Isola anterior instrumentation is indicated in idiopathic scoliosis patients, approximately 10 to 30 years of age, with thoracolumbar or upper lumbar curves of 40 to 65 degrees.

Procedural Considerations

The patient is positioned in a lateral decubitus position so that posteroanterior and lateral intraoperative radiographs can be taken. The anesthesia provider should ensure incomplete pharmacologic paralysis, to allow for intraoperative neurophysiologic monitoring. In addition to a major soft tissue set and laminectomy set, the Isola instrumentation and implants, a vascular set, and power equipment are needed.

Operative Procedure

1. The surgeon approaches the spine through a transthoracic retroperitoneal (or retropleural retroperitoneal) approach, resecting the rib two vertebral levels above the upper instrumented vertebrae.
2. The sympathetic chain is mobilized laterally with the psoas.
3. The segmental vessels are temporarily occluded and, provided that there are no monitoring changes, ligated.
4. The disks are exposed to the far side to allow a full annulectomy. The bodies, however, are not exposed much beyond the midline.
5. A full 360-degree diskectomy and annulectomy are done, exposing the posterior longitudinal ligament.
6. The surgeon places the screws in the vertebral body, placing the end screws first. Care is taken to place the longitudinal axis of the screw parallel to the endplate and at the apex of the vertebral body.

7. Screw placement is started with an awl and continued with a 5.5-mm tap, continuing until the tip just exits the far side of the cortex. The first one third of the hole is tapped with a 7-mm tap, and a 7-mm closed top screw with a washer is inserted. The screw must protrude through the opposite cortex by a thread or two. The same process is then repeated at the lower end vertebra.
8. The surgeon cuts the rod to the proper length and contours it to re-create the sagittal-plane angular position of the normal spine. It is then positioned in the end vertebra and used as a guide to locate the entry point for the intermediate screws.
9. Open-ended intermediate screws are inserted in a fashion similar to the end screws, taking care that their pathway is parallel to the end screws.
10. The rod is back-entered through the upper screw and then the lower screw, and seated into the intermediate open screws. The open screws are capped, and the rod is rotated to place the sagittal-plane contour of the rod in the sagittal plane. An intermediate set screw is tightened to secure the new position of the rod.
11. As the remaining screws are tightened about the rod, it is essential that the disk spaces be opened completely. A Cobb elevator can be used to pry the disk space open.
12. Rib corticocancellous autograft is used to completely fill the disk spaces. The surgeon obtains the graft from the tenth rib (the usual site of entry), the twelfth rib (taken from inside the chest), and the eighth rib (taken from outside the chest).
13. The disk spaces are compressed to provide anterior column load-sharing. Care should be taken to ensure that the set screws are visited at least twice for the end-closed connections and three times for the center-capped connections.
14. Closure is in the standard manner, using chest tubes if the chest has been entered or a retropleural Hemovac if a retropleural retroperitoneal exposure has been done.
15. Postoperative care consists of an overnight intensive care stay with the patient sitting out of bed the next morning. A cast or brace is used at the physician's discretion. Activities are restricted for 6 to 12 months, until there is clear indication of graft incorporation.

Artificial Disk Replacement for Degenerative Disk Disease

Degenerative disk disease (DDD) occurs when the intervertebral disk (IVD) is worn because of aging or trauma. Diskogenic back pain results from degeneration of the disk and is confirmed both by patient history and by radiographic studies. The IVD acts as the padding between the vertebrae. Once the IVD is worn out, pain, inflammation, and nerve impingement leading to numbness and muscle weakness can occur. Left untreated, nerve damage can be permanent. DDD occurs in 50% of people older than 40 years of age. Many patients are asymptomatic; however, those who are affected can be severely debilitated, changing their ability to cope with activities of daily living (ADLs) and affecting the quality of life. Artificial disk replacement (Figures 20-91 and 20-92) re-creates the natural disk function with preservation of spinal motion.

Procedural Considerations. The perioperative nurse and scrub person collaborate to ensure the availability of implants with the manufacturer's representative and reconfirm this during the preoperative verification process. Other considerations for this procedure include the use of a blood-salvaging system in both the

FIGURE 20-91 Three components of the ProDisc.

FIGURE 20-92 Assembled ProDisc.

intraoperative and postoperative periods. Templates of x-rays should be placed on the viewing box in the OR before the procedure. The patient is positioned supine on a Jackson bed with the right arm draped across the body. A C-arm is used to identify the disk or disks to be replaced in the marked areas. In many institutions, laminar airflow is used.

Operative Procedure. The two general anatomic routes for anterior exposure to the lumbar spine are retroperitoneal and transperitoneal.

The *retroperitoneal approach* can proceed from a variety of incisions, including vertical midline, paramedian, oblique, and transverse. This is determined by both the spinal level and the number of lumbar levels to be exposed. An infraumbilical transverse incision can accommodate most approaches to the L4-L5 and/or S1 disk levels, whereas a more obliquely oriented incision is favored for accessing disk levels above L4.

The *transperitoneal route* is not generally used except in extenuating circumstances (e.g., prior extensive retroperitoneal surgery or revisional spine surgery).

1. The surgeon creates a midline incision and places a fixed retractor system to move the small and large bowel out of the field and facilitate direct visualization of the abdominal cavity. Trendelenburg position can be used to assist with maintaining exposure.
2. For the L5-S1 level, the peritoneum superficial to the sacral prominence is incised.
3. The surgeon identifies the vascular structures, and uses blunt dissection to tease open the area of the facet of the disk.
4. The middle sacral vessels generally need to be divided to complete the exposure. Excessive electrocoagulation should be avoided to decrease the risk of injury to the sympathetic nerves.
5. After the exposure is complete the surgeon uses a #3 long handle with a #15 blade to make an incision into the disk body.
6. The diskectomy is completed using a rongeur and curettes to remove remaining disk tissue.
7. Correct sizing is determined using templates. Trial instrumentation is inserted and correct placement is verified with AP and lateral C-arm views.
8. The trial is centered in the AP plane, and the marker appears as a plus sign aligned with the spinous process. On the lateral x-ray, a hole in the trial represents the center of rotation.
9. After verifying correct placement of the trial, the surgeon uses an ESU to mark the midline of the superior vertebral body and removes the trial.
10. Next, the pilot driver is aligned with the midline ESU mark.
11. The pilot driver that corresponds to the chosen footprint is then carefully impacted to verify the ability to accurately place endplates.
12. During this process lateral C-arm imaging is used to accurately monitor the depths of the pilot driver.
13. After the correct depth is achieved, the surgeon uses the slap hammer, removing the pilot driver from the disk space.
14. The endplate insertion tips are then attached to the corresponding superior and inferior endplates.
15. The endplates are then carefully inserted into the disk space with the assistance of the guided impactor.
16. The insertion is monitored with fluoroscopy to accurately control the posterior depth and verify the appropriate lordotic angle.
17. With the superior and inferior endplates in place, the surgeon uses the spreading and insertion forceps to open the disk space.
18. After achieving appropriate distraction is achieved, the surgeon can use the size on the spacer to select the appropriate core trial.
19. The appropriate core insertion tip is loaded into the core insertion instrument, and the sliding core is inserted between the endplates.
20. The surgeon releases the distraction on the spreading forceps, which allows the endplates to close around and engage the sliding core.

FIGURE 20-93 Implanted ProDisc.

FIGURE 20-94 Implanted ProDisc with patient bending backward.

21. The core insertion instrument is removed and the final position verified using fluoroscopy (Figures 20-93 and 20-94).
22. The wound is irrigated and closed.

Vertebroplasty and Kyphoplasty

Vertebroplasty and kyphoplasty are used for the treatment of vertebral compression fractures attributable to osteoporosis or pathologic conditions. Bone cement is injected into the vertebral body to decrease back pain and prevent further vertebral body height loss (Ortiz, 2008).

Procedural Considerations. Patient selection is key in identifying appropriate candidates for this procedure. MRI is the most accurate radiologic diagnosis. Equipment includes C-arm, radiolucent procedure table, and x-ray vests for staff as well as vertebroplasty system and cement injection system. Bone biopsy needles should be available. The C-arm must provide a good quality image; all key bony landmarks should be clearly visible. Positioning of the patient requires careful vigilance to prevent skin breakdown and nerve damage. After the administration of anesthetic, the patient is positioned prone with hyperextension of the vertebral compression fracture on the radiolucent procedure table. The patient is then prepped and draped and the C-arm is positioned.

Operative Procedure

1. Confirmation of the level of the vertebroplasty (or kyphoplasty) is determined by fluoroscopy.
2. The surgeon inserts the appropriate gauge bone needle (11- to 13-mm gauge for vertebroplasty; 8- to 10-mm gauge for kyphoplasty) at the desired level and confirms the correct level with fluoroscopy (Figure 20-95, A).
3. For kyphoplasty:
   a. The inflatable balloon tamp is placed. Available tamps are 10, 15, or 20 mm in length, and styles include multi-, uni-, and bidirectional (see Figure 20-95, *B*).
   b. After placing the tamp the surgeon gradually inflates the balloon to 50 pounds per square inch (psi) and then continues inflation in increments of 25 psi until the desired pressure is achieved and either there is height restoration of the vertebral body or the tamp is in proximity to the cortical margin. Pressure is monitored by a manometer.
   c. Once the tamp has reach maximum inflation, the surgeon deflates the balloon. A cavity is left within the vertebral body.
4. Cement is mixed and then injected through the bone needle using a 1-mL syringe (see Figure 20-95) under fluoroscopic control.
5. The needle is removed and a dressing is applied.

KEY POINTS

- Preoperative preparation is key to prevent delays and cancellations on the day of surgery. This includes not only the patient and preoperative testing, paperwork, and education but also proper anticipation for the surgical procedure. Information regarding patient demographics, instrumentation and implants requested, and additional items such as bone grafts should be sent from the surgeon's office when the case is scheduled.
- All vendors should be notified of the scheduled cases to allow enough time to transport and properly sterilize instrumentation necessary for the surgery.
- Adherence to the Surgical Care Improvement Project (SCIP) guidelines for prevention of surgical site infection and venous thromboembolism is critical for this patient population.
- Patient positioning and padding is crucial in preventing nerve injury and maintaining skin integrity.
- Patients undergoing orthopedic surgery, as part of the preop evaluation, have discontinued all antiinflammatories 2 weeks prior to surgery. Care must be taken transporting and moving patients to prevent any additional pain.
- Trauma patients and their families need additional education and communication regarding the surgical process due to the critical nature of the surgery.

FIGURE 20-95 Vertebroplasty. **A,** Frontal fluoroscopic image shows multidirectional bone curette. **B,** Path of least resistance for subsequent balloon tamp inflation.

CRITICAL THINKING QUESTION

Reviewing the surgical schedule the day before surgery, you notice your first patient has been on Coumadin but was told to discontinue the medication 5 days before surgery. Lab work was done while the patient was still on Coumadin, but no additional testing has been ordered. The patient is scheduled to arrive at 6:00 AM for a 7:30 AM incision time. What is the first thing you should do regarding this patient? What needs to be done prior to surgery to ensure a safe procedure for this patient? Who should you notify? Should the OR schedule be changed?

evolve *The answers to the Critical Thinking Question can be found at http://evolve.elsevier.com/Rothrock/Alexander.*

REFERENCES

American Association of Tissue Banks (AATB): *Standards for tissue banking*, McLean, VA, 2011, The Association.

American Board of Orthopaedic Surgeons (ABOS): *History of the American Board of Orthopaedic Surgery*, available at www.abos.org/about/history.aspx. Accessed September 19, 2012.

Association of periOperative Registered Nurses (AORN): *AORN position statement on the role of the health care industry representative in the perioperative/invasive setting 2006*, available at www.aorn.org/PracticeResources/AORNPositionStatements/#axzz2H2NMgYK6. Accessed January 4, 2013.

Association of periOperative Registered Nurses (AORN): Recommended practices for transfer of patient care information. In *Perioperative standards and recommended practices*, Denver, 2013a, The Association.

Association of periOperative Registered Nurses (AORN): Recommended practices for patient skin antisepsis. In *Perioperative standards and recommended practices*, Denver, 2013b, The Association.

Association of periOperative Registered Nurses (AORN): Recommended practices for the use of the pneumatic tourniquet in the perioperative practice setting. In *Perioperative standards and recommended practices*, Denver, 2013c, The Association.

Association of periOperative Registered Nurses (AORN): Recommended practices for a safe environment of care. In *Perioperative standards and recommended practices*, Denver, 2013d, The Association.

Bertin KC, Rottinger H: Anterolateral mini-incision hip replacement surgery: a modified Watson-Jones approach, *Clin Orthop Rel Res* (429):248–255, 2004.

Denholm B: Tucking patient's arms and general positioning, *AORN J* 89(4):755–757, 2009.

Dorr LD et al: Outpatient total hip arthroplasty, *J Arthroplasty* 25(4):50–56, 2010.

Guido GW: *Legal and ethical issues in nursing*, ed 5, Upper Saddle River, NJ, 2010, Prentice-Hall.

Kleinert HE et al: Hand surgery. In Townsend CM, editor: *Sabiston textbook of surgery*, ed 19, Philadelphia, 2012, Saunders.

Miller MD: *Review of orthopaedics*, ed 6, Philadelphia, 2012, Saunders.

National Osteoporosis Foundation (NOF): *Bone health basics*, Washington, DC, National Osteoporosis Foundation, available at www.nof.org/learn. Accessed January 4, 2013.

Ortiz A: Vertebral body reconstruction: review and update on vertebroplasty and kyphoplasty, *Appl Radiol* 37(12):10–24, 2008.

Shigemura T et al: Acetabular liner revision using an anterolateral approach, *Orthopedics* 35(4): e570–e574, 2012.

Srivastav AK et al: Prophylactic use of antibiotic-loaded bone cement in primary total knee arthroplasty: justified or not, *Indian J Orthop* 43(3):259–263, 2009.

The Joint Commission (TJC): *Universal protocol*, 2012, available at www.jointcommission.org/standards_information/up.aspx. Accessed January 5, 2013.

CHAPTER 21

Neurosurgery

SARAH J. KRIZMAN GERMANOVICH

Neurosurgery is a very diverse, complex, and challenging specialty. Brain surgery is performed for head injury, tumors, vascular disorders, hydrocephalus, epilepsy, and Parkinson disease. Neurosurgery also treats disorders of the spine from trauma and fractures, spinal cord injury, spinal stenosis, spinal tumors, and disk disease. Advancements in the highly technical field of neurosurgery are constant.

The perioperative team who cares for neurosurgical patients are challenged by the need to have a working knowledge of neuroanatomy, function, and clinical presentations of the many neurologic conditions that require surgical interventions. Understanding the surgical procedure to be performed allows the perioperative nurse and scrub person, who may be a registered nurse or surgical technologist, to anticipate and respond to the intraoperative needs of the patient and neurosurgical team, and to surgical complications if they arise. Given the range and complexity of today's neurosurgical interventions, an understanding of highly sophisticated equipment and instrumentation is necessary. Like all patients undergoing surgery, the neurosurgical patient is often vulnerable secondary to the presenting pathologic condition. For perioperative personnel to deliver sensitive, humanistic care in this highly technical environment, they must recognize and appreciate the individual's emotional and spiritual state, whether it is manifested by fear, pain, or grief. Reaching out and making the human connection allay the fear, moderate the pain, and facilitate the patient's grieving process. Information in this chapter will assist those working in neurosurgery to provide optimal patient care.

Surgical Anatomy

The nervous system is the most complex and least understood of body systems. It is divided structurally into the central nervous system (CNS) consisting of the brain and spinal cord and the peripheral nervous system (PNS), which encompasses every neurologic structure outside the CNS, including the cranial and spinal nerves. The brain and spinal cord are protected by the skull and vertebral columns, respectively. The cranial nerves originate within the brain and emerge through openings in the skull to run peripherally. The spinal nerves that emerge from the spinal cord through the vertebral foramina also run peripherally.

The nervous system is divided functionally into a voluntary system and an autonomic, or involuntary, system. It provides a means of communication for the rest of the body. The functions of all body systems depend in part on nervous system function. In turn, the nervous system depends directly on circulatory system function to obtain life-sustaining glucose and oxygen. Nervous system functions include motor and sensory functions, orientation,

coordination, conceptual thought, emotion, memory, and reflex response.

Nervous system tissue is composed of vast amounts of neurons and far more neuroglial cells. Neurons are intercommunicating nerve cells that encode, conduct, and transmit information to other neurons, muscle, and glandular tissue (Figure 21-1). They are composed of a body or soma with branches or extensions, called dendrites and axons, which communicate with other cells at synapses. Dendrites are short branches that conduct impulses toward the soma. Cell bodies and dendrites are mostly confined to areas of gray matter in the CNS. Axons are long branches, often encased in a white myelin sheath, that conduct impulses away from the soma. Axons pass into bundles of nerve fibers that tend to form tracts or pathways and are referred to as white matter. Tracts that cross midline to create a communication pathway from each side of the body to the opposite side of the brain are called commissures. Neuroglial cells support the neurons by creating and maintaining an appropriate environment in which neurons can operate efficiently. Glial cells include astrocytes, oligodendrocytes, ependymal cells, and microglia. The mutation of these cells can form a glioma, one of the more common brain tumors.

This chapter divides the nervous system into logical divisions within the framework of neurosurgical techniques. The brain and adjacent structures include the cranial nerves of the PNS, which are commonly encountered during brain surgery. Discussion of the spine and spinal cord includes the adjacent spinal nerves and the disks and ligaments that support the spine. Surgically significant pathology is incorporated with the normal anatomy of structures.

Brain and Adjacent Structures

Scalp

Scalp layers (Figure 21-2) include skin, subcutaneous tissue, galea, and periosteum. Scalp skin is thick. The subcutaneous tissue, which is exceptionally dense, tough, and vascular, is firmly attached to the galea. Most of the blood vessels lie superficial to the galea. The subgaleal space contains loose areolar tissue that permits mobility of the scalp. It is in this bloodless plane that the standard craniotomy scalp flap is created. The pericranium, or outer periosteum of the skull, separates the galea from the cranium.

The arterial supply of the scalp comes from the external carotid artery through the superficial temporal, posterior auricular, occipital, frontal, and supraorbital branches. Most veins roughly follow the course of their corresponding arteries, except the emissary veins, which drain directly through the skull into the intracranial venous sinuses. The scalp, the extracranial arteries, and portions of the dura mater are the only pain-sensitive structures that cover the brain. The brain itself is insensate.

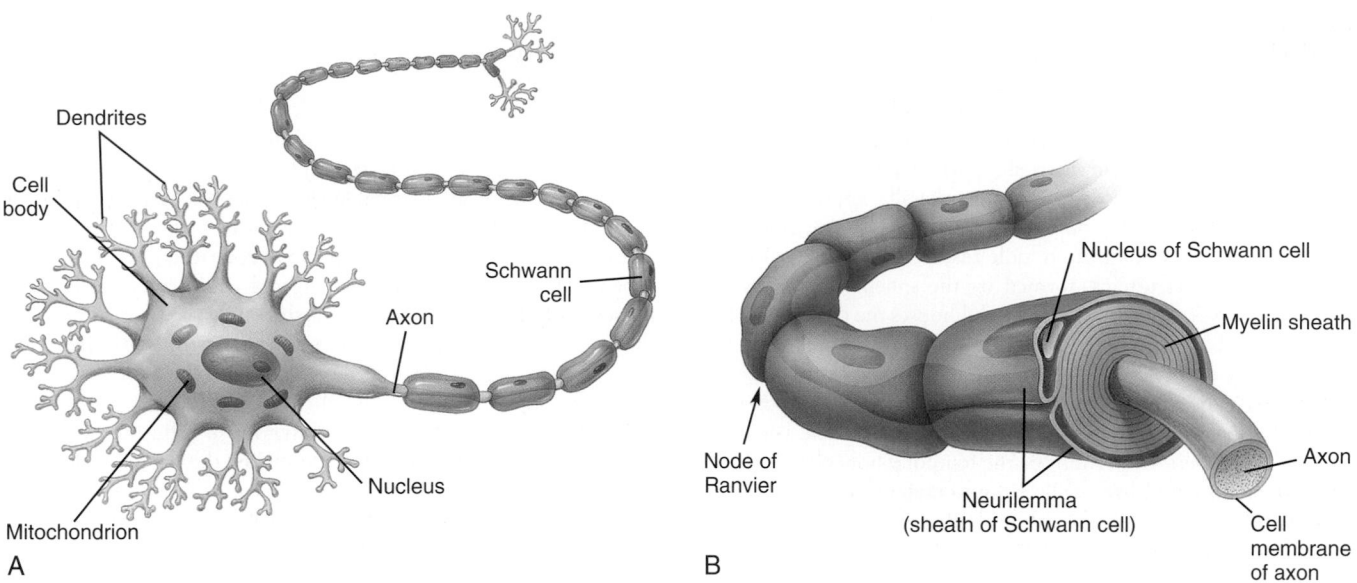

FIGURE 21-1 A, Many dendrites carry nerve impulses to the cell body, which then sends the nerve impulses along a single, long axon. Long axons are encased at intervals by a myelin sheath. **B,** A segment of myelinated fiber in cross section, showing myelin sheath composed of several layers of myelin, which insulate the axon.

FIGURE 21-2 Scalp is composed of the following layers: skin, subcutaneous tissue, galea, and periosteum. Skull bone has three tables: outer, diploë (or spongy layer), and inner. Dura mater lies beneath skull and completely encapsulates the brain. Other structures are identified for reference and are described in text.

Skull

The skull provides protection for the brain. It is formed by 28 bones, most of which are paired although some in the median plane are single. Many of the bones are flat bones, consisting of two thin plates of compact bone encasing a spongy layer of cancellous bone containing bone marrow (see Figure 21-2). Infants are born with two fontanelles. These are openings in the skull that are located both anterior and posterior to the parietal bones (Figure 21-3). The posterior fontanelle is generally closed by 2 months and the anterior by about 18 months after birth. The bones of the skull are joined by bony seams called *sutures.* Eight bones form the walls of the cranial cavity, which houses the brain. There are four single bones (frontal, occipital, ethmoid, and sphenoid) and four paired bones (temporal and parietal) (Figure 21-4). The sagittal suture lies in the medial plane and joins the two parietal bones. The coronal suture joins the frontal and parietal bones. The squamous sutures border the squamous part of the temporal bones. The lambdoid suture joins the occipital and parietal bones. Skull bones vary in thickness and tend to be thinner where they are covered in muscles, for example, in the temporal and posterior fossae. The skull articulates with the first cervical vertebra to allow for flexion and extension of the skull. The skeletal surface landmarks of the head can be palpated and are commonly used to plan surgical approaches (Figure 21-5).

The interior of the skull is anatomically divided into three cranial fossae: anterior, middle, and posterior. The anterior fossa is limited posteriorly by the sphenoid ridge, along which pituitary tumors and aneurysms of the circle of Willis are generally approached. The frontal lobes and olfactory bulbs and tracts lie in the anterior fossa. The temporal lobes lie in the middle fossa, which is shaped like a butterfly. The sella turcica, formed by the sphenoid bone, is the most central part of the middle fossa and houses the pituitary gland. The floor and lateral walls of the middle fossa are shaped from the greater wings of the sphenoid bone and parts of the temporal bone, which house the internal and middle ear structures. The posterior fossa, the largest and deepest fossa, is formed by the occipital, sphenoid, and petrous portions of the temporal bones; the cerebellum and brainstem lie here, as do many cranial nerves. The foramen magnum, the largest opening in the skull, provides passage for the

spinal cord to join the brainstem in the posterior fossa. Numerous other openings exist in the base of the skull for passage of arteries, veins, and cranial nerves (Figure 21-6).

Skull Fractures. The severity of skull fractures depends on the degree of resulting brain injury. Simple skull fractures can be serious if they cross major vascular channels in the skull. If vessels are torn, epidural or subdural hematomas may form. Depressed skull fractures require a surgical procedure to elevate the depressed bone. Open skull fractures should be irrigated copiously and closed to prevent infection. Basilar skull fractures may cause cerebrospinal fluid (CSF) rhinorrhea or otorrhea. A few patients with these CSF leaks require surgical repair if they do not resolve after 2 weeks.

Deformities of the Cranium. Craniosynostosis is the most common pediatric skull deformity seen and treated by the neurosurgeon. The phenomenon is a premature closure or lack of formation of cranial sutures, leading to cosmetic abnormalities, eventual life-threatening intracranial pressure (ICP) increases, and arrested brain development unless diagnostic and surgical interventions ensue. Cranial remodeling is most often undertaken during the first year of life, when brain capacity triples (see Chapter 26).

Meninges

The brain and spinal cord are completely enveloped by the meninges, which are three membranes that provide support and protection. The meningeal layers from superficial to deep are the dura mater, arachnoid mater, and pia mater (see Figure 21-2). The space superficial to the dura is known as the epidural space. The cranial meninges are located between the skull and the brain.

The dura mater is a tough, shiny, fibrous membrane that is close to the inner surface of the skull and folds to separate the cranial cavity into compartments. The largest fold is the falx cerebri—an arch-shaped, vertically placed, midline structure separating the right and left cerebral hemispheres (see Figure 21-2). A smaller fold of dura mater, the falx cerebelli, separates the cerebellar hemispheres vertically. A transverse fold, the tentorium cerebelli, forms the roof of the posterior fossa. The tentorium supports the temporal lobe

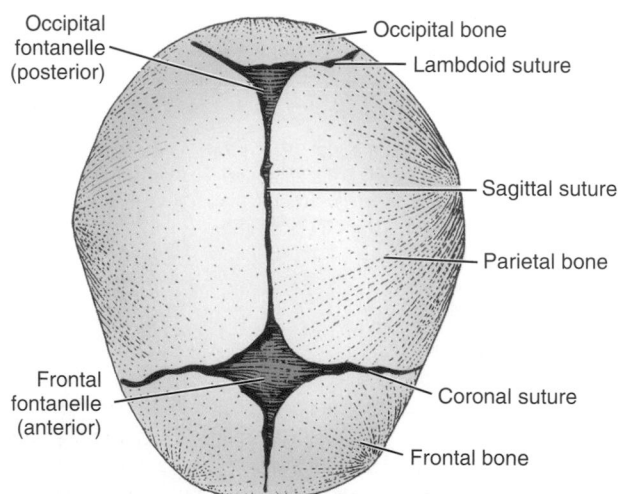

FIGURE 21-3 Skull at birth viewed from above.

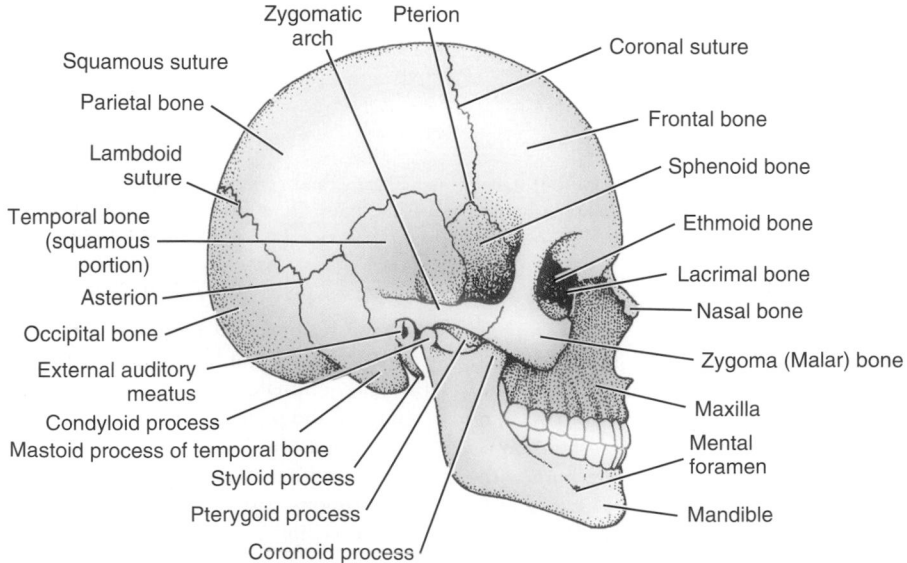

FIGURE 21-4 Skull viewed from right side.

and occipital lobes of the cerebral hemispheres. Below the tentorium lie the cerebellum and brainstem. Structures above the tentorium are referred to as *supratentorial* and those below as *infratentorial* (Figure 21-7). At margins of these dural folds lie large venous sinuses that drain blood from the intracranial structures into the jugular veins. Accidental breaching of a sinus during surgery can cause severe bleeding that is difficult to control and may put the patient at risk for a venous air embolism. Several arteries also lie within the layers of the dura. The largest is the middle meningeal, a source of serious epidural hemorrhage if torn by an overlying skull fracture. The rigid skull makes hemorrhage and swelling in the brain critical events. The volume of the intracranial cavity is fixed. Increasing the intracranial contents by a hemorrhage, tumor, or edema may lead to serious ICP problems. Pressure on brain tissue may cause irreparable damage.

Beneath the dura mater is a transparent membrane called the *arachnoid.* Although the outer layer of arachnoid closely approximates the dura mater, the space between is considered the subdural space. The inner arachnoid layer forms innumerable weblike filaments that bridge to the surface of the brain (see Figure 21-2). The arachnoid passes over the sulci and fissures of the brain, without dipping into them. The arachnoid is separated from the pia mater beneath it by the subarachnoid space, which is filled with CSF that bathes the brain. Around the base of the brain, particularly, this space becomes enlarged to form cisterns. The major intracranial nerves and blood vessels pass through these compartments. Intracranial approaches can be charted in terms of the basal cisterns.

The pia mater, the innermost membrane, closely follows the contours of the surface of the brain into the sulci and fissures. Only the microscopic subpial space separates the pia from the brain. The pia mater has a rich vascular network. Vascular fringes of pia mater project into the ventricles to form the choroid plexus of the ventricles, which produce CSF.

Brain

The anatomy of the brain, formally known as the encephalon, can be considered in multiple ways. Based on prenatal development, the principal divisions from rostral (head) to caudal (tail), descending toward the spinal cord, are the forebrain or prosencephalon, the midbrain or mesencephalon, and the hindbrain or rhombencephalon. The rhombencephalon is subdivided into the cerebellum, the medulla oblongata, and the pons. The prosencephalon includes the diencephalon and the telencephalon, or cerebrum. The medulla

FIGURE 21-5 Lateral aspect of the head: bones. *1,* Frontal. *2,* Parietal. *3,* Occipital. *4,* Bregma (anterior fontanelle). *5,* Lambda (posterior fontanelle). *6,* Greater wing of sphenoid. *7,* Squamous temporal. *8,* Pterion. *9,* Temporal lines. *10,* Zygomatic arch. *11,* Mastoid process. *12,* Styloid process. *13,* Glabella. *14,* External occipital protuberance.

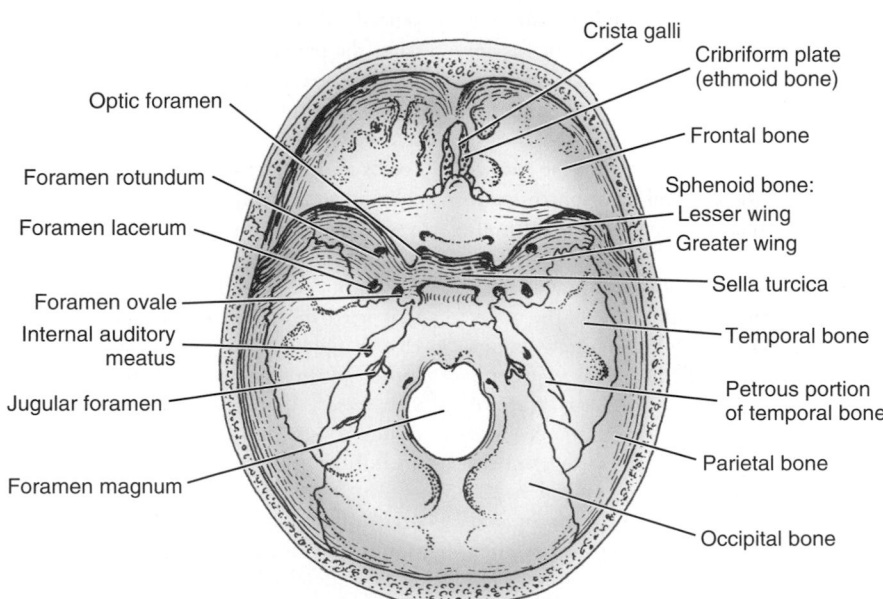

FIGURE 21-6 Floor of cranial cavity.

FIGURE 21-7 Sagittal section of head showing cerebrospinal fluid spaces and their relationship to venous circulation and their principal subdivision of the brain and its coverings.

oblongata, pons, and midbrain are collectively referred to as the brainstem (Figures 21-7 and 21-8).

Cerebrum. The right and the left cerebral hemispheres are the largest parts of the brain and occupy the anterior and middle fossae. Each hemisphere is divided into frontal, parietal, occipital, and temporal lobes. The two hemispheres are separated by the longitudinal fissure and the falx cerebri but remain connected underneath the falx by a large transverse bundle of nerve fibers called the corpus callosum (see Figure 21-8). Each of the cerebral hemispheres controls sensation and motor activity to and receives sensory stimuli from the opposite half of the body.

The convoluted surface of the cerebrum consists of gray matter, called the *cerebral cortex,* which contains the cell bodies of the many nerve pathways of the brain. The underlying white matter contains millions of myelinated nerve axons and is relatively avascular compared with the cortex. The nerve pathways, or fiber tracts, are of three types: (1) commissural fibers, which pass from one cerebral hemisphere to the other; (2) association fibers, which connect regions of gyri and lobes longitudinally within a cerebral hemisphere; and (3) projection fibers, including the great motor and sensory systems, which run vertically to connect the cortical regions with other portions of the CNS.

The surfaces of the hemispheres form convolutions called *gyri* and intervening furrows called *sulci,* which serve as anatomic landmarks. Two sulci of particular anatomic importance during surgery are: (1) the lateral sulcus, or sylvian fissure, which divides the temporal lobe from the frontal and parietal lobes, and (2) the central sulcus, or fissure of Rolando, which separates the frontal from the parietal lobe. The central sulcus also separates the motor cortex (precentral gyrus) from the sensory cortex (postcentral gyrus). The motor cortex lies anterior to the central sulcus, and the sensory cortex lies posterior to the central sulcus. Both the motor cortex and the sensory cortex can be represented by a topographically organized map called a homunculus that proportionately represents each body part at the area of the gyri that controls it. The diagrams illustrate how the number of neurons corresponds to the degree of motor and sensory control required. For example, areas that need more fine motor control, such as the fingers and face, have a higher concentration of neurons than other areas. The left motor and sensory cortices control the right side of the body and vice versa (Figure 21-9). Destruction of an area of motor cortex results in loss of voluntary motor function on the corresponding area of the opposite side of the body (Figure 21-10).

The frontal lobe is anterior to the central sulcus and controls the higher functions of intellect and abstract reasoning, along with movement, language, and personality. Posterior to the central sulcus is the parietal lobe, extending back to the parieto-occipital fissure. This area contains the final receiving and integrating station for sensory impulses, such as pain and touch, from the contralateral

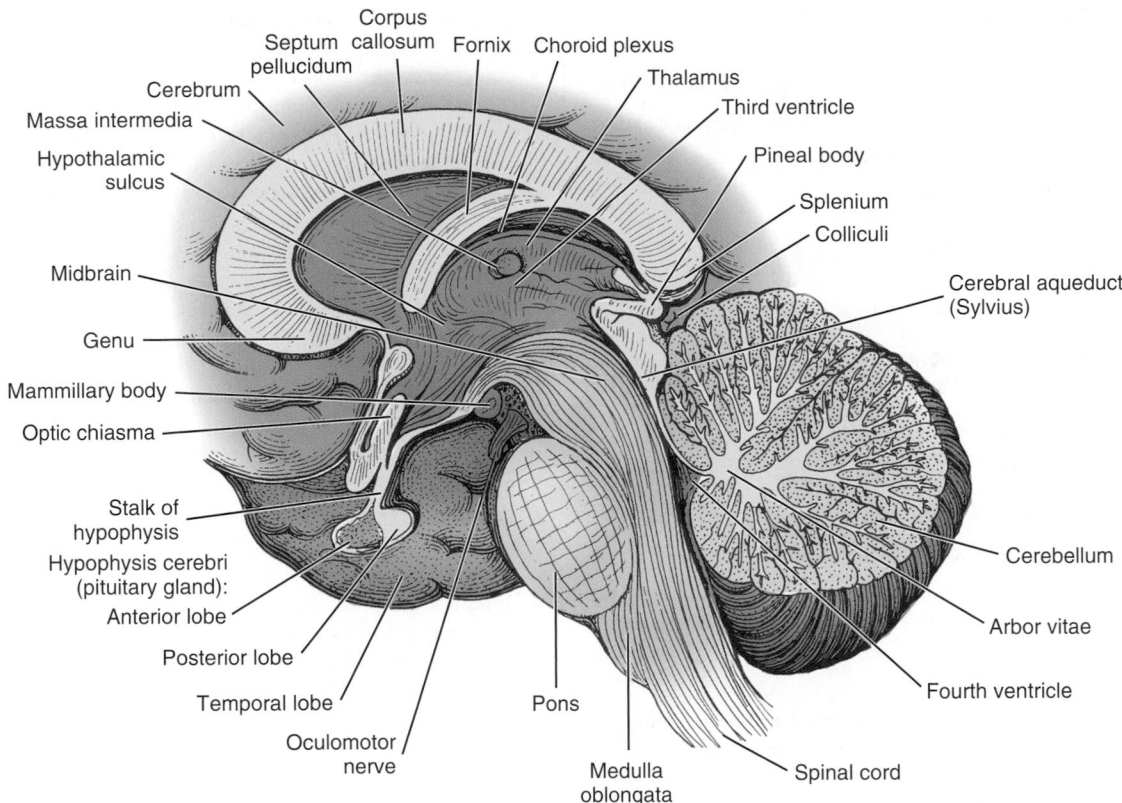

FIGURE 21-8 Sagittal section through midline of brain showing structures around third ventricle, including corpus callosum, thalamus, and hypothalamus.

FIGURE 21-9 Lateral view of cerebral hemisphere (showing lobes and principal fissures), cerebellum, pons, and medulla oblongata.

FIGURE 21-10 Principal functional subdivisions of cerebral hemispheres.

side of the body. It is also involved with special relationships and object identification. The occipital lobe lies posterior to the parieto-occipital fissure. It receives and integrates visual impulses and registers them as meaningful images (see Figures 21-9 and 21-10).

Inferior to the lateral sulcus, in the middle fossa, is the temporal lobe, which is involved with memory, speech, and smell. Lesions of the left temporal lobe in right-handed persons and in many left-handed persons may affect the comprehension and verbalization of words, resulting in aphasia. The insula (island of Reil) is an area of cortex that lies deep within the lateral sulcus and can be exposed when the upper and lower lips of the fissure are separated. The insula is believed to be involved with smell, taste, touch, and possibly language.

The limbic system consists of large parts of the cortex near the medial wall of the cerebral hemisphere (cingulate and parahippocampal gyri) along with the hippocampus, amygdala, and septum. It is closely and significantly connected with the hypothalamus. It has a diffuse distribution in the brain, and many components of the limbic system have overlapping functions. The hippocampus is critical for learning and memory. The amygdala regulates the

Gray matter
Anterior horn of lateral ventricle
Internal capsule
Globus pallidus
Midbrain
Pons
Medulla oblongata

White matter
Cerebral cortex
Corpus callosum
Head of caudate nucleus
Basal ganglia
Putamen
Thalamus
Subthalamic nucleus
Substantia nigra

FIGURE 21-11 Oblique coronal section through the cerebral hemisphere and brainstem showing the disposition of gray and white matter, the basal ganglia, and the internal capsule.

perceptive and expressive aspects of emotional and social behavior. The limbic system affects endocrine and autonomic functions of the body, recent memory, emotions, behaviors, and motivational and mood states. Restlessness and hyperactivity may result from lesions of this area.

The basal ganglia are subcortical collections of nuclei (gray matter) that include the caudate nucleus, putamen, and globus pallidus (collectively referred to as the *corpus striatum*); the substantia nigra (which is located in the midbrain); and the subthalamic nucleus (part of the diencephalon). The basal ganglia influence movement and behavior through projections to the thalamus and brainstem and subsequently the cortex (Figure 21-11). The basal ganglia function to promote and support patterns of behavior and movement that are appropriate in a given situation and to inhibit unwanted or inappropriate behavior and movements. Disorders of the basal ganglia are principally characterized by abnormalities of movement, muscle tone, and posture. Damage to these neural components may cause rigidity of the skeletal muscles and various types of spontaneous tremors.

Diencephalon. The diencephalon is composed of the thalamus, hypothalamus, epithalamus, and subthalamus and surrounds the third ventricle. The thalamus is the major relay station for incoming sensory stimuli. Except for some olfactory impulse transmission, all sensory information transmitted to the cerebral hemispheres is relayed through the thalamus. This is also true for motor pathways from the cerebellum and basal ganglia. Because of the central role of the thalamus in perception of body sensations, surgical lesions can be made in this area in an attempt to alleviate pain.

Along the floor of the third ventricle is the hypothalamus (see Figure 21-8), which is concerned principally with the autonomic regulation of the body's internal environment and is intimately connected with the pituitary gland. It controls fluid and electrolyte balance, appetite, reproduction, thermoregulation, immune response, and many emotional responses. It influences levels of attention and consciousness. The pituitary gland is suspended from the base of the hypothalamus by the pituitary stalk.

It secretes multiple hormones that are regulated by the hypothalamus. A pituitary tumor can result in a hormonal imbalance. It can also encroach on the optic chiasma, causing vision changes.

The subthalamus is a complex region of nuclear groups and fiber tracts, including the subthalamic nucleus, which is considered with the basal ganglia. The epithalamus consists of multiple nuclei and the pineal gland, an endocrine gland that regulates the circadian rhythm.

Brainstem. The brainstem consists of the midbrain, pons, and medulla oblongata. It is located in the posterior fossa and forms the floor of the fourth ventricle. It is the site of many ascending and descending fiber tracts that allow for communication among the structures of the brain and between the brain and spinal cord. All but 2 of the 12 cranial nerves attach to the brainstem. The short, stocky portion of the brain, between the cerebral hemispheres and pons, is the midbrain (see Figure 21-7), also referred to as the *mesencephalon*. It is composed of the cerebral peduncles, the substantia nigra, numerous nerve tracts and nuclei, and association centers that control the majority of eye movements. Immediately below the midbrain is the pons, which contains control areas for horizontal eye movement and face movement. The medulla oblongata is continuous with the spinal cord at the foramen magnum. It contains the vital cardiovascular and respiratory regulatory centers (see Figure 21-9). Damage to the brainstem is often devastating and life-threatening because it can affect movement, senses, consciousness, perception, and cognition.

Cerebellum. The cerebellum, which occupies most of the posterior fossa, forms the roof of the fourth ventricle (see Figures 21-8 and 21-12). It has two lateral lobes, or hemispheres, and a medial portion, the vermis. The fissures of the cerebellum are small and run transversely. The cerebellum is concerned principally with balance and coordination of movement. It has many complex connections with higher and lower centers and exerts its influence unilaterally—in contrast to the cerebral hemispheres, which act contralaterally. By splitting the vermis in the exact midline, a satisfactory exposure of tumors that lie in the fourth ventricle is obtained without sacrificing the important cerebellar functions.

Pathologic Lesions of the Brain. An estimated new 69,720 primary brain tumors are expected to occur in 2013 (American Brain Tumor Association [ABTA], 2012). Brain metastases outnumber primary neoplasms by at least 10 to 1, and are the most common brain tumor in adults. Unfortunately, the exact incidence is unknown, but it has been estimated that 100,000 to 170,000 new cases are diagnosed in the United States each year (ABTA, 2012).

Multiple factors are suspected of playing a role in the pathogenesis of intracranial neoplasms. Early diagnosis simplifies surgical treatment because increased ICP and severe neurologic changes are not usually present. Brain tumors are either malignant or benign, depending on the cell type. Primary tumors generally do not resemble the carcinomas and sarcomas found elsewhere in the body and rarely metastasize outside the CNS. Both primary and metastatic tumors of the brain and its membranes are included in the term *intracranial tumors.*

Traditionally, tumors are classified by cell type; however, classification of brain tumors is an evolving process. The widely used World Health Organization (WHO) system lists more than 120 types of brain tumors (National Cancer Institute [NCI], 2009). A brief description of a select list of brain tumors follows:

1. *Tumors of intraepithelial tissue* encompass gliomas, tumors believed to originate from neuroglial cells. Gliomas represent 30% of all brain tumors and 80% of all malignant tumors (ABTA, 2012).

   a. Astrocytomas represent 7% of all primary brain tumors (ABTA, 2012). They usually occur in the cerebellum of children and the cerebrum of adults. They are often cystic and discrete in children and infiltrating and ill-defined in adults. Astrocytomas are classified in the WHO system based on the principal cell type and on the degree of anaplasia as grade I to IV, with grade I being the more favorable type of tumor and grade IV being the most malignant. Glioblastoma multiforme (GBM), a grade IV astrocytoma, is an infiltrative, fast-growing, rapidly recurring cerebral tumor that occurs most frequently in the sixth and seventh decades of life. Glioblastomas represent 17% of all primary brain tumors, and account for about 54% of all gliomas (ABTA, 2012). It is one of the few tumors that is capable of invading both cerebral hemispheres by crossing the midline. Areas of necrosis are characteristic. Recent studies have consistently demonstrated the benefits of radical surgical resection. Postoperative radiation therapy significantly improves survival. Even with aggressive multimodality therapy, median survival is approximately 14.6 months and 2-year survival is about 30% (ABTA, 2012).

   b. Oligodendroglioma, typically found in the cerebral hemispheres, is usually infiltrating but occasionally moderately well defined. It frequently presents in middle age with seizure. The incidence of oligodendrogliomas is approximately 4% of all primary brain tumors, and represent 10% to 15% of all gliomas. Therapy usually consists of surgery followed by radiation therapy and chemotherapy (ABTA, 2012).

   c. Ependymoma occurs most frequently in children and is likely to arise in or near the ventricular walls. It commonly occurs in the fourth ventricle, where it abuts or involves vital medullary centers. It also frequently metastasizes into the subarachnoid spaces. This tumor accounts for 2% to 3% of gliomas in adults, and the fourth most common brain tumor in children. Surgical resection followed by radiation therapy is the usual treatment. With treatment survival rates are approximately 73%, however treatment in children may have significant side effects such as decreased intellect and learning problems (ABTA, 2012).

   d. Medulloblastoma is a fast-growing, rapidly recurring tumor of the vermis of the cerebellum and fourth ventricle that usually occurs in young children. It characteristically metastasizes into the subarachnoid spaces, usually spreading to the base of the brain by this route. It accounts for 15% to 20% of childhood intracranial brain tumors and is the most common malignant pediatric brain tumor.

2. *Tumors of the meninges (meningiomas)* have become the most common primary brain tumor, representing 34% of all primary brain tumors (ABTA, 2012). They are usually benign, circumscribed, slow-growing tumors, arising from arachnoid cells with secondary attachment to the dura. Various factors have been implicated in the development of meningiomas. They typically involve the cortex and bone of the skull with growth. They can be very vascular and may adhere to the dural venous sinuses or major arteries, making their complete removal challenging. However, meningiomas often can be totally surgically removed.

3. *Tumors of the cranial nerves (vestibular schwannomas)* are benign; they usually arise from the neurilemma sheath cells of the vestibular portion of the eighth cranial nerve within the auditory meatus. The term *acoustic neuroma* is a misnomer. These tumors grow slowly to fill the cerebellopontine angle and may indent the brainstem. Presenting symptoms include hearing loss, tinnitus, and disequilibrium.

4. *Hematopoietic neoplasms and lymphomas* occur most often in the cerebral hemispheres, but may also involve CSF, the eyes, or the spinal cord (ABTA, 2012). The main role for surgery is for tumor biopsy. Stereotactic techniques are well suited for these often-deep tumors. The standard treatment after biopsy is steroids to control brain swelling, chemotherapy, and radiation (ABTA, 2012).

5. *Germ cell tumors* occur in the midline (suprasellar and pineal region). Other than benign teratomas, all intracranial germ cell tumors are malignant and may metastasize by way of CSF and systemically. Tumors of the pineal region are very challenging to the neurosurgeon. Open microsurgery, endoscopy, and stereotactic biopsy are surgical options. Pineal region tumors often cause hydrocephalus. An endoscopic third ventriculostomy or a shunting procedure is routinely performed to alleviate the symptoms of hydrocephalus. Radiation therapy, chemotherapy, and radiosurgery are also treatment considerations.

   a. Germinoma is a neoplasm arising from germ cells. Survival with germinomas is much better than with nongerminomatous tumors (teratoma, embryonal cell carcinoma, choriocarcinoma).

   b. Teratoma is a congenital tumor containing embryonic elements.

   c. Embryonal cell carcinoma consists of a highly primitive group of neoplasms that arise in childhood. Predominantly large hemispheric masses involving deep supratentorial structures, these tumors are highly vascular and have poor prognoses. The primitive neuroectodermal tumor (PNET) is one such tumor.

   d. Choriocarcinoma is an extremely rare, very malignant neoplasm.

6. *Cysts and tumor-like lesions* include the following types:

   a. Epidermoid and dermoid cysts are developmental, benign tumors typically located in the suprasellar region.

   b. Colloid cysts are slow-growing benign tumors. They classically occur in the anterior third ventricle, blocking the foramen of Monro and causing obstructive hydrocephalus.

7. *Tumors of the sellar region* include the following types:

   a. Pituitary adenomas can be classified as nonfunctioning or functioning. *Nonfunctioning* pituitary adenomas account for approximately 30% of pituitary tumors, usually occur in people in the fourth and fifth decades of life, and do not cause clinical hormone hypersecretion. They are typically large and cause hypopituitarism or blindness from regional compression. The usual treatment is endoscopic or microscopic transsphenoidal removal of the tumor. Radiation therapy or stereotactic radiosurgery may also be used. *Functioning* pituitary adenomas secrete excess quantities of pituitary hormones, and account for 70% of pituitary tumors. The question of medical versus surgical treatment is ever present in the management of this group of patients. Adenomas may be further subdivided into microadenomas, which are less than 1 cm in diameter and may present with an increase in prolactin levels. Macroadenomas, which are larger than 1 cm, may present with an increase in growth hormone (ABTA, 2012).

(1) Chromophobe tumors are relatively common in the anterior pituitary glands of adults. They cause compression of the pituitary, adjacent optic chiasma, and hypothalamus. Compression of the hypothalamus may lead to diabetes insipidus.

(2) Eosinophilic adenomas are secretory, causing an excessive amount of growth hormone in the serum.

(3) Basophilic adenomas are responsible for the excessive secretion of corticotropic, gonadotropic, and thyrotropic hormones. Acromegaly or, less commonly, Cushing syndrome may occur and cause the patient to seek help long before the tumor has expanded sufficiently to compromise the optic chiasma.

(4) Prolactin cell adenoma exhibits considerable differences in clinical presentation, depending on the gender of the patient. In women of reproductive age, the onset of amenorrhea and galactorrhea with associated infertility is an obvious sign. The diagnosis of a prolactinoma is established early in the course. In men, the clinical endocrinal symptoms, which include decreased libido and impotence, are not as conspicuous and initially may be disregarded by the patient. As a result, male patients frequently do not seek medical attention until the tumors are large and have spread beyond the confines of the sella turcica.

b. Craniopharyngiomas account for 2.5% to 5% of adult intracranial tumors, and 5% to 10% of childhood brain tumors (ABTA, 2012). They arise from the region of the pituitary stalk and typically contain both solid and cystic components. Calcification above the sella turcica is often seen radiographically. In addition to headache, vertigo, vomiting, and papilledema, diabetes insipidus and visual field changes are common. Although complete surgical removal is often impossible if it adheres to the carotid artery or hypothalamus, a subtotal resection with radiation offers favorable results.

8. *Metastatic tumors* are the most common brain tumor seen clinically, making up about half of brain tumors. They usually arise from carcinomas, more rarely from sarcomas, and occasionally from melanomas and retinal tumors. The most common sources are lung and breast cancer. The management of brain metastasis is complex and controversial. The current principal options for treatment include whole-brain radiation therapy, surgery, and stereotactic radiosurgery. The most important prognostic variables are the extent of systemic disease and the patient's functional status and age. These factors, along with the size, number, and location of tumors, guide treatment decisions.

A brain lesion is diagnosed by history, neurologic examination, diagnostic studies (especially computed tomography [CT] scan and magnetic resonance imaging [MRI]), and biopsy. The manifestations of an intracranial tumor fall into two classes: those resulting from irritation or impairment of function in specific areas of the brain directly affected by the tumor and those resulting from diffuse increased ICP. The most common presentation of brain tumors is progressive neurologic deficit, usually motor weakness. Headache, seizures, vision loss, and hearing loss are also common presenting symptoms (ABTA, 2012).

Large left or bifrontal lobe tumors may cause striking personality changes and depressive symptoms. Lesions in the left frontotemporal region, where motor speech originates, lead to aphasia. Parietal lobe lesions may result in contralateral weakness and sensory changes, along with defects in the perception of objects. Occipital tumors produce hemianopic visual defects.

Cortical tumors frequently produce focal seizures of diagnostic value. The onset of epileptiform seizures in an adult is often associated with an intracranial neoplasm. Posterior fossa tumors often manifest their presence by blocking the CSF circulation, but they may also destroy cerebellar function, resulting in incoordination, ataxia, scanning speech, and deafness.

Treatment of brain tumors, although based on the characteristics of the tumor, can involve administration of steroids or antiepileptic medications, management of hydrocephalus, surgery, radiosurgery, radiation, and chemotherapy.

The presentation of multiple brain lesions in a patient is of grave concern, and an infective process should be considered along with the possibility of multiple tumors. Stereotactic biopsy of the lesion is most likely to provide a diagnosis. The operative team should use precautions to prevent the spread of an unknown infective process. Identification of the infective agent and process determines proper treatment.

Ventricular System and Cerebrospinal Fluid

Within the brain are four communicating cavities, or ventricles, filled with CSF. In the lower medial portion of each cerebral hemisphere lies a large lateral ventricle that resembles a wishbone and is separated anteriorly from its counterpart by a thin septum (Figure 21-12). Each lateral ventricle has a body and three horns: frontal, occipital, and temporal. Below the bodies of the lateral ventricles is a central cleft, or third ventricle. It communicates anteriorly with the lateral ventricles through the foramen of Monro and posteriorly with the fourth ventricle through the aqueduct of Sylvius—a long, narrow channel passing through the midbrain. The fourth ventricle is a cavity in the posterior fossa, between the cerebellum and the brainstem. In the roof of the fourth ventricle is the foramen of Magendie, an opening into the cisterna magna; at the lateral margins are the two foramina of Luschka, which open into the cisterna pontis. These cisterns are cavities that serve as reservoirs for CSF.

Much of the CSF originates in the choroid plexuses of the ventricles. These are tufted, vascular structures that allow certain fluid elements of the blood to pass through their ependymal linings. The choroid plexus is found along the floor in each lateral ventricle, on the roof of the third ventricle, and in the posterior portion of the fourth ventricle. Most of the fluid is formed in the lateral ventricles and flows through the interventricular foramen of Monro to the third ventricle and through the aqueduct of Sylvius to the fourth ventricle, where it escapes into the subarachnoid space of the basal cisterns through the foramina of Magendie and Luschka. From the basal cisterns the fluid flows around the spinal cord, over the cerebellar lobes, around the medulla and the base of the brain, and over the cerebral hemispheres in the subarachnoid space. The fluid is absorbed into the venous circulation through villi of the arachnoid (pacchionian granulations) into the great dural venous sinuses, particularly the superior sagittal sinus, and by diffusion through perivascular, perineural, and periradicular channels (see Figure 21-7).

Spinal fluid bathes the brain and spinal cord, helps support the weight of the brain, and acts as a cushion for the brain and spinal cord by absorbing some of the force of external trauma. By variation in its volume, it aids in keeping ICP relatively constant. If the brain atrophies, the amount of CSF increases to fill the dead space; if the

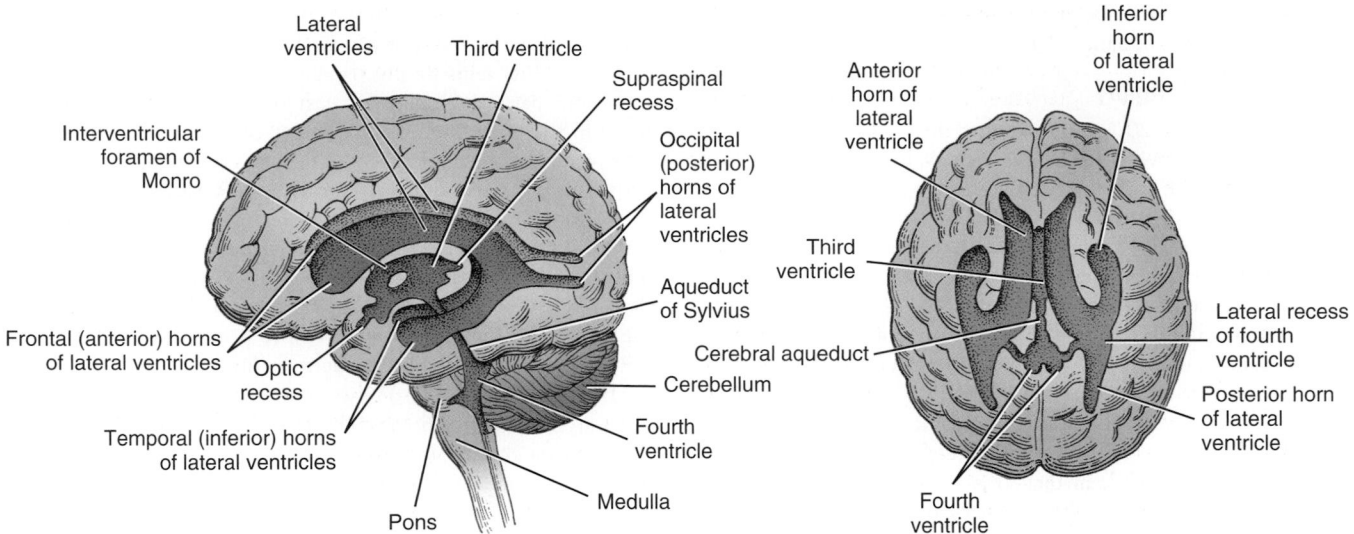

FIGURE 21-12 Ventricular system showing its relationship to various parts of brain.

brain swells, the amount of CSF decreases to compensate for the increase in brain mass. The fluid can carry certain drugs to diseased parts of the brain. It does not, however, play a significant role in supplying nutrition to the structures that it bathes. The total amount of circulating CSF averages 150 mL in the adult. The ventricles contain about 25 mL, and the remaining CSF circulates in the cranial and spinal subarachnoid space. CSF is secreted at a rate of between 21 and 24 mL/hr, or approximately 450 mL/24 hr. This means that in an adult, CSF is recirculated about three times each day.

Pathologic Conditions Related to CSF. CSF can be examined by the lab to provide diagnostic information. CSF is most commonly obtained by way of lumbar puncture (LP). Because the subarachnoid space surrounding the brain is freely connected to the subarachnoid space of the spinal cord, any abnormal increase in ICP will be directly reflected as an increase at the lumbar site. Tumors, infection, hydrocephalus, and intracranial bleeding can cause increased intracranial and spinal pressure. LP is contraindicated when ICP is increased from a suspected intracranial mass that is causing neurologic symptoms. In this situation the sudden reduction in pressure from the release of CSF could cause brain herniation. The ventricular fluid normally has a protein content of 5 to 15 mg/dL, whereas the protein content of spinal fluid is 25 to 45 mg/dL. These values may be considerably elevated in pathologic conditions of the CNS. The characteristics of normal spinal fluid are listed in Appendix A.

Elevations in CSF pressure can be caused by an expanding mass within the skull, such as a tumor, hemorrhage, or cerebral edema; an increase in formation or decrease in absorption of fluid, as in meningitis, encephalitis, and other febrile conditions; an increase in venous pressure within the skull from an obstruction to normal venous drainage; a blockage of absorption by inflammatory conditions of the arachnoid and perivascular spaces; any mechanical obstruction of the ventricular or subarachnoidal fluid pathways; or decreased absorption of CSF. These pathologic conditions can cause a dangerous increase in ICP, which ultimately could result in brain herniation and death.

The rate of absorption and production of CSF is related to the osmotic and hydrostatic pressures of the blood. Intravenous (IV) injection of hypertonic mannitol, commonly used with a nonosmotic diuretic, can be used to pull fluid from tissue to the vascular space for excretion by the kidneys, resulting in systemic diuresis and a decrease in ICP.

Hydrocephalus is a condition marked by an excessive accumulation of CSF, resulting in dilation of the intracerebral ventricles where CSF is synthesized and circulated. Enlargement of cerebral ventricles is the result of CSF blockage and interruption of CSF circulation or CSF reabsorption. The causes of hydrocephalus are many, including congenital conditions, aqueductal stenosis, tumors or cysts of the ventricular system, subarachnoid hemorrhage (SAH), posterior fossa tumors, or trauma with increased ICP. Noncommunicating (obstructive) hydrocephalus involves an obstruction of CSF pathways. In communicating hydrocephalus, the normal CSF pathways are open; however, there is an abnormality in CSF absorption with increased ICP. Normal-pressure hydrocephalus (NPH) is a chronic communicating adult-onset hydrocephalus that produces a normal pressure on random LP (Rosenberg, 2012). NPH most commonly develops in the elderly, probably because of abnormal CSF absorption; however, the cause may not be apparent. Symptoms of dementia, unsteady gait, and urinary incontinence are seen with normal pressure and chronic hydrocephalus. Those with acute hydrocephalus present with headache, nausea, vomiting, drowsiness, and papilledema.

The appropriate surgical procedure depends on the precise type of hydrocephalus. Whenever possible, an obstructing lesion that causes hydrocephalus should be surgically removed. For some cases of obstructive hydrocephalus, endoscopic third ventriculostomy may be possible. With endoscopic third ventriculostomy, CSF can be diverted by surgically creating an opening at the floor of the third ventricle, thus eliminating the need for a shunt. Commonly, treatment of hydrocephalus in the adult and pediatric population is by placement of a ventriculoperitoneal (VP) shunt; however, it may be necessary to revise the shunt periodically as the child grows (Karajannis et al, 2012). With acute symptoms, temporary placement of an external ventriculostomy catheter used to measure the

ICP and drain CSF may be preferred, thus postponing or eliminating the need for a permanent VP shunt.

Cerebral Blood Supply

The brain requires 20% more oxygen than any other organ to maintain its high level of metabolic activity. The arterial supply to the brain enters the cranium through the two internal carotid arteries anteriorly and the two vertebral arteries posteriorly. These communicate at the base of the brain through the circle of Willis (Figure 21-13), which ensures continuity of the circulation if any one of the four main channels is interrupted. However, these connections are extremely variable and do not always have functional anastomoses. The main branches for distribution of blood to each hemisphere of the brain from the internal carotid arteries are the anterior and middle cerebral arteries. Each artery nourishes a specific area of the brain (see Figure 21-13). The anterior cerebral artery supplies the anterior two thirds of the medial surface and adjacent region over the convexity of the hemisphere, thus including about half of the frontal and parietal lobes. The middle cerebral artery supplies most of the lateral surface of the hemisphere, including half of the frontal, parietal, and temporal lobes. The posterior cerebral artery, which originates at the basilar artery, supplies the occipital lobe and the remaining half of the temporal lobe, principally on the inferior and medial surfaces. The brainstem and cerebellum are supplied by branches of the basilar and vertebral arteries.

The cerebral veins do not parallel the arteries as the veins do in most other parts of the body. The external cortical veins anastomose freely in the pia mater, forming larger cerebral veins, and as such they pierce the arachnoid membrane, cross the subdural space, and empty into the great dural venous sinuses. A subdural hemorrhage after head trauma may arise from disruption of these bridging vessels; an epidural hemorrhage often results from lacerations of the middle meningeal artery—a branch of the external carotid artery that supplies the dura mater. The deep cerebral veins, which drain the interior of the hemispheres, empty principally into the great vein of Galen and the inferior sagittal sinus.

The blood transports oxygen, nutrients, and other substances necessary for the proper functioning of living tissue. The needs of the brain for oxygen and glucose are critical. The brain can store only small amounts of oxygen and energy-producing nutrients. Constant flow of blood to the brain must be maintained.

The brain uses oxygen in the metabolism of glucose—the chief source of energy. Protein and fat metabolism plays little part in energy production. In the face of an oxygen deficit, the survival time of CNS tissue is very short. In the presence of low levels of blood glucose, CNS function is compromised and unconsciousness results.

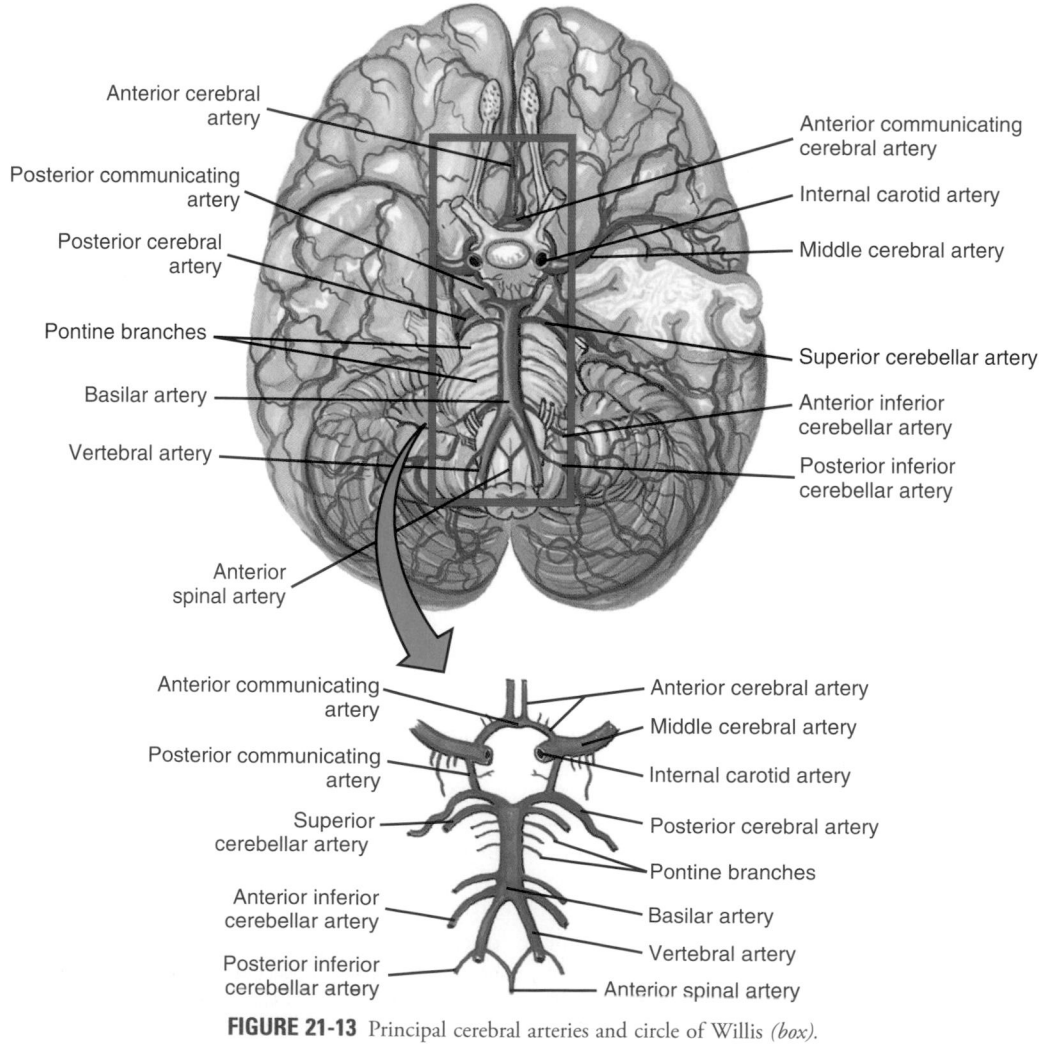

FIGURE 21-13 Principal cerebral arteries and circle of Willis (*box*).

Generally, all factors affecting the systemic blood pressure indirectly affect the cerebral circulation. The brain normally receives 20% of the cardiac output. The cerebral blood flow is kept constant by an autoregulation phenomenon such that increases in blood pressure lead to vasoconstriction of cerebral arteries and decreases in blood pressure cause cerebral vasodilation to maintain a relatively constant cerebral blood flow. When the mean arterial pressure falls below 60 mm Hg, the autoregulation mechanism usually fails.

Vascular Pathologic Conditions of the Brain. Vascular lesions of the brain are most often diagnosed in people who present with acute, spontaneous intracranial hemorrhage.

Aneurysms. Aneurysms arise from a complex set of circumstances involving a congenital anatomic predisposition and local or systemic factors that weaken the arterial wall, leading to dilation. The majority of these lesions occur at the branching points of large subarachnoid conducting arteries. The greatest vulnerability to aneurysmal development occurs at points of vessel bifurcation. Acute SAH in this setting can lead to vessel vasospasm (with greatest risk at 4 to 10 days after the SAH), cerebral ischemia, hydrocephalus, increased ICP, diabetes insipidus, syndrome of inappropriate antidiuretic hormone (SIADH), respiratory failure, brain injury, and risk of rebleeding. The vessels of the circle of Willis are most often implicated, including the posterior communicating artery, anterior communicating artery, middle cerebral artery, carotid artery, posterior inferior cerebellar artery, vertebral artery, and basilar artery. Surgical intervention techniques are based on the characteristics of the aneurysm. Small neck aneurysms may be occluded using coils placed by means of interventional radiology techniques. Aneurysmal clipping by way of a craniotomy approach is most often used to treat broad neck aneurysms.

Vascular Malformations. Vascular malformations of the CNS are characterized by congenital lesions that have the potential to produce symptoms any time during the life of an individual with the malformation. Types of vascular malformations include arteriovenous malformations (AVMs), cavernous malformations, capillary telangiectasias, and venous malformations. AVMs are complex lesions in which direct shunting of arterial blood to the venous system occurs. The vascular channels are tightly packed and have a propensity to hemorrhage. Capillary telangiectasias are small vascular malformations commonly seen in the pons. They rarely bleed. Cavernous malformations are cystic vascular spaces, similar to capillary telangiectasias but larger and with a tendency to bleed. Venous malformations are the most common type, comprising anomalous veins, a single tortuous vein, or a number of smaller veins joining at a single point. These are considered benign and rarely bleed. Surgical excision of the cavernous malformation and the AVM is recommended.

Hematomas. Hematomas are collections of blood that coagulate to form space-occupying lesions. An intracerebral hemorrhage, the cause of stroke in many hypertensive patients, results in hematoma formation most often in the basal ganglia, subcortical white matter, cerebellum, and brainstem. These hematomas compress vital structures, depress consciousness, and can be catastrophic. Intracerebral hematomas require emergent intervention or surgery to control the rising ICP. If the patient is unconscious prior to surgery, the mortality rate is approximately 45% (Biros and Heegaard, 2009).

Intracranial trauma (Research Highlight) can cause a shearing of arterial and venous vessels that results in hematoma collections in the epidural and subdural spaces. These space-occupying lesions raise ICP and often result in serious neurologic disruption (Figure

21-14). Epidural hematomas are often the result of a blow to the head causing a tear in the middle meningeal artery, which lies on the dura under the skull. These arterial hemorrhages can be life-threatening in that they can cause rapid deterioration in level of consciousness secondary to size of the bleed and brain displacement by the hematoma (Figure 21-15). In contrast to an epidural hematoma, a traumatic subdural hematoma usually results from venous bleeding and collects more slowly. Bridging veins in the subdural space are torn; blood escapes, dissecting a space between the dura

FIGURE 21-14 Types of intracerebral hemorrhage (in italics).

RESEARCH HIGHLIGHT

Impact of Head and Spinal Trauma

Prevention of head and spinal cord injuries has been a topic of public health officials for decades. It is estimated that it will cost more than $25 billion annually to treat people in the United States with head and spinal cord injuries. Researchers have found that these numbers will increase because the majority of injuries occur in adolescents and young adults. The mechanisms of injury include but are not limited to motor vehicle accidents, assaults, sports injuries, and falls. Most injuries are seen in males younger than age 35, and men are twice as likely to sustain a head or spinal injury than women. As of today, in the United States alone there are between 183,000 and 230,000 patients living with spinal cord injuries.

It is imperative that patients are evaluated as soon as possible for a neurologic injury once their cardiopulmonary status is stable. Head injury evaluations should also include a thorough assessment of the spine because 10% of individuals with severe head injuries also sustain a spinal cord injury. Assessments include using tools such as the Glasgow Coma Scale, the Medical Research Council Scale for Muscle Strength Grading, laboratory studies, and imaging studies. Once all of the pertinent data are obtained, a treatment plan can be outlined that may include medical therapy, observation, or surgical intervention.

Preventive measures that may be used to avert head and spinal cord injuries include appropriate seat belt use, helmet use for bicyclists/motorcyclists, and educational programs such as the ThinkFirst National Injury Prevention Foundation. Started in 1986 by the American Association of Neurological Surgeons and the Congress of Neurological Surgeons, ThinkFirst uses evidence-based programs across the country that are aimed at "helping people learn to reduce their risk for injury."

Modified from Karrar EE et al: Cranial and spinal trauma: current concepts, *Disease-A-Month* 57(10):543–57, 2011; *ThinkFirst*, National Injury Prevention Foundation, available at www.thinkfirst.org/About. Accessed December 18, 2012.

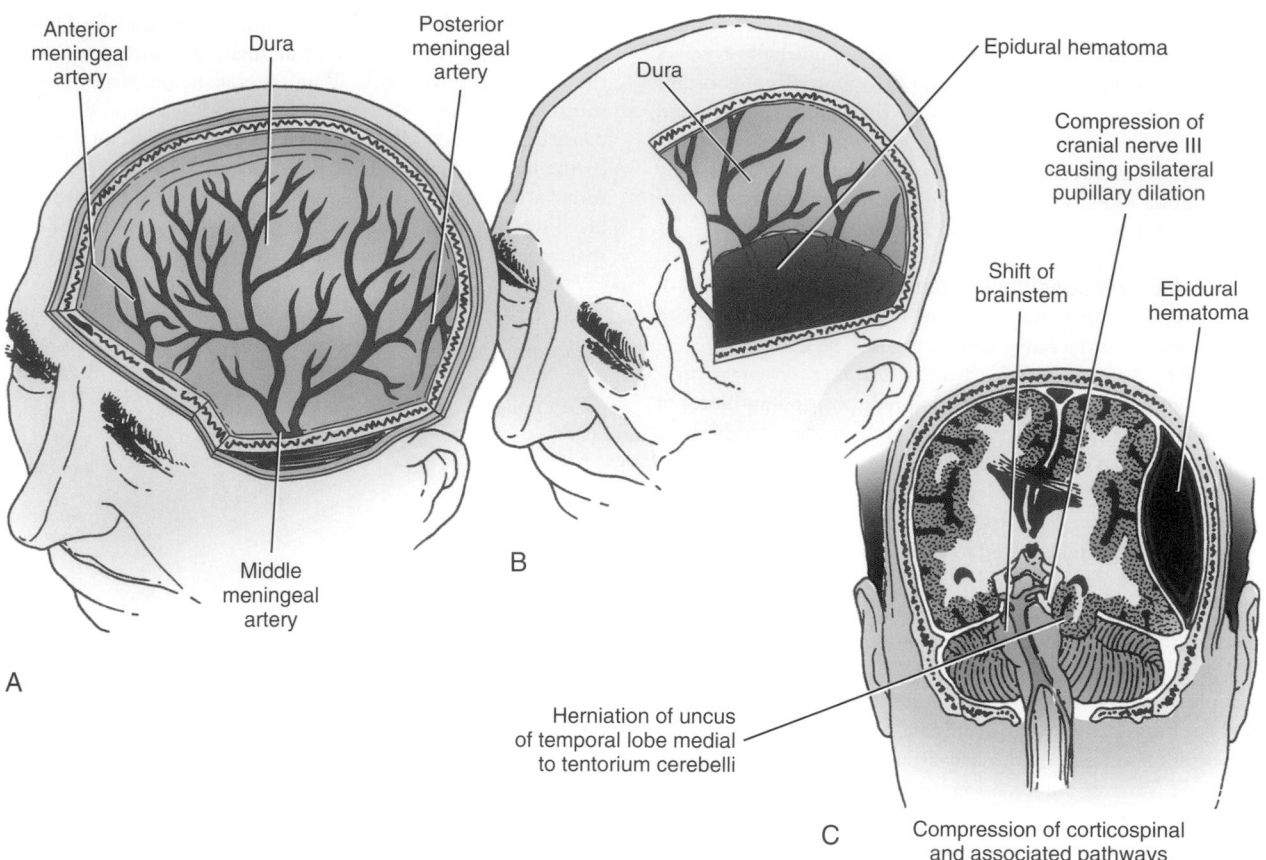

FIGURE 21-15 Epidural hematoma is typically caused by trauma resulting in laceration of the middle meningeal artery. **A,** The middle meningeal artery. The typical traumatic epidural hematoma is caused by a laceration of this vessel. **B** and **C,** A linear fracture of the squamous portion of the temporal bone has torn the middle meningeal artery, which has resulted in an epidural hematoma.

and the arachnoid, and collects over one cerebral hemisphere (Figure 21-16). Subdural hematomas may be acute, subacute, or chronic (Figure 21-17). Chronic hematomas can often be evacuated through burr holes, but acute hematomas may require a craniotomy to remove the clot and control bleeding.

Cerebral Ischemia. Any area of the brain can become ischemic from an arterial occlusion or embolization. Symptoms may be gradual or sudden. Intracranial plaques most commonly form at the bifurcation of the internal carotid artery, into the middle and anterior cerebral arteries. In select cases, extracranial-intracranial arterial microanastomosis can be performed. Carotid endarterectomy can be performed for extracranial lesions of the carotid artery (see Chapter 24).

Cranial Nerves

Twelve pairs of cranial nerves arise within the cranial cavity (Figure 21-18). Although they are part of the PNS, from a surgical standpoint they are considered with the head.

First Cranial Nerve. The olfactory nerve, a fiber tract of the brain, is located under the frontal lobe on the cribriform plate of the ethmoid bone. It transmits the sense of smell. Frontal lobe tumors, fractures of the anterior fossa of the skull, and lesions of the nasal cavity may affect the olfactory nerve.

Second Cranial Nerve. The optic nerve is a fiber tract of the brain. It originates in the ganglion cells of the retina and passes through

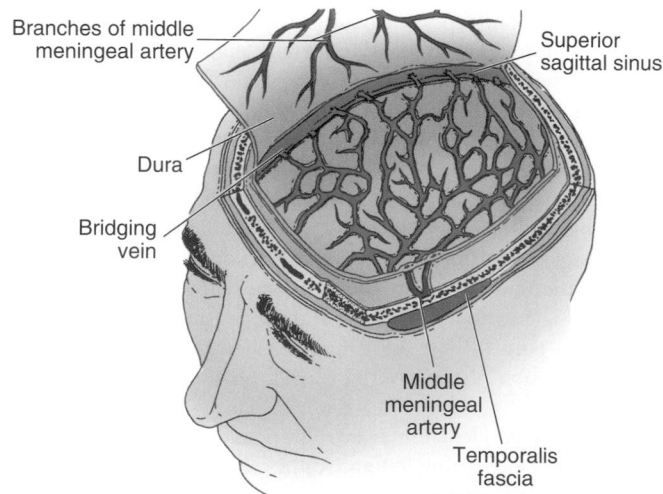

FIGURE 21-16 Veins are shown extending from the surface of the brain to the superior sagittal sinus. Differential movement of the brain within the skull at the time of injury may tear one or more of these veins, leading to the formation of a subdural hematoma.

the optic foramen in the apex of the orbit to reach the optic chiasma. A partial crossing of the fibers occurs there, so the fibers from the nasal half of each retina pass to the opposite side. Posterior to the chiasma, the visual pathway is called the *optic tract*. Still farther back it becomes the optic radiation. Lesions in various parts

Acute	Subacute	Subacute (later)	Chronic
Blood spreads widely over brain surface beneath the dura	Blood congeals; becomes darker, thicker, and "jellylike"	Clot breaks down	Formation of encasing membranes and enlargement

FIGURE 21-17 A subdural hematoma is liquid at first and subsequently clots. It is then reabsorbed or develops into a chronic subdural hematoma as a thick, vascular outer membrane. A thin, inner membrane develops around liquefying blood, starting about 2 weeks after injury. The chronic subdural hematoma enlarges as further bleeding occurs within it.

FIGURE 21-18 Ventral surface of brain showing attachment of cranial nerves.

of this pathway produce characteristic defects in the visual fields. For example, a lesion near the chiasma usually destroys the temporal vision of each eye (bitemporal hemianopsia), whereas a lesion of the occipital lobe produces impairment of vision (homonymous hemianopsia), affecting the right or left halves of the visual fields of both eyes.

Lesions that affect the optic nerve and are treated by neurosurgery include primary gliomas of the nerve, pituitary tumors that press on the optic chiasma, and occasionally meningiomas of the optic nerve sheath or in the region of the sella turcica and olfactory groove. The optic nerves and chiasma are best exposed through a frontal craniotomy along the floor of the anterior fossa or through a frontotemporal approach along the sphenoid ridge. Cranial base approaches using an orbital osteotomy or orbital-zygomatic osteotomies improve access and exposure of the optic system.

Third, Fourth, and Sixth Cranial Nerves. The third, fourth, and sixth cranial nerves are three pairs of nerves—the oculomotor, the trochlear, and the abducens, respectively. They are conveniently considered together because they are the motor nerves to the muscles of the eyes. They are affected by many toxic, inflammatory, vascular, and neoplastic lesions. The third nerve may be affected by aneurysms of the posterior communicating artery. Pressure against this nerve accounts for pupillary dilation when temporal lobe (uncal) herniation is present, resulting from increased ICP.

Fifth Cranial Nerve. The trigeminal nerve has two functions: (1) sensory supply to the forehead, eyes, meninges, face, jaw, teeth, hard palate, buccal mucosa, tongue, nose, nasal mucosa, and maxillary sinus; and (2) motor innervation of the muscles of mastication. The sensory fibers that arise from cells in the trigeminal ganglion travel along the medial wall of the middle cranial fossa and then extend peripherally in three divisions: ophthalmic, maxillary, and mandibular. Behind the ganglion the fibers enter the brainstem by way of the sensory root. The motor root, which originates from cells in the brainstem, follows the course of the larger sensory component (Figure 21-19).

Trigeminal neuralgia (tic douloureux) is characterized by excruciating, piercing paroxysms of pain, affecting one or more of the major peripheral divisions. The recurrent attacks are usually instigated by stimulation of trigger zones present about the face, nares, lips, and teeth. This condition, believed to be caused by a high incidence of vascular compression on the root entry zone of the nerve leading to demyelination, tends to occur unilaterally and in older persons. Medical treatment is frequently unsuccessful in the long term. Types of neurosurgical procedures currently recommended for trigeminal neuralgia include percutaneous rhizotomy using glycerol, radiofrequency, or balloon compression; radiosurgery; and microvascular decompression. Microvascular decompression requires a suboccipital craniotomy and is the most invasive of the techniques. However, it is the least destructive and probably the most durable treatment.

Seventh Cranial Nerve. The facial nerve supplies the musculature of the face and the sensation of taste for the anterior two thirds of the tongue. It originates in the brainstem, passes through the skull with the eighth nerve by way of the internal acoustic meatus, continues along the facial canal, and exits just posterior to the parotid gland. The nerve may be damaged by vestibular schwannomas (e.g., acoustic neuromas), fractures at the base of the skull, mastoid infections, and surgical procedures in the vicinity of the parotid gland.

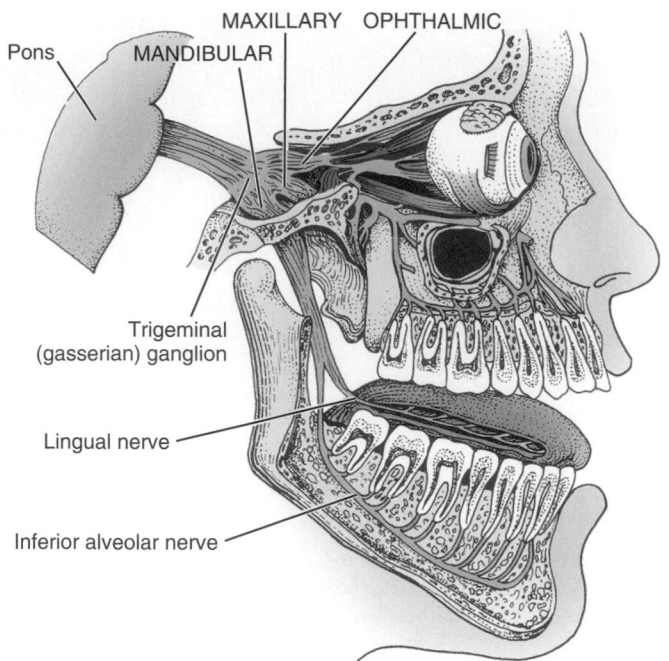

FIGURE 21-19 Trigeminal (fifth cranial) nerve and its three main divisions.

Bell palsy, a facial lower motor neuron paralysis, can affect the seventh nerve. It may last for a few weeks to a few months, but recovery usually takes place. When permanent interruption of the nerve occurs, useful operations for restoration of function include spinal accessory-facial anastomosis and hypoglossal-facial anastomosis. These operations are performed high in the neck behind the parotid gland by use of the operating microscope.

Eighth Cranial Nerve. The acoustic nerve has two parts, both sensory—the cochlear for hearing and the vestibular for balance. The former receives stimuli from the organ of Corti and the latter from the semicircular canals. The major surgical lesion of the eighth nerve is vestibular schwannoma (acoustic neuroma), a histologically benign tumor growing from the nerve sheath at its entrance into the internal auditory meatus. This tumor arises deep in the angle between the cerebellum and pons (cerebellopontine angle). Symptoms may include unilateral deafness, tinnitus, unilateral impairment of cerebellar function, numbness of the face from involvement of the fifth cranial nerve, and, late in the course, papilledema caused by increased ICP. The operative approach is usually through a retrosigmoid craniotomy, exposing the edges of the transverse and sigmoid sinuses. The surgeon must take great care to prevent injury to the pons and to preserve the facial nerve. Attempts are made to preserve the acoustic nerve with smaller tumors when hearing preservation is an option.

Meniere disease is an affliction of the eighth nerve characterized by a recurrent and usually progressive group of symptoms including dizziness and a sensation of fullness or pressure in the ears. When medical measures fail to alleviate the problem, sectioning of the eighth nerve may be a surgical option.

Ninth Cranial Nerve. The glossopharyngeal nerve supplies the sense of taste to the posterior third of the tongue, supplies sensation to the tonsils and pharyngeal region, partially innervates the

TABLE 21-1

Understanding Cranial Nerves

Cranial Nerve	Function	Origin	Structures Innervated	Assessment
I Olfactory	Sensory	Olfactory bulbs below frontal lobes	Olfactory mucous membranes	Ability to identify familiar odors
II Optic	Sensory	Diencephalon	Retina of eye	Visual acuity Visual fields
III Oculomotor	Motor	Midbrain	Medial, superior, and inferior rectus muscles of eye Inferior oblique eye muscles Sphincter of iris	Extraocular movements Pupillary reaction to light and accommodation
IV Trochlear	Motor	Midbrain	Superior oblique muscle of eye	Extraocular movements
V Trigeminal	Mixed	Pons	*Sensory:* Pain, touch, and temperature sensations in cheeks, jaw, and chin; corneal reflex *Motor:* Muscles of mastication	Sensation in forehead, cheeks, jaw, and chin Mastication
VI Abducens	Motor	Pons	Lateral rectus muscle of eye	Extraocular movement
VII Facial	Mixed	Pons	*Sensory:* Anterior two thirds of tongue *Motor:* Muscles of face, forehead, and eye	Taste for anterior two thirds of tongue Movement of facial muscles (smile) Facial symmetry
VIII Acoustic (vestibulocochlear)	Sensory	Pons	Cochlear organ of Corti Vestibule and semicircular canals	Hearing acuity Balance
IX Glossopharyngeal	Mixed	Medulla	*Sensory:* Posterior third of tongue *Motor:* Muscles of pharynx	Taste for posterior third of tongue Movement of pharynx Gag reflex
X Vagus	Mixed	Medulla	*Sensory:* Skin of external ear and mucous membranes *Motor:* Muscles of larynx, pharynx, and esophagus; thoracic and abdominal viscera	Swallowing Movement of pharynx Gag reflex Cough
XI Spinal accessory	Motor	Medulla	Sternocleidomastoid and trapezius muscles	Shoulder shrug Turn head
XII Hypoglossal	Motor	Medulla	Tongue	Movement and strength of tongue

pharyngeal muscles, and primarily innervates the carotid sinus. Stimulation of the baroreceptors of the carotid sinus causes slowing of the heart, vasodilation, and decreased blood pressure. Its sensory component can be sectioned to treat a hypersensitive carotid sinus, or it can be sectioned in conjunction with the fifth nerve to treat painful malignancies of the face, mouth, and pharynx. The ninth nerve lies near the eighth nerve in the posterior fossa and is exposed in a similar way.

Tenth Cranial Nerve. The vagus nerve has many motor and sensory functions, primarily including innervation of pharyngeal and laryngeal musculature, control of heart rate, and regulation of acid secretion of the stomach. In neck surgery the surgeon carefully avoids injury to the recurrent laryngeal branch because its injury results in vocal cord paralysis. In gastric surgery the surgeon could sever the vagus nerve at the lower end of the esophagus to treat a peptic ulcer. The neurosurgeon is also concerned with preventing damage to the vagus nerve during posterior fossa surgery.

Eleventh Cranial Nerve. The spinal accessory nerve is a motor nerve to the sternocleidomastoid and trapezius muscles. To restore mobility to the face, it may be anastomosed to the peripheral end of a damaged facial nerve.

Twelfth Cranial Nerve. The hypoglossal nerve innervates the musculature of the tongue. Its neurosurgical interest is similar to that of the spinal accessory nerve.

Table 21-1 lists the function, origin, structures innervated, and assessment of the cranial nerves.

Spine, Spinal Cord, and Adjacent Structures

Vertebral Column

The primary roles of the spine are maintaining stability, protecting the neural elements, and allowing range of motion. The vertebral column has four distinct curves: cervical lordosis (a backward bend), thoracic kyphosis (a forward bend), lumbar lordosis, and sacral kyphosis. The spinal column consists of 33 vertebrae: 7 cervical, 12 thoracic, 5 lumbar, 5 sacral (fused as 1 section), and 1 coccygeal, which may have 1 to 3 fused sections (Figure 21-20).

The first cervical vertebra, or atlas, supports the skull. The second cervical vertebra, or axis, can be identified by its odontoid process,

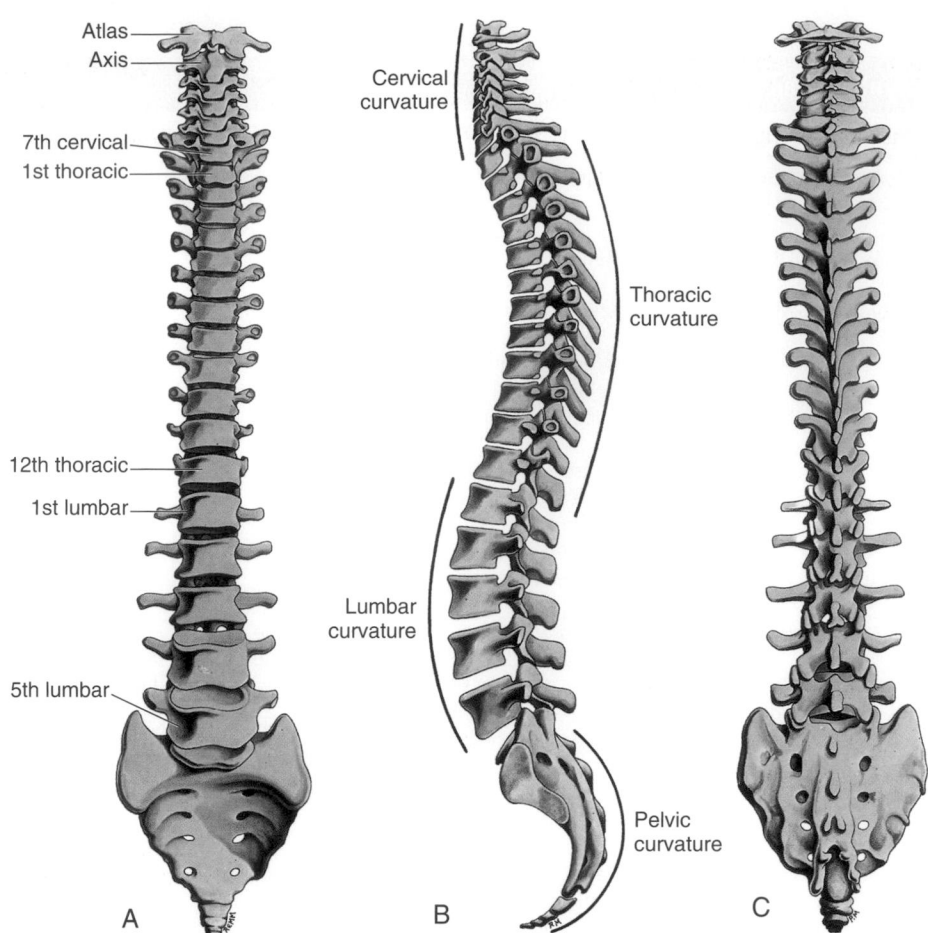

Atlas
Axis
7th cervical
1st thoracic
12th thoracic
1st lumbar
5th lumbar
A

Cervical curvature
Thoracic curvature
Lumbar curvature
Pelvic curvature
B

C

FIGURE 21-20 The vertebral column. **A,** Anterior aspect. **B,** Lateral aspect. **C,** Posterior aspect.

a vertical projection extending into the foramen of the atlas like a stick in a hoop. It rests against the anterior tubercle of the first cervical vertebra. Ligaments hold the two together but allow considerable rotational movement. The other cervical, thoracic, and lumbar vertebrae are more alike in structure. Each has a body, an oval block of bone situated anteriorly. An intervertebral disk, a fibrocartilaginous elastic cushion, separates one body from another (Figures 21-21 and 21-22). The spinal cord lies in a canal formed by the vertebral bodies, pedicles, and laminae. Articular surfaces or facets project from the pedicles and form joints with the facets of the vertebrae above and below. Transverse processes extend laterally and serve as hitching posts for muscles and ligaments. Spinous processes extend posteriorly and can be palpated in most people. The vertebrae are held together by multiple ligaments and muscles (see Figure 21-22). Motion of the spine occurs at the articular facets and through the elastic intervertebral disks. The intervertebral disks bond the adjacent surfaces of the vertebral bodies. Each disk consists of a fibrous outer annulus that contains the inner nucleus pulposus.

Spinal Cord

The spinal cord is protected by the bony framework of the spinal column. The dura mater is separated from its bony surroundings by a layer of epidural fat. Beneath the dura mater is the arachnoid, a continuation of the same structure in the head. The subarachnoid space contains CSF. A thin layer of pia mater adheres to the cord,

and CSF also circulates from the fourth ventricle into the central canal of the cord.

The spinal cord is a downward prolongation of the brainstem, starting at the upper border of the atlas and ending at the upper border of the second lumbar vertebra (Figure 21-23). The cord is oval in cross section. It is slightly flattened in the anteroposterior diameter. A cross section looks like a gray H surrounded by a white mantle split in the midline, anteriorly and posteriorly, by sulci (Figure 21-24).

The peripheral white matter carries long, myelinated motor and sensory tracts. The central gray matter consists of nerve cell bodies and short, unmyelinated fibers (see Figures 21-23 and 21-24). The principal long pathways are the laterally placed pyramidal tracts, carrying impulses down from the cerebral cortex to the motor neurons of the cord; the dorsal ascending columns, mediating sensations of touch and proprioception; and the antero-laterally placed spinothalamic tracts, carrying pain and temperature sensations to the thalamus—the sensory receiving station of the brain (Figure 21-25).

Spinal Nerves

At each vertebral level is a pair of spinal nerves, each consisting of an anterior and a posterior root (see Figure 21-24). The anterior, or motor, root contains cell bodies that lie in the anterior horn of the spinal gray matter. The posterior, or sensory, root contains cell bodies that lie in the spinal ganglia located in the intervertebral

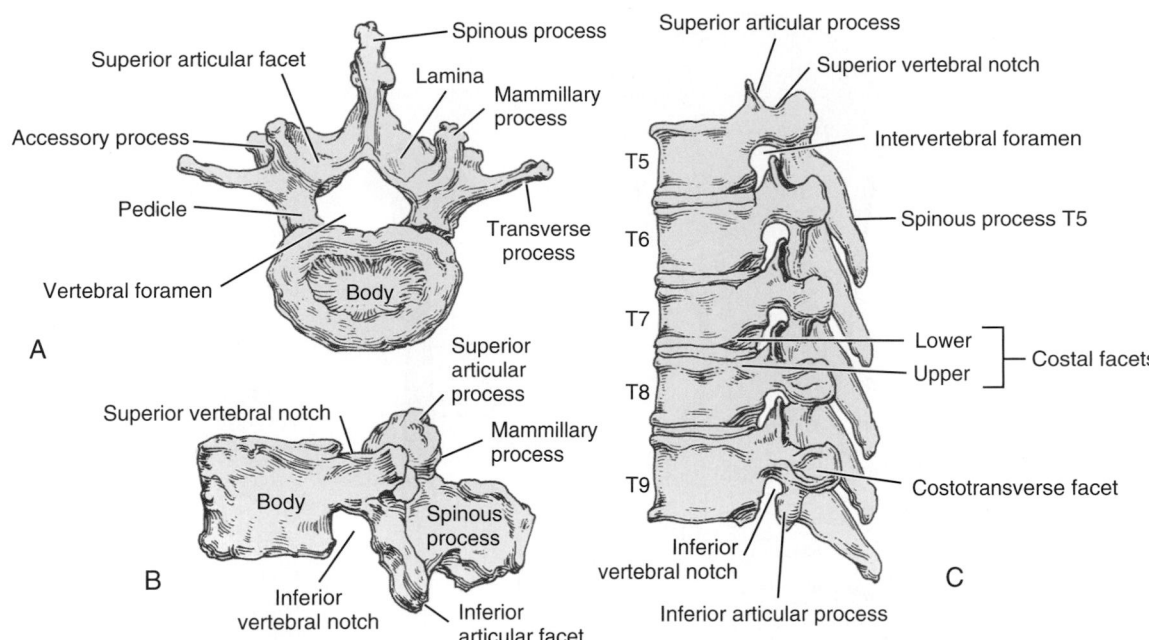

FIGURE 21-21 A, Fourth lumbar vertebra from above. **B,** Fourth lumbar vertebra from side. **C,** Fifth to ninth thoracic vertebrae, showing relationships of various parts.

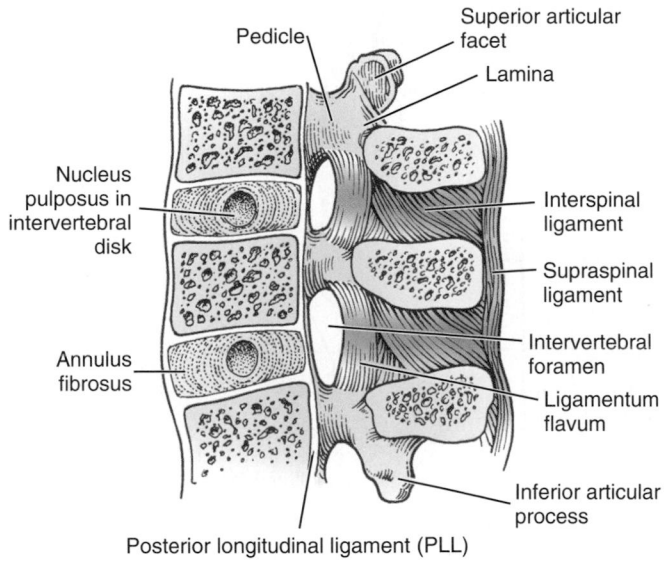

FIGURE 21-22 Median section through three lumbar vertebrae, showing intervertebral disks (nuclei pulposi).

foramina, the opening through which the nerves exit from the spinal canal and emerge from the cord. The course of the cervical nerves is horizontal, but at each lower level they assume an increasingly oblique and downward direction. In the lumbar region, the course of the nerves is nearly vertical, forming the cauda equina (see Figure 21-23). The normal segmental sensory distribution is valuable in the anatomic localization of sensory disorders (Figure 21-26).

Dermatomes are bands of skin innervated by a sensory root of a single spinal nerve. Knowledge of these dermatomes aids the practitioner in locating neurologic lesions (Figure 21-27).

Spinal Vasculature

The vasculature of the spinal cord and vertebral column is a rich, delicate network. The arterial blood supply to the spinal cord arises from the vertebral arteries as the anterior spinal artery and the posterior spinal arteries. These vessels branch and anastomose on both sides of the cord and within the substance of the cord. They also branch into anterior and posterior radicular arteries that form spinal rami as they accompany the spinal nerve roots through the intervertebral foramina.

A series of venous plexuses surround and innervate the spinal cord at each level in the vertebral canal. They anastomose with each other and form the intervertebral veins as they pass through the intervertebral foramina with the spinal nerves to join the intercostal, lumbar, and sacral veins. The lateral longitudinal veins near the foramen magnum empty into the inferior petrosal sinus and cerebellar veins. The venous network innervates the bony structures and musculature as well as the spinal cord and nerve roots. The perioperative nurse considers the possibility of venous bleeding during spinal surgery when planning care.

Pathologic Lesions of the Spinal Cord and Adjacent Structures

Surgery is performed to correct congenital malformations, traumatic injuries, tumors, abscesses, herniated and degenerative intervertebral disks, and intractable pain.

Meningocele. The most common congenital lesion encountered is a lumbar meningocele, or myelomeningocele—a failure of the union of the vertebral arches during fetal development. The fluid-filled, thin-walled sac often contains neural elements. This fetal anomaly is often diagnosed prenatally and is often seen with other CNS abnormalities, which include hydrocephalus, gyral abnormalities, and Chiari malformation of the hindbrain (see Chapter 26 for a discussion of the surgical treatment of meningocele).

Foramen magnum

Ventral fissure

Pyramidal decussation

Cervical

Lumbar enlarge-ment

Thoracic

Lumbar puncture area

Conus medullaris

Lumbar

Filum terminale

Sacral

Coccygeal (fused from four small vertebrae)

FIGURE 21-23 Posterior view of brainstem and spinal cord. **A,** Torso dissected from back is shown. Dura mater has been opened and cord exposed. Levels concerned can be easily determined by referring to ribs on left side of thorax. Cord proper terminates opposite body of second lumbar vertebra **(B)** as conus medullaris. **B,** Ventral surface of cord stripped of dura mater and arachnoid. It is symmetric in structure, two halves of which are separated by ventral fissure. This fissure stops at foramen magnum. Caudally, pia mater leaves conus medullaris as glistening thread, or filum terminale. **C,** Cord is exposed from lateral side. Dura mater has been opened. Because cord is shorter than canal and spinal nerves exit through intervertebral foramina, one at a time, lowest portion of canal is occupied only by a bundle-like accumulation of nerve roots—cauda equina. Caudal end of dural sac, enclosing spinal cord and cauda equina, lies somewhere between bodies of first and third sacral vertebrae. Size and position of the three views correspond, and elimination of major vertebral levels is indicated by transverse lines for all three figures.

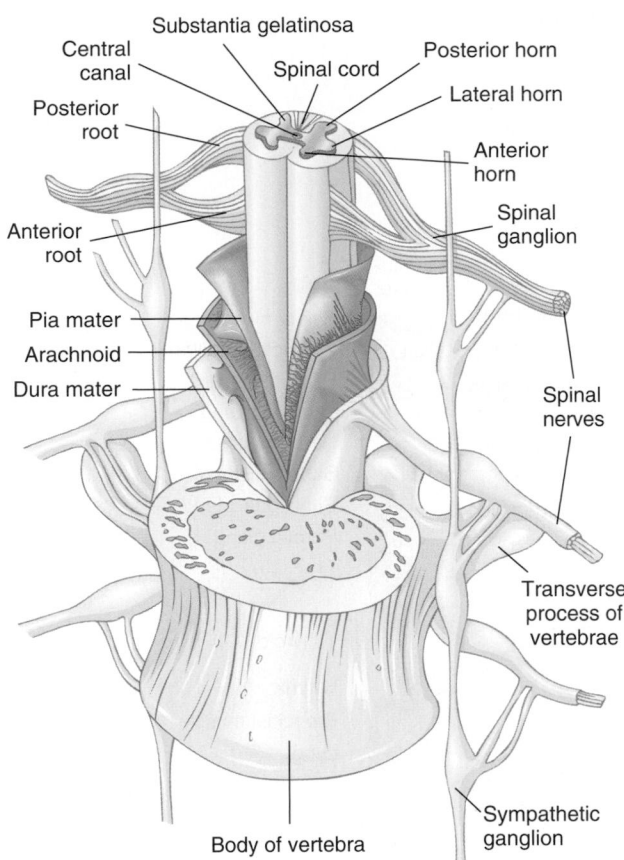

FIGURE 21-24 Spinal cord, showing meninges, formation of spinal nerves, and relationships to vertebra and to sympathetic trunk and ganglia.

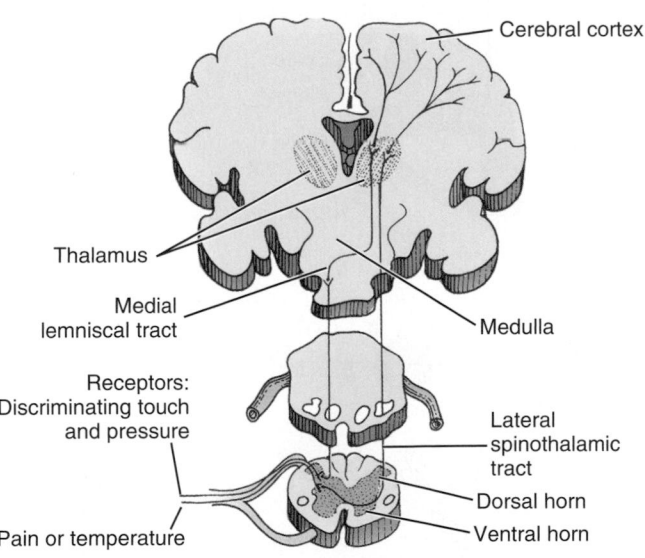

FIGURE 21-25 Lateral spinothalamic and medial lemniscal neural tracts.

Trauma. Trauma to the spine is most commonly caused by motor vehicle crashes and falls. Of all blunt trauma patients, 11.8% of patients sustain a vertebral column fracture. The cervical spine is the most vulnerable to injury, and encompasses one third of all traumatic vertebral column fractures (Martin and Meredith, 2012).

Standardized trauma care and transport, early diagnosis, and closed reduction with surgical stabilization as necessary are part of spinal care focused on minimizing cord trauma and maximizing cord recovery. Spinal decompression, stabilization, and traction are all common interventions performed in trauma centers.

Spine and Spinal Cord Tumors. The most frequently occurring tumors of the spine are metastatic, and the spine is the most common site for skeletal metastasis. Although it is estimated that between 5% and 10% of cancer patients develop *symptomatic* spinal metastasis, it is estimated that as many as 30% to 90% of cancer patients actually develop skeletal metastasis (Donthineni, 2009). Pain is the earliest and most prominent symptom, followed by weakness. Secondary spinal tumors most often originate from carcinomas of the lung, breast, prostate, and blood. Approximately 17% of patients with other primary tumors may experience cord compression as a result of spinal metastases. Metastases to the spine have a predilection toward the thoracic spine, followed by the lumbar and cervical areas (Donthineni, 2009). Treatment goals for metastatic tumors of the spine are pain relief and preservation or restoration of neurologic function. Options include radiation, surgery, or a combination of these. Surgery involves both decompression of the spinal cord and nerve roots and stabilization of the spinal column.

Spinal tumors are classified according to location as *extradural* (outside the dura mater) or *intradural* (inside the dura mater). Intradural tumors may be either *extramedullary* (outside the cord) or *intramedullary* (within the cord). Although most spinal tumors are benign, metastatic tumors may be found in each category, and are usually extradural. Other extradural lesions include lymphomas, lipomas, neurofibromas, chondromas, angiomas, abscesses, and granulomas.

Most intradural tumors are extramedullary and benign and, if diagnosed early before severe neurologic deficits occur, offer an excellent prognosis. They manifest their presence by pain of a radicular nature and various motor and sensory disabilities below their segmental locations. They are usually benign and originate from the dura mater and arachnoid surrounding the cord and from the root sheaths of spinal nerves. Schwannomas (neuromas) are especially common in the thoracocervical area and may be part of generalized neurofibromatosis. Meningiomas also commonly occur in intradural extramedullary locations. Less frequently, lipomas or other types of tumors are found. These tumors infiltrate the cord tissue and are much more difficult to remove than are extramedullary tumors. Of the intramedullary tumors, the most common are ependymomas and astrocytomas.

Cord tumors frequently produce spinal fluid blockage and can be pinpointed accurately with MRI. Intraspinal injection of contrast material (myelography) is another option for diagnosis. Often a standard laminectomy is used for exposure and removal.

Spinal Epidural Abscess. Spinal epidural abscess can develop from vertebral osteomyelitis, from infection originating at a distant source and transferred by the blood, or from direct inoculation caused by spinal surgery, LP, or epidural administration of anesthetic. Patients who are immunosuppressed are especially at risk for epidural abscesses. Clinical presentation involves spinal and radicular pain and muscle weakness that can progress to paralysis. Epidural abscess is most easily diagnosed by MRI and typically treated with surgical decompression, culture, and irrigation, along with 4 to 8 weeks of IV antibiotic therapy.

SURGICAL INTERVENTIONS

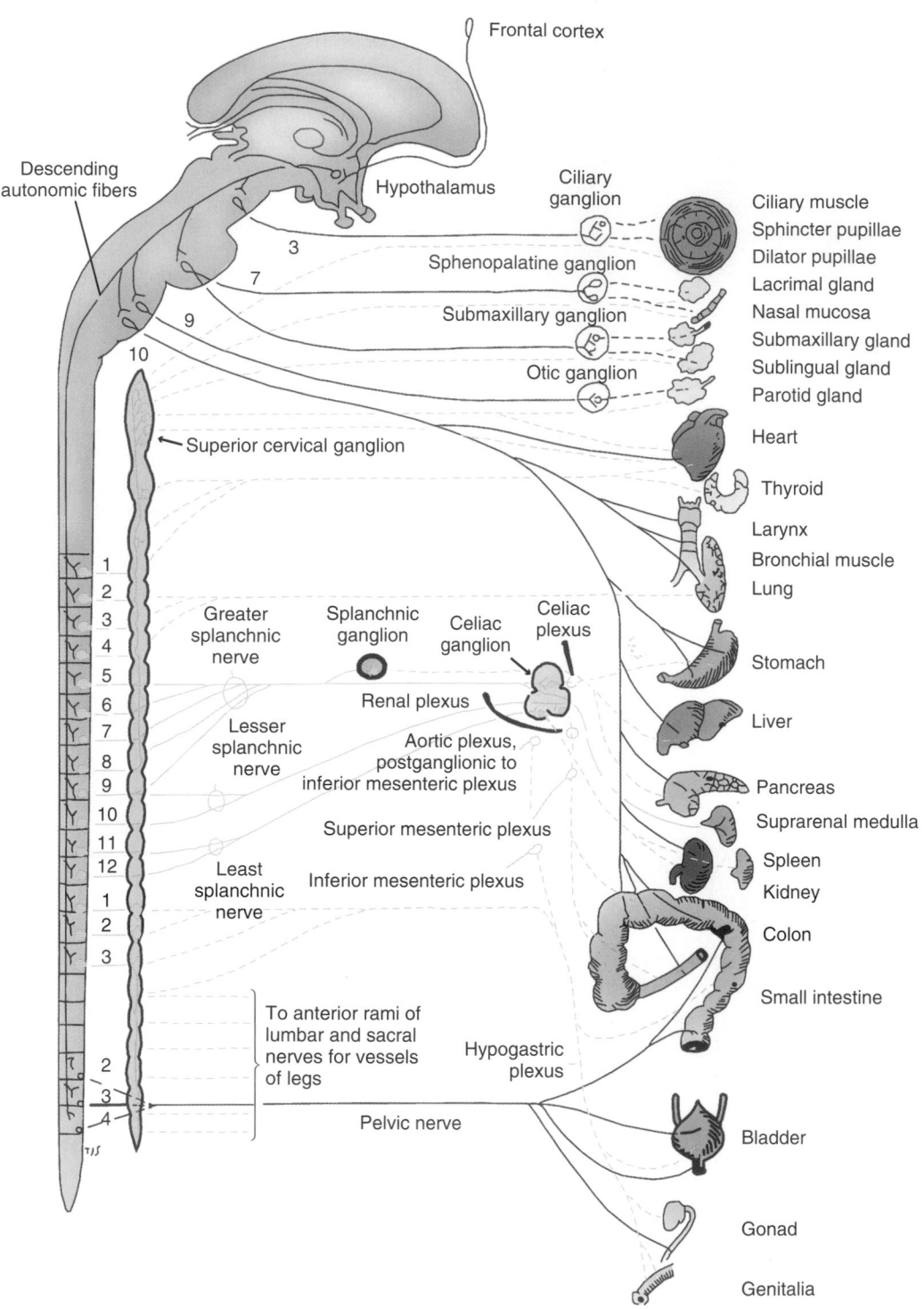

FIGURE 21-26 Sympathetic division of the autonomic nervous system.

Intervertebral Disk Disease. Intervertebral disk disease is the most frequently encountered neurosurgical problem. The axial skeleton bears both the body's weight and externally applied axial forces while maintaining mobility. Intervertebral disks serve as mechanical buffers that absorb axial loading, bending, and shear forces. Bipedal posture further stresses the intervertebral disks, leading to degenerative disk disorders. Disk rupture occurs with radial fissuring of the annulus. The nucleus pulposus then escapes, extending to the margin of the annulus and posterior longitudinal ligament. Once the nucleus pulposus protrudes beyond the perimeter of the disk

FIGURE 21-27 Dermatomes innervated by posterior nerve roots and their correlation on the body; both anterior and posterior views are shown. *C,* Cervical; *T,* thoracic; *L,* lumbar; *S,* sacral.

space into the epidural space, it results in nerve root compression and radiculopathy (pain produced by pressure or traction on the nerve roots) (Figures 21-28 and 21-29). Most disk protrusions occur at the L4-L5 and L5-S1 interspaces. Interventions include a medical trial of treatment with steroids and analgesics/narcotics, muscle relaxation, rest, epidural steroid injections, and, in failed cases, laminotomy or laminectomy with diskectomy. In far-lateral disk herniations, percutaneous lumbar diskectomy is often an alternative to laminotomy. This minimally invasive technique gains access to the disk space posterolaterally, using local anesthetic. The disk space is entered by way of a cannula. An aspiration probe may be used to remove the disk matter, or direct removal can be done microscopically or endoscopically.

Intractable Pain. Certain painful spinal lesions, usually of a malignant nature, can be controlled by use of epidural opiates, by use of fentanyl patches, or by temporary or permanent use of a medication pump. Another pain control procedure is to divide the pain fibers supplying the affected area. This may be accomplished by sectioning the sensory roots intraspinally (posterior rhizotomy) or by incising the spinothalamic tracts that carry pain and temperature impulses

(anterolateral cordotomy). Alternatively, spinal cord stimulation of the affected area can be achieved with the placement of electrodes in the epidural space. A laminectomy for exposure is necessary to perform these surgical procedures.

Peripheral Nerves. The PNS consists of those structures containing nerve fibers or axons that connect the CNS with motor and sensory, somatic and visceral, end-organs. The PNS includes the cranial nerves (III to XII), the spinal nerves, the autonomic nerves, and the ganglia.

The 31 pairs of spinal nerves are each numbered for the level of the spinal column at which they emerge: cervical, C1 through C8; thoracic, T1 through T12; lumbar, L1 through L5; sacral, S1 through S5; and coccygeal, 1. The first pair of cervical spine nerves emerges between C1 and the occipital bone. The eighth cervical nerves emerge from the intervertebral foramina between C7 and T1. The first thoracic nerves emerge between T1 and T2.

In the cervical and lumbosacral regions the spinal nerves regroup in a plexiform manner before they form the peripheral nerves of the upper and lower extremities. Those in the thoracic region form cutaneous and intercostal nerves. The principal nerves of the upper

FIGURE 21-28 Stages in the herniation of an intervertebral disk. **A,** Tearing of the rings of the annulus fibrosus. **B,** Protrusion of the disk against the nerve root. **C,** Extrusion of part of the nucleus pulposus, with further nerve root compression.

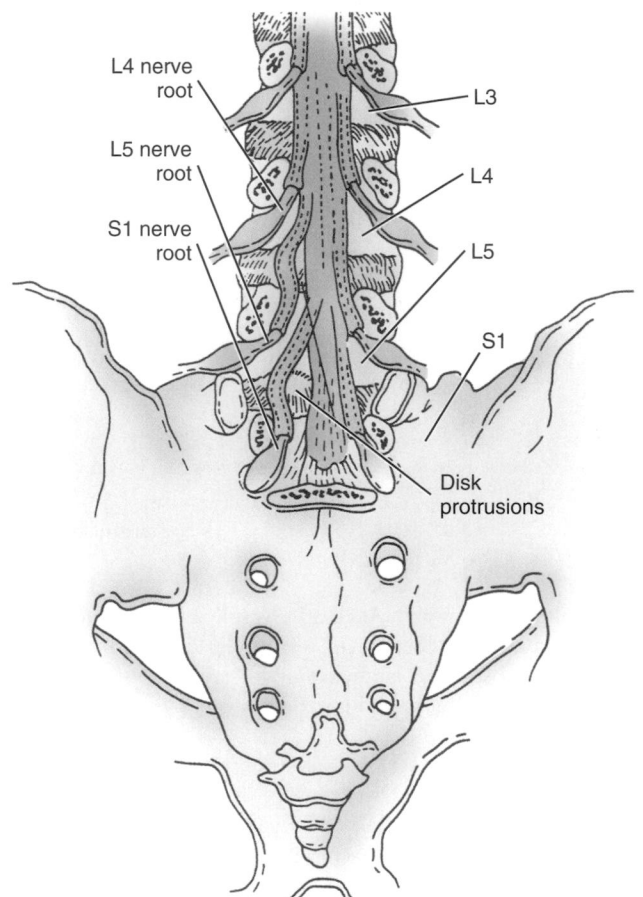

L4 nerve root

L5 nerve root

S1 nerve root

L3

L4

L5

S1

Disk protrusions

FIGURE 21-29 Posterior view of the lower lumbar spine. A disk protrusion at L4-L5 on the left results in compression of the L5 nerve root where it leaves the dural sac but before it exits the spinal canal.

plexus include the musculocutaneous, median, ulnar, and radial. Those of the lumbosacral plexus include the obturator, femoral, and sciatic.

Each spinal nerve divides into anterior, posterior, and white rami. Rami are primary divisions of a nerve. Anterior and posterior rami contain voluntary fibers; white rami contain autonomic fibers. Posterior rami further branch into nerves innervating the muscles, skin, and posterior surfaces of the head, neck, and trunk. Most anterior rami branch to the skeletal muscles and the skin of the extremities and anterior and lateral surfaces. In the process they form plexuses, such as the brachial and sacral plexuses. Spinal nerves contain sensory dendrites and motor axons; some have somatic axons, and some have axons of preganglionic autonomic motor neurons.

The autonomic (involuntary) nervous system consists of all the efferent nerves through which the cardiovascular apparatus, viscera, glands of internal secretion, and peripheral involuntary muscles are innervated (see Figure 21-26). There is a major anatomic difference between the somatic and autonomic nervous systems. In the somatic nervous system an impulse from the brainstem or spinal cord reaches the end-organ through a single neuron. In the autonomic nervous system an impulse passes through two neurons—the first ending in an autonomic ganglion and the second running from the ganglion to the end-organ. Some of the ganglia lie adjacent to the vertebral column to form the sympathetic trunks or chains; others are closely associated with the end-organs.

The preganglionic neurons from the brainstem (which traverse along the cranial nerves) and those from the second, third, and fourth sacral segments to the pelvic viscera end in ganglia in proximity to their end-organs; thus their postganglionic fibers are very short. This is known as the *parasympathetic,* or *craniosacral,* division of the autonomic nervous system. The preganglionic fibers from the thoracic and lumbar spinal cord terminate in the paravertebral ganglia, making up the sympathetic chain, and their postganglionic fibers are relatively long. This is termed the *sympathetic,* or *thoracolumbar,* division of the autonomic nervous system.

The two divisions are distinct anatomically and physiologically. The chemical substance mediating transmission of impulses at most postganglionic sympathetic nerve endings is *norepinephrine,* and the neurotransmitter at all parasympathetic and preganglionic sympathetic neurons is *acetylcholine.*

The majority of organs have dual innervation—part from the craniosacral division and part from the thoracolumbar division. The functions of these two systems are antagonistic. Together they work to maintain homeostasis. In general, the thoracolumbar division functions as an emergency protection mechanism, always ready to combat physical or psychologic stress. The craniosacral division functions to conserve energy when the body is in a state of relaxation.

Stimuli arising from internal organs or from outside the body traverse visceral and somatic afferent nerve fibers to make reflex connections with preganglionic autonomic neurons in the brainstem and spinal cord. Such stimuli trigger activity of these involuntary systems automatically. When these automatic mechanisms break down or overact, surgery may be indicated. Thoracolumbar sympathectomy was once performed in hypertensive patients as an attempt to decrease blood vessel tone and lower blood pressure. Vagotomy can be performed to decrease acid secretion to the stomach in patients with peptic ulcers. Lumbar sympathectomy is used to relieve vasospastic disorders of the legs. T2 ganglionectomy is done to relieve palmar hyperhydrosis (sweaty palms). See Chapter 23 for a discussion of thoracic ganglionectomy.

Perioperative Nursing Considerations

Assessment

Neurologic Assessment Tools. A familiarity with basic neurologic assessment tools gives the nurse the ability to perform a standardized neurologic assessment that can be compared with the patient's previous assessments and easily communicated to other healthcare professionals. These tools can be used preoperatively to establish a baseline assessment. Postoperatively they can be used to establish a return to baseline and to assess postoperative neurologic stability. The postoperative condition of a neurosurgical patient can quickly deteriorate, so an adequate baseline assessment is essential. The Glasgow Coma Scale is commonly used to assess patients with brain injury (Table 21-2). Three indicators of cerebral function—eye opening, verbal communication, and motor response to verbal and noxious stimuli—are assessed, and the appropriate number of points for each is assigned and totaled. The best possible score is 15, and the worst possible score is 3. The Medical Research Council (MRC) Scale for Muscle Strength Grading can be used to assess muscle strength in the upper and lower extremities of spinal cord injury patients or patients who are having spine surgery (Table 21-3).

Preparation for Surgery. Communication among the perioperative team is essential for planning care for the neurosurgical patient in the operating room (OR). Information the perioperative nurse needs before the arrival of the patient in the OR includes the following:

- The patient's age, height, weight, level of consciousness, physical disabilities resulting from neuropathologic or other conditions, stability of spine, and communication barriers
- Diagnosis, allergies, medical clearance for surgery, and nothing-by-mouth (NPO) status
- Planned and possible surgical procedures
- Surgical and anesthesia consent signed by the patient or person with power of attorney for medical decisions (if the patient is unable to provide consent)
- Surgical site marked by the surgeon or a representative to designate correct side of head, level of spine, or other surgical site
- Diagnostic and lab studies done and reports needed at the time of operation
- Specific surgical approach and position to be used
- Need for any special equipment, instruments, and supplies
- Amount of blood and blood products (fresh frozen plasma, platelets) ordered and available
- Need for radiologic support, neuromonitoring, intraoperative blood salvage unit, and image guidance
- Planned preliminary procedures, lumbar puncture, placement of lines (IV, central venous, arterial), and Foley catheter insertion
- Verification that all necessary personnel, equipment, and supplies are available
- A baseline, focused preoperative neurologic examination, which may include the following:
  - Mental status (level of consciousness, orientation, behavior, ability to follow commands)
  - Vision, pupil response, extraocular eye movements (EOMs), and hearing
  - Examination of sensation and motor strength of extremities
  - Area and intensity of pain

This information allows the perioperative nurse to properly plan and prepare for the surgery and to ensure the well-being of

---

TABLE 21-2

The Glasgow Coma Scale

	Points
Eye Opening	
Spontaneous	4
To speech	3
To pain	2
None	1
Verbal Communication	
Oriented	5
Confused conversation	4
Inappropriate words	3
Incomprehensible sounds	2
None	1
Motor Response	
Obeys commands	6
Localizes to pain	5
Withdraws to pain	4
Abnormal flexion	3
Abnormal extension	2
None	1

Modified from Palmieri RL: Assessment of the nervous system. In Ignatavicius DD, Workman ML, editors: *Medical-surgical nursing: patient-centered collaborative care*, ed 7, St Louis, 2013, Saunders.

TABLE 21-3

Medical Research Council Scale for Muscle Strength Grading

Grade	Strength
0	No muscle contraction
1	Trace of contraction
2	Active movement with gravity eliminated
3	Active movement against gravity
4	Active movement against gravity and resistance
5	Normal power

Modified from Daroff RB et al, editors: *Bradley's neurology in clinical practice*, ed 6, Philadelphia, 2012, Saunders.

the patient. Preoperative assessment data are also used during the postoperative period as a means of measuring progress toward outcomes.

Diagnostic Procedures. Most patients will have undergone diagnostic procedures before arriving in the OR. Radiologic and other diagnostic studies are of great significance to the surgical team. The nurse should ensure that any pertinent radiographic images are available in the OR before the procedure begins. The surgeon can refer to these images to locate the pathologic condition, verify the correct surgical site, and plan the appropriate surgical approach and procedure. Diagnostic studies include the following:

FIGURE 21-30 Lateral x-ray of the cervical spine. **A,** Anterior tubercle of the atlas (C1). **B,** Cervical body. **C,** Intervertebral disk. **D,** Spinous process of the axis (C2).

1. *Plain x-rays.* X-rays of the spine can be used initially to identify injury to the spinal column. They are referred to intraoperatively to verify that surgery to the spine is being done at the correct level (Figure 21-30).
2. *CT scan.* A CT scan uses x-ray studies, with or without instilled contrast medium, and computer technology to produce a sequential series of positive images of transverse sections of the brain and spinal cord in which differences in tissue density can be detected and deviations from normal identified. This study remains the criterion standard for evaluating acute head injury and is considered the first-line screening study.
3. *MRI.* Use of radiofrequency pulses in a powerful magnetic field yields high-resolution images of the human body and involves nonionizing radiation. Advances in MRI scanning provide enhancement of the scan with the use of gadolinium (contrast medium). A typical MRI study produces views of the brain featured as contiguous slices in three different planes. Axial cuts are from top to bottom. Coronal cuts are from front to back. Sagittal cuts are from side to side. The MRI is the gold standard for the diagnosis of tumors, abscesses, tissue/ligamentous injury, and disk herniation (Figures 21-31 and 21-32).
4. *Stereotactic MRI or CT scan.* Placement of a stereotactic head frame (frame-based system) or fiducials (frameless system) before receiving a CT scan or MRI produces information that is registered into a computer. The goal of stereotactic surgery is to localize a point or volume in three-dimensional space. The surgeon uses the frame-based system by using an arc system mounted on the bed frame. This system allows the surgeon to access the target by different trajectories (Gasco et al, 2012). The frameless system allows the neurosurgeon to see beyond the actual operative field by using an optical tracking device. This handheld device depicts in three planes on a computer screen where the surgeon is working in the brain relative to deeper structures beyond view.
5. *Magnetic resonance angiography (MRA).* MRA is a noninvasive means of studying the cerebral vasculature. An MRA study is capable of detecting carotid stenosis, post-traumatic carotid artery dissection, AVMs, and aneurysms.

FIGURE 21-31 Gadolinium-enhanced magnetic resonance image of a medial sphenoid wing meningioma in **(A)** axial, **(B)** coronal, and **(C)** sagittal planes.

FIGURE 21-32 Sagittal magnetic resonance image of **(A)** thoracolumbar spine and **(B)** cervicothoracic spine.

6. *Angiography (arteriography).* Injection of contrast medium into the brachial, carotid, vertebral, or femoral arteries is used to study the intracranial blood vessels for size, location, and configuration and to allow diagnosis of space-occupying lesions and vascular abnormalities.

7. *Digital subtraction angiography (DSA).* DSA is a computerized radiologic procedure. An IV rather than arterial injection is required; a contrast medium injection allows examination of selected arterial circulation. By using computer technology DSA provides an alternative to cerebral angiography for high-risk patients.

8. *Three-dimensional CT angiography.* Contrast-enhanced CT brain scan data are used to generate a three-dimensional image of the intracranial vasculature with minimal risk to the patient.

9. *Stereoscopic display of MRA.* Recent advances in MRI permit high-resolution imaging of blood flow. Projection angiograms can be produced to overcome the tomographic nature of conventional MRI scans. These angiograms are similar to plain x-ray films or digital subtraction angiograms in the demonstration of blood vessels, but the three-dimensional information inherent in them is partially lost in single projections. Stereoscopic image pairs allow the clinician to perceive the relative distance of vessels to one another. MRA permits perception of vascular anatomy in three dimensions.

10. *Myelography.* Contrast medium is injected into the spinal subarachnoid space and fluoroscopy is used to view the spinal cord, nerve roots, and spinal column and to demonstrate a defect involving these areas.

11. *Ultrasound.* Ultrasound is a noninvasive technique that uses high-frequency sound waves and a computer to create images of blood vessels, tissues, and organs. It is often used to assess the blood flow in the carotid artery. This procedure can be done in or out of the surgical suite. It can be used intraoperatively to localize intradural spinal cord tumors.

12. *Electroencephalogram (EEG).* An EEG is a procedure that records the brain's continuous electrical activity by means of electrodes placed on the scalp or intraoperatively on the brain.

13. *Evoked potentials (EPs).* Evoked potentials are procedures that record the brain's electrical response to visual, auditory, and sensory stimuli.

14. *Wada test (intracarotid amobarbital [Amytal] test).* The Wada test can be used before brain surgery to lateralize language, memory, and the dominant hemisphere. It can help lateralize seizure focus and assess the ability of the hemisphere with the lesion to maintain memory when isolated.

15. *Lumbar puncture.* A spinal needle is used to gain access to CSF in the subarachnoid space. Opening and closing pressures are measured to determine if there is increased pressure surrounding the brain and spinal cord. This can help diagnose hydrocephalus or a spinal tumor. CSF is sent to the lab to evaluate for blood, infection, malignancy, and other neurologic diseases. LP is contraindicated when an intracranial mass is known or suspected because it can cause herniation of the brain in the presence of increased ICP.

Nursing Diagnosis

Nursing diagnoses are developed from interpreting and analyzing patient information to determine whether there are specific (actual) or potential (risk for) problems that the perioperative nurse needs to consider in the plan of care. Nursing diagnoses are the basis on which nursing interventions are selected for patients. Neurosurgery patients share common problems that the perioperative nurse should address. Nursing diagnoses related to the care of patients undergoing neurosurgery might include the following:

- Anxiety related to surgery or surgical outcome
- Deficient Knowledge related to diagnostic tests and surgical procedures
- Risk for Ineffective Breathing Pattern related to location of tumor, surgical position, or effects of general anesthesia
- Risk for Hypothermia
- Risk for Perioperative Positioning Injury

Outcome Identification

Outcomes identified for the selected nursing diagnoses could be stated as follows:

- The patient will verbalize that anxiety is reduced or controlled.
- The patient or family will verbalize an understanding of the surgical procedure and postoperative plan of care.
- The patient will maintain effective breathing patterns.
- The patient will remain normothermic.
- The patient will be free from signs and symptoms of positioning injury.

Planning

Preparation can significantly reduce anesthesia time and intraoperative time for the patient, as well as physical and psychologic stress for the patient, surgeon, and perioperative nurse. Planning for the patient's care in the OR is based on the results of nursing assessment and the identification of relevant nursing diagnoses. The plan of care then identifies desired outcomes derived from the nursing diagnoses; priorities are set and nursing interventions are designed to assist the patient to reach the desired outcomes. Nursing interventions identified for the patient's plan of care may include reassessment, teaching, counseling, referrals, and specific interventions to assist the patient achieve patient care outcomes (Patient-Centered Care). A Sample Plan of Care for a patient undergoing a neurosurgical procedure is provided below.

Implementation

The perioperative nurse must determine that all personnel, equipment, instrumentation, and supplies necessary for a successful surgery are available. The nurse uses the information obtained through assessment of the patient and communication with the surgical team to provide individualized patient care. Neurosurgical patients vary in age from the very young to the very old. They often have special needs because of conditions such as mental status changes, spinal instability, spinal cord injuries, paralysis, other traumatic injuries, and pain. These conditions need to be considered at all times. Neurosurgery patients who seem to be unconscious may actually be aware of their environment and unable to voice their concerns. The perioperative nurse should always talk to the patient and explain what is happening. Showing compassion and attempting to relieve the fears of the patient and his or her family are essential.

Equipment. Neurosurgical procedures require an extensive amount of equipment. The nurse must analyze the arrangement of the

PATIENT-CENTERED CARE

The U.S. Department of Health and Human Services Health Resources and Services Administration defined health literacy as the degree to which individuals have the capacity to obtain, process, and understand basic health information and services needed to make appropriate health decisions. Neurosurgical patients are especially vulnerable if they are functioning at a decreased cognitive state secondary to their diagnosis. It is important that perioperative nurses do a thorough preoperative interview with the patient or the designated decision-maker to obtain their level of understanding of the diagnosis and treatment plan. Medical jargon should be avoided, and simple language explanations along with handwritten materials should be used. For example, a consent may read "endoscopic transsphenoidal resection of pituitary adenoma." The perioperative nurse should assess the level of understanding of patients or designees by asking them to state the procedure in their own words. They may reply by saying, "The surgeon is going to use a scope to look up my nose and remove a tumor from my pituitary gland." A response such as this is considered health literate and appropriate. If the response is, "The surgeon is taking out a tumor from somewhere," further discussion by all those involved in the care of the patient is essential.

Modified from Health Literacy, available at www.hrsa.gov/healthliteracy. Accessed January 27, 2013.

SAMPLE PLAN OF CARE

Nursing Diagnosis
Anxiety related to surgery or surgical outcome

Outcome
The patient's anxiety will be reduced or controlled.

Interventions
- Broadly classify intensity of the patient's anxiety.
- Determine the patient's coping skills.
- Provide listening, reassurance, and information.
- Provide ongoing opportunity for questions or expression of concerns or fears.
- Involve other support systems (e.g., family, friends, social worker, chaplain).
- Assist the patient to use personally effective coping skills.
- Use touch (if welcomed by the patient) and eye contact during communication.

Nursing Diagnosis
Deficient Knowledge related to diagnostic tests and surgical procedures

Outcome
The patient and family will verbalize an understanding of the surgical procedure and postoperative plan of care.

Interventions
- Determine knowledge level and desire for knowledge.
- Correct misinformation.
- Identify readiness and motivation to learn.
- Provide information regarding tests or surgery.
- Explain perioperative routine, postoperative recovery, and discharge plans.
- Base interventions on the patient's needs.

Nursing Diagnosis
Risk for Ineffective Breathing Pattern related to location of tumor, surgical position, or effects of general anesthesia

Outcome
The patient will maintain effective breathing patterns.

Interventions
- Provide appropriate positioning accessories, and assist in their placement.
- Collaborate with anesthesia provider and surgeon during positioning activities relevant to respiratory effectiveness.
- Determine the patient's comfort on the OR bed; provide comfort measures as appropriate.
- Maintain an open suction line.
- Observe respiratory rate, depth, and character.
- Encourage deep breaths and coughs.
- Communicate with the postanesthesia care unit (PACU) regarding respiratory needs.
- Check airway patency frequently during transport to the PACU.

Nursing Diagnosis
Risk for Hypothermia

Outcome
The patient will remain normothermic.

Interventions
- Provide warm ambient OR temperature during surgical intervention.
- Provide warmed intravenous (IV) fluids and blood products.
- Provide body-warming system (e.g., forced warm air) during surgery.
- Keep the head covered or wrapped when possible.

- Monitor temperature with the anesthesia provider.
- Cover the patient with warm blankets at end of the surgical intervention for transport to the PACU.

Nursing Diagnosis
Risk for Perioperative Positioning Injury

Outcome
The patient will be free from signs and symptoms of positioning injury.

Interventions
- Assess the patient's physical limitations before positioning; make accommodations.

- Carefully pad and protect all prominences and sites that are vulnerable to neurovascular injury.
- Check all positioning devices for cleanliness, working order, and freedom from sharp edges.
- Collaborate with the OR team in placing positioning devices to maintain patient safety.
- Assess the patient at completion of surgery for areas of redness, blanching, or bruising.
- Communicate any findings to the PACU nursing staff.
- Document findings and follow-up with the patient, as applicable.

FIGURE 21-33 A, Three-pin fixation skull clamp (Mayfield) for stabilizing head during neurosurgical procedures. **B,** Mayfield horseshoe headrest.

equipment in the OR to ensure that the sterile field is not compromised. Electrical equipment should be placed in proximity to electrical outlets, so that cords are out of high-traffic areas. Monitors should be in comfortable view of the surgeon. A microscope needs a clear path to the surgical field. The surgeon and surgical assistants may require specialized surgical chairs or sitting or standing stools to comfortably perform the surgery.

OR Table and Attachments. The nurse uses information about the proposed surgical procedure and desired surgical position to gather the proper OR bed, attachments, and positioning devices before the patient arrives in the OR suite. Perioperative nurses must anticipate needs that may arise during the surgery and prepare for them, considering questions such as the following: Is this the right OR bed in the right position with the right attachments? If fluoroscopy will be used, is the base of the OR bed in a position that will accommodate the C-arm? A specialized OR table, such as a Jackson table or Andrews table or frame, may be required for posterior spine surgery. Skull clamps, skull pins, and tongs are commonly used for craniotomies and posterior cervical spine surgeries

to stabilize the head and neck (Figure 21-33). Occasionally a patient may come to the OR in a halo that was placed for preoperative stabilization of the cervical spine. At least part of the halo will need to be removed so the surgical site can be accessed. Compatible wrenches must be available to accomplish this.

Basic Equipment. Neurosurgical procedures typically require one special neurosurgical overhead instrument table, such as the Mayfield table (Figure 21-34), or two large Mayo trays along with one long back table. Other basic equipment includes the following: an intermittent pneumatic compression device, a cooling-heating unit, one or two monopolar electrosurgical units (ESUs), a bipolar ESU, and a wall supply or tank of nitrogen with a special pressure gauge for operating air-powered instruments. Usually two suction units are required. Intraoperative blood salvage is used for most spine surgeries, unless infection or malignancy is suspected.

Neurosurgeons usually wear surgical loupes and a fiberoptic headlight, requiring a light source.

Operating Microscope. An operating microscope may be required for surgery on certain areas of the brain, spinal cord, and peripheral nerves. The operating microscope has revolutionized neurosurgery by providing intense light and magnification to areas that previously may have been inoperable or inaccessible. Microsurgery allows for greater surgical precision when operating in proximity to vital structures and has better surgical results. The perioperative nurse must be able to prepare the microscope for use in neurosurgery, and the surgeon must check it for focal length and focus before scrubbing. Disposable sterile drapes are available for the microscope, as are assistant and observer lenses. Cameras and closed-circuit television monitors are also available for use with the operating microscope.

Endoscopes. Surgeons use endoscopes to perform minimally invasive neurosurgery, such as endoscopic biopsy. The endoscope provides illumination and magnification of structures and an extended viewing angle. Perioperative nurses must be prepared to convert from a neuroendovascular procedure to an open procedure if it is determined that the surgery cannot be successfully completed endoscopically. An additional use for endoscopes is in open procedures to see areas that are otherwise visually inaccessible.

Radiologic Intervention. Radiology is commonly used intraoperatively for spine surgery. Typically a radiology technician operates the equipment. Lead aprons and thyroid shields must be worn or protective shields must be used by all staff in the OR as protection from radiation exposure. X-rays can be taken to check for proper positioning of the spine and to help the surgeon identify a specific level of the spine. This may be done before incision or after partial exposure of the spinous processes and laminae. In both cases an instrument or needle is used to mark a position on the spine, and an x-ray of the spine is taken. The x-ray enables the surgeon to identify the level of the spine that is marked. The surgeon uses that information to identify the correct surgical level. A postoperative x-ray is also taken to verify that the surgery was done to the correct level of the spine.

With fluoroscopy, also called direct image intensification, a C-arm (covered with a sterile drape) is used to take a continuous x-ray that is portrayed on a monitor. This gives the surgeon the ability to view the spine and to directly view screws as they are being placed during an instrumented fusion. This ensures that spinal instrumentation for fusion is properly positioned in the correct

levels. Fluoroscopy is also used for placement of nerve-stimulator electrodes in brain or spinal areas and stereotactic procedures.

Stereotactic and Image-Guided Equipment. Stereotactic and image-guided equipment is commonly used for neurosurgery. Either a frame-based (requiring a head frame skull attachment, see Figure 21-35) or a frameless system such as Brainlab or Stealth (using fiducials) can be used. Both systems use a computer to register points, based on information obtained from a stereotactic MRI or CT scan done preoperatively, to determine the least traumatic approach to the target (tumor, lesion, ventricle). Both systems have accompanying attachments and instruments that must be available. The frameless image-guided system requires a monitor to display views of the brain or spine in three different planes: axial, coronal, and sagittal (Figure 21-36).

FIGURE 21-35 Stereotactic procedure. Patient fitted with head frame before computed tomography (CT) or magnetic resonance imaging (MRI) scanning.

FIGURE 21-36 Frameless stereotactic image-guided navigation monitor showing the brain with tumor in three planes: coronal *(upper left),* sagittal *(upper right),* and axial *(lower left).*

FIGURE 21-34 Mayfield overhead instrument table.

Ultrasonic Aspirator. An ultrasonic aspirator (e.g., Cavitron Ultrasonic Surgical Aspirator, CUSA) may be used to emulsify and debulk a tumor with high-frequency sound waves. Various settings allow the surgeon to adjust the instrument to remove firm or calcified lesions, or soft masses. The ultrasonic aspirator provides hemostasis and spares adjacent nerves and vessels as it removes the tumor.

Audiovisual Equipment. The use of video cameras, recorders, and television monitors is invaluable to teach staff and enhance understanding of the surgical procedure by perioperative personnel who are otherwise unable to visualize the surgeon's actions directly. By viewing the operative field through the monitor, the experienced scrub person will be able to anticipate the neurosurgeon's next move and will therefore provide better assistance.

Intraoperative Monitoring Equipment. Equipment for intraoperative monitoring, such as EEG, EPs, ICP, and Doppler, may also be required.

Instrumentation, Implants, and Supplies. Typically instrumentation used in neurosurgery is added to basic surgical instrumentation to make neurosurgical-specific trays, such as a basic craniotomy tray or a laminectomy tray. Specialized trays, instruments, or implants can be added based on the surgical procedure.

Powered surgical instruments are commonly used in neurosurgery. Multiple drills, drill bits, and accessories are available. These tools may be powered by air, battery, or electricity and are operated by a hand control or foot pedal. All drills have a safety control that should be engaged at all times the instrument is not in use. The perioperative nurse should monitor the sterile field to ensure that drills and other power equipment are not left lying on the patient. The use of drills makes bone work easier and reduces operating time. Irrigating the tip of the drill while it is in use prevents overheating of the tissue. By changing drill bits and attachments, different drills can be used to make burr holes, craniotomies, craniectomies, and holes for dural tack-up sutures. They can be used to thin bone for a decompression, to perform decortication for spinal fusion, to harvest hip graft, to shape bone grafts, and to make holes for plating and fixation systems.

The Hall Surgairtome 200 (Figure 21-37) can be used for precision cutting, shaping, and repair of bone. Compressed nitrogen is the power source, as with other air-powered equipment. The Hall Surgairtome 200 can be used to widen the graft area in anterior fusions and to unroof the auditory canal in eighth cranial nerve surgery. For use in less accessible areas, such as the sphenoidal sinus, pituitary fossa, and vertebral bodies, attachments with 20- and 90-degree angles are available. A range of burrs and guards is available.

The craniotome offers a perforator drive for drilling burr holes. Both 12- and 7-mm perforators are available in disposable and reusable forms. The perforator driver attachment can be removed and a saw blade and dura guard attached to adapt the instrument for cutting a craniotomy bone flap. A cranioplasty burr and a skull contour burr as well as guards for each type of burr are available.

Another versatile pneumatic tool is the Midas Rex instrument (Figure 21-38). The variety of disposable cutting tools of this foot pedal–controlled instrument and its attachments provides the neurosurgeon with a versatile bone dissector capable of cutting bone by sawing through it or drilling it away. In addition, large craniotomy flaps can be turned with only a single burr hole. Manufacturers' precautions and instructions must be followed for all powered instruments.

A variety of suction tips, retractors, and retractor systems are required for visualization. A transsphenoidal tray and instruments are required for that specialized approach. Microneurosurgical instruments may be needed for delicate brain or spinal cord surgery. Dural grafts and substitutes may be required to repair the dura. Aneurysm instruments, aneurysm clips, or hemostatic clips may be needed for neurovascular surgery. Titanium plates or wire is used to replace a bone plate after a craniotomy. Spinal instrumentation (plating and fixation systems) may be implanted, and bone grafts and substitutes may be used to promote spinal fusion.

Specific surgeries may require shunts or CSF reservoirs, implantable stimulators or pumps, endoscopes and endoscopic instruments, endovascular instruments, catheters, and coils. These supplies must be available if they are to be placed or implanted during surgery.

The surgical nurse needs to assemble instrumentation with consideration for each individual surgery and according to each individual surgeon's preferences. The instrument list for each procedure and neurosurgeon should be documented, referenced, and frequently updated in collaboration with the surgeon. Specific instruments are mentioned in the surgical procedure descriptions that follow.

FIGURE 21-37 Hall Surgairtome 200 with attachments.

FIGURE 21-38 Midas Rex drill with attachments.

Preliminary Procedures. A number of procedures or therapeutic measures are performed before the primary surgery begins. It is important that the perioperative nurse anticipate these procedures, understand why they are done, and be prepared to facilitate them.

Anesthesia Concerns. The anesthesia provider collaborates with the surgeon and nurses to provide appropriate care to the patient. The anesthesia provider must be aware of and plan for situations in which the neurosurgery patient may need to be awake during the surgery for intraoperative assessment. Anesthesia agents must be adjusted if intraoperative monitoring of EPs is to be done. If the cervical spine is unstable or unable to extend, endotracheal intubation may need to be done while the patient is awake. The position of the bed in the OR should be communicated to the anesthesia provider. For surgery of the head, the bed may be turned 90 or 180 degrees away from the anesthesia machine to provide comfortable access to the surgical site. Anesthesia providers can prepare by having enough length on their tubing to make the turn while maintaining control of the patient's airway.

Anesthesia for neurosurgery requires sufficient IV access. The anesthesia provider may place a central line if peripheral IV lines are insufficient, or if the procedure requires the patient to be positioned in the sitting position. Increased risk of an air embolism during surgery exists when the patient is in a sitting position and when a venous sinus may be breeched. A precordial Doppler ultrasound or a pulmonary artery catheter may be placed to monitor for an air embolus. A catheter in the right atrium can be used to remove an air embolus in the heart. An arterial line may be placed for continuous monitoring of blood pressure and for drawing samples for arterial blood gas (ABG) analysis.

Antibiotic prophylaxis is administered within 60 minutes of incision time and continued at the appropriate dose schedule for at least 24 hours. The preoperative antibiotic dose is the most important dose in the prevention of postoperative infection. Generally a broad-spectrum cephalosporin is the antibiotic drug of choice, but this depends on the needs and allergies of the individual patient. In addition, antibiotics such as bacitracin can be added to the irrigation fluid. Preoperative steroids may be given to minimize inflammation and edema when surgery involves the brain or spinal cord. Diuretics may be added for brain relaxation during surgery and to decrease ICP. To prevent seizures, antiepileptic drugs are typically given when the cerebral cortex is manipulated. Coagulopathies must be identified and corrected preoperatively.

For all but minor surgeries, a Foley catheter is inserted into the bladder to monitor urinary output during the procedure. It is essential when procedures are expected to be prolonged, when excessive bleeding is anticipated, or when diuretics are to be given intravenously, so that the bladder does not become distended. A Foley catheter is needed by trauma patients for continual assessment of kidney function.

Stereotactic Image-Guided Navigation. To prepare for surgery on the brain, fiducials are placed on bony landmarks or points around the skull before a preoperative MRI or CT scan. Afterward the fiducials are left in place for entry into the OR. After the patient is anesthetized and positioned, a skull clamp is placed and an image-guided navigation arm is attached to the skull clamp. This provides a fixed point of reference. The arm should be out of the way of the surgical team to ensure that it will not be inadvertently bumped and moved from its fixed point during surgery, thus disrupting the navigation system and potentially making it useless. The location of the fiducials is registered into the computer, allowing the computer to align the preoperative images (of the CT scan or MRI) to the patient's head. The monitor then shows the location of the navigation probe (which is maneuvered by the surgeon) and its trajectory on all three planes (axial, coronal, and sagittal) of the CT or MRI (see Figure 21-36). This enables the neurosurgeon to plan the approach to the target area and to navigate the surgical area using the navigation probe. After the registration process is complete, the fiducials can be removed so that the area can be prepped for surgery. A sterile sleeve is placed over the navigation arm when draping. The navigation system is used to find the target (tumor, lesion, ventricle) using the least traumatic trajectory. It also helps to ensure that the desired amount of tissue is removed. The image-guided navigation system can also be used for spine surgery.

Neuromonitoring. An EEG can be used intraoperatively to view and record electrical activity by way of electrodes placed on the scalp or directly on the brain. It can be used to identify the location of seizure foci on the brain for possible resection. Nonconvulsive use of EEG monitors is used to monitor for burst suppression, which refers to a decrease in brain activity on the EEG monitor and may be related to hypoxemia-related hypoperfusion.

EPs record the brain's electrical response to visual, auditory, and sensory stimuli. They may be used intraoperatively to monitor hearing during resection of acoustic neuromas or to monitor somatosensory evoked potentials (SSEPs) during some spine surgery. SSEPs may also be used to localize the primary sensory cortex in anesthetized patients. SSEPs involve placing needles in significant muscles of the patient and recording a baseline reading before the surgical incision. A significant change in EPs can indicate surgical invasion of the spinal cord, peripheral nerves, brainstem, or midbrain. To avoid permanent injury to the patient, the patient's position may need to be adjusted, or the surgeon may need to adjust retractors or instrumentation, alter a surgical approach, or decide that a subtotal tumor resection is necessary.

Lumbar and Ventricular Drains. The neurosurgeon may place a lumbar drain in the subarachnoid space of the lumbar spine to allow for CSF removal and intraoperative brain relaxation during aneurysm or tumor exposure. It may also be placed to prevent (or postoperatively, to treat) a CSF leak, which is most likely to occur after posterior fossa or transsphenoidal procedures. Alternatively, surgeons may place a ventricular catheter through a burr hole into a ventricle of the brain. In addition to providing the ability to drain CSF, a ventriculostomy provides the most accurate method of monitoring ICP. A transducer-tipped catheter system is a less accurate but less invasive method for monitoring. It does not allow for CSF drainage. With both the lumbar drain and the ventricular catheter, the nurse must ensure that stopcocks and clamps are properly positioned to avoid overdrainage of CSF, which could result in brain herniation. A separate surgical prep and setup are required for placement of these ICP devices.

Positioning. Many of the basic body positions described in Chapter 6 and their modifications are used in neurosurgery. The perioperative nurse must collaborate with the surgeon before the procedure to ensure the appropriate OR bed, attachments, and supportive positioning devices are available. Positioning devices that may be needed include a headrest, pillows, blankets, gel pads, a safety belt, tape, a shoulder roll (supine), an axillary roll (lateral), a beanbag (lateral), and chest rolls (prone).

Specialized neurosurgical headrests and skull clamps are commonly used for craniotomies and posterior cervical spine surgeries to support and stabilize the head and neck. They can be used with any body position. The basic unit of the neurosurgical headrest

PATIENT SAFETY

Preventing Injury When Using an Intraoperative Head Fixation System

Specialized bed attachments in conjunction with a skull clamp create a mechanical support system that is often used in head and neck surgery when rigid cranial stabilization is desired. Features of this device include the base unit (which attaches to the OR bed), cross bars, a swivel adaptor (reticulating arm), and the skull clamp. Only properly trained OR staff should be permitted to operate these devices. Mounting instructions for the bed attachment vary by OR bed. The nurse must verify that the bed attachment is properly secured before the start of patient positioning.

Safe Application of the Skull Clamp

When the anesthesia provider has determined that the patient is ready for positioning, the designated member of the OR team will pin the patient's head with the skull clamp. The clamp consists of two skull pins in the rocker arm and one skull pin in the extension arm. When properly placed, the pins in the rocker arm are equidistant from the centerline of the patient's head and the single pin in the extension arm is exactly at the centerline. Improper positioning of the skull pins may cause serious injury to the patient. Special attention should be paid to avoiding the areas of the frontal sinus, temporal fossa, blood vessels, and nerves. The person securing the skull clamp must ensure that the pins are at a 90-degree angle, the necessary pounds of clamping force are applied, and the rocker arm is in the "CLOSED" position.

Safe Positioning

After the head is safely secured, the patient can be positioned for surgery. It is important that open communication exists among all members in the OR suite. Every member of the OR team plays a key role in the positioning process, and without good communication critical steps may be missed. Airway management is vital, and the anesthesia provider must have control of the patient's airway at all times. All movements of the patient's head and body must first be cleared by the anesthesia provider. There must be at least three people responsible for positioning the head. One member of the anesthesia team monitors the airway, one member of the surgical team holds the patient's head within the skull clamp, and one member secures the reticulating arm of the bed attachment to the skull clamp. All the components of the bed attachment have a starburst locking mechanism, and it is critical all teeth are engaged and locked securely. It is the responsibility of the team member holding the patient's head to do the final check to ensure all locking mechanisms are engaged properly. There should be no movement detected in any component of the system if secured properly. If even one component of the system is not properly engaged, the patient could be injured.

Postoperative Monitoring

Once the procedure is complete and it is time to remove the patient from the fixation system, the same safety measures go into effect. The anesthesia provider maintains control of the patient's airway while one member of the surgical team holds the patient's head within the skull clamp, and a second member of the surgical team releases all the locking mechanisms of the reticulating arm. At this time either the standard headpiece of the OR bed can be reattached or the patient can be moved to the postoperative bed or stretcher. When the skull clamp is released, the surgeon confirms that all three pins are extracted from the patient's head and secured. If bleeding is observed from the pin site, the surgeon may apply pressure to control the oozing, or may use a monofilament suture to close the hole.

Modified from Integra product information, available at www.integralife.com/Neurosurgeon/Neurosurgeon-Product-List.aspx?ProductLine=4&ProductLineName=Cranial%20Stabilization. Accessed December 18, 2012; PMI Pro Med Instruments product information, available at www.headrest.de/products/cranial-stabilization/doro-skull-clamps. Accessed December 18, 2012.

attaches to the frame of the OR bed after the standard OR bed headpiece has been removed. An articulated arm allows fine adjustments to the position of the head. A horseshoe-shaped headrest may be used. Alternatively, head clamps, skull pins, and tongs that are attached to the neurosurgical headrest bed attachment and provide maximum stability may be required (see Figure 21-33). A variety of manufacturers provide an array of skull clamps for intraoperative cranial stabilization. Standard skull clamps are molded of composite materials and stainless steel, and radiolucent skull clamps are made of a composite material that reduces artifact in procedures requiring x-ray (Integra, 2012).

Most skull clamps have three sterile pins that are placed in the skull clamp and covered with antibiotic or povidone-iodine ointment. Pins are available in adult and child sizes. Pins are not recommended for use in children less than 5 years of age, and it is at the discretion of the surgeon to determine which set of pins are appropriate for use on the patient (Integra, 2012). The surgeon or surgeon's assistant places the skull clamps on the patient's head after anesthetic is administered. The surgeon must place the skull clamp strategically in the skull to provide access to the surgical site and to avoid the frontal sinuses, the superficial temporal arteries, and the eyes. The pins on the clamp partially penetrate the outer table of the skull. If the prone position is used, the surgeon will place the skull clamp while the patient is supine. The surgeon supports the patient's head during the position change and adjusts the final head position after the patient is placed prone (Patient Safety).

After positional adjustments to the patient's body are complete, the skull clamp (and patient's head) is locked into the articulating arm of the headrest by someone other than the person who is supporting the head. The apparatus is tightened from proximal to distal and double-checked for security. After the patient's head is locked into place, no positional adjustments can be made to the patient's body without first releasing the head. Not doing so could cause injury to the patient's cervical spine. If necessary, an image-guided navigation arm can be attached to certain skull clamps, and the positions of the fiducials are registered into the system before the patient is prepped.

The skull clamp is detached from the basic headrest by loosening the arm from distal to proximal. Finally, while the head is being supported by another person, the skull clamp is loosened, allowing the pins to be released from the skull. Ointment can be applied to the pin sites. Bleeding may occur at the pin sites after the skull clamp is removed. It usually stops with digital pressure, but occasionally a stitch may be required.

The position of the patient's arms must also be considered. For cranial surgery, usually at least one arm is tucked so that the Mayo stand can be positioned over the patient. For cervical spine surgery, both arms are tucked so that the surgical site can be accessed from both sides of the bed. When the arms are tucked, the elbows are padded to protect the ulnar nerve, the palms face inward, and the wrist is maintained in a neutral position (Denholm, 2009). A drape secures the arms. It should be tucked snuggly under the patient, not under the mattress. This prevents the arm from shifting downward intraoperatively and resting against the OR bed rail.

For thoracic and lumbar spine surgery, armboards can usually be placed out of the way of the surgeon and radiology equipment. Armboards are maintained at less than a 90-degree angle to prevent brachial plexus stretch.

As always, the nurse identifies any potential hazards and takes precautions to prevent them. Intermittent pneumatic compression devices are applied before induction of anesthesia to prevent deep vein thrombosis (DVT) unless they are contraindicated because of a known DVT. Pressure points must be identified and relieved. Joints must be maintained in functional alignment with no pressure or tension on superficial nerves and vessels. A warming or cooling blanket is applied for temperature control. An occlusive dressing applied over the eyes protects them from chemical burns and corneal abrasions that may occur from solutions used to prep the head. Keeping the head positioned above the heart minimizes bleeding when operating on the head.

Supine position or some modification of it can be used for approaches to the frontal, parietal, and temporal lobes; the anterior cervical spine; and the anterior lumbar spine. Lateral position can be used for an approach to the cerebellopontine angle in the posterior fossa, for anterior thoracic and lumbar spine surgery, and for posterior spine surgery. It can be used for lumbar sympathectomies and for placements of nerve stimulators and pumps.

Prone position and modifications of it can be used for access to the posterior spine and for suboccipital and posterior fossa craniotomies. A laminectomy frame or chest rolls are commonly used for prone position. The Jackson table permits access of the C-arm for intraoperative fluoroscopy of the spine. The Andrews table or frame can be used for a modified knee-chest position, which is useful for posterior lumbar spine surgery. The patient's hips and knees are flexed so that the lower body is supported primarily by the knees. The Hicks spinal surgery frame may be used to support this position and allow the abdomen to hang free. The chest is supported on a chest roll. Advantages of this position include decreased bleeding because of the collapse of epidural veins, better exposure resulting from hyperflexion of the spine, absence of pressure on the vena cava, and increased ease of ventilation. Operating time is usually reduced when this position is used. Disadvantages of the knee-chest position include the difficulty of maintaining physical stability on the OR bed, the increased possibility of patient hypotension, and the pooling of blood in the lower extremities.

The Fowler (sitting) position is used for some craniotomies involving a posterior or occipital approach. Advantages of this position include optimum visibility of the operative field and decreased blood loss because of the lowered arterial and venous pressures. Disadvantages are the potential for orthostatic hypotension and air embolism. In the sitting position the venous pressure in the head and neck may be negative, predisposing the patient to air embolism. Other potential problems with this position include neck flexion with airway compromise and difficulty in achieving and maintaining functional alignment (see Chapter 6 for more information on the previously mentioned positions).

Skin Preparation. Prevention of infection is a primary concern in neurosurgery. An antiseptic skin prep is performed by the perioperative nurse, surgeon, resident, or surgical assistant. General principles and precautions cited in Chapter 4 apply to neurosurgical preps. Although studies have shown that shaving the surgical site can contribute to the possibility of infection, usually some hair removal is necessary when operating on the head and posterior cervical spine.

Hair removal from the head causes a disturbance in body image and can be upsetting to patients. A discussion and often a compromise regarding hair removal should take place between the surgeon and patient before the surgery, and an understanding should be reached as to how much hair will be removed. Hair that is removed is the property of the patient. It should be placed in a container, labeled with the patient's name, and kept with the patient after surgery.

Hair removal should be done as close to the time of skin incision as possible to decrease the possibility of surgical site infection. Whenever possible, minimal hair removal is recommended. It is possible to shave a 1- to 2-cm-wide area along the length of some craniotomy incisions after the hair is parted at the incision site. After the minimal shave, the hair can be combed away from the incision and held back with prepping solution or antimicrobial ointment. However, other craniotomies require more extensive hair removal. Electric hair clippers are preferred to razors because they are less irritating and less likely to nick the skin, which would predispose the area to infection. After hair removal the nurse should inspect the patient's skin carefully for any signs of inflammation or infection. If any such signs are noted, they should be reported to the surgeon immediately. The head and hair surrounding the planned incision can be prepped, even though the hair will be draped out of the operative field.

For surgery on the cervical spine it is possible to secure long hair on top of the head and remove neck hair with clippers to a level even with the top of the ears or to the occipital protuberance. Postoperatively, patients with long hair can comb it down over the shaved area until the hair regrows. Patients undergoing thoracic or lumbar spine surgery may not need to be shaved. If a bone graft from the hip will be taken for spinal fusion, that area must be prepped as well as the spinal incision area.

Many neurosurgeons mark the incision line with a marking pen or a marking solution and wooden stick. If a marking solution is used, indigo carmine, gentian violet, or brilliant green is recommended. Methylene blue should never be present in a neurosurgical OR because it produces an inflammatory reaction in CNS tissue. Because the markings tend to wash off during the prep, some surgeons may scratch the scalp along the planned incision with a sharp sterile needle. This increases the risk of infection and should only be done if there is danger of harming the patient by varying from the planned line of incision.

Draping. In neurosurgical procedures, the right or left side of the head and the level of the spine must be specified. The surgical team should also check that the marking (initials) made to the surgical site in the holding area are in the operative field.

Draping for some neurosurgery procedures is complex and requires the cooperation of the surgeon, assistant, and scrub person. Four or more towels are placed around the operative site. They may be secured by disposable skin staples, small towel clips, or silk sutures on a cutting needle.

Draping for a craniotomy is challenging. If a minimal shave was done, an adhesive drape with staples placed around the shaved area near the incision can help to keep hair out of the incision. Towels can be contoured to the prepped area of the head and held in place with staples, leaving the operative site exposed. A craniotomy drape can then be placed over the towels. A sterile drainage bag below the incision will help to catch irrigation and blood and drain it into a suction canister. If a stereotactic head frame is used, the team confirms that the drapes do not interfere with the head frame attachments.

Prepping a hip graft incision site may need to be done with spinal fusion surgery. Two areas may need to be prepped and squared off with towels, which can be held in place with an adhesive drape. A partially unfolded three-quarters drape can be placed between the two planned incision sites before the universal or laparotomy drape is placed. A clamp can be placed over the prepped hip area to positively identify it. The drape can be cut over the prepped area, being sure not to cut an area of the drape that covers a nonsterile area. A second adhesive drape can hold the cut drape in place (see Chapter 4 for general draping procedures).

Hemostasis and Visualization. A few minutes before making the incision, the surgeon may inject the incision site with a local anesthetic agent, such as lidocaine or bupivacaine. Lidocaine has a more rapid onset and shorter duration of action than bupivacaine. Along with decreasing the effect of the stimulus of the skin incision, infiltration of the solution will apply pressure within the tissues and decrease bleeding at the time of incision. Using a local anesthetic that also contains epinephrine will constrict blood vessels to further minimize bleeding.

Meticulous hemostasis is particularly important in neurosurgery. Many methods are incorporated to limit blood loss. A major consideration is control of hemorrhage from the highly vascular scalp. Skin edges along the wound are compressed with gauze sponges and fingers during the initial incision. Usually, this is followed by application of disposable scalp clips (Figure 21-39). An automatic clip gun may be used to apply clips to include the galea and skin edge. The clips limit bleeding by applying pressure to the scalp edges. They remain in place until closure. Placement of self-retaining retractors also helps to control bleeding of the scalp.

Retraction is required for visualization. Self-retaining retractors such as cerebellar or Gelpi retractors can be used to retract skin, subcutaneous tissue, muscle, or the scalp. Suture can be used to retract the scalp or the dura of the brain or spinal cord. Blunt, malleable retractors are used on brain tissue. Table-mounted self-retaining retractor systems such as the Greenberg help the surgeon to see deep into the brain and may be used with a microscope.

Electrosurgery is routine for neurosurgical procedures. Perioperative nurses must understand the uses and hazards of the ESU and be familiar with the safety measures. Electrocoagulation current seals the blood vessels. To be effective the electrocoagulating current must contact the vessel in a dry field. For this reason, suctioning is necessary to remove blood as the contact is made between the instrument carrying the current and the bleeding point. A monopolar current is used to cut and coagulate tissue. It can be applied to forceps, a metal suction tip, or another instrument, which acts as a conducting tool. Monopolar electrosurgery is safe to use on the epidermis, dermis, galea, periosteum, muscle, and bone. It is used extensively for exposure of the posterior spine.

Bipolar ESUs provide a completely isolated output with negligible leakage of current between the tips of the forceps, permitting use of electrocoagulating current in proximity to structures where ordinary monopolar electrocoagulation would be hazardous (Figure 21-40). It is safe to use the bipolar ESU to control bleeding on the dura of the brain and spinal cord and near vital nerves and vessels. The bipolar ESU can be used to maintain hemostasis and to dissect tissue in the brain. Ringer's or normal saline solution irrigation is often used during bipolar electrocoagulation to minimize tissue heating, shrinkage, drying, and adherence to the forceps. Some bipolar units have built-in irrigating systems. The use of the bipolar electrocoagulation technique allows hemostasis of almost any size

FIGURE 21-39 Automatic clip gun, with disposable scalp clips and cartridge.

FIGURE 21-40 Malis bipolar coagulator and bipolar cutter, with irrigation module.

vessel encountered. Vessels as large as the superficial temporal artery, as well as those too small for suture or clip ligation, may be coagulated with bipolar units.

Suction is necessary to evacuate blood, CSF, and irrigation solution from the surgical site. Metal suction tips in multiple sizes, such as the Sachs, Frazier, and Adson, are used not only because they keep the wound dry but also because they can conduct electrocoagulation current from a monopolar unit to the bleeding point. Suction applied directly on normal neural tissue may be harmful and is avoided. Instead, a cottonoid patty may be placed between the suction tip and neural tissue for protection. Suction can be used to aspirate necrotic or traumatized brain tissue or soft brain tumors after a sample has been obtained for pathologic examination. It is also useful in evacuating abscess cavities, removing fluid from a ventricle or the subarachnoid space, holding a solid tumor during its removal, and applying compression to a bleeding vessel.

Bone wax is a hemostatic material that should be available for all cranial and spinal cord operations. Bone wax may be applied with the surgeon's fingertip or with the tip of an instrument such as a Freer or Penfield elevator. The surgeon firmly rubs or packs the wax into the bleeding surfaces of bone. Bone wax is commonly used in burr holes, along the edges of a craniotomy, and on the cut edges of the spine.

Soft goods (e.g., gauze sponges) are used to control bleeding before the skull or spinal canal is entered; however, they are coarse and can injure fragile tissues such as the brain and spinal cord. Instead, compressed, absorbent patties made of rayon or cotton (cottonoids) are used to control bleeding beneath the skull and around the spinal cord. Patties are also placed over delicate neural tissue for protection. It is far less traumatic to suction on a patty than directly on the tissue. Patties are available in a variety of sizes, both squares and strips, ranging from 4 inch to 6 inches long and from ¼ inch to 1 inch wide (Figure 21-41). A supply of various sizes is typically moistened with irrigation solution or thrombin and offered to the surgeon on a waterproof surface. Patties have x-ray–detectable markers and strings attached and are included in the standard soft goods count.

Cotton balls moistened with irrigation solution or thrombin may be used as a temporary pack or tamponade in a bleeding tumor

bed after a tumor has been removed. The gentle pressure of the cotton balls along with time and patience on the part of the surgeon may stop bleeding not controllable by other means. Cotton balls also have x-ray–detectable strings and are included in the soft goods count.

A variety of hemostatic clips are available and used by neurosurgeons to occlude both superficial and deep vessels. Unlike clips that were used in the past, hemoclips and Ligaclips are made of an alloy that is compatible with the MRI scanner. The scrub person removes the clips from a special cartridge with the appropriate applicator and passes them to the surgeon for application to a vessel. Such clips enable the surgeon to occlude vessels in areas difficult to reach by other means and to ligate superficial vessels of the brain before cutting them and without destroying any surrounding tissues. Clips are available in a variety of sizes. Numerous types of special clips are used for permanent or temporary occlusion of vessels or an aneurysm neck in the surgical treatment of an intracranial aneurysm (Figure 21-42).

Neurosurgeons almost routinely use certain hemostatic agents in addition to mechanical hemostasis (Surgical Pharmacology). An absorbable gelatin sponge (Gelfoam) can be applied to an oozing surface, either dry or saturated with irrigation solution or topical thrombin. Larger pieces can be cut into a variety of sizes of strips and squares. Gelfoam is often followed by a patty, which enables the surgeon to maneuver and compress it once it is in the surgical site. Gelfoam is absorbable and can be left in the body.

Oxidized regenerated cellulose is available in two forms: a rayon-like gauze (Surgicel) and a cotton-like form (Fibrillar). These are also absorbable hemostatic agents that are used to control bleeding from oozing surfaces, vessels, and sinuses in the brain. These hemostatic substances are presented in various sizes and shapes and are offered to the surgeon dry. The hemostatic material adheres to the bleeding area with gentle pressure.

Thrombin is a drug that can be topically applied to bleeding surfaces to achieve hemostasis. Typically, Gelfoam or patties are saturated with thrombin and placed on the oozing surface.

Irrigating the wound helps the surgeon identify active bleeding points and may facilitate hemostasis. A syringe with an angiocatheter tip may be used to deliver irrigation for microsurgery. Many neurosurgeons irrigate surgical wounds with an antibiotic solution before wound closure. The antibiotic is mixed with irrigation

FIGURE 21-41 Cottonoid patties.

FIGURE 21-42 Standard aneurysm clips and appliers.

SURGICAL PHARMACOLOGY

Hemostatic Agents

Achieving hemostasis in delicate areas can be a challenge for the neurosurgeon. In addition to using meticulous technique to prevent bleeding, topical agents are routinely used as an adjunct to hemostasis. The perioperative nurse must be familiar with the agents used in this setting.

Medication/Category	Dosage/Route	Purpose/Action	Adverse Reactions	Nursing Implications
Topical thrombin/ hemostatic agent	Bovine-derived thrombin: 1000 to 2000 units/mL applied directly to the source of bleeding or in conjunction with absorbable gelatin sponges	Catalyzes conversion of fibrinogen to fibrin	May cause fever or allergic-type reactions	Product is for external use only; not for intravenous use.
Gelatin matrix (FloSeal)/hemostatic agent	Gelatin matrix granules and topical thrombin packaged as a kit with syringes and mixing bowl. Available in 5- and 10-mL kits. FloSeal is applied directly to the source of bleeding	Matrix particles form a composite clot that seals bleeding site; thrombin component converts fibrinogen in patient's blood to fibrin	Anemia, atrial fibrillation, infection	Product reaches maximum expansion at approximately 10 min. Excess product should be removed with gentle irrigation. Not for intravascular use.
Absorbable gelatin sponge (Gelfoam)/ hemostatic agent	Film, powder, and compressed sponge forms. Can be cut to the desired size and used directly at the site of bleeding	Absorbs and holds blood and fluid within its interstices; exerts physical hemostatic effect	Local infection and abscess formation	Should not be used in closure of skin incisions because it may interfere with healing of skin edges. Often moistened with saline or topical thrombin before use.
Collagen hemostat (Avitene, Helistat, Instat)/hemostatic agent	Available in powder, sheets, or sponges. Powder is available in 0.5-, 1-, and 5-g containers. Applied directly to the site of bleeding	When in contact with a bleeding surface, attracts platelets that aggregate into thrombi, initiating formation of a physiologic platelet plug	Adhesion formation, allergic reaction, foreign-body reaction, inflammation, potentiation of infection	Apply dry. Excess material should be removed with irrigation and suction.
Oxidized regenerated cellulose (Surgicel)/ hemostatic agent	Fibrous, knitted, or sheer weave fabric. Can be cut to the desired size and used directly at the site of bleeding	Allows platelets and aggregates of thrombin and particulate blood elements to cling and form a coagulum that can act as a patch	Encapsulation of fluid, foreign-body reactions	Store at room temperature.

Modified from LexiComp Online, available at www.crlonline.com/crlsql/servlet/crlonline. Accessed January 27, 2013; FloSeal package insert product information, available at www.baxter.com/downloads/healthcare_professionals/products/Floseal10ml_IFU_r3.pdf. Accessed January 13, 2013; Gelfoam package insert product information, available at www.pfizer.com/files/products/uspi_gelfoam_plus.pdf. Accessed January 13, 2013.

solution according to the surgeon's preference so that it is ready for use when needed.

Suture. Required suture will vary according to the surgery, the condition of the wound and patient, and the surgeon's preference. Suture can be used for retraction of the scalp for a craniotomy flap. Dura of the brain and spinal cord may be retracted, tacked up, and closed with braided nylon suture. In general, high tensile strength is needed for closure of the galea of the scalp and the fascia and subcutaneous tissue of the back. Braided, absorbable suture can be used in interrupted stitches to close these layers. Skin may be closed with subcuticular absorbable suture, with either a continuous or an interrupted suturing technique using a monofilament, nonabsorbable suture material such as nylon; alternatively, skin can be closed with staples. Whatever technique is used for skin closure, skin edges should be everted. A drain may be secured to the skin with a nonabsorbable suture such as nylon. In an environment of infection, monofilament, nonabsorbable suture is preferred.

Dressings. Applying dressings to wounds on the head is challenging, especially if a minimal shave was done. For larger incisions in particular, a head wrap can be the best alternative. A wrap helps to keep the nonadherent dressing in place over the incision site and provides compression to prevent the formation of a postoperative hematoma. A smaller dressing can sometimes be held in place with a transparent dressing or tape. Applying a liquid adhesive, such as Mastisol, to the skin before application of the dressing can help to hold it in place.

Evaluation

The identified outcomes from the established nursing diagnoses and interventions are evaluated on an ongoing basis throughout the perioperative period, and adjustments to the plan are made as necessary. Before leaving the OR, the nurse assesses the patient's postoperative skin integrity and performs a postoperative neurologic assessment for comparison with the preoperative assessment. In addition, the patient's outcomes from the identified nursing diagnoses are evaluated. If the outcomes were met, they may be communicated as follows:

- The patient expressed feeling less anxious, coped with perioperative routines adequately, and verbalized an understanding of the planned procedure or procedures.
- The patient or family verbalized knowledge of diagnostic and surgical procedures and had realistic expectations of tests, routines, and postoperative care.
- The patient maintained effective breathing patterns; ventilation was maintained, ABGs were within normal limits, and breath sounds were bilateral.
- The patient will continue to maintain a normal body temperature or undergo rewarming.
- The patient exhibited no signs and symptoms of pressure injury; sensation and motion were the same as preoperative functional levels; and respiratory status and blood pressure were maintained within expected parameters.

After the surgical procedure is completed, the team transports the patient to the intensive care unit (ICU) or postanesthesia care unit (PACU). The perioperative nurse provides the intraoperative documentation and a verbal report to the nurse receiving the patient.

Patient and Family Education and Discharge Planning

Patient and family education is the key to helping the patient return to his or her optimal quality of life. As soon as the need for surgery is identified, a multidimensional education program should begin and include the patient's family. Teaching should address the psychosocial as well as the physiologic aspects of the patient's life. The plan should offer opportunities for the patient to develop new skills, coping mechanisms, and behaviors to adapt to aspects of temporary or permanent neurologic deficit.

Neurosurgery patients may experience a variety of deficits involving vision, hearing, swallowing, speech, motor, sensation, and mental status. Depending on the patient's pathologic condition and surgery, other physicians may observe the patient postoperatively along with the neurosurgeon. Neurologists, ophthalmologists, endocrinologists, cardiologists, radiologists, oncologists, and infectious disease physicians may be involved with managing the medical care of neurosurgery patients. Rehabilitation, physical, occupational, and speech therapists are instrumental in the recovery of neurosurgery patients. They also teach the patients and their families how to cope with temporary and lifelong deficits and how to improve their quality of life. Some patients may benefit from time spent in a rehabilitation facility before returning home. Patients with severe alterations in neurologic function may require long-term care.

The nurse plays an important role in teaching patients and family members how to look for and recognize potential postoperative complications, such as changes in mental status or behavior, progressive weakness, seizure activity, increasing pain, and signs and symptoms of infection. Routine discharge instructions should include information about newly prescribed medications and their potential side effects in addition to treatment options for postoperative and chronic pain (Patient and Family Education). The nurse should also ensure the patient has instructions for the use of cervical collars, braces for spinal stability, and wound dressing changes when applicable.

The entire healthcare team is responsible for planning the transition from the acute care center to the patient's home or to a skilled nursing or rehabilitation facility. The patient and family need to be involved in every aspect of the neurosurgery patient's care and should be encouraged to ask questions and voice their concerns and opinions.

Surgical Interventions

Minimally Invasive and Specialized Neurosurgery Techniques

Microneurosurgery

Adaptation of the operating microscope for neurosurgery has resulted in improvement of many neurosurgical procedures and made new procedures possible. For years, neurosurgeons have worn magnifying loupes to see small structures. Loupes usually have a magnification of 2× or 3.5×. The microscope has a variety of magnifications ranging from 6× to 40×, providing flexibility and precision. The coaxial illumination overcomes the difficulties of lighting neurosurgical wounds.

Use of the microscope restricts the surgeon's field of vision and mobility; therefore, the scrub person and surgical assistant must be actively engaged in the procedure and must be proficient. The operative field, unless video monitoring is available, cannot be seen. Surgical personnel must understand the surgical procedure and the corresponding anatomy, know the names and uses of all microinstruments, and be proficient at passing the instruments to the surgeon without delay. Each time the surgeon must look away and then back to the surgical field, open wound time and anesthesia time are increased while the surgeon becomes reoriented to the field. Therefore, the assistance the scrub person gives the surgeon saves time and directly benefits the patient.

Microsurgical instruments have been modified and adapted to the requirements of neurosurgery. These instruments often possess the following characteristics: bayonet shape, so that the surgeon's hand remains outside the line of vision and the beam of the microscope light; finely sprung and fluted grip; long length for access to deep structures; and slender and delicate tips that occupy as little space as possible. Microneurosurgical instruments are expensive and fragile. Instructions for handling, cleaning, sterilizing, and storing these instruments should be followed. An instrument that is sprung, bent, dulled, hooked, or in any way damaged must never be handed to a surgeon for use but must be repaired or replaced. Instruments must be kept free from blood and tissue during use because the microscope also magnifies debris on the instruments, occluding the structure the surgeon is about to approach. Very fine microsutures are available.

Microsurgical techniques have been applied to cranial, spinal, and peripheral nerve operations. Some procedures in which microsurgery is of value are explorations of the posterior fossa, especially for tumors of the fourth ventricle or cerebellopontine angle, and removal of small acoustic neuromas, with resulting preservation of the facial nerve. Small-vessel endarterectomy, cerebral arterial bypass, cerebral aneurysm clipping, and excision of AVMs are performed using the microscope for visualization of the surgical site. Microsurgery also has advantages in the treatment of tumors and AVMs of the spinal cord.

Neuroendoscopy

Neuroendoscopy is a rapidly evolving field of minimally invasive surgery, where the goal is to minimize collateral damage without compromising the intended goal of surgery (Baehring and Hochberg, 2012). The endoscope provides illumination and

PATIENT AND FAMILY EDUCATION

Discharge Planning for Spinal Surgery

When discharging patients, ensure that all postoperative instructions are clear and legible, including proper phone numbers for the surgeon and nurse. The nurse should reinforce all written instructions, and ask the patient and caregivers to verbalize and demonstrate a clear understanding of the instructions.

Home Care

- Stress the importance of follow-up care. Advise patients when to schedule a follow-up appointment with the surgeon, and when to begin physical therapy.
- Review the signs or symptoms of infection that warrant immediate notification to the surgeon. They include a temperature of 101° F (38° C) or greater; increased swelling, redness, or tenderness around the incision site; and any drainage originating from the incision.
- Instruct the patient to seek immediate medical attention if he or she experiences the onset of a sudden and/or severe headache, weakness of the extremities, or changes in bowel or bladder function.

Wound Care

- Ensure that patients and caregivers are instructed on proper cleaning, inspecting, and dressing of the wound. Assure them that a small amount of swelling is normal and should continually decrease. Instruct patients to avoid soaking the wound, to shower only when cleared by the surgeon, and to discontinue the use of any lotions or oils on or near the incision site.
- Educate patients on the risk factors that contribute to delayed wound healing such as smoking, obesity, advanced age, diabetes, chronic steroid use, and malnutrition.

Activity

- Walking and climbing stairs are typically encouraged. Activity tolerance is generally patient specific and should be personalized as necessary.

- Patients will have activity restrictions that typically include the following: prolonged travel or driving; sitting for longer than 30 minutes at a time; occupational limitations; strenuous exercise; lifting more than 10 pounds; and bending or twisting at the waist.

Pain Management

- Discuss how much pain, soreness, and stiffness are expected and the importance of contacting the surgeon if the pain is excessive. Over several months, back and leg pain should decrease, depending on the severity of pain preoperatively.
- Review all prescriptions and proper dosing. Discuss which over-the-counter medications, such as acetaminophen, are appropriate. Advise patients that the use of aspirin and NSAIDs, such as ibuprofen, may not be indicated for several weeks because they can cause bleeding.
- Offer pain-reducing activities such as exercise, and relaxation techniques.

Diet

- Proper nutrition promotes wound healing.
- Fluids, fruits, and fiber can help prevent constipation.

Special Instructions and Follow-Up Care

- Provide instructions for use of any braces or supports. Generally a brace should be worn at all times, except when showering and sleeping, until told otherwise by the surgeon.
- Advise patients to resume all preoperative medications unless otherwise noted.
- Provide prescriptions for new x-rays, CT scans, and MRIs according to the physician's orders.
- Discuss smoking cessation when appropriate. Stress the connection between smoking and delayed would healing, and offer resources for smoking cessation.

CT, Computed tomography; *MRI,* magnetic resonance imaging; *NSAIDs,* nonsteroidal antiinflammatory drugs.
Modified from Albert T et al: Discharge instructions for lumbar fusion surgery, available at www.spineuniverse.com/treatments/surgery/lumbar/discharge-instructions-lumbar-fusion-surgery. Accessed January 13, 2013.

magnification of structures and an extended viewing angle. The surgical team must be prepared to convert from a neuroendovascular procedure to an open procedure if it is determined that the surgery cannot be successfully completed endoscopically.

Indications for neuroendoscopic surgery are many. Endoscopic tumor removal or CSF diversion through endoscopic fenestration, such as a third ventriculostomy, can be done for the treatment of hydrocephalus and can eliminate the need for a shunt. Interventricular tumors may be removed endoscopically. In addition, the endoscope can be used to assess adequacy of tumor removal and to identify tumor portions left behind or adherent to vital structures. Stereotactic and image-guided surgery is often used with neuroendoscopy successfully. The endoscope is commonly used in the transsphenoidal approach for pituitary and sellar tumor resection (possibly in collaboration with an otolaryngology surgeon), for microvascular decompression, and for endoscopic biopsy of a lesion.

Endovascular Procedures

Several neurovascular disorders are amenable to endovascular intervention. The endoscopic approach is considered minimally invasive, and is therefore a reasonable option for patients who are not candidates for open surgical procedures because of age, health status,

medical condition, or location of the lesion. Interventional neuroradiology uses fluoroscopy to gain access to the intracranial circulation by way of a percutaneous transfemoral catheter.

The endovascular approach to the treatment of both ruptured and unruptured cerebral aneurysms is endosaccular occlusion (Evidence for Practice). This is an excellent technique for aneurysms that are complex, have a neck that is too short for clipping, or are difficult to reach via traditional craniotomy. A flexible platinum coil is fed through the transfemoral catheter and is coiled within the body of the aneurysm, conforming to the aneurysm's shape. The coil is then detached from the catheter. The coil blocks blood flow to the site, thereby preventing rupture or re-rupture, both of which can be fatal.

Although surgical excision is still the standard treatment for intracranial AVM, surgical morbidity may be decreased by using endovascular embolization preoperatively in select cases. A specialized microcatheter is guided directly into the AVM via angiography. The abnormal blood vessels in the AVM are occluded from the inside by means of embolization. Several materials are used to cause embolization, including fibered titanium coils, polyvinyl alcohol particles, and fast-drying biologically inert glues. The AVM may effectively be devascularized and reduced in size

EVIDENCE FOR PRACTICE

Surgical/Endovascular Treatment of Ruptured Aneurysms

The Stroke Council of the American Heart Association (AHA) has formulated recommendations for the surgical/endovascular treatment of ruptured aneurysms. These guidelines are intended to serve as a framework for the treatment of ruptured aneurysms.

- Endovascular coil occlusion of the aneurysm is appropriate if the aneurysm is deemed treatable by either endovascular coiling or surgical clipping.
- Reasonable consideration of the individual characteristics of the patient and aneurysm must be used in deciding the best means of repair.
- The patient should be managed in a surgery center offering both techniques.
- Either procedure should be performed to reduce the risk of rebleeding after the initial aneurysmal subarachnoid hemorrhage (SAH).

Clipping

The surgeon performs a craniotomy (opening of a portion of the skull) and separates the aneurysm from the surrounding tissue. A small titanium clip, whose features are similar to those of a clothespin, is then placed across the base of the aneurysm. Once the clip is secured, blood can no longer enter or exit the aneurysm sac. By using a needle to drain the remaining blood from the aneurysm, the sac should empty and eventually collapse. The procedure is ideally performed within 72 hours of diagnosis. It is important to note that following rupture there is a 40% chance of death and 80% chance of disability. Early detection and treatment offer the best chances of survival.

Coiling

Also known as endovascular therapy, coiling is a less invasive treatment option. Especially for those patients who are in poor health, surgical intervention may pose a greater threat than the aneurysm itself. Coiling has proven to be a safe alternative to the traditional treatment of a craniotomy. This procedure does not involve opening of the skull, and is performed from inside the blood vessel. A catheter is inserted into the patient's groin, and is guided up toward the brain under fluoroscopy. A wire is then threaded into the catheter and directed into the aneurysm. Once inside the aneurysm the wire twists into small coils and continues filling the aneurysm sac until eventually the aneurysm is occluded (Zuccarello and Ringer, 2010).

Previous studies, such as the International Subarachnoid Aneurysm Trial (ISAT) in 2002, found that patients who were initial candidates for both types of procedures had better outcomes 1 year after endovascular coiling as opposed to surgical clipping. In 2010 a study of 205 aneurysm patients concluded that the less invasive nature of endovascular coiling was more favorable for older patients and those with comorbid medical problems (Gonzalez et al, 2010).

Modified from Bederson BJ et al: Guidelines for the management of aneurysmal subarachnoid hemorrhage: a statement for healthcare professionals from a special writing group of the Stroke Council, *Stroke* 40:994–1025, 2009; Gonzalez NR et al: Endovascular coiling of intracranial aneurysms in elderly patients: report of 205 treated aneurysms, *Neurosurgery* 66:714–721, 2010; Zuccarello M, Ringer A: *Aneurysm clipping*, Mayfield Clinic & Spine Institute, University of Cincinnati Neuroscience Institute, 2010, available at http://mayfieldneuro.com/PE-Clipping.htm. Accessed January 13, 2013.

through endovascular embolization, and when combined with microsurgery or stereotactic radiosurgery, the AVM may be completely eradicated.

Endovascular embolization is also advantageous when used as a preoperative treatment for select intracranial tumor resections. Highly vascular tumors, as well as tumors that are inopportunely positioned, can be devascularized using techniques similar to those used in the treatment of AVMs, thus decreasing blood loss and risk of hemorrhage during resection.

Intracranial stenosis has been deemed a high-risk disease in need of alternative therapies. Successful use of balloon angioplasty has been documented in mostly academic, high-volume centers, performed by highly skilled and experienced physicians. Although the results are encouraging, the technically demanding nature of the procedures carries substantial risk. The Wingspan stent has been approved by the U.S. Food and Drug Administration (FDA) to treat symptomatic patients with intracranial stenosis greater than 50% that is refractory to medical therapies. The stent is implanted using the Wingspan technique. Following balloon angioplasty, a self-expanding nitinol stent is placed across the atherosclerotic lesion in the brain. Although the Wingspan system appears to be a viable treatment option, a high rate of restenosis has been reported, and its value is not yet firmly established (American Association of Neurological Surgeons [AANS], 2009).

Intra-arterial thrombolysis for the treatment of acute ischemic stroke is a consideration for patients who have missed the 3-hour window for therapeutic IV thrombolysis. The endovascular route is used to deliver a high concentration of a thrombolytic agent directly to the site of the offending thrombus in combination with mechanical clot extraction. Intra-arterial thrombolysis is still being studied for its long-term value. It is recommended for selected patients with major ischemic stroke of less than 6-hours' duration caused by occlusion to the middle cerebral artery, and who are being treated at hospitals with appropriate facilities (Biller et al, 2012).

Mechanical clot extraction is an endovascular technique that may be used alone or in conjunction with intra-arterial thrombolysis. Success rates are improved when both modalities are used. Several retrieval devices are approved by the FDA for extraction of thrombi from occluded intracranial arteries. A typical retrieval device consists of a coil that is delivered to the thrombus site via endovascular microcatheter and screwed into the clot like a corkscrew to extract the clot. The coils are available in different shapes and configurations to accommodate the specific thrombus. Mechanical clot extraction shows its best use for cerebral arteries demonstrating large or irregularly shaped clot burdens (Meyers et al, 2009).

Stereotactic Radiosurgery

In stereotactic radiosurgery, stereotactic localization is coupled with delivery of ionizing radiation to destroy a lesion in the brain. Radiosurgery is technically noninvasive and has a low associated morbidity. The use of radiosurgery has increased, and success of treatment has improved with advancements in neuroimaging (CT and MRI) and computer technology. The goal of radiosurgery is to obliterate a relatively small intracranial target with a high irradiation dose while sparing adjacent and distant tissues. Radiosurgical instruments include the Gamma Knife, the Novalis, and the CyberKnife. With any of these techniques, using a stereotactic head frame along with the radiation delivery system allows for great precision (Baehring and Hochberg, 2012).

Radiosurgery can be used to treat AVMs, tumors, and trigeminal neuralgia. Best results are achieved for lesions smaller than 35 mm.

Larger lesions or lesions involving or near cranial nerves can be successfully treated with a fractionated approach in which the radiation is precisely delivered in small daily fractions. This technique, called fractionated stereotactic radiotherapy (FSR), has been particularly useful for preserving vision and hearing. Patients with larger lesions often have symptoms of mass effect that are generally not improved with radiosurgery. Radiosurgery and FSR techniques have successfully sterilized a variety of intracranial lesions often with far less morbidity than a surgical approach.

Stereotactic Procedures

The goal of stereotactic surgery is to target a point or volume in three-dimensional space (Gasco et al, 2012). This is accomplished with coordinate systems that provide a constant frame of reference. Radiographic modalities (CT, MRI) are used to navigate three dimensionally and locate and destroy target structures. Predetermined anatomic landmarks are used as guides.

Originally, special head-fixation devices were developed for stereotactic brain surgery (see Figure 21-35). Since the early 2000s, frameless systems have surpassed frame-based techniques in popularity and versatility. These systems use fiducial markers that either affix temporarily to the skin or are implanted into the outer table of the skull, thereby eliminating the need to mount a frame on the patient's head. These markers are visible on the imaging modality being used.

Both frame-based and frameless stereotactic systems use radiography, fluoroscopy, CT scans, or MRI to permit accurate placement of a probe directed at the target area. The preoperative images are aligned to the patient's head during surgery so that the surgeon has a better idea of the target area.

The many common applications for cranial stereotactic surgery include craniotomies, transsphenoidal approaches, endoscopic surgery, needle biopsies, and therapeutic aspiration. It is also used for catheter placement and third ventriculostomy surgery. Spinal stereotactic surgery is used for screw placement and spinal cord lesions. Common target areas for the stereotactic approach include tumors, infectious lesions, vascular malformations, the basal ganglia, the thalamus, and anterolateral spinal tracts. Target areas can undergo biopsy, be destroyed by chemical or mechanical means, or be electrically stimulated (Research Highlight). Stereotactic procedures are also done to place electrodes in various regions of the brain to determine the site of origin of seizures.

Procedural Considerations.
As in most image-guided surgery (IGS), carts with a monitor and computer, along with accessory equipment and supplies, are required. A variety of stereotactic frame systems are available. The nurse must be familiar with the system in place at his or her institution. Frameless stereotactic surgery triggered a new era in surgical navigation and information delivery. This technology provides three-dimensional visualization of anatomic features with real-time localization information (see Figure 21-36).

Operative Procedure
1. The surgeon places the patient's head into a halo head frame with a stereotactic cage before the surgery (framed stereotaxy). Alternatively, fiducials are placed on the patient's skull (frameless stereotaxy).
2. The patient is then transported for a CT or MRI scan of the brain. The target is identified, and computer coordinates are determined and recorded.

3. After the scan the nurse takes the patient to the OR with the frame or fiducials left in place. The stereotactic coordinates are registered or entered into the computer, and the surgeon performs the procedure through a burr hole. The stereotactic probe is guided by the computer, directing the surgical approach and trajectory (see Figure 21-35).
4. The surgeon may introduce hollow cannulae, coagulating electrodes, cryosurgical probes, wire loops, and other lesion-producing or biopsy instruments through the burr hole for the destruction of areas in the brain. Temporary and permanent nerve-stimulator electrodes may also be introduced to augment the pain-control function of the CNS.

Surgical Approaches to the Brain

Burr Holes

A burr hole is the minimum exposure that can be made to gain access to the brain.

Burr holes are necessary for many neurosurgical procedures. They are placed in the skull to remove a localized fluid collection secondary to head trauma that results in an epidural or subdural hematoma. A burr hole can be used to access the intracerebral ventricles for the following reasons: placement of a ventricular catheter to drain obstructed CSF; measurement of ICP; or establishment of a ventricular shunting system. Burr holes are often placed for many stereotactic procedures, such as stereotactic biopsy or placement of electrodes. Additionally, burr holes are also made before turning the bone flap in preparation for a craniotomy procedure.

Craniotomy

A craniotomy is the removal of a section of the cranium referred to as a bone flap. One or more burr holes are placed, and the dura is dissected away from the cranium. A craniotome with a dura guard attachment is used to excise a section of the cranium, exposing an area of the brain. The surgeon replaces the bone flap to its original location and secures it with wire or titanium plates and screws.

Multiple types of craniotomy incisions are used to expose different parts of the brain. Depending on the location of the pathologic condition, a craniotomy may be frontal, parietal, occipital, temporal, or a combination of two or more of these approaches. The pterional craniotomy is an extremely versatile approach to the anterior and middle fossae. It is useful to access lesions of the frontal or temporal lobes near the sylvian fissure or skull base. A craniotomy may be performed to evacuate intracranial hematomas not accessible through a burr hole, to control bleeding, to debulk or resect tumors, to excise or clip vascular lesions, to aspirate abscess formation, and to decompress cranial nerves.

When turning a scalp flap for a craniotomy, the surgeon may peel the scalp back off the pericranium. The surgeon elevates the bone flap with the overlying muscles still attached (osteoplastic) or strips the periosteum off the skull before the bone flap (free flap) is turned. The bone plate may be separated from the soft tissues, removed from the skull, and set aside for replacement at the end of the procedure. It is placed in an antibiotic solution and remains on the sterile field. The scrub person ensures that the bone flap stays separate from other items on the sterile field and alerts the perioperative circulating nurse and any relief scrub persons of its location to prevent it from being inadvertently discarded. If the bone is not separated from the soft tissues, it is reflected with the temporal muscle and soft tissues. If intracranial swelling is a major concern or the purpose for the craniotomy, the bone plate may not be replaced. If it is not replaced, it may be preserved by means of deep freezing, preservation in bactericidal solutions, sterilization, and preservation in a subgaleal pouch. A recent study found that the technique of storing the craniotomy graft in a subcutaneous location on the patient reduces graft devitalization, and provides the best cosmetic outcome (Morina et al, 2011).

Craniectomy

Craniectomy is the permanent removal of a section of the cranium using burrs and rongeurs to enlarge one or more burr holes. The surgeon performs a craniectomy to gain access to the underlying structures. This procedure may be required to remove tumors, hematomas, and infection of the bone. A suboccipital craniectomy, done with the patient in prone or lateral position, allows access to the posterior fossa. Titanium mesh may be used to repair the cranial defect. Craniectomy is also indicated as treatment for craniosynostosis in infants and young children. Severe head injuries with increased ICP can be treated with a craniectomy to give the brain room to swell.

Transsphenoidal Approach

The transsphenoidal route to the pituitary fossa is a less invasive means of removing tumors than the transcranial route. The approach can be performed via a small incision through the nose or through the gingiva under the upper lip. More recently, an endoscope has been used to assist with access through the sphenoid sinus into the pituitary fossa. Tumors of the parasellar region may also be accessed using this technique.

Surgery of the Brain and Cranium

Ventricular Catheter and Shunt Placement for Hydrocephalus

Hydrocephalus is a condition marked by an excessive accumulation of CSF resulting in dilation of the ventricular system (where CSF is manufactured and circulated) and increased ICP. Conditions that result in the development of hydrocephalus and CSF obstruction in both children and adults include congenital hydrocephalus, spina bifida, tumors, intracranial/intraventricular hemorrhage, aqueductal stenosis, and Chiari malformations. Hydrocephalus is treated by accessing the lateral ventricles for the insertion of a ventricle shunting system. The most commonly used methods to divert CSF from the ventricles are the externalized ventriculostomy catheter and the internalized VP shunt.

Placement of an externalized ventriculostomy catheter requires that a burr hole be made to access either the right or the left lateral ventricle. The ventricular catheter is passed into the ventricle. Flow of CSF is verified. The distal end of the catheter is tunneled beneath the scalp, posterior to the burr hole, externalized, and secured to the scalp with suture. The externalized end of the catheter is connected to an external drainage system, which allows for controlled CSF drainage and for ICP measurement. This system has allowed for temporary shunting in patients with elevated ICP and hydrocephalus from any cause. It is an invaluable adjunct in the clinical assessment and management of head trauma with increased ICP.

For more permanent control of hydrocephalus, an internalized ventricular shunt is placed. The type of shunt and the site of insertion are determined by the neurosurgeon. Three approaches for ventricular insertion are frontal, parietal, and occipital. Although the most common drainage site for an internalized shunting system is the peritoneum by way of open dissection or percutaneous trocar, there are other options. If drainage in the peritoneum is inappropriate because of infection or adhesions, other possible shunting techniques include ventriculovenous, ventriculoatrial, ventriculopleural, and lumboperitoneal (Korley, 2010).

The VP shunt system components are a ventricular (proximal) catheter, a reservoir, a valve, and a peritoneal (distal) catheter. A unitized shunt has fewer separations and connections. The reservoir, if used, is inserted between the catheter and the valve. Access to the system through the reservoir enables the practitioner to assess the patency of the shunt, to obtain CSF for laboratory analysis, to introduce contrast medium for radiologic studies, and in some specific cases to inject medication into the shunt. The one-way valve system directs flow of CSF out of the ventricular system. Valves are available in a variety of different pressure and flow settings. Nonprogrammable valves and shunts are pressure controlled and open to release flow whenever the actual pressure exceeds the pressure that the valve is designed to open (the opening pressure). Some valves are flow controlled and attempt to maintain a constant flow despite pressure changes. Programmable valves and shunts allow adjustments to the opening pressure after the shunt is implanted, avoiding surgical procedures to change valves.

Procedural Considerations. The patient is placed in a modified supine position with a shoulder roll. The head is turned to the opposite side and supported on a donut. Hair is removed from the site where the burr hole will be made to behind the ear and down to the neck. The burr hole site must be prepped, along with the neck, chest, and abdomen on the side of the shunt insertion.

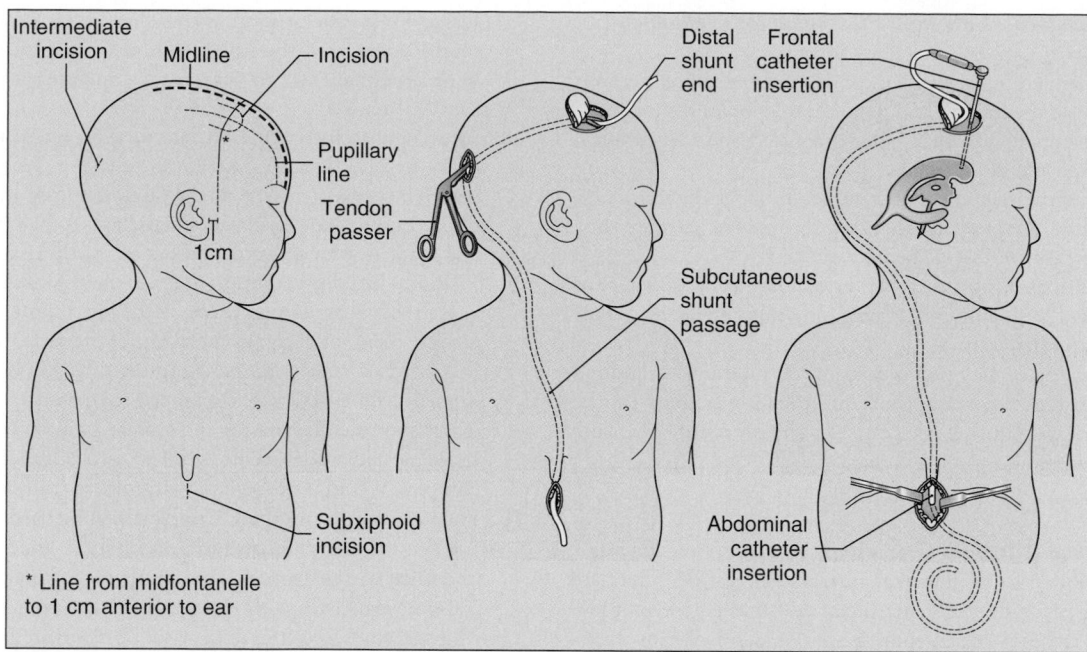

FIGURE 21-43 Placement of a frontal ventriculoperitoneal (VP) shunt. The technique is similar for adult and pediatric patients. The patient is positioned, and coordinates are marked. The shunt is passed subcutaneously. The ventricular catheter and then the peritoneal catheter are inserted.

The shunt unit should be handled with extreme care. As with all implantable devices, each manufacturer's specific instructions must be followed and care taken to keep the assembly free of lint, powder, or other foreign bodies that could cause a reaction in the patient's tissues. Lubricants are never used. Blood should be kept clear from the lumen of the catheter to prevent clotting and obstruction. The scrub person soaks the unit in normal saline and antibiotic solution and primes it at the surgeon's direction before implantation. Air trapping in the valve assembly should be avoided. The valve must be properly oriented to facilitate CSF flow from the ventricles to the peritoneum.

The surgeon may use an endoscope or stereotactic image-guided navigation system to locate small ventricles or to fenestrate the septum between ventricles, thus avoiding the necessity to place multiple ventricular catheters. Surgical technique for VP shunt placement is basically the same for adults and children (Figure 21-43).

Operative Procedure

1. The surgeon makes a horseshoe-shaped incision to the right or left of midline, along the papillary line.
2. Scalp bleeding is controlled, and the skin flap is retracted.
3. The surgeon uses a periosteal elevator to clean the periosteum from the skull.
4. Next the surgeon uses a drill or cranial perforator to create a 1- to 2-cm burr hole. The dura is coagulated and incised. The surgeon uses the bipolar ESU to electrocoagulate the pia at the catheter insertion site.
5. The ventricular catheter with an introducer is inserted perpendicularly into the lateral ventricle approximately 4.5 cm in the infant and 6.5 cm in the adult. When the ventricle is penetrated, the surgeon removes the introducer, verifies the CSF flow, and attaches and secures the reservoir and valve with 2-0 silk ties.

6. A subcutaneous tunnel is created from the burr hole to a neck incision, where the peritoneal catheter is then connected.
7. The surgeon makes a subxiphoid or lateral abdominal incision and exposes the peritoneum.
8. Further tunneling is performed from the neck to the chest and abdomen, avoiding the nipples and umbilicus. The surgeon passes the catheter through the tunneling device to the abdominal incision. After spontaneous distal flow of CSF is verified, the distal end of the peritoneal catheter is passed into the peritoneal cavity, leaving enough length to allow for growth in the child and movement in the adult.
9. The catheter is secured to the peritoneum with a purse-string suture. All incisions are closed, with care taken not to puncture the shunt system with a suture needle.

Shunt failure can occur at any time, requiring any single portion of the shunt system or the entire system to be replaced. Obstruction, disconnection, malfunction, and infection are routine causes of shunt failure. Revising a shunt typically involves a troubleshooting process. Therefore, it is best to prep and drape the patient to provide access to any and all portions of the shunt system. An infected shunt may be externalized until the infection is treated.

Evacuation of Epidural or Subdural Hematoma

After trauma, decompression of the brain, as well as removal and drainage of blood clots and collections of liquefied blood from above or beneath the dura mater, may be required. The need for hematoma evacuation is primarily determined by a declining neurologic status in the patient. Depending on the severity of the injury, evacuation can be accomplished through burr holes or a craniotomy. If elevated ICP is a major concern, the craniotomy plate may be temporarily removed from the skull to allow for swelling and prevention of brain herniation.

Operative Procedure—Burr Hole Placement for Evacuating a Hematoma

1. The surgeon makes at least two linear or small horseshoe incisions over the site of the lesion. Two or more burr holes are made.
2. The surgeon enlarges the burr hole with a Kerrison rongeur until adequate exposure is obtained.
3. If the hematoma is subdural, the surgeon incises the dura.
4. Clot and fluid are evacuated, and hemostasis is accomplished with the ESU or the use of hemostatic clips.
5. The surgeon irrigates through the burr holes using catheters or bulb syringes. Large amounts of irrigating solution are used until the return appears clear.
6. A drain or catheter may be inserted in the subdural or epidural space for postoperative drainage. Additional burr holes can be made as necessary during the course of the procedure to ensure complete evacuation.

Craniotomy

Procedural Considerations. Craniotomy is a technique for exposure of the brain to surgically treat intracranial disease. There are multiple types of craniotomy incisions. A key element of these operative approaches is patient positioning, which facilitates exposure, allowing complex procedures to be done through small bony windows with limited dural opening and minimum cortex exposure. A skull fixation device provides head stability and allows for rotation, flexion, and extension in the final head positioning. If frameless stereotactic image-guided navigation is used, registration of fiducials must be done. Careful planning of the incision is imperative for adequate exposure. As a rule, flaps that create a vascular pedicle should be avoided and linear or sigmoid (S-shaped) flaps should be used. This is particularly true for patients with malignant brain tumors who will be treated with radiation, steroids, and chemotherapy. A pedicle flap compromises the blood supply to the incision and, with these other treatments, increases the likelihood of wound infection.

Operative Procedure—Craniotomy for Tumor Resection

1. The surgeon infiltrates the incision site using a local anesthetic with epinephrine.
2. The surgeon and the assistant apply digital pressure along the skin edges as the surgeon incises the skin through the galea.
3. Raney scalp clips are applied to skin edges, and/or self-retaining retractors are placed. The ESU is used on the major scalp vessels for hemostasis.
4. The scalp flap is reflected in the subperiosteal plane with periosteal elevators or with the monopolar device to divide muscle attachments. It is retracted up using devices that may include retractors, towel clips, suture, or rubber bands and supported with a scalp roll.
5. The surgeon places burr holes to expose the dura and are then widened with curettes and Kerrison rongeurs. The dura is dissected from the cranium using Woodson, Penfield, or Adson dissectors.
6. The surgeon creates the craniotomy using a craniotome loaded with the footplate attachment as the assistant irrigates to cool the bone. The bone flap is carefully elevated from the dura and placed in irrigating solution on the back table.
7. Bone dust is irrigated away from the wound, and hemostasis is established. Bleeding edges of bone are waxed, and bleeding vessels in the dura are electrocoagulated with the bipolar ESU or occluded with thrombin-soaked Gelfoam and patties. The

surgeon places hemostatic agents and patties around the craniotomy edges, and then places dural tacking sutures that will remain permanently to prevent postoperative epidural hematoma formation.
8. After hemostasis is achieved, the surgeon opens the dura with a #11 or #15 blade. A dural suture may be placed in the dura before incising it. This tents the dura, ensuring that the surface of the brain is not inadvertently nicked. A Woodson dissector and blade or Metzenbaum scissors are used to extend the dural incision. Bleeding from transected dural vessels can be prevented by coagulating them with the bipolar ESU before cutting them, or to avoid shrinking of the dura, hemoclips can be placed or vessels can be compressed with a hemostat.
9. The surgeon places a self-retaining retractor system. Cortical dissection is achieved using the bipolar ESU, microscissors, and suction, and the specific surgical procedure is completed. Samples of tumor are sent for pathologic study if applicable.
10. Hemostasis is established. Irrigation can be used to find bleeding sites in the brain. A resection cavity is lined with Surgicel and filled with irrigation. The anesthesia provider produces the Valsalva maneuver with the ventilator to verify hemostasis.
11. The surgeon closes the dura with a 4-0 suture (braided nylon or silk). Gaps in the dura can be repaired using muscle, pericranium, dural substitute, or pericardium. A central dural tacking suture may be placed, and Gelfoam may be placed over the dura.
12. The bone plate is fitted with titanium plates and screws and reconnected to the cranium, or it may be wired into place depending on the surgeon's preference.
13. Muscle/fascia is reapproximated and galea is closed with interrupted absorbable sutures. Skin is closed with suture or staples.

Operative Procedure—Pterional Craniotomy

1. The skin incision for the pterional craniotomy extends from the zygoma to the midline, curving gently just posterior to the hairline (Figure 21-44).
2. The surgeon and the assistant apply digital pressure over folded sponges on both sides of the incision line. The skin and galea are incised in segments, with the length of each segment being equal to that over which the finger pressure is applied. The tissue edges are held with 6-inch toothed forceps as scalp clips are placed on the flap edges. Any remaining active arterial bleeding is controlled with the ESU. If the incision extends into the temporal area, bleeding in the temporal muscle is managed by electrocoagulation, hemostats, tamponade, or suture ligature. Mayo scissors can be used to incise temporal muscle and fascia.
3. The surgeon uses sharp or blunt dissection or electrodissection to remove the soft tissue off the periosteum. The scalp flap is reflected over folded sponges and retracted by use of small towel clips and rubber bands or by muscle hooks on rubber bands. In either case, the traction is maintained by securing the rubber band to the drapes with heavy forceps. The flap may be covered with a moist sponge or Telfa strips and a sterile towel. Bleeding is controlled with the ESU (Figure 21-45).
4. When a free bone flap is planned, the muscle and periosteum are incised. Muscle and periosteum are elevated with the skin-galea flap, reflected, and retracted as a unit, as described previously.
5. The surgeon incises the periosteum and muscle with a scalpel or ESU knife except at the inferior margins, which are left

FIGURE 21-44 The skin incision for a pterional craniotomy.

FIGURE 21-46 The pterion craniotomy is performed with power instruments so that three burr holes are placed. The bone is cut as shown, exposing the frontal and temporal dura and the sphenoid ridge.

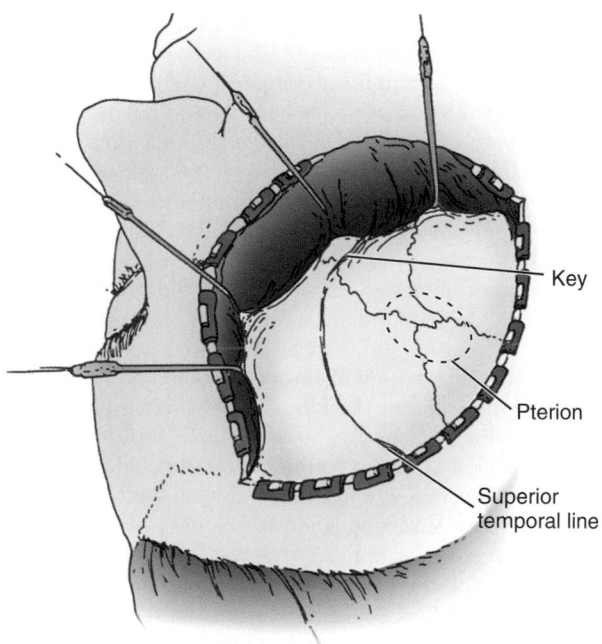

Key

Pterion

Superior
temporal line

FIGURE 21-45 A commonly used means of opening the scalp involves incision of the skin, galea, temporalis fascia, and muscle with reflection of the resultant flap in a single layer.

intact to preserve the blood supply to the bone flap. The periosteum is stripped from the bone at the incision line with a periosteal elevator. Bone wax is used to control bleeding.

6. The scalp edges and muscle are retracted from the bone incision line by a Sachs or Cushing retractor. Two or more burr holes are placed (Figure 21-46). A great deal of heat is generated by the friction of the perforator or burr against the bone. The

assistant must irrigate the drilling site to counteract the heat and remove bone dust, which collects as the holes are made. A large-gauge suction tip is used to remove both irrigating solution and debris from the field. As the inner table is perforated and the dura exposed, tamponade of the burr hole may be achieved temporarily with bone wax or a cottonoid strip or patty. Each hole is eventually debrided by a #0 or #00 bone curette or small periosteal elevator. The dura mater is freed at the margins with a #3 Adson elevator, #3 Penfield dissector, or right-angle Frazier elevator or similar instrument. The hole is irrigated and suction applied simultaneously. Active bleeding points in the bone are identified, and bone wax is applied.

7. When all burr holes have been made, the surgeon separates the dura mater from the bone with a dural separator, such as a #3 Penfield dissector. Dural separation is done to prevent tearing of the dura mater, especially over venous sinuses. An air craniotome or Midas Rex drill can be used for cutting the bone flap. Irrigation and suction are required as the bone flap is cut. Soft tissue edges are retracted with Sachs or Cushing retractors.

8. The surgeon lifts the bone flap (with muscle attached) off the dura mater with two periosteal elevators. Bleeding from the bone is controlled with bone wax. The bone flap is covered with a moist sponge, cottonoid material, and then a clean sterile towel and is retracted in the same manner as the scalp flap.

9. The dura mater is irrigated. Moist patties may be inserted between the dura mater and bone and folded back to cover the exposed bone edges. Epidural tack-up sutures are usually placed around the edge of the craniotomy defect to close the epidural dead space. Sterile towels may be placed around the operative site.

10. The surgeon opens the dura (Figure 21-47). A dura hook or a dural stitch may be used to elevate the dura mater from the brain, and a small nick is made in the dura mater with a #15 blade. Alternatively, a small opening may be made in the dura

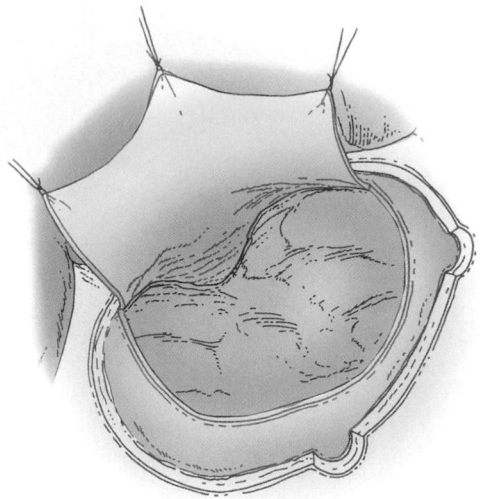

FIGURE 21-47 The dura is opened and reflected back with stay sutures.

mater without elevating it, after which the dural edges are grasped with two forceps with teeth and are elevated. A narrow, moist cottonoid strip is inserted with smooth forceps (bayonet or Cushing) into the opening to protect the brain as the dura mater is incised and elevated. The dural incision can be made with Metzenbaum scissors, special dura scissors, or a Rayport dura knife. Usually traction sutures are placed at the outer edge of the dura mater and are tagged with small bulldog clamps or mosquito hemostats. Sometimes the tag instruments are attached to the drapes to increase traction and keep tension on them. As the dural veins are approached during dural opening, the surgeon ligates or coagulates them before cutting. Ligation is done with hemostatic clips such as Weck hemoclips, McKenzie clips, or Ligaclips. The brain surface is protected by moist cottonoid patties.

11. The surgeon appropriately places cottonoid patties and brain retractors, both self-retaining and manual, while working toward visualizing the particular pathologic entity.

12. Pituitary rongeurs as well as the Cavitron Ultrasonic Surgical Aspirator (CUSA) may be needed for tumor removal. Also, a selection of dissectors, bayonet and Gerald forceps, and a bipolar ESU are used. Completely filled irrigating syringes and a full range of moist cottonoid patties and strips must be within easy reach of the surgeon and the assistant. After correction of the pathologic condition and control of bleeding, the brain may be irrigated with an antibiotic solution of the surgeon's choice.

13. The surgeon closes the dura mater using running or interrupted sutures of absorbable suture or black braided nylon. If necessary a dural graft may be used if a defect is present.

14. The bone flap is replaced and fixated with titanium plates and screws.

15. Periosteum and muscle are approximated with 2-0 or 3-0 absorbable suture. The galea is closed with the same sutures. Skin closure can be interrupted or continuous suture or skin staples.

Surgery for Intracranial Aneurysm

An aneurysm is a vascular dilation usually caused by a local defect in the arterial vascular wall, particularly at points of bifurcation.

Vessels at risk within the brain involve those of the major circulation within and around the circle of Willis. Aneurysms are believed to arise from a complex set of circumstances involving a congenital anatomic predisposition enhanced by local and systemic factors. Aneurysmal rupture and hemorrhage into the subarachnoid space are frequently the first sign of an aneurysm, resulting in a sudden, severe headache described as "the worst headache ever." Current neurosurgical techniques have made operations on intracranial aneurysms more feasible; however, the mortality rate is still as high as 40%. Furthermore, 66% of survivors have long-term cognitive impairment (The Brain Aneurysm Foundation [TBAF], 2012). Hemorrhage and the cascade of ensuing cerebral trauma are the greatest hazards of the condition and of the operation. To minimize this, control of blood pressure as well as vascular supply to the region beyond the limits of the lesion may be required. Occasionally, control of the cerebral circulation at the level of the cervical carotid artery is desired. The artery may be exposed and controlled by means of preplaced ligatures or clamps that can be tightened to occlude the vessel if bleeding occurs at the aneurysm site during the operation. This is a separate preliminary surgical procedure.

Procedural Considerations. Aneurysm clips and appliers of the surgeon's choice must be included with the instrumentation. A variety of aneurysm clips are available; most are spring loaded (Figure 21-42 illustrates a few of clips and appliers). Clips may be classified as temporary or permanent, and both must be available with a minimum of two appliers for each type of clip. Temporary clips are commonly used to control giant aneurysms where it may be necessary to evacuate clot and debris before permanent occlusion can be accomplished (Figure 21-48). Temporary clips may also be used to establish the best position for the permanent clip. Temporary clips should be discarded after use. Permanent clips are used to occlude the neck of the aneurysm. Aneurysm clips should not be compressed between the fingers. Clips should be compressed only by the surgeon when seated in their appliers. Once a clip has been compressed, it should be discarded. Clips that have been compressed may be sprung and may slip, causing complications such as bleeding or compression of another vessel or a nerve.

The full armamentarium of aneurysm-occlusion tools should be available for the surgeon. Besides clips, fast-setting aneuroplastic resinous material, a piece of temporal muscle, ligature carriers, or any other material requested by the surgeon should be in the room and ready to use. Fine silk ligatures and hemostatic clips, with or without bipolar electrocoagulation of the neck of the aneurysm, have also been used successfully.

A basic craniotomy setup is required in addition to the special items mentioned. Supplementary suction must be immediately available on the field to prevent hemorrhage from obscuring the surgeon's vision if the aneurysm dome ruptures during the operation. A blood salvage unit should be available for reprocessing blood for replacement when significant blood loss is expected.

Interventional radiology plays an important role in the management of intracranial aneurysms. Intravascular balloon occlusion and coiling of aneurysms by interventional radiologists are considerations in the treatment of aneurysms that meet the criteria for endoscopic therapy. The coils, composed of a soft platinum alloy, allow conformability to the dome of the aneurysm. A guide catheter is introduced into the femoral artery under fluoroscopy and advanced from the aorta into the vessel specific to the aneurysm. Coils are first introduced to outline the border of the aneurysm,

FIGURE 21-48 Temporary arterial occlusion is often necessary in repairing complex large or giant aneurysms. **A,** Temporary clips are placed on the feeder vessels. **B,** The aneurysm sac is opened to allow evacuation of debris and thrombus. **C,** Permanent clip in place.

and then smaller coils are added to fill the center of the aneurysm. Gradually, blood flow will be reduced, allowing the aneurysm to thrombose. Both the neurosurgeon and the radiologist work closely to diagnose and treat these life-threatening anomalies.

Operative Procedure

1. A frontal, pterional, or bifrontal craniotomy may be done to approach an aneurysm in the area of the circle of Willis. The bifrontal approach requires extra scalp clips and hemostatic forceps. All aneurysm instruments preferred by the surgeon must be included.
2. After the dura mater has been opened, the surgeon places a self-retaining brain retractor and exposes the optic nerve and

subarachnoid cisterns. The olfactory nerve may be electrocoagulated and divided with a long scissors for better exposure.
3. The scrub person and perioperative nurse position the operating microscope as directed by the surgeon. Microinstruments, including a micropolar bayonet, are used.
4. Bridging veins are coagulated with bipolar electrocoagulating forceps. Irrigation, which may be a part of the bipolar ESU, is necessary during bipolar electrocoagulation.
5. The surgeon uses microdissectors, hooks, elevators, scissors, knives, forceps, a diamond microknife, and an irrigating bipolar ESU to dissect the covering arachnoidal webs.
6. Careful dissection of the arachnoid and clear visualization of the neck of the aneurysm without rupture of the dome are the aims of the surgeon.
7. The surgeon identifies and frees the parent arteries so that they can be occluded with a temporary clip if necessary. Other structures, such as the optic chiasma and optic nerves, are identified.
8. As the surgeon works slowly toward the dome and neck of the aneurysm, the anesthesia provider may lower the patient's blood pressure for easier control of hemorrhage, should the aneurysm rupture. If the neck of the aneurysm can be isolated, the surgeon places a clip across it. Clips such as the Sundt-Kees and Heifetz have Teflon linings and can be used to approach the aneurysm from a 180-degree angle to avoid excessive manipulation and traction of the parent vessel, if the neck is on the underside of the vessel. These clips support the vessel and serve as a clip graft.
9. Following clip placement, the surgeon may check the aneurysm sac by puncturing it with a needle to see if the clip pressure is adequate to stop blood flow to the aneurysm or to aspirate the aneurysmal contents.
10. As soon as the aneurysm has been occluded, the anesthesia provider returns the patient's blood pressure to normal and the surgeon checks the aneurysm site for bleeding. When the surgeon is satisfied that the operative field is dry, wound closure is begun.

Surgery for Arteriovenous Malformation

An AVM consists of thin-walled vascular channels that connect arteries and veins without the usual intervening capillaries. These vascular lesions may be microscopic or massive. AVMs are rare, affecting only about 300,000 people in the United States (National Institute of Neurological Disorders and Stroke [NINDS], 2009). Malformations vary widely in size, area of involvement, and structure. Arteriovenous fistulas may be congenital or may result from trauma or disease. Vascular anomalies may also lead to subarachnoid or intracerebral hemorrhage or may have extensive irritative effects and cause focal or generalized seizures.

Procedural Considerations. AVMs are difficult to treat successfully. Feeding vessels can be clipped with or without partial removal of the lesion. Total removal, when possible, gives best results. Microsurgical techniques have made total removal without devastating injury to surrounding brain tissue and vessels possible in many cases.

Other methods of treating these malformations include stereotactic radiosurgery with the Gamma Knife. Another method is preoperative embolization, which makes dissection much easier. Surgical glue, such as *N*-butyl cyanoacrylate and tantalum powder, is delivered by means of a catheter into the blood vessels before surgery. During the surgery, the glue is removed along with the AVM.

Operative Procedure

1. A supratentorial or infratentorial craniotomy is performed, depending on the location of the lesion.
2. The surgeon exposes the feeding arteries distant from the malformation, traces toward it, and then occludes the feeders by clipping, electrocoagulation, ligation, or laser beam coagulation.
3. The malformation is dissected out with suction and bayonet forceps. Additional vessels are clipped or coagulated along the way. Usually one or more draining veins are left to be ligated as the last step in the removal. Closure and dressing are as described for craniotomy.

Craniotomy for Suprasellar and Parasellar Tumors (Pituitary Tumor, Craniopharyngioma, Meningioma, Optic Glioma)

Procedural Considerations. The preferred approach for pituitary tumors and some parasellar tumors is the less invasive transsphenoidal approach. However, for large and complex pituitary and parasellar tumors, a craniotomy may be indicated. A craniotomy setup is used with these additional pituitary instruments: Ray curettes (ring, sharp); angulated suction tips, right and left; large and small spinal needles, #22 or #24; curettes, small, #0 through #4-0; and a Luer-Lok syringe, 10 mL.

Extreme caution must be used in removing fluid from the capsule of a craniopharyngioma because the fluid is extremely irritating and may cause chemical leptomeningitis. Calcified pieces of tumor are dissected and removed in the same manner as the capsule of a pituitary adenoma. This is an extremely difficult procedure because of deposits on the carotid arteries, optic nerves, and optic chiasma. The tumor capsule is often left behind on the hypothalamus to avoid stripping off blood vessels supplying this structure. Many moist cottonoid patties are used to protect the surrounding areas from the cystic contents.

Suprasellar meningiomas usually arise from the tuberculum sellae just anterior to the optic nerves and chiasma. Tumor removal is similar to that of a pituitary adenoma except that the electrosurgical cutting loop may be used to excavate the interior of the tumor. After the tumor has been removed, the site of its attachment to the dura is thoroughly electrocoagulated to prevent recurrence. Other meningiomas arising at the base of the skull are treated by similar techniques.

Operative Procedure—Craniotomy for Pituitary Tumor Resection

1. The surgeon makes either a bifrontal or a unilateral incision into the frontal or frontotemporal region. Most unilateral approaches are carried out from the right side.
2. Wet brain retractors over moist cottonoids are inserted for exposure of the optic chiasma and the pituitary gland. The frontal and often the temporal lobes are retracted. The olfactory nerve may be coagulated and divided with scissors.
3. A DeMartel, Yasargil, or Greenberg self-retaining retractor is placed to maintain exposure. Aneurysm clips and applicators should be available to control unexpected bleeding from major vessels. The microscope may be moved into place.
4. The surgeon uses the bipolar ESU for hemostasis around the tumor capsule and incises it with a #11 blade on a long knife handle; the tumor is removed with a pituitary rongeur or cup forceps.
5. Small stainless steel, copper, or Ray curettes, as well as suction, may be used during tumor removal.

6. A wide clip may be applied to the stalk of the pituitary, which may then be cut distally. A long angulated scissors is especially helpful for this.
7. If the tumor capsule is to be removed the surgeon uses bayonet forceps, cup forceps, nerve hooks, and suction to aid in the dissection.
8. Closure and dressing are as described for craniotomy.

Suboccipital Craniectomy for Posterior Fossa Exploration

The posterior occipital bone is perforated and removed using a drill and rongeurs, and the foramen magnum and arch of the atlas are exposed to remove a lesion in the posterior fossa (Figure 21-49). Posterior fossa lesions include lesions in the cerebellum, the fourth ventricle, and the brainstem; posterior fossa meningiomas; and nerve sheath tumors.

Procedural Considerations. Depending on the type and size of the lesion, the exposure may be unilateral or bilateral. The operation may include the removal of the arch of the atlas. This approach gives the surgeon access to the fourth ventricle, the cerebellum, the brainstem, and the cranial nerves.

The prone position with the head of the OR table elevated is the preferred position, but other positions may also be used. An extra-high instrument table or two Mayo stands and standing stool are necessary for the scrub person.

Operative Procedure

1. Before the initial surgical incision, the surgeon may make an occipital burr hole for placement of a ventricular catheter. This can be done as a separate procedure or concurrently with the procedure.
2. The incision may be made from mastoid tip to mastoid tip, in an arch curving upward 2 cm above the external occipital protuberance. Alternatively, a posterior midline incision can be used.
3. Scalp bleeding is controlled, and the skin flap is retracted with Weitlaner retractors.
4. The surgeon uses a periosteal elevator to free the muscles, and then divides them with an electrosurgical blade. The incision is deepened. A self-retaining retractor is used. The laminae of the first two or three cervical vertebrae may be exposed.
5. One or more holes are drilled in the occipital bone. A Midas Rex or Anspach drill is used to perform the craniectomy.
6. The surgeon frees the dura from under the bone. A double-action rongeur, Raney punch, Kerrison punch, or Leksell rongeur is used to enlarge the hole and smooth the edges.
7. Osseous and cerebellar venous bleeding is controlled at each step with bone wax, Gelfoam, and electrocoagulation to prevent air embolism.
8. Using a small brain spoon or cottonoid patty to protect the brain, the surgeon extends the initial nick with scalpel or scissors. The dural incision is continued until the cerebellar hemispheres, the vermis, and the cerebellar tonsils can be visualized. Hemostatic clips are used on the dura mater as necessary. Dural traction sutures are placed.
9. The cisterna magna is opened, emptied of spinal fluid, and protected with a cottonoid strip.
10. The surgeon inspects the cerebellar hemispheres and controls bleeding with the bipolar ESU. A needle may be introduced through a small, coagulated incision into the cerebellar hemisphere in an attempt to palpate or tap a deep lesion.

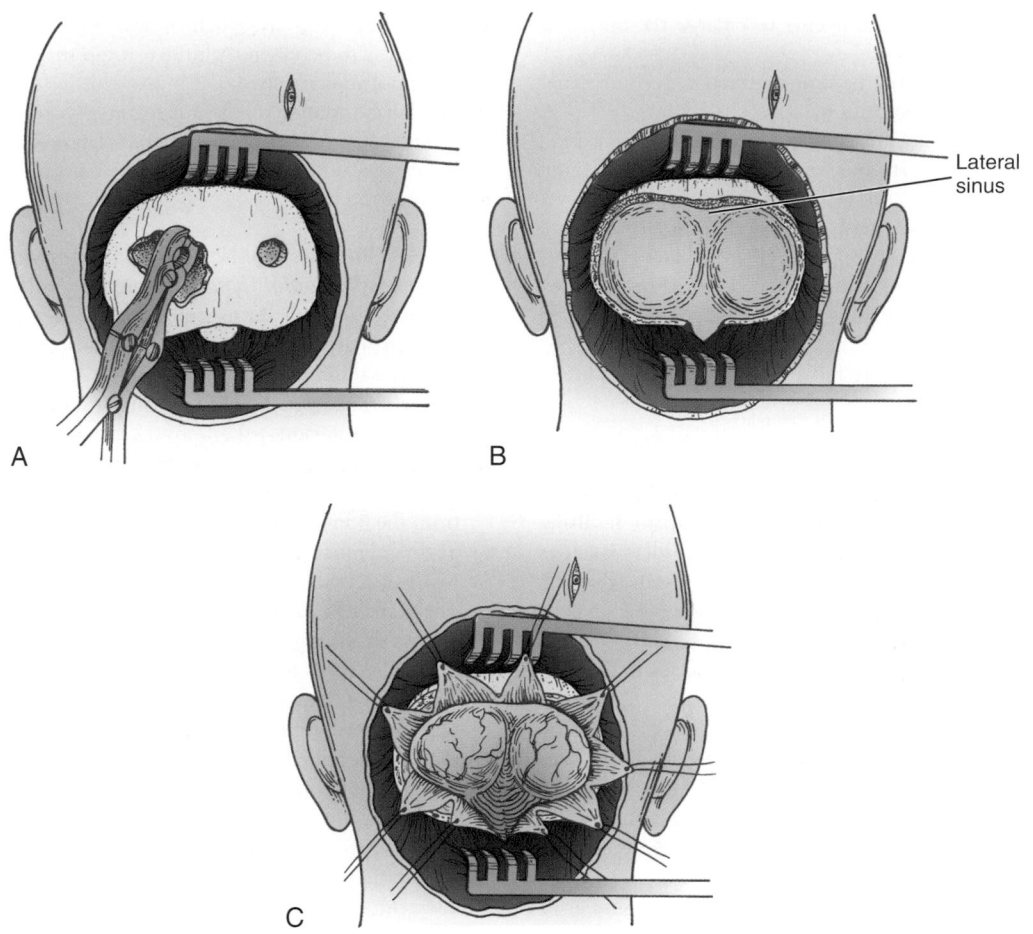

FIGURE 21-49 Suboccipital craniectomy. **A,** Craniectomy being performed. **B,** Dura exposed. **C,** Dura incised and cerebellum exposed.

11. Brain retractors over cottonoid patties are placed for exposure. The handle of the retractor must be kept dry to avoid slippage in the surgeon's hand. However, the inserted edge should be wet to prevent damage or tears in the brain surface. These retractors may be positioned in areas that control respiration or other vital functions, so every effort must be made to avoid jarring these instruments in the operative field. When the pathologic entity is identified, a self-retaining retractor may be placed.

12. Long bayonet forceps, bayonet cup forceps, pituitary forceps, suction, and the electrosurgical loop tips may be used to remove the lesion. Clips may be used to aid in hemostasis. A nerve stimulator may be used to identify cranial nerves; EPs for brainstem monitoring are becoming routine practice.

13. After the lesion has been removed and bleeding controlled, the surgeon checks to ensure adequate hemostasis has been achieved. The anesthesia provider generates the Valsalva maneuver to increase venous pressure in the patient's head and facilitate identification of bleeding vessels.

14. The dura mater may be partially or completely closed. The cranial defect may be repaired with titanium mesh. The muscle, fascia, and skin are closed. A dressing is applied.

15. The patient must remain anesthetized until the supine position is achieved and the prongs of the headrest are removed. Particular attention must be given to the patient's head when these prongs are removed to prevent tearing the scalp or damaging the eyes.

Retromastoid Craniectomy for Microvascular Decompression of the Trigeminal Nerve

Trigeminal neuralgia (tic douloureux, fifth cranial nerve pain) is a condition characterized by brief, repeated attacks of excruciating, lancinating pain in the face. The etiology of this facial pain is believed to be the compression of the trigeminal nerve at its exit from the pons by an adjacent artery that has elongated over time to become wedged against the nerve, resulting in demyelination. Pain distribution follows one or all of the trigeminal nerve branches. It is characteristically severe, with sudden onset, short duration, and paroxysmal nature. Triggers often precipitate the pain, such as touching the face, chewing, and talking. When pharmacologic measures fail, surgery to decompress the nerve is undertaken. Frequently more than one treatment is necessary during the course of the disease. Newer options include Gamma Knife radiosurgery.

Procedural Considerations. The patient is in the supine, lateral, or sitting position, depending on the surgeon's preference. An endoscope can be used along with the microscope to improve visualization.

Operative Procedure

1. The surgeon makes a vertical retromastoid incision.
2. The soft tissue is freed from the bone with a periosteal elevator. The bone exposure is maintained with a self-retaining retractor.
3. A burr hole is created, and the dura mater is freed.

4. The surgeon uses a drill and rongeurs to enlarge the burr hole to a diameter of about $2\frac{1}{2}$ inches.
5. Using a moist brain retractor, the surgeon retracts the dura mater overlying the pons and cerebellum.
6. A self-retaining brain retractor is placed deeper into the wound to retract the cerebellum. The microscope is used to provide light as well as magnification.
7. The surgeon identifies the pons, the superior cerebellar artery, and the trigeminal nerve.
8. Additional blunt dissection frees the vessel from the nerve. A synthetic microsponge is inserted between the vessel and nerve to maintain the separation.
9. The dura and cranial defect are repaired, the incision is closed, and dressings are applied.

Transsphenoidal Hypophysectomy

Endocrine pituitary disorders (such as Cushing syndrome, acromegaly, malignant exophthalmos, and hypopituitarism resulting from intrasellar tumors) as well as nonpituitary disorders (such as advanced metastatic carcinoma of the breast and prostate, diabetic retinopathy, and uncontrollable severe diabetes) have been successfully treated by transsphenoidal hypophysectomy (TSH). A transnasal or a sublabial incision can be used for rapid access to the sella turcica.

Endoscopy has been used to assist with access through the sphenoid sinus into the pituitary fossa. Otorhinolaryngologic surgeons can be consulted to assist the neurosurgeon with this approach. The endoscope and instrumentation access the sphenoid sinus by the transnasal route. Endoscopic transsphenoidal surgery eliminates the need for an incision and the need for a microscope. When the sphenoid sinus is reached, instruments and technique are similar to the microsurgical technique. Stereotactic image-guided navigation can also be used with the transsphenoidal technique.

All these approaches produce similar results. Complete extracapsular enucleation of the pituitary in cases of hypophysectomy and possible complete removal of small pituitary tumors, with the remaining normal portion of the gland left intact, can be achieved. Patients are relatively free from pain after surgery. No visible scar remains.

Procedural Considerations—Microsurgical Approach for Transsphenoidal Hypophysectomy. General endotracheal anesthetic, combined with a local anesthetic is used. The surgical team places the patient in a semi-sitting position, with the head against the headrest. The surgeon may use a subnasal midline rhinoseptal approach or a transnasal route, both exposing the sphenoid bone, the sphenoid sinus behind the bone, and the sella containing the tumor. Frequently an otorhinolaryngologist assists the neurosurgeon in gaining access to the surgical site.

The face, mouth, and nasal cavity are prepped with an antiseptic solution. The surgeon infiltrates the patient's nasal mucosa and gingiva with a local anesthetic such as lidocaine with epinephrine with a concentration of $1:100,000$ to initiate submucosal elevation and diminish oozing from the mucosa. A sterile adhesive plastic drape is applied to the entire face, with additional sterile drapes to ensure a relatively sterile operative field. Sterile soft goods (sponges) are placed in the patient's mouth so that only the upper gum margin is exposed.

Although sterile technique is used, this approach through the nose or mouth is technically not a sterile procedure. Therefore, a separate sterile field and instruments must be maintained for adjunct procedures. The thigh or abdomen is prepped if a muscle or fat graft is to be taken. A lumbar drain may be placed preoperatively or postoperatively.

Specialized transsphenoidal instruments are required. The operating microscope is used for the cranial portion of the procedure. A fluoroscopy unit with C-arm may be used to verify the anatomic location of the sella.

Operative Procedure—Microsurgical Approach for a Transsphenoidal Hypophysectomy

1. Using the biopsy setup on a separate small Mayo table, the surgeon may take a small piece of muscle from the previously prepared thigh or a fat graft from the abdomen to be used later in the procedure. This is kept in a moist sponge or soaked in antibiotic solution.
2. The surgeon creates an incision in the middle of the upper gum margin. The soft tissues of the upper lip and nose are elevated from the bone with an elevator, and the nasal septum is exposed. The nasal mucosa is elevated from either side of the nasal septum, which is flanked by the blades of a Cushing bivalved speculum. The transnasal approach avoids the sublabial incision, instead operating through a bivalve speculum inserted directly through the nares. The inferior third of the anterior cartilaginous septum and osseous vomer are resected, as is the floor of the sphenoidal sinus, exposing the sinus cavity. The floor of the sella turcica can then be identified.
3. The surgeon opens the floor with a sphenoidal punch, and incises the dura mater. The hypophyseal cavity should be opened only in patients undergoing surgery for pituitary adenoma. In these patients the gland is explored and the tumor is identified and removed.
4. The extracapsular cleavage plane is identified, and the superior surface of the pituitary is dissected until the stalk and the diaphragmatic orifice are found. Cotton pledgets are applied for exposure, hemostasis, and protection of structures.
5. Using a sickle knife, the surgeon sections the pituitary stalk and uses an enucleator to dissect the lateral posterior and inferior surfaces of the gland.
6. The gland is removed, and the sellar cavity may be packed to prevent CSF leakage. The packing is accomplished with muscle obtained previously from the thigh or with the fat graft previously obtained from the abdomen or thigh. The floor is reconstructed with cartilage from the nasal septum.
7. Antibiotic powder may be used and nasal packing introduced for 2 days. If a gingival incision is used, it is closed with suture of the surgeon's preference.
8. Some surgeons prefer to perform this operation by means of a lateral rhinotomy with a transantral-transsphenoidal approach.

Cranioplasty

Cranioplasty is performed for repair of a skull defect resulting from trauma, malformation, or a surgical procedure. The purpose of cranioplasty is to relieve headache and local tenderness or throbbing, to prevent secondary injury to the underlying brain, and for cosmetic effect.

Procedural Considerations. Repair of a skull defect may be performed acutely in clean cases. In contaminated cases, 6 months should pass before repair is attempted (Connolly et al, 2009). When a bone plate is removed for control of elevated ICP, it can be repaired following resolution of ICP issues. If the patient's bone

plate was preserved, it could be replaced with microplates and screws.

The most common materials used for cranioplasty include titanium mesh and/or methylmethacrylate. Commercially prepared cranioplastic synthetics that supply the needed chemicals and mixing containers have simplified the procedures of shaping and molding the prosthesis. Sometimes heavy wire mesh is cut to the shape of the defect, and the methylmethacrylate is molded over the mesh.

Recent technologic advancements use CT scans to produce a computer-generated duplication of the defect. A properly sized prosthesis can be produced and sterilized before the surgery. After the defect is exposed, minor adjustments in the shape of the prosthesis can be made with a burr to achieve an optimal fit.

Operative Procedure—Cranioplasty Using Computer-Generated Prosthesis

1. Typically the old incision is reopened.
2. Keeping in mind that there is no bony protection between the scalp and the brain, the surgeon carefully elevates the scalp flap from the underlying scar, dura, and brain.
3. Bone edges are exposed with a curette, and the prosthesis is fitted to the defect using a burr. Debris is irrigated out of the wound.
4. The surgeon uses microplates and screws to secure the prosthesis in place.
5. The incision is closed as usual for craniotomy.

Operative Procedure—Cranioplasty Using Cranioplastic Material

1. A scalp flap is turned, and the bony defect is exposed.
2. The surgeon trims the edges of the defect, forming a ledge to seat the prosthesis.
3. After the bone defect has been prepared so that it is slightly saucerized, the methylmethacrylate is mixed by combining one volume of liquid monomer with one volume of the powdered polymer. When this has formed a doughy mass, it is dropped into a sterile polyethylene bag. The soft plastic is then rolled on a flat surface into the desired shape, leaving the thickness to the approximate depth of the skull edges. A sterile test tube, syringe barrel, or other round object can be used, although a stainless steel roller is preferred because of its weight and ease of use.
4. The soft cranioplastic material in the bag is placed over the skull defect and, through light pressing with the ends of the fingers, is fitted into the missing skull area. Assistants stretch the plastic bag as the surgeon molds the plate into the defect and forms an overlapping bevel edge. This overlapping fringe keeps the plate from falling inside the skull, in the same manner as the skull saucerization.
5. When the heat of the chemical reactions is evident, the surgeon lifts the plate out of the bony wound and removes it from the polyethylene bag. Cool saline should be used on the flap while the exothermic reaction takes place.
6. When the plate is cool enough to handle, the surgeon trims excess material and bone using rongeurs or a saw and places the plate in the cranial defect to check for fit.
7. The surgeon uses a craniotome to smooth the rough spots and bevel the edges so that the plate will blend gradually with the skull.
8. Mixing and fitting the plate take about 7 minutes, the same time needed for the cranioplastic material to harden. Sutures may be used to hold the plate in place, generally at three or more points.

Surgery of the Spine

Surgery of the spinal column is also discussed in Chapter 20.

Anterior Cervical Decompression and Fusion

Anterior cervical decompression and fusion (ACDF) is performed to treat cervical disk herniation or cervical spondylosis (degeneration in the spine) with myelopathy (disorder of the spinal cord) or radiculopathy (disorder of the nerve roots). Symptoms include pain in the neck, shoulders, arms, and hands; and weakness of the upper extremity. An ACDF entails a corpectomy (removal of a vertebral body), diskectomy, and fusion of the vertebral bodies. Bone grafts for the fusion are obtained from the patient's iliac crest (autograft) or from a bone bank (allograft).

Procedural Considerations. Awake endoscopic intubation may be required if the patient's neck is unstable or does not readily extend. Neurologic monitoring is commonly used to prevent further injury during surgery. The patient is placed in the supine position, with a small shoulder roll placed horizontally for mild neck extension. The perioperative nurse ensures the patient's arms are tucked, and the hip is elevated for exposure if bone graft is to be taken from the iliac crest (Figure 21-50). Intraoperative x-ray may be used to confirm the correct surgical site and verify placement of the graft and related hardware.

Operative Procedure

1. The surgeon may harvest the iliac crest bone graft before the neck procedure begins, or after exposure of the anterior cervical spine. An incision is made over the iliac crest, at least 3 cm posterior to the anterosuperior iliac spine. The skin and subcutaneous tissues are retracted with a Weitlaner retractor.
2. Soft tissue is dissected until the crest is reached and exposed.
3. The surgeon uses an osteotome or oscillating saw to remove the bone graft. The graft is soaked in antibiotic solution and set aside. The perioperative nurse initiates a sponge and sharps count for this portion of the procedure. Following verification of a correct count, the surgeon irrigates and closes the wound and covers it with a sterile towel.
4. A transverse or horizontal skin incision is made on one side of the neck, directly over the involved cervical level.
5. A Weitlaner retractor is placed, and the surgeon uses sharp dissection to divide the platysma.
6. The medial edge of the sternocleidomastoid muscle is defined with the scissors by blunt and sharp dissection.
7. Using blunt finger dissection, the surgeon creates a vertical plane of dissection between the carotid artery laterally and the trachea and esophagus medially. This plane is held open with retractors.
8. The anterior surface of the spine is identified, and the long muscles of the neck are peeled off the anterior surface of the spine with periosteal elevators or peanut dissectors. The bipolar ESU is used for hemostasis.
9. A 20-gauge spinal needle is inserted a short distance into the disk space, and the location is confirmed radiographically.
10. Self-retaining retractors are inserted into the neck incision. Care is used to protect the carotid artery and the esophagus. A combination of sharp and dull blades is used to acquire the best retraction. If a toothed blade is used, the teeth are carefully hooked beneath the long muscle of the neck.

FIGURE 21-50 Anterior cervical decompression and fusion. **A** and **B,** A bone graft from the iliac crest or fashioned from bank bone is tailored to fit the site of corpectomy, resting on the vertebral endplates. **C** and **D,** An anterior spinal plate and screws are secured to the vertebral bodies above and below the spanned segment to stabilize and promote a stable fusion.

11. The surgeon uses a #15 or #11 blade on a #7 knife handle to incise the disk space; a pituitary rongeur is used to remove the disk material, which may be saved as a specimen. A vertebral spreader may be inserted into the vertebral space to widen the area. Residual disk material is removed with the rongeur (Kerrison or pituitary) or small curettes (angled or straight, #0 to #4-0) until the entire surface of both vertebrae is clean. A small burr may also be used until complete anterior decompression of the nerve root or dural sac is obtained. Nerve hooks may be used for demonstration of adequate decompression.
12. A depth gauge and caliper measure the size of the interbody defect. The bone graft is cut to the appropriate size and placed into the defect with a tamp and a mallet.
13. The anterior cervical plate and screws are secured to the vertebral bodies above and below the bone graft.
14. Lateral x-ray or fluoroscopy is done to confirm location, degree of distraction, and alignment.
15. Hemostasis is obtained, and the wound is irrigated. A drain may be placed. The platysma is closed with absorbable suture.

A subcuticular closure of the skin is done, and wound closure strips are applied.
16. A cervical collar is placed before the patient awakens.

Posterior Cervical Approach

The posterior cervical approach is used for laminectomy for decompression, intradural tumor removal, cordotomy, diskectomy, and fusion (Connolly et al, 2009).

Procedural Considerations. A patient with severe spondylosis may require fiberoptic intubation. Intraoperative neurologic monitoring should be used to detect a change in neurologic status. The patient is positioned prone with a three-pin skull clamp. The OR bed is positioned in slight reverse Trendelenburg position to encourage venous drainage. The patient's arms are tucked. If autograft bone graft is desired for fusion, the posterior iliac crest will be prepped. A cervical collar may be required postoperatively.

Operative Procedure

1. The surgeon palpates the cervical spinous processes as landmarks before creating a midline incision.
2. Soft tissue dissection is done, and a clamp is placed on the spinous process to verify the correct level with x-ray.
3. After placing self-retaining retractors to help to gain exposure, the surgeon performs a subperiosteal dissection to the lateral margins of the involved facets using the Bovie, suction, and a cervical Cobb elevator.
4. Hemostasis is maintained with the bipolar ESU, Gelfoam, and patties.
5. A laminectomy is performed using a drill, Leksell rongeurs, curettes, a nerve hook, and Kerrison punch rongeurs.
6. The surgeon removes the disk with pituitary rongeurs and curettes.
7. If a fusion is required, instrumentation and allograft or autograft may be needed.
8. The wound is irrigated. A drain may be placed.
9. Bupivacaine may be injected into the paraspinal muscles and subcutaneous tissue for postoperative pain.
10. Absorbable sutures are used to close the fascia and subcutaneous layers. Suture or staples are used for the skin.

Anterior Thoracic Approach

A transthoracic thalamotomy is done to access the spine for a thoracic diskectomy, burst fracture, osteomyelitis, and metastatic disease (Connolly et al, 2009). Usually a thoracic or trauma surgeon assists the neurosurgeon in obtaining adequate exposure.

Procedural Considerations. The anesthesia provider may need to place a double-lumen endotracheal tube to allow for deflation of the lung for exposure of the higher thoracic levels. Lateral position with a beanbag is preferred. If intraoperative fluoroscopy is necessary, a Jackson table is needed. A beanbag interferes with fluoroscopy. For T1 to T4, a right-sided approach is preferred to avoid the aortic arch and heart. For T5 to T12, a left-sided approach is preferred because the aorta is safer to manipulate than the vena cava (Connolly et al, 2009). If allograft is desired for fusion, prep the iliac crest.

At times, an anterior thoracic surgery is performed in combination with a posterior thoracic surgery. In this case the patient is repositioned prone after the completion of the anterior portion of the surgery. The posterior surgical site is prepped and draped, and the posterior portion of the surgery is completed.

Operative Procedure

1. The surgeon creates a thoracotomy incision and transects the latissimus dorsi and other muscles. A rib may be resected with a rib cutter to gain exposure.
2. The parietal pleura is opened, and a thoracotomy retractor is placed. If necessary, the anesthesia provider manually deflates the patient's lung.
3. A localization x-ray is done to verify the correct level. The parietal pleura is incised further onto the vertebral body and cleared with blunt dissection. Segmental vessels are ligated as necessary with hemoclips and transected to mobilize the aorta.
4. For diskectomy or decompression, a drill, rongeurs, and curettes may be needed. For spinal fusion, instrumentation and autograft or allograft may be used.
5. The wound is irrigated, and a chest tube is placed. The ribs are reapproximated with a rib approximator and sutured with heavy absorbable suture.
6. The fascia and subcuticular layers are closed.

Laminectomy

Laminectomy is removal of one or more of the vertebral laminae to expose the spinal canal. Laminectomy, hemilaminectomy, and the interlaminar approach are performed to reach the spinal canal and its adjacent structures to treat compression fracture, dislocation, herniated nucleus pulposus, and cord tumor, as well as for spinal cord stimulation. Section of the spinal nerves, including cordotomy and rhizotomy, requires similar surgical exposure.

Procedural Considerations. Laminectomy is performed with the patient in the prone or lateral position. It is performed on the cervical, thoracic, or lumbar spine. Laminectomy instruments include the basic neurosurgical set, the retractor of the surgeon's choice, and an assortment of specialty rongeurs.

Operative Procedure—Laminectomy for Spinal Stenosis

1. The surgeon makes a midline vertical incision at the operative site.
2. Two self-retaining retractors (Cone, Weitlaner, or Beckman-Adson) are inserted for exposure.
3. The fascia is incised in the midline with Mayo scissors, electrosurgical cutting tip, or a scalpel.
4. The surgeon uses sharp dissection to expose both sides of the spinous processes.
5. Correct surgical level is verified by lateral spine x-ray film.
6. The paraspinous muscles and periosteum are stripped off the laminae with sharp periosteal elevators. Dissection with the ESU may be used.
7. As each area is stripped, the surgeon packs radiopaque soft goods around the bony structures with a periosteal elevator to aid in further blunt dissection of muscles from the laminae and to tamponade bleeding.
8. A laminectomy retractor is then placed. A Scoville (with a blade on the tissue side and a slightly shorter hook on the bone side), Tower, Crank, or Adson-Beckman retractor can be used.
9. Cottonoid patties may be placed in the extremes of the field for hemostasis.
10. The surgeon removes the spinous processes over the involved area with a rongeur. The bone edges are waxed.
11. The ligamentum flavum is cut with a scalpel, Metzenbaum scissors, or a rongeur. Cottonoid patties are passed through this incision to protect the underlying dura, and a window is cut into the flaval ligament with a #15 blade on a #7 knife handle.
12. Additional ligaments in the lateral gutter of the spinal canal may be removed with a large curette or a Cloward rongeur after first protecting the dural sac.
13. The surgeon controls bleeding from the epidural veins by packing the area with narrow cottonoid patties and if necessary, by careful coagulation with the bipolar ESU.
14. Various rongeurs are used to remove the laminae after edges are defined with a curette. Bone drills are commonly used to reduce bone down to epidural fat, saving time and wear on the surgeon's hands.
15. Rongeurs—straight and angled, narrow and wide—are used to remove further bony areas until the cord with its dural covering is exposed and decompressed.
16. The surgeon uses a blunt nerve hook to explore the nerve roots and extradural space.
17. If no further stenosis is felt, hemostasis is secured.
18. The cottonoid patties are removed from the epidural space, and the area is further irrigated. Retractors are removed, and the wound is closed.

Operative Procedure—Laminectomy for Intradural Spinal Cord Tumor

1. The surgeon creates a midline fascial incision, dissects both sides of the spinous processes, and reflects the bilateral paraspinous muscles, one side at a time. The level is confirmed with x-ray.
2. One or more Gelpi or Adson-Beckman self-retaining retractors are placed to maintain the bony exposure.
3. The surgeon performs a midline laminectomy and excises the spinous processes. Various rongeurs (e.g., Leksell) are used to remove the laminae after the edges are defined with a curette. A Midas Rex drill may also be used. The bone edges are waxed for bleeding.
4. The remaining flaval ligament is removed with scissors, scalpel, and a Kerrison rongeur. Epidural fat is removed so that the dura mater is fully exposed.
5. The surgeon places a wide, moist cottonoid patty over the superficial soft tissues and muscle down to the bone bordering the exposed dura mater to provide additional hemostasis.
6. Intraoperative ultrasound may be used to verify the tumor's exact location beneath the dura.
7. The surgeon elevates the dura mater with a small hook and nicks it with a #15 blade. A grooved director is inserted beneath the dura mater, and the dural incision is extended over it using long forceps and fine scissors. Alternatively, the surgeon may lengthen the incision with Metzenbaum scissors. Traction sutures of 4-0 silk or braided nylon on dura needles are placed in the dural edges, and the cord is exposed (Figure 21-51). The operating microscope may be used.
8. The cord is explored for the pathologic area. Aspiration through a #22 needle on a plain-tipped syringe may be carried out. Whenever possible, the tumor mass is dissected free and removed using suction, the dissecting scissors, the bipolar forceps, small (pituitary) scoops, curettes, pituitary rongeurs, or an ultrasonic aspirator. Bleeding is controlled with moist cottonoids, hemostatic clips, gelatin gauze, and topical hemostatics. Bipolar electrocoagulation is used around the nerves and spinal cord.
9. The surgeon irrigates the wound and obtains hemostasis, being careful to protect the spinal cord.

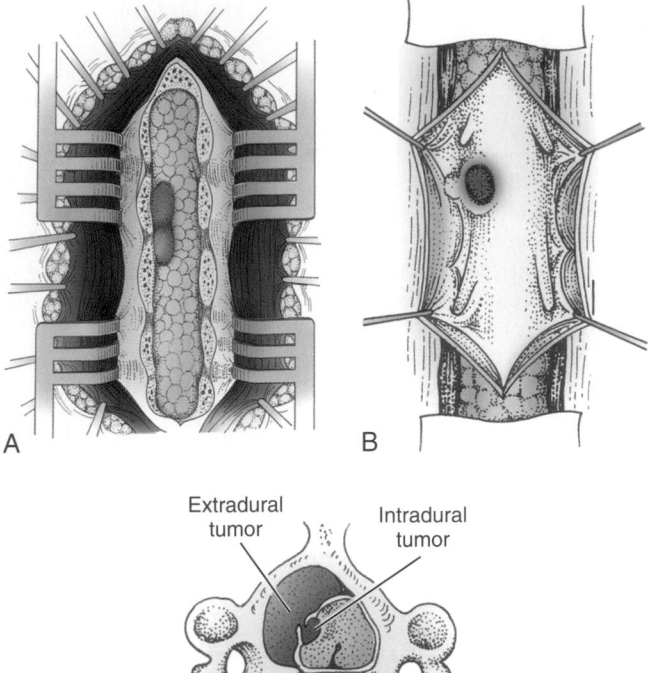

Extradural
tumor   Intradural
                        tumor

C

FIGURE 21-51 A, Laminectomy completed: dura mater and tumor exposed. **B,** Dura mater incised and retracted, revealing pia arachnoid over spinal cord and part of tumor. **C,** Diagram of cross section of tumor site and location of extradural and intradural pathologic areas.

10. The dura mater is closed with a braided nylon or polytetrafluoroethylene (PTFE) suture.
11. The incision is checked for further bleeding, and the paraspinous muscles are approximated with absorbable suture. The remainder of the wound is closed.

    NOTE: In the case of extradural tumors, invasion of the dura is avoided. Once the dura is opened from a tear or an incision, the surgeon may require that the patient remain flat for 24 hours or longer to allow healing of the dura.

Laminotomy

Laminotomy is the traditional approach to posterior microdiskectomy at the cervical, thoracic, and lumbar levels. Laminotomy is performed on the symptomatic side with resection of a small portion of the medial facet. The goal of this surgery is the resolution of leg pain with little to no residual back pain and a return to preinjury activity and lifestyle. The operating microscope has improved this surgical approach by offering magnification and illumination, which allows for smaller incisions and less tissue dissection. This surgical procedure is associated with less postoperative discomfort and shorter hospital stays. The majority of patients who undergo this procedure can be discharged home on the same day (Ambulatory Surgery Considerations). See Chapter 20 for a full description of the surgical procedures for a discussion of diskectomy, disk replacement, and microdiskectomy.

Spinal Cord Stimulators

A spinal cord stimulator (SCS) is an implantable, nondestructive medical device used to treat chronic intractable pain of the trunk

Microdiskectomies

Microdiskectomies are one of several spinal surgeries performed to relieve pain caused by disk herniations. Patients selected for this specific procedure typically complain of leg pain longer than 6 weeks in duration, and receive minimal relief from prescribed pain medications. An magnetic resonance image scan confirming the level of nerve root compression as well as a detailed history and physical will determine if the patient is a candidate for surgery.

Ambulatory surgeries are designed for patients who have a nominal health history and pose minimal risk for operative complications. Microdiskectomies have the flexibility of being performed either in a same-day surgery center or in a hospital OR suite. The procedure is typically performed using a general or spinal anesthetic, depending on the needs of the patient. After the anesthesia provider has control of the airway, the patient is positioned prone for maximum operative accessibility. Positioning may take time, and it is essential that every precaution is taken to prevent patient injury. If the patient is awake, talking should be kept to a minimum, and OR traffic should be closely monitored by the perioperative nurse. Before making the incision the surgeon may inject a local anesthetic containing epinephrine into the lumbar spine to minimize bleeding intraoperatively.

The procedure is approximately 2 hours in duration, and many patients are able to return home the same day. Postoperative pain relief is maximized by the use of intraoperative topical steroids on the nerve root, local anesthetics, and prescribed oral pain medications.

Possible complications include bleeding, infection, and, on rare occasions, nerve damage. On discharge the patient is instructed to keep the surgical site clean, restrict activity, and notify the surgeon immediately if he or she experiences excessive pain, swelling, or discharge from the incision site. Follow-up appointments are generally scheduled 2 weeks following the procedure, and most patients can return to work after 4 to 6 weeks.

and limbs. The device generates an electrical impulse to the epidural space, which produces a tingling sensation that masks the perception of pain.

The goal of the stimulation is to lower the perception of pain, reduce medication use, increase function, and improve quality of life. Patients who are considered good candidates for a spinal cord stimulator placement undergo a trial to check for efficacy prior to permanent implantation. During the trial a temporary percutaneous lead is placed and connected to an external pulse generator for approximately 3 to 7 days. The patient must experience at least 50% improvement in pain to be considered a candidate for permanent lead placement. The trial is generally performed in the OR using monitored anesthesia care (MAC) or general anesthesia.

The permanent spinal cord stimulator lead is implanted into the epidural space, and the impulse generator (IPG), which is the device battery, is implanted in the abdomen or buttocks. The lead is positioned at a specific level of the spinal cord. The targeted level is determined by the individual patient's symptoms, and by information obtained from the trial. A thoracic spinal cord stimulator is placed for lower back and leg pain. A cervical spinal cord stimulator is placed for upper extremity pain. Peripheral nerve stimulators are an alternative or conjunctive neuromodulation technique that targets peripheral nerves.

Procedural Considerations. Lead placement must be assessed during the surgery. This can be done by waking the patient during the surgery and asking where the stimulation is felt. To secure the airway, lateral position is used with this method. Alternatively, electromyogram (EMG) monitoring may be used while the patient is under general anesthesia to verify motor responses in the targeted muscle groups. Fluoroscopy is also used to verify lead placement.

The surgeon determines the battery site and directs the patient's position accordingly. The prone position is used if the battery will be inserted into the subcutaneous tissue of the buttocks. The lateral position is used if the battery is placed in the subcutaneous tissue of the abdomen, or if the patient will be awakened during surgery. The perioperative nurse ensures that the SCS system, the product representative, and the fluoroscopy unit are available, and that the OR bed is compatible with fluoroscopy. The surgeon marks the operative site before the patient is prepped. The surgical prep includes the entire area from the lead placement site to the IPG site.

Operative Procedure

1. The surgeon makes a midline incision at the proper level over the spine and uses sharp and dull dissection through the subcutaneous tissues to reach the fascia.
2. Paravertebral muscles are then dissected off the spinous process and lamina. A self-retaining retractor is placed to provide a visual field.
3. Instruments such as punches and rongeurs are then used to perform a surgical laminectomy. The stimulator lead is placed in the epidural space. Proper placement is confirmed by testing with the stimulator programmer while waking and assessing the patient's perception of the stimulation, or while using EMG monitoring. Lead placement is also verified with fluoroscopy or x-ray. Once testing is complete, the surgeon anchors the lead with a 4-0 nonabsorbable suture.
4. The surgeon creates a pocket in the subcutaneous tissue of the buttocks or the abdomen for IPG placement.
5. Using a tunneling device the surgeon tunnels the lead from the lead site to the battery location. The IPG is attached. Excess wire is protected by placing it beneath the IPG.
6. The IPG is anchored with 2-0 nonabsorbable suture to prevent migration.
7. Both incisions are irrigated and closed.
8. An abdominal binder is applied to compress the battery site.
9. A postoperative x-ray is obtained to confirm lead placement.

Intrathecal Pump Therapy

An intrathecal pump (ITP) is a specialized device that offers precise, targeted, and adjustable medication treatment for patients with spasticity and/or chronic pain. It delivers medication directly into the CSF via a small catheter attached to a pump.

The pump is controlled via a radiotelemetry link from an external programmer. This controls the rate and mode of infusion. The pump reservoirs are refilled with medication in the physician's office. Baclofen for spasticity or morphine sulfate for pain is most commonly used.

All patients are carefully screened for specific criteria, such as ineffective results or intolerable side effects with oral medication, limited functional abilities, no significant addiction history, and a diagnosed pathology. Contraindications for ITP therapy include active or frequent infections, medication allergy, failed screenings, and lack of patient reliability, resources, or support. ITP complications can include:

- Infection
- Mechanical failure
- CSF leak
- Overdose or adverse drug reactions

Each patient undergoes a trial injection that lasts 6 to 8 hours. Positive results must be noted before final implantation. Trials are performed in the physician's office; final implantation is performed in the OR using MAC or general anesthesia.

Procedural Considerations. The nurse ensures the availability of the intrathecal pump system and the prescribed intrathecal medication before the procedure. A representative from the manufacturer should be present to assist with pump programming. Intraoperative fluoroscopy is used to verify proper placement of the catheter, so a compatible OR bed is necessary. The surgeon will determine the patient's preference for pump placement (right or left abdomen) and mark the abdomen and back incisions. The back incision is typically marked at the area of L3-4. The abdominal incision is marked strategically to avoid the belt line, umbilicus, and the iliac crest. The perioperative nurse assists with placing the patient in the lateral position, using pillows and side braces as positioning aids. The surgical prep extends from the posterior incision site to the abdominal pump site.

Operative Procedure

1. The surgeon makes an incision in the patient's back and extends it through the subcutaneous tissue to the fascia. Hemostasis is obtained with the ESU.
2. A Tuohy needle is inserted paraspinally and at a 30-degree angle through the fascia into the intrathecal space, usually at L3-4. The surgeon confirms proper needle placement by removing the inner stylet of the Tuohy needle and visualizing a flow of CSF through the outer cannula.
3. The surgeon threads the catheter through the needle and feeds it to the proper level of the spine. This is determined by the patient's symptoms and the type of medication that will be administered. The catheter placement is verified under fluoroscopic visualization and is secured with anchors and a 4-0 nonabsorbable suture.
4. The abdominal incision is made to create a pocket approximately 2.5 cm deep subcutaneously for pump placement.
5. Using a tunneling device the surgeon tunnels the catheter from the back to the abdominal pocket. The flow of CSF is once again verified through the catheter before it is connected to the pump. The pump is placed in the abdominal pocket and secured with 2-0 nonabsorbable suture to prevent migration.
6. Both the back and abdominal incisions are irrigated and closed.
7. Dressings are applied to both incisions, and an abdominal binder is secured. In the recovery room, the pump is set with the external programmer.

Additional spine techniques are covered in Chapter 20.

KEY POINTS

- Perioperative nurses and scrub persons who care for neurosurgical patients are challenged by the need to have a working knowledge of neuroanatomy, function, and clinical presentations of the many neurologic conditions that require surgical interventions.
- The nervous system is divided functionally into a voluntary system and an autonomic, or involuntary, system.
- The nervous system is divided structurally into the central nervous system (CNS) consisting of the brain and spinal cord

and the peripheral nervous system (PNS), which encompasses every neurologic structure outside the CNS, including the cranial and spinal nerves.

- The brain and adjacent structures include the cranial nerves of the PNS, which are commonly encountered during brain surgery. Discussion of the spine and spinal cord includes the adjacent spinal nerves and the discs and ligaments that support the spine.
- Surgical procedures to address disorders of the brain and spine are the cornerstone of the specialty. Brain surgery is performed to excise tumors, address trauma, and correct congenital and acquired conditions. Spinal surgery is performed to correct congenital malformations, traumatic injuries, tumors, abscesses, herniated and degenerative intervertebral disks, and intractable pain.
- Neurosurgical patients often have special needs because of conditions such as mental status changes, spinal instability, spinal cord injuries, paralysis, other traumatic injuries, and pain.

CRITICAL THINKING QUESTION

While interviewing Mr. J, who is scheduled for a right craniotomy and tumor resection, you discover that he is having a hard time answering your questions. He does not remember talking to the surgeon, or exactly what he was told about the treatment plan. You notice that Mr. J signed his surgical consent a month ago, and find the anesthesia provider is at the bedside assessing Mr. J and obtaining the anesthesia consent. You feel uneasy about Mr. J's level of understanding. What should you do?

evolve *The answer to the Critical Thinking Question can be found at http://evolve.elsevier.com/Rothrock/Alexander.*

REFERENCES

American Association of Neurological Surgeons (AANS): *Endovascular surgery*, 2009, available at www.neurosurgerytoday.org/what/fact/endo_vascular.pdf. Accessed January 13, 2013.

American Brain Tumor Association (ABTA): *Brain tumor facts*, 2012, available at www.abta.org/news/brain-tumor-fact-sheets. Accessed October 16, 2012.

Baehring JM, Hochberg FH: Cancer and the nervous system: management of primary nervous system tumors in adults. In Daroff RB et al, editors: *Bradley's neurology in clinical practice*, ed 6, Philadelphia, 2012, Saunders.

Biller J et al: Vascular diseases of the nervous system: ischemic cerebrovascular disease. In Daroff RB et al, editors: *Bradley's neurology in clinical practice*, ed 6, Philadelphia, 2012, Saunders.

Biros MH, Heegaard WG: Head injury. In Marx JA et al, editors: *Rosen's emergency medicine*, ed 7, St Louis, 2009, Mosby.

Connolly ES et al: *Fundamentals of operative techniques in neurosurgery*, ed 2, New York, 2009, Thieme.

Denholm B: Tucking patient's arms and general positioning, *AORN J* 89(4):755–757, 2009.

Donthineni R: Diagnosis and staging of spine tumors, *Orthop Clin North Am* 40:1–7, 2009.

Gasco J et al: Neurosurgery. In Townsend CM et al, editors: *Sabiston textbook of surgery*, ed 19, Philadelphia, 2012, Saunders.

Integra: Products for the neurosurgeon, 2010-2012, available at www.integralife.com/Neurosurgeon/Neurosurgeon-Product-List.aspx?ProductLine=4&ProductLineName=Cranial%20Stabilization. Accessed December 5, 2012.

Karajannis MA et al: Cancer and the nervous system: management of primary nervous system tumors in infants and children. In Daroff RB et al, editors: *Bradley's neurology in clinical practice*, ed 6, Philadelphia, 2012, Saunders.

Korley FK: Management of increased intracranial pressure and intracranial shunts. In Roberts JR, Hedges JR, editors: *Clinical procedures in emergency medicine*, ed 5, Philadelphia, 2010, Saunders.

Martin RS, Meredith JW: Management of acute trauma. In Townsend CM et al, editors: *Sabiston textbook of surgery*, ed 19, Philadelphia, 2012, Saunders.

Meyers PM et al: Indications for the performance of intracranial endovascular neurointerventional procedures, a scientific statement, *Circulation* 119: 2235–2239, 2009.

Morina A et al: Cranioplasty with subcutaneously preserved autologous bone grafts in abdominal wall-experiences with 75 cases in post war Kosova, *Surg Neurol Int* 2:72, 2011.

National Cancer Institute (NCI): *Adult brain tumors treatment*, available at www.cancer.gov/cancertopics/pdq./treatment/adultbrain/HealthProfessional/page3. Accessed January 13, 2013.

National Institute of Neurological Disorders and Stroke (NINDS): *NINDS arteriovenous malformation information page*, 2009, available at www.ninds.nih.gov/disorders/avms/avms.htm. Accessed February 4, 2013.

Rosenberg GA: Brain edema and disorders of cerebrospinal fluid circulation. In Daroff RB et al, editors: *Bradley's neurology in clinical practice*, ed 6, Philadelphia, 2012, Saunders.

The Brain Aneurysm Foundation (TBAF): *Understanding: brain aneurysm statistics and facts*, 2012, available at www.bafound.org/node/124. Accessed December 18, 2012.

CHAPTER 22

Reconstructive and Aesthetic Plastic Surgery

THERESA FINK AND ROBERT M. BLUMM

Derived from the Greek word *plastikos,* which means to mold or give form, plastic surgery is a medical specialty that restores or gives shape to the body. There are two different subspecialties of plastic surgery. *Cosmetic surgery* restores or reshapes normal structures of the body, to modify or improve appearance. *Reconstructive surgery* treats abnormal structures of the body caused by birth defects, developmental problems, disease, tumors, infection, or injury to restore function and correct disfigurement or scarring. As a surgical specialty plastic surgery owes much of its heritage to knowledge gained from the wars of the twentieth century.

Despite the economic downturn, 14.6 million cosmetic surgical procedures were performed (by surgeons certified by the American Society of Plastic Surgeons [ASPS]) in 2012, a 5% increase in both minimally invasive and surgical procedures. The top five surgical procedures were breast augmentation, nose reshaping, liposuction, eyelid surgery, and facelift. The top five minimally invasive procedures were Botulinum toxin type A injections (e.g., Botox), soft tissue filler injection/insertion, chemical peels, laser hair removal and microdermabrasion. Many cosmetic procedures are performed in outpatient settings (Ambulatory Surgery Considerations). Reconstructive plastic surgery, which improves function and appearance, was up 5%. The top five reconstructive procedures were tumor removal, laceration repair, maxillofacial surgery, scar revision, and hand surgery. Breast reconstruction increased 8% over the previous year with more than 68,000 procedures performed (ASPS, 2012a).

Surgical Anatomy

Plastic and reconstructive surgery is not limited to a single anatomic or biologic system. It is based on thorough understanding of the anatomy and biology of tissue. Operative techniques are complex and staged to achieve the expected results. The surgery also involves removing, reducing, enlarging, and recontouring tissue, as well as camouflaging scars into existing skin lines (Figure 22-1). The tissues of the body can be transferred to use as various types of flaps. Free flaps are the transfer of tissue along with its vascular pedicle. When nerve is anastomosed with these flaps, they are called neurovascular free flaps. Flaps are used to cover defects or create new structures such as breasts, digits, or facial structures. Body parts can also be transplanted. By improving the patient's deformity, the patient's self-esteem will improve and the patient will feel more comfortable in public and social activities. The body changes as we age. The patient's concern with aesthetics, the variety of acquired defects, the diversity of operative techniques, and the psychologic responses of patients offer unique learning experiences and challenges for perioperative nursing care.

Perioperative Nursing Considerations

The prospect of surgery, even elective, can produce anxiety and fear. Because it is so often associated with body image and self-esteem, plastic and reconstructive surgery can trigger these emotions, especially when the proposed surgery is associated with potential disfigurement because of disease or trauma. Even a planned (desired) change in body image can be stressful. Many cosmetic patients lack the traditional support system one comes to expect during illness and recuperation because of a desire for confidentiality or because cosmetic surgery is elective and may be viewed by friends or family as nonessential. In these situations the sensitivity of the perioperative nurse is critical.

In general, the nurse creates a therapeutic environment in the following ways: introducing self and other members of the surgical team; explaining all perioperative events and any sensations likely to be experienced; determining the patient's normal coping patterns; communicating with the patient in a calm, unhurried, and reassuring manner; encouraging the patient to verbalize feelings and concerns, and listening attentively; reducing distracting stimuli in the perioperative environment; providing reassurance and information about the progress of surgery (for awake patients); communicating progress reports to family; providing comfort measures (e.g., warm blankets, soft music of patient preference); and encouraging and assisting the patient to use personally effective coping strategies (e.g., meditation, guided imagery, relaxation) (Patient-Centered Care).

Appropriate candidates for plastic surgery include those who have positive self-image but are bothered by a physical aspect that they would like to improve; after surgery these patients maintain their positive self-image. Another category of appropriate surgical candidates includes patients who have a physical defect or cosmetic flaw that has lowered their self-esteem over time; these patients require time to adjust (rebuild confidence) postoperatively and generally their self-esteem is strengthened, even dramatically. Patients who may not be suitable for plastic surgery include those in crisis or with unrealistic expectations; those who have an unwillingness to learn risks or unwillingness to change the behavior that led to the problem (e.g., a liposuction patient who continues to overeat) and those who are mentally ill/psychotic, delusional, or paranoid (ASPS, 2012b).

The nursing process is dynamic, fluid, and complex. The nature of plastic and reconstructive surgery is rarely simple, routine, or predictable, and the nursing care must mirror that fact. It must include thorough and ongoing assessment, establishment of nursing diagnoses and outcomes, fastidious planning, superior implementation, and thoughtful evaluation. The perioperative nurse's goal is to produce positive, high-quality outcomes in an environment that is safe and nurturing and will facilitate physical and emotional healing.

AMBULATORY SURGERY CONSIDERATIONS

Patient Choices in Facility

There has been a dramatic shift toward encouraging patients to be more involved and informed in all of their healthcare decisions. Many organizations are focusing on active participation of patients in their own care. One aspect of this is choosing the outpatient facility for their plastic surgery. In keeping with this trend, the American Society of Plastic Surgeons (ASPS) has developed a brochure, with an excerpt available online, to help patients choose a facility. The brochure includes the following information:

- *Types of facilities:* For ambulatory (discharge same day as surgery) procedures, the facility may be part of the surgeon's office, a surgical suite adjacent to the office, a free-standing facility, or part of a hospital.
- *Choice and benefits:* Some patients prefer no overnight stay at a hospital. Cost savings and convenience along with added privacy and personalized care may be factors.
- *Accreditation:* As a result of the strict guidelines for equipment, staff, anesthesia services, and hospital access, patients are encouraged to determine if a facility is accredited because it could indicate the quality of the facility. (All ASPS member surgeons are required to operate in an accredited medical facility.)
- *Insurance:* Accreditation also affects financial aspects. Although facility fees are typically not covered by insurance providers for elective procedures, facility fees for reconstructive procedures may be covered. Reimbursement may be expedited for facilities that carry accreditation because the accreditation ensures that certain quality standards are met at that facility. Also similar services at a hospital generally cost more than in an ambulatory facility.
- *Individual considerations:* Each patient must discuss the options with his or her surgeon. Depending on medical history and condition requiring surgery, ambulatory surgery may not be appropriate for everyone.

Modified from American Society of Plastic Surgeons: *Guide to safe plastic surgery, patient safety, surgery at a accredited facility,* available at www.plasticsurgery.org/articles-and-galleries/patient-and consumer-information/patientsafety.html. Accessed November 27, 2012.

Assessment

As part of a holistic assessment, perioperative nurses consider physical and emotional factors of the planned procedure. A comprehensive review of the patient's chart is the first step. The presence of a signed and witnessed informed consent, a systems review and health history, pertinent laboratory and diagnostic data, interdisciplinary planning, anesthesia evaluation, and the surgical plan disclose vital information necessary to begin the assessment process. Visual assessment should include the patient's overall physical condition, the condition and integrity of the skin, nutritional status, and physical limitations. The next step is the patient interview, which includes checking patient identification, explaining the perioperative nursing role, and verifying the patient's understanding of the planned procedure. The perioperative nurse must be skilled in establishing communication quickly to create an instant relationship. Greeting the patient by name in a calm, comforting manner, perhaps with a gentle, caring touch (if welcomed by the patient), and maintaining good eye contact will help establish the rapport needed to assess emotional status, body image disturbances, and anxiety level. Asking the patient questions will help reveal any barriers to communication or learning; religious, cultural, or other preferences;

A

B

FIGURE 22-1 The surgeon adheres to several principles when planning skin incisions, one of which is to reduce the amount of tension across the wound, thus minimizing scarring. Elective incisions should preferably parallel relaxed skin tension lines (RSTLs) in the face **(A)** and the body **(B).** These lines are also referred to as Langer lines.

mental status; and insight into compliance. Other vital pieces of knowledge the nurse must obtain include the presence of realistic expectations and motivation for surgery, as well as support systems available to the patient.

An important component of the assessment phase of nursing care involves communication with the surgeon and anesthesia provider to determine the need for special equipment, supplies, sutures, or implants. The perioperative nurse should verify the procedure

PATIENT-CENTERED CARE

Creating a supportive patient-centered environment for care is especially important for the specialty of plastic surgery, in which patients may lack traditional support systems or are struggling with body image changes. An important consideration for patient-centered care is the relationship between healthcare providers and their patients. This relationship, as well as the patient's perceived healthcare provider's empathy, can greatly influence treatment outcomes and the patient's satisfaction with the care provided.

Clinical empathy (CE) is a tool that can be used to foster patient-centered care. Adams (2012) notes that empathy and sympathy are similar but different; both are capacities and compassionate acts result based on feeling. Sympathy refers to an individual's ability to share an emotion being experienced by another. In CE, more imaginative insight is required for the healthcare provider to understand what suffering from a particular pathology actually means from the patient's perspective. Halpern (2012), states:

> "When possible, invite the patient to tell you his or her own story, from its beginning to its imagined ending. Try to pause when the patient is obviously processing an emotional issue. Practice patience by becoming more aware of your own embodied reactions, and if you feel anxious, take breaths or otherwise relax yourself, to give the patient the message you are truly present and not in a rush. Your tone and gestures will convey your genuine emotional resonance, but be wary of making overreaching statements like, 'I know how you feel.' When a patient says something contradictory or seemingly irrational, avoid correcting him or her and ask instead, 'Tell me what I'm missing.'"

Clinical empathy is beneficial for patients, but also for health providers. It helps with professional self-development, increased work satisfaction, and as cited in Adams (2012), "the meaning of what practitioners do is found through and in those they treat."

Modified from Adams R: Clinical empathy: a discussion on its benefits for practitioners, students of medicine and patients, *J Herb Med* 2:52–57, 2012; Halpern J: Gathering the patient's story and clinical empathy, *Perm J* 16:52–54, 2012; Rickert J: *Patient centered care: what it means and how to get there*, Jan 24, 2012, available at http://healthaffairs.org/blog/2012/01/24/patient-centered-care-what-it-means-and-how-to-get-there. Accessed March 5, 2013.

and position and, in the case of multiple procedures on the same patient, identify the planned order of surgeries.

Clear and effective hand-off communication is critical to patient safety. According to The Joint Commission (TJC), communication is the top contributing factor to medical error and at least 65% of sentinel events. At least half those incidents occurred as responsibility for the patient was transferred from one team of care providers to another. In the perioperative suites, hand-offs occur as patients move to and from the operating room (OR), involving many different care providers for one patient (Association of periOperative Registered Nurses [AORN], 2012). TJC addresses communication in their *National Patient Safety Goal 2* (Improve staff communication) (TJC, 2013) and through recommendations around effective hand-offs. The primary objective of a hand-off is to provide information about a patient's, client's, or resident's general care plan, treatment, services, current condition, and any recent or anticipated changes (TJC, 2012). Whatever form the hand-off communication takes at each facility, it must be standardized and provide a thorough discussion of patient history, issues, special needs, and precautions for safety, with opportunity for the receiving provider to ask questions.

Nursing Diagnosis

Nursing diagnoses related to the care of the patient undergoing plastic and reconstructive surgery might include the following:
- Anxiety related to surgical interventions or outcomes
- Risk for Infection related to operative/invasive plastic/reconstructive procedure
- Deficient Knowledge related to perioperative process
- Disturbed Body Image related to congenital or acquired defect or developmental abnormality
- Risk for Ineffective Peripheral Tissue Perfusion related to surgical intervention
- Impaired Comfort related to surgical/invasive procedure
- High Risk for Impaired Skin Integrity and injury related to positioning during surgical procedure
- High Risk for Altered Body Temperature related to procedure

Outcome Identification

Nursing diagnoses lead to the formulation of desired or expected patient outcomes. These are desirable and measurable patient states, including biologic or physiologic states; psychologic, cultural, and spiritual aspects; and the knowledge, behavior, or skills related to these states. As such, the patient outcome indicates progress toward or resolution of the nursing diagnosis. Outcomes should be mutually formulated with the patient, family, and other healthcare providers. Such formulations should be realistic, involve consideration of the patient's present and potential capabilities and resources, and provide direction for continuity of care, as well as determine satisfaction with that care. Outcomes identified for the selected nursing diagnoses could be stated as follows:
- The patient will verbalize management of anxiety.
- The patient is free from signs and symptoms of infection.
- The patient participates in decision-making affecting the perioperative plan of care.
- The patient will acknowledge feelings about altered structure or function.
- The patient has wound/tissue perfusion consistent with or improved from baseline level established preoperatively.
- The patient demonstrates knowledge of pain management.
- The patient will be free of injury and have intact skin integrity at the end of the procedure.
- The patient will maintain adequate body temperature.

Planning

The perioperative nurse designs a plan of care using critical thinking to integrate knowledge gained from prior steps with the plastic surgical patient. The nurse should seek to create and maintain a culture and environment of safety for the patient, the OR, and all members of the surgical team during the planning process. A Sample Plan of Care for a patient undergoing plastic and reconstructive surgery is on pages 826-827.

Implementation

The implementation phase typically begins with preparation of the OR and requires a thorough understanding of the procedure and the special needs of the patient, surgeon, and anesthesia provider. The perioperative nurse must continually monitor and reassess the patient as well as the needs of the perioperative team, implementing and documenting the delivery of care. Constant consideration is given to the safety of the patient and the perioperative environment during this phase.

SAMPLE PLAN OF CARE

Nursing Diagnosis
Anxiety related to surgical intervention or outcome

Outcome
The patient will verbalize management of anxiety.

Interventions
- Broadly classify the patient's anxiety (mild, moderate, severe).
- Try to understand the patient's perception of the stressors or stressful situation or event.
- Identify contributing factors.
- Introduce self and other members of the surgical team.
- Explain all perioperative events and any sensations likely to be experienced.
- Determine the patient's normal coping patterns.
- Communicate with the patient in a calm, unhurried, reassuring manner.
- Encourage the patient to express feelings and concerns; listen attentively.
- Reduce distracting stimuli in the perioperative environment.
- Provide reassurance and information about the progress of the surgery (if the patient is awake); implement mechanism for family progress reports also.
- Provide comfort measures (e.g., warm blankets, soft music that the patient prefers).
- Use touch as appropriate (e.g., softly stroking the hand).
- Encourage and assist the patient to use personally effective coping strategies (e.g., meditation, guided imagery, relaxation).

Nursing Diagnosis
Risk for Infection related to surgical/invasive plastic/reconstructive procedure

Outcome
The patient is free of signs and symptoms of infection.

Interventions
- Assess susceptibility for infection and risk for inadvertent hypothermia.
- Assess nutritional habits and patterns.
- Implement thermoregulation measures and aseptic technique (create and maintain a sterile field, prevent contamination of open wounds, and isolate the operative site from the surrounding physical environment).
- Minimize the length of invasive procedure by planning care (coordinate team members' efforts to set priorities and efficiently accomplish the tasks necessary to achieve a common goal).
- Perform skin preparations.
- Administer prescribed antibiotic therapy and prophylactic treatments, verifying surgeon orders.
- Protect from cross-contamination; maintain continual surveillance.
- Record devices implanted during the operative or invasive procedure (according to federal regulations for tracking).
- Administer care to wound sites and invasive device sites.
- Monitor for signs and symptoms of infection.
- Encourage deep-breathing and coughing exercises.
- Evaluate response to thermoregulation measures and progress of wound healing.

Nursing Diagnosis
Deficient Knowledge related to the perioperative process

Outcome
The patient demonstrates knowledge of the expected responses to the operative or other invasive procedure.

Interventions
- Determine knowledge level (assess knowledge and comprehension of new information and ability to apply in self-care activities); assess readiness to learn (evaluate factors that may affect abilities to learn or demonstrate knowledge).
- Provide instruction based on age and identified needs; identify barriers to communication and adapt instructions to these.
- Evaluate environment for home care; identify expectations of home care.
- Explain expected sequence of events related to perioperative care; include family members in preoperative teaching; identify family members' knowledge and provide education and support.
- Assess knowledge; provide and evaluate response to instructions (e.g., about wound care and phases of wound healing) (evaluate patient's/family members' understanding of instruction regarding perioperative experience and ongoing care, listening to explanations and observing return demonstrations, techniques of wound care, and signs and symptoms to report).
- Provide information and explain Patient Self-Determination Act.
- Include patient and family members in discharge planning, including resources available to facilitate the rehabilitation process.
- Initiate institution's checklist policy for correct site surgery.
- Verify surgical consent with OR schedule and patient's statement of planned surgery.
- Solicit the patient's questions; answer or refer questions as appropriate.
- Explain the sequence of perioperative events and their purpose, as appropriate (e.g., holding area, OR attire, insertion of lines and attachment of monitoring devices, type of anesthesia, PACU, protocols).
- Provide sensory (what the patient will hear and feel, using lay terms) as well as factual procedure-related information.
- Provide printed material to reinforce patient education (e.g., preoperative routines, explanations of surgical intervention, postoperative management of pain, discharge instructions).

Nursing Diagnosis
Disturbed Body Image related to disease, congenital or acquired deformity, developmental abnormality

Outcome
The patient will acknowledge feelings about altered structure or function and identify effective, optimistic coping options.

Interventions
- Identify psychosocial status; elicit perceptions of surgery.
- Identify individual values and wishes concerning care.
- Assess coping mechanisms.
- Implement measures to provide psychologic support.
- Maintain patient's dignity and privacy (e.g., keep OR doors closed, only expose body as needed for care).
- Assist patient to identify and discuss feelings, stressors, and perception of physical deformity.
- Provide environment (e.g., privacy, supportive listening) conducive to expression of feelings.
- Help patient identify significance of culture, religion, gender, and age on perceived changes in body structure or function or image.
- Determine patient's body image expectations and whether expectations are realistic; clarify unrealistic expectations or misconceptions.
- Convey sense of respect for abilities and strengths in coping with problems or concerns.

SAMPLE PLAN OF CARE—cont'd

- Assist patient to separate physical appearance from feelings of personal worth, self-concept, and self-esteem (as appropriate).
- Refer the patient to other health professionals (e.g., clergy, social worker, psychiatric liaison) or support groups as appropriate.

Nursing Diagnosis
Risk for Ineffective Peripheral Tissue Perfusion related to surgical intervention

Outcome
The patient has wound/tissue perfusion consistent with or improved from baseline levels established preoperatively.

Interventions
- Assess factors related to risks for ineffective tissue perfusion (e.g., presence of diabetes, immunosuppression); assess history of previous radiation exposure.
- Evaluate postoperative tissue perfusion.
- Identify factors associated with an increased risk for hemorrhage or fluid and electrolyte loss (e.g., patients with recent traumatic injury, abnormal bleeding or clotting time, extensive surgical procedure, complicated renal/liver disease, and major organ transplant).
- Implement hemostasis techniques (provide supplies, instrumentation, and appropriate surgical techniques as needed to control hemorrhage).
- Frequently reevaluate intraoperatively for signs and symptoms of physical injury to skin and tissue (positioning).
- Note any sensory or perceptual alterations in the affected body part, and document them.
- Maintain body temperature with the use of warming device or reflective blankets, for example.
- Warm intravenous fluids, blood and blood products, and irrigating fluids.
- Increase the temperature in the OR as indicated.
- Collaborate with anesthesia provider in monitoring the patient's core temperature.
- Apply compression stockings and antiembolic devices as indicated.
- Monitor tissue perfusion (e.g., by assessing blanching and capillary refill; using Doppler ultrasound), as prescribed; record results.
- Note any swelling, change in color or temperature, or drainage from graft sites before discharge from the OR.
- Provide warm blankets for the patient at the conclusion of the surgical procedure.
- Teach the patient or the family how to care for the incision, including signs and symptoms of infection and graft failure (as applicable).

Nursing Diagnosis
Impaired Comfort related to surgical procedure

Outcome
The patient demonstrates knowledge of pain management.

Interventions
- Assess pain control using validated pain scale.
- Identify cultural and value components related to pain (e.g., stoicism, alternative therapy, verbalization, meditation).
- Implement pain guidelines; provide pain management instruction (purpose, administration, and desired, side, and adverse effects of prescribed medications and nonpharmacologic techniques for managing pain).
- Evaluate response to pain management instruction and instruction about prescribed medications.
- Collaborate in initiating patient-controlled analgesia.
- Evaluate response to pain management interventions (physiologic parameters and subjective and objective findings) and response to medications.
- Implement alternative methods of pain control (diversified activities, therapeutic touch, meditation, breathing, and positioning to augment pain control methods).

Nursing Diagnosis
High **Risk for Impaired Skin Integrity** and injury related to positioning during surgical procedure

Outcome
The patient will have intact skin and be free from injury.

Interventions
- Make sure all bony prominences are well padded with use of positioning devices.
- Monitor patient's extremities every 30 minutes during procedure.
- Maintain extremities in anatomic alignment during surgical procedure.

Nursing Diagnosis
High **Risk for Imbalanced Body Temperature** related to procedure

Outcome
The patient will maintain adequate body temperature during surgical procedure.

Interventions
- Provide warm blankets prior to anesthesia induction.
- Monitor body temperature during surgical procedure with use of temperature probe.
- Use forced-air warming unit during procedure.
- Cover undraped parts of body during surgical procedure.
- Increase operating room temperature prior to anesthesia induction and before extubation.

Preparation of the OR Suite. Before transporting the patient to the OR, the perioperative nurse will assemble all necessary medical and surgical supplies, equipment, suture material, positioning aids, implantable devices, and medications. The nurse is responsible for ensuring that equipment is in working order, that emergency supplies are present, and that compressed gases are adequate. Depending on the procedure to be performed, the OR bed may need to be configured differently from the standard room setup. To minimize inefficiencies during the procedure the nurse should confirm with the surgeon and anesthesia provider the position of the bed and any proposed intraoperative changes to the bed, room temperature, or

room configuration. Plastic and reconstructive surgeons frequently use preoperative photographs of the patient when attempting to restore or modify appearance. These photographs help the surgeon maintain perspective because features may change as a result of surgical positioning. The nurse should collaborate with the surgeon to determine the best placement of these photographs for intraoperative viewing.

Equipment and Special Mechanical Devices. Essential equipment for any OR includes a fully functional bed that may be positioned for any number of special needs and also has accessory

FIGURE 22-2 Powered Brown dermatome.

FIGURE 22-3 Manual skin graft meshing device.

attachments, such as headrests and aids for extremity positioning. The room must also have well-positioned and numerous electrical outlets, good overhead lighting, suction equipment, mounted x-ray view boxes, and computer terminals for those facilities using electronic medical records. Stepstools, tables, chairs, hand tables, tourniquets, microscopes, and intravenous (IV) poles should be in appropriate supply and accessible.

Instrumentation. Basic instrument trays are available for the plastic surgery OR. A local procedure tray may include Bishop Harmon and Adson tissue forceps (with and without teeth); straight and curved iris, Stevens, and Metzenbaum scissors; fine mosquito forceps; and skin hooks. Minor and major trays for plastic surgery may contain a range of tissue forceps, scissors, hemostats, and retractors. With the addition of instruments for specific surgeries and surgeons, these trays usually suffice for all plastic surgery operations. Adequate instrumentation should be available to avoid immediate use sterilization. Plastic surgeons all have their own instrument preferences that should be discussed and available prior to the procedure.

Dermatomes. Dermatomes are used for removing split-thickness skin grafts (STSGs) from donor sites; they are of three basic types: knife, drum, and electric and air driven (Figure 22-2). Sterile mineral oil and a tongue blade should be available when STSGs are being obtained.

Skin Meshers. Several types of skin meshers are available, each designed to produce multiple uniform slits in a skin graft, approximately 0.05 inch apart. These multiple apertures in the graft can then expand, permitting the skin graft to stretch and cover a larger area. Meshing also facilitates drainage through the graft, preventing fluid accumulation under a graft. The graft is placed on the carrier and passed through the mesher (Figure 22-3). The manufacturer supplies sterile carriers for meshers. They are usually available in several sizes, which determine the expansion ratio of the skin graft.

Pneumatic-Powered Instruments. Pneumatic-powered instruments use an inert, nonflammable, and explosion-free compressed gas as their power source. The motor may be activated by a foot pedal or hand control. The various attachments should be sterilized

as recommended by the manufacturer to prolong instrument life and ensure effective sterilization. The following attachments may be used in plastic surgery:
- Wire driver and bone drill
- Oscillating saw
- Derma-Tattoo (used with reciprocating-saw handpiece)
- Reciprocating saw
- Dermabrader
- Sagittal saw

A pneumatic tourniquet with an inflatable cuff is used in most hand surgery procedures as well as in other upper and lower extremity surgical interventions. Safe use of the tourniquet is described in Chapter 20.

Hemostatic Devices and Equipment. Monopolar and bipolar electrosurgical units (ESUs) are commonly used in plastic surgery. The functionality of ESUs and the safety precautions to observe during their use are described in Chapter 8.

Harmonic ultrasonic devices are cutting instruments used during surgical procedures to simultaneously cut and coagulate tissue. They are similar to ESUs but superior in that they can cut thicker tissue, and create less toxic smoke with less thermal damage.

Tissue fusion devices provide a combination of pressure and energy to create vessel fusion. They permanently fuse vessels up to and including 7 mm in diameter and tissue bundles without dissection or isolation an average seal cycle of 2 to 4 seconds. Seals withstand three times normal systolic blood pressure.

Lasers. A variety of lasers are used for plastic surgical procedures. The perioperative nurse must ensure that the laser safety accessories specific to the type of laser being used are available. Laser safety is discussed in Chapter 8.

FIGURE 22-4 Loupes from Carl Zeiss, used for magnification.

Fiberoptic Instruments. Examples of fiberoptic instrument attachments used in plastic surgery are a headlight for rhinoplasties, augmentation mammoplasties, and other procedures; a mammary retractor for augmentation mammoplasties; a rhytidectomy retractor; abdominoplasty retractors; and endoscopic face and forehead fiberoptic instrumentation.

Loupes. Loupes (Figure 22-4) are magnifying lenses used by many plastic surgeons for microvascular surgery and nerve repairs and for numerous other instances in which cosmetic results are improved by the magnification effect. The nurse should inquire about the use of loupes before the surgeon dons a headlight because adjustments will need to be made to the headlight alignment if the loupes are required in midprocedure. Adjusting or removing the headlight in midprocedure has the potential to contaminate the sterile field.

Microscope. The microscope is frequently used in nerve repairs and microsurgical anastomoses; the nerves or vessels to be repaired, such as in hand surgery, and the suture used to do so (sometimes 9-0, 10-0, or even 11-0 size) can be finer than human hair and thus requires magnification. Although each microscope has different features, an important matter to avoid confusion is whether the surgeon control overrides the assistant view, or if each can separately adjust the field of view.

Wood Lamp. The Wood lamp is an ultraviolet lamp used in a darkened room to determine the viability of skin flaps. After IV injection of fluorescein, the blood vessels appear bright purple (the skin appears yellow). Sodium fluorescein is excreted in the urine, and patients should be informed of this.

Special Supplies. Surgeon-specific and procedure-specific special supplies are frequently added to instrument setups for plastic and reconstructive procedures. These commonly include the following: sterile marking pen or methylene blue; ruler; local anesthetic of choice for injection, with syringes and needles; and ESU, with active electrode (pencil) and tip of choice, with tip cleaner.

Sutures. Sutures range from permanent to absorbable and include monofilament and multifilament materials. The perioperative nurse should be a good steward of costly resources and verify the type and number of sutures needed before opening suture packages, as well as needle preference, to prevent waste. Many plastic surgical procedures have multiple techniques, each of which necessitates very specific suture choices. See Chapter 7 for further discussion and explanations.

Dressings. Dressings are an essential part of the operative procedure in plastic surgery and may contribute to the ultimate outcome of the surgical intervention. Dressings are usually applied while the patient is still anesthetized. In general, the dressing should accomplish the following five goals:

1. Immobilize the surgical part.
2. Apply even pressure over the wound.
3. Collect drainage.
4. Provide comfort for the patient.
5. Protect the wound.

Pressure dressings may be used to eliminate dead space, to prevent seroma and hematoma formation, and to prevent third spacing associated with liposuction and reconstructive procedures involving transfer of large muscle or tissue flaps. In some cases pressure can be achieved by the use of catheters or drains placed within the operative site and connected to closed-wound suction devices. In smaller wounds a Penrose drain or a butterfly cannula may be inserted into the operative site, with the needle end placed into a red-top tube, such as a blood collection tube, that has a vacuum (evacuated tube).

The perioperative nurse should be familiar with common general dressings and supplies available in sterile form and various sizes.

In some instances, such as a free flap, transparent dressings are used so that the flap can be monitored and observed for vascular flow. Compression garments and support devices are also frequently used by plastic surgeons. Proper fit is essential to minimize vascular compromise. Compression garments are typically applied over a light dressing. A proper garment is selected based on its characteristics (e.g., fabric, stretch, softness, antimicrobial properties) and proper sizing according to measurement instructions. Educating patients of the needs and benefits of compression garment use as well as providing hints for their proper application (avoid ripping with long nails, instructions on how to don the garment) promotes comfort and compliance (Gladfelter, 2007).

Implant Materials. The range of materials available for implantation and augmentation in the specialty of plastic and reconstructive surgery has benefited from ongoing research and includes prosthetic and natural materials. Perioperative nurses are responsible for complying with tracking regulations for implantable materials and devices (Patient Safety).

Biologic materials (autogenous grafts) are preferred when available. Autologous human tissue successfully used includes fat, solid dermis, and collagen. A cellular collagen (AlloDerm regenerative tissue matrix) is a material that allows for a strong intact repair in breast reconstruction post-mastectomy procedures by providing soft tissue reinforcement or replacement. Human cadavers are used as a source for AlloDerm (Figure 22-5). This product is available in various sizes of sheeting and must be rehydrated in several steps. AlloDerm integrates with the body's tissue and helps prevent rejection over the long term, which allows for a safe and clinically optimal outcome (Life Cell Corporation, 2012).

Implant failure may be directly linked to bacterial contamination; therefore meticulous aseptic technique with minimal handling is essential when using implants of any sort. Most alloplastic implants are presterilized from the manufacturer.

Anesthesia. A variety of anesthetic techniques are used with plastic surgery procedures. Local, regional, tumescent, conscious sedation, deep sedation, and general anesthesia may be used, depending on the type of procedure, the patient's anesthetic history, the American

PATIENT SAFETY

Tracking Medical Devices

A variety of implantable devices are used in aesthetic and reconstructive plastic surgery procedures. Tracking these devices is
critical to patient safety. The device's manufacturer must have a
mechanism to locate implantables after they have been distributed. Devices may be recalled for sterility issues, malfunction, or
any event that is found to pose a serious health risk.

The U.S. Food and Drug Administration (FDA) regulates the
process of tracking medical devices and directs the tracking of
devices whose failure would result in serious, adverse health
consequences; devices that are intended to be implanted in the
human body for more than 1 year; and devices that are life-
sustaining and life-supporting and are used outside of a facility
such as a hospital, nursing home, or ambulatory surgery center.

The perioperative nurse plays an important role in the accurate
documentation of implantable devices for tracking purposes. Information that the nurse typically will gather for tracking purposes
includes:

- Device identification (i.e., lot, batch, model number, serial
  number)
- Date of manufacture and shipping
- Name, address, telephone number, and social security
  number of the patient who received the device
- Location the device was implanted
- Name, address, and telephone number of the surgeon who
  is caring for the patient, if different from the prescribing
  physician

If an implantable device is sterilized within the sterile processing
department of the facility, monitoring requirements include the use
of a process challenge device containing a biologic indicator. The
load should be quarantined until the result of the biologic indicator
is determined. Documentation should include a record of the sterilizer load identification number on the patient's medical record, or
the patient's name on the load record. Lot identification provides
a method for tracing problems in the event of a recall. Immediate-
use sterilization of implantable devices is not recommended.

Patients have the right to refuse tracking of their devices and
may refuse to have their social security number used for tracking.
The patient's consent for tracking should be obtained before the
procedure. If the patient refuses to have the device tracked, the
nurse will document the refusal along with the required product
information and report this information to the manufacturer.

Under the Safe Medical Device Act, institutions must also report
any incident of death or serious injury relating to the use of a medical
device. The FDA has classified and identified more than 1700 different devices that must be reported if the device is suspected of
causing serious injury or death to an individual. Nurses should work
within their institutional policies to report these incidents.

Modified from Association for the Advancement of Medical Instrumentation: *Comprehensive guide to steam sterilization and sterility assurance in health care facilities*, Arlington,
VA, 2012, AAMI; Denholm B: Clinical issues, *AORN J* 93(2):296–298, 2011; U.S. Food
and Drug Administration: *Medical device tracking, guidance for industry and FDA staff*,
available at www.fda.gov/downloads/MedicalDevices/DeviceRegulationandGuidance/
GuidanceDocuments/UCM95266.pdf. Accessed December 2, 2012; U.S. Food and Drug
Administration: *Medical device reporting*, available at www.fda.gov/MedicalDevices/
Safety/ReportaProblem/default.html. Accessed December 2, 2012.

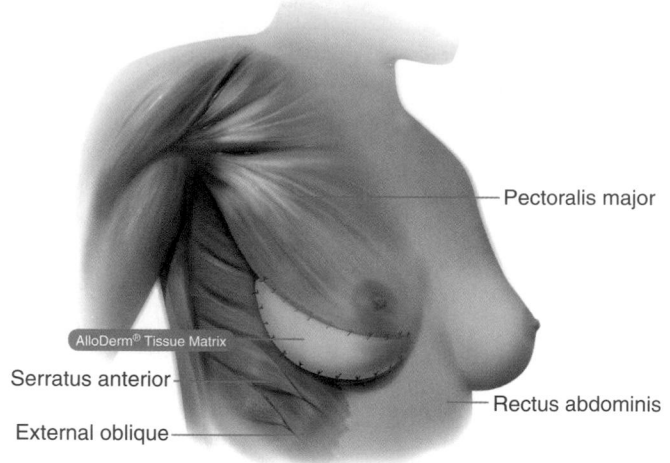

Pectoralis major

AlloDerm® Tissue Matrix

Serratus anterior

Rectus abdominis

External oblique

FIGURE 22-5 AlloDerm.

(E_TCO_2) pressure if indicated. When using oxygen on a head and
neck procedure, oxygen must be temporarily shut off while the ESU
is being used due to its flammability. If a local or regional anesthetic
is used without an anesthesia provider, appropriate staffing should
be determined based on patient assessment and nurse competency.
The presence of a perioperative registered nurse whose sole responsibility is to monitor the patient may be warranted, depending on
clinical assessment and patient behavior. This nurse must be sufficiently skilled in assessment and knowledgeable about the agents
being used so that changes in the patient's status can be promptly
reported and appropriate interventions to prevent complications
can be initiated (AORN, 2013a).

Injectable anesthetics are frequently used, not only for strictly
local cases but also in conjunction with regional, sedation, and even
general anesthesia. Local anesthetics (e.g., lidocaine, bupivicaine,
prilocaine) act by reversibly blocking nerve impulses—they stop
nerve conduction by blocking sodium channels in the axon membrane. When combined with a vasoconstrictor such as epinephrine,
local blood flow is decreased and systemic absorption of the anesthetic delayed. This prolongs anesthesia time and reduces the risk
of toxicity. Sodium bicarbonate also can be combined with local
anesthetics to decrease pain during injection by changing the pH
of the solution. In addition, infiltration of a local anesthetic can
help define tissue planes through hydrodissection. Use of epinephrine is contraindicated in areas with limited vascularity, such as
digits, the penis, nasal tip, and ears. Additional information about
the use of local anesthetics is found in Chapter 5.

Topical anesthetics used by the plastic surgeon include tetracaine
(Pontocaine) 2% ophthalmic drops (for blepharoplasty or before
application of eye shields), EMLA (eutectic mixture of local anesthetics) for penetration on intact skin (associated with laser surgery),
and cocaine solution applied on neurosurgical patties for mucous
membranes (for rhinoplasty).

Preoperative Skin Preparation. Most surgical interventions
require that the operative site and adjacent areas be cleansed with
an antibacterial soap before surgery. The surgeon may prescribe that
the patient carry out this treatment before surgery. Special attention
is given to the fingernails for patients undergoing hand surgery; to

Society of Anesthesiologists (ASA) physical status classification, and
the surgeon's preference. Regardless of the type of anesthesia,
patients should have baseline vital signs recorded and fully monitored, including blood pressure, heart rate, respirations, cardiac rate
and rhythm, oxygen saturation, and end-tidal carbon dioxide

hair for surgery of the head, face, or neck; and to oral hygiene for surgery in or near the mouth. The perioperative nurse should verify with the patient that the prescribed regimens have been performed. All body jewelry that pierces the skin should be removed before the skin prep. The operative site should be inspected for any rashes, bruises, open sores, cuts, or other skin conditions. Hair should only be removed if it interferes with the procedure. Shaving is avoided and clippers, not a razor, are used if needed, because shaving creates an access for the entry of bacteria into the operative site (AORN, 2013b). The eyebrows and eyelashes, in particular, are left intact to preserve facial appearance and expression. The surgical site is marked before surgery by the surgeon to designate the correct site and to define landmark areas. Either a povidone-iodine solution, an iodine-alcohol mixture, chlorhexidine gluconate (CHG), or another broad-spectrum agent may be selected for the antimicrobial skin prep. The use of CHG should be avoided around the ears and eyes. It is important to place shields on the eyes and/or eye ointment if prepping the periorbital site or performing an extensive head and neck prep, and to place plugs in the ear canals, and prevent pooling of the prep agent. The perioperative nurse should query the patient regarding any allergies to antimicrobial agents. If indicated, the plan of care should be changed to avoid the use of these products. When prepping for a skin graft procedure, separate skin prep setups are needed for the graft and donor sites.

Positioning and Draping. The OR bed must be positioned so that the remaining space in the room can comfortably accommodate anesthetic equipment, members of the surgical team, instrument tables, and any adjunct equipment (hand table, drills, microscope, laser) to be used. The patient is carefully positioned on the OR bed so that all operative sites may be appropriately exposed and the airway easily observed and accessed.

Before implementing any positioning changes, the perioperative nurse should verify the appropriate placement of the OR bed and the desired patient position. Adequate numbers of personnel and supportive positioning devices must be present. No changes should begin until the anesthesia provider gives permission. Whereas a majority of plastic surgical procedures are performed in the supine position, many also take place with the patient prone or lateral. Liposuction and post-bariatric body contouring procedures may also require repositioning one or more times during surgery. Abdominal procedures may start supine and usually require repositioning to facilitate closure. With each new position, reassessment and documentation of the position and devices used to stabilize the patient should occur. Chapter 6 reviews patient positioning and appropriate safety measures for the supine, lateral, and prone positions, all of which may be used during plastic surgical patient care. The perioperative nurse pays particular attention to the patient's arms during positioning to ensure that they are placed on padded armboards with the palms up and fingers extended (for the supine position). Armboards are maintained at less than a 90-degree angle to prevent brachial plexus stretch. If there are surgical reasons to tuck the arms at the side, the elbows are padded to protect the ulnar nerve, the palms face inward, and the wrist is maintained in a neutral position (Denholm, 2009). A drape secures the arms. It should be tucked snugly under the patient, not under the mattress. This prevents the arm from shifting downward intraoperatively and resting against the OR bed rail.

Correct draping procedures depend on the location of the operative site or sites. Disposable drapes (see Chapter 4) are often used because of their barrier qualities, ease of handling and storage, and versatility in adapting to a variety of plastic surgery procedures. Three frequently used draping techniques in plastic surgery are the head drape, chest drape, and hand drape. These draping techniques have the goal of providing maximum mobility of the operative part. The head drape includes a fluid-resistant drape that encircles the head and the addition of a drape to cover the remainder of the body. The following techniques represent methods of obtaining maximum accessibility and sterile coverage for facial surgery:

1. A barrier sheet, folded in half, and two towels are placed beneath the patient's head with the towels uppermost. The folded barrier sheet covers the headrest or head portion of the OR bed. One towel is brought around the patient's head on each side to cover all hair, leaving the entire face (and ears, as necessary) exposed; the towel is then secured with nonpenetrating towel clamps. For craniofacial procedures a towel folded lengthwise in quarters may be placed under the head to assist with moving the head from side to side. Two additional towels are then placed diagonally across the neck, just under the chin; they are secured to each other (with nonpenetrating towel clamps) in the middle over the neck and are secured on each side to the towel around the head. A full sheet is then added to cover the patient from neck to feet.

2. After the head portion of the drape is placed, a split, or U, drape is added to cover the patient from neck to feet.

Additional Considerations. Preparation is a key ingredient in success. Having backup supplies or equipment, sometimes as elementary as an extra bulb for the light source, can mean the difference in a positive outcome for the patient. Occasionally during the course of a procedure, a flap may become congested and fail, the anatomy may dictate a change in the surgical plan, or perhaps a preselected implant just may not be right. Flexibility, meticulous preparation, and a willingness to improvise and innovate will always serve the perioperative nurse well when working with plastic surgeons.

Evaluation

During the surgical intervention the perioperative nurse is constantly evaluating the patient's response to nursing interventions, anesthesia, and the surgery itself. Progress or lack of progress toward the identified patient outcomes is continually assessed. The results of this ongoing evaluation enable the perioperative nurse to reassess the patient, reorder priorities of patient care, establish new patient outcomes, and revise the perioperative plan of care.

At the conclusion of the surgical intervention the perioperative nurse reviews whether identified patient outcomes have been achieved. The patient's skin integrity is assessed; dressings are applied and their integrity is established before discharge from the OR. Any drains or tubes incorporated in the dressing should be noted. Infusion sites are inspected, and the type of infusing solution, flow rate, and amount infused are noted in the patient record. Local anesthetics, sedatives, or other medications received by the patient are similarly documented. The patient's response during the perioperative period is noted; any unusual or untoward responses are reported to the nurse in the recovery unit. The transport vehicle is obtained; any special equipment needed for patient transport is also obtained and checked for proper functioning. Warm blankets may be provided, and the patient is gently moved to the transport vehicle. The patient who is recovering from general anesthesia is placed in a safe position on the vehicle; the awake patient should be assisted to a position of comfort.

The perioperative nurse, in collaboration with the anesthesia provider, should give the hand-off report to the nurse in the post-anesthesia care unit (PACU). Areas requiring ongoing patient observation should be noted in this report; the patient's preoperative, intraoperative, and immediate postoperative statuses are also reported. Using the Sample Plan of Care introduced earlier in this chapter, the perioperative nurse may give part of the report based on patient outcomes. If they were achieved, they may be stated as listed under the Outcomes section.

Patient and Family Education and Discharge Planning

Education of the plastic surgery patient begins at the time of consultation. Anxiety inhibits the retention of information; therefore, it is always helpful to have written information or other tools for the patient to use as a reference source, beginning with the preoperative instructions as well as postoperative information. The approach to teaching should lend itself to the patient's preferred learning style (e.g., auditory, visual). Specifics that should be addressed include pain management, self-care, diet, exercise, care of incisions and drains, return to the clinic for follow-up appointments, signs and symptoms of infections or complications, and how to reach the surgeon in case of an emergency.

Benefits of an effective education intervention are numerous; it serves to decrease anxiety, improves compliance, reduces the incidence of complications, empowers the patient to become an active participant in his or her own care, and maximizes independence, allowing the patient to more quickly return to an optimal state of health. The patient's readiness to learn, needs, and styles of learning must be assessed. A teaching plan should be individualized based on the desired outcomes of all parties. The teaching should be implemented with respect to the most effective methods of learning for the individual, taking into account cultural, psychologic, physical, and cognitive limitations.

Surgical Interventions

Reconstructive Plastic Surgery

Reconstructive plastic surgery seeks to restore or improve function after trauma, disease, infection, congenital anomalies, or acquired defects while trying to approximate an aesthetic appearance.

Removal of Skin Cancers

The estimated number of new skin cancer cases diagnosed in 2012 was 2 million (National Cancer Institute [NCI], 2012). The three most common skin cancers are basal cell, squamous cell, and melanoma (McCance, 2012). Basal cell cancer accounts for approximately 70% of all skin cancers (Figure 22-6, *A*). If basal cell cancer is left untreated, it will grow locally, but rarely metastasizes (Box 22-1). Treated early, it may be cured by simple excision and closure (with pathologic diagnosis to ensure disease-free margins). The second most common form of cancer is squamous cell carcinoma. Squamous cell skin cancers are considered more aggressive (see Figure 22-6, *B*). Surgical treatment is the same as that for basal cell carcinomas. Melanoma accounts for the smallest percentage of skin cancers but it is treated much more aggressively because of its high mortality rate, with an estimated 9480 deaths to occur in 2013 (NCI, 2013) (see Figure 22-6, *C*). Excision of melanoma may involve sentinel node mapping and excision. Early diagnosis of melanoma is imperative to successful treatment (Evidence for Practice).

Procedural Considerations. Consideration must be given to the type of skin cancer to be excised and the anticipated closure technique. Simple excision and closure with adjacent tissue is the simplest technique, requiring a local plastic tray accompanied by skin markers and an ESU, and usually involving use of a local anesthetic with epinephrine. A simple excision may be performed with the patient administered a local or general anesthetic or after induction of sedation. If additional procedures will be performed (e.g., reconstruction with skin graft, flap, or sentinel node mapping), refer to those sections for additional procedural considerations.

Operative Procedure—Simple Excision

1. The site is marked, prepped, and draped.
2. The surgeon infiltrates the site with a local anesthetic.
3. The lesion is curetted or excised and may be sent for frozen section or pathologic diagnosis.
4. Hemostasis is obtained.
5. The surgeon closes the wound if necessary.

Mohs Surgery

Mohs surgery is a specialized excision used to treat basal and squamous cell skin cancers. The procedure involves excising the lesion layer by layer and examining each layer under the microscope until all the abnormal tissue is removed.

Procedural Considerations. Mohs surgery is usually completed on an ambulatory basis with the patient administered a local anesthetic. The procedure can be very time-consuming to accomplish, but it typically results in the preservation of the surrounding healthy tissue. Because the procedure is lengthy, patient preparation and comfort are essential to facilitate cooperation during the procedure. A minor plastic surgery set is required, along with fine (5-0 or 6-0) suture material.

Operative Procedure. Current procedures involve removal of all visible portions of the skin cancer lesion. A horizontal layer of tissue is removed and divided into sections that are color-coded with dyes. A map of the surgical site is then drawn. Frozen sections are immediately prepared and examined microscopically for any remaining tumor. If tumor is found, the location or locations are noted on the map and another layer of tissue is resected. The procedure is repeated as many times as necessary to completely remove the tumor. The patient may be referred to a plastic surgeon for reconstruction of the defect after completion of the Mohs procedure.

Burn Surgery

A majority of burns result from exposure to high temperatures, which injures the skin. Flame, scalding, or direct contact with a hot object may cause thermal skin injury. Similar destruction of skin can result from contact with chemicals such as acid or alkali or contact with an electrical current. The latter, however, often involves extensive destruction of the underlying tissue and physiologic systems in addition to the skin. Approximately 450,000 burn injuries receive medical treatment yearly; 40,000 patients are hospitalized in the United States for burn injuries, with 30,000 of those admitted to the 127 hospitals with specialized burn centers (American Burn Association [ABA], 2012).

Intact skin provides protection against the environment for all underlying tissues and organs. It aids in heat regulation, prevents water loss, and is the major barrier against bacterial invasion. The tissue injury resulting from a burn disrupts this normal protective

FIGURE 22-6 **A**, Basal cell carcinoma. **B,** Squamous cell carcinoma. **C,** Melanoma.

BOX 22-1

Important Trends for Skin Cancer

Incidence
More than 1 million cases per year, with the majority being the highly curable basal or squamous cell cancers, accounting for more than 50% of all cancers; not as common is the most serious malignant melanoma, with an estimated 76,250 cases per year.

Mortality
Total estimated deaths for 2012 were 9180 from malignant melanoma and 12,190 from other skin cancers.

Risk Factors
- Excessive exposure to ultraviolet radiation from the sun, including history of sunburns, tanning booths
- Fair complexion
- Occupational exposure to coal tar, pitch, creosote, arsenic compounds, and radium
- Exposure to human papillomavirus and human immunodeficiency virus
- Skin cancer negligible in African Americans because of heavy skin pigmentation

Warning Signals
Any unusual skin conditions, especially a change in the size or color of a mole or other darkly pigmented growth or spot; a sore that doesn't heal. Changes that occur over a month or so should be evaluated.

Prevention and Early Detection
Avoid sun when ultraviolet light is strongest (e.g., 10:00 AM to 3:00 PM); use sunscreen preparations, especially those containing ingredients such as *para*-aminobenzoic acid (PABA). Basal and squamous cell cancers often form a pale, waxlike, pearly nodule or a red, scaly, sharply outlined patch; melanomas are usually dark brown or black pigmentation; they start as small molelike growths that increase in size, change color, become ulcerated, and bleed easily from a slight injury.

Treatment
The four methods of treatment are excisional surgery, electrodesiccation (tissue destruction by heat), radiation therapy, and cryosurgery (tissue destruction by freezing). For malignant melanomas, wide and often deep excisions and removal of nearby lymph nodes are required.

Survival
For basal cell and squamous cell cancers, cure is virtually ensured with early detection and treatment. Malignant melanoma, however, is more likely than other skin cancers to spread to other parts of the body. The 5- and 10-year survival rates for people with melanoma are 91% and 89%, respectively.

Modified from American Cancer Society (ACS): *Cancer facts and figures 2012,* Atlanta, 2012, The Society; Nicol NH, Huether SE: Structure, function, and disorders of the integument. In Huether SE, McCance KL: *Understanding pathology,* ed 5, St Louis, 2012, Mosby.

EVIDENCE FOR PRACTICE

Melanoma Awareness, Prevention, and Detection

It is estimated that more than 76,000 men and women were diagnosed with melanoma in 2012, according to the American Cancer Society. Melanoma is more common in men than women, with 12,190 estimated deaths from melanoma in 2012. Although the exact cause of developing a melanoma is not known, certain risk factors have been identified:
- *Ultraviolet (UV) radiation:* Sunlight, tanning beds
- *Moles:* More than 50 = greater risk
- *Fair skin:* Fair skin, freckling, red or blond hair
- *Family history:* 10% have a relative with melanoma
- *Immune system compromise:* Taking antirejection medications after organ transplantation surgery
- *Age:* Increased risk in older adults
- *Gender:* Men more than women
- *Previous melanoma:* Increased risk for having another melanoma

Prevention
Limit UV radiation exposure:
1. Wear protective clothing (tight weave) and a hat with a broad brim.
2. Avoid too much sunlight; remember that it reflects off water, sand, concrete, and snow. Shade is good.
3. Use sunscreen—SPF 15 or higher (daily use); apply 20 to 30 minutes before sun exposure; reapply every 2 hours; protect your lips.
4. Do not forget your eyes—look for sunglasses with 99% UV absorption.
5. Stay away from tanning beds and lamps—try using self-tanning lotions.
6. Protect children with sunscreen—their skin is fragile; most damage to skin is acquired before the age of 18 years.
7. Take an inventory—know your moles and what they normally look like so you can detect changes if and when they occur.

Know Your A-B-C-D-Es
Asymmetry—one half of the lesion looks different from the other side.
Border irregularity—instead of a smooth edge, the border is ragged or irregular.
Color—the color is usually irregular as well; may have a number of different hues and colors.
Diameter—lesions larger than 6 mm have a greater chance of being a melanoma.
E—enlargement and elevation.

Melanoma Awareness, Prevention, and Detection—cont'd

Malignant melanomas. Note presence of "ABCDE" characteristics (*a*symmetry, irregular *b*order, variation in *c*olor, *d*iameter >6 mm, *e*nlargement and *e*levation). **A,** Superficial spreading melanoma. **B,** Nodular melanoma. **C,** Lentigo malignant melanoma.

Modified from American Cancer Society (ACS): *Cancer facts and figures 2012,* Atlanta, 2012, The Society.

function, resulting in local and systemic effects (Box 22-2). Burn patients are therefore some of the most acutely ill patients brought to the OR. The greater the degree of injury to the skin, expressed in percentage of total body surface area (BSA) and depth of burn, the more severe the injury. One method of measuring BSA in adults is by use of the "rule of nines" (Coffee, 2013) (Figure 22-7).

Partial-thickness (first- and second-degree) burns heal by regeneration of skin from dermal elements that remain intact. First-degree burns involve the epidermis, which appears pink or red; sunburn is usually a first-degree burn. Second-degree burns, also called partial-thickness burns, involve the epidermis and some of the dermis. Full-thickness (third-degree) burns (Figure 22-8) involve the epidermis, the entire dermis, and the subcutaneous tissues; they require skin grafting to heal because no dermal elements remain intact. Both partial- and full-thickness burns may require debridement of necrotic tissue (eschar) before healing can occur by skin regeneration or grafting. An allograft may be used to cover the burned area during the initial healing process. However, the allograft must be carefully tested for immunodeficiency diseases. A xenograft (e.g., pig skin) may also be used for covering the burned area.

BOX 22-2

Pathophysiology of Burn Injuries

Thermal and chemical injuries disrupt the normal protective function of the skin, causing local and systemic effects. The extent of these effects depends on the type, duration, and intensity of exposure to the causative agent. With electrical burns, heat is generated as the electrical current passes through body tissues, causing thermal burns along the path taken by the current. Local damage is marked by histamine release and severe vasoconstriction, followed in a few hours by vasodilation and increased capillary permeability, which allows plasma to escape into the wound. Damaged cells swell and platelets and leukocytes aggregate, causing thrombotic ischemia and escalating tissue damage. Systemic effects, which are caused by vascular changes and tissue loss, include hypovolemia, hyperventilation, increased blood viscosity, and suppression of the immune system. The severity of the burn determines the extent of local and systemic effects. Severity is judged by the depth of the burn and the quantity of tissue involved. The depth of the burn is classified by degree. First-degree (superficial) burns affect the epidermis only; second-degree burns (split thickness) affect the epidermis and dermis; third-degree burns (full thickness) affect all skin layers and extend to subcutaneous tissue, muscle, and nerves; fourth-degree burns involve all skin layers, plus bone. The percentage of body surface area (BSA) system of the American Burn Association classifies quantity as follows:

- *Minor burn:* Full-thickness burns over less than 2% of BSA; partial-thickness burns over less than 15% of BSA
- *Moderate burns:* Full-thickness burns over 2% to 10% of BSA; partial-thickness burns over less than 15% to 25% of BSA
- *Major burns:* Full-thickness burns over 10% or more of BSA; partial-thickness burns over 25% or more of BSA; any burn to face, head, hands, feet, or perineum; inhalation and electrical burns; burns complicated by trauma or other disease processes

Modified from Jeschke M et al: Burns. In Townsend CM et al, editors: *Sabiston textbook of surgery: the biological basis of modern practice*, ed 19, Philadelphia, 2012, Saunders.

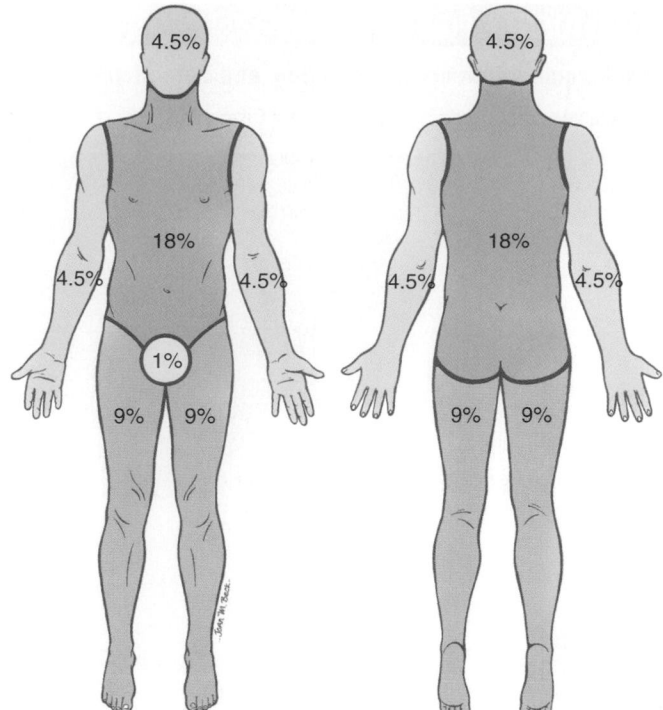

FIGURE 22-7 The "rule of nines." The amount of skin surface burned in an adult can be estimated by dividing the body into 11 areas of 9% each.

FIGURE 22-8 Full-thickness thermal injury.

Procedural Considerations.

The essentials of skin grafting are discussed later in this chapter. This section therefore deals only with the procedure for debridement of burn wounds.

A basic plastic instrument set is required, plus a knife dermatome, an ESU, topical thrombin solution, a pneumatic tourniquet for isolated extremity burns, and a topical antimicrobial agent of choice.

Because patients who have sustained burns are vulnerable to hypothermia from the loss of BSA, the perioperative nurse should ensure the temperature and humidity in the OR are increased and exposure is limited only to the areas related to the planned surgical event. Anesthesia is often induced while the patient is on the burn unit bed; transfer to the OR bed is done carefully and gently, with attention to maintaining the airway. Most burn patients arrive in the OR with dressings covering their wounds. The dressings are removed after the patient has been anesthetized to minimize pain and loss of body heat through the open burn wounds. Throughout the procedure, the temperature in the OR is constantly monitored to prevent hypothermia. The OR team caring for burn patients coordinates activities to prevent any delays in obtaining required equipment or supplies. The perioperative nurse will need to collaborate with the anesthesia provider in determining fluid replacement requirements. A variety of topical agents are used to dress wounds.

Perioperative nurses must be familiar with these agents and their uses (Surgical Pharmacology).

Operative Procedure

1. The surgeon excises only affected damaged nonviable tissue down to underlying muscle fascia.
2. An alternative method is tangential excision of the burn wound, which is performed with a knife dermatome. This type of excision is usually carried down only to the bleeding subcutaneous fat, rather than to fascia.
3. Hemostasis is obtained with the ESU or use of topical thrombin solution.
4. Dressings saturated with the topical antimicrobial agent of choice are applied.

Although skin grafting may be done at the time of wound debridement, it is usually performed several days later, particularly in extensive burns.

SURGICAL PHARMACOLOGY

Topical Medications Used in Burn Therapy

Medication and Category	Dosage and Route	Purpose and Action	Adverse Reactions	Nursing Implications
Petroleum-based antimicrobials (bacitracin, polymyxin B, Neosporin)	Topical (500 units/g): Apply 1 to 5 times a day as directed	Partial-thickness burns Provides barrier protection to wound Has broad-spectrum antimicrobial action against gram negative, gram-positive, and candida organisms Minor skin abrasions, superficial infections, prophylactic postsurgical wounds	Rash, burning, inflammation, pruritus	Gently cleanse wound prior to application; evaluate for hypersensitivity reaction.
Silver sulfadiazine (Silvadene)	Topical: Apply 1 or 2 times a day as directed	Deep partial to full-thickness burns Wound infection	Burning, stinging at treatment site; fungal superinfections may occur; toxic nephrosis possible with significant systemic absorption	Apply to cleansed, debrided burns using sterile gloves; keep burns covered with silver sulfadiazine at all times.
Mafenide acetate (Sulfamylon)	Topical cream (1 g): 2 or 3 times daily 11.1% cream: Penetrates thick eschar and cartilage 5% solution: Antimicrobial solution used to treat and prevent wound infections	Deep partial to full-thickness burns Wound infection Is bacteriostatic against gram-negative and gram-positive bacteria Diffuses through devascularized areas, is absorbed, and rapidly converts to a metabolite	Pain on application, metabolic acidosis, hypersensitivity rash, fungal growth	Discontinue when eschar no longer present; may need pain management during application.
Silver nitrate (5% solution)	Topical: Apply 2 or 3 times per week for 3 weeks	Deep partial to full-thickness burns Wound infection Has poor penetration of eschar Is bacteriostatic against gram-negative and gram-positive organisms	Skin discoloration, pain on application, staining of clothes and linens, decreases in electrolytes	Apply with cotton-tipped applicator; treat only affected areas.

Modified from Hodgson BB, Kizior RJ: *Saunders nursing drug handbook 2013*, St Louis, 2013, Saunders.

Excisional Debridement

Excisional debridement is the act of removing dead or devitalized tissue to promote healing. Plastic surgeons use debridement in conjunction with treatment of injuries, trauma, and infection. Additional information on wound debridement may be found in Chapter 9.

Treatment of Pressure Ulcers

Pressure ulcers result from prolonged compression of soft tissues overlying bony prominences (Figure 22-9). However, whether excessive pressure is sufficient to create an ulcer depends on the intensity and duration of the pressure as well as on tissue tolerance. Prevention is the key; avoiding pressure on bony prominences is most important in immobilized or paralyzed patients. Factors that contribute to pressure ulcer development are immobility, sensory and motor deficits, reduced circulation, anemia, edema, infection, moisture, shearing force, friction, and nutritional debilitation (McGrath and Pomeranz, 2012). The most common sites of

pressure ulcers are the sacrum, the ischium, the trochanter, the malleolus, and the heel; these are called decubitus ulcers. These ulcers are different from chronic ulcers such as vascular, diabetic, and neurogenic ulcers. Surgical interventions for pressure ulcers are usually based on ulcer staging (also referred to as *grading*). In stage I the ulcer involves the epidermis and has soft tissue swelling that is irregular and ill-defined; heat and erythema at the ulcer site are characteristic. A stage II ulcer involves the epidermis and dermis but not the subcutaneous fat. Stage III ulcers show full-thickness skin loss with injury to underlying tissue layers and may contain necrotic material. Thorough excisional debridement is performed, and IV antibiotic therapy is instituted. Although debrided stage III ulcers often heal on their own, surgical excision and closure may be done to prevent a lengthy spontaneous closure, which may result in a weak, unstable scar with resultant recurrence. Stage IV ulcers are the deepest, requiring more radical excisional debridement. Adequate soft tissue cover may be obtained by either split-thickness or full-thickness skin grafting or tissue flaps (Figure 22-10). Tissue expansion may be used when there is not enough tissue adjacent to the ulcer site to provide flap coverage.

The use of a CO_2 laser minimizes blood loss and possibly reduces infection rates in the presence of gross contamination. Although many techniques and flaps are surgical options, basic principles apply to all pressure ulcer closure procedures. The following procedure is for an adjacent flap.

FIGURE 22-9 Pressure ulcers often appear after blood flow to an area slows or is obstructed because of pressure on bony prominences. Infections often follow because lack of blood flow causes tissue damage or death.

Procedural Considerations. A basic plastic instrument set is required, as well as assorted sizes of osteotomes (straight and curved), a mallet, the Gigli saw and handle, assorted curettes, a Key periosteal elevator, a duckbill rongeur, bone wax, the dermatome of choice, the ESU, a sterile marking pen, and a closed-wound drainage system. The patient is positioned and draped so that the pressure ulcer, adjacent flap donor site, and skin graft donor site are well exposed.

Operative Procedure

1. The area to be excised and the local flap are outlined.
2. The surgeon excises the ulcer along with the underlying bony prominence. Avascular bone is debrided using rongeurs, rasps, osteotomes, and curettes.
3. Large drains are placed into the defect left by excision of the ulcer and beneath the flap.
4. The flap is sutured in place.
5. A split-thickness skin graft generally is used to resurface the flap donor site.
6. A stent dressing is placed over the skin graft, and gauze dressings or a plastic spray dressing is applied over the suture lines of the flap.

Skin and Tissue Grafting

Skin grafting provides an effective way to cover a wound if vascularity is adequate, infection is absent, and hemostasis is achieved. Skin from the donor site is detached from its blood supply and placed on the recipient site, where it develops a new blood supply from the base of the wound. Color match, contour, and durability of the graft are all considerations in selection of an appropriate donor area. Other types of grafts that are available for surgical reconstruction include bone, cartilage, nerve, tendon, and autologous fat grafts.

FIGURE 22-10 A, Rotational flap from abdomen for pressure sore coverage. **B,** Placement of flap. **C,** Completed coverage with flap placement.

Split-Thickness and Full-Thickness Skin Grafts. Skin grafts can be either split-thickness (STSGs) or full-thickness grafts (FTSGs) (Figure 22-11). An STSG (or partial-thickness graft) contains epidermis and only a portion of the dermis of the donor site; its thickness varies. Although this type of graft becomes vascularized more rapidly and the donor site heals more rapidly than a full-thickness graft, it may exhibit postgraft contraction, be minimally resistant to surface trauma, and be least like normal skin in texture, suppleness, pore pattern, hair growth, and other characteristics. An STSG may be meshed (Figure 22-12); meshed grafts can expand to many times their original size. Meshing allows the graft to be placed on an irregular recipient area; however, its appearance may be aesthetically undesirable. An FTSG contains both epidermis and dermis; any remaining subcutaneous tissue is trimmed before the FTSG is applied to the graft site. The advantages of this type of graft are that it causes minimal contracture, can be used in areas of flexion, has a greater ability to withstand trauma, can add tissue where a loss has occurred or where padding is required, and is aesthetically more acceptable than an STSG. The donor site can be closed primarily, leaving a minimal defect.

The donor site for an STSG heals by regeneration of epithelium from dermal elements that remain intact. Thus only a dressing is

FIGURE 22-11 Split-thickness and full-thickness skin grafts.

placed over this donor site. Because no dermal elements remain when an FTSG is taken, this donor site does not heal spontaneously. It heals either when the wound edges of the donor site are sutured together (primary closure) or when an STSG is applied over it. A scar remains at the donor site of a skin graft; therefore, donor sites that are covered by clothing are generally chosen.

For a graft to survive, the vascularity of the recipient area must be adequate, contact between the graft and recipient bed must be maintained, and the graft-bed unit must be adequately immobilized.

Color, temperature, signs of infection, blanching of the skin, excessive pain and discomfort, edema, vasoconstriction, and venous congestion should be noted and any change documented and reported to the surgeon.

A stent or tie-over dressing is often placed over a skin graft (Figure 22-13). This exerts even pressure, ensuring good contact between graft and recipient site. It also eliminates potential shearing forces at the graft and recipient site interface that might disrupt new blood vessels growing into the graft.

Procedural Considerations. A plastic local procedure instrument set is required, with the addition of a dermatome of choice, a skin mesher, sterile tongue blades, mineral oil, and a sterile marking pen. The patient is positioned so that both donor and recipient sites are well exposed. Both areas are prepped and draped to maintain adequate exposure and mobility, as required.

Operative Procedure

1. The recipient site is prepared as necessary. This step may involve excision of a benign or malignant skin tumor, debridement of an open wound, or release of a scar contracture.
2. Careful planning and marking before harvesting the graft from the recipient site are essential. Patterns matching intended recipient site and the donor site are outlined with a sterile marking pen.
3. STSGs are harvested with a knife dermatome or powered dermatome of the surgeon's choice (Figure 22-14).
4. Counted soft goods moistened in normal saline, an antibiotic solution, or a solution of 20 mg of phenylephrine HCl (Neo-Synephrine) per 1000 mL of normal saline may be applied to the donor sites to aid hemostasis. Medication labels indicating

FIGURE 22-12 A, Split-thickness skin is meshed and used to cover a marginal wound. Minimal expansion is used, and the holes provide drainage. **B,** Appearance of the graft after healing.

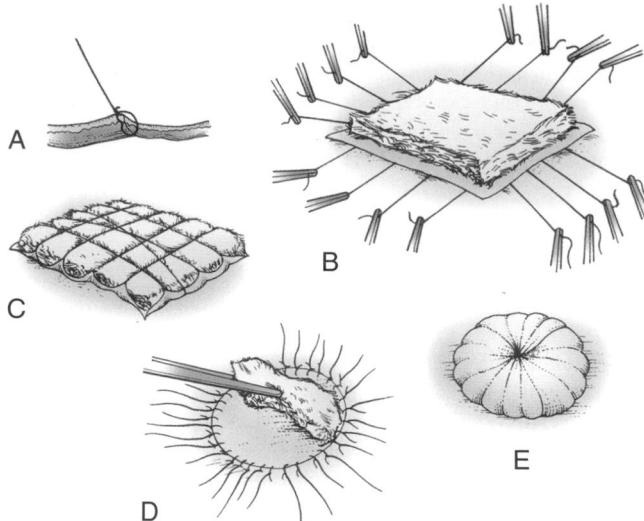

FIGURE 22-13 A, Method of fixation of skin graft to edges of wound. **B,** Nonadherent dressing is applied over skin graft, on top of which is placed a generous pad of acrylic fiber. **C,** Long ends of suture are tied over fiber to produce area of pressure between graft and base. **D,** Similar dressing is applied to circular graft. **E,** Long suture ends are tied over circular graft (often called *stent dressing*).

FIGURE 22-14 Harvesting a split-thickness skin graft (STSG) with the Humby knife.

strength are placed on all solutions to further identify all solutions on the sterile field. The soft goods are removed, the count reconciled, and the donor site covered with the surgeon's preference, which could include Biobrane, xeroform, scarlet red, or OpSite.

5. If the graft is to be meshed, it is now applied to the skin mesh carrier.

6. The scrub person, who may be a registered nurse or surgical technologist, should ensure that the graft is kept on the carrier and covered with moist gauze sponges to prevent drying and inadvertent loss of the graft. Meshed skin should not be removed from its carrier until it is applied directly to the recipient site. Whether applied as a sheet or meshed, the STSG may be sutured

or stapled with a skin stapler. Nonadherent gauze is usually applied as the first layer of dressing over a graft. Moist dressings should be applied to all meshed grafts to prevent desiccation and loss of the graft.

7. Fat adherent to the graft is trimmed. The graft is applied to the recipient site and usually sutured at the edges, and these sutures are left long to tie over a stent dressing. Blood clots beneath the graft are removed by saline irrigation before the dressing is applied.

Composite Graft. Composite grafts are composed of skin and underlying tissues that are completely separated from the blood supply of the donor site and transplanted to another area of the body. The survival of a composite graft depends on ingrowth of new blood vessels from the recipient site around the periphery of the graft. Therefore, composite grafts are usually small so that no portion of the graft is more than 1 cm from its periphery. An example of compound tissues used as composite grafts is hair transplants, composed of skin, fat, and hair follicles, which are used to treat male pattern baldness. The term *composite* thus indicates a defect that requires a graft be transferred to the area to meet more than one type of tissue deficiency.

Procedural Considerations. A plastic local instrument set is required, plus a sterile marking pen. The patient is positioned, prepped, and draped such that adequate exposure of both donor and recipient sites is achieved.

Operative Procedure

1. When feasible, the surgeon makes a pattern of the recipient site and transfers it to the donor site.

2. The surgeon excises the composite graft and closes the donor site by approximating its skin edges or leaving it unsutured if appropriate.

3. Meanwhile, the composite graft is kept in a moist sponge until it is sutured to the edges of the recipient site.

4. Dressings of choice are applied to the composite graft and donor site.

Replacement of Lost or Absent Tissue

When coverage for a defect cannot be achieved through skin grafting, plastic surgeons rely on other techniques to replace tissue. Just as the flap has evolved, other techniques for tissue restoration through biologic tissue engineering have also evolved. In 1987, the National Science Foundation bioengineering panel defined that tissue engineering was "the application of the principles and methods of engineering and the life sciences toward the development of biologic substitutes to restore, maintain, or improve function. The use of biologic dressings as well as scaffolds, stem cell therapy and gene therapy are a few examples of tissue engineering, in which new tissues are created rather than transferred" (Leona and Phillips, 2012). A discussion of flap techniques follows.

Flaps. The term *flap* refers to tissue that is detached from one area of the body and transferred to the recipient area with either part or all of its original blood supply intact. Because flaps carry their own blood supply, they generally are used to cover recipient sites that have poor vascularity and full-thickness tissue loss. Flaps are used for reconstruction or wound closure. They are useful for covering exposed bone, tendon, or nerve. They may be used if surgery through the wound may be necessary at a later date to repair underlying structures. Flaps containing skin and subcutaneous tissue retain more properties of normal skin and shrink less than skin grafts. Flaps, however, have some disadvantages, such as bulky appearance, failure to match tissue of the recipient site in texture or color, and the possibility of requiring multiple operations and prolonged hospitalization.

Flaps may be classified according to blood supply. *Random pattern flaps* consist of skin and subcutaneous tissue vascularized by random perforators with limited length-to-width ratio. *Axial pattern flaps* have a well-defined arteriovenous supply along the long axis; they can be comparatively long in relation to width. Flaps may also be classified according to position or how they are rotated after elevation. *Advancement flaps* are cut and advanced to reconstruct a nearby defect. *Transposition flaps* are advanced along an axis that forms an angle to the flap's original position. *Rotation flaps* are similar to transposition flaps but are semicircular and rotate along a greater axis. *Island flaps* of isolated sections of skin and subcutaneous tissue are tunneled beneath the skin to new sites. *Pedicle flaps* were the forerunners of muscle and musculocutaneous flaps. These consist of skin and underlying muscle; they are very mobile and can be rotated into distant defects. *Free flaps* are actually a form of tissue transplantation. Using microvascular techniques, a defined amount of skin, muscle, or bone can be isolated, totally detached, and reattached at the recipient site by microvascular anastomoses between recipient site blood vessels and the major vessels that supply the flap. The vascular pedicle may contain functional nerves, yielding sensory flaps to provide protective sensation or motor flaps to restore function. Bone and joints may be transplanted as free flaps, as in the case of toe-to-thumb site transfers.

Procedural Considerations. The perioperative nurse should consult with the surgeon in advance of the procedure to determine the donor site, the patient's position(s), and the surgical sequence of the procedure. Generally the surgical site and flap area are marked preoperatively with the patient in a functional position because landmarks and aesthetics are influenced by surgical positioning. If marking is undertaken on the anesthetized and surgically positioned patient, inaccuracies in tissue placement could occur. Flap procedures may involve two teams of surgeons working simultaneously: one raising the flap and closing the resulting defect, and the other preparing the site, repositioning the flap in its new site, and, in the case of a free flap, microscopically reanastomosing the blood vessels. For any lengthy procedure, a Foley catheter, intermittent pneumatic compression device, warming units, and positioning aids that are safe for the skin are needed. Skin grafts are sometimes used to achieve closure of the flap donor site; if this is anticipated, then the nurse and scrub person should add appropriate instrumentation for harvesting a skin graft. A plastic instrument set and surgeon's preference of dermatome and skin mesher should be available as well as any other equipment requests.

Operative Procedure—Advancement, Transpositional, Rotational, Island, and Pedicle Flaps

1. The recipient site is prepared in the same manner as for a skin graft.
2. Patterns matching the recipient and donor sites are drawn or marked.
3. The surgeon incises, elevates, and transfers the flap to the recipient site.
4. The edges of the flap are sutured to the periphery of the recipient site.
5. The surgeon repairs the flap donor site by approximating the skin edges directly or by covering the defect with a skin graft or another flap.
6. Drains are usually placed under flaps.

7. Dressings are applied with particular attention given to immobilization of the flap, which may require a stockinette, padding, or plaster of paris.

NOTE: Before a pedicle flap is detached from the donor site, the surgeon may want to determine the adequacy of circulation within the flap. One method to check circulation involves placing rubber-shod clamps across the base of the pedicle and injecting sodium fluorescein intravenously. After 10 minutes have elapsed, all lights in the OR are turned off and a Wood lamp is held over the flap to determine the presence or absence of fluorescence within the flap. Fluorescein may be injected locally for the same purpose.

Operative Procedure—Free Flaps. See Operative Procedure for free TRAM flap described under Reconstructive Breast Surgery.

Reconstructive Breast Surgery

According to the U.S Department of Labor (DOL), The Women's Health and Cancer Rights Act of 1998 (WHCRA) mandates financial coverage of all breast reconstruction–related procedures (DOL, 2012).

The loss of a breast because of cancer may have a devastating effect on a woman. Fortunately the option of breast reconstruction is available to virtually any woman who loses her breast to cancer. Reconstruction has the ability to offer hope and a return to wholeness and normalcy. Normal, of course, is subjective, and although breasts may be reconstructed, there is a wide range of outcomes, and it must be stressed that breast reconstruction is not a onetime surgery. Revisions are the rule, not the exception. Techniques and options continue to evolve and improve, and women have many options. Breast reconstruction may be offered at one of many times during this process—initially, at the time of mastectomy; before or after adjunct therapy; or even many years later. The important fact is that each woman and her oncologic status are individual, so the decision for reconstruction must be made according to the woman's wishes coupled with her most favorable circumstances. Reconstruction has no known effect on the recurrence of breast cancer. Breast reconstruction options include alloplastic (artificial materials such as breast implants), autogenous (flaps), or a combination of both. Flaps may be pedicle-based or free flaps, requiring microsurgical techniques for their reconstruction.

Breast Reconstruction Using Tissue Expanders and Permanent Implants. Mastectomy may leave a shortage of skin that prevents creation of a breast mound. For these patients, extra tissue can be created locally with the use of tissue expanders (Figure 22-15). Tissue expansion is a technique used to stretch normal tissue that is adjacent to a defect, mechanically creating redundancy of normal tissue to correct the defect. For breast reconstruction, the expander resembles the shape of a breast prosthesis. The expander has a metal-backed, self-sealing silicone valve at its dome. Another type of expander used less frequently has a small, dome-shaped reservoir with a fill tube that is positioned subcutaneously at a distance from the expander but connected to it. Following surgery, the tissue expander is gradually filled with percutaneous injections of normal saline during routine office visits. The expander may be filled as often as weekly, or it may remain unused until chemotherapy or radiation is completed. Once the tissue expander is filled to the appropriate volume, it may be removed and replaced with a permanent reconstructive mammary prosthesis, either saline or silicone, as an ambulatory surgical procedure. Silicone can be used for breast augmentation for patients older than 22 years. If silicone is chosen,

FIGURE 22-15 Tissue expanders are inflatable plastic reservoirs of various shapes and volumes that are implanted under the skin. The skin over the expander is stretched during a period of several weeks as the expander is gradually filled by percutaneous injection of saline into an incorporated part of the remote-fill port. Expanders are useful for breast reconstruction.

FIGURE 22-16 While discussing options in the surgeon's office, samples of tissue expanders, textured and smooth saline and silicone implants, are shown to patients for their selection.

both the surgeon and the patient must participate in an adjunct clinical study at this time; the patient may opt out. Another option is the use of combination tissue expander and breast prosthesis, which remains in place once the desired amount of saline has been sequentially added. The benefit of this prosthesis is the ability to add or remove saline in case an adjustment proves necessary. The recent introduction of allografts helps to achieve better shape and fast expansion and is less painful. A direct-to-implant or "one step" approach can make it possible for some patients to undergo immediate reconstruction of the breast. A mastectomy that conserves a large amount of breast skin is best for this approach. The permanent saline or silicone implant is placed behind the pectoralis major muscle. AlloDerm (collagen sheeting) is placed from below to provide coverage for the implant. Sometimes nipple sparing can also be accomplished depending on the location of the breast mass. Planning between the plastic and general surgeon preoperatively will determine the best procedure to be performed.

Procedural Considerations. A basic plastic set may be used with the addition of fiberoptic breast retractors. Positioning is usually supine with both arms extended on armboards. Both inframammary folds are marked preoperatively, and both sides of the chest should be prepped and draped. The breast shape expander and sizers are supplied in a sterile package from the manufacturer and are available in a variety of sizes. If permanent saline or silicone implants are used, they will be ordered by the surgeon ahead of time. Meticulous sterile technique is required, and the expander/implant should be handled as little as possible. This procedure may be performed immediately following mastectomy or at a later date. Drains are usually placed to prevent hematoma and seroma formation, the latter of which could cause rotation or malposition of the tissue expander. If a surgical bra is used, care must be taken that it is not too tight and does not compromise circulation to the skin flaps. A breast band may also be used to hold the implant down and in place postoperatively.

Operative Procedure

1. Skin flaps are assessed for adequate blood supply, and then the pectoralis fascia is incised along its lateral border. The surgeon creates a submuscular pocket for the temporary expander or permanent implant by undermining the muscle over the sternal attachments and down over the lower ribs.

2. Allograft material may be used to bridge the gap created from the elevated pectoral and serratus muscles to the inframammary fold.

3. The tissue expander is tested before insertion for watertight integrity. The surgeon inspects the implant for defects.

4. After hemostasis is achieved, the surgeon checks the expander for integrity and then inserts it into the pocket. Muscle coverage is assessed, and if adequate the reservoir is positioned subcutaneously and connected, the wound is closed, and the expander is filled with sterile saline solution until slight blanching of the skin is achieved. The amount is recorded on the patient record.

Second-Stage Tissue Expander Breast Reconstruction. Once the tissue expander has been expanded to the desired size, the patient is taken back to surgery for the next stage of her breast reconstruction. This is a relatively minor procedure in which the tissue expander is deflated and replaced with a permanent mammary prosthesis (Figures 22-16 and 22-17, *A* and *B*). At this time, if there is asymmetry of the contralateral breast, surgery may be performed to create bilateral symmetry. The patient may require correction of breast ptosis through mastopexy, with or without the addition of a breast implant; alternatively, a reduction mammoplasty may be needed on the opposite breast. This procedure is usually performed on an outpatient basis in which the patient is administered a general anesthetic.

Breast Reconstruction Using Myocutaneous Flaps. Flaps are described by the types of tissue they contain, the blood supply of the tissues, and the method by which the flaps are moved from the donor site to the recipient site. Options may include the latissimus dorsi, and transverse rectus abdominis myocutaneous (TRAM) flap procedures, which are detailed in the following sections. An additional option is the superior gluteal artery perforator (SGAP) flap, which has become more refined. Some women choose to use their own tissue for reconstruction because they prefer what they consider more realistic, supple breasts that would not need to be replaced or removed as is possible with implants. The SGAP flap does require microsurgical skills and is not offered at all institutions. Factors for

FIGURE 22-17 A, Tissue expander is used to create extra tissue after mastectomy so a breast mound can be created. **B,** Postoperative result after tissue expander replaced with breast prosthesis.

FIGURE 22-18 Latissimus dorsi flap for breast reconstruction. **A,** Preoperative view. **B,** Healed bilateral back incisions. **C,** Postoperative view with nipple reconstruction.

choosing reconstructive options include the patient's size and availability of appropriate abdominal or gluteal tissue. Even very thin patients generally have enough skin and fat for the SGAP procedure, and the consistency of the buttock fat (thicker than abdominal) provides the more supple result. Positioning is especially challenging, and some operative efficiency may be achieved by using two OR beds (Edwards et al, 2009).

Latissimus Dorsi Flap. The latissimus dorsi myocutaneous flap is used during reconstruction of the breast after mastectomy. This procedure may be staged. Because the flap consists of skin fat and muscle, it is described as *myocutaneous*. This flap is used when significant tissue deficiency occurs after a mastectomy or when TRAM flap reconstruction is not an option. The latissimus dorsi muscle is a wide, flat muscle extending over the midthoracic portion of the back and inserting into the humerus. Its blood supply comes from the thoracodorsal artery and from perforators of the upper lumbar arteries and intercostal vessels. This rich vascularity allows the surgeon flexibility in orienting and positioning the flap to the pattern of the deficit on the anterior chest wall. Latissimus dorsi flaps are usually used in conjunction with a reconstructive breast prosthesis, in order to create a more natural breast mound (Figure 22-18).

Procedural Considerations. The surgeon marks the donor site of the latissimus dorsi with its skin island, along with the intended recipient site, before surgery with the patient in a sitting position. In the OR the patient is placed in a lateral position, donor side up, with the arm extended and safely supported. The perioperative nurse should assemble extra padding and positioning aids in

preparation for the patient's arrival. After the donor muscle has been mobilized and exteriorized through the area of defect, the back incision is closed and the patient repositioned supine with the arm extended on an armboard. Instrumentation should include a basic plastic instrument set, fiberoptic breast retractor, vascular instruments, sterile marking pens, suction, and long tissue forceps and scissors, and a Doppler probe should be available.

Operative Procedure

1. Initially the island of skin is incised transversely across the back, being careful to ensure that a bra or bathing suit will cover the resulting scar.
2. The surgeon frees the muscle, subcutaneous fat, and fascia from the overlying skin by undermining so that part or all of the muscle may be mobilized.
3. The skin island and the muscle are then tunneled under the axilla to the chest wall. The insertion of the muscle on the humerus and accompanying blood vessels are left undisturbed. The latissimus dorsi muscle fills the space left by the missing pectoralis muscle.
4. The island of skin is oriented to the recipient site, and the surgeon sutures both into place.
5. A permanent mammary prosthesis is placed under the muscle before suturing to reconstruct the breast mound.
6. The wound is drained via a closed-wound drainage system
7. The surgeon may reconstruct the nipple-areola complex by sharing the nipple on the unaffected side or by using groin, adjacent tissue, thigh, or auricular tissue. This can be done at the time of reconstruction or at a later date as a minor procedure with the patient administered a local anesthetic.
8. Dressings are applied. If a surgical bra is used, care must be taken not to compromise blood supply to the flap.

Transverse Rectus Abdominis Myocutaneous Flap. TRAM flaps are pedicle-based flaps used for breast reconstruction. The rectus muscle is the broad, wide abdominal muscle that reaches from under the ribs to the pubis, and either one or both sides of the muscle may be used for reconstruction. The blood supply (superior epigastric artery and vein) is carried within the muscle pedicle. The muscle along with its pedicle is severed at its most distal origins and pulled through a subcutaneous tunnel to the chest to form a breast. Although this procedure has the added benefit of an abdominoplasty, if there is inadequate abdominal tissue the patient may require a small mammary prosthesis.

The several types of TRAM techniques are based on blood supply, but the procedure still follows a basic format. As with other types of breast reconstruction, TRAM flaps may be performed immediately following mastectomy or planned for a later stage in the patient's recuperative phase.

Procedural Considerations. The surgeon marks the surgical landmarks preoperatively with the patient in a standing position. A basic plastic instrument set is used as for the latissimus dorsi flap. The patient is positioned supine with arms extended on armboards. Positioning the patient for this procedure is particularly difficult because of the need to promote closure of the abdominal wound, support circulation to the flap, and protect the patient from injury. The OR bed is often flexed; additional padding of the lower extremities may be required. The skin prep should extend from the lower neck to midthigh.

Operative Procedure

1. The surgeon excises the skin from the mastectomy scar and makes the abdominal incision. The abdominal flap is dissected with care being taken not to shear the skin and subcutaneous tissue from its underlying muscle attachments (Figure 22-19, *A*).
2. The transverse rectus abdominis muscle is divided from its inferior-most attachment (see Figure 22-19, *B*).
3. The flap is rotated and passed through to its new location on the chest wall (see Figure 22-19, *C* and *D*) and sutured medially;

the thinnest portion of the flap is superior and medial, and the thickest portion is inferior and lateral.

4. Because of the amount of tissue available, an implant is often unnecessary (see Figure 22-19, *E*).

Free Transverse Rectus Abdominis Myocutaneous Flap. The free TRAM flap is indicated when there is concern about the absence of one or both of the rectus muscles following the procedure or when there are concerns about vascularity, either with the pedicle used in the standard TRAM flap or with any other factors that may compromise vascularity of the flap. A newer technique of the free TRAM (deep inferior epigastric perforator procedure) has the advantage of not requiring the entire rectus muscle, because only a small portion of the rectus muscle that carries a segment of the deep inferior epigastric perforator vessels is needed to move with the fat and skin to its new location. It is also used when the buttock tissue (superior gluteal perforator flap) is planned to replace the absent breast or breasts.

Procedural Considerations. Care of the patient undergoing a free TRAM procedure is identical to that of patients undergoing pedicle TRAM flaps with the addition of the surgical microscope. Refer to the Procedural Considerations under TRAM. Two surgical teams may be used—one for harvesting and one for site preparation. Meticulous attention must be paid to positioning and protection from pressure injuries because of the length of the procedure. During the preoperative verification process, the perioperative nurse should determine if the patient has made preoperative autologous blood donations and if the appropriate blood work has been performed.

Operative Procedure

1. The site is prepped, and the recipient site blood vessels are identified for anastomosis.
2. The surgeon dissects and isolates the recipient vessels.
3. Donor vessels are selected based on pedicle length, and the flap is prepared.
4. The anesthesia provider administers heparin to prevent clotting and vasospasm.
5. When the recipient vessels are ready, the surgeon severs the flap.
6. The microscope is positioned in place and draped with a sterile drape.
7. The free flap is transferred to the recipient site, and the surgeon anastomoses the blood vessels.
8. The breast mound is shaped and sutured in place.
9. The donor site is closed, covering with a skin graft if necessary.

Nipple Reconstruction. Although nipple reconstruction can be performed at the time of breast reconstruction or replacement of the tissue expander with a mammary prosthesis, some surgeons prefer to wait and let the new breast tissues "settle" and mature to reconstruct the new nipple in the most accurate anatomic position. Generally this may take a minimum of 6 to 8 weeks. Tissue for the new nipple can be recruited locally by raising a flap or be grafted from the opposite nipple. The areola is reconstructed with skin grafting from the groin, buttock crease, or auricle (Figure 22-20). The areolar skin may be tattooed to create a very pleasing nipple-areolar complex (Figure 22-21, *A* and *B*).

Microsurgery

The term *microsurgery* was coined on experimental anastomosis of 1- to 2-mm vessels at the American College of Surgeons meeting in 1960 by Jacobsen and Suarez (Pederson, 2011). Reconstructive microsurgical procedures include, but are not limited to, replantation of amputated body parts, repair of facial nerves, repair of

FIGURE 22-19 Transverse rectus abdominis myocutaneous (TRAM) flap for postmastectomy breast reconstruction (see text for procedure).

lacerated nerves and blood vessels, treatment of extensive trauma to extremities and hands, reconstruction following removal of extensive cancers, and female-to-male transsexual reassignment. Today's surgeons skilled in microsurgery can successfully anastomose the ends of a vessel measuring less than 1 mm in diameter. The surgeon's use of an operating microscope or loupes for microsurgical procedures depends on the procedure to be performed, condition of the tissue, and personal preference. Endoscopic harvesting of tissues for microsurgical grafting is possible in some circumstances. Factors contributing to the success of microsurgery include (1) the individual and collective experiences of the surgical team and the members' ability to work together, relieving each other as necessary during long operations; (2) the surgeon's knowledge of the physiology of the microcirculation; (3) many hours of practice in the

laboratory by the surgical team; and (4) the availability of proper microscopes, microvascular instruments, and microvascular suture.

Replantation of Amputated Body Part. Replantation is an attempt to reattach a completely amputated digit or other body part. Revascularization is the procedure performed on incomplete amputations, when the part remains attached to the body by skin, artery, vein, or nerve. Good candidates for replantation are those with the following amputations: (1) thumb, (2) multiple digits, (3) distal portion of hand at palm level, (4) wrist or forearm, (5) elbow and above the elbow, and (6) almost any body part of a child.

The success of digital replantation depends primarily on the microsurgical repair of one digital artery and two digital veins. Replantation of an amputated part is ideally performed within 4 to

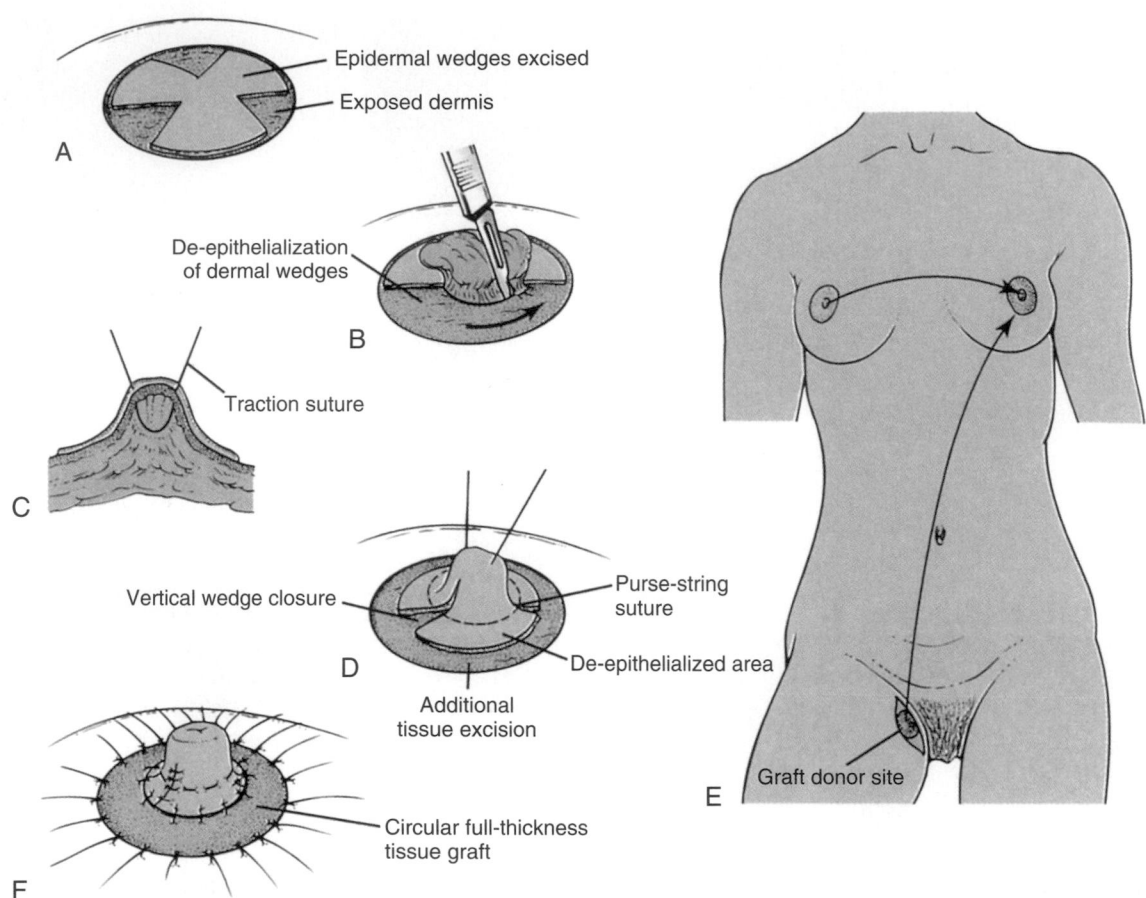

FIGURE 22-20 A, Circumferential demarcation of the nipple periphery with removal of dermal wedges. **B,** Dermal wedges are de-epithelialized from the rim toward the center. **C,** A traction suture is used to elevate the central future nipple tip. **D,** Traction is applied to the future nipple tip as the wedges are approximated to create a permanent projected surface. A purse-string suture is placed, and excess tissue is excised. **E,** Possible full-thickness donor site areolar color match may be found in the labial folds. **F,** The donor graft is measured, cut, and secured to the dermal ring of the neonipple-areolar complex.

6 hours after injury, but success has been reported up to 24 hours after injury if the amputated part has been cooled. Proper care of the amputated body part or parts before surgery is vital to successful replantation. The ultimate aim of replantation is the restitution of function beyond that provided by a prosthesis.

Procedural Considerations. A regional anesthetic is usually given to replantation patients if the anticipated length of surgery permits. Because of the length of these surgeries (12 to 16 hours), positioning is important. The perioperative nurse ensures the OR bed and armboards are carefully padded with pressure-reducing materials to support the supine patient. The surgeon may request the room temperature increased before the patient arrives because the warm room will reduce vasoconstriction in the extremities. A warming device, such as a forced–air warming blanket, is usually applied to maintain the patient's core body temperature. The surgeon usually brings the amputated part to the OR before the patient arrives to ensure ample time for preparation of the amputated part for replantation. The amputated body part should be maintained by wrapping it in saline-soaked gauze, placing it in an occlusive bag, and immersing it in a container of iced saline. If radiographs of the amputated body part and amputation site have not been taken before the patient's arrival in the OR, the perioperative nurse should arrange for these to be taken. Radiographic films are crucial to determine bone trauma and loss.

The hand drape (described later in this paragraph) can be applied to either upper or lower extremities, as required by the surgical procedure. Before a hand drape is placed, a pneumatic tourniquet cuff is often applied to the upper arm over padding. The patient is positioned supine on the OR bed, with the affected arm extended and supported on a hand table. While an assistant holds the patient's arm with both hands around the tourniquet cuff, the skin prep solution is applied from fingertips to tourniquet cuff. Care is taken to keep the cuff dry and free of solution. Then two folded barrier sheets are used to cover the hand table. The first sheet is placed with the folded edge nearest the patient (thus forming a cuff). A double-thickness, 4-inch stockinette is used to cover the extremity, and the edge is rolled over the tourniquet. The upper arm and upper half of the body are covered by a folded sheet, with the folded edge placed across the part of the stockinette that covers the tourniquet cuff. A small, non-perforating towel clamp that grasps the edge of the folded top sheet, the stockinette, and the edge of the cuff of the bottom sheet is placed on each side of the arm. This excludes the tourniquet cuff from the sterile field. The remainder of the body is covered with one or two additional sheets. A commercially prepared extremity drape that has an aperture incorporated into the drape also may be used.

Instrumentation includes a plastic hand instrument set, microvascular instruments, a Kirschner wire driver, Kirschner wires, an operating microscope, and a bipolar ESU.

A

B

FIGURE 22-21 A, Breast nipple reconstruction. *1* and *2* represent wing flaps raised from side and wrapped around *3;* the central flap was raised superiorly; *4* represents areolar skin created with skin grafted either from pigmented groin skin or from opposite areolar skin by tattooing. **B,** Areolar tattoo.

Operative Procedure

1. The surgeon shortens the bone ends to eliminate tension on vascular anastomoses to be done later; the bone is stabilized by means of internal fixation with Kirschner wires.
2. Flexor and extensor tendon repairs are usually performed next.
3. The digital nerves are repaired with the aid of loupes or the operating microscope.
4. Using microsurgical instruments and techniques, the surgeon repairs the two digital veins followed by repair of one digital artery. If ischemic time has been prolonged, digital vessel repair may precede repair of tendons and nerves.
5. The skin is sutured.
6. A bulky supportive hand dressing is applied. A posterior splint may be placed.

Toe-to-Hand Transfer. The reconstructive procedure of toe-to-hand transfer involves surgical removal of a single toe or multiple toes and anastomosis of the vessels of the toes to those on the hand to restore finger and thumb functions. It is lengthy surgery (12 to 16 hours) and entails a two-team approach; one team is at the foot for toe removal, and one team is at the recipient site—the hand.

Procedural Considerations. The patient is placed in the supine position on the OR bed. The anesthesia provider administers an anticoagulation regimen during the anastomosis procedure. Two tourniquets are needed—one on the thigh of the operative foot and one on the operative arm. Both extremities are separately prepped and draped. Instrumentation includes a plastic hand set, microvascular instruments, power Kirschner wire driver, and Kirschner wires. Additional equipment includes the operating microscope, two tourniquet power sources, two bipolar ESUs, a sterile marking pen, and an Esmarch bandage.

Operative Procedure

1. The surgeon preparing the hand determines adequate blood flow and vessel location on the thumb site (Figure 22-22, *A*). This may prevent a needless amputation of the toe.
2. Appropriate skin flaps are incised to expose the veins on the dorsum of the hand and clamped with vessel microclips.
3. The radial artery or its branches are dissected out and prepared for anastomosis.
4. The surgeon locates and transfixes the flexor and extensor pollicis longus tendons.
5. The bone at the base of the thumb is prepared for the toe.
6. The nerves to the thumb are dissected out with adequate length for suturing without tension.
7. Using a racket-shaped incision the surgeon circumscribes the toe (see Figure 22-22, *B*). Next, the veins are isolated through the dorsal aspect and clamped with vessel microclips.
8. The extensor tendon is dissected proximally and transected over the base of the metatarsal.
9. The dorsalis pedis artery is dissected to the digital vessels with ligation of all branches of that vessel to prepare for the anastomosis.
10. On the plantar surface the digital nerves and flexor tendons are transected at levels of adequate length for anastomosis (see Figure 22-22, *C*).
11. The surgeon transects the toe at the level previously determined for adequate length of the thumb.
12. The toe vessels are anastomosed microsurgically to the thumb vessels. The toe is attached to the thumb area by Kirschner wires (see Figure 22-22, *D*).

An aesthetic and functionally effective hand can be achieved through this procedure (see Figure 22-22, *E*).

Reconstructive Maxillofacial Surgery

The need for maxillofacial surgery results from blunt or penetrating trauma, disease, or congenital anomaly. Regardless of the cause, the principles are the same: establishment of preinjury/predisease/normal anatomic dental occlusion, anatomic reduction, stabilization of the fracture, and healing for functional results. The technique and approach must be individualized to optimize the visual reduction (or reconstruction) of the procedure as well as minimize facial scarring and nerve injury, whether it be a mandibular free flap tissue and bone reconstruction or open reduction and internal fixation of any number and combination of facial fractures. In addition to midface fractures, other common facial fractures include nasal, orbital (blow-out) floor, zygomatic, and mandibular fractures.

Procedural Considerations for Maxillofacial Surgery. The perioperative nurse should ask the surgeon about the precise injuries and the expected surgical treatment plan: open or closed reduction; intraoral or extraoral approach; the order of multiple procedures; need for intraoperative x-rays; and type, number, and sizes of screws and compression plates to be placed if rigid fixation is to be used. Orbital fractures may require alloplastic implant material. Wire is used less frequently for immobilization because of the greater degree of stability afforded by plating systems. The patient's head should be immobilized and stabilized in a gel-type head ring; the position

FIGURE 22-22 Toe-to-hand transfer. **A,** Preoperative appearance of hand. **B,** Harvest of toe. **C,** Identification of vessels and nerves. **D,** Transfer of toe to thumb site. **E,** Postoperative view of toe-to-thumb site transfer.

is almost always supine. Both eyes should be protected, and care must be taken not to displace endotracheal tubes. Instrumentation needs include a plastic surgery set, periosteal elevators, power drill for plating systems, bone hooks, Rowe disimpaction forceps (for maxillary fractures), an ESU, sterile marking pens, and suction. For application of arch bars, the nurse should assemble arch bars, wires, elastics, wire cutters, wire twisters, and dull retractors for good exposure of the teeth. A set of wire cutters should be sent to PACU with patient and kept at the bedside in the event emergent access to the patient's airway becomes necessary.

Reduction of Nasal Fracture.
Usually a closed reduction of the bony nasal fragments is performed by digital and instrumental manipulation. Occasionally an open reduction with interosseous wire fixation of nasal bone fragments is necessary. A nasal fracture may involve a fracture of the nasal bones or cartilage (including the septum). Closed reduction of a nasal fracture is most often performed with the patient administered topical and local anesthetics. Procedural considerations and the surgical intervention are described in Chapter 19.

Reduction of Orbital Floor Fractures.
The orbital floor is the eggshell-thin bone on which the eye and periorbital tissues rest. It separates the orbit from the maxillary antrum. Orbital floor fractures usually occur in combination with fractures of the infraorbital rim (maxillary and zygomatic fractures). An isolated depressed

orbital floor fracture with an intact infraorbital rim is called a *blow-out* fracture.

Fractures of the walls of the orbit may be caused by direct blows or by extension of a fracture line from adjacent bones. Isolated orbital floor, or blow-out, fractures usually occur after injury to the region of the eye by an object the size of an apple or an adult's fist (Figure 22-23). Orbital contents herniated into the maxillary sinus, and the inferior rectus or inferior oblique muscle, may become incarcerated at the fracture site. A Caldwell-Luc antrostomy may be done with reduction of the fracture from below, or the fracture site may be approached directly through the lower lid along the orbital floor; the prolapsed tissue is reduced, the orbital floor is reduced, and the orbital floor defect is bridged with bone grafts, molded metal implants, or plastic material.

Procedural Considerations. A graft set may be used for implantation of autogenous graft or synthetic graft materials of various sizes and thicknesses, along with a flexible narrow-width retractor. Interosseous wiring may be required for fractures of the frontozygomatic junction. Microplates and screws to stabilize fractures involving the fragile facial and orbital bones also may be used. A general anesthetic is usually administered.

Operative Procedure

1. The surgeon tests the maximum ocular rotation by exerting traction with a forceps on the tendon of the inferior rectus muscle to determine if the inferior muscle sling is trapped in the fracture.

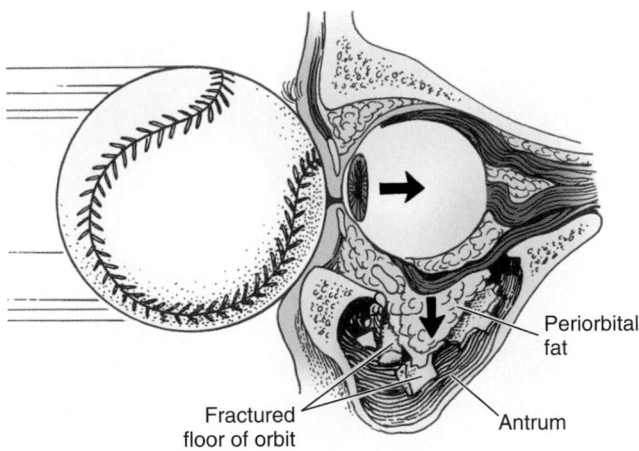

FIGURE 22-23 Ball has struck rim of orbit and has pressed orbital contents backward, displacing fragments of bone into maxillary sinus. Inferior rectus muscle is incarcerated in fracture. Inferior oblique muscle may also be involved.

2. To distribute tension over the lower lid and stretch the orbicularis muscle, the surgeon inserts a traction suture through the lower lid margin.

3. With a #3 knife handle and a #15 blade, the surgeon incises the lower lid in the lid fold above the orbital rim.

4. The skin is separated from the orbicularis muscle, and the orbital septum is identified by blunt dissection. Dissection is continued down to the periosteum of the orbital rim by means of scissors, loop retractors, elevators, and forceps.

5. The periosteum of the orbital rim is incised with a #15 blade. With periosteal elevators, the floor of the orbit is exposed and explored. When the fracture site is identified, bone spicules (needle-shaped bone fragments) are removed and the herniated contents are freed from the maxillary antrum. The contents of the orbit are elevated by means of narrow-width, flexible retractors. A 4-0 traction suture is placed around the tendon of the inferior rectus muscle.

6. An autogenous graft is taken from the iliac crest, or an alloplastic material of proper size is used to repair the bony defect. The material may or may not be anchored to the orbital rim by wire sutures.

7. The periosteum is carefully closed with 4-0 absorbable sutures.

8. The skin is closed with 6-0 nonabsorbable sutures, and a pressure dressing is applied.

Reduction of Zygomatic Fractures. Fractures of the zygoma (the cheek or malar bone) are corrected by either closed or open reduction. The two most common types of zygomatic fractures are depressed fractures of the arch and separation at or near the zygomaticofrontal, zygomaticomaxillary, and zygomaticotemporal suture lines, which constitutes a trimalar fracture. Although fractures of the zygoma can interfere with the ability to open and close the mouth properly, their chief consequence is a flattening of the cheek on the involved side, which results from a depressed trimalar or zygomatic arch fracture. Treatment is directed toward elevating the depressed fracture and maintaining the reduction. Closed reduction is the procedure used for treatment of zygomatic arch fractures, whereas most trimalar fractures are reduced by means of open reduction with internal fixation.

Procedural Considerations. A plastic instrument set, a Suraci zygoma hook-elevator, and a jaw hook are required for a closed reduction. A basic plastic instrument set, along with the following instruments and supplies, is required for an open reduction: a Hall II air drill; stainless steel wires (#26, #28, and #30); the Suraci zygoma hook-elevator; a jaw hook; a Kerrison rongeur; two Blair retractors; a bipolar ESU; a sterile marking pen; epinephrine 1:200,000 for injection; and a mini-plating rigid fixation set. The patient is placed in the supine position on the OR bed. A head drape is used.

Operative Procedure. The surgeon performs a closed reduction by elevating the depressed fracture with a percutaneous bone hook. Stabilization of a trimalar fracture may then be achieved by inserting a transantral Kirschner wire from the fractured side to the normal side.

The technique of open reduction of a trimalar fracture is as follows:

1. Incisions are marked along the lateral area of the eyebrow and lower eyelid over the zygomaticofrontal suture line and zygomaticomaxillary suture line (infraorbital rim) fractures, respectively.

2. After injection with epinephrine 1:200,000 for hemostasis, the surgeon incises along the premarked lines down to bone, and suture lines are identified and exposed.

3. The depressed zygoma is elevated with a Kelly hemostat or periosteal elevator placed behind the body of the zygoma through the lateral eyebrow incision. Bone hooks placed percutaneously or at the fracture sites may be used instead.

4. The surgeon drills holes into bone on each side of the fracture lines. Stainless steel wires are passed through the hole and twisted down tightly to maintain the reduction (reduction and stabilization of two of the three fractures are sufficient). Alternative methods of stabilization of the fractures are interosseous wiring of the zygomaticofrontal fracture and placement of a transmural Kirschner wire or stabilization with micro/mini plates and screws.

5. Using a subcuticular technique, the surgeon closes the incisions.

6. An eyepatch dressing may be applied.

Reduction of Maxillary Fractures. Midface fractures are usually classified according to a system developed in the early 1900s by Dr. Rene Le Fort: (1) Le Fort I, or transverse maxillary, fracture—this horizontal fracture includes the nasal floor, septum, and teeth; (2) Le Fort II, or pyramidal maxillary, fracture (unilateral or bilateral)—this type often involves the nasal cavity, hard palate, and the orbital rim; and (3) Le Fort III, or craniofacial dysjunction, fracture—this type includes fractures of both zygomas and the nose (Kelman, 2010) (Figure 22-24). Like a mandibular fracture, a maxillary fracture also produces malocclusion. In addition, depending on the severity of the fracture, it may produce considerable deformity of the middle of the face, usually perceived as a flattening or smashed-in appearance.

Closed reduction with intermaxillary fixation suffices for treatment of Le Fort I and some Le Fort II fractures. The more severe Le Fort II and all Le Fort III fractures require open reduction in addition to intermaxillary fixation.

Procedural Considerations. The basic plastic instrument set is required as well as an air drill; stainless steel wires (#25, #26, and #28); Rowe maxillary forceps, right and left; a Brown fascia needle; polyethylene buttons (for suspension wire pull-through for Le Fort

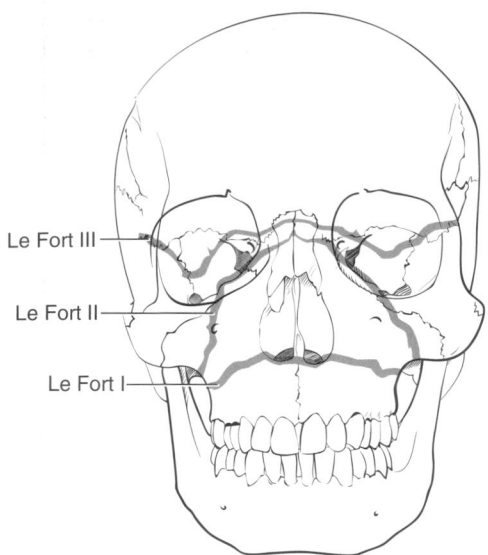

FIGURE 22-24 Le Fort classification of fractures.

FIGURE 22-25 Teeth in occlusion with arch bars in place. Tongs on arch bars will accept latex bands, which maintain occlusion for several weeks (wires around tongs are shown).

III repair); a small foam-rubber pad; a sterile marking pen or methylene blue; an ESU; epinephrine 1:200,000 for injection; periosteal elevators; and a rigid fixation system. A separate Mayo setup for the application of arch bars is required, as described for reduction of mandibular fractures. The patient is placed in the supine position on the OR bed. A head drape is used.

Operative Procedure. The surgeon will apply arch bars either before or after the open reduction, or in some cases use them as the only mode of treatment in closed reduction. In addition to ligating the maxillary arch bar to the teeth, it must also be suspended from stable bones superior to the fractured maxilla (which is unstable). In Le Fort I fractures, suspension may be around both zygomatic arches by passage of percutaneous wires. In Le Fort II and Le Fort III fractures, the surgeon may place suspension wires through holes drilled bilaterally into the zygomatic process of the frontal bone. This requires incisions into both lateral eyebrow areas. The following description pertains to open reduction of Le Fort II and Le Fort III fractures:

1. After injection of epinephrine 1:200,000 for hemostasis, the surgeon makes bilateral incisions to expose the infraorbital rims and zygomaticofrontal suture lines.
2. The surgeon applies Rowe maxillary forceps intranasally and intraorally to disimpact and reduce the maxilla. Holes are drilled into bone on each side of fracture lines along the infraorbital rim (and zygomaticofrontal area for Le Fort III fractures, after reducing the zygomatic fractures).
3. Stainless steel wires are passed through these holes and twisted down tightly to maintain the reduction.
4. Suspension wires are passed from the eyebrow incisions, behind the zygomatic arches, and into the mouth with the Brown fascia needle. A pullout wire is looped through each suspension wire within the eyebrow incision, brought out through the skin near the hairline, and tied down over a polyethylene button and foam-rubber padding. Self-tapping screws, mini compression plates, and bone grafts may also be used, based on the surgeon's preference. Incisions are closed.
5. When indicated, reduction of a nasal fracture is then performed.

Reduction of Mandibular Fractures. The purpose of treatment for a mandibular fracture is to restore the patient's preinjury dental occlusion. With some types of fractures, a closed reduction with immobilization by means of intermaxillary fixation is sufficient for treatment. With a majority of mandibular fractures, however, an open reduction with wire fixation is necessary, plus supplemental intermaxillary fixation to achieve adequate immobilization for healing.

Intermaxillary fixation is most often accomplished when arch bars are applied to the maxillary and mandibular teeth. The surgeon places stainless steel wires (#24 or #25) around the necks of the teeth and ligates the wire around the arch bars to hold the latter in place. Latex bands are attached to the tongs on the maxillary and mandibular arch bars to fix the teeth in occlusion (Figure 22-25). If the patient is edentulous, arch bars are attached to dentures or specially fabricated dental splints. The dentures or splints are held in place by means of wires placed around the mandible (for the mandibular arch bar) and through the nasal spine and around the zygomatic arches (for the maxillary arch bar). Wire cutters must be sent with the patient to the PACU.

Procedural Considerations—Open Reduction. In addition to a basic plastic instrument set, the following instruments and supplies are needed for an open reduction of a fractured mandible: a Hall II air drill, two Dingman bone-holding forceps, a nerve stimulator, a sterile marking pen, stainless steel wires (#24, #26, and #28), an ESU, epinephrine 1:200,000 for injection, and a rigid fixation system.

For the application of arch bars or other types of interdental wiring techniques, a separate Mayo setup with the following instruments and supplies is required: a set of coil arch bars and latex bands; stainless steel wire (#25 or #26); wire suture scissors; a wire twister; Wieder tongue depressors, large and small; a Brown fascia needle (if dentures or splints are used); a Freer septal elevator; and a small drain.

If arch bars are applied before the open reduction is performed, this former setup must be kept completely separate from the instruments used for the open reduction. Because the mouth is a contaminated area, a complete change of gowns, gloves, and drapes is necessary after the intraoral procedure.

Operative Procedure

1. The surgeon may apply the arch bars before or after the open reduction.
2. A line inferior and parallel to the lower border of the mandible at the fracture site is marked, and the area is infiltrated with epinephrine 1:200,000 for hemostasis.
3. The surgeon places the incision to expose the inferior border of the mandible. The nerve stimulator may be used to aid in identification of the marginal mandibular branch of the facial nerve in fractures of the posterior body and angle of the mandible.
4. The fracture is reduced by manipulation. The surgeon drills holes into the mandible on each side of the fracture line with the Hall II air drill while an assistant holds the reduced fracture with the aid of Dingman bone-holding forceps.
5. Stainless steel wire is inserted through the holes and twisted tightly to secure the fracture fragments in anatomic alignment.
6. In the event that rigid fixation is desired with the use of plates and screws, the appropriate drill bit, tap, and depth gauge are chosen. With these items the surgeon places the proper-size prosthesis, and the fracture is approximated, aligned, and placed in anatomic position.
7. A small drain may be placed into the wound, and the wound is closed in layers (periosteum, platysma muscle, and skin).
8. The latex bands may be applied to the arch bars at this time but more frequently are applied later, after the patient is fully awake and reactive.
9. A moderate compression dressing is applied to cover the submandibular wound and drain.

Elective Orthognathic Surgery. A large number of patients have either acquired or congenital facial defects that affect the maxilla, the mandible, or both. The condition of many of these patients can be improved dramatically with orthodontic care; however, many also require surgical rearrangement of the maxilla or mandible.

Procedural Considerations. Psychosocial and functional deficits are related to abnormalities of the maxilla and mandible. Surgical correction of these defects can improve patients' quality of life. Surgery is usually delayed until an adequate number of permanent teeth are in place for postoperative immobilization. Coordinated preoperative and postoperative planning is of great importance to the success of these procedures. Meticulous oral hygiene is extremely important to prevent tooth decay and gum inflammation caused by food buildup between the wires and the teeth. Thorough tooth brushing with a child-sized soft-bristled toothbrush is recommended for cleaning. A home dental irrigator can also be useful in loosening food and debris trapped between the wires and elastic bands of the arch bars. A liquid diet that is high in protein and calories is recommended. A blender or food processor will be necessary to prepare meals. The arch bars will be in place for 4 to 6 weeks. Commercial nutritional supplements are a convenient way to increase calories and protein because it is difficult to maintain weight on a liquid diet. An over-the-counter liquid multivitamin supplement is also recommended.

Operative Procedure

1. The surgeon applies arch bars for postoperative immobilization.
2. Intraoral incisions are made to provide exposure to the maxilla or mandible.
3. Using a saw, the surgeon cuts the maxilla or mandible as indicated by the patient's diagnosis.

4. Bone is advanced or set back to a predetermined position.
5. Bones are wired in place, with grafts placed in defects as needed.

Gender Reassignment

Transsexualism is defined as the condition in which an individual with chromosomes and internal and external organs normal to one gender identifies psychologically and socially with attributes of the opposite gender. Reassignment of gender by means of surgery is the last step to be taken in treatment of transsexuals. It is performed only after the patient has been treated with hormones of the opposite gender, has experienced a period of cross-gender living, and has had intensive psychiatric evaluation. Most institutions performing this type of surgery have gender-identity teams who evaluate and treat transsexuals. These teams usually include a variety of professionals: psychiatrist, psychologist, endocrinologist, plastic surgeon, urologist, gynecologist, and social worker.

The surgical techniques for assignment of male to female are technically easier. A breast augmentation may be performed if hormone therapy has not sufficiently changed breast size. Construction of the neovagina includes radical penectomy, bilateral orchiectomy, urethroplasty, perineal dissection, creation of a neovaginal vault, vaginoplasty, and vulvoplasty.

The surgical technique for female to male is technically more difficult and requires multiple surgical procedures. Considerations that must be addressed are twofold: the neophallus must be constructed to: (1) allow the patient to stand to void, and (2) permit stimulation of a sexual partner during intercourse. This may require a radial artery forearm free flap with a later-stage surgical insertion of a penile prosthesis for attaining an erection.

Aesthetic Surgery

Aesthetic surgery may be performed after induction of general anesthesia, monitored anesthesia care, or local anesthesia with moderate sedation. The perioperative nurse must be qualified and prepared to monitor the patient during the procedure according to AORN Perioperative Standards and Recommended Practices (AORN, 2013a). Baseline vital signs should be recorded in the OR record. A blood pressure cuff, pulse oximeter, and cardiac monitor electrodes should be placed (with staff capable of interpreting cardiac data). IV fluids should be administered. The OR should be kept quiet and patient privacy protected. Care should be taken to avoid conversation that could be misinterpreted by the patient.

Scar Revision

Scar revision involves the rearranging or reshaping of an existing scar so that the scar is less noticeable. The simplest form of scar revision is excision of an existing scar and simple resuturing of the wound. This may improve scars that are wide.

The Z-plasty is the most widely used method of scar revision (Figure 22-26). It breaks up linear scars, rearranging them so that the central limb of the Z lies in the same direction as a natural skin line. Scars that are parallel to skin lines are less noticeable than scars that are perpendicular to skin lines. A contracted scar line can also be lengthened with a Z-plasty.

Procedural Considerations. A plastic local instrument set and a sterile marking pen are required. The procedure may be performed with the patient administered a local or general anesthetic. The patient is positioned, prepped, and draped so that the scar that is to be revised is well exposed.

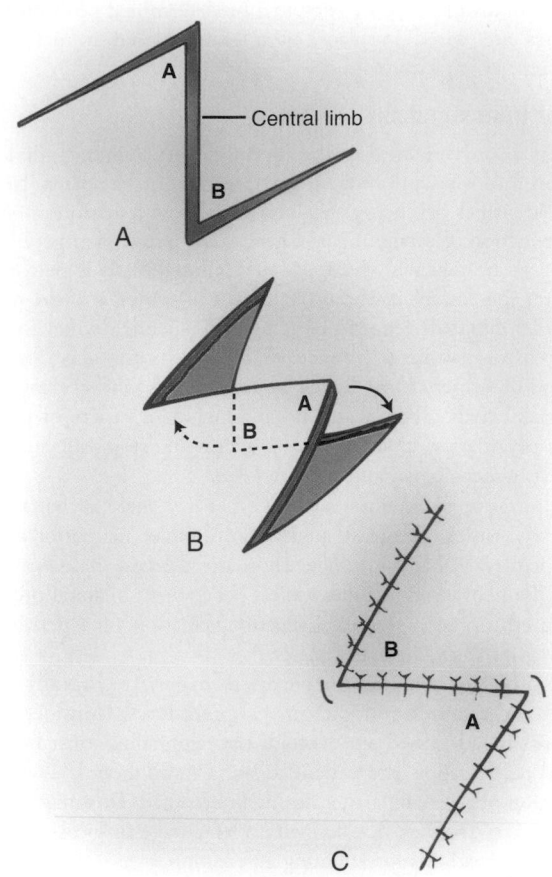

FIGURE 22-26 Z-plasty for scar revision. **A,** The central limb of the Z-plasty is over the scar that needs to be revised. **B,** Two other limbs are incised—each equal in length to the central limb and diverging from it at an equal angle. The flaps are then transposed. **C,** Flaps transposed, and original Z rotated 90 degrees and reversed.

Operative Procedure

1. The surgeon marks the pattern for the planned revision and injects local anesthesia.
2. The scar is excised.
3. The surrounding tissue is undermined, and the wound edges are approximated according to the surgeon's markings.
4. Dressings may or may not be applied.

Endoscopic Brow Lift

The aging process affects the area above the eyes and brows in several ways. Loss of skin elasticity can cause the appearance of a heavy brow and emphasize hooding of the upper eyelids. Repetitive muscle action results in horizontal forehead lines and furrows as well as creases between the brows. The goal of endoscopic brow/forehead surgery is to minimize the heaviness of the brow and improve the frown lines of aging, reduce upper eyelid hooding, reposition the eyebrows if necessary, and create a more youthful, refreshed appearance of the forehead and brow area, all through multiple, short incisions in the scalp.

Procedural Considerations. Positioning the patient at the very top of the OR bed is necessary for good utilization and mobility of the endoscopic instruments. For patients with medium to long hair, the hair may be sectioned and tied with sterilized rubber bands to minimize interference with the planned incision. The surgeon marks the patient's incision lines and anatomic landmarks before the surgery. The entire head (scalp, face, ears, and neck) should be prepped and draped with impervious drape material. The patient's eyes may be protected with ointment and shields for the duration of the procedure; ear canals may also be protected from pooling of prep solution by using sterile cotton balls. During preparation of the room, the perioperative nurse and scrub person perform a check of all endoscopic equipment to ensure it is functioning properly. Endoscopic instrumentation includes elevators, scissors, clamps, needle holders, camera, and light sources. Depending on the method of fixation, screws and accompanying instrumentation may be necessary.

Operative Procedure

1. The surgeon injects a local anesthetic and places three to five small incisions in the scalp (one midline and one or two paramedian).
2. Using blunt dissection, the surgeon elevates the forehead skin.
3. The endoscope is placed to allow visualization of muscles, vessels, nerves, and tissues.
4. Using endoscopic instruments the surgeon dissects the corrugator and procerus muscles and soft tissues. The area is redraped to produce a smoother appearance and desired repositioning of brows.
5. The surgeon places screws in the outer table of the cranium at designated points, and then places sutures through the galea. These sutures are tied around the screws to facilitate elevation of the brow and forehead.
6. The surgeon staples or sutures the scalp incisions for closure.

Rhytidectomy (Facelift)

As the aging process progresses, the skin of the face and neck may become loose and redundant. This is particularly noticeable in the "jowl" areas and just beneath the chin. A facelift may be performed to correct the sagging skin. The typical facelift addresses the face and neck and involves removal and redraping of excess skin of the face and neck after repositioning of the underlying muscle and platysma has been performed. The result is a smooth, rested appearance, without unnatural tightness or distortion of facial features (Figure 22-27). Rather than excising the redundant skin directly, incisions adjacent to or within hairlines are used so that the scars are virtually indiscernible.

Procedural Considerations. The perioperative nurse assists with positioning the patient supine with the head and shoulders slightly elevated. Attention should be given to safety by using proper positioning to prevent pressure injuries, using intermittent pneumatic compression devices, forced-air warming unit, and preventing eye injuries by using shields or eye ointment. Sterile kitners or cotton may be used in the ears to keep blood and fluids from entering. They should be included in the surgical soft goods count. Depending on the complexity of the procedure and planned surgical time, the nurse may insert an indwelling urinary catheter.

Specialized scissors of varying lengths should be available, along with smooth and toothed tissue forceps and various sizes of needle holders. A fiberoptic lighted retractor is standard for facelifts. To avoid immediate use steam sterilization, contact with the surgeon or office staff should be initiated before the day of surgery to discuss

FIGURE 22-27 A, Preoperative and **B,** postoperative rhytidectomy.

special requests and ensure that instrumentation is prepared according to AORN standards and facility guidelines.

There are numerous techniques for rhytidectomy, and a well-prepared perioperative nurse will ask the surgeon about the specific technique in order to have the appropriate suture material and special needles available. The underlying superficial muscular aponeurotic system (SMAS) may be repositioned, the cheek may be elevated independently, the midface may be lifted, and there may or may not be accompanying liposuction. Facelift procedures are customized specific to the anatomic needs of the individual patient. The entire head, neck, ears, and scalp are prepped and draped.

Operative Procedure

1. The surgeon marks bilateral incision lines from the temporal scalp, around the earlobe, around the posterior margin of the auricula, and into the occipital scalp (Figures 22-28 and 22-29).
2. The incision lines, both temples, cheeks, upper neck, and the submental area are injected with the local anesthetic agent.
3. The surgeon may inject wetting solution (e.g., tumescent) and perform liposuction on the neck, jowls, or cheeks before placing the incisions. The tumescent can assist in undermining the tissue (see Liposuction section, p. 855).
4. After the incisions are made, the surgeon elevates the temporal and cheek skin. The SMAS is plicated cephalad and caudally, elevating and tightening the SMAS and platysma.
5. The surgeon elevates and repositions the malar pad; it is then anchored with suture.
6. The facial skin flap is then elevated in a superior and slightly posterior direction and tacked, and excess skin is trimmed at the flap edges.
7. Through a submental incision, the surgeon undermines the neck, and identifies and plicates the platysmal bands. Excess tissue is trimmed and tacked postauricularly. Small drains are placed beneath the skin flaps and secured.

FIGURE 22-28 Rhytidectomy: line of incision and undermining. **A,** Traction sutures of 4-0 silk placed into auricle; temporal incision curved posteriorly for better support of upward pull. **B,** Incision carried under earlobe and then curved posteriorly upward and then caudad toward midline. **C,** Skin undermined almost to nasolabial fold, to area of mental foramen, and to midline of neck as far down as thyroid cartilage. Care is taken to avoid injury to submandibular branches of facial nerve and facial artery.

FIGURE 22-29 Rhytidectomy: removal of superfluous skin. **A,** Skin drawn upward to proper degree of tension, and incision made along posterior margin of clamp. **B,** Incision continued upward around posterior margin of auricle and then backward to excise skin specimen.

FIGURE 22-30 A, Preoperative and **B,** postoperative blepharoplasty.

8. Incisions are closed in one or two layers. Fibrin sealant and/or a drain may be used prior to closure to aid in hemostasis.
9. The patient's hair is cleaned prior to the application of the dressing. A moderate pressure dressing is applied depending on surgeon preference.

Blepharoplasty

The aging process causes a sagging or relaxation of eyelid skin and the orbital septum. As the latter becomes weaker, it allows periorbital fat to bulge. These changes are perceived as baggy eyelids, which give the patient a chronically tired appearance. The goal of blepharoplasty is to improve the patient's appearance by removing excess eyelid skin, removing or repositioning bulging periorbital fat, and tightening and smoothing the muscles under the eye (Figure 22-30). The upper eyelid skin can be so redundant that it encroaches on the patient's field of vision, and removal of excessive hooding of the upper eyelid skin may even improve peripheral vision. The upper eyelid crease may also be enhanced. Not all patients need removal of skin; for selected individuals, CO_2 skin resurfacing may be the procedure of choice to achieve a smoother appearance of the lower eyelid skin. Incisions in the subconjunctival mucosa of the lower lids are sometimes used for this group of patients if resection or repositioning of the periorbital fat is also indicated. Blepharoplasty is often performed with rhytidectomy. Blepharoplasty may be performed on both the upper and lower lids, upper lids only, or lower lids only.

Procedural Considerations. A plastic local instrument set is required. Delicate, short instruments are used, with special attention to scissors (curved Kaye blepharoplasty); fine Adson forceps with teeth; calipers; and fixation forceps. Webster needle holders are frequently desired. A bipolar ESU unit may be used. A needle tip for the active electrode may be requested if the monopolar ESU is used. (With the monopolar ESU, a lower setting is used. The perioperative nurse should verbally repeat back the settings requested by the surgeon.) Blepharoplasty is usually performed using a local anesthetic with monitored anesthesia care. The patient is in the supine position on the OR bed. The patient's face is prepped, and the head drape is used. Corneal shields may be used to protect the cornea.

Operative Procedure—Upper Lids

1. The surgeon marks the lines of incision and injects local anesthetic.
2. The incision is placed, and excess skin is removed. Hemostasis is obtained (Figure 22-31, *A* to *C*).
3. The surgeon trims the orbicularis oculi muscle and identifies and excises the septum orbitale. Excess periorbital fat is trimmed and coagulated.
4. Upper lid incisions are closed; and the surgeon repeats the procedure for the opposite upper lid.
5. Finely crushed ice on moist gauze 4 × 4 pads may be applied to the periorbital region; other means of reducing swelling, such as

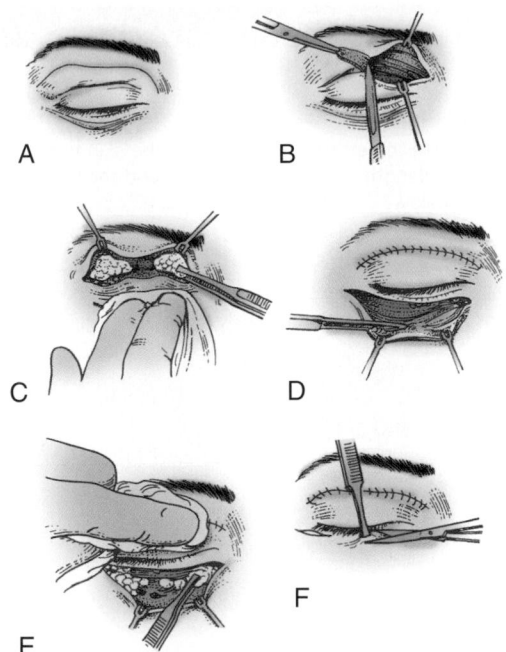

FIGURE 22-31 Blepharoplasty for drooping eyelids. **A,** Areas of proposed skin excision marked with methylene blue or a sterile marking pen. **B,** Strip of skin excised from upper lid; fat pad shining through orbital fascia and orbicular muscle of eye. **C,** Orbital fascia opened in two places (medially and laterally). Pressure on eyeball causes fat pads to bulge. They are eased out meticulously. **D,** Upper lid incision sutured with continuous 6-0 suture material of choice. Orbital muscle fibers of lower lid are separated from skin. **E,** Orbital fascia opened; fat pads bulge because of digital pressure and are teased out meticulously. **F,** Skin tailored to fit and sutured.

cold compresses or a mechanical cold mask, may be similarly applied. Compresses are changed as often as they become warm.

Operative Procedure—Lower Lids

1. The surgeon marks the lines of incision and injects local anesthetic.
2. A subciliary incision (1 mm below eyelashes) is made and brought out in a natural line in the outer canthal skin.
3. The skin-muscle flap is raised, leaving a 3-mm strip of muscle attached to the tarsus (see Figure 22-31, *D*).
4. The skin-muscle flap is dissected down below the level of the orbital rim.
5. The surgeon incises the arcus marginalis, and redundant fat with the overlying septum orbitale is draped over the orbital rim (see Figure 22-31, *E*) and sutured.
6. Hemostasis is obtained. Skin is redraped in an upward and outward fashion with attention to prevention of ectropion.
7. Excess skin is trimmed (see Figure 22-31, *F*).
8. Lateral muscle is sutured to periosteum.
9. The surgeon closes the lower lid incision, and repeats the procedure for the opposite lower lid.
10. Compresses are applied as described in the upper lid procedure.

Rhinoplasty

Deformities of the external nose and nasal septum may be congenital or secondary to previous trauma. The goal of rhinoplasty is to improve the appearance of the external nose. This is accomplished

by reshaping the underlying framework of the nose, which allows the overlying skin and subcutaneous tissue to redrape over the new framework. Reshaping the nasal skeleton usually includes use of a rasp for dorsal hump reduction, partial excision of lateral and alar cartilages, shortening of the septum, and osteotomy of nasal bones. A procedure to alter the nasal septum—septoplasty, or submucous resection (SMR)—often accompanies rhinoplasty. The goal of SMR is to improve the nasal airway by resecting a segment of septal cartilage. Septoplasty reshapes the existing septal cartilage; it may aid in altering the appearance of the nose or in improving the airway. Rhinoplasty may be performed as an open procedure by making an external incision across the base of the columella, or it may be performed entirely through the nares by using internal incisions. Small external incisions at the alar bases are used to narrow the nares, and internal incisions placed alongside the base of the nasal bones are used to narrow the entire nose once the hump is removed or dorsum is incised. A full description of rhinologic procedures may be found in Chapter 19.

Laser Surgery

Several different types of lasers are commonly used in plastic and reconstructive surgery (Box 22-3). One of the most popular types of laser is the skin resurfacing, or CO_2, laser. The laser is attracted to the water in the skin cells and ablates the cells at a predetermined depth. The collagen material is also heated, resulting in smoother and slightly tighter skin. This treatment has virtually replaced dermabrasion, because it is much more consistent in terms of depth of penetration and less dependent on user technique or skill.

Tattoo removal and destruction of vascular lesions, such as facial telangiectasias, spider veins, and hemangiomas, may be achieved with the use of other types of lasers. Whether using lasers for skin resurfacing or tattoo removal procedures, the areas must first be numbed with a local anesthetic. Use of sedation depends on the anxiety level of the patient as well as the total surface area to be treated. Vascular lesions may be treated without local anesthesia, although there is some temporary discomfort with each pulse of the laser. Laser safety and procedures are described in great detail in Chapter 8.

Liposuction

Liposuction is a surgical technique designed to remove excess deposits of fat and improve the contour of the body (Figure 22-32). It is not a treatment for obesity or simply a weight reduction procedure; rather, the ideal candidate is of normal weight and desires to remove localized fat that has proved resistant despite diet and exercise. By extension, liposuction patients must adhere to lifestyle changes (e.g., proper nutrition, adequate exercise) to maintain optimal results (Logan and Broughton, 2008). Although most often associated with contour correction, liposuction may also be used for treatment of gynecomastia or to remove lipomas. Areas that may be suctioned include face, neck, back, breasts (not a replacement for reduction mammoplasty, only contour correction), waist, abdomen, midriff, flanks, upper arms, hips, medial and lateral thighs, knees, and ankles (Figures 22-33 and 22-34).

Multiple techniques have been developed to enhance the final results as well as ease the removal of the fat. These techniques are not always used in isolation of each other; rather, some may be combined both to achieve the best possible outcome and to address the surgeon's preferences. Each procedure has specific equipment needed for that technique and often has highly specific

Text continued on p. 859

BOX 22-3

Lasers in Plastic Surgery

Common uses for lasers in plastic surgery include exfoliation, treatment of vascular malformations, removal of hair and tattoos, and tightening of collagen fibers in aging skin. A variety of lasers are available; selection of the appropriate laser depends on the patient's diagnosis because the effect of the laser on the skin tissue is dependent on its wavelength. The types of lasers and their common uses are described below.

Laser	Use
CO_2	Desiccation of benign lesions of skin, skin resurfacing, cutting tissue
Excimer	Eye surgery, psoriasis
Argon	Hemangiomas, telangiectasias
Nd:YAG	Benign pigmented lesions and red tattoos
Candela dye	Tattoos, pigmented benign lesions, hemangiomas
Helium-neon	Biostimulation, wound healing alleviation, acupuncture
Diode	Hair removal, tattoo removal
Ruby	Nevi removal, dark tattoos
Erbium:YAG	Rhytides
Q-Switch	Benign pigmented lesions and dark tattoos

ND:YAG, Neodymium Yttrium Aluminum Garnet; *YAG,* Yttrium Aluminum Garnet.

A, Laser removal of large facial telangiectasia. **B,** Laser removal of photoaging and lentigines on hands of woman in her 60s.

BOX 22-3

Lasers in Plastic Surgery—cont'd

C, Laser removal of multicolored tattoo on the posterior shoulder. **D,** Laser hair removal. **E,** Laser skin resurfacing and wrinkle tightening.

Modified from Choi JE et al: Treatment of Becker's nevi with a long-pulse alexandrite laser, *Dermatol Surg* 35:1105–1118, 2009; Kono T et al: Long-pulsed neodymium:yttrium-aluminum-garnet laser treatment for hypertrophic port-wine stains on the lips, *J Cosmet Laser Ther* 11(1):11–13, 2009; Krupashankar DS: Standard guidelines of care: CO_2 laser for removal of benign skin lesions and resurfacing, IADVL Dermatosurgery Task Force, *Indian J Dermatol Venereol Leprol* 74(Suppl):S61–S67, 2008; Mendonca DA et al: Venous malformations of the limbs: the Birmingham experience, comparisons and classification in children, *J Plast Reconstr Aesthet Surg* 64:383–389, 2010; Onesti MG: Surgical and laser treatment of Sturge-Weber syndrome, *Aesthet Plast Surg* 33:666–668, 2009.

FIGURE 22-32 **A,** Normal appearance of excess fat. **B,** Removal of deep fat by larger-diameter cannulae. **C,** Corrected contour following removal of excess fat by liposuction. **D,** Removal of superficial fat involves using narrower-gauge cannulae.

FIGURE 22-33 Submental liposuction. **A,** Preoperative. **B,** Postoperative.

FIGURE 22-34 Female 43-year-old patient. **A,** Before and **B,** 6 months after liposuction of the abdomen and buttocks.

cannulae and other instrumentation. Because multiple areas are usually treated, the perioperative nurse should determine the sequence of liposuction the surgeon prefers to be prepared for positioning.

Procedural Considerations. Immediate preoperative preparation includes asking the patient to stand while the area of deformity is outlined. The surgeon usually draws two lines on the skin surface—one delineating the major area of defect and the other placed a short distance outside the first area. These lines make it easier for the surgeon to make a smooth transition toward the normal tissue by adjusting the amount of fat removed from the center to the periphery of the deformity. The patient may remain standing and be prepped circumferentially with a spray bottle of antimicrobial skin solution. The perioperative nurse provides for the patient's privacy and uses appropriate measures to protect the patient from hypothermia.

Preoperative patient education should include a discussion of the compression garment, which is typically worn for 2 to 4 weeks postoperatively. Patients should also be informed about the likelihood of the puncture sites leaking tumescent solution during the first 24 hours of the postoperative period. Absorbent dressings are required to minimize soiling of clothing and bedding during this period as well as to maintain the cleanliness of the compression garment.

Depending on the areas targeted for liposuction, draping may require a good deal of innovation. Minimal instrumentation is necessary. A knife handle, towel clips, tissue forceps, scissors, clamps, and needle holder are used along with the suction cannulae specific to the proposed liposuction technique. A general anesthetic, moderate sedation, or epidural anesthetic may be used. However, the surgeon typically injects a medicated wetting solution into the fatty areas before removal because of concerns about large fluid volume shift and blood loss after lipectomy. The wetting solution contains IV fluid (e.g., lactated Ringer's), lidocaine, and epinephrine. Using more than 70 mL/kg of wetting solution for infiltration can lead to fluid overload; this may present as increased blood pressure, jugular vein distention, bounding pulses, cough, dyspnea, lung crackles, and pulmonary edema. For safety issues the nurse needs to communicate and verify with the surgeon the total lipoaspirate and volume of wetting solution used. Additionally, it is imperative that warmed wetting solution be used for suction-assisted lipectomy (Logan and Broughton, 2008).

In the tumescent technique, large volumes of this solution are administered. The "super-wet" technique uses less solution; usually the amount of fluid injected approximates the amount of fat to be removed—thus the name, which refers to the swollen and firm ("tumesced") state of the tissues when they are filled with solution. The perioperative nurse should inquire if the surgeon will be infiltrating tumescent solution and, if so, what ingredients are used for his or her technique. Also the nurse should ask whether the surgeon uses internal or external ultrasound (sound waves that liquefy fat) or power-assisted liposuction. One of the newer techniques is the use of VASER-Assisted Liposuction, which incorporates thermal energy to liquefy the fat, thus aiding greatly in its removal.

Operative Procedure
1. The surgeon places stablike incisions in concealed areas to access sites to be liposuctioned.
2. The tumescent solution is infused.

3. Depending on technique, at this point either internal or external ultrasound or the VASER technique is performed at predetermined settings and length of time.
4. Liposuction is performed with the use of various sizes and lengths of cannulae. The cannula is attached to large-bore, firm suction tubing and connected to an aspirating unit. The high vacuum pressure caused by the unit causes the fat cells to emulsify so that they can be suctioned through the vacuum opening near the rounded tip of the cannula. Areas are usually cross-suctioned to achieve the best outcomes. Stab wounds may be closed with absorbable suture or left open to drain.
5. The patient's skin is cleaned, and bulky dressings and compression garments are applied.

Abdominoplasty

Abdominoplasty is particularly useful in improving the appearance (and to a certain extent, function) of persons who have lost a great deal of weight or who suffer from laxity of abdominal skin following pregnancy. Obesity produces distention and stretching of the skin of the abdomen. Weight loss reduces the volume of the underlying fat; however, it does not produce concomitant reduction in the excess surface area of the overlying skin, which results from destruction or insufficiency of elastic fibers in the skin. The rectus abdominis fascia is also stretched in obese patients, and weight loss does not restore its integrity.

There are several versions of the abdominoplasty procedure, and the choice of which technique to use depends on the degree of deformity of the abdominal skin and muscle. All techniques are designed to improve the appearance of the abdomen by tightening the abdominal area (abdominal wall/rectus muscles) and removing excess skin or fullness.

If there is minimal to no laxity of the skin and mostly fullness of the lower abdomen, then a "mini-abdominoplasty" may be indicated. With this technique it is not necessary to relocate or incise the umbilicus and a short incision, resembling a Pfannenstiel, may be effectively used. However, if there is laxity of the periumbilical and upper and lower abdominal skin accompanied by protrusion of the abdominal wall with diastasis (separation) of the rectus muscle, then full abdominoplasty is the procedure of choice. This version requires relocation of the umbilicus and an incision that stretches from hip to hip. Endoscopic abdominoplasty is another option if only muscle repair (correction of the diastasis deformity or shortening of the rectus muscles) is needed.

Procedural Considerations. A basic plastic instrument set is required, as well as extra retractors and clamping instruments, an ESU, and a sterile marking pen. Frequently tumescent anesthetic solution is added to minimize bleeding, reduce postoperative discomfort, and aid in dissection. The perioperative nurse should ask the surgeon about the use of tumescent as well as preference for ingredients. A lighted fiberoptic retractor should be available. Intermittent pneumatic compression devices or antiembolism hose are usually in place or applied in the OR. The patient is in the supine position with slight flexion at the hips. Draping is such that the entire abdomen, lower costal margins, upper thighs, and both anterior iliac spines are exposed.

Operative Procedure
1. The surgeon makes a low transverse abdominal incision across both inguinal areas laterally and the superior border of the mons pubis in the midline down to fascia.

2. A large flap of skin and subcutaneous tissue is elevated away from the fascia of the anterior abdominal wall.

3. The umbilicus is circumscribed and left in its normal position.

4. The surgeon elevates the abdominal flap until the xiphoid process of the sternum and the lower costal margins are reached.

5. If diastasis of the rectus abdominis fascia is present, the surgeon plicates it with suture from the xiphoid process to the mons pubis.

6. The flap of abdominal skin and subcutaneous tissue is pulled inferiorly, and excess tissue is excised.

7. A small incision is made in the midline of the flap to accommodate the umbilicus, which is then sutured peripherally to the flap.

8. Drains are inserted, followed by closure of the lower abdominal incision in layers.

9. Postoperatively the patient is placed in the hospital bed in high Fowler position.

Post-Bariatric Surgery Body Contouring

Successful bariatric surgery produces significant weight loss. The weight loss may result in a trunk that lacks waist and hip definition; ptosis of the mons pubis; and various degrees of skin, fat, and abdominal wall laxity. Upper and lower back rolls accompany the anterior truncal deformities; the buttocks are lower and lack fullness. Upper arms and thighs exhibit similar deformities.

Treatment is aimed at removing the excessive skin and creating a desirable body contour. Most patients are candidates for some form of circumferential recontouring (belt lipectomy) (Figure 22-35) in combination with any number of other recontouring procedures: brachioplasty (Figure 22-36), thigh lifts (Figure 22-37), and mastopexy. For the perioperative nurse, these surgeries offer a logistical challenge because of the combination of procedures and positioning required. The malabsorptive effects of the original bariatric surgery may compromise postoperative wound healing after body contouring procedures. The perioperative nurse must be familiar with the complications relating to post-bariatric surgery body contouring to provide comprehensive care for this unique group of patients (Research Highlight).

Procedural Considerations. Extensive measuring and marking are performed by the plastic surgeon in the preoperative area. The perioperative nurse should inquire about the ordering of the procedures and positioning. If more than one procedure is planned, intermittent pneumatic compression devices and a Foley catheter should be used once the patient arrives in the OR. During prepping and draping, attempts should be made to preserve the patient's body temperature. Repositioning is a standard part of these procedures. Pressure points should be well padded with appropriate positioning aids to maintain functional alignment and stable positioning. With each repositioning activity the patient must be reassessed for

FIGURE 22-35 Belt lipectomy and thigh liposuction. The patient was a 40-year-old woman 40 months after gastric bypass surgery with a weight loss of 269 pounds.

FIGURE 22-36 Brachioplasty.

FIGURE 22-37 Thigh lift.

RESEARCH HIGHLIGHT

Body Lift Complications

Lower body reconstructive procedures after bariatric surgery have increased in popularity since 2000 according to the American Society of Plastic Surgeons, who reported 207 cases in the year 2000 compared with 7163 cases in 2012. Although in high demand, these procedures are associated with a high complication rate.

Kitzinger and colleagues conducted a prospective study to identify the complications and possible risk factors for a lower body lift, including a belt lipectomy and thigh lift in a single procedure. Study criteria included patient age ≥65 years, body mass index (BMI) ≤35 kg^{-2}, an excess weight loss (EWL) of at least 66%, and a stable body weight for at least 12 months. Study participants were followed postoperatively at 1 week, 2 weeks, 4 weeks, 8 weeks, 12 weeks and 6 months after the lift procedure.

Fifty patients were in the study group (44 females and 6 males). Of the group, 35 (70%) developed at least one complication,

including 18 who had two or more complications. Five patients (10%) had to undergo surgical revisions. The most common complication was wound dehiscence followed by seroma. Other complications included infection and hematoma. Analysis showed the two most important risk factors were BMI maximums and the age of the patient. Amount of weight lost by the patient and the weight of the specimen were also cited as possible risk factors.

The researchers note that the overall complication rate of 70% is comparable with rates in other well-known high risk groups such as patients with cancer, those undergoing transplantation, obesity, and severe burns and recommend that the massive weight loss patient be assigned to a high-risk group in terms of complications. Regarding their finding of higher complications in older patients, they recommend avoiding the procedure on patients older than 55 years of age noting that recovery in older patients with ongoing arthritis and/or joint replacement to be difficult and protracted.

Modified from Kitzinger HB et al: Prospective study on complications following a lower body lift after massive weight loss, *J Plast Reconstr Aesthet Surg* 66:231–238, 2013; American Society of Plastic Surgeons, *2012 Cosmetic plastic surgery statistics,* available at www.plasticsurgery.org/Documents/news-resources/statistics/2012-Plastic-Surgery-Statistics/Cosmetic -Procedure-Trends-2012.pdf. Accessed March 3, 2013.

safety in terms of skin and nerve compression and competence of the grounding pad, Foley catheter, and all monitoring devices. A basic plastic surgery instrument set with additional towel clamps is used. Other supplies include a stapler for skin approximation, multiple drains, and an ESU. The surgeon may choose to use tissue adhesive products in combination with suture material to reduce the incidence of seroma. Compression garments may be applied, but care must be taken not to compromise the vascularity of the skin flaps.

Operative Procedure—Belt Lipectomy. Sites addressed are the abdomen, including mons pubis; upper and lower back; lateral trunk skin; buttocks; and lateral upper thighs.

1. The surgeon infuses dilute tumescent solution to aid in hemostasis and facilitate undermining of flaps.
2. Incisions are made and taken down to the level of the fascia, and flaps are elevated to previously marked margins. Liposuction cannulae without vacuum attachments may be used for undermining.
3. Liposuction is used if indicated for contouring only.
4. Muscle plication is performed when indicated.
5. The surgeon approximates and sutures the superficial fascia with permanent sutures.
6. Skin flaps are approximated, and excess skin is excised.
7. Closed-wound suction drains are inserted and secured with suture.
8. The patient is repositioned; depending on position at the start of the procedure, this could be lateral decubitus or supine.
9. Similar techniques are used for defects in areas presented by the new position and repeated until all areas are addressed, including relocation of the umbilicus.
10. The patient's skin is cleaned, incisions are dressed, and compression garments are applied at the surgeon's preference.
11. The patient is transferred to a stretcher or bed and placed in the flexed position.

Breast Surgeries

A variety of surgical procedures are available to enhance the aesthetic appearance of the breasts. Patients may choose to enlarge, reduce, and change the position of their breasts.

Augmentation Mammoplasty. Breast augmentation is performed for correction of hypomastia, to correct breast asymmetry, and to re-create the breast after mastectomy. A prosthesis is inserted to enlarge or form the breast mound.

Breast Implants. The two basic types of breast implants are saline filled and silicone gel filled. Both are approved by the U.S. Food and Drug Administration (FDA) for elective breast augmentation; in November 2006 the FDA approved the use of silicone gel filled breast implants for breast augmentation and breast reconstruction and revision surgeries. Of the total breast implants performed in 2011 about half used saline-filled implants and half used silicone implants (FDA, 2011).

Implants are configured into round or teardrop (also known as anatomic) shapes and may have a smooth or textured surface. The surfaces are designed to minimize capsular contracture and migration. The choice to use a round or an anatomic implant is based on the shape and form of the existing breast.

Procedural Considerations. The perioperative nurse verifies style and size of implant and handles the implant according to the manufacturer's recommendations. Handling implants as little

| A | **Submuscular** with more fullness above | B | **Submammary** with more superior slope |

FIGURE 22-38 A, Augmentation mammoplasty implant under muscle. **B,** Implant under breast tissue.

as possible assists in efforts to reduce the potential for implant contamination. A basic plastic instrument set is used, plus lighted fiberoptic retractors. The breast implants are packaged in sterile containers from the manufacturer and given to the scrub person when breast size is determined. Breast implants should only be filled with sterile injectable saline using a closed system designed for that purpose. The patient is supine. The arms may be extended on armboards to approximately 60 degrees. Prepping and draping are carried out in the routine manner to expose the operative site.

Operative Procedure. The surgeon may perform augmentation mammoplasty through circumareolar, inframammary, axillary, or transumbilical incisions using an open or endoscopic approach. Depending on the anatomy of the patient and the surgeon's preference, breast implants may be placed subglandularly, subpectorally (Figure 22-38), or biplanarly (partial muscle coverage).

Operative Procedure—Unfilled Saline Implants

1. The surgeon may inject local anesthetic to decrease bleeding and provide analgesia.
2. An incision is made, the pocket is dissected, and hemostasis is achieved.
3. The surgeon may use breast implant sizers (gel or saline) to evaluate the size of the pocket and determine the size of the final implant.
4. With the sizers in place, the anesthesia provider elevates the patient to the 90-degree position so the surgeon can evaluate the appearance from various angles and plan for any adjustments or revisions to the pocket.
5. The sizers are removed, and the surgeon finalizes the pocket.
6. The perioperative nurse verifies the implant type and size again with the surgeon and dispenses it to the sterile field.
7. The surgeon rolls the implant into a cylindric shape in preparation for insertion.
8. The pocket is irrigated with saline or antibiotic solution.
9. The surgeon inserts the implant and unrolls it, and once it is properly positioned, the surgeon inflates the implant with an appropriate amount of saline.
10. The procedure is repeated for the opposite breast.
11. The incision is closed in two layers.

12. The patient is cleaned, and bandages and a surgical bra are applied.

Capsulotomy. Capsule contracture occurs when the normal envelope of fibrous tissue around an implant gets thicker or tighter so that the implant no longer feels soft and pliant. If the degree of capsular contracture is great, there can be pain, distortion, and palpability or distortion of the implant. Capsular contracture occurs in approximately 15% of patients, and it is not possible to predict who will develop it or take preventive measures (McGrath and Pomeranz, 2012). Depending on the extent of the contracture, an open capsulotomy may be used to release the constrictive tissue, or a capsulectomy may be indicated to actually remove the tissue. Although patients receive education about capsule contracture as part of the informed consent process for breast augmentation, the actuality of the event may cause emotional distress for the patient. The patient may verbalize disappointment over the results and express fear related to additional postoperative changes in the appearance and functioning of the breast. In addition, the patient now faces the surgical and anesthetic risks associated with a second surgical procedure and may also be struggling with a possible financial burden because these procedures may not be covered by the patient's health plan. An empathic and understanding approach is paramount to easing the patient's anxiety.

Procedural Considerations. The patient is prepared, positioned, and draped in the same manner as for breast augmentation.

Operative Procedure

1. The surgeon incises the skin and exposes the capsule.

2. The capsule is scored in multiple areas to achieve the desired release. Depending on the degree of contracture, circumferential incisions may be necessary to release the contracture.

3. If capsulotomy is not effective in releasing the capsule, a partial or full capsulectomy may be required to physically remove all or a portion of the capsule.
   a. The capsule is excised, and the breast implant is removed.
   b. The breast implant may be replaced in the same area, exchanged and replaced, or placed in a new pocket.

4. The site is irrigated with antibiotic solution. Drains are placed if a capsulectomy was performed.

5. The surgeon closes the incision in two layers.

6. The patient's skin is cleaned, and dressings are applied.

Reduction Mammoplasty. Reduction mammoplasty is indicated for the patient with macromastia with resulting back pain, intertrigo (chronic skin infection), or deep grooving in the shoulders from bra straps because of the weight of the breasts (Patient and Family Education) (Research Highlight) (Figure 22-39, *A*). The procedure may also be performed to achieve symmetry after a mastectomy on the contralateral side. Excessive breast tissue and its overlying skin are excised, with reconstruction of the breast contour, size, shape, and symmetry (see Figure 22-39, *B*).

Procedural Considerations. A basic plastic instrument set is used with the addition of a "cookie cutter" areola marker or a "keyhole" pattern marker, a sterile marking pen, skin stapler, tape measure, baby Deaver retractors, and two closed-wound suction systems. An ESU and a scale for weighing specimens should also be available, and tissue from each side should be carefully weighed and marked appropriately. The perioperative nurse should ensure the scale is calibrated correctly before weighing any tissue. Numerous blades will be used if deepithelializing breast skin. If the nipple is removed and placed as a free nipple graft, extra suture will be

FIGURE 22-39 A, Preoperative view of reduction mammoplasty. **B,** Postoperative view.

necessary for tie-over bolsters. There are numerous choices in the reduction mammoplasty technique; therefore, before opening suture or other supplies, the perioperative nurse should ask the surgeon which technique will be used. The surgeon will mark the skin to be excised and the new site for the nipple preoperatively with the patient in a sitting position.

The patient is supine with arms slightly extended on padded armboards. The hips should be positioned at the break in the OR bed so that the patient may be raised to a sitting position if necessary. Standard prepping and draping are done. Care should be taken not to remove the preoperative markings.

Operative Procedure. The standard reduction mammoplasty procedure is described below. If the surgeon is using the "short scar" technique, the breast tissue is incised and removed according to the technique chosen. The nipple pedicle technique, wherein the nipple is mobilized and secured in a new position, may be chosen, or a free nipple graft may be used.

1. The surgeon incises and removes the skin between the new and the old nipple sites, with the nipple remaining attached to the underlying breast tissue. On patients with very large breasts, the nipples are removed and then reapplied as free grafts when the reduction is complete.

PATIENT AND FAMILY EDUCATION

Patient Education for Breast Reduction

General Information

Women with very large, pendulous breasts (a condition known as macromastia) can experience a number of physical and emotional problems. Macromastia is generally defined as excessive breast size, usually a bra cup size of D or larger. This condition is seen in young girls to middle-aged women. The condition probably is caused by hormonal factors but is also associated with obesity. Often there is a family pattern of large breasts.

Common Signs and Symptoms

- Breast size that is out of proportion to the torso and larger than the accepted norm
- Upper back and neck pain
- Shoulder pain
- Arm pain
- Breast pain
- Rashes and sometimes infections of the skin under the breasts
- Shoulder grooving from bra straps
- Hyperpigmentation (dark marks) in the bra strap lines
- Difficulty in finding bras or clothing that fits
- Possibly shyness or other personality changes because of appearance and the effects of excessively large breasts

Diagnosis

The surgeon will confirm the diagnosis of macromastia by examining the breasts carefully and relating the findings of the patient's history.

Treatment

- Women with large breasts have often tried custom bras and weight loss as a way of reducing breast size or adding support. Physical therapy and pain medications may also be used in an effort to relieve symptoms. After trying these methods without success, many women seek surgical help in the form of breast reduction surgery. Technically, breast reduction surgery is known as reduction mammoplasty.
- The best candidates for breast reduction usually have at least two of the symptoms listed in the aforementioned Common Signs and Symptoms section.
- Breast reduction surgery should be delayed if weight gain or loss is anticipated. The patient's weight should be stable at the time of the procedure.
- The aims of the operation are the following:
  - To remove enough breast tissue to be able to construct a normal-appearing breast mound
  - To reposition the nipple-areola complex in a suitable position in the "new" breast

There are many operations to reduce large breasts. A common technique is shown in the figures.

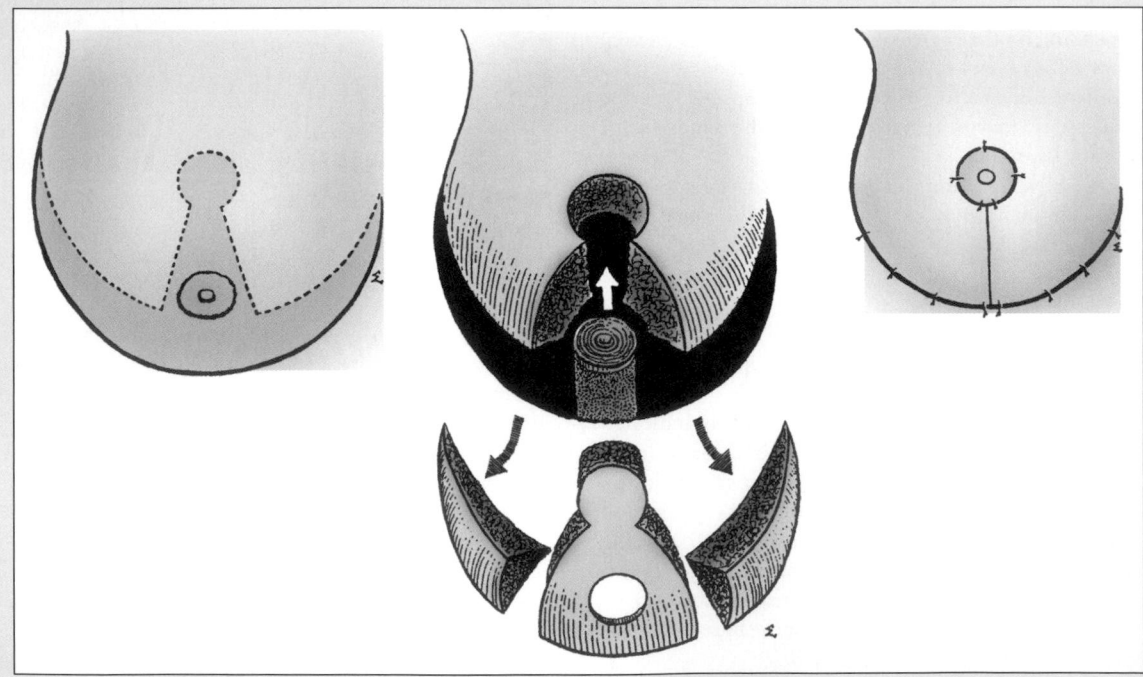

Preparing for the Operation

- The surgeon will examine and measure the breasts and will probably photograph the patient for reference during the surgery and afterward.
- A mammogram may be ordered if patient is 35 years or older or there is a family history of breast cancer.
- The patient should avoid smoking completely for at least 1 month before surgery. Smoking affects the blood vessels in the skin and can slow healing. A drug and alcohol consumption history should also be obtained prior to surgery (can be done during the history and physical).
- The surgeon may instruct the patient to avoid taking aspirin, nonsteroidal antiinflammatory drugs (ibuprofen [Motrin]), vitamin E, fenfluramine, or phentermine at least 2 weeks before surgery. These substances may interfere with normal blood clotting or with the ability to heal after surgery.

PATIENT AND FAMILY EDUCATION

Patient Education for Breast Reduction—cont'd

- Before surgery the patient may want to do the following:
  - Wash hair (will not be able to shower or bathe immediately after surgery).
  - Arrange for temporary care for any house pets or children.
  - Move "daily use" items within arm's reach.
  - Fill any prescriptions from the surgeon.
- Following are common after this operation:
  - The sensation in the nipples probably will be decreased.
  - Patient may not be able to breastfeed.
  - Reading the mammogram may become more difficult for the physician because of the scarring inside the breast.
  - The scars from the operation may be prominent.
- On the day of the operation, the places where the incisions will be made on the breasts and the new position of the nipple-areola complex will be marked with dissolving ink while patient is in a sitting position.
- Patient may be given medicine that will make the patient feel drowsy before being taken to the OR.

The Operation

- Most women have general anesthesia (going to sleep) for breast reduction. Some surgeons may perform the procedure with a local anesthetic and sedation.
- The operation generally takes 3 to 4 hours.

After Your Operation

- You will be taken to a recovery room and observed. When blood pressure, pulse, and breathing are stable, you will be taken to a regular hospital room.
- You will be wrapped in elastic bandages or a surgical bra over gauze. Small plastic tubes called drains may be coming from the breast incisions and will be connected to small plastic bulbs. They drain any extra fluid that needs to come out.
- Many breast reduction surgeries are done as outpatient procedures, in which case you will go home after you wake up from the anesthesia and the pain is under control. In some cases you

may stay in the hospital after surgery for a short period (1 or 2 days).

- Recovery is different for every patient, but bed rest may only be needed for 1 or 2 days after the procedure. Even in the first 24 to 48 hours after surgery it is important for you to get out of bed and walk around every 2 hours during the day and early evening. Coughing, deep breathing, and incentive spirometry are also important to prevent atelectasis and pneumonia. Continuous bed rest after surgery may increase your risks for pneumonia or blood clots.
- As with any operation, complications are always possible. With this type of operation, they can include bleeding, infection, delayed wound healing, abnormal scarring, and shape irregularities.

Home Care

You will want to take it easy at first, but may walk about as you wish, even climb stairs, but should not overdo things. Avoid heavy exercise, heavy lifting, or stress on the upper body for 1 month. Items that can be helpful as you recover include the following:

- A body or sitting support pillow
- Cordless phone
- Variety of easy-to-cook or precooked meals
- Two or three loose-fitting robes or housedresses with snaps in the front and large pockets
- Slip-on shoes
- Soft sponge for bathing before showering is allowed
- Small containers for drinks (gallon containers are very heavy)
- A listing of physicians, pharmacy, and caregivers/helpers with telephone contact information. You should call the surgeon if any of the following occurs:
  - The incisions become red and inflamed, or have abnormal pain or excessive swelling.
  - You develop a temperature higher than 101.5°F (38°C).
  - You have any questions.

Modified from *Consumer's guide to breast reduction,* available at www.plasticsurgery.org/Patients_and_Consumers/Procedures/Reconstructive_Procedures/Breast_Reduction/Consumers_Guide_to_Breast_Reduction.html. Accessed November 27, 2012; McGrath MH, Pomeranz J: Plastic surgery. In Townsend CM et al, editors: *Sabiston textbook of surgery: the biological basis of modern practice,* ed 19, Philadelphia, 2012, Saunders.

RESEARCH HIGHLIGHT

Quality of Life After Breast Reduction Surgery

Macromastia can be the source of both health and emotional problems for women. Large breasts may impair a woman's ability to lead an active life and may result in back and shoulder pain. Emotional discomfort and self-consciousness are other issues faced by women with large breasts. These factors often prompt women to seek reduction mammoplasty in an effort to improve their quality of life.

This study sought to determine if there was an improvement in the quality of life for patients undergoing reduction mammoplasty and if the breast volume or patient size influenced the hypothesis that breast reduction surgery has a high satisfaction rate among patients regardless of the amount of tissue removed.

Researchers used a retrospective chart review on 600 patients to gather their study group. They mailed the Breast Q questionnaire

to the participants to complete and then entered demographic, surgical, and clinical data into a database. The Breast Q questionnaire asks patients to rate satisfaction with their breasts, overall outcome, and process of care, as well as psychosocial, physical, and sexual well-being.

The response rate for the questionnaire was 29.6% with 178 questionnaires returned. Survey results demonstrated that more than 95% of patients were satisfied with their breast surgery. The mean response was 2.8 with a standard deviation of 0.47 (where 1, disagree; 2, somewhat disagree; and 3, definitely agree). Patient body mass index (BMI) and total amount of breast tissue removed had a statistically significant positive correlation (0.479; $P < 0.0001$). There was no statistically significant difference between the total breast tissue removed and patient response ($P = 0.57$). The same respondents indicated they would have the surgery again.

Modified from Gonzales MA et al: Quality of life after breast reduction surgery: a 10-year retrospective analysis using the Breast Q questionnaire: does breast size matter?, *Ann Plast Surg* 69:361–363, 2012; American Society of Plastic Surgeons: *Breast reduction surgery: health and beauty for life,* 2013, available at www.plasticsurgery.org/reconstructive-procedures/breast-reconstruction.html?sub=How%20much%20will%20breast%20reconstruction%20surgery%20cost? Accessed March 3, 2013; Pusic AL et al: Development of a new patient-reported outcome measure for breast surgery: the BREAST-Q, *Plast Reconstr Surg* 24:345–353, 2009.

FIGURE 22-40 Mastopexy. **A,** Preoperative view. **B,** Postoperative view; ptosis corrected.

2. The redundant segment of breast tissue inferior to the nipple is excised through an inverted-T incision. Tissue from each breast is weighed and kept separate.
3. The surgeon mobilizes the nipple and adjacent tissue and sutures them in place.
4. The medial and lateral skin edges are approximated in a vertical suture line inferior to the nipple.
5. The inframammary elliptic incision is trimmed and closed transversely. Closed-wound suction catheters may be placed. The wound is dressed.

Mastopexy. Breast ptosis is corrected by moving the nipple to a more normal position and removing excess breast skin (Figure 22-40). With mastopexy surgery there is usually minimal to no removal of breast tissue, although it may be necessary to add a breast implant to achieve the desired result.

Procedural Considerations. The surgeon marks the patient before surgery. Positioning is similar to that used for breast augmentation. Skin incision choices are periareolar only; periareolar combined with a vertical (known as a short scar or vertical mastopexy); the classic inverted T, which adds an inframammary incision to the previous incision; or the horizontal inframammary, which combines the periareolar and inframammary, leaving out the vertical component. Mastopexy may involve reduction of the skin envelope only or combine skin removal with glandular reshaping and placement in a more desirable position.

Operative Procedure

1. Incisions are placed; one or more of the following techniques are used:
   a. Excess skin is removed.
   b. The breast cone is reshaped by invagination of lower mid-breast tissue.
   c. The lower submammary breast tissue pedicle is advanced below the breast tissue and tacked superiorly to the pectoral muscle.
   d. Lower midbreast tissue is incised and overlapped.
   e. A superiorly based (on the nipple-areolar complex pedicle) wedge tissue flap is created, turned under, and superiorly attached.
   f. The upper pole of breast tissue is mobilized and advanced superiorly and tacked to the pectoral muscle fascia.
2. The breast may be sutured entirely at this time or approximated, and the same procedure is applied to the opposite breast, closing both at the end of the procedure.
3. The operative area is cleaned, dressings of choice are applied, and a surgical bra is applied.

Excision of Gynecomastia. Gynecomastia is a relatively common pathologic condition that consists of bilateral or unilateral enlargement of the male breast. It occurs primarily during puberty or after age 40 years. Although it may be produced by a variety of diseases or be the result of side effects related to certain medications, it is usually related to excessive hormone production or alterations in hormonal balance. It may also be seen in elderly men and in men after excessive use of marijuana. All subareolar fibroglandular tissue is removed, and the resultant defect is surgically closed (Figure 22-41). The patient may be positioned in a supine position or semi-Fowler position, according to the surgeon's preference. Supplies and equipment needed are the same as those for a simple mastectomy, plus a basic plastic instrument set. Because suction-assisted lipectomy (SAL) may be used for contouring, suction cannulae, associated supplies, and an aspirator should also be available. All breast tissue removed should be weighed and then sent for pathologic examination. Although infrequent, men are not immune from breast cancer.

Operative Procedure

1. The surgeon instills local anesthetic and makes a stab wound incision for introduction of the liposuction cannula.
2. Liposuction is performed. If satisfactory removal of breast tissue is accomplished, the incision is closed and a compression garment applied.
3. If additional surgery is required, the surgeon makes a periareolar incision. Through this incision the fibrous and ductal attachments of the underlying glandular tissue to the nipple are divided.
4. A cuff of fatty tissue is left attached to the underlying nipple surface to protect the blood supply.
5. The surgeon dissects the breast tissue mass. Carrying the dissection to the pectoralis fascia is usually necessary to remove the entire mass.
6. Hemostasis is achieved.
7. Closure is performed, the area cleaned, and a compression garment applied.

FIGURE 22-41 A, Preoperative view of gynecomastia. **B,** Postoperative view after excision of gynecomastia.

KEY POINTS

- There are two subspecialties in plastic surgery. Cosmetic surgery restores or reshapes normal structures of the body; reconstructive surgery treats abnormal structures of the body caused by birth defects, developmental problems, disease, tumors, infection, or injury.
- Plastic surgery is not limited to a single anatomic location or biologic system.
- Procedures involve removing, reducing, enlarging, recontouring tissue and camouflaging of scars. Microsurgical techniques are often utilized.
- The top five cosmetic procedures performed in 2012 were breast augmentation, nose reshaping, liposuction, eyelid surgery, and facelift.
- The top five reconstructive procedures performed in 2012 were tumor removal, laceration repair, maxillofacial surgery, scar revision, and hand surgery.

CRITICAL THINKING QUESTION

You are caring for a female patient who is undergoing tumescent liposuction of her abdomen, hips, and thighs under general anesthesia. About 30 minutes into the procedure the anesthesia provider notes that the patient is tachycardic with a widened PR interval and is hypertensive. As he informs the surgeon of these findings, the patient experiences a tonic-clonic seizure. What is the likely cause of the patient's clinical deterioration? How should the nurse intervene?

⊖volve *The answers to the Critical Thinking Question can be found at http://evolve.elsevier.com/Rothrock/Alexander.*

REFERENCES

American Burn Association (ABA): *Burn incidence and treatment in the U.S.,* 2012, available at www.ameriburn.org/resources_factsheet.php. Accessed March 3, 2013.

American Society of Plastic Surgeons (ASPS 2012a): *ASPS annual statistics: plastic surgery in 2012,* February 19, 2013, available at www.plasticsurgery .org/news-and-resources/14-million-cosmetic-plastic-surgery-procedures -performed-in-2012.html. Accessed March 2, 2013.

American Society of Plastic Surgeons (ASPS 2012b): *Physician's guide to cosmetic surgery overview,* 2012, available at www.plasticsurgery.org/for-medical -professionals/resources-and-education/publications/physicians-guide-to -cosmetic-surgery/physicians-guide-to-cosmetic-surgery-overview.html. Accessed March 2, 2013.

Association of periOperative Registered Nurses (AORN): *Patient hand off tool kit,* 2012, available at www.aorn.org/practiceresources/toolkits/patienthand offtoolkit. Accessed March 2, 2013.

Association of periOperative Registered Nurses (AORN): Recommended practices for managing the patient receiving local anesthesia. In *Perioperative standards and recommended practices,* Denver, 2013a, The Association.

Association of periOperative Registered Nurses (AORN): Recommended practices for preoperative patient skin asepsis. In *Perioperative standards and recommended practices,* Denver, 2013b, The Association.

Coffee T: Care of patients with burns. In Ignatavicius DD, Workman ML, editors: *Medical-surgical nursing: patient-centered collaborative care,* ed 7, St Louis, 2013, Saunders.

Denholm B: Tucking patients' arms and general positioning, *AORN J* 89(4):755–757, 2009.

Edwards C et al: The SGAP flap for the postmastectomy patient, *OR Nurse* 3(3):28–34, 2009.

Gladfelter J: Compression garments 101, *Plast Surg Nurs* 27(2):73–77, 2007.

Kelman RM: Maxillofacial trauma. In Flint PW et al, editors: *Cummings otolaryngology head and neck surgery,* ed 5, Philadelphia, 2010, Mosby.

Leona M, Phillips LG: Wound healing. In Townsend CM et al, editors: *Sabiston textbook of surgery: the biological basis of modern practice,* ed 19, Philadelphia, 2012, Saunders.

Life Cell Corporation: *AlloDerm 2012,* available at www.lifecell.com/health -care-professionals/lifecell-products/allodermr-regenerative-tissue-matrix/ allodermr-tissue-matrix-defined. Accessed October 5, 2012.

Logan JM, Broughton G: Plastic surgery: understanding abdominoplasty and liposuction, *AORN J* 88(4):587–600, 2008.

McCance KL: Cancer epidemiology. In Huether SE et al, editors: *Understanding pathophysiology,* ed 5, St Louis, 2012, Mosby.

McGrath MH, Pomeranz J: Plastic surgery. In Townsend CM et al, editors: *Sabiston textbook of surgery: the biological basis of modern practice,* ed 19, Philadelphia, 2012, Saunders.

National Cancer Institute, U.S. National Institutes of Health (NCI): *Skin cancer,* 2012, available at www.cancer.gov/cancertopics/types/skin. Accessed July 20, 2012.

National Cancer Institute, U.S. National Institutes of Health (NCI): *Melanoma,* 2013, available at www.cancer.gov/cancertopics/types/melanoma. Accessed March 3, 2013.

Pederson WC: Principles of microsurgery. In Wolfe SW et al, editors: *Green's operative hand surgery,* ed 6, Philadelphia, 2011, Churchill Livingstone.

The Joint Commission (TJC): *Joint Commission introduces new, customized tool to improve hand-off communications,* 2012, available at: www.joint commission.org/issues/article.aspx?Article=RZlHoUK2oak83WO8RkCmZ 9hVSIJT8ZbrI4NznZ1LEUk%3D. Accessed March 2, 2013.

The Joint Commission (TJC): *Hospital national safety goals,* 2013, available at www.jointcommission.org/assets/1/6/2013_HAP_NPSG_final_10-23.pdf. Accessed March 2, 2013.

U.S. Department of Labor (DOL): *Your rights after a mastectomy, women's health and cancer rights act of 1998 (WHCRA),* 2012, available at www.dol.gov/ ebsa/publications/whcra.html. Accessed March 3, 2013.

U.S. Food and Drug Administration (FDA): *Medical devices: update on the safety of silicone gel-filled breast implants-executive summary,* 2011, available at www .fda.gov/MedicalDevices/ProductsandMedicalProcedures/Implantsand Prosthetics/BreastImplants/ucm259866.htm. Accessed March 3, 2013.

CHAPTER 23
Thoracic Surgery

MARIA ARLENE GAPAC LEMIN

Thoracic surgery, like other specialties, has evolved with the increased understanding of pathophysiology, and development of improved surgical techniques and treatments. The thoracic specialty extends beyond the surgical arena into infectious disease, trauma, and oncology. Improved technology and the determination to treat diseases previously considered untreatable with operative and other invasive procedures continue to improve the recovery rate for patients experiencing thoracic diseases. As the ability to treat thoracic disease has improved, the responsibilities of the perioperative nurse have expanded, resulting in accomplishments throughout the years that have provided an extensive knowledge base and specialized perioperative practitioners.

Surgical Anatomy

The skeletal framework of the thorax is formed anteriorly by the sternum and costal cartilages, laterally by the 12 pairs of ribs, and posteriorly by the 12 thoracic vertebrae (Figure 23-1). This airtight compartment is enclosed in the root of the neck by Sibson fascia and is separated from the abdomen by the diaphragm.

The sternum forms the anterior thoracic wall in the midline. It consists of three parts: (1) the upper part, or manubrium; (2) the body, or gladiolus; and (3) the lower cartilage, or xiphoid process. The manubrium articulates with the clavicles and the first two ribs on each side; the gladiolus articulates with the remaining true ribs by separate costal cartilages; and the xiphoid fuses with the gladiolus in early development and is attached to the diaphragm by the substernal ligament.

Normally the lateral walls of the thorax are formed by the 12 pairs of ribs. Posteriorly, each pair of ribs articulates with its corresponding thoracic vertebrae. Anteriorly, the first seven ribs articulate with the sternum. The eighth, ninth, and tenth ribs articulate with the costal cartilages of the rib above; however, the eleventh and twelfth ribs are not fixed to the costal arch (see Figure 23-1).

The muscles of each hemithorax (Figures 23-2 and 23-3) include the 11 external and 11 internal intercostal muscles, which fill the spaces between the ribs. An intercostal artery, vein, and nerve accompany each intercostal muscle. The arteries communicate with the internal thoracic artery anteriorly and arise from the aorta posteriorly. The intercostal veins follow the course of the arteries and communicate with the mammary veins anteriorly and with the azygos and hemiazygos veins posteriorly.

During surgery great care is taken to prevent injury to the intercostal nerve, which passes forward and alongside the posterior intercostal artery and shares the intercostal groove on the inferior edge of the corresponding rib with the superior branch of the artery.

When the nerve must be disturbed, an anesthetic agent may be injected to prevent postoperative pain.

The thoracic outlet is a junction bound anteriorly by the manubrium, anterolaterally by the first ribs, and posteriorly by the first thoracic vertebrae and posterior angles of the first ribs of the space. The great vessels of the head, neck, and arm pass through this space. Compression of these structures may cause thoracic outlet syndrome.

The mediastinum is divided into anterior, middle, and posterior compartments. The anterior mediastinum is bound anteriorly by the sternum and posteriorly by the pericardium and great vessels. It contains the thymus gland, lymph nodes, and pericardial fat. The middle mediastinum is bound anteriorly by the pericardium and great vessels and posteriorly by the anterior border of the vertebral bodies. The posterior mediastinum is bound anteriorly by the vertebral bodies and extends posteriorly to the chest wall.

The chest cavity is subdivided into the right and the left pleural cavities, which contain the lungs separated by the mediastinum, which lies medially between the two pleural membranes. The parietal pleura, the membrane that lines the inner surface of each hemithorax, is adjacent to the inner surfaces of the ribs posteriorly and the mediastinum medially and covers the surface of the diaphragm except at the central portion. Part of the parietal membrane is reflected back at the root of each lung to form a sac around it. This reflection is called the *visceral pleura.* The pleural space normally holds about 50 mL of pleural fluid, a serous secretion that provides lubrication between these two membranes to minimize friction during inspiration and expiration (Brashers, 2012).

FIGURE 23-1 Bony thorax.

Dome of
pleura
Thyrohyoid
muscle
Sternocleidomastoid muscle
Middle scalene muscle
Anterior scalene muscle
Trapezius muscle
Brachial plexus
Deltoid muscle
Subclavian artery
and vein
External intercostal muscle
Internal intercostal muscle
Pectoralis major muscle
Internal mammary
artery and vein
Subscapularis muscle
Rectus abdominis muscle
Latissimus dorsi muscle
Serratus anterior muscle
Diaphragm
External oblique muscle
Transverse muscle
Internal oblique muscle

FIGURE 23-2 Anterior view of thorax and contiguous portions of base of neck and anterior abdominal wall. *Right half,* Superficial layer of muscles and fascia; *left half,* relations of deep muscles of neck and abdomen to rib cage, intercostal muscles, diaphragm, and internal mammary vessels; relations of muscles, nerves, and vessels with first rib; and anterior relations of lung.

Splenius capitis muscle
Levator muscle of scapula
Trapezius muscle
Trapezius muscle
Infraspinatus muscle
Rhomboid muscle
Latissimus dorsi muscle
Serratus anterior muscle
Teres major muscle
Intercostal muscles
Rhomboid muscle
Sacrospinalis muscle
Latissimus dorsi muscle
Diaphragm
Internal oblique muscle
External oblique muscle
Latissimus dorsi muscle

FIGURE 23-3 Posterior view of thorax and contiguous portions of neck and abdominal wall. *Left half,* Superficial muscles; *right half,* deeper muscles.

The lungs are the essential organs of respiration. The base of each lung rests on the diaphragm, whereas its apex (upper end) projects into the base of the neck at a level above the first rib. The bronchus, the nerves, the lymphatics, and the pulmonary and bronchial vessels enter and leave the lung on the mediastinal surface in a structure known as the *hilum,* or *root,* of the lung. Deep fissures divide the spongy, porous lung into lobes. The primary bronchi divide and then subdivide into each lobe and eventually become bronchioles. The right lung has an upper, a middle, and a lower lobe; the left lung has only an upper and a lower lobe (Figure 23-4). However, the lungs are similar in that each is composed of 10 major segments (Figure 23-5). Each segment extends to the pleural surface, expanding in

volume from its center to its peripheral edges. Each segment also has its own bronchus and branches of the pulmonary artery and vein.

The bronchial arteries, arising from the aorta, supply nourishment to the lungs. They vary in their number and course. The arrangement may include two branches to the left lung and one branch to the right lung, which later branches into two, or there may be one or two branches for each lung. The pulmonary arteries carry the blood to the pulmonary parenchyma, and the pulmonary veins transport the oxygenated blood to the left atrium.

The nerves of the lungs are a part of the autonomic nervous system (see Chapter 21). They regulate constriction and relaxation of the bronchi and of the blood vessels within the lungs.

Although the thoracic cavity is an airtight space, the lungs receive outside air through the nasal passages, trachea, and bronchi. The main function of the lungs is to exchange carbon dioxide for oxygen. Normally, as the thorax expands, the lungs also expand as air is drawn in; during expiration, the thorax relaxes and the lungs passively contract as air is forced out. Inspiration normally takes place when the intrathoracic pressure is slightly below atmospheric pressure (76 cm Hg, or 760 mm Hg) and when a partial vacuum exists between the parietal and visceral pleural (intrathoracic) surfaces. As the muscles of inspiration contract to enlarge the chest cage, the lungs passively follow the diaphragm and chest wall because of decreased intrathoracic pressure. The acts of inspiration and expiration are the result of air moving in and out of the lung, causing pressure to equalize with that of the atmosphere at the end of expiration.

The normal intrapleural pressure varies from −9 to −12 cm H_2O during inspiration and from about −3 to −6 cm H_2O during expiration. The greatest amount of air that can be expired after a maximum inspiration is termed the *vital capacity*, and the volume of gas remaining in the lungs after maximal expiration is *residual volume*. Size, age, gender, and pulmonary disease of the patient influence vital capacity. Any condition that interferes with the normally negative intrapleural pressure affects respiratory function.

Perioperative Nursing Considerations

Assessment

During assessment the perioperative nurse gathers information that is important to planning patient care. Signs and symptoms demonstrated by the patient are confirmed by the perioperative nurse during the admission assessment. The nurse may begin data collection by identifying the patient and confirming the correct surgical site. A thorough review of the patient's medical record, including results of the history, physical examination, laboratory tests, other diagnostic workups, and the nursing history and assessment, is critical for subsequent care planning. It is valuable to assess the patient's understanding of the disease process and of the anticipated procedure. In addition to assessing the patient's knowledge and understanding of the proposed surgical procedure and outcomes, the perioperative nurse ensures that the patient has adequate support to assist the patient through the surgical experience and recovery. The nurse should also assess emotional status because patients with a possible diagnosis of carcinoma may be very anxious. A focused assessment of the respiratory system should be included during the physical assessment. The nurse questions the patient or otherwise

FIGURE 23-4 Organs of thoracic cavity. Part of pericardium has been removed to expose heart.

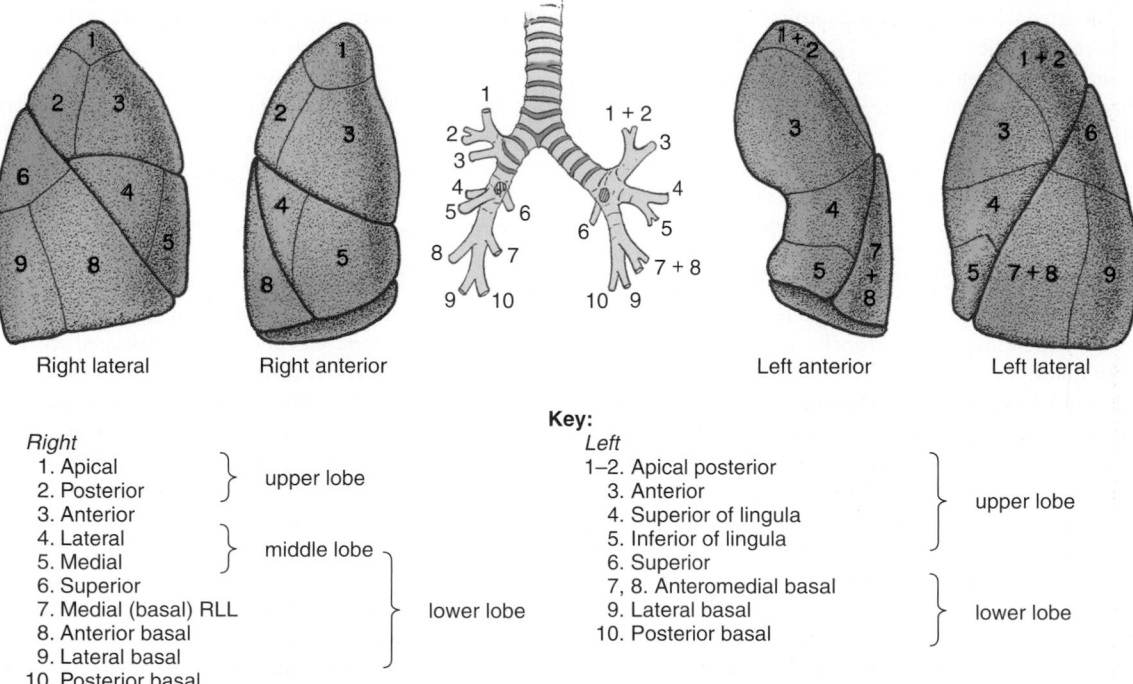

Right
1. Apical } upper lobe
2. Posterior
3. Anterior
4. Lateral } middle lobe
5. Medial
6. Superior
7. Medial (basal) RLL } lower lobe
8. Anterior basal
9. Lateral basal
10. Posterior basal

Key:

Left
1–2. Apical posterior } upper lobe
3. Anterior
4. Superior of lingula
5. Inferior of lingula
6. Superior } lower lobe
7, 8. Anteromedial basal
9. Lateral basal
10. Posterior basal

FIGURE 23-5 Segments of the pulmonary lobes. *RLL,* Right lower lobe.

TABLE 23-1

Pulmonary Function Tests

Test	Purpose
FVC (forced vital capacity): Records maximum amount of air that can be exhaled as quickly as possible after maximum inspiration	Provides an indication of respiratory muscle strength and ventilatory reserve. Often reduced in obstructive disease (because of air trapping) and in restrictive disease
FEV$_1$ (forced expiratory volume in 1 second): Records maximum amount of air that can be exhaled in first second of respiration	Effort dependent and declines with age; reduced in certain obstructive and restrictive disorders
FEV$_1$/FVC: Ratio of expiratory volume in 1 second to FVC	Provides a more sensitive indicator of obstruction to airflow. Ratio is normal or increased in restrictive disease, but decreased in obstructive disease.
FEF$_{25-75\%}$: Records forced expiratory flow over 25%-75% volume (middle half) of FVC	This measure provides a more sensitive index of obstruction in smaller airways.
FRC (functional residual capacity): Amount of air remaining in lungs after normal expiration	Increased FRC indicates hyperinflation or air trapping, which may result from obstructive disease.
TLC (total lung capacity): Amount of air remaining in lungs at end of maximum inhalation	Increased TLC indicates air trapping associated with obstructive pulmonary disease. Decreased TLC indicates restrictive disease.
RV (residual volume): Amount of air remaining in lungs at end of a full, forced exhalation	RV is increased in obstructive pulmonary disease, such as emphysema.
DL$_{co}$ (diffusion capacity of carbon monoxide): Reflects surface area of alveolocapillary membrane	DL$_{co}$ is reduced when alveolocapillary membrane is diminished, such as in emphysema, pulmonary hypertension, and pulmonary fibrosis.

From Pagana KD, Pagana TJ: *Mosby's diagnostic and laboratory test references*, ed 10, St Louis, 2012, Mosby; Rees HC: Assessment of the respiratory system. In Ignatavicius DD, Workman ML, editors: *Medical-surgical nursing: patient-centered collaborative care*, ed 7, St. Louis, 2013, Saunders.

confirms the presence of an increased frequency of cough, increase in sputum production, recurrent hemoptysis, malaise, shortness of breath, substernal chest discomfort, weight loss, poor appetite, status of nutrition, and hypoxia. The results of the physical examination of the chest should be reviewed; the perioperative nurse may auscultate the chest and confirm the presence of crackles or wheezes on inspiration or expiration, which should be documented on the medical record.

The review of diagnostic and laboratory tests may include the chest x-ray films, sputum analysis obtained during bronchoscopy, cytology reports, arterial blood gas (ABG) results (Appendix A), and pulmonary function studies (Table 23-1). Laboratory tests including the complete blood count (CBC) should be within normal limits but may indicate anemia. The chest x-ray film remains an indispensable diagnostic tool and is needed in the operating room (OR). This film outlines the lesion, if any is present, and defines its shape and space-occupying nature (e.g., tracheal shift). The presence of air in the hilar region, pleural effusion, or atelectasis may also be confirmed by radiologic evidence. Sputum analysis for culture and sensitivity may alert the perioperative nurse to an infectious process; cytologic examination may confirm a malignancy. The patient may have already undergone diagnostic bronchoscopy or mediastinoscopy; if so, the findings for acid-fast bacillus smear, culture, bronchial washing, and biopsy should be reviewed. Pulmonary function tests with a forced expiratory volume in 1 second (FEV$_1$) less than 1 L indicate the patient is at extremely high risk for pulmonary complications in the postoperative period. Computed tomography (CT) scans of the chest, as well as of the brain, liver, and abdomen, may reveal the presence or absence of metastasis, pleural calcification, thickening, or plaque. Radioisotope scans may have been done for similar reasons as the CT. Magnetic resonance imaging (MRI) detects vascular relationships to masses or vascular lesions. Positron emission tomography (PET) is a noninvasive study demonstrated to be highly accurate in diagnosing malignant pulmonary nodules and lymphadenopathy. MRI and PET are sometimes performed to rule out metastasis of the lesion. Transbronchial needle aspiration

is useful in diagnosing mediastinal lymphadenopathy and staging lung cancer. Ventilation and perfusion studies show the distribution of each function in the lung. These results assist the perioperative nurse in collaborating with the surgical team to maintain effective gas exchange during the surgical intervention. The results are also valuable in predicting postoperative respiratory function and metabolic responses. Patients hospitalized for surgery related to carcinoma may have received chemotherapy or radiation therapy before surgery. Assessment of the skin and the patient's general condition is important in preventing perioperative complications. The nurse should also assess the patient's pain tolerance to determine necessary teaching or tools that will assist in achieving positive postoperative outcomes.

The nurse should assess the patient's smoking history (including the use of cigars, pipes, tobacco, or controlled substances) and any exposure to secondhand smoke within the home and workplace. The nurse should also reinforce the need to abstain from tobacco following surgery (Rees, 2013). Patients might be sensitive about smoking history because of the assumed relationship between smoking and lung disease. The nurse should phrase questions in a way that will not result in guilt about smoking habits or assumptions that the diagnosed condition is associated with smoking.

After a general and focused review of the patient's medical record and patient interview, the perioperative nurse formulates nursing diagnoses. These statements reflect problems that require perioperative nursing intervention, either independently or collaboratively with other members of the surgical team. Nursing diagnoses should be individualized and prioritized for each patient.

Nursing Diagnosis

Nursing diagnoses related to the care of patients undergoing thoracic surgery might include the following:

- Impaired Gas Exchange related to surgical intervention
- Risk for Impaired Skin Integrity related to surgical positioning, length of surgical intervention, or use of chemical antimicrobial agents on the skin

- Risk for Imbalanced Fluid Volume related to decreased surface area of the lung for perfusion and to administration of intravenous (IV) fluids during surgery
- Risk for Infection at surgical site related to inadequate secondary defenses (presence of existing disease process) and surgical disruption of tissues
- Impaired Comfort related to pain following surgical intervention

Outcome Identification

Outcomes identified for the selected nursing diagnoses could be stated as follows:

- The patient will experience adequate gas exchange during the surgical procedure.
- The patient's skin integrity will be maintained.
- The patient will maintain appropriate fluid balance.
- The patient will be free from postoperative surgical site infection.
- The patient's pain will be monitored and managed.

Planning

A Sample Plan of Care for a patient undergoing thoracic surgery is shown below.

Implementation

During implementation of the plan of care the perioperative nurse is concerned with both preparatory patient considerations (e.g., procedure explanation and teaching for the patient; verification of the patient, surgical procedure, and site; positioning; presurgical diagnostic interventions; draping) and the requirements of the surgical intervention (e.g., medication delivery; instrumentation equipment, and supply availability). These patient care needs are coordinated with the other nursing interventions identified in the specific patient's plan of care.

Positioning. The type of position used in thoracic surgery is determined by the operative procedure planned. Bronchoscopy is usually performed in the supine position, commonly with a shoulder roll. Thoracotomy can be performed with the patient in one of three common positions: (1) lateral for the posterolateral approach, (2) semilateral for the anterolateral approach (Figure 23-6), and (3) supine for the median sternotomy approach. Arms are placed on padded armboards with the palms up and fingers extended. Armboards are maintained at less than a 90-degree angle to prevent brachial plexus stretch. If there are surgical reasons to tuck the arms at the side, the elbows are padded to protect the ulnar nerve, the palms face inward, and the wrist is maintained in a neutral position (Denholm, 2009). A drape secures the arms. It should be tucked snuggly under the patient, not under the mattress. This prevents the arm from shifting downward intraoperatively and resting against the OR bed rail. A beanbag can be used to support the patient in the lateral decubitus position.

The prone position also can provide access in some procedures (see Chapter 6 for safe positioning interventions). Adequate padding and safe transfer should be implemented to prevent pressure injury.

SAMPLE PLAN OF CARE

Nursing Diagnosis
Impaired Gas Exchange related to surgical intervention

Outcome
The patient will experience adequate gas exchange during the surgical procedure.

Interventions
- Determine the preoperative status of gas exchange by reviewing laboratory results and assessing the patient; report deviations from preoperative laboratory values and patient assessment findings.
- Obtain chest x-ray films for the intraoperative period.
- Verify that a double-lumen endotracheal tube with a soft, inflatable cuff is available for the anesthesia provider.
- Collaborate in obtaining equipment for and monitoring arterial blood gases (ABGs); document results.
- Obtain equipment for and assist with patient preparation for hemodynamic monitoring: electrocardiogram (ECG), CO_2 analyzer, pulse oximeter, arterial pressure line, and central venous pressure line; collaborate with the anesthesia provider in evaluating results provided by these monitoring devices during the procedure.
- Apply thermal unit (forced-air warming device or other device as available in institution); check equipment before procedure; monitor and note patient temperature during procedure.
- Collaborate in positioning the patient to provide access to the endotracheal tube, enable efficient ventilatory function, and prevent injury.
- Obtain and label specimens (e.g., ABG, blood count) to be sent to laboratory; document specimens sent, and evaluate results.

Report abnormal values to the anesthesia provider and surgical team.

Nursing Diagnosis
Risk for Impaired Skin Integrity related to surgical positioning, length of surgical intervention, or use of chemical antimicrobial agents on the skin

Outcome
The patient's skin integrity will be maintained.

Interventions
- Assess skin integrity and condition of the skin preoperatively. Document findings; report the presence of any lesions, rashes, cuts, nicks, or reddened areas.
- Determine presence of preexisting conditions that could compromise skin integrity (e.g., age, obesity, diabetes, allergies, radiation therapy).
- Apply principles of positioning for efficient circulatory function for lateral or supine position during the procedure; pad and protect vulnerable neurovascular bundles and dependent pressure areas:
  - *Lateral position:* Ear, acromion process, iliac crest, greater trochanter, medial and lateral condyles, malleolus
  - *Supine position:* Occiput, scapula, olecranon, sacrum, ischial tuberosity, calcaneus
- Position the patient in the best possible body alignment to allow visualization of the operative field.
- Assess for preexisting conditions (e.g., joint implants, arthritis, restricted movement) to prevent patient injury during positional maneuvers.

Continued

SAMPLE PLAN OF CARE—cont'd

- Stabilize the patient in lateral position (e.g., beanbag, sandbag, soft shoulder roll, pillows between knees); check for tape sensitivity if adhesive tape is used. Flex the upper arm slightly (not exceeding 90-degree extension) above the head on a raised, padded armboard, or support on padding.
- Use adequate number of individuals to position the patient for the lateral position.
- Assess the area where the electrosurgical dispersive pad will be placed; clip the area if necessary. Document assessment and pad placement on the intraoperative record.
- If hair must be removed from the operative site, use clippers or a depilatory (check patient sensitivity); shave the patient with wet shave if a razor must be used.
- Prevent pooling of skin prep solutions at the bedline, site of ECG electrodes, and electrosurgical dispersive pad.
- Decrease surgical time by anticipating needs of the patient and surgical team.
- Observe and document skin integrity and condition postoperatively; compare with preoperative status.

Nursing Diagnosis

Risk for Imbalanced Fluid Volume related to decreased surface area of the lung for perfusion and to administration of intravenous (IV) fluids during surgery

Outcome

The patient will maintain appropriate fluid balance.

Interventions

- Insert indwelling urinary catheter; use aseptic technique.
- Position drainage bag off the floor, where it is readily observable.
- Monitor urinary output hourly during the procedure; report output less than 30 mL/hr.
- Provide access for administration of IV fluids; assist with fluid administration and insertion of lines. Keep lines protected and patent during positional changes.
- Monitor results of hemodynamic parameters; document and report appropriately.
- Monitor blood loss during the procedure; document and report appropriately.
- Provide blood (including autologous) or blood products for fluid replacement; assist in replacement therapy and patient monitoring.
- Observe for signs of shock (e.g., hypotension, abnormal ECG); report signs, and initiate corrective nursing actions.
- Observe for signs of excess blood loss (e.g., rapid, weak pulse; rapid respirations; cool, moist skin; early, slight rise in blood pressure); report signs, and initiate corrective nursing actions.
- Observe for signs of fluid excess (e.g., tachycardia, increased blood pressure); report signs, and initiate corrective nursing actions.
- Have available and administer furosemide (Lasix) and other diuretic agents as prescribed; monitor for therapeutic results.

Nursing Diagnosis

Risk for Infection at surgical site related to inadequate secondary defenses (presence of existing disease process) and surgical disruption of tissues

Outcome

The patient will be free from surgical site infection.

Interventions

- Create and maintain a sterile field immediately before use; monitor the sterile field, and take corrective action if breaks in technique occur.
- Administer preoperative antibiotics at least 1 hour before the procedure.
- Do not remove hair preoperatively unless the hair at or around the incision site will interfere with the surgical procedure. If hair must be removed, it should be done immediately before the surgical procedure, preferably using a means other than a razor.
- Practice aseptic technique when opening supplies, moving around the sterile field, catheterizing the patient, inserting IV lines, completing skin preparation, and draping the surgical site.
- Complete skin preparation at the incision site and point of insertion of monitoring lines to decrease microbial contamination. Use an appropriate antiseptic agent, applied in concentric circles moving toward the periphery. The prepped area should be extensive enough to extend the incision or create new incisions or drain sites.
- Monitor traffic patterns; limit the number of people entering and leaving the OR.
- Administer prescribed antibiotics for irrigation and IV administration; check for patient allergies; record all medications administered by the perioperative nurse or scrub person at the sterile field.
- Decrease surgical time by anticipating patient and surgical team needs.
- When visible soiling with blood or other body fluids of surfaces or equipment occurs during the procedure, use an Environmental Protection Agency (EPA)–approved hospital disinfectant to wipe the affected area (confine and contain).
- Correctly classify the surgical wound according to the institution's wound classification system on completion of the surgical procedure.
- Using sterile gloves, apply sterile dressings to the surgical site before the drape is removed.

Nursing Diagnosis

Impaired Comfort related to pain following surgical intervention

Outcome

The patient's comfort will be assessed, monitored, and managed.

Interventions

- Teach the pain assessment scale preoperatively.
- Provide education to the patient regarding the physiology of pain and the importance of treating pain before it becomes unmanageable.
- Discuss pain management techniques and options (i.e., oral, intramuscular [IM], IV medications, patient-controlled analgesia [PCA], epidural use, intercostal blocks).
- Assist anesthesia provider in initiating pain control methods (i.e., epidural placement, nerve blocks).
- Assess pain before and following administration of pain medication or use of comfort measures (e.g., repositioning, applying support devices).
- Monitor the effects of pain management strategies, and document.
- Assess verbal and nonverbal cues during procedures requiring monitored anesthesia care and administration of local anesthesia.
- Teach pain control methods and medication uses and side effects before discharge.

FIGURE 23-6 Positions for thoracotomy incisions. **A,** Lateral position for posterolateral incision. **B,** Semilateral position for axillary or anterolateral position.

Draping. Draping may be minimal for bronchoscopic procedures. The principles of draping for other procedures (see Chapter 4) are followed in all other thoracic procedures. Drapes may consist of a fenestrated sheet or single sheets surrounding the incision site. To prevent instruments from falling from the field, the scrub person may place a magnetic pad on the drapes below the incision site when the patient is placed in lateral position. The perioperative nurse ensures a forced-air warming blanket is placed on the patient before draping to maintain normothermia. Intermittent pneumatic compression devices are often applied also to prevent the development of deep vein thrombosis (DVT).

Instrumentation. Bronchoscopy instruments are designed to directly inspect and observe the larynx, trachea, and bronchi; to remove secretions; to obtain washings or tissue for bacterial and cytologic studies; or to remove tissue. They are also designed to remove foreign bodies. Both rigid and flexible bronchoscopes are available, with the rigid bronchoscope being better suited for removing foreign bodies. Instrumentation for thoracic surgery includes the laparotomy instrument set (see Chapter 11) and specialty items. Instruments used for a thoracotomy or chest procedure include a combination of delicate and heavy instruments. Stapling equipment is commonly used. These devices require staplers and staple reload of appropriate sizes. The delicate instruments are used to cut tissue and vessels or to clamp tissue in an atraumatic manner. The heavier instruments are used for bone cutting, dissecting, or retracting. Instrumentation must also be available for hemostasis and suturing of all types of tissue.

The scrub person, who may be a registered nurse or surgical technologist, should determine the arrangement of items on the instrument table and Mayo stand; this arrangement should be an

effective standard method that applies principles of work simplification and thorough knowledge of procedures. The possibility always exists that any incision may need to be extended to accommodate a more extensive procedure than was originally planned. Therefore, the practice of performing an initial count is recommended for all procedures, including minimally invasive procedures such as laparoscopy or thoracoscopy (Association of periOperative Registered Nurses [AORN], 2013). Lengthy incisions are often required for thoracic procedures; therefore, it is critical that an instrument count be performed before closure.

Equipment. In thoracic surgery a variety of equipment is used, including a forced-air warming unit, fiberoptic headlights, fiberoptic light sources, video equipment, intermittent pneumatic compression devices, and anesthesia supplies. To deflate the operative lung and ventilate the nonoperative lung, double-lumen endotracheal tubes are commonly used for thoracotomies.

The neodymium:yttrium-aluminum-garnet (Nd:YAG) or CO_2 laser can be used for treating tracheobronchial lesions with use of a bronchoscope. Obstruction of the mainstem bronchus and trachea caused by benign and malignant lesions can also be effectively treated with laser therapy. Use of laser equipment requires a thorough understanding of the equipment, the safety issues, the responsibilities (see Chapter 8), and the planned surgical procedure.

Monitoring. Monitored anesthesia care, local anesthesia, or topical anesthesia may be used during some bronchoscopic procedures. General anesthesia also may be used for bronchoscopic procedures as well as other thoracic procedures. Team members work in cooperation to constantly monitor laboratory results (e.g., ABGs), oxygenation, temperature, blood loss, and urine output. Monitoring intermittent pneumatic compression device settings and patient position also is important in providing safe patient care. Results are communicated with other team members and documented for continuity of care.

Blood Replacement. Blood replacement therapy during or after the procedure may be required because of extensive tissue dissection in a highly vascular area. The patient may have autologous blood ordered; however, the diagnosis or urgency of the procedure may prohibit patient donation of his or her own blood. The patient's blood type and amount of blood ordered should be noted before the procedure and its availability confirmed. During the procedure every effort should be made to control and monitor bleeding. If blood collection or reinfusion systems are used, the manufacturer's instructions and institutional protocols should be followed. Bloodless surgery programs are available at some institutions and can help minimize the need for allogeneic or autologous blood use.

Chest Drainage Systems. Chest tube and chest drainage system management represents an important intervention for perioperative nurses. In the presence of restrictive and obstructive pulmonary disease, the lung may not fully expand or contract, causing a reduction in alveolar ventilation with resultant hypoxia. Other conditions that interfere with respiratory function are excessive accumulation of mucus, pleural effusions, a foreign body in a bronchus, closed pneumothorax (simple and tension types), open pneumothorax, hemothorax, and multiple rib injuries that produce paradoxical motion of the thoracic cage, or flail chest (Figure 23-7).

The normal function of the lungs is supported by elasticity and negative intrapleural pressure. Collapse of the normal lung follows

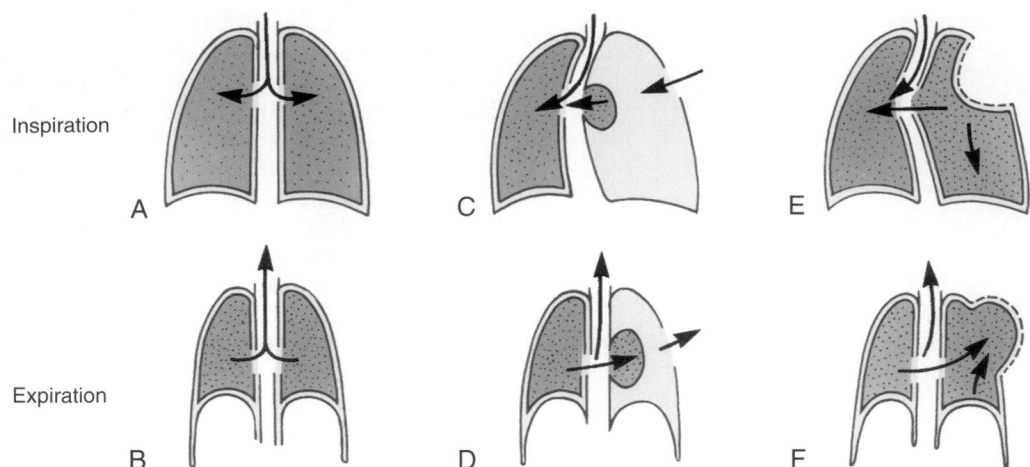

Inspiration

Expiration

A B C D E F

FIGURE 23-7 Pathophysiology of severe chest injuries. **A** and **B,** Normal physiology of inspiration and expiration. **C** and **D,** Open (sucking) wound of thorax. On inspiration, air at atmospheric pressure rushes in through defect **(C),** collapsing lung. Next, positive pressure causes mediastinum to shift, compressing opposite lung. On expiration **(D),** air from lung on uninjured side reenters collapsed lung and is rebreathed in next inspiration. Impaired cardiopulmonary function in presence of sucking wound of chest is caused by: (1) collapse of lung on injured side, (2) partial collapse of opposite lung, (3) increased functional dead space caused by rebreathing of unoxygenated air from collapsed lung, and (4) diminished venous return to right side of heart. **E** and **F,** Primary effect of paradoxical motion resulting from flail or stove-in chest is diminution of pulmonary ventilation and extensive rebreathing from one lung to the other. Venous return to right side of heart is impaired. Appropriate treatment requires intubation of trachea and use of volume-limited ventilator.

any condition that reduces or eliminates the negative intrapleural pressure if the lung is not adhering to the chest wall. When the pleural space is filled with air, the lung collapses due to the loss of negative pressure. This action may cause complete collapse if the pressure within the intrathoracic (pleural) space becomes positive.

A diminished negative pressure or the occurrence of actual positive pressure in one pleural space may cause the mediastinum or trachea to shift toward the opposite side. When this occurs, not only does the affected lung collapse because of a positive pressure in the pleural space, but also the function of the lung on the opposite side may be impaired as a result of compression by the mediastinal shift. Tension pneumothorax can produce serious effects as air continues to escape from the lung into the intrapleural space. The air cannot return to the bronchi to be exhaled, thereby increasing the intrapleural pressure. As the positive pressure continues to build, venous return to the heart is impaired and hemodynamic collapse may occur. When a large opening in the chest wall allows direct communication of the pleural space with atmospheric pressure, it may cause death if the mediastinum becomes mobile.

Paradoxical motion of the chest results from severe instability of the chest wall because of multiple and often bilateral rib fractures; with inspiration, partial collapse of the thoracic space occurs. The blunt injury that caused the multiple rib fractures also causes severe contusion of the lung itself. This contusion contributes to impairment of lung function by affecting gas exchange, which may result in severe, life-threatening hypoxia.

One or more chest catheters (tubes) may be inserted for postoperative closed-chest drainage. The chest tubes provide a conduit for drainage of air, blood, and other fluid from the intrapleural or mediastinal space and reestablishment of negative pressure in the intrapleural space (Patient Safety). Drainage systems use three mechanisms to drain fluid and air from the pleural cavity: positive expiratory pressure, gravity, and suction. The chest tubes are connected to a sterile water-seal or gravity drainage system. Water-seal suction may be necessary when a persistent air leak cannot be controlled by drainage alone. Several compact, disposable units are available. The disposable units have three or four compartments for drainage, water seal, and suction. The first chamber collects the drainage from the intrapleural space, the second chamber provides the water seal, and the third provides the suction control determined by the level of water (Figure 23-8). If two chest tubes are inserted, they may be attached by a Y connector to a single drainage unit or may be attached individually to two separate units. Chest tubes may be removed when the air leak has been resolved and the volume of drainage remains at an acceptable level for 24 hours (Nason et al, 2010).

Documentation. The nurse's documentation of perioperative care includes a summary of preoperative assessment information that supports formulated nursing diagnoses, nursing interventions, and postoperative evaluation. Documentation for a patient undergoing a thoracotomy specifically addresses patient assessment information related to position of the patient, positioning aids used, medications administered, results of laboratory tests completed, special equipment used, urine output, blood replacement, insertion of chest tubes and drainage systems, and postoperative evaluation of patient care outcomes.

Transfer Report. The patient is transferred from the OR to the postanesthesia care unit (PACU) after thoracotomy. The report to the PACU nurse is often a collaborative effort of the nurse and anesthesia provider. The perioperative nurse reports the procedure performed, particularly if it varies from the anticipated or scheduled procedure, and describes the patient's preoperative status, including anxiety level and understanding of the procedure, to assist the PACU nurse in meeting the emotional and educational needs of the patient. The nurse's description of the patient's position during the procedure provides criteria for assessment and evaluation of mobility. Results of immediate postoperative assessment, including skin integrity, location and type of dressing applied, location and

PATIENT SAFETY

Chest Tube Safety

The use of chest tubes is almost synonymous with thoracic surgery. Effective strategies for the management of chest tubes and chest tube drainage systems promote reduction of risk to patients for this aspect of thoracic surgery.

According to the Agency for Healthcare Research and Quality (AHRQ), major sources of adverse outcomes include breaks in sterile technique, inadequate anesthesia, incorrect insertion techniques, and inadequate self-protection by clinicians. The agency issued the following findings:

- Trying to perform multiple procedures concurrently is a major source of error.
- Equipment trays should be positioned near the surgeon's dominant hand.
- A patient's discomfort can make it difficult to perform a sterile procedure. Although adequate anesthesia is important, the patient may also need verbal and physical comforting. If a patient's movements cannot be controlled, the anesthesiology team should be called.
- Correct techniques can prevent damage to the lung and surrounding tissue, wound contamination, and fluid leakage.
- Universal Precautions against bloodborne infections are crucial to protect clinicians and their patients. In U.S. urban trauma centers, HIV rates among trauma patients are as high as 10%, and hepatitis C rates are as high as 15%; therefore, Universal Precautions should be practiced for all chest tube insertions.
- Additional management strategies include the following:
  - Ensure that the dressing on the chest around the tube is tight and intact. Palpate the area for puffiness or crackling that may indicate subcutaneous emphysema.
  - Assess for difficulty breathing.
  - Assess breathing effectiveness by pulse oximetry.
  - Check alignment of the patient's trachea.
  - Keep the drainage system lower than the patient's chest.
  - Keep the chest tube as straight as possible, avoiding kinks and dependent loops; do not "strip" the chest tube.
  - Ensure the chest tube is securely taped to the connector and the connector is taped to the tubing that enters the collection chamber.
  - Assess bubbling in the water-seal chamber; gentle bubbling should occur on patient's exhalation, forceful cough, position changes.
- The physician or rapid response team should be notified when the following are observed:
  - Tracheal deviation
  - Sudden onset or increased intensity of dyspnea
  - Oxygen saturation less than 90%
  - Drainage greater than 70 mL/hr
  - Visible eyelets on the chest tube
  - Chest tube falls out of the patient's chest or disconnects from the drainage system

HIV, Human immunodeficiency virus.
Modified from Problems and Prevention: *Chest tube insertion. Patient safety: findings in action*, AHRQ Publ No. 06-P024, Sept 2006, Agency for Healthcare Research and Quality, Rockville, MD, available at www.ahrq.gov/legacy/qual/chesttubes.htm. Accessed April 7, 2013; Workman ML: Care of patients with noninfectious lower respiratory problems. In Ignatavicius DD, Workman ML, editors: *Medical-surgical nursing: patient-centered collaborative care*, ed 7, St Louis, 2013, Saunders.

FIGURE 23-8 Commercial chest drainage system.

type of drains, blood loss, fluid replacement, medications administered, and laboratory results obtained during the procedure, are reported by the nurse and anesthesia provider as a baseline control for assessment in the PACU. The perioperative care plan should be reviewed and patient outcomes reported.

Postprocedural Concerns. The patient's endotracheal tube may remain in place to maintain an adequate gas exchange. Gas exchange and effective ventilation are two immediate clinical needs after thoracotomy. Chest tubes are often connected to suction, except for post-pneumonectomy procedures. The thoracotomy is considered a painful procedure and, when coupled with muscle injury, affects functional capacity. Anesthesia providers frequently use postprocedure epidural catheters for pain management to improve the comfort level of the patient because postoperative activities are encouraged.

Fluid volume overload can lead to acute life-threatening respiratory disease syndrome that should be avoided. Monitoring urine output is important, but post-thoracotomy patients should be maintained in a state of hydration that does not require a fluid bolus for low urine output.

Patients are often anxious about their limitations, the environment, and the results of the procedure. Patients and families will benefit from preoperative teaching about pain management techniques and use of the institution's pain assessment tool. Patients and families should also be encouraged to discuss their feelings and needs both before and after the surgical procedure. The perioperative nurse should facilitate notification of the patient's status to the family members during and as soon as possible after the procedure.

Evaluation

At the completion of the surgical procedure, perioperative nursing goals are evaluated. They may be restated as brief outcomes. For the goals identified for the patient undergoing thoracic surgery, outcomes could be stated as follows:

- The patient's gas exchange was unimpaired; ventilation/perfusion ratios were adequate as evidenced by laboratory results, and vital signs were within normal limits; skin, nailbeds, and mucosa were pink; lung fields were clear bilaterally; and chest excursion was normal.
- The patient's skin integrity was maintained; reddened or discolored skin and other signs of altered tissue perfusion were not present.
- Fluid balance was maintained; there were no fluid excesses or deficits; mental orientation was consistent with preoperative level; serum electrolytes and ABGs were within normal limits; urinary output was adequate.
- A postoperative surgical site infection will not be experienced; the incision site will remain approximated and dry, without redness, drainage, or undue tenderness. (This is a long-term goal, and its evaluation requires the collaboration of the nurse in the patient care unit.)
- Comfort will be managed and pain levels assessed.

Patient and Family Education and Discharge Planning

Discharge status is determined by the type of procedure being performed and the patient's overall state of health. General patient concerns might include mobility and activity levels or restrictions, pain management, wound care, dietary recommendations, medication regimens, follow-up appointments, and any prescribed outpatient care or referrals. Both the patient and the family need specific instructions for discharge that relate to the specific procedure. Patients and their families are encouraged to partner with the healthcare team and to ask appropriate questions and establish lines of communication (Patient-Centered Care). The nurse fosters patient autonomy and reviews all information verbally and provides it in written form, with verification of understanding and time for questions and concerns.

Patients are discharged within hours of a bronchoscopy. Their main concerns might be the results of biopsy and diagnosis. The patient and family should be aware of the length of time until results will be available and the method used to obtain those results. Patients should also be reminded of the need to rest for 2 to 3 days after the procedure. Side effects might result from medications used for moderate sedation or untoward intraoperative outcomes (e.g., the patient may experience bloody sputum, difficulty breathing). In addition, patients should be reminded that their throats might feel numb 2 to 3 hours after the procedure and difficulty with swallowing will subside (Ambulatory Surgery Considerations).

After a surgical procedure such as thoracoscopy or thoracotomy, vigorous pulmonary toileting is encouraged, including use of a spirometer, deep breathing, and turning and coughing every 1 to 2 hours while awake. Patients will transfer to the chair or ambulate on the day of surgery; length of time until discharge might be a few days to 1 week or more. Patients who progress without difficulty after a thoracoscopy or thoracotomy will be monitored for drainage from the chest tubes and for pain management or complications. Postoperative air leaks or pulmonary infections will delay discharge from the healthcare setting.

In-home nursing care may be initiated to monitor oxygen levels, wound care needs, and pain management. The patient may be discharged with supplemental oxygen (Patient and Family Education). This requires that the patient be weaned and demonstrate satisfactory ambulatory SaO_2 (i.e., percent saturation of arterial

---

PATIENT-CENTERED CARE

Various healthcare organizations have emphasized the importance of patient safety considerations. Since 2002, The Joint Commission (TJC) and the Centers for Medicare & Medicaid Services have encouraged patient participation through the Speak Up initiative as detailed below:

Speak up if you have questions or concerns. If you still don't understand, ask again. It's your body and you have a right to know.

Pay attention to the care you get. Always make sure you're getting the right treatments and medicines by the right health care professionals. Don't assume anything.

Educate yourself about your illness. Learn about the medical tests you get, and your treatment plan.

Ask a trusted family member or friend to be your advocate (advisor or supporter).

Know what medicines you take and why you take them. Medicine errors are the most common healthcare mistakes.

Use a hospital, clinic, surgery center, or other type of healthcare organization that has been carefully checked out. For example, TJC visits hospitals to see if they are meeting TJC's quality standards.

Participate in all decisions about your treatment. You are the center of the healthcare team.

Suggestions include basics of speaking up about any questions or concerns, emphasizing the right to know information about one's own care, and the importance of asking again if one does not understand explanations given.

Various initiatives are intended to help prevent errors, such as avoiding mistakes during surgery, preventing infection, and accurately administering medications. Patients are encouraged to know their rights, understand instructions from healthcare providers, and be active in their pain management plan. A majority of healthcare institutions using the initiatives add value to accreditations and certification processes; in fact, some institutions even advertise their accreditation status.

Besides patient information, nurses need to be actively engaged in activities promoting safety; this influence can be exercised in many ways. Siefert (2008) notes: "One of the simplest and most effective [ways] is to verbalize that something does not seem right. Motivate novice nurses to articulate concerns, encourage experts to scrutinize assumptions, and promote a workplace that respects curiosity and inquiry. The question not asked may lead to an error not prevented." Speaking up might take the form of strictly adhering to institutional policies concerning time-outs, patient identification, or soft goods and instrument counts or even questioning a medication order.

Modified from Seifert PC: Want to improve safety? Ask questions, *AORN J* 88(5):707–708, 2008; The Joint Commission: *Speak up: facts about speak up initiatives,* 2013, available at www.jointcommission.org/assets/1/18/Facts_Speak_Up.pdf. Accessed April 4, 2013.

---

oxygen) rates of 88% to 90%, which will most likely be supervised by home-care nurses.

Surgical Interventions

Endoscopy (Diagnostic or Therapeutic)

Endoscopy refers to examination of hollow body organs or cavities with instruments that permit visual inspection of their contents and walls. The endoscopic procedures pertinent to thoracic surgery are bronchoscopy, esophagoscopy, mediastinoscopy, and thoracoscopy.

AMBULATORY SURGERY CONSIDERATIONS

Ambulatory Thoracic Surgery

The concept of ambulatory surgical procedures is not new to the thoracic specialty; patients undergoing bronchoscopy or endoscopic sympathectomy have often completed their procedures on an outpatient basis. With the increased trend toward more minimally invasive procedures and improved technology to accomplish those procedures, the indications for ambulatory thoracic surgery are growing. Proper patient selection is key to the success of an ambulatory thoracic program. The surgeon must weigh the risks and benefits of performing surgery on a patient and allowing a discharge to home within several hours of the procedure. Anesthesia risk can be assessed according to the individual patient's American Society of Anesthesiologists (ASA) physical status classification (see Chapter 5). The surgeon considers the complexity of the surgery, the patient's medical and surgical history, and other factors on a case-by-case basis before surgery to ensure the most appropriate patients are selected for outpatient procedures. Because the majority of thoracic procedures entail entering the chest, the patient's level of pain, amount of chest tube output, presence or absence of an air leak, and pneumothorax status must be closely monitored before the final determination for discharge that same day.

Many ambulatory surgical centers in the United States offer an array of thoracic services. Mediastinoscopies, endoscopic, and minimally invasive procedures on the lungs and nerves of the mediastinum are the most frequently performed thoracic surgeries on an outpatient basis. Through proper patient selection, excellent surgical technique, and exceptional postoperative care the majority of patients treated at these centers can safely be discharged to home the day of surgery. Essential teaching points to cover with the patient and caregiver include pain control, respiratory treatments (to include deep breathing and coughing as ordered by the surgeon), and activity. Because the chest wall has been entered, the nurse must emphasize the importance of seeking emergency care if the patient experiences difficulty breathing, sudden chest pain, palpitations, uncontrollable cough, or bloody sputum.

Though they do not meet the standard definition of outpatient surgery, there is a movement toward programs to fast-track thoracic patients to earlier discharge to reduce inpatient stays. These fast-track programs usually operate, recover, and discharge a patient within a few days of being admitted. The postoperative recovery periods at these centers focus on pain relief and advances in chest tube management. Patients are often able to be discharged home safely with chest tubes in place using either a Heimlich valve or a portable drainage collection system. As more fast-track programs evolve and are able to demonstrate successful outcomes, new indications for outpatient care are likely to evolve.

Modified from Ansari D et al: Fast-track surgery: procedure-specific aspects and future direction, *Langenbecks Arch Surg* 398(1):29–37, 2013; Cerolio R, Brant AS: Does minimally invasive thoracic surgery warrant fast tracking of thoracic surgical patients? *Thorac Surg Clin* 18:301–304, 2008; Molins L et al: Outpatient thoracic surgery, *Thorac Surg Clin* 18:321–327, 2008.

PATIENT AND FAMILY EDUCATION

Patient Education and Home Care Teaching for Oxygen Therapy

General Information
- Review the physician's order for the type of delivery system and liter flow or percentage of oxygen to be delivered.
- Give the patient and the caregiver both *oral* and *written* instructions. Provide them with the name and telephone number of the physician to call if questions arise. Use visual aids to assist in instruction.
- Explain the purpose for oxygen therapy and how it will be delivered to the patient, and review the three commonly used methods to deliver oxygen as appropriate to the surgeon's order:
  - *Nasal cannula*. This is a two-pronged device inserted in the nostrils that is connected to tubing carrying the oxygen. The tubing can rest on the ears or be attached to the frame of eyeglasses.
  - *Mask*. People who need a high flow of oxygen generally use a mask.
  - *Transtracheal catheter*. Transtracheal oxygen therapy requires the insertion of a small, flexible tube (catheter) in the windpipe (trachea). This catheter is held in place by a necklace. Because transtracheal oxygen bypasses the mouth, nose, and throat, a humidifier is absolutely required at flow rates of 1 LPM or greater.
- Review that shortness of breath is not always from a lack of oxygen. If the patient's oxygen level is not the cause of the shortness of breath, taking oxygen will not help.
- Explain the importance of maintaining the appropriate flow rate because high flow rates in patients with chronic obstructive pulmonary disease can suppress the respiratory drive.
- Discuss that when the patient no longer needs oxygen, his or her physician will have the oxygen discontinued. Inform the patient that oxygen is not addicting or habit-forming.

Safety Tips
Review the following safety tips for using oxygen:
- Never smoke while using oxygen. Oxygen does not burn or explode, but materials will burn faster in the presence of oxygen.
- Keep a fire extinguisher close by. Let your fire department know that you have oxygen in your home.
- Warn visitors not to smoke near you when you are using oxygen. Put up "no smoking" signs in your home where you most often use the oxygen.
- Ask to be seated in the nonsmoking section when you go to a restaurant with your portable oxygen source.
- Stay at least 5 feet away from gas stoves, candles, lighted fireplaces, or other heat sources.
- Do not use materials that burn easily (flammable) while using your oxygen.
- Make sure your oxygen cylinder is secured to some fixed object or in a stand. If you use an oxygen concentrator, call your electric company so you will be given priority if there is a power failure. Avoid using extension cords, if possible.

Home Care
Discuss important factors the patient needs to consider when using oxygen in the home:
- Do not change the flow of oxygen unless directed by your caregiver.

Continued

Each surgeon has preferences regarding the type of endoscope, positioning of the patient, type of anesthetic, and equipment. Invasive diagnostic or therapeutic measures enhance the decision to pursue surgical intervention by providing information related to the disease process, including histologic characteristics, location of the lesion, and lesion extent. Therapeutic endoscopy provides treatment by removal of the lesion or foreign body.

Standard Bronchoscopy Using a Rigid Bronchoscope

Standard bronchoscopy is the direct visualization of the mucosa of the trachea, the main bronchi and their openings, and most of the segmental bronchi. It also includes removal of material for microscopic study if necessary.

Bronchoscopy is an integral part of the examination of patients with pulmonary symptoms such as persistent cough or wheezing, hemoptysis, obstruction, and abnormal roentgenographic changes. Common causes of bleeding (hemoptysis) are bronchiectasis, carcinoma, and tuberculosis. Congenital anomalies and suspected presence of a foreign body, especially in infants and children, are responsible for emergency examination of the respiratory tract.

The surgeon performs bronchoscopy to determine the presence of a lesion in the tracheobronchial passages, to identify and localize that lesion accurately, and to observe periodically the effects of therapy. It can be completed for dilating structures, debriding tumors, obtaining biopsies of masses, or evacuating clots. In suspected carcinoma, the aspirated secretions obtained by bronchoscopy may contain malignant cells.

Procedural Considerations. Flexible bronchoscopy on an adult patient may be completed after induction of local (topical) anesthesia or monitored anesthesia care; a child usually receives a general anesthetic. Patients undergoing rigid bronchoscopy should be paralyzed and ventilation continued to minimize trauma. The adult patient administered a local anesthetic may experience discomfort and anxiety. To reduce anxiety, the perioperative nurse should introduce members of the surgical team, explain intraoperative activities, and provide reassurance to the patient (Patient and Family Education, p. 881). The oral structures, including the teeth and lips, should be assessed for integrity. Loose teeth may require removal before or during the procedure.

The anesthesia provider or nurse providing moderate sedation may administer IV sedatives or analgesics during the procedure. See Chapter 5 for perioperative nursing considerations when the patient is receiving local or monitored anesthesia care. The topical (or local) anesthetic setup should include a headlight for visualization, laryngeal mirrors of various sizes, a lingual spatula, sprays with straight and curved cannulae, and anesthetic drugs, as ordered. Other items include the laryngeal syringe with straight and curved cannulae, Jackson cross-action forceps, and the Schindler pharyngeal anesthetizer, if desired. Luer-Lok 10-mL syringes and 20- and 22-gauge needles are needed for transtracheal injection. The scrub person ensures that all requested instrumentation is available to avoid delays and ensure the procedure is performed efficiently for the patient.

Anesthetic drugs frequently used for local or topical anesthesia are lidocaine (Xylocaine), procaine (Novocain), and tetracaine (Pontocaine, Cetacaine) with or without epinephrine. Pauses of 3 to 4 minutes are taken between applications of the anesthetic agent to the tongue, palate, and pharynx and then to the larynx and to the trachea. The surgeon or anesthesia provider applies the anesthetic agent by means of a spray or laryngeal syringe with a straight or curved cannula.

Some physicians prefer to have the patient sit upright and gargle with the topical anesthetic mixture, rinse it around in the mouth, and then expectorate it, thereby producing a partial anesthesia of the buccal mucosa and pharynx.

For direct bronchoscopy, the surgeon or anesthesia provider uses a long metal cannula attached to a syringe to apply the anesthetic agent to the surface of the vocal cords; then the agent is injected through the anesthetized glottis into the trachea. This act causes the patient to produce a sharp, sudden cough. For intrabronchial anesthesia, a portion of the anesthetic agent is introduced through the bronchoscope.

The patient may be positioned either in the supine position—with the shoulders elevated on a small roll, gel pad, or a sandbag to gently extend the head and neck—or in the sitting position.

The setup includes the bronchoscope, telescopes of desired types, fiberoptic light cords, and the fiberoptic light source. Each standard scope requires a fiberoptic light carrier, cord, and light source. The scrub person ensures that duplicates of each, along with the appropriate replacement light bulbs for the light source, are available for immediate use. The light source should be tested periodically and immediately before use. To test the fiberoptic light carrier and telescope, the instrument should be held vertically by the ocular

Patient Education and Teaching for Bronchoscopy with Patient-Administered Local Anesthetic

Preprocedural Teaching
- Review the physician's explanation of the procedure and the reason for it; encourage the patient to ask questions and to discuss any fears or anxieties.
- Discuss who will perform the procedure and where it will take place.
- Instruct the patient to have someone available after the procedure to drive the patient home.
- Review the following information about the procedure:
  - Medications may be given to relax you, dry up your secretions, and to control coughing. The medication that dries up secretions will make your mouth very dry.
  - Local anesthetics (medications) are given to numb your mouth, nose, throat, and voice box.
  - Your breathing is not blocked during this procedure. You will be able to breathe normally during the procedure.
  - If tissue samples (biopsies) are needed in the outer portions of the lung, sometimes a special type of x-ray (fluoroscopy) is required.
  - Abnormal areas will be brushed or biopsied for examination under a microscope. If any bleeding occurs from these areas, a drug may be used to make the blood vessels smaller (constrict) to stop or decrease the bleeding.
  - You may receive a chest x-ray following the procedure to make sure the lungs have not collapsed (pneumothorax).

Postprocedural Teaching
- Explain that after the procedure the patient's vital signs will be monitored frequently; discuss the need to maintain nothing-by-mouth (NPO) status until the gag reflex returns to prevent tissue injury and aspiration.
- Provide explanations about any temporary hoarseness and sore throat. Lozenges and throat gargles can be provided after the gag reflex returns.
- Review the signs and symptoms that should be reported immediately to a physician or nurse:
  - Lightheadedness
  - Shortness of breath
  - Fainting
  - Chest pain
  - Hemoptysis

Modified from MD Consult Patient Education: *Bronchoscopy*, 2012, available at www.mdconsult.com/das/patient/body/407108860-4/0/10089/59019.html?tab=eng. Accessed April 4, 2013.

end. The endoscope should always be tested immediately before passage into the patient. The light-intensity dial should be set at the proper level, as specified by the manufacturer. The light source should be switched on and off to test its function. During a procedure, the perioperative nurse switches the light source to standby mode whenever it is not in active use to conserve the life of the bulb and promote cooling. The light source should be kept away from any flammable materials (e.g., radiopaque soft goods and drapes) to avoid creating a fire hazard.

Other supplies that will be needed are suction tubing, aspirating tubes, specimen collectors, soft goods carriers, and the desired type of forceps. The metal soft goods carrier consists of two parts: an inner rod, which has two jaws protruding from its distal end; and an outer band, which is screwed down on the inner rod so that a soft good can be held securely within the jaws. Small gauze soft goods are used to keep the field dry, remove secretions, and apply topical anesthetic agents. Cytologic specimen collectors, such as the Clerf or Lukens, are used to hold secretions as they are obtained. Aspirating tubes of different lengths and designs are used to remove secretions and collect material for microscopic examination and culture(s). The straight aspirating tube with one or two openings at the distal end is used to remove material from the pharynx, larynx, and esophagus. The curved aspirating tube with a flexible tip is used to remove secretions from the upper and dorsal orifices of the bronchi.

The surgeon uses various types of forceps to remove foreign bodies or tissues for histologic study. Biting-tip forceps may be used to secure tissue for pathologic study. Forceps with jaws that veer laterally at about a 45-degree angle from the instrument's axis permit visualization during the biopsy maneuver. Bronchoesophageal forceps consist of a stylet, a cannula with a handle, a screw, a locknut, and a setscrew. Forceps for laryngeal and bronchial regions are designed to remove tissue specimens. The nurse should prepare several specimen containers with the identifying patient information label, along with laboratory slips for specific requests. If brush specimens are collected, slides and alcohol are required.

The standard bronchoscope is a rigid speculum used for visualizing the tracheobronchial tree. The rigid bronchoscope might be selected for biopsy of a large central mass, for removal of a foreign object, or to control hemorrhage during biopsy of a vascular mass. The rigid bronchoscope remains the instrument of choice for removal of foreign bodies in infants and children. A fiberoptic light carrier is inserted into the bronchoscope to illuminate the distal opening. A side channel is incorporated into the bronchoscope to permit aeration of the lungs with oxygen or anesthetic gases. An additional device, the Sanders Venturi system, which is available to the anesthesia provider, provides adequate patient ventilation during bronchoscopies and laryngoscopies.

The surgeon risks contamination in the presence of communicable diseases. For this reason, the surgeon and assistants should wear facemasks and eye protection or a transparent shield attached to a headband (see Chapter 4 for specific Transmission-Based Precautions). With increasing numbers of patients with tuberculosis, particulate respirators are recommended as protective devices. Aseptic technique is used to prevent cross-contamination.

Operative Procedure
1. The patient's head is placed in position for visualization of the bronchus—to the left when the right main bronchi are inspected and to the right when the left bronchi are inspected. The head is lowered for inspection of the middle lobe.
2. The surgeon places a tooth guard to protect the patient's teeth. The bronchoscope is inserted over the surface of the tongue, usually through the right corner of the mouth. The patient's lip is retracted from the upper teeth with a finger of the surgeon's left hand. The epiglottis is identified and elevated with the tip of the bronchoscope.
3. The surgeon passes the distal end of the scope through the true vocal cords of the larynx, and views the upper tracheal rings. A small amount of anesthetic solution may be sprayed through the tube on the carina of the trachea and into the bronchus with the bronchial atomizer or spray. The patient's head is moved to the left to obtain a view of the right bronchi. The right-angle telescope is inserted with the light adjusted into the bronchoscope.

4. The segmental bronchial orifices of the upper right lobe bronchi are viewed, and the telescope is removed. The surgeon uses suction and aspirating tubes to clear the field of vision and remove accumulated secretions.

5. The surgeon inserts an oblique 45-degree-angle telescope or right-angle telescope and advances it to inspect the middle lobe branches. The patient's head is lowered to view the right middle lobe or turned to the right to view the left main bronchus.

6. Secretions are aspirated by the surgeon for study. Biopsy forceps are used if indicated; foreign bodies are removed with forceps.

7. The bronchoscope is removed, and the patient's face is cleansed.

The nurse encourages patients who have undergone bronchoscopy after administration of a local anesthetic to sit on the edge of the OR bed before transfer to the stretcher. An emesis basin and tissues should be provided for the patient's use. Assistance and support are provided to the patient to prevent a fall.

Postprocedural Concerns. Patient safety during and after endoscopy using topical anesthetics, local anesthetics, or monitored anesthesia care is a concern attributable to the medications administered. The gag reflex may not return for 2 to 3 hours. The patient may be positioned on his or her side or with the head of the bed elevated to promote secretion drainage. The patient should be restricted from any oral intake until the gag reflex has returned. During bronchoscopy, particularly with a rigid bronchoscope, teeth could be loosened or oral structures damaged. The lips, teeth, and oral mucosa should be examined to ensure undisturbed integrity. Patients are often anxious to know the results of the procedure, and they benefit from the perioperative nurse's openness and willingness to discuss when results might be available, as well as the patient's feelings and concerns.

Bronchoscopy Using a Flexible Bronchoscope

Flexible bronchoscopy is performed to view structures that cannot be observed with a rigid scope. It is often the first choice for routine pre- and postoperative examination of the airways. Flexible bronchoscopy may be performed in addition to a standard rigid bronchoscopy or as an independent procedure. If performed independently, the patient may remain on the transporting stretcher during the procedure. Flexible bronchoscopy is completed for the same reasons as rigid bronchoscopy. Flexible fiberoptic telescopes permit visualization of the upper, middle, and lower lobe bronchi. They can be passed in patients with a jaw deformity or cervical bone rigidity with less difficulty than the rigid scope. A flexible bronchoscope can also be passed through the nares in an awake patient. Flexible fiberoptic bronchoscopes are more frequently used, as is video endoscopy.

Procedural Considerations. Patient considerations are as described for rigid bronchoscopy. Instruments and equipment used include the flexible bronchoscope, fiberoptic light source, flexible biopsy forceps, flexible brush (optional; if used, slides and alcohol are necessary to collect specimen), labeled specimen collectors, pathology requests, syringe for wash, and suction tubing with collection tube attached to collect the wash specimen.

Operative Procedure

1. The lubricated bronchoscope is passed through the adapter on the endotracheal tube, which is held secure by the anesthesia provider. If local or monitored anesthesia care is used for the procedure, the lubricated bronchoscope may be passed nasally.

2. The suction tube is positioned with the specimen collector attached for collection of bronchial washings. When indicated, the suction tubing is connected to the bronchoscope; the container for collection is held securely in an upright position to prevent loss of the specimen through the suction.

3. The surgeon or scrub person injects approximately 5 mL of saline solution into the channel. Suction is quickly reapplied. This procedure may be repeated as necessary.

After completion of the procedure, the perioperative nurse sends the specimens to the laboratory for analysis.

Mediastinoscopy

Mediastinoscopy is the direct visualization and possible biopsy of lymph nodes or tumors at the tracheobronchial junction, under the carina of the trachea, or on the upper lobe bronchi or subdivisions. Mediastinoscopy may precede an exploratory thoracotomy in known cases of lung carcinoma or may be completed to assist in accurately staging the patient's lymph node status. Patients with positive findings may be treated with radiation or chemotherapy, as indicated. The mediastinoscope is a hollow tube with a fiberoptic light carrier. A fiberoptic light source with a light-intensity dial provides power and control of illumination.

Procedural Considerations. The setup for mediastinoscopy includes a set of instruments for incising, cutting, retracting, and suturing similar to those needed for a minor procedure. In addition, the desired type of mediastinoscope, fiberoptic light cords, fiberoptic light source, suction tubing, aspirating tubes, biopsy forceps, electrosurgical unit (ESU), and an 8-inch, 20-gauge endocardiac needle are required. Depending on institutional policy, a thoracotomy tray may be in the OR on standby in the event of uncontrolled bleeding after biopsy.

The anesthesia provider administers a general anesthetic agent and assists with positioning the patient as described for a tracheostomy (see Chapter 19).

Operative Procedure

1. The surgeon makes a short (approximately 2 cm) transverse incision above the suprasternal notch, and exposes and incises the pretracheal fascia.

2. Using blunt (digital) dissection, the surgeon tunnels anteriorly along the trachea into the mediastinum.

3. The surgeon introduces the mediastinoscope under direct vision deep to the fascial plane and advances it anterior to the trachea toward the mediastinum.

4. The scope is manipulated to visualize the tracheal bifurcation, bronchi, aortic arch, and associated lymph nodes.

5. Lymph node tissue is located for biopsy and aspirated with a small-gauge needle and syringe to verify that it is a nonvascular structure.

6. The surgeon inserts a biopsy forceps through the scope, and obtains a tissue specimen. Pressure can be applied to the excision site with a bronchus soft good on a holder. The mediastinum is reinspected for bleeding.

7. The mediastinoscope is withdrawn.

8. Subcutaneous tissue is sutured with absorbable sutures. The surgeon closes the skin with absorbable material on a small cutting needle.

9. A small dressing is applied.

Video-Assisted Thoracic Surgery

Video-assisted thoracic surgery (VATS) is a minimally invasive operative technique that has evolved since 2003. It uses an endoscopic approach to visualize the thoracic cavity for diagnosis of pleural disease or treatment of pleural conditions, such as cysts, blebs, and effusions; to biopsy mediastinal masses; to perform wedge resections, lobectomy, pericardectomy, lung volume reduction surgery, and cervical sympathectomy; to obtain hemostasis; and to evacuate blood clots or divide adhesions. Pleurodesis with instillation of talc, tetracycline, or other sclerosing treatment can be accomplished through the thoracoscope (Surgical Pharmacology). VATS has many benefits, including the elimination of a thoracotomy incision, decreased pain, shortened hospital stay, and reduced morbidity. VATS also may be used in conjunction with robotically assisted thoracic procedures such as robotic lobectomy.

Procedural Considerations. Endoscopic instrumentation and equipment used for a thoracoscopy include 5- and 10-mm telescopes, light cord, camera, graspers, dissectors, scissors, ligators, and endoscopic soft tissue instruments (scissors, hemostats, suction tips, retractors) and stapling devices. It is also advisable to have thoracic instrument trays set up in the event there is a need to convert to a thoracotomy. Accessory equipment for video (television monitors, recorder, printer, light source for camera and scope, slave television monitor) and insufflation is also used. The perioperative nurse will assist in positioning the patient supine, semilaterally, or laterally, depending on the anatomic structures involved.

Operative Procedure

1. The surgeon creates a 2- to 3-cm incision between the fifth and seventh intercostal spaces for insertion of the 10- or 12-mm trocar. The zero-degree telescope is inserted to view the site so that the approach can be determined.
2. If the procedure can be completed by thoracoscopy, the surgeon creates additional puncture sites for insertion of additional trocars to allow instrument manipulation. The size of trocars and types of instruments vary for the diagnosis.
3. After the selected procedure, the surgeon inserts a chest tube through one of the surgical puncture sites and secures it to the skin. Trocar sites are closed, and small dressings or adhesive skin tapes are applied.

SURGICAL PHARMACOLOGY

Agents for Chemical Pleurodesis

Pleurodesis is undertaken as a treatment for malignant pleural effusion and for unresolved T-type spontaneous pneumothorax. A variety of chemical agents are used to cause adherence of the pleural layers. Adherence of the pleural layers is thought to prevent the accumulation of pleural fluid in the case of pleural effusion and to prevent subsequent pneumothoraces. Commonly used agents for chemical pleurodesis are listed. Other agents may be used according to the surgeon's preference, surgical region, and agent availability. Perioperative nurses should consult with the surgeon before the procedure to determine the agent used.

Medication/Category	Dosage (Intrathoracically)	Purpose/Action	Adverse Reactions	Nursing Implications
Talc	5-10 g in 250 mL of sodium chloride	Stimulates mesothelial cells to coordinate an inflammatory response	Pain, infection, ARDS, pulmonary edema	May be administered as a poudrage, aerosol, or slurry. Facial talc is unsterile, contains asbestos, and requires stringent sterilization technique. Commercially available sterile talc is preferable.
Antineoplastics	Bleomycin: 60 units mixed with 100-200 mg of lidocaine	Chemical pleural irritation and fibrosis of pleural surfaces	Pain, fever, neutropenia	Antineoplastics require special handling to reduce personal exposure. Nurses should follow hospital policies and procedures for safe medication handling procedures.
Cyclines	Minocycline: 7 mg/kg Doxycycline: 500 mg in 30-50 mL of sodium chloride	Indirectly stimulate pleural macrophages, activating pleural mesothelial cells; low pH initiates an inflammatory reaction, causing fibrosis	Pain, fever, hemothorax, neutropenia	Determine if patient is allergic to cycline medications before procedure.
Silver nitrate	20 mL of 0.5% silver nitrate	Coagulates cellular protein to form pleural eschar	Pain, fever	Handle with care. Solution stains skin and clothing. Not commonly used for pleurodesis.
Quinacrine	500 mg in 200 mL of saline	Causes systemic inflammatory response	Pain, fever	Not available in United States or Canada.
Iodopovidone	20 mL of 10% iodopovidone in 80 mL of saline	Mechanism of action unknown	Severe pain, hypotension	Assess patient for allergies to iodine.

ARDS, Acute respiratory distress syndrome.
Modified from Colt HG, Davoudi M: The ideal pleurodesis agent: still searching after all these years, *Lancet Oncol* 9(10):912–913, 2008; Khaleeq G, Musani AI: Emerging paradigms in the management of malignant pleural effusions, *Respir Med* 102:939–948, 2008; Rodriguez-Panadero F, Montes-Worboys A: Mechanisms of pleurodesis, *Respiration* 83(2):91–98, 2012; Yrndamuri S et al: Malignant pleural and pericardial effusion. In Selke FW et al, editors: *Sabiston & Spencer surgery of the chest*, ed 8, Philadelphia, 2010, Saunders.

Endoscopic Thoracic Sympathectomy

Hyperhidrosis is defined as excessive sweating, usually affecting the palms, axillae, and soles of the feet. It may also affect the face, groin, or legs. Patients with severe hyperhidrosis may produce 40 times the normal amount of sweat compared with patients without hyperhidrosis. Hyperhidrosis affects approximately 1% to 3% of the general population, with most of these individuals projected to have axillary hyperhidrosis and a small percentage to have sweating that is intolerable or interferes with daily activities. Familial history of hyperhidrosis is implicated in approximately 5% cases (Cerfolio et al, 2011). Endoscopic thoracic sympathectomy (ETS) is a thoracoscopic intervention used to surgically treat hyperhidrosis. To treat palmar hyperhidrosis, the surgeon interrupts the sympathetic chain at the T2 level. Compensatory sweating, defined as increased sweating in other areas following the procedure, is the most common side effect of this procedure. The incidence of compensatory sweating varies from 3% to 98% and may be classified as mild, which occurs in small amounts and is tolerable; moderate, which is defined as sweat that coalesces into flowing droplets; and severe, which is characterized by flowing sweat necessitating a change of clothing several times a day (Cerfolio et al, 2011). Many patients who undergo ETS do so on an ambulatory basis or require only an overnight stay. The procedure can produce dramatic and immediate results and is associated with a positive outcome for the patient.

ETS may also be used to surgically treat pain syndromes (e.g., complex regional pain syndrome), facial blushing, and Raynaud syndrome.

Procedural Considerations. The patient is positioned supine, and the anesthesia provider inserts a double-lumen endotracheal tube. The patient may be repositioned into a lawn chair or upright position depending on the surgeon's preference. Video monitors are placed on each side of the patient to allow the surgeon an unobstructed view from either side, because the procedure is performed bilaterally.

Operative Procedure

1. The anesthesia provider deflates the patient's lung as directed by the surgeon.
2. The surgeon uses the blade to make a small (2 mm or less) incision between the patient's second and third ribs in the axillary plane.
3. A disposable thoracic port is inserted through the incision, and the surgeon inserts a small (2 or 5 mm) telescope through the port.
4. The surgeon identifies the sympathetic chain at the T2 level (Figure 23-9, *A* and *B*), and uses endoscopic scissors to open the pleura.

FIGURE 23-9 A, Thoracoscopic view of right superior posterior mediastinum. The sympathetic chain runs over the anterior surface of the posterior rib heads. The first rib is not visualized but can be palpated. **B,** Schematic diagram. The first rib is outlined. The sympathetic ganglion and its rami are seen just below the respective rib level. **C,** Sympathectomy over the right second and third ribs. The ganglia themselves are spared. *a,* Artery; *n,* nerve; *R1,* first rib; *R2,* second rib; *R3,* third rib; *SVC,* superior vena cava; *Symp,* sympathetic.

5. The nerve is grasped with a bipolar forceps and divided with bipolar ESU (see Figure 23-9, *C*). Alternatively, clips may be applied to the nerve.
6. The port is removed, and a small thoracic catheter is inserted through the incision.
7. The surgeon closes the incision, and the lung is reexpanded. As the air is forced out of the pleural cavity, the catheter is removed and wound closure is completed.
8. The procedure is repeated for the opposite side.
9. Adhesive skin tapes are placed over the incision sites.
10. A postoperative chest x-ray film is obtained in the PACU to rule out any residual pneumothorax.

Robotic-Assisted Surgery

Robotic-assisted thoracic procedures enhance the accuracy and safety of VATS. During traditional thoracotomy the surgeon's view is hampered by the size of the incision and rigidity of the chest wall. An advantage to the robotic-assisted approach is the superior three-dimensional view of the operative field and thoracic cavity, allowing the surgeon superior visualization, increased magnification, and better maneuverability. Smaller incisions are used for robotic surgery, so patients experience less postoperative pain and morbidity (Figure 23-10). A variety of robotic-assisted procedures are performed by specially trained surgeons, including mediastinal tumor resection, lobectomy, and sympathectomy. Continued advances in technology will allow for the development of additional applications and procedures within the thoracic specialty (Research Highlight). The procedure for robotic-assisted lobectomy is described below.

Procedural Considerations. Refer to Chapter 8 for a general discussion of the equipment and instrumentation (e.g., robotic console,

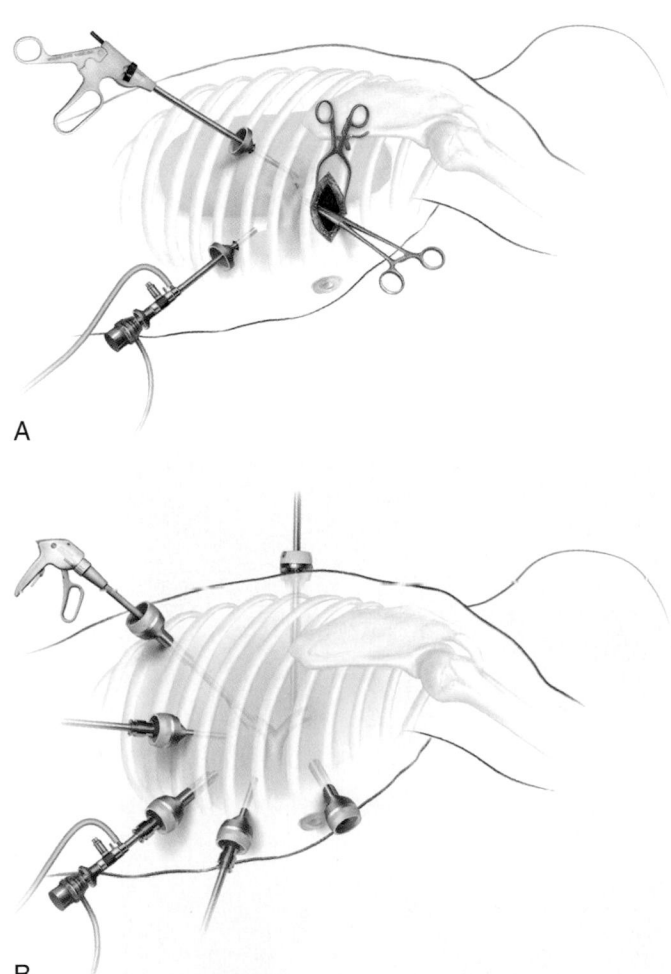

FIGURE 23-10 Comparison of VATS lobectomy to robotic lobectomy. The two patients shown are undergoing hilar dissection. **A,** VATS resection. Three incisions are shown: one for the videoscope and the other two for the right-angle clamp and stapler. The manipulation of the instrumentation and the arcs of rotation occur outside of the chest. The fulcrum of the instrumentation occurs at the chest wall, compressing and distending the intercostal nerves. **B,** Robotic resection. The arcs of rotation and management of the instrumentation for dissection are within the chest, allowing surgical dissection to occur in small spaces.

chassis) used for the procedure. In addition to preparing for the robotic procedure, the perioperative nurse and scrub person ensure that they have also gathered instrumentation and supplies to convert to an open procedure in the event an emergency arises or the surgeon is unable to complete the procedure through the minimally invasive approach. The nurse assists the anesthesia provider with inserting a double-lumen endotracheal tube and helps to position the patient in the lateral position with the operative side up. After the patient is prepped and draped, the anesthesia provider places the patient in reverse Trendelenburg position. The nurse assists with positioning the robot, video monitors, and three-dimensional vision console equipment.

Operative Procedure

1. The surgeon consults the patient's preoperative CT scans to determine the placement of the thoracoports based on the location of the lesion.
2. The surgeon incises the skin at the seventh to eighth intercostal space along the midposterior axillary line and inserts the 12-mm thoracoport.
3. The robotic system is positioned, and the surgeon inserts a 30-degree scope through the thoracoport and connects the scope to the camera arm.
4. The surgeon incises the skin at the sixth to seventh, fourth to fifth, and fifth to sixth intercostal spaces; inserts the remaining thoracoports; and passes the dissecting instruments through the ports and connects them to the instrument arms.
5. A combination of blunt and sharp dissection is used by the surgeon around the hilar structures to gain exposure to the pulmonary vessels.

6. The surgeon ligates the pulmonary vein and artery using suture and/or robotic clips.
7. The surgeon dissects the lobar bronchus and nodes.
8. A 3.5-mm endostapler is passed through the appropriate thoracoport, clamped, and fired to complete the bronchial transection.
9. The specimen is placed in a sterile removal bag and removed via the port site.
10. The surgeon tests the bronchial stump for leaks under water.
11. The pleural space is vented and the surgeon places a closed suction drain before closing the incisions.
12. Dressings are applied.

Lung Surgery

Thoracotomy

Thoracotomy involves an incision in the chest wall through a median sternotomy or a lateral or posterolateral incision for the purpose of operating on the lungs. Thoracotomy may be performed for a variety of benign and malignant conditions. Lung cancer (Figure 23-11) is a common diagnosis for which a thoracotomy may be required. Patients with lung cancer may have specific treatment based on their tumor, node, and metastasis (TNM) characteristics. The TNM system defines tumor (T) as the size, location, and spread (pulmonary or extrapulmonary). The designation of nodes (N) refers to spread to a lymph node or group of lymph nodes. Metastasis (M) relates to metastatic tumor activity in distant organs (e.g., brain, liver) (Box 23-1). Staging is based on TNM findings (Figure 23-12). Intraoperative patient care is similar for various thoracotomy procedures, with consideration of the patient's history and disease

FIGURE 23-11 Lung cancer. **A,** Squamous cell carcinoma originating from the main bronchus. **B,** Peripheral adenoma. **C,** Small cell carcinoma.

BOX 23-1

Tumor, Node, and Metastasis (TNM) Definitions and Staging for Lung Cancer

T (Tumor) Descriptors

T0 No visible primary tumor

T1 Tumor <3 cm in diameter and completely surrounded by lung tissue. No evidence of tumor in main lung airways.

T1a Tumor <2 cm in diameter

T1b Tumor >2 cm and <3 cm in diameter

T2 Tumor with one of the following characteristics:
1. >3 cm and <7 cm in diameter
2. Present in mainstem airway and >2 cm from where trachea divides to form the mainstem bronchi (main carina)
3. Invades the surface covering of the lung
4. Causes partial collapse or inflammation of the lung

T2a Tumor >3 cm but <5 cm in diameter

T2b Tumor >5 cm but <7 cm in diameter

T3 Tumor >7 cm

Tumor invades any of the following:
1. Chest wall
2. Diaphragm
3. Mediastinal surface
4. Heart surface

Tumor in the mainstem bronchi within 2 cm of but not involving the main carina

No whole lung collapse or lung inflammation

Separate tumor in same lobe of lung as primary cancer

T4 Tumor of any size that invades any of the following:
1. Mediastinum
2. Heart
3. Great vessels
4. Trachea
5. Esophagus
6. Spine
7. Carina

Separate tumor in different lobe of lung but on same side as primary cancer

N (Node) Descriptors

N0 No lymph node involvement

N1 Tumor involvement of hilar lymph nodes on the same side as the primary cancer

N2 Tumor involvement of subcarinal or paratracheal lymph nodes on the same side as the primary cancer

N3 Tumor involvement of paratracheal lymph nodes on the opposite side of the primary cancer

M (Metastasis) Descriptors

M0 No distant metastasis

M1 Distant metastasis

M1a Separate tumor in opposite lung
Tumor in pleural fluid
Tumor in pericardial fluid
Tumor nodules on lung surface

M1b Tumor in non-lung organs

Biopsy Methods for the Staging and Diagnosis of Lung Cancer

Biopsy Method	Accessible Lymph Node Stations
Endobronchial ultrasonography–guided fine needle aspiration	2, 3, 4, 7, 10, 11
Endoscopic ultrasonography–guided fine needle aspiration	4, 5, 7, 8, 9
Cervical mediastinoscopy	1, 2, 3, 4, anterior 7
Anterior mediastinoscopy	5
Extended cervical mediastinoscopy	6
Video-assisted thoracoscopic surgery	Ipsilateral mediastinal lymph nodes

Anatomic Stage/Prognostic Groups

Occult carcinoma	TX	N0	M0
Stage 0	Tis	N0	M0
Stage IA	T1a	N0	M0
	T1b	N0	M0
Stage IB	T2a	N0	M0
Stage IIA	T2b	N0	M0
	T1a	N1	M0
	T1b	N1	M0
	T2a	N1	M0
Stage IIB	T2b	N1	M0
	T3	N0	M0
Stage IIIA	T1a	N2	M0
	T1b	N2	M0
	T2a	N2	M0
	T2b	N2	M0
	T3	N1	M0
	T3	N2	M0
	T4	N0	M0
	T4	N1	M0
Stage IIIB	T1a	N3	M0
	T1b	N3	M0
	T2a	N3	M0
	T2b	N3	M0
	T3	N3	M0
	T4	N2	M0
	T4	N3	M0
Stage IV	Any T	Any N	M1a
	Any T	Any N	M1b

Modified from American Cancer Society: *Lung cancer staging, 2009,* available at www.cancerstaging.org/staging/posters/lung12x15.pdf. Accessed April 4, 2013; Ankaru M et al: Lung cancer: surgical treatment. In Selke FW et al, editors: *Sabiston & Spencer surgery of the chest,* ed 8, Philadelphia, 2010, Saunders; Rusch VW et al: The IASLC lung cancer staging project: a proposal for a new international lymph node map in the forthcoming seventh edition of the TNM classification for lung cancer, *J Thorac Oncol* 4(5):568–577, 2009; Tan WW: Non-small cell lung cancer, *eMedicine,* 2013, available at http://emedicine.medscape.com/article/279960-overview. Accessed April 4, 2013.

process, planned procedure, and individualized patient needs. Basic thoracic instrumentation is used and may include a sternal saw and stapling devices. Preparation by the anesthesia provider with careful monitoring of the patient is a priority. Insertion of a double-lumen endotracheal tube, an arterial line for monitoring ABG samples, and a central venous line to ensure patent access for fluids are procedures performed by the anesthesia provider. An epidural catheter may be inserted for intraoperative and postoperative pain management. Patient preparation by the surgical team includes positioning, placement of devices for prevention of complications (e.g., intermittent pneumatic compression devices, thermal-regulating blanket, electrosurgical dispersive pad), insertion of a urinary catheter, and ongoing evaluation and communication of the patient's status to the family throughout the procedure.

| A | Stage I disease | B | Stage I disease | C | Stage I disease | D | Stage II disease | E | Stage III disease |

FIGURE 23-12 Staging of lung cancer by the tumor, node, and metastasis (TNM) system. **A** and **B,** Stage I disease includes tumors classified as T1 with or without metastasis to the lymph node in the ipsilateral hilar region. **C,** Also included in stage I are tumors classified as T2 but having no nodal or distant metastases. **D,** Stage II disease includes those tumors classified as T2, with metastasis only to the ipsilateral hilar lymph nodes. **E,** Stage III includes all tumors more extensive than T2 or any tumor with metastasis to the lymph nodes in the mediastinum with distant metastasis.

Pneumonectomy

Pneumonectomy is the removal of an entire lung, usually to treat malignant neoplasms. Other reasons for this procedure include removal of an extensive unilateral bronchiectasis (e.g., irreversible dilation of the bronchi) involving the greater part of one lung, drainage of an extensive chronic pulmonary abscess involving portions of one or more lobes, removal of selected benign tumors, and treatment of any extensive unilateral lesion. Other resections are often combined with pneumonectomy, such as resection of mediastinal lymph nodes, resections of portions of the chest wall or diaphragm, and removal of parietal pleura.

Operative Procedure

1. The surgeon incises the skin, subcutaneous tissue, and muscle with a blade and an ESU. Hemostasis is attained. If a rib is to be excised, bone instruments are required.
2. The ribs and tissue are protected with moist soft goods; the rib retractor is placed (Figure 23-13) and opened slowly and gently.
3. The surgeon frees any peripheral adhesions to mobilize the lung and divides the pulmonary ligament. Dissection to the hilum of the involved lobe is carried out.
4. The superior pulmonary vein is gently retracted, and the pulmonary artery is dissected.
5. The surgeon clamps the branches of the pulmonary artery and vein of the involved lobe, places double ligatures, and divides them with fine right-angled vascular clamps, scissors, and nonabsorbable suture. Alternatively, a stapling device may be used to ligate the vessels.
6. The inferior pulmonary vein is exposed by incising the hilar pleura and retracting the lung anteriorly. The inferior pulmonary vein is clamped, doubly ligated, and divided.
7. The surgeon applies a bronchus clamp and divides the bronchus near the tracheal bifurcation. The stump is closed with atraumatic nonabsorbable mattress sutures or bronchus staples. If staples are applied, the blade is used to complete division of the bronchus. The lung is removed from the chest.
8. The scrub person supplies normal saline to irrigate the pleural space and check for hemostasis and air leaks during positive-pressure inspiration.

FIGURE 23-13 Rib retractor placed for thoracotomy.

9. A pleural flap may be created and sutured over the bronchial stump. Other methods of securing the bronchus (such as placement of an intercostal flap) might be used.
10. Hemostasis is ensured in the pleural space.
11. Chest tubes (28-French [F] to 30F) are inserted into the pleural space and exteriorized through a stab wound at the eighth or ninth interspace near the anterior axillary line (Figure 23-14). An upper tube is inserted through a second stab wound if indicated to evaluate leaking air. The tubes are secured with heavy sutures and connected to water-seal drainage after closure of the pleural space.
12. The surgeon places the rib approximator (Figure 23-15) and begins closure with interrupted sutures.
13. The muscle, subcutaneous tissue, and skin are closed. Drains are anchored to the chest wall with suture.
14. The dressing is applied.

FIGURE 23-14 A, Introduction of chest drainage tube through a stab wound. **B,** Placement of apical and basal drainage tubes after upper and middle lobectomy.

FIGURE 23-15 A, Rib approximator placed for closure of incision. **B,** Heavy-gauge suture used for closure of ribs.

15. Chest tube connections are secured with Parnham bands or tape and labeled (anterior or posterior).

Lobectomy

Lobectomy is excision of one or more lobes of the lung. It is performed when the primary tumor is located in a particular lobe or to remove metastatic lesions when the tumor is peripherally located and hilar nodes are not involved. Other conditions affecting the lung and treated by lobectomy might be bronchiectasis; giant emphysematous blebs or bullae; large, centrally located benign tumors; fungal infections; and congenital anomalies.

Procedural Considerations. Basic thoracic instrumentation is used. The perioperative nurse assists with placing the patient in a lateral position for a posterolateral approach; the supine position

may be used for upper- and middle-lobe resections. The procedure varies with the specific lobe to be removed depending on the anatomic structure.

Operative Procedure

1. The surgeon incises the skin, subcutaneous tissue, and muscle using a blade and an ESU. Hemostasis is attained. If a rib is to be excised, bone instruments are required.
2. The ribs and tissue are protected with soft goods. The rib retractor is placed and opened slowly and gently.
3. The surgeon enters the pleura and frees the peripheral adhesions with scissors, blunt dissection, or small folded soft good on a forceps.
4. The hilar pleura is incised and separated.
5. The branches of the pulmonary arteries and veins are isolated, clamped, doubly ligated, and divided with fine, right-angled vascular clamps, scissors, and nonabsorbable suture. A stapling device may be used to divide the vessels as an alternative.
6. The surgeon identifies the main trunk of the pulmonary artery and the fissure between the lobes.
7. The bronchus clamp is applied. The remaining lung is inflated to identify the line of demarcation. The bronchus is divided with a blade or heavy scissors.
8. Bronchial secretions are suctioned.
9. The surgeon closes the bronchus with atraumatic nonabsorbable mattress sutures or bronchus staples. If staples are applied, a blade is used to complete division of the bronchus.
10. Incomplete fissures are divided between hemostats with fine Metzenbaum scissors. Edges may be sutured closed.
11. A pleural flap may be created and sutured over the bronchial stump (other methods of securing the bronchus might be used).
12. The pleural cavity is thoroughly irrigated with normal saline, and hemostasis is ensured. The remaining lobes are inflated to check for air leaks, and the degree of expansion of the remaining lobes is assessed.
13. The pleural space is irrigated, and the procedure is completed as described for a pneumonectomy.

Segmental Resection

Segmental resection is removal of one or more anatomic subdivisions of the pulmonary lobe. It conserves healthy, functioning pulmonary tissue by sparing remaining segments. Segmental resection is indicated for any benign lesion with segmental distribution or diseased tissue affecting only one segment of the lung with compromised cardiorespiratory reserve. The most common cause for removal is bronchiectasis. Other conditions requiring removal include chronic, localized inflammation and congenital cysts or blebs.

Procedural Considerations. Basic thoracotomy instrumentation is used. The perioperative nurse assists the surgical team in placing the patient in the lateral position.

Operative Procedure

1. The surgeon incises the skin, subcutaneous tissue, and muscle using a blade and an ESU.
2. The parietal pleura is incised with a blade and scissors. Adhesions are divided with sharp or blunt dissection.
3. The segmental artery is identified to provide accurate identification of the bronchus of the diseased segment.

FIGURE 23-16 A, Staple suturing of bronchus. **B,** Conventional suturing of bronchus; application of bronchus clamp and incision; closure of stump. **C,** Staple suturing of pulmonary vessels. **D,** Staple suturing of lung tissue (wedge resection or lung biopsy).

4. The surgeon ligates the segmental pulmonary vein and branches.
5. The surgeon clamps the bronchus with the bronchus clamp, and the remaining lung is inflated. The intersegmental boundary is confirmed, and proper placement of the clamp is ensured.
6. The visceral pleura is incised around the diseased segment, beginning anterior to the hilum and progressing toward the periphery. Exposure is facilitated with a malleable or other type of retractor. The intersegmental vessels are clamped with thoracic hemostats and ligated.
7. The surgeon transects the segmental bronchus and closes the stump with atraumatic nonabsorbable mattress sutures or bronchus staples (Figure 23-16).
8. Dissection is continued to separate segmental surfaces, and vessels are ligated as needed. The segment of the lung is removed.
9. The anesthesia provider reinflates the lung and the surgeon irrigates with normal saline. Bleeding is controlled with ligatures or hemoclips.
10. The procedure is completed as described for pneumonectomy.

Wedge Resection

Wedge resection is removal of a wedge-shaped section of parenchyma that includes the identified lesion, without regard for intersegmental planes. The resection is also used for removal of small, peripherally located benign primary tumors and peripherally located inflammatory disease, as well as for biopsy in patients with chronic, diffuse lung disease.

Procedural Considerations. Thoracic instrumentation is used. The team positions the patient to allow access to the operative site with consideration of the area of lung to be resected.

Operative Procedure
1. The surgeon incises the skin, subcutaneous tissue, and muscle using a blade and an ESU.
2. The rib retractor is placed.
3. The wedge is outlined for excision, with a margin of normal tissue left, using one of the following techniques:
   a. Long hemostatic clamps are applied in three rows to outline the wedge. Excision is accomplished with a blade. The tissue

FIGURE 23-17 Wedge resection. Clamps applied to edge of lung tissue to be excised with blade and sutured with a running suture and oversewn.

is sutured with a running absorbable suture behind the clamps before removal. The edges of the tissue are oversewn with a continuous or interrupted suture (Figure 23-17). The surgeon controls bleeding and secures the small bronchi with clamps and ligature. Large bronchi are ligated or sutured to prevent persistent air leak.

b. The lobe is grasped with a lung clamp, and the thoracic stapling instrument is applied to the parenchymal portion of the lung. Staples are applied, and the wedge is excised with the blade. Staples are reapplied to the opposite side of the lesion adjoining the staple lines.

4. The specimen is removed. The surgeon checks for air leaks by irrigation and inspection. Bleeding is controlled with ligation or hemoclips. The procedure is completed as described for pneumonectomy.

Lung Volume Reduction Surgery

Lung volume reduction surgery (LVRS) is an alternative surgical treatment for patients with chronic pulmonary emphysema (Figure 23-18). The surgery is intended to increase expiratory airflow, maximal exercise capacity, and respiratory muscle strength, thereby relieving dyspnea. The procedure may also be referred to as *lung volume reduction,* or *pneumoplasty.* Candidates for the procedure are those who have progressive, severe dyspnea secondary to pulmonary dysfunction; those whose medical management is ineffective; and those in whom disease distribution is limited to target areas of severity (Evidence for Practice). The two most common operative approaches for LVRS are median sternotomy and VATS. Median sternotomy provides excellent bilateral exposure and flexibility, whereas the VATS approach has the advantage of a shorter hospitalization, fewer days of postoperative air leaks, and fewer days on the ventilator (Puc, 2010). Patients undergoing LVRS participate in vigorous pulmonary rehabilitation as a standard practice in preparation for surgery. Pulmonary rehabilitation programs not only improve airway clearance and diaphragmatic function but also ensure that optimal conditioning is achieved, which improves surgical outcomes, improves tolerance for surgery, and decreases postoperative complications. An alternative procedure, bronchoscopic lung volume reduction (BLVR), using either an implanted valve system or a distributed sclerosant, continues to be studied and evaluated (Taneja, 2013) (Research Highlight, p. 894).

Procedural Considerations. The basic thoracotomy setup and instrumentation are used, along with stapling devices, chest tubes,

and a water-seal drainage system. A laser may be required, as may other materials for sealing the resected edges (e.g., bovine pericardium, collagen). Positioning is a particular concern for this patient population, who are often malnourished and are at increased risk for positioning injury. The perioperative nurse must collaborate with the surgeon and anesthesia provider to ensure that the best possible positioning practices are implemented.

Operative Procedure

1. The surgeon exposes the patient's lungs through a transverse anterior thoracotomy incision using the sternal saw to separate the sternum. Adhesiotomies are performed, and the inferior pulmonary ligaments are incised.

2. The anesthesia provider deflates the patient's lungs to allow for visualization of the portions of the lung where air is trapped in emphysematous lung tissue.

3. A lung-grasping forceps is used to hold the portion of the lung to be excised. A surgical stapling device is lined with bovine pericardium and positioned on either side of the lung. The stapling of emphysematous lung tissue continues, and staple lines are overlapped to prevent air leaks. Alternative means of sealing the resection line include the use of a pleural flap or the application of collagen.

4. The anesthesia provider reinflates the lung to identify air leaks. If air leaks are found, the lung is deflated and the stapling procedure continues.

5. One or two chest tubes are placed into each pleural space. The chest tubes are connected to water-seal drainage systems without suction.

6. The surgeon reapproximates the ribs and sternum using stainless steel surgical wire. The muscle layer, subcutaneous tissue, and skin are closed, and dressings are applied.

Lung Biopsy

Lung biopsy is the resection of a small portion of the lung for diagnosis. The biopsy allows removal of relatively large specimens for microscopic examination of the lung tissue. Indications include (1) failure of closed methods (needle biopsy) for diagnosis and (2) the presence of small, localized lesions that can be removed by biopsy.

Procedural Considerations. In addition to the basic instrument setup, a rib retractor, a lung-grasping forceps, dissecting scissors, a chest tube and water-seal system, and an endostapling device are

FIGURE 23-18 Airway obstruction caused by emphysema, chronic bronchitis, and asthma. **A,** The normal lung. **B,** Emphysema enlargement and destruction of alveolar walls with loss of elasticity and trapping of air; *(left)* panlobular emphysema showing abnormal weakening and enlargement of all air spaces distal to the terminal bronchioles (normal alveoli shown for comparison only); *(right)* centrilobular emphysema showing abnormal weakening and enlargement of the respiratory bronchioles in the proximal portion of the acinus. **C,** Chronic bronchitis: inflammation and thickening of mucous membrane with accumulation of mucus and pus leading to obstruction; characterized by cough. **D,** Bronchial asthma: thick mucus, mucosal edema, and smooth muscle spasm causing obstruction of small airways; breathing becomes labored, and expiration is difficult.

▌EVIDENCE FOR PRACTICE

Determining Candidates for Lung Volume Reduction Surgery

Although lung volume reduction surgery (LVRS) is considered an effective procedure to treat patients with emphysema, successful outcomes depend on factors such as appropriate patient selection, surgical technique, and surgeon experience. After the reintroduction of LVRS to the medical community in 1995, there was a resurgence of interest in the technique. However, surgical interventions were accompanied by significant morbidity and mortality. As a result, the Health Care Financing Administration (HCFA) organized a clinical trial (the National Emphysema Treatment Trial [NETT]) to identify factors that contribute to successful outcomes. The NETT suggests the following criteria as patient eligibility for LVRS:

- High-resolution computed tomography evidence of moderate to severe bilateral heterogeneous emphysema or moderate to severe bilateral homogeneous emphysema; if emphysema is homogeneous, additional physiologic criteria may be required
- Target zones of poorly perfused lung

- Nonsmoker (tobacco products) for a minimum of 4 months before interview for screening, with willingness to sustain nonsmoking status
- Body mass index less than 31.1 kg/m^2 (men) or less than 32.3 kg/m^2 (women)
- No previous laser surgery or LVRS
- No giant bulla (one third or more of the volume of the lung in which the bulla is located)
- No previous coronary artery bypass surgery
- Oxygen requirement of 6 L/min or less to keep saturation at 90% or higher during an oxygen titration assessment
- No cardiac dysrhythmia that, in the judgment of the supervising physician, might pose a risk to the patient during exercise testing or training
- Postbronchodilator total lung capacity (TLC) at 110% or more of predicted

Determining Candidates for Lung Volume Reduction Surgery—cont'd

- Postbronchodilator residual volume (RV) at 220% or more of predicted
- Postbronchodilator forced expiratory volume in 1 second (FEV₁) at 45% or less of predicted and, if age 70 years or older, postbronchodilator FEV₁ at 15% or more of predicted

- FEV₁ postbronchodilator increase of 30% or less, or 300 mL or less
- DL_{co} (lung diffusing capacity for carbon monoxide) at 70% or less of predicted
- Consent for screening and patient registry
- Consent for pulmonary rehabilitation

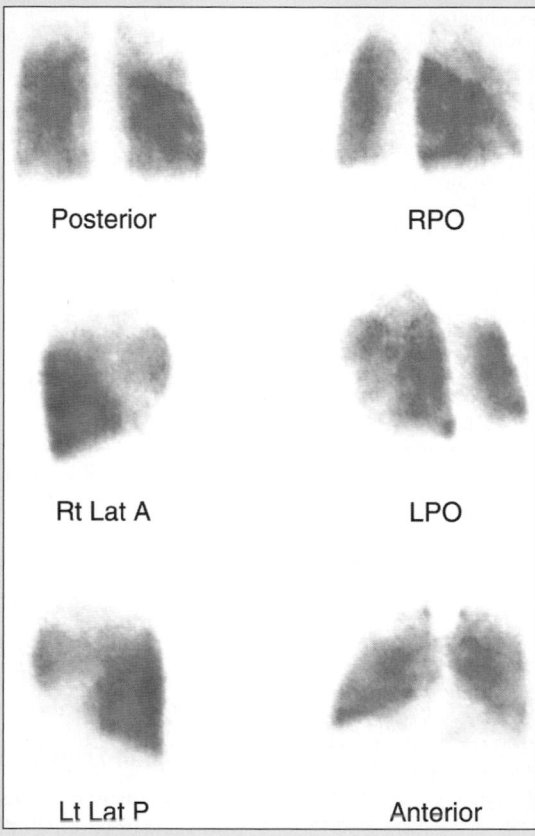

Pulmonary perfusion scintigraphy demonstrating typical upper lobe predominant emphysema that is viewed as the most suitable morphology for lung reduction surgery. (From Selke FW et al, editors: *Sabiston & Spencer surgery of the chest,* ed 8, Philadelphia, 2010, Saunders.)

Modified from Edwards MA et al: The National Emphysema Treatment Trial: summary and update, *Thorac Surg Clin* 19(2):169–185, 2009; Meyers BF et al: Surgery for emphysema. In Selke FW et al, editors: *Sabiston & Spencer surgery of the chest,* ed 8, Philadelphia, 2010, Saunders; Centers for Medicare & Medicaid Services: *Medicare national coverage determinations,* Revision 240.1 of pub. 100–03, available at www.cms.gov/Regulations-and-Guidance/Guidance/Transmittals/downloads/R3NCD.pdf. Accessed April 4, 2013.

required. More than one specimen container may be needed. The patient is positioned in a semilateral position for an anterolateral incision.

Operative Procedure
1. A short incision (approximately 5 cm) is made at the fifth intercostal space. The surgeon incises the pleura and retracts the ribs. Alternatively, a VATS approach may be used.
2. The lung is secured and exteriorized using a Duval lung clamp.
3. Using a Satinsky clamp or a stapling device, the surgeon segments the tissue to be biopsied. The tissue to be removed is excised with a blade. After application of the clamp, tissue edges are approximated with absorbable suture. If a larger piece of tissue is desired, a stapling device may be used as described under Wedge Resection.

4. Bleeding is controlled by the application of moist soft goods at the incision site. The area is irrigated and inspected for air leaks.
5. The chest tube (28F to 30F) is inserted and connected to suction.
6. The incision is closed, the chest tube is anchored to the chest wall, and a dressing is applied.

Decortication

Decortication of the lung is removal of any fibrinous deposit, cancer, or restrictive membrane on the visceral and parietal pleura that interferes with pulmonary ventilatory function. It may also be done in conjunction with a pleurectomy for patients with pleural-based tumors, such as mesothelioma. The procedure can result in significant blood loss and trauma to the lung. The objective is to allow full expansion of the lung in order to maximize its function.

RESEARCH HIGHLIGHT ┃┃

Bronchial Valve Treatment for Emphysema

Chronic obstructive pulmonary disease (COPD) is the third leading cause of death in the United States behind heart disease and cancer (Hoyert and Xu, 2011). Treatment of COPD is primarily medical, but surgical options do exist. Lung volume reduction surgery (LVRS) is the primary option for COPD; however, not all patients meet the criteria established by the National Emphysema Treatment Trial, so researchers have been incented to investigate other less invasive surgical options such as bronchoscopic LVRS. Taneja (2013) notes there are five main categories of bronchoscopic LVRS: unidirectional endobronchial valves (EBVs), airway bypass stents, biologic and polymeric LVRS, thermal vapor ablation, and endobronchial coils. EBVs are the most widely studied technique. These are one-way valves and can be placed and removed via flexible or rigid bronchoscopy. Side effects include COPD exacerbation, hemoptysis, and pneumonia. Benefit is maximum if complete lobe occlusion and atelectasis are achieved (Taneja, 2013).

Two types of EBVs, the Zephyr valve and the Spiration IBV, have been investigated in the United States and Europe. Sterman and colleagues (2010) conducted a multicenter pilot study of the IBV to evaluate its safety and effectiveness. The IBV is placed bilaterally in the upper lung lobes.

The Sterman trial enrolled 91 patients from 11 sites over a 12-month period. All patients had severe obstruction hyperinflation and upper lobe predominant COPD. Bronchoscopy was used to place 609 IBVs. The primary outcome of safety was measured by valve migration, procedure complications, and other severe adverse effects such as pneumothorax, exacerbation of COPD, pneumonia, respiratory failure, bleeding or hemoptysis, and death. There were no procedure-related deaths and no instances of valve migration or erosion. Seven patients experienced adverse effects. Effectiveness was measured via the health-related quality of life (HRQL) questionnaire, pulmonary function testing and exercise testing, lung perfusion scans, and quantitative computed tomography (QCT). Results showed a clinically significant improvement in HRQL scores of 51% at 1 month, increasing to 57% at 12 months. Pulmonary function, arterial blood gases at rest, airflow rates, and oxygen use did not demonstrate significant or sustained changes, but the QCT measurements of regional lung volume demonstrated significant decrease in volume, which correlated to symptom improvement seen in the HRQL scores. Lung perfusion scans showed a shift from upper lobe perfusion to lower zone perfusion at 6% and 9% at 1 and 3 months, respectively.

Previously reported hypotheses for the mechanisms for improvement with bronchial valve treatment are lobar atelectasis emulating volume reduction and reduction of dynamic hyperinflation. Sterman also postulates that bronchial valve treatment redirects ventilation to the untreated, healthier lung parenchyma and represents a viable option in the treatment of COPD.

Modified from Hoyert DL, Xu J: Deaths: preliminary data for 2011, *Natl Vital Stat Rep* 61:6, available at www.cdc.gov/nchs/data/nvsr/nvsr61/nvsr61_06.pdf. Accessed April 7, 2013; Taneja A: Bronchoscopic interventions in the management of chronic obstructive pulmonary disease, *Curr Opin Pulm Med* 19(2):145–151, 2013; Sterman DH et al: A multicenter pilot study of a bronchial valve for the treatment of severe emphysema, *Respiration* 79(3):222–233, 2010.

Procedural Considerations. The basic thoracic instrumentation is used. The perioperative nurse assists with positioning the patient in a lateral position for a posterolateral incision.

Operative Procedure

1. The surgeon incises the skin, subcutaneous tissue, and muscle using a blade and an ESU.

FIGURE 23-19 Separation of muscles of rib with a periosteal elevator and rib stripper.

2. A rib, usually the fifth or sixth, is stripped (Figure 23-19) and resected.
3. The scrub person provides moist soft goods (e.g., sponges) to protect the ribs and tissue. The rib retractor is placed and slowly and gently opened.
4. Parietal adhesions are divided to the margins of the lung, mediastinal surface, and pericardium with thoracic scissors, forceps, and a moist small folded soft good on forceps.
5. The fibrous membrane is incised and separated from the visceral pleura using blunt and sharp dissection, handling the tissues gently (Figure 23-20). The procedure is completed as described for pneumonectomy.

Drainage of Empyema

The accumulation of pus in the pleural space might be associated with acute or chronic infection. Acute empyema may result from a lung abscess, pneumonia, or infection after thoracotomy. Parapneumonic effusions occur in 20% to 60% of patients hospitalized for bacterial pneumonia; 5% to 10% of these parapneumonic effusions progress to empyema. The occurrence of empyema is more prevalent in older or debilitated patients (Nason et al, 2010). Empyema (other than a pure tuberculous type) must be drained to prevent fibrothorax, and patients with empyema may require further treatment with decortication. When the infection is not extensive or organized, it can be managed by placing a chest tube under a local anesthetic. Prolonged intrapleural infection results in chronic empyema, which can result in the formation of loculations and create additional complications such as mediastinal shift, swallowing difficulties, respiratory limitations, bronchus erosion, and chest deformity. Postoperative empyema or empyema occurring in immunosuppressed patients can be effectively treated with a rib resection and drainage.

Procedural Considerations. If the patient is administered a general anesthetic, the basic thoracic instrumentation is used. The team positions the patient in a lateral position for an anterolateral incision. If a pleurodesis is to be performed for a simple pleural effusion, a catheter for instillation of the sclerosing agent is required. The

FIGURE 23-20 Decortication. Methods of separating fibrous membrane from visceral pleura.

chest cavity is irrigated profusely during and on completion of the procedure.

Operative Procedure

1. The surgeon incises the skin and tissues with a blade to expose the affected area of the lung. Suction is used to prevent spillage of drainage from the chest.
2. The adjacent rib may be resected, and the intercostal neurovascular bundle is divided.
3. The underlying thickened pleura is incised and gross pus is evacuated. An inflammatory response might be created by stripping the parietal pleura from the visceral pleura by sharp or blunt dissection.
4. A large-bore catheter (46F) is inserted, and the sclerosing agent is instilled when indicated.
5. The surgeon closes the incision site as described for other thoracotomy procedures.
6. A dressing is applied.

Open Thoracostomy—Partial Rib Resection

Partial rib resection is removal of a portion of selected rib or ribs through an open thoracostomy incision to allow healing and reinflation of an infected lung. The procedure is performed for treatment of chronic empyemic lesions to establish a mechanism for continuous drainage.

Procedural Considerations. The basic thoracic instrument set and bone-cutting instruments are used. An ESU, chest tube, and

FIGURE 23-21 Chest x-ray showing large right pleural effusion outlined by arrows.

water-seal drainage system are required, as are culture tubes for aerobic and anaerobic laboratory analysis. The patient is placed in a lateral position for a posterolateral incision. The surgical procedure can be completed with the patient administered a local anesthetic, but is most commonly performed under general anesthesia.

Operative Procedure

1. The surgeon incises the skin, subcutaneous tissue, and muscle using a blade and an ESU.
2. The rib is resected, and the pleura is incised. Suction is used to control anticipated drainage.
3. Aerobic and anaerobic swabs for culture and sensitivity are obtained. The chest cavity is irrigated.
4. A large chest tube may be inserted through the pleural opening. The incision is packed open.
5. The chest tube is secured with a suture of heavy-gauge material on a cutting needle.
6. The chest tube is connected to a water-seal drainage system, and connections are secured.
7. A dressing is applied. A number of layers of dressing may be necessary to absorb drainage.

Closed Thoracostomy—Intercostal Drainage

Closed thoracostomy is insertion of a chest catheter through an intercostal space for establishment of closed drainage. The procedure provides continuous aspiration of air, blood, or infectious fluid from the pleural cavity. It is indicated for treatment of spontaneous pneumothorax, traumatic hemothorax, pleural effusion, and acute empyema. Malignant pleural effusions (Figure 23-21) may be managed by drainage and chemical pleurodesis by way of the thoracostomy tube.

Procedural Considerations. The thoracostomy may not take place in an OR setting. The procedure is usually done with monitored anesthesia care and local anesthesia. A local anesthesia set, including syringes, needles, and an anesthetic agent of choice for local injection, is needed. The minor instrument set is used, in addition to disposable chest catheters, water-seal drainage system, two aspirating needles, and culture tubes. The patient is placed in a lateral or sitting position. Despite the administration of local anesthetic, thoracostomy can be uncomfortable for the patient. Administration of IV narcotic agents at the time of the procedure may help prevent pain during performance of the procedure. The perioperative nurse should provide explanations and emotional support to the patient during the procedure.

Operative Procedure

1. The surgeon estimates the correct depth of insertion and marks the catheter. The operative site is anesthetized.
2. An aspirating needle attached to a syringe is introduced into the chest cavity to verify the presence of purulent drainage, air, or blood.
3. The surgeon incises the skin and introduces a clamp through the incision into the intercostal space and pleural cavity.
4. Next, the surgeon inserts a catheter through the incision site and clamps it to prevent egress of air as it is inserted into the cavity.
5. The incision site is sutured, and the catheter is secured.
6. The catheter is attached to water-seal drainage, and the tubing is secured. The clamp is removed, and a dressing is applied.

Decompression for Thoracic Outlet Syndrome

Thoracic outlet syndrome is a compression of the subclavian vessels and brachial plexus at the superior aperture of the thorax (Figure 23-22). The first rib is the usual cause of the compression, because of either a congenital deformity or a traumatic injury that results in anatomic changes. Fibromuscular bands may also form between the cervical rib and other structures (i.e., scalenus tubercle) and cause compression. Symptoms depend on whether nerves, blood vessels, or both are compressed at the thoracic outlet. Decompression is accomplished through partial or entire removal of the rib using an open technique or video-assisted endoscopic techniques.

Procedural Considerations.
Soft tissue and bone instrumentation is used. An ESU is required. The patient is positioned in a lateral decubitus position.

Operative Procedure—Open Technique

1. The surgeon incises the skin, subcutaneous tissue, and muscle using a blade and an ESU. Soft tissue dissection continues to identify the neurovascular bundle.
2. The first rib is meticulously dissected subperiosteally using the periosteal elevator. A rib elevator, stripper, and rib raspatories may be required. Undue traction on the brachial plexus and damage to the subclavian artery or vein are avoided during the dissection.
3. A wedge is taken from the midportion, or the rib is removed in its entirety using rib shears.
4. A drain is placed, and the incision is closed. A dressing is applied.

Excision of Mediastinal Lesion

Excision of a mediastinal lesion involves removal of a lesion from the anterior, middle, and posterior sections of the mediastinum. Identifying the compartment is important for planning a surgical approach to the resection, for optimal exposure and access. Typically preoperative imaging will determine the location of the lesion. A mediastinoscopy may be a useful adjunct to help determine the diagnosis of an anterior mediastinal lesion. Indications for excision of a mediastinal lesion include miscellaneous cysts and tumors, thymoma, lymphoma, and neurogenic tumor.

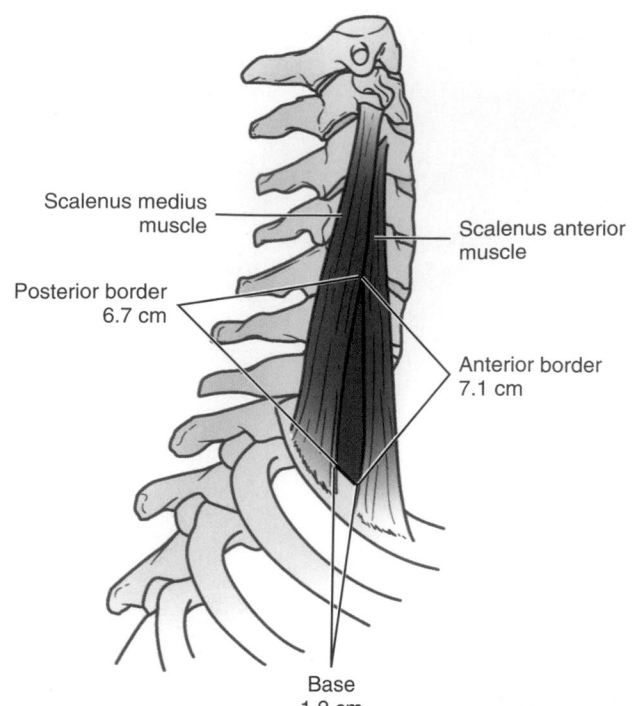

FIGURE 23-22 The scalene (anterior) triangle showing its measurements and the narrow space through which the neurovascular bundle passes.

Procedural Considerations.
The thoracic instrumentation set is used. A procedure on the superior mediastinum might require use of thyroid instruments (see Chapter 16). An ESU and bone wax are needed. The perioperative nurse assists with placing the patient in a supine position for a median sternotomy incision (alternatively, lateral position may be used).

Operative Procedure—Thymectomy

1. The surgeon incises the skin, subcutaneous tissue, and muscle using a blade and an ESU.
2. The sternum is transected with a power saw or sternal knife. Bleeding is controlled at the bone edges with bone wax. Alternatively, a transcervical approach may be used. Some surgeons have also used VATS or robotic-assisted approaches.
3. The thymus gland is dissected; vessels are clamped, ligated, and divided. The gland is removed.
4. The incision is closed. The sternum is reapproximated and closed with heavy wire. The skin is sutured closed. A dressing is applied.

Lung Transplantation

Since 1988 more than 25,000 lung transplants have been performed (Organ Procurement and Transplantation Network, 2013). Indications for single-lung transplantation (SLT) include restrictive lung disease, emphysema, pulmonary hypertension, and other nonseptic end-stage pulmonary diseases. Double-lung transplantation (DLT) can be performed for many of these indications and is specifically indicated for patients with cystic fibrosis or patients with a chronic infection in end-stage pulmonary failure. The procedure involves the allografting of one or both lungs from a cadaver or donor who has met clinical criteria for brain death. Developments in SLT include donor contribution from living relatives for patients who have chronic disease and a high risk for death while waiting on the donor transplantation list. Contraindications for transplantation include multisystem disease other than the lung, history of carcinoma or sarcoma, current infection, significant renal or hepatic dysfunction, cigarette smoking within 3 or 4 months, drug or alcohol abuse, psychologic instability, or poor medication compliance. Although the surgical technique is increasingly successful, the application of lung transplantation techniques may be limited by donor supply. As the field of lung transplantation continues to evolve, questions will need to be answered regarding quality of life after transplantation and whether the single or double procedure is ultimately best for patients with chronic obstructive lung disease and primary pulmonary hypertension. Issues include the shortage of suitable donors, improved methods for early detection of chronic rejection, and improved immunosuppressive agents and regimens.

Procedural Considerations. Selection of the donor and recipients, preservation of the lung, and administration of anesthetic agents are considerations in this procedure. The nursing plan of care is modified considerably for each patient because nursing personnel are caring for two patients with different needs. Recipient patients will have been started preoperatively on immunosuppressive therapy and infection prophylaxis. The patient's positioning will vary for the techniques being used. The instrumentation is similar to that used for a thoracotomy. Cardiopulmonary bypass (CPB) may be required, as described in Chapter 25, along with the ESU, cold perfusion solution, and surgical stapling devices. The perioperative nurse will need to collaborate with the anesthesia provider because continuous hemodynamic monitoring, oximetry, and ventricular function assessment by transesophageal echocardiography (TEE) are all performed intraoperatively.

Operative Procedure—Single-Lung Transplantation
Donor Harvesting
1. The patient's skin is prepped from chin to knees and laterally to the midaxillary line. A median sternotomy incision is most commonly used. A thoracotomy may also be used.
2. The surgeon opens the pleura longitudinally posterior to the sternum, and divides the pericardium back to the hilum on both sides. The inferior pulmonary ligament is dissected, pleural adhesions are incised, and the proximal pulmonary arteries are dissected at their origin.
3. After heparinization and hypotensive anesthesia, the superior vena cava is ligated and divided and heavy silk ties are placed around each vessel.
4. The surgeon dissects the aortic arch free, and divides the ligamentum arteriosum. The anterior and inferior margins of the pulmonary artery are separated from the main artery and ascending aorta. Umbilical tapes are placed around the pulmonary artery and aorta. A purse-string suture is placed for infusion of the cardioplegia solution in the heart.
5. After cardioplegia and pulmoplegia are established, the heart is prepared for removal; veins and arteries are separated, and the heart is removed and placed in cold preservation solution.
6. Using blunt and sharp dissection, the surgeon dissects the pulmonary arteries free from the mediastinum to the hilum anteriorly and then posteriorly to the anterior aorta and hilum. The trachea is dissected free. The lungs are inflated before stapling and dissection. The lungs are removed and immersed in cold preservation solution.

Recipient Preparation and Transplantation
1. The perioperative nurse assists with positioning the patient laterally for single lung transplants or in the supine position for bilateral lung transplants. The nurse also performs a wide skin prep for exposure of the chest and abdomen (nipple line to knees).
2. An incision is made. Usually a thoracotomy is created for single lung transplants. Bilateral lung transplants may be performed through bilateral thoracotomies, median sternotomy, or a clamshell incision. The conduct of the procedure depends on which lung is to be removed. If the right lung is being removed, the pulmonary vein is isolated extrapericardially; the pulmonary artery is isolated as close to the lung as possible. The surgeon may ligate and divide the azygos vein for additional exposure; the pulmonary artery is dissected.
3. If the left lung is being removed, the ligamentum arteriosum is divided.
4. The anesthesia provider collapses the lung to be removed, and the proximal pulmonary artery is occluded. If instability occurs after occlusion, cardiopulmonary bypass may be required. In some cases femoral bypass is initiated. If the patient remains stable, the pneumonectomy is performed.
5. Pulmonary veins are divided extrapericardially. The first branch of the pulmonary artery and descending branch are separated. The blood supply to the bronchus is preserved by not dissecting tissue around the bronchus.
6. The surgeon divides the bronchus and removes the lung. The pericardium is opened around the pulmonary veins to allow room for the atrial clamp.
7. Inferior and superior pulmonary veins are incised and joined.
8. Three anastomoses are completed for a single-lung transplant: bronchus to bronchus, pulmonary artery to pulmonary artery, and recipient pulmonary veins to donor atrial cuff. Techniques used to minimize bronchial anastomotic complications include shortening the donor bronchial stump, reinforcing the anastomosis with a vascularized tissue pedicle such as omentum or intercostal muscle pedicle flap, or using an intussuscepting bronchial anastomosis technique.
9. After anastomoses and restoration of circulation, the lung is fully inflated and observed. Chest tubes are placed and secured.
10. After closure of the chest the surgeon performs a bronchoscopy to remove secretions and to ensure that the anastomosis is intact.

KEY POINTS
- Patients undergoing thoracic surgery are at risk for impaired gas exchange, imbalanced fluid volume, infection, and impaired comfort.
- Supine and lateral positioning are used most often to accommodate the different approaches for thoracic surgery.
- Correction of pneumothorax is an essential component of thoracic surgery. Perioperative nurses must be familiar with the physiology of pneumothorax and chest tube technology to provide safe patient care.
- Thoracic surgery may be accomplished via open or minimally invasive approaches; the use of robotic-assisted technology is evolving. Diagnostic endoscopy often precedes thoracic surgery.
- Malignant and nonmalignant conditions are treated with thoracic surgery.

CRITICAL THINKING QUESTION

You have just completed an ETS procedure on Ms. N., a 21-year-old who was diagnosed with severe palmar hyperhidrosis. No intraoperative complications were noted. The surgeon evacuated the air from Ms. N.'s chest cavity with a catheter at the end of the procedure and closed the incision. The anesthesia provider confirmed that Ms. N. had bilateral breath sounds and extubated her shortly after the team transferred her to the transport vehicle. While en route to the PACU, Ms. N. becomes agitated and complains she "can't breathe." On arrival at the PACU, the anesthesia provider notes that Ms. N. no longer has breath sounds on the right and orders a chest x-ray. What actions should you prepare for next?

℮volve *The answers to the Critical Thinking Question can be found at http://evolve.elsevier.com/Rothrock/Alexander.*

REFERENCES

Association of periOperative Registered Nurses (AORN): Recommended practices for prevention of retained surgical items. In *Perioperative standards and recommended practices*, Denver, 2013, The Association.

Brashers VL: Structure and function of the pulmonary system. In Huether S, McCance K, editors: *Understanding pathophysiology*, ed 5, St Louis, 2012, Mosby.

Cerfolio RJ et al: The Society of Thoracic Surgeons expert consensus for the surgical treatment of hyperhidrosis, *Ann Thorac Surg* 91(5):1642–1648, 2011

Denholm B: Tucking patient's arms and general positioning, *AORN J* 89(4):755–757, 2009.

Nason K et al: Chest wall, lung, mediastinum, and pleura. In Brunicardi FC et al, editors: *Schwartz's principles of surgery*, ed 9, New York, 2010, McGraw-Hill.

Organ Procurement and Transplantation Network (OPTN): *Transplants by donor type 1988 to date*, available at http://optn.transplant.hrsa.gov/latestData/rptData.asp. Accessed April 7, 2013.

Puc MM et al: Early outcomes after bilateral thoracoscopy versus median sternotomy for lung volume reduction, *Innovations (Phila)* 5(2):97–102, 2010.

Rees HC: Assessment of the respiratory system. In Ignatavicius DD, Workman ML, editors: *Medical-surgical nursing: patient-centered collaborative care*, ed 7, St Louis, 2013, Saunders.

Taneja A: Bronchoscopic interventions in the management of chronic obstructive pulmonary disease, *Curr Opin Pulm Med* 19(2):145–151, 2013.

CHAPTER 24
Vascular Surgery

PATRICIA WIECZOREK

Atherosclerosis continues to be one of the leading causes of death and disability in the Western world. It is estimated that peripheral atherosclerosis, including carotid, mesenteric, renal, and peripheral arterial disease (PAD) (also referred to as peripheral arterial occlusive disease [PAOD]), affects about 8 million people in the United States. The prevalence of PAD is approximately 12% of the adult population, with men being affected slightly more than women (Ferreria and Macedo, 2010). This is particularly striking, given that by the year 2030 the percentage of the U.S. population older than 65 years will increase to 20% (Federal Interagency Forum on Aging-Related Statistics, 2012). Many of these people will require interventions for the syndromes of peripheral ischemia, aneurysm, and venous disease.

Interventional therapy for peripheral atherosclerosis has become common. Aortic procedures are now routinely performed with minimal mortality. Carotid endarterectomy has also proven to be safe and effective. Peripheral angioplasty and bypass have a high initial success rate, but restenosis, graft failure, and progression of distal disease still lead to limb loss in certain patients after several years. Thus emphasis has been placed on decreasing morbidity and hospital stay associated with revascularization. Minimally invasive methods and strategies, including endovascular aortic aneurysm repair (Schwarze et al, 2009), carotid artery stenting (Liu et al, 2009) (Research Highlight), stenting for lower-limb ischemia, and percutaneous transluminal angioplasty (Zeller et al, 2009), have been developed, and their application and popularity continue to increase. New technologies, such as miniature shavers and laser

---

RESEARCH HIGHLIGHT

Carotid Revascularization Using Endarterectomy or Stenting Systems (CaRESS): 4-Year Outcomes

The prospective nonrandomized study compares the 4-year outcomes of carotid revascularization using endarterectomy or stenting systems. With the continued evolution of endovascular techniques, carotid artery stenting (CAS) has become an option in high-risk patients. A cohort of 397 symptomatic (33%) and asymptomatic (64%), broad-risk patients with carotid stenosis underwent carotid endarterectomy (n = 254) or CAS (n = 143). The 4-year outcome results suggest that the risk of death or stroke following CAS is equivalent to endarterectomy and there appeared to be no differences in mortality when comparing high-risk and non–high-risk patients. The authors did see a twofold higher restenosis rate with carotid stenting compared with carotid endarterectomy surgery after 4 years. Further studies are recommended on symptomatic patients as well as additional long-term follow-up.

Modified from Zarins CK et al: Carotid revascularization using endarterectomy or stenting systems (CaRESS): 4-year outcomes, *J Endovasc Ther* 16(4):397–409, 2009.

---

arthrectomy devices for arterial plaque, continue to be developed (Kolakowski et al, 2009). Perioperative nurses must be prepared for the demands of patient care in vascular surgery. This chapter reviews surgical anatomy, perioperative nursing considerations, and surgical interventions for a variety of vascular procedures.

Surgical Anatomy

Basic knowledge of anatomy is essential when caring for perioperative patients with a vascular disorder. Figure 24-1 depicts the principal arteries and veins of the body. Arteries and veins have three layers:

- Tunica intima (innermost layer)
- Tunica media (muscular middle layer)
- Tunica adventitia (fibrous outer layer)

Arteries differ from veins in function and slightly in structure (Figure 24-2). Structurally, arteries have a thicker muscle layer and more elastic fibers than veins. The properties of elasticity and distensibility enable arteries to compensate for changes in blood pressure and volume. Because of the thicker muscle layer, severed arteries are capable of contracting and constricting enough to stop hemorrhage. In contrast, veins are more fragile than arteries, and whether its cause is traumatic or iatrogenic, venous bleeding may be difficult to control. Another difference is the presence of semi-lunar intimal folds, or valves, in veins that prevent backflow. Veins and arteries are nourished by a tiny network of vessels (the vasa vasorum), as well as from the intraluminal blood flow. Both are regulated by the autonomic nervous system, with veins having fewer nerve fibers than arteries. The two systems are connected (except for the pulmonary artery and pulmonary venous system): major arteries carry oxygenated blood, they branch into smaller arteries and arterioles, and then blood moves into capillaries to venules and to veins. The work of exchanging nutrients and metabolic waste is done at the capillary level.

Blood flow is a complex process that depends on many factors. Blood flows through arteries such that the blood in the center of the vessel moves faster than the blood at the periphery. Because the movement of the blood is in parallel lines, it is referred to as *laminar*. When flow is disrupted by an obstruction, stenosis, curve, or bifurcation, the particle motion is referred to as *turbulent*. Turbulence may be evidenced by the presence of a bruit (e.g., turbulent noise), detected by auscultation, or detected by a characteristic Doppler signal. Flow depends on blood viscosity, vessel wall resistance, and the peripheral resistance of the arterioles. There must be a difference in pressures, or a pressure gradient, to allow blood to flow. The gradient is provided by the contraction of the left ventricle. The negative pressure created by the relaxed right ventricle assists in

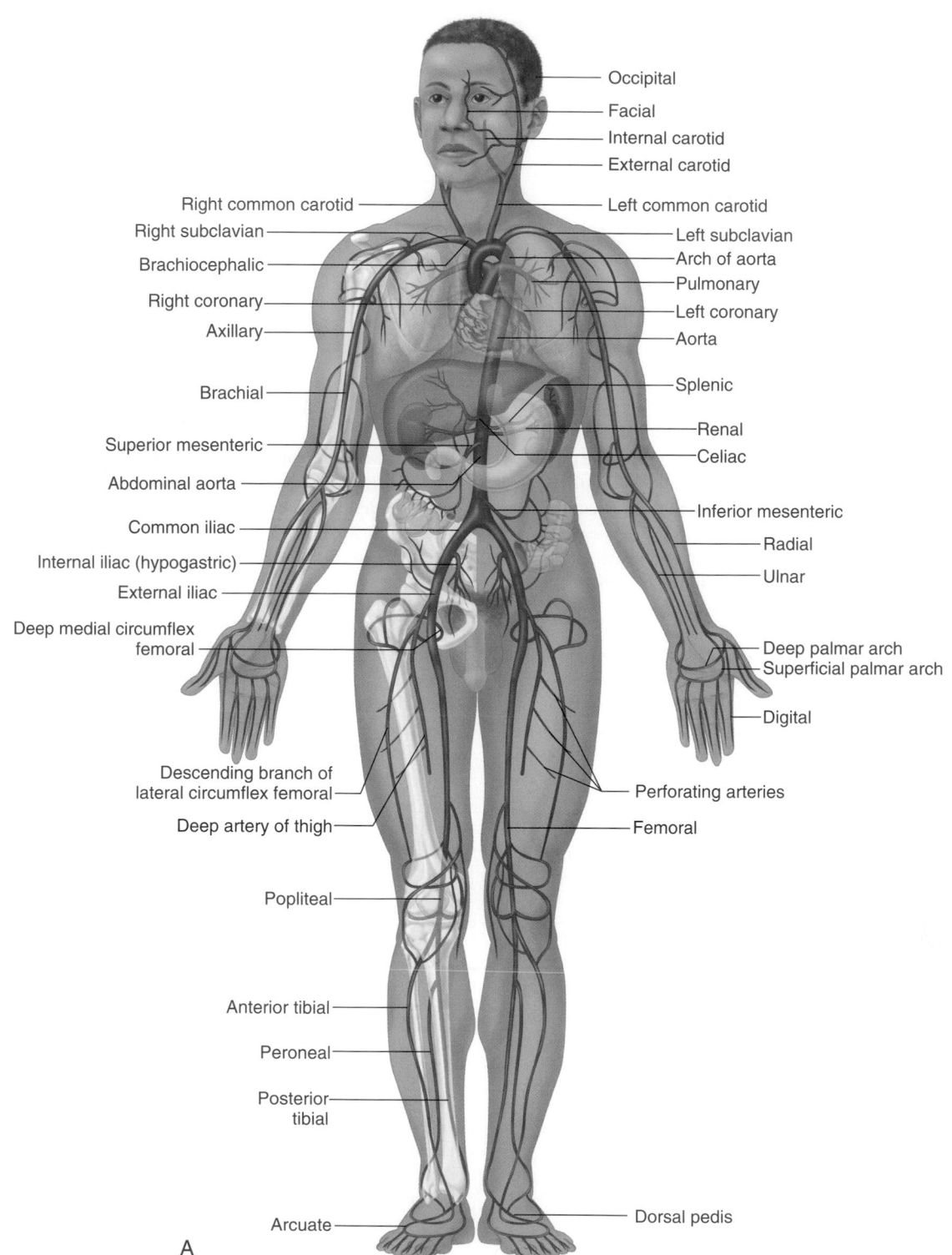

Occipital
Facial
Internal carotid
External carotid
Right common carotid — — Left common carotid
Right subclavian — — Left subclavian
Brachiocephalic — — Arch of aorta
— Pulmonary
Right coronary — — Left coronary
Axillary — — Aorta
Brachial — — Splenic
— Renal
Superior mesenteric — — Celiac
Abdominal aorta — — Inferior mesenteric
Common iliac — — Radial
Internal iliac (hypogastric) — — Ulnar
External iliac —
Deep medial circumflex
femoral — — Deep palmar arch
— Superficial palmar arch
— Digital
Descending branch of
lateral circumflex femoral — — Perforating arteries
Deep artery of thigh — — Femoral
Popliteal —
Anterior tibial —
Peroneal —
Posterior
tibial —
Arcuate — — Dorsal pedis

A

FIGURE 24-1 A, Principal arteries of the body.

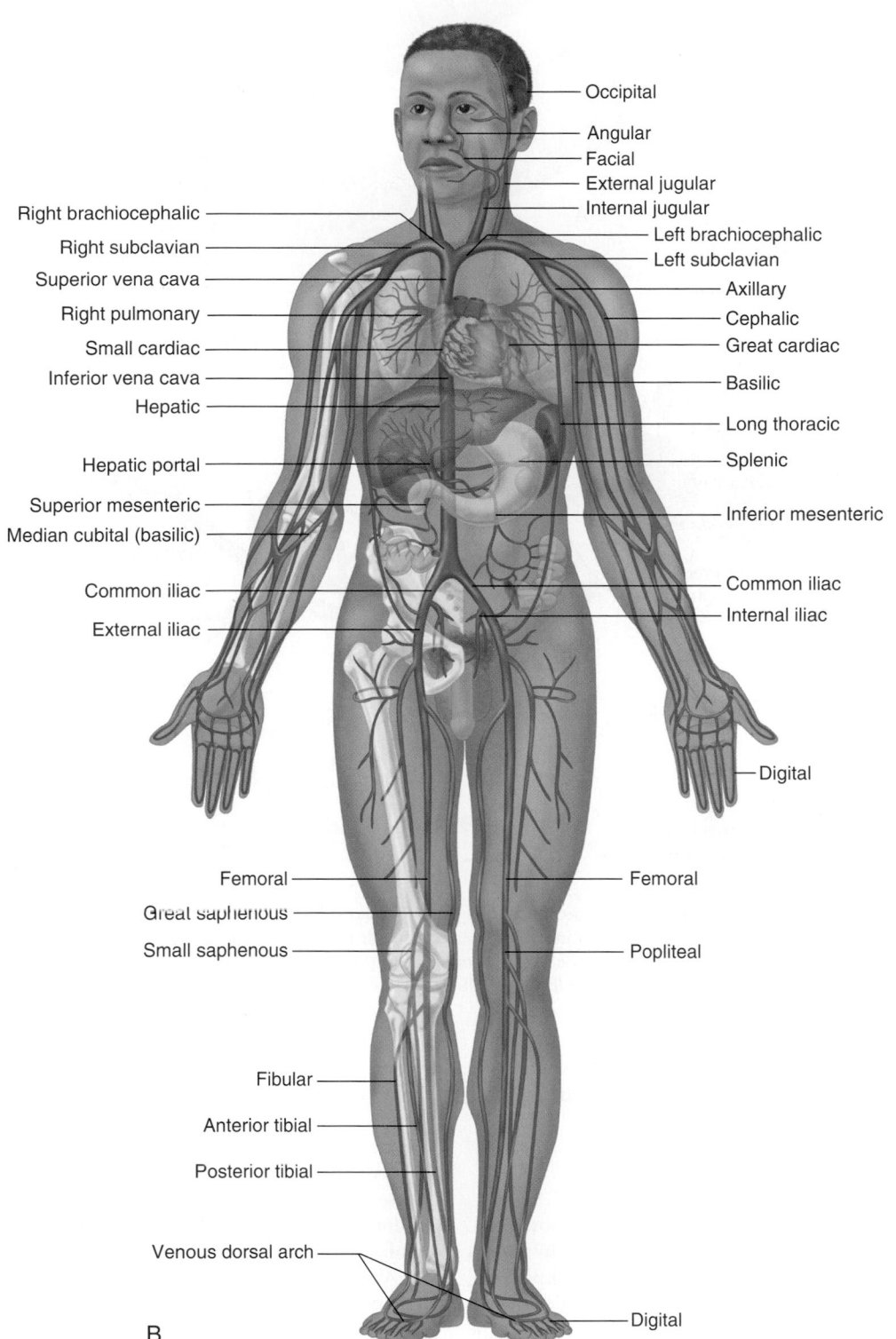

FIGURE 24-1, cont'd B, Principal veins of the body.

Tunica adventitia
(connective tissue)

Tunica media
(smooth muscle
and elastic tissue)

Tunica intima
(endothelium)

A

Capillary

Arteriole

Capillaries

Precapillary
sphincters

Venule

B

Arteriole

FIGURE 24-2 A, Layers of artery and vein. Drawings of a sectioned artery and vein show the three layers of large vessel walls. **B,** Microcirculation. The smaller blood vessels—arterioles, capillaries, and venules—cannot be observed without magnification. Note that the control of blood flow through any particular region of a capillary network can be regulated by the relative contraction of precapillary sphincters in the walls of the arterioles *(inset).* Note also that capillaries have a wall composed of only a single layer of flattened cells, whereas the walls of the larger vessels also have a smooth layer.

venous return by creating a suctioning effect, and the skeletal and visceral muscles help propel venous return toward the heart.

Arterial Disease

Aneurysmal Disease

The most common cause of an arterial aneurysm is atherosclerotic degeneration of the arterial wall. The pathogenesis is a multifactorial process, involving atherosclerosis along with genetic predisposition, aging, inflammation, and localized activation of proteolytic enzymes (Sawabe, 2010). A true aneurysm is a dilation of all layers of the artery wall. A dissecting aneurysm results from a tear in the artery wall, allowing blood to dissect between the layers of the vessel wall. A false aneurysm, or pseudoaneurysm, is not an aneurysm but a disruption through all the layers of a vessel wall with the escaping blood being contained by the perivascular tissues. False aneurysms may result from trauma, infection, or disruption of an arterial

suture line after surgery. True aneurysms are most frequently found in the abdominal aorta but are also found in the thoracic aorta and iliac, femoral, and popliteal arteries. More men than women are affected, and aneurysmal disease tends to be a disease of older adults. As early as 1977, a familial tendency was observed that subsequent research verified; as many as 18% of patients with abdominal aortic aneurysms have a first-degree relative with a similar diagnosis (Sawabe, 2010).

Abdominal aortic aneurysms (AAAs), which account for most aneurysms, occur primarily between the renal arteries and the aortic bifurcation (Little, 2013). An aneurysm involves intimal damage of the aorta and weakening of the tunica media (Sawabe, 2010) or elastic portion (collagen and elastin defects) of the arterial wall. Gradually the vessel wall in the damaged area expands and atheroma develops within the aneurysm sac (Figure 24-3). An AAA has minimal symptoms and is generally discovered on routine history and physical examination. In men, the diameter of the infrarenal

FIGURE 24-3 Abdominal aortic aneurysm. **A,** External view, gross photograph of a large aortic aneurysm that ruptured *(arrow)*. **B,** Opened view. The wall of the aneurysm is thin and the lumen is filled with a large quantity of thrombus. The probe indicates the track of the rupture.

RESEARCH HIGHLIGHT

Population-Based Outcomes Following Endovascular and Open Repair of Ruptured Abdominal Aortic Aneurysms

The purpose of this study was to evaluate national outcomes after endovascular and open surgical repair of ruptured abdominal aortic aneurysms (rAAA). A nationwide sample to identify all repairs between 2000 and 2005 for rAAAs was interrogated using ICD-9 codes. A total of 28,429 patients were identified; 2323 underwent an endovascular repair and 26,106 had open procedures. The outcomes studies showed the overall mortality rate was 41%: 33% and 41% for endovascular repair versus open repair, respectively. The length of hospital stay was shorter after endovascular repair (7 vs. 9 days) and respiratory complications (8% vs. 4%) and acute renal failure (30% vs. 23%) was more common in the open repair group. Endovascular repairs increased more rapidly at high-volume centers, and those centers saw a lower mortality rate than low-volume centers.

The authors concluded that mortality associated with rAAAs may be improved by using the endovascular technique. The study also supports the referral of this patient population to high-volume centers for both open and endovascular repair of rAAAs.

Modified from Giles KA et al: Population-based outcomes following endovascular and open repair of ruptured abdominal aortic aneurysms, *J Endovasc Ther* 16(5):554–564, 2009.

aorta normally measures between 14 and 24 mm and in women it measures between 12 and 21 mm. An AAA is diagnosed if the diameter is 3 cm or larger for men or 2.6 cm or larger for females. Mortality is low with elective repair of the aneurysm. Dissection and rupture of the aneurysm (aortic dissection) dramatically increase operative mortality because of the abrupt and massive hemorrhagic shock that accompanies the rupture (Research Highlight). Aortic dissection is believed to arise from a sudden tear in the aortic intima, opening the way for blood to enter the aortic wall.

Acute Arterial Insufficiency

Arterial insufficiency may result from an acute occlusion, as in embolic disease, or from the rupture of an unstable atherosclerotic plaque, causing acute thrombosis of the vessel. Emboli usually arise from the heart as a result of atrial fibrillation but may occasionally result from a myocardial infarction (MI), where a clot forms on the endocardium (the lining of the heart) in an area of muscle damage. Atherosclerotic plaque can also break loose from other areas and result in an acute arterial blockage. Patients with acute arterial occlusion usually present with the onset of the six *P*'s: sudden severe *p*ain, *p*ulselessness, *p*aresthesia, *p*aralysis, *p*allor, and *p*oikilothermia (coolness) of an extremity (Little, 2013). Heparin is the mainstay to prevent the enlargement of emboli while allowing time for collateral blood flow to develop. However, in the threatened limb there are basically two options: surgical removal of the clot (embolectomy) or chemical removal of the clot with the use of a thrombolytic medication. If the limb reaches the point where the muscle is rigid, the limb is not salvageable and amputation is a lifesaving procedure.

Chronic Arterial Insufficiency

Chronic arterial insufficiency occurs because of the deposition of calcium and cholesterol within the wall of the artery. Arteriosclerosis is a natural part of the aging process and occurs when the walls

of the arterial vasculature undergo changes such as increased thickness and hardening, reducing the elasticity of the arteries. The decrease in elasticity should not be confused with atherosclerosis obliterans, which is a pathologic process that affects the intimal layer of the artery with the buildup of a fibrous plaque of lipids that can calcify and necrose. Atherosclerosis is the most common cause of PAD, the probable mechanism being initial damage to the intima and subsequent activation and aggregation of the body's platelets. Inflammation follows, with the deposition of lipoproteins forming an atheroma. Calcification of this lesion leads to the development of an atherosclerotic plaque, resulting in inadequate muscle perfusion and ischemia (Zeller et al, 2009). The process is a gradual one, and a localized lesion usually indicates systemic disease. The body develops a network of collateral vessels as an adaptive mechanism to supply the tissues with oxygenated blood. Many theories have been postulated to explain the process of atherogenesis. The inflammatory process of intimal injury, as just described, seems to be the current and most widely accepted hypothesis. Box 24-1 presents risk factors for atherosclerosis. A large number of vascular surgical procedures revolve around the results of chronic arterial insufficiency.

Arterial Insufficiency: Cerebrovascular Disease and Stroke

Cerebrovascular accident (CVA or stroke) is a leading cause of death in the United States and most industrialized countries. In the United States, approximately 795,000 people experience a new or recurrent stroke each year (Roger et al, 2012). Cerebrovascular disease may manifest itself as a transient ischemic attack (TIA) or as a major or minor stroke. A TIA is an episode of neurologic dysfunction that resolves in 24 hours. It may be caused by atheromatous debris or a thromboembolism from a carotid artery or the vertebral basilar system. Vascular lesions in the carotid artery occur primarily at the bifurcation of the common carotid artery into the internal and the external carotid arteries. The internal carotid artery

Risk Factors for Atherosclerosis

Firmly Established Factors
• Hypercholesterolemia
• Cigarette smoking
• Hypertension
• Diabetes mellitus

Relative Factors
• Advanced age
• Male gender
• Hypertriglyceridemia
• Hyperhomocysteinemia
• Sedentary lifestyle
• Family history

supplies the brain with needed oxygenated blood. Obstruction in this arterial vessel leads to cerebrovascular insufficiency.

The right and the left carotid and vertebral arteries supply the brain (Figure 24-4). The first major branch of the internal carotid artery is the ophthalmic artery. Thromboembolic events that affect this artery may result in visual disturbances, ocular TIAs, or "amaurosis fugax" (complete or partial loss of vision). Patients often describe amaurosis fugax as a curtain over a partial field of vision, usually the top. Clinical conditions that generally indicate the need for a carotid endarterectomy (CEA) are transient cerebral ischemia, asymptomatic severe stenosis, and stable strokes. Carotid disease may recur after a CEA. Redo surgery for restenosis poses the same complication risks as the original procedure.

Arterial Insufficiency: Peripheral Vascular Disease

The initial and most important symptom of vascular disease in the aortoiliac vessels and distal arteries is intermittent claudication. The term *claudication* is derived from the Latin word *claudicare,* which means "to limp." This is the most common symptom of lower-extremity PAD and occurs distal to the arterial obstruction while the patient is exercising. Many patients are asymptomatic and do not experience pain. When this symptom does occur, it is typically located in the working muscle, occurs with the same amount of exercise each time, and is relieved with rest. This is referred to as functional ischemia; blood flow is adequate at rest but inadequate to sustain exercise. The increased muscle demand for oxygen with exercise cannot be met distal to the arterial obstruction. Anaerobic metabolism occurs, and muscle cramping develops. Walking difficulties are often seen in the elderly patient with PAD (Patient-Centered Care). Surgery is not usually performed for claudication unless it is unusually disabling.

The second symptom—rest pain, which is located in the foot—develops as the vascular disease progresses (Oka et al, 2012). At this stage the ischemia is termed *critical.* Rest pain occurs without exercise and is a constant discomfort, often aggravated at night. The body is now unable to meet the oxygen needs of distal tissues even at rest. Rest pain may be somewhat relieved by analgesics or by lowering the legs off the bed. Gravity assists in increasing the tissue perfusion and oxygen supply to decrease the pain. Unless the vascular disease is corrected, nonhealing ulcers and gangrene can develop. Gangrene occurs when the arterial vessels are unable to meet the oxygen needs of distal tissues even at complete rest.

Peripheral artery disease (PAD) is a manifestation of atherosclerosis that is most prevalent in the elderly population. Risk factors of PAD include hypertension, diabetes, obesity, and physical inactivity. Patients with PAD often report walking difficulties due to the symptoms of the disease process resulting in a decreased quality of life. To help improve the quality of life for this population, a 24-month patient-centered behavioral change study was done. The study examined the impact of PAD risk reduction program, targeting exercise and diet on walking and the quality of life.

The significance of using a patient-centered approach allows for collaboration between the healthcare provider and the patient. Problems are identified and prioritized with the patient's input. The collaborative approach helps identify strategies to barriers to ensure success with a diet and exercise program (Oka et al, 2012). Problem-solving techniques are shared, and active participation in the program improves compliance. This approach can also be applied to patients undergoing surgery to ensure success with their postoperative plan of care. The nurse facilitates this collaboration through the use of open-ended questions to elicit a more thoughtful response from the patient versus a yes or no answer. For example, the nurse might say, "We've talked about how important diet and exercise are going to be during your recovery. Can you tell me what you think you will do with this information to make sure you're doing everything to improve the chances of this surgery helping your PAD?"

Modified from Oka RK et al: Efficacy of optimal long-term management of multiple cardiovascular risk factors (CVD) on walking and quality of life in patients with peripheral artery disease (PAD): protocol for randomized controlled trial, *Vasc Med* 17(1):17–28, 2012.

Venous Disease

Acute Venous Insufficiency

Acute venous insufficiency is caused by a clot in the deep venous system, or deep vein thrombosis (DVT). Such venous insufficiency can be a diagnosis of DVT, phlebitis, thrombophlebitis, or phlebothrombosis, which merely indicates that there is a clot, usually in the lower extremity. Virchow, a pathologist, identified the three elements that trigger venous thrombosis. Referred to as Virchow's triad, these elements, or risk factors, are endothelial injury, venostasis, and hypercoagulability (Little, 2013). The cause of hypercoagulability is sometimes unknown but is seen in patients with tissue trauma (e.g., surgery, burns, or stroke), malignancy, sepsis, pregnancy or estrogen use, and diabetes mellitus. The patient may be asymptomatic or present with limb swelling, pain, and a skin color change. The danger lies in the potential emboli migrating to the right ventricle and proceeding to the lungs. A pulmonary embolus (PE) can be fatal. The majority of pulmonary emboli cases are caused by DVT. The majority of these originate in the lower extremities. The use of heparin and bed rest is the usual medical treatment. In cases that preclude the use of systemic heparin or in which heparin is ineffective, surgical insertion of a vena cava filter may be indicated.

Chronic Venous Insufficiency

Patients with chronic venous insufficiency (CVI) have not been treated surgically as often as patients with arterial disease for several reasons. CVI is generally not life- or limb-threatening. Improved imaging techniques (e.g., duplex ultrasonography) allow better diagnoses of the precise problem. The treatment of the majority of

FIGURE 24-4 Arteries at the base of the brain. **A,** Diagram shows the cerebral arterial circle (of Willis) and related structures on the base of the brain. Note the arterial anastomoses. **B,** Origins of blood vessels that form the cerebral arterial circle. **C,** Magnetic resonance image of the cerebral arterial circle.

venous disorders is nonsurgical and aimed at increasing venous return and decreasing edema. CVI, which presents with stasis ulcers from postphlebitic syndrome, usually occurs in one leg. The leg is usually very swollen with a cyclic edema, which does not change visibly after overnight leg elevation. Stasis ulcers and hyperpigmentation usually are found in the "gaiter" area (e.g., midcalf to about 1 inch above the medial malleolus) on the leg. The condition is caused by incompetent perforator valves. The perforating veins connect the superficial and deep venous systems. The usual management is to apply 20 to 30 mm Hg of external pressure by means of special pressure stockings. Surgical interventions such as valvuloplasty (direct repair of the valve), valve transposition or transplantation (moving a valve from the arm to the leg), or perforator interruptions are occasionally performed but have had limited success. Patient selection is critical, and long-term results are mixed.

Diabetic and Vascular Foot Conditions

The severity of these conditions is conveyed by diagnoses and sequelae (e.g., necrotizing fasciitis, gas gangrene, ascending cellulitis, and infection with systemic toxicity or metabolic instability). Because patients with diabetes mellitus may have peripheral neuropathies, they may not feel and therefore not notice any tenderness or early signs of infection. These foot infections can lead to hospitalization and eventual lower extremity amputation for patients with preexisting ulcerations; surgical management is often required for the severe infections. The experienced surgeon determines when and how to intervene. Main principles for management include stabilization of the patient; adequate debridement along with antibiotic therapy; vascular evaluation and revascularization as necessary; delayed soft tissue reconstruction; and postoperative information and intervention for medical and surgical issues. In addressing all these aspects, the surgeon optimizes the possibility for limb salvage. This overview serves as a reminder to emphasize the importance of overall adherence in managing diabetes mellitus to prevent further complications (Aragón-Sánchez et al, 2011).

These complex patients are best handled with multidisciplinary consultations to coordinate care and determine optimal timing for soft tissue reconstruction. Primary closure may not be an option and secondary healing is not necessarily reliable. The proactive surgical approach aims to salvage the diabetic limb by improving overall health and to provide a stable, mechanically sound limb that will resist further breakdown once the patient is able to walk again. Patients need ongoing support and validation to prevent complications. Hospital care focuses on dressing changes, wound care, physical therapy, limb position, and laboratory testing. Postoperative nursing care should provide instruction for follow-up and frequency of monitoring of the surgical results, ambulatory status, work and social restrictions, and bathing. Especially important for the perioperative nurse to review with the patient are identification of infection and ways of contacting the surgical team if problems arise (Aragón-Sánchez et al, 2011).

Perioperative Nursing Considerations

Assessment

Nursing Responsibilities. A preoperative assessment is necessary for an adequate understanding of the patient's disease, the patient's response, and the proposed surgical procedure. Knowledge of vascular disease and its progression assists the perioperative nurse in performing a critical review of the comprehensive assessment and

---

BOX 24-2

Review of Patient's Medical Record

The perioperative nurse should review the patient's medical record, confirming or obtaining information for the following items:
- Correct and current medical record/chart
- Surgical consent
- History and physical examination
- Baseline vital signs (including height and weight)
- Mental status
- Medications
- Allergies or adverse reactions to drugs, topical agents, or other substances (e.g., latex)
- Skin tone and integrity
- Physical limitations
- Laboratory data (e.g., prescribed bloodwork, electrocardiogram [ECG] report, urinalysis, ultrasound or x-ray studies, other pertinent tests)
- Religious, cultural, ethnic preferences
- Nursing plan of care or other notations from transferring nurse
- Presence or disposition of prosthetic devices (e.g., hearing aids, dentures, glasses)

---

developing a plan of care for patients undergoing vascular surgical procedures.

The perioperative nurse should assess the patient, reviewing an already completed, current nursing assessment for the development and extent of vascular symptoms. The nurse must assess medical conditions—including cardiac, renal, and pulmonary disease; coagulation status; and allergies (Box 24-2)—to ensure that the patient can tolerate a possible angiogram, because the contrast medium is toxic and increased fluid volumes are needed if angioscopy or intraoperative angiography is planned. This is a shared responsibility of the nursing, surgical, and anesthesia providers. The patient's nutritional status, the patient's use of alcohol and tobacco, and the existence of any skin lesions should also be noted. Preoperative location, grading, and marking of distal peripheral pulses assist the perioperative nurse with intraoperative and postoperative assessment of tissue perfusion. The nurse shares pertinent information gathered during the assessment phase with the rest of the surgical team, including the scrub person (who may be a surgical technologist or registered nurse), as appropriate.

The nurse greets the patient by name and verifies identification using two unique identifiers. When possible, the patient should confirm such identification. Identification must also be confirmed by the name band, medical record, surgical consent, operating room (OR) schedule, and marked surgical site. Safety is always the first priority. The surgical procedure must be confirmed and the patient's understanding of the procedure and associated risks assessed; inaccuracies or misconceptions must be clarified before proceeding with surgery. Written consent is designed to protect the patient by providing written clarification of the proposed procedure. The National Quality Forum (NQF) identified Safe Practice 10 for informed consent, recommending that each patient (or legal surrogate) be asked to "teach-back" what he or she has been told during the informed consent discussion (Fink et al, 2010). Consents that are valid and obtained freely from a competent person remain in effect for as long as the person still agrees to the surgery or procedure. This may vary by institutional modification.

FIGURE 24-5 Digital subtraction angiography.

The nurse assesses patient comfort before continuing the interview and assessment. This reflects caring and will promote nurse-patient rapport and facilitate obtaining accurate and complete information. The acuity of the patient's condition will also affect the order of priority of the assessments and interactions. After reviewing the results of the patient's physical examination, the perioperative nurse should verify signs and symptoms of vascular disease that need to be considered during intraoperative care. Muscle and skin atrophy, the presence of tissue ulceration or necrosis, pain, neurovascular status, skin color and temperature, and other integumentary changes should be noted. Elderly, cachectic, or obese patients are at increased risk for pressure injuries.

The perioperative nurse should assess the patient's mental status and determine the level of understanding and emotional response to the surgery. Patients with vascular disorders usually have systemic disease, and the fear of a stroke (if the patient is having a carotid procedure), amputation (if the patient has an ischemic limb), or other complications may be a realistic concern. A skin assessment should include notation of color, integrity, pain, and pulses. Any musculoskeletal problems that preclude patients moving themselves to the OR bed and any weaknesses that may have resulted from a stroke or that would modify the positioning for surgery should be noted. Correction of misunderstandings is possible only if the perioperative nurse identifies the patient's current level of knowledge. Identification of the patient's fears and concerns helps with planning supportive nursing interventions.

Vascular surgery can be lengthy. The nurse must consider the effects of hypothermia during long procedures. The patient's extremities should be assessed for color, temperature, and strength of pedal pulses before the surgical procedure so that baseline data will be available for comparison with perioperative assessment data. This assessment evaluates tissue perfusion distal to the arterial obstruction.

Preoperative Tests. A variety of tests may be required to plan for surgical interventions. Segmental pressure measurements give partial anatomic information in that they assist in locating lesions.

Hemodynamic tests provide information on the flow of blood, such as that to the brain or an extremity, and the effects on flow caused by a vascular lesion.

Angiography. Invasive diagnostic tests may be performed preoperatively to identify the extent and location of the patient's peripheral vascular disease (Oka et al, 2012). The introduction of a contrast medium through a catheter into the arterial or venous system of the patient facilitates this visualization. Angiography also involves injecting a contrast medium into the patient's arterial system and taking serial radiographs of the movement of the dye through the arteries. Digital subtraction angiography (DSA) is one such technique that uses a computer along with contrast medium injection to make the image (Figure 24-5). Usually one side of the film shows the bone for orientation, and the other side subtracts the density of the bone and soft tissue to allow a clearer view of the vessels. Arteriography provides information on arterial anatomy and the location of stenotic or occluded vessels and assists the surgeon in planning bypass procedures. A venogram (contrast venography) is performed to show venous abnormalities in extremities, the vena cava, and the hepatic and renal systems. Ascending venography can differentiate between acute and chronic thrombosis and can define anatomy. Descending venography assesses valve competence of the lower extremities.

Doppler Scanning. The Doppler effect is the change in the frequency of echo signals that occurs whenever there is a change in the distance between the sources of a sound and the receiving object. The probe, or transducer, is aimed toward the blood vessel at an angle of 45 to 60 degrees. This directs an ultrasound beam that is reflected back to the probe by moving red blood cells (RBCs). The velocity of the flow of cells is converted into an audible signal heard through a speaker. The signal is described as a swishing sound. The sound is called a signal, not a pulse. The tip of the probe is made of an element called a ceramic piezoelectric crystal, which can send, receive, and convert signals when an electric current is applied. The element becomes thicker and thinner, thus resulting in a pressure wave converted to an audible signal. The simplest form is the continuous wave (CW) Doppler probe. It has two elements: one sends a high-frequency wave, and the other receives it. In a pulsed Doppler probe, the same element sends and receives signals. The pulsed Doppler probe has the advantage of being able to differentiate among vessels of different depths. A normal arterial Doppler signal is either biphasic or triphasic. The first sound corresponds to systolic flow and is forward-moving and of high velocity. The second sound is related to early diastole and has a lesser reversal of flow. The third sound is later diastole and is smaller, forward-flowing, and of a lower velocity. The pitch is described as rising quickly in systole and dropping quickly in early diastole. An abnormal signal, indicating stenosis or occlusion is heard as low-pitched and monophasic. These abnormal arterial signals may sound like venous signals.

The Doppler probe can provide information in three forms: the audible signal, a visible graph printout similar to an electrocardiogram (ECG) tracing, and a spectral analysis that appears on a screen and may be recorded on paper as well. The Doppler transducer is the most widely used instrument for vascular study. It has the advantages of being readily available, inexpensive, and easy to use. A small, portable battery unit is durable and can be transported and stored easily. When the probe is used on intact skin, a water-soluble gel is needed to conduct a signal. Probes can be used directly on a vessel intraoperatively. The probes are heat sensitive and must either be sterilized according to manufacturer's instructions or be inserted into a sterile sleeve or probe cover. If they are handled gently, the probes have a reasonable life span. Care must be taken to protect the sensitive tip from being dropped or crushed. The biggest drawback of the Doppler probe is a negative finding in the presence of a stenotic lesion pronounced enough to produce a flow disturbance resulting in an altered signal.

A bruit is a sound disturbance that is sometimes described as a low-pitched, blowing sound. It can be heard through a stethoscope over an area of blood flow turbulence that occurs at points of vessel stenoses. Bruits do not provide information on the extent of a lesion—only that an abnormal flow may exist. They occur at points of significant stenosis and are not heard when severe flow restriction or total flow occlusion occurs. The Doppler probe is noninvasive and painless for patients.

Ultrasonography. Ultrasonography is done to obtain information about structures through the emission of high-frequency sound waves. These sound waves are reflected, or bounced back, to the probe or transducer that emits them and are electronically transformed into an image.

B-Mode Ultrasonography. B-mode is brightness modulation, a technique in ultrasound imaging that projects a two-dimensional image on an oscilloscope screen. The image appears as dots from the echoes of the signal. The strength of the echo is shown by the intensity and brightness of the dots on the screen.

Duplex Ultrasonography. A duplex ultrasound machine is a combination of the pulsed Doppler image and the so-called real-time B-mode image ultrasonogram. "Real time" simply refers to the image projecting current, undelayed information. B-mode image is best when the probe is perpendicular to the vessel, but the Doppler probe does not pick up signals at a perpendicular angle. Some manipulation of the probe angle is required to obtain the best results. Color duplex imaging converts the detected signals caused by blood flow into a color, depending on the direction of flow. Flow toward the probe may be displayed as red, away from the probe as blue, and turbulence as multiple colors. This imaging provides both hemodynamic and anatomic information. The technology is also used in transesophageal echocardiography (TEE) and is the diagnostic method of choice for venous insufficiency.

Pulse Volume Recording (PVR) or Sequential Volume Plethysmography. A plethysmograph measures and records the changes in the sizes and volumes in extremities by measuring the blood volumes at blood pressure cuffs placed at intervals along the extremity. The methods include electrical impedance, mercury in Silastic strain gauges, and air or fluid displacement. This test, which is used to determine the location of an arterial lesion and estimate the severity of the disease, requires careful limb positioning and a cooperative patient. A negative study is a good predictor of low risk for PE.

This test is inexpensive, has good predictive value, and is accurate in detecting thrombosis. It has the disadvantage of a high rate of false-positive results in the presence of old DVT, congestive heart failure (CHF), and external compression.

Magnetic Resonance Imaging. Magnetic resonance imaging (MRI) measures the behavior of atoms in a strong magnetic field. This test provides detailed and three-dimensional images of anatomy for evaluation of carotid, aortic, and lower-extremity disease (Oka et al, 2012). An MRI provides more detail than ultrasonography or computed tomography (CT) scan and avoids the complications of contrast medium injection and exposure to x-rays. MRI is contraindicated for patients with preexisting implantable devices.

Nursing Diagnosis

Nursing diagnoses related to the care of patients undergoing vascular surgery might include the following:

- Anxiety related to the surgical intervention and its outcomes
- Hypothermia related to surgical exposure and anesthesia
- Risk for Deficient Fluid Volume related to loss of body fluids
- Risk for Impaired Skin Integrity and Ineffective Tissue Perfusion related to surgical positioning, presence of vascular disease, and vascular clamping

Based on the perioperative nurse's assessment, identification and prioritization of nursing diagnoses aid in the development of an individualized plan of care.

Outcome Identification

Outcomes identified for the selected nursing diagnoses could be stated as follows:

- The patient will have all questions answered, will verbalize decreased anxiety and understanding of surgical procedure and perioperative routines, and will exhibit increased relaxation as shown by facial expression or other body language.
- The patient's body temperature will remain within normal limits as evidenced by postoperative temperature equivalent to preoperative level and absence of postoperative shivering.
- Fluid balance will be maintained as evidenced by postoperative pulses equivalent to preoperative level, hourly urine output of at least 30 mL, and good skin turgor.
- Skin integrity will be maintained. Skin temperature and color will be within normal limits. No skin injury lesions will be evident, and the electrosurgical unit (ESU) dispersive pad site will be intact.

Planning

Before the patient is transported to the OR, the perioperative nurse should procure the necessary supplies and equipment for the intended surgical intervention. Because the need for intraoperative arteriography or fluoroscopy for endovascular procedures is a possibility, the patient with a vascular disorder should be positioned on an appropriate OR bed with x-ray capabilities. The perioperative nurse needs to coordinate the availability of x-ray department personnel. Appropriate contrast media, catheters, and impermeable sterile x-ray covers must be available. Radiation-protection devices, such as lead aprons and shields, should be used for the patient when possible and for surgical team members. A typical plan of care for a patient undergoing vascular surgery, using the suggested nursing diagnoses, is seen in the Sample Plan of Care below.

Arterial procedures, especially those that involve the aorta, may place the patient at risk for significant blood loss. The perioperative nurse should confirm the availability of ordered blood-replacement products. The use of rapid infusion systems or blood salvage equipment should be determined and planned.

Implementation

Site Verification: Time-Out. Patient safety is of utmost importance. It is the entire surgical team's responsibility to verify that the correct patient is receiving the correct procedure on the correct site immediately before the start of any surgical procedure. The surgical

---

SAMPLE PLAN OF CARE

Nursing Diagnosis
Anxiety related to the surgical intervention and its outcomes

Outcome
The patient will have all questions answered. The patient will verbalize decreased anxiety and understanding of surgical procedure and perioperative routines. The patient will exhibit increased relaxation as shown by facial expression or other body language.

Interventions
- Include the family, significant others, or both in explanations of perioperative routines.
- Allow time for patient's questions; provide explanations, or make appropriate referral.
- Observe verbal and nonverbal indications of anxiety; assist the patient with anxiety-reducing/coping techniques that have proven effective in the past, such as meditation, prayer, rhythmic breathing, music, self-guided imagery, massage, and relaxation.
- Encourage expression of concerns and fears; clarify any misperceptions, and reinforce information provided by other members of the healthcare team.
- Provide emotional support and comforting nursing measures (e.g., touch, a warm blanket).
- Demonstrate warmth, calmness, and acceptance of the patient's anxiety.
- Maintain a quiet environment; minimize distractions.
- Document patient's reactions.

Nursing Diagnosis
Hypothermia related to surgical exposure and anesthesia

Outcome
The patient's body temperature will remain within normal limits as evidenced by postoperative temperature equivalent to preoperative level and absence of postoperative shivering.

Interventions
- Limit the patient's physical exposure; expose only those body surfaces required for skin preparation.
- Cover the patient's head with a blanket or cap.
- Use a warming device (e.g., a forced-air warming unit).
- Provide the anesthesia provider with a fluid warmer.
- Consult with the anesthesia provider regarding the patient's temperature.
- Use warm saline for irrigation.
- Provide warm blankets at the end of the surgical procedure.

Nursing Diagnosis
Risk for Deficient Fluid Volume related to loss of body fluids

Outcome
The patient's fluid balance will be maintained as evidenced by postoperative pulses equivalent to preoperative level, hourly urine output of at least 30 mL, and good skin turgor.

Interventions
- Determine the availability of replacement blood or blood products.
- Assist with the insertion of intravenous (IV) lines and fluid replacement therapy. Keep IV lines patent.
- Estimate blood loss on sponges and drapes; communicate to the anesthesia provider and surgeon.
- Initiate autotransfusion or use of an autologous blood salvage unit as required.
- Record the amount of irrigation used.
- Document the contents of the suction canisters.
- Monitor and document hourly urine output (as applicable); communicate results of measurements.
- Collaborate with the collection and interpretation of intraoperative blood analyses.

Nursing Diagnosis
Risk for Impaired Skin Integrity and **Ineffective Tissue Perfusion** related to surgical positioning, presence of vascular disease, and vascular clamping

Outcome
The patient's skin integrity will be maintained. Skin temperature and color will be within normal limits. No skin injury lesions will be evident, and the electrosurgical unit (ESU) dispersive pad site will be intact.

Interventions
- Assess and document the patient's preoperative skin condition and tissue perfusion.
- Position the patient on a pressure-reducing mattress on the OR bed.
- Collaborate with the anesthesia provider in modifications of surgical position required for access to airway and monitoring devices.
- Keep OR bed sheets dry and wrinkle-free.
- Pad all bony prominences.
- Maintain body alignment.
- Place restraining straps snugly but not tightly.
- Protect vulnerable neurovascular bundles from compression.
- Monitor and record tissue perfusion (e.g., color, temperature, pulses) as required.
- Elevate drapes off the patient's toes; use appropriate positioning accessories.
- Implement safety precautions for proper use of ESU.
- Reassess and document the patient's postoperative skin condition and tissue perfusion.

site needs to be marked and visible after draping if laterality is involved. The time-out is a requirement of The Joint Commission. During the time-out, the patient's name, procedure, site verification, and laterality are reviewed. Other items that may be discussed include the consent, anesthesia plan/concerns, the patient's allergies, antibiotics ordered, the patient's position, required instruments and special equipment, availability of blood, and anticipated length of the procedure. Such briefings improve team communication and intraoperative patient care (Johnson and Kimsey, 2012).

Intraoperative Monitoring.

Intraoperative monitoring for patients with vascular disorders includes the use of the basic ECG, pulse oximeter, and blood pressure cuff. For patients undergoing saphenous vein stripping or amputation, these are usually adequate. For lengthy procedures, such as arterial bypass or reconstruction, the anesthesia provider usually places an arterial line into the radial artery. This line is kept open by a pressurized heparin drip line attached to a transducer, and a waveform monitor reads the systolic and diastolic pressures. The monitor calculates the mean arterial pressure (MAP), which aids in the evaluation of the perfusion of systemic and cardiac circulation. This arterial line also allows easy access for collecting specimens for arterial blood gas (ABG) analysis. Continuous assessment of the patient's arterial pressure is a critical part of the surgical procedure. Pulmonary capillary wedge pressure, as an index of left atrial pressure (LAP), may be monitored depending on the patient's physiologic status. A general anesthetic may be administered and the patient intubated; local or regional anesthesia may also be used, depending on the surgical intervention. Epidural catheters may be placed to provide intraoperative anesthesia that can be augmented to accommodate increased surgical time, as opposed to a spinal anesthetic, which provides a finite period of anesthesia. Epidural catheters may be left in place postoperatively for pain management as well. Because many patients undergoing vascular surgery have generalized atherosclerotic disease, the perioperative nurse should be constantly alert for cardiac dysrhythmias and blood pressure changes. Acid-base balance and pulmonary gas exchange are assessed from the ABG analysis.

The anesthesia provider may also place a central venous pressure (CVP) catheter or pulmonary artery (PA) catheter, usually by way of the right internal jugular vein. The CVP line allows assessment of blood volume and vascular tone. The PA catheter monitors cardiac output, fluid balance, and the cardiac response to medications. PA catheters are commonly used for patients undergoing aortic surgery or for patients with cardiac disease.

TEE may be used to monitor the heart noninvasively during aortic surgery. The device looks similar to a bronchoscope and can be passed down the esophagus to provide an ultrasonic image. The cardiac structures, blood flow, wall motion, and great vessels can be observed. Use of TEE requires highly skilled personnel and may not be available in all surgical settings.

Electroencephalographic (EEG) monitoring is used for patients undergoing a carotid endarterectomy and allows for immediate observation of the slowing of brain waves caused by cerebral ischemia or reduced perfusion. The surgeon may elect to place a temporary shunt in the artery if this occurs during clamping, potentially reducing the chances of perioperative stroke.

The perioperative nurse inserts a urinary catheter for many procedures, including the following: if the proposed procedure involves the renal arteries or clamping of the aorta above the renal arteries; if considerable blood loss is anticipated; if the planned procedure time is lengthy; or whenever spinal or epidural anesthesia is used,

because they delay the patient's ability to void voluntarily. Urinary catheterization facilitates accurate hourly measurements of urine during and after the surgical procedure and assists in the assessment of renal perfusion and fluid status.

Positioning.

Positioning of the patient undergoing vascular surgery is of particular importance because of restricted circulation distal to the area of arterial obstruction and a generalized state of poor circulation. Particular care must be exercised in positioning elderly patients (see Chapter 27). Awareness of joint range-of-motion limitations attributable to immobility or joint surgery is critical even for a procedure as routine as urinary catheter insertion. Again, preoperative assessment can prevent injury and decrease OR time. Whenever possible, the perioperative nurse should have the patient demonstrate the ability to assume the position for the proposed procedure and provide feedback. A footboard may be applied to the OR bed to prevent the weight of drapes resting on the patient's lower extremities. A head support may be used to position the head. A roll may be placed between the scapulae. For surgical procedures involving a lower extremity, the patient's thigh may be externally rotated and abducted with the knee flexed. A small bolster may be used under the knee to support the patient's leg. Proper skeletal alignment during surgery prevents injury to the neuromuscular system. The nurse pays close attention to the skin overlying bony prominences, especially the heels, sacrum, and elbows, and uses the proper supports and pads to prevent pressure and potential positioning injury to the patient. If the procedure will be lengthy, a pressure-reducing mattress or pad can be placed on the OR bed to help prevent patient injury. Arms are placed on padded armboards with the palms up and fingers extended. Armboards are maintained at less than a 90-degree angle to prevent brachial plexus stretch. If there are surgical reasons to tuck the arms at the side, the elbows are padded to protect the ulnar nerve, the palms face inward, and the wrist is maintained in a neutral position (Denholm, 2009). A drape secures the arms. It should be tucked snuggly under the patient, not under the mattress. This prevents the arm from shifting downward intraoperatively and resting against the OR bed rail. During the procedure the perioperative nurse and scrub person continually monitor the sterile field to ensure heavy instruments and drapes do not rest on the patient's body and cause pressure injuries.

Skin Preparation and Draping.

Skin preparation for vascular surgery may be extensive. The patient's hair should be removed preoperatively only if it interferes with the procedure; if hair removal is necessary, it should be done immediately before the surgical procedure using clippers (Evidence for Practice), not a razor. For carotid surgery, the patient is prepped from the ear and chin on the affected side to below the clavicle (Figure 24-6, *A*). For abdominal aortic surgery, the patient's skin is prepped from the nipple line to the midthigh area (see Figure 24-6, *B*). For peripheral vascular surgery on the lower extremities, the patient is prepped from the umbilicus to the feet. The patient's legs are prepped circumferentially. It is important that alcohol-based prep solutions are allowed to dry completely before applying the surgical drapes and starting the surgical procedure.

Draping should permit the surgeon free access to involved areas. For example, abdominal surgery may also require exposure of the groin region for possible exploration of the femoral arteries. A femoral-popliteal bypass on one leg may require access to the other leg for saphenous vein harvesting. Impervious drapes should be used

FIGURE 24-6 Surgical skin prep (**A**) for carotid endarterectomy and (**B**) for abdominal aortic aneurysm procedures.

to prevent contamination of the surgical field from blood and irrigation fluids.

Medications and Solutions. In vascular surgery, several medications may be present on the sterile field at any given time (Surgical Pharmacology). These may include heparin, heparinized saline, protamine sulfate, and papaverine hydrochloride, as well as local anesthetic medications and contrast dye. All medications and solutions on and off the sterile field must be labeled (Brown-Brumfield and DeLeon, 2010). Heparin is the most common medication used in vascular surgery and may be given as an intravenous (IV) bolus

---

▍ EVIDENCE FOR PRACTICE

Reducing the Risks of Surgical Site Infections: Preoperative Hair Removal

Surgical site infections (SSIs) can be devastating to patients. An infection may mean a prolonged hospital stay, additional surgical procedures, or even death in an extreme case. A systematic literature review showed that clinical studies done in the early 1990s indicated that shaving with a razor increased the frequency of SSIs and that using clippers is the preferred method for hair removal when hair removal is deemed necessary. The increased SSI risk associated with shaving versus clipping is attributed to microscopic cuts in the skin that later serve as foci for bacterial multiplication. The Centers for Disease Control and Prevention (CDC) developed guidelines to reduce the risks of surgical site infections using this evidence of best practice from the literature. Following the CDC's recommended guidelines for hair removal to reduce the risks of SSIs equates to providing optimal patient care.

Modified from Sparkes D, Rylah B: The World Health Organization surgical safety checklist, *Br J Hosp Med* 71(5):276–280, 2010; Mangram A et al: Guidelines for prevention of surgical site infection, *Infect Control Hosp Epidemiol* 20(4):247–278, 1999, available at www.cdc.gov/hicpac/pdf/guidelines/SSI_1999.pdf. Accessed October 26, 2012.

SURGICAL PHARMACOLOGY

Medications Used in Vascular Surgery

Medication/ Category	Dosage/Route	Purpose/Action	Adverse Reactions	Nursing Implications
Heparin/anticoagulant	5000 units intravenous injection (IV) for systemic anticoagulation during a surgical procedure (IV bolus), followed by maintenance infusion based on activated clotting times (ACTs)	Prevention of blood clot formation by inactivating thrombin and preventing the conversion of fibrinogen to fibrin	Hemorrhage, thrombocytopenia, abnormal liver function tests, hypersensitivity, allergic reaction	Increased bleeding.
Protamine sulfate/ antiheparin agent	IV: 1 mg of protamine neutralizes not less than 100 USP heparin units given over a 10-min period	Neutralization of heparin	IV administration may cause sudden decrease in blood pressure, bradycardia, and anaphylactic reactions. This medication must be infused slowly.	Patients with a fish allergy may develop hypersensitivity to protamine. Overdose may cause increased bleeding.
Papaverine hydrochloride (HCl)/alkaloid	IV or intramuscular IV: 1-4 mL (30 mg/mL)	Smooth muscle relaxant, reduces vasospasm	Slight rise in blood pressure, increase in heart rate, excessive sedation, skin rash, abdominal discomfort, nausea, vomiting, weakness	Should be used with caution in patients with glaucoma.

USP, United States Pharmacopeia.
Modified from *Physicians' Desk Reference,* available at www.pdr.net/drugpages. Accessed November 15, 2012.

by the anesthesia provider for systemic anticoagulation. When administered parenterally, heparin has a rapid onset of action, peaks in minutes, and has a 2- to 6-hour duration. Because it is metabolized in the liver and excreted by the kidneys, the effects of heparin may be prolonged in patients with liver and renal disease. The anticoagulant effects may be monitored by measurement of the activated partial thromboplastin time (APTT) or partial thromboplastin time (PTT). Patients are given anticoagulants just before the placement of a vascular clamp to prevent a thromboembolic event. The effects of systemic heparin may or may not need to be reversed at the end of the surgical procedure. Monitoring the activated clotting time (ACT) intraoperatively provides useful data for judging the need for reversal or additional medication. The effects of heparin can be reversed by the administration of protamine sulfate.

Because protamine sulfate is derived from fish sperm and testes, caution is advised when administering it to patients who are allergic to fish or who have received protamine-containing insulin. One milligram of protamine neutralizes 100 mg of heparin. The dose should be calculated to offset half of the last dose of heparin. Protamine must be given slowly, at a maximum rate of 50 mg in 10 minutes, or dyspnea, flushing, bradycardia, and severe hypotension may occur. Another reason for monitoring heparin dose is that protamine, given in the absence of circulating heparin, acts as an anticoagulant and could delay hemostasis intraoperatively.

Heparinized saline solution is often used during vascular surgery for irrigation. It may be used to irrigate a blood vessel lumen during surgery, usually after the patient has been systemically heparinized. It is also commonly used to flush the lumen of tubes used to shunt blood. The strength of the heparin solution will vary according to the manufacturer's recommendations for certain implant devices or by the surgeon's preference. A reasonable range is 250 to 1000 units in 250 mL of normal saline.

Surgeon preferences differ regarding solutions with which to distend, irrigate, or store vein grafts. Some surgeons prefer a cold solution to decrease the metabolic demands of the vessel, whereas others believe this may lead to spasm. Spasm may be of particular concern when working with the small vessels of the distal leg or foot. Papaverine hydrochloride (HCl) may be added to a heparinized saline solution for its direct antispasmodic effect on the smooth muscle of the vessel wall and for its vasodilating properties. A reasonable dose is 120 mg in 250 mL of saline. The pressure of a handheld syringe to distend vein grafts has been viewed as a potential cause of graft failure or graft stenosis because this causes endothelial damage. Papaverine HCl, as a smooth muscle relaxant, allows distention at a lower pressure and may decrease the risk of injury. Concentrations for infiltration range from 0.05 to 0.6 mg/mL, or 12.5 to 150 mg per 250 mL of solution.

Topical hemostatic agents may be needed. Absorbable hemostatics are effective by creating an environment that promotes the adhesion of platelets. For example, an absorbable gelatin sponge may be applied to a bleeding surface to provide a matrix into which clots form. It may be applied dry, moistened with saline, or soaked in a topical thrombin-saline solution; 100 to 2000 National Institute of Health (NIH) units of thrombin per 1 mL of saline or blood may be applied to control bleeding.

Infections of prosthetic vascular grafts are rare but are extremely serious. Infection may be life-threatening for patients with aortic grafts or may be limb-threatening in lower-extremity procedures. Protecting the prosthetic graft from contact with the skin is essential to prevent bacterial contamination. Prophylactic IV antibiotics that provide coverage for any likely organisms to be encountered in the procedure should be administered within 1 hour before the surgical incision (Zaidi et al, 2009). In some institutions medical staff–approved protocols are available for selection of the appropriate antibiotic.

Vascular Prostheses. Vascular grafting materials and techniques are of major importance to the field of vascular surgery for bypass procedures and reconstruction. The understanding, study, and comparison of new prosthetic grafts; utilization and preparation of autogenous grafts; and knowledge of long-term patency rates are critical to improving patient outcomes. Grafts are made in various sizes and configurations; they may be straight, tapered, or Y-shaped (i.e., bifurcated); or they may be pieces of material cut for use as a patch. The arteriotomy from a carotid endarterectomy may be closed primarily or with a patch of either vein or synthetic fabric. In aortic surgery a straight tube or a bifurcated synthetic graft is used. Dacron (polyester) grafts are the usual choice and have been used successfully for many years. Large vessels, such as the aorta, have high flow rates and thus have a low incidence of thrombus formation and excellent graft-patency rate. Desirable characteristics for vascular grafts are that they are reasonably priced, readily available in a variety of sizes, suitable for use anywhere in the body, biocompatible and hypoallergenic, and able to survive repeated sterilizations. Grafts should be easy to handle and last a lifetime while permitting blood passage without clotting or infection.

Prosthetic grafts are nonantigenic; tissue incorporates well, which helps prevent infection, and such grafts generally resist thrombosis. For years, knitted polyester grafts were preferred over woven polyester because they were easier to handle, although they had to be preclotted because of their high porosity. Woven grafts are somewhat stronger and bleed less through the fabric interstices but can be less flexible. Newer grafts have been developed to incorporate the best of both by using velour polyester. They are often impregnated with albumin, collagen, or gelatin to provide ease in handling without the need to preclot. The scrub person ensures the graft is preclotted by submerging it into a basin containing a small quantity of the patient's own blood collected before systemic heparinization. This makes the graft impervious by allowing fibrin to fill in the fabric spaces.

The other popular prosthetic material is polytetrafluoroethylene (PTFE), which is available in straight, tapered, and bifurcated styles of varying lengths and may have external support rings to prevent compression. These grafts do not stretch, and needle-hole bleeding may be troublesome.

Cryopreserved saphenous vein grafts are commercially available for patients who have no veins available because of previous bypass procedures, saphenous vein stripping, or poor quality or size of available veins. The nurse and scrub person must follow the manufacturers' instructions for rinsing these grafts to remove all traces of preservative.

Volumes have been written about vascular grafts, and the reader should consider this chapter an introduction only. The American National Standards Institute (ANSI), the U.S. Food and Drug Administration (FDA), and the Association for the Advancement of Medical Instrumentation (AAMI) are a few of the organizations active in setting standards and regulating usage and development of grafts.

Autogenous vein grafting for infrainguinal bypass is considered the criterion standard. Undamaged endothelial cells inhibit the clotting mechanism by the natural release of fibrinolytic substances and plasminogen factors. Two methods of grafting veins have been

FIGURE 24-7 Valve incision with valvulotome.

A

B

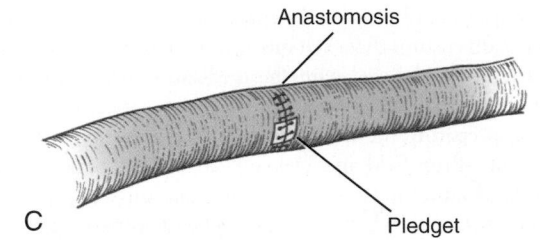

C

FIGURE 24-8 Pledgetted suture. **A,** Double-armed vascular suture prepared with pledget. **B,** Technique for surgeon to add pledget to suture already in use. **C,** Appearance of suture line with pledget in place.

extensively studied, and the results are not totally conclusive that one method is better than the other. These are the in situ graft and the reversed vein graft. The in situ method leaves the vein in its place, side branches are ligated to prevent arteriovenous fistulas, and the valves that would impede arterial flow are disrupted with instruments specifically designed to cut valves, called *valvulotomes* (Figure 24-7). Reoperation is more frequent with the in situ method because of missed valves and residual arteriovenous fistulas. Reversal of a vein graft is performed per the surgeon's preference or when it must be harvested from the contralateral limb. Vein grafts are used in below-knee (BK) bypass procedures. Above-knee (AK) bypasses may use PTFE or other synthetic grafts for vein sparing, or they may be used in high-risk patients who may not tolerate the longer vein harvesting or have a life expectancy of less than 3 years. *Atraumatic* clamps with rubber, plastic, or hydrostatic jaw clamps are used to protect vein grafts from injury. Distal bypasses, particularly those in patients with diabetes, are more successful today as a result of improved tissue handling. The surgeon may also use the pneumatic tourniquet as an alternative to clamping the vessels.

Sutures. Most vascular sutures are made of synthetic nonabsorbable materials, such as Dacron, polyester, PTFE, and polypropylene. Vascular sutures have swaged-on needles of various sizes and are available in sizes 0 to 10-0. The suture may be single-armed or double-armed (i.e., a needle on one or both ends). The size and curve of the needle depend on the vessel and its location. Teflon felt or leftover pieces of graft material (synthetic or vein) may be used as pledgets or buttresses under a suture. They are used when tissue is friable to keep the suture from tearing through or when an anastomosis leaks and needs a better seal. The pledget may be loaded onto the vascular suture or added by the surgeon to a suture already in use. The pledget remains on the suture line (Figure 24-8).

Vascular Monitoring Equipment. Assessing blood flow through diseased vessels by palpation is often difficult. Physical assessment of the patient's hemodynamic status during surgery can be further complicated by spasm of the vessel walls, the cool environment of the OR, and alterations in blood pressure caused by hemorrhage. Therefore, the surgeon often uses vascular monitoring equipment to evaluate tissue perfusion and flow. The Doppler device is critical when pulses cannot be palpated. With a coupling gel, the unsterile

Doppler probe can be placed on the patient's skin distal to the surgical site. Some probes can be sterilized and used within the sterile field to assess the flow in an arterial graft or determine whether the blood supply to the intestines or other structures is intact after aortic surgery. Besides providing an audible signal, the Doppler probe can provide a permanent record of the sound if a recorder is attached.

An EEG accurately determines reduced cerebral perfusion during a CEA. This enables the surgeon to decide whether to use a temporary shunt in the carotid artery or if the patient can tolerate clamping. Sterile IV tubing connected to an arterial transducer can also be used to check pressure gradients intraoperatively. The stump pressure of unclamped carotid arteries before thromboendarterectomy can also determine the need for intraoperative shunting. Trained personnel are necessary to operate this equipment.

Instrumentation. Most vascular procedures begin with a basic laparotomy set (for scissors, clamps, and retractors) and a vascular set. Items specific to each surgical procedure are then added. For abdominal surgery, a large self-retaining retractor should be added. Additional individually wrapped, sterile aortic clamps; some long clamps (cystic duct and right angle); and long forceps for larger patients should be available in the OR. Smaller vascular clamps and vascular bulldog clamps should also be kept sterile in the OR. For peripheral procedures, a variety of Weitlaner self-retaining retractors should be available. Carotid surgery requires carotid shunt clamps, shunts, microforceps, and dissectors for peeling plaque from the artery. The surgeon may use the saphenous vein as a graft conduit by removing and reversing it or by using it in situ. A variety of instruments are available for disrupting the valves to permit arterial flow in the in situ procedure. Amputations do not require vascular instrumentation. A minor basic set and appropriately sized bone instruments are needed.

Documentation. During the implementation of perioperative nursing care, documentation of patient problems and nursing actions addressing these identified problems is important. Every patient is identified and assessed for allergies; the surgical procedure is verified; and any other interventions performed by the nurse for patient safety and mandated by institution policy are documented. A brief mental status and neurologic assessment are especially important for vascular patients who are at risk for stroke. For a patient undergoing vascular surgery, documentation may include the preoperative and postoperative assessment of the integrity of the patient's skin, the presence or absence of peripheral pulses, the surgical position and positioning devices used, fluid intake and output measurements, and the achievement of patient goals. During surgery various local anesthetic medications and irrigating solutions, such as thrombin, antibiotic, and heparin solutions, may be used. The scrub person ensures that each medication or solution container on the sterile field is labeled with the medication name, strength, and amount. Labels should be verified by two qualified individuals if the person preparing the medication is not the person administering it (Brown-Brumfield and DeLeon, 2010). The perioperative nurse maintains an accurate record of the solutions used and the amounts administered. The recording of ischemic times is captured when vascular clamps are applied and removed from arteries. The type, size, and serial and lot numbers of vascular implants should be documented according to institutional policy and procedure.

Evaluation

Evaluation is an ongoing process during which the perioperative nurse determines the extent to which the patient goals are met. Patient evaluation is continuous as the perioperative nurse assesses, observes, and appraises the results of nursing interventions. The conclusion of the intraoperative phase is the transfer of the care of the vascular surgical patient to colleagues in the postanesthesia care unit (PACU) or the intensive care unit (ICU). A nursing hand-off report should be given, which includes identification of the patient, the surgical procedure performed, any allergies or special needs, location of surgical wounds and drains, and the achievement of patient outcomes.

Some of the desired patient outcomes are achieved at the end of the intraoperative phase of surgical patient care. Others require ongoing evaluation during the postoperative phase. Because perioperative nursing practice is collaborative, the perioperative nurse develops a plan of care that extends from the admission to the surgical suite through safe recovery from surgery. Some goals can be measured immediately on discharge from the OR; others require the collaboration of the PACU or unit nurse for final evaluation. The perioperative nurse thus develops and contributes to a comprehensive, holistic plan of patient care. Such planning and measurement of outcomes provide evidence of quality patient care and provide a mechanism of communication and continuity of care with other healthcare professionals.

Outcomes identified for the stated nursing diagnoses could be stated as follows:

- The patient verbalized an understanding of the surgical procedure and routines. All questions were answered to the patient's

satisfaction. The patient appeared calmer as evidenced by facial expression and other body language.
- The patient's temperature remained within normal limits.
- The patient's fluid balance was maintained. Intake and output measurements were documented.
- The patient's skin remained intact, with no lesions or reddened areas; skin color, temperature, and turgor were adequate.

Patient and Family Education and Discharge Planning

All surgical patients need basic instruction on care of their wounds, identification of the signs and symptoms of infection, review of medications (Patient Safety), schedule of follow-up appointments, and procedure for contacting healthcare providers. Proper hand-washing should be reviewed and emphasized to prevent wound infection. Patients who have undergone a lower-extremity arterial bypass are most interested in information that will assist them in recognizing, preventing, and managing complications. They need

---

PATIENT SAFETY

Teaching the Patient Discharged Home with Prescribed Anticoagulant Therapy

Anticoagulant therapy is prescribed to prevent the formation of blood clots. The length of time a patient is prescribed anticoagulant therapy depends on the underlying condition for which it is prescribed. It can be of short duration or lifelong. The patient and family or other caregiver should be provided with both verbal and written instructions. These should include the condition requiring anticoagulation therapy; reasons and benefits of therapy; name of the anticoagulant prescribed along with dosage, time of administration, and side effects; importance of follow-up monitoring; compliance issues; potential for any drug interactions; and safety precautions. After the patient and family member or other caregiver are instructed, they should "teach-back" information in their own words. In this way the nurse can verify their understanding. Additional helpful information to provide includes the following:

- Use only an electric razor or hair removal cream; do not use a straight razor.
- Take precautions to avoid injury. For example, do not use tools such as saws or hammers, which could lead to an accident. Avoid contact sports and other hazardous activities that can increase the risk of tissue injury.
- Report any signs and symptoms of bleeding, such as excessive bleeding from cuts; blood in urine, stool, or vomit; nosebleeds; bleeding from the gums; excessive menstrual bleeding; unusual bruising for unknown reasons; a change in mental status; dizziness; severe headache; or blurred vision.
- Take the prescribed dose of medication at the precise time it is prescribed to be taken.
- Do not stop taking the medication abruptly; the surgeon usually tapers this medication gradually.
- Carry or wear a MedicAlert bracelet or tag, and carry information in your wallet naming the specific medication.
- Avoid eating foods high in vitamin K, such as tomatoes, dark leafy vegetables, bananas, and fish.
- In the event of a missed dose, do not make up for any missed dose or double-up on doses. Call your physician if you are unsure about what to do in the event of a missed dose.

Modified from Little TK: Care of patients with vascular problems. In Ignatavicius DD, Workman ML, editors: *Medical-surgical nursing: patient-centered collaborative care*, ed 7, St Louis, 2013, Saunders.

instruction on incision care and bathing to optimize incision healing. Many have had experience with slow healing of wounds because of their arterial disease. Pain, sleep disturbances, and fatigue have been identified as important topics for instruction. Patients are often capable of identifying their discharge learning needs in the preoperative period. Patients should be taught to manage the discomfort of incisions and leg swelling to prevent sleep disturbances. The need to balance activity and rest should be emphasized. Patients in the immediate postoperative period are often receptive to counseling on risk-factor modification such as cessation of smoking and control of hypertension, diabetes, and stress (Oka et al, 2012).

Assisting the patient in setting realistic goals without overwhelming demands is usually most productive. Patients must believe that their efforts will make a difference in improving their quality of life for lifestyle changes to be sustained.

Patient and family education related to postoperative activities and discharge planning for vascular procedures varies. Following an integrated care pathway improves efficiency and length of stay. Major vascular procedures, such as the resection of an AAA, have different educational concerns than peripheral vascular surgery. Patient and family education and discharge teaching for various procedures are presented in the Patient and Family Education box.

PATIENT AND FAMILY EDUCATION

Education for Various Vascular Procedures

Abdominal Aortic Aneurysm Resection

Postoperative care procedures include the following:

- Maintain intubation and ventilation for 12 hours (varies with setting and surgeon preference).
- Monitor cardiac, respiratory, and renal function.
- Maintain nothing-by-mouth (NPO) status and nasogastric tube placement until bowel signs and flatus return; diet is advanced as tolerated.
- Perform hourly assessment of lower-extremity perfusion.
- Assess pain: Provide pain relief via epidural and/or patient-controlled analgesia (PCA); provide periods of rest.
- Prescribe bed rest, with the patient out of bed on postoperative day 1 and ambulating on postoperative day 2.

Discharge planning education includes the following instructions to the patient:

- Feelings of fatigue are normal and take weeks to resolve.
- Incision care: Showering is permitted; use soap and water only, and pat dry. Protect incision from oils, lotions, and powder. If wound closure strips are in place, showering is permitted. The strips will peel away in about 5 to 7 days.
- Activity is allowed with specific restrictions per surgeon:
  - Avoid lifting more than 5 to 10 pounds for 6 weeks to allow abdominal healing.
  - Walk to increase strength and improve circulation; progress gradually.
  - Climb stairs and walk outside as desired.
  - Avoid sitting for more than 1 or 2 hours.
  - Avoid crossing legs.
  - Obtain permission from surgeon before driving. Driving is usually permitted after first office visit and when pain medication is discontinued.
- Smoking should be stopped because it has a profound effect on vascular disease and wound healing.
- The surgeon's instructions regarding dietary recommendations and medication use should be followed.
- Antibiotics may be prescribed before any endoscopic procedures, surgery, or dental procedures.
- The patient should notify the surgeon of the following: Changes in wound (e.g., redness, swelling, increased tenderness, bleeding, drainage), fever, change in bowel habits.

Endovascular Abdominal Aortic Aneurysm Repair

Postoperative care procedures include the following:

- Transfer the patient from the OR to the postanesthesia care unit (PACU).
- Monitor cardiac, respiratory, and renal function.

- Assess peripheral pulses every 15 minutes for 1 hour, every hour ×4, every 2 hours ×4, and then every 4 hours (in general).
- Assess the presence of abdominal or back pain, sensation, and movement in the lower extremities.
- Provide pain management as ordered (encourage the patient to request pain medication).
- Transfer to a general nursing unit within 2 hours.
- Advance the patient from clear liquid to regular diet the first evening after surgery. The patient is NPO after midnight for ultrasound examination on day 2, with regular diet resumed after the examination.
- Perform gradual ambulation three times on day 1 (within 4 to 6 hours after surgery) and ambulation at will on day 2.
- Discharge to home generally on day 2.

Discharge planning education includes the following instructions to the patient:

- Showers are permitted; tub soaks are not.
- Intercourse is permitted as comfortable, with no restrictions.
- No driving is permitted until cleared by surgeon.
- No lifting more than 5 pounds is allowed for 6 weeks.
- Soap and water on sterile wound closure strips is permitted; strips will gradually fall off.
- Stair climbing is permitted.

Arterial Reconstructive Procedures of the Lower Extremity

Patient and family education and discharge planning include the following instructions to the patient:

- Diabetes and hypertension control is very important.
- Smoking should be stopped because it has a profound effect on vascular disease and wound healing.
- Signs and symptoms of graft failure may include the absence of a pulse in the extremity.
- Implement a foot care program as noted below:
  - Inspect daily (use mirror-assistive methods, or have a family member help).
  - Observe for cracks, ulcers, blisters, rashes, or discoloration.
  - Trim nails properly for prevention of ingrown toenails.
  - Shoes must fit properly (avoid walking barefoot).
  - Avoid tight socks or hose.
  - Incision care is essential for avoiding infection and promoting wound healing.
- ACE wraps for leg swelling (normal after surgery) should be applied per surgeon's instructions.
- Sleep disruption and fatigue are normal after surgery. Ongoing pain management is important; pain levels should decrease gradually.

Continued

- Driving with the surgeon's approval is usually allowed after follow-up office visit (approximately 2 weeks postoperatively).
- No heavy lifting, vigorous exercise, or prolonged upright sitting is allowed; walking, stair climbing, and going outside are permissible as able.
- Gentle range-of-motion exercise of leg prevents flexion contractures.
- Showering is permitted.
- Diet: Resume previous diet; follow special diets (e.g., diabetic, low salt, low fat) per surgeon's instructions.
- The surgeon should be called for any of the following: Return of preoperative symptoms; wound changes (e.g., redness, swelling, drainage, pain); fever; change in color, temperature, sensation, or use of leg, foot, or toes.
- Antibiotics may be recommended before any dental or endoscopic procedures if a synthetic graft was implanted.

Carotid Endarterectomy

- Teach the patient about possibility of reperfusion headaches (patients may fear that they are having recurrent symptoms unless they know about this possibility).
- Explain that if there are no postoperative complications, discharge to home will occur within 24 to 48 hours after surgery.
- Explain that activity may return to normal as tolerated and driving may be resumed when neck discomfort no longer restricts range of motion and the surgeon has examined patient 2 weeks postoperatively.
- Explain that fatigue for 4 to 6 weeks after surgery is normal.
- Explain incision care: Keep the incision clean and dry; may shower with transparent dressing in place. Remove transparent dressing in 3 or 4 days. Wash the incision with soap and water; pat gently to dry. Avoid the use of powder and lotion. Do not shave over the incision until it is well healed.
- Explain that numbness around the incision and extending to the ear is normal, as well as mild swelling.
- Teach the patient about any cranial nerve deficits that may be the result of manipulation of nerves during surgery. Assist the patient in understanding the difference between an intraoperative stroke and cranial nerve deficits; that is, nerve injury or trauma from surgical manipulation occurs on the same side as

surgery except for eye symptoms. Use diagrams and pictures to review pertinent anatomy.

- Encourage relevant lifestyle changes as indicated (e.g., low-cholesterol diet, review of diabetic diet, smoking cessation).
- Teach the patient and family to observe for and report any new symptoms, transient ischemic attacks (TIAs), mental status changes, personality changes, or speech difficulties.
- If a synthetic patch is in place, explain that the patient will need antibiotics before dental procedures or endoscopic procedures. Instruct the patient to notify dentists and other healthcare providers of this need.
- Explain that if a vein was used for a patch, occasional swelling in the leg may occur. If this occurs, elevate leg above the level of the heart. Swelling may take 4 to 6 weeks to completely resolve.

Vena Cava Filter Insertion (Inferior Vena Caval Interruption)

Postoperative patient teaching for vena cava filter insertion includes the following:

- For a femoral vein insertion site, do not bend leg for about 8 hours.
- Avoid strenuous activity or lifting more than 5 pounds.
- Expect that bruising of the insertion site may occur because this is common in patients who are or have been receiving anticoagulant therapy.
- Inspect the incision site for bleeding; apply pressure using appropriate method if bleeding at insertion site occurs.
- Report signs of local infection or significant bleeding.
- Elevate the affected leg and wear elastic stockings to relieve lower-extremity swelling, which may be a temporary side effect of the underlying deep vein thrombosis (DVT).
- Understand the purpose of and proper way to wear support stockings.
- Report sudden or severe leg swelling.
- Follow instructions for DVT prophylaxis.

Varicose Vein Surgery

- Provide instruction on the proper way to wrap an ACE bandage, the timing of rest and leg elevation, and how to apply manual pressure if bleeding occurs.
- Remind the patient that walking is permitted, but sitting should be limited as should standing in one place. Legs should be elevated when sitting.

Surgical Interventions

Arterial Surgical Interventions

Abdominal Aortic Aneurysm Resection

Abdominal aortic aneurysmectomy is surgical obliteration of an aortic aneurysm, which may or may not include the iliac arteries, with insertion of a synthetic prosthesis to reestablish functional continuity. The majority of AAAs begin below the renal arteries (infrarenal), and many extend to involve the bifurcation and common iliac arteries. Severe back pain, along with symptoms of hypotension, shock, and distal vascular insufficiency, usually indicates rupture and represents a true emergency condition. The prime surgical consideration when a rupture occurs is the control of hemorrhage by occlusion of the aorta proximal to the point of rupture. AAAs are usually asymptomatic and are found on routine physical examination. They occur more frequently in men than in women.

Aneurysmal disease is caused by a disruption of the tunica media, which structurally weakens the aortic wall. Aneurysmal aortas are found to have a significantly decreased amount of collagen and elastin in the vessel wall. Rupture carries less than a 50% death rate for patients in stable condition with a contained rupture. Risks from AAA surgery include massive hemorrhage and hypotension, injury to the ureters, renal failure, spinal cord ischemia, and death. Because peripheral vascular disease is a manifestation of a systemic disorder, it is not surprising that patients with aneurysms often have concomitant coronary artery disease. Patients are at risk of myocardial ischemia, MI, hypotension, and hypertension. MI is the leading cause of death after AAA repair; therefore, it is imperative that a patient with cardiac symptoms or ECG abnormalities have a thorough preoperative cardiac assessment.

The perioperative nurse must be alert to the fact that at the time the aortic clamp is released to permit distal flow, "declamping shock" or severe hypotension may occur. This may be attributable to the presence of inadequate volume replacement, the sudden reestablishment of flow to dilated distal vessels, or the release of acidic metabolites. Declamping shock and hemorrhage have been proposed as causes of renal failure from acute tubular necrosis.

Procedural Considerations. The patient is placed in the supine position. General endotracheal anesthesia is used. The anesthesia provider inserts a central venous catheter and arterial line. After inserting the urinary catheter, the perioperative nurse preps the fields for a midline abdominal incision, and the scrub person assists with draping to permit access to the groin region for possible exploration of femoral arteries. The nurse ensures the patient's pedal pulses are marked before the beginning of the procedure so that they may be located easily when the surgeon requests a check of the pulses. This assessment of pulses can be done manually or with a Doppler probe.

Operative Procedure—Transperitoneal Approach

1. The surgeon makes a long midline abdominal incision (Figure 24-9, *A*) from the xiphoid process to the symphysis pubis and achieves hemostasis.
2. An abdominal self-retaining retractor is inserted into the wound. The surgeon and assistant retract the patient's small bowel, including the duodenum, to the right; they may place it outside the abdomen and cover it with moist laparotomy packs for better exposure.
3. The retroperitoneum overlying the aneurysm is incised and extended superiorly to expose the aneurysm and also inferiorly over the bifurcation and beyond the iliac arteries. Metzenbaum scissors, smooth forceps, and hemostats are used.
4. Careful blunt and sharp dissection is used to expose the aorta above the aneurysm to permit placement of an aortic clamp while avoiding the renal artery and ureters. The surgeon inspects the iliac vessels and bifurcation for evidence of small aneurysms, thrombosis, and calcification.
5. The anesthesia provider administers a dose of heparin intravenously, and the surgeon applies and closes an aortic clamp such as a DeBakey, Fogarty, or Satinsky around the aorta. Distal runoff vessels are also clamped. Opening of the aneurysm is undertaken with a scalpel or electrosurgical blade and heavy scissors (see Figure 24-9, *B*).
6. The aneurysm is completely opened, and all atheromatous and thrombotic material is removed. The aneurysm walls may be excised but usually are left in place for eventual coverage of the prosthesis. In either case, the posterior aspect of the aorta is left intact (see Figure 24-9, *C*). The surgeon controls bleeding, especially from the lumbar vessels, which enter posteriorly, by oversewing their orifices with vascular suture.
7. At the direction of the surgeon, the scrub person prepares the prosthetic graft of appropriate size for insertion. If the aneurysm does not involve the aortic bifurcation, a straight tubular graft is used; otherwise, a bifurcated or Y-shaped graft is necessary. Preclotting of a knitted graft may be accomplished by immersing the graft into a small quantity of the patient's own blood before systemic heparinization, or a manufactured graft impregnated with collagen, albumin, or gelatin may be used.
8. The aortic cuff is prepared for anastomosis by irrigating it with heparinized saline solution and by removing all fibrotic plaques. One or two vascular sutures (double-armed) are used to accomplish the anastomosis by a through-and-through continuous suture (see Figure 24-9, *D*). Additional interrupted

sutures may be needed if the anastomosis leaks on completion. A strip of Teflon felt may be used along the suture line for reinforcement.

9. The surgeon opens and inspects the distal vessels for backbleeding, and may inject heparinized saline solution to prevent clotting.
10. Each limb of the graft is anastomosed to the iliac artery, using a smaller vascular suture and similar technique (see Figure 24-9, *E*). After the first side of the anastomosis has been completed, blood is permitted to circulate and the remaining limb of the graft is clamped to prevent leaking during the last part of the anastomosis.
11. The aneurysm may be closed over the graft.
12. The peritoneum is closed to exclude contact of the intestine with the graft, and the abdominal wound is closed.

Endovascular Abdominal Aortic Aneurysm Repair

Endovascular aneurysm repair (EVAR) differs from open surgical repair in that the surgeon introduces the prosthetic endograft or stent-graft into the aneurysm through a surgically exposed femoral artery and fixes it in place to the nonaneurysmal infrarenal neck and iliac arteries with self-expanding or balloon-expandable stents rather than sutures (Figure 24-10). A major abdominal incision is thus avoided, and patient morbidity related to the procedure is much reduced. The benefits of this procedure are a hospital stay of 1 to 2 days, a rapid return to normal physical activity, and a reduction in the mortality and complication rates compared with those of the conventional surgical procedure (Lederle et al, 2009). The procedure may also be applicable to high-risk patients.

A number of commercially manufactured stent-grafts have been developed since the first EVAR was carried out in 1991, using a Dacron graft sutured onto balloon-expandable Palmaz stents. Early tubular grafts have largely been replaced by modular bifurcated grafts that have expanded the applicability of this therapy. Different graft configurations, depending on the anatomic problem, are available. For patients with an AAA that is limited to the aorta and in whom there is both a neck between the renal arteries and the aneurysm and a neck between the lower portion of the aneurysm and the iliac bifurcation, a graft of tubular configuration is available. For those patients in whom the abdominal aneurysm extends to the iliac bifurcation, a bifurcated or Y-shaped graft is available. For those patients who have both an AAA and an aneurysm of one or both iliac arteries, a tapered tube graft that excludes both the aortic aneurysm and one iliac aneurysm is usually selected. The technical details of endovascular repair vary with each specific device, but the general principles are similar. Candidates for this procedure include patients with a proximal infrarenal neck at least 1 to 2 cm in length and common iliac arteries for proximal and distal fixation of an endograft, without excessive tortuosity and with appropriate iliofemoral access. Long-term follow-up data are ongoing, and patients undergoing this procedure should understand that prolonged follow-up with periodic imaging will be required and that reintervention may become necessary. Nonetheless, the future of endoluminal grafting continues to evolve and has the potential of significant rewards (Giles et al, 2009).

Procedural Considerations. The team positions the patient supine on a radiolucent OR bed with a special marker board. The board has remotely controlled radiopaque cursors that are used to fluoroscopically detect proximal and distal positions for graft deployment. An ample supply of lead gowns needs to be available. The anesthesia

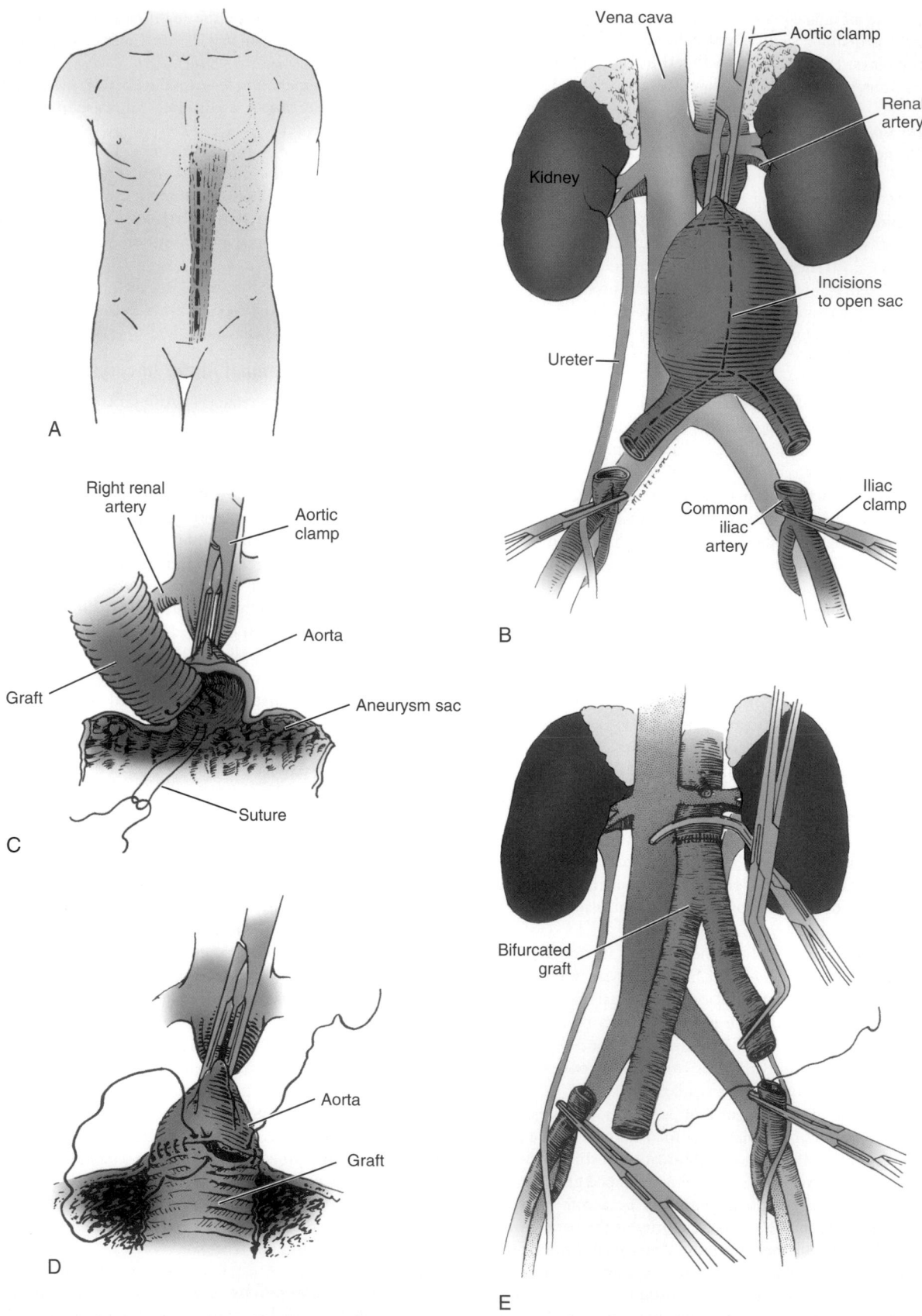

FIGURE 24-9 Resection of abdominal aortic aneurysm. **A,** Midline abdominal incision. **B,** Aneurysm sac is opened. **C,** Prosthetic graft is sewn to back wall of aorta, creating a cuff. **D,** Completion of aortic graft anastomosis. **E,** Iliac artery anastomosis.

FIGURE 24-10 Endovascular abdominal aortic aneurysm repair involves aneurysm exclusion with an endoluminal aortic stent-graft introduced remotely, usually through the femoral artery. An endovascular graft extends from the infrarenal aorta to both common iliac arteries, preserving the flow to the internal iliac arteries. *CIA,* common iliac artery; *EIA,* external iliac artery; *IIA,* internal iliac artery; *IN,* infrarenal aortic neck; *LK,* left kidney; *RK,* right kidney; *SA,* Suprarenal aorta.

provider may administer a general anesthetic or an epidural anesthetic. If an epidural anesthetic is used, mechanical ventilation is available in case conversion to the traditional surgical procedure is required. The anesthesia provider inserts a central venous catheter and an arterial catheter for hemodynamic monitoring. The perioperative nurse inserts a urinary catheter, and ensures that the patient's abdomen and groin areas are prepped and draped to allow conversion to the traditional surgical technique if necessary.

Operative Procedure

1. The surgeon performs bilateral groin cutdowns and dissects both common femoral arteries.
2. After the anesthesia provider administers IV heparin, the surgeon clamps the right common femoral artery, performs an arteriotomy, and introduces an 8-French (8F) sheath into the right external iliac artery.
3. The left femoral artery is punctured, and the surgeon places a 12F sheath into the left external iliac artery. An angiocath is inserted, and an arteriogram is obtained to clearly mark the renal arteries and aortic bifurcation. The final length of the device to cover the aorta from the renal arteries to a suitable section of the common iliac arteries is chosen.
4. A snare is introduced into the aorta through the left femoral artery, and a pull wire is introduced into the aorta by way of the right femoral artery. The pull wire is snared above the aortic bifurcation and retracted into the left iliac artery. This step is done to help position the limbs of the graft into the iliac arteries.
5. The surgeon inserts the grafting device into the right femoral artery, advances it into the proximal part of the aorta, and

positions it above the aortic bifurcation. Fluoroscopy is used to determine proper position of the stent.
6. The device is exposed by retracting a covering jacket, and the graft limbs are positioned in the iliac arteries. The hooks of the graft become attached to the walls of the aorta and the iliac arteries as the attachment systems are deployed.
7. The balloon on the device is inflated to secure the proximal attachment system to the aorta and the contralateral and ipsilateral systems to the iliac arteries.
8. An arteriogram is obtained to confirm proper positioning and complete exclusion of the AAA. Ideally, the graft is positioned to occlude the inferior mesenteric artery to prevent persistent blood flow within the aneurysmal sac.
9. After all the sheaths are removed, the surgeon closes the wounds with subcuticular sutures.

Percutaneous Transluminal Angioplasty

Percutaneous transluminal angioplasty (PTA) is performed with a local anesthetic and minimal sedation, as a same-day surgery admission. Although initially performed only in the common iliac artery for stenosis, PTA is routinely used to treat short-segment occlusions as well as external iliac lesions. Iliac artery PTA may be particularly useful to help improve inflow before a more distal surgical reconstruction.

The use of iliac artery stents has also begun to play an increasing role in the management of patients with aortoiliac occlusive disease. Iliac artery stents are most useful after initial suboptimal results from PTA. However, they are used primarily in the treatment of complex lesions. When PTA is not an option, a number of surgical alternatives are available. Depending on the condition of the patient and the patient's pathologic anatomy, the options include aortobifemoral bypass, aortoiliac thromboendarterectomy, axillofemoral bypass, iliofemoral bypass, and femorofemoral bypass.

Femoropopliteal and Femorotibial Bypass

Femoropopliteal bypass is the restoration of blood flow to the leg with a graft bypassing the occluded section of the femoral artery. The bypass may be a saphenous vein or straight synthetic graft. The patient must have a patent outflow artery for a successful bypass procedure. If popliteal patency is doubtful, artery exploration is necessary as the first procedure. Involvement of the popliteal artery may necessitate the exposure and use of the tibial vessels for the lower anastomosis. If this occurs, the procedure could require the use of microvascular instruments and technique.

Procedural Considerations. The patient is placed in a supine position. The hip is externally rotated and abducted with the knee flexed. Prepping and draping include the entire groin and leg. The instrument setup includes the basic minor and vascular sets, plus the following: Gelpi retractors, Garrett or Weitlaner retractors, a device to tunnel, and supplies and equipment for operative arteriograms.

Operative Procedures
Exploration of Common Femoral Artery

1. A vertical incision, extending downward about 3 to 5 inches along the medial aspect of the thigh, is made by the surgeon over the femoral artery below the inguinal area, and the field is exposed with a self-retaining retractor.
2. The surgeon locates the common femoral artery and dissects it in both directions for complete exposure.

3. The scrub person supplies moist umbilical tapes or vessel loops, which the surgeon passes around the common femoral, the superficial femoral, and the deep femoral arteries.

Exploration of Above-Knee Popliteal Artery

1. The surgeon makes a vertical incision along the medial aspect of the lower area of the thigh. If the popliteal artery is diseased, an additional incision below the knee is made to expose the distal popliteal artery.

2. A Weitlaner retractor is used to retract the muscles and expose the artery.

3. The surgeon flexes the patient's knee, dissects the popliteal artery, and passes a moist umbilical tape around the popliteal artery. Arteriograms may be performed at this time if doubt exists about the patency of the popliteal artery or distal arterial tree.

4. The saphenous vein is exposed via joined femoral and popliteal incisions the length of the thigh or through multiple short incisions along the medial area of the thigh. If the vein is suitable, the surgeon resects the necessary length or prepares it for in situ grafting. If a prosthesis will be used, the surgeon determines the length and size and the scrub person preclots the graft as previously described.

5. The surgeon ligates the side branches of the saphenous vein with fine silk. Finally, because of venous valves, the vein is reversed so that the end originally in the groin is anastomosed to the popliteal artery.

6. If a synthetic graft is used, the surgeon passes a tunneling device beneath the sartorius muscle from the popliteal fossa to the groin.

7. The graft is carefully pulled through the tunnel and positioned to prevent kinks or twists.

8. The anesthesia provider administers IV heparin to the patient before the surgeon applies a vascular clamp to the femoral artery. An incision is made into the femoral artery with a #11 blade and extended with a Potts angulated scissors.

9. The graft is anastomosed to the artery with fine vascular sutures.

10. The patient's knee is flexed, and the surgeon places vascular clamps on the popliteal artery at the site of the distal anastomosis.

11. An incision is made into the popliteal artery as explained for femoral arteriotomy.

12. The graft is sutured to the popliteal (or tibial) artery, and before completion the femoral occluding clamp is momentarily opened to eliminate air and debris.

13. All occluding clamps are removed, and the graft is assessed for anastomotic leaks.

14. The incision is closed as described previously.

Femoropopliteal Bypass In Situ

In situ femoropopliteal bypass is the restoration of blood flow to the leg, bypassing an occluded portion of the femoral artery with the patient's saphenous vein, which remains in place. The procedure includes incising the venous valves and interrupting the venous tributaries. The adequacy of the patient's saphenous vein may be validated before the surgical procedure by an ultrasound duplex scan. Varicose veins or a previous saphenous vein ligation and stripping are contraindications to the procedure. The advantages of a vein-bypass procedure include increased graft availability and improved patency. A disadvantage is the time-consuming aspect of this technique.

Procedural Considerations. The surgeon uses microvascular scissors, a valvulotome, or a leather in situ valve cutter kit to incise the valves within the vein. An angioscope may be used to monitor the lysis of valve leaflets.

Operative Procedure

1. The procedure is similar to that for a femoropopliteal bypass. The surgeon extends the groin incision downward over the course of the saphenous vein. A skin bridge may be left between the groin and the popliteal incisions.

2. The saphenous vein is exposed and divided at its proximal and distal ends. Venous tributaries are occluded with vessel clips, such as hemoclips, or fine nonabsorbable sutures.

3. The surgeon passes a valvulotome from below to the top, usually through side branches. The valvulotome is used to incise the internal valve (see Figure 24-6). In angioscopically assisted bypass, valve lysis is done under direct vision.

4. The saphenous vein is distended with heparinized saline, papaverine, or heparinized blood to identify any valvular obstruction or open venous tributary. Another pass of the valve cutter alleviates the obstruction. Open branches of the saphenous vein can also be ligated with vessel clips or fine nonabsorbable sutures.

5. The incompetent saphenous vein is used to bypass the occluded segment of the femoral artery (see steps 8 through 14 of the femoropopliteal bypass procedure described under Exploration of Above-Knee Popliteal Artery).

Femorofemoral Bypass

Femorofemoral bypass is an extra-anatomic (a route that is outside the normal path) bypass that is performed to restore blood flow to one leg when an inflow procedure is necessary but a major aortic procedure is not desired. This type of bypass procedure is also used when the surgical risks for the patient are high because of a complicated medical condition or there are technical problems with the procedure (Figure 24-11). Studies continue to examine the long-term patency rate and outcomes for this patient population. Severe cardiac or pulmonary disease may prevent the patient from undergoing a more extensive procedure. Subcutaneous vascular grafting is an option in these conditions because the procedure bypasses normal vascular anatomy and can be performed using a local anesthetic with adjunct moderate sedation and analgesia. The patient must have one good iliac artery for inflow for a femorofemoral bypass to be considered. Another extra-anatomic procedure that can be done in these instances is an axillofemoral bypass involving the subcutaneous placement of a prosthesis from the axillary artery to the femoral artery on the same side (Figure 24-12).

Procedural Considerations. The perioperative nurse assists with positioning the patient supine on the OR bed with a small pad placed under each knee. The area prepped for surgery extends from the umbilicus to midthigh area. The patient's genitalia are covered with a sterile towel.

Operative Procedure

1. A longitudinal incision is made by the surgeon over each femoral artery from the inguinal ligament to just below the femoral bifurcation.

2. Each common femoral artery, superficial femoral artery, and deep femoral artery is dissected free, mobilized, and secured with umbilical tapes or vessel loops.

FIGURE 24-11 Femorofemoral bypass to restore blood flow to left leg. **A,** Left iliac artery occlusion and right femoral artery exposure. **B,** Exposure of the right and left femoral arteries: tunneling device creating a path for the graft in the subcutaneous tissue. **C,** Femorofemoral bypass graft in place.

FIGURE 24-12 Axillofemoral bypass graft for right iliac artery occlusion.

3. The surgeon creates a graft tunnel between the two femoral arteries across the symphysis pubis in the subcutaneous tissue with digital dissection, scissors dissection, or the passage of a clamp or tunneling device across the preperitoneal space.
4. A Dacron or PTFE vascular graft is passed through the subcutaneous tunnel with care to prevent kinking of the graft.
5. The anesthesia provider administers IV heparin, and the surgeon places vascular clamps on the common femoral, superficial

femoral, and deep femoral arteries. A longitudinal arteriotomy is made in the common femoral artery.
6. The surgeon performs an end-to-side anastomosis using nonabsorbable vascular sutures to join the graft with the common femoral artery. A similar anastomosis is done on the other side.
7. After the clamps are released and flow is restored, the patient's pulses are checked with a sterile Doppler; the perioperative nurse may be asked to assess the patient's feet for warmth and color.
8. The femoral incisions are closed.

Arterial Embolectomy

Arterial embolectomy entails an incision made in the affected artery to remove thromboembolic material and restore blood flow. Emboli may be clot particles, a foreign body, air, fat, or a tumor that circulates through the bloodstream and becomes lodged as the vessel decreases in size. More often the direct source is a cardiac mural thrombus, associated with cardiac or vascular disease. Pain or numbness distal to the obstruction is the initial symptom, accompanied by other signs of vascular occlusion, such as pallor and absence of pulses.

Procedural Considerations. The patient is placed in the supine position, the skin area is prepped, and draping is completed to permit access to the affected area. The instrument setup includes the basic instrument and vascular sets, including embolectomy catheters and irrigation catheters. Heparinized saline is required.

Operative Procedure—Femoral Embolectomy
1. After making a groin incision the surgeon exposes the femoral artery to permit the application of vascular clamps (Figure 24-13, *A* and *B*).
2. An incision is made into the artery with a #11 blade and a Potts scissors. The surgeon carefully inserts an embolectomy catheter through the incision beyond the point of clot proximally and distally. The balloon is inflated, and the catheter is withdrawn along with the detached clot (see Figure 24-13, *C* and *D*).
3. As backflow is obtained, the surgeon applies a vascular clamp below the arteriotomy.
4. The artery may be flushed by injection of heparinized saline solution through a small irrigating catheter. Angioscopy or an arteriogram may be requested at this time (see Figure 24-13, *E*).
5. The arterial closure is completed with vascular sutures (see Figure 24-13, *F*). The wound is closed, and dressings are applied.

Amputation

Amputations involving the lower extremity are performed to eliminate ischemic, gangrenous, necrotic, or infected tissue; relieve pain; and promote maximum independence. Amputations may be necessary because of trauma or malignancy or when the lower limb cannot be salvaged by arterial reconstruction. In the immediate postoperative period, patients may experience phantom limb pain, described as shooting, burning, throbbing, stabbing, or squeezing. Phantom limb pain, which is pain in the area where the limb has been amputated, may recur, but less frequently, in the months following surgery (Chapman, 2011).

Procedural Considerations. It is critical to verify the correct limb for this procedure. Because amputations are often performed with the patient administered a regional anesthetic, the perioperative nurse must be sure that the patient does not witness the wrapping or transport of the amputated limb. Toes or partial foot amputations

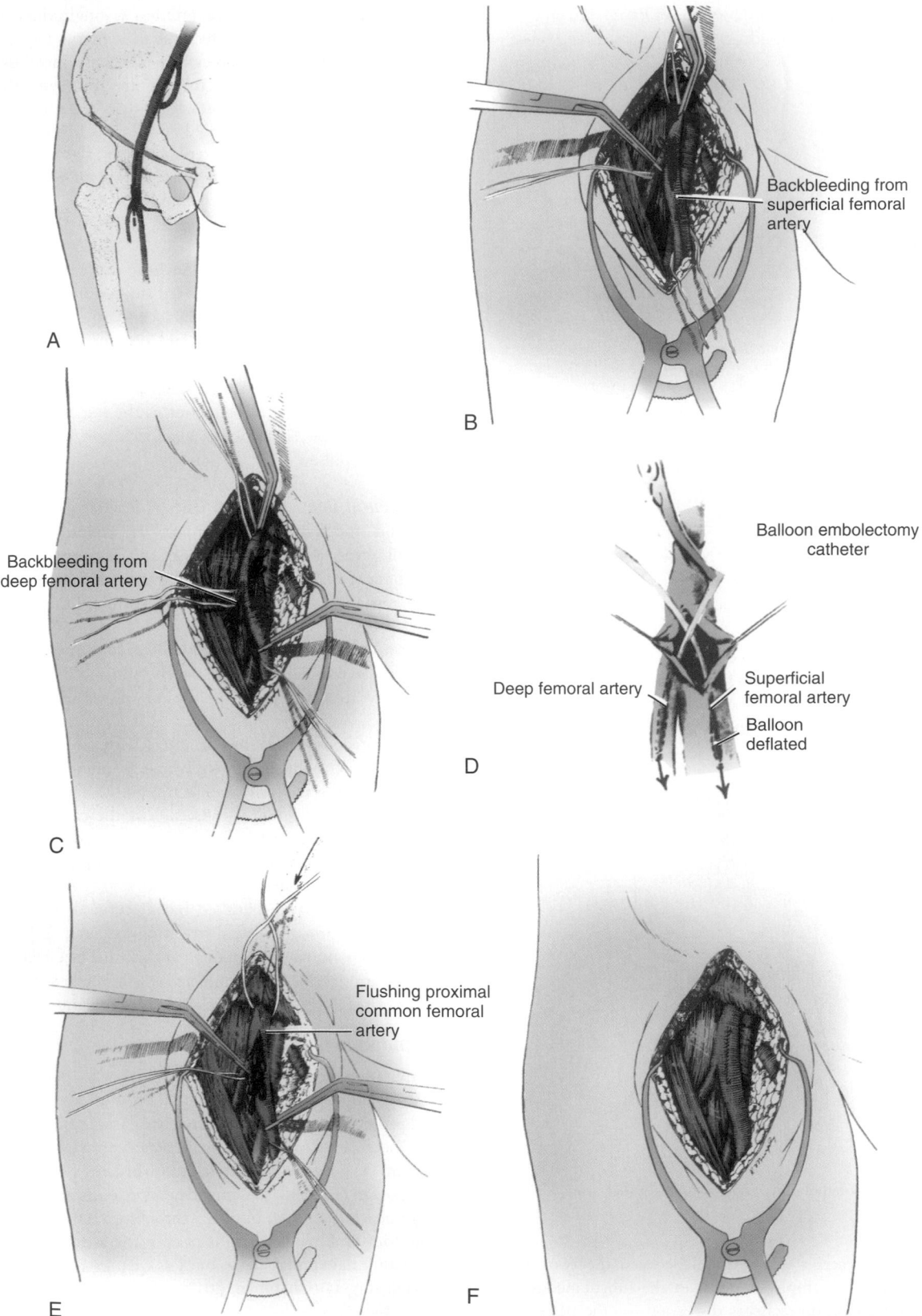

A

B

Backbleeding from
superficial femoral
artery

C

Backbleeding from
deep femoral artery

D

Balloon embolectomy
catheter

Deep femoral artery

Superficial
femoral artery

Balloon
deflated

E

Flushing proximal
common femoral
artery

F

FIGURE 24-13 Femoral embolectomy. **A,** Femoral arteriotomy. **B,** Clamp on common femoral and deep femoral (profunda femoris) arteries. Backflow of blood from superficial femoral artery (SFA) is checked. **C,** Clamp on common femoral artery and SFA. Backflow of blood from deep femoral artery is checked. **D,** Balloon embolectomy catheters are passed into SFA and profunda. **E,** Proximal (common femoral) artery is unclamped and flushed. **F,** Arteriotomy is closed.

may be done in certain instances, but often a BK or AK amputation is indicated. A Syme amputation, through the ankle, is seldom performed because of improved prosthetics and rehabilitation that favor midcalf amputation. The level is based on the health of the patient, level of vascularity, and potential for healing and rehabilitation. Severe infection or bacteremia may require amputation as a lifesaving procedure. Operative risks for amputation are higher than those for reconstruction, possibly because of more extensive vascular disease. BK amputations are best done at the junction of the upper and middle thirds of the lower leg. This allows for an immediate postoperative prosthesis, aids in better healing, and may reduce phantom limb pain. AK amputations may be at the middle or lower third of the thigh. Flaps are tailored to provide fascial and skin coverage to cushion the smoothed end of the bone. Meticulous hemostasis and drainage are needed to decrease hematoma formation because healing is both problematic and critical in these patients. Individuals with diabetes are at highest risk for amputation because of their neuropathy, altered response to infection, and vascular insufficiency.

Operative Procedure

1. The surgeon determines the level of amputation, and marks the incision line to create a long posterior flap for a BK amputation. For an AK amputation, the anterior and posterior flaps are fairly equal in size (Figure 24-14).
2. Blood loss may be reduced by using a sterile tourniquet after the leg is raised to drain venous blood. The tourniquet is inflated

and the surgeon makes the incision and divides the muscle and soft tissue. The periosteum is raised with an elevator.
3. The surgeon cuts the bones—the tibia with a Gigli or oscillating saw and the fibula with a bone cutter—and bevels their anterior aspect and smoothes them with a rongeur and rasp. The specimen is handed off the field.
4. The stump is gently irrigated, and hemostasis is achieved.
5. A closed-wound drainage system may be inserted.
6. Fascia is closed with interrupted sutures.
7. Skin is approximated and closed with interrupted suture or staples.
8. An immediate postoperative stump dressing may be applied to prevent flexion contracture.

Carotid Endarterectomy

CEA is the removal of an atheroma (plaque) at the carotid artery bifurcation to increase cerebral perfusion and decrease the risk of embolization and consequent stroke (Liu et al, 2009). In most settings the patient is discharged on the first postoperative day. Lessening the likelihood of any transient or permanent neurologic deficit is a major concern during a CEA. The use of a temporary carotid artery shunt (Figure 24-15), such as an Argyle or Javid shunt, allows for continuous blood flow through the carotid artery and to the brain. Some disadvantages in using this temporary device are that additional dissection is necessary for its placement and that there is a possibility of dislodging debris when the shunt is inserted. Also it is difficult to view the endarterectomy endpoint and suturing a patch is more difficult.

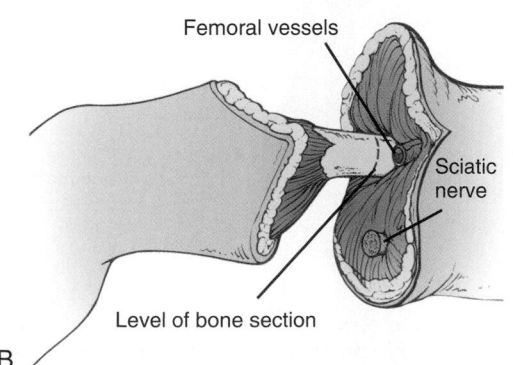

FIGURE 24-14 Leg amputation, above knee, through the middle third of the thigh. **A,** Level of skin incision. **B,** Level of bone resection.

FIGURE 24-15 Examples of temporary carotid artery shunts that are used to permit blood flow during carotid endarterectomy procedures.

Two techniques that facilitate continual assessment of cerebral perfusion are the use of a cervical plexus block for anesthesia and the use of EEG. A conscious patient with a cervical plexus block can be observed for neurologic deficits encountered during the procedure. The patient who is administered a general anesthetic can be monitored with an EEG. If either method demonstrates reduced cerebral perfusion, the surgeon may decide to use a temporary carotid artery shunt. The shunting device should always be available and sterile at the beginning of the procedure.

Procedural Considerations. The perioperative nurse assists with positioning the patient supine on the OR bed with the head supported on a head support. The head is turned away from the operative side, and the neck may be slightly hyperextended. A roll may be placed between the scapulae.

Operative Procedure

1. The surgeon makes a longitudinal incision over the area of the carotid bifurcation (Figure 24-16, *A*) and places a Weitlaner self-retaining retractor for exposure.

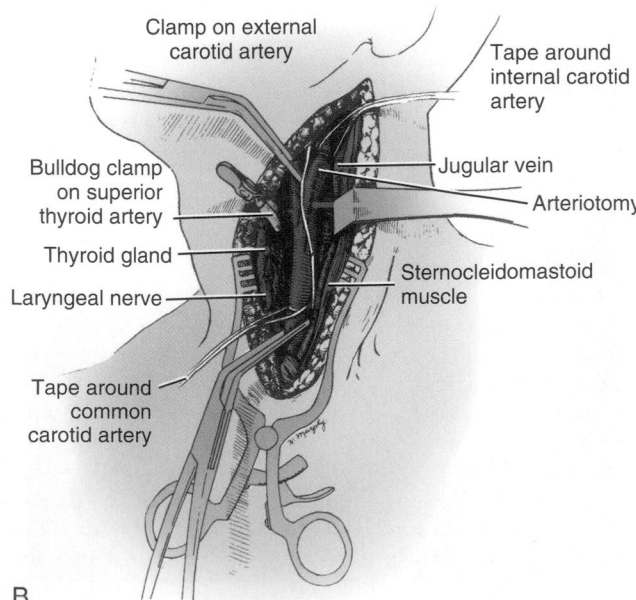

2. With Metzenbaum scissors, the surgeon dissects the soft tissue to expose the carotid artery and its bifurcation (see Figure 24-16, *B*).
3. A moistened umbilical tape or vessel loop is passed around the vessel for ease of handling. Systemic heparin is given to the patient by the anesthesia provider.
4. The surgeon clamps the external, common, and internal carotid arteries.
5. The surgeon uses a #11 blade to create an arteriotomy over the stenotic area and lengthens the incision with a Potts angulated scissors to expose the full extent of the occluding plaque.
6. Using a blunt dissector, the surgeon dissects the plaque or plaques free from the arterial wall. Heparin solution is used as an irrigant to clean the intima.
7. The surgeon closes the arteriotomy with fine vascular sutures. A synthetic (polyester or PTFE) or autogenous (vein) patch graft may be used to restore the arterial lumen if it is small (Figure 24-17). Before complete closure, blood flow is temporarily restored through the arteries to wash away any free plaques, air, or thrombi. For this to be done, the occluding clamps are opened and closed individually, with flushing of any debris away from the internal carotid artery. The closure of the arteriotomy is completed (Figure 24-18).
8. The occluding clamps are removed from the external and common carotid arteries; the internal carotid artery clamp is removed last. This sequence ensures that any minor debris missed will be flushed harmlessly into the external rather than the internal carotid artery.
9. Additional interrupted sutures may be needed to control leakage.
10. A closed drainage system is inserted by way of a separate stab incision.
11. The wound is closed, and dressings are applied.

Carotid Endarterectomy with Shunt

Operative Procedure.

1. Steps 1 through 5 of the carotid endarterectomy procedure are performed.

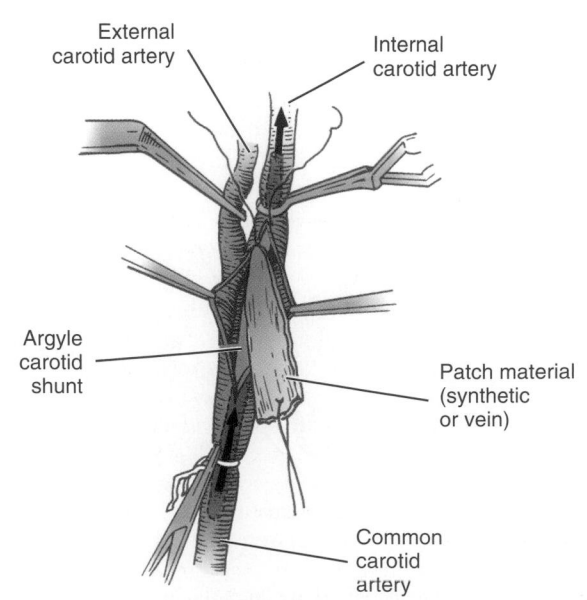

FIGURE 24-16 Left carotid endarterectomy. **A,** Incision and anatomy. **B,** Exposure of carotid bifurcation.

FIGURE 24-17 Left carotid endarterectomy illustrating initial placement and suturing of a patch (a shunt is in place).

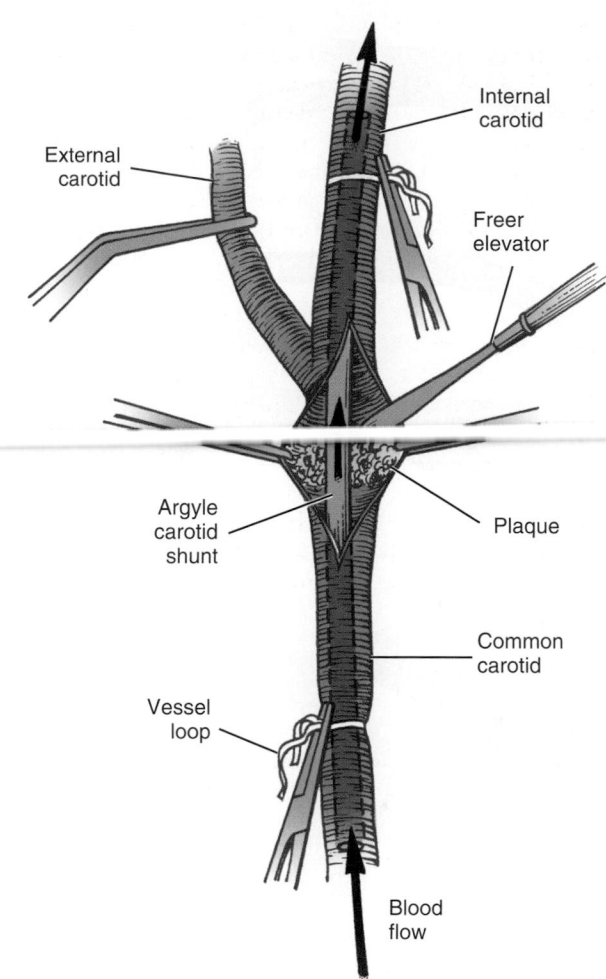

FIGURE 24-18 Left carotid endarterectomy (patch angioplasty) with patch sewn in place. Arrows show the direction of blood flow.

2. To maintain cerebral blood flow the surgeon inserts either a piece of tubing (polyethylene or Silastic) with a suture tied around its center or a commercially prepared shunt device into the common carotid artery and the internal carotid artery. The surgeon then stabilizes the tube or shunt with vessel loops or shunt clamps (Figure 24-19).
3. The surgeon removes the plaque as described for carotid endarterectomy and the arteriotomy is closed with or without a patch.
4. Before the arteriotomy closure is completed, the surgeon releases the shunt clamp or vessel loop on the internal carotid artery and removes the shunt. The external carotid occluding clamp is removed, followed by the common carotid artery clamp, and, last, the internal carotid artery occluding clamp.
5. The wound is closed, and dressings are applied.

Arteriovenous Fistula

Arteriovenous fistulas—direct connections between an artery and a vein—are the standard means of vascular access for long-term renal dialysis (Capurro et al, 2012). The dilated vein can then be used for direct cannulation with large-bore needles for hemodialysis. This method is preferable to an external shunt, which carries a high risk of thrombosis and infection. The best access is achieved using the patient's own vessels and creating a subcutaneous connection between the artery and vein, referred to as an arteriovenous shunt, or bridge fistula. Other choices include using a bovine carotid artery, a human umbilical vein graft, or a synthetic vascular graft, usually PTFE. Four anastomoses that can be created between the artery and vein are side of artery to side of vein, end of artery to side of vein, end of vein to side of artery, and end of vein to end of artery (Capurro et al, 2012) (Figure 24-20). The Brescia-Cimino fistula is a connection between the radial artery and cephalic vein at the wrist (Figure 24-21). A basic principle of creating a fistula is to start in the distal arm and move proximally with subsequent fistulas. These include ulnar artery to basilic vein and brachial artery to brachial or cephalic vein (Figure 24-22).

Arteriovenous shunts are indicated for long-term renal dialysis access. Patients with end-stage renal disease have their creatinine

FIGURE 24-19 Left carotid endarterectomy. Argyle carotid shunt in place to allow blood flow to the brain. Stenotic plaque being removed with Freer elevator.

clearance levels observed. When the creatinine clearance level falls to 10 mL/minute, a Cimino fistula may be created in anticipation of the need for dialysis. A Cimino (or Brescia-Cimino) type of fistula has proved to have the longest patency and lowest infection rate. It is created to connect the patient's artery to a vein that will dilate and become thick-walled (its muscle layer hypertrophies). This occurs from the high rate of blood flow delivered by the connection to the artery. The arterialization, or maturation process, necessary to allow the fistula to withstand the repeated needle punctures of dialysis takes about 3 weeks.

Bridge fistulas do not need to mature and therefore are available for immediate dialysis use. For connections between an artery and a vein that are in proximity, a U-shaped graft is placed. Grafts that are far apart require a straight or slightly curved graft. Although the saphenous vein, an umbilical vein graft, and the bovine carotid artery are often used, PTFE grafts work the best and are most commonly used for bridge fistulas. Some surgeons prefer to use a specially designed PTFE step-graft, or tapered graft. These have a short segment of 4 mm in diameter at one end and the majority of the graft with a 7-mm diameter. This graft may avoid an output or flow rate that is so high it causes cardiac overload. Primary sites for bridge fistulas include the upper arm between the brachial artery and axillary vein and the forearm between the brachial artery and antecubital vein or between the brachial artery and basilic vein (Figure 24-23).

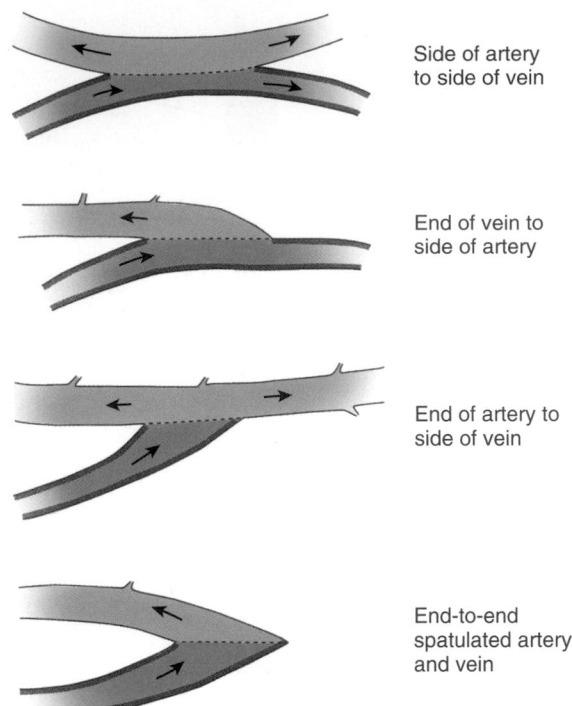

FIGURE 24-20 Four types of anastomoses between radial artery and cephalic vein.

Side of artery to side of vein

End of vein to side of artery

End of artery to side of vein

End-to-end spatulated artery and vein

Arteriovenous anastomosis

Completed fistula with distal vein ligated

FIGURE 24-21 Arteriovenous anastomosis. The artery is anastomosed to the vein.

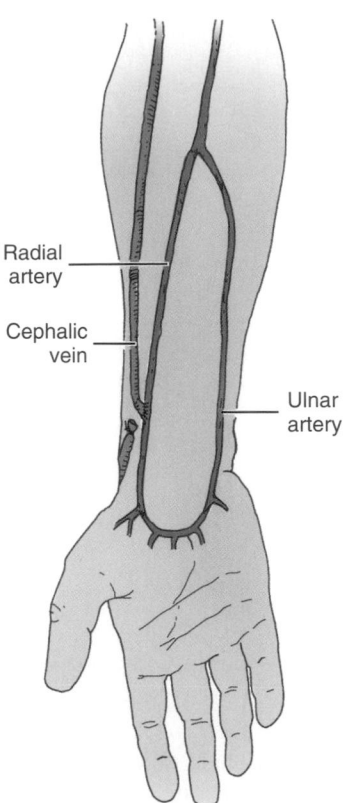

Radial artery

Cephalic vein

Ulnar artery

FIGURE 24-22 End of the cephalic vein anastomosed to the side of the radial artery at a site superior to the usual location of the radiocephalic fistula. This technique can be useful if the distal radial artery is small or the cephalic vein at the wrist is thrombosed.

FIGURE 24-23 An example of a loop fistula. A synthetic graft has been used to create a loop brachiocephalic fistula.

The axillofemoral graft for dialysis is reserved for those patients who have exhausted other fistula sites. A regular-walled (versus a thin-walled) graft is placed from the axillary artery to the common femoral vein. PTFE grafts can be used immediately, but it may be better to wait 2 weeks for anastomotic healing to occur.

The side-to-side fistula was the original subcutaneous method introduced by Brescia in 1966. The side-to-side fistula is technically the easiest to perform and creates the highest flow rate. The arterial end-to-vein side fistula has a lower flow rate. The arterial side-to-vein end fistula is technically more difficult to create but has a lower incidence of venous hypertension. The end-to-end construction has the lowest rate of venous hypertension but also has the lowest flow rate. There is a trend toward performing fewer side-to-side fistulas and more artery side-to-vein end fistulas.

Because the patency of fistulas is limited, dialysis patients return for revision or embolectomy in attempts to salvage their function. Unfortunately the success rate for salvage is low and access may be better managed by the creation of another site or a bridge fistula. Risk factors for complications include female gender, African American race, increased age (older than 65 years), and presence of diabetes. Treatment for the most common complication, stenosis, is surgery. Stenosis usually results in thrombosis. Stenosis most often involves the venous anastomosis, and a patch angioplasty is usually performed to revise a thrombosed fistula. Other complications include aneurysm and pseudoaneurysm formation, infection, subclavian steal syndrome, and high-output CHF.

Venous Surgical Interventions

Vena Cava Filter Insertion

Vena cava filter (VCF) insertion entails the partial occlusion of the inferior vena cava with an intravascular filter, such as a Greenfield filter, inserted under fluoroscopy using a local anesthetic or moderate sedation and analgesia (monitored anesthesia care). VCFs are generally placed in the OR or angiography suite with fluoroscopic guidance. The Greenfield device offers the option of jugular or femoral vein insertion, and the correct kit must be selected. Box 24-3 gives indications for a caval filter (Meisner et al, 2012). Several types of filters have been used, as illustrated in Figure 24-24. The Greenfield filter is the most successful and widely used device, and the mortality and morbidity have been extremely low. The device has progressed from an early design that required an incision and venotomy to the current percutaneous titanium VCF. The filter maintains a patent vena cava but prevents PE by trapping the emboli at the apex of the device.

Procedural Considerations. The perioperative nurse assists the patient to the supine position on a radiopaque OR bed to permit fluoroscopic visualization at the level of the renal veins. This

---

BOX 24-3

Indications for a Vena Cava Filter

- Recurrent thromboembolism despite "adequate" anticoagulation
- Deep venous thrombosis in a patient with contraindications to anticoagulation
- Chronic pulmonary embolism and resultant pulmonary hypertension
- Complications of anticoagulation
- Propagating iliofemoral venous thrombus in anticoagulation

FIGURE 24-24 Vena cava filters. **A,** Actual filters. **B,** Radiographic images. *Left to right,* Kimray-Greenfield, titanium Greenfield, Simon nitinol, Gianturco bird's nest, and Vena Tech.

procedure may be performed in the OR, radiology suite, or ICU for critical patients. The head is turned to the left for jugular vein insertion, or the groin is exposed for femoral vein insertion. The right femoral vein is preferred over the left because the anatomy of the left vein often makes threading the filter more difficult. The nurse ensures that local anesthetic, heparinized saline to flush the device, and contrast media are available.

Operative Procedure

1. The right groin area is prepped and draped and infiltrated with local anesthetic.
2. An 18-gauge entry needle is used for right femoral venotomy.
3. The surgeon inserts the guidewire and advances it to a level above the renal veins under fluoroscopic guidance.
4. The sheath or dilator is inserted over the guidewire after all device lumens have been flushed with heparin solution.
5. The surgeon removes the sheath, and inserts and advances the introducer catheter to the implantation site.
6. The introducer catheter carries the preloaded, radiopaque carrier capsule. The sheath is retracted, the filter is discharged, and the sheath is removed.
7. Pressure is applied to the puncture site for approximately 5 minutes or until hemostasis is achieved.

Varicose Vein Excision and Stripping

Varicose veins are enlarged and distended veins that are visible and palpable beneath the skin. Varicose veins are described as primary or secondary. Primary varicose veins are more prevalent and are not associated with a pathologic condition of the deeper venous system, that is, post-thrombotic syndrome or a history of DVT. Secondary varicose veins are believed to be a result of insufficiency of the deep venous system. Disease may prevent the normal functioning of these valves, resulting in distention; as the vein wall weakens and dilates, venous pressure increases and the valves become incompetent. The

veins gradually become dilated. Veins in the lower extremities are most frequently affected, particularly the long saphenous vein. Risk factors include female gender, increased age, pregnancy, geographic location, and race (more prevalent in Caucasians).

Dilation of the saphenous vein produces venous stasis, which may be followed by secondary complications, such as stasis ulcers. Venous obstruction causes an increase in venous pressure, which leads to an increase in capillary pressure. This causes fluid to leak from the capillaries and produce edema. The objective of surgical intervention is to remove the diseased veins, thus preventing ulceration, secondary edema, pain, and fatigue in the extremity.

Procedural Considerations. Before sedation or entrance into the OR, the patient should stand and the varicose veins should be marked with an indelible marker. This ensures adequate visualization for complete removal of the varicosities because the patient is often placed in the Trendelenburg position intraoperatively to decrease venous congestion, which could interfere with visualization of the varicosities. The perioperative nurse assists with positioning the patient on the OR bed in a supine position with the legs slightly abducted. Ligation or stripping of the lesser saphenous veins and branches may require placing the patient in the prone position. In the stab avulsion technique, multiple small (2 to 3 mm) incisions are made over the identified varicosities, and the affected vein segments are removed (Figure 24-25). Stripping indicates removal of a long segment of vein by means of a special device (Figure 24-26). Drapes are placed to enable flexing and lifting at the knee. Instruments include a basic minor instrument setup, plus the following: Weitlaner self-retaining retractors, #11 blades, skin hooks, mosquito hemostats, vein strippers with various tips available, and elastic bandages. Endovenous laser ablation (EVLA) is an innovative nonsurgical procedure for varicose veins and offers patients an alternative treatment to surgical vein stripping (Ambulatory Surgery Considerations).

FIGURE 24-25 Technique of stab avulsions of varicosities.

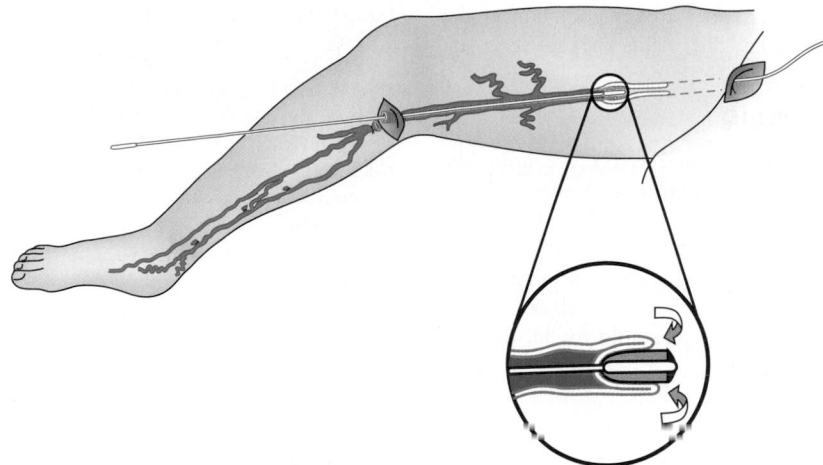

FIGURE 24-26 Inversion stripping of the saphenous vein for superficial venous reflux caused by an incompetent saphenofemoral junction.

AMBULATORY SURGERY CONSIDERATIONS

Postdischarge Follow-Up: Endovenous Laser Ablation for Varicose Veins

Endovenous laser ablation (EVLA) is an innovative nonsurgical procedure for varicose veins that offers an alternative treatment to the often painful surgical ligation (or stripping) of veins, which is performed with the patient administered a general anesthetic and often has a long recovery time. During EVLA, by delivering laser energy through a fiberoptic catheter a particular vein is sealed to prevent blood flow. The catheter is inserted into the vein with ultrasound guidance. The entire procedure can be done in 1 hour as an ambulatory surgery procedure with the patient administered a local anesthetic. Once the procedure is completed, the skin puncture site is approximated with an adhesive strip. A graduated compression stocking or wrap is applied to the affected extremity from the base of the toes to the groin; it is constantly kept in place for 2 weeks and thereafter for 6 weeks when ambulatory to help maintain occlusion of the vein. Immediate and frequent ambulation is encouraged to decrease the incidence of DVT formation.

An important consideration for vascular procedure patients in the ambulatory setting is postoperative and discharge education. Patients need detailed instructions regarding recovery and convalescence because this phase is not complete on discharge. These instructions should include possible complications, activity level, wound care, pain management, and the plan for follow-up. Postoperative phone calls, 24 to 48 hours after discharge, have proven beneficial to identify any adverse events and answer patient questions. In a study by Vinoles and colleagues (2011), postoperative phones calls following ambulatory surgery provided greater patient satisfaction and better outcomes. Although all patients received detailed education, new questions arose. The postdischarge phone call can stress the importance of wearing the compression stocking or wrap to prevent complications.

Modified from Sadek M et al: Update on endovenous laser ablation: 2011, *Perspect Vasc Surg Endovasc Ther* 23(4):233–237, 2011; Vinoles et al: Predicting recovery at home after ambulatory surgery, *BMC Health Serv Res* 11(1):269–280, 2011.

Operative Procedure

1. The surgeon makes an incision in the upper area of the thigh, parallel to the crease in the groin, and clamps and ligates any bleeding vessels.
2. The saphenous vein is identified and isolated. Margins of the wound are separated with a Weitlaner self-retaining retractor.
3. The surgeon double ligates the saphenous vein branches with black silk ties, or they are transfixed, clamped, and divided. The proximal stump is dissected upward to the point at which it enters the femoral vein, where it is carefully ligated.
4. If the saphenous vein is to be excised, the surgeon makes an incision at its distal portion at the ankle, and the vein is identified, ligated, and divided.
5. A vein stripper is inserted and advanced to the proximal end of the vein in the groin, where it is secured with a heavy suture, and the tip is attached.
6. As the surgeon pulls the stripper up the leg, external compression is applied by the assistant or scrub person.
7. Tributaries may be excised through numerous small incisions along the course of the vein.
8. The surgeon closes the groin wound in layers, and other small incisions are closed with skin sutures or staples. Dressings and circular compression bandages are applied.

KEY POINTS

- Atherosclerosis continues to be one of the leading causes of death and disability in the Western world. It is estimated that peripheral arterial disease (PAD) affects about 8 million persons in the United States.
- The prevalence of PAD is approximately 12% of the adult population. This is particularly striking, given that by the year 2030 the percentage of the U.S. population older than 65 years will increase to 20% (Federal Interagency Forum on Aging-Related Statistics, 2012).
- Many of these people will require surgical interventions for the syndromes of peripheral ischemia, aneurysm, and venous disease.
- Perioperative nursing assessments should take into consideration risk factors of PAD including hypertension, diabetes, obesity and physical inactivity and use this information to plan the intra and postoperative plan of care.

- Also of importance, is to maintain skin integrity during the surgical skin prep to reduce the risks for surgical site infections.

CRITICAL THINKING QUESTION

Your first case is an elective carotid endarterectomy. During the preoperative assessment you note the patient is a 68-year-old male who states he has been in good health and is very active. His medical history includes mild hypertension and smoking. The patient expresses he has tried to stop smoking on his own without success. He has normal range of motion of all extremities as well as his neck. Based on your assessment, what information would you incorporate into your postoperative teaching plan?

evolve *The answer to the Critical Thinking Question can be found at http://evolve.elsevier.com/Rothrock/Alexander.*

REFERENCES

Aragón-Sánchez J et al: The role of a specialized approach for patients with diabetes, critical ischemia and foot ulcers not previously considered for proactive management, *Diabet Med* 28(10):1249–1252, 2011.

Brown-Brumfield D, DeLeon A: Adherence to medication safety protocol: current practice for labeling medications and solutions on the sterile field, *AORN J* 91(5):610–617, 2010.

Capurro F et al: The middle arm arteriovenous fistula is an additional option to expand autogenous hemodialysis access, *J Vasc Access* 13(2):208–214, 2012.

Chapman S: Pain management in patients following limb amputation, *Nurs Stand* 25(19):35–40, 2011.

Denholm B: Tucking patient's arms and general positioning, *AORN J* 89(4):755–757, 2009.

Federal Interagency Forum on Aging-Related Statistics: *Older Americans 2012: key indicators of well-being.* Federal Interagency Forum on Aging-Related Statistics, Washington, DC, June 2012, U.S. Government Printing Office. Available at www.agingstats.gov/agingstatsdotnet/Main_Site/Data/2012_Documents/Docs/EntireChartbook.pdf. Accessed October 22, 2012.

Ferreria AC, Macedo FY: A review of simple, non-invasive means of assessing peripheral artery disease and implications for medical management, *Ann Med* 42(2):139–150, 2010.

Fink AS et al: Enhancement of surgical informed consent by addition of repeat back: a multicenter randomized control clinical trial, *Ann Surg* 252(1):27–36, 2010.

Giles KA et al: Population-based outcomes following endovascular and open repair of ruptured abdominal aortic aneurysms, *J Endovasc Ther* 16(5):554–564, 2009.

Johnson H, Kimsey D: Patient safety: break the silence, *AORN J* 95(5):591–601, 2012.

Kolakowski S et al: Is infrainguinal percutaneous atherectomy better suited for certain arteries than others, *Vasc Endovasc Surg* 43(5):462–466, 2009.

Lederle FA et al: Outcomes following endovascular vs. open repair of abdominal aortic aneurysm: a random trial? *JAMA* 302:1535–1542, 2009.

Little JK: Care of patients with vascular problems. In Ignatavicius DD, Workman ML, editors: *Medical-surgical nursing: patient-centered collaborative care*, ed 7, St Louis, 2013, Saunders.

Liu Z et al: Carotid artery stenting versus carotid endarterectomy: systematic review and meta-analysis, *World J Surg* 33:586–596, 2009.

Meisner RJ et al: Review of indications and practices of vena cava filters at a large university hospital, *Vasc Endovascular Surg* 46(1):21–25, 2012.

Oka RK et al: Efficacy of optimal long-term management of multiple cardiovascular risk factors (CVD) on walking and quality of life in patients with peripheral artery disease (PAD): protocol for randomized controlled trial, *Vasc Med* 17(1):17–28, 2012.

Roger VL et al: Heart disease and stroke statistics—2012 update: a report from the American Heart Association Statistic Committee and Stroke Statistics Committee, *Circulation* 125:188–197, 2012.

Sawabe M: Vascular aging: from molecular mechanism to clinical significance, *Geriat Gerontol Int* 10:S213–S220, 2010.

Schwarze ML et al: Age related trends in utilization and outcome of open and endovascular repair of abdominal aortic aneurysm in the United States, *J Vasc Surg* 50:722–729, 2009.

Zaidi N et al: Perioperative use of antibiotics in elective surgical patients: timing of administration, *J Periop Pract* 19(7):225–227, 2009.

Zeller T et al: New techniques for endovascular treatment of peripheral artery disease with focus on chronic critical limb ischemia, *Vasa* 38(1):3–12, 2009.

CHAPTER 25
Cardiac Surgery

PATRICIA C. SEIFERT

Cardiac surgery is increasingly moving toward interventional procedures that use minimally invasive approaches and percutaneous access routes. The introduction of coronary angioplasty in the 1970s accelerated interventional technology and stimulated perioperative clinicians to expand both traditional and innovative treatment options. These changes have also encouraged individuals to refine anastomotic techniques, investigate new routes to achieve cardiopulmonary bypass and vascular repair, design more tissue-friendly instrumentation, and create operative arenas that embrace aspects of both the typical operating room (OR) and the newer interventional suites. These newer, "hybrid" ORs have stimulated cardiac clinicians to expand their skill sets, develop closer working relationships with colleagues in the cardiac catheterization and electrophysiology laboratories, and reassess how these changing technologies can strengthen the delivery of patient-focused care (Weisse, 2011). Other advances have included the growth of precise, three-dimensional diagnostic images; improved monitoring of neurologic and renal function; effective blood conservation strategies; refined anesthetic and cardiac drugs; and an overall greater understanding of the causes and treatment of glucose abnormalities, antibiotic-resistant infections, and other abnormalities that affect patient outcomes (Hatton et al, 2011; Nalla et al, 2012; Nussmeier et al, 2009; Teirstein and Lytle, 2012).

Other trends that have significantly affected cardiac surgery include heightened emphases on safety, education, quality outcomes, staff competence, and cost effectiveness (Speir et al, 2009). The use of a simple checklist to ensure correct identification of the patient or that performance of a central line insertion is in a manner that eliminates or minimizes the risk of a catheter-based infection (Lipitz-Snyderman, 2011) are among the many safety initiatives that produce better patient outcomes.

This chapter describes both traditional and newer, innovative treatment options for coronary artery disease (CAD), valvular dysfunction, thoracic aneurysms, conduction disturbances, heart failure, and end-stage cardiac disease. Therapeutic interventions may use laser, radiofrequency, or cryothermal energies. Stem cell therapy, used to induce cardiac neorevascularization at the cellular level (Jeevanantham et al, 2012), and "destination" mechanical assist devices (which remain implanted)—or devices that can result in the "recovery" of the ventricle—are among the newer areas of investigation showing great promise (Acker and Jessup, 2012).

Surgical Anatomy

The heart (Figure 25-1) is a four-chamber muscular pump that propels blood into the systemic and pulmonary circulatory systems. It sits within a pericardial sac within the mediastinum, which lies between the lungs, posterior to the sternum, and anterior to the vertebrae, esophagus, and descending portion of the aorta. The location of the diaphragm is below the heart (Figure 25-2). The heart bears attachments at the aorta, pulmonary artery, superior and inferior venae cavae, and the pulmonary veins; the ventricles are relatively mobile, enabling the surgeon to rotate the walls of the ventricles and the apex of the left ventricle in order to assess (and graft) coronary arteries to the lateral and posterior aspects of the myocardium.

The cardiac wall consists of three layers: the epicardium or outer lining; the myocardium or muscular layer, an important functional layer; and the endocardium or inner lining (Figure 25-3). The left ventricular muscle layer has the most depth (i.e., thickness) of the four chambers and can generate the greatest pressure, required to pump blood into the circulatory system.

Two thirds of the heart are to the left of the midline, and the remaining one third is to the right. Although functionally divided into right and left halves, the heart sits rotated to the left, with the right side anterior and the left side relatively posterior. Injury to the anterior chest (e.g., from blunt force or stab wounds) is likely to damage the right ventricle. This may prove significant for myocardial repair because the right ventricle has lower pressures than the left, thus allowing additional time for repair before exsanguination.

Each half of the heart contains an upper and a lower communicating chamber—the atrium and ventricle, respectively. The right atrium (RA) receives desaturated blood from the inferior and superior venae cavae and from coronary circulation via the coronary sinus. The left atrium (LA) receives oxygenated blood from the lungs by way of the pulmonary veins. From both atria, blood then flows through the atrioventricular (AV) valves into the ventricles.

The left ventricle (LV) pumps oxygenated blood into the major vessels of the *systemic circulatory system* by way of the aorta and its main branches to the head, upper extremities, abdominal organs, and lower extremities. The right and left internal mammary arteries (IMAs) (thoracic), used as grafts during coronary bypass surgery, branch off the subclavian arteries and course behind and parallel to the edges of the sternum. The arteries of the circulatory system subdivide into arterioles and eventually into capillaries and the individual cells, where internal respiration and metabolic exchange occur. From the cells and capillary beds, desaturated blood flows into the venules and veins and finally returns to the RA.

In the *pulmonary circulatory system*, blood pumps from the right ventricle (RV) through the pulmonary valve into the main pulmonary artery (PA). The PA divides into the right and left pulmonary arteries, which further subdivide into the arterioles and capillaries of the lungs. External respiration occurs in the capillary beds and the alveoli, wherein carbon dioxide exchanges for oxygen. Freshly oxygenated blood from the lungs then flows through the pulmonary veins into the LA.

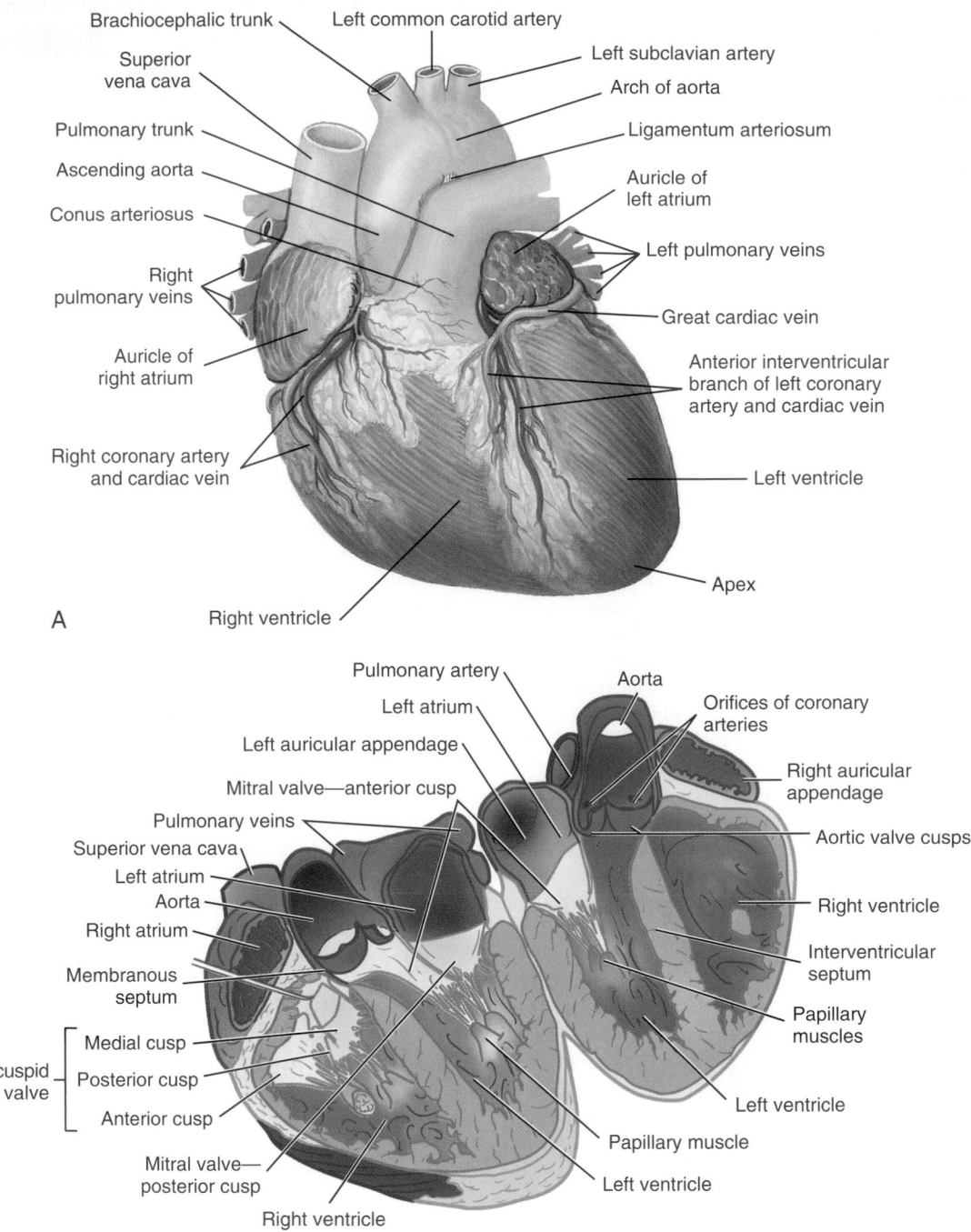

FIGURE 25-1 A, Anterior view of heart illustrates major vessels and chambers. **B,** Drawing of a heart split perpendicular to the interventricular septum illustrates the anatomic relationships of the leaflets of the atrioventricular and aortic valve, and the receiving chambers (atria) and the pumping chambers (ventricles). Systemic venous blood returns to the heart by way of the inferior and superior venae cavae. It enters the right atrium, flows through the tricuspid valve into the right ventricle, and ejects through the pulmonic valve (not shown) into the pulmonary circulation. The blood oxygenates in the lungs and returns to the left atrium through the pulmonary veins. From the left atrium it flows through the mitral valve into the left ventricle, where it ejects through the aortic valve into the aorta and systemic circulation.

Coronary circulation (Figure 25-4) supplies oxygen and nutrients to, and removes metabolic waste from, the myocardium; internal respiration occurs in the *myocytes*. The heart receives its blood supply from the left and right coronary arteries, which originate in the corresponding left and right sinuses of Valsalva behind the cusps of the aortic valve in the ascending aorta. The left main coronary artery divides into the left anterior descending (LAD) coronary artery and the circumflex coronary artery; with the right coronary artery (RCA), these arteries are the three main vessels of the coronary arterial system.

In coronary arteries affected by CAD, focal or diffuse atherosclerotic plaques develop and progressively enlarge, diminishing myocardial blood flow and oxygenation, which produces ischemic pain in many, but not all, cases. Occlusion of a coronary artery by

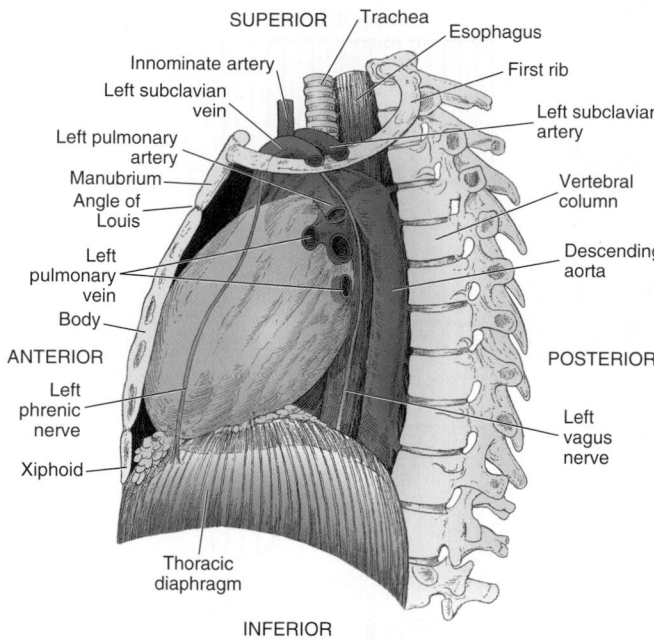

FIGURE 25-2 Regions of the mediastinum.

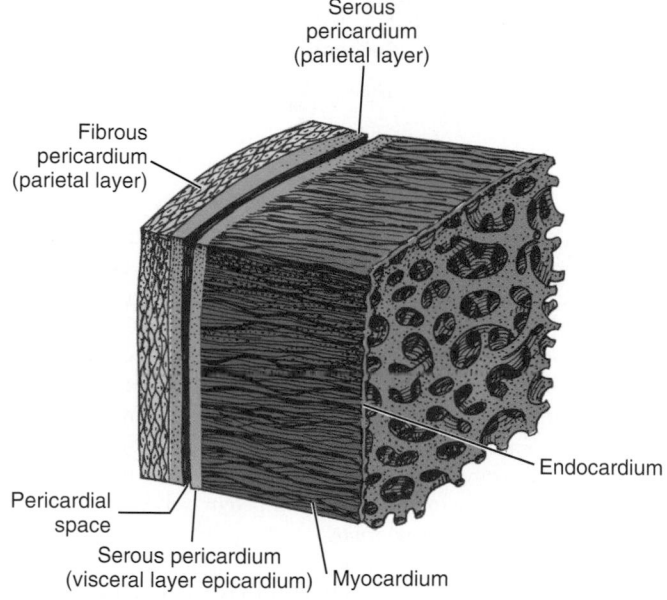

FIGURE 25-3 Cross section of cardiac muscle showing its three layers (endocardium, myocardium, epicardium) and pericardium.

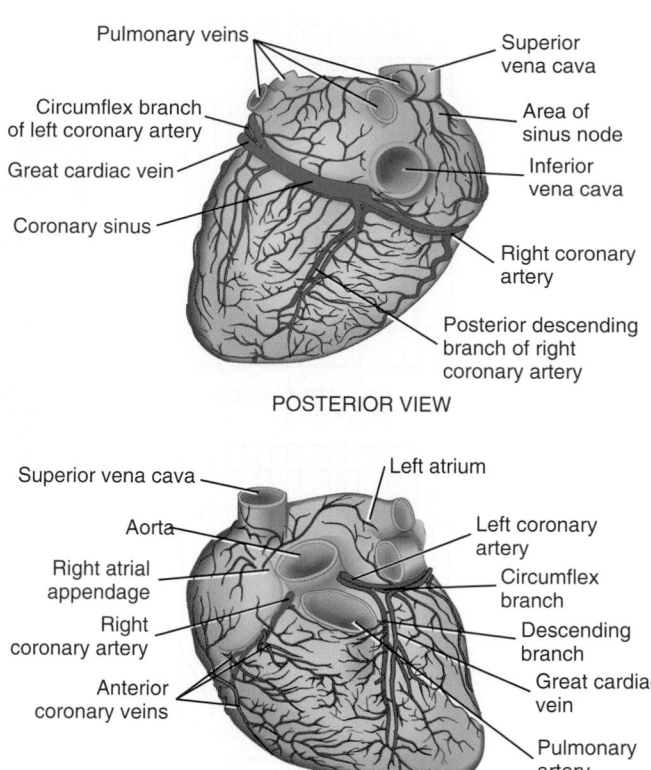

FIGURE 25-4 Anterior and posterior surfaces of the heart, illustrating the location and distribution of the principal coronary arteries and veins.

expanding atherosclerotic lesions causes myocardial infarction (MI) and irreversible damage to the region of the myocardium perfused by the obstructed artery. Coronary artery bypass procedures increase blood flow to the affected ischemic areas by attaching a bypass graft conduit to the artery distal to the narrowed portion of the artery. A totally occluded (infarcted) artery does not benefit from bypass surgery because the myocardial injury is irreversible if not treated (e.g., via revascularization) within 6 hours (Jneid et al, 2012). The main coronary arteries sit in the epicardium, which facilitates accessibility during coronary bypass procedures. From these arteries arise the septal perforators and other branches that penetrate the entire

myocardium. The cardiac veins empty into the RA by way of the coronary sinus; the thebesian veins, prominent in the walls of the RA and the RV, open directly into these chambers.

From the medulla oblongata, nerve impulses to the heart travel along the middle cervical nerve, composed of sympathetic fibers, and the vagus nerve, composed of parasympathetic fibers. Sympathetic fibers increase the force and rate of contraction, whereas parasympathetic fibers control heart rate. Running vertically along the right and left sides of the pericardium are major branches of the phrenic nerve, which innervate the diaphragm and stimulate it to contract. In order to protect the diaphragm, identifying the phrenic nerve is important in procedures that involve incision or excision of the lateral pericardium. Within the myocardium itself, certain areas of tissue undergo natural modification to form a *conduction system* (Figure 25-5). The process of excitation and contraction originates in the sinoatrial (SA) node, located in the area where the superior vena cava (SVC) meets the RA. The impulse spreads to the atria through internodal pathways and travels to the AV junction (which contains the AV node) located medial to the entrance of the coronary sinus in the RA, close to the tricuspid valve. From the AV junction, the impulse spreads to the bundle of His, which extends down the right side of the interventricular septum. The bundle of His divides into the right and left bundle branches, which terminate in a network of fibers called the *Purkinje system*. Purkinje fibers are spread throughout the inner surface of both ventricles and the papillary muscles, which when stimulated produce contraction of the heart muscle. Thus the location of conduction tissue is clinically significant during surgical repair of atrial or ventricular septal defects.

FIGURE 25-5 Heart with normal conduction pathways and transmembrane action potential of sinoatrial *(SA)* node, **A;** atrioventricular *(AV)* node (AV junction), **B;** bundle branches, **C;** and ventricular muscle, **D.**

During myocardial contraction and relaxation, spiral fibers of the heart contract and relax (Figure 25-6, *A*). To prevent regurgitation of blood, the four cardiac valves (see Figure 25-6, *B* and *C,* and Figure 25-7) open and close to maintain unidirectional blood flow. The AV valves are between the atria and the ventricles. The right AV valve is called the *tricuspid valve* and contains three leaflets (or cusps). The left AV valve, called the *mitral valve,* consists of two leaflets (see Figure 25-6). Each AV valve is a complex system consisting of a fibrous annulus surrounding the valve orifice, the valve leaflets, the chordae tendineae, the atrium, and the papillary muscles, which anchor the valve to the inner ventricular wall (see Figure 25-1). The mitral valve annulus is a dynamic structure with a three-dimensional "saddle" shape, which has stimulated the design of newer prosthetic annuloplasty rings (Silbiger, 2012). When the ventricle contracts, these muscles and the chordae tendineae, connected to the valve leaflets, prevent the leaflets from everting into the atrium. All parts of the system must function for the valve to work properly. If the shape of the ventricle has been changed by dilation or hypertrophy, for example, the altered geometry of the ventricle impairs ventricular function. Conditions such as hypertension, myocardial injury, and aortic stenosis promote a pathologic *remodeling* of the heart that can lead not only to valvular dysfunction but also heart failure and malignant dysrhythmias (Gopaldas, 2012).

The semilunar valves are at the outlets of the LV and RV. These valves are known as the *aortic* and *pulmonic* valves, respectively. They have fewer components than the AV valves, and they open and close passively with cyclic fluctuations in blood pressure and volume that occur during systole and diastole.

Abnormalities such as stenosis, insufficiency, or a combination of both impair the mechanical function of the valves. Stenosed valves have leaflets that are fibrous and stiff, with uneven and adherent margins. Regurgitant, insufficient, or incompetent valves, such as those with leaflet degeneration or perforations, dilated annuli, or ruptured chordae tendineae, produce regurgitation of blood into the originating chamber. These conditions, or a combination of stenosis and insufficiency, strain the myocardium by increasing intracardiac pressure, volume, and workload. The sound of blood flowing through a narrowed or incompetent valve produces an abnormal sound called a *murmur.*

Any of the four valves may be deformed congenitally. Acquired valvular heart disease most commonly affects the mitral and aortic valves and appears to worsen with increased stress associated with the higher pressures within the left chambers of the heart. Although rare, primary tumors of the heart may impair valve function by partially occluding a valve orifice, causing incomplete closure of the leaflets. Portions of the tumor may break off and embolize. Most tumors are benign; the most common is the cardiac myxoma. Diagnostic imaging can identify many of these lesions, but the lesion may not cause symptoms to motivate a person to seek medical treatment (McManus, 2012).

Perioperative Nursing Considerations

Specialized nursing considerations that apply to thoracic surgery (see Chapter 23) and to vascular surgery (see Chapter 24) often also

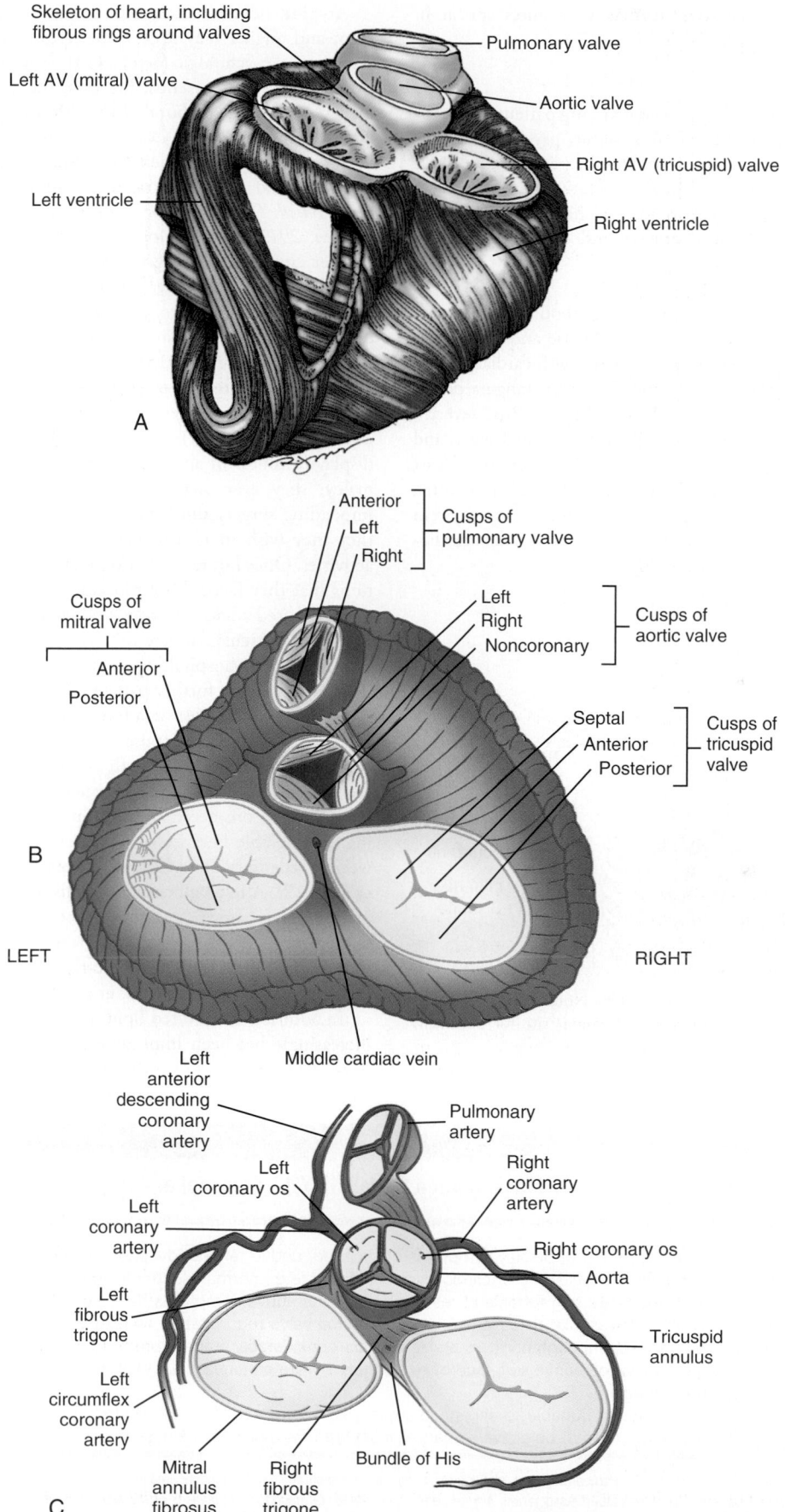

FIGURE 25-6 A, Location of the heart valves in relation to the spiral fibers of the myocardium. **B,** Superior view of cardiac valves: pulmonary *(top);* aortic *(middle);* mitral *(bottom left);* and tricuspid *(bottom right).* **C,** Superior view of valves in relation to coronary arteries and conduction tissue. *AV,* Atrioventricular.

apply to cardiac surgery. Pediatric cardiac procedures appear in Chapter 26.

Assessment

As the severity of pathologic changes varies among patients throughout the life span, knowledge of physical status, psychosocial concerns, and functional health patterns enables the perioperative nurse to plan and manage patient care. The perioperative nursing data set should include the patient's biopsychosocial history, the physical examination, and results from laboratory and diagnostic imaging tests.

History. The history includes information about the patient's health status as well as the response to the disease and the recommended intervention or interventions. Patients with cardiac disease may display such symptoms as ischemic chest pain (angina pectoris), fatigue, dyspnea, and syncope. Depending on their severity, these *subjective* symptoms affect the patient's functional status and ability to engage in activities of daily living; the New York Heart Association's Functional Classification System (Box 25-1) is often used to assess functional ability. Updates to the classification system also include *objective* measurements such as x-rays and echocardiograms (American Heart Association [AHA], 2012 a,b).

FIGURE 25-7 Anatomic position of cardiac valves. Note relationship of left ventricular apex to fourth and fifth ribs—a frequent site for minimally invasive incisions.

Atypical ischemic chest pain is more likely in women than in men, and angina may arise from vasospastic angina, mitral valve prolapse, or psychologic factors. CAD is unusual in premenopausal women; after menses ends, however, the risk is similar to that of men (AHA, 2013; Caboral, 2013; Mosca et al, 2011; Roger et al, 2012; Wenger, 2012). Controversy exists regarding menopausal hormone therapy. Estrogen hormone replacement therapy is not recommended in postmenopausal women, according to the *Evidence-Based Guidelines for Cardiovascular Disease Prevention in Women: 2011 Update* (Mosca et al, 2011) (Evidence for Practice). Greater emphasis is being placed on effectiveness of interventions as well as on the evidence supporting those interventions; effective control of blood pressure, diabetes management, and maintenance of optimal lipid levels are significant risk reduction interventions for women (Caboral, 2013).

Women undergoing coronary artery bypass graft (CABG) also have some unique challenges and experiences. According to Banner and colleagues (2011), some women may minimize any public display of illness in an attempt to preserve the appearance of normalcy; they even may hesitate to tell significant others about impending surgery until the day before admission. Postoperatively they may wish to return home early in order to resume regular activities. Once home, some women were unprepared for the limitations that they faced, both physical and social; the authors recommend focused advice, support, and education (Banner et al, 2011).

A cardiovascular disease risk factor profile (Box 25-2) is helpful to plan care for hospitalization and discharge by focusing on areas that might require further patient education. For example, diabetes is a risk factor because it affects the vascular system, may retard healing, and may predispose the patient to infection. Of special concern is the epidemic growth of type 2 diabetes in particular and the role of hyperglycemia in general. Although type 2 diabetes formerly was considered an adult-onset disease, children are increasingly vulnerable because of a greater incidence of increased body weight, sedentary lifestyle, and accelerated insulin resistance (Roger et al, 2012). Altered glucose metabolism (absent diagnosed diabetes mellitus) has shown a significant correlation to atherosclerosis; control of hyperglycemia during coronary bypass surgery is an important strategy to reduce the risk of adverse clinical outcomes (Hillis et al, 2011; Nussmeier et al, 2009).

In addition to elevated lipid or cholesterol levels, inflammation increasingly has been implicated in the development of CAD. In

---

BOX 25-1

New York Heart Association's Functional Classification System (NYHA Classes) and Associated Objective Evidence*

Class I   Patients with cardiac disease do not display symptoms of syncope, undue fatigue, dyspnea, or anginal pain with ordinary physical activity; no objective evidence of cardiovascular disease (e.g., normal electrocardiogram).

Class II   Patients with cardiac disease are comfortable at rest but display the above symptoms during ordinary physical activity; objective evidence of minimal cardiovascular disease (e.g., minimal mitral valve regurgitation on echocardiography).

Class III   Patients with cardiac disease, although comfortable at rest, are considerably limited functionally and display symptoms with less-than-ordinary exercise; objective evidence of moderately severe cardiovascular disease (e.g., ischemic electrocardiographic changes).

Class IV   Patients with cardiac disease are unable to engage in any physical activity without discomfort and may have symptoms of cardiac insufficiency even at rest; objective evidence of severe cardiovascular disease (e.g., enlarged heart shadow on x-ray).

*Objective evidence refers to measurements such as electrocardiograms, stress tests, x-rays, echocardiograms, and diagnostic images.
Modified from The Criteria Committee of the New York Heart Association: *Nomenclature and criteria for diagnosis of diseases of the heart and great vessels*, ed 9, Boston, 1994, Little, Brown.

EVIDENCE FOR PRACTICE

Women and Cardiovascular Disease

Guidelines and interventions that may be useful for preventing cardiovascular disease (CVD) in women:

Lifestyle Interventions

- Avoid smoking and environmental tobacco smoke
- Engage in at least 150 minutes of exercise per week
- Consume diet rich in fruits and vegetables, high-fiber foods, fish; avoid or limit high-saturated fats or *trans*-fatty acids, cholesterol, alcohol, sodium, and sugar
- Maintain body mass index (BMI) of <25 kg/m²

Major Risk Factor Interventions

- Maintain close to optimal blood pressure of 120/80 mm Hg
- Use appropriate pharmacotherapy to control hypertension, diabetes mellitus, renal disease, and high level of lipids and lipoproteins

Guidelines and interventions that may *not* be useful or that may be *harmful* in preventing CVD in women:

Menopausal Therapy

- Hormone therapy should not be used for the primary or secondary prevention of CVD
- Antioxidant supplements
  - Vitamin supplements (e.g., vitamins E, C, and beta carotene) should not be used for prevention of CVD
- Folic acid
  - Should not be used for primary or secondary prevention of CVD
  - Folic acid supplementation should be used in the childbearing years to prevent neural tube defects
- Aspirin for MI in women younger than 65 years of age
  - Routine use of aspirin in healthy women older than 65 years of age may be useful to prevent ischemic stoke and MI if the use outweighs the risk of gastrointestinal bleeding

- May be useful in women with certain forms of AF and who have a contraindication to warfarin

Guidelines and interventions that may be useful in women undergoing CABG:

Use of Internal Mammary Artery (IMA)

- IMA associated with significant reduction in mortality (compared with CABG using venous conduits alone); less use of IMA in women
- At least one IMA used to bypass stenotic coronary artery; bilateral IMA associated with reduced morbidity and mortality

Use of Off-Pump CABG

- Less use of off-pump CABG in women
- Comorbid conditions in women affecting surgical intervention
  - Greater incidence of diabetes mellitus, hypertension, hyperlipidemia, chronic renal insufficiency, COPD
  - Increased risk of bleeding
  - Women tend to be older at time of surgery
  - Hyperglycemia increases risk in women
  - Greater incidence of concomitant valvular disease
- Surgical outcomes: equivocal
  - Perioperative mortality may differ depending on studies (when data adjusted for age and comorbidities)
  - Perioperative morbidity may differ depending on studies (when data adjusted for age and comorbidities)
  - Evidence that women use more resources than men: intra-aortic balloon counterpulsation, vasopressors, mechanical ventilation, dialysis, blood products
- Women less likely to be completely revascularized
- Women tend to have smaller body surface area and hearts, smaller coronary arteries.

AF, Atrial fibrillation; *CABG,* coronary artery bypass graft; *COPD,* chronic obstructive pulmonary disease; *MI,* myocardial infarction.
Modified from Mosca L et al: Effectiveness-based guidelines for the prevention of cardiovascular disease in women—2011 update: a guideline from the American Heart Association, *Circulation* 123:1243–1262, 2011; Banner D et al: Women's experiences of undergoing coronary artery bypass graft surgery, *J Adv Nurs* 68(4):919–930, 2011; Hillis LD et al: 2011 ACCF/AHA guideline for coronary artery bypass graft surgery: a report of the American College of Cardiology Foundation/American Heart Association Task Force on Practice Guidelines, *J Am Coll Cardiol* 58(24):e123–e210, 2011, available at http://content.onlinejacc.org/article.aspx?articleid=1147818. Accessed March 19, 2013; Newby LK, Douglas PS: Cardiovascular disease in women. In Bonow RO et al, editors: *Braunwald's heart disease: a textbook of cardiovascular medicine,* ed 9, Philadelphia, 2012, Saunders; Wenger NK: Women and coronary heart disease: a century after Herrick, *Circulation* 126:604–611, 2012; Caboral MF: Update on cardiovascular disease prevention in women, *Am J Nurs* 113(3):26–33, 2013.

BOX 25-2

Risk Factors for Coronary Artery Disease

Nonmodifiable

- Age
- Male (but postmenopausal women have risk similar to that of men)
- Heredity, genetic makeup, family history
- Race
- Menstrual status (estrogen levels may be modifiable; postmenopausal women have risk similar to that of men)

Modifiable

- Elevated levels of serum cholesterol and other lipids
- Hypertension
- Cigarette smoking
- Obesity, metabolic syndrome
- Diabetes mellitus

- Psychologic stress
- Personality type
- Physical inactivity

Newer, Novel Contributing Factors

- Elevated homocysteine levels (increase platelet aggregation)
- Inflammation (the atherosclerotic process is associated with inflammation)
- High C-reactive protein level (CRP is a marker for inflammation associated with atherogenesis)
- Periodontal disease (a marker for inflammation and possible infection)
- Atrial and ventricular natriuretic peptides (hormones secreted by the atria and ventricles in response to volume expansion and fluid retention; predictive of a variety of cardiac problems)

Modified from Bachmann JM et al: Association between family history and coronary heart disease death across long-term follow-up in men: The Cooper Center Longitudinal Study, *Circulation* 125:3092–3098, 2012; Bonow RO et al, editors: *Braunwald's heart disease: a textbook of cardiovascular medicine,* ed 9, Philadelphia, 2012, Saunders; The Emerging Risk Factor Collaboration: C-reactive protein, fibrinogen, and cardiovascular disease prediction, *New Engl J Med* 367(14):1310–1320, 2012; Yang Q et al: Trends in cardiovascular health metrics and associations with all-cause and CVD mortality among US adults, *JAMA* 307(12):1273–1283, 2012.

particular, elevated homocysteine levels (which increase platelet aggregation) and high C-reactive protein (CRP) levels have been implicated (CRP is a biologic marker for inflammation and is associated with increased risk for CAD) (Horak et al, 2011). Additional recognized risk factors include metabolic syndrome (central obesity, hypertension, insulin resistance, and dyslipidemia) and obesity (Hillis et al, 2011; Roger et al, 2012). Hypertension and obesity increase the workload of the heart; obesity may also increase the risk for postoperative infection because adipose tissue vascularizes poorly. Additionally, a growing percentage of the population is aging. Age, in and of itself, rarely contraindicates intervention, but comorbidities often associated with older individuals constitute additional risk factors and areas—for example, cognitive impairment, depression, and decision-making capacity—that may require investigation (Chow et al, 2012).

Among the newer biomarkers denoting cardiovascular diseases are the *natriuretic peptides*—cardiac hormones synthesized and secreted by the atrium (atrial natriuretic peptide [ANP]) and the ventricle (B-type natriuretic peptide [BNP]). Discovered in 1981, natriuretic peptides have a regulatory effect that causes myocardial relaxation in response to acute increases in ventricular volume. Measurement of circulating peptides is increasingly used to identify heart failure and sudden cardiac death. Another biomarker under intensive study as a risk factor is lipoprotein(a) (Lp[a]), which has been identified from genetic studies as a causal link to MI; niacin has been shown to reduce the level of Lp(a) in some individuals (Hall, 2010).

Genetic risk factors for CAD and other cardiac disorders have been identified and are undergoing extensive study (Judge, 2012). Genetic studies have created a burgeoning body of knowledge about genetic mutations associated with risk factors such as CRP and possible pathways linking inflammatory processes with CAD (Kim et al, 2011; Roberts and Stewart, 2012a). Genetic risk variants mediate their risk in multiple ways; researchers have discovered that there are more unknown mechanisms than known mechanisms such as those associated with hypertension or lipids (Roberts and Stewart, 2012b). Soon an integral component of the preoperative assessment likely will include a genetic profile.

The risk for complications and major adverse cardiac events (MACEs) after cardiac surgery also appears to vary somewhat depending on gender (Hillis et al 2011; Newby and Douglas, 2012; Wenger, 2012). Investigations of risk factors in men and women for sternal wound infection have identified three significant risk factors that occur at significantly different rates in men and women: smoking, use of a single IMA, and age more than 70 years. Smoking and the use of a single IMA for bypass grafting are more common risk factors in men compared with women; women tend to be older than men at the time of surgery (Newby and Douglas, 2012). Fewer MACEs arose in women undergoing coronary bypass surgery without the use of cardiopulmonary bypass (CPB)—"off-pump" procedures—compared with surgery with CPB; however, malignant ventricular dysrhythmias (e.g., ventricular tachycardia), a calcified aorta, and preoperative renal failure are poor prognostic signs in women (Newby and Douglas, 2012). These findings should be incorporated into patient and family teaching plans with recommendations for lifestyle changes as indicated.

In addition to health status and risk factors, the perioperative nurse reviews patient medication history with particular attention to vasoactive drugs, anticoagulants, and other medications that can affect surgery. Nurses should note that patients taking aspirin and other antiplatelet drugs (such as 2b/IIIa inhibitors) may require intraoperative replacement of platelets. Lipid-lowering drugs (statins) have shown cardiovascular benefits, but in high doses (i.e., 80 mg, compared to moderate doses of 40 mg), they have been associated with new onset diabetes mellitus (Preiss et al, 2011). Patients taking herbal medicines may be at risk for increased bleeding, hypoglycemia, or other complications, depending on the specific side effects of some herbal drugs (see Chapter 30).

Patient knowledge and understanding of cardiovascular disease and related risk factors and their effect on functional, physiologic, and psychologic status should also be part of the perioperative nursing assessment. The patient's personal strengths, external resources, and coping strategies are important subjects to consider. The perioperative nurse also notes any cultural, ethnic, spiritual, or religious beliefs that appear relevant to perioperative patient care.

Physical Examination. Physical assessment provides the perioperative nurse with baseline information about potential problems that might require intervention. Normal, age-specific changes in very young and elderly populations must be differentiated from pathologic conditions. Chapters 26 and 27 provide extensive age-related considerations.

In addition to age-specific changes, a growing number of adults with acquired heart disease underwent surgery in childhood to repair congenital cardiac lesions (Webb et al, 2012). For example, patients with a previous Blalock-Taussig shunt for tetralogy of Fallot (see Chapter 26) may have altered pulmonary and subclavian artery anatomy. Likewise, patients with a mechanical closure device inserted for an atrial septal defect may be at risk for endocardial injury if the heart is retracted or otherwise manipulated too forcefully. The nurse must be aware that anatomic anomalies associated with the original congenital defect, or its subsequent repair, may mandate alteration of the current surgical plan. Consultation with the surgeon can alert the cardiac team to anticipate different anatomy (and surgical landmarks), special supplies and prosthetic materials, and potential complications.

Before beginning a review of systems, it is helpful to assess the patient's functional capacity. How are activities of daily living accomplished? What are the barriers that make independent living difficult? How are activities performed when there are disabilities? What support systems are available? What educational resources are available? These and other questions will alert the clinician to the need for referrals and other resources to help the patient achieve optimal outcomes.

A systems review often starts with the skin. The appearance of the skin offers clues to cardiovascular status. Dryness, coolness, diaphoresis, paleness, edema, poor capillary refill, bruising, and petechiae may reflect impaired cardiovascular function. Visual problems and headaches may relate to inadequate cardiac output, atherosclerotic disease, peripheral vascular disease, aortic valve stenosis, or medications such as digitalis. The presence of chronic or local infection must be identified; if untreated, these are potential sources of postoperative infection. Nutritional status assessment (including metabolic syndrome) helps to determine increased risk for infection, skin breakdown, impaired wound healing, and other complications.

The patient's level of consciousness, memory, comprehension, and emotional status require assessment. Confusion, restlessness, slurred speech, numbness, and paralysis may signal impaired perfusion. The perioperative nurse should note their presence preoperatively and communicate this to nurses receiving the patient postoperatively.

During respiratory assessment the perioperative nurse should note the use of accessory muscles or nostril flaring and should auscultate breath sounds. Adventitious sounds such as crackles and wheezes may point to pulmonary edema. Orthopnea, shortness of breath, or dyspnea may require elevation of the head of the stretcher and assistance during transfer onto the OR bed. If the patient is receiving oxygen, the flow rate and method of administration should be observed.

Alleviating pain is a prime consideration in the care of the cardiovascular patient because pain is a myocardial stressor. A patient with angina may arrive in the OR after nitroglycerin tablets have been administered or transdermal patches applied. Cold also increases the workload of the heart because the shivering that accompanies chilling elevates the metabolic rate; the patient should be kept warm.

Heart sounds, murmurs, and friction rubs provide clues to congenital, ischemic, valvular heart disease, or pericarditis. The patient may experience palpitations. Apical, radial, and femoral pulses also reflect cardiac function, and their rate, rhythm, and quality should be determined. The presence of cyanosis or peripheral edema should be noted.

Blood pressure is an important assessment consideration. The hypertensive patient may have left ventricular hypertrophy, and the hypotensive patient may display changes in neurologic, gastrointestinal, and renal function. Blood pressures should be checked bilaterally. Unequal pressures in the arms may be a contraindication for the use of the IMA as a bypass graft on the side of the lower blood pressure, where perfusion may not be optimal. Radial and ulnar artery pulses should be checked bilaterally when the radial artery is to be used as a bypass graft. Patients with dissections or aneurysms may have unequal carotid, femoral, brachial, or radial artery blood pressures when the lesion occludes one or more of these vascular branches.

Cardiac function affects all the body's organ systems; therefore, assessment of the patient should be comprehensive whenever possible. A thorough assessment also alerts the physician and perioperative nurse to the need for special diagnostic tests and laboratory procedures.

Diagnostic Studies. Most patients referred for surgery have had clinical evaluations, including invasive and noninvasive studies (Box 25-3). After the history and physical assessment, a resting electrocardiogram (ECG) follows. An exercise ECG (stress test) is often undertaken because ST-segment changes indicating myocardial ischemia may be apparent only during or after exercise. In patients with intractable dysrhythmias, electrophysiology (EP) studies may help locate irritable atrial or ventricular foci that can be surgically ablated, excised, or controlled with pharmacologic therapy. EP studies also may determine the need for internal defibrillators or antitachycardia devices. Bradycardia may indicate the need for pacemaker insertion.

Chest radiography provides information about the size of the cardiac chambers, thoracic aorta, and pulmonary vasculature as well as the presence of calcium in valves, pericardium, coronary arteries, and aorta (Figure 25-8). Lateral chest radiographs of patients with prior sternal surgery show the chest wires and extent of pericardial adhesions. Magnetic resonance imaging (MRI) enables assessment of myocardial viability and also can image vascular structures with MRI angiograms that provide great clarity (Figure 25-9, *A*). In patients with suspected aortic or other vascular abnormalities, a computed tomography (CT) scan of the chest with intravenous

---

BOX 25-3

Diagnostic Tests Commonly Performed for Cardiovascular Disorders

Noninvasive*
- Resting ECG
- Exercise ECG (stress test)
- Chest radiography
- Echocardiogram (TTE, TEE)
- Epiaortic ultrasound (sternum already opened)
- Carotid Doppler echocardiogram
- Resting MUGA
- Exercise thallium
- Exercise MUGA
- CT scan
- PET scan with stress
- CMRI, MRA

Invasive
- Aortography
- Arteriography
- Digital subtraction angiography
- Electrophysiology
- Cardiac catheterization
- Ventriculography
- Endomyocardial biopsy

*When dye is injected into the vascular system, the test is considered semi-invasive.
CT, Computed tomography; *CMRI,* cardiovascular magnetic resonance imaging; *ECG,* electrocardiogram; *MRA,* magnetic resonance angiogram; *MUGA,* multiple uptake gated acquisition; *PET,* positron emission tomography; *TEE,* transesophageal echocardiogram; *TTE,* transthoracic echocardiogram.
Modified from Bonow RO et al, editors: *Braunwald's heart disease: a textbook of cardiovascular medicine,* ed 9, Philadelphia, 2012, Saunders; Pagana KD, Pagana TJ: *Mosby's diagnostic and laboratory test reference,* ed 11, St Louis, 2012, Mosby.

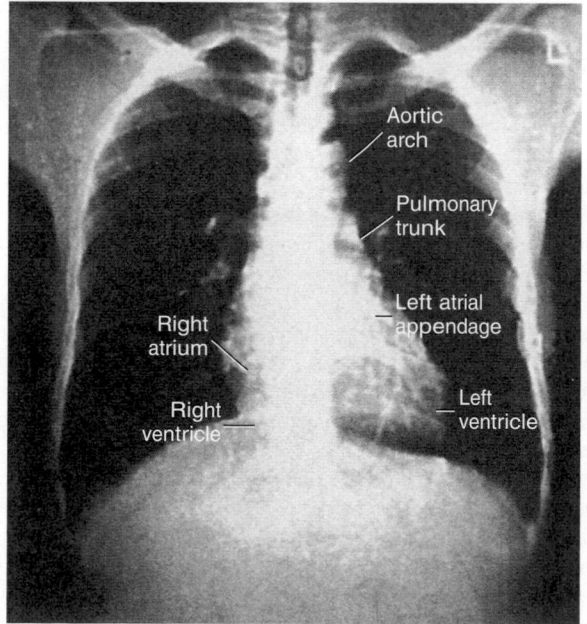

FIGURE 25-8 Anteroposterior chest radiograph (normal).

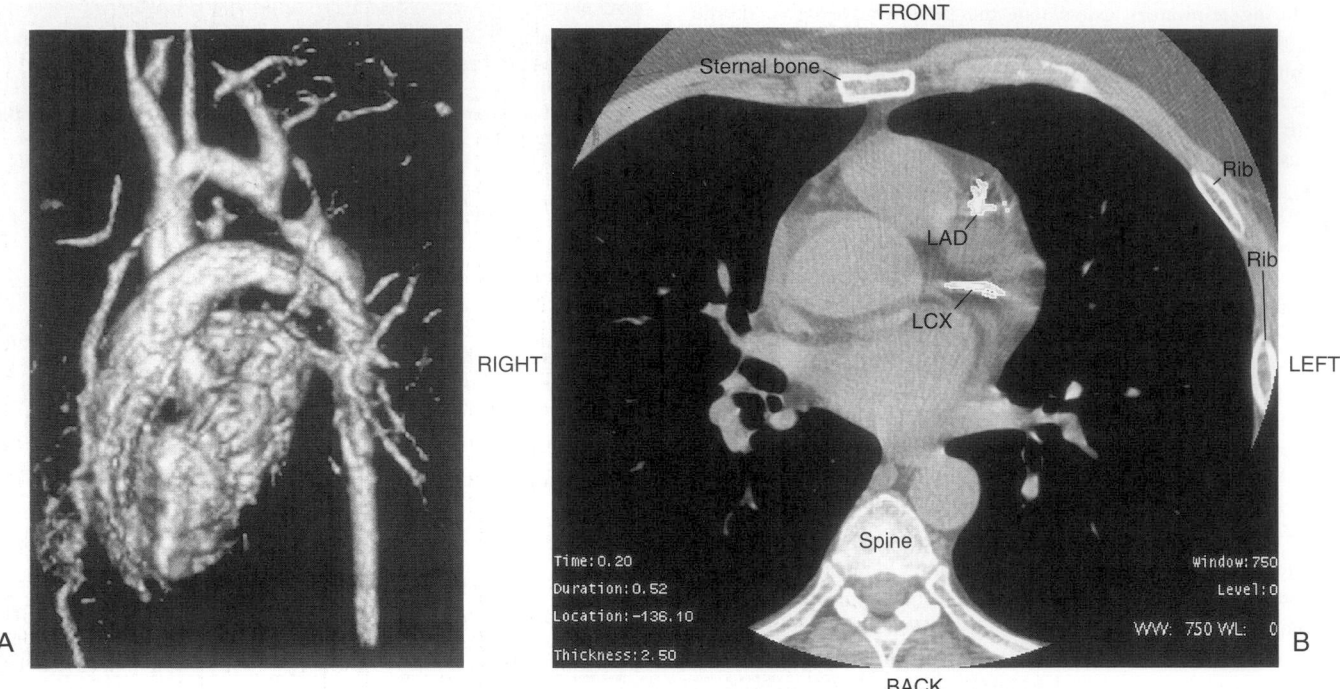

FIGURE 25-9 A, Three-dimensional reconstruction of a contrast medium–enhanced magnetic resonance angiogram of the thoracic aorta, illustrating a severe coarctation (narrowing) of the aorta. **B,** High-resolution cross-sectional computed tomography (CT) scan of the heart, illustrating calcification within the left anterior descending *(LAD)* coronary artery and left circumflex *(LCX)* coronary artery.

injection of a contrast medium creates x-ray serial "slices" of the body area under study (see Figure 25-9, *B*). CT angiography is especially useful to image the aorta and the great vessels. CT images of the coronary arteries are used increasingly to identify areas of coronary calcification (shown in Figure 25-9, *B*), a recognized CV risk factor. One study demonstrated the value of coronary artery calcium scoring to identify patients who may be asymptomatic for CAD, but are at risk for increased mortality (Tota-Maharaj et al, 2012).

CT scans may be contraindicated in very unstable patients because their position in the tubelike scanner makes patient access difficult. Less frequently performed is arteriography with radiographic contrast dye to determine the size and location of the lesion and the site of the intimal tear in aortic dissections (Figure 25-10); digital subtraction angiography (DSA) provides clear images and requires less contrast material.

Echocardiography is a noninvasive test that evaluates both the structure and the function of the heart by transmitting sound waves to the heart and measuring those sound waves reflected back to the transducer (Figure 25-11). Sound waves undergo processing by the transducer, which creates visual images of the structure's movements. This test enables assessment of ventricular and valvular function before, during, and after surgery, and determination of the degree of valvular stenosis or regurgitation. It can also demonstrate a tumor, thrombus, or air in the ventricular or atrial cavities. Two-dimensional and color-flow Doppler techniques have greatly enhanced functional assessment of valvular performance and carotid artery stenoses. Echocardiography is the gold standard to diagnose mitral stenosis, and its use to assess other valvular disorders and congenital heart disease is widespread. Transesophageal echocardiography (TEE) also allows evaluation of the effectiveness of valve repairs and other surgical procedures (Table 25-1).

FIGURE 25-10 Aortogram of ascending aortic dissection, with aortic valve insufficiency. Note regurgitation of dye into left ventricle.

FIGURE 25-11 Two-dimensional echocardiography showing two views of the cardiac chambers. *LA,* Left atrium; *LV,* left ventricle; *MV,* mitral valve; *RA,* right atrium; *RV,* right ventricle.

FIGURE 25-12 Right anterior oblique (RAO) view of left coronary artery injection demonstrating high-grade stenosis of the left anterior descending coronary artery *(arrow)* at the lead of the first septal perforator.

Radionuclide imaging illustrates wall motion and blood flow through the heart and quantifies cardiac function. Patients generally tolerate these noninvasive techniques well, especially when they may be too unstable to withstand a cardiac catheterization. These techniques may also serve as a complement to catheterization.

Cardiac catheterization provides definitive information about the extent and location of ischemic heart disease, acting as an adjunct to echocardiography to diagnose valvular heart disease (Kern, 2011). A radiopaque plastic catheter is inserted retrograde through the aortic valve into the left side of the heart by a percutaneous puncture or a cutdown to the vessels of the brachial artery (Sones technique) or the femoral artery (Judkins technique). The right side of the heart is approached percutaneously by the superior or inferior vena caval route. To perform coronary angiography that demonstrates intracoronary anatomy, a contrast medium is injected into the coronary ostia. Obstructions (Figure 25-12), flow, and distal perfusion are assessable. Ventriculography illustrates contractile weaknesses of the ventricles as well as shunting and regurgitation of blood. These studies enable assessment of the degree of myocardial dysfunction and planning for interventions such as CABG, valve repair or replacement, repair of congenital anomalies, and cardiac transplantation. The cardiologist can compute the orifice of a stenosed valve or determine the degree of regurgitation of an incompetent valve.

Ventricular, atrial, and pulmonary pressures are recorded, and cardiac output and ejection fraction estimated (Box 25-4 and Table 25-2). Oxygen saturation of cardiac chambers and the ratio of pulmonary to systemic blood flow (Q_p/Q_s) are calculated for patients with shunts and congenital or acquired defects. Cinearteriograms record the movement of the heart, and cut films or digitized versions of the cines may be displayed during surgery.

The cardiac catheterization laboratory also performs percutaneous coronary interventional (PCI) therapies for evolving and acute MIs (Morrow and Boden, 2012). Coronary thrombolysis with fibrinolytic drugs can dissolve fresh blood clots and reopen (i.e., recanalize) the artery; prescription of antiplatelet agents such as aspirin, dipyridamole, and clopidogrel often can block platelet aggregation that otherwise can lead to restenosis. Percutaneous transluminal coronary angioplasty (PTCA) followed by insertion of intracoronary (bare metal or drug-eluting) stents is often performed to dilate and maintain the patency of the recanalized artery. In many

---

TABLE 25-1

Echocardiograpy Findings

Transesophageal Echocardiography (TEE)

Monitoring hemodynamic function	Assess ventricular, valve function, thoracic aorta; diastolic dysfunction; identify retained intracardiac air (to guide removal); guide insertion of intra-aortic balloon pump, ventricular assist device
Intraoperative evaluation	Valve function, cardiac structures, thoracic aorta; identify calcium and/or atheromas in area of aortic arterial cannulation site; guide cannulation entry into aorta; evaluate post-repair/replacement valve function, valve regurgitation
Measurement	Blood flow velocity

Modified from Bonow RO et al, editors: *Braunwald's heart disease: a textbook of cardiovascular medicine,* ed 9, Philadelphia, 2012, Saunders; Nussmeier NA et al: Anesthesia for cardiac surgical procedures. In Miller RD et al, editors: *Miller's anesthesia,* ed 7, Philadelphia, 2009, Churchill Livingstone.

BOX 25-4

Hemodynamic Concepts

Afterload: Impedance, or resistance, the heart must overcome to pump blood into the systemic circulation; left ventricular wall tension during systole; systemic vascular resistance.

Cardiac index (CI): Cardiac output corrected for differences in body size.

Cardiac output (CO): Amount of blood (in liters) ejected by left ventricle per minute; product of heart rate times stroke volume.

Contractility: Inotropic state of the heart; ability of the ventricle to pump.

Ejection fraction (EF): Percentage of end-diastolic volume ejected into systemic circulation; indicator of ventricular function.

Preload: Volume and pressure of blood in the ventricle at the end of diastole. Central venous pressure (CVP) measures right-sided heart preload; pulmonary artery wedge pressure (PAWP) indirectly measures left-sided heart preload.

instances these interventions may obviate the need for surgical bypass grafting, although the progressive nature of CAD may eventually lead to patients requiring surgical revascularization.

EP studies enable diagnosis of conduction disturbances and allow therapeutic interventions, such as radiofrequency or cryologic ablation of foci producing atrial fibrillation or accessory pathways seen in Wolff-Parkinson-White syndrome. Insertion of a pacemaker for bradydysrhythmias or an internal cardioverter defibrillator for ventricular tachydysrhythmias commonly occurs in EP laboratories. Insertion of these devices, however, may require an OR when percutaneous access is unfeasible or when concomitant cardiac surgery is performed.

Laboratory Tests. Preoperative laboratory tests enable assessment of physiologic function (see Appendix A). Hematologic tests include a detailed coagulation profile to uncover hemorrhagic disorders. In patients who have been taking aspirin or dipyridamole, platelet activity is decreased; this alerts the perioperative nurse to anticipate prolonged bleeding, which will require replacement.

TABLE 25-2

Cardiac Catheterization Data

Hemodynamic Data	Normal Values		
Flow			
Cardiac output (CO)	3-6 L/min		
Cardiac index (CI)	2.8-4.2 L/min/m^2		
Ejection fraction (EF)	60%-70%		
Left ventricular end-diastolic volume (LVEDV)	90-180 mL		
Stroke volume (SV)	60-130 mL/beat		
Stroke volume index (SVI)	35-70 mL/beat/m^2		
	Systolic	**Diastolic**	**Mean**
Resistances (Wood Units)			
Systemic vascular resistance (SVR)	<20		
Total pulmonary resistance	<3.5		
Pulmonary vascular resistance (PVR)	<2.0		
Shunts (Q_p/Q_s)			
Pulmonary flow/systemic flow		1:1	
% Oxygen Saturation			
Venae cavae		70	
Right atrium		70	
Right ventricle		70	
Pulmonary artery		70	
Pulmonary veins		97	
Left atrium		97	
Left ventricle		97	
Aorta		97	
Valve Orifices (Adult) (cm^2)			
Aortic	2-4		
Mitral	4-6		
Tricuspid	10		
Pressures (mm Hg)			
Venae cavae			0-5
Right atrium (RA)			2-6
Right ventricle (RV)	20-30	0-5	
Pulmonary artery (PA)	15-28	5-16	10-15
Pulmonary artery wedge pressure (PAWP)			4-12
Left atrium (LA)			4-12

TABLE 25-2

Cardiac Catheterization Data—cont'd

	Systolic	Diastolic	Mean
Left ventricle (LV)	90-140	0-5	
Left ventricular end-diastolic pressure (LVEDP)			4-12
Aorta	120-140	60-80	70-90
Brachial artery	90-140	60-90	
Femoral artery	125	75	

	Findings
Angiographic Data	
Coronary arteries	Anatomy/function of coronary vascular bed; distal coronary flow; arteriovenous (AV) fistula; atherosclerosis; anomalous origin of coronary arteries
Ventriculography	Anatomy/function of ventricles and associated structures; LV aneurysm; congenital abnormalities; valvular stenosis/regurgitation; shunts
Valvular angiography	Intact mitral/tricuspid complex; valvular incompetence/stenosis/regurgitation
Pulmonary angiography	Pulmonary embolism; congenital abnormalities
Aortography	Patency of aortic branches; normal mobility, competence, and anatomy of aortic valve; aneurysms: saccular, fusiform; origin of aortic dissection; shunts or anomalous connections; congenital defect or obstructions

Modified from Pagana KD, Pagana TJ: *Mosby's diagnostic and laboratory test reference*, ed 11, St Louis, 2012, Mosby; Bonow RO et al, editors: *Braunwald's heart disease: a textbook of cardiovascular medicine*, ed 9, Philadelphia, 2012, Saunders; Kern MJ: *Cardiac catheterization handbook*, ed 5, Philadelphia, 2011, Saunders; Nussmeier NA et al: Anesthesia for cardiac surgical procedures. In Miller RD et al, editors: *Miller's anesthesia*, ed 7, Philadelphia, 2009, Churchill Livingstone.

After determination of the patient's blood type, an appropriate order to the blood bank follows. The blood undergoes testing for viral contamination and for cold antibodies that could produce agglutination of the patient's blood during surgery and after patient cooling to hypothermic temperatures. A monitored blood refrigerator stores blood brought to the OR suite before surgery. Although autotransfusion techniques have reduced the use of blood bank products, the occasional, emergent need for blood requires immediate availability of blood bank packed red blood cells.

Liver and kidney function test results may be abnormal in patients with chronic heart failure, possibly because congestion related to right heart failure in the former and reduced blood flows in the latter occur with some frequency. Progressive improvement in hepatic and renal function often follows successful operative intervention. The use of statins and other cholesterol-reducing drugs that can adversely impair hepatic function also alerts the nurse to review liver function laboratory results (Pagana and Pagana, 2012). Blood glucose levels require testing, monitoring, and control, especially in patients with impaired glucose metabolism and both type 1 and type 2 diabetes.

Additional perioperative laboratory examinations may include arterial blood gases and enzyme biomarkers of myocardial damage (e.g., troponin I and troponin T; creatine kinase MB isoenzyme, known as *MB bands*), particularly with persistent angina (Canty, 2012). Troponin levels are the focus of a revised definition of MI. This new definition incorporates specific troponin levels and at least one of the following criteria: symptoms of ischemia, new ST-/T-wave changes or left bundle branch block on the ECG, pathologic Q waves on ECG, evidence of loss of viable myocardium or regional wall motion on diagnostic images, and documentation of an intra-coronary thrombus (Thygesen et al, 2012). This new definition differentiates between infarction and injury. The distinction is important to plan treatment; it also may affect the ability to obtain insurance and participate in secondary prevention (Mitka, 2012).

Pulmonary function tests may help determine baseline data and plan postoperative care. The use of extracorporeal circulation and associated inflammatory responses, as well as the stasis of lung secretions that accompany prolonged surgery, may impair postoperative respiratory function.

Nursing Diagnosis

After a comprehensive review of individual patient data, the perioperative nurse identifies relevant nursing diagnoses, from which the perioperative plan for patient care derives (Sample Plan of Care on pages 944-945).

Nursing diagnoses related to the care of patients undergoing cardiac surgery might include the following (Association of peri-Operative Registered Nurses [AORN], 2013; Petersen, 2011; Seifert, 2008, 2013):

- Decreased Cardiac Output related to emotional (fear), sensory (pain), or physiologic (electrical, mechanical, or structural) factors
- Risk for Infection related to surgical incision(s), catheters and intravascular lines, and altered cardiac function
- Risk for Perioperative Positioning Injury related to, for example, preexisting musculoskeletal malformation, insecure attachment to OR bed
- Risk for Contamination related to break in aseptic technique, preexisting infection, self-contamination (e.g., contamination by patient's own groin material)
- Risk for Bleeding related to surgical incision(s), tissue dissection, altered coagulation function, and inadvertent hypothermia
- Deficient Knowledge related to physiologic effects of the cardiac disorder, proposed surgical procedures, and immediate perioperative events
- Risk for Impaired Tissue Integrity (myocardial, peripheral, renal, and cerebral) related to surgery, hypothermia, CPB, or surgical particulate or air emboli

SAMPLE PLAN OF CARE

Nursing Diagnosis
Decreased Cardiac Output related to emotional (fear), sensory (pain), or physiologic (electrical, mechanical, or structural) factors

Outcome
The patient's cardiac function will be consistent with or improved from baseline levels established preoperatively as evidenced by hemodynamic indicators (blood pressure, oxygenation, ECG) within expected range; warm, dry skin; and urine output more than 30 mL/hr.

Interventions
- Identify baseline cardiac status.
- Use monitoring equipment to assess cardiac status.
- Identify and report the presence of implantable cardiac devices.
- Institute anxiety-reduction measures, address fear-producing concerns, clarify misconceptions, and answer questions.
- Measure pain level with pain scale; provide comfort measures and pharmacologic interventions as ordered; confirm and document degree of pain relief, measures used, and any medications administered.
- Check results of clotting function, coagulation profile, and electrolyte values; report abnormalities.
- Monitor blood pressures (arterial, central venous pressure [CVP], pulmonary artery wedge pressure [PAWP]) and ECG.
- Maintain an adequate supply of and assist with administration of replacement blood or blood products.
- Follow institutional protocol for allergic blood reaction; document same according to institutional protocol.
- Have inotropic and antidysrhythmic medications available; assist with administration; document same according to institutional protocol.
- Monitor, report, and record urine output and chest tube drainage; keep tubes and catheters patent.
- Have available defibrillator (with appropriate internal and external paddles and settings), fibrillator, external pacemaker, temporary epicardial pacemaker leads, and appropriate ECG cables for cardioversion and intra-aortic balloon pump.
- Evaluate postoperative cardiac status.

Nursing Diagnosis
Risk for Infection related to surgical incision(s), catheters and intravascular lines, and altered cardiac function

Outcome
The patient will be free from signs and symptoms of infection at the surgical or other incisional sites as evidenced by absence of redness, edema, purulent incisional drainage, or untoward postoperative temperature elevation.

Interventions
- Administer prescribed prophylactic treatments.
- Verify that prescribed preoperative prophylactic antibiotic has been administered within 1 hour of the surgical incision; document same according to institutional protocol.
- Assess individual patient risk factors for infection.
- Encourage teaching and reinforce previous teaching regarding deep-breathing and coughing exercises.
- Classify surgical wound; document same according to institutional protocol.
- Implement and maintain aseptic technique.
- Initiate and maintain traffic control.
- Minimize the length of an invasive procedure by prioritizing, organizing, and planning care.
- Completely drape central line insertion sites.
- Dress all invasive arterial and venous lines.
- Perform skin preparation, using care to prevent pooling of solution; implement fire safety precautions during prepping. Prepare anatomic area to knees (or lower if leg vein needed) with antimicrobial antiseptic agent; document same according to institutional protocol.
- Use depilatories or electric clippers to remove hair at the surgical site; avoid shaving with razors.
- Monitor aseptic technique; correct breaks; accurately reclassify surgical wound on perioperative nursing record if a break in technique occurs.
- Have available prescribed topical antibiotics; document their administration according to institutional protocol.
- Manage culture specimen collection as indicated; use safe specimen management practices. Document specimens collected according to institutional protocol.
- Protect from cross-contamination.
- If the OR bed is raised, lowered, or turned from side to side, take measures to maintain sterility of field.
- Protect sterility of closed urinary drainage system.
- Maintain continuous surveillance.
- Provide or apply surgical dressings to the wound and invasive device sites.
- Maintain sterility of instrument setup until patient is discharged from the OR.
- During patient rewarming, avoid excessive heat loss: cover exposed areas, irrigate with warm solutions, and increase room temperature.
- Use forced-air warming systems before and after period of induced hypothermia.
- Monitor for signs and symptoms of infection.

Nursing Diagnosis
Risk for Perioperative Positioning Injury

Outcome
The patient will be free from signs and symptoms of injury related to surgical position as evidenced by the absence of acquired neuromuscular impairment and tissue necrosis.

Interventions
- Obtain and prepare appropriate positioning accessories; verify that these are clean and in working order.
- Identify any physical alterations that require additional precautions for procedure-specific positioning.
- Verify the presence of prosthetics or corrective devices; document same according to institutional protocol.
- Position the patient, maintaining proper body alignment.
- Pad and protect vulnerable neurovascular bundles and dependent pressure areas.
- Prevent pooling of skin preparation agents at bedlines.
- Pad thermia blanket to prevent direct contact with patient skin.
- Keep all OR bed surfaces dry and wrinkle-free.
- Ensure patency and security of peripheral and central lines, catheters, and ESU dispersive pad on positional changes.
- Have adequate personnel to assist with patient transfer to and from the OR bed and positional changes; lift (do not pull) patient during all positioning maneuvers.
- Safely secure patient to OR bed; ensure that safety straps are not too tightly placed yet maintain patient stability.
- Confirm correct position during time-out.
- Evaluate for signs and symptoms of injury as a result of positioning.

Nursing Diagnosis
Risk for Contamination related to break in aseptic technique, pre-existing infection, self-contamination (e.g., contamination by patient's own groin material).

Outcome
The patient will be free from signs and symptoms of contamination as evidenced by maintenance of aseptic technique, timely treatment

SAMPLE PLAN OF CARE—cont'd

for preexisting infection, separation of "clean" and "dirty" areas of the field, confirmation of integrity of implants (e.g., prosthetic heart valves, vascular grafts).

Interventions

- Monitor asepsis; correct as indicated (e.g., change contaminated glove).
- Identify patient infection (e.g., methicillin-resistant *Staphylococcus aureus* [MRSA]).
- Confirm that antibiotics have been infused before incision.
- Assess patient concerns or fears about postoperative infection prevention practices.
- Confine and contain instruments used in the groin or leg.
- Change gown and gloves when moving from lower extremities to chest or after moving from one side of OR bed to other side (e.g., after holding the heart).
- Confirm that temperature-sensing package inserts have not changed (indicating ambient temperatures too high or too low for proper prosthesis storage).
- Document implants according to institutional protocol.

Nursing Diagnosis

Risk for Bleeding related to surgical incision(s), tissue dissection, altered coagulation function, and inadvertent hypothermia

Outcome

The patient will be free from excessive bleeding as evidenced by chest tube drainage less than 100 mL/hr, dressings dry and intact, normal coagulation function studies (or undergoing replacement treatment for deficient clotting factors), and normal body temperature.

Interventions

- Review results of clotting function and coagulation profile; report abnormalities.
- Check patient history for use of anticoagulant medication and other drugs affecting bleeding time and clotting function.
- Measure and report blood loss (e.g., suction, sponges).
- Use autotransfusion system per protocol.
- Have topical hemostatic agents available.
- Monitor, report, and record chest tube drainage; keep tubes patent.
- Before postoperative transfer, alert surgeon to chest tube drainage in excess of 100 mL/hr.
- Maintain adequate supply and assist with administration of replacement blood, blood products, and clotting factors.
- Follow institutional protocol for allergic blood reaction.
- Adjust room temperature as needed; room temperature should be warm (68° to 75° F [20° to 24° C]) before and after completion of cardiopulmonary bypass.
- Apply dressings to all incision sites (chest incision, conduit excision sites, and central line insertion sites).
- Monitor for development of inadvertent hypothermia.
- Evaluate for signs and symptoms of excessive bleeding.

Nursing Diagnosis

Deficient Knowledge related to the physiologic effects of the cardiac disorder, proposed surgical procedures, and immediate perioperative events

Outcome

The patient will demonstrate knowledge of the physiologic responses to the cardiac disorder (at his or her level of understanding), the proposed surgical treatment, and the immediate postoperative events as evidenced by verbalization of disease state, purpose of surgery, sequence of events, anticipated outcomes, and recovery process.

Interventions

- Explain or describe the following events; solicit feedback from patient:
  - Purpose and expectations of surgery
  - Disease state producing need for surgery
  - Sequence of events during perioperative period
  - Recovery and rehabilitation process
  - Nothing-per-mouth (NPO) status
  - Administration and effects of preoperative medication
  - Transport to OR
  - Preoperative unit
  - Insertion of peripheral, arterial, and venous lines
  - OR environment (temperature, room furniture and equipment, sounds of monitors and other machines, staff functions, induction of anesthesia)
  - Skin preparation
  - Anticipated length of surgery
  - Minimally invasive versus standard cardiac procedures
  - Surgical ICU and patient status (e.g., unable to talk while intubated and plans for alternative methods of communication)
- Assess knowledge regarding wound care and phases of wound healing.
- Provide information about wound care and anticipated phases of wound healing.
- Determine patient's desire for additional knowledge (respect denial).
- Answer questions; clarify misperceptions.
- Know where family or significant others will be waiting during surgery; provide communication per institutional protocol.
- Evaluate response to information about wound care and phases of wound healing.

Nursing Diagnosis

Risk for Impaired Tissue Integrity (myocardial, peripheral, renal, and cerebral) related to surgery, hypothermia, CPB, surgical particulate, or air emboli

Outcome

The patient's myocardial, peripheral, renal, and cerebral tissue integrity will be adequate or improved as evidenced by absence of new electrocardiograph manifestations of infarction, the presence of palpable peripheral pulses, adequate urine output, and a clear or improving sensorium postoperatively.

Interventions

- Identify baseline tissue perfusion.
- Assess factors related to risks for ineffective tissue perfusion.
- Place padded thermia blanket on OR bed.
- Preoperatively, provide warm blankets as required.
- Expose only those body areas required for surgical intervention.
- Use forced-air warming systems during period requiring normothermia (keep patient warm before and after arrest; warm throughout for "warm heart" surgery).
- Monitor patient's temperature (esophageal, pulmonary, rectal, bladder, or ventricular septal).
- Adjust room temperature as needed.
- Inspect cardiopulmonary bypass lines for patency and presence of particulate matter; alert the surgeon as indicated.
- Use solutions of appropriate temperature when irrigating the heart (cold during hypothermia arrest; warm before and after arrest); warm throughout for warm heart surgery.
- Avoid large ice particles on heart.
- Evaluate postoperative tissue perfusion.
- Evaluate progress of wound healing as applicable.

CPB, Cardiopulmonary bypass; *ECG,* electrocardiogram; *ESU,* electrosurgical unit; *ICU,* intensive care unit.

Outcome Identification

Outcomes identified for the selected nursing diagnoses could include:

- The patient's cardiac function will be consistent with or improved from baseline levels established preoperatively as evidenced by hemodynamic indicators (blood pressure, oxygenation, ECG) within expected range; warm, dry skin; and urine output more than 30 mL/hr.
- The patient will be free from signs and symptoms of infection at the surgical or other incisional sites as evidenced by absence of redness, edema, purulent incisional drainage, or untoward postoperative temperature elevation.
- The patient will be free from signs and symptoms of injury related to surgical position as evidenced by the absence of acquired neuromuscular impairment and tissue necrosis.
- The patient will be free from signs and symptoms of contamination as evidenced by maintenance of aseptic technique, timely treatment for preexisting infection, separation of "clean" and "dirty" areas of the field, and confirmation of integrity of implants (e.g., prosthetic heart valves, vascular grafts).
- The patient will be free from excessive bleeding as evidenced by chest tube drainage less than 100 mL/hr, dressings dry and intact, normal coagulation function studies (or undergoing replacement treatment for deficient clotting factors), and normal body temperature.
- The patient will demonstrate knowledge of the physiologic responses to the cardiac disorder (at his or her level of understanding), the proposed surgical treatment, and the immediate perioperative events as evidenced by verbalization of disease state, purpose of surgery, sequence of events, anticipated outcomes, and recovery process.
- The patient's myocardial, peripheral, renal, and cerebral tissue integrity will be adequate or improved as evidenced by absence of new electrocardiograph manifestations of infarction, the presence of palpable peripheral pulses, adequate urine output, and a clear or improving sensorium postoperatively.

Additional nursing diagnoses based on individual patient assessment should have a corresponding outcome statement. The outcome should be measurable, with criteria by which to evaluate achievement. For example, for the outcome "The patient's cardiac function will be consistent with or improved from baseline levels established preoperatively as evidenced by blood pressure within expected range; warm, dry skin; and urine output more than 30 to 50 mL per hour," the perioperative nurse might identify criteria such as vital signs and hemodynamic status consistent with or better than preoperative parameters; fluid and electrolyte balance consistent with preoperative levels; adequate urine output; normal temperature and pink mucosa; absence of rate, rhythm, or conduction disturbances; absence of iatrogenic injury to the heart; and normal levels of clotting parameters. Each criterion evidences achievement of the outcome. Outcome evaluations should be documented in the perioperative record. Some outcome achievements will occur after the surgical procedure; others will require ongoing evaluation in the postoperative period for adequate measurement. The evaluation section affirmatively mandates ongoing goal measurement by the use of the word "will" rather than stating the outcome as "having been" achieved.

The nursing interventions in the Sample Plan of Care incorporate data elements from AORN's Perioperative Nursing Data Set (PNDS) (Petersen, 2011). With increasing emphasis on correlating patient outcomes with clinical interventions, the PNDS is a valuable resource by which to demonstrate the nurse's ability to influence positive patient outcomes.

Planning

After establishing the diagnoses and outcomes, the perioperative nurse devises a plan of care (see Sample Plan of Care) to achieve the goals set. Patient and family needs, elicited from interviews when possible, are integrated into the planning. The perioperative nurse should then identify criteria specific to the patient for each of the stated outcomes in the Sample Plan of Care.

Implementation

Additional considerations may prove useful to implement the perioperative plan of care for patients undergoing cardiac surgery.

Safety Considerations. The safety of the perioperative patient is a primary responsibility of the nurse. Among important National Patient Safety Goals (NPSGs) is compliance with "briefing," "debriefing," and other components of The Joint Commission's (TJC) Universal Protocol (TJC, 2013). The protocol consists of a checklist that addresses critical components (i.e., patient identification, confirmation of surgical procedure, availability of anticipated devices such as heart valves) that form the basis of a safe operation. Of special importance is promotion of a work culture that encourages asking questions and sharing information.

Equipment must function properly and undergo routine testing by the biomedical engineering department. Supplies should be used according to manufacturers' instructions, and instruments should be regularly scrutinized to ensure that there are no burrs that could injure tissue, that the jaws of vascular and other clamps align properly, and that small items are accounted for at the end of surgery. Toxic material, such as the glutaraldehyde storage solution of bioprosthetic valves, should be thoroughly rinsed before implantation. Monitoring aseptic practices of team members as well as visitors is important to safety.

Staff safety is also important. Protective personal equipment should be worn consistently and properly. Gloves should be used by personnel whenever contact may occur with blood or other body fluids. Injury from inadvertent effects of electrical, chemical, and other potentially hazardous materials within the OR can be minimized by reinforcing safe practices.

Special Facilities. The OR must be large enough to accommodate bulky, highly specialized equipment while maintaining aseptic technique. Multiple electrical outlets, auxiliary lighting, and additional suction outlets should be available. Ceiling-mounted, mobile booms for housing electrosurgical units (ESUs), headlight sources, suction, medical gases, electrical outlets, and other items can reduce floor clutter and enhance the safety of the environment for patients and staff.

A growing number of hybrid suites have been designed that combine the traditional surgical controlled environment and the fluoroscopic imaging capabilities of interventional cardiology laboratories. A typical hybrid procedure may consist of a surgical coronary anastomosis under direct vision or with a robot, combined with percutaneously inserted coronary artery stents under fluoroscopy. Endovascular aneurysm (of the thoracic and abdominal aorta) and percutaneous aortic valve insertion via fluoroscopic imaging are among other procedures performed in hybrid ORs (Kpodonu, 2012).

Instrumentation and Equipment. The basic setup described for thoracic procedures (see Chapter 23) is used, along with specialized cardiovascular instruments and equipment.

Vascular clamps, designed to occlude blood flow partially or completely, must be maintained in good condition if they are to prevent fracture of the delicate tunica intima of the blood vessels and still retain their specific holding qualities. There are many variations in construction of vascular instruments. Jaws may consist of single or double rows of fine, sharp, or blunt teeth or special crosshatching or longitudinal serrations. The working angles of the clamps also vary. All clamps are designed to hold vessels securely, without causing trauma (Figure 25-13).

Minimally invasive procedures require special instrumentation to access the heart through smaller incisions in the anterior and lateral aspects of the chest wall (Figure 25-14). Retractors, dissecting instruments, suturing devices, coronary artery stabilizers, and vascular clamps are available.

Sternal and rib retractors are available to meet specific needs. IMA retractors expose the retrosternal artery bed by elevating the sternal border (Figure 25-15). Some sternal retractors have attachments to provide improved exposure of the LA during mitral valve replacement (MVR) (Figure 25-16). Handheld retractors can also expose the left or RA or the aortic root. Special rib spreaders provide exposure for mini-thoracotomy procedures. Coronary artery stabilizer systems with left ventricular apical suction retractors are widely used for beating heart coronary bypass surgery (described later).

Other equipment commonly used (or available) for cardiac surgery may include the following:

- Sternal saw and motor
- Irrigation fluid cooling/warming machine
- Autotransfusion/cell saver system
- Electrical fibrillator
- Direct current (DC) defibrillator with internal paddles (Figure 25-17) and adhesive external pads
- Thermia unit (mattress or forced-air warming)
- External and internal pulse pacemaker generator (single and dual chamber)
- Epicardial pacemaker leads (temporary)
- Pump oxygenator/CPB machine
- Fiberoptic headlight and light source
- Intra-aortic balloon pump (IABP)
- Mechanical ventricular assist devices (VADs)
- Cryothermal energy ablation source (for atrial fibrillation surgery)
- Radiofrequency energy ablation source (for atrial fibrillation surgery)

FIGURE 25-13 Cardiovascular clamps *(top to bottom):* Semb suture passer, Fogarty cross-clamp (angled), Beck partial occlusion clamps (medium and small), Lambert-Kay partial occlusion clamp.

A   B

FIGURE 25-14 A, Transthoracic DeBakey vascular clamps, designed to pass through the chest wall by way of smaller incisions for minimally invasive procedures. **B,** Close-up views of minimally invasive needle holder, trocar/suture puller, and knot slider.

FIGURE 25-15 Retractor used to elevate sternal border for exposure of the internal mammary artery.

FIGURE 25-16 Sternal self-retaining retractor with attachments for left atrial retraction during mitral valve replacement.

FIGURE 25-17 Internal defibrillator paddles are available in an array of sizes and designs: the paddles may be activated through the handles or by pressing the button on the defibrillator. Smaller internal paddles are used for infants and children.

FIGURE 25-18 Technique for wire closure of the sternum. A variety of closing mechanisms are available. These may consist of monofilament wire (shown), twisted wire cables, or (in some instances) plates and screws. In selected patients in whom disruption may be anticipated, such as elderly, obese, or malnourished patients, two or more heavy bands of nylon may be passed around the sternum and secured by a twisted stainless steel wire in addition to the wire sutures. Use of a figure-of-eight technique is also possible.

- Ultrasonic cutting/coagulation device (Harmonic scalpel)
- TEE probe and monitor
- Endoscopic, video-assisted vein-harvesting system
- Thoracoscopic equipment
- Video equipment
    Lasers (for transmyocardial laser revascularization) and robots (for valve repair) may also be found in a cardiac OR.

Suture Materials. A variety of nonabsorbable cardiovascular sutures with atraumatic needles are available from most suture manufacturers. Synthetic sutures of Teflon, Dacron, polyester, or polypropylene are usually selected for insertion of prostheses and for vascular anastomoses. Most sutures are double armed with a needle on each end. Given the numerous stitches required for prosthetic valve repair and replacement, alternately colored suture and slotted, numbered suture holders may help avoid confusion. Polytetrafluoroethylene (PTFE) sutures can be used for replacement of mitral valve chordae. Vessel loops and umbilical tapes are commonly used to identify and to retract blood vessels and other structures. Wire (monofilament or twisted cable) commonly is used to approximate the sternum (Figure 25-18), with plastic, metal, or nylon bands occasionally added to reinforce fragile bone. Skin staplers may be used to close skin incisions; a staple remover must accompany the patient to the postanesthesia area if staples have been used to close the chest.

Supplies. The following supplies are used in most cardiac procedures. Depending on the surgeon's preference, other items may be added or substituted.

- Rubber shods (placed on the tips of hemostats to protect suture clamped by the hemostat)
- Pill sponges (small gauze dissectors; also called peanuts, pushers, kitners)
- Various-sized Silastic or polyvinyl chloride tubing
- Tourniquet catheters
- Disposable drapes
- Foot-controlled and hand-controlled ESU pencils, ultrasonic scalpel
- Adapters, connectors, stopcocks
- Extra syringes and needles for injections, infusions, and blood samples
- Sterile marking pen to identify anastomotic sites and mark grafts
- Cotton gloves (worn by assistant to retract heart and expose target coronary artery); some surgeons prefer a sling to pull up the heart to expose the coronary arteries
- Suture organizer (to keep valve sutures in correct order)
- Irrigation cannulae
- Disposable vascular (bulldog) clamps
- Coronary occluders and stabilizers
- Autotransfusion supplies
- Chest tubes, chest drainage system
- Topical hemostatic agents
- Femoral arterial blood pressure supplies (hypodermic needle, guidewire, stopcocks, pressure tubing)
- IABP insertion supplies (hypodermic needle, guidewire, vascular dilators, stopcocks, pressure tubing, IABP catheter)
- CPB and myocardial protection cannulae, tubing, connectors, stopcocks

Prosthetic Material. In addition to these general supplies, special supplies are needed to repair or replace cardiovascular structures. Intracardiac patches, heart valves, and synthetic grafts should be handled with care to prevent damage or the introduction of foreign materials. Teflon, a fluorocarbon fiber, and Dacron, a polyester fiber, come in a variety of meshes, fabrics, felts, tapes, and sutures, and it is possible to combine them with other materials in prosthetic heart valves (Figure 25-19).

Teflon patches are made in a variety of forms for intracardiac and outflow tract use. Varying degrees of firmness, thickness, and porosity are available for specific uses. Low reactivity, strength retention, and tissue acceptance are important considerations when selecting such patches.

Use of Dacron arterial tube grafts is common in cardiac surgery, although reinforced expanded PTFE grafts are also available. There are two types of Dacron grafts: knitted and woven. Woven prosthetic grafts are usually used when the patient has been fully heparinized because the interstices of woven grafts are tighter than those in knitted grafts and bleeding is usually less. Compared with woven grafts, the advantages of knitted grafts are that they do not fray as readily, they are easier to handle, and they reendothelialize more quickly. Grafts come in a variety of sizes and may be straight or bifurcated (Figure 25-20). Knitted and woven grafts impregnated with collagen to reduce interstitial bleeding are useful in the

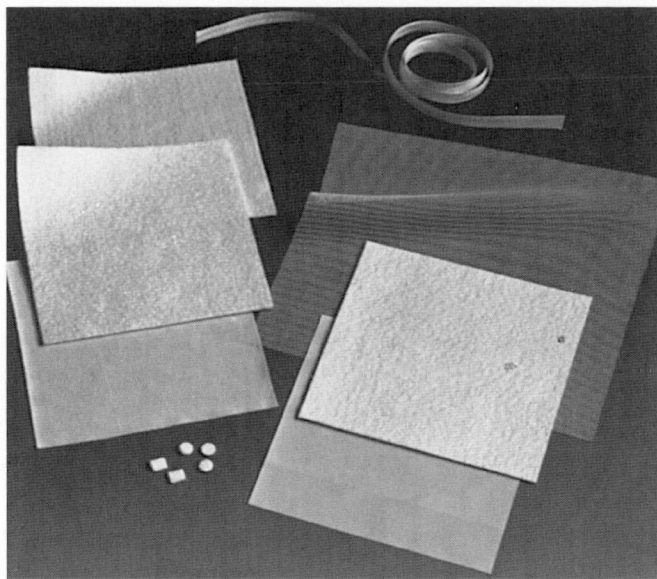

FIGURE 25-19 Assorted prosthetic materials to repair intracardiac and extracardiac defects: tapes, Teflon and Dacron patches, and pledgets.

FIGURE 25-20 Straight and bifurcated arterial tube grafts.

thoracic aorta and do not have to be preclotted, even when the patient is fully heparinized for cardiopulmonary bypass. Graft sizers are available to determine correct size.

Specially designed tube grafts for the aortic arch incorporate prosthetic branches for the head vessels (bracheocephalic, left common carotid, and subclavian arteries); and tube grafts for replacement of the aortic root and ascending aorta are available with preformed sinuses of Valsalva incorporated into the prosthesis (David, 2009).

Endovascular, expandable stented tube grafts are available for both the abdominal aorta and the descending portion of the thoracic aorta (Figure 25-21). The endovascular graft is inserted percutaneously into the femoral artery and advanced to the desired position in the abdominal or descending thoracic aorta, where the prosthesis is opened, implanted, and secured (Thompson and Bertling, 2009; Tinkham, 2009).

FIGURE 25-21 Thoracic aortic endovascular stented prosthesis made from expanded polytetrafluoroethylene (PTFE). Insertion of the compressed device is percutaneous through the femoral artery by a delivery catheter, guided to the desired position in the thoracic aorta under fluoroscopy. Following confirmation that its position is correct, the device expands automatically on deployment from the delivery catheter. The delivery catheter is then withdrawn, and hemostasis of the femoral incision site follows.

FIGURE 25-22 St. Jude Medical bileaflet tilting disk valve prosthesis.

FIGURE 25-23 Carbomedics supra-annular aortic prosthesis, designed for the small aortic root.

Valve Prostheses. Valve prosthesis selection depends on multiple factors: hemodynamics, thromboresistance, durability, ease of insertion, anatomic suitability, and patient acceptability; cost, patient outcome, and value are also important (Manji et al, 2012; Rahimtoola, 2010, 2011). Most mechanical prostheses use a tilting disk design. The ball-and-cage prosthesis was the first mechanical valve implanted in the anatomic position but is no longer available. Prosthetic valves allow complete closure with slight regurgitation to prevent stasis of blood (Figures 25-22 to 25-24). Prosthetic valves are manufactured with an attached annular sewing ring (often made of Dacron). The surgeon places sutures into the native valve annulus and then into the prosthesis sewing ring. The sewing ring occupies space within the valvular orifice and may affect the amount of flow through the valve orifice. This is especially significant in the small aortic root (the location of the valve annulus). Aortic prostheses, especially in the smaller sizes (e.g., 21 mm), tend to have minimal sewing ring material to avoid taking up space so as to minimize cardiac reduction of cardiac output that can flow through the prosthetic orifice. When blood flow through the prosthetic valve fails to meet metabolic demands, a *prosthesis-patient mismatch* is said to exist (Daneshvar and Rahimtoola, 2012; Head et al, 2012; Rahimtoola, 2011). The deleterious effect of such a mismatch eventually produces deterioration of cardiac function. Surgeons, increasingly aware of the problem, select the prosthesis with the best hemodynamics for the patient. If a suitable prosthesis is unavailable, the surgeon may opt to perform a procedure to enlarge the aortic root in order to insert a larger, more hemodynamically suitable valve.

Bioprostheses derive from porcine, bovine, or equine tissue (Figures 25-25 to 25-27). Porcine valves consist of an aortic valve from a pig that can be sutured to a Dacron-covered stent (Figure 25-25, *A*); alternatively, the porcine aortic valve may be "stentless" (without a sewing ring) to enhance the hemodynamics, especially in patients with a small aortic root (see Figure 25-25, *B*). The bovine (calf) (see Figure 25-26) pericardial bioprosthesis is created by cutting leaflet-shaped pieces from the pericardium and sewing them onto a Dacron ring; more recently, a newer bovine pericardial prosthesis (Kocher et al, 2013) can be rapidly deployed by sliding the valve into position in the aortic annulus and inflating the frame

FIGURE 25-24 **A,** Medtronic-Hall tilting disk valve prosthesis. **B,** Double-ended sizing obturators for the Medtronic-Hall prosthesis *(left and center)* and probe *(right)* to test leaflet movement. All valve prostheses have sizing obturators specific to the prosthesis itself.

FIGURE 25-25 **A,** Medtronic Mosaic porcine aortic *(top)* and mitral *(bottom)* bioprostheses. **B,** Stentless porcine aortic valve. The absence of a stent and sewing ring provides a greater orifice area through which blood can flow.

to sit firmly in place (three commissural stitches also help to anchor the prosthesis). The equine (horse) (see Figure 25-27, *A*) pericardial prosthesis is created by cutting pieces of the pericardium, shaping the pieces into a tube, and attaching the prosthesis to a ring of Dacron material. The advantage of these biologic valves is that administration of long-term anticoagulants is not necessary in most patients. Obturators to size prosthetic valves as well as valve holders are specific to the prostheses (see Figures 25-24, *B,* and 25-27, *B*). Tables 25-3 and 25-4 compare mechanical and biologic prosthetic heart valves. Tissue-engineered heart valves may offer a future potential cure for valvular heart disease (Rahimtoola, 2011).

Transcatheter, percutaneously inserted aortc valves come from bovine pericardium (Figure 25-28). These may be inserted in a hybrid OR with fluoroscopy.

Aortic valve allografts (homografts) pose little or no risk of thromboembolism, offer optimal hemodynamic function, require no anticoagulation drugs, and raise virtually no risk of sudden catastrophic failure. Moreover, they demonstrate a lower incidence of infective endocarditis than that found in mechanical or biologic valves, and their long-term durability is comparable with that of bioprostheses. Allograft root replacement is also a valuable technique in the context of prosthetic valve endocarditis. The entire

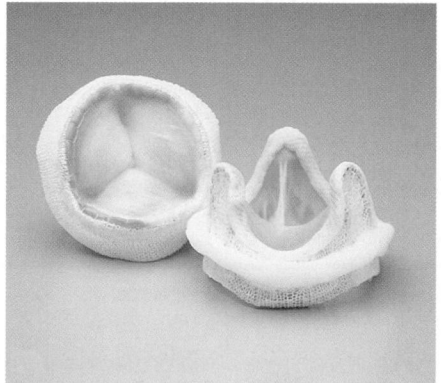

FIGURE 25-26 Carpentier-Edwards bovine pericardial aortic bioprosthesis.

A

B

FIGURE 25-27 A, ATS Medical equine pericardial aortic prosthesis. **B,** Obturators for ATS Medical 3f prosthesis.

ascending aorta and valve (Figure 25-29) or the valve alone (Figure 25-30) may be inserted. Allografts are cryopreserved and must be thawed in saline according to the vendor's protocol before implantation. Because stentless aortic valves (see Figure 25-25, *B*) are more easily available than allografts, they are increasingly preferred for aortic root replacement.

Conduits consisting of mechanical or biologic aortic valves attached to a tube graft (Figure 25-31) are used in procedures such as repair of aortic dissections requiring replacement of the aortic valve and ascending aorta. If vein grafts must be inserted into the conduit or if a direct coronary ostial anastomosis is required, the surgeon uses an electrocoagulator to make the opening into the graft and at the same time heat-seals the cut edges of the prosthesis. Conduits with *biologic* valves interposed between tube graft materials may be used when patients are at increased risk for bleeding complications associated with the need for chronic anticoagulation therapy. Allograft conduits may be used for these procedures as well.

Although allografts and stentless bioprostheses may minimize prosthesis-patient mismatch and avoid the complications associated with prosthetic mechanical valve replacement, valve repair rather than replacement is preferred, particularly for mitral and tricuspid valve lesions. Numerous mitral valve rings and bands are available for both surgical and interventional percutaneous reparative procedures. Consult with the surgeon about the intended prosthesis as well as alternative devices should another prosthesis be required (Otto and Bonow, 2012). When repairing the native valve with an annuloplasty ring, obturators specific to various kinds of annuloplasty rings are used to size the annulus (Figure 25-32, *A, B, C*). Ensure that the sizers appropriate for the desired prosthesis are available.

Additional safety considerations include storing prosthetic materials in a clean, protected environment and using them according to manufacturers' instructions. Before implantation, biologic valves

TABLE 25-3
Mechanical Valve Prostheses*

| | Tilting Disk | |
	Medtronic-Hall, Omniscience	St. Jude Medical, Carbomedics
Model/description	Spherical (single) tilting disk	Bileaflet tilting disk
Advantages	Long-term durability	Long-term durability
	Good hemodynamics in all sizes	Good hemodynamics in all sizes
	Low profile	Low profile
		Low TE rate for mechanical valve
Disadvantages	Anticoagulation required	Anticoagulation strongly recommended
	Potential for sudden thrombosis	Potential for sudden thrombosis
	Noisy	Some noise
	Higher risk of TE in mitral position	Higher risk of TE in mitral position
	If warfarin (Coumadin) must be discontinued, there is increased risk of catastrophic thrombosis	If warfarin (Coumadin) must be discontinued, there is increased risk of catastrophic thrombosis
Special considerations	Sizers and handles specific to prosthesis; must be sterilized	Sizers and handles specific to prosthesis; must be sterilized
		Frequently used in children needing mechanical prosthetic valve

*All prostheses should be stored in a cool, dry, contamination-free area. Resterilization is no longer recommended. The Starr-Edwards ball-and-cage valve is no longer available; clinicians occasionally still may encounter a patient with a ball-and-cage valve.

TE, thromboembolism.

Modified from Otto CM, Bonow RO: Valvular heart disease. In Bonow RO et al, editors: *Braunwald's heart disease—a textbook of cardiovascular medicine,* ed 9, Philadelphia, 2012, Saunders; Rahimtoola SH: Choice of prosthetic heart valve in adults: an update, *J Am Coll Cardiol* 55(22):2413–2426, 2010; Rahimtoola SH: The year in valvular heart disease, *J Am Coll Cardiol* 58(12):1197–1207, 2011.

TABLE 25-4

Biologic Valve Prostheses

	Heterograft (Xenograft)			
	Heterograft/Xenograft		**Allograft**	**Transcatheter Heterograft Valve**
	Stentless Porcine Bioprostheses	**Stented Porcine Heterograft; Bovine and Equine Pericardial Valve Prostheses**	**Allograft (Homograft; Human Cadaver Valve)**	**Transcatheter Aortic Valve Replacement (Bovine, Porcine or Equine)**
Model/ description	For use in aortic position Stentless (aortic): no sewing ring; includes porcine aortic root valve with coronary ostial branches	Pericardial valve used in aortic position; porcine heterograft used in aortic, mitral, and tricuspid positions Porcine heterograft (from excised pig aortic valves; leaflets attached to sewing ring) Aortic bovine and equine pericardium (cut and shaped into trileaflet valve)	Aortic valve allograft (cadaver, organ donor, excised cardiomyopathic heart from transplant recipient; mitral valve allograft also available)	For use in aortic position; trileaflet bovine pericardial valve mounted within a frame and placed into a delivery catheter; inserted via the femoral artery (occasionally through the subclavian artery) and guided fluoroscopically with TEE into the aortic position Two types: Self-expanding device placed into a nitinol frame (see Figures 25-28, 25-67); balloon-expandable device placed into a chromium frame see (Figure 25-68)
Advantages	Incidence of TE very low; anticoagulation rare after AVR Stentless has excellent flow, especially in small aortic annulus (≤21 mm) No hemolysis Excellent hemodynamics; use may avoid need for aortic root enlargement	Incidence of TE very low; anticoagulation rare after AVR No hemolysis Good hemodynamics in all sizes	Incidence of TE very low; anticoagulation rare; used for AVR and MVR No hemolysis Excellent hemodynamics (especially with stentless technique)	Suitable for elderly (e.g., >80 years old) patients with severe aortic stenosis deemed unsuitable for surgical therapy No hemolysis Good hemodynamics
	Central flow Gradual failure allows elective reoperation Little residual gradient; durability good after age 60 years Stentless graft has many advantages of allograft valves	Central flow Gradual failure allows elective reoperation Residual gradient minimal Slower rate of calcification in patients 60 years or older	Central flow Gradual failure allows elective reoperation No residual gradient	Central flow Gradual failure Little residual gradient
Disadvantages	Durability may be less than 15 years	Durability not yet established In small aortic root of large body, may produce prosthesis-patient mismatch	Limited availability Insertion technique more complex than stented valve Possible immunologic reaction (current decellularization process strips cells from graft and reduces immune response)	Long-term durability not yet established; outcomes beyond 2 or more years not known; insertion technique more complex; potential injury to access vessels; higher stroke rate; paravalvular leak a problem with newer sewing cuffs
	Accelerated fibrocalcific degeneration in children, patients with hypertension, or patients needing chronic renal dialysis Cross-clamp time and CPB longer than those for insertion of stented valve because of greater complexity of subcoronary insertion	Accelerated calcification may be a problem in children, renal patients, or those with hypertension		Requires fluoroscopy; requires radiation protection (lead aprons, etc.); long-term durability not yet established; significant initial learning curve

Continued

TABLE 25-4

Biologic Valve Prostheses—cont'd

	Heterograft/Xenograft		Heterograft (Xenograft) Allograft	Transcatheter Heterograft Valve
	Stentless Porcine Bioprostheses	**Stented Porcine Heterograft; Bovine and Equine Pericardial Valve Prostheses**	**Allograft (Homograft; Human Cadaver Valve)**	**Transcatheter Aortic Valve Replacement (Bovine, Porcine or Equine)**
Special considerations	Sizers and handles specific to prosthesis; must be sterilized before insertion; must be rinsed in saline to remove storage solution before insertion; follow manufacturer's instructions for rinsing; frequent irrigation recommended to prevent drying	Sizers and handles specific to prosthesis; must be sterilized before insertion; must be rinsed in saline to remove storage solution before insertion; follow manufacturer's instructions for rinsing; frequent irrigation recommended to prevent drying	No specific sizers; may use sizers for heterografts; cryopreserved allograft must be thawed per protocol; used for aortic or mitral valve replacement; stent can be attached if indicated for use in other positions	No specific sizers; sizing via fluoroscopic imaging; potential radiation risks to patient and staff; need fluoroscopy, trained staff to run fluoroscopic machine, contrast media, and radiation protection
	Diets low in calcium recommended for children, renal patients	Diets low in calcium recommended for children, renal patients		

AVR, Aortic valve replacement; *CPB,* cardiopulmonary bypass; *MVR,* mitral valve replacement; *TE,* thromboembolism; *TEE,* transesophageal echocardiography.

Modified from Gilard M et al: Registry of transcatheter aortic-valve implantation in high-risk patients, *N Engl J Med* 366(18):1705–1715, 2012; Kodali SK et al: Two-year outcomes after transcatheter or surgical aortic valve replacement, *N Engl J Med* 366(18):1686–1695, 2012; Otto CM, Bonow RO: Valvular heart disease. In Bonow RO et al, editors: *Braunwald's heart disease: a textbook of cardiovascular medicine,* ed 9, Philadelphia. 2012, Saunders; Rahimtoola SH: Choice of prosthetic heart valve in adults: an update, *J Am Coll Cardiol* 55(22):2413–2426, 2010; Rahimtoola SH: The year in valvular heart disease, *J Am Coll Cardiol* 58(12):1197–1207, 2011.

A   B

FIGURE 25-28 Percutaneous aortic valve. **A,** Diagram of bioprosthesis situated in the aortic valve annulus. **B,** Valve frame with implanted bioprosthesis.

FIGURE 25-29 Aortic allograft with aortic valve and arch vessels attached.

FIGURE 25-31 Valved conduit with Medtronic-Hall tilting disk valve prosthesis.

FIGURE 25-30 Aortic valve allograft.

FIGURE 25-32 A, Carpentier-Edwards "classic" tricuspid and mitral annuloplasty rings, sizers, and sizer handle. The tricuspid rings bear notches in the area corresponding to conduction tissue in the tricuspid annulus to avoid suture injury. **B,** Cosgrove annuloplasty ring. **C,** Ring attached to ring holder and handle.

(including the biologic valves within transcatheter aortic valve implantation [TAVI] systems) must be rinsed in three saline baths to remove the glutaraldehyde (or other) storage solution. The prescribed number of baths, the amount of physiologic fluid in each rinsing bath, and the recommended rinsing time for each bath vary among bioprosthetic manufacturers (Table 25-5). Adhere to the specific manufacturer's instructions for each prosthesis. Some bioprostheses do not require rinsing because their storage is in a physiologically neutral solution (i.e., not glutaraldehyde). However, before and during insertion, all bioprostheses should be kept moist with saline. Mechanical valves should be protected from scratching and other injury as well.

Preinduction Care. After patient transfer to the OR suite, a focused preoperative assessment commences, and the perioperative nurse reviews the chart for a duly signed and witnessed informed consent

TABLE 25-5

Valve-Rinsing Procedures for Biologic Heart Valves

Glutaraldehyde storage solution is used for many (but not all) bioprostheses, and rinsing procedures for its removal vary among bioprosthetic heart valve manufacturers. The amount of rinsing solution in each rinse basin, the number of basins, and the time for each rinse (and the total time of the rinsing baths) should be followed according to each manufacturer's instructions. Some manufacturers recommend a *fourth* basin for storing the bioprosthesis until implantation. The following sampling of rinsing processes reflects the differences among manufacturers' recommended rinsing procedures. The person rinsing the valve should collaborate with the circulating nurse when following the instructions for that particular valve. Given the wide variation in the following procedures, it is critical to check the manufacturers' instructions every time a bioprosthetic valve requires preparation for implantation.

Description	Number of Rinse Basins	Amount of Fluid in Each Basin	Rinse Time per Basin	Comments/Additional Information
Pericardial (equine) aortic valve (ATS Medical)	4	Minimum 500 mL physiologic saline	30 sec in first 3 basins (total: 90 sec/1.5 min)	Allow bioprosthesis to remain in fourth basin until required by surgeon.
Pericardial (bovine) valve (Sorin Mitroflow)	3	Minimum 300 mL physiologic saline	2 min in the 3 basins (total: 6 min)	Allow bioprosthesis to remain in third basin until required by surgeon.
Pericardial (bovine) valve (St. Jude Medical EPIC)	3	Minimum 500 mL physiologic saline	10 sec in each of the first 2 basins (total: 20 sec)	Allow bioprosthesis to remain in third basin until required by surgeon.
Pericardial (bovine) valve (Edwards Lifesciences Perimount Magna)	2	Minimum 500 mL physiologic saline	1 min in each of 2 basins (total: 2 min)	Allow bioprosthesis to remain in second basin until required by surgeon.
Porcine valve (Medtronic Mosaic)	2	Minimum 500 mL physiologic saline	15 sec in each of 2 basins (total: 30 sec)	Allow bioprosthesis to remain in second basin until required by surgeon.
Porcine valve (Medtronic Hancock)	2	Minimum 500 mL physiologic saline	15 sec in each of 2 basins (total: 30 sec)	Allow bioprosthesis to remain in second basin until required by surgeon.
Porcine stentless valve (Medtronic Stentless FreeStyle)	3	Minimum 500 mL physiologic saline	2 min in each basin (total: 6 min)	Allow bioprosthesis to remain in third basin until required by surgeon.
Pericardial (bovine) valve (Sorin Freedom Solo)	None; rinsing not required because prosthesis not stored in glutaraldehyde	Not applicable	Not applicable	Although bioprosthesis does *not* require rinsing, it should be kept moist with physiologic saline to prevent drying.
Pericardial (bovine) Transcatheter Heart Valve (Edwards Lifesciences *Sapien*)	2	Minimum 500 mL physiologic saline	1 min in each basin (total: 2 min)	This is a bioprosthetic valve used for transcatheter aortic valve implantation (TAVI) in patients at high risk for open chest surgery. Keep bioprosthesis moist with physiologic saline to prevent drying.
Pericardial (Porcine) Transcatheter Heart Valve (Medtronic *CoreValve*)	3	Minimum 500 mL physiologic saline	2 min in each basin (total: 6 min)	This is a bioprosthetic valve used for TAVI in patients at high risk for open chest surgery. Keep bioprosthesis moist with physiologic saline to prevent drying.

form, advance directives, laboratory results, diagnostic data, and other pertinent information. The nurse also confirms the identity of the patient and the intended operation, including identification and confirmation of site and side, and required position, all as applicable. Verification of which leg (i.e., right or left) will serve for vein harvest in bypass patients may not be necessary if this decision depends on the surgeon's preference, rather than on a specific clinical indication. Some institutions, however, may require site marking of bypass harvesting sites, and the nurse should comply with institutional policy.

Preoperatively, cardiac surgical patients may exhibit more stress and anxiety than other surgical patients. Perioperative nurses should anticipate and prepare for this because stress and anxiety increase myocardial oxygen consumption. Efforts to reduce the family's

stress and anxiety level are also important and may result in less communication of stress and anxiety to the patient. Often patients and family members ask questions about the surgery and the immediate postoperative appearance of the patient. It is helpful to prepare the family for some of the physical changes (e.g., edema, multiple tubes and lines) they can expect to see in their loved one postoperatively, and to encourage talking and touching the patient—even if the patient seems unable to respond (Patient-Centered Care).

In addition to communication with the patient, members of the team prepare the patient by ensuring vascular access for pressure monitoring and medication infusion. They insert a peripheral arterial pressure line and venous infusion lines. They may use a local anesthetic at insertion sites and may inject an IV sedative. Occasionally a patient's response to sedation results in impaired respiration,

PATIENT-CENTERED CARE

The patient, a 50-year-old male, is accompanied by his wife and two teenage children. They are in the cardiac surgery preoperative area. Teenage children are very focused and protective about their loved one. You should initially recognize and answer any questions of the spouse, and be also alert to the children's concerns and fears. They will ask very direct and pointed questions that must be answered as truthfully and candidly as possible. When there is no answer (e.g., "Is my dad going to die?"), avoid making claims that you cannot substantiate. Allow the questioner to talk about specific fears, and address them; if there is a specific medical question, contact the physician (surgeon, anesthesia provider) to respond to the questioner. You can also discuss some of the precautions taken to protect the loved one (e.g., sterile technique, having the necessary supplies, safe positioning). The OR remains foreign territory for many people.

The following is a possible scenario when the nurse provided patient-centered care:

RN: "Hello Mr. Jones, my name is Trish Seifert and I am a registered nurse. I will be in your room during surgery. Is this your family?" (nods toward older woman and a teenage male and female)

PATIENT: "Yes, my wife, Susan, my daughter Beth and son Jack."

RN: "Hello Mrs. Jones…Beth…Jack." [addressing children primarily] "Your dad will be in the OR for a few hours [confirms surgeon's time estimation]; we will call you if that time changes. Sometimes there are delays and we don't want you to worry if you don't hear from us when you expect to hear. I also want to tell you a bit about what your dad will look like when you see him after surgery. As we discussed before, we cool the body during surgery and use medication that keeps your dad comfortable and somewhat unconscious. When you see him right after surgery, he is going to look pale and feel cool and clammy. And he'll be *wired for sound*; there will be lots of tubes and catheters in your dad. These are important because they give us important information about what is going on inside his body. Most of these tubes will be gone in about 48 hours. Don't let his appearance and all the tubes stop you from touching your dad—patting his arm or hand. To us he looks beautiful, but to you he is going to look quite different. Also don't hesitate to talk to your dad; he will be medicated but the hearing—last to go—is the first sense to come back. So he may not respond to your words, but I am sure that it will be a positive experience for him, and for you both. And don't hesitate to ask any questions. The nurses in the intensive care unit are terrific and can answer most of your questions. And if they can't, they'll find someone who can. I have worked with these nurses for many years and they are terrific. We'll all take good care of your dad."

---

as evidenced by shallow respirations, decreased oxygen saturation, and a reduced respiratory rate (e.g., eight breaths per minute or less) (Nussmeier et al, 2009; Reich et al, 2011). The nurse noticing these respiratory changes can call a rapid response team (RRT) to assess the patient and initiate treatment before the patient develops more serious reactions, such as cardiopulmonary arrest. In this situation the RRT may consist of the anesthesia providers and staff in the immediate preoperative area rather than a specific hospital-wide RRT. For patients awaiting transfer from the preoperative area to the OR for cardiac surgery, the concept of a clinician acting promptly on changes in a patient's status and initiating a "rapid response" is an important aspect of enhancing a culture of patient safety.

Admission to the OR. Depending on the patient's response to sedative medications received preoperatively, the patient may require assistance onto the OR bed. Warm blankets should be provided for comfort and to reduce shivering; the nurse should ensure that the blanket temperature does not produce thermal injury.

After application of the ECG leads and the pulse oximeter finger cot, padding of the hands, elbows, and feet follows. The perioperative nurse confirms that the peripheral arterial pressure line functions properly, may reposition the arm as necessary in collaboration with the anesthesia provider, and confirms that pulse oximetry functions properly. Additional monitoring devices appear in Table 25-6. A time-out commences to comply with TJC's Universal Protocol (see Chapter 2).

Anesthesia Induction. The choice of anesthetic agent or agents depends on the cardiovascular effects of the anesthetic, the patient's hemodynamic status and general health, and the anticipated length of stay in the surgical intensive care unit (SICU). Newer, fast-acting anesthetic agents are used to "fast-track" patients postoperatively, whereby the patient may undergo extubation in the OR or very shortly after admission to the SICU, to speed recuperation (Kaplan et al, 2011; Nussmeier et al, 2009).

The period of induction, one of the most critical elements during the procedure, requires close monitoring of the patient, especially for patients with ventricular ischemia from congenital or acquired disease. Anesthetic management focuses on maintaining an adequate cardiac output by keeping myocardial oxygen demand low and oxygen supply high (Kaplan et al, 2011; Nussmeier et al, 2009) (see Chapter 5 for additional considerations related to anesthesia care monitoring).

Medication Safety. In addition to anesthetic medications, anesthesia providers use many other drugs to produce vasodilation or vasoconstriction, to enhance heart rate and contractility, to promote anticoagulation, to effect diuresis, and to provide antibiotic prophylaxis. Antibiotic prophylaxis to prevent infection in the cardiac patient is an important consideration, and the nurse should confirm that antibiotic infusion has occurred before surgical incision.

An additional safety precaution is ensuring the labeling of all medications on the field (including irrigating fluids and H_2O). Of particular importance are heparinized solutions, papaverine (to reduce spasm in IMA and radial artery conduits), saphenous vein infusions, and topical hemostatics (Achneck et al, 2010; Barnard and Millner, 2009; DeAnda et al, 2009; Spotnitz, 2012). Containers and syringes are labeled, and the circulating nurse and scrub person visually and verbally should confirm drug name, dose, route, strength, and end date of every medication passed onto the field (Hodgson and Kizior, 2013) (Surgical Pharmacology).

Monitoring. Extensive monitoring of hemodynamic and other variables is the norm during cardiac surgery (see Table 25-5). After intubation (or before, depending on the anesthesia provider's preference), insertion of additional pressure lines to measure central venous pressure (CVP) and pulmonary artery pressures (PAPs) may follow. Central line arterial bloodstream infections (CLABSIs) have lessened with adherence to practices that minimize infection (e.g., maximal barrier draping during insertion) (Patient Safety).

TABLE 25-6

Perioperative Patient Monitoring

Monitoring Device	Location	Measures
Electrocardiogram (ECG)	Lateral, posterior electrode placement	Electrical activity of heart
Arterial line	Peripheral radial artery	Arterial blood pressure (direct)
	Central femoral artery	
	Aorta (with needle attached to pressure tubing, or with sensor in bypass circuit or IABP)	
Blood pressure (BP) cuff	Upper arm	Arterial BP (indirect)
Central venous pressure (CVP)	Right atrium (RA)	RA pressure (e.g., CVP)
Pulmonary artery (PA) catheter (Swan-Ganz)	RA (proximal port)	RA pressure (e.g., CVP)
	Right ventricle (RV) (midline port)	RV pressure
	Distal PA (distal port)	PA and pulmonary artery wedge pressure (PAWP)
		Indirect measure of left atrial and left ventricle (LV) pressure
		Cardiac output
Left atrium (LA) line	Left atrium	LA, LV pressure
Pulse oximeter	Finger, earlobe	Oxygen saturation of arterial hemoglobin
Urinary drainage catheter	Urinary bladder	Urine output, renal perfusion/function, temperature
Temperature probes	Esophagus	Temperature (core and peripheral)
	Nasopharyngeal	
	Urinary bladder	
	Rectum	
	Ventricular septum	
	Bypass circuit	
	Tympanic	
	Face/forehead (adhesive patch)	
Neurologic monitoring	Head	
Electroencephalogram (EEG)		Electrical activity of brain; awareness
Transcranial Doppler		Detects cerebral arterial emboli
Bispectral index (BIS)		Detects anesthesia awareness
Cerebral oximetry		
Transesophageal echocardiogram (TEE)	Esophagus	Measures cerebral tissue oxygen saturation with sensors placed bilaterally on patient's forehead
		Cardiac function, presence of air, integrity of valve repair
Epiaortic ultrasound	Ascending aorta	Amount of calcium within aorta (assists with location of calcium-free area for placement of aortic cross-clamp)

IABP, Intra-aortic balloon pump.
Modified from Kaplan JA et al: *Kaplan's cardiac anesthesia: the echo era,* ed 6, Philadelphia, 2011, Saunders; Nussmeier NA et al: Anesthesia for cardiac surgical procedures. In Miller RD et al, editors: *Miller's anesthesia,* ed 7, Philadelphia, 2009, Churchill Livingstone.

SURGICAL PHARMACOLOGY

Medications Commonly Used During Cardiac Surgery

Medication/Category	Dosage/Route	Purpose/Action	Adverse Reactions	Nursing Implications
Heparin	For institution of CPB: 300-400 units/kg (bolus) injected via central line or injected directly into RA For irrigation: 5000 units (per mg) in 500 mL of 0.9% NS	Systemic anticoagulation; prevents thrombosis of blood in CPB circuit; blocks activation of thrombin (and intrinsic clotting cascade) Topical irrigation	Excess heparin can increase bleeding; possible allergic reaction	Ensure that heparin is infused before initiating CPB; if resuming CPB after reversal of heparin with protamine sulfate, confirm that patient has been reinfused with heparin; maintain ACT greater than 500 seconds.

SURGICAL PHARMACOLOGY

Medications Commonly Used During Cardiac Surgery—cont'd

Medication/Category	Dosage/Route	Purpose/Action	Adverse Reactions	Nursing Implications
Protamine sulfate	Can vary from 1-1.3 mg to 4 mg for every 100 units of heparin; infused through IV line	Reverse heparin; heparin antagonist	Potential for allergic reaction	If the patient's hemodynamic status requires reinstituting CPB, confirm that heparin has be reinfused; in some patients who are sensitive to protamine sulfate, heparin reversal proceeds without protamine; should have been administered slowly (over 5 min or more); heparin can rebound and may require additional protamine and/or blood tests to check platelet and fibrinogen levels.
Papaverine	For IMA: 30 mg/mL in injectable NS; injected directly into IMA by surgeon For radial artery: 60 mg in 45 mL autologous blood; injected by person harvesting artery	Antispasmodic (used to minimize spam in IMA)	Potential for allergic reaction	Use a blunt-tipped needle to prevent injury to the artery.
Bacitracin (or other topical antibiotic)	50,000 units in 1 L of NS Topical: Poured or applied with bulb syringe onto surgical site	Antibiotic (antibacterial) used for prophylaxis	Potential for allergic reaction	May be poured or applied with bulb syringe.
Hemostats: *Mechanical*	Gelatin, collagen, cellulose, polysaccharide: applied topically	Compresses tissue and absorbs blood; provides scaffold for clots to form; promotes hemostasis; halts bleeding in presence of active flowing blood; used for diffuse bleeding	Potential for allergic reaction	Examples: Gelfoam, Surgicel, Oxycel; has little hemostatic effect on heparinized patients.
Hemostats: *Active*	Bovine or human pooled thrombin; applied topically	Promotes platelet activation and initiation of clotting cascade	Potential for allergic reaction	Example: FloSeal
Hemostats: *Flowable*	Bovine gelatin and human plasma; porcine gelatin; applied topically	Initiates clotting cascade through activation on contact with blood	Potential for allergic reaction	Examples: Gelfoam, thrombin; gelatin has little hemostatic effect on heparinized patients
Hemostats: *Fibrin sealant*	2- or 5-mL packages; human pooled plasma; applied topically	Mixes fibrinogen, thrombin, and clotting factors to generate a clot; emulates final stages of clotting cascade	Potential for allergic reaction	Examples: Tisseel, Hemaseel; effective in patients with coagulopathies or who are on anticoagulants
Sealants: *Polyethylene glycol (PEG)*	Becomes a gel and seals bleeding site; applied topically	Creates barriers to prevent leakage from tissues; used for vascular reconstruction	Potential for allergic reaction	Examples: CoSeal, FocalSeal
Adhesives: *Cyanoacrylate*	Cyanoacrylate; applied topically	Adjunct to sutures or staples; used to attach tissues to each other	Potential for allergic reaction (especially in patients with bovine or glutaraldehyde allergies)	Example: Dermabond

Continued

SURGICAL PHARMACOLOGY

Medications Commonly Used During Cardiac Surgery—cont'd

Medication/Category	Dosage/Route	Purpose/Action	Adverse Reactions	Nursing Implications
Adhesive: *Albumin and glutaraldehyde*	Bovine serum albumin and 10% glutaraldehyde; applied topically	Glutaraldehyde and albumin form a strong adhesive	Potential for allergic reaction	BioGlue
Vein solution	1000 mL Plasma-Lyte, 4000 units heparin, 120 mg papaverine; injected into vein graft	Provides physiologic solution for distending vein graft	Potential for allergic reaction	Ensure that solution is clear of particulate matter when transferring to field.

ACT, Activated clotting time; *CPB,* cardiopulmonary bypass; *IMA,* internal mammary artery; *IV,* intravenous; *NS,* normal saline; *RA,* right atrium

Modified from Achneck HE et al: A comprehensive review of topical hemostatic agents: efficacy and recommendations for use, *Ann Surg* 251(2):217–228, 2010; DeAnda A et al: Improving outcomes through the use of surgical sealants for anastomotic sealing during cardiovascular surgery, *J Card Surg* 24:325–333, 2009; Barnard J, Millner R: A review of topical hemostatic agents for use in cardiac surgery, *Ann Thorac Surg* 88:1377–1383, 2009; Hodgson BB, Kizior RJ: *Saunders nursing drug handbook 2013,* Philadelphia, 2013, Saunders; Kaplan JA, et al: *Kaplan's cardiac anesthesia: the echo era,* ed 6, Philadelphia, 2011, Saunders; Nussmeier NA et al: Anesthesia for cardiac surgical procedures. In Miller RD et al, editors: *Miller's anesthesia,* ed 7, Philadelphia, 2009, Churchill Livingstone; Spotnitz WD: Getting to hemostasis: general and thoracic surgical challenges, *Texas Heart Inst J* 39(6):868–870, 2012.

PATIENT SAFETY

Preventing Central Line–Associated Bloodstream Infections (CLABSIs)

Cardiac surgery patients routinely undergo insertion of central venous lines to monitor cardiac function and to infuse medications. Unfortunately central venous catheters have been associated with significant bacterial colonization, local infection at the site of insertion, and bloodstream infection. As early as 2006, Pronovost and colleagues described preliminary results of a simple but effective five-step intervention to reduce CLABSIs:
1. Handwashing
2. Skin cleansing with chlorhexidine gluconate
3. Avoiding the femoral (inguinal) area whenever possible
4. Using maximal barriers for draping the insertion site
5. Removing catheters as soon as possible.

In 2009 Dr. Carolyn Clancy, director of the Agency for Healthcare Research and Quality, reported that 250,000 CLABSIs occurred annually in U.S. hospitals, adding $36,000 in additional cost per patient. The study sites of Pronovost's underlying 2006 research, demonstrated remarkable results, as reported by Lipitz-Snyderman and associates (2011). The authors explored and quantified how long ICUs could sustain zero CLABSIs in 80 ICUs within 57 hospitals, predominantly in Michigan: 60% of ICUs had no CLABSIs for 12 months or more, and 26% of the ICUs had zero CLABSIs for 24 months or more. These results illustrate the effectiveness of infection prevention strategies to reduce not only morbidity and mortality associated with CLABSIs, but also the high financial and personal costs of infection. The findings of this and similar studies provide valuable evidence for improving patient safety.

Modified from Lipitz-Snyderman A et al: The ability of intensive care units to maintain zero central line-associated bloodstream infections, *Arch Int Med* 171(9):856–858, 2011; Clancy CM: Reducing central line-related bloodstream infections, *AORN J* 89(6):1123–1125, 2009; Pronovost P et al: An intervention to decrease catheter-related bloodstream infections in the ICU, *N Engl J Med* 355:2725–2732, 2006.

Peripheral and central arterial and venous pressures usually are monitored directly via transducer and oscilloscope. Perioperative nurses may need to collaborate in central line(s) preparation and placement; they then should observe ECG monitors for signs of ventricular irritability, such as ectopy or tachycardia, and be prepared to assist with defibrillation of the patient if necessary. If the patient cannot be resuscitated, the chest must be opened rapidly and internal cardiac massage performed to decompress the heart and to perfuse the circulatory system.

An indwelling urinary catheter is inserted to measure urine output and to monitor renal function, especially during and after CPB. The urinary catheter may contain a thermistor temperature probe. Placement of other temperature probes, usually in the esophagus, nasopharynx, or rectum, or on the forehead, is common. Temperatures also can be secured from the pulmonary artery catheters and the arterial infusion line of the bypass circuit. Ventricular septal temperatures can be recorded by insertion of a needle probe while the patient's heart is arrested. Monitoring cerebral oxygenation and the level of anesthesia awareness frequently occurs.

The skin requires careful inspection before placement of ECG and ESU dispersive pads. Bony prominences, such as the coccyx and the back of the head, need padding to prevent pressure necrosis from hypoperfusion and hypothermia during bypass. Elderly patients are especially vulnerable to skin breakdown and require additional precautions to avoid pressure injuries (Kaplan et al, 2011). Monitoring aseptic practice is an important infection control strategy.

Positioning. The supine position provides optimal exposure for CPB and surgery to repair the heart and great vessels. In addition, respiratory impairment and discomfort lessen with this approach (Teirstein and Lytle, 2012). When using supine position, the hands and arms are tucked along either side of the body. The legs may be "frog-legged" slightly to provide access to the femoral arteries for insertion of pressure lines and IABP lines or to excise the saphenous vein. Measures to avoid pressure injury (especially in the elderly, debilitated, or obese patient) include padding the coccyx and applying heel protectors. Measures to protect the occipital area from pressure ulcers include placing pillows under the head and repositioning the head during surgery. Significant factors associated with the development of pressure ulcers include preexisting diabetes mellitus; lower preoperative hemoglobin, hematocrit, and serum albumin levels (Kaplan et al, 2011); and the presence of intra-aortic balloon pumps.

A semilateral position may prove optimal for thoracoabdominal aneurysms in order to expose both the descending thoracic aorta and the abdominal aorta. A thoracotomy position is common for some minimally invasive procedures including surgery on the descending thoracic aorta. For minimally invasive surgery, elevation of the right or left side of the chest with a roll or other positioning device provides adequate exposure for one or more small thoracotomy incisions. The presence of severe mediastinal adhesions may also necessitate this approach in some repeat valve operations. For newer percutaneous, fluoroscopically guided endovascular repairs of descending thoracic lesions, patient positioning in the *supine position* is the norm (and not in the lateral position traditionally used for open procedures). Thoracotomy positioning aids should be available to position arms and legs per the surgeon's selected protocol (see Chapter 6 for a discussion of positioning).

Prepping and Draping. For procedures requiring excision of the saphenous vein, prep extends from the jaw to the toes and includes the anterior (or lateral) area of the chest, abdomen, groin, and legs. Prep of legs and feet occurs circumferentially and, as to the chest and abdomen, from bedline to bedline.

In procedures without saphenous vein excision, prep extends to a level below the knees to give the surgeon access to the femoral artery or saphenous vein in the thigh area. Some surgeons nevertheless prefer to have both legs prepped circumferentially for all cardiac procedures. Femoral artery access may be required for arterial pressure monitoring or insertion of an intra-aortic balloon. Saphenous vein exposure facilitates access if need for a bypass conduit appears. In lateral position, the patient is prepped bedline to bedline, anteriorly and posteriorly at least to the knees.

A study of nurses' error recovery in the cardiovascular OR focused on nursing surveillance and its role in detecting—and preventing—error (Yang et al, 2012) (Research Highlight). The most incidents or errors related to surgical prep and aseptic technique. Some other types of error related to counting, positioning, patient transfer, and skin or tissue injury.

After prep, patient draping follows so that anterior areas of the chest, abdomen, and inguinal area are accessible. The perineum is

covered, and a towel folded lengthwise creates a "belt," which is placed across the umbilicus to connect the side drapes. When excising the saphenous vein, both legs remain exposed, with only the feet covered. When draping, the perioperative nurse should consider placement of bypass lines so that they remain securely attached and do not become contaminated. A small drape or towel may cover the groin when access to it is not immediately necessary. If the femoral artery needs to be accessed, the drape or towel can be discarded. Similarly, placement of towels over the legs after saphenous vein excision reduces inadvertent cooling.

Incisions. Surgeons use a variety of incisions. The standard median sternotomy is most common, but mini-sternotomy, minithoracotomy, or full thoracotomy incisions are frequent alternatives, depending on surgeon preference and the specific procedure (Figure 25-33).

Median Sternotomy. The skin incision for full sternotomy extends from the sternal notch to the linea alba below the xiphoid process (Figure 25-34). Occasionally a shorter sternal incision is made for aortic valve replacement (see Figure 25-33, *E*). Nurses should realize that some women (and men) may be unprepared for a sternal scar (King et al, 2009); nurses may wish to help patients prepare for their postoperative appearance by briefly asking what the patient knows about the postoperative scar, and clarifying concerns. Such an occasion represents an opportunity for nurses to consult with female patients to prepare for the effect of a sternal scar, to encourage them to initiate discussions early in their recuperation, and to differentiate between objective and subjective perceptions and concerns of the patient.

For mini-sternotomy, the surgeon partially divides the sternum with a saw, starting from either the sternal notch or the xiphoid process (depending on the cardiac structures to be exposed), and a sternal retractor is then inserted. If the IMA or the saphenous vein will be used, it is made available at this time. The pericardium is incised and the pericardial edges retracted with six to eight sutures sewn to the subcutaneous tissue; this technique enhances exposure by elevating the heart and creates a well to contain irrigation solutions.

In repeat sternotomy, adhesions from a previous cardiac operation require dissection. The surgeon divides the sternum with an oscillating saw and dissects retrosternal tissue free. Increased risk of fibrillation from manipulation of the heart and bleeding and laceration of the RV provides the rationale for exposing the axillary artery or groin vessels (i.e., femoral vein and artery) before sternotomy. Further, authorities suggest that perfusion be in the OR during opening in the event that rapid initiation of CPB becomes necessary (Roselli, 2011). In addition, disposable defibrillation patches, applied preoperatively to the left lateral chest and the right upper posterior chest, can be activated for defibrillation if the heart has not been exposed. Sterile external paddles may also be available.

Three-dimensional CT scans of the chest in real time illustrate various chest structures, extent of retrosternal adhesions, previous bypass grafts, and number of chest wires to be removed. Anteroposterior and lateral chest radiographs also may be available.

These images assist the surgeon and other members of the surgical team to anticipate and prepare for rescue interventions (Roselli, 2011). The preoperative briefing is important to confirm not only the "usual" plan, but also to consider specific interventions unique to the patient's history of surgeries.

On occasion a patient presents for repeat mitral valve surgery. If the original repair was through a thoracotomy incision, sternal

---

RESEARCH HIGHLIGHT

Error Recovery in Cardiac Surgery

In a study describing the role of perioperative cardiac nurses in promoting patient safety in the OR, researchers assessed the types of actual or potential errors identified and recovered from, by the circulating nurse during surgical procedures on patients undergoing CABG or valve surgery. The researchers observed 18 operations and noted an average of 11.11 (61%) errors or incidents per procedure. Seventy-seven percent of the incidents were intercepted and in the remaining 23%, outcomes were improved; there were no adverse outcomes. AORN's PNDS (Petersen, 2011) interventions from the safety domain were selected to guide the observers. The most common errors related to breaks in sterile technique (56/28%) or the surgical prep (36/18%); other possible errors included potential for infection and preventive measures (19/10%), counting (16/8%), and skin or tissue injury (16/8%). Of the incidents, 94% were considered potentially significant, 75% considered definitely preventable, and 20% considered probably— or probably not—preventable. This study illustrates the importance of alert surveillance by perioperative nurses to detect, avoid, or recover from errors. Nurses play a significant role in protecting patients, and their participation in collecting data, identifying potential errors, and preventing injury contributes to safer care and is critical to proper and safe care of the patient in cardiac surgery.

CABG, Coronary artery bypass graft; *PNDS*, Perioperative Nursing Data Set.
Modified from Yang YT et al: The circulating nurse's role in error recovery in the cardiovascular OR, *AORN J* 95(6):755–762, 2012.

A

B

C

D

E

F

FIGURE 25-33 Schematic representation of traditional incision and sternotomy (**A**) compared with a variety of less-invasive incisions (*dotted lines* represent chest wall incisions). Limited skin incision/full sternotomy (**B**) is gaining popularity arising from improved cosmesis and reduced trauma from more limited chest wall retraction. The parasternal approach (**C**) is used less frequently because a residual chest wall defect can result. Partial lower or upper sternotomy (**D** and **E**), respectively, has been used, predominantly in valve procedures. Right anterior thoracotomy (**F**) is a useful approach, particularly in mitral valve reoperations.

FIGURE 25-34 Median sternotomy with sternal saw.

adhesions may prove minimal or nonexistent, and the special precautions associated with repeat sternotomy may be unnecessary. Conversely, if the original chest incision was a sternotomy, a right or left lateral thoracic incision may provide better exposure because fewer adhesions are likely.

Mini-Thoracotomy. For minimally invasive cardiac procedures, a variety of smaller incisions (up to approximately 4 to 8 cm) and ports can be used. These include anterolateral chest incisions small enough for the insertion of specially designed instruments (see Figure 25-14), including video cameras and robotic arms. Performance of minimally invasive cardiac procedures using smaller incisions under direct visualization or, increasingly, by means of video assistance, is common.

Cardiopulmonary Bypass. The temporary substitution of a pump oxygenator for the heart and lungs permits the surgeon to stop the heart to perform cardiac procedures under direct vision in a relatively dry, motionless field. It also allows the surgeon to manipulate the heart with no attendant risk to produce ventricular fibrillation or reduced cardiac output that otherwise could jeopardize perfusion to the myocardial, peripheral, and cerebral tissues.

A   B   C   D   E

FIGURE 25-35 Arterial and venous perfusion cannulae. **A,** Venous return cannula, dual-stage. **B,** Malleable venous return cannula. **C,** Pediatric venous cannula. **D,** Sarns Soft-Flow aortic cannula with suture flange. **E,** Aortic cannula "Soft Flow"—extended. Venous cannulae have a larger bore compared to aortic cannulae in order to facilitate gravity drainage into the bypass machine. Venous cannulae often have wire-reinforced walls in order to prevent crimping of the cannula (which would cause an immediate drop in venous return and subsequent reduction in cardiac output).

Under some circumstances it is possible to access the anteroapical portion of the heart without excess manipulation of the heart. Special retraction and stabilization devices (see Figure 25-17) allow the surgeon to create CABGs to the anterolateral coronary arteries without the use of CPB and induced cardiac arrest. This enables surgery to be performed on a beating heart (discussed later).

In traditional CPB circuits, systemic venous return to the heart flows by gravity drainage through cannulae (Figure 25-35) placed in the superior and inferior venae cavae (Figure 25-36) or through a single two-stage cannula in the RA (Figure 25-37) into tubing connected to the bypass machine. Blood is oxygenated, filtered, warmed or cooled, and pumped back into the systemic circulation through a cannula placed in the ascending aorta or occasionally in the femoral artery (Figure 25-38) or the axillary artery (Grocott et al, 2011). As the CPB machine (Figure 25-39) oxygenates blood, the lungs need not function and may be deflated to provide better exposure of the mediastinal structures.

A percutaneous method to institute femoral vein–femoral artery CPB is possible for minimally invasive (or conventional open) procedures (Figure 25-40) and for emergencies in which the environment is not conducive to traditional CPB methods (e.g., in the cardiac catheterization laboratory, the intensive care unit, and the emergency department). The system uses thin-walled, wire-reinforced catheters inserted into the femoral vein or artery, or both. Resistance of the small-bore cannula used in the femoral vein can impede gravity drainage; to overcome this, a centrifugal pump can siphon blood actively to the pump oxygenator. Other advances include the use of heparin-bonded bypass circuits and tubing; this

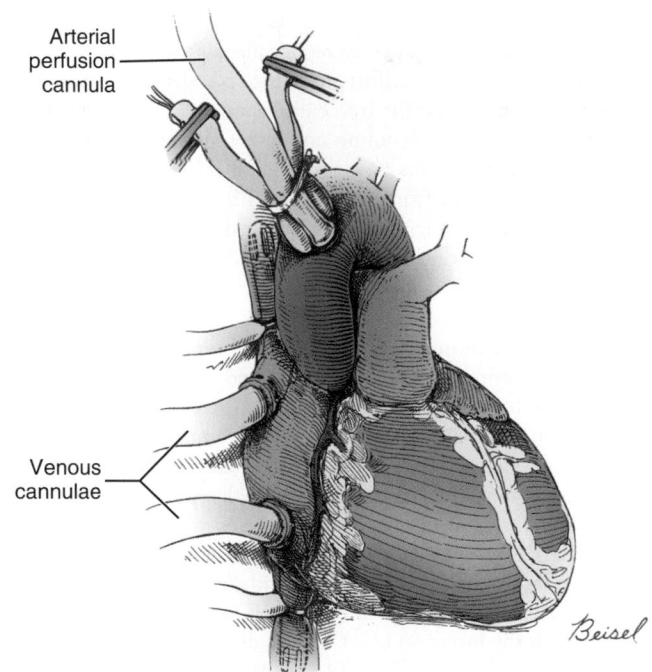

Arterial perfusion cannula

Venous cannulae

Beisel

FIGURE 25-36 Bicaval cannulation of the superior and inferior venae cavae; aortic cannulation.

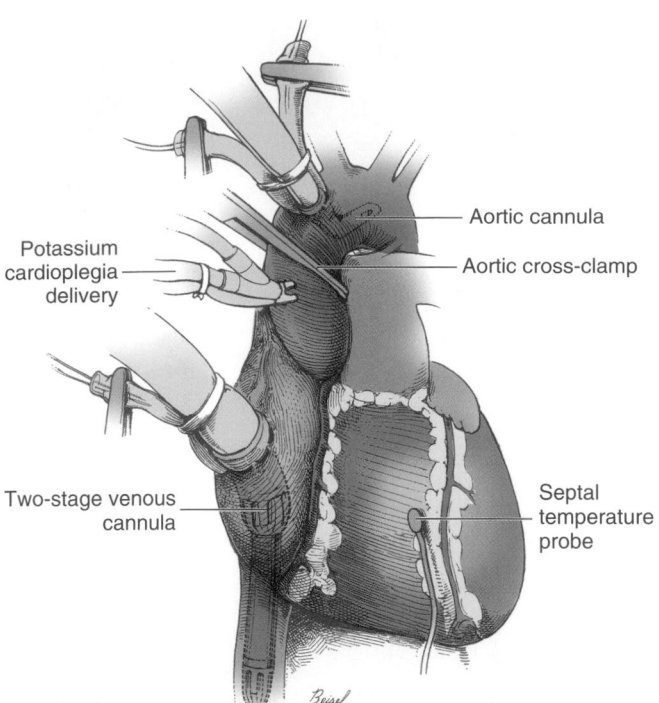

FIGURE 25-37 Diagram showing aortic and venous cannulae during aortic cross-clamping. Also shown is antegrade cardioplegic solution delivery catheter in the aorta, proximal to the cross-clamp, and temperature probe. The single (two-stage) venous cannula has openings in the distal end of the cannula to drain the inferior vena cava; the openings in the midportion (right atrial area) of the cannula drain the superior vena cava and the coronary sinus venous return.

FIGURE 25-38 Cardiopulmonary bypass circuit. Venous blood drains by gravity from the right atrium or venae cavae into an oxygenator that incorporates a blood reservoir and a heat exchanger, which warms or cools the blood as needed. The ventilating gas flowing into the oxygenator removes carbon dioxide and adds oxygen to the blood. Saturated blood leaves the oxygenator and is pumped from the reservoir into the arterial system by the use of a centrifugal pump. Filters and monitors incorporate into the circuit. Additional roller pumps suction shed blood from the pericardial well and the intracardiac chambers (cardiotomy suckers); the blood then returns to the cardiotomy reservoir. A roller pump delivers cardioplegia.

reduces (but does not obviate) the heparin required to achieve systemic anticoagulation and can reduce bleeding and the associated need for blood products. Efforts to reduce platelet destruction and the inflammatory response by coating components of the CPB circuits with phosphorylcholine and other newer materials have shown encouraging results (Grocott et al, 2011).

By diverting blood from the heart, CPB also decompresses the ventricles, thereby reducing myocardial wall tension, a significant determinant of myocardial oxygen demand. This effect is evident with CPB or other means of ventricular support aiming to "rest" the heart. Further decompression results by venting the LV to remove air and accumulated thebesian and bronchial venous return as well as systemic return flowing around the venous cannulae (Figure 25-41). Insertion of the venting catheter is into the LV via the right superior pulmonary vein or, less commonly, through the left ventricular apex. The venting line connects to the suction lines of the bypass machine. Insertion of a small venting catheter into the ascending aorta to remove air is also possible. Occasionally a vent is inserted into the pulmonary artery. The aim of venting is to reduce the incidence of gaseous microemboli. Ambient air removal is also achievable in cases when the heart is opened (e.g., in valve surgery) with the insertion of a CO_2 gas diffuser; the gas insufflates into the pericardial well. The CO_2 gas dissolves in blood about 25 times faster than room air; CO_2 retained within the cardiac chambers is better tolerated than ambient air and potentially less harmful to tissue. Specifically, CO_2 insufflation use aims to decrease gaseous microemboli in the circulation; a study by Chaudhuri and associates (2012) showed no difference in neurocognitive outcomes, but their

FIGURE 25-39 Cardiopulmonary bypass pump.

A

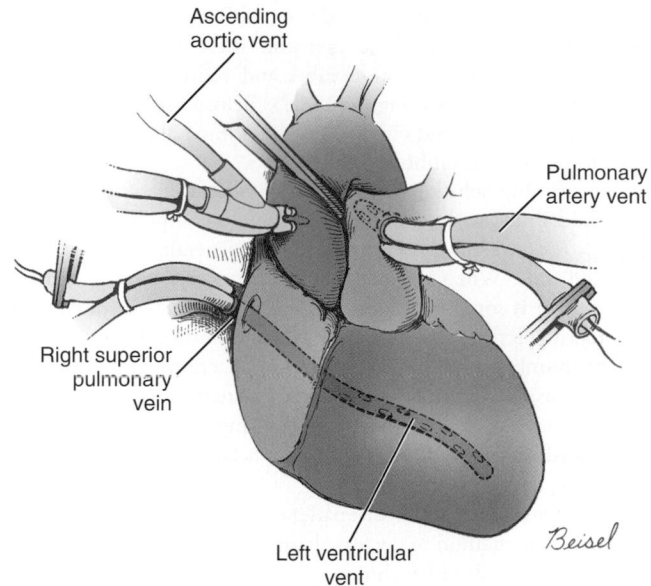

FIGURE 25-41 Types of venting catheters.

B

FIGURE 25-40 A, Venous endovascular cannula. **B,** The catheter tip inserts into the femoral vein and threads into the right atrium; the distal tip is positioned in the superior vena cava (SVC) to drain the upper body.

research did show fewer gaseous emboli and a shortened period of de-airing (at least 3 minutes shorter).

Improved bypass technology also reduces the incidence of bypass-related microemboli and cellular injury with the use of finer filters for air and particulate emboli and moderation of siphoning pressure strength (Groom et al, 2009). Membrane oxygenators incorporated

into the bypass circuit (see Figure 25-38) perform gas exchange (CO_2 removal and oxygen addition to the blood) more efficiently and less traumatically. Gases diffuse through a semipermeable membrane that separates the oxygenating gas and the venous blood. Although membrane oxygenators preserve platelet and red blood cell function better than older "bubble" oxygenators, there remains considerable morbidity associated with the use of CPB. Extracorporeal circulation causes fluid retention and intercompartmental fluid shifts, multiple organ dysfunction, showers of microemboli, inflammatory responses, and unique bleeding complications (Groom et al, 2009). The mechanisms of injury likely relate to exposure of the blood to abnormal surfaces of the bypass circuit, hypothermia, shear forces, and altered blood flow. These can initiate a systemic inflammatory response (complement activation), which releases vasoactive substances. Attempts to minimize inflammatory reactions have focused on modifying the activation of platelets and blood factors that play a major role in initiating the response (Kaplan et al, 2011). To avoid complications associated with CPB, clinicians have stimulated greater use of "beating heart" ("off-pump") techniques for myocardial revascularization. It should be noted, however, that off-pump techniques do not apply to procedures requiring the heart to be opened (e.g., mitral valve surgery, left ventricular aneurysm repair) because air within the opened chamber would embolize to the brain. CPB enables the heart to be isolated from systemic circulation so that after repair completion (and before cross-clamp removal), various venting techniques can remove residual air effectively.

Two pumps are available: roller pumps and centrifugal pumps. Roller pumps have roller heads that propel blood forward by compressing blood-filled tubing against a smooth metal housing. Centrifugal pumps use cones or blades that rotate at high speed to produce forward flow. Both pumps produce some hemolysis from turbulence and shear forces, but careful calibration and minimal use of connectors can provide relatively atraumatic flow for short periods (e.g., less than 6 hours). Arterial blood flow on bypass is largely nonpulsatile, although modifications to the pump can simulate phasic (systolic/nonsystolic) flow (Grocott et al, 2011); arterial blood pressure usually appears as a mean arterial waveform on the oscilloscope during CPB.

Suction lines, ordinarily used during CPB, return shed blood to the venous reservoir and the oxygenator. These lines may combine conventional handheld suction tubes and ventricular decompression lines or sumps (see Figure 25-41). Before initiation of CPB, the entire extracorporeal circuit must be primed and rendered free of air to prevent air emboli.

The priming solution is usually a combination of colloid and crystalloid fluids with a balanced electrolyte component. Priming volumes (i.e., within the CPB circuit) are generally between 1400 and 2000 mL. When the patient's blood volume mixes with the prime, there is some hemodilution and a subsequent reduction of hematocrit (Hct) level. Advantages of hemodilution include reducing the number of homologous serum reactions and providing better perfusion of capillary beds, a result of reduced blood viscosity. Hct levels as low as 25% may suffice during CPB, but once CPB ends, transfusion of red blood cells may need to follow to enhance the blood's oxygen-carrying capacity.

Low-weight, low-hematocrit patients may not tolerate hemodilution well. One method to decrease hemodilution is to use the *rapid-autologous-prime* (RAP) technique. First, the perfusionist shortens the length of bypass tubing to reduce the volume of prime solution in the CPB circuit. The surgeon then inserts an arterial cannula into the aorta and connects it to the arterial tubing leading to the bypass machine. Before initiation of bypass, the perfusionist allows a predetermined amount of the patient's arterial blood to drain from the line to fill part of the bypass circuit and then clamps the circuit; unclamping follows at bypass initiation (Grocott et al, 2011).

The amount and kind of drugs used in the priming solution vary among institutions, but addition of heparin to block clot formation in the bypass circuit is routine. Anticoagulation monitoring is usual during bypass as is adding more heparin as needed to maintain an activated clotting time (ACT) that exceeds 600 seconds. Addition of other ingredients to maintain normal pH and electrolytes is also common.

Finally, team members must estimate arterial blood flow rates according to the patient's height, weight, and body surface area. Arterial and venous pressure values and the results of blood gas determinations dictate flow adjustments.

Myocardial Protection. Improving cardiac surgery results are attributable in great part to progress made in protecting the myocardium. Coronary circulatory interruptions, ischemia, and hypoperfusion accompanying induced cardiac arrest are often necessary to permit the surgeon sufficient time to repair cardiac lesions under direct vision. Without measures to protect the myocardium during these periods, irreversible damage can result. The main protective strategies are cooling the heart (and the rest of the body) to reduce metabolic demand, rapidly arresting the heart to preserve myocardial energy resources, and restoring intracellular homeostasis (e.g., by correcting pH, oxygen, and electrolyte imbalances) to avoid postischemic reperfusion injury (Kaplan et al, 2011).

Hypothermia. Hypothermia in cardiac surgery is the deliberate reduction of body temperature for therapeutic purposes. A moderate degree of hypothermia, to 82.4° F (28° C), permits reduction of oxygen consumption by 50%. At 68° F (20° C) there is a further reduction of about 25%. The heat exchanger of the heart-lung machine achieves systemic circulatory cooling. When very cold temperatures (less than 68° F [20° C]) are desired for myocardial protection in prolonged, complex cases, additional surface cooling of the heart with topical application of cold saline/slush or continuous irrigation of the pericardial wall come into play. Avoiding large

ice chips in pericardial irrigating fluids prevents injury to the phrenic nerve within the right and left lateral pericardium and other cardiac tissue. Insulation pads placed behind the heart can reduce heat conduction from relatively warmer organs. Transmural cooling of the heart is achieved with cardioplegia (discussed later).

Ventricular fibrillation can occur during the cooling process, although it is less likely at temperatures greater than 89.6° F (32° C). Other complications relate to adverse effects that hypothermia has on coagulation and wound healing; this may delay hemostasis after heparin reversal and affect recuperation (Kaplan et al, 2011).

Cardioplegic Arrest. Rapidly arresting the heart during diastole is beneficial because an arrested heart uses less energy than a fibrillating or beating heart. Cardioplegia with hypothermia can reduce energy requirements even further. Providing a warm terminal bolus of cardioplegia helps to avoid reperfusion injury (caused by oxygen free radicals and lactic acid buildup) by providing oxygen and other nutrients to the heart.

Cardioplegia Delivery. Cardioplegic arrest occurs by infusing the coronary arteries with a 39.2° to 50° F (4° to 10° C) solution containing potassium (2 to 50 mEq/L) and buffering agents to counteract ischemic acidosis. Potassium acts to depolarize the myocardial cell membrane and arrests the heart in diastole.

Delivery of the solution may be by antegrade or retrograde routes (Figures 25-42 and 25-43). Antegrade delivery requires insertion of a needle into the aortic root proximal to the aortic cross-clamp; the cardioplegic solution infuses under pressure to close the aortic valve leaflets. The only remaining route for the solution is into the right and left coronary arteries and the coronary circulation (see Figure 25-37). If the aortic valve does not close properly, the cardioplegic solution will flow preferentially into the left ventricular chamber, causing distention. In such cases, direct cannulation of the coronary ostia is performed. Direct infusion into vein grafts protects the myocardium distal to coronary lesions and enhances transmural cooling. Retrograde infusion requires placement of a catheter transatrially into the coronary sinus; perfusate enters the coronary venous system and flows through the myocardial circulation, leaving through the coronary ostia. Retrograde infusion is especially useful when coronary artery obstructions and left ventricular hypertrophy are present.

When the heart sufficiently arrests, the ECG reflects a straight line; when electrical activity appears on the monitor (as fine fibrillation), the cardioplegic solution is reinfused to continue cooling as desired (about every 15 to 20 minutes).

Minimally invasive techniques for myocardial protection also have been developed (described under Cardioplegia Delivery). Percutaneously inserted catheters can infuse antegrade cardioplegic solution through a catheter threaded into the aortic root; likewise, a catheter inserted into the internal jugular vein and then passed into the SVC, the RA, and the coronary sinus can infuse retrograde cardioplegic solution.

Circulatory Arrest. In highly complex procedures, such as those involving the aortic arch, it may be impossible to place an occluding clamp across the aorta. In these cases circulatory arrest may be used to maintain a dry operative site. Because all blood flow will be interrupted, protection of myocardial, cerebral, and other tissue from ischemia requires additional measures.

The patient undergoes cooling with the heat exchanger to about 65° F (18° C), at which point team members turn off the bypass pump. Incision and repair follow. A suction catheter can remove the small amount of collateral drainage entering the field. With repair complete, air removal follows.

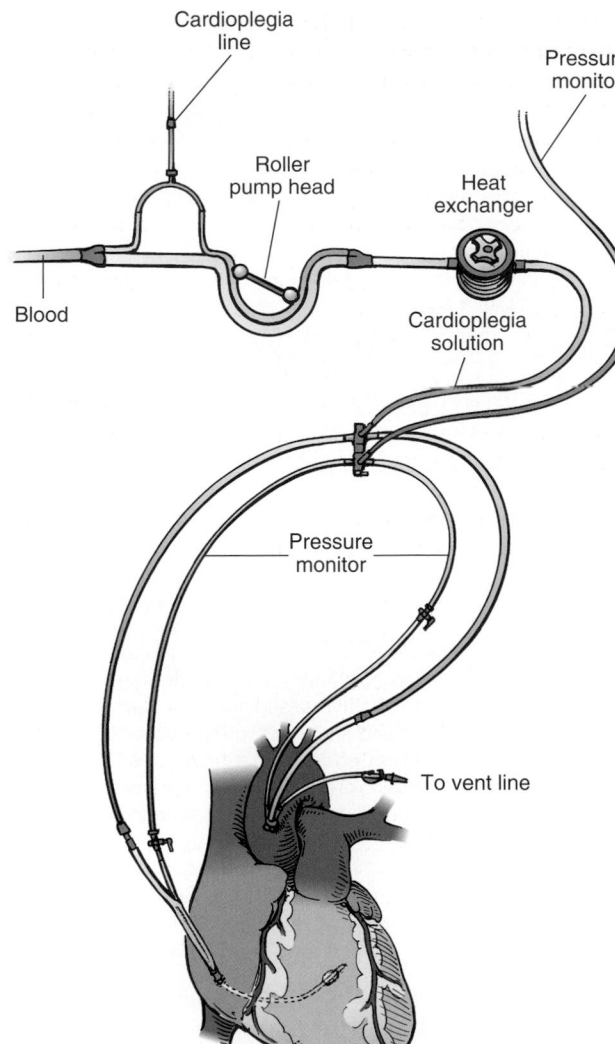

FIGURE 25-42 Antegrade-retrograde cardioplegia system. The antegrade cardioplegia catheter inserts into the aorta proximally to the cross-clamp; the catheter is Y-ed into a vent line and into the retrograde cardioplegia catheter, which inserts transatrially into the coronary sinus. The coronary sinus pressure is monitored; its pressure should remain less than 50 mm Hg.

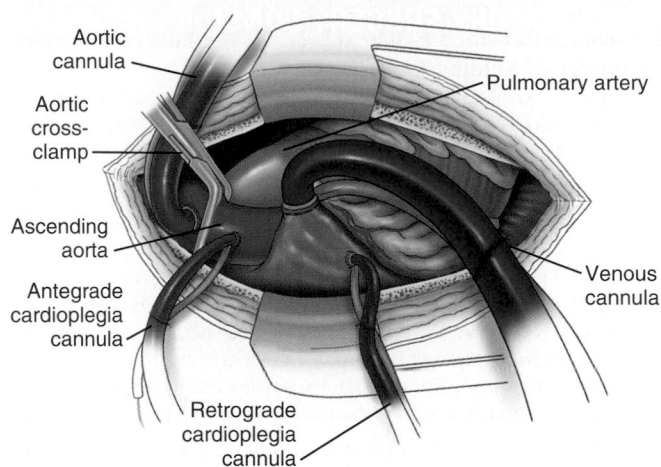

FIGURE 25-43 View of cannulated heart from surgeon's perspective. The cross-clamp isolates the aortic root and coronary blood vessels from the systemic circulation. This creates a closed circuit and allows the administration of cardioplegia without allowing systemic blood to wash cardioplegia out of coronary circulation during induced arrest. This enables the surgeon to create a bloodless field.

Cerebral Perfusion. Circulatory arrest also poses risk to the brain. Cerebral protection, cerebroplegia, is by infusion of oxygenated blood to the brain. *Antegrade* cerebral perfusion occurs via insertion of cannulae directly into the innominate artery, the right common carotid artery, or another branch of the aortic arch. *Retrograde* cerebral perfusion is by use of a cannula that has been Y-ed to the superior vena cava drainage cannula that connects to the arterial infusion line. Once blood flow stops (during circulatory arrest), the venous line is clamped, the connection to the arterial line opened, and the retrograde cerebral perfusion line infuses cerebroplegia into the head vessels. Blood returning from the head (through the carotid or vertebral arteries) is suctioned from the field.

Termination of CPB. Near the end of the repair, the heart is allowed to rewarm while the perfusionist rewarms the patient systemically with the oxygenator's heat exchanger. Air is evacuated from the LV and the proximal portion of the aorta. Removal of the cross-clamp

follows. The heart often converts spontaneously to sinus rhythm, but internal (or external) defibrillation may be necessary. Temporary epicardial pacing wires may be sutured to the right atrial appendage or the RV; these remain postoperatively if the patient has transient bradycardia, supraventricular tachycardia, or other dysrhythmias. Atrial fibrillation (AF) is a common postoperative complication associated with a greater risk of embolic events and increases length of stay (Bojar, 2011).

When the heart is contracting, and the lungs are being ventilated, the patient undergoes gradual weaning from CPB. Reduction of venous flow is gradual, accomplished by reduced clamping of the venous line or lines, and the perfusionist effects a commensurate reduction in arterial flow. When heart action is sufficient and systemic, and pulmonary blood pressures stabilized, the bypass terminates and the cannulae removed.

Active measures to promote body heat retention and to enhance clotting mechanisms, immune function, and oxygenation follow. There is authority to suggest that maintenance of normothermia after termination of CPB reduces the risk of postoperative infection (Grocott et al, 2011).

Closing. After achieving hemostasis a team member inserts catheters into the pericardium to drain mediastinal shed blood. Entry into either or both pleurae requires the insertion of chest tubes to drain shed blood entering from the pericardium and to create negative intrapleural pressure to facilitate lung expansion. The tubes connect to a water-seal drainage system or an autotransfusion drainage system by using straight or Y connectors. Chest tube drainage of greater than 100 mL/hr requires investigation of possible causes (Bojar, 2011). The clinician anticipates such excess drainage by ordering possible blood studies in advance to determine whether clotting factors require replacement, hemostasis of anastomoses is present, or bypass conduits require exploration. Reopening the chest may be necessary to control bleeding.

Chest closure in median sternotomy requires wire sutures (see Figure 25-18). The wire sutures are twisted, excess wire is cut, and

AMBULATORY SURGERY CONSIDERATIONS

Excision of Keloid Scar

Postcardiac surgery patients may develop a keloid scar: a nonmalignant, abnormal proliferation or overgrowth of dense, fibrous tissue that extends beyond the borders of the original wound. Keloid scars affect both sexes, but tend to appear more often in individuals with greater pigmentation of the skin. Keloids are considered a proliferative disorder, in which the control mechanism regulating tissue repair and regeneration distorts. Therapy includes compression, corticosteroids, and occlusive dressings; excisional surgery is possible, but this usually is only partially successful. Laser therapy is increasingly used to treat keloids. The procedure usually takes place in the ambulatory surgery setting. If anesthesia is indicated, topical lidocaine generally suffices. Laser pulses are delivered over the entire scar area. The size, thickness, location, and color determine the number of laser sessions required.

Modified from Jansen DA et al: Keloids, *Medscape Reference*, updated January 30, 2012, available at http://emedicine.medscape.com/article/1298013-overview. Accessed March 19, 2013; Nouri K et al: Laser treatment of scars and stria distensae, *Medscape Reference*, updated May 21, 2012, available at http://emedicine.medscape.com/article/1120673 -overview. Accessed March 19, 2013.

the wire ends are buried into the sternal periosteum. Some surgeons use small metal crimpers to approximate and hold the wires (rather than twisting and burying the wire ends). In a frail sternum, a long sternal closing wire may be threaded longitudinally along the right and left lateral margins of the sternum; the crossed sternal wires insert through the longitudinal wires and then are approximated to close the sternum. This reinforces the sternal closure and reduces the possibility of sternal dehiscence.

In some thin patients with little subcutaneous tissue over the sternum, one (or more) of the sternal wires may continue to cause irritation and discomfort after the sternum has fully healed. For these patients the surgeon may remove the wire during an ambulatory (outpatient) procedure. The surgeon makes a small incision over the wire, dissects down to the wire, cuts it on the anterior surface, pulls it out of the sternum, and closes the incision.

An ambulatory procedure to remove a keloid, an overgrown, elevated, and rounded scar, is possible (Jansen and Molnar, 2012; Nouri and Elston, 2012). Patients may choose plastic repair if scarring poses personal or professional concerns (Ambulatory Surgery Considerations).

Closure of the linea alba is with suture. Placement of a layer of sutures approximates the fascia over the sternum, and closure of subcutaneous tissue and skin follows. If metal staples are used on the skin, a staple remover should accompany the patient to the recovery area. The clinician closes thoracotomy incisions in standard fashion.

Before transferring the patient, the perioperative nurse transfers information to the receiving unit, usually the cardiovascular SICU and telephones a report to the recovery area. Figure 25-44 lists commonly supplied information. The patient's special concerns and fears, as well as significant physiologic alterations, should be communicated (Seifert, 2012).

Improving cardiac patient safety by using evidence-based practices between and among cardiac surgery clinicians has been the subject of an American Heart Association Scientific Statement (Wahr et al, 2013). Among recommended practices are checklists,

RESEARCH HIGHLIGHT ‖

Communication and Teamwork

Few studies identify perioperative nurses' interventions to reduce error and improve safety in the cardiac OR. Communication and teamwork are two critical factors that must be considered. Preventable errors are often due to cognitive, system, or teamwork failures. In particular, human factors such as the *nontechnical skills* of communication (communication failures underlie many adverse events), cooperation, coordination, and leadership are necessary components of effective teamwork. Adverse events often occur even absent optimal nontechnical skills. Additionally, a rigid hierarchical and disruptive culture works against effective teamwork and communication. *Physical environment* is also important because poor layout can impede communication (e.g., a perfusionist speaks to the surgeon's back) and noise levels (e.g., monitoring alarms) increase distractions.

The American Heart Association's *Scientific Statement on Patient Safety in the Cardiac Operating Room* is a multidisciplinary work by surgeons, anesthesiologists, perfusionists, human factors experts, and a nurse that identifies risks to patient safety and interventions based on evidence to reduce risks and errors in cardiac surgery. Among the recommendations supported by research studies are the following: those that address teamwork training, implementation of briefings/debriefings, formal hand-off protocols, questions and answers, and safety culture standards.
- Implement briefings and checklists in the cardiac OR
- Establish team training efforts and studies using tools (e.g., Oxford Non-Technical Skills [NOTECHS] system) to address safety attitudes, compliance with recommended practices, communication skills
- Establish and adhere to hand-off protocols (e.g., situation, background, assessment, recommendation [SBAR])
- Crisis and disaster team training
- Implement policies to address, deal with and minimize disruptive behavior

The statement is an important contribution to the safety literature because it addresses many hard-to-measure areas (e.g., teamwork, leadership), but have a powerful influence within the perioperative work culture. Further research to identify and implement improvements to safe patient care remains to be done and is strongly recommended.

From Wahr JA et al: American Heart Association: scientific statement on patient safety in the cardiac operating room: human factors and teamwork, *Circulation*, August 5, 2013, doi 10.116/CIR.06013e3182a38efa.

briefings, structured team training processes, communication protocols, and other essential behaviors (Research Highlight).

Perioperative documentation follows the standard protocol and includes a description of the procedure performed and identification of medications and all implanted material (with lot and serial numbers). Following hospital policy should ensure compliance with the Safe Medical Devices Act.

Postoperative complications associated with cardiac surgery appear in Table 25-7.

Excessive or sudden hemorrhage producing cardiac tamponade usually requires a rapid response team to control hemorrhage and to achieve hemostasis (Lemmer and Vlahakes, 2010; Bojar, 2011).

Evaluation

Evaluation of perioperative care includes determination of whether the patient met the outcomes identified in the plan of care. Such

Patient Transfer Report

PROCEDURE (include source of autogenous grafts)   on-pump _____   off-pump _____

                                        Endoscopic vein harvest yes ___ no ___ N/A ___

MONITORING DEVICES (LOCATION)

CVP _____   Arterial Line_____   SWAN _____   Peripheral _____

LA _____   Other_____

HEMODYNAMICS

BP _____   PAP _____   PAD _____   PAWP _____   CO _____   CI _____   CVP _____   Svo$_2$ _____

INTRAOPERATIVE OCCURRENCES

BLOOD LOSS _____   URINE _____   DYSRHYTHMIAS _____   BYPASS

PROBLEMS _____   DEFIB X's _____   LO TEMP _____   HI TEMP_____

CROSS-CLAMP TIME _____   PUMP TIME _____

BLOOD: GIVEN _____   AVAILABLE _____   AUTOTRANSFUSION TOTALS: _____ mL _____ Units

COMPONENTS: FFP _____   PLATELETS _____   CRYO _____

ADDITIONAL ORDERED (TYPE) _____

MEDICATIONS

NEO _____   DOPAMINE _____   DOBUTAMINE _____   LIDOCAINE _____   NITRO _____

LEVOPHED _____   EPINEPHRINE _____   NITROPRUSSIDE _____   INOCOR _____

DDAVP _____   OTHER _____

TUBES/DRAINS: MEDIASTINAL _____   PLEURAL (Rt/Lt) _____

EPICARDIAL LEADS: ATRIAL _____   VENTRICULAR _____

PACING: YES/NO   RATE_____

LABS:

K+ _____   Na+ _____   Glu _____   Hgb _____   Hct _____

PATIENT CONCERNS _____

ADDITIONAL INFORMATION _____

ICU BED # _____   ETA _____

REPORTED BY _____

To _____   TIME _____

BP, Blood pressure; *CI*, cardiac index; *CO*, cardiac output; *CRYO*, cryoprecipitate; *CVP*, central venous pressure; *DDAVP*, 1-deamino-8-*D*-arginine vasopressin (e.g., desmopressin), *ETA*, estimated time of arrival; *FFP*, fresh frozen plasma; *Glu*, glucose; *Hct*, hematocrit; *Hgb*, hemoglobin; *K+*, potassium; *LA*, left atrium; *Na+*, sodium; *NEO*, Neo-Synephrine; *NITRO*, nitroglycerin; *PAD*, pulmonary artery diastolic pressure; *PAP*, pulmonary artery pressure; *PAWP*, pulmonary artery wedge pressure; *Svo$_2$*, percent saturation of mixed venous blood; *SWAN*, Swan-Ganz (pulmonary artery) catheter.

FIGURE 25-44 Patient transfer report.

evaluation assists perioperative nurses to determine whether nursing interventions designed for a specific patient were successful. This type of data collection becomes the basis for development of future plans of care for similar patients. Documentation of the evaluation should appear in the perioperative record. For the nursing diagnoses and the subsequent plan of care presented in this chapter, outcome statements might be as follows:

• The patient's cardiac function is consistent with or improved from baseline levels established preoperatively, as evidenced by blood pressure within expected range; warm, dry skin; and urine output more than 30 mL/hr.

• The patient is free from signs and symptoms of infection at the surgical site or sites as evidenced by absence of redness, edema, purulent incisional drainage, or untoward elevation of temperature postoperatively.

• The patient is free from signs and symptoms of injury related to surgical position as evidenced by the absence of acquired neuromuscular impairment and tissue necrosis.

• The patient is free of contamination from external and internal sources; there are no documented lapses in sterile technique, no preexisting infections, or no other episodes of contamination.

• The patient is free from excessive bleeding as evidenced by chest tube drainage less than 100 mL/hr, dressings dry and intact, normal coagulation function studies (or undergoing replacement treatment for deficient clotting factors), and normal body temperature.

• The patient demonstrates knowledge of the physiologic responses to the cardiac disorder (at his or her level of understanding), the proposed surgical treatment, and the immediate perioperative events as evidenced by verbalization of disease state, purpose of

TABLE 25-7

Complications of Cardiac Surgery

Body System	Complication	Treatment Measures
Cardiovascular	Bleeding	Transfusion
		Replacement of clotting factors
		Control of hypertension
		Maintenance of normothermia
		Possible return to OR for exploration and hemostasis
	Cardiac tamponade	Release of constricting blood via chest tube insertion or operative exploration
	Myocardial ischemia/infarction	Monitor ECG for ischemic changes
		Measure serum enzymes
		Minimize oxygen demand
		Administer medications to reduce cardiac workload and dysrhythmias
		Insertion of an IABP
	Dysrhythmias	Administer antidysrhythmic drugs
		Correct electrolyte imbalances
		Correct acid-base, hypovolemia
		Use pacemaker therapy
		Cardiovert or defibrillate as necessary
		Maintain adequate CO
Pulmonary	Hemothorax/pneumothorax	Maintain chest tube patency
		Check chest tubes for air leaks
		Insert additional chest tube (pleural or mediastinal)
	Atelectasis/pneumonia	Check ventilator settings and endotracheal tube
		Suction endotracheal tube
		Monitor breath sounds
		Monitor pulse oximetry
		Obtain chest x-ray film
		Elevate head of bed
		Ensure proper function of NG tube
		After extubation, encourage mobilization and use of incentive spirometry
		Frequent staff handwashing
	Pulmonary embolus	Frequent patient mouth care
		Use compression stockings
		Assess for acute chest pain and SOB
		Perform radiologic examination
		Possible surgical embolectomy
	Failure to wean from ventilator	Maintain aggressive pulmonary toilet
		Elevate head of bed 30 degrees
		Monitor pulse oximetry
		Frequent mobilization (even while on ventilator)
		Pain and anxiety management
		Incentive spirometry once extubated
		Possible tracheostomy
Kidneys	Renal insufficiency/failure	Promote adequate CO, renal perfusion
		Monitor urine output
		Diuretics for oliguria
		Administer volume (vs. drugs) to increase renal perfusion
		Possible dialysis
Gastrointestinal (GI)	Ileus	Assess bowel sounds and distention
		Maintain NG tube function
		Progress diet slowly
	GI bleeding	Maintain NG tube function to differentiate upper and lower GI bleeding
		Stress ulcer prophylaxis
		Monitor complaints of nausea
		Use extra caution with anticoagulants
Neurologic	Stroke	Avoid hypotension
		Assess neurologic function
		Restart preoperative antidepressant drugs
	Neurocognitive dysfunction/ postcardiotomy delirium	Avoid hypoperfusion
		Correct metabolic derangements
		Avoid hypoxemia
		Orient frequently to time and place
		Discontinue medications that may promote delirium
		Ensure a safe environment

TABLE 25-7

Complications of Cardiac Surgery—cont'd

Body System	Complication	Treatment Measures
Immune	Hospital-acquired infection	Frequent staff handwashing
		Strict aseptic technique
		Dressing care, urinary catheter care
		Early removal of central lines, urinary catheters, chest tubes
		Administer antibiotics
	Mediastinitis	Strict aseptic technique
		Administration of antibiotics
Metabolic	Hyper-/hypoglycemia	Limited blood transfusion
		Glucose (hyperglycemic) control
		Possible return to OR for debridement and muscle flap repair
		Avoid hyperglycemia (maintain glucose at less than 200 mg/dL)
		Avoid hypoglycemia
		Monitor for potential rebound from insulin administered during surgery

CO, Cardiac output; *ECG,* electrocardiogram; *IABP,* intra-aortic balloon pump; *NG,* nasogastric; *SOB,* shortness of breath.
Modified from Babb M: Clinical risk assessment: identifying patients at high risk for heart failure, *AORN J* 89(2):273–288, 2009; Bojar RM: *Manual of perioperative care in adult cardiac surgery,* ed 5, Oxford, 2011, Wiley-Blackwell; Lemmer JH, Vlahakes GJ: *Handbook of patient care in cardiac surgery,* ed 7, Philadelphia, 2010, Lippincott Williams & Wilkins; Seifert PC: Care of the cardiac surgical patient. In Odom-Forren J, editor: *Drain's perianesthesia nursing: a critical care approach,* ed 6, St Louis, 2013, Saunders.

surgery, sequence of events, anticipated outcomes, and recovery process.

- The patient's myocardial, peripheral, and cerebral tissue integrity are adequate: there are no new electrocardiographic manifestations of infarction, peripheral pulses are palpable, and sensorium is improving after extubation in the OR.

In addition to clinical outcomes, healthcare professionals scrutinize the costs of various cardiac procedures (Gelsomino et al, 2011; Speir et al, 2009). For example, Vassileva and colleagues (2012) found that the cost of mitral valve repair and replacement increases in patients with preoperative comorbidities (e.g., MI, heart failure, renal disease, neurologic deficits), emergency admission, and postoperative complications. Perioperative nurses, normally very familiar with resource utilization, can and should participate actively in cost saving initiatives.

Patient and Family Education and Discharge Planning

The cardiac service admits many patients on the day of surgery; teaching sessions therefore are scheduled appropriately before admission, along with preoperative laboratory testing. Perioperative nurses should include details about the surgical procedure, sights and sounds that the patient may face, and anesthesia care. With hospital lengths of stay shortened from 1 week or more to 3 to 5 days, patient education and preparation for home care maintenance has become even more critical to enhance positive patient outcomes. The perioperative nurse acts to reinforce, review, clarify, and add to important information and instructions the patient and family or significant others need to plan for surgery, recovery, and discharge. Although patients undergoing repeat operations have some experience with cardiac surgery, they often continue to have unmet educational and emotional needs. Changes in the patient's disease, alterations in surgical techniques, and the introduction of newer devices may require changes in expectations. Articles about endovascular thoracic repairs, endoscopic vein harvesting, and percutaneous aortic valve replacement, in less technical language, are available widely online; technology-savvy consumers can download information about many aspects of cardiac surgery, and

nurses should be prepared to answer questions and clarify common misconceptions.

The *AORN Journal* initiated a "Patient Education" page to accompany many clinical articles in order to assist perioperative nurses in their cardiovascular patient teaching activities (see Cochico, 2012; Tinkham, 2009). The *Journal of the American Medical Association* (JAMA) and other journals offer patient education. An area of currently intense patient interest is minimally invasive surgery and comparisons of "on-pump" and "off-pump" techniques (Patient and Family Education).

Postoperative education also plays an important role in reducing hospital readmissions. An innovative program employed physician assistants (PAs) to perform home visits to postoperative cardiac surgery patients. The PAs used educational techniques as well as clinical judgments to manage the patients' medication use, wound healing, and patient or family concerns; the program demonstrated a 25% reduction in hospital readmissions (Nabagiez et al, 2013). Such a program would be appropriate especially for advanced practice registered nurses to influence patient outcomes and expand opportunities to apply their skill sets.

Additional electronic and peer support resources can supplement traditional education tools. An expanding array of Internet sites developed by professional organizations offer numerous examples of patient information. The American College of Surgeons (ACS, 2013), the American Heart Association (AHA, 2012 a,b; 2013), the American Society of Anesthesiologists (ASA, 2013), the Society of Cardiovascular Anesthesiologists (SCA, 2012), and the Society of Thoracic Surgeons (STS, 2013) all have cardiac-related materials for consumers as well as clinical staff. Support groups such as the Mended Hearts (www.mendedhearts.org) provide education, support, and social networking among cardiac surgical patients. Email is an increasingly popular form of communication between patients and caregivers, and some cardiac surgical practice groups as well as healthcare institutions offer interactive websites.

In addition to specific information about the perioperative period, the cardiac patient's preoperative state of mind is worthy of consideration. Having the patient complete a preoperative mental

PATIENT AND FAMILY EDUCATION

Patient Teaching Considerations for Minimally Invasive Surgery (On-/Off-Pump)

	Beating Heart/Off-Pump	Arrested Heart/On-Pump
Definition	CABG without CPB or induced cardiac arrest; HR and contractile force may be pharmacologically reduced; stabilizer used at anastomotic site; apical retractor used to expose lateral and posterior coronary arteries	CABG with CPB and endovascular technique for CPB and induced cardiac arrest
Indications	Multiple-vessel disease, angioplasty contraindicated, medical problems, poor anatomy, accessible target arteries, previous CABG with blocked grafts	Multiple-vessel disease, angioplasty contraindicated, need to stop heart to enhance technical precision, accessible target arteries, valve or other cardiac disease requiring entry into a heart chamber
Contraindications	Intramyocardial lesions, hemodynamic instability	Highly complex lesions, posterior targets
Incisions	Sternotomy or mini-sternotomy (cephalad or caudad); 1 to 3 small right or left rib or submammary incisions	1 to 4 small rib incisions, 1 or 2 groin incisions, 1 or 2 neck incisions
CPB	No, available on standby	Yes
Cardioplegia	No	Yes
Procedure time	2 hr or more	2 hr or more
Hospital LOS	2-5 days (vs. 4-6 days for sternotomy)	3-5 days (vs. 4-6 days for sternotomy)
Advantages	Avoids CPB, ischemic arrest, and hypothermia; may enable more complete revascularization with postoperative insertion of intracoronary stents into posterolateral coronary arteries in cardiac catheterization laboratory ("hybrid" procedure); may reduce MACE in patients with LMCAD	Allows repair of more complex lesions without technical challenge of a moving heart; better able to produce more complete revascularization; significantly reduces air embolism as a result of opening cardiac chambers
Potential complications and disadvantages	Learning curve technically more challenging; may cause VF; may have to revert to standard sternotomy with CPB and induced arrest; may be more technically challenging in females	Learning curve technically more challenging; may have to revert to standard sternotomy; potential for endovascular injury to cannulated blood vessels
Discharge planning	Anticipated faster recovery of 1-2 wk (vs. 4-12 wk for sternotomy), earlier ambulation, need to identify reportable signs and symptoms (angina, difficulty breathing, infection)	Anticipated faster recovery of 1-2 wk (vs. 4-12 wk for sternotomy), earlier ambulation, need to identify reportable signs and symptoms (angina, difficulty breathing, infection)

CABG, Coronary artery bypass graft; *CPB,* cardiopulmonary bypass; *HR,* heart rate; *LMCAD,* left main coronary artery disease; *LOS,* length of stay; *MACE,* major adverse cardiac event; *VF,* ventricular fibrillation.

Modified from Sarin EL et al: Off-pump coronary bypass grafting is associated with reduced operative mortality and in-hospital adverse events in patients with left main coronary artery disease, *Innovations* 4(2):80–85, 2009; Grocott HP et al: Cardiopulmonary bypass management and organ protection. In Kaplan JA et al, editors: *Kaplan's cardiac anesthesia: the echo era,* ed 6, Philadelphia, 2011, Saunders; Morrow DA, Boden WE: Stable ischemic heart disease. In Bonow RO et al, editors: *Braunwald's heart disease: a textbook of cardiovascular medicine,* ed 9, Philadelphia, 2012, Saunders.

health status questionnaire, or being aware of the results of a previously completed questionnaire, can provide insight into the patient's frame of mind and serve as an opportunity to change pessimistic attitudes to a more positive state of mind. Patient attitudes can be affected negatively by the anticipation of pain, as well as by hesitation to complain of pain or to request pain medication. Perioperative nurses need to anticipate these normal fears and encourage patients to ask for pain medications in order to facilitate early postoperative ambulation, deep breathing and coughing, and other activities that promote recovery. Sharing such information with staff in the receiving unit during the hand-off report is entirely proper and good practice (see Figure 25-44).

The hand-off report should include specific information to optimize recuperation. For example, patients undergoing prosthetic (e.g., mechanical) valve replacement need to know they will require long-term anticoagulation therapy. Important information includes drug dosage, reportable signs and symptoms of complications and side effects (e.g., bleeding, poor healing), and a follow-up protocol to monitor bleeding times.

Assessment of the patient's ability to cough and to breathe deeply is important; further, the patient needs instruction to use a cough pillow or splinting techniques. The patient also needs to know about required lifestyle changes and to express feelings about these modifications. The perioperative nurse should verify that the patient knows reportable signs and symptoms associated with the specific procedure and understands prescribed medications, including medication dosages, potential side effects, and signs and symptoms of complications (see Table 25-6). Any misconceptions should be corrected or referred to an appropriate source. The family or significant others' ability and willingness to assist the patient in home care maintenance should be queried; referrals to an agency for assistance at home may be appropriate.

Quality of life is an important concern for patients. Although objective measures are often used by clinicians to determine the patient's level of satisfaction with the quality of care received, measuring the patient's quality of life after surgery has been largely limited to evaluating angina relief and return to work. Other important variables, however, may affect quality of life positively or negatively, and nurses can assist patients with recovery and recuperation by incorporating these variables into the discharge plan. For example, quality of life for family caregivers also is an important consideration because shortened lengths of stay may force patients to depend more heavily on others to assist them with recuperation. Thus support for caregivers is an important adjunct to patient recovery.

Nurses can help patients to set realistic postoperative goals and develop strategies for appropriate lifestyle changes. The subjective perceptions of patients usually accurately reflect the patient's quality of life. At times when the quality of life is perceived as less than optimal (e.g., during a difficult recuperative period), the nurse can reassure patient and family that physical, emotional, and psychologic improvement is a progressive process. A patient's perception and the clinical indications for treatment may not be the same, but clinicians should recognize that the patient's definition of quality of life is valid in its own right and should be addressed whenever feasible.

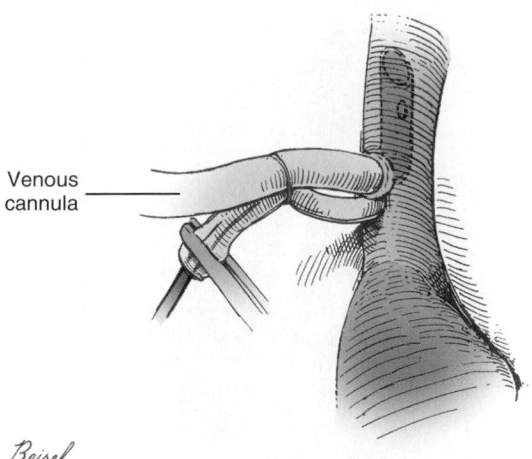

FIGURE 25-45 Right-angle cannula in superior vena cava.

Surgical Interventions

The following section describes surgery for acquired forms of heart disease. It describes both traditional "open" procedures and minimally invasive techniques. Performance of open procedures is through a median sternotomy incision using aortocaval CPB (see Figures 25-37 and 25-38) and antegrade-retrograde cardioplegia (see Figures 25-42 and 25-43) with routine chest drainage and closure. Minimally invasive procedures include descriptions of CPB, saphenous vein harvesting, CABG, AF, and MVR. Performance of these procedures may be through a median sternotomy or an anterior left or right thoracotomy; approaches for some lesions, however, may be via cephalad or caudal mini-sternotomy.

Extracorporeal Circulation Procedures

Operative Procedures

Aortocaval Cannulation by Sternotomy

1. The surgeon makes a longitudinal pericardial incision, and retraction of the pericardial edges is by suture to the chest wall.
2. If the aorta is to undergo cannulation for arterial blood return to the patient, the surgeon partially dissects it from the pulmonary artery.
3. The surgeon next places purse-string sutures in the aorta (twice) and RA (or both venae cavae) for eventual placement of perfusion cannulae. Tourniquets are placed over the suture ends and held with a hemostat.
4. For ascending aortic cannulation, the aorta is incised inside the purse-string sutures with a knife (the surgeon places a finger over the aortotomy); the cannula is inserted, and the purse-string sutures are firmly secured with the tourniquet. It is important to have the distal end of the cannula clamped before it is inserted into the aorta to prevent backbleeding from the aorta. To prevent air emboli, the arterial connection is made under a saline drip or by having the perfusionist slowly pump priming solution out of the arterial line. Arterial cannulation generally occurs before caval cannulation so that direct access for blood replacement is available if needed.
5. Venous cannulation occurs in one of the following ways:
   a. *Single, two-stage cannulation for venous return to the pump-oxygenator:* An incision is made into the right atrial appendage, and the two-stage cannula (see Figure 25-38) is inserted

into the atrium. Placement of the distal end of the cannula is into the inferior vena cava (IVC). A tourniquet secures the purse-string suture, and the catheter is permitted to fill partially with blood before being connected to the venous line.
   b. *Double cannulation:* Double cannulation requires a second incision into the atrial wall within the purse-string suture, and the cannulae are placed in the inferior and superior venae cavae (see Figure 25-36). To force all venous return into the cannulae, umbilical tapes with tourniquets may be placed around each cava and then tightened. This forces systemic venous return to enter the cannulae, producing total CPB (see Figure 25-36).
6. In procedures requiring greater exposure of the RA (e.g., tricuspid valve surgery or closure of atrial septal defects in adults), a right-angle cannula may be inserted into the SVC (Figure 25-45).

Femoral Vein–Femoral Artery Cannulation

1. A vertical or oblique incision is made into the femoral triangle, exposing the femoral vein and artery. Umbilical compression tapes are passed around the vessels, above and below the proposed venotomy and arteriotomy. Vascular clamps may be applied above and below the incision into each vessel.
2. A purse-string suture is placed in the femoral artery. A needle inserted into the artery is followed by a guidewire. The needle is removed and dilators thread over the guidewire to enlarge the artery. After removal of the dilators, a perfusion catheter (occluded distally with a tubing clamp) is inserted retrograde into the arteriotomy as release of the proximal clamp or tourniquet occurs. The proximal tourniquet is tightened (Figure 25-46). The cannula is connected to the arterial line.
3. The surgeon incises the femoral vein, and a venous catheter is inserted into the vein as the proximal clamp or tourniquet is released. After the cannula is in place, the proximal tourniquet is tightened to prevent bleeding from the venotomy. Occlusion of the cannula at the distal end with a tubing clamp occurs to prevent bleeding from the cannula. Connection of the cannula is made to the venous line, and the tubing clamp removed.

Minimally Invasive Cannulation. Femoral cannulation techniques apply here. Femoral arterial cannulation is as just described. Venous drainage is with an extended catheter inserted into the exposed femoral vein, and the distal tip advanced to the SVC to the inferior portion of the RA (see Figure 25-41). Side ports along

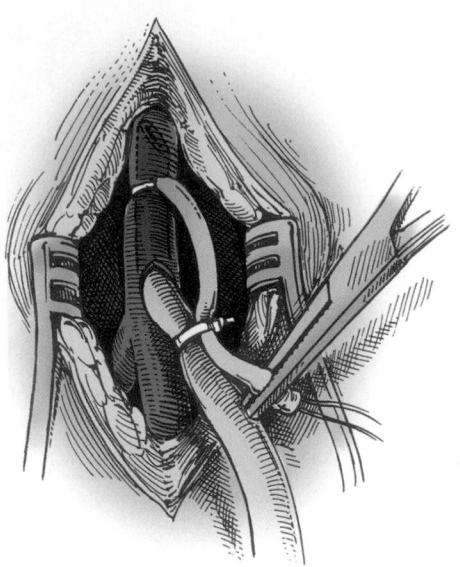

FIGURE 25-46 Cannulation of femoral artery.

the distal portion of the cannula allow drainage of blood from the SVC, the RA, and the IVC. Given higher resistance to drainage flow compared to right atrial cannulation, a centrifugal pump or vacuum-assisted drainage incorporated in the CPB circuit augments venous drainage. These minimally invasive techniques also apply to newer percutaneous procedures (e.g., catheter-based aortic valve replacement).

Pump-Oxygenator Preparation. After completion of arterial and venous connections and securing of lines, bypass slowly begins and the desired flow rate gradually is achieved. Arterial infusion calibration matches venous outflow in order to maintain consistent cardiac output and blood volume. Perfusion flow adjustments follow as required throughout the operation (Grocott et al, 2011).

Axillary Artery Cannulation. Although infrequently used for arterial perfusion, the right axillary artery (AA) is a useful cannulation site when the ascending aorta cannot undergo cannulation due to aneurysm or dissection or when circulatory arrest is necessary for surgery on the aorta. Another use occurs in the presence of acute or chronic aortic dissection, when retrograde flow through the femoral artery may produce femoral artery dissection and malperfusion of the central organs (e.g., the kidneys). The AA is usually free of atherosclerosis and has excellent collateral flow from the thyrocervical trunk to the suprascapular and transverse cervical arteries, which helps to avoid upper extremity ischemia during cross-clamping (Grocott et al, 2011). Use of the AA for cannulation also facilitates antegrade cerebral perfusion during hypothermic arrest. The artery can undergo direct cannulation, but the risk of dissection favors indirect cannulation via an 8- to 10-mm Dacron tube graft anastomosed to the artery.

Positioning of the patient is supine with a roll under the shoulders to enhance access to the artery; tilting the OR bed to the left provides better exposure of the artery during cannulation. Positioning of the right arm is next to the body with the elbow flexed slightly; extension of the arm is proper in some procedures, depending on surgeon preference. Avoidance of severe traction and manipulation is the norm in order to prevent injury to the brachial plexus.

Cannulation Procedure

1. Exposure of the right axillary (or subclavian) artery is by a small incision below and parallel to the midportion of the right clavicle. The tissue is dissected toward the insertion of the pectoralis minor muscle and the deltopectoral groove; the pectoralis major muscle is dissected and divided, and the axillary vein and underlying artery exposed and gently mobilized for about 2 cm.
2. The brachial plexus is located (cephalad to the vessels); manipulation is avoided to protect the plexus during cannulation and the operative procedure.
3. A partial occlusion clamp is applied to the artery and an 8- to 10-mm Dacron tube graft is anastomosed end-to-side to the artery with 4-0 or 5-0 polypropylene suture.
4. A straight arterial cannula is inserted through the graft and a heavy silk tie or umbilical tape is tied around the graft over the cannula to prevent bleeding.
5. A slow initiation of arterial flow follows. Comparison of blood pressures via both the right and left radial arteries must confirm the absence of a pressure gradient; after confirmation, arterial flow is increased to the initial desired rate of 2.2 to 2.8 L/min/m^2.
6. Completion of bypass and removal of the AA cannula: After CPB ends, the arterial cannula is gradually withdrawn and the AA graft is clamped (or ligated with two large metal clips); the graft is cut a few millimeters above the artery and oversewn with polypropylene suture. The surgeon carefully avoids narrowing the AA or leaving a graft "stump" (which could become a source of emboli) during closure.

Cardioplegic Delivery

Antegrade Cardioplegia. Placement of a purse-string suture and tourniquet is into the anterior ascending aorta proximal to the aortic cross-clamp, followed by insertion of a needle-tipped catheter. Flushing of both the catheter and the cardioplegic tubing removes residual air. The catheter tubing is Y-ed into a vent line so that alternatively the needle can infuse the cardioplegic solution into the aortic root or vent air and blood from the aorta and LV. Individual lines incorporated into the antegrade infusion system can infuse the coronary bypass graft or grafts selectively. Handheld cardioplegic cannulae can infuse cardioplegic solution directly into the coronary ostia, but the risk of injuring ostial tissue usually favors this technique when retrograde delivery cannot be achieved.

Retrograde Cardioplegia. A purse-string suture is placed into the lateral wall of the RA, and a tourniquet applied to the suture. The surgeon makes a stab wound into the atrium, and insertion and palpation of the retrograde catheter into the coronary sinus follow. Blood is aspirated from the catheter, and the catheter is connected to the flushed retrograde infusion line and to a pressure line. Infusion pressure should be between 20 and 45 mm Hg (Grocott et al, 2011). Because a full RA facilitates insertion of the catheter, insertion occurs before initiation of CPB when possible. If the patient is already on CPB, the surgeon can fill the atrium by clamping the venous drainage line momentarily, thereby diverting blood into the heart.

Minimally Invasive Endovascular Antegrade-Retrograde Cardioplegia. A system of endovascular multilumen catheters designed to infuse solutions, vent air and blood, measure intravascular pressures, and occlude the aorta may be used (Figure 25-47). Fluoroscopy or TEE confirms proper catheter placement.

The intravascular aortic catheter has three lumens. The first lumen has an inflatable balloon at the tip that when inflated inside the vessel, occludes the aorta and serves as an internal "cross-clamp."

FIGURE 25-47 A, Endovascular cardiopulmonary bypass and myocardial protection system (see text). **B,** Intracardiac placement of catheters.

The second lumen either infuses antegrade cardioplegic solution or vents the ventricle. The third lumen measures aortic root pressure. The catheter is introduced into the femoral artery and advanced into the ascending aorta. Either the femoral artery used for arterial inflow or the contralateral femoral artery is used.

A triple lumen coronary sinus retrograde cardioplegic catheter inserts percutaneously through the jugular vein into the SVC. Fluoroscopy guides the catheter into the coronary sinus. One lumen allows manual catheter balloon inflation, another lumen infuses retroplegic solution, and the third lumen measures coronary sinus pressure.

A third catheter serves as a venting and decompression device. It inserts into the jugular vein (through a separate sheath from the retrograde catheter) and advances into the main pulmonary artery.

These catheter systems allow surgeons to use minimally invasive techniques to treat lesions, such as mitral valve stenosis, that cannot be performed safely with a beating heart.

Termination of Cardiopulmonary Bypass

1. After the intracardiac procedure ends, evacuation of all air from the LV follows. A warm dose of cardioplegic solution may be given, after which the cross-clamp is removed. The warm solution dilates the coronary vascular bed and enhances coronary perfusion after removal of the cross-clamp.
2. Defibrillation is often spontaneous with removal of the aortic cross-clamp and the entry of warm blood into the coronary circulation. If fibrillation persists, internal defibrillation is necessary. Endovascular minimally invasive procedures require

external defibrillation with sterile external paddles or patches. Temporary epicardial pacing wires attached to the atrium and to the ventricle adjust the heart rate and optimize cardiac output.
3. Venous flow to the pump is reduced. Arterial flow is also reduced to equal the reduced venous return. When heart action is sufficient and systemic arterial blood pressure stabilizes, venous return further reduces and the patient is taken off bypass by clamping all lines and stopping the pump.
4. On removal of the cannulation catheters, the purse-string sutures are tightened and tied. Hemostasis may require additional sutures.
5. Chest tubes are inserted into the pericardium (and the pleural cavity if the pleura has been opened).
6. Administration of protamine sulfate, a heparin antagonist, follows.
7. The pericardium is usually left open so that accumulating drainage does not produce cardiac tamponade.

Closure of Femoral Incisions

1. The femoral catheters are removed, and the arteriotomies are closed with nonabsorbable cardiovascular suture. Removal of any compression tapes and bulldog clamps, if used, follows.
2. Closure of the incision is with absorbable sutures and of the skin, with interrupted or continuous sutures. Closure is performed in multiple layers (e.g., fascia, subcutaneous tissue) in order to avoid seroma formation.
3. All incisions receive dressings.

Pericardiectomy

Pericardiectomy is partial excision of an adhered, thickened fibrotic pericardium to relieve constriction of compressed heart and large blood vessels. Adhered portions of a scarred, thickened pericardium restrict diastolic filling and myocardial contractility. As the pericardial space is obliterated and calcification of the pericardium occurs, the heart is further compressed. Ascites, elevated venous pressure, decreased arterial pressure, edema, and hepatic enlargement result. In most patients etiology is unknown, although there are documented cases caused by chronic pericarditis, which may be of tubercular, rheumatic, viral, or neoplastic origin. Either the supine position or the left lateral position may be used for a left anterolateral thoracotomy.

Procedural Considerations

The use of CPB is rare for pericardiectomy, but the surgeon on occasion may request it on a standby basis. Dissection of extensive adhesions contributes to increased bleeding, and packed red blood cells should be readily available. Supplies and instruments for bypass should be available accordingly.

Operative Procedure

1. The team hypoinflates the lungs to enhance exposure of the heart. Identification and protection of the right and left phrenic nerves follow. The surgeon incises the pericardium.
2. Removal of the outer, thickened pericardium is as indicated. Cartilage scissors are available as required. The surgeon carefully dissects fibrous portions adhering to the atria and ventricles with dry dissectors and scissors. The surgeon must exercise caution to prevent perforation of the atria and RV; thus the result may be small islands of retained, adherent pericardium.
3. Dissection continues, exposing and freeing the large blood vessels as indicated.
4. Placement of drainage catheters is near the heart or through the pleural spaces; connections to the water-seal drainage system follow.

Surgery for Coronary Artery Disease

The growth of minimally invasive surgical techniques (including off-pump CABGs) and PCIs is most evident in the treatment of CAD. When compared to PCI with stent insertion, CABG remains the standard of care for patients with left main or three-vessel CAD (Patel et al, 2012); an observational study to determine the comparative effectiveness of PCI and CABG showed a survival advantage in older CABG patients with multivessel CAD (Weintraub et al, 2012). Additionally, a randomized trial by Farkouh and colleagues (2012) demonstrated CABG to be superior to PCI in patients with advanced CAD and diabetes mellitus; CABG reduced both the rates of MI and death, but demonstrated a higher stroke rate.

Revascularization procedures for ischemic myocardium also include an expanding array of options, such as port-access, robotic, endoscopic, and video-assisted procedures using smaller thoracic or sternal incisions (Table 25-8). A combination of both traditional CABG surgical techniques and fluoroscopically guided PCI are appropriate in *hybrid* ORs. Hybrid ORs are also appropriate for transcatheter aortic valve implantation (see following), arrhythmia surgery (e.g., for atrial fibrillation), and congenital surgery (Chikwe et al, 2011).

Off-pump CABG is gaining popularity as are procedures using CPB with minimally invasive systems (Morrow and Boden, 2012;

Sarin et al, 2009). Revascularization procedures can be performed using a variety of on- or off-pump techniques and approaches (see Table 25-7). Advantages of minimally invasive techniques, with or without CPB, include more cosmetic incisions, less perioperative bleeding, fewer surgical wound infections, and earlier postoperative ambulation.

A number of studies related to off-pump CABG show apparently conflicting results. The ROOBY (Randomized On/Off Bypass) trial showed increased repeat revascularization and fewer grafts compared with the on-pump group (Shroyer et al, 2009). A newer study, the CORONARY (CABG Off or On Pump Revascularization Study) trial showed more positive results (Lamy et al, 2012, 2013). Some reasons offered for the differences include fewer experienced surgeons (residents were frequently the primary surgeon), more MIs and coronary reintervention, and fewer bypass grafts in the ROOBY trial (Grover, 2012). Some early advantages in the off-pump group demonstrated in the CORONARY trial were that surgeons were experienced with off-pump techniques, and more high-risk patients were included (e.g., older females, patients with aortic calcification or renal disease); long-term data should make the relative advantages and disadvantages more evident (Grover, 2012).

In patients with ST-elevation myocardial infarction (STEMI), CABG surgery within 6 hours of symptom onset may be appropriate in patients who are not in cardiogenic shock and are not candidates for fibrinolysis or PCI; on-pump or off-pump techniques and temporary mechanical assistance demonstrate improved survival rates. In the acute phase of STEMI, the efficacy of CABG may prove limited (O'Gara et al, 2013).

Standard surgical treatment of CAD includes myocardial revascularization with CABG by use of the left or right thoracic IMA, greater saphenous vein, radial artery, and other autogenous arterial and venous conduits. CABG can alleviate angina pectoris and prolong life in patients with CAD of the left main and left anterior descending coronary arteries (Farkouh et al, 2012; O'Gara et al, 2013). Selection of the IMA demonstrates excellent long-term patency (Nasso et al, 2012); this result has promoted the use of arterial conduits such as bilateral IMAs (Dorman et al, 2012), and the radial artery, especially in diabetic patients. Use of both IMAs has not been widespread in obese and diabetic patients due to fears of deep sternal infections (Puskas, 2012), but Dorman and colleagues (2012) demonstrated no increased morbidity and mortality in diabetic patients receiving bilateral mammary grafts.

The saphenous vein nevertheless remains an effective conduit when the need for multiple grafts appears. Endoscopic saphenous vein harvest occurs frequently (Williams et al, 2012); emergency surgery may preclude the endoscopic technique in favor of the faster, traditional "open" excision of the vein, but more recently trained clinicians may have learned only the endovascular technique and hence are able to perform rapid vein endoscopic harvesting (Aranki, and Shopnick, 2011; Dacey, 2012).

Performance of radial artery excision via endoscopic techniques is more frequent. Use of the radial artery as a second graft in conjunction with the IMA has shown benefits in older (e.g., greater than 70 years old) patients (Habib et al, 2012) and in both men and women, although a long-term survival advantage was relatively lower in women (Schwann et al, 2012). The increasing number of reoperations for CAD has also stimulated use of alternative conduits (Box 25-5).

Distal and proximal anastomotic devices offer the potential for easier bypass procedures; these devices may use grasping hooks that attach the vein to the aorta, magnets, or coupling systems.

TABLE 25-8

Thoracic Incisions

Incision	Position	Possible Indications	Special Patient Needs
Median sternotomy: Incision along center of sternum (sternal notch to xiphoid process)	Supine	Most adult cardiac procedures except those on branch pulmonary arteries, distal transverse aortic arch, and descending thoracic aorta; OPCAB	Padding for hands, elbows, feet/ heels, back of head, dependent bony prominences
Mini-sternotomy: Partial upper or lower sternal incision starting either from sternal notch or from xiphoid process and extending to midportion of sternum; lower-end sternal splitting (LESS)	Supine	MAS, or OPCAB procedures	Same as median sternotomy
Parasternotomy: Resection of right or left costal cartilages (from second to fifth cartilage, depending on surgical target)	Supine; small roll may be placed under affected side	Left: MAS CABG Right: MAS CABG, valve procedures	Same as median sternotomy; risk of postoperative chest wall instability
Anterolateral thoracotomy: Curvilinear incision along subpectoral groove to axillary line	Supine with pad or pillow under operative site; arm supported in sling or overarm board; arm on unaffected side may be tucked along side	MAS, MIDCAB, trauma to anterior pericardium and left ventricle; repeat sternotomy	Padding for extremities; pillow or other device to elevate affected side; armboard or sling for arm on affected side
Left anterior mini-thoracotomy; right anterior mini-thoracotomy: One or more small incisions (or ports) on left or right side	Supine with small roll under affected side	Left: MAS, MIDCAB, port access for robotic surgery Right: MAS valve procedures, surgery for atrial fibrillation ("mini-maze"); port-access for robotic surgery	Same as anterolateral thoracotomy
Lateral thoracotomy: Curvilinear incision along costochondral junction anteriorly to posterior border of scapula	Placed on side with arms extended and axilla and head supported; knees and legs protected	Lung biopsies; first-rib resection; lobectomy	Armboard, overarm board, axillary roll, padding for extremities, pillow between legs; sandbags, straps, wide tape, or other devices to support torso
Posterolateral thoracotomy: Curvilinear incision from subpectoral crease below nipple, extended laterally and posteriorly along ribs almost to posterior midline below scapula (location of intercostal incision depends on surgical site); used less frequently with availability of VATS techniques	Lateral with arms extended and axilla and head supported; knees and legs protected	First-rib resection; lobectomy	Similar to needs for lateral thoracotomy
Transsternal bilateral anterior thoracotomy ("clamshell"): Submammary incision extending from one anterior axillary line to the other across sternum at fourth interspace	Supine	Bilateral lung transplant; emergency access to heart when sternal saw not available	Same as median sternotomy; requires transection of left and right IMA
Subxiphoid incision: Vertical midline incision from over xiphoid process to about 10 cm inferiorly (may divide lower portion of sternum to enhance exposure)	Supine	Pericardial drainage, pericardial biopsy, attachment of pacemaker electrodes, MAS	Same as median sternotomy
Thoracoabdominal incision: Low curvilinear incision on left side extended to anterior midline, continued vertically down abdomen	Anterior thoracotomy with chest at 45-degree angle to table; abdomen supine	Thoracoabdominal aneurysm	Same as anterolateral thoracotomy

CABG, Coronary artery bypass graft; *IMA,* internal mammary artery; *MAS,* minimal access surgery; *MIDCAB,* minimal access direct coronary artery bypass; *OPCAB,* off-pump coronary artery bypass; *VATS,* video-assisted thoracoscopic surgery.

Modified from Bojar RM: *Manual of perioperative care in adult cardiac surgery,* ed 5, Oxford, 2011, Wiley-Blackwell; Roselli EE: Reoperative cardiac surgery, *Texas Heart Inst J* 38(6):669–671, 2011; Walton-Geer PS: Prevention of pressure ulcers in the surgical patient, *AORN J* 89(3):538–548, 2009.

FIGURE 25-48 View of internal mammary artery (IMA) and accompanying veins during dissection. Vascular clips on the IMA side and electrocoagulation on the sternal side control bleeding from side branches. A no-touch technique is important to achieve an atraumatic harvest of the vessel. Dilute solution of papaverine sprayed onto or into the lumen of the IMA dilates the artery and reduces muscular spasm. The IMA pedicle, placed in the pleural cavity, remains there until needed for anastomosis.

Clampless devices or "no-touch" techniques may reduce the risk of disrupting aortic atherosclerotic plaque, which can dislodge and embolize after application of a vascular occlusion clamp (Morrow and Boden, 2012).

Dysrhythmias and AF in particular are common after CABG, and these can lead to hemodynamic compromise, systemic embolism, the need for extended anticoagulation therapy (with attendant risk of bleeding), cardiac pacing, patient discomfort and anxiety, and increased cost and length of stay. Preoperative administration of beta-blockers is effective to reduce incidence of postoperative AF; beta-blockers should be reinstituted (absent contraindications) after CABG as soon as possible to reduce the effects of AF. Giving amiodarone may reduce the incidence of AF in patients with contraindications for beta-blockers or in those at high risk for postoperative AF (Hillis et al, 2011).

Increasing recognition of gender differences in the planning, treatment, and outcomes in men and women are apparent in a growing number of practice guidelines for CABG (Hillis et al, 2011; Mosca et al, 2011; Newby and Douglas, 2012) (see Evidence for Practice). In particular, guidelines for women focus on use of the IMA, glycemic control, avoidance of anemia and hypothyroid states, avoidance of hormone replacement therapy, and use of off-pump CABG techniques.

Other ischemia-related disorders (including heart failure) that can benefit from surgery include postinfarction ventricular septal defect, mitral regurgitation (MR), and certain ventricular (e.g., tachycardia) and supraventricular (e.g., AF) dysrhythmias (O'Gara et al, 2013).

Coronary Artery Bypass Grafts with Arterial and Venous Conduits

Operative Procedure. Coronary artery instruments supplement the basic setup for cardiac surgery.

1. Performance of a median sternotomy is as described previously.
2. Conduit preparation:
   a. *IMA.* A special retractor, such as the one shown in Figure 25-15, elevates the sternum to expose the IMA. The surgeon dissects the IMA from its retrosternal bed to obtain the necessary length (Figure 25-48). Heparin is administered, after which the surgeon clamps the exposed artery, cuts the IMA caudal to the clamp, and confirms that blood flow through the IMA is adequate. The surgeon may inject papaverine (or another antispasmodic drug) into the IMA lumen with a blunt-tipped needle and then occlude the tip

of the IMA with a small bulldog clamp. The surgeon may wrap the pedicle with a papaverine-soaked sponge and store the vessel in the left (or right) pleural space until needed. Ligation of the remaining clamped portion of the distal IMA is with a tie to prevent backbleeding. Increasingly, both right and left IMAs are used, even in patients with diabetes due to improved glucose control in this population. Heparin is given before clamping and cutting arterial grafts in order to prevent intraluminal thrombosis.

   b. Endoscopic IMA dissection can occur through thoracic ports (see Table 25-8) inserted into the left anterior thorax at the level of the fourth intercostal space. Ligation of arterial branches and venous tributaries is with hemostatic clips and electrocoagulation.

   c. *Radial artery.* Generally the surgeon takes the artery from the patient's nondominant arm; adequate blood flow through the ulnar artery must be confirmed, commonly by Doppler. The surgeon may remove the artery endoscopically or through a longitudinal incision beginning 3 cm distal to the elbow crease lateral to the biceps tendon and ending 1 cm before the wrist crease (Figure 25-49). The surgeon then exposes and mobilizes the artery with a vessel loop, and then harvests it as a free graft with adjacent veins and fatty tissue. Ligation of the artery occurs proximally and distally after systemic heparinization. Injection of papaverine into the lumen reduces spasm. The surgeon closes the arm incision; team members may dress it, reposition the arm along the patient's side, and apply more drapes to maintain sterility of the field.

   d. *Gastroepiploic artery.* Rarely used but when need for an additional arterial conduit appears, the surgeon may choose to use the gastroepiploic artery, although required entry into the peritoneum to dissect the artery increases the risk of postoperative complications (Figure 25-50).

   c. *Saphenous vein.* Harvesting of the necessary length of saphenous vein is from one or both legs, either with video-assisted

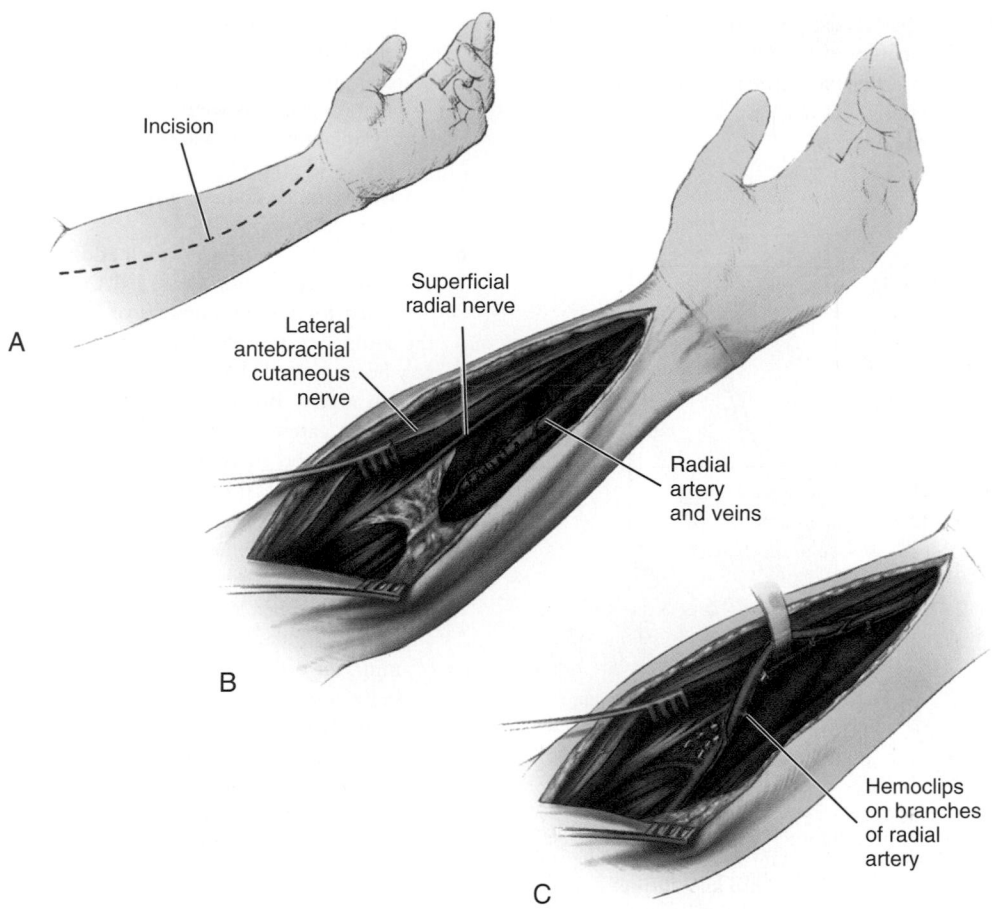

A Incision

Lateral antebrachial cutaneous nerve

Superficial radial nerve

Radial artery and veins

B

Hemoclips on branches of radial artery

C

FIGURE 25-49 Dissection of radial artery. Before removal of the radial artery, an Allen test ensures that the ulnar artery will provide sufficient blood flow to the hand if the radial artery is excised: compression of the radial and ulnar arteries produces blanching of the hand. The ulnar artery is released while compression is maintained on the radial artery. The skin on the palm should immediately become red as blood flow returns through the ulnar artery to the hand. **A,** Incision line. **B,** Deep forearm dissection exposes the radial artery and vein pedicle. **C,** Radial artery pedicle is mobilized, and the multiple side branches clipped. The artery is removed and may be irrigated with a vasodilator. A continuous intravenous infusion of diltiazem helps prevent vasoconstriction of the artery.

endoscopic techniques or, less commonly, by traditional open incision (Figure 25-51). Tributaries on the leg side undergo ligation, electrocoagulation, or clipping. After dissection frees the saphenous vein, the surgeon removes it and ligates tributaries on the vein side. The distal end of the vein is identified to place the vein in a reversed position so that the semilunar valves do not interfere with blood flow. The vein undergoes flushing with heparinized blood or saline and must remain moist until needed.

3. With the endoscopic technique, saphenous vein harvesting is through one to three incisions over the vein at the knee and at the ankle and groin if necessary. The surgeon locates the vein under direct vision; excision of the remaining length of vein is with a 5-mm angled endoscope and endoscopic scissors. An endoscopic clip applier and bipolar electrocoagulation can seal tributaries on the leg side. Once removal of the vein is complete, the surgeon ligates the vein tributaries with silk ties. Wrapping of the leg with a pressure bandage follows in order to reduce postoperative tunnel dead space and to minimize fluid accumulation.

4. CPB with mild hypothermia begins. Antegrade-retrograde cardioplegic solution is infused after the aorta is cross-clamped.

A   **B**

FIGURE 25-50 Right gastroepiploic artery mobilization. **A,** Branches to the stomach are divided with clamps and ties; omental branches may be divided with a staple gun. The gastroepiploic pedicle is isolated proximally to its origin from the gastroduodenal artery. **B,** The pedicle is brought up into the pericardium and anastomosed to the right coronary artery (shown here). The artery can also be grafted to the distal right and left anterior descending coronary arteries.

(NOTE: If CABG is performed without CPB, there is no patient cooling; CPB standby is usually available.)

5. Coronary anastomoses using the saphenous vein, free arterial grafts, and in situ arterial grafts (e.g., IMA and gastroepiploic artery) follow as described below.

   a. The surgeon identifies the affected coronary artery, makes a small incision into the artery, and bevels the graft conduit to approximate the incision (side-to-side jump grafts may be appropriate as well).

   b. Completion of anastomoses is with fine cardiovascular sutures (Figure 25-52). Before completing each anastomosis, the surgeon may probe the distal coronary artery to ensure patency.

6. Steps 5a and 5b repeat for each additional anastomosis.

7. The distal anastomosis of the IMA to the coronary artery is as described for the anastomosis of the saphenous vein graft to the coronary artery. No aortic (proximal) anastomosis is necessary because the IMA remains attached proximally to the subclavian artery. Because the IMA has demonstrated superior long-term patency—and the LAD coronary artery is a critical source of blood to the LV—the surgeon commonly attaches the IMA to the LAD coronary artery.

8. Aortic anastomoses:

   a. Proximal aortic anastomoses may be with a partial occlusion clamp, but more often performance of the anastomoses occurs during a single aortic cross-clamping to avoid excessive manipulation of the aorta that could lead to intimal injury or dislodgement of atherosclerotic material. Increasingly, assessment of the aorta is with epiaortic ultrasound before beginning the anastomoses in order to identify proximal anastomotic sites relatively free of atherosclerotic plaque. After completion of the proximal anastomoses, the team removes the aortic cross-clamp and defibrillates the heart. Assessment of the aorta is especially helpful during *beating heart surgery* (usually through a median sternotomy) that requires proximal aortic anastomoses (with saphenous vein or other free graft) to be completed while the heart is contracting. After identification of a suitable site (i.e.,

FIGURE 25-51 Excision of greater saphenous vein. **A,** Traditional open incision. **B,** Incision sites (ankle, knee, groin) for video-assisted endoscopic vein harvesting. **C,** Endoscope inserted into medial knee incision and used to dissect the vein. **D,** Venous tributaries may be divided, and electrocoagulated or clipped, on the leg side; silk ties are commonly used on the vein side.

FIGURE 25-52 A, End-to-side coronary anastomosis with bypass graft conduit. Side-to-side coronary anastomosis with bypass graft conduit. **B,** Arteriotomy made with #11 blade is shown. **C,** Double-ended suture used to create anastomosis. **D,** Completed anastomosis. Side-to-side anastomoses are used to make more than one attachment of a conduit to an artery, especially when there may be insufficient available conduit material.

FIGURE 25-53 Proximal anastomosis of bypass graft. A partial occlusion clamp isolates the portion of the ascending aorta where the aortotomy is to be made with the punch.

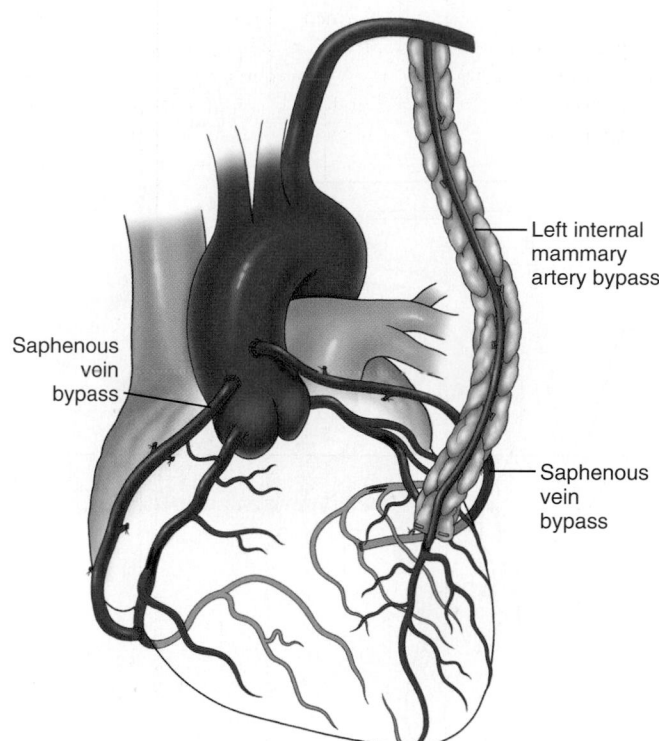

FIGURE 25-54 Coronary artery bypass grafts with reversed saphenous vein grafts and the left internal mammary artery.

relatively free of plaque), the proximal anastomoses may follow with a partial occlusion clamp. An angled vascular clamp partially occludes the aorta, and the surgeon resects a small segment (approximately the diameter of the vein graft). The surgeon performs the aortotomy with a knife blade and enlarges the opening with a punch (Figure 25-53).

b. Anastomosis of the conduit is end-to-side to the aorta with fine vascular sutures (Figure 25-54). Removal of the partial occlusion clamp (if used) follows, so that the proximal portion of the vein graft can fill with blood. Needle aspiration of the vein graft prevents air from entering the coronary circulation.

c. When performing proximal anastomoses during a single period of cross-clamping, aspiration from the grafts removes air before removal of the cross-clamp.

9. Marking the aortic anastomoses of the vein grafts with radiopaque clips or rings may follow in order to aid future identification.

10. Cardiopulmonary bypass ends and closure of the sternum follows.

11. Minimally invasive procedures:

a. Performance of minimally invasive direct coronary artery bypass (MIDCAB) occurs, albeit less frequently, in patients with lesions (e.g., narrowings in the LAD and diagonal coronary arteries) that are easily accessible through an anterior thoracotomy. Beating heart procedures performed through a median sternotomy allow surgeons to access lateral and posterior arteries. When using endovascular CPB and cardioplegic solution, it is possible to graft more lateral and posterior arteries (e.g., obtuse marginal and right coronary arteries) because ventricular fibrillation secondary

to stimulation of the heart obviates with induced cardioplegic arrest. The surgeon may call for insertion of a double-lumen endotracheal tube to hypoventilate the left lung to enhance visualization of the LAD (and the IMA) while ventilating the right lung sufficiently to oxygenate pulmonary blood flow.

b. With off-pump CABG, cardiac contraction may pose technical difficulty for the surgeon to create a precise anastomosis. Coronary stabilizers reduce the motion of the heart in the vicinity of the anastomosis (Figure 25-55). These stabilizing attachments fit onto the retractor, thereby freeing the surgeon's hands to suture the anastomosis. Left ventricular apical suction cups allow retraction of the apex, thereby exposing lateral and posterior coronary arteries (see Figure 25-55). Beta-blockers and adenosine have achieved successful pharmacologic cardiac motion reduction, but the newer stabilizers have reduced the need for these drugs. Bleeding from the arteriotomy, resulting from the heart's continued beating, obscures the field; to counteract this, the surgeon may use a fine mist of humidified CO_2 gas sprayed over the anastomotic site, elastic coronary artery tourniquets, or Silastic shunts to control bleeding.

c. Thoracic port-access procedures are performable with a robot and endovascular catheters. Anastomoses are with video-assisted thoracoscopic techniques. If the surgeon desires or requires better visualization, conversion to a median sternotomy is an option.

Laser Transmyocardial Revascularization

In patients with chronic, severe angina who are not amenable to revascularization with either coronary bypass surgery or PCI, laser

FIGURE 25-55 Coronary anastomotic site stabilizer used during beating heart bypass surgery. The vacuum-assisted horseshoe-shaped foot reduces the movement of the beating heart and isolates the target coronary artery site for anastomosis. The apical suction cup enables apical retraction.

transmyocardial revascularization (TMR) has become an option. The surgeon creates channels in the left ventricular wall with laser energy (e.g., CO_2, Holmium : yttrium-aluminum-garnet [Ho : YAG]) to increase blood flow to the myocardium. In a collaborative study by the U.S. Food and Drug Administration, the Society of Thoracic Surgeons, and the Duke Clinical Research Institute (Tavris et al, 2012), researchers found poor outcomes with isolated TMR. TMR performed with CABG (in areas of the myocardium that could not be revascularized with traditional bypass techniques) demonstrated improved clinical outcomes. The authors recommend further research, noting that laser safety precautions are mandatory.

Ventricular Aneurysmectomy

Left ventricular aneurysmectomy (LVA) is excision of the aneurysmal portion of the LV and its reinforcement with synthetic patch material. LVA is a form of left ventricular reconstruction undertaken to optimize cardiac function. An aneurysm of the LV occasionally develops after a severe MI; the aneurysm consists of thin scar tissue that replaces part of the myocardium and may rupture spontaneously. The LV undergoes *remodeling* when the scar stretches as a result of left ventricular pressure and forms an aneurysm (Teirstein and Lytle, 2012). The aneurysm usually adheres to the pericardium; it may not be possible to dissect it free until CPB commences.

Procedural Considerations. Patient positioning is supine. Setup is the same as that described for open-heart surgery, with the addition of synthetic patch material, Teflon felt pledgets, and 0, 3-0, and 4-0 cardiovascular sutures. Occasionally additional Teflon felt strips

bolster the suture lines. Patch closure of the ventriculotomy (endo-aneurysmorrhaphy) is more common than traditional excision, plication, and oversewing of the ventricular tissue because patch closure better preserves the geometry of the LV; mortality remains very high at approximately 30% (Teirstein and Lytle, 2012).

Operative Procedure
1. The surgeon performs a median sternotomy, and CPB begins as previously described.
2. Excision of scar tissue of the ventricle follows as well as careful removal of any clot (Figure 25-56, *A* and *B*).
3. The surgeon leaves a circular cuff of scar tissue and places a purse-string suture with felt pledgets through the rim of the scar (see Figure 25-56, *C*).
4. The surgeon then sews a patch of woven Dacron to the rim with interrupted sutures (see Figure 25-56, *D*) and may place a second (internal) patch of pericardium for hemostasis.
5. A running suture reinforces the edge of the patch (see Figure 25-56, *E*).
6. A catheter inserted into the right superior pulmonary vein may vent the LV; after de-airing the ventricle, removal of the catheter and closure of the incision follow to end the procedure.

Postinfarction Ventricular Septal Defect. Ventricular septal or free-wall rupture is a catastrophic complication of MI, creating an acute left-to-right shunt and cardiac failure requiring early surgical repair. Use of a prosthetic patch or pericardial tissue (Figure 25-57) to close the defect follows. Felt strips and plicating sutures can reinforce the suture line. Insertion of percutaneous occlusion devices is via the transcatheter route in the cardiac catheterization laboratory (Sayfo et al, 2012).

Surgery for Heart Failure

Patients with heart failure associated with ischemic coronary disease may benefit from CABG (compared with medical treatment) (Velazquez et al, 2011). Additional interventions include mitral valve repair (see following section) for ischemic mitral regurgitation, mechanical and biologic support, and cardiac transplantation (described later) (Acker and Jessup, 2012).

Surgery for the Mitral Valve

Mitral *stenosis* (MS) is a narrowing of the valve orifice that impedes forward blood flow. It is often caused by rheumatic fever, especially in poor and developing countries (Shrestha et al, 2012). The normal orifice area of the valve is about 5 cm². As the disease progresses, the mitral valve becomes a narrow slit in a fibrotic plaque, severely limiting blood flow into the LV. MS causes a rise in pressure and dilation of the LA. This pressure transmits throughout the pulmonary vascular bed, with subsequent pulmonary hypertension, right ventricular hypertrophy, and possible tricuspid valve regurgitation (Otto and Bonow, 2012). The major symptoms of MS are dyspnea, fatigue, and orthopnea. Late findings are severe pulmonary congestion and right ventricular failure. A diastolic murmur is characteristic, and AF is not unusual. Thromboembolism may result from stasis of blood in the left atrial appendage.

MR occurs when the valve leaflets do not close properly or when the leaflets perforate and blood escapes back into the LA during ventricular systole. Isolated MR is most commonly associated with posterior leaflet prolapse (Gillinov and Mihaljevic, 2012). Common causes of MR are myxomatous degeneration and as a secondary result of aortic valve stenosis. Other causes of MR are degenerative,

A

Ventricular aneurysm

B

Purse-string suture

C

Dacron felt patch

D

E

FIGURE 25-56 Repair of left ventricular aneurysm. **A,** Left ventricular apical aneurysm. **B,** Intracavitary clot is removed. **C,** Pledgeted sutures placed around the edge of the excised ventricular tissue. **D,** A patch is inserted. **E,** Completed repair.

Ventriculotomy

Patch

Felt buttress

FIGURE 25-57 Patch repair of acute ventricular septal defect after myocardial infarction.

ischemic, and dilated cardiomyopathy. During ventricular diastole, blood regurgitated into the LA augments blood volume entering the LV. MR may accompany MS or be attributable to leaflet tears, annular dilation, or elongated or ruptured chordae. Ischemic heart disease may produce papillary muscle dysfunction, which prevents sufficient anchoring of the leaflets in the closed position. Symptoms are primarily dyspnea on exertion and easy fatigability related to pulmonary congestion.

The surgeon's selection of the procedure (repair or replacement) depends on mitral valve anatomy, stage of disease, presence or absence of calcification, history of thromboembolism and dysrhythmia, the patient's ability to tolerate long-term anticoagulation therapy (required after insertion of a mechanical valve prosthesis), and the patient's willingness to undergo reoperation if a bioprosthesis deteriorates. Improvements in imaging capabilities with two-dimensional, three-dimensional, and color-flow Doppler echocardiography have enabled surgeons to diagnose more precisely and subsequently identify the most appropriate repair procedure. Improved imaging has also fostered development of a consistent nomenclature to describe specific segments of the mitral valve leaflet anatomy. Building on the classic study of Carpentier (1983), surgeons commonly divide each mitral leaflet into an alpha-numeric system: (1) The *anterior* leaflet is divided into three sections that are designated from the lateral to the medial position (left to right): *A1* (lateral), *A2* (middle), and *A3* (medial); and (2) the *posterior* leaflet is divided into three sections that are designated (left to right): *P1* (lateral), *P2* (middle), and *P3* (medial) (see mitral valve in Figure 25-6, *B*). The goal of this system is to provide consistent descriptions for planning, performing, and documenting care for this highly variable, complex, and dynamic structure.

Consistency in description also promotes reproducibility of the reparative procedures performed to preserve the native valve. Mitral valve repair is widespread because the complications associated with prosthetic replacement and anticoagulation therapy do not arise. The technique selected must be tailored to the unique pathophysiologic findings; therefore, the surgeon carefully evaluates the leaflets and related structures at the time of surgery before deciding which procedure to perform. Because there is a possibility that the valve may have to be replaced, instruments (and prostheses) for replacement as well as repairs must be available. Also included are atrial handheld or self-retaining retractors, obturators to size prosthetic rings and valves, sizer or prosthesis handles, and special sutures if requested. Surgeons often use bicaval cannulation to enhance exposure of the operative field and decompress the heart (see Figure 25-37). TEE establishes a cardiac functional baseline and confirms efficacy of the repair both after the cross-clamp is removed and the heart resumes beating and after the bypass is discontinued. TEE used intraoperatively assesses left ventricular function and detects the presence of air (seen as white specks) within the cardiac chambers.

Mitral Valve Repairs

Open Commissurotomy of the Mitral Valve for Mitral Stenosis.
Open commissurotomy is separation of fused, adherent leaflets of the mitral valve.

Procedural Considerations. The patient is positioned supine for a median sternotomy. Setup is the same as that described for open-heart procedures, with addition of mitral valve instruments.

Operative Procedure

1. The surgeon performs a median sternotomy, and bicaval cannulation follows for CPB.
2. The surgeon incises the LA and inspects the valve; in some cases the surgeon may use a transseptal approach (RA to LA).
3. Using vascular forceps and scissors or a knife, the surgeon separates fused leaflets (Figure 25-58) and can use a dilator to enlarge the mitral valve orifice.
4. Reinspection of the valve for any resultant insufficiency occurs.
5. The surgeon may insert an annuloplasty ring to reinforce the repair.
6. Closure of the LA is with a continuous cardiovascular suture.

Mitral Annuloplasty for MR.
Mitral annuloplasty is reduction of a dilated annulus by inserting a prosthetic ring. Although clinicians commonly assumed that only the posterior leaflet was subject to annular dilation, it now has been demonstrated that the anterior portion also can be affected. Prostheses are available to repair the entire circumference of the annulus (see Figure 25-32, *A*) or only the posterior leaflet (see Figure 25-32, *B*). The techniques (and associated prostheses) introduced in the 1980s by Carpentier and others continue to expand.

Operative Procedure

1. The surgeon incises the LA, after which sump suctions inserted into the atrial cavity remove blood.

Stenotic mitral valve

FIGURE 25-58 Mitral commissurotomy.

2. Inspection of the annulus, leaflets, chordae, and the rest of the mitral complex follows.
3. If generalized annular dilation appears, the surgeon inserts an annuloplasty ring; a *C*-shaped ring may address dilation affecting the posterior leaflet (see Figure 25-32, *B*). An obturator determines the appropriate-size ring (Figure 25-59, *A*). The surgeon places interrupted sutures in the valve annulus and then into the corresponding position in the ring (see Figure 25-59, *B*). As the stitches are tied, excess annular tissue of the posterior leaflet draws up evenly against the prosthesis (see Figure 25-59, *C*).
4. The surgeon inspects the valve for competency; use of a bulb syringe filled with saline to distend the ventricle confirms competence of the valve leaflets. Closure of the LA follows.

Mitral Valvuloplasty Repairs for MR.
Mitral valvuloplasty is repair of the valve leaflets or related structures. Selection of the appropriate repair for perforated or redundant valve leaflets or for shortened or elongated chordae tendineae requires careful assessment and evaluation of the abnormalities present. Historically most mitral valve repairs have focused on the posterior leaflet, but a number of anterior leaflet repairs have developed (see steps 5 to 8 in the following Operative Procedure).

Operative Procedure

1. The surgeon can patch perforated leaflets with pericardium.
2. Redundant, prolapsed *posterior* leaflet tissue is resectable (Figure 25-60). The surgeon sews cut edges of the posterior leaflet together, and plicates the corresponding annular segment. An annuloplasty ring, inserted to reinforce the leaflet repair, also reduces annular dilation.
3. Shortened, fused chordae tendineae can be lengthened and mobilized by dividing them into secondary chordae or by incising the tip of the papillary muscles.
4. The surgeon can also implant redundant tissue of elongated chordae into the papillary muscle head or, rarely, fold it over itself, secured with a suture.

FIGURE 25-59 Mitral valve annuloplasty. Redundant mitral valve leaflet tissue is resected and the cut edges reapproximated.

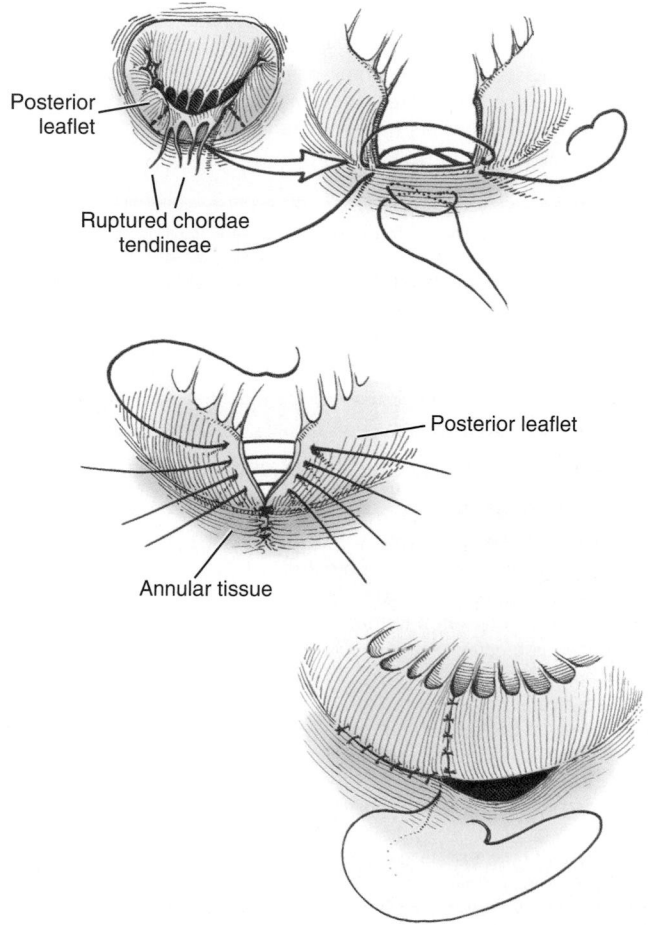

FIGURE 25-60 Quadrangular resection of nonsupported posterior leaflet tissue caused by ruptured chordae tendineae. A similar technique can be used to resect *redundant* tissue causing mitral regurgitation.

5. *Anterior* leaflet prolapse is a greater challenge and traditionally has indicated valve replacement. A small triangular resection of the anterior leaflet (reinforced with annuloplasty ring insertion) can be performed as well.
6. PTFE suture can replace elongated or ruptured chordae (Figure 25-61).
7. Surgical use of a chordal flip procedure (Figure 25-62) can reestablish chordal attachment to the *anterior* leaflet. The surgeon

FIGURE 25-61 Chordal replacement with polytetrafluoroethylene (PTFE).

cuts a section of the posterior leaflet with attached chordae, swings it over to the anterior leaflet, and sews it onto the anterior leaflet. Closure of the remaining posterior leaflet defect with suture follows (see step 2).
8. The edge-to-edge technique (Alfieri technique) is used to repair mitral valves with bileaflet prolapse (i.e., both the *anterior* and *posterior* leaflets are incompetent, producing severe MR). The surgeon approximates the free edges of the mitral leaflets, then places a figure-of-eight suture (or percutaneously delivered clip) in the central portion of the apposed leaflets. This creates a double-orifice mitral valve that often significantly reduces MR and preserves the native valve. Frequently an annuloplasty ring supplements the Alfieri technique (Otto and Bonow, 2012).

Recently investigators have experimented with percutaneous mitral valve repair using various devices and delivery methods. In a transcatheter procedure that echoes the Alfieri technique, the interventionalist implants a clip that approximates the edges of the mitral leaflets (Feldman et al, 2011). Although a number of innovative percutaneous techniques have been developed—and succeeded in, for example, aortic valve replacement (see following)—the complex nature of the mitral valve apparatus, consisting of the annulus, leaflets, chordae tendineae, papillary muscles, and LV, poses particular challenges to successful percutaneous mitral valve repair and, conversely, to avoiding injury to the valve components and other cardiac structures (Otto and Verrier, 2011; Tesler, 2012).

FIGURE 25-62 Chordal flip procedure. Although portions of the posterior leaflet are resectable with success, the same is not true of the anterior leaflet because resection alters the shape of the valve and coaptation margin. **A,** When there are ruptured chordae of the *anterior* leaflet of the mitral valve, the flip procedure can reestablish chordal support for the anterior leaflet. **B,** A portion of normal posterior leaflet tissue with attached chordae is cut, swung over, and sewn onto the flail segment of the anterior leaflet.

Mitral Valve Replacement

MVR is excision of the mitral valve leaflets and replacement with a mechanical or biologic prosthesis. Bioprostheses are increasingly the choice for valve replacement due to three improvements: improved bioprosthetic durability, fewer valve-related complications, and a decrease in mortality associated with reoperative valve replacement (McCarthy and Malaisrie, 2009).

During replacement, the surgeon often retains the mural (posterior) leaflet, and associated chordae and papillary muscles, to maintain left ventricular configuration (i.e., geometry), thereby enhancing postoperative ventricular function. If possible, the surgeon also may retain the anterior leaflet if it does not interfere with prosthetic function and is not too heavily calcified.

Surgeons choose to perform median sternotomy in most cases, but right thoracotomy incisions are useful in selected cases (e.g., reoperation, especially in patients with CABG IMA and vein grafts to the left ventricular coronary circulation). Minimally invasive (and robotic) procedures on the mitral valve can also use right and left thoracotomy incisions or ports (Cook et al, 2011; Kypson and Chitwood, 2009).

Procedural Considerations. Although the surgeon may intend to implant a specific type of prosthesis, patient-related factors (Box 25-6) or prosthetic valve complications (Box 25-7) may compel modification of the plan. Additionally there is a greater focus on patients' ideas about the ideal prosthetic heart valve (Box 25-8) (Rahimtoola, 2010). Nurses can incorporate all these ideas into their patient teaching.

A complete range of the surgeon's preferred valves should be available, as well as saline to rinse the glutaraldehyde storage

---

BOX 25-6

Patient-Related Factors and Risks for Valve Surgery

- Age
- Gender
- Residence
- History of atrial fibrillation
- Endocarditis (preoperative)
- Connective tissue disorders (e.g., myxomatous changes)
- Congenital anomalies (e.g., bicuspid aortic valve)
- Enlarged left atrium
- Left atrial thrombus
- Coronary artery disease
- Left ventricular function (e.g., functional class, myocardial infarction, heart failure)
- Syncope
- Mismatch between native valve orifice and patient body size (insufficient cardiac output for metabolic demands)
- Anticoagulation therapy compliance
- Comorbid conditions, preexisting medical problems (e.g., diabetes mellitus, hypertension, hepatic or renal disease)
- Valve lesion, anatomic anomalies
- Previous cardiac surgery

Modified from Otto CM, Bonow RO: Valvular heart disease. In Bonow RO et al, editors: *Braunwald's heart disease: a textbook of cardiovascular medicine*, ed 9, Philadelphia, 2012, Saunders; Rahimtoola SH: Choice of prosthetic heart valve in adults: an update, *J Am Coll Cardiol* 55(22):2413–2426, 2010.

BOX 25-7

Valve-Related Risks and Complications

- Thromboembolism, stroke
- Anticoagulation-related hemorrhage
- Prosthetic valve endocarditis
- Mismatch between prosthetic valve orifice and patient body size (inadequate cardiac output)
- Periprosthetic leak
- Perivalvular regurgitation
- Prosthetic failure
- Injury to heart or vascular access vessel (for percutaneous, transcatheter valve devices)

Modified from Gilard M et al: Registry of transcatheter aortic-valve implantation in high-risk patients, *N Engl J Med* 366(18):1705–1715, 2012; Kodali SK et al: Two-year outcomes after transcatheter or surgical aortic valve replacement, *N Engl J Med* 366(18):1686–1695, 2012; Otto CM, Bonow RO: Valvular heart disease. In Bonow RO et al, editors: *Braunwald's heart disease: a textbook of cardiovascular medicine*, ed 9, Philadelphia, 2012, Saunders; Rahimtoola SH: Choice of prosthetic heart valve in adults: an update, *J Am Coll Cardiol* 55(22):2413–2426, 2010; Peltz M: Surgery for valvular heart disease. In Antman EM, Sabatine MS, editors: *Cardiovascular therapeutics—a companion to Braunwald's heart disease*, Philadelphia, 2012, Saunders.

---

solution from biologic prostheses, if used. Pledgeted sutures of alternating colors are used, and suture holders may be available as well to keep the stitches in correct order. Venting catheters and aspirating needles remove air from the heart and ascending aorta. The surgeon may choose to use a small dental mirror after implanting a bioprosthesis to ensure that sutures are not caught in the struts of the valve.

BOX 25-8

Patients' Ideas of the Ideal Heart Valve

The prosthesis should:
- Cure the valve disease
- Function like a normal valve
- Improve the patient's lifestyle
- Last as long as the patient

The valve replacement operation should be:
- Performed with low morbidity and mortality
- Nondamaging to other components of the cardiovascular system
- Associated with a short hospital stay
- Affordable
- Possible via the percutaneous route

Follow-up requirements should:
- Require minimal laboratory testing and procedures
- Require minimal therapy

Modified from Rahimtoola SH: Choice of prosthetic heart valve in adults: an update, *J Am Coll Cardiol* 55(22):2413–2426, 2010.

Operative Procedure. Double venous cannulation is used.

1. With the aorta first cross-clamped, infusion of cardioplegic solution through the aortic root or retrograde through the coronary sinus follows.

2. The surgeon incises the LA along the interatrial groove to expose the mitral valve (Figure 25-63, *A*).

3. The surgeon carefully assesses the valve and excises the anterior leaflet. Retention of the posterior leaflet and occasionally the anterior leaflet enhances ventricular configuration and postoperative function. Rongeurs are available to debride heavy calcification; loose debris is removed. The surgeon retains a margin of the valve annulus to insert fixation sutures to the prosthesis (see Figure 25-63, *B*).

4. A valve sizer determines the correct size of the prosthesis, which then is delivered to the field.

5. The surgeon places nonabsorbable cardiovascular sutures (15 to 20 or more) in the annulus of the valve and then into the sewing ring of the prosthesis.

6. The sutures are held taut (and moistened with saline) as the surgeon guides the prosthesis into position and secures it; the sutures are tied and cut (see Figure 25-63, *C*).

7. Partial closure of the atriotomy is with continuous nonabsorbable sutures. Team members place the patient in Trendelenburg position and inflate the lungs to remove air from the pulmonary veins and atrium. Air aspiration from the LV is through a hypodermic needle inserted into the left ventricular apex or through the vent catheter, and completion of the atrial closure follows.

Endoscopic, video-assisted, robotic mitral valve surgery has progressed from technical curiosity to acceptable method, albeit with a significant learning curve, for intracardiac, telemanipulated valve repair. Surgeons have performed both mitral valve repair and replacement with these techniques (Figure 25-64), as well as procedures to correct other intracardiac structural lesions (Bailey, 2012; Peltz, 2012).

Surgery for the Tricuspid Valve

Significant aortic or mitral valve disease necessitates most tricuspid valve surgery (Cook et al, 2011; Duran, 2009). When right-sided pressures have increased significantly due to chronic tricuspid regurgitation, the surgeon will look for a patent foramen ovale and the potential for a right-to-left shunt, which could allow an air embolus to travel to the LV (Cook et al, 2011).

Among the treatment options for tricuspid valve disease are suture annuloplasty, ring annuloplasty, and valve replacement with either a biologic or a mechanical prosthesis. Percutaneous approaches are under investigation in the experimental setting (Cook et al, 2011; Duran, 2009; Peltz, 2012).

Like the mitral valve, the tricuspid annulus is saddle-shaped, and clinicians considering techniques to repair the valve also must consider this anatomic configuration for optimal repair. Annuloplasty ring insertion is preferable to suture annuloplasty (which does not offer the support provided by the annuloplasty ring) (Duran, 2009).

Tricuspid Valve Annuloplasty

Tricuspid valve annuloplasty reduces a dilated annulus with a prosthetic ring. Tricuspid valve regurgitation may arise from bacterial or viral endocarditis, the presence of a pacemaker or defibrillator lead through the valve annulus, or the functional result of mitral or aortic valve disease. After mitral valve correction, tricuspid valve function may return to normal, although this theory is subject to question (Duran, 2009). Preoperatively, if the tricuspid annular dilation is diagnosed as severe, ring repair (similar to mitral annuloplasty) or valve replacement may be appropriate. The surgeon must take care to avoid injury to the conduction tissue in the area of the AV node. The nurse should be aware that a pulmonary artery pressure catheter may not be inserted in order to avoid interference with the surgical site (and potentially be caught in the right atrial suture line); insertion of the PA pressure line may follow completion of surgery.

Patients with significant tricuspid stenosis or regurgitation, failed tricuspid annuloplasty, or significant leaflet damage may require insertion of a prosthetic biologic or mechanical valve (Duran, 2009; Peltz, 2012). There are no specific tricuspid prosthetic valves; rather, implantation is with a mitral prosthesis.

Operative Procedure

1. Double venous cannulae are inserted so that they do not cross one another in the RA, and occluding tapes are tightened around the cavae and cannulae to prevent venous return from entering the RA and obscuring the surgical site. A right-angled venous cannula may be placed into the superior vena cava to enhance exposure.

2. The surgeon opens the RA longitudinally to expose the tricuspid valve. Inserted sump suctions remove coronary sinus drainage.

3. For ring annuloplasty, insertion of a prosthetic ring in a manner similar to that used for mitral valve annuloplasty follows (see Figure 25-59).

4. For valve replacement, the surgeon selects the desired prosthesis and inserts it in a manner similar to that for mitral valve replacement (see Figure 25-63).

5. Saline injected into the ventricle tests competence of the repair, with TEE also used.

6. Closure of the RA is with nonabsorbable suture.

Surgery for the Pulmonary Valve

Adult pulmonary valve surgery is unusual, although patients with genetic deformities or those who have undergone repair of congenital pulmonary valve or right ventricular outflow tract obstruction

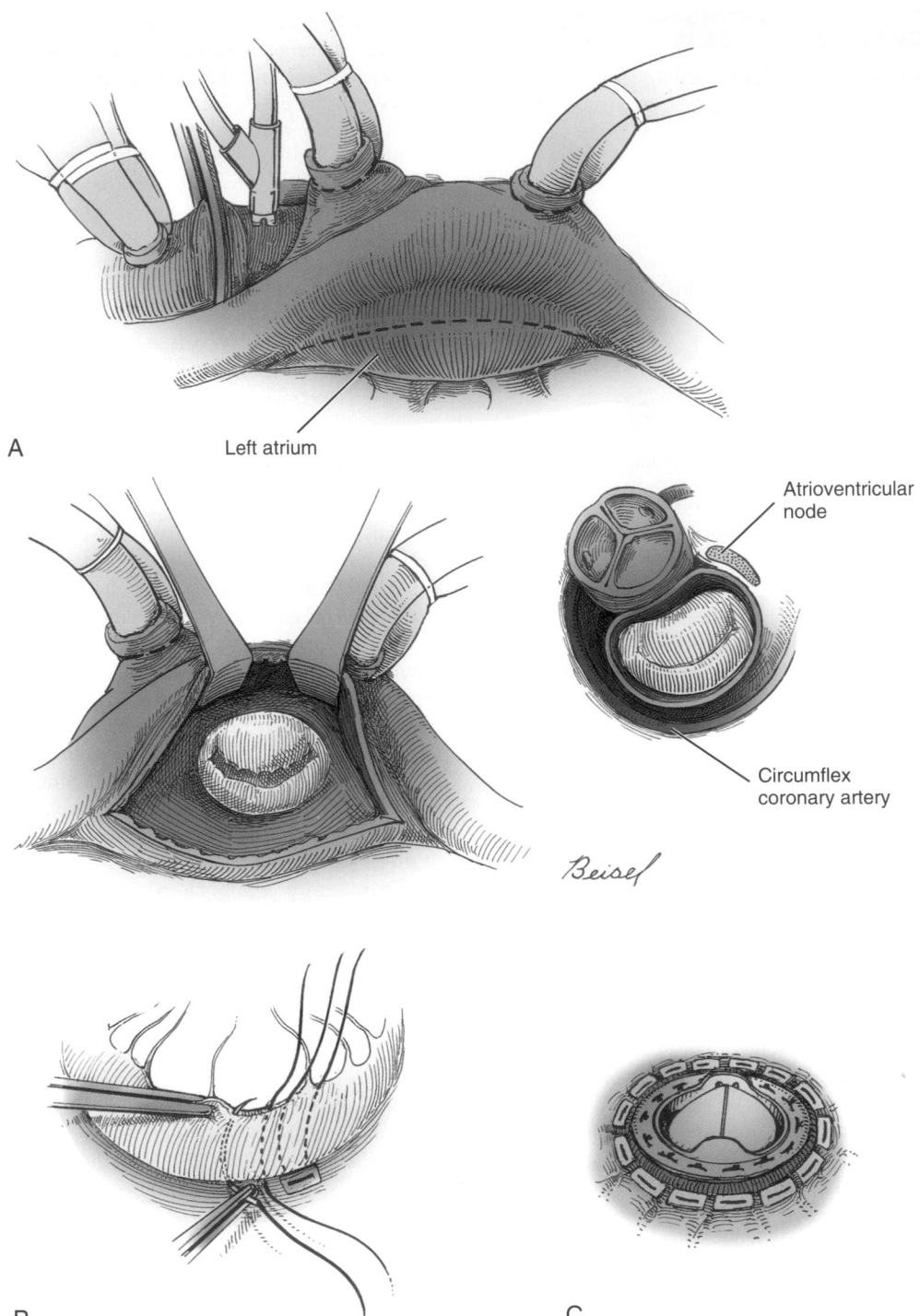

Left atrium

Atrioventricular node

Circumflex coronary artery

Beisel

A

B

C

FIGURE 25-63 Mitral valve replacement. **A,** Line of incision and cannulation for bypass, anatomic relationship between mitral and aortic valves with location of conduction node, and exposure of valve. **B,** Placement of pledgeted double-armed sutures in native valve annulus. **C,** Completed valve replacement.

may present with significant pulmonary valve disease (Otto and Bonow, 2012). Generally mild or moderate pulmonary stenosis (PS) produces few symptoms. For patients with severe PS, treatment options include valvulotomy or valve replacement via percutaneous or standard surgical techniques. Generally surgeons insert an aortic bioprosthesis or an allograft for valve replacement.

Surgery for the Aortic Valve

Aortic *stenosis* (AS) produces obstruction to left ventricular outflow. Whether caused by rheumatic fever, a congenital bicuspid valve, or calcification, the fused valve leaflets present increasing resistance to left ventricular outflow, thus increasing pressure inside the LV. Recent histopathologic and clinical data suggest that calcified AS

FIGURE 25-64 The 1-cm robotic instrument arms are placed through the chest wall. A transthoracic retractor arm elevates the interatrial septum toward the sternum. The three-dimensional camera is placed through a 4-cm incision, which also serves as a working port for the assistant.

is not a "degenerative" passive process, but rather an active and possibly inflammatory disease process (Carabello, 2012; Otto and Bonow, 2012) with genetic association (Thanassoulis et al, 2013).

To compensate for the increased pressure load, the ventricle hypertrophies so that it can generate sufficient pressure to eject blood through the narrowed opening. When disease is severe, large pressure gradients are often measured during cardiac catheterization, with differences in systolic pressures between the ventricle and the aorta reaching 50 mm Hg or more. In early stages of the disease, a systolic ejection murmur may be heard, but patients are rarely symptomatic. Eventually, fatigue, exertional dyspnea, angina pectoris, syncope, and congestive heart failure may develop, presenting a grave prognosis. Although infrequent, sudden death may be the first sign of AS in asymptomatic patients who are not well monitored (Bailey, 2012; Cook et al, 2011; Otto and Bonow, 2012).

In developing countries aortic *insufficiency* (AI), a form of regurgitation, often arises from rheumatic fever or aortic root disease (for example, aortic dilation preventing leaflet coaptation); other causes include calcific AS in older patients (the fixed lesion prevents complete closure of the stiffened leaflets), infective endocarditis (causing perforation of one or more leaflets), and trauma. Although *repair* of the aortic valve is challenging because of the precise closing mechanism of the valve leaflets, aortic valve reparative techniques have proved successful in selected patients (Otto and Bonow, 2012). Total valve excision and replacement with a prosthesis or an allograft are common. Transcatheter aortic valve implantations occur increasingly in a hybrid OR as do mini-sternotomy incisions performed for isolated aortic valve replacement (Bailey, 2012).

Prosthetic selection depends on achieving appropriate hemodynamic function in relation to body size. The small aortic root (e.g., less than 21 mm) presents challenges to provide an adequate cardiac output. In patients with a small aortic annulus and large body mass (analogous to patient/prosthesis mismatch), the surgeon selects a prosthesis that will provide flow adequate to meet the body's needs. The stentless aortic valve (see Figure 25-25, *B*) is advantageous because there is little sewing ring to reduce output, thereby offering excellent hemodynamic function. Patch enlargement of the small aortic root is another option (described in the following Operative

Procedure), and the patient's own pulmonary valve can be used as an autograft to replace the aortic valve; replacement of the pulmonary valve is with an allograft. Allografts may replace the aortic valve as well (David, 2009; Otto and Bonow, 2012).

Aortic Valve Replacement (AVR)

The surgeon excises the aortic valve and replaces it with a mechanical or biologic prosthesis or an aortic valve allograft or autograft. Insertion of a percutaneous valve may be with fluoroscopic guidance.

Procedural Considerations—Traditional AVR. To the basic setup, the following may be added:
- Aortic valve instruments
- Aortic valves, sizers, and holders
- Coronary sinus retrograde-infusion cannula and venting catheters
- Saline and three basins to rinse the glutaraldehyde storage solution from bioprostheses
- Saline bath to thaw frozen allografts

Operative Procedure
1. After institution of CPB (a two-stage venous cannula is often used), insertion of a left ventricular vent is through a stab wound into the right superior pulmonary vein, with the tip then advanced into the LV. Insertion of a retrograde cardioplegia catheter into the coronary sinus follows (Figure 25-65, *A*).
2. The aorta is cross-clamped. If aortic insufficiency is present, the initial bolus of cardioplegic solution infuses retrogradely; subsequent cardioplegic infusions are also given retrogradely. Occasionally direct coronary perfusion (see Figure 25-65, *B*) is given if insertion of a retrograde catheter is not possible; the surgeon refrains from direct perfusion, however, when possible, to avoid the risk of injuring the coronary endothelium. If aortic stenosis is present, infusion of the initial bolus of cardioplegic solution may be by needle through the aorta into the aortic root. After arrest of the heart, the surgeon opens the aorta.
3. The surgeon first inspects the native valve and then carefully excises it to avoid injury to the annulus and underlying structures (see Figure 25-65, *C*). Calcium is debrided from the annulus with scissors or rongeurs, or both. Narrow packing used in the LV can confine any small, loose, calcified fragments that could subsequently embolize. Team members frequently wipe instruments clean with a moist sponge.
4. After sizing the annulus, selection of the proper prosthesis follows, as does attachment of a prosthesis holder.
5. a. If the surgeon has selected a biologic valve, it is delivered to the field and rinsed typically in three saline baths in accordance with the manufacturer's instructions. Biologic valves should be kept moist with frequent saline rinsing, but they should *not* be immersed in antibiotic solution.
   b. If using an allograft, once delivered to the field, it thaws in saline baths according to protocol.
   c. If using a mechanical valve, the team protects it from scratches or other damage.
6. a. Implantation of the new valve follows, using a technique similar to that earlier described for MVR (see Figure 25-65, *D* and *E*).
   b. If the aortic annulus is too small to accept a prosthesis of adequate size, enlargement of the annulus and proximal portion of the ascending aorta is possible. The surgeon places

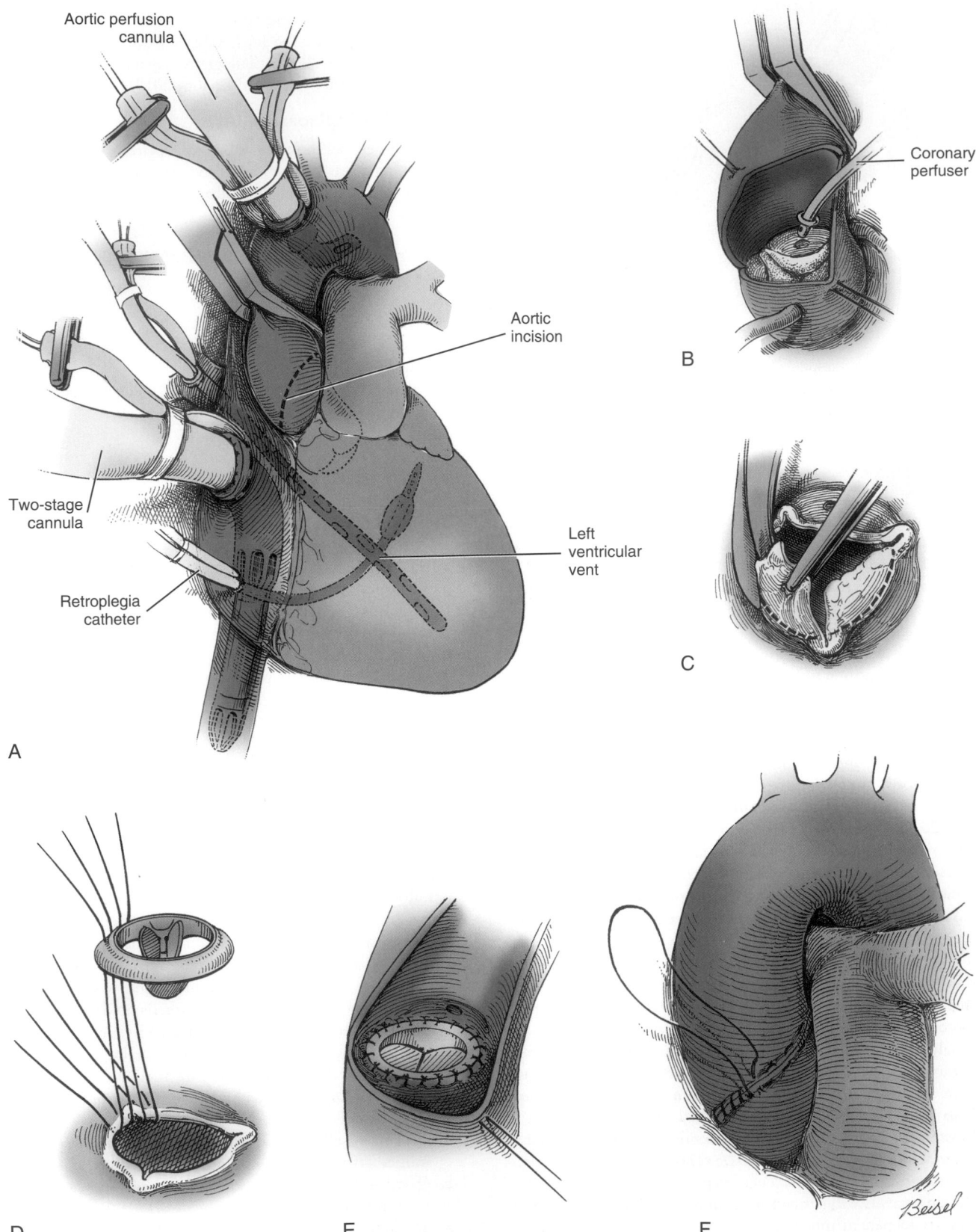

FIGURE 25-65 A, Cannulation, retrograde cardioplegia, and vent sites for aortic valve procedures. Note incision line. **B,** If retrograde cardioplegia is not used, handheld coronary ostial catheters can deliver antegrade cardioplegic solution. **C,** Diseased valve is completely excised. **D,** Sutures are placed in the valve annulus and the prosthetic sewing ring. **E,** Stitches are tied and cut. **F,** Closure of the aortic suture line.

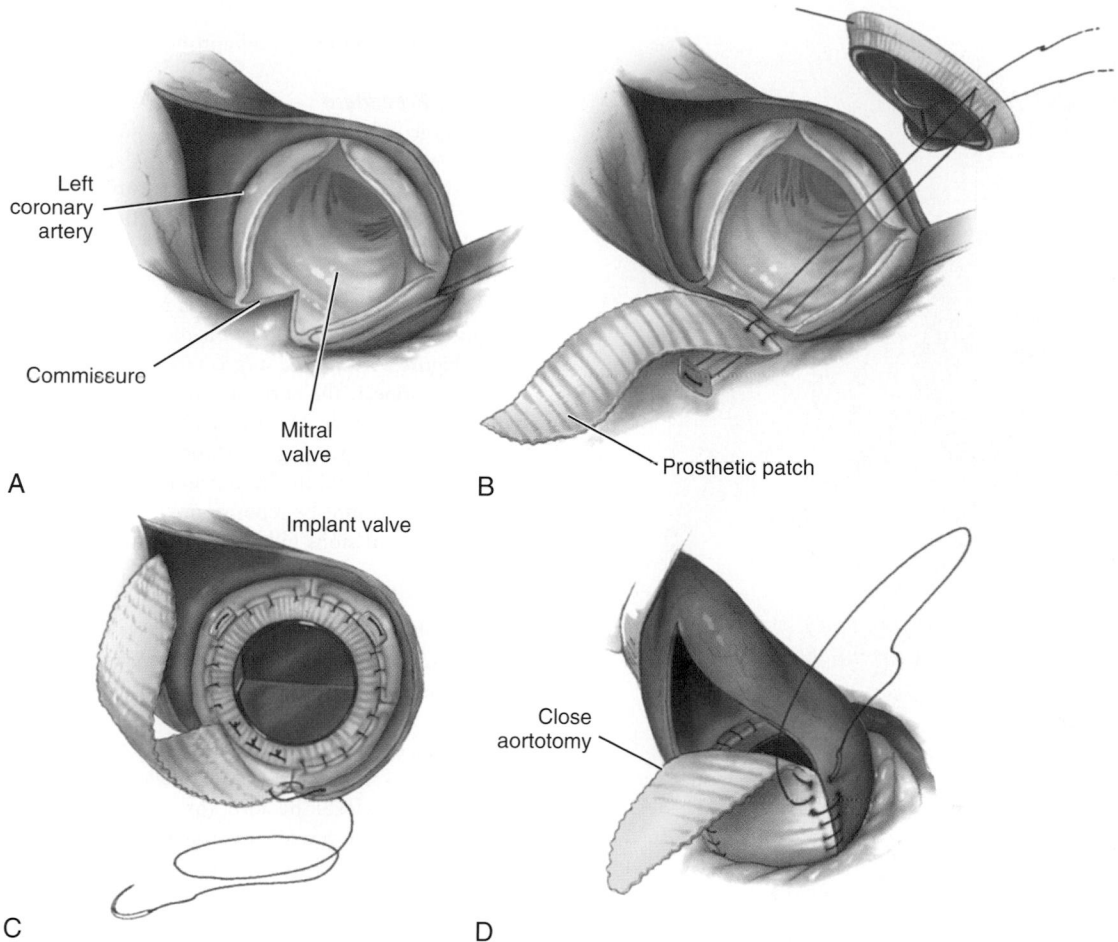

Left coronary artery

Commissure

Mitral valve

A

Prosthetic patch

B

Implant valve

C

Close aortotomy

D

FIGURE 25-66 Technique for aortic enlargement (Nicks-Nuñez operation). **A,** The aortotomy is extended through the commissure separating the left and noncoronary cusps. **B,** A prosthetic patch is sewn into the cut portion of the aorta and into the prosthetic valve. **C,** The prosthetic valve is seated, and the stitches are tied and cut. **D,** The patch is incorporated into the aortotomy closure.

a patch of bovine pericardium or Dacron graft longitudinally in the proximal anterior ascending aorta where the aortic annulus has been incised (Figure 25-66, *A* and *B*). Suturing of the valve prosthesis is to the natural annulus and then to the patch (see Figure 25-66, *C*). The surgeon then sutures the patch to the remaining edges of the aortotomy (see Figure 25-66, *D*).

7. The surgeon closes the aorta with nonabsorbable sutures; removal of the cross-clamp follows.

8. The left side of the heart de-airs by vent, by moving the OR bed side to side, or by other maneuvers chosen by the surgeon. The team places the patient in Trendelenburg position, and lung inflation follows. The heart is not allowed to eject blood until the surgeon is satisfied that no air remains within the LV. TEE identifies residual air. The team defibrillates the heart if it does not resume beating spontaneously.

9. Rewarming of the heart continues, removal of the venting catheter or catheters follows, and the surgeon or other clinician closes the chest in the routine manner.

Procedural Considerations—Transcatheter Aortic Valve Replacement. Patients with severe, symptomatic aortic stenosis, who have comorbid conditions that pose a high risk for open chest

surgery, are candidates for this procedure (Bailey, 2012). Formerly referred to as transcatheter aortic valve Implant (TAVI), the name for the percutaneous insertion of an aortic valve has evolved into transcatheter aortic valve replacement (TAVR). Performance of TAVR is via femoral access obtained in a hybrid OR or cardiac catheterization laboratory with fluoroscopy and intravascular ultrasound (IVUS) available. CT images should be available also for immediate review. If there is severe iliac or femoral tortuosity, atherosclerosis, or calcification, an axillary or LV transapical approach may prove appropriate (Bailey, 2012).

Basic TAVR setup includes the following:

• Endovascular aortic valve instruments

• Femoral access instruments

• Percutaneous aortic valve (e.g., bovine [see Figure 25-28], equine, or porcine pericardial prosthesis compressed either into a self-expanding system [see Figures 25-28 and 25-67]) or a balloon-expanding system [Figure 25-68]); the perioperative nurse confirms the valve size required by the surgeon in timely fashion.

• Valve deployment accessories

• Lubricants for catheters (follow manufacturer's instructions for proper use of lubricants)

• Guidewires and other catheters

- Contrast media
- X-ray protection (e.g., lead aprons)

Operative Procedure

1. The surgeon inserts a cannula over a guidewire into the femoral artery and threads the catheter up the aorta to the aortic valve.
2. The surgeon checks and confirms landmarks fluoroscopically.
3. The aortic valve is inserted through the catheter and threaded to the area of the aortic valve.
4. The surgeon positions the valve in the aortic annulus; depending on the type of device the valve is released and self-expands (see Figures 25-28 and 25-67), or, the balloon expands the device (see Figure 25-68). The surgeon then looks for perivalvular leaks. If leaks appear, the surgeon can adjust the self-inflating valve device (see Figures 25-28 and 25-67); if the balloon-expanding device is used (see Figure 25-68), another device of the same type is placed within the previously inserted device (currently this device cannot be repositioned).
5. Closure of incisions follows.

Combined Surgery

When combining CABG with aortic valve replacement, the procedure usually occurs in the following order:

1. The diseased valve is excised, the annulus is sized, and the prosthesis is selected.
2. The surgeon performs distal coronary anastomoses.
3. Insertion of the prosthetic valve follows.
4. The surgeon closes the aorta (or LA in MVR).
5. Insertion of the proximal coronary anastomoses into the aorta follows, after which the aortic cross-clamp is removed.

FIGURE 25-67 Transcatheter self-expanding aortic valve in the aortic root.

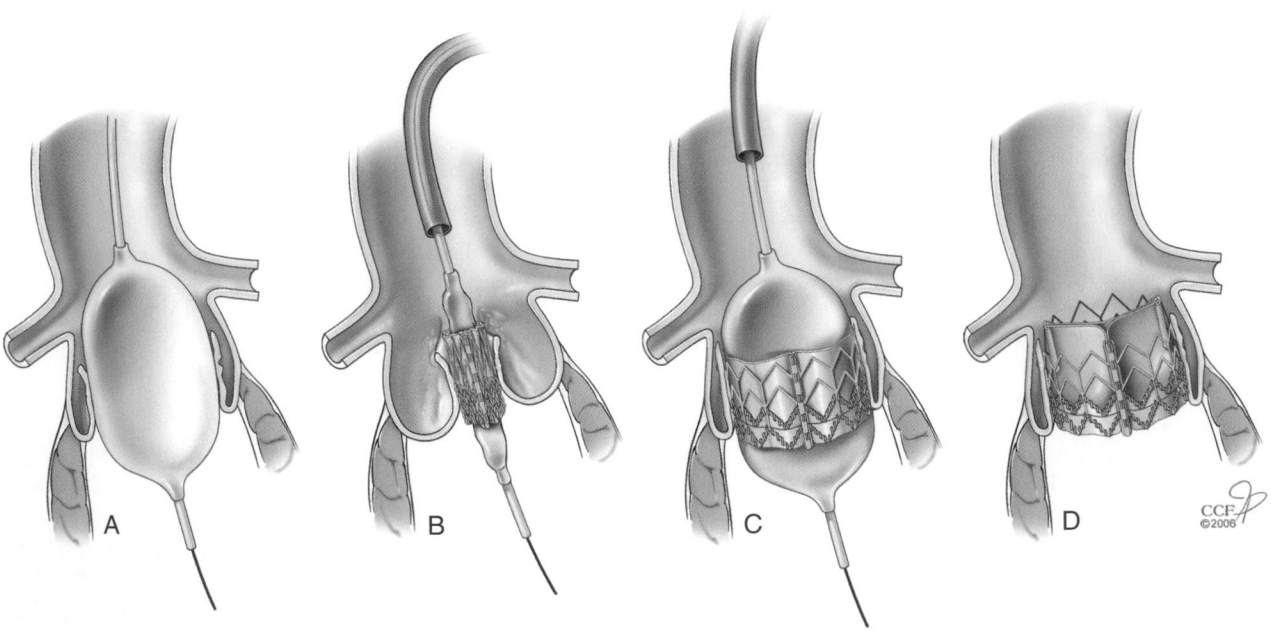

FIGURE 25-68 A, Percutaneous insertion of balloon-expandable transcatheter aortic valve. **B,** The compressed valve is delivered to the aortic root with a delivery catheter via a major artery (e.g., the femoral artery). **C,** A balloon expands the valve prosthesis and seats it into the aortic root. **D,** The balloon is deflated and removed, leaving the aortic valve prosthesis in place.

Double Valve Replacement

When *both the aortic and mitral valves are to be replaced,* the surgeon first excises the valves and sizes the annuli. The surgeon implants the mitral valve prosthesis first and then implants the aortic valve prosthesis. Otherwise, if the aortic prosthesis were inserted first, the firm prosthetic aortic annular ring might cause cardiac injury and make insertion of a mitral prosthesis more difficult. Closure of the aorta follows, and after sufficient de-airing of the LV, the clinician closes the LA.

Surgery for the Thoracic Aorta

Aneurysms may result from atherosclerosis, trauma, infection, or cystic medial degeneration (David, 2009; Szeto and Bavaria, 2009). *Atherosclerosis* affects large and medium arteries with tunica intima deposits of plaques containing cholesterol, lipoid material, and lipophages. Atherosclerosis generally affects the smaller arteries, rather than the aorta. *Arteriosclerosis* is a condition characterized by loss of elasticity and by thickening and hardening of the arteries. Both conditions may lead to aneurysm formation within an artery.

Thoracic aortic aneurysmectomy is excision of an aneurysmal portion of the ascending aorta, aortic arch, or descending thoracic aorta and replacement with a prosthetic graft or valve-graft conduit.

Collagen-impregnated grafts have significantly reduced interstitial bleeding and obviated the need for preclotting techniques. It is also possible to use an allograft (cadaver segment of aorta) or an autograft (patient's own PA) to replace the affected aorta (a graft replaces the PA).

Aortic *dissection* is a unique condition related to a tear in the tunica intima of the aorta that exposes underlying degenerative changes in the tunica media layer of the artery. Intraluminal blood flow penetrates and flows through the tear, resulting in subsequent dissection of the tunica media (David, 2009). As blood passes between the layers of the wall, it forms a false channel; as the channel extends and enlarges, it can obstruct blood flow through the aorta and its branches, or the aorta can rupture, causing severe hemorrhage (Figure 25-69, *A* and *B*). Surgical intervention becomes necessary when presenting symptoms indicate a compromised circulation or danger of rupture. Generally, medical management with hypotensive agents to reduce stress on the vessel is the preferred initial treatment until surgical repair can be performed. Increasingly, aneurysms and dissections of the descending thoracic aorta undergo repair with endovascular prostheses (Desai et al, 2011).

Aneurysms are characterized morphologically as follows: (1) saccular—a sac type of formation with a narrowed neck projecting from the side of the artery; or (2) fusiform—a spindle-shaped formation with complete circumferential involvement of the artery. *Dissections* can be characterized in at least two systems according to type, origin, and extent of the lesion (Table 25-9).

Procedural Considerations. Several methods of surgical treatment appear in the classic study by Crawford (1990). When an ascending aortic aneurysm or aortic dissection produces annular dilation with

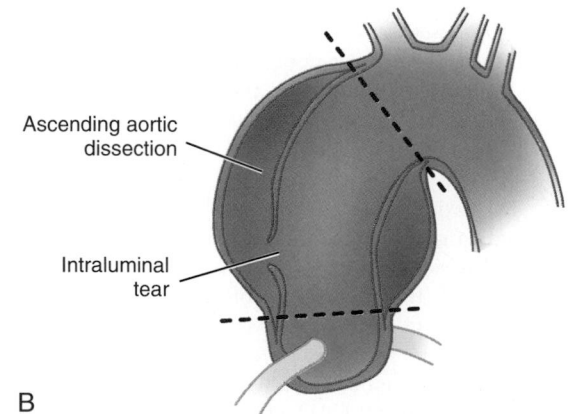

FIGURE 25-69 Aortic dissection. **A,** Proposed mechanism of the initiation of an aortic dissection (*A* = adventitia; *M* = media; *I* = intima). **B,** Intimal tear in the ascending aorta causing a dissection.

TABLE 25-9

Commonly Used Classification Systems to Describe Aortic Dissection

Type	Site of Origin and Extent of Aortic Involvement
Debakey	
Type I	Originates in ascending aorta and extends at least to aortic arch and often beyond it distally
Type II	Originates in and is confined to ascending aorta
Type III	Originates in descending aorta and extends distally down aorta or, rarely, retrograde into aortic arch and ascending aorta
Stanford	
Type A	All dissections involving ascending aorta, regardless of site of origin
Type B	All dissections not involving ascending aorta
Descriptive	
Proximal	Includes DeBakey types I and II or Stanford type A
Distal	Includes DeBakey type III or Stanford type B

Modified from David TE: Surgery of the aortic root and the ascending aorta. In Sellke FW et al, editors: *Sabiston and Spencer's surgery of the chest,* ed 8, Philadelphia, 2009, Saunders; Szeto WY, Bavaria JE: Endovascular therapy for thoracic aortic aneurysms and dissections. In Sellke FW et al, editors: *Sabiston and Spencer's surgery of the chest,* ed 8, Philadelphia, 2009, Saunders; Harris KM et al: Correlates of delayed recognition and treatment of acute type A aortic dissection: the International Registry of Acute Aortic Dissection (IRAD), *Circulation* 124(18):1911–1918, 2011; Hiratzka L et al: 2010 ACCF/AHA/AATS/ACR/ASA/SCA/SCAI/SIR/STS/SVM Guidelines for the diagnosis and management of patients with thoracic aortic disease, *Circulation* 121:e266–e369, 2010.

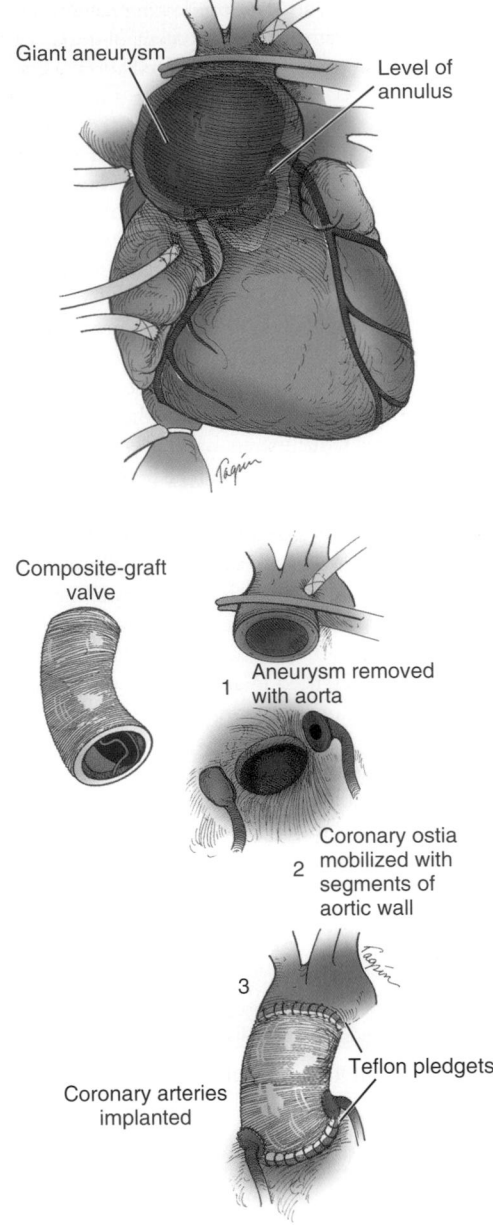

FIGURE 25-70 Bentall-DeBono procedure (see text).

Labels in figure: Giant aneurysm; Level of annulus; Composite-graft valve; 1 Aneurysm removed with aorta; 2 Coronary ostia mobilized with segments of aortic wall; 3 Coronary arteries implanted; Teflon pledgets

consequent aortic valve insufficiency, clinicians may use a modified Bentall-DeBono procedure with a composite graft-valve conduit, and reimplantation of the coronary ostia may be performed to replace the aortic valve and the aneurysmal aorta (David, 2009) (Figure 25-70). Retrograde cardioplegia is usually used to arrest the heart; if necessary, selective coronary infusion is an option. The Bentall-DeBono procedure requires reimplanting the right and left coronary ostia into the prosthetic graft; in patients with documented CAD, the surgeon may anastomose vein grafts to the affected coronary artery and attach them proximally to the prosthetic graft.

Positioning, instrumentation, and the type of CPB depend on the location of the aneurysm or dissection. Often patients with dissections present emergently, requiring immediate intervention.

The perioperative nurse can minimize delays by asking some basic questions to presage appropriate preparation and intervention in order to promote an effective outcome.

To initiate CPB, the atrium undergoes cannulation for venous return and use of the femoral or axillary artery affords arterial inflow because the weakened ascending aorta cannot be cannulated safely. Deep hypothermia with circulatory arrest and cerebroplegia offer protection of the heart and brain during procedures to address particularly complex lesions of the aortic arch, where placement of a cross-clamp is difficult. If used, cerebral oximetry monitors oxygenation of the brain.

Traditionally, during open repair of descending thoracic aortic aneurysms, the heart is not arrested; it continues beating to perfuse the upper body. It is possible to institute a femoral bypass to perfuse the kidneys and lower extremities; however, normothermia usually continues. Hypothermic CPB is available to repair complex descending and thoracoabdominal aneurysms in order to provide protection against paralysis and renal, cardiac, and visceral organ system failure. Increasingly, clinicians use an endovascular stent (see Figure 25-21 for aneurysms and dissections (Desai et al, 2011; Ehrlich et al, 2013); insertion of the prosthesis is through the femoral artery, guided under fluoroscopy to the area of the descending aortic aneurysm or dissection.

In complex lesions involving the ascending aorta, arch, and descending aorta, clinicians may repair the ascending aorta and arch using an open technique. Repair of the descending aorta may be achieved with an endovascular graft (Coselli and Green, 2012; David, 2009).

Repair of Ascending Thoracic Aortic Aneurysm or Dissection

Procedural Considerations. To the basic setup are added aneurysm instruments. Valve instruments, coronary instruments, and an array of tube grafts, valves, or valved conduits should be available. Preference is for bicaval cannulation, but if the cavae cannot be accessed safely due to increased risk of injury to the enlarged aneurysm, the femoral vein affords initial venous drainage. Once control of the aneurysm is at hand, the femoral venous line can be Y-ed to a vena caval cannula.

Operative Procedure
1. The patient's position is for median sternotomy.
2. Cannulation for CPB follows.
3. The surgeon opens the sternum and inspects the aneurysm.
4. The surgeon assesses the condition of the aortic annulus.
   a. If the aortic annulus is not involved, the surgeon may incise the aneurysm longitudinally and anastomose a woven graft proximally and distally to the healthy aorta (Figure 25-71). Felt strips incorporated into the anastomosis can bolster friable tissue.
   b. If the aortic annulus is involved, the surgeon incises the ascending aorta to the annulus and then excises the aneurysm. Excision of the valve leaflets follows, and the annulus is measured. The proximal end of a valved conduit is inserted. The surgeon uses an electrocoagulator to create openings in the graft at the location of the right and left coronary ostia, which are then mobilized and anastomosed to the graft. If there is concomitant CAD, saphenous vein grafts are inserted. The surgeon sutures the distal end of the conduit to healthy aorta.
5. Bypass ends, and closure of all incisions follows.

FIGURE 25-71 Resection and graft repair of ascending aortic aneurysm.

Repair of Aortic Arch Aneurysm

Procedural Considerations. Aneurysm instruments and woven grafts are available. If the surgeon chooses deep hypothermia, the patient's head may be covered with bags of ice at the beginning of the procedure to reduce cerebral oxygen demand. Precautionary measures (e.g., padding) to prevent frostbite are in place. The location of the aneurysm determines positioning. Access to aneurysms of the proximal arch is through median sternotomy; distal arch aneurysms may require a modified thoracotomy position to optimize exposure. Selective cerebral perfusion may be used during circulatory arrest to perfuse the brain. *Retrograde* cerebral perfusion is via the superior vena caval venous line Y-ed off the arterial line; arterial blood slowly infuses through the SVC line into the cerebral circulation while the surgeon anastomoses the distal aorta. *Antegrade* cerebral perfusion occurs by infusing arterialized blood through one or more catheters into aortic arch vessels (i.e., brachiocephalic artery and left common carotid artery).

Operative Procedure

1. The team cannulates the RA and femoral or axillary artery.
2. After cooling the patient to the desired temperature, cross-clamping of the arch vessels individually follows (Figure 25-72,

Aortic arch aneurysm

A

B

C

D

FIGURE 25-72 Repair of aortic arch aneurysm. **A,** Incision. **B,** Distal anastomosis. **C,** Anastomosis of graft to common origin of arch vessels. **D,** Proximal anastomosis.

A and B) (if circulatory arrest is indicated, a cross-clamp is not used). The surgeon incises the aneurysm, selects a tube graft (with or without side branches), and anastomoses it to the descending aorta. Depending on the pathoanatomy, the surgeon may add individual branch grafts to the main graft (Coselli and Green, 2012).

3. After making an opening into the side of the graft, the surgeon anastomoses the graft to the common origin of the brachiocephalic, left carotid, and left subclavian vessels. Alternatively, when using a graft with side branches, the surgeon creates individual anastomoses to the head vessels. The graft is cross-clamped proximally to the arch and de-aired (see Figure 25-72, *C*).

4. The surgeon anastomoses the proximal aorta to the graft while the patient rewarms. After de-airing the graft, the patient undergoes weaning from bypass (see Figure 25-72, *D*).

5. Closure of all incisions follows.

Repair of Descending Thoracic Aortic Aneurysm

Procedural Considerations. *Endovascular* repair (see Figure 25-21) of descending aortic aneurysms and dissections largely has supplanted the traditional open technique, although anatomic considerations may increase the difficulty of placing the straight endovascular tube graft into the angled portion of the proximal descending aorta (just distal to the left subclavian artery) (Hughes, 2012). Additionally, endovascular insertion requires nondiseased tissue for implantation of the device in the areas proximal and distal to the lesion (the "landing zones"); in patients with diffuse atherosclerotic disease or extensive dissection, viable tissue may not exist (Ehrlich et al, 2013). It is not unusual to deploy more than one graft in order to cover the lesion. Setup includes endovascular instruments, guidewires, introducer sheaths, pigtail catheters, intravascular dye, dilators, catheters, an array of stent graft sizes, and deployment devices. Performance of the procedure occurs with fluoroscopy, usually on an OR bed that allows imaging without extensive manipulation of the bed. Radiation precautions apply. The guidewires may be more than 6 feet in length; the scrub person therefore must protect sterility of the distal portion of the guidewire by anchoring it with towels or other sterile objects when not being used. The postoperative period is considerably shorter than that for a thoracotomy approach. Potential complications include bleeding and migration of the device (requiring adjustment and/or insertion of another device) (Ehrlich et al, 2013). There is some evidence (Luozzo et al, 2013) that open repair (described following) may be preferable to endovascular repair in patients younger than 60 years.

For *open* repair, thoracotomy instruments and supplies are added to the basic setup, plus additional long aortic cross-clamps may be needed. Prosthetic grafts are available. Positioning of the patient is for a left posterolateral thoracotomy. Use of femoral vein–femoral artery bypass perfuses the lower body. In this situation, the heart perfuses the upper body proximal to the aneurysm, and normothermia continues.

If the surgeon uses hypothermic CBP with circulatory arrest, instruments and supplies per the surgeon's request should be available. Protective coverings for the patient's head, face, and extremities avoid frostbite.

Operative Procedure—Endovascular Repair

1. The surgeon secures access to one or both femoral arteries via percutaneous (Seldinger) or cutdown technique. A hypodermic needle inserts into the femoral artery. A guidewire passes through the needle and threads into the aorta. Fluoroscopy images the

FIGURE 25-73 Resection and graft replacement for descending thoracic aortic aneurysm.

aortic lumen and measures targeted segments of the aorta. The hypodermic needle is removed and a sheath inserted, through which the device will insert.

2. Insertion of a delivery catheter housing the graft is into the descending aorta.

3. A monitoring device inserted through the contralateral femoral artery can measure intraluminal pressures.

4. Using fluoroscopy, the surgeon guides the graft into position and deploys it into the aorta (see Figure 25-21). The device self-expands; a balloon can inflate against the inside of the graft to secure the prosthesis against the aortic lumen.

5. Fluoroscopy images the aorta and confirms exclusion of the aneurysm/dissection.

6. Removal of deployment devices and other intraluminal catheters and wires follows as does closure of all incisions.

Operative Procedure—Open Repair

1. Cannulation for femoral vein–femoral artery bypass commences.

2. The surgeon makes a thoracotomy incision, exposes the aneurysm, and inspects the surrounding structures. Occasionally the surgeon may make two thoracotomy incisions for better access to, and control of, the aorta. Assessment of renal involvement follows; if indicated, the surgeon directs institution of measures to protect the kidneys (e.g., local cooling).

3. Normothermic femoral bypass is initiated.

4. Incision of the aneurysm is longitudinal, and aorta sizing follows.

5. The surgeon inserts a woven graft (Figure 25-73) and wraps any aneurysmal remnants around the graft.

Assisted Mechanical Circulation

Mechanical circulatory support has been available for more than three decades, expanding the treatment for heart failure into a rapidly growing specialty that also includes coronary artery revascularization, left and right ventricular reconstruction, circulatory assist device implantation, and cardiac transplantation (Bowdish et al, 2010; Gregoric, 2012). Formerly, ventricular assist devices were reserved only for those patients who could not be weaned from

CPB after open-heart operations or who had end-stage cardiomyopathy. Current indications and choices have expanded and a variety of active and passive devices are available to support circulation for short-, intermediate-, and long-term use (Bogaev et al, 2011; Gregoric, 2012). Use of VADs is not only for "destination" therapy (i.e., implanted permanently) and as a "bridge to transplantation," but also for recovery (Bowdish et al, 2010). The evolution of mechanical circulatory support (MCS) and the success of MCS devices for destination therapy (especially continuous flow devices) have enabled mechanical devices to compete with cardiac transplantation (Kirklin et al, 2012).

Intra-Aortic Balloon Pump

The most widely used short-term device is the IABP, a percutaneously inserted device. The IABP (Figure 25-74) uses the principle of counterpulsation to increase coronary blood flow and decrease afterload (i.e., the resistance the ventricle must overcome to open the aortic valve).

Operative Procedure

1. The clinician passes a flexible guidewire through a percutaneous needle into the femoral artery. After removing the needle, the clinician inserts graduated dilators over the guidewire to dilate the overlying tissue and the artery wall.

2. The IABP catheter (with furled balloon) inserts into the artery and advances to a position just distal to the left subclavian artery. The surgeon marks the catheter at the proximal end with a silk tie to measure the distance the catheter should be inserted.

3. The clinician unfurls the balloon and activates it.

Ventricular Assist Device

An expanding array of VADs are available. Their position may be internal or external, they may be electrically or pneumatically powered, they may be pulsatile or nonpulsatile, and they may require warfarin anticoagulation. Most devices allow ambulation and some enable the patient to be discharged from the hospital (Bogaev et al, 2011). As designed, VADs augment cardiac output from the left (LVAD), right (RVAD), or both (biventricular [BiVAD]) ventricles and decrease workload of the heart by diverting blood from the ventricle or ventricles to an artificial pump that maintains systemic perfusion. Patients with an LVAD benefit from the resulting enhanced anabolism, ambulation, and improved organ function. Complications (e.g., bleeding, thromboembolism, infection, device failure) persist, but they have lessened with the newer VADs (Gregoric, 2012).

Among designs are the axial flow pump, which inserts into the LV to propel blood flow (Figure 25-75). The distal end anastomoses to the descending aorta. Miniaturized centrifugal pumps, totally

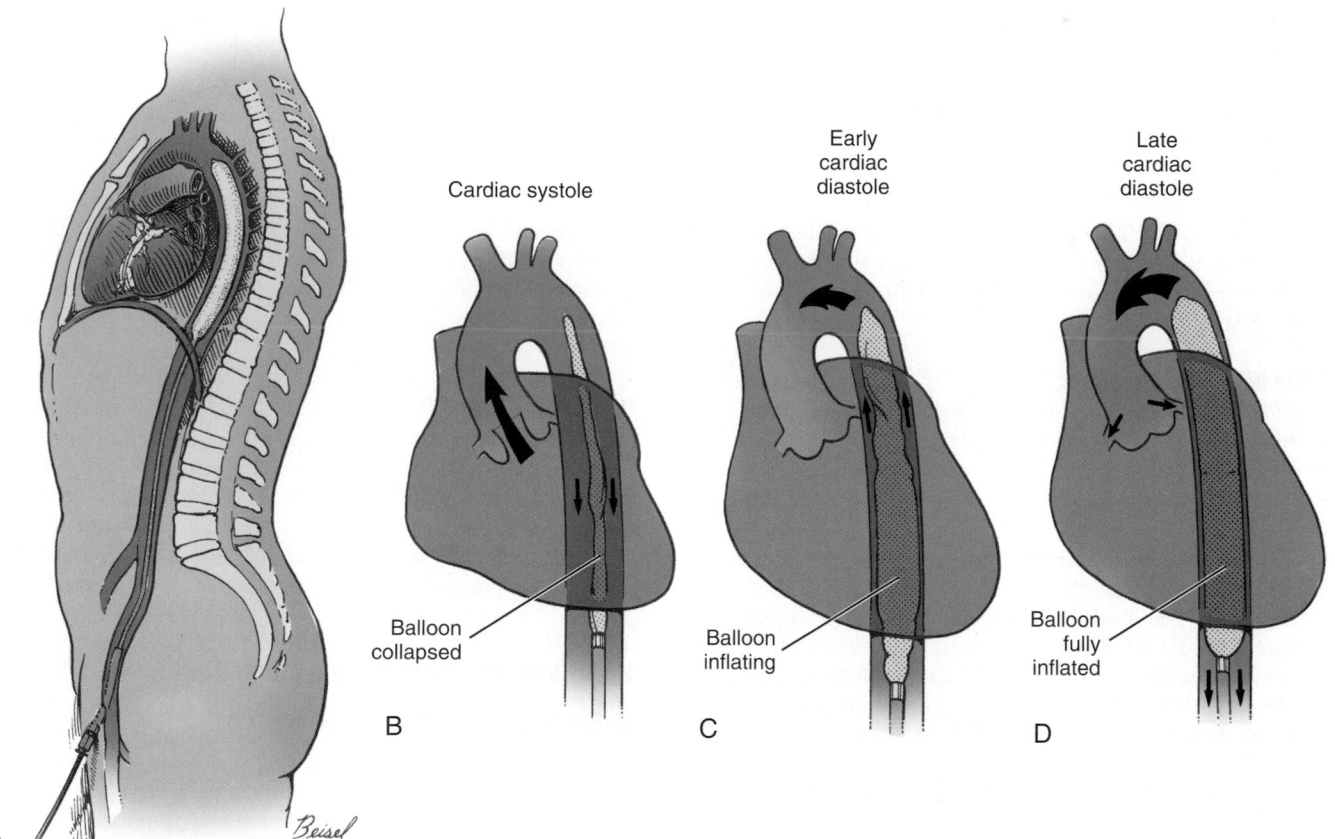

FIGURE 25-74 Phases of balloon pumping. **A,** Balloon inflation occurs from closure of aortic valve to end of diastole. Inflation causes retrograde flow of blood in aorta, increasing coronary perfusion pressure without increasing myocardial work or oxygen demand. Inflation also causes antegrade flow, increasing mean arterial pressure, renal flow, and cerebral flow. **B,** Balloon deflation occurs from just before opening of aortic valve to closure of aortic valve. Deflation encourages antegrade flow, decreasing afterload or resistance to left ventricular ejection. Deflation also decreases oxygen required by left ventricle, shortens systolic ejection, and increases stroke volume. **C** and **D,** When the balloon reinflates, the cycle repeats anew.

FIGURE 25-75 Axial flow left ventricular device. Based on the principle of Archimedes screw, the device contains a propeller that propels blood from the left ventricle into the systemic circulation via the ascending aorta, thereby reducing the workload of the heart while enhancing perfusion to the body.

implantable pulsatile devices incorporating a transcutaneous energy transmission (and power regeneration) system, and artificial hearts are additional devices used to treat heart failure (Bogaev et al, 2011; Naidu, 2011).

Procedural Considerations. Insertion of an assist device may be indicated for patients who cannot be weaned from CPB, or device insertion may be scheduled. Depending on the system, components of the system must be collected and prepared according to the manufacturer's instructions. Device components may include external centrifugal pumps, internally powered assist devices (Figure 25-76), or wholly implantable systems with transcutaneous, rechargeable power sources.

The LVAD described in the following section is approved for support of the LV when right ventricular function is normal. Prosthetic valves incorporated into the circuit maintain unidirectional blood flow. All VADs differ, and preparation should be specific to the particular device. In preparation for VAD insertion, perioperative nurses should discuss VAD type, insertion considerations, possible complications, and trouble-shooting scenarios with the surgeon in advance. Preclotting and availability of topical hemostatic agents are also topics to discuss with the surgeon (see Surgical Pharmacology).

Operative Procedure
Thoratec Heartmate LVAD

1. The surgeon makes a median sternotomy incision, extended to the umbilicus (see Figure 25-76, *A*).

2. The surgeon next makes a preperitoneal pouch for placement of the assist device.
3. CPB commences and the aorta is cross-clamped. The surgeon inspects the atrial septum for defects (or a patent foramen ovale), which are closed if found.
4. Anastomosis of a Dacron graft is to the aorta (see Figure 25-76, *B*).
5. The surgeon mobilizes the left ventricular apex and creates an opening in the apex (see Figure 25-76, *C*).
6. The surgeon inserts a connector into the apex and sews the flange to the surrounding left ventricular myocardium with pledgeted sutures. Attachment of the inflow conduit is to the apical connector (see Figure 25-76, *D* to *G*).
7. The surgeon then makes an opening into the diaphragm near the location of the apical connector and inflow conduit. Passed through the diaphragm, the conduit undergoes attachment to the assist device.
8. Attachment of the aortic graft is to the outflow conduit, which is connected to the assist device (see Figure 25-76, *H* and *I*).
9. Tunneling of the percutaneous driveline runs to the left lower quadrant, where it exits through the skin. The driveline connects to the drive console (shown) or to a battery pack (not shown). Blood flows from the left ventricular apex, to the device, and back into the body through the aortic conduit (see Figure 25-76, *J*).
10. CPB ends, and closure of incisions follows.

To remove or replace the pump, the patient returns to the OR, the surgeon reopens the sternotomy and removes the cannulae, and then removes or replaces the device.

Total Artificial Heart

The total artificial heart (TAH) continues to undergo refinement and implantation in patients with end-stage biventricular failure. Complications associated with thromboembolism and infection have lessened, but not ended, with technical and material refinements of VAD systems. Use of long-term RVADs or LVADs has increased as a bridge to cardiac transplantation by supporting circulation until a suitable donor heart appears (Mehra and Griffith, 2012).

Two examples of the TAH are the AbioCor TAH and the CardioWest SynCardia (Bogaev et al, 2011; Mehra and Griffith, 2012). The AbioCor TAH uses a centrifugal pump powered by an internal battery (rechargeable via transcutaneous energy source). The CardioWest TAH uses two pneumatically driven pumps containing mechanical tilting disk valves. This TAH requires a chest anteroposterior diameter of at least 10 cm and a large body surface area, so the device is appropriate only for larger patients (Mehra and Griffith, 2012).

Heart and Heart-Lung Transplantation

Heart Transplantation (Figure 25-77)

Orthotopic transplantation (replacing one heart with another) is most commonly performed; less common are heterotopic (piggyback) and combined heart-lung procedures. Important considerations continue to be recipient and donor selection, immune response, and infection control. Older recipients and donors (older than 65 to 70 years) have demonstrated acceptable morbidity and survival (Acker and Jessup, 2012). There also is a growing need of transplantation in patients who reach adulthood with congenital heart disease (CHD). Although adults with CHD demonstrate a

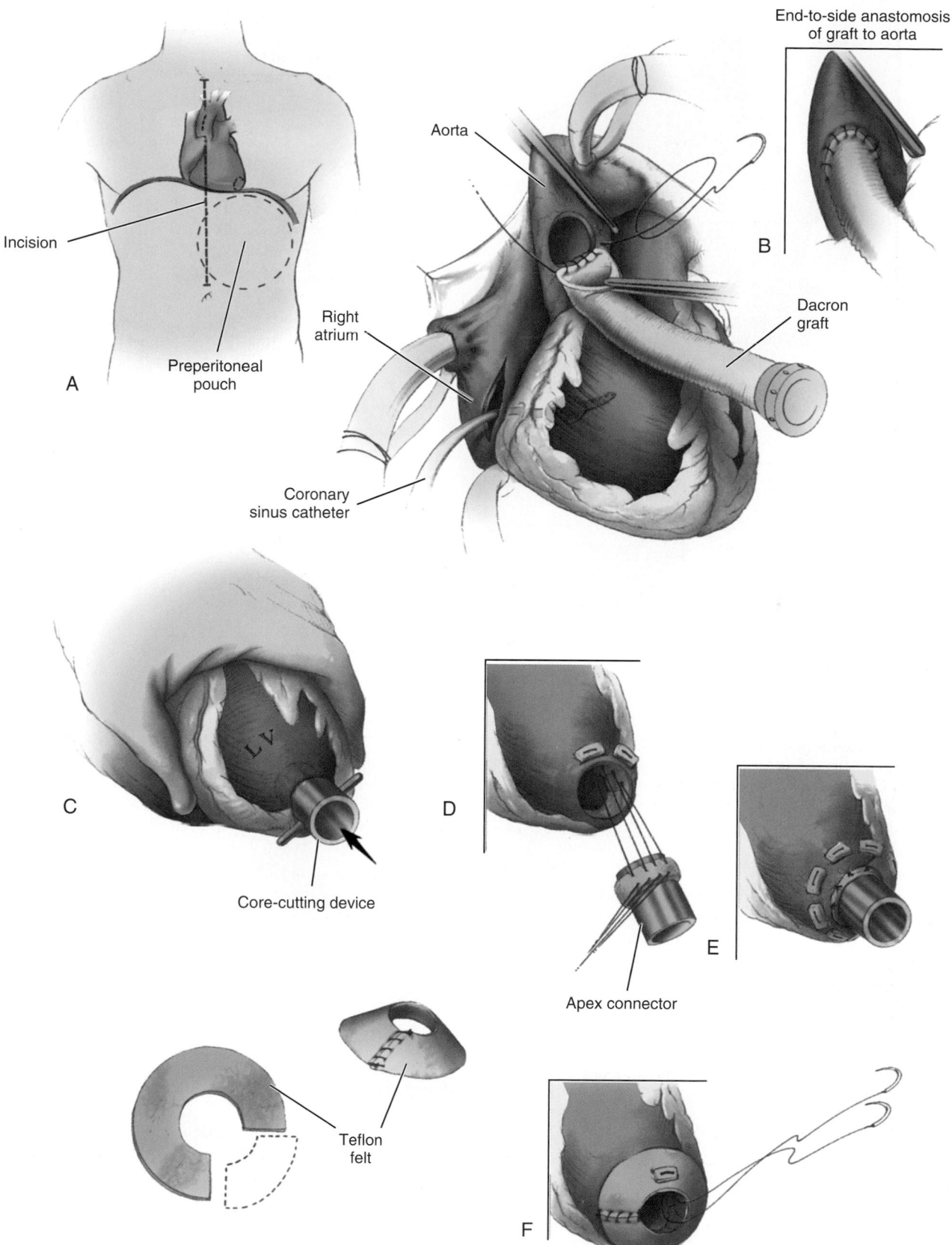

End-to-side anastomosis of graft to aorta

Incision

Preperitoneal pouch

A

Aorta

Right atrium

Coronary sinus catheter

B

Dacron graft

C

Core-cutting device

LV

D

Apex connector

E

Teflon felt

F

FIGURE 25-76 Left ventricular assist device.

Continued

Secure inflow conduit
to apex connector

H

G

HeartMate left
ventricular assist device

I

Secure outflow conduit
to aortic graft

Drive line

Drive
console

J

Completed implant

FIGURE 25-76, cont'd Left ventricular assist device.

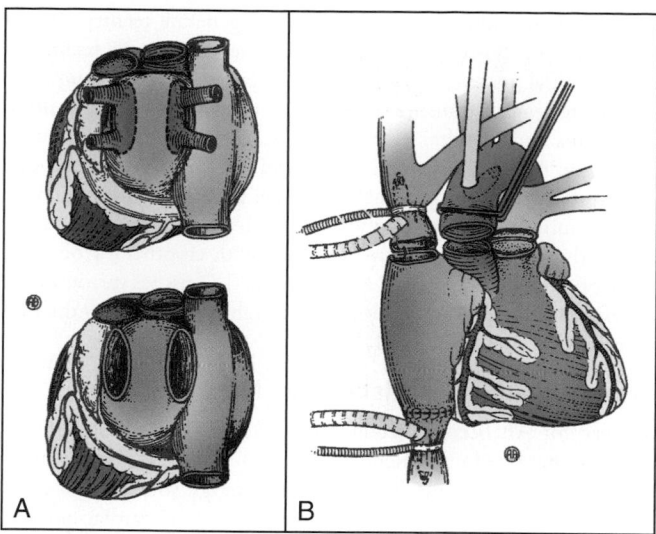

FIGURE 25-77 A, Heart transplantation with pulmonary venous anastomoses on right or left side, and caval anastomoses at the superior and inferior vena cavae. **B,** Aorta and pulmonary artery are joined last.

FIGURE 25-78 Traditional atrial anastomosis for heart transplantation.

high 30-day mortality, they have better long-term late survival (Davies et al, 2011). For CHD transplants, perioperative nurses should review medical and surgical history and discuss the proposed surgery with the surgeon in order to anticipate anatomic anomalies related to CHD and its surgical correction.

Modification of traditional transplantation technique (i.e., atrial-atrial anastomoses or *biatrial technique*) developed to reduce dysrhythmias and tricuspid valvular dysfunction associated with traditional transplantation. This modification, the *bicaval technique,* consists of end-to-end anastomoses between the donor and recipient SVC and the donor and recipient IVC, producing a more physiologic atrial contribution to ventricular filling and less distortion of the mitral and tricuspid annuli (Bowdish et al, 2010). If there is tricuspid insufficiency, ring annuloplasty may be performed on the donor heart. Performance of pulmonary artery and aortic anastomoses is in the traditional manner.

Procedural Considerations. Donor and recipient each require individual instrument setups.

Operative Procedure
Donor Heart. Exposure of the donor heart is through median sternotomy. The surgeon dissects the aorta, pulmonary artery, and venae cavae. After occlusion of the venae cavae, the surgeon opens the LA to decompress the ventricle, after which rapid cooling and arrest of the heart follow.

Heart excision is by incision of the SVC and the IVC, the LA, the aorta, and the pulmonary artery. The team immediately places the donor heart into cold saline and transports it to the site where the recipient will receive it. If other organs (e.g., lungs, liver, kidneys, pancreas) are to be procured simultaneously, heart procurement team members must coordinate removal of other organs with their respective colleagues (Bowdish et al, 2010).

Recipient Heart. The recipient undergoes bypass with cannulation of the IVC and the SVC; caval tapes are placed around the cavae. Cooling of the patient is to about 89.6° to 93.2° F (32° to 34° C), followed by tightening of the caval tapes. The surgeon

dissects the pulmonary trunk and aorta immediately above their respective semilunar valves; incises the LA to leave intact portions of the left atrial wall and the atrial septum of the recipient; incises the RA, retaining the SVC and IVC for anastomosis to the donor heart; and then removes the recipient's heart.

The team places the donor heart in the pericardial well. The surgeon next performs pulmonary anastomoses (see Figure 25-77, *A*). The SVC and IVC are anastomosed with running cardiovascular sutures (see Figure 25-77, *B*). Similar joinders of the donor and recipient aortas and pulmonary arteries are next. Removal of air from the left side of the heart follows. Before suturing the pulmonary artery, the surgeon carefully inspects all caval and atrial suture lines for significant bleeding areas, after which the cross-clamp is removed. Figure 25-78 illustrates the traditional (but less frequently anastomosed) right atrial suture line; aortic and pulmonary anastomoses are similar to the technique just described.

A single direct-current shock usually is effective to defibrillate the ventricles. A needle vent in the ascending aorta allows residual air to escape. The patient then gradually undergoes weaning from the bypass. Cannulae are removed from the venae cavae and the aorta. Incision closures are as described previously.

Heart-Lung Transplantation

Newer techniques for lung and heart-lung transplantation incorporate the bicaval anastomoses used for orthotopic heart transplantation and also use bibronchial anastomosis to reduce bleeding and to enhance airway integrity. To maximize allocation of scarce donor organs, transplant procedures for the lungs may use a single lung or bilateral lungs; heart-lung transplantation is relatively rare, largely due to increased frequency of lung transplantation (Quinlan et al, 2011). Preservation of the *donor's* sinus node and the *recipient's* recurrent laryngeal, vagus, and phrenic nerves is an important surgical consideration.

Operative Procedure. The recipient's diseased heart and lung(s) undergo excision separately or en bloc, during which care must be taken not to injure the major nerves previously listed. The recipient's RA, SVC, and IVC are saved to create bicaval attachments to the donor heart. As the surgeon transects the bronchi, the team brings the donor heart and lungs onto the field. Placement of the right lung is in the right pleural space and of the left lung in the left pleural space. The surgeon performs bronchial and the bicaval anastomoses, and rewarming begins. Aortic anastomosis follows; the aorta is de-aired and the cross-clamp is removed.

Surgery for Conduction Disturbances

Disturbances of the conduction system affect the rate, rhythm, and effectiveness of the contracting heart. Clinicians and researchers have developed surgical techniques to treat a variety of supraventricular dysrhythmias (e.g., AF and Wolff-Parkinson-White reentry tachycardia) and both ischemic and nonischemic ventricular tachydysrhythmias (e.g., ventricular tachycardia or fibrillation). Preprocedural electrophysiologic mapping of the patient's conduction pathways identifies and locates aberrant pathways, tachydysrhythmias, and the existence of additional pathways, as well as the effects of medications on a particular dysrhythmia. Indications for pacemaker implantation (including resynchronization therapy) and antitachycardia-antifibrillation devices have been expanded. Many (but not all) pacemaker and internal cardioverter defibrillator (ICD) insertions now occur in the EP laboratory or the cardiac catheterization suite (Cheng et al, 2011).

Ablation procedures for AF normally happen in the EP laboratory. Depending on the anticipated locus of the problem, the electrophysiologist inserts a catheter percutaneously into the femoral vein or artery and threads the catheter retrograde to the RA or LA and ventricle. The electrophysiologist tests various areas of the heart in an attempt to reproduce the dysrhythmia and then ablates the area of the heart where the rhythm disturbance originates. Postoperative considerations are similar to those for atrial fibrillation surgery. Surgical correction normally occurs in the OR.

AF is the most common sustained cardiac dysrhythmia, with a prevalence in the United States ranging from approximately 2.7 to 6.1 million in 2010; AF is expected to rise in prevalence to between 5.6 and 12 million by 2050 (AHA, 2012b; Judge, 2012; Go et al, 2013). AF was considered a "benign" condition in the past, but serious consequences associated with the dysrhythmia have made it the subject of intense study. AF interferes with the atrial kick (which contributes a significant amount of "preload") and the dysrhythmia can lead to insufficient cardiac output. Moreover, the stasis of blood within the atria promotes the formation of thrombus (clotting), which leads to cerebrovascular accident or pulmonary embolism.

Although *intermittent* AF commonly follows CABG, it is potentially preventable by treatment with amiodarone, beta-blockers, angiotensin-converting enzyme (ACE) inhibitors, and nonsteroidal antiinflammatory drugs. Treatment includes restoration of sinus rhythm (when possible), control of ventricular rate, and administration of anticoagulants (Bainbridge and Cheng, 2011).

New techniques to treat *continuous* AF have arisen based on research demonstrating that the pulmonary veins are an important source of ectopic beats that can initiate paroxysms of AF (Haissaguerre et al, 1998). Surgical interventions for AF have expanded beyond Cox's original maze procedures (Cox et al, 1991), in which the surgeon sutured extensive atrial incisions to create a maze through which electrical impulses were directed from the SA node to the AV node. Early research by Cox (Cox et al, 1991) demonstrated that electrical impulses are unable to cross incised and

sutured tissue and consequently cannot regenerate reentry circuits producing the dysrhythmia. Cox revised the cut-and-sew technique of the initial maze procedures with a cryosurgical technique to ensure creation of transmural lesions in the vicinity of the pulmonary veins and in other areas of the heart that generate impulses producing AF. The clinician can perform this "mini-maze" through a sternotomy or via a minimally invasive thoracic route; the mini-maze requires placement of fewer lesions in the left and right atria. Currently, focus is on selective ablation (with cryotherapy or ultrasonic or radiofrequency [RF] energy sources) of tissues surrounding, for example, the pulmonary veins to reestablish normal conduction pathways (Cheng et al, 2011).

Surgery for Atrial Fibrillation (The Maze Procedure)

Surgery for AF occurs through open sternotomy or right minithoracotomy incisions (Cheng et al, 2011). The perioperative nurse ensures appropriate supplies (including energy sources) are available. By creating small areas of scar tissue in the cardiac muscle, electrical impulses—unable to cross scar tissue—must follow an alternative conduction path, or maze.

Operative Procedure—Sternotomy

1. The surgeon performs a midline sternotomy.
2. Cannulation of the superior and inferior venae cavae follows for total cardiopulmonary bypass.
3. The surgeon occludes the ascending aorta, and cardioplegic solution infuses through the aortic root and into the coronary arteries.
4. After performance of a right atriotomy, ablation of the first set of lesions in the RA occurs (Figure 25-79, *A*).
5. A left atriotomy follows, as does ablation of the left atrial lesions (see Figure 25-79, *B*).
6. After closure of the atriotomies, the aorta is unclamped.
7. Cardiopulmonary bypass discontinues, followed by removal of the cannulae.
8. The team inserts chest tubes and pacing wires, and the wound is closed.

Operative Procedure—Mini-Thoracotomy (Figure 25-80)

1. The patient's position is supine, but tilted slightly to the left with a roll under the right rib cage; placement of the right arm is on an armboard at a right angle.
2. The surgeon makes a 5- to 7-cm incision in the right submammary area in the fourth intercostal space and another incision for exposure.
3. Exposure of the right femoral vein and artery for CPB is by groin incision.
4. The anesthesia provider deflates the right lung and the surgeon opens the pericardium and tacks the pericardial edges to the chest wall.
5. The surgeon accesses the IVC and SVC.
6. The surgeon cannulates the femoral vein and artery; and then places a purse-string suture into the SVC, followed by a venous cannula through the purse-string into the SVC.
7. Before instituting CPB, the surgeon creates the right atrial lesions.
8. After the surgeon completes the right atrial lesions, the perfusionist initiates CPB; the surgeon then cross-clamps the aorta and arrests the heart (with a retrograde cardioplegia catheter inserted through the right atrial wall into the coronary sinus).

FIGURE 25-79 A, First lesion set for maze procedure. **B,** Second lesion set for maze procedure.

9. The surgeon makes the left atrial lesions.
10. CPB discontinues and the cannulae are removed.
11. Chest tubes and pacing wires are inserted and the incisions closed.

Postoperative Considerations. Postoperatively, patients undergo monitoring for heart rhythm problems. In patients treated for AF, it may take up to 3 months for the heart to resume beating normally. Additional postoperative considerations include monitoring for bleeding, infection, and other potential complications related to heart surgery (Cheng et al, 2011).

Insertion of Permanent Pacemaker

A permanent pacemaker (pulse generator and electrodes) initiates atrial or ventricular contraction, or both. Complete heart block and bradydysrhythmias (i.e., slow heart rates) are the most common indications for pacemaker implantation. A temporary pacemaker is also possible to remedy acute forms of heart block and dysrhythmias that occasionally occur during and after cardiac surgery (Cheng et al, 2011).

Insertion of Transvenous (Endocardial) Pacing Electrodes

Positioning of the patient is supine and the anesthesia provider monitors the ECG. Because lethal dysrhythmias can occur, a defibrillator must be available. Because the procedure requires fluoroscopy, either a portable image intensifier is needed, or the procedure occurs in the special studies section of the radiology or cardiac catheterization department. Setup requires a minor set of instruments with vascular dissecting and tunneling instruments, as well as an introducer set, testing instruments, and supplies (e.g., alligator cables). Often the pacemaker representative will bring a pacing system analyzer (PSA).

Using local anesthetic, the surgeon puts the patient in Trendelenburg position in order to engorge the vein for easier access and to avoid air emboli, and makes a skin pocket close to the subclavian vein. A venotomy is performed and a guidewire threaded to the desired cardiac chamber, after which the needle is removed. The pacing electrode inserts through a dilator and advances under direct fluoroscopic vision into the RA, through the tricuspid valve, and into the RV. The surgeon places the electrode in the trabeculae carneae cordis of the right ventricular apex and tests the electrode with alligator test cables and the PSA to confirm proper placement and function. If insertion is of a dual-chamber pacemaker, the surgeon entraps the second lead in the right atrial appendage. Attachment of the electrode(s) is to the pulse generator, which is placed into the pocket. A tunneling device can thread the electrode to the pocket. Closure of the incision is in layers with absorbable sutures.

Insertion of Myocardial (Epicardial) Pacing Electrodes

A subxiphoid left anterior thoracotomy approach or sternotomy approach is appropriate. The subxiphoid process and left upper quadrant area are infiltrated with an anesthetic agent. The surgeon makes a small transverse incision below the xiphoid process and extends it down to the linea alba. Creation of a tunnel is under the xiphoid process to the pericardium, incised to expose the heart. The pacing electrode, mounted on its carrier, screws into the ventricular myocardium, followed by removal of the carrier. The remainder of the procedure is the same as that described for insertion of the endocardial electrode.

FIGURE 25-80 Mini-thoracotomy position and incisions for minimally invasive maze procedure.

For the sternotomy approach, the surgeon opens the mediastinum for the concomitant cardiac procedure and chooses an area of myocardium to place the pacing electrodes. The electrode tips either screw into or are sutured to the myocardium and attached by an appropriate cable to an external pulse generator or PSA for testing. Creation of the pocket and subcutaneous tunnel is as described for insertion of the endocardial electrode.

Cardiac Resynchronization Therapy

Dual-site pacing of both the RV and LV is another treatment for patients with dilated cardiomyopathy and heart failure (Stone et al, 2011). *Cardiac resynchronization therapy* (CRT) uses leads placed on the RA and the RV. An electrode introduced transvenously into the coronary sinus and extended into the great cardiac vein (or a tributary) to a position in the left side of the heart achieves left ventricular pacing; this electrode functions as the second ventricular lead. The three electrodes connect to the pacemaker generator. Resynchronization improves the mechanical pumping action between the RV and LV and optimizes AV synchrony; as a result, hemodynamic function improves in heart failure patients.

The *transvenous* or the *epicardial* approach may be used to place the electrodes. The transvenous route is most common because it does not require a major thoracotomy or a general anesthetic and is therefore safer for high-risk patients. Permanent epicardial electrodes may be placed during cardiac operations when the chest is opened and the heart is exposed; if a permanent pacemaker is required, however, it is likely to be inserted transvenously during the postoperative period (temporary electrodes placed during surgery achieve pacing). To avoid opening the sternum, a subxiphoid approach to place epicardial leads is possible.

Insertion of Implantable Cardioverter Defibrillator

Surgery or pharmacologic intervention may not prevent malignant ventricular dysrhythmias (ventricular fibrillation and ventricular tachycardia) in people who survive sudden cardiac death. The implantable cardioverter defibrillator (ICD) is an electronic device designed to monitor cardiac electrical activity and deliver prompt defibrillator shocks. The ICD differs from a pacemaker in that the ICD senses ventricular tachycardia or fibrillation, whereas the pacemaker senses asystole. ICD models are capable of tiered therapy, whereby increasingly stronger impulses are delivered depending on the underlying dysrhythmias; some devices can also terminate AF. These devices are capable of pacing as well as defibrillating (pacing cardioverter defibrillators [PCDs]). Although the purposes of pacemakers and ICDs differ, their respective surgical procedures are similar (e.g., transvenous access, testing).

The ICD device consists of a generator and sensing and defibrillator electrodes. Many ICD electrodes consist of transvenous electrodes inserted into the generator much like a transvenous pacemaker system. Addition of myocardial or thoracic subcutaneous patches is possible if transvenous catheters alone can not defibrillate the heart adequately. Patients with previously applied defibrillator patches may present for patch removal; perioperative nurses should prepare for emergency intervention if excessive bleeding or lethal dysrhythmia appears. EP studies performed before and after insertion enable diagnosis of the dysrhythmia and evaluation of device function, respectively.

The transvenous route with fluoroscopy is common, and insertion is similar to that described for transvenous pacemaker insertion. Tunneling of the free ends of the lead system is to the generator, implanted in a subcutaneous pocket in the chest wall.

After testing the device, closure of the incisions concludes the procedure.

KEY POINTS

- Cardiac surgery is increasingly moving toward interventional procedures that use minimally invasive approaches and percutaneous access routes.
- Therapeutic interventions may use laser, radiofrequency, and cryothermal energies.
- The heart is a four-chamber muscular pump that propels blood into the systemic and pulmonary circulatory systems. It sits within a pericardial sac within the mediastinum, between the lungs, posterior to the sternum, and anterior to the vertebrae, esophagus, and descending portion of the aorta.
- Each half of the heart contains an upper and a lower communicating chamber—the atrium and ventricle, respectively.
- The pulmonary circulatory system pumps blood from the RV through the pulmonary valve into the main PA.
- The coronary circulation supplies oxygen and nutrients to, and removes metabolic waste from, the myocardium.
- To prevent regurgitation of blood, the four cardiac valves open and close to maintain unidirectional blood flow. Any of the four valves may be deformed congenitally or subject to acquired valvular heart disease.
- Because the severity of pathologic changes varies among patients throughout the life span, knowledge of physical status, psychosocial concerns, and functional health patterns enables the perioperative nurse to plan and manage patient care.
- In addition to health status and risk factors, the perioperative nurse reviews patient medication history with particular attention to vasoactive drugs, anticoagulants, and other medications that can affect surgery.
- After a comprehensive review of individual patient data, the perioperative nurse identifies relevant nursing diagnoses, from which the perioperative plan for patient care derives.
- The safety of the cardiac surgery patient is a primary responsibility of the perioperative nurse.

CRITICAL THINKING QUESTION

When the on-call nurse receives a page to "come in for an aneurysm" (often at night), some of the immediate questions that come to mind concern types of aneurysm (or dissection), comorbid conditions, location, and treatment options relative to these factors. One of the first considerations is *location,* because that can affect positioning, instrumentation, tissue perfusion, and other interventions. The differences among types of aneurysms and dissections are crucial.

The location can be in the ascending aorta, the aortic arch, the descending aorta, or a combination of sites. It is important to prepare for the patient and set up the OR appropriately, promptly, and efficiently. Communication with the surgeon is essential for optimal outcomes. Describe the instrumentation, equipment, prosthesis, and accessory items or supplies you would anticipate for an ascending aortic aneurysm, an aortic arch aneurysm, and a descending thoracic aortic aneurysm. What comorbid conditions would you consider important to your plan of care? Review extracorporeal support for each of these types of patients along with your plans for the surgical position, skin prep, and draping. What infection prevention strategies and special safety considerations would you implement for each type of patient? What are essential items to include in your hand-off report?

⊖volve *The answers to the Critical Thinking Question can be found at http://evolve.elsevier.com/Rothrock/Alexander.*

REFERENCES

Achneck HE et al: A comprehensive review of topical hemostatic agents: efficacy and recommendations for use, *Ann Surg* 251(2):217–228, 2010.

Acker MA, Jessup M: Surgical management of heart failure. In Bonow RO et al, editors: *Braunwald's heart disease: a textbook of cardiovascular medicine*, ed 9, Philadelphia, 2012, Saunders.

American College of Surgeons (ACS): *Patient education*, available at www.facs.org/Patienteducation/Index.html. Accessed March 18, 2013.

American Heart Association (AHA) (2012a): *For patients*, available at w.heart.org/HEARTORG/General/Consumer-And-Patient-Education-Materials_UCM_314813_Article.Jsp. Accessed March 18, 2013.

American Heart Association (AHA): *Heart disease and stroke statistics—2013* update, 2012b, available at http://circ.ahajournals.org/Content/Early/2012/12/12/CIR.0b013e31828124ad.Citation. Accessed March 18, 2013.

American Heart Association (AHA): *Women's statistical fact sheet*: 2013 update, available at http://my.americanheart.org/Idc/Groups/Heart-Public/@Wcm/@Sop/@Smd/Documents/Downloadable/Ucm_319576.Pdf. Accessed March 18, 2013.

American Society of Anesthesiologists (ASA): *Patient education*, 1995-2013, available at https://ecommerce.asahq.org/C-8-Patient-Education.Aspx. Accessed March 18, 2013.

Aranki SF, Shopnick B: Demise of open vein harvesting (editorial), *Circulation* 123:127–128, 2011.

Association of periOperative Registered Nurses (AORN): *Perioperative standards and recommended practices*, Denver, 2013, The Association.

Bailey SR: Percutaneous treatment for valvular heart disease. In Antman EM, Sabatine MS, editors: *Cardiovascular therapeutics—a companion to Braunwald's heart disease*, Philadelphia, 2012, Saunders.

Bainbridge D, Cheng DCH: Postoperative cardiac recovery and outcomes. In Kaplan JA et al, editors: *Kaplan's cardiac anesthesia: the echo era*, ed 6, Philadelphia, 2011, Saunders.

Banner D et al: Women's experiences of undergoing coronary artery bypass graft surgery, *J Adv Nurs* 68(4):919–930, 2011.

Barnard J, Millner R: A review of topical hemostatic agents for use in cardiac surgery, *Ann Thorac Surg* 88:1377–1383, 2009.

Bogaev RC et al: Circulatory assist devices in heart failure. In Mann DL, editor: *Heart failure—a companion to Braunwald's heart disease*, ed 2, Philadelphia, 2011, Saunders.

Bojar RM: *Manual of perioperative care in adult cardiac surgery*, ed 5, Oxford, 2011, Wiley-Blackwell.

Bowdish ME et al: Cardiac transplantation and mechanical circulatory devices. In Runge MS et al, editors: *Netter's cardiology*, ed 2, Philadelphia, 2010, Saunders.

Caboral MF: Update on cardiovascular disease prevention in women, *Am J Nurs* 113(3):26–33, 2013.

Canty JM: Coronary blood flow and myocardial ischemia. In Bonow RO et al, editors: *Braunwald's heart disease: a textbook of cardiovascular medicine*, ed 9, Philadelphia, 2012, Saunders.

Carabello BA: Valvular heart disease. In Goldman L, Schafer AI, editors: *Goldman's Cecil medicine*, ed 24, Philadelphia, 2012, Saunders.

Carpentier A: Cardiac valve surgery: the "French Correction." *J Thorac Cardiovasc Surg* 86(3):323, 1983.

Chaudhuri K et al: Carbon dioxide insufflation in open-chamber cardiac surgery: a double-blind, randomized clinical trial of neurocognitive effects, *J Thorac Cardiovasc Surg* 144:646–653, 2012.

Chikwe JO et al: Procedures in the hybrid operating room. In Kaplan JA et al, editors: *Kaplan's cardiac anesthesia: the echo era*, ed 6, Philadelphia, 2011, Saunders.

Cheng A et al: Cardiac electrophysiology: diagnosis and treatment. In Kaplan JA et al, editors: *Kaplan's cardiac anesthesia: the echo era*, ed 6, Philadelphia, 2011, Saunders.

Chow WB et al: Optimal preoperative assessment of the geriatric surgical patient: a best practices guideline from the American College of Surgeons National Surgical Quality Improvement Program and the American Geriatrics Society, *J Am Coll Surg* 215(4):453–466, 2012.

Cochico SG: Propofol allergy: assessing for patient risks, *AORN J* 96(4):399–405, 2012.

Cook DJ et al: Valvular heart disease: replacement and repair. In Kaplan JA et al, editors: *Kaplan's cardiac anesthesia: the echo era*, ed 6, Philadelphia, 2011, Saunders.

Coselli JS, Green SY: Open aortic arch surgery: doomed to extinction? *Texas Heart Inst J* 39(6):836–837, 2012.

Cox JL et al: The surgical treatment of atrial fibrillation, iii—Development of a definitive surgical procedure, *J Thorac Cardiovasc Surg* 101(4):569–583, 1991.

Crawford ES: The diagnosis and management of aortic dissection, *JAMA* 264(9):2537–2541, 1990.

Dacey LJ: Endoscopic vein-graft harvest is safe for CABG surgery, *JAMA* 308(5):512–513, 2012.

Daneshvar SA, Rahimtoola SH: Valve prosthesis-patient mismatch (VP-PM), *J Am Coll Cardiol* 60(13):1123–1135, 2012.

David TE: Surgery of the aortic root and the ascending aorta. In Sellke FW et al, editors: *Sabiston and Spencer's surgery of the chest*, ed 8, Philadelphia, 2009, Saunders.

Davies RR et al: Listing and transplanting adults with congenital heart disease, *Circulation* 123:759–767, 2011.

DeAnda A et al: Improving outcomes through the use of surgical sealants for anastomotic sealing during cardiovascular surgery, *J Card Surg* 24:325–333, 2009.

Desai ND et al: Thoracic endovascular repair: evolution of therapy, patterns of use, and results in a 10-year experience, *J Thorac Cardiovasc Surg* 142(3):587–594, 2011.

Dorman MJ et al: Bilateral internal mammary artery grafting enhances survival in diabetic patients: a 30-year follow-up of propensity score-matched cohorts, *Circulation* 126:2935–2942, 2012.

Duran CMG: Surgical treatment of the tricuspid valve. In Sellke FW et al, editors: *Sabiston and Spencer's surgery of the chest*, ed 8, Philadelphia, 2009, Saunders.

Ehrlich MP et al: Midterm results after endovascular treatment of acute, complicated type B aortic dissection: the Talent thoracic registry, *J Thorac Cardiovasc Surg* 145:159–165, 2013.

Farkouh ME et al: Strategies for multivessel revascularization in patients with diabetes, *New Engl J Med* 367(25):2375–2384, 2012.

Feldman T et al: Percutaneous repair or surgery for mitral regurgitation, *New Engl J Med* 364:1395–1406, 2011.

Gelsomino S et al: Cost and cost-effectiveness of cardiac surgery in elderly patients, *J Thorac Cardiovasc Surg* 142:1062–1073, 2011.

Gillinov AM, Mihaljevic T: The future of mitral valve surgery, *Texas Heart Inst J* 39(6):840–841, 2012.

Go AS et al: On behalf of the American Heart Association Statistics Committee and Stroke Statistics Subcommittee. Heart disease and stroke statistics—2013 update: a report from the American Heart Association, *Circulation* 127:E127-E245, 2013, available at http://circ.ahajournals.org/content/127/1/e6.full.pdf+html. Accessed August 2, 2013.

Gopaldas RR et al: Acquired heart disease: coronary insufficiency. In Townsend CM et al, editors: *Sabiston textbook of surgery*, ed 19, Philadelphia, 2012, Saunders.

Gregoric ID: Mechanical circulatory support in acute heart failure, *Texas Heart Inst J* 38(6):854–855, 2012.

Grocott HP et al: Cardiopulmonary bypass management and organ protection. In Kaplan JA et al, editors: *Kaplan's cardiac anesthesia: the echo era*, ed 6, Philadelphia, 2011, Saunders.

Groom RC et al: Detection and elimination of microemboli related to cardiopulmonary bypass, *Circ Cardiovasc Qual Outcomes* 2:191–198, 2009.

Grover FL: Current status of off-pump coronary-artery bypass, *New Engl J Med* 366(16):1541–1543, 2012.

Habib RH et al: Late effects of radial artery versus saphenous vein grafting in patients aged 70 years or older, *Ann Thorac Surg* 94:1478–1484, 2012.

Haissaguerre M et al: Spontaneous initiation of atrial fibrillation by ectopic beats originating in the pulmonary veins, *N Engl J Med* 339(10):659–666, 1998.

Hall JE: *Guyton and Hall textbook of medical physiology*, ed 12, Philadelphia, 2010, Saunders.

Hatton KW et al: Integrating evidence-based medicine into the perioperative care of cardiac surgery patients, *J Cardiothorac Vasc Anesth* 25(2):335–346, 2011.

Head SJ et al: The impact of prosthesis-patient mismatch on long-term survival after aortic valve replacement: a systematic review and meta-analysis of 34 observational studies comprising 27,186 patients with 133,141 patient years, *Eur Heart J* 33:1518–1529, 2012.

Hillis LD et al: ACCF/AHA guideline for coronary artery bypass graft surgery: a report of the American College of Cardiology Foundation/American Heart Association Task Force on Practice Guidelines developed in collaboration with the American Association for Thoracic Surgery, Society of Cardiovascular Anesthesiologists, and Society of Thoracic Surgeons, *J Am Coll Cardiol* 58(24):E123–E210, 2011.

Hodgson BB, Kizior RJ: *Saunders 2013 nursing drug handbook*, Philadelphia, 2013, Saunders.

Horak J et al: Assessment of cardiac risk and the cardiology consultation. In Kaplan JA et al, editors: *Kaplan's cardiac anesthesia: the echo era*, ed 6, Philadelphia, 2011, Saunders.

Hughes GC: Endovascular repair will be the best option for thoracoabdominal aortic aneurysm in 2020, *Texas Heart Inst J* 39(6):834–835, 2012.

Jansen DA, Molnar JA: *Keloids, Medscape Reference*, updated January 30, 2012, available at http://emedicine.medscape.com/Article/1298013-Overview. Accessed March 19, 2013.

Jeevanantham V et al: Adult bone marrow cell therapy improves survival and induces long-term improvement in cardiac parameters: a systematic review and meta-analysis, *Circulation* 126:551–568, 2012.

Jneid H et al: ACCF/AHA focused update of the guideline for the management of patients with unstable angina/non–ST-elevation myocardial infarction (updating the 2007 guideline and replacing the 2011 focused update): a report of the American College of Cardiology Foundation/American Heart Association Task Force on Practice Guidelines, *J Am Coll Cardiol* (7):645–681, 2012.

Judge DP: The complex genetics of atrial fibrillation, *J Am Coll Cardiol* 60(13):1182–1184, 2012.

Kaplan JA et al: *Kaplan's cardiac anesthesia: the echo era*, ed 6, Philadelphia, 2011, Saunders.

Kern MJ: *Cardiac catheterization handbook*, ed 5, Philadelphia, 2011, Saunders.

Kim L et al: Impact of genetic insights into mendelian disease on cardiovascular clinical practice, *Circulation* 123:544–550, 2011.

King KM et al: A descriptive examination of the impact of sternal scar formation in women, *Eur J Cardiovasc Nurs* 8(2):112–118, 2009.

Kirklin JK et al: Long-term mechanical circulatory support (destination therapy): on track to compete with heart transplantation? *J Thorac Cardiovasc Surg* 144(3):584–603, 2012.

Kocher AA et al: One-year outcomes of the surgical treatment of aortic stenosis with a next generation surgical aortic valve (TRITON) trial: a prospective multicenter study of rapid deployment aortic valve replacement with the Edwards Intuity Valve System, *J Thorac Cardiovasc Surg* 145:110–116, 2013.

Kpodonu J: Hybrid cardiovascular suite: evolving into the future of cardiovascular surgery, *Cath Lab Digest* 20(3):30–34, 2012.

Kypson AP, Chitwood WR: Robotic cardiac surgery and novel visualization systems. In Sellke FW et al, editors: *Sabiston and Spencer's surgery of the chest*, ed 8, Philadelphia, 2009, Saunders.

Lamy A et al: Off-pump or on-pump coronary-artery bypass grafting at 30 days, *N Engl J Med* 366(16):1489–1497, 2012.

Lamy A et al: Effects of off-pump and on-pump coronary-artery bypass grafting at 1 year, *N Engl J Med*, March 11, 2013, available at www.nemj.org. Accessed March 19, 2013.

Lemmer JH, Vlahakes GJ: *Handbook of patient care in cardiac surgery*, ed 7, Philadelphia, 2010, Lippincott Williams & Wilkins.

Lipitz-Snyderman A et al: The ability of intensive care units to maintain zero central line–associated bloodstream infections, *Arch Intern Med* 171(9):856–858, 2011.

Luozzo GD et al: Open repair of descending and thoracoabdominal aortic aneurysms and dissections in patients aged younger than 60 years: superior to endovascular repair? *Ann Thorac Surg* 95:12–19, 2013.

Manji RA et al: Porcine bioprosthetic heart valves: the next generation, *Am Heart J* 164:177–185, 2012.

McCarthy PM, Malaisrie SC: Mitral valve repair and replacement, including associated atrial fibrillation and tricuspid regurgitation. In Otto CM, Bonow RO, editors: *Valvular heart disease—a companion to Braunwald's heart disease*, ed 3, Philadelphia, 2009, Saunders.

McManus B: Primary tumors of the heart. In Bonow RO et al, editors: *Braunwald's heart disease: a textbook of cardiovascular medicine*, ed 9, Philadelphia, 2012, Saunders.

Mehra MR, Griffith BP: Assisted circulation in the treatment of heart failure. In Bonow RO et al, editors: *Braunwald's heart disease: a textbook of cardiovascular medicine*, ed 9, Philadelphia, 2012, Saunders.

Mitka M: New definition of myocardial infarction puts biomarkers front and center, *JAMA* 308(15):1511–1512, 2012.

Morrow DA, Boden WE: Stable ischemic heart disease. In Bonow RO et al, editors: *Braunwald's heart disease: a textbook of cardiovascular medicine*, ed 9, Philadelphia, 2012, Saunders.

Mosca L et al: Effectiveness-based guidelines for the prevention of cardiovascular disease in women—2011 update: a guideline from the American Heart Association, *Circulation* 123:1243–1262, 2011.

Nabagiez JP et al: Physician assistant home visit program to reduce hospital readmissions, *J Thorac Cardiovasc Surg* 145(1):225–233, 2013.

Naidu SS: Novel percutaneous cardiac assist devices, *Circulation* 123:533–543, 2011.

Nalla BP et al: Update on blood conservation for cardiac surgery, *J Cardiothorac Vasc Anesth* 26(1):117–133, 2012.

Nasso G et al: Impact of arterial revascularization in patients undergoing coronary bypass, *J Cardiac Surg* 27(4):427–433, 2012.

Newby LK, Douglas PS: Cardiovascular disease in women. In Bonow RO et al, editors: *Braunwald's heart disease: a textbook of cardiovascular medicine*, ed 9, Philadelphia, 2012, Saunders.

Nouri K, Elston DM: *Laser treatment of scars and stria distensae*, Medscape Reference, updated May 21, 2012, available at http://emedicine.medscape.com/Article/1120673-Overview. Accessed March 19, 2013.

Nussmeier NA et al: Anesthesia for cardiac surgical procedures. In Miller RD et al, editors: *Miller's anesthesia*, ed 7, Philadelphia, 2009, Churchill Livingstone.

O'Gara PT et al: 2013 ACCF/AHA guideline for the management of ST-elevation myocardial infarction: a report of the American College of Cardiology Foundation/American Heart Association Task Force on Practice Guidelines, *Circulation* 127:529–555, 2013.

Otto CM, Bonow RO: Valvular heart disease. In Libby P et al, editors: *Braunwald's heart disease*, ed 9, Philadelphia, 2012, Saunders.

Otto CM, Verrier ED: Mitral regurgitation—what is best for my patient? *New Engl J Med* 364:1462–1463, 2011.

Pagana KD, Pagana TJ: *Mosby's diagnostic and laboratory test reference*, ed 11, St Louis, 2012, Mosby.

Patel MR et al: Appropriate use criteria for coronary revascularization focused update: a report by the American College of Cardiology Foundation Appropriate use criteria task force, Society for Cardiovascular Angiography and Interventions, Society of Thoracic Surgeons, American Association for Thoracic Surgery, American Heart Association, American Society of Nuclear Cardiology, and the Society of Cardiovascular Computed Tomography. Endorsed by the American Society of Echocardiography and the Heart Rhythm Society, *J Am Coll Cardiol* 59:857–881, 2012.

Peltz M: Surgery for valvular heart disease. In Antman EM, Sabatine MS, editors: *Cardiovascular therapeutics—a companion to Braunwald's heart disease*, Philadelphia, 2012, Saunders.

Petersen C, editor: *Perioperative nursing data set*, ed 3, Denver, 2011, Association of periOperative Registered Nurses, Inc., The Association.

Preiss D et al: Risk of incident diabetes with intensive-dose compared with moderate-dose statin therapy, *JAMA* 305(24):2556–2564, 2011.

Puskas JD: Why did you not use both internal thoracic arteries? (editorial) *Circulation* 126:2915–2917, 2012.

Quinlan JJ et al: Anesthesia for heart, lung, and heart-lung transplantation. In Kaplan JA et al, editors: *Kaplan's cardiac anesthesia: the echo era*, ed 6, Philadelphia, 2011, Saunders.

Rahimtoola SH: Choice of prosthetic heart valve in adults, *J Am Coll Cardiol* 55(22):2413–2426, 2010.

Rahimtoola SH: The year in valvular heart disease, *J Am Coll Cardiol* 58(12):1197–1207, 2011.

Reich DL et al: Monitoring of the heart and vascular system. In Kaplan JA et al, editors: *Kaplan's cardiac anesthesia: the echo era*, ed 6, Philadelphia, 2011, Saunders.

Roberts R, Stewart AFR: Genes and coronary artery disease, *J Am Coll Cardiol* 60(18):1715–1721, 2012a.

Roberts R, Stewart FR: Genetics of coronary artery disease in the 21st century, *Clin Cardiol* 35(9):536–540, 2012b.

Roger VL et al, on behalf of the American Heart Association Statistics Committee and Stroke Statistics Subcommittee: *Heart disease and stroke statistics—2012 update: a report from the American Heart Association*, *Circulation* 125:E2–E220, 2012.

Roselli EE: Reoperative cardiac surgery, *Texas Heart Inst J* 38(6):669–671, 2011.

Sarin EL et al: Off-pump coronary bypass grafting is associated with reduced operative mortality and in-hospital adverse events in patients with left main coronary artery disease, *Innovations* 4(2):80–85, 2009.

Sayfo S et al: Management of recurrent leaks following postinfarction ventricular septal defect repairs, *J Cardiac Surg* 27(5):576–580, 2012.

Schwann TA et al: Comparison of late coronary artery bypass graft survival effects of radial artery versus saphenous vein grafting in male and female patients, *Ann Thorac Surg* 94:1485–1491, 2012.

Seifert PC: Nurses in perioperative settings. In Moser DK, Riegel B, editors: *Cardiac nursing—a companion to Braunwald's heart disease*, St Louis, 2008, Saunders.

Seifert PC: Implementing AORN recommended practices for transfer of patient care information, *AORN J* 96(5):475–493, 2012.

Seifert PC: Care of the cardiac surgical patient. In Odom-Forren J, editor: *Drain's perianesthesia nursing: a critical care approach*, ed 6, St Louis, 2013, Saunders.

Shrestha NR et al: Rheumatic heart disease revisited: patterns of valvular involvement from a consecutive cohort in eastern Nepal, *J Cardiovasc Med* 13:755–759, 2012.

Shroyer AL et al: On-pump versus off-pump coronary-artery bypass surgery, *N Engl J Med* 361:1827–1837, 2009.

Silbiger JJ: Anatomy, mechanics, and pathophysiology of the mitral annulus, *Am Heart J* 164(2):163–176, 2012.

Society of Cardiovascular Anesthesiologists: *FAQs (frequently asked questions)*, available at http://test2.societyhq.com/Sca3/FAQ.Shtml. Accessed December 16, 2012.

Society of Thoracic Surgeons (STS): *STS patient information*, available at www.sts.org/Sections/Patientinformation. Accessed March 19, 2013.

Speir AM et al: Additive costs of postoperative complications for isolated coronary artery bypass grafting patients in Virginia, *Ann Thorac Surg* 88:40–46, 2009.

Spotnitz WD: Getting to hemostasis: general and thoracic surgical challenges, *Texas Heart Inst J* 39(6):868–870, 2012.

Stone ME et al: New approaches to the surgical treatment of end-stage heart failure. In Kaplan JA et al, editors: *Kaplan's cardiac anesthesia: the echo era*, ed 6, Philadelphia, 2011, Saunders.

Szeto WY, Bavaria JE: Endovascular therapy for thoracic aortic aneurysms and dissections. In Sellke FW et al, editors: *Sabiston and Spencer's surgery of the chest*, ed 8, Philadelphia, 2009, Saunders.

Tavris DR et al: Long-term outcomes after transmyocardial revascularization, *Ann Thorac Surg* 94:1500–1508, 2012.

Teirstein PS, Lytle BW: Interventional and surgical treatment of coronary artery disease. In Goldman L, Schafer AI, editors: *Goldman's Cecil medicine*, ed 24, Philadelphia, 2012, Saunders.

Tesler UF: Mitral valve repair: historical evolution and what lies ahead, *Texas Heart Inst J* 38 (6):862–865, 2012.

Thanassoulis G et al: Genetic associations with valvular calcification and aortic stenosis, *New Engl J Med* 368(6):503–512, 2013.

The Joint Commission: *National patient safety goals 2013*, available at www.Jointcommission.Org/Assets/1/6/2013_HAP_NPSG_Final_10-23.Pdf. Accessed March 19, 2013.

Thompson J, Bertling G: Endovascular leaks: perioperative nursing implications, *AORN J* 89(5):839–846, 2009.

Thygesen K et al: The writing group on behalf of the joint ESC/ACCF/AHA/WHF Task Force for the Universal Definition of Myocardial Infarction. Third universal definition of myocardial infarction, *Circulation* 126:2020–2035, 2012.

Tinkham MR: The endovascular approach to abdominal aortic aneurysm repair, *AORN J* 89(2):289–302, 2009.

Tota-Maharaj R et al: Coronary artery calcium for the prediction of mortality in young adults <45 years old and elderly adults >75 years old, *Eur Heart J* 33:2955–2962, 2012.

Vassileva CM et al: Cost analysis of isolated mitral valve surgery in the United States, *Ann Thorac Surg* 94:1429–1437, 2012.

Velazquez EJ, et al: Coronary-artery bypass surgery in patient with left ventricular dysfunction, *New Engl J Med* 364(17):1607-1616, 2011.

Wahr JA et al: American Heart Association scientific statement on patient safety in the cardiac operating room: human factors and teamwork, *Circulation*, August 5, 2013. doi 10.116/CIR.0b013e3182a38efa.

Webb GD et al: Congenital heart disease. In Bonow RO et al, editors: *Braunwald's heart disease: a textbook of cardiovascular medicine*, ed 9, Philadelphia, 2012, Saunders.

Weintraub WS et al: Comparative effectiveness of revascularization strategies, *New Engl J Med* 366(16):1467–1476, 2012.

Weisse AB: Cardiac surgery: a century of progress, *Tex Heart Inst J* 38(5):486–490, 2011.

Wenger NK: Women and coronary heart disease: a century after Herrick, *Circulation* 126:604–611, 2012.

Williams JR et al: Association between endoscopic vs open vein-graft harvesting and mortality, wound complications, and cardiovascular events in patients undergoing CABG surgery, *JAMA* 308(5):475–484, 2012.

Yang YT et al: The circulating nurse's role in error recovery in the cardiovascular OR, *AORN J* 95(6):755–762, 2012.

CHAPTER 26
Pediatric Surgery

LEIGH ANN DIFUSCO

Pediatrics is a specialty focused on the health and well-being of neonates, infants, children, and adolescents. The pediatric patient often needs surgery for congenital anomalies that threaten life or the child's ability to function. Trauma also affects a child's health far more often than an adult's; injury is a common reason for surgical intervention. Pediatric surgery is an area of practice unto its own because the pediatric patient is so different from an adult. The field is even further subdivided into all the surgical specialties. It is important to recognize that the difference between pediatric care and adult care is not just a size issue; from birth onward, the body and organs exist in a continual state of development, and multiple physiologic changes occur with age. Major areas of distinction are the airway and pulmonary status, cardiovascular status, temperature regulation, metabolism, fluid management, and psychologic development. A thorough knowledge of these differences is integral to the provision of nursing care for the pediatric patient in the operating room (OR).

Advances in surgical interventions for children have been phenomenal for many reasons. The advancement of improved diagnostic and interventional technology, the development of new anesthetics and pharmacologic agents for pain management, and the creation of even smaller and more delicate instrumentation have revolutionized perioperative care of the pediatric population. Numerous pediatric surgeries that were once performed as open cavity procedures are now being done endoscopically with minimally invasive techniques, resulting in shorter hospital stays and faster recovery times. Improvements in the transport of critically ill children and the intensive care management of neonatal and pediatric patients as well as the development of new surgical procedures are also saving more lives yet presenting medical professionals with a new and unique set of problems as complex, medically fragile children are now surviving into adulthood.

Pediatric Surgical Anatomy

Airway and Pulmonary Status

Respiratory mechanics alter dramatically from infancy to adulthood, resulting from increases in airway size, transformations in the rigidity of airway and chest structures, and major changes in neuromuscular status. A proportionally large head, a short neck, and a large tongue in relation to jaw size create more of a challenge for airway management. The glottis is very anterior, moving from the level of the second cervical vertebra to the level of the third or fourth vertebra in the adult. The epiglottis is floppy and more curved, and the vocal cords are slanted anteriorly. The airway forms an inverse cone with the narrowest portion at the cricoid cartilage until 8 years of age; endotracheal tube size is therefore very important because a tube that passes easily through the glottis may be too tight at the subglottic area, compromising the child's airway in the immediate postoperative period because of swelling. The infant is an obligate nasal breather, and the chest wall of an infant is very compliant, leading to increased work of breathing with any type of airway compromise. Infants also have type 2 respiratory muscle fibers until age 2 years, which fatigue more easily than type 1 muscle fibers. Premature infants are at risk for postanesthetic apnea until 60 weeks after conception age. There is a depression in the CO_2 response curve in infants; compared with an adult, the respiratory rate does not increase as readily in response to a rising CO_2 level, although all ages undergo a CO_2 response depression related to inhalational agents and narcotics. One of the most important considerations is that children have a much smaller pulmonary functional residual capacity; a child becomes hypoxic more quickly if the airway is lost. Alveolar maturation is not complete until 8 years of age. Smaller airways have higher resistance; airway resistance decreases approximately 15 times from infancy to adulthood, again with a major change occurring around 8 years of age. It is important to note that smaller airways can become compromised with even a minor amount of swelling. An additional consideration in the pediatric setting is loose teeth. Loose teeth are common in children ages 5 to 14 years; a dislodged tooth is a potential airway foreign-body risk.

Cardiovascular Status

The most dramatic changes in the cardiovascular system occur at birth with the transition from fetal circulation. Even in full-term infants, persistent transitional circulation may occur. Heart rate is the predominant determinant of cardiac output in infants and children; bradycardia drastically decreases cardiac output and requires swift intervention. There is a decreased cardiac compliance because of a lower proportion of muscle to connective tissue until age 1 to 2 years, making infants preload insensitive. Young children are predisposed to parasympathetic hypertonia (increased vagal tone), which can be induced by painful stimuli such as laryngoscopy, intubation, eye surgery, or abdominal retraction. Attention to blood loss in young patients is very important because the patient's total blood volume is very small. Blood volume in neonates is 80 to 90 mL/kg; at 1 to 6 years it is 70 to 75 mL/kg; and at age 6 years to adult it is 65 to 70 mL/kg. At birth, 70% to 90% of the hemoglobin is fetal hemoglobin with a high affinity for oxygen. It is normal for hemoglobin levels to fall at about 2 to 3 months of age (physiologic anemia) to a hematocrit level of 29% and a hemoglobin level of 10 mg/dL as the infant's body begins to produce its own blood cells. A cardiology evaluation is essential if a murmur is auscultated. A murmur can be from a patent foramen ovale, which normally closes at 3 to 12 months; a patent ductus arteriosus, which can be present for up to 2 months; a previously undetected cardiac anomaly; or an innocent flow murmur. The evaluation is critical because anesthetic agents cause vasodilation and potentiate cardiac dysrhythmias.

Temperature Regulation

Infants and young children are most at risk of hypothermia because of their increased body surface area-to-weight ratio and thin fat layer. Cold stress leads to increased oxygen consumption, resulting in hypoxia, respiratory depression, acidosis, hypoglycemia, and pulmonary vasoconstriction. Hypothermia alters drug metabolism, prolongs the action of neuromuscular blockers, and delays emergence from anesthesia. The child's temperature must be monitored continuously throughout the intraoperative experience. An axillary temperature probe is acceptable for short procedures in healthy children; an esophageal or rectal temperature probe provides more accurate monitoring of the child's temperature for longer cases. Hyperthermia should also be avoided because it leads to increased oxygen consumption and increased fluid losses.

It is vital to maintain normothermia in children, and the easiest way to do this is by exposing only the area on which surgery is being performed. Additional thermoregulatory interventions include altering the room temperature before the child enters the room, using a water-filled temperature-regulating blanket under the patient, or using a forced-air warming blanket over nonsurgical areas of the child. An overhead heater can be used during the anesthetic induction and patient preparation period immediately before prepping and draping. The anesthesia ventilation circuit can be heated and humidified, as can insufflated carbon dioxide during minimally invasive surgical procedures. For surgical procedures with large areas of exposure, warmed solutions should be available for use instead of room temperature solutions. Intravenous (IV) solutions can also be warmed before administration.

Metabolism

Infants have a higher basal metabolic rate than adults, and it is greatest at 18 months. Most importantly, children younger than age 2 years have immature liver function; pharmacologic response is altered, and there is slower hepatic clearance, decreased hepatic enzyme function, and decreased protein binding. Medication distribution is different in neonates and infants compared with older children and adults because of an increased percentage of total body weight and extracellular body fluid. Infants have an immature blood-brain barrier and decreased protein binding, which results in an increased sensitivity to sedatives, opioids, and hypnotics.

Fluid Management

Renal function at birth is immature, and the ability of the kidneys to concentrate urine is limited, so the infant is much more prone to dehydration. Complete maturation of renal function occurs at about 2 years. Compared to an adult, a child has a higher body water weight, a higher body surface area, and an increased metabolic rate, resulting in increased fluid requirements per kilogram of body weight. Despite these significant points, it is also important to remember that the body weight of the child, the length of time without fluids, and surgical losses are the primary factors in the calculations of the child's hydration needs.

Psychologic Development

A child's comprehension of and responses to the environment are based on developmental age. A key factor is that a child's developmental age does not necessarily match the chronologic age. Nursing care should be tailored to the developmental age of the child to optimize the child's ability to understand the situation, to minimize the child's and family's stress and anxiety, and to facilitate the development of a trusting and supportive medical relationship. The types of fears are also related to the child's level of psychologic development. Predictable stages mean predictable behaviors. The stages of growth have been described from a variety of different aspects; Dr. Jean Piaget described the stages by changes in cognition and the ability to think, and Dr. Erik Erikson based the stages on psychosocial and emotional needs. Their work provides an excellent guideline for assessing the pediatric patient's developmental level in order to use appropriate interventions (Table 26-1).

Perioperative Nursing Considerations

Assessment

The initial patient assessment provides information necessary to develop a plan of care specific to the needs of each pediatric patient related to age, developmental level, and diagnosis. The unique aspects of care of the pediatric surgical patient revolve around the fact that the child is constantly growing and changing. The perioperative nurse must have a good understanding of the normal physical and psychologic parameters for pediatric patients and be able to recognize and act on deviations from these parameters. Table 26-2 presents normal vital sign ranges for infants and children.

In addition, the perioperative nurse must be familiar with normal growth and developmental factors for each age group. During any given day, the perioperative nurse may care for a variety of pediatric patients ranging from neonates through adolescents. In some instances, children undergoing an ambulatory surgical procedure may visit the OR complex and ambulatory surgery area with their families 1 to 2 weeks before surgery, depending on the child's developmental level and the availability of a preoperative pediatric education program. If the child has a complex medical history or an extensive surgical procedure is planned, the child and family members will meet with a member of the anesthesia team during this advance visit. A tour may be provided by a child life specialist (Patient and Family Education), along with pictures and age-appropriate explanations of what the child will see and experience. Visiting before the day of surgery can help decrease the anxiety related to the novelty of the experience.

Occasionally the child's history and physical, surgical consent, and any necessary tests or lab work are done in advance in the surgeon's office setting, and the child and family have no introduction to the surgical experience until the day of surgery. Information related to the child's scheduled procedure is either sent home with the family from the surgeon's office or mailed to the family the week before the surgery is scheduled. The surgical facility contacts the family the day before surgery to inform them when the child should arrive at the facility and to review preoperative eating and drinking instructions. In these instances, the initial interview performed by the perioperative nurse is especially crucial to provide a thorough, documented assessment of the child's growth (height and weight), current physical status (vital signs, heart and breath sounds, skin integrity), current medication history, allergies, nothing by mouth (NPO) status, recent illnesses, current medical concerns, and behavioral responses to the interview process. The perioperative nurse confirms the intended surgical procedure with the child and family as it is written on the surgical consent as well as their understanding of the operation. This information is critical to the intraoperative nursing team's plan of care during the surgical procedure.

TABLE 26-1

Developmental Stages

Approximate Ages	Piaget's Stage	Erikson's Stage	Developmentally Based Fears	Appropriate Nursing Interventions
Infancy to 1 yr (Erikson) Infancy to 2 yr (Piaget)	Sensorimotor Uses senses and motor skills to understand world Develops memory; begins to imitate others	Trust vs. mistrust—develops belief that world can be counted on to meet basic needs Who to trust? Identifies strangers at 7-8 mo	Separation	Use soothing voice; sing, hold child, give child objects to hold to provide distractions. Meet child, family without touching child at first. Allow personal item into OR for comfort/security.
Toddlerhood	Preoperational Use of symbols, creative play (can pretend) Is very egocentric	Autonomy vs. shame, doubt Develops free will; increasing control of their bodies Feels regret, sorrow for inappropriate behavior	Separation Forced dependence	Give only simple choices; involve child in actions when possible, use distractions, sing songs child may recognize. Allow personal item into OR for comfort/security.
Early childhood, preschool	Preoperational	Initiative vs. guilt Begins to explore, imagine Feels remorse for actions Thinking dominated by perceptions—distorted reasoning	Separation Body mutilation	Magical thinkers—use stories during induction. Likes colorful Band-Aids. Allow child to handle unfamiliar objects to decrease stress (e.g., mask, pulse oximeter probe). Allow personal item into OR for comfort/security.
Middle childhood, elementary school age (Erikson) Ages 7-11 yr (Piaget)	Concrete operations Uses symbols, logic, principles to solve problems Classifies, sorts everything	Industry vs. inferiority Beginning to understand time and unseen body functions Is cooperative; desires recognition for achievements	The unknown Body mutilation Inadequate performance	Provide simple information to decrease stress. Be honest at all times. Do not expect child to act like an adult yet. Allow personal item into OR for comfort/security.
Adolescence, puberty	Formal operations Uses logical and abstract thinking Understands hypothetical concepts	Identity vs. role diffusion Peer group has increased importance Body image, clothing, activities help define identity	Altered body image Death	Query patient about concerns; offer information to decrease fears. Provide as much privacy as possible if disrobing is necessary. Use mental imagery to decrease stress. Offer to hold hand to provide comfort; personal item still permitted.

Modified from Taylor E: Providing developmentally based care for toddlers, *AORN J* 87(5):992–999, 2008; Taylor E: Providing developmentally based care for school-aged and adolescent patients, *AORN J* 90(2):261–269, 2009; *Stages of social-emotional development in children,* available at http://childdevelopmentinfo.com/child-development/erickson.shtml. Accessed February 1, 2013.

TABLE 26-2

Pediatric Vital Signs

Age	Heart Rate (Beats/min)	Respirations (Breaths/min)	Systolic Blood Pressure (mm Hg)
Newborn	100-150	30-55	50-70
Infants to 2 years	80-120	25-40	70-88
2-6 years	70-110	20-30	88-94
6-10 years	60-95	16-22	94-102
10-16 years	60-85	12-20	80-111

From Ball JW, Bindler RC: *Principles of pediatric nursing: caring for children,* ed 5, Upper Saddle River, NJ, 2012, Pearson Prentice Hall.

Children may undergo surgery at ambulatory surgery facilities or in a hospital setting. Certain criteria must be met for children to qualify for surgery at an ambulatory facility (Ambulatory Surgery Considerations). Children who are inpatients may be visited by a perioperative nurse in the hospital on the day before surgery. The nurse reviews the patient's chart, giving particular attention to the patient's age, developmental level, diagnosis, and intended surgical procedure. Current nursing diagnoses and the ongoing plan of care are examined. A discussion with the primary nurse can facilitate data collection, assist in providing continuity of care, and provide the perioperative nurse with information regarding preoperative education previously provided. The perioperative nurse can meet the child and any family members present at the time of the visit. The interview can be used to gather information helpful to developing the intraoperative plan of care and to decreasing the anxiety related to the child's impending surgery by providing a familiar face on the day of the procedure. The focus of this visit is to discuss the perioperative process, not always to provide preoperative education regarding the surgery. In pediatric centers in the inpatient setting, preoperative education may be provided by the primary nurse, child life therapist, or clinical nurse specialist. During the preoperative visit the perioperative nurse can explain, at a developmentally appropriate level, what the child will experience in the preoperative, intraoperative, and postoperative phases of care. The perioperative nurse may briefly describe the roles of various staff members who

PATIENT AND FAMILY EDUCATION

The Role of the Nurse Educator and Child Life Specialist in Supporting Education

In the pediatric setting, patient and family education is accomplished through many avenues. Patient and family education manuals contain teaching and information inserts that include but are not limited to explanations of conditions, procedures, diagnostic studies, and home management techniques. These manuals also contain lesson plans that a provider can access before providing teaching to a patient or family at the bedside or in a family learning center.

Many institutions have family learning centers onsite that adapt teaching and learning techniques to suit both inpatient and outpatient clients and their families. A patient may be referred to the family learning center in preparation for discharge, so that medical care can be effectively managed at home. Family learning centers promote learning in a safe, quiet environment with one-to-one instruction by a nurse educator. Care is simulated using mannequins, models, and other realistic tools and validated by return demonstration from the patient or caregiver. In addition, patients and caregivers are provided with feedback and additional materials to support the management of medical care in the home environment.

Institutions may also assign child life specialists to pediatric units and floors. Child life specialists are experts in child development who promote effective coping through play, preparation, education, and self-expression activities. They provide emotional support for families, and encourage optimum development of children facing a broad range of challenging experiences, particularly those related to healthcare and hospitalization. Understanding that a child's well-being depends on the support of the family, child life specialists provide information, support, and guidance to parents, siblings, and other family members. They also play a vital role in educating caregivers, administrators, and the general public about the needs of children under stress.

FIGURE 26-1 Perioperative nurse and parent verify that the surgical site marking on a pediatric patient matches consent.

AMBULATORY SURGERY CONSIDERATIONS

Guidelines for Pediatric Ambulatory Surgery

Candidates for ambulatory surgery in a pediatric institution should:
- Be categorized as either class I or class II in accordance with the American Society of Anesthesiologists (ASA) guidelines; in some cases, patients who are categorized as class III may be eligible for ambulatory surgery with the approval of the medical director or attending surgeon
- Be older than 6 months of age; patients older than the age of 18 who are followed by a physician on staff may have surgery at the ambulatory surgery center with the approval of the medical director and surgeon-in-chief

Procedures that are eligible for scheduling in ambulatory surgical settings should:
- Be no more than 4 hours in duration and have a total 4 hours of direct supervised recovery unless exceeded by patient condition demands that cannot be anticipated before surgery
- Be able to be performed using local or regional anesthetics, monitored anesthesia care (MAC), or general anesthetic with a duration of less than 4 hours
- Be able to be performed without the risk of extensive blood loss, major prolonged invasion of body cavities, or direct involvement of major blood vessels

Modified from Children's Hospital of Philadelphia: *Ambulatory surgery policy and procedure manual*, 5.2.1 approved surgical procedures for ambulatory surgical centers; *Ambulatory surgery policy and procedure manual*, 2.1.1 patient selection criteria for the ambulatory surgery center, Philadelphia, 2011.

will be a part of the team responsible for the child's care in the OR. Common concerns that families express are the length of time that they will be separated from their child and their child's pain management. Explanations to children should be provided within a developmental framework, taking into account each child's cognitive and psychosocial abilities. Medical play items, audiovisual aids, puppets, and photographs are all helpful in the education process.

The perioperative nurse who will be participating in the intraoperative care of the child will review the patient's information and meet with the patient and the family before the child is transferred to the OR. In addition to reviewing the documentation, the nurse validates the patient's identification using two patient identifiers, confirms that the surgeon has marked the child's surgical site per institutional protocol, and seeks verbal verification from the patient, parent, or legal guardian about the scheduled procedure, making sure that it matches what is written on the surgical consent (Figure 26-1). If implants are to be used, availability must be confirmed before the patient's transport to the surgical suite. Frequently children will be given a premedication 20 to 45 minutes before their transportation to the OR. A premedication such as midazolam can greatly decrease a child's anxiety, minimizing the stress of separation for both child and family. The surgeon and anesthesia provider will each meet with the child and family, usually while the OR is being prepared for the patient. The perioperative nurse will assess the

child's psychologic state, review the intended surgical procedure with the child and family, and ensure that they have no additional questions or concerns. A final communication among the anesthesia provider, surgeon, and nursing staff for the room confirms the team's state of readiness for the delivery of care before the nurse transports the child to the OR.

Informed Consent. Informed consent must be obtained prior to administering anesthesia or performing surgery. For children

---

BOX 26-1

Clinical Manifestations of Child Abuse and Neglect

Skin Injuries

Skin injuries are the most common and easily recognized signs of maltreatment of children. Human bite marks appear as an ovoid area with tooth imprints, suck marks, or tongue thrust marks. Multiple bruises in inaccessible places are indications that the child has been abused. Bruises in different stages of healing may indicate repeated trauma. Bruises that take the shape of a recognized object are generally not accidental.

Traumatic Hair Loss

Traumatic hair loss occurs when the child's hair is pulled or used to drag or jerk the child. The result of the pulling on the scalp can cause the blood vessels under the skin to break. An accumulation of blood can help differentiate between abusive and nonabusive loss of hair.

Falls

If a child is reported to have experienced a routine fall but appears to have severe injuries, the inconsistency of the history with the trauma sustained indicates suspected child abuse.

External Head, Facial, and Oral Injuries

Cuts, bleeding, redness, or swelling of the external ear canal; facial fractures; tears or scarring of the lip; oral, perioral, and/or pharyngeal lesions; loosened, discolored, or fractured teeth; dental caries; tongue lacerations; unexplained erythema or petechiae of the palate; and bilateral black eyes without trauma to the nose may all indicate abuse.

Deliberate or Unexplained Thermal Injuries

Immersion burns, with a clear line of demarcation; multiple small circular burns, in varying stages of healing; iron burns (show iron pattern); diaper area burns; and rope burns suggest intentional harm.

Shaken Baby Syndrome

A shaken baby may suffer only mild ocular or cerebral trauma. The infant may have a history of poor feeding, vomiting, lethargy, and/or irritability that occurs periodically for days or weeks before the initial healthcare consult. In 75% to 90% of cases, unilateral or bilateral retinal hemorrhages are present but may be missed unless the child is examined by a pediatric ophthalmologist. Shaking produces an acceleration-deceleration (shearing) injury to the brain, causing stretching and breaking of blood vessels that results in subdural hemorrhage. Subdural hemorrhage may be most prominent in the interhemispheric fissure. However, cerebral edema may be the only finding. Serious insult to the central nervous system may result, without evidence of external injury.

Unexplained Fractures and Dislocation

Posterior rib fractures in different stages of healing, spiral fractures, or dislocation from twisting of an extremity may provide evidence of intentional injury in children.

Sexual Abuse

Abrasions or bruising of the inner thighs and genitalia; scars, tearing, or distortion of the labia/hymen; anal lacerations or dilation; lacerations or irritation of external genitalia; repeated urinary tract infections; sexually transmitted disease; nonspecific vaginitis; pregnancy in young adolescent; penile discharge; and sexual promiscuity may provide evidence of sexual abuse.

Neglect

The symptoms of neglect reflect a lack of both physical and medical care. Manifestations include failure to thrive without a medical explanation, multiple cat or dog bites and scratches, feces and dirt in the skinfolds, severe diaper rash with the presence of ammonia burns, feeding disorders, and developmental delays.

Modified from Betz CL, Sowden LA: *Mosby's pediatric nursing reference*, ed 6, St Louis, 2008, Mosby.

---

younger than age 18, consent must be obtained from one of the following individuals: a legal parent (biologic parent whose parental rights have not been terminated) or an adoptive parent who has completed the adoptive process. Foster parents of children in the custody of a child and youth agency (CYA) are not permitted to give consent. Rather, consent should be obtained from the CYA social worker. Legal guardians should be encouraged to bring any supporting documentation of legal guardianship or ability to consent for the child's medical care on the day of surgery. Perioperative nurses should review the chart for documentation of legal guardianship and ensure that each document is signed by the appropriate individual.

When emergency situations arise and the need for treatment is immediately necessary to prevent serious or permanent impairment of the patient's health or to preserve the life of a patient, surgery may be performed without consent of the legal parent. In the event that a legal parent is unable to be located or unable or unwilling to provide informed consent, a court order may be obtained to permit treatment. A pediatric patient who is an emancipated minor (e.g., legally under the age of consent but recognized as having the legal capacity to consent), can give valid consent for him- or herself. It is important for children to develop a trusting relationship with medical professionals and that these older children are in agreement (within their developmental capabilities) with their family's decision

regarding surgery. Risk management and legal departments can assist in clarifying questions or conflicts specific to informed consent.

Child Abuse and Neglect. Perioperative nurses are obligated to screen all pediatric patients for abuse or neglect. Child abuse and neglect results from any of the following: physical injury, sexual abuse or exploitation, negligence or maltreatment (Betz and Sowden, 2008). Child abuse is found in all segments of society, crossing cultural, ethnic, religious, socioeconomic, and professional groups. The perioperative nurse is in a unique situation to assess for the presence of abuse because the patient will be disrobed in the OR. Box 26-1 lists the clinical manifestations of child abuse. Every state has a child abuse law that dictates legal responsibility for reporting abuse and suspicion of abuse, and nurses are mandated reporters. Failure to report suspected child abuse could result in a fine or other punishment, according to individual statutes (Betz and Sowden, 2008).

Nursing Diagnosis

Nursing diagnoses related to the care of pediatric patients undergoing surgery might include the following:
- Anxiety related to separation from family and friends
- Fear related to developmental level (fear of the unknown, fear of painful procedures and surgery)

- Risk for Infection related to surgical intervention and other invasive procedures
- Risk for Imbalanced Fluid Volume related to invasive surgery and accompanying blood loss
- Risk for Hypothermia related to loss of body surface heat to environment and immature temperature-control mechanism

Outcome Identification

Perioperative nursing care is predicated on relevant nursing diagnoses and their corresponding desired outcome. Outcomes should be measurable with criteria by which to judge their attainment. Thus for the desired outcome, "The patient will demonstrate some ability to manage anxiety," measurable criteria (e.g., the child will have posture, facial expressions, gestures, and activity levels that reflect decreased anxiety and will demonstrate increased focus) might be identified.

Outcomes identified for the selected nursing diagnoses for the pediatric patient could be stated as follows:

- The child will demonstrate some ability to manage anxiety.
- The child will verbalize less fear.
- The child will remain free from signs and symptoms of surgical site and invasive procedure site infection.
- The child will be maintained in a state of fluid and electrolyte balance.
- The child will be maintained in a state of normothermia.

Planning

Assessment data, combined with information about the planned surgical procedure, enable perioperative nurses to anticipate requirements for surgical positioning, instrumentation, equipment and supplies, medications, and activities necessary for the provision of safe, competent care for the pediatric patient. Knowledge of the child's developmental level allows the nurse to plan her or his approach and interactions with the child and family (Figure 26-2). The perioperative nurse identifies criteria appropriate to the child and surgical setting for each of the desired outcomes (Sample Plan of Care). A Sample Plan of Care is shown for the pediatric patient on pages 1014-1015.

FIGURE 26-2 Perioperative nurse engages in play with a toddler during preoperative assessment.

The perioperative nurse must also develop a trusting relationship with the child and his or her parents, family, or legal guardians. The nurse must explain the events of surgery in a way that allows the child and accompanying adults to better understand what to expect on transfer to the OR (Patient-Centered Care).

Implementation

Age-appropriate communication is important in implementing the pediatric nursing plan of care. Implementation begins during the perioperative nursing assessment and continues through discharge to the postanesthesia care unit (PACU) or other area. The presence of a parent during much of the preoperative period, including during anesthesia induction in the OR and after anesthesia emergence in the PACU, can help decrease anxiety for both young children and their families and facilitates family-centered care (Evidence for Practice).

Infants, reliant on family to meet their basic needs, are difficult to pacify when NPO for surgery. The facility should provide rocking chairs, pacifiers, warm blankets, and simple distractions such as music or toys. Preoperative teaching should include telling the family to provide fluids for the infant until the deadline for NPO status. Unnecessary delays should be avoided at all costs. Parents may need reassurance and support during the period immediately before surgery.

The toddler or preschooler fears parental separation and abandonment. Toddlers fear, among other things, strangers, the dark, and machines. They attribute lifelike qualities to inanimate objects, believing that the objects, like them, have feelings. Thus a blood pressure cuff that squeezes the child's arm may be perceived to be doing so because it is angry with the toddler. Toddlers may also believe that their body is held together by their skin; anything that violates the skin integrity is feared. For this reason, bandages are very important. Toddlers and preschoolers interact with the environment using their senses. To integrate this into the patient's care, the perioperative nurse should give the toddler the opportunity to touch and play with objects that he or she will encounter. An example is to give the child a small anesthesia mask to put on his or her teddy bear. Sensory information should be provided in a soft, gentle voice (i.e., what the toddler will see, feel, touch, and hear). A security object is extremely comforting. The OR should be quiet; background noise should be controlled. Instruments that are frightening should be kept from view. To allow quick induction of anesthesia the toddler should be transferred into the surgical suite when the room and staff are completely prepared.

The school-age child may still perceive hospitalization or surgery as a punishment but can evaluate painful intrusive actions in terms of logical function (e.g., getting an IV line hurts, but then I can get medicine in it to make me feel better). Feelings of inadequacy may be associated with something the child thinks he or she should be expected to do or know. Fear of body injury or mutilation, loss of control, and fear of the unknown characterize this developmental stage. These children benefit from simple, concrete explanations in familiar terms; a book or other teaching aid can be helpful. The concepts of time and unseen body functions can now be incorporated in the explanations. The child should be allowed to make choices when possible (e.g., letting the child decide in which hand to place the IV line or which flavor to add to the anesthetic mask).

Adolescents may fear altered body image, peer rejection, disability, and loss of control or status. The fear of death is more prevalent in this age-group than any other, and adolescents may find explanations of monitoring and safety measures reassuring.

SAMPLE PLAN OF CARE

Nursing Diagnosis
Anxiety related to separation from family and friends

Outcome
The child will demonstrate some ability to manage anxiety; a toy or other comfort/security object will remain with the child, and he or she will cooperate with requests.

Interventions
- Provide an atmosphere of warmth and acceptance for both child and family members.
- Maintain a calm and relaxed manner; try to smile at the child. Talking with the child, being calm, and smiling can provide comfort.
- Explain to the child when he or she will be reunited with the parents.
- Speak softly and slowly. When speaking, try to get down to the child's eye level so he or she can see your face. Do not assume you were understood. Repetition may be necessary.
- Allow the child to keep familiar security objects (e.g., toy, blanket).
- Administer preoperative sedation as prescribed; note effects.
- Encourage parents to stay with the child as long as permitted and according to their wishes.
- Encourage parents to hold child until child falls asleep, if desired (may vary according to institution policy).
- Touch the child, and hold his or her hand.

Nursing Diagnosis
Fear related to developmental level (fear of the unknown, fear of painful procedures and surgery)

Outcome
The child will verbalize less fear; he or she will respond in an age-appropriate manner to comfort measures and recognize that the perioperative nurse is present to help.

Interventions
- Assess the child's growth and development, noting any variations from expected normal age-appropriate maturational levels.
- Provide preoperative education for the child and family, using audiovisual aids such as photographs, drawings, items for medical play, or a tour of the surgical suite.
- Provide explanations according to the child's level and the parent's level of understanding; use age-appropriate terminology that is familiar to the child, such as for body function.
- Place unfamiliar equipment out of the child's view to decrease fear.
- Encourage the child to handle items that may seem strange or threatening.
- Reassure the child that certain body parts can be removed without producing harm (e.g., blood, tonsils, appendix).
- Provide ongoing age-appropriate explanations for procedures/events during the perioperative period. Do not try to explain everything at once; explain procedure-by-procedure.
- Allow choices whenever possible, such as wearing pajamas or clothing to the OR.
- Respect need for modesty; expose only those body parts necessary.
- Provide diversional activities to decrease fear.
- Use pain assessment questions if the child is fearful of procedures.
- Be honest about the possibility of pain or discomfort; do not lie to the child.
- Reassure the child that you are there to help.

Nursing Diagnosis
Risk for Infection related to surgical intervention and other invasive procedures

Outcome
The child will remain free from signs and symptoms of infection at the surgical site and invasive procedure sites; the surgical site will heal by first intention, and white blood cell count and differential will remain within normal limits.

Interventions
- Administer antibiotic prophylaxis as prescribed.
- Follow Standard Precautions.
- Maintain aseptic technique, and monitor members of the surgical team for breaks in technique.
- Teach family members signs and symptoms of surgical site infection:
  - Redness
  - Swelling
  - Warmth
  - Tenderness
  - Pain
- Teach family members the importance of and proper handwashing techniques.
- Apply dressing to the surgical site before sterile drapes are removed to prevent contamination of incision.

Nursing Diagnosis
Risk for Imbalanced Fluid Volume related to invasive surgery and accompanying blood loss

Outcome
The child will maintain fluid balance as evidenced by blood pressure within expected/acceptable range, palpable peripheral pulses, moist mucous membranes, and absence of peripheral edema.

Interventions
- Maintain and protect patency of intravenous lines.
- Review laboratory analyses for results of total blood volume.
- Calculate estimated total blood volume using formula of 85 to 90 mL/kg of body weight if total blood volume has not been determined by laboratory tests.
- Provide gram scales for weighing sponges discarded from operative field; weigh sponges, and report estimated loss.
- Provide suction units with reservoirs that measure in 5- to 10-mL increments.
- Measure and record the quantity of irrigating fluid used.
- Provide appropriate amounts of intravenous fluid replacement (e.g., 250-mL containers).
- Measure and record urinary output and output from other drainage tubes.
- Send laboratory specimens for analysis as indicated; review the results indicating fluid status.

Nursing Diagnosis
Risk for Hypothermia related to loss of body surface heat to environment and immature temperature-control mechanism

Outcome
The child will maintain normothermia as evidenced by body temperature within normal limits/expected range.

Interventions
- Adjust room temperature approximately 1 hour before arrival of the child: 78.8° to 80.6° F (26° to 27° C) for infants and newborns; 73.4° to 75.2° F (23° to 24° C) for older children.

SAMPLE PLAN OF CARE—cont'd

- Keep the child covered as much as possible.
- Consider wrapping lower extremities in soft gauze or stockinette and encasing in a plastic bag for newborns and infants.
- Provide a radiant heat lamp for use during placement of monitoring lines, induction of anesthesia, positioning, skin prep, and draping.
- Warm blankets, skin prep solutions (according to manufacturer's instructions), and irrigation and other solutions to body temperature before use.

- Use warmers during administration of intravenous fluids and blood products; temperature settings should not exceed 100.4° F (38°C).
- Monitor body temperature by rectal, esophageal, tympanic membrane, or other automatic temperature-monitoring device.
- Document temperature at prescribed intervals; take appropriate action for temperature extremes.

PATIENT-CENTERED CARE

A perioperative nurse can describe what to expect in the first minutes after entering the OR for an umbilical hernia repair to a preschooler in the following way:

"You and I are going to take a ride on the stretcher to the OR. (The word stretcher can be replaced with a vehicle specific to child interests, e.g., spaceship, princess chariot, race car.) When we get there you'll meet some of my friends, and we will help you move onto a different bed. We will give you stickers that tell us how fast your heart is beating and give your arm a hug with a special sleeve that tells us how strong your heart is. You will breathe air that might smell funny and then fall asleep. While you are sleeping the doctor is going to fix your belly button so that it does not stick out so much. You will not feel the doctor fixing your belly button, but will wake up with a bandage on it. You may feel sleepy and your belly may hurt for a while, but you can have medicine when you wake up to take the pain away. Your caregivers [parents, family, legal guardians) will be waiting for you in a place with other grown-ups and will be well cared for. We will bring them to you a few minutes after you leave the OR."

EVIDENCE FOR PRACTICE

Safe Patient Handling in the Pediatric Perioperative Population

The Handle with Care Campaign was launched by the American Nurses Association (ANA) in 2004 with the intent of promoting injury prevention strategies and campaigns across the healthcare industry (deCastro, 2004). The Centers for Disease Control and Prevention (CDC) cite nurses as having the highest rate of back and shoulder injuries, 2012). The greatest risk factor associated with these injuries result from manual moving and positioning patients (CDC, 2012). High-risk perioperative tasks include (Ogg, 2011):

- Transferring patients to and from OR beds
- Repositioning patients on OR beds
- Lifting and holding a patient's extremities
- Standing for long periods
- Lifting and carrying supplies and equipment
- Pushing, pulling, and moving equipment on wheels

Patient handling injuries are not specific to adult healthcare facilities. Pediatric hospitals must also consider safe patient handling initiatives. Increasing patient weights, unpredictable movements, awkward postures and positions, and developmental disabilities contribute to the risk of injury not only to healthcare providers, but to patients as well (Haglund et al, 2010). Handling injuries in the pediatric population can result from pulling off items of clothing, lifting a child by the feet or ankles to change a diaper, or being manually restrained when emerging from anesthesia.

The following measures may be taken to prevent handling injuries in the pediatric perioperative population:

- Clustering patient care activities—if a patient needs to be rolled to the side to assess skin on the back, take advantage of the opportunity to remove soiled linens or place/remove a grounding pad
- Considering extra supportive devices to reduce pressure from taping or safety belts

- Using size-appropriate devices and supplies when delivering patient care

Pediatric hospitals that strive to develop Safe Patient Handling programs may consider:

- Emphasizing the importance of proper body mechanics
  - Use a wide base of support, keeping legs shoulder-width apart.
  - Maintaining straight posture, using legs as much as possible.
  - Supinate the arms when moving patients on a drawsheet.
  - Maintaining an even height of transfer surfaces.
  - Designating a manual lift limit (one person for every 16 kg of patient body weight).
- Emphasizing safe patient handling:
  - Use wide-spread fingers to support patients during transfer.
  - Avoid pulling on the patient's extremities.
  - Support the patient's limbs and back with the forearm instead of grasping.
  - Hold the patient close to the joint as opposed to at the end of an extremity.
- Designating the caregiver positioned at the patient's head as the director of the patient transfer:
  - Use a count-down method—"on the count of 3, we will move"—to ensure that everyone helps at the same time.
- Using transfer devices to protect both the patient and healthcare provider from handling injuries:
  - Transfer boards
  - Air-assisted lateral patient transfer devices
  - Overhead lift systems

Modified from Centers for Disease Control and Prevention (CDC): *Safe patient handling,* 2012, available at www.cdc.gov/niosh/topics/safepatient. Accessed December 14, 2012; de Castro AB: Handle with care: the American Nurses Association's campaign to address work-related musculoskeletal disorders, *Online J Issues Nurs,* 9(3), manuscript 2, 2004, available at www.nursingworld.org/MainMenuCategories/ANAMarketplace/ANAPeriodicals/OJIN/TableofContents/Volume92004/No3Sept04/HandleWithCare.aspx. Accessed December 14, 2012; Haglund K et al: Pediatric safe patient handling, *J Pediatr Nurs* 25(2):98–107, 2010; Ogg M: Introduction to the safe patient handling and movement series, *AORN J* 93(3):331–333, 2011.

They need as much privacy as possible, and their attempts to be independent should be respected (e.g., walking into the OR instead of being wheeled in on a stretcher if the patient has not been sedated). The adolescent may not wish to show any fear; questions might not be asked while the parents are present. Information and explanations should be provided as reasonably and truthfully as possible. If appropriate, some choices should be allowed, such as wearing underwear to the OR. Patient care procedures that violate privacy, such as hair removal, skin preparation, or insertion of an indwelling urinary catheter, should be conducted after the patient is anesthetized.

Key points in providing perioperative care to pediatric patients include remaining alongside the child until the child is anesthetized, keeping the room quiet during induction, accepting a child's need to express fear and fearful behaviors (e.g., crying), and using simple words without double meanings to explain care. Security objects should remain with the child until induction has been completed. A child's behavior during induction is likely to be the same during emergence; thus all attempts should be made to provide calm, reassuring care. Parents should be alerted to delays in the surgery schedule; in some instances, the child may be allowed to have fluids if the surgery is delayed by several hours.

Implementing the nursing plan of care includes continual reassessment of the patient's needs as well as the efficient execution of activities that facilitate the surgical intervention. Remaining with the child during induction, positioning, and prepping the surgical site; creating and maintaining a sterile field; collecting, documenting, and disposing specimens; and administering medications are all part of helping to provide a safe environment for the pediatric surgical patient. Making sure that the pediatric patient's family receives regular updates of the child's status is also a part of the perioperative nurse's responsibilities and will decrease their anxiety and help foster a sense of trust in the healthcare professionals caring for their child.

Instrumentation. The same types of instruments used in adult surgery are used in pediatric surgery. However, pediatric instruments are usually shorter, have more delicate or less pronounced curves, and are smaller. A complete range of instrument sizes is necessary to make the appropriate size available to each child because pediatric patients can range in size from less than 1 to more than 100 kg. Fewer instruments are normally required because incisions in children are shorter and shallower than those in adults. Use of basic instrument sets, grouped according to types of surgery performed (e.g., minor, major), facilitates instrument counts. Instrument sets may also be grouped according to categories of patient size (e.g., infant, pediatric, adolescent, and adult). These sets are easily adapted to the patient's needs as well as the surgeon's preferences and eliminate unnecessary instruments from the sterile field.

Sutures. A variety of sutures are used with the pediatric population because of the wide range of patient size; needles from size 0 to 7-0 are routinely stocked. Both absorbable and nonabsorbable sutures on cutting and tapered needles are used. The most frequently used sizes are 3-0 to 5-0 with ½- and ⅜-circle needles. Staples, both pediatric and regular sizes, are occasionally used. Many skin incisions are closed with subcuticular techniques, over which adhesive strips or cyanoacrylate glue is then applied. The use of tape to apply dressings is done conservatively because of the delicate nature of children's skin; frequently, either a small transparent or an elastic net dressing is used to hold gauze dressings in place.

TABLE 26-3

Recommended Sizes of Oral Endotracheal Tubes Based on Age and Weight

Age	Weight (kg)	Internal Diameter of Uncuffed Endotracheal Tube (mm)	Internal Diameter of Cuffed Endotracheal Tube (mm)
Premature	Less than 1.5 kg	2.5-3	NA
Premature	1.5-2.5 kg	3-3.5	3-3.5
Newborn	3.5 kg	3.5	3.5
1 year	10 kg	4	3.5-4
2-3 years	15 kg	4.5	4-4.5
4-6 years	20 kg	5	4.5-5
7-9	30 kg	NA	5.5
10-12 years	40 kg	NA	6
13-15 years	50 kg	NA	6.5
Greater than 16 years	Greater than 60 kg	NA	7

Modified from Gottlieb EA, Andropolous DB: Pediatrics. In Miller RD, Pardo MC, editors: *Basics of anesthesia*, ed 6, Philadelphia, 2011, Churchill Livingstone; Stackhouse RA: Airway management. In Miller RD, Pardo MC, editors: *Basics of anesthesia*, ed 6, Philadelphia, 2011, Churchill Livingstone.

Anesthetic Considerations. Anesthesia is approached differently in pediatric patients than it is in adults. The equipment and supplies are scaled down to match the size of the patient, and different anesthesia circuits and delivery systems may be used. Adult facilities that provide anesthesia to pediatric patients should consider developing a mobile pediatric intubation cart that houses the appropriate sized equipment and devices necessary to care for the anesthetized child.

The most common technique used in the pediatric population is a general inhalational anesthetic administered by facemask, laryngeal airway, or endotracheal tube. Selection of the endotracheal tube involves several considerations; the tube must be large enough to permit ventilation but small enough to minimize damage to the trachea while maintaining a seal to prevent aspiration. Table 26-3 provides a guide to choosing endotracheal tube sizes for pediatric patients. Depth of insertion to the lip is calculated by multiplying the inner diameter of the endotracheal tube by 3 (Gottlieb and Andropolous, 2011).

Microdrip IV tubing and burettes are commonly used to avoid the administration of excess fluids in pediatric patients younger than 8 years, and only 500-mL bags of IV solution are used. The patient's IV line is usually started in the OR after induction with mask anesthesia, depending on the patient's diagnosis and medical history. Patients who require emergency surgery who have not been NPO; have increased intracranial pressure, an unusually difficult airway, or neuromuscular disease; or have been diagnosed with malignant hyperthermia require an IV placement before anesthesia induction. If the IV line is started before induction, measures should be taken to lessen the discomfort, such as an intradermal injection of 1% buffered lidocaine or saline at the site or the application of topical anesthetic creams. If possible, the surgical team should allow the child the option of sitting up or lying down during IV placement; if developmentally appropriate, hold the child's hand and tell the child about each step in the placement of an IV line.

Preoperative sedation is generally accomplished by the oral administration of midazolam. Midazolam is the most commonly used pediatric premedication in the United States and can be given orally, nasally, rectally, intramuscularly, or intravenously. Oral midazolam should be administered in a flavored base to mask the bitter taste. Relaxation is noted 15 to 45 minutes after administration; the child should be kept in a safe, observable environment after being medicated. Other agents used for premedication include fentanyl and, infrequently, ketamine.

Depending on institutional policy, a parent may be present during induction to comfort the child and decrease the child's anxiety. The perioperative nurse should provide the parent an explanation of how the OR will appear and who will be present in the OR, how the child's anesthesia induction will be performed, and how the child will appear as the anesthetic takes effect. An additional staff person, such as a parent services' provider or child life therapist, should be present to escort the parent to and from the OR so that the perioperative nurse can focus on providing care for the patient once the child has been anesthetized.

Distraction methods during the induction of anesthesia can help minimize a child's stress and anxiety. Singing softly, telling a story, and, for the older child, providing a relaxing mental image are effective diversion techniques.

Malignant hyperthermia (MH), although very rare, may be more prevalent in the pediatric population as a result of the administration of inhalational anesthetics and succinylcholine. In addition, physiologic conditions present in some pediatric patients are associated with a higher risk of MH. These conditions include congenital myopathies such as central core disease and King-Denborough syndrome (Gottlieb and Andropolous, 2011). Careful assessment of family history is essential to identify patients at risk for developing MH. The management of an MH crisis is described in Chapter 5.

Pain Management. In the past, many common fallacies existed about pain in the pediatric population. Some of these mistruths were that infants do not feel pain; children have better pain tolerance than adults; children cannot tell the healthcare provider where they hurt; children always tell the truth about pain; children become accustomed to pain or painful procedures; and narcotics are more dangerous for children than they are for adults. Research into this important area has revealed that infants do demonstrate behavioral and physiologic indicators of pain. Compared with adults, children have less pain tolerance; their pain tolerance increases as they mature. Children are able to indicate pain, and children as young as 3 years can use pain-rating scales. Often children may not admit to having pain; they may believe that others know how much they hurt, or they fear receiving an injection. Children may also feel that pain and suffering are punishment for some misdeed, or they may not know what the word *pain* means. Children do not become accustomed to pain or painful procedures. They actually may demonstrate increased behavioral signs of pain with repeated procedures. Many factors, such as developmental level, culture, coping ability, temperament, and activity levels, influence the behavioral manifestations of pain exhibited by the patient. Narcotics are no more dangerous for children than they are for adults and are not excluded as a treatment modality. The evaluation of a pediatric patient's level of pain is performed using a variety of assessment tools (pain scales) that are based on the age and developmental level of the child. Often these scales are tested for reliability and validity. In infants and nonverbal children, evaluation is based on physiologic changes and observation of behaviors. Children with verbal skills are able to articulate pain. One assessment strategy to use with pediatric patients is the *QUESTT* method:

Question the child.
Use pain-rating scales.
Evaluate behavior and physiologic changes.
Secure the parents' involvement.
Take cause of pain into account.
Take action, and evaluate results.

Questioning the child provides the most reliable indicator of pain. Children may not be familiar with the word *pain* and may be more comfortable with words like "ouch," "hurt," or "owie." It may also be helpful to ask the child to point to where it hurts. The FACES pain scale uses cartoon faces with a variety of expressions ranging from happy to crying. The child selects the face that best describes his or her pain (see Chapter 10). The Oucher scale has a numeric component and a component similar to the FACES scale but uses actual photographs of children. The adolescent pediatric pain tool (APPT) is a line drawing of a body; the child marks the drawing where he or she has pain. Other tools include Likert-type scales rating pain on a score of 0 (no pain) to 10 (worst pain) or incorporate several components of pain assessment (subjective and objective data).

Physiologic indicators of pain, such as increased blood pressure, respirations, and heart rate and restlessness, are the same for children as for adults but may not be as reliable, except in neonates and nonverbal children. These indicators may also reflect anxiety or fear and should not be the sole indicator used to determine pain. Children may also tug or hold painful areas or show preference to a painful extremity.

Parental involvement in pain management is important. Parents know their child's normal behavior and can provide input into the behaviors being exhibited in the perioperative setting. Parents should be queried about the child's previous experiences with pain and be taught the nonverbal behaviors that may indicate pain.

Nurses should investigate all complaints of pain or discomfort and be sensitive to behavioral and nonverbal cues to determine treatment. Postoperative pain should be assessed after all surgical procedures, regardless of their nature. It is also critical to assess and document the child's response to the interventions provided for relief of pain.

Effective pain management requires a willingness to use a variety of methods and modalities to achieve optimal results. Pharmacologic methods include the administration of analgesics, both narcotic and non-narcotic. Patient-controlled analgesia (PCA) is an option for children. Children as young as 5 years have the cognitive and physical capabilities to successfully use this modality with appropriate instruction and support (Wetzel, 2011). Nonpharmacologic methods include distraction, relaxation, guided imagery, behavioral contracting, and cutaneous stimulation. Nonpharmacologic methods should never be used as substitutes for appropriate medication administration but instead to enhance pain management.

Evaluation

The perioperative nurse evaluates care provided throughout the perioperative period. At the conclusion of the surgical intervention, the skin is inspected, especially at dependent pressure points and at the site of the electrosurgical dispersive pad. Inspection is carried out to detect any reddened, irritated areas or evidence of compression injury. If povidone-iodine or chlorhexidine gluconate preparations were used for skin prep, the area needs to be checked for any signs of chemical irritation. The patient's temperature is reassessed. The cardiopulmonary status is closely monitored as the child emerges from anesthesia. The perioperative nurse should assist the anesthesia team during emergence, remaining at the patient's bedside. Warm blankets are provided; hydration status is evaluated as replacement fluids continue to be administered, and fluid output is noted. The child is transferred to and positioned on the stretcher, crib, neonatal intensive care unit (NICU) warmer, or ICU bed; the airway and respiratory effort are reassessed before departing the OR. Tubes, IV lines, drains, and drainage devices must be carefully protected during the move from the operating bed. Supplemental oxygen is always given during transport from the OR to the PACU for pediatric patients.

The perioperative nurse provides a hand-off report to the PACU nurse, focusing on the condition of the child, the response to surgery and anesthesia, the presence of catheters and drains, the quality and amount of wound drainage, a description of the dressings applied, and any special needs. Part of this report should focus on the outcomes established in the perioperative plan of care. For the plan of care presented in this chapter, they might be as follows:

- The patient demonstrated decreased anxiety.
- The patient responded in an age-appropriate manner to comfort measures and exhibited decreased fear.
- The patient was protected from infection related to operative intervention; principles of asepsis and infection control were maintained.
- The patient remained hemodynamically stable and did not exhibit fluid volume deficit.
- The patient's temperature was maintained in the desired range during the perioperative period.

The perioperative nurse may receive further feedback on the child's progress after the child is discharged from the PACU; information may be relayed by the surgeon, unit nurse, or anesthesia provider. This type of informal feedback helps the perioperative nurse collect additional data regarding effectiveness of the plan of care, providing information about the achievement of identified outcomes.

Patient and Family Education and Discharge Planning

Patient and family teaching varies significantly based on the type of surgery performed. Some hospitals provide special preoperative teaching and hospital tours for pediatric patients and their parents to help them prepare for the surgical experience. Sometimes information is discussed with the child and family at the time of the office visit, when the surgery is scheduled. For same-day procedures, the day-surgery nursing staff might teach postoperative care immediately before patient discharge. Basics of postoperative care are reviewed with the parents at this time. In some cases, written material may be provided (Box 26-2). Parents should be advised to be alert for certain signs and symptoms during the postoperative recovery period that could indicate an infectious process, such as fever, pain, nausea, redness around the incision area, drainage from the wound, or difficulty breathing. These signs and symptoms may develop days or even weeks after surgery. It is important that parents understand the necessity of not ignoring any of these signs and symptoms and of reporting them to the surgeon promptly so that an early diagnosis can be made and treatment prescribed. Although discharge information depends on the type of surgery performed, it typically includes recommendations about activity restrictions, return to school or daycare, wound care, bathing or showering, diet, and follow-up appointments. The printed discharge instructions are

---

BOX 26-2

Sample Discharge Instructions

- Leave the wound open to the air.
- Do not apply any creams or ointments to the wound for 14 days.
- Starting the day of surgery, clean the incision three times a day using a paper towel, mild soap, and water. Do this three times a day for 2 weeks, then just daily. Do not rub the incision. Gently clean the area in a circular motion with mild pressure. Remove the soap with a wet paper towel and pat dry. Do not use terry cloth washcloths. The fabric loops may snag and pull on stitches.
- Do not allow the incision to be under water for the first 2 weeks after surgery.
- Your child may shower the day after surgery.
- If the stitches are clear, they will dissolve and do not need to be removed. If they are blue or black, they need to be removed about 10 to 14 days after the surgery. Your surgeon will tell you how long they need to be in.
- Call the surgeon's office soon after going home if you need an appointment for stitch removal.
- You will also need to schedule a follow-up appointment in 4 to 6 weeks for a postprocedure visit.
- Check the wound daily. It is normal to have some redness around the stitch holes or on the incision line. Call the surgeon's office if you notice that the area around the outside of the incision is red, hot, or tender or has pus draining from it. Also call if your child has a fever greater than 101.5° F (38° C).

Modified from Children's Hospital of Philadelphia, 2012.

---

reviewed with the parents, and their understanding is verified. This time should provide the family with an opportunity to ask questions or seek clarification of the instructions. Phone numbers for the surgeon and the main hospital are provided in case the family has concerns or questions during the child's recovery period at home. An appointment for the child's follow-up visit may be made before discharge, or the parents are instructed to call the physician's office to schedule an appointment.

Surgical Interventions

As mentioned, children require surgery for congenital malformations, an acquired disease, or trauma. The field of pediatric surgery is further subdivided into all the specialties. Several surgical procedures that may be designated pediatric are presented in previous chapters of this text under particular specialty headings. The surgical interventions presented here represent procedures that are most commonly performed on children.

Vascular Access

Vascular access in pediatric patients may be established intraoperatively for short-term (weeks) or long-term (months, years) use. Examples of short-term use include peripherally inserted central catheters (PICC lines) for antibiotic therapy. Central venous lines or implanted ports are placed for long-term access to provide parenteral nutrition, chemotherapy, bone marrow transplantation, or multiple IV access lines for the critically ill patient. Neonates and children born at low birthweights are at highest risk for catheter-associated infections as a result of their compromised immune status (Curry et al, 2009). National and consumer organizations are exerting pressure on hospitals to implement practices aimed at reducing and eliminating catheter-associated infections in all patients (Wheeler et al, 2011).

Central Venous Catheter Placement

The preferred site of placement for central venous access is the external jugular vein. The internal jugular vein may be chosen if the external jugular vein has been used or is too small. From the cannulation site the catheter is tunneled under the skin about 5 to 10 cm. This is done to inhibit contamination of the bloodstream from frequent dressing changes. Subcutaneous ports are placed in a similar fashion. In cases in which the internal or external vein sites are unavailable, the catheter may be placed into the external iliac vein by way of a cutdown in the greater saphenous vein. In these cases, the catheter is tunneled into the abdominal wall.

Procedural Considerations. The manufacturer's instructions for handling and preparing the catheter must be followed. The catheter must not contact lint, glove powder, or other foreign matter. Before insertion the catheter is flushed and filled with heparinized saline (1 unit of heparin to 1 mL of saline) to prevent air bubbles from entering the circulatory system and to eliminate blood clots in the catheter lumen. Fluoroscopy is used to confirm proper placement of the catheter; lead shielding must be provided for patient and staff, with appropriate warning signs placed on room doors. The use of a lead shield for the patient should be documented in the perioperative record.

The child is appropriately positioned as dictated by the site chosen for cannulation, and organs are protected with a lead shield. The area is prepped and draped.

Operative Procedure—External Jugular Vein Site

1. The surgeon uses a needle and syringe to puncture the external jugular and aspirates to confirm blood flow.
2. The syringe is removed from the needle, and a guidewire is fed through the needle into the vein. An intraoperative x-ray is taken to confirm correct position.
3. Once the position is confirmed, the surgeon makes an incision over the insertion site. A silver probe or tendon passer is used to create a tunnel beneath the skin to the desired exit site of the catheter. A second incision is made over the tip of the probe or passer.
4. The implantable end of the catheter is attached to the end of the passer or probe and pulled through the subcutaneous tunnel. The catheter is cut to a desired length.
5. The needle is removed from the vein, leaving the guidewire in place. An obturator is placed over the guidewire, and the wire is removed. The catheter is placed through the obturator into the vein, and an intraoperative x-ray is taken to confirm position.
6. The catheter is secured at the exit site on the chest wall with nonabsorbable sutures, flushed with a "super flush" of heparinized saline (10 units of heparin to 1 mL of saline in children younger than 12 months or 100 units of heparin to 1 mL of saline in children older than 12 months), and clamped.
7. An occlusive transparent dressing is placed over the catheter site. The catheter is coiled under this dressing to avoid tension on the line and accidental displacement.

Minimally Invasive Surgery

Improvements in instrumentation and the development of equipment in smaller sizes have resulted in the evolution of minimally invasive surgery (MIS) from that of a rapidly growing field to one of routine practice in the pediatric surgical arena. Much like the adult population, many traditional "open" pediatric surgical procedures are being replaced by MIS procedures. Because the field of pediatric MIS is relatively new, surgeons are at an advantage because they are able to combine virtual reality techniques and robotics with the most current technology and instrumentation (Harrington et al, 2008). Advantages of MIS include diminished postoperative pain, improved cosmetic results, decreased prevalence of adhesion formation, and accelerated recovery periods and shorter hospital stays.

Despite the technical congruence with adult MIS procedures, the pediatric populations undergoing these procedures have specific needs that must be satisfied in order to promote positive outcomes. Anesthesia providers must take the size and age of the patient into consideration because of the risk of physiologic compromise related to insufflation. Likewise, steps are taken intraoperatively to decrease the likelihood of intra-abdominal injury, such as insertion of an appropriate size Foley catheter to decompress the bladder or application of thromboembolic hose or sleeves to prevent deep vein thrombosis.

Common pediatric MIS procedures for general surgery include diagnostic laparoscopy, pyloromyotomy, splenectomy, gastric fundoplication, and cholecystectomy. Thoracoscopic approaches may be used for correction of pectus excavatum, lung biopsy, sympathectomy, and closure of a patent ductus arteriosus (PDA). Procedures that are currently less common but increasing in prevalence include pancreatectomy for focal lesion, choledochal cyst excision, lobectomy for congenital cystic adenomatoid malformation (CCAM), and repair of congenital diaphragmatic hernia (CDH) and tracheoesophageal fistula (TEF). Minimally invasive procedures in other disciplines include (but are not limited to) ventriculoscopy, which can be used to view the ventricles of the brain; functional endoscopic sinus surgery (FESS); and nephrectomy and pyeloplasty, both of which may involve the use of a surgical robotic system.

Laparoscopic Pyloromyotomy for Pyloric Stenosis

Pyloric stenosis (Figure 26-3) is the most common cause of gastric outlet obstructions in children and is the most common condition requiring surgery in the newborn. Signs and symptoms of high gastrointestinal (GI) obstruction appear at 2 to 6 weeks of age. The first sign is bile-free projectile vomiting after feeding. The infant usually fails to gain weight adequately, and there may be a severe loss of body fluids and electrolyte imbalance, evidenced as hypochloremic, hypokalemic metabolic alkalosis. Once the diagnosis of hypertrophic pyloric stenosis is made, either through physical examination or by imaging techniques, surgical intervention is planned. Electrolyte imbalances must be corrected before surgery. The Fredet-Ramstedt pyloromyotomy for pyloric stenosis is an open procedure that involves the incision of the muscles of the pylorus to treat congenital hypertrophy of the pyloric sphincter that is obstructing the stomach. However, laparoscopic pyloromyotomy has replaced the open procedure as the standard for repair. The laparoscopic procedure is described in the following Operative Procedure.

Procedural Considerations. The stomach is emptied just before induction of anesthesia, and the nasogastric tube is removed to guard against reflux of gastric contents around the tube during induction. The patient is positioned transverse on the OR bed so that the operating surgeon stands at the patient's feet. A video monitor is positioned above the patient's head. The abdomen is prepped in the usual manner, and trocar sites are injected with a

FIGURE 26-3 Pyloric stenosis.

FIGURE 26-4 Laparoscopic pyloromyotomy.

local anesthetic. The perioperative nurse must consider the location of the incision and position the patient in a fashion that facilitates maximum exposure of the surgical site. Appropriate-sized instrumentation and sterile supplies must be available, along with imaging equipment. Insufflation flow rate should be set to the lowest acceptable level for achieving pneumoperitoneum and increased slowly to prevent adverse physiologic effects (decreased end-tidal CO_2, decreased SpO_2, tachycardia, cyanosis, arrhythmias) associated with CO_2 embolism.

Operative Procedure

1. The surgeon makes a small incision in the umbilicus and places a 3- or 5-mm trocar through it to accommodate the telescope. Insufflation tubing is attached to this trocar and the abdomen is insufflated (maximum pressure of 10 mm Hg).
2. Using a #11 blade, the surgeon makes a small stab incision laterally, slightly above the umbilicus on each side.
3. The 3-mm laparoscopic instruments are passed directly through the stab incisions.
4. The surgeon makes an incision in the serosa on the anterior wall of the pyloric mass from the duodenal junction proximally to a point proximal to the area of hypertrophied muscle using an arthroscopic knife and laparoscopic grasper. The circular muscle is spread with the 3-mm laparoscopic pyloric spreader on the submucosal base so that all muscle fibers are completely divided (Figure 26-4).
5. The anesthesia provider injects 60 to 120 mL of air into the stomach through an orogastric (OG) tube to ensure that there are no air bubbles at the pyloric incision.
6. The umbilical incision is closed using absorbable suture and cyanoacrylate glue applied to each incision.

Laparoscopic Nissen Fundoplication

Nissen fundoplication is indicated for infants and children who experience severe gastroesophageal (GE) reflux. The cause of GE reflux in these patients is believed to be an inadequate antireflux barrier. The antireflux barrier normally consists of a combination of anatomic and physiologic factors, including sufficient amount and strength of muscle fibers located in the lower esophageal sphincter, adequate length of the abdominal esophagus, and a high-pressure zone in the lower esophagus. An incompetent antireflux barrier can result in life-threatening complications, including obstructive apnea, aspiration pneumonia, esophagitis, and failure to thrive. GE reflux can be medically or surgically managed. Medical management relies on proton pump inhibitors (PPIs) to reduce the production of stomach acid. With successful medical management of GE reflux, surgery to correct the antireflux barrier may be avoided.

In certain cases, however, surgical intervention outweighs the benefit of medical management. Children who are more likely to benefit from surgical management of GE reflux include those suffering from erosive esophagitis or volume regurgitation, patients who have had an adverse reaction to PPIs, or those who wish to avoid long-term drug therapy (Bulsiewicz and Madanick, 2012). Surgical management of GE reflux is accomplished by open or laparoscopic Nissen fundoplication. The goal of the Nissen fundoplication is to create a competent antireflux barrier. There are several types of laparoscopic fundoplications, encompassing full and partial wraps. The partial laparoscopic wrap (Toupet) is described in the following Operative Procedure.

Procedural Considerations.

The patient is positioned supine for induction of general anesthesia. The anesthesia provider inserts an OG tube, which serves as a stent for the wrap during the procedure. Once the endotracheal tube location is confirmed and secured, the patient is moved to the foot of the OR bed and positioned in low lithotomy position using stirrups and protective padding. The operating surgeon stands in the area between the patient's legs. A video monitor is positioned above the patient's head. The abdomen is prepped in the usual manner, and trocar sites are injected with local

FIGURE 26-5 Laparoscopic Nissen fundoplication, 270-degree (Toupet) wrap.

FIGURE 26-6 Repair of pectus excavatum. **A,** Preoperative. **B,** Postoperative.

anesthetic. The perioperative nurse must consider the location of the incision and position the patient in a fashion that facilitates maximum exposure of the surgical site. Appropriate-sized instrumentation and sterile supplies must be available, along with the appropriate imaging equipment. Insufflation flow rate should be set to the lowest acceptable level for achieving pneumoperitoneum and increased slowly to prevent adverse physiologic effects (decreased end-tidal CO_2, decreased SpO_2, tachycardia, cyanosis, arrhythmias) associated with CO_2 embolism.

Operative Procedure

1. Using a #15 blade the surgeon creates a tiny fasciotomy, places a trocar, and insufflates the abdomen with CO_2 gas. After insufflation the abdomen is inspected for gross abnormality. Additional fasciotomies and trocars are placed to accommodate camera, telescope, and instrumentation.
2. A Colorado clamp is used to elevate the liver away from the stomach, and gastrohepatic connections are cut from the right crus. The crus is carefully dissected away from the esophagus, taking care to preserve the integrity of the peritoneum.
3. Any adhesions on the left side of the stomach are taken down in order to mobilize the fundus and provide access to the left crus.
4. The surgeon uses a blunt dissector to create a retroesophageal tunnel for the esophageal length. The hiatus is reapproximated and tightened using endoscopic suturing devices.
5. A 270-degree (Toupet) wrap is completed. Two sutures incorporate the esophagus, stomach, and crus at the 10 o'clock and 2 o'clock positions on the diaphragmatic hiatus. Four sutures create intra-abdominal esophageal length with stitches anchored at the GE junction, giving the fundoplasty the appearance of a "hot dog in a bun" (Figure 26-5).
6. The OG tube is removed, and a final barrel suture is placed at the posterior portion of the wrap to anchor it to the right crus and keep it from unwrapping.
7. The stomach is inspected again to rule out gross abnormality or injury, then desufflated. Incisions are closed in layers using absorbable suture and sealed with cyanoacrylate glue.

Endoscopic Correction of Pectus Excavatum—Nuss Procedure

Pectus excavatum (funnel chest) is a visually obvious defect of the sternum, seen as a deep depression on the chest as a result of posterior displacement of the sternum (Figure 26-6). It is usually associated with kyphosis. The defect may be asymmetric, most often deeper on the right side, with sternal angulation. In a majority of cases surgical treatment is cosmetic; impaired cardiorespiratory function is the underlying reason for surgical intervention in fewer cases. The procedure is most commonly performed in patients between 10 and 16 years of age, when children become embarrassed to undress in front of peers. Rigid fixation has become a choice for correction of the defect, wherein a metal bar and retaining stabilizer are inserted to gain chest wall stability and prevent recurrence. The bar and stabilizers are maintained for approximately 3 years (Varela et al, 2010. Other treatments may cosmetically correct the situation over the short term but usually result in progressive retraction of the sternum.

Procedural Considerations. Adolescent endoscopic instrumentation is used along with a camera, telescopes, corresponding thoracic instrumentation, and a fixation rod. The patient is positioned supine with the arms positioned along the sides and the elbows flexed 90 degrees and propped so that they are anterior to the chest. The hands are propped so that they are anterior to the elbows. The upper chest is elevated on a soft roll or sheets. A Foley catheter may be placed, and the patient is prepped and draped in sterile fashion.

Operative Procedure

1. The surgeon measures the patient's chest to determine the size of the stabilization bar to be used, and bends an aluminum template to the desired shape of the chest. A stainless steel bar is bent to match the aluminum template using plate benders.
2. Two lateral chest incisions are made in-line with the deepest part of the pectus using a #15 blade, and subcutaneous pockets are created.
3. A port is placed into the left chest through which gentle insufflation takes place.
4. An incision is made via the subcutaneous pocket in order to pass the Lorenz introducer. The introducer is positioned through one

side of the chest, across the mediastinum, and out the other side guided by thoracoscopic visualization techniques.

5. A doubled tracheostomy tape is placed at the end hole of the Lorenz introducer and brought through the anterior mediastinal tunnel. The tracheostomy tape is then tied to the stainless steel bar, which is brought through the chest using the same tunnel and flipped using a flipping device. Chest configuration is checked for correction, contour, and symmetry.

6. A side bar (strut) is placed on each side of the bar and a stainless steel wire is wrapped around the main bar both medially and laterally. Two sutures are placed between the chest wall and the end holes of the side and main bars. The suture knots are buried within the holes, and the thoracic cavity may be irrigated with antibiotic irrigation.

7. The wounds are closed in layers using absorbable suture, and a chest x-ray is obtained postoperatively to rule out pneumothorax.

Video-Assisted Thoracoscopic Surgery for Patent Ductus Arteriosus

Although thoracoscopy was first described in 1910 (Rao, 2011), the application of video-assisted thoracoscopic surgery (VATS) to the pediatric population for cardiovascular repairs was slower to evolve. The procedure requires thoracoscopic equipment and supplies, including 0- and 30-degree, 4- and 2.7-mm thoracoscopes, depending on the surgeon's preference and the patient's age and size. The endoscopic instruments, made smaller for the pediatric patient, include an electrocoagulation hook; Castroviejo-type scissors; graspers and right-angle clamps; fan lung retractors of varying sizes, either medium or medium-large; large endoscopic clip appliers; trocars with ports; and suction tip, preferably one that has a porthole to occlude when suction is required. Instrumentation for closure of PDA by thoracotomy is also set up in case the thoracoscopy fails or a complication arises and the chest needs to be opened emergently.

Procedural Considerations. Before the procedure the television cameras are set up on either side of the OR bed. The patient is placed in a right lateral position.

Operative Procedure

1. Usually four small incisions are made along the line of the posterolateral thoracotomy incision and ports are introduced.
2. The surgeon inserts the thoracoscope. The first assistant holds the lung retractor while the second assistant holds the camera. Some institutions use a mechanical articulating arm.
3. A grasper is used to elevate the pleura overlying the aorta near the insertion of the PDA and pulmonary artery, and careful dissection is begun with electrocoagulation. Suction is required to keep the area of dissection clear to enhance the surgeon's vision.
4. When the ductus has been clearly identified, a right-angle clamp may first be introduced and a tie applied to the duct. The clip applier is then inserted, and clips are applied.
5. Transesophageal or transthoracic echocardiography is usually performed by a cardiologist before closure of the porthole incisions to ensure closure of the ductus. Also a chest tube is inserted into the pleural space, the lungs are inflated, and the chest tube is removed; alternately, a chest tube may be left in place before porthole incision closures.

Bariatric Surgery

More than 17% of children and adolescents are obese, a prevalence that has more than tripled since 1990 (Centers for Disease Control and Prevention [CDC], 2013). Obesity in adolescents is defined as having a body mass index (BMI; kg/m²) greater than the 95th percentile for age and weight. Obesity contributes to many medical conditions such as hypertension, diabetes, sleep apnea, and skeletal deformities. Overweight and obese children also suffer from social isolation, bullying, and discrimination. The long-term outlook for morbidly obese children is guarded due to the high risk of premature cardiovascular disease and peripheral vascular disease (Ingelfinger, 2011).

Bariatric surgery is gaining popularity as a treatment option for obesity in some adolescents. The timing of the surgical procedure is critical. The patient must be physically mature. Skeletal maturation is generally complete by age 13 to 14 years in girls and age 15 to 16 years in boys. Bariatric surgery can be safely performed once the child has attained more than 95% of adult stature. Candidates undergo psychologic evaluation before surgery to ensure they are cognitively mature enough to participate in decision making and to comply with postoperative regimens. Box 26-3 describes qualifications for bariatric surgery in adolescent patients.

Procedural Considerations. The bariatric procedure most commonly performed in adolescents is the laparoscopic Roux-en-Y gastric bypass. The adjustable gastric band (i.e., lap band) has not been approved by the U.S. Food and Drug Administration (FDA) for use in adolescents (Research Highlight). The perioperative nurse must plan carefully for this surgical intervention with an emphasis on obtaining the appropriate-sized transport vehicle and monitoring devices (e.g., larger blood pressure cuff, possibly longer electrocardiogram [ECG] leads to accommodate placement on a larger

---

BOX 26-3

Qualifications for Bariatric Surgery in Adolescent Patients

- Body mass index (BMI) of at least 40 with coexisting medical conditions
- BMI of at least 50 in patients with no coexisting medical conditions
- Patient has reached physical maturity (Tanner stage 4 or 5)
- Patient evidences cognitive maturity
- Patient evidences emotional maturity
- Well-documented and at least temporarily successful weight loss attempts have been made.
- Family support, presence, and commitment are present.
- Patient is motivated and has good insight
- Patient has realistic expectations
- Family is compliant with healthcare commitments
- Family and patient understand long-term lifestyle changes are needed
- No major psychiatric disorders that may complicate postoperative regimen adherence are present.
- No major conduct/behavioral problems are present.
- Patient has had no substance abuse in preceding years
- Patient has no plans for pregnancy in upcoming 2 years

Modified from Ingelfinger J: Bariatric surgery in adolescents, N Engl J Med [serial online] 365(15):1365–1367, 2011.

RESEARCH HIGHLIGHT

Short-Term Results of Laparoscopic Adjustable Gastric Banding in Adolescents

Gastric bypass surgery is the most common weight-loss surgery performed in the United States. Laparoscopy lowers the morbidity of these procedures and yields safer and more successful procedures. In 2001, the U.S. Food and Drug Administration (FDA) approved laparoscopic adjustable gastric banding (LAGB) for obese adults. Although LAGB in adolescents has not received FDA approval, a device exemption was obtained from the FDA and approval was garnered by the Columbia University Institutional Review Board to allow for a study of short-term results in LAGB surgery in 100 adolescents (69 female, 31 male, mean age at operation 17.0).

Adolescent patients who were referred for LAGB surgery provided their age, height, and weight in a telephone screening prior to meeting with the pediatric surgeon. Candidates were required to complete a screening questionnaire detailing previous weight loss attempts as well as medical, family, and psychologic history; they also submitted a statement describing their purpose for pursuing weight-loss surgery. Each candidate had to meet evidence-based best practice guidelines for adolescent bariatric surgery.

After enrollment, participants were evaluated by a pediatric endocrinologist, exercise specialist, and nutritionist and underwent laboratory and imaging studies. They were followed on a monthly basis for 3 to 6 months by a nurse practitioner and nutritionist. Additionally participants were assigned to walk 5000 steps three times a week as measured by a pedometer. Height and weight measurements were obtained at each visit to determine whether they met criteria for excess weight (weight higher than 85th percentile as defined by the study team). Those who met the criteria were approved by the team and offered LAGB.

Participants who chose to undergo LAGB met with the surgeon, endocrinologist, nutritionist, and anesthesia provider 2 weeks prior to surgery. The participants were measured, underwent baseline serum testing, and were given instructions for maintaining a liquid diet throughout the preoperative period. They underwent LAGB in the OR and were observed overnight. They were maintained on sips of water, progressing to a liquid diet through discharge, and underwent a contrast swallow study on postoperative day 1.

On discharge, participants were monitored by the pediatric endocrinologist at 2 weeks postoperative, then every 3 months for 18 months postsurgery. Participants were monitored monthly for 6 months and every 6 months thereafter by the surgical team and nutritionist. At 6 months postsurgery, participants completed a psychologic questionnaire.

Results of the adolescent LAGB study are reflective of a study population ages 14 to 19 that weighed an average of 136.7 kg (body mass index [BMI] 48.7) with comorbid medical conditions. Of the 87 patients who were followed for a minimum of 6 months, average weight loss was 12.4 kg and average change in BMI was 4.4. These results depict a lower average weight loss than other adolescent reports, largely due to dramatic contrast between the success of some patients and failure of others. There was no correlation between the number of pre- or postoperative visits and weight loss outcome. There is unexplained significance in the difference of weight loss between the sexes, which has encouraged the study team to review their selection process to determine whether any factors have emerged as reliable predictors of success or failure. Gastric bypass, LAGB and gastric sleeve resections have proven to be helpful in assisting adolescents who have had minimal success with diet and weight loss programs to lose weight. Although long-term studies must be conducted to assess safety and lasting benefits of bariatric surgery in adolescents, LAGB can be effective in highly motivated adolescents.

Modified from Zitsman JL et al: Laparoscopic adjustable gastric banding in adolescents: short-term results, *J Pediatr Surg* 46(1):157–162, 2011.

patient), an OR bed rated for the patient's weight, and appropriate-length instruments in case conversion to an open procedure is necessary. Obesity places this patient group at risk for deep vein thrombosis (DVT); the nurse should ensure that elastic stockings and pneumatic intermittent compression devices are available.

Operative Procedure. The operative procedure is described in Chapter 11.

Fetal Surgery

The expansion of prenatal diagnosis centers for mothers with problem pregnancies has resulted in earlier detection of fetal malformations, such as CDH, myelomeningocele (MMC), and twin-to-twin transfusion syndrome (TTTS). One of the most significant advances in pediatric surgery is in the field of fetal surgery, which includes closed (percutaneous), minimally invasive (fetoscopic), open and ex utero intrapartum therapy (EXIT) procedures (a specialized delivery technique originally developed to deliver babies who have undergone tracheal occlusion for CDH). Research has been, and continues to be, a cornerstone of the fetal surgery discipline because performing fetal interventions without supporting research puts both the mother and fetus at higher risk for morbidity or mortality.

The type of anomaly and its immediate danger to the fetus determines the options for the pregnancy available to the family: allow nature to take its course and deliver at term, fetal surgery when the anomaly is life-threatening or when significant morbidity exists such as in MMC, or interruption of the pregnancy before 24 weeks' gestation. Criteria for consideration of fetal intervention include (Partridge and Flake, 2012):

1. Ability to accurately establish a prenatal diagnosis
2. Evidence of a well-defined natural history of the disorder
3. Presence of a correctable lesion that, if left untreated, could result in fetal demise, irreversible organ dysfunction prior to birth, or severe postnatal morbidity
4. Absence of severe associated anomalies
5. Acceptable risk-to-benefit ratio to both the mother and the fetus

Descriptions of some defects that can be repaired prenatally are described in Table 26-4.

Procedural Considerations. The most important factor to consider when preparing for fetal surgery is that two patients are undergoing surgery: the mother (an innocent bystander) and the fetus. The perioperative nurse must understand the maternal and fetal anatomy and pathophysiology as well as the entire operative procedure and potential risks to both patients in order to respond to emergencies such as fetal bradycardia, placental abruption, or other maternal-fetal complications. According to Scully and colleagues the mother has a mature airway that is easily accessible, viable lungs, and good vascular access, the fetus does not, and this leaves little

TABLE 26-4

Defects That May Be Repaired Prenatally

Diagnosis	Definition	Treatment Modality
Congenital cystic adenomatoid malformation (CCAM)	*Microcystic*: Solid appearing *Macrocystic:* Grossly cystic; less predictable growth pattern can grow rapidly Fetal hydrops and placentomegaly may jeopardize maternal health ("maternal mirror" syndrome, in which the mother's condition mirrors that of the sick fetus).	Microcystic CCAM with hydrops may be effectively managed with steroids. If steroids do not correct hydrops, open resection is offered. Macrocystic CCAM may respond to thoracocentesis, thoracoamniotic shunting, or open lung resection.
Giant neck mass	A large tumor in the neck that can compress the fetus's airway (e.g., cervical teratoma) Lymphangioma May compress esophagus, leading to polyhydramnios and preterm labor	EXIT procedure. For babies at or near term, cesarean section to resection, postnatal sclerotherapy
Hypoplastic left heart syndrome (HLHS)	A range of congenital cardiac malformations that have in common underdevelopment of the left-sided heart structures Malformations include aortic valve atresia and stenosis with associated hypoplasia or absence of the left ventricle.	Laparotomy without hysterotomy for percutaneous fetal aortic valvuloplasty continues to be studied.
Sacrococcygeal teratoma (SCT)	Fetal sacrococcygeal teratoma may be cystic, solid, or mixed in its sonographic appearance (due to mixed areas of tumor necrosis, cystic degeneration, hemorrhage, or calcification). Prenatally diagnosed sacrococcygeal teratoma associated with fetal hydrops (excess fluid retention from high-output cardiac failure) can be rapidly fatal in utero; high-output cardiac failure is related to "vascular steal" from the high blood flow through the tumor. Fetal hydrops and placentomegaly may jeopardize maternal health (maternal mirror syndrome, in which the mother's condition mirrors that of the sick fetus).	Steroid therapy can help manage the effects of preterm delivery. Sulindac can help manage hydrops Cyst decompression Fetal surgery or EXIT procedure in cases in which increasing continuous cardiac output (CCO) and placentomegaly (due to vascular steal and resulting high output failure) is present For babies at or near term, cesarean section to resection, postnatal sclerotherapy
Myelomeningocele (MMC)	Failure of the neural tube to close, resulting in protrusion of spinal cord and surrounding nerves from the open vertebrae The developing spinal cord and nerves are continuously exposed to amniotic fluid and friction over the course of gestation, which results in progressive neurologic injury.	Fetal surgery or postnatal surgery options dependent on selection criteria
Twin reversed arterial perfusion (TRAP) sequence	A rare complication of identical twinning in which one twin lacks a functioning cardiac system and is dependent on the twin with the fully functioning cardiac system (the "pump" twin) "Reversed perfusion" occurs when blood enters the acardiac/acephalic twin through its umbilical artery and exits through the umbilical vein (opposite of normal blood supply) The pump twin sustains increased cardiac demands that result in increased cardiac output, overproduction of urine, and ultimately, polyhydramnios.	Fetoscopy to gain access to the fetus Bipolar cord coagulation (BCC) or radiofrequency ablation (RFA) to nonviable twin
Twin-to-twin transfusion syndrome (TTTS)	A rare and serious complication in identical twins who share a placenta that has abnormal connections between the two twins' blood vessels. The smaller (donor) twin pumps blood to the larger (recipient) twin. The recipient twin produces excess urine and is at risk for polyhydramnios and hydrops. The donor twin produces less urine and is at risk for oligohydramnios and a small or absent bladder.	Amnioreduction Fetoscopic placental laser surgery Selective reduction by BCC or RFA as a last option when the at-risk twin faces imminent demise; protects the co-twin from neurologic impairment or demise

EXIT, Ex utero intrapartum therapy.
Modified from McElhinney DB et al: Current status of fetal cardiac intervention, *Circulation* 121:1256–1263, 2010; Partridge EA, Flake AW: Maternal-fetal surgery for structural malformations, *Best Pract Res Clin Obstet Gynaecol* 26:669–682, 2012; Children's Hospital of Philadelphia (CHOP): *Center for fetal diagnosis and treatment: fetal intervention and diagnosis,* available at www.chop.edu/service/fetal-diagnosis-and-treatment/fetal-diagnoses. Accessed December 24, 2012.

room for error (2012). Perioperative nurses must also possess knowledge of fetal resuscitation medications as they prepare the field for any emergency.

Preparation of the fetal surgery OR is extensive, and usually involves multiple setups and specialized instrumentation and equipment. The concept of teamwork is of utmost importance because the multidisciplinary approach to care extends into the OR. Multiple attending surgeons participate in the very small surgical field, and the procedures are performed within a short window of operating time. EXIT procedures necessitate an additional scrub and circulator team, who assume responsibility for supporting the fetal airway during bronchoscopy, intubation, and tracheostomy.

Similar to any surgical procedure, perioperative team members who care for patients undergoing fetal surgery must be able to demonstrate critical judgment, organization, and prioritization skills. Circulating nurses and scrub persons who choose to participate in fetal surgery cases receive additional, specialized, simulation-based training that is both case and equipment specific. Precepted experiences in the circulating and scrub role are beneficial in promoting skill acquisition and competency achievement for fetal surgeries, which are considered a low-volume, high-risk surgery.

Minimally Invasive Fetal Surgery

TTTS can be treated by amnioreduction and placental laser ablation. Bipolar cord coagulation (BCC) and radiofrequency ablation (RFA) are used to treat TTTS when the at-risk twin faces imminent demise. Regardless of the type of fetoscopic procedure, mothers who have fetuses with TTTS receive monitored anesthesia care (MAC; light intravenous sedation), antibiotics and an infiltration of a local anesthetic at the surgery site. Surgery is performed using continuous ultrasound guidance.

When TTTS is treated using selective placental laser coagulation, the recipient twin undergoes amnioreduction by needle aspiration prior to inserting a fetoscopic sheath. The fetoscopic sheath is attached to a rapid fluid infusion warmer or pump and has a side port that accommodates a diode laser fiber. The fetoscope is inserted into the amniotic cavity of the recipient twin and is directed to the placental cord insertion site using ultrasound guidance. The branching vessels are followed in the direction of the donor twin until the collapsed inter-twin membrane is identified. Blood vessels crossing from the donor side across the collapsed inter-twin membrane are mapped. Vascular anastomoses with the recipient twin side are laser photocoagulated on continuous power with 0.5- to 1-second power bursts. After completion of the first pass, the region is remapped and reevaluated to identify additional anastomoses, and the process is repeated until no additional anastomoses are identified. The laser is removed and amnioreduction is completed on the recipient twin. Antibiotics are infused into the amniotic space, and the insertion site on the uterine wall is assessed for bleeding and membrane separation. The maternal stab wound is approximated and closed with cyanoacrylate glue and covered with a transparent dressing. Postoperatively, fetal heartbeats are confirmed and assessed in both twins using ultrasound and Doppler velocimetry.

Fetal intervention continues to be studied in fetuses with cardiac conditions such as aortic stenosis (AS) with evolving hypoplastic left heart syndrome (HLHS) (Tworetsky et al, 2004). The complexity of the procedure determines whether IV sedation with local infiltration at the surgery site or general anesthesia is used. A mini-laparotomy without hysterotomy provides imaging or access to perform an aortic valvuloplasty to alter the in utero history of AS with evolving HLHS (McElhinney et al, 2010). The end

result of percutaneous intervention alters left heart physiology and growth and allows postnatal survival with biventricular circulation (McElhinney et al, 2010). Postnatal repair of HLHS is described in a later section of this chapter detailing surgery for congenital heart disease.

The type of surgery and degree of intervention dictate how long a mother remains hospitalized after surgery. For example, typically a 4-day length of stay is incurred after open fetal surgery, whereas for a fetoscopic procedure, mothers stay overnight, then stay at a nearby facility such as a local Ronald McDonald House and return in a week. If all is well, they are then discharged to home. After discharge the mother is instructed to remain on bed rest for 2 weeks, and activity is restricted for an additional 3 to 4 weeks. Activity may be gradually increased if there are no concerns noted during follow-up appointments. Mothers are provided with discharge instructions including information regarding medications, preterm labor, and recovery.

Open Fetal Surgery

Mothers undergoing open fetal surgery or an EXIT procedure require deep general anesthesia in order to provide uterine relaxation to prevent placental abruption. These mothers also receive antibiotics and an epidural prior to incision. Examples of diagnoses in which open fetal surgical procedures may be indicated include CCAM in the presence of hydrops, sacrococcygeal teratoma (SCT) with high-output cardiac failure, and MMC (Figures 26-7 and 26-8) (Research Highlight). CCAMs grow primarily between 20 and 28 weeks' gestation, and may jeopardize maternal health ("maternal mirror" syndrome), in which the mother's condition mirrors that of the sick fetus. In cases of maternal mirror syndrome, the only cure is delivery. Frequent ultrasound follow-up provides critical information about growth of the mass and is able to detect early development of hydrops. The CCAM volume ratio (CVR) can determine the likelihood of hydrops developing (Box 26-4). If the mass remains large, but no hydrops develops then an EXIT procedure or cesarean section to mass resection may be warranted. Postnatal repair of SCT and MMC are described later in this chapter.

Open fetal surgery is performed using a low, transverse maternal laparotomy to expose the uterus. A sterile ultrasound probe is then used to map the placental edges to identify the uterine hysterotomy

FIGURE 26-7 The exposed fetal myelomeningocele.

FIGURE 26-8 Completed fetal myelomeningocele repair.

BOX 26-4

Congenital Cystic Adenomatoid Malformation (CCAM) Volume Ratio (CVR)

The CVR is a measurement of prolate ellipse first described at the Children's Hospital of Philadelphia. Today it is used throughout the United States to determine the likelihood of hydrops for CCAM.

$$CVR = CCAM\ volume\ (length \times width \times height \times 0.52)/\\ head\ circumference\ (all\ measurements\ in\ cm)$$

A CVR less than 1.6 predicts a low likelihood of developing hydrops. A CVR greater than 1.6 is associated with a 75% chance of developing hydrops.

From Partridge EA, Flake AW: Maternal-fetal surgery for structural malformations, *Best Pract Res Clin Obstet Gynaecol* 26:669–682, 2012.

RESEARCH HIGHLIGHT

Fetal Myelomeningocele Repair

Myelomeningocele (MMC) is the most serious form of spina bifida. Beginning in the late 1980s and early 1990s fetal surgeons set out to test the hypothesis whether fetal MMC repair would improve postnatal morbidity including hydrocephalus, bowel and bladder problems, and mobility. Animal models were created to elucidate the mechanical issues and toxic effects of amniotic fluid and whether the sequelae associated with MMC were ameliorated by fetal surgery. Simultaneously, postnatal outcomes were followed for those babies undergoing postnatal repair. Experimental work showed hindbrain herniation or the Arnold-Chiari malformation to be reversed, obviating the need for a ventriculoperitoneal (VP) shunt. Once rigorous animal studies demonstrated an improvement in outcome after fetal surgery, and clinical follow-up described the natural history of MMC, healthy women of selected fetuses with MMC in whom a benefit could be shown were offered fetal surgery. After reporting positive outcomes for this fetal surgery, a multi-center trial was funded.

The Management of Myelomeningocele Study (MOMS), funded by the Eunice Kennedy Shriver National Institute of Child Health and Human Development (NICHD), was designed to compare the outcomes of two approaches to treating MMC: prenatal surgery and postnatal surgery. Three clinical centers participated in the MOMS trial: Children's Hospital of Philadelphia (CHOP), Vanderbilt University, and University of California San Francisco (UCSF) Medical Center. George Washington University served as the data coordinating center. All other U.S. prenatal diagnosis and treatment centers who considered performing fetal surgery for MMC intervention agreed not to perform this surgery until the trial was completed.

Any woman (age 18 or older) interested in learning more about the study contacted the coordinating center. Once educated about the trial, determining eligibility, and deciding to participate, these women were referred to a MOMS clinical center in their geographic region. Each subject was required to enroll in the study by her twenty-fifth week of pregnancy and was randomly assigned to fetal or postnatal surgery. Proposed study enrollment was 200 subjects, with the intent to enroll 100 subjects in each group.

After evaluation at one of the clinical centers was completed, and the women agreed to participate, they were randomized to either the prenatal or postnatal group. Mothers assigned to the prenatal intervention group underwent fetal surgery for MMC repair between the nineteenth and twenty-fifth completed week of gestation at the assigned MOMS center. Mothers assigned to the postnatal intervention group returned home and received care from their regular obstetrician until 37 weeks' gestation, at which time they returned to their assigned MOMS center for cesarean delivery after lung maturity was confirmed, but delivery occurred no later than 37 weeks. Babies born to mothers in the postnatal group underwent closure of MMC by the MOMS neurosurgeon. Postnatal repair of myelomeningocele is described in the Neurosurgery section of this chapter.

All participants agreed to return to their assigned MOMS center at 12 and 30 months for follow-up. A psychosocial questionnaire was administered, and motor function and developmental progress were evaluated as well as bladder, kidney, and brain development in order to determine whether the outcome was better with prenatal or postnatal surgery. Follow-up assessments for both groups were done by a team of specialists blinded to the assignment of each participant and independent from the clinical centers.

The MOMS trial was stopped due to efficacy on December 7, 2010, after 183 of the planned 200 patients were randomized and underwent either prenatal or postnatal repair. The authors found that 40% of children whose deformity was corrected with fetal surgery required a VP shunt for hydrocephalus during the first 12 months of life, compared with 82% of children who received surgery postnatally. Moreover, by 30 months, 42% of children who had undergone fetal surgery were able to walk without orthotics or assistive devices as opposed to 21% of children in the postnatal repair group. Although prenatal surgery reduced the need for VP shunting and improved motor outcomes at 30 months, there is significant maternal risk. Ongoing work with the MOMS trial subjects will report bladder and bowel outcomes as well as neurocognitive development at 6 to 9 years of age.

Modified from Adzick N et al: A randomized trial of prenatal versus postnatal repair of myelomeningocele, *N Engl J Med* 364(11):993–1004, 2011.

FIGURE 26-9 Specially designed stapler used to quickly open the uterus during fetal surgery.

site. The uterine hysterotomy is performed using a uterine stapling device that has absorbable staples and allows the thickened mid-gestation uterus to be opened bloodlessly (Figure 26-9). (This type of incision requires a cesarean section delivery for this and all subsequent pregnancies.) Fetal oxygen saturation is monitored using pulse oximetry on the exposed limb. The fetus receives an IV line and an intramuscular shot of muscle relaxant and narcotic. Throughout the surgery the uterine cavity is continually filled with lactated Ringer's solution warmed to 98.6°F (37°C). A rapid infusion warmer and pump is used to maintain adequate uterine volume and to prevent umbilical cord compression and potential placental abruption. Postoperatively, preterm labor is of great concern, and uterine contractions, fetal heart rate, and fetal ECG are continually monitored. Tocolytic medications are titrated to control uterine contractions. The mother is educated in self-monitoring of uterine contractions, and tocolytic therapy is continued on an outpatient basis. Frequent fetal ultrasounds are performed postoperatively to monitor fetal well-being, amniotic fluid volume, and the adequacy of surgical repair.

Ex Utero Intrapartum Treatment

In cases in which the prenatal diagnosis confirms difficulty in obtaining a fetal airway (such as in giant neck masses) or difficulty ventilating a baby (such as in large CCAMs), the EXIT procedure may be warranted. After placing the epidural, the anesthesia provider administers antibiotics and deep general anesthesia. The surgeon then performs a maternal laparotomy and hysterotomy. Every attempt is made to use a stapling device to create an extended low-transverse incision. (This type of incision allows the mother to deliver vaginally for subsequent deliveries.)

Only the affected area of the fetus is delivered through the hysterotomy—the entire fetus is not entirely exposed. Fetal oxygen saturation is monitored using pulse oximetry on the exposed limb. The fetus receives an IV line and an intramuscular shot of muscle relaxant and narcotic. Fetuses are generally able to be maintained on placental circulation for approximately 45 to 60 minutes (Howell et al, 2002; Partridge and Flake, 2012), which allows time to obtain, establish, and secure the fetal airway and place umbilical arterial and venous lines. In emergent situations, resection of the tumor may be completed (Howell et al, 2002) before dividing the

cord and delivering the baby (Laje et al, 2012). The placenta is removed and residual blood clots are cleared, the hysterotomy and the maternal laparotomy are closed, and a sterile dressing is applied. After the baby is removed from placental support, he or she is taken to a stabilization room for resuscitation or to the adjacent OR for immediate surgical mass resection specific to diagnosis and related condition.

General Surgery—Gastrointestinal Procedures

Repair of Atresia of the Esophagus

Esophageal atresia is a congenital anomaly that may develop between the third and sixth weeks of fetal life. Several types are recognized, the most common being an upper segment of esophagus ending in a blind pouch and a lower segment of esophagus communicating by a fistula with the trachea (esophageal atresia with TEF). Ideally this defect is recognized in the first hours of life, but more often the diagnosis is made in the first 36 to 48 hours of life. Hallmark indicators of esophageal atresia include excessive salivation, choking during feeds, and the inability to pass a suction catheter more than 10 cm into the esophagus (Broemling and Campbell, 2011). Prompt surgical intervention allows the child to breathe and eat without the danger of aspirating mucus, saliva, feedings, or stomach contents. Atresia of the esophagus is repaired through a right retropleural thoracotomy, with closure of the TEF and anastomosis of the segments of the esophagus.

Procedural Considerations. A bronchoscopy is performed to promote accurate placement of the endotracheal tube before surgical repair. Additionally a gastrostomy may be done first to decompress the air-distended stomach, thus facilitating chest movement and ventilation and preventing reflux of stomach contents into the trachea. The team then positions the patient for a right thoracotomy (sometimes rather posteriorly) and preps, and drapes. The major instrument set and a thoracotomy set are required with the appropriate size of chest tube and infant chest drainage system.

Operative Procedure

1. The surgeon enters the chest through the fourth intercostal space. Removal of the rib is not necessary (Figure 26-10, *A*).
2. The pleura is gently dissected off the chest wall (see Figure 26-10, *B*).
3. As the dissection proceeds posteriorly, the azygos vein is identified, which is reflected inferiorly after its highest intercostal branches are divided to expose the fistula beneath (see Figure 26-10, *C*).
4. The surgeon passes an umbilical tape or vessel loop under the fistula to apply traction gently (see Figure 26-10, *D*). Dissection of the mediastinum begins with the TEF and distal end of the esophagus. The vagus nerve is an important landmark for the distal end of the esophagus.
5. The fistula is clamped and transected, leaving a thin cuff of esophageal tissue on the tracheal side to allow closure of the trachea without narrowing it and compromising the lumen of the airway (see Figure 26-10, *E*).
6. To close the fistula, three or four interrupted atraumatic sutures of 5-0 nonabsorbable suture are used.
7. The upper esophageal pouch is dissected; passage of a nasogastric tube by the anesthesia provider aids in its identification. The proximal pouch is identified and dissected as needed to allow it to reach the distal esophageal segment with minimal

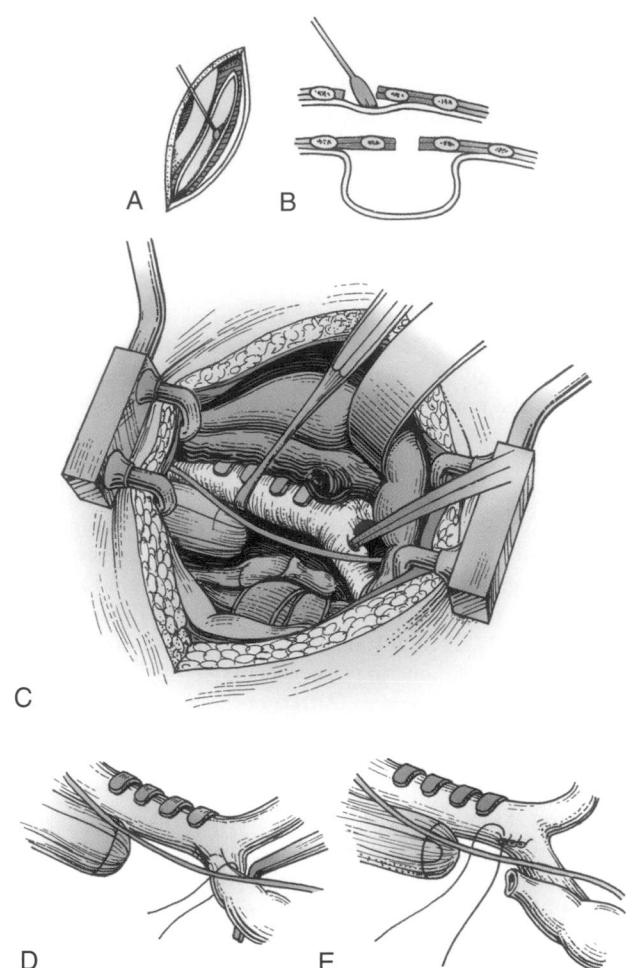

FIGURE 26-10 Repair of atresia of the esophagus. **A,** Incision at fourth intercostal space. **B,** Dissection of pleura off chest wall. **C,** Identification and division of azygos vein to expose fistula beneath. **D,** Traction applied to fistula. **E,** Transection of fistula leaving 3-mm cuff on trachea.

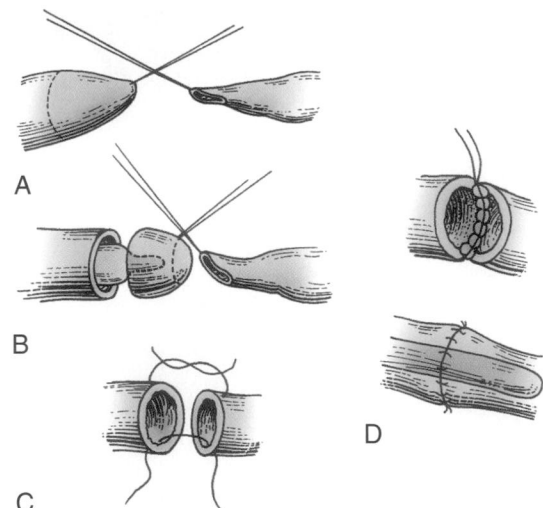

FIGURE 26-11 Primary repair of atresia of the esophagus: single-layer repair. **A,** Traction applied to proximal and distal portions of esophagus. **B,** Blind proximal pouch transected. **C,** Full-thickness bites of anterior and posterior borders. **D,** Repair completed with Replogle tube in place to allow adequate lumen of esophagus.

FIGURE 26-12 Haight anastomosis. Mucosal layer of proximal pouch sutured to full thickness of distal esophagus. Muscular sleeve of upper pouch pulled down over inner anastomosis and sutured to muscle of distal esophagus.

tension for anastomosis. At this point the surgeon decides whether to attempt primary anastomosis. If primary anastomosis is impossible, the distal esophagus is closed and tacked high on the prevertebral fascia. Infrequently the gap between the proximal and distal portions of esophagus is so long that esophageal replacement is required. In these cases the upper pouch is brought out to the neck in the form of a cervical esophagostomy.

8. Primary anastomosis is performed with 5-0 or 6-0 nonabsorbable suture, taking full-thickness bites along anterior and posterior borders (Figure 26-11). Some surgeons prefer the Haight, or two-layer, anastomosis (Figure 26-12). The inner layer is composed of the upper pouch mucosa sutured to the full thickness of the distal esophagus. The muscular sleeve of the upper esophagus is then pulled down over the inner anastomosis and sutured to the muscular layer of the inferior esophagus. The incision is irrigated with saline.

9. Some surgeons place a 14 French (F) or 16F extrapleural chest tube near the anastomosis through a posterior stab wound. It is secured with sutures to prevent it from putting direct pressure on the anastomosis.

10. Muscle layers and fascia are closed with nonabsorbable suture.
11. The skin is closed with a continuous absorbable suture. The incision is approximated with cyanoacrylate glue or topical skin adhesive and wound closure strips.
12. The extrapleural chest tube is water-sealed after ensuring that the number of centimeters of water and the suction-control chamber are appropriate for the size of the infant. A postoperative chest x-ray is obtained.

When the child reaches 1 year of age, esophageal replacement is attempted through colon interposition or construction of a reverse gastric tube (Figure 26-13).

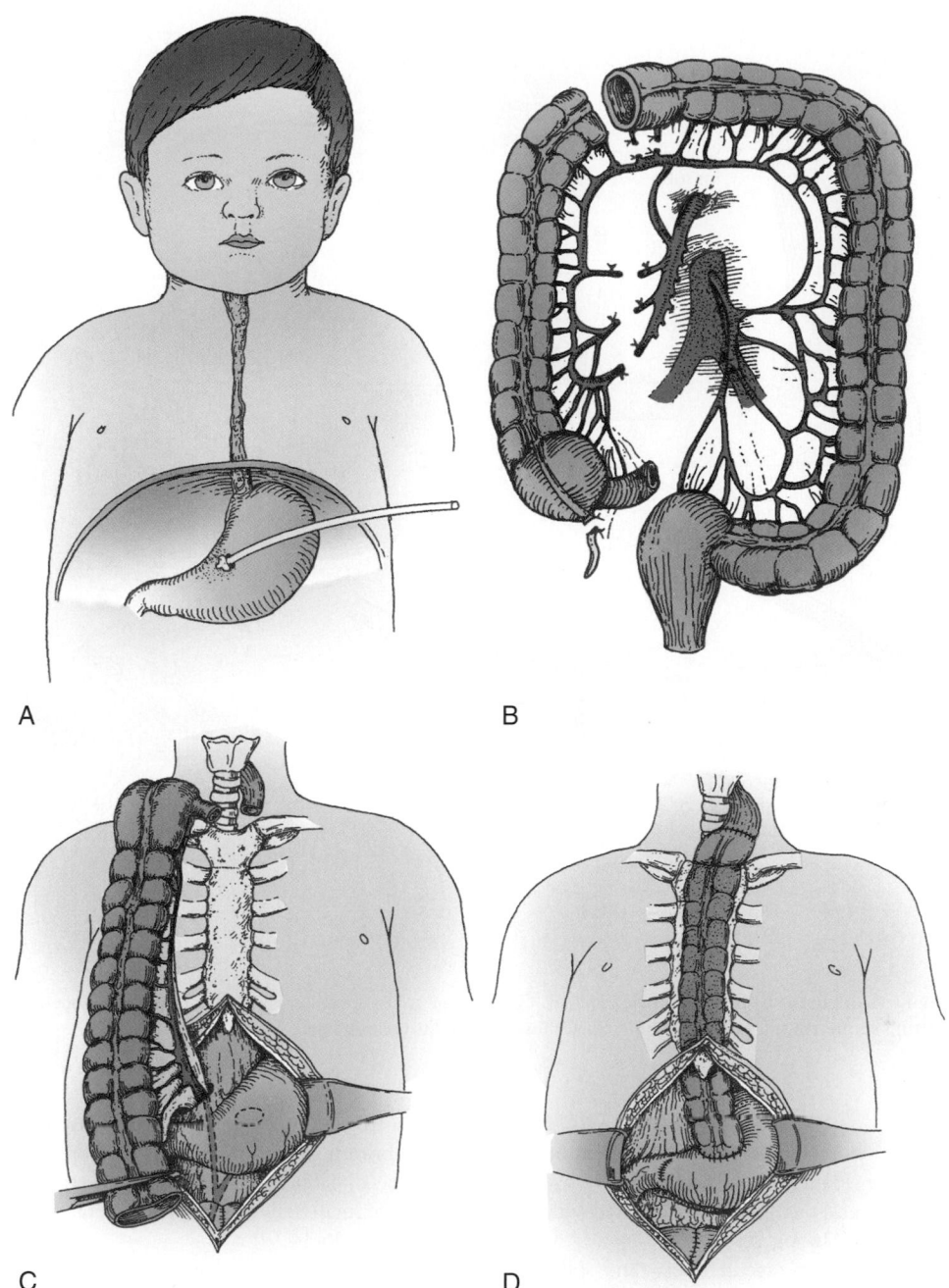

A

B

C

D

FIGURE 26-13 Esophageal replacement. **A,** Gastrostomy. **B,** Isolation of right colon and ileum. **C,** Colon pedicle prepared for anastomosis. **D,** Anastomosis.

Gastrostomy

Gastrostomy is establishment of a temporary or permanent channel from the gastric lumen to the skin to permit gastric emptying, liquid feeding, or retrograde dilation of an esophageal stricture. The procedure may be completed as a separate procedure or be performed with other surgical procedures to facilitate care of the patient after surgery. A growing number of surgeons are inserting low-profile (e.g., button, Gastroport) devices on initial creation of the gastrostomy because these are preferred for children receiving long-term feedings through the device. Low-profile devices, which protrude slightly from the abdomen, are more cosmetically acceptable and

allow more mobility for the child. A gastrostomy tube can be placed in the OR as an open or laparoscopic procedure, or it can be performed as a percutaneous procedure under fluoroscopy; both require the patient to receive a general anesthetic. The open surgical procedure is described in the following section.

Procedural Considerations. A minor instrument set is required, plus a gastrostomy feeding catheter (generally a 14F or 16F for infants, or an 18F, 20F, or 22F for older children) and a #11 blade on a knife handle. A variety of latex-free gastrostomy catheters are available.

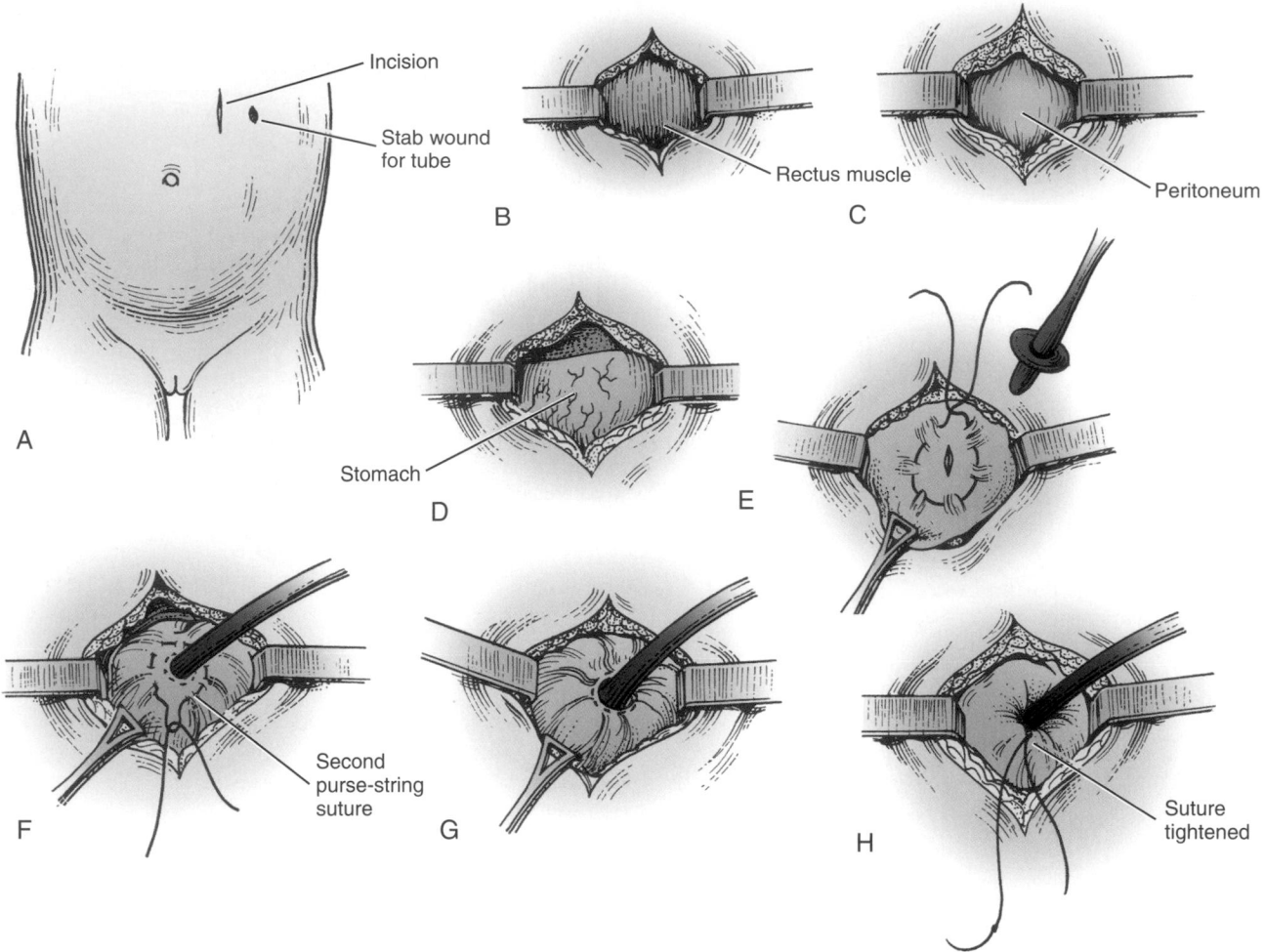

FIGURE 26-14 Gastrostomy. **A,** Incision. **B,** Rectus muscle exposed. **C,** Posterior rectus sheath exposed. **D,** Peritoneum opened. **E,** Purse-string suture placed. **F,** Second purse-string suture placed. **G,** Mushroom catheter inserted. **H,** Suture tightened.

Operative Procedure

1. The surgeon makes a short incision over the outer border of the left rectus muscle (Figure 26-14, *A*).
2. The subcutaneous tissues and rectus fascia are exposed with two small retractors (see Figure 26-14, *B*).
3. The surgeon opens the anterior rectus fascia, and splits the rectus muscle for exposure of the posterior rectus sheath (see Figure 26-14, *C*).
4. The peritoneum is opened for exposure of the liver edge and the greater curvature of the stomach (see Figure 26-14, *D*).
5. The surgeon pulls the stomach out through the wound with Babcock forceps. A circular, nonabsorbable purse-string suture is placed: in the center of this a very small incision is made with the #11 blade through the gastric wall (see Figure 26-14, *E*).
6. A second purse-string suture is placed outside the first one, and the same needle is then taken through the peritoneum and the posterior surface of the rectus fascia to place the stomach against the peritoneum and thus prevent leaks (see Figure 26-14, *F* and *G*).
7. The feeding catheter is inserted into the stomach through the small incision, and the purse-string suture is tied (see Figure 26-14, *H*). Some surgeons may choose to use a dilator kit to assist with proper insertion of the tube. When inserting a

gastrostomy tube with a balloon, sterile water and water-based lubricant should be used to avoid breakdown of the tube itself.
8. The surgeon exteriorizes the catheter through the skin by way of a small stab wound left, lateral to the skin incision (see Figure 26-14, *A*).
9. The stomach wall adjacent to the gastrostomy site is tacked to the undersurface of the peritoneum with interrupted nonabsorbable sutures.
10. Routine abdominal closure is performed. The gastrostomy tube is left open to straight drainage at the end of the surgical procedure.

Reduction of Intussusception

Intussusception is the telescopic invagination of a portion of intestine into an adjacent part, with mechanical and vascular impairment (Figure 26-15). The most common site for intussusception is the ileocecal junction. Intussusception in most children is idiopathic; in others, causes may include Meckel diverticulum, polyps, or hematoma of the bowel. Intussusception is the most common cause of small bowel obstruction in children (Fraser et al, 2009). It is relieved by reduction of invaginated bowel by the hydrostatic pressure of a barium enema or by laparotomy and manual manipulation. Laparoscopy may prove effective in some cases (Fraser et al,

FIGURE 26-15 Operative view of intussusception.

FIGURE 26-16 Manual reduction of intussusception.

2009). Early diagnosis and reduction are essential to bowel viability.

Procedural Considerations. The child is prepped for surgery as described previously. Reduction by barium enema is attempted only with the collaboration of the radiologist, surgeon, and pediatrician, with the OR team on standby. If reduction is unsuccessful, a surgical reduction by laparotomy or laparoscopy must be performed. The open procedure requires a major instrument set and pediatric bowel clamps.

Operative Procedure

1. The surgeon makes a right lower quadrant transverse or right paramedian incision and enters the peritoneum.
2. The cecum and ileum are identified; the intussusception is located and elevated with fingers.
3. If there is no evidence of bowel compromise, the bowel immediately distal to the intussusception is occluded with one hand and stripped proximally with the other in an attempt to achieve manual reduction (Figure 26-16). If the serosa splits during

attempted reduction or if the mass cannot be reduced, bowel resection is done.
4. The abdomen is closed in layers, and the wound is dressed.

Bowel Resection and Colostomy for Necrotizing Enterocolitis

Necrotizing enterocolitis (NEC) is a condition that manifests with death of intestinal lining and sloughing of corresponding tissues. Its exact cause is unknown, but it is suspected that NEC may result from two mechanisms: decreased blood flow to the bowel, which prevents the bowel from secreting the protective mucus that protects the GI tract; or bacteria within the intestine (Medline Plus Medical Encyclopedia, 2011). NEC primarily affects premature newborns. When surgical intervention is needed, the patient undergoes a bowel resection and ostomy procedure. The type of ostomy created depends on the location of the necrotic bowel. The procedures for bowel resection and colostomy are described in the following sections.

Procedural Considerations. The major instrument set and pediatric bowel clamps are required. The infant is positioned supine, and routine prepping and draping of the abdomen are done.

Bowel Resection

Operative Procedure

1. The surgeon makes an abdominal incision.
2. The intestines are explored to determine the location of the obstruction. The surgeon must examine the entire bowel to rule out multiple areas of involvement in patients with atresia or stenosis. If aganglionosis of the colon is suspected, sequential biopsy specimens are sent fresh immediately to the pathology laboratory to determine the segment of large bowel to be resected.
3. Resection is performed as indicated.

Colostomy

Operative Procedure

1. A transverse incision usually is preferred, and the abdomen is entered in the right upper quadrant for a transverse colostomy or the left lower quadrant for a sigmoid colostomy.
2. The loop of colon is freed of peritoneal attachments until it can be brought easily through the abdominal wall without tension.
3. The surgeon sutures the edges of the mesentery to the parietal peritoneum, and the serosa of the colonic loop is sutured with fine absorbable suture materials to the peritoneum and fascia as well as to the skin.
4. The colostomy may be sutured immediately. Some surgeons prefer to close the skin under a colostomy loop; others prefer to suture mucosa directly to skin edges. This decision may depend on the location of the colostomy. An important point is that each layer must be securely attached to the serosa of the colon to prevent evisceration and prolapse. The posterior wall of a loop colostomy may be divided by electrosurgery several days after surgery.

Resection and Pull-Through for Hirschsprung Disease (Reconstruction)

Hirschsprung disease is characterized by the absence of ganglion cells in a distal portion of the bowel. The distal colon is more frequently involved, but the disease may encompass the entire colon, with a less favorable prognosis. The absence of ganglion cells results in a lack of peristalsis. The normal proximal colon becomes dilated with stool because intestinal contents do not pass through the involved segment normally. The child presents with an abnormally distended abdomen. Barium enema reveals proximal distention of the colon and then a transition zone where the bowel appears funnel-shaped, followed by the distal aganglionic segment, which is narrowed. The child is taken to the OR for a leveling colostomy (a colostomy placed at the level at which ganglion cells begin and where there are no hypertrophic nerves). Multiple frozen-section biopsy specimens from the muscularis of the proximal portion of the colon are taken to determine the presence of ganglion cells. The colostomy is performed at the most distal portion of the colon that contains ganglion cells. Some surgeons prefer a routine right transverse colostomy at this time and delay frozen-section biopsy specimens until the time of the definitive procedure. Resection and pull-through for Hirschsprung disease, the definitive surgical procedure, consists of the removal of the aganglionic portion of the bowel and anastomosis of the normal colon to the anus. The child is returned to the OR for the definitive repair at 1 year of age if clinical and nutritional status permits.

Several surgical techniques have been devised. The procedure may be done laparoscopically or by an open approach. The Soave procedure of endorectal pull-through uses internal bypass of the involved segment. The internal sphincter muscle of the anus is kept intact for continence.

Procedural Considerations. The patient is prepped and draped from the nipples down to and including the buttocks, genitalia, perineal area, and upper thighs to permit positioning for the perineal stage without redraping. (Before prepping, the rectum may be irrigated with warm saline solution.) An indwelling catheter is inserted to keep the bladder empty during the operation. The major instrument set, a minor instrument set, and pediatric intestinal clamps are needed.

Operative Procedure

1. A left paramedian incision that includes the sigmoid colonic stoma, if present, is made.
2. The surgeon frees the stoma from the abdominal wall, and mobilizes the left portion of the colon. (If there is no sigmoid colonic stoma, the extent of aganglionic intestine is established by biopsy and frozen section, and all involved colon is excised. If a stoma is present and the area has already been established as normal, the colon above it constitutes the proximal end of the resection.)

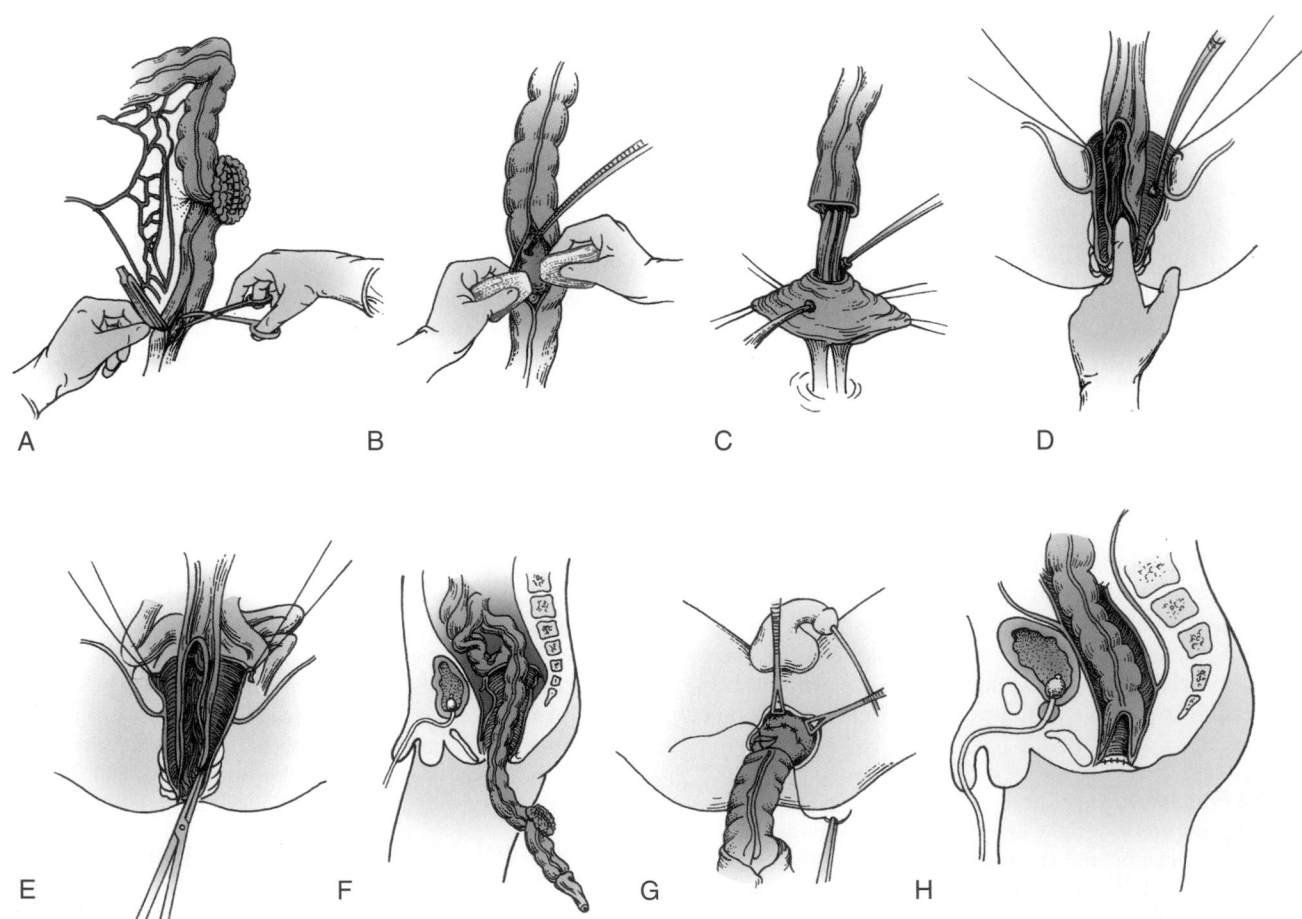

FIGURE 26-17 Pull-through for Hirschsprung disease. **A,** Dissection of mucosal tube begun through longitudinal incision. **B,** Blunt dissection with sponges used to dissect entire circumference of tube. **C,** Muscular sleeve transected. **D,** Depth of dissection determined by insertion of finger into anus. **E,** Circumferential incision made. **F,** Mucosal tube and proximal portion of colon and stoma pulled through rectal muscular cuff. **G,** Anastomosis performed among all layers of colon and anal mucosa. **H,** Anastomosis completed.

3. The mesocolon and the vessels of the intestine to be resected are divided close to the intestine, with care taken to preserve the blood supply to the rectum (Figure 26-17, *A*).

4. The mucosal tube is freed from the outer muscular layers by sharp dissection with Metzenbaum scissors and blunt dissection (see Figure 26-17, *B*).

5. A muscular sleeve is transected, and 4-0 nonabsorbable traction sutures are placed on the distal edge (see Figure 26-17, *C*). The mucosa is stripped down to the anus. The depth of the dissection may be checked by inserting a finger into the anus (see Figure 26-17, *D*).

6. When the mucosa is adequately freed, the perineal phase is started and the perineal instrument table is used.

7. The surgeon dilates the anus and retracts it with Allis forceps. A circumferential incision is made, and the mucosal stripping is completed (see Figure 26-17, *E*).

8. The proximal portion of the intestine is pulled through the rectal muscular sleeve and out the anus (see Figure 26-17, *F*). If the portion of colon to be resected is large, it is excised abdominally before the proximal portion of the intestine is pulled through the anus.

9. Absorbable sutures are used to secure the seromuscular layers of the intussuscepted colon to the rectal muscular cuff. The surgeon divides the colon into axial or longitudinal quadrants, and an anastomosis is performed with 3-0 absorbable sutures (see Figure 26-17, *G*).

10. Gowns and gloves are changed, and abdominal instruments are used. The abdominal phase of the operation is completed by approximating the proximal edge of the muscular cuff to the seromuscular layer of the colon with 4-0 nonabsorbable sutures (see Figure 26-17, *H*). The abdomen is closed in the routine manner, without the use of drains.

Repair of Imperforate Anus

Congenital imperforate anus (Figure 26-18) presents in a variety of forms, classified as low, intermediate, and high lesions, depending on how far the pelvis descends into the rectum. Baby girls commonly have low lesions, and baby boys primarily exhibit intermediate or high lesions. A covered anus and anovulvar fistula is an example of a low lesion. Intermediate and high lesions consist of a blind rectal pouch, a "flat bottom," and a posterior urethral fistula or a fistula to the bladder. This type is the most prevalent and the most difficult to repair. An imperforate anus is repaired by establishing colorectoanal continuity through the external anal sphincter and closure of fistulas, if present.

Repair of Low Imperforate Anus in a Girl—Anal Transposition
Procedural Considerations. The patient is placed in the lithotomy position. A Foley catheter is inserted, and the perineum is prepped and draped. The major instrument set is required, with the addition of both a nerve and a muscle stimulator. The anesthesia provider must avoid the use of neuromuscular blocking agents for the nerve and muscle stimulator to work during the surgical procedure.

Operative Procedure
1. An electrical stimulator is applied to elicit muscle contractions and serve as a guide to the midline of the anus. The goal is to leave equal innervated tissue on both sides of the anus so that the child will be continent of stool.

2. Stay sutures are placed in the fistula, and it is excised using an oval incision (Figure 26-19, *A*).

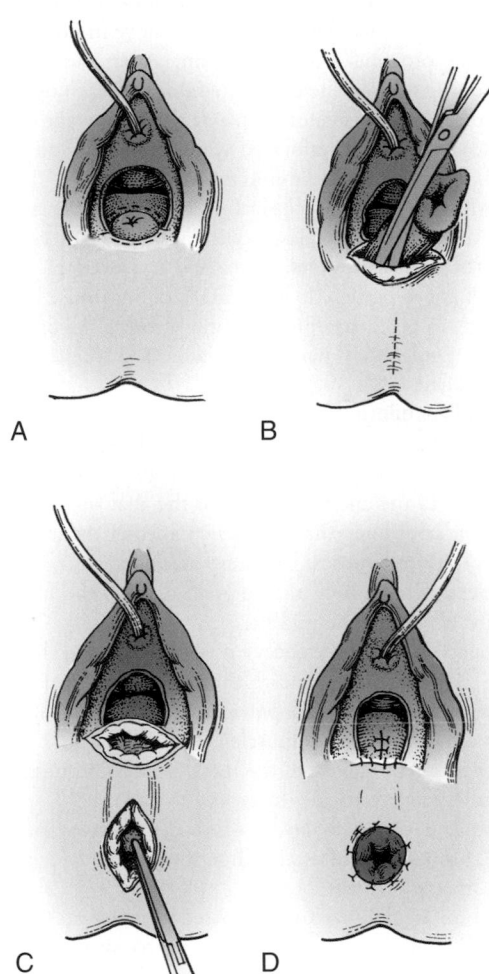

FIGURE 26-19 Anal transposition. **A,** Fistula excised by means of oval incision. **B,** Dissection of bowel from surrounding structures. **C,** Vertical midline incision at site of true anus; identification of external sphincter fibers; mobilized rectum pulled down through subcutaneous tissue to new location. **D,** External sphincter sutured to rectal mucosa; new anus constructed with interrupted sutures through all layers.

FIGURE 26-18 Imperforate anus.

3. The surgeon dissects the bowel free from surrounding structures, taking care not to damage the vagina (see Figure 26-19, *B*).
4. When the dissection is complete, a vertical midline incision is performed at the opening of the true anus and the fibers of the external sphincter are identified (see Figure 26-19, *C*).
5. The mobilized rectum is pulled down through the subcutaneous tissue to its new location.
6. The surgeon amputates the end of the fistula. Using 4-0 nonabsorbable interrupted sutures, the surgeon sutures the external sphincter to the rectal serosa.
7. Using 4-0 absorbable suture, the surgeon constructs a new anus with interrupted sutures through all layers (see Figure 26-19, *D*).
8. A drain may or may not be placed in the anterior incision before it is closed in layers with interrupted 4-0 absorbable sutures.
9. Using a Hegar dilator, the surgeon calibrates the size of the new anus after closure.

Repair of Intermediate or High Imperforate Anus—Posterior Sagittal Anorectoplasty.

When an intermediate or high imperforate anal anomaly presents, surgical intervention is indicated within 24 to 48 hours of birth. A transverse or sigmoid colostomy is performed to irrigate the hiatal lumen and to remove meconium plugs while allowing proximal colon function. After the colostomy, further diagnostic studies, such as cystograms and vaginograms, are done. The posterior sagittal anorectoplasty (PSARP) is the definitive surgical procedure and is performed when the condition and size of the child permit—usually around 1 year of age.

The PSARP is a highly technical procedure that uses electrostimulation throughout and may require position changes.

Procedural Considerations. The child is placed in jackknife position with the hips flexed. Adequate padding must be placed under the hips to avoid compression injury to the femoral nerves. The major instrument set, nerve stimulator, and intestinal instruments are required.

Operative Procedure (Figure 26-20)

1. The surgeon uses the electrostimulator to locate the true anus, and makes a midsagittal incision through the skin from the midsacrum to the anterior border of the anal site.
2. Dissection continues through subcutaneous tissue until the external sphincter muscle layers are identified.
3. With electrostimulation, the surgeon dissects the fibers midsagittally, exactly in the midline.
4. A midsagittal split of the coccyx is performed, and the striated muscle complex found beneath the coccyx is incised sagittally, along with the visceral endopelvic fascia. Electrostimulation is used to aid in identifying muscle complexes.
5. Next, the surgeon identifies the rectal pouch and urethra, and incises the bowel vertically to expose the fistulas.
6. The fistula is closed in layers—first the mucosa with interrupted absorbable sutures and then the muscle layer with 5-0 nonabsorbable sutures.
7. The rectum is mobilized and tapered to allow its placement within the muscle complexes. Tapering consists of excising a wedge of bowel from either the ventral or the dorsal surface. The edges are approximated, and the mucosal layer is closed with 5-0 absorbable interrupted sutures. The muscularis layer is closed with interrupted 5-0 nonabsorbable sutures.
8. Again using electrostimulation, the tapered rectum is placed deep within the muscle complex. Then 5-0 nonabsorbable sutures are used to reconstruct the muscles. The seromuscular

layer of the bowel is incorporated into these sutures to keep it securely positioned within the muscle complex.
9. The external sphincter muscles and coccyx are reapproximated.
10. Excess bowel is trimmed before it is secured to the skin edges of the anus.
11. The surgeon closes the skin with running absorbable subcuticular sutures.

In cases of very high rectal pouches and fistulas, an abdominal approach may be required. After the midsagittal incisions and dissections are completed, a rubber drain is placed through the pelvis with one end in the peritoneal cavity and the other through the center of the anus to the skin, where it is temporarily sutured. The child is then turned supine, and an abdominal incision is made. The rectal pouch is mobilized, and the fistula is closed. The bowel is tapered as described previously, and the terminal portion is attached to the rubber tube, which then is used to pull the rectum through the anal orifice. The bowel is sutured to the muscle complex, and reapproximation of the coccyx and external sphincter muscle is done as described earlier.

General Surgery—Hernias

Umbilical Hernia Repair

Umbilical hernias are frequently seen in pediatric populations and are more common in African American children and low-birthweight children (Carlo, 2011). These hernias are also common in premature infants and are corrected by repair of the defect where the intestine protrudes at the umbilicus. An umbilical hernia is always covered by skin. Small umbilical hernias may be left untreated. They usually close within a few months to 1 year. If surgical repair is required in a large fascial defect, it may be delayed until the child is at least 2 years of age; some surgeons delay repair until 5 years of age.

Procedural Considerations. Surgical correction of umbilical hernia may be an ambulatory surgical procedure. A general anesthetic is used. A minor instrument set is required. Several variations in technique have been used; an infraumbilical approach is most common, and its description follows.

Operative Procedure

1. An incision is made below the umbilicus through the skin and subcutaneous tissue.
2. Flaps of skin and subcutaneous tissue are mobilized and held back with small retractors to expose the rectus fascia and hernial protrusion.
3. The hernia sac, which is between the rectus muscle sheaths in the midline, is completely freed from all surrounding structures.
4. The hernia sac may be invaginated, dissected free and ligated, or excised.
5. The surgeon closes the peritoneum with interrupted suture. Each suture is tagged, and then closed all at once.
6. The two edges of the rectus fascia are approximated using interrupted 3-0 nonabsorbable sutures.
7. Using a fine absorbable suture, the surgeon performs a subcuticular closure of the skin and applies a pressure dressing.

Inguinal Hernia Repair with Laparoscopic Exploration of Contralateral Side

An inguinal hernia is a protrusion into the inguinal canal of a sac that contains the intestine. The testis develops high on the posterior

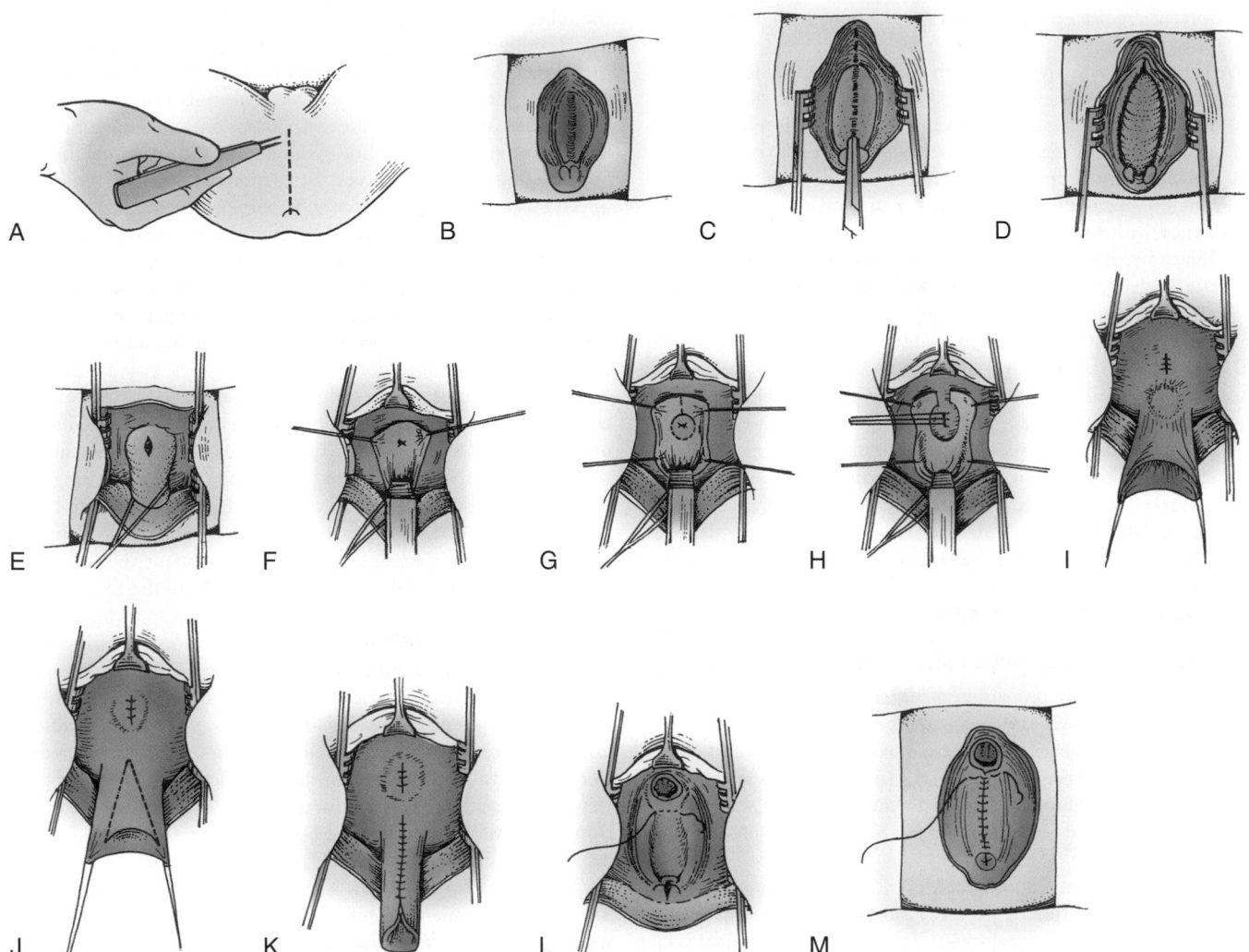

FIGURE 26-20 Posterior sagittal anorectoplasty. **A,** Line of incision and electrical stimulation to determine appropriate anal site. **B,** Midsagittal incision through coccyx and external sphincter fibers of anus, showing striated muscle complex deep to anal site; subcutaneous external sphincter extending about halfway to coccyx; superficial external sphincter inserting on coccyx; levator deeper in midline. **C,** Right-angled forceps beneath levator ani. **D,** All layers of striated muscle partially retracted laterally to expose visceral endopelvic fascia. **E,** Sagittal incision in terminal bowel after proximal dissection around rectum and placement of tape around rectum proximally. **F,** Retracted rectotomy showing fistula site. **G,** Semicircumferential incision through mucosa-submucosa for placement of first sutures to close fistula. **H,** Completed closure of fistula orifice. **I,** Stippled area where muscular bowel wall is left in place and clear area above where peritoneum may be encountered. **J,** Extent of anterior wedge resection for tapered repair of rectum *(dotted line)*. **K,** Approximation of tapered edges of rectum. **L,** First and deepest suture for approximation of levators to establish beginning of canal. **M,** After reapproximation of levator ani to coccyx, interrupted sutures are placed in edges of superficial external sphincter muscle.

wall of the abdomen. It gradually descends into the scrotum. Before the testis enters the inguinal canal, the processus vaginalis projects downward but retains a communication with the peritoneal cavity. The upper part of the processus does not project downward; the remaining sac constitutes an indirect inguinal hernia. In a female child, a similar hernial sac is contiguous with the round ligament.

Procedural Considerations. A minor instrument set is used. A laparoscope may be used to visualize the contralateral side, as it is not uncommon for inguinal hernias to occur bilaterally. The patient is positioned supine, and routine prepping and draping procedures are followed.

Operative Procedure

1. The surgeon makes an incision over the inguinal area in the direction of the skin crease.
2. The subcutaneous tissue is opened, and hemostats are placed on bleeding vessels, which are then ligated or electrocoagulated.
3. Right-angle retractors are placed inferiorly and medially.
4. The surgeon identifies the external ring, and uses small Metzenbaum scissors to free and clean the external oblique fascia.
5. Using a #15 blade, the surgeon opens the external oblique fascia and frees the upper flap. The lower flap is freed to expose the inguinal ligament.

6. Cord structures are opened at the upper end of the cord. Two forceps are used to grasp tissues at the same level and to separate them.
7. The hernia sac is grasped with a hemostat, and structures of the cord are peeled downward and away from the sac with forceps until the sac is freed. Care is taken to protect the spermatic cord and major vessels as the sac is freed.
8. After the sac is opened, the surgeon's index finger is inserted and the sac is pulled upward. The upward traction is maintained with two or three hemostats.
9. If laparoscopic exploration of the contralateral side is indicated, the 20-gauge IV catheter is inserted over the opposite inguinal area. The insufflation tube is connected, and CO_2 instilled. The contralateral side is explored using a 2.7-mm telescope.
10. The sac is ligated with 3-0 nonabsorbable suture, and excess sac is removed. Repair of the inguinal canal may be done with nonabsorbable sutures.
11. The subcutaneous tissue is closed with interrupted fine sutures; closure of the skin is with fine nonabsorbable subcuticular sutures. Cyanoacrylate glue or wound closure strips are applied.
12. If a bilateral hernia is diagnosed, steps 1 through 10 are repeated on the contralateral side.

General Surgery—Abdominal Procedures

Gastroschisis Repair and Omphalocele

An omphalocele is the protrusion of abdominal viscera outside the abdomen through a defect in the umbilical ring into a sac of amniotic membrane and peritoneum at the base of the umbilical cord. There is no skin covering (Figure 26-21). Gastroschisis is the protrusion of the viscera through a defect in the abdominal wall to the right of the umbilical cord. No amniotic membrane or peritoneum covers the defect.

Omphalocele occurs during the eleventh week of fetal life when the viscera fail to withdraw normally from the exocoelomic position to occupy the peritoneal cavity. The resulting abdominal wall defect can vary in size from 2 to 15 cm. The sac may contain only a few loops of bowel, or nearly all the intestines and the liver and spleen. Associated anomalies can include disorders of the cardiac, musculoskeletal, genitourinary, and nervous systems, along with malrotation and abnormal fixation of the bowel. Gastroschisis, on the other hand, is generally not associated with major congenital defects other than intestinal atresia (Verklan, 2012) (Figure 26-22).

Direct closure is the treatment of choice for both gastroschisis and omphalocele (Henrich et al, 2008). Treatment consists of inserting a nasogastric tube to prevent distention and aspiration, and beginning IV access with fluid resuscitation and antibiotic therapy. Surgical intervention is necessary to prevent rupture of the sac, infection, or both. If intrauterine rupture of the sac has occurred, the newborn is kept warm, and the bowel is inspected for perforation and torsion. In certain cases a petroleum gauze dressing may be applied to the defect, but care must be taken to keep it moist.

Omphaloceles and gastroschisis are repaired by placement of the viscera in the abdominal cavity, with reconstruction of the abdominal wall. Surgical procedures for omphaloceles may be primary (Shuster procedure) or staged (giant omphaloceles). Mesh may be used as a barrier to create tension that helps to push the internal organs into the abdominal cavity. In some cases of gastroschisis, a silo is applied to the defect. The silo is made of a flexible ring that sits inside the abdomen and its size is gradually decreased to facilitate movement of the organs back to the abdominal cavity. Silo material may be prepackaged and kept at the patient's bedside if the patient is unable to tolerate an immediate trip to the OR.

Procedural Considerations. Particular attention to maintaining body temperature is essential because of the massive exposed surface area from which body heat can be lost. The use of nitrous oxide as an anesthetic agent is avoided during this procedure because it causes increased gas in the intestine, which in turn makes the reduction of abdominal contents into the peritoneal cavity very difficult. Repeated rectal irrigation with warm saline to evacuate meconium from the bowel may be carried out before the abdominal prep to aid in bowel decompression.

The major instrument set is required. The patient is positioned supine; the abdomen, umbilical cord, and sac are gently prepped with a povidone-iodine solution.

Gastroschisis Repair with Silo Placement

Procedural Considerations. A major instrument set is required. The patient is positioned supine for the procedure. The abdomen, umbilical cord, and sac are gently prepped with povidone-iodine.

FIGURE 26-21 Newborn with giant omphalocele containing liver and intestine.

FIGURE 26-22 Gastroschisis. A large amount of small intestine has eviscerated through a defect to the right of a normal-appearing umbilical cord. No sac is visible, and the intestine is thickened, edematous, and ischemic in areas.

FIGURE 26-23 Operative view of silo for the intestines.

Operative Procedure

1. The surgeon examines the bowel and measures the size of the defect to determine silo size. The silo is applied so that the flexible ring is positioned inside the abdomen (Figure 26-23).
2. The patient returns to the OR every 48 hours for a reduction of the silo, which is accomplished by decreasing the size of the ring to help guide the contents back into the abdominal cavity.
3. The height of bowel in the silo and length of reduction are measured with each procedure. When the amount of bowel remaining in the silo is 1 cm or less, the patient is transferred to the OR for closure of the defect.
4. The silo is trimmed and the spring-loaded ring is removed. The wound site and bowel are inspected and cleaned with surgical prep material.
5. The surgeon closes the defect using synthetic purse-string sutures or, if the defect is too large, running sutures that begin at each end of the wound and meet in the middle to preserve the umbilical cord stump.
6. The inferior aspect of skin is wrapped around the stump and secured with absorbable suture. Any redundant skin is trimmed and the stump is ligated using nonabsorbable suture.
7. A subcutaneous drain may be left in place, and a dry, sterile dressing is applied.

Omphalocele Repair

Procedural Considerations. The patient is positioned supine for the procedure and the abdomen is prepped as described for silo placement.

Operative Procedure

1. The surgeon dissects the amnion of the omphalocele circumferentially from the dermis.
2. The umbilical vein is identified and ligated with absorbable suture. Umbilical cord structures and arteries are dissected and ligated with absorbable suture, and then oversewn with nonabsorbable suture.
3. Organs connected to the omphalocele are dissected, reduced (if necessary), and mobilized, and the internal mucosal layer is closed with running nonabsorbable suture.
4. The outer muscular layer is closed with interrupted nonabsorbable suture, organs are returned to the peritoneal cavity, and fascia is closed with interrupted nonabsorbable suture.
5. If necessary, an umbilicoplasty may be performed using interrupted absorbable suture. Dry, sterile dressings are placed over the incision.

In certain cases in which the defect is of medium to large size, a primary closure may not be accomplished. In these situations a staged procedure is done using prosthetic reduction. In the first stage the patient is taken to the OR and positioned and prepped as previously described. Then the following steps are performed:

1. The sac is excised, and the umbilical vein and arteries are ligated.
2. A gastrostomy may be performed at this time.
3. A barrier is then created with Silastic mesh. The mesh is secured through all layers of the edge of the defect using a continuous locking nonabsorbable suture. The open end of the barrier is closed in the same manner.
4. The surgeon closes the open end of the cylinder with umbilical tape or, alternatively, attaches to a specifically designed roller clamp.
5. The mesh barrier suture line and edge of the defect are wrapped with roller gauze dipped in an iodophor solution. The patient is transferred to an open Isolette, and the silo is suspended from the top of the Isolette. Plastic wrap is applied to the barrier to prevent heat loss. The patient is then transported to the NICU, where daily reduction of abdominal contents is performed by adding a lower tie of umbilical tape or by adjusting the roller clamp. The abdominal viscera are gradually reduced over several days, taking care to avoid respiratory compromise from abdominal distention. When reduction has successfully approached skin level, the patient is returned to the OR for the final stage of repair.
6. The mesh barrier is removed, and the remaining abdominal contents are brought into the peritoneal cavity. The peritoneal fascia is closed with interrupted nonabsorbable sutures. The skin is closed with interrupted nonabsorbable suture. In an attempt to create the appearance of an umbilicus, a purse-string suture is used to close the inferior 2 cm of incision.

Correction of Biliary Atresia—Hepatic Portoenterostomy (Kasai Procedure)

Biliary atresia is a congenital defect that results from nonpatent extrahepatic bile ducts. Bile is unable to drain from the liver to the small intestine, leading to eventual cirrhosis and death. The Kasai procedure is the construction of a bile drainage system by use of an intestinal conduit. This procedure is indicated in patients with extrahepatic biliary atresia who are younger than 3 months. All atretic segments of the existing bile ducts are removed. An intraoperative cholangiogram and frozen-section biopsy of the hepatic duct remnant are included in the surgical procedure.

Procedural Considerations. The patient is positioned supine over a radiographic plate, or fluoroscopy is used. Both a major instrument set and bowel clamps are required, as well as radiopaque dye and a 6F or 8F catheter for the cholangiography.

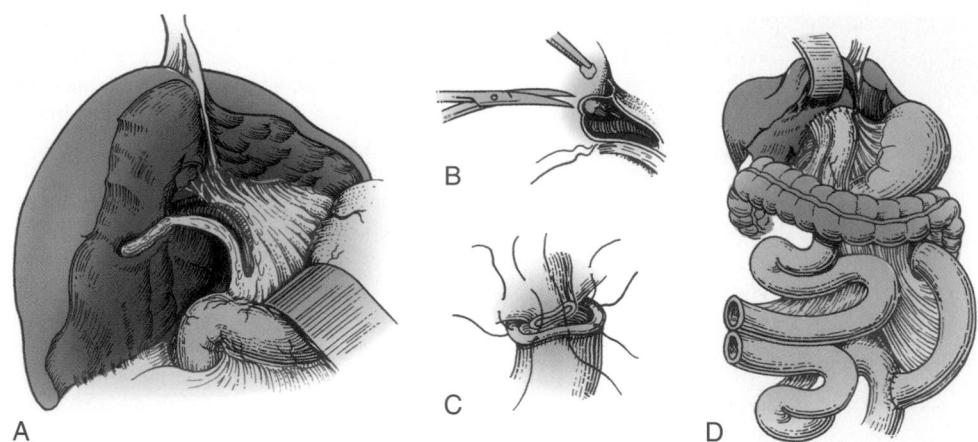

FIGURE 26-24 Kasai procedure. **A,** Exploration of hepatoduodenal ligament and ligation of drainage structures. **B,** Transection of hepatic duct remnant using frozen-section biopsy specimens as a guide. **C,** Anastomosis of jejunal conduit at porta hepatis. **D,** Exteriorization of conduit using double-barreled Roux-en-Y approach.

Operative Procedure

1. The surgeon makes a right upper quadrant incision and exposes the gallbladder.
2. A small catheter is placed into the gallbladder and secured with a purse-string suture. Radiopaque dye is instilled into the gallbladder, and an x-ray examination is done. The surgeon observes for free flow of the dye through the ducts and into the duodenum, which occasionally is seen. These patients are then categorized as having correctable biliary atresia. In such situations, a liver biopsy is performed and the incision is closed. The majority of patients with correctable biliary atresia demonstrate progressive improvement. More commonly, however, there is a very small amount of flow or none at all, for which the Kasai procedure is performed.
3. The intra-abdominal organs are thoroughly inspected because of the high prevalence of associated anomalies.
4. The hepatoduodenal ligament is explored, and all drainage structures are ligated (Figure 26-24, *A*).
5. The hepatic duct remnant is identified and traced to the liver hilum. The remnant is transected as high as possible using frozen-section biopsy specimens as a guide. Frozen-section biopsy specimens are also obtained at the porta hepatis to denote the presence of ductules. Precise identification of this location is essential (see Figure 26-24, *B*).
6. The proximal portion of the jejunum is generally used as the intestinal conduit. A meticulous anastomosis is performed at the porta hepatis as previously identified, using a single running layer of absorbable sutures (see Figure 26-24, *C*).
7. The conduit is exteriorized with a double-barreled Roux-en-Y approach (see Figure 26-24, *D*).
8. A liver biopsy is then performed.
9. A drain is placed, and the incision is closed in layers.

The procedure just described is one approach of many. Others include exteriorization of the jejunal conduit as a cutaneous jejunostomy and use of double Roux-en-Y loops, avoiding any need for an enterostomy. If none of these procedures is successful, the patient may be a candidate for liver transplantation.

Repair of Congenital Diaphragmatic Hernia

A CDH is repaired by replacement of the displaced viscera into the abdominal cavity with surgical correction of the diaphragm

FIGURE 26-25 Defect in the posterolateral aspect of the left diaphragm (diaphragmatic hernia).

defect (Figure 26-25). The conventional surgical repair is through the abdomen, though some cases of CDH can be repaired using a thoracic approach. The concurrence of intra-abdominal abnormalities is somewhat high in infants with diaphragmatic hernia; therefore, treatment is facilitated with an abdominal approach. It is technically easier to extract the viscera from below than to push them out of the thorax. The abnormal intrathoracic intrusion of the abdominal viscera usually causes severe compromise of intrathoracic pulmonary and vascular activities. Therefore, urgent restoration of more normal intrathoracic and intra-abdominal relationships is the rule in these newborns. The lung may be hypoplastic because of prolonged compression in utero by the displaced abdominal viscera. A residual intrapleural space usually remains for a few days after surgery.

Procedural Considerations. Direct suturing of the margins of the defect is usually possible. Insertion of prosthetic Silastic sheeting is occasionally required and should be available. The major instrument set is required. The patient is positioned supine.

Operative Procedure

1. The surgeon makes a subcostal incision on the side of the defect, going through all muscle layers.

2. The abdominal viscera are withdrawn from the chest and held downward through the abdominal wound. Because abnormalities of abdominal viscera, such as malrotation, are associated with diaphragmatic hernia, the organs are carefully inspected at this time. If a malrotation is found, the surgeon may repair it if the patient's clinical condition is amenable to the procedure.

3. The defect is then carefully inspected, including a search for a hernia sac, which is present in less than 5% of cases. If a sac is identified, it is excised.

4. The surgeon identifies the posterior and anterior rims of the diaphragm, and primary closure is performed with mattress sutures of nonabsorbable material. If the rim of tissue is too small for mattress sutures, ample nonabsorbable sutures are used. Occasionally, reinforced Silastic sheeting may be needed if sufficient diaphragm is not available for primary closure.

5. The abdominal wall is then closed, followed by subcutaneous tissue and skin closure. If the musculature cannot accommodate the abdominal viscera, it is left open and the skin is closed to leave a ventral hernia. In severe cases the patient may be given extracorporeal membrane oxygenation (ECMO) for several days before repair of the defect. The patient is returned to the OR within 7 days for repair of the ventral hernia.

Pancreatectomy

Pancreatectomy is the treatment for several disorders, including congenital hyperinsulinism (HI) and pancreatitis. Congenital HI is a condition in which the release of insulin is not properly regulated and insulin (beta) cells of the pancreas secrete too much insulin at the wrong time (Children's Hospital of Philadelphia [CHOP], 2013). Treatment of HI is focused on regulating the blood glucose level to reduce the risk of brain damage. Surgical intervention is recommended when medical management of HI proves unsuccessful. A pancreatectomy may be total, meaning that the entire pancreas is removed. In some cases, the common bile duct, spleen, gallbladder, and portions of the small intestine and stomach may be removed along with it. Pancreatectomies may also be partial—only the body and tail of the pancreas are removed. The procedure for a total pancreatectomy for congenital HI is described in the following section.

Procedural Considerations. Multiple specimens are sent to the pathology laboratory for frozen-section analysis throughout the procedure in order to confirm the extent of the disease. The patient is positioned supine with the hips elevated.

Operative Procedure

1. The surgeon makes a transverse supraumbilical incision using a #15 blade. The Denis-Browne retractor is placed.

2. The body and tail of the pancreas are exposed for biopsy for analysis by frozen section.

3. The hepatic flexure of the colon and the duodenum are exposed for additional biopsy and frozen section.

4. If results indicate the need for total pancreatectomy (large nuclei in islet cells), the dissection is begun at the pancreatic tail, and then extended to the body and head.

5. A vessel loop is used to isolate the common bile duct and care is taken to preserve duodenal blood supply to the pancreatic head during dissection. Once the uncinate process is mobilized from behind the superior mesenteric vessels and the common bile duct is dissected away from its entry point into the duodenum, the pancreatic head is freed.

6. A pancreatectomy is performed and blood supply to the duodenum is evaluated. In the event that a pancreatic remnant remains, it is ligated using nonabsorbable interrupted horizontal mattress sutures. Omentum is tacked down to the dissected area, and the gallbladder is milked to evaluate patency and test for bile leak.

7. In certain cases, a gastrostomy tube may be placed.

8. The abdominal incision is closed in layers using nonabsorbable suture for fascia and absorbable sutures for subcutaneous and subcuticular tissue. The incision is dressed with cyanoacrylate glue or topical skin adhesive and wound closure strips.

General Surgery—Resection of Tumors

Nearly two thirds of childhood cancers occur as solid tumor malignancies. As is always the case, the therapy administered depends on the type of tumor. Examination and judicious investigation of all unusual masses are imperative. Thorough diagnostic workup and prompt definitive treatment may result in cure, even if the tumor is malignant. Chemotherapy and radiation therapy are adjuncts to surgical excision of tumors.

Resection of Wilms Tumor

Wilms tumor, also known as nephroblastoma, is the most common intra-abdominal childhood tumor. It presents as a painless mass whose enlargement may laterally distend the abdomen (Figure 26-26). The child may be asymptomatic or may have weight loss, malaise, or abdominal pain. Nephroblastomas may cause obstruction of the vena cava, hepatic veins, or renal veins.

FIGURE 26-26 A CT scan of the abdomen shows a large right-sided Wilms tumor *(arrow)* **(A)** in an infant who subsequently underwent biopsy. **B,** The tumor was not primarily resected secondary to size and adherence to surrounding structures.

Procedural Considerations. The child is positioned supine with a roll under the affected side. Both chest and abdomen are prepped. Infrequently the tumor extends into the inferior vena cava as well as the right atrium of the heart, and in such cases cardiopulmonary bypass (CPB) should be readily available. Lines are placed into the arms and neck to facilitate clamping of the inferior vena cava if needed. Separate sterile gloves and instruments should be available for inspection of the contralateral kidney. Careful attention should be given when handling tumor and lymph nodes to avoid tumor spillage.

Operative Procedure. If the tumor is operable, the following aspects are important:

1. The transabdominal approach, which may be extended to a combined transabdominal-transthoracic approach, is used to inspect abdominal contents and clamp the vessels of the renal pedicle before tumor dissection.
2. All suspicious lymph nodes are removed, placed into separate containers, and labeled. If no suspicious nodes are present, biopsy specimens are obtained of those in adjacent areas.
3. The surgeon explores the opposite kidney before dissecting the tumor.
4. The extent of the tumor can be marked with hemostatic clips to facilitate radiation therapy.
5. The entire primary tumor is removed if doing so does not place the patient in jeopardy.
6. Any residual tumor is marked with clips.
7. Because of its proximity to the kidney, the adrenal gland is usually removed.
8. The abdominal cavity and viscera are thoroughly inspected for evidence of tumor extension or metastases. Extensive surgery may include partial colectomy or partial resection of the diaphragm.
9. The abdominal incision is closed in layers using nonabsorbable suture for fascia and absorbable sutures for subcutaneous and subcuticular tissue. The incision is dressed with cyanoacrylate glue or liquid adhesive and wound closure strips.

Resection of Neuroblastoma

Neuroblastoma is responsible for approximately 6% of all childhood cancers and is the third most common childhood cancer after leukemia and brain and nervous system cancers (American Cancer Society [ACS], 2012). It arises from neural crest tissue and can develop anywhere sympathetic nerve tissue is found; the most common sites are the retroperitoneum and adrenal medulla. The mass is usually firm, irregular, and nontender. It is a silent tumor in its early stages and metastasizes rapidly, often to the lymphatics, liver, skin, bone marrow, lung, brain, or orbits. Treatment includes an operation to ligate the tumor's blood supply and remove as much of the tumor as possible, as well as chemotherapy and radiation.

Resection of Sacrococcygeal Teratoma

An SCT is a tumor that originates early in embryonic cell division. The tumor consists of cell types from more than one embryonic germ layer. Teratomas range from benign, well-differentiated cystic lesions to solid, malignant lesions. They are the most common tumor in newborns, occurring in 1:40,000 live births (Barakat et al, 2011). The sacrococcygeal area is the most common extragonadal site of teratoma, usually presenting as a large protuberance rising from that site (Figure 26-27). It may be irregular or symmetric, may vary in size, and may be pedunculated.

FIGURE 26-27 Infant with large sacrococcygeal teratoma.

An SCT is usually resectable but may undergo malignant changes if not removed early in life. Sacrococcygeal teratomas can be resected prenatally using fetal surgery techniques (see p. 1025) or postnatally. Tumors resected in the newborn period show microscopic evidence of malignant cells, but surgical cures have been achieved. Early surgical resection is important because these tumors are not sensitive to irradiation and are only temporarily responsive to chemotherapy.

The tumor is in the area of the sacrum and coccyx but may extend into the pelvis or abdomen. Resection is usually feasible by placing the patient in the jackknife position and excising the tumor mass and coccyx en bloc. In cases in which the tumor extends high into the pelvis, an abdominal incision also may be required.

Genitourinary Surgery

Pediatric Cystoscopy

Pediatric cystoscopy is endoscopic examination of the lower urinary tract of pediatric patients. The major difference between adult and pediatric cystoscopy is the size of the instruments used and consideration of the small, delicate orifices of the pediatric patient. Indications for pediatric cystoscopy include urinary tract infections, enuresis, urethral valves, vesicoureteral reflux, diverticula, bladder neck contractures, bladder tumors, and urinary tract obstructions.

Procedural Considerations. The cystoscopy setup has the same type of components as those for the adult cystoscopy patient (see Chapter 15), except that the size of the cystourethroscope system is specific to the pediatric patient's needs.

Each pediatric cystourethroscope is designed to fit specific component parts and is very delicate. Therefore, the perioperative nurse must be familiar with the proper use of the system and handle the components carefully. The resectoscope loop is commonly used to resect urethral valves and occasionally bladder tumors. The cold knife (cutting blade without electrosurgery) may be used with the resectoscope to cut urethral strictures and occasionally resect a urethral valve.

The most common type of anesthesia used for the pediatric patient is general anesthesia. After induction of anesthesia, the child is placed in a lithotomy or frog-leg position and prepped and draped according to established procedure.

Operative Procedure. The pediatric cystourethroscope is lubricated and inserted through the urethra into the bladder. The light cord and irrigation tubing are attached to the telescope and cystoscope, and the examination is performed. Most commonly the interior of the bladder is viewed on a video monitor by means of a camera attached to the cystoscope.

Circumcision

Circumcision is the excision of the foreskin (prepuce) of the glans penis. Circumcision may be done for therapeutic reasons or for perceived prophylactic benefits; it may also be done for religious reasons, as is required in specific faiths. Provision should be made to observe the religious needs and preferences of the parents.

Therapeutic indications include correction of phimosis or paraphimosis or treatment of balanoposthitis. Phimosis is a condition in which the orifice of the prepuce is stenosed or too narrow to permit easy retraction behind the glans. Balanoposthitis is characterized by an inflamed glans and mucous membrane with purulent discharge and may require circumcision. Paraphimosis is a recurrent condition in which the prepuce cannot be reduced easily from a retracted position.

Procedural Considerations. Newborns are generally positioned on a specially constructed board that facilitates restraint by immobilizing the limbs and exposing the genitalia. Although it was once thought that circumcision caused infants little pain, the neonatal foreskin contains mature nerve endings that allow for the transmission of pain. Measures to ameliorate the pain of the procedure include local dorsal penile nerve block, a ring block with buffered lidocaine and bupivacaine, or the topical application of a eutectic mixture of local anesthesia (EMLA) cream. Older children require general anesthesia.

For infants, the setup includes fine plastic surgery instruments. A Gomco clamp of the appropriate size, a Plastibell, or the Hollister disposable circumcision device may be used. The Hollister device includes sutures that are sealed in a sterile packet ready for use. The Plastibell technique uses a plastic ring and suture tied around the foreskin like a tourniquet. The excess tissue is trimmed, and in about 5 to 8 days the ring falls off. For older patients a circumcision clamp is not needed, and only a plastic surgery instrument set is used. Petrolatum gauze for dressing should be available.

Operative Procedure (Figure 26-28)

1. If the prepuce is adherent, the surgeon may use a probe or hemostat to break up adhesions. The prepuce is clamped in the dorsal midline and incised toward the coronal mucosa margin, leaving about 5 cm of coronal mucosa intact. A similar procedure is performed ventrally. The two incisions are then joined circumferentially. Alternatively, a superficial circumferential incision is made in the skin with a scalpel at the level of the coronal sulcus and mucosa at the base of the glans. The redundant skin is undermined between the circumferential incisions and removed as a complete cuff.
2. Bleeding vessels are coagulated or clamped with mosquito hemostats and tied with fine absorbable ligatures. Before closure the area may be cleansed with an appropriate antiseptic solution.
3. The surgeon approximates the raw edges of the skin incision to a coronal cuff of mucosal prepuce, generally with interrupted 4-0 or 5-0 absorbable sutures on fine plastic cutting or GI needles. The wound is usually dressed with petrolatum gauze or an antibiotic ointment. A penile block with bupivacaine is often done for immediate postoperative pain, thus providing a more comfortable emergence from anesthesia.

Hypospadias Repair

Hypospadias is a developmental anomaly characterized by a urethral meatus that opens onto the ventral surface of the penis proximal to the end of the glans (Figure 26-29). There are varying degrees of hypospadias. The meatus may be on the ventral surface of the glans, on the corona, anywhere along the shaft, in the scrotum, or even in the perineum. The more proximal the opening, the greater the degree of chordee (downward curvature of the penis). Chordee is caused by fibrous bands that extend from the hypospadiac urethral meatus to the tip of the glans and represent the abnormally developed urethra and its investing layer of Buck fascia, dartos, and skin. In some cases of clinical curvature, however, these fibrous bands may not be present. Although these curvatures are still termed *chordee,* they are not true fibrous chordee.

The principal methods of hypospadias repair are meatoplasty and glanuloplasty, orthoplasty (release of chordee, thereby straightening the penis), urethroplasty (reconstruction of the urethra), skin cover, and scrotoplasty. These may be done in one- or two-stage repairs depending on the extent of the condition. Efforts have increased to relocate the meatus to the apex of the glans, especially in the more extensive one-stage repair.

One complication of hypospadias repair is urethral fistula formation, which can be repaired without much difficulty. Correction of strictures is more troublesome.

Procedural Considerations. The patient (the majority are infants and young children) is placed in the supine position with legs apart. Urine may be diverted with a urethral catheter intraoperatively. The instrument setup varies according to the surgeon's preference. However, a minor set with fine plastic surgery instruments is generally required. Owens gauze, Elastomull, Coban, and Elastoplast, as well as adhesive tape, are generally required for the dressing, which is an important part of the hypospadias repair.

Meatoplasty and Glanuloplasty Incorporated (MAGPI) Procedure

Operative Procedure

1. The surgeon makes a subcoronal circumferential incision about 8 mm proximal to the meatus and corona. The skin is stripped

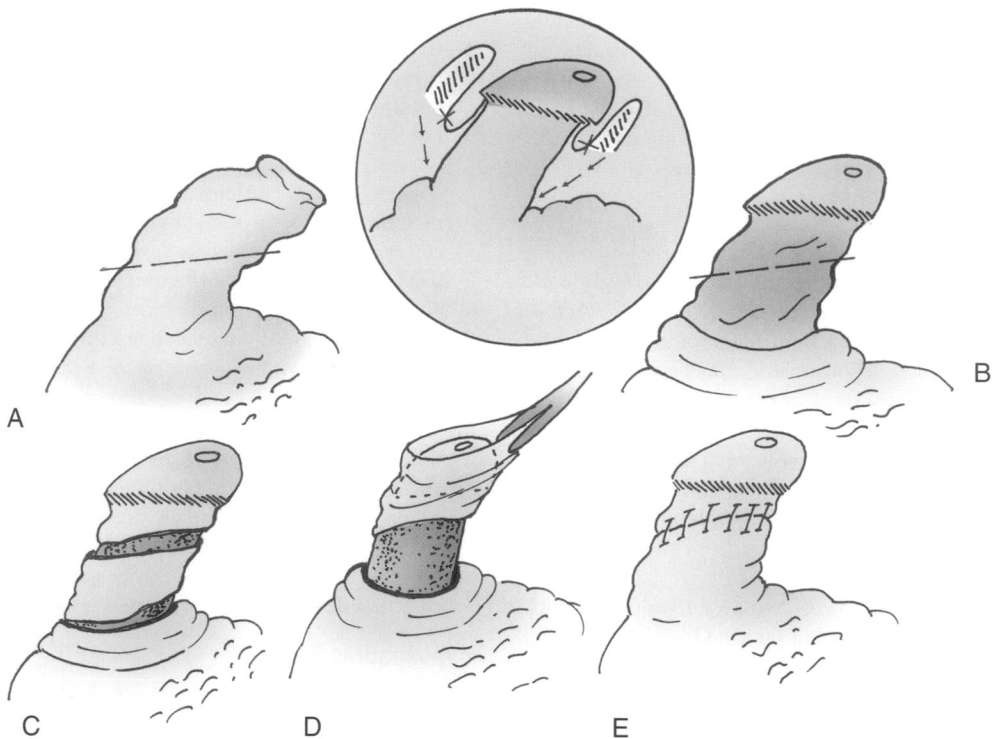

FIGURE 26-28 Circumcision. **A,** Initial incision made in the shaft. **B,** Second incision made in subcoronal sulcus. **C,** Amount of tissue to be removed. **D,** Removal of tissue. **E,** Shaft skin sutured to subcoronal skin.

FIGURE 26-29 Hypospadias.

FIGURE 26-30 Meatal advancement and glanuloplasty.

back from the phallus by subcutaneous dissection (Figure 26-30).

2. A bridge of tissue between the meatus and glanular groove is made, with a transverse closure of the dorsal (upper) meatal edge to the distal glanular groove.

3. Three traction sutures are placed where the foreskin stops, at the apex of the ventral meatus (on the lower side) and lateral areas of the glans.

4. The surgeon sutures the edges of the glans together ventrally in a V configuration, and the redundant edges are excised. Vertical mattress sutures are used to approximate the glans beneath the meatus.

5. If foreskin is excessive, it may be trimmed, followed by a sleeve style of reapproximation of the penile skin. If a ventral skin defect is present, a rotational skin flap closure is used.

6. An indwelling catheter is placed, and the wound is dressed.

Orthoplasty. Orthoplasty is the proper designation for the plastic procedure performed to straighten the penis. Chordee repair is the more common term used. In true fibrous chordee the penis is curved downward, with the meatus and glans in proximity to one another.

Artificial erection is achieved by injecting 0.9% preservative-free injectable saline solution into the corpus cavernosum. Both corporal bodies fill, making it possible to determine the degree of curvature before and after the resection of the fibrous bands.

Operative Procedure

1. The surgeon makes a circumferential incision around the corona and carries it distally to the urethral meatus and well below the glans cap (Figure 26-31, *A*). Dissection continues to the level of the tunica albuginea of the corpora cavernosa.
2. With proximal dissection the adherent fibrous plaque is freed, working in a side-to-side fashion. The urethra is elevated from the corpora during this process (see Figure 26-31, *B*).
3. The chordee generally surrounds the urethral meatus and often extends for some distance. It is important to free it completely along the entire penile shaft to the penoscrotal junction or, in severe cases, into the scrotum or perineum.

4. After release of the chordee, the glans penis is closed with 4-0 absorbable sutures in a circular manner (see Figure 26-31, *C*).
5. If urethroplasty is either delayed or unnecessary, excess dorsal skin is excised (see Figure 26-31, *D*) and the incision is closed along the dorsal midline with interrupted absorbable mattress sutures (see Figure 26-31, *E*). The wound is dressed according to established protocol.

Urethroplasty. Many procedures are described for reconstruction of a urethra. They may be divided into three general groups: adjacent skin flaps, free skin grafts, and mobilized vascular flaps. There are also many combinations of these procedures. In all the procedures, some type of temporary urinary diversion, such as a perineal urethrostomy, may be used.

The procedural considerations are the same as those for chordee repair.

Adjacent Skin Flap. It is possible to tubularize skin adjacent to the meatus to create a neourethra in a one-stage repair. Transfer of dorsal skin to the ventrum will also provide graft material close to

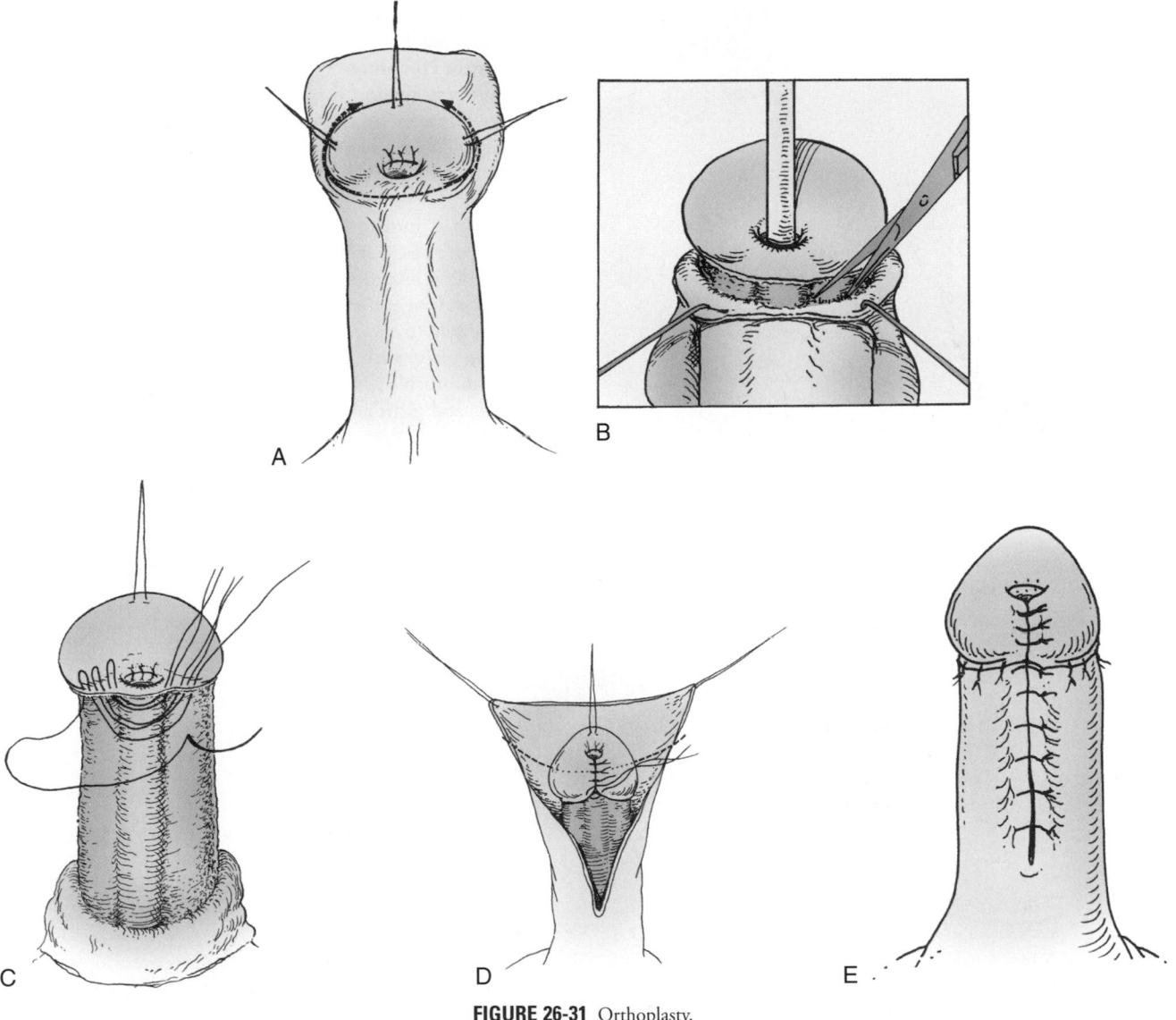

FIGURE 26-31 Orthoplasty.

the meatus. However, this is generally done in two stages, and the vascularity of this thin rotational flap is less than optimum, with results that are prone to complication.

Operative Procedure

1. The surgeon places traction sutures in the tip of the penis and in the glans wings for stabilization and exposure.
2. The distance between the glans tip and the lower edge of the meatus is measured. An outline of the proposed incision is drawn on the penile shaft (Figure 26-32, *A*). In a one-stage approach the distal length must be increased to compensate for the added penile length after chordee release.

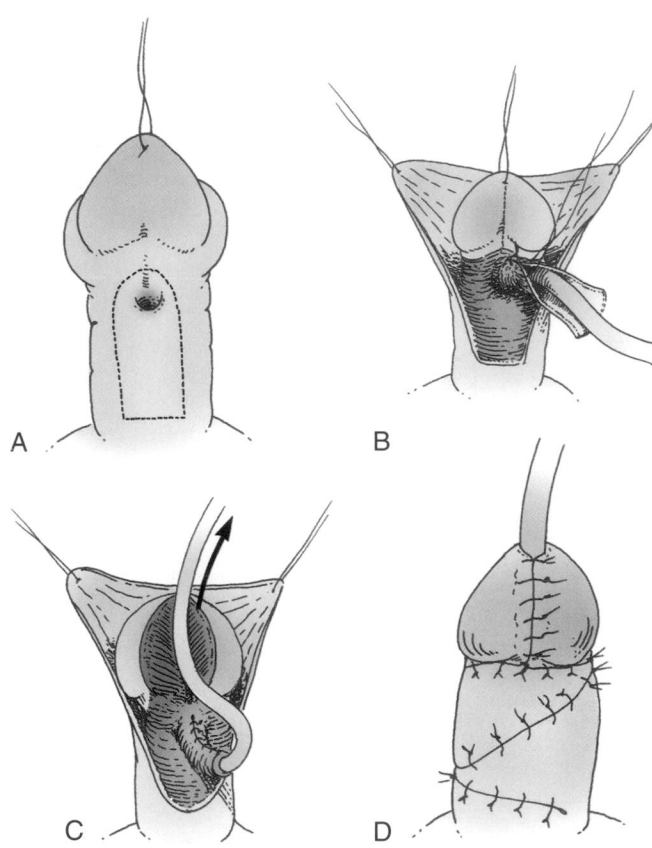

FIGURE 26-32 Urethroplasty with adjacent skin flap.

3. An incision is made around the outlined flap and carried proximally to a point on the shaft that corresponds to the distance required to reach the glans tip. A flap width of 14 to 16 mm is usually sufficient to ensure good circumference of the neourethra.
4. Once incised, the tube is rolled over an 8F or 10F catheter (see Figure 26-32, *B*) with an inverted running stitch of 4-0 or 5-0 absorbable suture.
5. Next, the surgeon incises the glans penis and the glans wings are undermined and freed. The neourethra is carried to the distal portion of the glans and sutured in place (see Figure 26-32, *C*).
6. The glans wings are sutured around the neourethra with absorbable interrupted mattress sutures. The redundant foreskin is split down the midline, and the flaps are transposed in a Z-plasty manner (see Figure 26-32, *D*).
7. A dry, sterile pressure dressing is applied. The patient can often be discharged on the same day, without the need for an indwelling catheter.

Free Skin Graft. Free skin grafts should be of full thickness. Because the free graft must be revascularized, it is important that it have a perfect skin cover of dorsal preputial penile skin that is well vascularized. This type of graft is generally used with a one-stage hypospadias repair.

Operative Procedure

1. A V-shaped incision is made on the glans, and the penile skin is mobilized after the chordee is released (Figure 26-33, *A*).
2. Glans wings are developed in a triangular fashion, and ventral preputial skin is used for the full-thickness free graft (see Figure 26-33, *B*).
3. The graft is formed into a neourethra over a stenting catheter (see Figure 26-33, *C*).
4. The surgeon anastomoses the graft proximal to the urethra with the suture line of the graft next to the corpora. The middle glans dart is fixed to the corpora (see Figure 26-33, *D*).
5. A meatoplasty with the dorsal glans dart is accomplished.
6. Fine absorbable interrupted sutures are placed around the meatus and glans and along the dorsal penile shaft (see Figure 26-33, *E*).
7. The wound is dressed according to established protocol.

Mobilized Vascularized Flaps. Vascularized flaps of preputial penile skin may be mobilized to the ventrum by leaving them attached to the outer surface of the prepuce or as an island flap. One modification is the transverse preputial island-flap neourethra

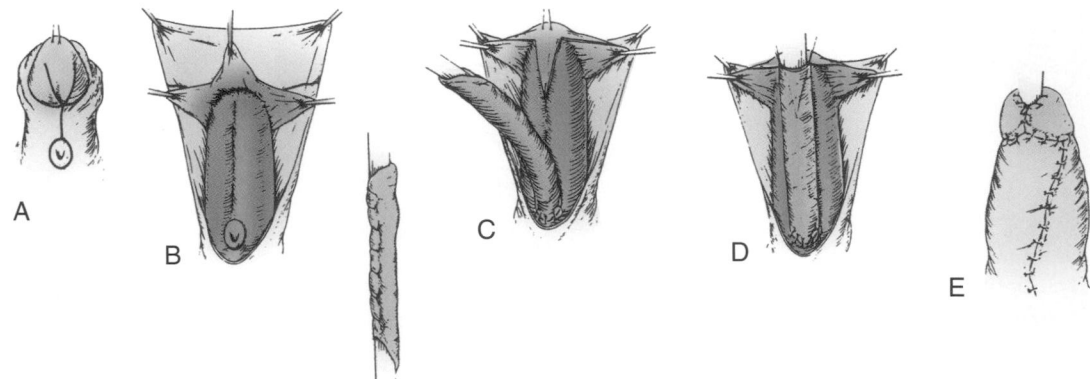

FIGURE 26-33 Urethroplasty with free graft.

with glans-channel positioning for the meatus. Preputial skin is often preferred because of its rich, reliable blood supply.

Operative Procedure

1. The chordee is released (Figure 26-34, *A*).
2. Ventral preputial skin is dissected free and fanned out (see Figure 26-34, *B*).
3. The rectangle of skin is rolled into the neourethra and measured (see Figure 26-34, *C*).
4. The surgeon develops an island flap by dissection of the subcutaneous tissue from the dorsal penile skin (see Figure 26-34, *D* and *E*).
5. A glans channel is created with fine scissors in a plane just above the corpora. The glans tissue is removed with the 14F channel, and the island-flap urethra is spiraled to the ventrum (see Figure 26-34, *F*).
6. The surgeon anastomoses the neourethra proximal to the urethra (see Figure 26-34, *G*).
7. The neourethra is carried to the tip of the glans (see Figure 26-34, *H*).
8. The dorsal penile flaps are transposed laterally to the midline, and excess skin is excised. The surgeon closes the wound with

fine absorbable interrupted mattress sutures around the glans and down the penile shaft (see Figure 26-34, *I*).
9. Dressings are applied according to established protocol.

Skin Cover. After orthoplasty and urethroplasty, the penis must be resurfaced with skin. Abundant excess dorsal foreskin is usually adequate to achieve the desired results.

Operative Procedure

1. Preputial tissue is transposed through a small buttonhole opening in the midline (Figure 26-35, *A*).
2. The vasculature is spread laterally, and the glans penis is delivered through the hole (see Figure 26-35, *B*).
3. The surgeon sutures the skin flap with fine absorbable interrupted mattress sutures (see Figure 26-35, *C*).

Epispadias Repair

An epispadias is a congenital anomaly characterized by a urethral opening on the dorsum of the penis. The surgical procedures used in the correction of epispadias depend on the extent of the deformity. In mild, incomplete defects the repair is the same as a simple hypospadias repair. Complete deformity is always associated with

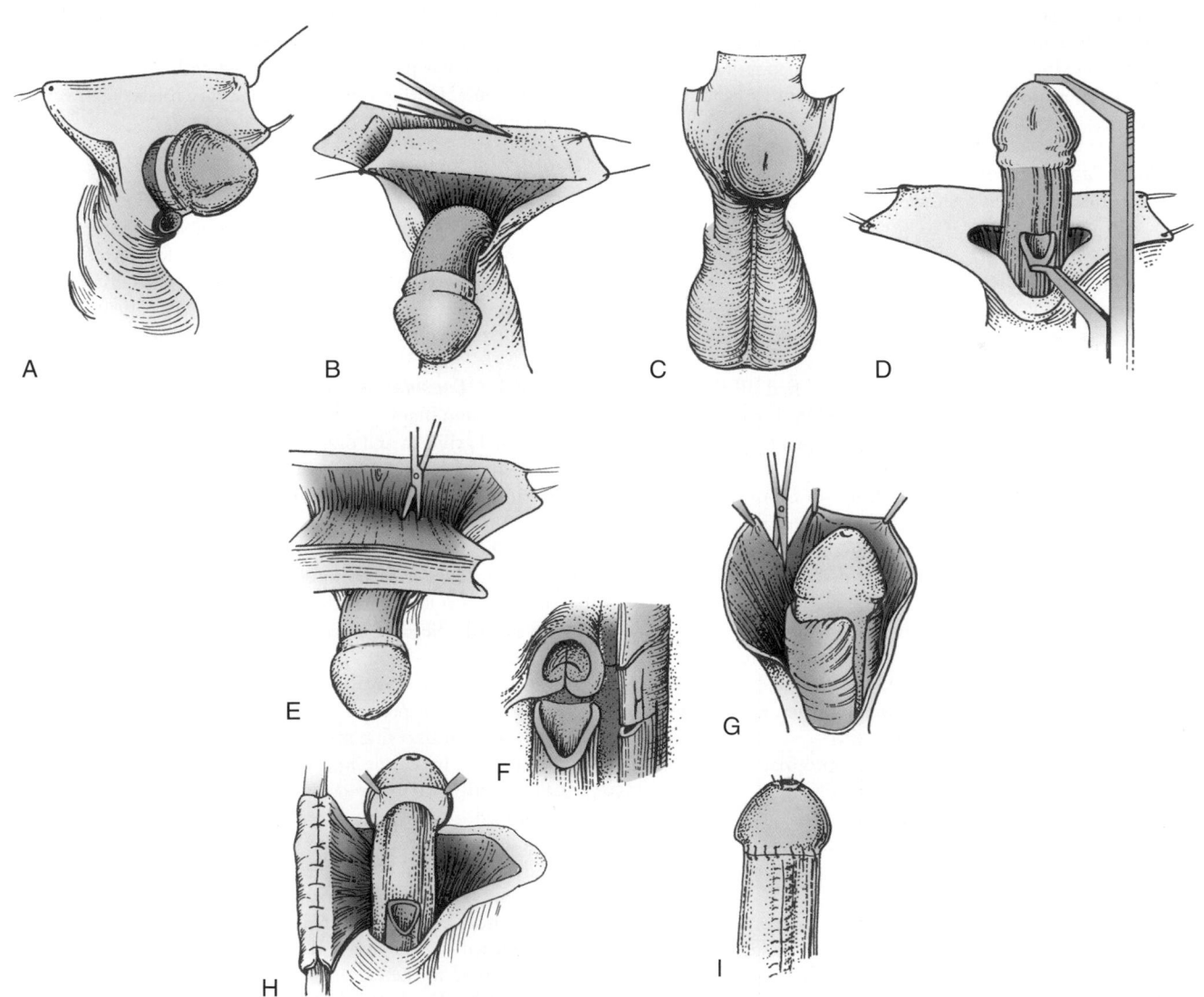

FIGURE 26-34 Urethroplasty, island flap.

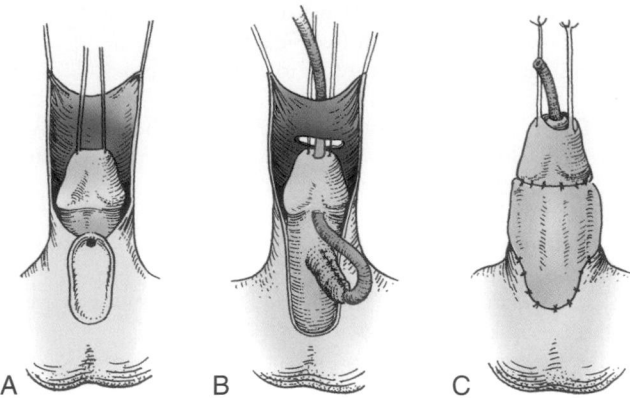

FIGURE 26-35 Skin cover procedure.

urinary incontinence because of little or no development of the bladder neck; thus the operation is much more involved. The least severe forms of the exstrophy-epispadias complex are (1) balanic epispadias, in which the urethra opens on the dorsum of the glans, and (2) penile epispadias, in which the urethra opens on the shaft of the penis. The more severe variety, which occurs when the urethra opens on the proximal end of the shaft or in the penopubic position, is generally associated with severe dorsal chordee and urinary incontinence.

Procedural Considerations. The setup for an epispadias repair is the same as that described for hypospadias repair.

Operative Procedures
First-Stage Epispadias Repair
1. The surgeon makes a vertical incision distal to the epispadial meatus and extends it circumferentially to the dorsal coronal margin.
2. The foreshortened dorsal urethral strip is lifted off the corpora cavernosa, and the ventral prepuce (foreskin) is rotated dorsally to cover the dorsal skin defect created by penile straightening.

Second-Stage Epispadias Repair
1. A vertical suprapubic incision is made to expose the anterior bladder wall and widened vesical neck. A wedge section of the anterolateral prostatic urethra is removed on either side so that when it is reconstructed, a more normal-caliber prostatic urethra is formed.
2. The roof of the membranous urethra is removed.
3. The surgeon closes the prostatic urethra, including muscle that is sutured together in the midline, with absorbable sutures. The bladder is closed so that an indwelling suprapubic catheter is left. The abdomen is closed in layers.
4. The anterior urethra is closed after an appropriate size of octagonal strip of dorsal penile skin is outlined.
5. The remainder of the repair—the creation of the urethra and its coverage with lateral penile skin—is the reverse procedure of a second-stage hypospadias repair.

Bladder Exstrophy Repair

Bladder exstrophy repair corrects a more severe form of epispadias, in which the anterior bladder wall as well as the roof of the urethra is absent. Bladder exstrophy is always accompanied by wide separation of the rectus muscles of the lower abdominal wall and by diastasis of the pubic bone with anterior displacement of the anus. Repair of bladder exstrophy requires an adequate size of bladder for ultimate continence to be achieved. It is preferable to perform this procedure in the neonatal period.

Procedural Considerations. The patient is placed in a supine position, and the abdomen and thighs are prepped and draped. Instruments are the same as those required for hypospadias repair.

Operative Procedure
1. The surgeon makes an incision around the exposed bladder medial to the paravesical neck mucosa. The incision is carried distally across the epispadial urethra distal to the verumontanum. The paravesical mucosa is preserved for urethral lengthening. The bladder is then freed from the rectus fascia and the peritoneum. The dorsal chordee is released, and the mobilized paravesical mucosa is apposed in the midline and sutured to the proximal end of the urethra just distal to the verumontanum.
2. The bladder wall is closed vertically in two layers with 3-0 absorbable sutures, and a suprapubic tube is inserted for drainage.
3. The bladder neck is loosely reconstructed by approximating the interpubic ligament, which extends between the proximal end of the phallus and the pubic bone.
4. The symphysis pubis is approximated with a heavy nonabsorbable suture. During this step the assistant rotates the iliac bones anteriorly.

Hydrocelectomy

A hydrocele is an abnormal accumulation of fluid contained within the tunica vaginalis of the scrotum. Excessive secretion or accumulation of hydrocele fluid may be the result of infection or trauma. A hydrocelectomy is the excision of the tunica vaginalis of the testis to remove the enlarged fluid-filled sac. In older patients the procedure is performed through a scrotal incision.

Procedural Considerations. The patient is positioned supine. Preparation and draping of the patient include routine cleansing of the external genitalia and draping with a fenestrated sheet. A minor instrument set is required, plus a small drain; a 30-mL syringe with a 20-gauge, 2-inch aspirating needle; and a suspensory dressing.

Operative Procedure
1. The surgeon makes an anterolateral incision in the skin of the scrotum over the hydrocele mass with a #10 or #15 blade (Figure 26-36, *A*). Bleeding is controlled with an electrosurgical unit (ESU).
2. Small retractors may be placed, after which the fascial layers are incised to expose the tunica vaginalis (see Figure 26-36, *B*). The surgeon uses fine scissors, forceps, and blunt dissection to dissect the hydrocele and deliver it through the incision (see Figure 26-36, *C*). The sac is opened, and the fluid contents are aspirated.
3. The surgeon inverts the sac so that it surrounds the testis, epididymis, and distal cord. Excess tunica vaginalis is excised, and the edges of the tunica are sutured with a continuous 4-0 absorbable suture behind the testicle (see Figure 26-36, *D*). The testicle is "bottled" by the inverted tunica vaginalis, and this may then be returned to the sac.
4. A drain is placed within the scrotum and exteriorized through a stab wound in the most dependent portion of the scrotum.

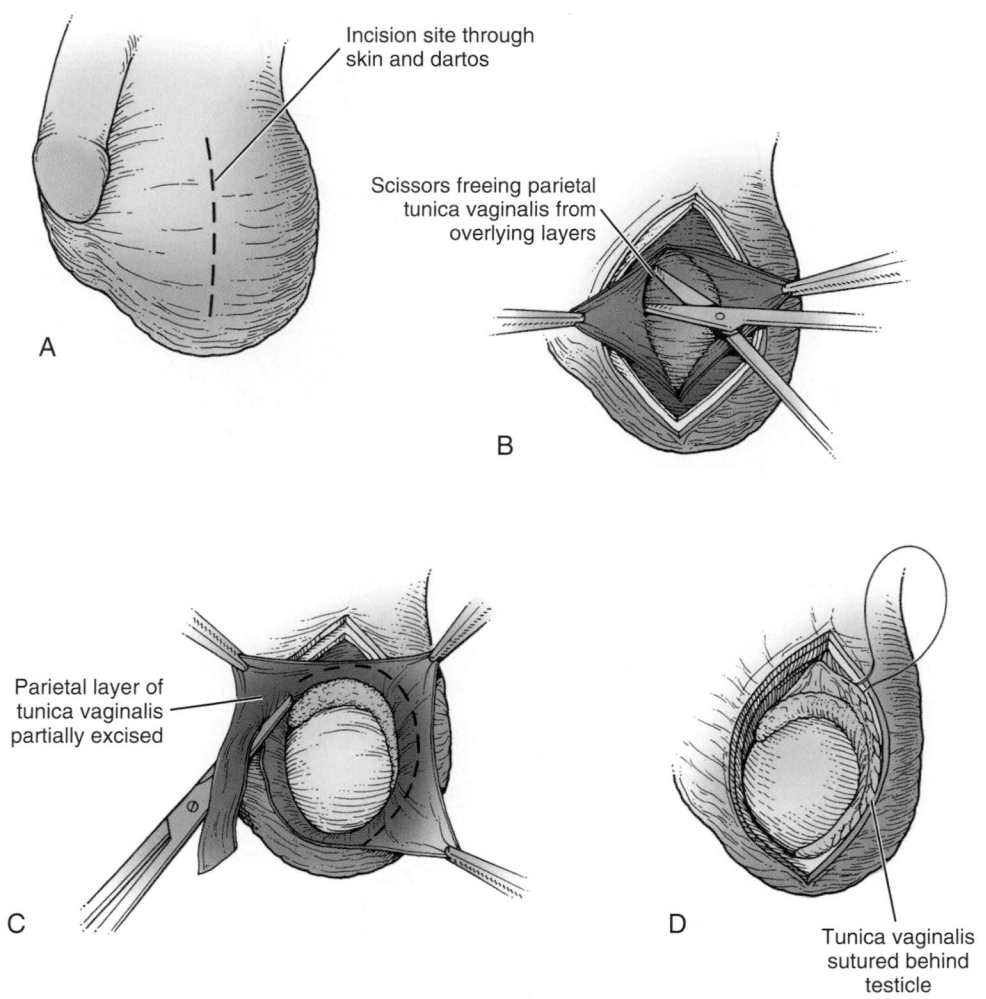

Incision site through
skin and dartos

A

Scissors freeing parietal
tunica vaginalis from
overlying layers

B

Parietal layer of
tunica vaginalis
partially excised

C

D

Tunica vaginalis
sutured behind
testicle

FIGURE 26-36 Hydrocelectomy.

The scrotal incision is closed in layers with 3-0 and 4-0 absorbable sutures. A fluff compression dressing contained in a scrotal support (suspensory) helps reduce postoperative scrotal edema.

Orchiopexy

An orchiopexy is the surgical placement and fixation of the testicle in a normal anatomic position in the scrotal sac. If the testis fails to descend into the scrotum during gestation, it is considered undescended. An undescended testis becomes arrested somewhere along its normal path of descent. If it is palpable in a position other than its normal path of descent, its position is considered to be ectopic.

A retractile testis has fully descended into the scrotum but retracts out of the scrotum as a result of contraction of the cremaster muscle. Gentle manipulation allows replacement of the testis in the most dependent portion of the scrotum. Retractile testes require no surgical or hormonal treatment.

All testes that are undescended after 1 year, including those that are unresponsive to hormone injections, require surgical placement in the scrotum for optimum maturation. Laparoscopic exploration may also be used to determine position, existence, or size of a "hidden" testis.

Procedural Considerations. The setup is the same as that described for hydrocelectomy. Prepping and draping include the lower abdomen, genitalia, and thighs. Because this operation is usually performed on children, a setup containing small, delicate instruments and sutures is required.

Operative Procedure

1. An inguinal incision is generally used for exploration of undescended testes (Figure 26-37, *A*). Most undescended testes are located in the superficial inguinal pouch or inguinal canal.
2. The external oblique aponeurosis is opened through the external inguinal ring to expose the inguinal canal; the gubernacular attachments of the undescended testis are dissected free as high as the internal inguinal ring or into the abdominal cavity (see Figure 26-37, *B*).
3. The surgeon frees all adhesions and the associated inguinal hernia sac to lengthen the cord so that the testis is allowed to reach the scrotal cavity (see Figure 26-37, *C*). The hernia sac is transected, twisted, and ligated with sutures.
4. To draw vessels into the inguinal canal, more proximal to the scrotum, the floor of the inguinal canal may have to be divided at the internal ring (see Figure 26-37, *D*).
5. The lateral portion of the internal ring is closed to prevent herniation. A scrotal pocket is created, and the testis is anchored in a normal anatomic position within the scrotum with absorbable sutures (see Figure 26-37, *E* to *K*).

FIGURE 26-37 Orchiopexy.

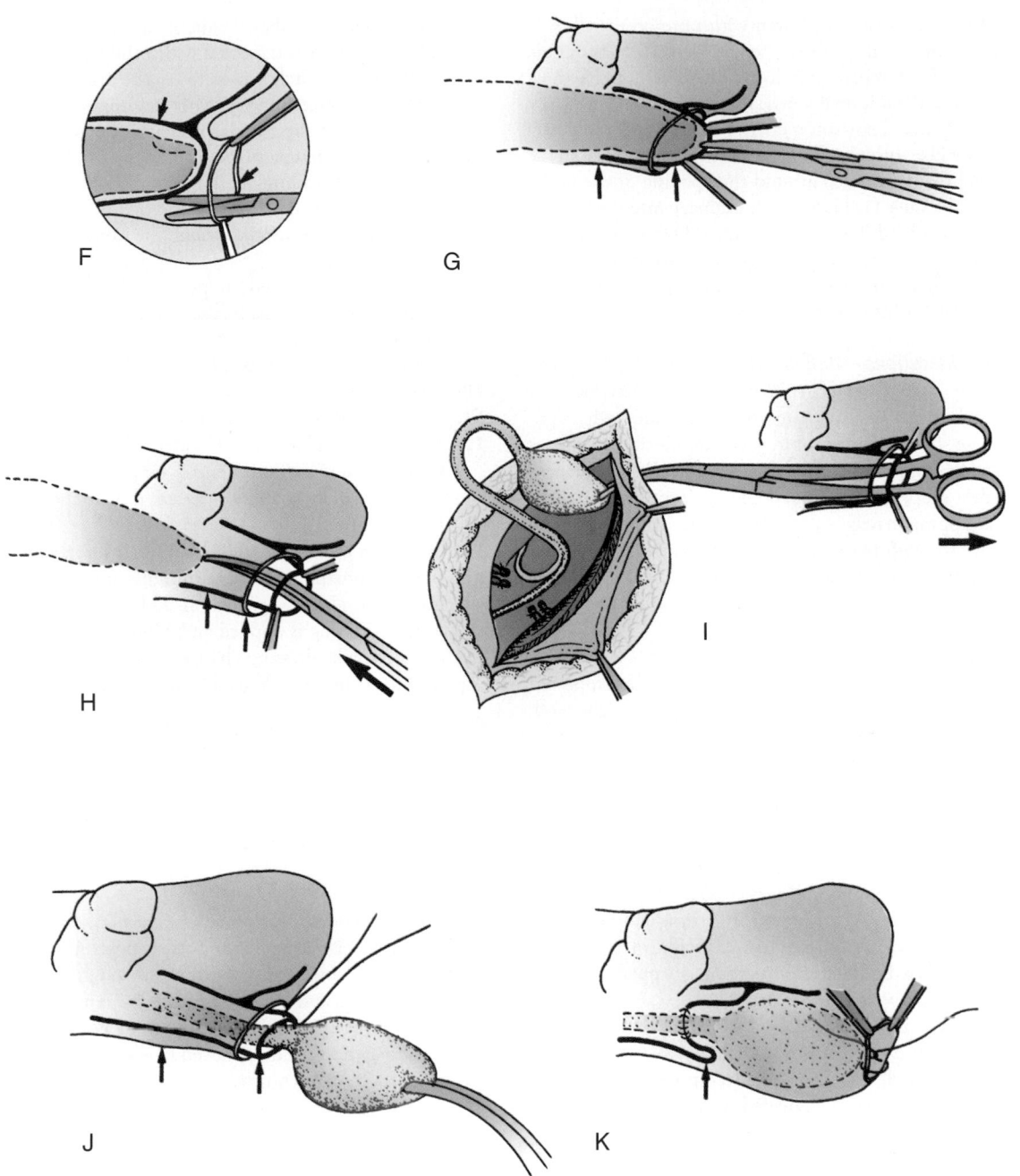

FIGURE 26-37, cont'd Orchiopexy.

Orchiopexy may be accomplished by several surgical methods. The dependent portion of the undescended testis may be sutured to the base of the scrotum with absorbable or nonabsorbable sutures exteriorized through the scrotal wall and tied over a peanut dissector or pledget. The most popular method is to anchor the testis into a dissected subdartos pouch. In this procedure a small midtransverse scrotal incision is made, and the skin and dartos muscle are dissected to create a pouch. The testis is then moved through a small hole in the dartos into the subdartos pouch and anchored in position by the traction suture. The overlying skin of the subdartos pouch is closed with fine absorbable suture material. The inguinal incision is repaired in layers with 3-0 absorbable suture. The skin is closed with a subcuticular suture, and cyanoacrylate glue is used for dressing.

Repair of Vesicoureteral Reflux

Vesicoureteral reflux (VUR) is defined as the retrograde flow of urine from the bladder to the ureter and even to the kidney pelvis. Children are usually initially diagnosed with the occurrence of a febrile urinary tract infection (UTI). The workup for reflux includes a renal bladder ultrasound with prevoid and postvoid views as well as a voiding cystourethrogram (VCUG). The VCUG is used to grade the reflux, with grade I being the least and grade V being the most extensive reflux. Children with VUR are given prophylactic antibiotics and checked yearly. Children with unresolved reflux or breakthrough infections will probably require repair of the reflux. There are two types of repair. For lower-grade reflux the most common approach is the minimally invasive approach of cystoscopy with injection of Deflux (dextroanomer/hyaluronic acid copolymer) at the ureteral orifice into the bladder wall). Deflux is a sterile biodegradable gel that is injected around the opening of the ureter to create a valve. The valve facilitates urine drainage into the bladder while preventing backward flow into the ureter. Deflux is gradually replaced by body tissues, so the integrity of the valve is maintained over time. If the reflux is more severe, the child may require reimplantation of the ureter into the bladder wall.

Procedural Considerations—Deflux. The setup for Deflux injection includes the same basic instrument setup as described for cystoscopy including a 10F offset cystoscope, light cord with a light source, cystoscopy fluid delivery tubing, Deflux needle, syringe of Deflux, and camera and monitor for the surgeon to view the procedure. The offset scope is the key to a good injection because the lens is offset at approximately a 45-degree angle, and the port to insert the needle through the scope comes straight off the end of the scope. The patient is placed in dorsal lithotomy position for the procedure.

Operative Procedure

1. The surgeon lubricates the pediatric offset cystourethroscope and inserts it through the urethra into the bladder. The light cord, camera, and irrigation tubing are attached to the cystoscope, a urine specimen for culture is obtained, and an examination is performed.
2. The bladder is partially filled, to allow for visualization.
3. The irrigation fluid is jetted into the ureteral orifice, opening it wide (hydrodistention), then the needle is introduced under the mucosa of the midureteral tunnel at the 6-o'clock position. The needle tip is positioned just under the urothelium and is advanced 4 to 5 mm in the submucosal plane of the ureter. Deflux is then injected until a prominent bulge appears, and the orifice has assumed a volcano-like shape.
4. The needle is kept in position for 15 to 30 seconds after the injection to prevent extravasation of Deflux.
5. The needle is removed, the bladder is decompressed, the scope is removed, and the patient is returned to the supine position.

Procedural Considerations—Reimplantation of the Ureter. Reimplantation of the ureter is indicated in children with high-grade VUR. The patient rarely requires a cystoscopy before the operative procedure. A Foley catheter is placed intraoperatively. The patient is placed in the supine position.

Operative Procedure

1. The surgeon makes a Pfannenstiel incision.
2. The anterior rectus fascia is opened transversely, and then flaps are developed superiorly and inferiorly above the muscle using blunt dissection.
3. The rectus muscle is separated at the midline along the linea alba.
4. The bladder is exposed and then opened in the midline approximately 2 cm above the bladder neck. The bladder is decompressed and then packed with radiopaque soft goods.
5. A Denis-Browne retractor is placed, and the trigone is exposed.

6. The surgeon identifies the ureter and places a 6F or 8F feeding tube; the ureter is dissected with minimal tissue handling and an absorbable stitch is used to tag the orifice. The ureter is then further dissected sharply with tenotomy scissors, completely freeing it from the bladder wall and allowing it to move freely.
7. The original ureteral orifice is then used to begin the dissection for a tunnel leading to the new outlet between the bladder mucosa and the detrusor muscle.
8. The suture tag is passed through the tunnel, bringing the ureter to its new outlet.
9. The ureter is sutured in place with interrupted absorbable stitches circumferentially, and the feeding tube is removed from the ureter. If ureteral catheters are left in place, they are exteriorized through the bladder and skin and sutured in place.
10. The soft goods are removed from the bladder.
11. The Denis-Browne retractor is removed from the field.
12. The surgeon closes the bladder with a running absorbable suture (a suprapubic tube may be placed during the closure). A Penrose drain may be inserted and stitched in place with a nylon suture.
13. The fascia is closed with a running absorbable suture, and the skin is approximated with a running subcuticular closure. Cyanoacrylate glue is applied. If a drain is used, an absorbent wound dressing is applied and Montgomery straps are used in order to make dressing changes easier for the child, using twill tape to string in shoelace-like fashion to close the dressing.

Otorhinolaryngologic Procedures

Three common otorhinolaryngologic procedures in the pediatric population include myringotomy with insertion of pressure equalizing tubes, tonsillectomy, and adenoidectomy. These procedures are explained in greater detail in Chapter 19.

Foreign-Body Removal

In the normal course of exploration and play, children often ingest foreign objects or place objects in their noses or ears. Most foreign bodies that are ingested pass safely through the digestive tract without incident and do not need to be removed. If the foreign body is sharp, is caustic (i.e., batteries), or becomes lodged (Figure 26-38), it may need to be removed by esophagoscopy (see Chapter 19) or through an open procedure.

The external ear canal and nose are other areas of interest to curious children. Common objects placed in the nares and external ear canal are dried beans, buttons, plastic objects, metals, food, erasers, nuts, seeds, and button batteries. Items placed in the ear can cause bleeding and difficulty with hearing. A high index of suspicion should be raised in the child with unilateral rhinorrhea, nasal crusting, and air outflow obstruction because these symptoms are often caused by a nasal foreign body. Foreign bodies in the nose and ear may require removal in the OR setting with conscious sedation or a general anesthetic.

The most significant risk of foreign-body ingestion is aspiration. Children are more prone to aspiration than adults because their laryngeal sphincters are immature, they do not have molars to chew all foods adequately, and they often run, shout, and play with objects in their mouths. Commonly aspirated food items include candy/gum, peanuts and other nuts, seeds, popcorn, hot dogs, vegetable matter, meat matter, and fish bones. Commonly aspirated nonfood items include coins, toy parts, crayons, pen tops, tacks, nails, needles, pins, beads, and screws. Aspiration may produce a complete or partial airway obstruction (Figure 26-39). Foreign

FIGURE 26-38 **A,** Anteroposterior view of coin trapped in esophagus. **B,** Lateral view.

FIGURE 26-39 Foreign body causing partial airway obstruction.

objects in the respiratory tree are removed by means of rigid or flexible bronchoscopy (see Chapter 23).

Excision of Branchial Cleft Cyst/Remnant/Sinus Tract

Congenital branchial cleft anomalies are remnants of the branchial arch apparatus that failed to disappear during early embryologic development. At approximately 5 weeks' gestation, the branchial arches are associated with an external cleft of ectodermal origin and an internal pouch of endodermal origin. Anomalies that remain from incomplete resolution can be in the form of a branchial cleft cyst, a sinus, or a fistula. The location of branchial cleft anomalies ranges from the preauricular area (type 1) to the lateral neck along

the sternocleidomastoid muscle (types 2, 3, and 4). A cyst may not become apparent until later in childhood, typically during times of acute infection or possible abscess formation, and can occur anywhere along the course of a branchial sinus tract or fistulous tract. A sinus tract usually has an external opening to the neck, generally along the anterior border of the sternocleidomastoid muscle. A fistula has both an external opening and an internal opening; the internal opening is usually in the area of the pyriform sinus near the tonsil on that side. Excision of the branchial cleft anomaly is indicated if it is cystic or if it has become infected. The infection must be treated before surgical excision; if an abscess is present an incision and drainage may be needed.

Procedural Considerations. Imaging studies (computed tomography [CT], magnetic resonance imaging [MRI]) are helpful to determine the presence of an associated tract. The patient is positioned supine with a roll under the shoulders to slightly extend the neck. A surgical drain, such as a rubber band, is frequently placed. Antibiotics are usually given intraoperatively before surgical incision. Description of a branchial cyst (type 2) excision follows.

Operative Procedure

1. A transverse skin crease overlying the lesion and 1.5 cm below the margin of the mandible is selected. The surgeon injects the proposed incision line with 1% lidocaine with 1:100,000 epinephrine.
2. The surgeon makes the skin incision with a #15 blade through the skin and subcutaneous tissues.
3. The platysma muscle is divided with an ESU.
4. The tissues overlying the cyst are gently dissected with fine forceps and small scissors or a small gauze peanut.
5. The cyst is gently grasped with a Babcock clamp. Surrounding tissue is dissected free from the cyst using small scissors to spread between the cyst capsule and surrounding tissue and then to cut through fibrous attachments.

6. If a pedicle or fibrous tract is identified, it is followed as far cephalic as possible before it is clamped, cut, and tied with 3-0 absorbable suture.

7. A small rubber band drain is usually placed to prevent accumulation of fluid or blood in the dissected cavity. A safety pin or suture is attached to the distal end of the drain; the drain is removed within 24 hours.

8. The surgeon closes the wound in layers, finishing with subcuticular sutures, and adhesive strips.

Neurosurgical Procedures

Neuropathologic conditions requiring surgical intervention can be found in any age group. The most common problems requiring neurosurgical procedures in infants and children include meningocele, myelomeningocele, encephalocele, craniosynostosis, hydrocephalus, brain tumors, and trauma. The surgical approach, instruments, and equipment required for brain tumors and trauma are relatively similar to those required for adults; consequently, the majority of these procedures are as described in Chapter 21.

Myelomeningocele and Meningocele Repair

Myelomeningocele (Figure 26-40) is a form of spina bifida and is always associated with Chiari type II malformations. It occurs because of a congenital flaw in neural tube closure at approximately 8 to 12 days after conception. The failure of the neural tube to close correctly causes a defect in the posterior elements of the lumbar vertebrae, fascia, and dura, allowing the meninges, spinal cord, and nerve roots to protrude out in a sac or cyst through the skin. The developing spinal cord and nerves are continuously exposed to amniotic fluid over the course of gestation, which results in progressive neurologic injury. There is always some degree of paralysis and loss of sensation below the defect. The amount of disability depends on the vertebral level of the spina bifida and frequently includes loss of bladder and bowel function and hydrocephalus. Meningoceles are similar to myelomeningoceles but not as neurologically devastating: meninges and cerebrospinal fluid (CSF) protrude into the defect but not the spinal cord.

Procedural Considerations. Infants born with either of these defects need to be given broad-spectrum antibiotics immediately after birth and taken to the OR within 24 hours for closure of the defect. Nursing care includes ensuring the area of the defect is covered with sterile gauze kept moistened with normal saline solution; positioning the infant so that the defect is not compressed; and maintaining the infant's body temperature, a more difficult task because of the need to keep the exposed defect moist. A very high

FIGURE 26-40 Examples of meningocele and myelomeningoceles. **A,** Meningocele. Lesion is covered by skin and meninges. **B,** Myelomeningocele. Neural component evident at central strip of lesion. **C,** Thoracolumbar myelomeningocele. **D,** Severe myelomeningocele. Neural tissue in center represents the open spinal canal.

percentage of children with this defect develop an allergy to latex; surgical closure and all subsequent surgical procedures should be performed in a latex-free environment. Repair of myelomeningocele may occur prenatally or postnatally. Concepts specific to prenatal repair are discussed in the Fetal Surgery section. The postnatal repair is described below.

Operative Procedure

1. The surgeon makes an elliptical incision around the defect with a #15 blade.
2. Metzenbaum scissors are used to remove the pearly epithelial tissue around the neural placode. Retention of the epithelial tissue can lead to formation of a postoperative epidermoid.
3. Using the Metzenbaum scissors, the surgeon performs blunt dissection following the nerve tissue on the ventral side of the placode down to the spinal canal.
4. The dura is then separated from the fascia with the Metzenbaum scissors.
5. Using 4-0 braided nylon suture, the surgeon closes the dura over the neural placode.
6. A #11 blade and Metzenbaum scissors are used to free the fascia from the muscle layer.
7. Braided nylon suture is used to close the fascial layer over the dura.
8. The muscle layer is then closed, followed by skin closure.

Craniectomy for Craniosynostosis

Craniosynostosis is the premature fusion of one or more cranial sutures. The condition can occur as part of a syndrome or as an isolated process. Craniosynostosis is characterized as "simple" when only one suture line is involved and "compound" when two or more suture lines are involved. The defect occurs in utero, and the exact etiology remains unknown. The purpose of the cranial sutures is to allow the calvaria to bend during the birth process and to allow the skull to expand to accommodate normal brain growth during infancy. The normal brain is finished growing by 2 years of age; at this time fusion of the cranial sutures normally begins. The fusion process is complete by 8 years of age.

Sagittal synostosis accounts for approximately 50% to 58% of all the synostoses with equal distribution between males and females (Sheth et al, 2012). The sagittal suture runs in the midline of the skull, connecting the anterior fontanelle to the posterior fontanelle. Premature closure of this fontanelle produces an elongation of the skull in the anteroposterior plane. Surgical intervention involves a linear strip craniectomy to excise the sagittal suture line from the anterior fontanelle to the lambdoidal suture line. Surgery is generally performed on the infant between 6 weeks and 6 months of age, with the best cosmetic results coming from the earlier repair. A craniectomy for sagittal synostosis is described.

Procedural Considerations.
The patient is positioned supine using a cerebellar headrest. Additional measures are needed to maintain the patient's normal body temperature; room temperature should be elevated, and a forced-air warming blanket should be used. An overbed warmer should be used during anesthesia induction and IV placement.

Operative Procedure

1. A sinusoidal incision is made midway between the anterior and posterior fontanelles from ear to ear, just posterior to the pinna.

2. The surgeon elevates the scalp off the skull anteriorly and posteriorly to expose the anterior fontanelle, posterior fontanelle, and asterion. Care is used to leave the pericranium attached to the skull to minimize bleeding.
3. A burr hole is made on each side of the sagittal suture on the lambdoidal suture.
4. A craniotome is used to cut anteriorly to the anterior fontanelle on each side of the sagittal suture. The surgeon uses a Leksell or Lempert rongeur to cut across the sagittal suture and connect the burr holes.
5. A Cobb periosteal elevator is used to carefully dissect the sagittal suture off the underlying dura.
6. A burr hole is placed at the asterion on each side. The craniotome is used to make a curvilinear cut just posterior to the coronal suture.
7. The parietal bone is then "greensticked" (fractured but leaving the periosteum intact) laterally.
8. The skin is closed with 3-0 and 4-0 absorbable sutures.

Ventriculoatrial and Ventriculoperitoneal Shunt Insertion

Hydrocephalus is characterized by excess production of CSF or is associated with a blockage in the ventricular drainage system. Early intervention is indicated in infants to prevent cranial distortion caused by the increasing size of the ventricles (Figure 26-41).

The two most widely used pediatric surgical procedures to divert excessive CSF from the ventricles to other body cavities from which it can be absorbed are ventriculoatrial (ventriculocardiac) (Figure 26-42) and ventriculoperitoneal shunts. See Chapter 21 for complete information related to these two procedures.

Orthopedic Procedures

Pediatric orthopedic surgery may encompass the following areas: spine disorders, sports medicine, cerebral palsy, musculoskeletal tumors and injuries, foot and ankle disorders, limb length discrepancy, hip disorders, hand surgery, limb deficiency (amputations), thoracic insufficiency, and trauma. The majority of instrumentation, equipment, and procedural considerations are similar to those described in Chapter 20. Nonetheless, there are treatment

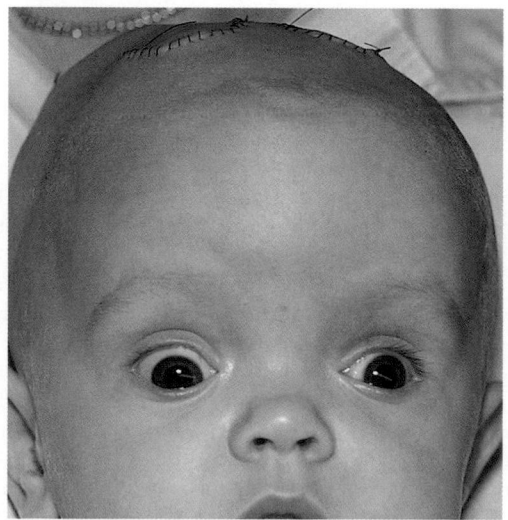

FIGURE 26-41 Infant with hydrocephalus.

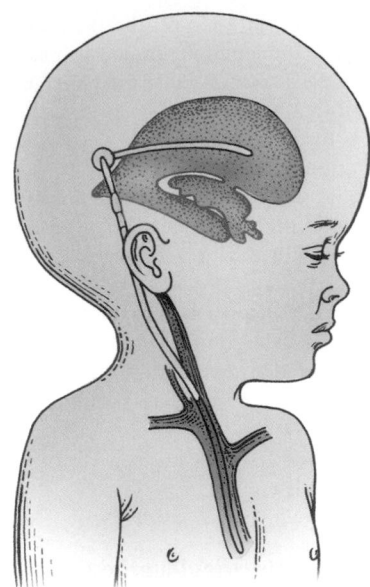

FIGURE 26-42 Placement of ventriculoatrial shunt.

FIGURE 26-43 Pavlik harness.

modalities and procedures that are more commonly performed in the pediatric population than in the adult population. Procedures for developmental dysplasia of the hip, abductor and adductor tenotomy, and variations of clubfoot are described in this section.

Repair of Developmental Dysplasia of the Hip

Until recently, dislocation of the hip seen in newborns was referred to as congenital dislocation of the hip. Developmental dysplasia of the hip (DDH) has replaced the former name to reflect the evolutionary nature of hip problems in the first few months of life. DDH is a progressive condition in which the hip structures fail to develop adequately. Because the pathologic process leading to hip dysplasia may not be present or identifiable at birth, periodic exams of every infant's hips are essential at each routine baby examination until the child is 1 year old. About 1% of infants have dislocated, dislocatable, or subluxatable hips: 60% of DDH cases occur in females, and 60% of all cases involve only the left hip (Curry et al, 2012). DDH encompasses the entire spectrum of abnormalities involving the growing hip, ranging from simple dysplasia to dysplasia with subluxation or dislocation of the hip joint. The goal of DDH management is to achieve and maintain a concentric reduction of the femoral head within the acetabulum, in order to provide the optimal environment for the normal development of both structures. When proper alignment is disrupted, soft tissue and bony changes cause contractures of the hip muscles, a shallow acetabulum, and possibly a deformed femoral head. Treatment of congenital dislocation of the hip varies depending on the age of the patient and the stability of the hip. A Pavlik harness (Figure 26-43) is the most commonly used nonoperative device in infants. If the Pavlik harness fails, the patient is taken to the OR and anesthetized for a closed reduction of the hip (proper positioning of the femur head within the acetabulum) confirmed by intraoperative arthrogram and fluoroscopy, with application of a spica cast. Failure of closed reduction and immobilization necessitates an open reduction with an adductor tenotomy to allow adequate abduction to reduce the femoral head; after surgery, children younger than 2 years are then placed

in a postreduction spica cast. For children older than 3 years the surgeon may need to perform a shortening varus femoral osteotomy (derotational osteotomy) to facilitate reduction of the femoral head into the acetabulum. In addition, if the acetabulum coverage is inadequate, a pelvic realignment (pelvic osteotomy) procedure may be necessary. Many of the pediatric orthopedic plating systems offer congenital dysplastic hip implants, which can be used in the reconstruction.

Procedural Considerations. The patient most often is in the lateral position for these procedures. An anterior incision is usually made for open reduction, whereas a lateral incision is made for the subtrochanteric femoral osteotomy. A soft tissue set and bone set (appropriate for age) are required as well as an oscillating saw, a wire driver, Steinmann pins, blade plate implants, and instrumentation.

Operative Procedures
Open Reduction for Developmental Dysplasia of the Hip (Figure 26-44)
1. The surgeon opens the hip joint and excises the soft tissue in the acetabulum.
2. The femoral head is then reduced into the acetabulum and held by suturing of the capsule.

Derotational Osteotomy for Developmental Dysplasia of the Hip. A derotational osteotomy is performed when the femoral head is improperly seated in the acetabulum.
1. The femur is placed in internal rotation and divided.
2. The distal fragment is rotated externally to place the knee and foot straight ahead.
3. If the patient is a young child, the osteotomy is frequently performed in the supracondylar region, and the patient is immobilized in a plaster spica cast.

FIGURE 26-44 Repair of congenital hip disorder using open reduction. **A,** T-shaped incision of capsule. **B,** Capsulotomy of the hip and locating the true acetabulum. **C,** Removal of tissue from the depth of the acetabulum. **D,** Capsulorrhaphy.

4. For an older child, the osteotomy is frequently done in the subtrochanteric region and the osteotomized fragments are held with an osteotomy blade plate or an intermediate compression screw. Immobilization may not be necessary.

Pelvic Osteotomy for Developmental Dysplasia of the Hip

1. A complete division of the wing of the ilium is made by an osteotomy from the sciatic notch to the anterior margin of the ilium, superior to the acetabulum.
2. The ilium is then wedged down to increase the depth of the acetabulum when the osteotomy site is opened and a bone graft is inserted.
3. The surgeon uses heavy suture to close the capsule and applies a spica cast for postoperative immobilization.

Tenotomy and Lengthening Surgery

Tenotomies and lengthening procedures are commonly recommended for children with cerebral palsy to treat contractures or because the spasticity of these muscles makes mobility and abduction and adduction of the extremities difficult (Curry et al, 2012). These procedures also may be recommended as treatment for groin injuries when traditional medical treatment has failed. Once the tendons are cut, the affected extremity may be immobilized in a cast, brace, or splint to allow for healing and promote normal growth patterns. In other cases, a dressing may be applied without immobilization. The procedure may be performed open (as described here) or using percutaneous techniques.

Procedural Considerations. The patient is positioned supine for the procedure with the affected extremity or extremities draped free for prepping and draping.

Operative Procedure

1. The surgeon makes a medial groin incision and lengthens the adductor longus, gracilis, and adductor brevis to improve hip abduction.
2. The pectineus adductor brevis interval is exposed to locate the iliopsoas tendon. The iliopsoas tendon is divided to correct hip flexion contractures.
3. Wounds are irrigated and closed using absorbable suture; cyanoacrylate glue is applied to each incision line.

Clubfoot Repair

Clubfoot is a complex deformity that is diagnosed prenatally through ultrasound or at birth. According to the American Academy of Orthopedic Surgeons (AAOS), clubfoot may occur unilaterally or bilaterally and may be idiopathic or one in a combination of other syndromes with associated anomalies (AAOS, 2007). The general characteristic for all cases includes inversion of the foot such that the anterior foot is located in the typical position of the posterior foot. Often there is a deep crease in the midfoot. Each case of clubfoot differs in severity, but all require treatment. Treatment options include nonsurgical methods such as taping, bracing, physical therapy, or continuous passive motion exercise using a machine. When clubfoot is treated surgically, the following procedures are required: release of soft tissue and joint contractures, tendon lengthening, and temporary pin fixation of the joints in the foot. Many variations of surgical intervention exist, one of which is described in the following Operative Procedure.

Procedural Considerations. The patient is positioned supine for induction of anesthesia and surgical repair. A tourniquet cuff is applied to the affected leg. The leg is prepped and draped free.

Operative Procedure

1. The surgeon makes an incision through the skin, subcutaneous tissue, and scar tissue posteriorly and medially on the affected foot with a #15 blade and dissects the tissue to locate the Achilles tendon.
2. The Achilles tendon is lengthened by tenotomy, and scar tissue is removed.
3. The surgeon identifies the peroneal tendons and lengthens them via tenotomy. Dissection is carried around to the medial aspect of the foot.
4. The posterior subtalar capsule is identified and divided, and scar tissue is removed.
5. The posterior aspect of the ankle is identified, divided, and debrided of scar tissue. The surgeon carries the dissection around medially to the posterior tibialis tendon, taking care to isolate and protect the neurovascular bundle. The posterior tibialis tendon is released.

6. Next, the medial aspect of the talonavicular joint is released. Foot flexion and rotation are verified and the surgical incision is irrigated and closed using absorbable suture.

7. A bulky dressing and cast are applied to the affected foot, and the tourniquet cuff is deflated.

Plastic and Reconstructive Surgery

Cleft Lip Repair

The normal upper lip is composed of skin, underlying orbicularis oris muscle, and mucosa. Two skin ridges are situated near the midline of the central philtrum of the lip. The vermilion (red portion of the lip) peaks at the philtral ridge on each side and gently curves downward as it reaches the midline to form Cupid's bow. A deficiency in tissue (skin, muscle, and mucosa) along one or both sides of the upper lip or, rarely, in the midline results in a cleft at the site of this deficiency. The deficiency of tissue present with a cleft lip results in distortion of Cupid's bow, absence of one or both philtral ridges, and distortion of the lower portion of the nose. Cleft lip is usually associated with a notch or cleft of the underlying alveolus and a cleft of the palate.

Cleft lip repair is most often performed when the infant is about 3 months of age. Timing of the repair follows the "rule of 10": the infant is 10 weeks of age, weighs 10 pounds, and has a hemoglobin level of 10 g/dL. Early surgical correction aids in feeding and infant-parent bonding. Lip repair is directed toward rearrangement of existing tissues to approximate the normal lip as closely as possible. Some considerations also may be given to correcting the nasal deformity at the time of the cleft lip repair.

Procedural Considerations. A plastic surgery local instrument set is required, plus the following special instruments: Brown lip clamps; calipers; a Foment retractor; Beaver blades, #64 and #65; and a Logan bow. The OR bed is usually reversed to create more knee room if the surgeon prefers to sit during the surgery. The patient is placed in the supine position, with the head at the edge of the OR bed. The face is prepped, and the head drape is used. The surgeon may stand or sit at the patient's side or just above the patient's head during the operation.

Operative Procedure. Many techniques for cleft lip repair are in common use. One type is illustrated in Figure 26-45. The following steps are applicable to all lip repairs:

1. Normal landmarks are identified and marked or tattooed. Precise measurements, taken with calipers and a ruler, are made so that corresponding points can be marked along the cleft.
2. The surgeon may infiltrate the lip with epinephrine 1:200,000, or lip clamps may be used to aid hemostasis.
3. Incisions are made along the markings for the repair.
4. The surgeon dissects the abnormal musculature.
5. Additional dissection along the maxilla and nose may be performed.
6. Closure is accomplished in three layers: muscle, skin, and mucosa. Adhesive strips may be used. A metal Logan bow is applied to the cheeks with tape strips, and elbow restraints are placed.

Cleft Palate Repair

The palate is composed of the bony or hard palate anteriorly and the soft palate posteriorly. The alveolus borders the hard palate. A separation or cleft of the palate occurs in the midline and may

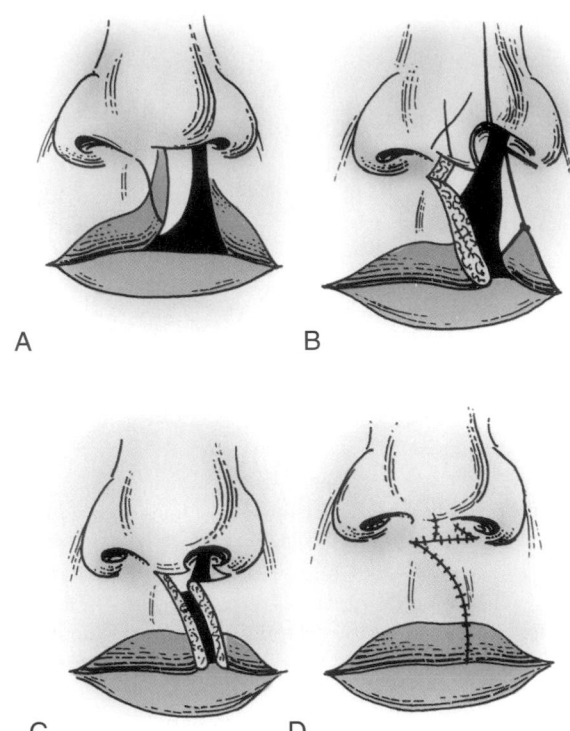

FIGURE 26-45 Rotation-advancement method to correct complete unilateral cleft of lip. **A,** Rotation incision marked so that Cupid's bow–philtral dimple component will rotate down into normal position; flap advances into columella to form nostril sill. **B,** Dimple component has dropped down; second flap has advanced into columella. **C,** Flap is being advanced into rotation gap, while skin-roll flap is interdigitated at mucocutaneous junction line. **D,** Scar is maneuvered into strategic position where it is hidden at nasal base and floor and at philtrum column; then it is interdigitated at mucocutaneous junction.

involve only the soft palate or both hard and soft palates. The alveolus may be cleft on one or both sides.

The major function of the soft palate is to aid in the production of normal speech sounds. An intact hard palate is necessary to prevent escape of air through the nose during speech and to prevent the egress of liquid and food from the nose.

Cleft palate repair is usually performed when the child is 6 months old and should be completed before the beginning of speech. Variable factors, including the child's weight and the possibility of other disease processes, can affect surgery timing. The various operations used to achieve surgical closure of the palate all use tissue adjacent to the cleft (in the form of flaps), which is shifted centrally to close the defect.

Procedural Considerations. A basic plastic surgery instrument set is required, plus the following special instruments: Dingman mouth gag with assorted blades; Blair palate hook; palate knives; Blair palate elevators; and Fomon lower lateral scissors, short and long. The patient is placed in the supine position, with the head at the edge of the OR bed. The head drape is used. Many surgeons sit just above the patient's head and cradle the head on their lap (with the patient's neck hyperextended).

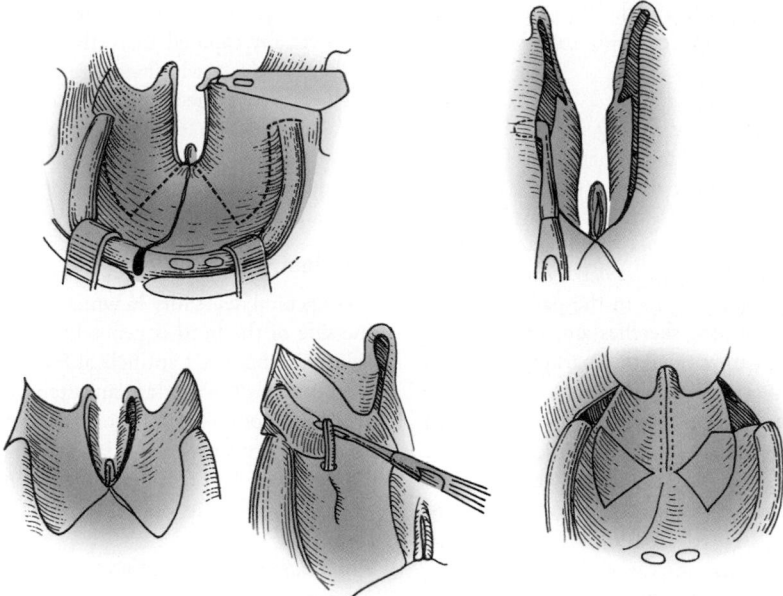

FIGURE 26-46 Closure of cleft of soft palate by V-Y (Wardill-Kilner) palatoplasty. A V-shaped incision is made on oral side of palate; mucoperiosteal flaps are elevated on oral and nasal sides, with preservation of blood vessels; Y-shaped closure (in three layers) closes cleft and lengthens palate.

Operative Procedure. One of the most frequently used cleft palate repairs is illustrated in Figure 26-46. The following steps are common to all palate repairs:

1. The Dingman mouth gag is inserted. Maintenance of the position of the endotracheal tube is crucial at this point. The surgeon may also insert a throat pack to absorb blood that may drain into the throat.
2. The outlines of the palatal flaps are marked.
3. The palate is injected with 1% lidocaine with epinephrine 1 : 100,000 for hemostasis.
4. The flaps are incised and elevated.
5. Closure is in three layers: nasal mucosa, muscle, and palatal mucosa.
6. The surgeon places a large horizontal mattress traction suture through the body of the tongue. If the patient experiences upper airway obstruction after extubation, traction is placed on this suture to pull the tongue forward, rather than insert an airway that might harm the palate repair. The throat pack is removed.

Creation of a Pharyngeal Flap

When abnormal speech (velopharyngeal insufficiency) results despite a cleft palate repair, a secondary surgical procedure may be necessary to improve speech. Primarily an excess of air escaping through the nose during speech characterizes typical "cleft palate speech." This hypernasality often results from insufficient bulk or movement of the muscles of the soft palate. To decrease or eliminate this problem, tissue from the pharynx, in the form of a pharyngeal flap, is added to the soft palate. This flap also reduces the size of the opening between the oropharynx and nasopharynx, thus decreasing or eliminating the nasal escape of air during speech.

A pharyngeal flap repair may be done at any age, but most are done before the patient is 14 years old. A pharyngeal flap also may be part of primary cleft palate repair.

Procedural Considerations. Positioning, draping, and instruments are the same as those described for cleft palate repair, with the addition of two 12F red rubber catheters.

Operative Procedure

1. The Dingman mouth gag is inserted. A throat pack may be inserted.
2. The surgeon injects the palate and posterior wall of the pharynx with 1% lidocaine with epinephrine 1 : 100,000 for hemostasis.
3. The palate is incised, and the pharyngeal flap is incised and elevated.
4. The pharyngeal wall donor site may be sutured or left open.
5. The pharyngeal flap is sutured to the palate, and the palate is closed.
6. A traction suture is placed through the body of the tongue. The throat pack is removed.

Total Ear Reconstruction

An absent external ear presents the surgical team with the objective of developing or restoring a part of the appearance that will help with self-esteem and confidence in daily interactions as well as enhance hearing because the external ear funnels sound waves from the environment into the inner ear. Emotional support is a key aspect of the plan of care for these patients.

The external ear consists of skin, subcutaneous tissue, and cartilage. The surgical procedure to create an external ear involves the retrieval of rib cartilage, carving the cartilage, placing the newly fashioned ear on the side of the patient's head, and skin grafting and dressing of the operative sites, with continual assessment and reassessment of the preoperative sketches made of the patient's ear with relation to facial structure. This can be accomplished as a one-stage procedure or as a sequence of surgeries. For congenital defects, the ideal time for initiating the procedure is between 6 and 10 years of age. In the case of traumatic loss of the external ear (as from burns), the time is individually determined. The use of tissue expanders may be considered in some cases to stretch the skin surface required to cover the ear.

Procedural Considerations. A basic plastic surgery instrument set is required, with the addition of rib graft instrumentation for autologous rib cartilage retrieval in total ear reconstruction. A sterile Doppler probe with sterile conduction gel should be available for intraoperative use. The surgeon creates preoperative sketches of the ear using unexposed x-ray film placed over the ear. Symmetric and anatomic landmarks are vital considerations in the patterns developed for the reconstruction. When the sketches are complete, the films are sterilized, with care not to remove the markings made by the surgeon. The patient is positioned supine with the arms tucked securely at the sides. Appropriate padding and protection of vulnerable neurovascular bundles and pressure sites are critical. Use of a pneumatic intermittent compression device and a forced-air warming unit over the lower half of the patient's body should be considered because of the anticipated length of the procedure. Before the skin prep the surgeon assesses the vascular integrity of the temporoparietal flap with an unsterile Doppler probe and conduction gel and marks the incision sites. Infiltration of the operative sites with local anesthetic with epinephrine 1:200,000 can be used for hemostasis. Epinephrine in higher concentrations (e.g., 1:100,000) is not recommended for use in the area of the flap because of the possible obliteration of the vascular complexes present. The perioperative nurse preps the patient's face, torso, and an additional site if a skin graft is anticipated. A standard head drape and a split drape (or U drape) for the patient's torso allows the team access to the auricular area and chest, respectively. Usually two instrument tables are used, with one designated for carving the rib cartilage. Because the procedure is lengthy (6 to 8 hours on average), rolling sitting stools should be provided for the sterile team members. The nurse ensures the patient's family receives periodic progress reports of the procedure.

Operative Procedure

1. The surgeon lifts a temporoparietal fascia flap, and uses a sterile Doppler probe to assess the vascular integrity of the flap.
2. The chest wall is incised, and the rib cartilage segments are removed, taking care to preserve the perichondrium. This encourages bone growth and helps prevent a chest wall defect. The assessment of intact pleura is critical before closure of the chest. Instillation of saline into the wound is done; if bubbles appear, the pleura is not intact; a chest tube is then inserted and attached to a chest drainage system. If the integrity of the pleura is in question, an intraoperative chest x-ray film may be taken to assess for a pneumothorax. If the pleura is intact, the surgeon closes the wound and injects 0.25% bupivacaine into the intercostal incision area.
3. While one team closes the chest, another team begins the process of carving the rib cartilage for the ear reconstruction. The previously marked radiographs are crucial aids for the artistic abilities of the surgeon, providing a blueprint for the sculpting phase of the procedure. Surgical wire is used to connect the carved pieces of rib cartilage as it is shaped to resemble the external ear.
4. A skin graft is taken, and the donor site is covered with a dressing of choice.
5. Hemostasis is maintained with an ESU, topical thrombin, and infiltration of local anesthetic with epinephrine.

6. The flap covers the sculpted ear, and the skin graft is used to cover any exposed areas (this is a technique used especially with burn patients who have less available skin for coverage).
7. Next, the surgeon places drains and attaches them to closed-wound suction, or gauze stents wrapped with nonadherent gauze are sutured in place behind the ear. Soft, bulky dressings are applied to the ear and secured with a head wrap of rolled gauze. Standard dressings are applied to the chest wall.

Otoplasty

A congenital deformity in which the ear protrudes abnormally from the side of the head is generally the result of an absent or insufficiently pronounced antihelical fold of the external ear. The various methods of otoplasty are an attempt at correction by creating an antihelical fold that positions the ear more normally (Figure 26-47). Protruding ears may be unilateral or bilateral. An otoplasty is generally performed for children who are uncomfortable or self-conscious about the deformity, usually in the elementary-school years.

Procedural Considerations. A plastic surgery instrument set is needed. The patient is placed supine on the OR bed, and a head drape is used, leaving both ears well exposed. The patient's head is turned with the affected ear up and with the lower ear well padded to avoid pressure injury.

Operative Procedure

1. The antihelical fold is created when the external ear is bent backward. The surgeon marks the position of the antihelical fold by placing 25-gauge or straight needles through the ear from anterior to posterior, applying methylene blue to the tips of the needles, and withdrawing them to mark the cartilage within.
2. An ellipse of skin is excised from the posterior surface of the ear after it has been infiltrated with 1% lidocaine with epinephrine 1:100,000.

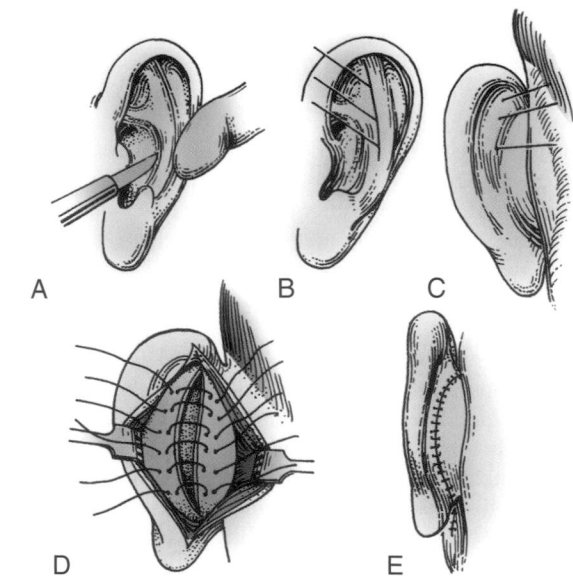

FIGURE 26-47 Otoplasty for correction of protruding ears. **A,** Antihelix defined by application of pressure to ear. **B,** Position of antihelical fold marked by the passage of straight needles through ear. **C,** Needle points visible along posterior surface of ear with ellipse of skin to be excised marked. **D,** Section of ear cartilage incised and scored or excised with sutures placed to hold cartilage back. **E,** Posterior ear incision sutured.

3. The ear cartilage is usually incised near the antihelical fold, and the anterior surface of the cartilage is scored to allow it to bend backward.
4. Next, the surgeon places sutures to hold the cartilage in its new position.
5. The skin incision is closed.
6. A drain may be placed to aid in the skin's adherence to the cartilage framework beneath.
7. A nonadherent dressing, such as petroleum gauze or cotton coated with antibiotic ointment, is usually placed in front of and behind the ear, followed by fluffed gauze and a bulky dressing made of rolled gauze to exert moderate compression on the ear.

Repair of Syndactyly

Syndactyly refers to a congenital webbing of the digits of the hands or feet. It is occasionally seen in association with other abnormalities, such as extra fingers or toes (polydactyly), or with bony abnormalities. In syndactyly with normal digits, most commonly seen, a web of skin joins adjacent fingers (Figure 26-48) but each finger has its own tendons, vessels, nerves, and bony phalanges. Although the skin web may appear loose, a deficiency in skin is always present when surgical separation is performed. Plans for taking a skin graft (usually full thickness) should always be made. Surgical separation of syndactyly is performed at any time, usually after approximately 12 months of age.

Toe syndactyly is less often treated surgically than finger syndactyly because proper function of the foot does not require fine movements of individual toes. Although the setup and description that follow are for the repair of finger syndactyly, they can also be applied to the repair of toe syndactyly.

Procedural Considerations. A plastic surgery local instrument set is required, plus a sterile marking pen, sterilized unexposed x-ray film, a pediatric pneumatic tourniquet, and an Esmarch bandage. The patient is placed supine on the OR bed with the affected arm extended on a hand table. A hand drape is used, and the affected hand and wrist are prepped and draped as well as both inguinal areas (donor sites for full-thickness skin grafts). Some surgeons prefer to use the wrist or forearm as donor sites.

Operative Procedure

1. The surgeon incises the skin and elevates small flaps at the sides of fingers and in the web.
2. After the flaps have been sutured into position, patterns of areas of absent skin on the sides of fingers are made and transferred to the skin-graft donor site.
3. The skin graft is taken; if a full-thickness skin graft is used, it must be defatted before the graft is sutured in place.
4. Skin grafts are sutured to fingers.
5. Stent dressings are placed over the skin grafts. The entire hand is immobilized in a bulky dressing or in a long arm cast.

Orbital-Craniofacial Surgery

Some congenital anomalies involve the orbital-craniofacial skeleton. These include hypertelorism, in which the distance between the orbits is increased as seen in Crouzon disease and Apert syndrome. Crouzon disease (Figure 26-49) is characterized by premature closure of the cranial sutures, resulting in an abnormally shaped skull, exophthalmos and hypertelorism, parrot's beak nose, and maxillary hypoplasia. Apert syndrome (Figure 26-50) includes the same craniofacial deformities as Crouzon disease as well as syndactyly or other hand anomalies. Advances in plastic surgery make surgical correction of some of these deformities possible.

Binocular vision is normal in humans. It involves the coordinated use of both eyes to obtain a single mental impression of objects. Binocular vision is usually absent in craniofacial anomalies because of the increased distance between the orbits. The purposes of orbital-craniofacial surgery are to provide the patient with binocular vision by moving the orbits closer together and to provide the patient with a more acceptable appearance by moving the bones of the orbital-craniofacial skeleton into a more normal position. Correction of the deformity seen in Crouzon disease and Apert syndrome involves a surgically created Le Fort III maxillary fracture.

Although an extracranial approach may be used, an intracranial approach is used in most cases; therefore, a neurosurgeon and a plastic surgeon perform these operations through a bifrontal (coronal) craniotomy. A tracheostomy may be done before the start of the procedure. Bone grafts from hips or ribs are necessary to

FIGURE 26-48 Syndactyly involving third and fourth fingers.

FIGURE 26-49 Crouzon disease.

FIGURE 26-50 Apert syndrome.

augment areas of bone deficit, which result from movement of the craniofacial skeleton.

Procedural Considerations. These operations are usually performed on children. They are very extensive procedures, often lasting 12 to 14 hours. Blood loss is considerable. Postoperative complications, such as cerebral edema or meningitis, can be formidable. The perioperative nurse must pay particular attention to the following important details: (1) insertion of a Foley catheter into the patient's bladder before the operation is started, (2) positioning of the patient on the OR bed so that all bony prominences are well padded, and (3) availability of accurate means for measuring blood loss. Use of a pneumatic intermittent compression device and forced-air warming units should also be anticipated.

A basic plastic surgery instrument set, craniectomy instruments and supplies (see Chapter 21), plastic hand instrumentation, and tracheostomy instruments and supplies are required. A high-speed drill, saws, and general orthopedic instrumentation are also needed. A separate setup is necessary for obtaining the bone graft.

The patient is positioned, prepped, and draped as described for bifrontal craniotomy (see Chapter 21). The entire face is left exposed, however, and may temporarily be covered with a plastic drape until the portion of the operation requiring access to the face is reached. The bone-graft donor site is also prepped and draped so that both iliac crests and the lower ribs are exposed.

Operative Procedure

1. Tracheostomy, if required, is performed first, followed by application of arch bars (when indicated as in Crouzon disease and Apert syndrome).
2. The bifrontal craniotomy with craniectomy is performed.
3. Bilateral orbital osteotomies (Figure 26-51, *A*) into the anterior cranial fossa are performed. Bilateral conjunctival (lower eyelid) and labiogingival sulcus incisions (for Crouzon disease and Apert syndrome) are made for orbital and maxillary osteotomies.
4. The surgeon moves the bones of the orbital-craniofacial region (see Figure 26-51, *B*), based on measurement of the intercanthal distance (in hypertelorism) or occlusion of the teeth (in Crouzon disease and Apert syndrome).
5. Bone grafts may be taken from the calvaria, ribs, or hips to augment areas of bone deficit, which result from movement of the craniofacial skeleton.

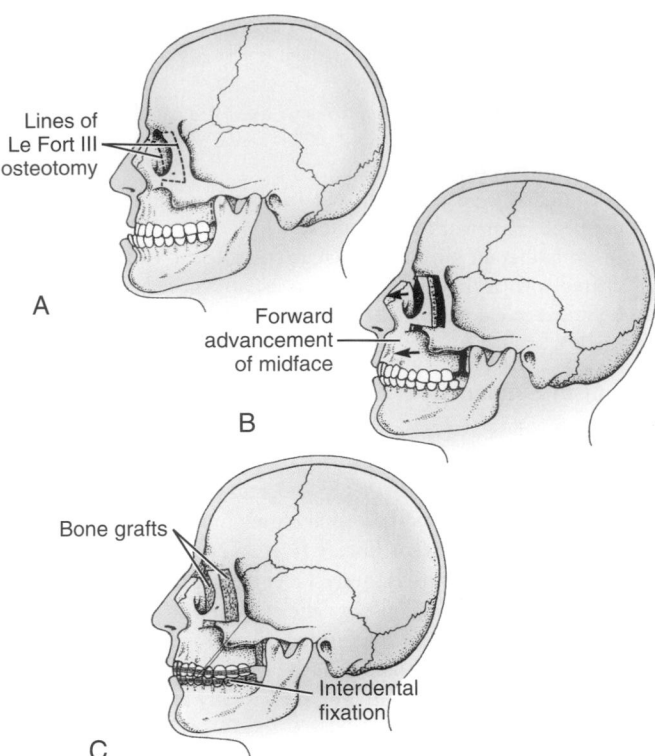

FIGURE 26-51 Steps in surgical correction of Crouzon disease deformities.

6. Bone grafts are fixed in place with interosseous wires and by means of intermaxillary fixation applied to arch bars (for Crouzon disease and Apert syndrome) (see Figure 26-51, *C*). Rigid plate-and-screw fixation is another option.
7. The craniotomy, conjunctival, intraoral, and bone-graft donor site incisions are closed and dressings applied.

Pediatric Ophthalmic Surgery

Although the anatomy of the eye remains the same (refer to Chapter 18), children experience different eye conditions from adults that are specifically related to vision development in the brain. Vision develops in the brain until approximately 9 years of age. It is affected by eyes that are not straight or do not focus correctly. Therefore, it is imperative that any vision problems are detected and corrected early.

Pediatric ophthalmologists participate in specific programs of study that focus on examination and care of childhood vision problems and structural disorders of the eye. Their scope of practice includes not only examination and treatment, such as vision testing and treatment of eye infections, but also surgical management of disorders such as congenital nasolacrimal duct obstruction, pediatric cataracts, ptosis, strabismus, pediatric glaucoma, and eye injuries (American Association for Pediatric Ophthalmology and Strabismus [AAPOS], 2012). It is not uncommon for pediatric ophthalmology to be subdivided into specialty categories. The field of oculoplastics was first identified in 1966. Oculoplastics encompasses the merging of plastic surgery and ophthalmology in attempt to treat or repair the oculo-orbital region of the face, be it structural (drainage problems) or cosmetic (Whitaker, 2002). Surgeons may also focus their practice on corneal disorders, retinal disorders, or neuro-ophthalmology.

A   B

FIGURE 26-52 Forniceal incisions for strabismus surgery. All six muscles can be isolated from these two incisions. **A,** Inferotemporal incision: isolates the lateral rectus, inferior rectus, and inferior oblique muscles. **B,** Superonasal incision: isolates the medial rectus, superior rectus, and superior oblique muscles.

BOX 26-5

Types of Strabismus

- *Esotropia*: Inward turning of one or both eyes
- *Exotropia*: Outward turning of one or both eyes
- *Hypertropia*: One eye higher than the other
- *Hypotropia*: One eye lower than the other

Eye Muscle Surgery for Strabismus (Figure 26-52)

Any misalignment of the eyes is called strabismus. Strabismus is further subdivided into the categories listed in Box 26-5. Strabismus occurs as a result of poorly controlled neuromuscular eye movements. Any child can suffer from strabismus, but disorders that affect the brain (cerebral palsy, hydrocephalus, Down syndrome, brain tumors) are associated with an increased prevalence of the disorder. Additionally, strabismus may occur in conjunction with traumatic brain, nerve, or ocular injury.

The goal for treatment of strabismus is to straighten the eyes so that binocular vision functions appropriately. Nonsurgical treatments may include eyeglasses and eye exercises. Surgery may be recommended to change the alignment of the eyes relative to each other by strengthening, weakening, or repositioning the eye muscles. If a child presents with strabismus in addition to another eye disorder (e.g., ambylopia, cataract, or ptosis), the other condition will be treated before corrective surgery.

Skin incisions are not necessary to repair strabismus. Instead the surgeon uses a lid speculum to retract the eyelid and incises the conjunctiva to expose the muscles. Box 26-6 differentiates between the methods of muscle repair. The repaired muscles are sutured using a standard knot or adjustable suture. Adjustable sutures consist of temporary knots (bow or slip) placed in an accessible position so that eye alignment can be altered approximately 24 hours after surgery. The lateral rectus recession and lateral rectus resection procedures are described below.

Procedural Considerations. The patient receives a general anesthetic, and the full face above the nose is prepped with half-strength povidone-iodine. Both eyes are prepped so that the repair can be measured against the contralateral eye for symmetry.

BOX 26-6

Methods of Muscle Repair

Recession
- Is a weakening procedure
- Alters the attachment site of the eye muscle on the eyeball
- Muscle is cut from the surface of the eye and reattached at a point farther back from the front of the eye

Resection
- Is a strengthening procedure
- Extraocular muscle is reattached to the eyeball at its original site.
- A section of the muscle is removed and a stitch is placed in the muscle at the intended new attachment site.
- The segment of muscle between the stitch and the eyeball is removed.
- The shortened muscle is reattached to the eye.

Operative Procedure—Lateral Rectus Recession

1. A lid speculum is placed in the affected eye and the unaffected eye is taped closed.
2. The surgeon grasps the infratemporal limbus using Moody locking forceps, then rotates the eye superonasally.
3. A conjunctival fornix incision is made posterior to the limbus in the infratemporal quadrant.
4. Tendons and episclera are dissected until bare sclera is reached, and the lateral rectus is isolated with a Green muscle hook.
5. The surgeon passes a suture through the original insertion of the lateral rectus muscle and locks it on superior and inferior aspects. The muscle is then cut from its insertion on the globe using Aebli scissors.
6. Calipers are used to mark a location posterior to the insertion point, and the surgeon passes a suture through the sclera using the "crossed swords" technique.
7. The muscle is pulled up firmly to the globe and tied into position. The location is measured again using calipers.
8. Conjunctiva is closed using plain gut suture.
9. The surface of the eye may be covered in neomycin/polymyxin/dexamethasone and tetracaine ointment.

Operative Procedure—Lateral Rectus Resection

1. Steps 1 through 4 of the Lateral Rectus Recession procedure are performed.
2. A suture is passed through the original insertion of the lateral rectus muscle and locked on superior and inferior aspects. The central sutures are tied together, and a resection clamp is placed anteriorly.
3. The surgeon cuts the muscle anterior to the resection clamp, then cuts the remaining muscle stump from its original insertion point.
4. The suture needles are passed through the original insertion in a perpendicular fashion and tied together.
5. The muscle is pulled up firmly to the globe and tied into position.
6. Conjunctiva is closed using plain gut suture.
7. The surface of the eye may be covered in neomycin/polymyxin/dexamethasone and tetracaine ointment.

Ptosis (Blepharoptosis) Surgery

Defined as a droopy eyelid, ptosis is either congenital or acquired. Congenital ptosis (Figure 26-53) is usually a result of a deficit in the levator palpebri muscle in the upper eyelid. Acquired ptosis occurs as a result of neurologic conditions that affect the nerves of the eye (myasthenia gravis, Horner syndrome, third nerve paralysis). It also can manifest in conjunction with movement disorders,

resulting in double vision. Ptosis also may result from orbital tumors.

Ptosis is treated with corrective lenses if amblyopia with astigmatism is present. Surgery is indicated for cases in which the droopy eyelid is blocking normal vision or causes the child to position the head with the chin up in an attempt to compensate for the block in vision. The goal of surgery is to create as perfect an anatomic result as possible by elevating the position of the lid, creating a lid fold, and preserving the contour and symmetry of both lids (Figure 26-54). The Fasenella-Servat procedure is indicated for mild congenital ptosis (less than 2 mm of lid droop) with good levator function. Variations of this procedure are favored over other types of repair, including Werb procedure (Heher and Katowitz, 2002).

Procedural Considerations. The patient is positioned supine with the head on a gel ring. The eyes are prepped with half-strength povidone-iodine (1 : 1 povidone-iodine and normal saline solution). The patient is draped to expose both eyes for comparison during the procedure. Ointment is applied to the contralateral eye, and the eye is taped shut for protective purposes during surgery.

Operative Procedure

1. The surgeon places a scleral shell into the affected eye to protect the globe.

FIGURE 26-53 Simple congenital ptosis. **A,** Unilateral. **B,** Bilateral.

FIGURE 26-54 Modified Fasenella-Servat procedure. **A,** Preoperative. **B,** Six months postoperative.

2. The upper lid is everted and two curved hemostats are placed at the upper tarsal border and adjusted so that the tips are centrally located (Figure 26-55, *A*).
3. Traction sutures are passed through the tissue at the nasal and temporal end, approximately 3 mm below the clamps (see Figure 26-55, *B*).
4. The tissue between the two clamps and traction sutures is excised using a #15 blade (see Figure 26-55, *C*) or sharp scissors (see Figure 26-55, *D*).
5. A nylon suture is passed through the end of the lid crease out through the apex of the incision and run in a "serpentine" fashion. The suture reconnects the conjunctiva and Müller muscle to the cut edge of the tarsus (see Figure 26-55, *E* to *G*).
6. At the opposite end of the incision, the suture is passed through the apex of the incision and out through the crease, then buried beneath the conjunctival surface (see Figure 26-55, *H* and *I*).
7. The surgeon removes the traction sutures and returns the lid to its normal position. A lid plate is used to smooth the incision line by pressing directly on the skin surface to flatten the tissues against the plate (see Figure 26-55, *J*).
8. The nylon suture is tied snugly over the skin and remains in place approximately 1 week following surgery to allow for lid adjustment (see Figure 26-55, *K*).
9. The surgeon removes the scleral shell and applies ophthalmic antibiotic to the eye and suture line. A dressing may be applied to the surgical site.

Cataract Surgery

Cataracts occur in approximately 3 out of 10,000 children and are primarily classified as nuclear, posterior subcapsular, anterior polar, posterior polar, lamellar, or traumatic (AAPOS, 2012) (Box 26-7). If a cataract causes significant vision loss, it must be removed as soon as possible. An intraocular lens (IOL) may be used in order to replace the focusing power once the natural lens is surgically removed. These devices have not been approved by the FDA for younger populations. Sometimes IOL use is in the best interest of the patient, and in these cases, a surgeon can use the IOL "off-label." Other options include wearing glasses or contact lenses to correct the deficit.

Corneal Surgery

The cornea is only about 0.5 mm thick and consists of many layers. The stroma is the thickest part of the cornea. Diseases of the cornea include, but are not limited to, allergies, conjunctivitis (pink eye), corneal infections, dry eye, herpes zoster (shingles), ocular herpes, pterygium, and Stevens-Johnson syndrome. In some cases corneal surgery or a corneal transplant is necessary, particularly when high pressure from glaucoma allows fluid to accumulate in the stroma. Once this occurs, it may lead to a cloudy cornea.

Trabeculotomy for Glaucoma

The pathophysiology of glaucoma is markedly different for infants and children than in adults, and its occurrence is rare, occurring in

FIGURE 26-55 Modified Fasenella-Servat procedure. **A,** Hemostats at upper tarsal border. **B,** Passage of traction sutures. **C,** Excision of tissue using blade. **D,** Excision of tissue using sharp scissors.

Continued

FIGURE 26-55, cont'd **E** to **G,** Reconnection of conjunctiva and Müller muscle to edge of tarsus. **H** and **I,** Suture passed through apex of incision and out through crease. **J,** Smoothing incision line with lid plate. **K,** Nylon suture allows for lid adjustment.

Types of Cataracts

- *Nuclear:* Cloudiness in the center part of the lens
- *Lamellar:* Cloudiness between the nuclear and cortical layers of the lens
- *Traumatic:* Results from blunt or penetrating force that damages the lens
- *Posterior subcapsular:* Affects the back surface of the lens cortex, inside the capsule
- *Anterior polar:* Central opacity of the front part of the lens capsule; do not grow during childhood and do not require surgical management
- *Posterior polar:* Central opacity of the back of the lens

TABLE 26-5

Categories of Glaucoma

Category	Age at Presentation	Symptoms at Presentation
Congenital	Glaucoma present at birth	Excessive tearing Light sensitivity Large, cloudy cornea Dull-appearing iris
Infantile	Glaucoma presents between 1 and 24 months of age	Excessive tearing Light sensitivity Large, cloudy cornea Dull-appearing iris
Juvenile	Glaucoma presents after 36 months of age	No obvious symptoms; presents similar to adult-onset glaucoma

TABLE 26-6

Stages of Retinopathy of Prematurity (ROP)

Stages	Description	Intervention
Stage 1	Mildly abnormal growth of retinal vessels	Usually does not require treatment, no long-term affects
Stage 2	Moderately abnormal growth of retinal vessels	Usually does not require treatment, no long-term affects
Stage 3	Severely abnormal growth of retinal vessels	May require treatment Children with stage 3 ROP have a higher risk of long-term vision problems
Stage 4	Partial retinal detachment	Usually requires treatment May lead to long-term vision problems or blindness
Stage 5	Complete retinal detachment	Requires treatment May lead to long-term vision problems or blindness

management of the disease typically requires multiple examinations and procedures.

Retinal Disorders

Retinal diseases include retinopathy of prematurity (ROP). ROP is one of the most common causes of visual loss in childhood and can lead to lifelong vision impairment and blindness, and is classified according to stage (Table 26-6). The most effective proven treatments for ROP are laser therapy or cryotherapy. Both laser treatments and cryotherapy are performed only on infants with advanced ROP. Severe cases (stage V) of this disorder are treated with scleral buckle and posterior vitrectomy (see Chapter 18).

Trauma

Principles governing surgical care of trauma patients are discussed in Chapter 28. However, when caring for the pediatric trauma patient in surgery, the perioperative nurse must possess additional knowledge to develop a detailed plan of action that effectively drives the delivery of safe patient care. During all episodes of patient care, it is necessary for the perioperative nurse to communicate with members of the surgical and interdisciplinary team in a fashion that best supports positive patient outcomes. The urgency of injury will dictate the timeliness of surgical intervention—in some instances, pediatric trauma patients may require transfer to a level I trauma center. The criteria for transfer are outlined in Box 26-8. The perioperative nurse should be prepared to administer care to any type of injury in a safe and effective manner that is appropriate across all age levels.

Trauma is the leading cause of death in children from 1 to 14 years of age. Each year another 100,000 children experience disability from trauma. Several factors, such as age, gender, behavior, and environment, influence the risk of traumatic injury. For instance, infants and toddlers are more prone to falls resulting in severe injury, which may be related to the pliable nature of their skeletal system. If broken bones are present, a severe force of injury must be assumed. Older children and adolescents are at higher risk for bicycle-related and motor vehicle—related injuries. In this age group, blunt injuries resulting from motor vehicle accidents or

approximately 1 in 10,000 births (AAPOS, 2012). Pediatric glaucoma is categorized according to age of onset (Table 26-5). Cases of glaucoma are classified as primary (without specific identifiable cause) or secondary (occurring in conjunction with another disorder, medication use, or eye trauma). Children with glaucoma could have other eye abnormalities in addition to the glaucoma, including opacities of the cornea (Peters anomaly, for example).

Pediatric glaucoma is treated by a combination of medical and surgical intervention because the goal of treatment is more than simply lowering intraocular pressure. Children diagnosed with congenital or infantile glaucoma often develop myopia and require glasses. There is also an increased occurrence of strabismus and amblyopia in children with glaucoma. Extreme cases may result in vision loss, supporting the need for early diagnosis and management of the disorder.

Pediatric glaucoma is commonly evaluated by examining under anesthesia (EUA). At this time the ophthalmologist measures intraocular pressure, corneal length, axial diameter, and refractive error and assesses corneal clarity and the optic nerve. If the intraocular pressure is elevated, it can be treated medically or surgically. The majority of primary pediatric glaucoma cases are treated surgically.

The most common surgical approach is trabeculotomy with goniometry, which opens the drainage canal and facilitates aqueous drainage. Other options, such as trabeculotomy with tube placement, create a bypass route to shunt aqueous drainage. Laser procedures are also effective in some cases of glaucoma. Successful

BOX 26-8

Trauma Transfer Criteria for Pediatric Patients Less Than or Equal to Age 14

Consider Transfer to Pediatric Trauma Center
- Nonoperative management of solid organ injury
- Assessment of any of the following "negative points" on the pediatric trauma scale:
  - Weight less than 10 kg
  - Unstable airway
  - Blood pressure less than 50 mm Hg (systolic)
  - Coma
  - Major open, penetrating wound
  - Open, multiple fractures
- Injury severity score greater than 9
- Victim of nonaccidental injury that requires intervention from child protective team or other resources
- Anticipated complexity of care exceeds the capabilities of local resources at adult trauma center

Transfer to Pediatric Trauma Center
- Persistent physiologic demise (the decision to transfer should be consistent with best practices in trauma care)
- Traumatic brain injury
- Intubation and mechanical ventilation with no expectation to wean within 24 hours
- Children with special needs or other comorbid conditions

Modified from Pennsylvania Trauma Systems Foundation: *Adult trauma center accreditation, Appendix C: transfer guidelines: adult trauma centers (level I, II, and III) to pediatric trauma centers,* Mechanicsburg, PA, 2010.

PATIENT SAFETY

Child Passenger Safety

Motor vehicle crashes are the number one killer of children older than the age of 4. Parents and caregivers should be encouraged to follow these best-practice recommendations to reduce the risk of injury or death for children who ride in motor vehicles:

1. All infants and toddlers should ride in a rear-facing car safety seat (CSS) until they are 2 years of age *or* until they reach the highest weight or height allowed by the manufacturer of their CSS.
2. All children older than 2 years *or* children younger than 2 years who have outgrown the rear-facing weight or height limit for their CSS should ride in a forward-facing CSS with a harness for as long as possible, up to the highest weight or height allowed by the manufacturer of their CSS. The lowest maximum weight limit currently available in forward-facing CSSs is 40 pounds, but some seats can accommodate children up to 80 pounds.
3. All children whose height or weight is more than the forward-facing limit for their CSS should use a belt-positioning booster seat until the vehicle lap and shoulder seat belt fits properly (approximately 4 feet 9 inches in height and between 8 and 12 years of age).
4. Children who are old enough and large enough to use vehicle seatbelts should use lap and shoulder seat belts for optimal protection.
5. All children younger than 13 years of age should be restrained in the rear seats of vehicles for optimal protection.

Modified from Durbin D: Child passenger safety, *Pediatrics* 127(4):788–793, 2011.

TABLE 26-7

Pediatric Modification of Glasgow Coma Scale

Glasgow Coma Scale	Pediatric Modification
Eye Opening	
Birth to 1 Year	**12 Months or Older**
4 Spontaneous	4 Spontaneously
3 To shout	3 To verbal command
2 To pain	2 To pain
1 No response	1 No response
Best Motor Response	
Birth to 1 Year	**12 Months or Older**
6 Purposeful movements	6 Obeys command
5 Localizes pain	5 Localizes pain
4 Flexion, withdrawal	4 Flexion, withdrawal
3 Flexion, abnormal	3 Flexion, abnormal
2 Extension, rigidity	2 Extension, rigidity
1 No response	1 No response

Best Verbal Response

Birth to 1 Year	1 to 5 Years	Older than 5 Years
5 Babbles, coos appropriately	5 Age-appropriate words, phrases	5 Oriented and converses
4 Cries, but consolable	4 Confusion, inappropriate words, phrases (for age)	4 Confused or disoriented conversation
3 Inconsolable crying	3 Cries, screams	3 Inappropriate words
2 Grunts	2 Grunts	2 Incomprehensible sounds
1 No response	1 No response	1 No response

Modified from Lerner JT, Giza CC: Traumatic brain injury in children. In Swaiman KF et al, editors: *Swaiman's pediatric neurology,* ed 5, Philadelphia, 2012, Saunders; Kleigman RM et al, editors: *Nelson textbook of pediatrics,* ed 19, Philadelphia, 2012, Saunders.

direct blows (as with contact sports or child abuse) along with falls are the most common mechanisms of injury (Moore et al, 2009). It is not uncommon for pediatric traumatic injuries to occur in the home environment, stressing the importance of community awareness and education as it relates to trauma prevention. Some of the most significant prevention strategies focus on car seat safety as a means of preventing injury from motor vehicle accidents (Patient Safety).

Throughout the pediatric population neurologic injuries are the most common cause of traumatic death in children; their head is proportionately larger in relation to their body mass and especially vulnerable to injury. Table 26-7 provides guidelines for using the Glasgow Coma Scale for infants and children. Because children have a much smaller reserve than adults, once a decline in vital functions is noted, demise is rapid. Information about commonly used medications in pediatric resuscitation is noted in the Surgical Pharmacology box.

IV access is often difficult in the pediatric patient, and an intraosseous line may be inserted by emergency rescue personnel before arrival at the hospital or in the emergency department (ED). These lines are inserted by use of an intraosseous needle or bone marrow aspiration needle and are placed slightly below the knee on the anterior aspect of the tibia at a 90-degree angle (Figure 26-56). Stabilization of the line may be difficult, but the line can remain for up to 24 hours and provides rapid access when other routes are

SURGICAL PHARMACOLOGY

Medications Used in Pediatric Resuscitation

Perioperative nurses must always be prepared in the event of a compromising cardiac or respiratory event in the pediatric patient. The information contained in this section provides several commonly used medications, their mode of action, and nursing implications for pediatric resuscitation.

Medication/Category	Dosage/Route for Infants and Children	Purpose/Action	Adverse Reactions	Nursing Implications
Adenosine *Pharmacotherapeutic:* Antiarrhythmic	IV: 0.1 mg/kg. If not effective, give 0.2 mg/kg. Do not exceed 6 mg in first dose and 12 mg in successive doses.	Treatment of paroxysmal supraventricular tachycardia (PSVT)	• AV block, chest pain, facial flushing, hypotension • Dizziness, headache • GI discomfort, nausea • Dyspnea • Diaphoresis • Asystole, atrial fibrillation, bradycardia, bronchospasm (rare, but life-threatening)	Possible exacerbation of asthma in asthmatic patients. Follow by rapid saline flush.
Amiodarone *Pharmacotherapeutic:* Antiarrhythmic	IV bolus/IO: 5 mg/kg	Pulseless ventricular fibrillation or ventricular tachycardia	• AV block, bradycardia, cardiac arrhythmia, edema, hypotension • Dizziness, headache • Slate-blue skin discoloration • Abdominal pain, abnormal salivation • Coagulation abnormalities • Phlebitis with concentrations greater than 3 mg/mL • Acute intracranial hypertension, acute renal failure, acute respiratory distress syndrome (rare, but life-threatening)	Administer slowly in patients with diminished cardiac function.
Atropine sulfate *Pharmacotherapeutic:* Antiasthmatic/ anticholinergic	IV/IT: 0.02 mg/kg, minimum dose 0.1 mg, maximum single dose 0.5 mg in children and 1 mg in adolescents. May repeat in 5-minute intervals to a maximum of 1 mg in children or 2 mg in adolescents.	Treatment of sinus bradycardia	• Arrhythmia, hypotension, tachycardia • Ataxia, coma, disorientation • Urticaria • Delayed gastric emptying, nausea • Urinary retention • Weakness • Dyspnea, laryngospasm, pulmonary edema • Anaphylaxis	Monitor heart rate.
Calcium gluconate *Pharmacotherapeutic:* Electrolyte supplement	IV: 30-100 mg/kg	Treatment of cardiac disturbances of hypocalcemia	• Arrhythmia, bradycardia, cardiac arrest, hypotension, syncope, vasodilation • Hypercalcemia • Tingling sensation	Contraindicated in ventricular fibrillation during cardiac resuscitation.
Epinephrine *Pharmacotherapeutic:* Adrenergic agonist agent	IV/IO: 0.01 mg/kg of 1:10,000 solution, maximum single dose 1 mg ETT: 0.1 mg/kg of 1:1000 solution, maximum single dose of 2.5 mg. Repeat every 3-5 minutes as needed to a maximum total dose of 10 mg.	Treatment of bradycardia, asystole, or pulseless arrest	• Cardiac arrhythmia, chest pain, flushing, hypertension • Cerebral hemorrhage, restlessness • Nausea and vomiting • Dyspnea, pulmonary edema • Diaphoresis	Protect drug from light (do not use discolored or precipitated solutions); unstable in alkaline solution. Most useful drug during cardiac arrest.

Continued

SURGICAL PHARMACOLOGY

Medications Used in Pediatric Resuscitation—cont'd

Medication/Category	Dosage/Route for Infants and Children	Purpose/Action	Adverse Reactions	Nursing Implications
Lidocaine *Pharmacotherapeutic:* Antiarrhythmic agent	IV/IO/ETT: Loading dose 1 mg/kg. May repeat in 10-15 minutes times 2 doses. After loading dose, start IV continuous infusion 20-50 mcg/kg/min. Use 20 mcg/kg in patients with shock, hepatic disease, cardiac arrest, or mild congestive heart failure.	Treatment of ventricular arrhythmias from myocardial infarction or cardiac manipulation	• Bradycardia, hypotension, arrhythmias • Agitation, lethargy, seizures • Nausea and vomiting • Thrombophlebitis • Muscle twitching, paresthesias • Dyspnea, respiratory depression or arrest	For ETT administration, dilute with 1-2 mL normal saline prior to ETT administration.
Sodium bicarbonate *Pharmacotherapeutic:* Alkalizing agent	IV push: 1 mEq/kg initially, may repeat with 0.5 mEq/kg in 10 minutes once as indicated by acid-base status. Rate of administration should not exceed 10 mEq/min.	Management of metabolic acidosis or life-threatening hyperkalemia	• Cerebral hemorrhage, edema • Tetany • Gastric distention • Hypernatremia, hypocalcemia, hypokalemia • Pulmonary edema	Patient should be adequately ventilated before administering sodium bicarbonate in cardiac arrest.

AV, Atrioventricular; *ETT,* endotracheal tube; *GI,* gastrointestinal; *IV,* intravenous; *IT,* intratracheal; *IO,* intraosseous.
Modified from the *Children's Hospital of Philadelphia emergency medication dosing book,* 2011, available at www.crlonline.com/lco/action/doc/retrieve/docid/chiphi_f/381007. Accessed December 11, 2012.

too time-consuming or difficult to access. Fluid resuscitation levels for children experiencing hemorrhage, as well as types and dosages of medications, are based on body weight because weight provides a better mechanism of accuracy when calculating dosage.

Because of the nature of the trauma, it may be difficult for the healthcare team to obtain the patient's exact body weight. In these instances, body weight can be estimated using Broselow tapes or palmar methods. The body size of the patient determines the type of instrumentation required. Pediatric trauma instrument sets, including vascular clamps and retractors, and suture supplies should be available and organized in a fashion that promotes easy and timely access when urgent situations arise. Creative problem solving may be required of the perioperative nurse in adaptation of feeding tubes, drains, and other equipment.

Maintenance of body temperature is of utmost concern in the pediatric population, and undue skin exposure should be avoided. Fluids for irrigation and IV infusion may be warmed, depending on the preferences of the surgeon and the status of the child. Whenever possible, room temperature is elevated. Warming blankets and head coverings (stockinettes) may be used to prevent heat loss; this is especially critical with children who have sustained burns.

Traumas are graded based on the severity of injury (Table 26-8). The perioperative nurse should attempt to obtain a trauma history from ED personnel or the family if the patient comes directly to the OR. Initial vital signs should be obtained and compared with those obtained during prehospital care or in the ED; Box 26-9 gives a formula for blood pressure estimation. When obtaining the initial assessment it is important to use a developmental approach to pediatric trauma patients, who respond differently from adults. During traumatic events it is also imperative to consider the well-being of patients, families, and caregivers. The perioperative nurse plays an integral role in preparing those associated with the child for outcomes associated with trauma surgery and may help facilitate consults from the departments of child life, social work, and clergy.

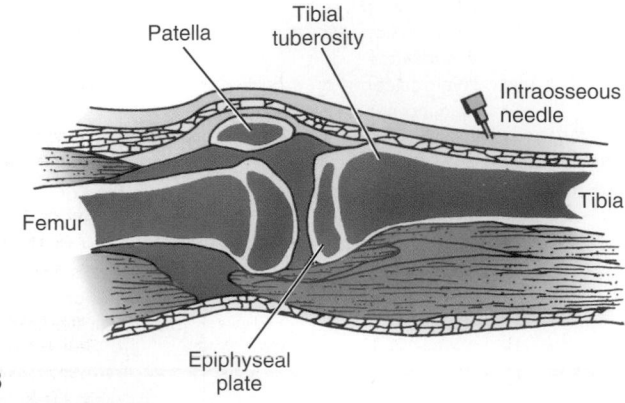

FIGURE 26-56 **A,** Intraosseous infusion technique. **B,** Insertion.

TABLE 26-8

Trauma Grading

Level	Physiologic Considerations	Anatomic Considerations
Level I: Life-threatening injuries, unstable vital signs	Respiratory distress Artificial airway/unstable airway Cardiac arrest Hemodynamic instability Severe uncontrolled hemorrhage Systolic blood pressure (SBP) less than 80 mm Hg that does not respond to fluid resuscitation Glasgow Coma Scale (GCS) score ≤8 Lateralizing neurologic signs or worsening neurologic exam	Airway compromise Severe maxillofacial trauma Major vascular injury including significant crush or amputation above the elbow or knee with a high probability of operative intervention Significant penetrating injury to the head, neck, or torso Burns ≥25% total body surface area with or without inhalation injury Spinal cord injury with neurologic signs or symptoms Unstable vertebral fractures
Level II: Potentially life-threatening injuries, hemodynamically stable	GCS ≥9 and ≤13 Hypotension before transport, resolved during transport Transient neurologic changes	Blunt abdominal trauma with abnormal exam Blunt chest trauma with ≥2 rib fractures Significant penetrating trauma to upper extremities or distal to groin Significant crush or amputation distal to elbow or knee with high probability of operative intervention

Modified from Children's Hospital of Philadelphia: *2012-2013 Trauma program resident/fellow manual,* Philadelphia.

BOX 26-9

Estimating Blood Pressure for the Pediatric Patient

Systolic BP (mm Hg) = (2 × age in years) + 80
Diastolic BP (mm Hg) = $\frac{2}{3}$ systolic BP

Airway and breathing are part of the primary survey for pediatric trauma victims. Anatomic variations of the upper airway related to age must be considered. Airway patency must be assessed and secured. Initial assessment for all pediatric trauma patients may best be obtained by application of the head tilt–chin lift or jaw-thrust method, depending on the age of the child and the nature of the injury. When the integrity of the spinal cord is questionable, in-line cervical traction should be applied. Collars and stabilizing devices must remain in place until cervical fracture has been ruled out and the spine "cleared," or declared free of injury by a radiologist. Airway equipment sizes may be selected based on age as well as whether the child is breathing spontaneously and whether the child is unconscious. An assessment of relevant systems will be performed on stabilization of the pediatric airway, and surgery will progress as planned.

Surgery for Congenital Heart Disease

Congenital heart disease (CHD) occurs in approximately 5 to 8 of every 1000 live births. Structural abnormalities of the heart and great vessels result in an embryologic failure in septation, malalignment, failure to develop, or failure to progress.

The etiology of CHD varies, although certain factors are associated with increased prevalence. For example, risk of CHD is increased secondary to environmental factors: rubella during the first 8 weeks of gestation may result in patent ductus arteriosus and pulmonary artery stenosis (along with other syndromes). Other risk factors include maternal chronic illnesses such as diabetes or poorly controlled phenylketonuria (PKU), alcohol consumption, and exposure to environmental toxins. The incidence of CHD is increased also in certain chromosomal defects; for example, atrial

BOX 26-10

Classification of Congenital Cardiac Defects

Acyanotic with Increased Pulmonary Blood Flow
- Patent ductus arteriosus
- Atrial septal defect
- Ventricular septal defect
- Atrioventricular septal defect

Acyanotic Obstructive Lesions
- Coarctation of the aorta
- Aortic stenosis
- Pulmonary stenosis

Cyanotic with Decreased Pulmonary Blood Flow
- Tricuspid atresia
- Tetralogy of Fallot
- Pulmonary atresia with intact ventricular septum

Cyanotic with Increased Pulmonary Blood Flow
- Total anomalous pulmonary venous connection (return)
- Truncus arteriosus
- Hypoplastic left heart syndrome

Cyanotic with Variable Pulmonary Blood Flow
- Transposition of the great arteries
- Double-outlet right ventricle
- Double-outlet left ventricle
- Single ventricle

---

septal defects are seen in children with trisomy 21 (Down syndrome). In addition, an increased prevalence is seen in small-for-gestational-age (SGA) babies and in children who have a positive family history of CHD (that is, those families with a sibling or parent who has CHD).

Congenital cardiac abnormalities are classified as cyanotic or acyanotic as well as by their effect on pulmonary blood flow (Box 26-10). Of the acyanotic lesions, there are those that increase pulmonary blood flow, such as patent ductus arteriosus (PDA), atrial septal defect (ASD), ventricular septal defect (VSD), and atrioventricular canal (AVC) defects. With these abnormalities, blood flows from the high-pressure left side of the heart to the low-pressure right side of the heart because of an abnormal connection either between the septum or in the great arteries. The resultant increase in pulmonary blood flow causes the right side of the heart and lungs to become overloaded. Congestive heart failure (CHF) may develop, pulmonary vascular resistance may increase, and the pulmonary vessel walls may thicken; if left untreated, the condition may become irreversible.

Acyanotic obstructive lesions, such as aortic stenosis, pulmonary stenosis, or coarctation of the aorta, increase the workload of the chamber that pumps against the obstruction (increases afterload). Cardiomegaly and ventricular hypertrophy may be seen in response to the increased workload, and if the obstruction is severe, heart failure may ensue.

The presence of cyanosis implies that one of the following conditions is present: right-sided heart obstruction with blood traveling right to left without passing through the lungs; mixing of venous and arterial blood within the heart or great vessels; or incorrect positioning of the great vessels. The degree of cyanosis depends on pulmonary blood flow and intracardiac mixing of blood through a shunt. This classification of lesions includes, but is not limited to, tetralogy of Fallot (TOF), pulmonary atresia with intact ventricular septum (PA/IVS), tricuspid atresia (TA), transposition of the great arteries (TGA), total anomalous pulmonary venous return (TAPVR), and HLHS. Treatment goals for these lesions include managing pulmonary blood flow or arterial oxygen saturation.

Repair of Atrial Septal Defect

ASDs are one of the most common forms of CHD (Ferdman et al, 2011). The classification within this group of defects is based on anatomic location and associated abnormalities (Figure 26-57). The ostium secundum defect is located in the superior and central portions of the septum. The ostium primum defect is located in the lower portion of the atrial septum and is associated with other defects in the AVC, usually with a cleft of the mitral valve or occasionally of the tricuspid valve. An accompanying VSD may also be present. The sinus venosus defect is located at the right atrium–superior vena cava junction and is associated with partial anomalous pulmonary venous return.

An ASD results in a left-to-right atrial shunt whose direction and magnitude are determined by the size of the defect and relative resistance to flow into the ventricles and great vessels (Figure 26-58). ASDs are often tolerated well with no symptoms during childhood, especially if the defect is small. However, if the defect is large or of the ostium primum type, with a pronounced shunting of blood, the workload of the right side of the heart is increased. On assessment, there is a characteristic systolic pulmonary murmur at the second intercostal space at the left sternal border; a fixed splitting of the second heart sound also may be heard. The right side of the heart and the pulmonary artery and its branches become enlarged. The vascularity of the lung field is increased, with resulting pulmonary hypertension and subsequent failure of the right side of the heart. At this point the shunt may reverse. The initial symptoms may include fatigue, retardation of normal weight gain, and increased susceptibility to respiratory tract infections. Later signs and symptoms include those of failure of the right side of the heart and cyanosis with a reverse shunt. Asymptomatic children whose ASD is left unrepaired until adulthood may develop right atrial and right ventricular hypertrophy, atrial dysrhythmias, CHF, embolic events, and pulmonary vascular disease. The defect is common in children with Down syndrome.

Procedural Considerations. ASDs are closed, under direct vision, by a simple suture technique (primary closure) or by insertion of a synthetic prosthetic patch or pericardial patch.

The child is placed in the supine position for a median sternotomy or in a right anterior oblique position for an anterolateral thoracotomy. The instrument setup is the same as that described for basic open-heart surgery (see Chapter 25), with consideration given to the age and size of the child; intracardiac patch material, 2×2 inches or larger, also may be required.

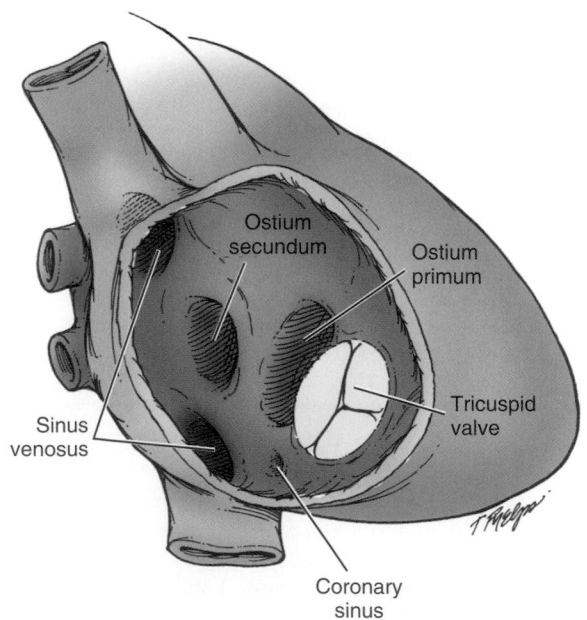

FIGURE 26-57 Various types of atrial septal defects (ASDs) viewed through the right atrium (ostium secundum, ostium primum, sinus venosus). An unroofed coronary sinus may also act as an ASD.

FIGURE 26-58 Atrial septal defect.

Operative Procedure (Figure 26-59)

1. The surgeon opens the chest with a median sternotomy incision and institutes CPB. (Infrequently, a right anterolateral incision is performed.) Many bypass strategies can be used. With bicaval cannulation, the child remains on bypass during the repair and blood is directed away from the right atrium through cannulae in the superior and inferior venae cavae. Occasionally with this method the cannulae may obstruct the view of the ASD. With single venous cannulation, a cannula is placed into the right atrium and the child remains on bypass during the repair. With this technique the venous line is clamped immediately before the right atrium is incised and pump suctions are placed into the inferior and superior venae cavae during ASD closure. Deep hypothermic circulatory arrest is sometimes used in more complicated repairs, such as ostium primum ASD or sinus venosus defects associated with anomalous pulmonary venous return.

2. The right atrium is incised, and the pathologic defect is determined.

3. The defect is closed with a continuous suture, or a patch of pericardium or prosthetic material may be used. By filling the atrium with blood before the atriotomy is completely closed, the surgeon can express air from the atrium. For the ostium primum defect with a cleft mitral valve, repair of the cleft is accomplished by approximation, with use of interrupted (possibly pledgeted) sutures.

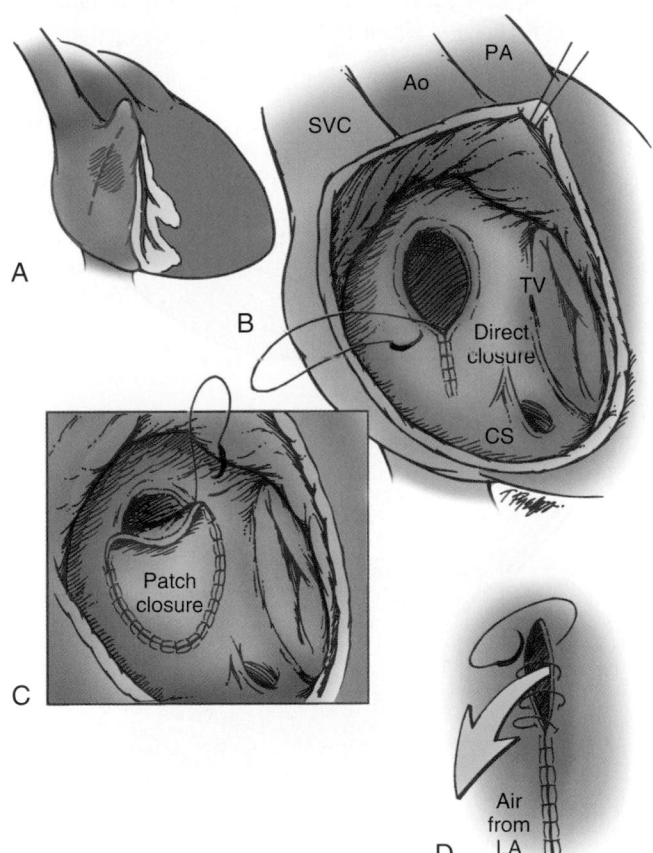

FIGURE 26-59 Surgical procedure for atrial septal defect (ASD) closure. **A,** Incision through right atriotomy. Direct suture closure, **B,** and patch closure, **C,** of secundum ASD. **D,** De-airing of the left atrium. *Ao,* Aorta; *CS,* conduction system; *LA,* left atrium; *PA,* pulmonary artery; *SVC,* superior vena cava; *TV,* tricuspid valve.

Repair of Ventricular Septal Defect

One of the most common congenital cardiac anomalies, VSDs (Figure 26-60) occur in approximately 2% to 7% of live births, with as many as 60% closing spontaneously (Ramaswamy et al, 2011). Most VSDs are small with little physiologic importance. As with ASDs, the classification of VSDs depends on location and associated lesions (Figure 26-61). Perimembranous VSDs (also called conoventricular, subaortic, infracristal, or membranous) are most commonly found. These defects occur directly adjacent to the membranous septum and the fibrous trigone of the heart, where the aortic, mitral, and tricuspid valves are in fibrous continuity. The tricuspid valve tissue sometimes forms an aneurysm of the membranous septum, which may be a mechanism of defect closure for this type of defect. Subpulmonary VSDs (also referred to as supracristal, infundibular, intracristal, outlet, conoseptal, or conal) are located above the crista supraventricularis within the outlet septum and border the semilunar valves. Muscular-type VSDs can be located anywhere in the muscular septum, including apical, anterior, or posterior, or in the midseptum inlet and outlet. Malalignment-type VSDs are created by a malalignment between the infundibular septum and the trabecular muscular septum. Canal-type or inlet defects are located posteriorly within the area confined by the tricuspid valve septal leaflet papillary muscles. The defect borders the tricuspid valve annulus.

The hemodynamics depend on the size and location of the defect as well as the pulmonary vascular resistance (PVR) and systemic vascular resistance (SVR). Newborns are often asymptomatic until the PVR decreases—then a left-to-right shunt occurs, and the corresponding murmur is auscultated. Small defects with moderate shunt and increased pulmonary blood flow but not increased pulmonary pressure may not produce any symptoms. A large VSD, however, may produce high pulmonary flow under high pressure and contribute to CHF. In this case the patient is at risk of developing pulmonary hypertension (Figure 26-62). Surgical closure of the defect should be performed to prevent increased pulmonary

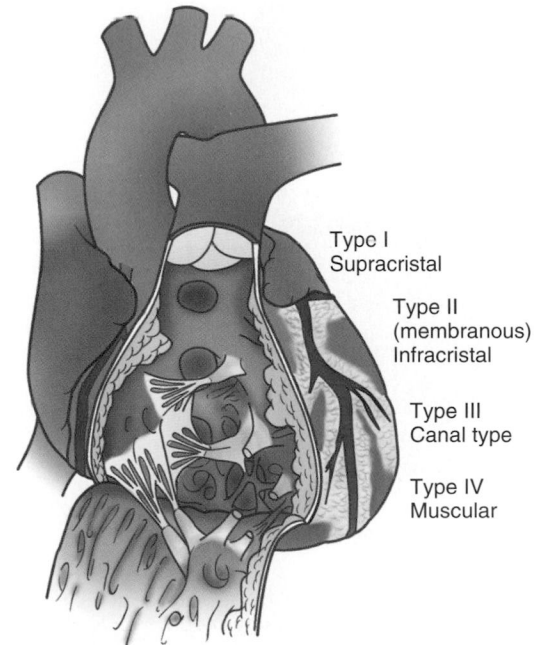

FIGURE 26-60 Ventricular septal defects: anatomic classification.

FIGURE 26-61 Various types of ventricular septal defects viewed within the right ventricle. **A,** Infundibular (supracristal). **B,** Membranous. **C,** Inlet (AV canal). **D,** Muscular (trabecular).

FIGURE 26-62 Ventricular septal defect.

hypertension. If PVR further increases and rises above SVR, shunt reversal (Eisenmenger syndrome, or shunting from right to left) and cyanosis may occur.

Operative Procedure. Under direct vision a congenital defect in the ventricular septum (Figure 26-63) is closed by a simple suture technique or, in most instances, by insertion of a synthetic prosthetic or pericardial patch.

1. A median sternotomy is performed, and CPB is instituted.
2. The location of the defect determines the location of the incision. For membranous and canal defects, an incision is usually made in the right atrium, the atrium is retracted, and the VSD is identified by use of a pump suction through the tricuspid valve into the right ventricle. For supracristal VSDs, an incision is usually made in the pulmonary artery and may be extended into the right ventricle. A muscular VSD may require a ventriculotomy.
3. A patch (synthetic or pericardium) is most frequently used to close the defect. To place the patch, the surgeon uses a continuous 6-0 or 5-0 nonabsorbable suture on a small needle or an

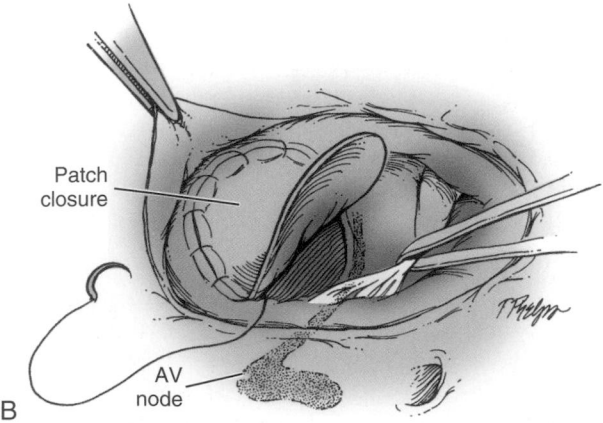

FIGURE 26-63 Ventricular septal defect *(VSD)* closure through the tricuspid valve *(TV)*. **A,** Open site. **B,** Partial closure. *Ao,* Aorta; *AV,* atrioventricular; *CS,* conduction system; *PA,* pulmonary artery; *SVC,* superior vena cava.

Pulmonic stenosis

Overriding aorta

Ventricular septal defect

Right ventricular hypertrophy

FIGURE 26-64 Tetralogy of Fallot.

interrupted suture with or without pledgets. Rarely is the defect closed primarily.

4. CPB is discontinued, and the sternum is closed.

Correction of Tetralogy of Fallot

TOF, described initially in the early nineteenth century, includes the association of four anatomic findings: VSD, subpulmonic stenosis, aortic override of the ventricular septum, and right ventricular hypertrophy (RVH) (Figure 26-64). Occurring in approximately 10% of congenital heart defects, TOF is actually the result of a single anatomic abnormality: anterior malalignment of the infundibular septum with the muscular septum (Verklan, 2012).

The preoperative hemodynamics or physiology depends mainly on the degree of pulmonary stenosis. In patients with minimal obstruction to pulmonary blood flow, the physiology is similar to that of a VSD with left-to-right shunting. These patients have pulmonary overcirculation and symptoms of CHF. Occasionally labeled as "pink tets," these patients have little to no right-to-left shunting and do not exhibit cyanosis.

At the other end of the spectrum of this particular type of heart defect are children with severe pulmonary stenosis, who may have significant right-to-left shunting at the VSD level and exhibit hypoxemia with oxygen saturations in the 60% to 80% range. Cyanosis, as seen in the superficial vessels of the skin, is the result of shunting unoxygenated blood into the systemic circulation. Other clinical manifestations may include episodes of acute dyspnea with cyanosis, retarded growth, clubbing of extremities, reduced exercise tolerance, and increased prevalence of "tet," or hypercyanotic spells. A systolic murmur and secondary polycythemia are usually present in the cyanotic child. Echocardiography is performed to confirm the diagnosis of TOF; occasionally a cardiac catheterization and angiography may be necessary in delineating other anatomic abnormalities, such as with the coronary arteries, before surgical repair.

The selection of a palliative or corrective procedure is based on the age and general condition of the child and the severity of the pulmonary stenosis. The treatment of choice is primary repair;

contraindications for primary repair include anomalous origin of the anterior descending coronary artery and presence of pulmonary atresia. Complete or primary repair consists of closure of the VSD and repair of the pulmonic stenosis under direct vision.

Procedural Considerations. The child is placed on the OR bed in a supine position. The setup is the same as that described for open-heart surgery, with consideration given to the child's age and size. Additional items to be added to the basic open-heart setup include the following: intracardiac patch, 2 × 2 inches; outflow cardiac patch, 2 × 2 inches; and a felt or Gore-Tex patch, 4 × 4 inches.

Operative Procedure

1. A median sternotomy is performed, and CPB with hypothermia is instituted.
2. A vertical ventriculotomy over the infundibular area may be performed (Figure 26-65, *A*).
3. The surgeon identifies the VSD. Closure requires an intracardiac patch in almost all instances. This can be of a synthetic material or a piece of pericardium.
4. Interrupted or continuous cardiovascular sutures are placed in the septum with caution because of the danger of suturing a branch of the neuroconductive system.
5. The surgeon excises the hypertrophied infundibular muscle as completely as possible, from the right ventricular outflow tract. If the pulmonic valve is stenosed, the fused commissures are incised.
6. An estimate is made about whether the right ventricle can be closed primarily or if a patch is necessary. If the pulmonic stenosis cannot be relieved adequately by valvulotomy and infundibulectomy, an outflow patch of synthetic material or pulmonary homograft tissue may be needed to enlarge the outflow tract (see Figure 26-65, *B*). If the pulmonary artery or valve annulus is quite small, it may be necessary to extend the patch across the valve ring to the proximal portion of the pulmonary artery (see Figure 26-65, *C*).
7. CPB is discontinued, and the sternum is closed.

Closure of Patent Ductus Arteriosus

PDA occurs because of persistence of the fetal ductus arteriosus, which connects the pulmonary artery to the aorta. The condition is common in premature infants. In fetal life, blood bypasses the lungs, traveling directly to the systemic circulation through the PDA. This vessel normally closes shortly after birth as a result of the onset of respiration causing an increase in PaO_2 level and the release of circulating humoral substances. However, if this does not occur, the ductus arteriosus remains open (Figure 26-66), creating a shunt from the aorta through the ductus into the pulmonary circulation. This increases the workload of the heart and causes subsequent enlargement and hypertrophy of the left atrium and ventricle. However, when persistent patency of the ductus is associated with other malformations such as TOF and extreme stenosis of the pulmonary orifice, it is a means of maintaining life. Surgery is not performed if the PDA is serving in a compensatory capacity.

Many children have few symptoms because of the small size of the shunt. A frequent clinical sign associated with this condition is a harsh, continuous murmur. Because the blood passing through the shunt is oxygenated, there is no cyanosis, clubbing, or reduction in peripheral arterial oxygen saturation. However, growth is retarded in children who have a large ductus. Other signs and symptoms

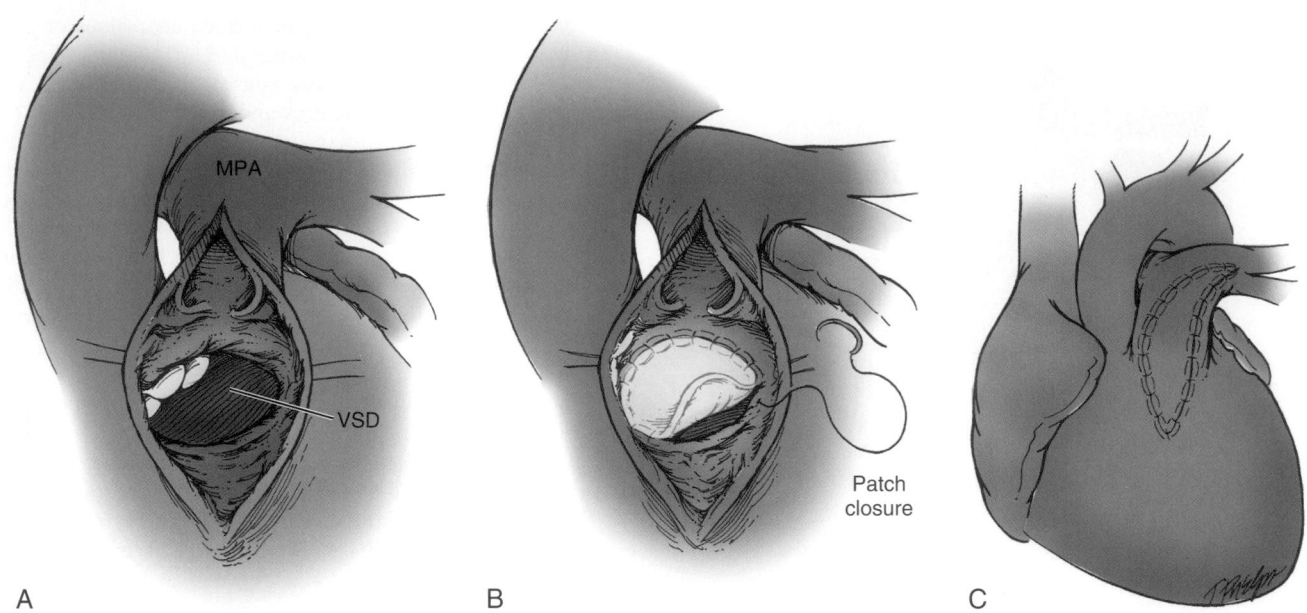

A   B   C

FIGURE 26-65 A, The most common ventricular incision used for repair of tetralogy of Fallot is vertical so that it can be extended as shown from the right ventricle across the pulmonary valve annulus and onto the main pulmonary artery *(MPA)*. It is possible to gain adequate exposure to the ventricular septal defect *(VSD)* by extending the incision a short distance beyond the infundibular septum. This "limited ventriculotomy" may help preserve late right ventricular function yet enable adequate enlargement of the hypoplastic area in the right ventricular outflow tract. **B,** The VSD is closed with a prosthetic patch. Right ventricular outflow obstruction is relieved when the outflow tract is enlarged with a patch as shown. **C,** In some cases it may be necessary to extend the incision onto the left pulmonary artery and to taper the patch at its most distal extent.

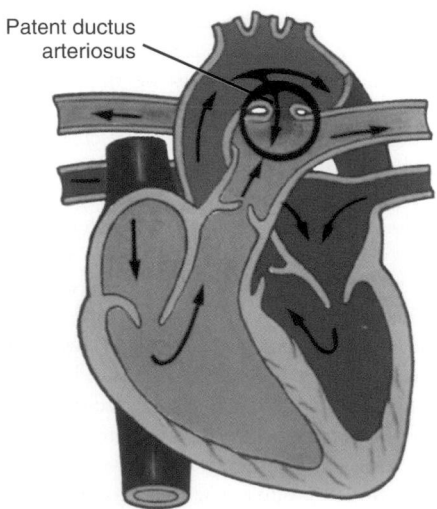

FIGURE 26-66 Patent ductus arteriosus.

may include dyspnea, frequent upper respiratory tract infections, palpitations, limited exercise tolerance, and cardiac failure.

Procedural Considerations. Closure of the PDA is achieved by suture ligation or by division of the ductus. For newborns, the surgeon and anesthesia provider may elect to perform this procedure in the intensive care nursery bed because the operation is short. However, after the newborn period, the surgery is done in the OR. The child is placed in a right lateral position. The setup is the same as that described for open-heart surgery, but with special patent ductus clamps and without items for CPB. Generally a left

posterolateral approach is used; in some cases, however, a left anterolateral approach is used.

Operative Procedure

1. The incision is carried through the muscles over the fourth interspace. The chest wall is entered through the third or fourth intercostal space, with use of items as described for thoracotomy (see Chapter 23). The wound edges are protected and retracted with a Finochietto rib spreader.
2. The surgeon incises the pleura with Metzenbaum scissors, and the left lung is protected and retracted with a moist pack and a malleable retractor.
3. The mediastinal pleura is opened between the phrenic and vagus nerves over the region of the ductus. The pleura is retracted by insertion of stay sutures. The recurrent laryngeal nerve is identified and protected. The aortic arch and pulmonary artery are dissected with fine scissors and dry dissectors. Fine arterial branches are divided and ligated with curved Crile or mosquito hemostats and nonabsorbable ligatures and cardiac suture ligatures.
4. The parietal pleura overlying the ductus is dissected with fine vascular forceps and scissors. Stay sutures may be inserted to facilitate retraction.
5. The surgeon dissects the adventitial layer of the ductus. A small portion of the obscure posterior ductus is carefully freed to admit a right-angle clamp.
6. The final step is performed in one of the following ways:
   a. For the suture-ligation method (Figure 26-67, *A*), two ligatures are placed around the ductus—one near the aorta and the other near the pulmonary artery side, both of which are tied in place. Between these two ligatures, two transfixion sutures may be inserted.

FIGURE 26-67 Surgical correction of patent ductus arteriosus *(PDA).* **A,** Ligation of ductus arteriosus. **B,** Division of ductus arteriosus. *Ao,* Aorta; *PA,* pulmonary artery.

FIGURE 26-68 Hypoplastic left-sided heart syndrome.

b. For the division of the ductus method, the patent ductus clamps are applied as close to the aorta and pulmonary artery as possible. The ductus is divided halfway through and partially sutured with mattress cardiovascular sutures and continued back over the free edge with an over-and-over whip suture (see Figure 26-67, *B*). After both openings are sutured, a sponge is held on the area for compression while the patent ductus clamps are removed.

c. In premature infants only a hemoclip may be applied to the ductus because of the friable nature of the ductal tissue. The mediastinal pleura is closed with interrupted sutures. The lung is reexpanded, and a chest catheter may be inserted to establish closed drainage. In newborns reexpansion of the lung may be accomplished by gradual withdrawal of a catheter during closure; no chest drainage tube is required unless there is oozing. The chest wall is closed in layers, and dressings are applied.

Repair of Hypoplastic Heart Syndromes

Hypoplastic heart syndromes can occur on both the left and right side. Patients with hypoplastic right heart syndrome (HRHS) falling on the milder end of the spectrum may respond to biventricular repair, whereas those with more severe hypoplasia are managed with univentricular palliation or transplantation (McElhinney et al, 2010). Because HLHS (Figure 26-68) is one of the most common forms of single ventricle malformation, it is described in further detail.

HLHS describes a range of congenital cardiac malformations that have in common underdevelopment of the left-sided heart structures, which include aortic valve atresia and stenosis with associated hypoplasia or absence of the left ventricle. The ascending aorta and arch are usually only a few millimeters in diameter and are functionally a branch of the ductus arteriosus–thoracic aorta continuum, with blood flowing retrograde through the aortic arch and into the small ascending aorta to the coronary arteries. Mitral valve atresia or stenosis also is present. Survival in the newborn period depends on a PDA to maintain systemic circulation; therefore, these infants are maintained on an infusion of prostaglandin E_1 (PGE_1) to maintain ductal patency before surgical intervention.

Newborns with HLHS typically present with cyanosis, respiratory distress, and variable degrees of circulatory collapse during the first few days of life. If left untreated, a majority of these neonates will die within the first month of life; without surgical intervention, HLHS is fatal.

It was not until the development of the Fontan procedure—a surgical correction for another form of single ventricle malformation (tricuspid atresia)—that long-term survival in patients with HLHS was considered possible. However, because of the neonate's high PVR, the Fontan procedure is not a surgical option in the newborn period. A palliative repair (stage I) was developed in the late 1970s by Norwood to prepare the heart for the Fontan procedure.

Two surgical options for patients with HLHS exist: a series of reconstructive procedures or heart transplantation. The series of reconstructive procedures usually involves three stages. Stage I is performed during the newborn period. The goals of stage I are to (1) maintain systemic perfusion, (2) preserve the function of the only ventricle, and (3) allow normal maturation of the pulmonary ventricle. The first goal is met by creating an unobstructed communication between the right ventricle and the systemic circulation. This is accomplished by transecting the main pulmonary artery and creating a neoaorta from the main pulmonary artery, native aorta, and pulmonary homograft tissue. The other two goals are met by creating a right modified Blalock-Taussig (BT) shunt and a nonrestrictive interatrial communication. These measures allow for adequate pulmonary blood flow and for the PVR to decrease as the child grows while the volume interposed on the single ventricle is limited.

The modified Fontan procedure was initially performed on a child at approximately 18 months of age. However, since 1989 a staged approach to the Fontan procedure has been undertaken to minimize the effect of rapid changes in ventricular configuration and diastolic function that can be associated with a primary Fontan procedure and its accompanying postoperative complications. In the stage II procedure (hemi-Fontan or the bidirectional Glenn shunt), superior vena cava (SVC) blood flow is directed to the lungs, and inferior vena cava (IVC) blood flow continues to flow to the right ventricle. The third and final stage, the modified Fontan

procedure, separates the systemic and pulmonary circulations. These same procedures can be carried out for patients with HRHS.

Procedural Considerations. Additional items for the open-heart setup include the following:
- *Stage I*: Polytetrafluoroethylene (PTFE) tube graft, 3.5 or 4 mm, and pulmonary homograft tissue
- *Stage II*: Oscillating saw and pulmonary homograft tissue
- *Stage III*: Oscillating saw and PTFE tube graft, 10 mm; a higher-than-usual supply of blood should be available

Operative Procedure
Stage I (Norwood Procedure) (Figure 26-69)
1. The surgeon opens the chest with a median sternotomy incision. The aortic cannula is placed into the main pulmonary

FIGURE 26-69 Stage I Norwood procedure. **A,** Transection points of the main pulmonary artery *(PA)* and ductus arteriosus. **B,** Atrial septectomy to avoid pulmonary venous hypertension. Patch closure of the distal main PA. Division and ligation of the ductus arteriosus. **C** and **D,** Construction of a "neoaorta" with use of the proximal main PA, diminutive ascending aorta, and vascular allograft. **E,** Pulmonary blood flow supplied by a right modified Blalock-Taussig shunt connecting the right subclavian artery to the right PA. *Ao,* Aorta; *LV,* left ventricle; *RV,* right ventricle.

artery rather than the diminutive aorta, and the venous cannula is placed into the right atrium. CPB is instituted, and the right and left pulmonary arteries are immediately occluded with tourniquets to force the blood through the ductus arteriosus to the systemic circulation.

2. When deep hypothermic circulatory arrest is about to be instituted, the innominate and left carotid arteries are occluded with tourniquets. The venous and aortic cannulae are removed.

3. The septum primum is excised through the venous cannulation site; occasionally a right atriotomy is necessary to facilitate the atrial septectomy.

4. The main pulmonary artery is transected immediately before the bifurcation of the right and left pulmonary arteries.

5. The surgeon closes the distal pulmonary artery with a small patch of homograft tissue.

6. The ductus arteriosus is then exposed and closed using a 2-0 nonabsorbable tie. The tie is left long to better expose the thoracic aorta. The ductus is transected.

7. At the point where the ductus was attached to the aorta, the thoracic aorta is opened 1 to 2 cm, and the aortic arch and ascending aorta are opened to a point adjacent to the main pulmonary artery.

8. A gusset of homograft tissue is joined to the aorta starting at the thoracic end, and the pulmonary artery is incorporated at the proximal end of the ascending aorta. A continuous monofilament suture is used. Occasionally interrupted sutures are used to attach the main pulmonary artery to the aorta.

9. To perform a right BT shunt, the innominate artery is cross-clamped and incised and a 3.5- or 4-mm PTFE tube graft is interposed.

10. CPB is instituted, and the pulmonary end of the shunt is performed by incising the pulmonary artery and interposing the distal end of the tube graft.

11. Immediately after the shunt is completed, the surgeon occludes it with a bulldog clamp until termination of bypass.

Stage II (Hemi-Fontan Procedure) (Figure 26-70)

1. The surgeon opens the previous chest incision using an oscillating saw to create the sternotomy. An oscillating saw is used for safety because it allows the surgeon to gradually cut through the sternum and avoid any adhesions that may be present from the previous surgery.

2. The aorta, right atrium, and right BT shunt are exposed.

3. CPB is instituted, and the shunt is immediately occluded with a clip.

4. The surgeon exposes the branch pulmonary arteries.

5. Depending on the surgeon's preference, deep hypothermic circulatory arrest may be instituted.

6. An incision is made in the confluence of the pulmonary arteries, extending to the pericardial reflections.

7. An incision is made in the dome of the right atrium, extending to the SVC.

8. The surgeon anastomoses the pulmonary artery to the SVC–right atrial junction.

9. The pulmonary arteries are augmented with a gusset of homograft tissue. In the hemi-Fontan procedure part of the homograft tissue is incorporated intra-atrially as a dam between the common atrium and the vena cava–pulmonary artery anastomosis. In the Glenn shunt, there is no intra-atrial incorporation.

10. CPB is reinstituted until the patient is normothermic. CPB is then discontinued, and chest closure is completed.

Stage III (Modified Fontan Procedure) (Figure 26-71)

1. A median sternotomy is performed with an oscillating saw.

2. The surgeon exposes the aorta and right atrium.

3. CPB is instituted.

4. Deep hypothermic circulatory arrest may be used.

5. A lateral incision is made in the right atrium.

6. A 10-mm PTFE tube graft is cut in half lengthwise and placed intra-atrially by suturing the inferior end of the graft around the orifice of the IVC and up the right lateral free wall of the right atrium to the superior dome of the right atrium. This creates a tunnel in which the inferior blood flow is directed to the pulmonary arteries. The superior vena cava blood flow was directed to the pulmonary arteries during the stage II repair. (The surgeon may perform variations on this procedure, such as excluding a hepatic vein or performing a fenestrated Fontan by making a series of small openings in the PTFE tube graft or a single 4-mm opening with an aortic punch in the graft material.)

7. The atria are closed, and CPB is reinstituted until the patient is normothermic. CPB is then discontinued, and chest closure is completed.

Extracorporeal Membrane Oxygenation

ECMO is a therapy used on pediatric patients who have reversible pulmonary or cardiac disease. Many patients are neonates with respiratory disease syndrome (RDS), persistent pulmonary hypertension (PPH), meconium aspiration (MA), or CDH requiring adequate tissue oxygenation and waste removal from the body. In the cardiac patient it also may be used as a bridge to heart or lung transplantation until donor organs are available. To perform ECMO, a facility must have an established ECMO service.

Most of the time patients are placed on ECMO in the ICU. For venoarterial ECMO the surgical approach is usually through the right carotid artery and internal jugular vein. For the cardiac patient after surgical repair, cannulation of the carotid artery and jugular vein provides good venous drainage of the right atrium, and the incision site is remote from the sternotomy wound. However, the surgeon may choose to reopen the sternum on postoperative patients and cannulate the aorta and right atrium. In the OR, for a patient who cannot be successfully weaned from bypass after surgery, the patient's bypass circuit may be switched to an ECMO circuit and the patient may be transferred on ECMO to the ICU.

Procedural Considerations. An area by the patient's bedside should be provided for the ECMO pump, surgical table and instrumentation, ESU, surgeon's headlight, and defibrillator with external and sterile internal paddles. A wall suction outlet should be available. Appropriate surgical attire must be provided for everyone involved with the procedure, and traffic should be limited.

Operative Procedure

For Neck Cannulation. A shoulder roll is placed under the patient, and the neck and chest to the nipple line are prepped and draped. The ears should also be exposed and prepped for use as reference points.

1. An incision is made in the neck, and the right common carotid artery and right internal jugular vein are exposed for venoarterial ECMO.

2. The surgeon may cannulate the vessels through a purse-string suture and then reconstruct these vessels at the time of decannulation.

FIGURE 26-70 Hemi-Fontan procedure in a patient with hypoplastic left-sided heart syndrome. **A** and **B,** Ligation of the systemic-to-pulmonary artery shunt and side-to-side anastomosis of the superior vena cava *(SVC)* to the confluence of the pulmonary artery *(PA)* with allograft augmentation. **C** to **E,** Placement of a dam to close the junction of the atrium with the SVC so that saturated pulmonary venous blood mixes in the common atrium with desaturated blood draining from the inferior vena cava. Pulmonary blood flow is supplied exclusively through the SVC.

3. After insertion of the arterial and venous cannulae, the clamped cannulae are connected to the ECMO circuit. All the air is eliminated (Figure 26-72).
4. The cannulae are secured to the skin. The neck incision is closed and dressed. The surgical instruments are kept sterile until proper positioning of the venous and arterial cannulae is confirmed by x-ray examination.
   For Median Sternotomy Cannulation. The patient is prepped from neck to umbilicus and draped.
1. The patient has usually had a prior sternotomy incision, and so the sternum is opened with wire cutters.

2. A chest retractor is inserted, and purse-string sutures for cannulation are placed in the aorta and right atrium.
3. The surgeon inserts the aorta and venous cannulae and clamps them.
4. The clamped cannulae are connected to the ECMO circuit. All the air is eliminated.
5. The sternum is left open to prevent kinking of the cannulae and ECMO pump tubing. The wound is closed with a synthetic patch sutured to the skin. An antibiotic ointment may be applied and an "Open Chest" sign placed on top of the outer dressing to serve as a warning related to potential chest compressions.

KEY POINTS

- Children require surgery for congenital malformations, an acquired disease, or trauma. The field of pediatric surgery is further subdivided into all the specialties.
- The difference between pediatric care and adult care is not just a size issue; from birth onward, the body and organs exist in a continual state of development, and multiple physiologic changes occur with age. Major areas of distinction are the airway and pulmonary status, cardiovascular status, temperature regulation, metabolism, fluid management, and psychologic development.
- Medical play items, audiovisual aids, puppets, and photographs are helpful in the perioperative education process. Tailor interventions to suit the developmental level of the pediatric patient.
- Remaining with the child during induction, positioning, and prepping the surgical site; creating and maintaining a sterile field; collecting, documenting, and disposing specimens; and administering medications contribute to a safe environment for the pediatric surgical patient.
- Ensuring that the pediatric patient's family receives regular updates of the child's status will decrease their anxiety and help foster a sense of trust in the healthcare professionals caring for their child.
- For children younger than age 18, consent must be obtained from one of the following individuals: a legal parent (biologic parent whose parental rights have not been terminated) or an adoptive parent who has completed the adoptive process. Foster parents of children in the custody of a child and youth agency (CYA) are not permitted to give consent. Rather, consent should be obtained from the CYA social worker. Legal guardians should be encouraged to bring any supporting documentation of legal guardianship or ability to consent for the child's medical care on the day of surgery.
- Every state has a child abuse law that dictates legal responsibility for reporting abuse and suspicion of abuse, and nurses are mandated reporters. Laws may differ from state to state.

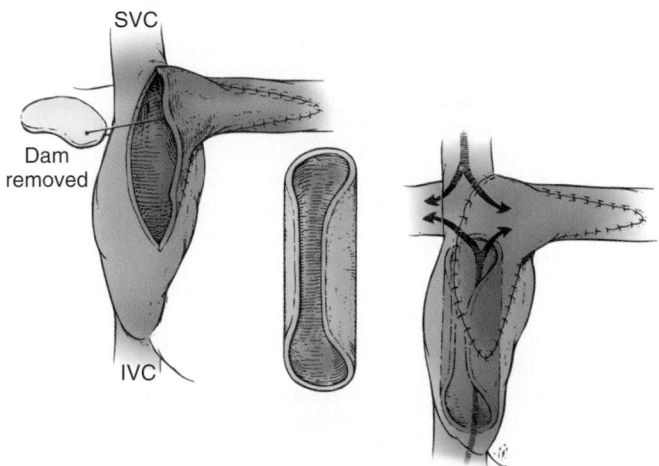

FIGURE 26-71 Conversion of hemi-Fontan to completion of Fontan. Excision of the dam between the right atrium and the superior vena cava–pulmonary artery anastomosis. Inferior vena cava flow is directed to the inlet of the superior vena cava–pulmonary artery anastomosis by a baffle. *IVC,* Inferior vena cava; *SVC,* superior vena cava.

FIGURE 26-72 Extracorporeal membrane oxygenation (ECMO) circuit.

• Pediatric instruments are usually shorter, have more delicate or less pronounced curves, and are smaller. A complete range of instrument sizes is necessary to make the appropriate size available to each child because pediatric patients can range in size from less than 1 kg to more than 100 kg.

CRITICAL THINKING QUESTION

Several unique situations may arise when providing perioperative care to pediatric patients. Consider the following scenarios and determine the actions you would take:

• Short-acting premedications are often administered to the pediatric patient before transfer from the preoperative area to the OR. What must the perioperative nurse consider when premedicating a patient?
• What is the most appropriate way to facilitate parental presence in the OR for induction?
• Some implants and devices are not approved for use in children by the FDA. How can perioperative nurses ensure that implants and devices are approved for use?
• In the pediatric population, medications are dosed based on weight in kilograms. What are some strategies that perioperative nurses can use to streamline medication administration in the pediatric population?

evolve *The answers to the Critical Thinking Question can be found at http://evolve.elsevier.com/Rothrock/Alexander.*

REFERENCES

American Academy of Orthopedic Surgeons (AAOS): *Children's clubfoot: treatment with casting or operation*, 2007, available at http://orthoinfo.aaos.org/topic.cfm?topic=A00296. Accessed February 1, 2013.

American Association for Pediatric Ophthalmology and Strabismus (AAPOS): *Eye terms and conditions*, 2012, available at www.aapos.org/terms. Accessed December 3, 2012.

American Cancer Society (ACS): *Neuroblastoma*, Atlanta, 2012, The Society, available at www.cancer.org/cancer/neuroblastoma/detailedguide/neuroblastoma-key-statistics. Accessed February 1, 2013.

Barakat M et al: Sacrococcygeal teratoma in infants and children, *Acta Neurochir* 153(9):1781–1786, 2011.

Betz CL, Sowden LA: *Mosby's pediatric nursing reference*, ed 6, St Louis, 2008, Mosby.

Broemling N, Campbell F: Anesthetic management of congenital tracheoesophageal fistula, *Paediatr Anaesth* 21(11):1092–1099, 2011.

Bulsiewicz WJ, Madanick RD: Antireflux surgery in the proton pump inhibitor era, *Cleve Clin J Med* 79:273–281, 2012.

Carlo WA: The umbilicus. In Kleigman RM et al, editors: *Nelson textbook of pediatrics*, ed 19, Philadelphia, 2011, Saunders.

Centers for Disease Control and Prevention (CDC): *Overweight and obesity: data and statistics*, 2013, available at www.cdc.gov/obesity/data/childhood. Accessed February 1, 2013.

Children's Hospital of Philadelphia (CHOP): *Congenital hyperinsulinism center*, available at www.chop.edu/service/congenital-hyperinsulinism-center/home.html. Accessed February 1, 2013.

Curry MR et al: The child with musculoskeletal or articular dysfunction. In Hockenberry MJ, Wilson D, editors: *Wong's essentials of pediatric nursing*, ed 9, St Louis, 2012, Mosby.

Curry S et al: Catheter-associated bloodstream infections in the NICU: getting to zero, *Neonat Netw* 28(3):151–155, 2009.

Ferdman D et al: Common atrium and pulmonary vascular disease, *Pediatr Cardiol* 32(5):595–598, 2011.

Fraser J et al: Laparoscopic management of intussusception in pediatric patients, *J Laparoendosc Adv Surg Tech A* 19(4):563–565, 2009.

Gottlieb EA, Andropolous DB: Pediatrics. In Miller RD, Pardo MC, editors: *Basics of anesthesia*, ed 6, Philadelphia, 2011, Churchill Livingstone.

Harrington S et al: Pediatric laparoscopy, *AORN J* 88(2):211–236, 2008.

Heher KL, Katowitz JA: Pediatric ptosis. In Katowitz JA, editor: *Pediatric oculoplastic surgery*, New York, 2002, Springer.

Henrich K et al: Gastroschisis and omphalocele: treatments and long-term outcomes, *Pediatr Surg Int* 24(2):167–173, 2008.

Howell LJ et al: Management of fetal airway obstruction an innovative strategy, *MCN Am J Matern Child Nurs* 27(4):238–244, 2002.

Ingelfinger J: Bariatric surgery in adolescents, *N Engl J Med* 365(15):1365–1367, 2011.

Laje, P, et al: Ex utero intrapartum treatment in the management of giant cervical teratomas, *J Pediatr Surg* 47(6):1208–1216, 2012.

McElhinney DB et al: Current status of fetal cardiac intervention, *Circulation* 121:1256–1263, 2010.

Medline Plus Medical Encyclopedia: *Necrotizing enterocolitis*, 2011, available at www.nlm.nih.gov/MEDLINEPLUS/ency/article/001148.htm. Accessed February 1, 2013.

Moore M et al: The imaging of paediatric thoracic trauma, *Pediatr Radiol* 39(5):485–496, 2009.

Partridge EA, Flake AW: Maternal-fetal surgery for structural malformations, *Best Pract Res Clin Obstet Gynaecol* 26:669–682, 2012.

Ramaswamy P et al: *Ventricular septal defect, general concepts*, 2011, available at http://emedicine.medscape.com/article/892980-overview. Accessed February 1, 2013.

Rao PS: *Tricuspid atresia*, 2011, available at www.emedicine.com/PED/topic2550.htm. Accessed February 1, 2013.

Scully SM et al: Fetal myelomeningocele repair: a new standard of care, *AORN J* 96:176–192, 2012.

Sheth RD et al: *Craniosynostosis*, 2012, available at: http://emedicine.medscape.com/article/1175957-overview. Accessed February 1, 2013.

Tworetzky W et al: Balloon dilation of severe aortic stenosis in the fetus, *Circulation* 110:2125–2131, 2004.

Varela P et al: A simple technique for removing the Nuss bar with one stabilizer: the lateral approach, *J Laparoendosc Adv Surg Tech A* 20(1):91–93, 2010.

Verklan MT: Hemolytic disorders and congenital abnormalities. In Lowdermilk DL et al, editors: *Maternity and women's health care*, ed 10, St Louis, 2012, Mosby.

Wetzel RC: Anesthesia, perioperative care, and sedation. In Kleigman RM et al, editors: *Nelson textbook of pediatrics*, ed 19, Philadelphia, 2011, Saunders.

Wheeler D et al: A hospital-wide quality-improvement collaborative to reduce catheter-associated bloodstream infections, *Pediatrics* 128(4):e995, 2011.

Whitaker L: Foreword. In Katowitz JA, editor: *Pediatric oculoplastic surgery*, New York, 2002, Springer.

CHAPTER 27

Geriatric Surgery

MARYANN PAPANIER WELLS AND ALLISON LINDSEY FLANAGAN

The elderly contingent is growing in leaps and bounds in today's population, and consequently perioperative nurses must be proficient in meeting the needs of geriatric patients. As a geriatric patient, a different set of variables becomes important to maintain one's lifestyle. First and foremost, the older adult generation wants to live independently, care for themselves, and keep their quality of life intact.

Aging is a process that can be described in chronologic, physiologic, and functional terms. Human aging from a physiologic perspective has changed little in the past 300 years. In general, we age neither faster nor slower than we did in Colonial America. Chronologic age, the number of years a person has lived, is an easily identifiable measurement. Average or median life span, or life expectancy, is the age at which 50% of a given population survives. Maximum life span potential (MLSP) is the age of the longest-lived member or members of the population or species. Although the number of people living beyond their 90s has increased more recently, the MLSP, estimated at 125 years for women and somewhat less for men, has not changed significantly in recorded history. Chronologic age or MLSP may not be the most meaningful measurement of age, however. Nevertheless, many people who have lived a long time remain physiologically and functionally young, whereas others are chronologically young but physiologically and functionally old (Wold, 2012).

Many aspects of our society will be affected by the growth of the population that is 65 years old or older. Policymakers, families, businesses, and healthcare providers will be challenged to meet the needs of this growing age group. With the aging of the baby-boomers (born between 1946 and 1964), the gerontology boom will occur somewhere between 2010 and 2030, producing the most rapid increase in the older population. Individuals older than 85 years now make up 4% of the entire U.S. population and represent the fastest growing segment of the older population. Economics will play a factor because individuals born before 1937 will still qualify for full Social Security benefits at age 65 with incremental increases regarding benefit age for everyone born after that time. Those born in 1960 or after will have to wait until age 67 to qualify for full benefits, with reduced benefits calculated for individuals who apply for benefits after age 62 but before the specified retirement age (Wold, 2012). Nearly 36 million people 65 years and older lived in the United States in 2003, accounting for more than 12% of the total population, and they can be divided into four subgroups (Box 27-1). The population considered oldest-old (age 85 years and older) increased from just more than 100,000 in 1900 to 4.2 million in 2000. In 2011 baby-boomers (born between 1946 and 1964) started turning 65 years old; this segment of the population will increase at such a rate that the 2030 population is projected to be twice as large as it was in 2000. The 65-year and older population

will increase from 35 million to 72 million, representing nearly 20% of the total U.S. population. In 2012 there were 40 million people age 65 and older, accounting for 13% of the total population (Federal Interagency Forum on Aging-Related Statistics [FIFARS], 2012). The growth rate for this age-group is expected to stabilize at around 20% of the population after 2030, when the last of the boomers join the older population ranks. After 2030 the baby-boomers will move into the oldest-old population (age 85 and older), which will grow accordingly (FIFARS, 2012; Figure 27-1 provides population data). The U.S. Census Bureau estimates that the population age 85 and older could grow from 5.7 million in 2008 to nearly 19 million by 2050 (Wold, 2012). The proportion of the older population (65 and older) varies by state. This proportion is partly affected by the state fertility and mortality levels and partly by the number of older and younger people who migrate to and from the state. In 2010 Florida had the highest proportion of people ages 65 years and older at 17%. Maine, Pennsylvania, and West Virginia also had high proportions: more than 15%. The proportion of the population 65 years and older varies even more by county. In 2010 43%% of Sumter County, Florida, was 65 years and older, the highest proportion in the United States. In several Florida counties the proportion was more than 30%. At the other end of the spectrum was Aleutians West Census Area, Alaska, with only 3.5% of its population 65 years and older (FIFARS, 2012). As in most countries of the world, older women outnumber older men in the United States, and the proportion that is female increases with age. In 2010 women accounted for 57% of the older population and for 67% of the population 85 years and older. The United States is fairly young by comparison with other countries, with just more than 13% of its population age 65 years and older. In most European countries the older population comprised more than 15% of the population, and it included nearly 20% of the population in both Germany and Italy in 2010 (FIFARS, 2012). Mirroring the total U.S. population, the elder population is more racially diverse

---

BOX 27-1

Categorizing the Aging Population

- 65 to 74 years of age: The young-old
- 75 to 84 years of age: The middle-old
- 85 to 99 years of age: The old-old
- 100 years of age or more: The elite-old

From Ignatavicius DD: Common health problems of older adults. In Ignatavicius DD, Workman ML, editors: *Medical-surgical nursing: patient-centered collaborative care*, ed 7, St Louis, 2013, Saunders.

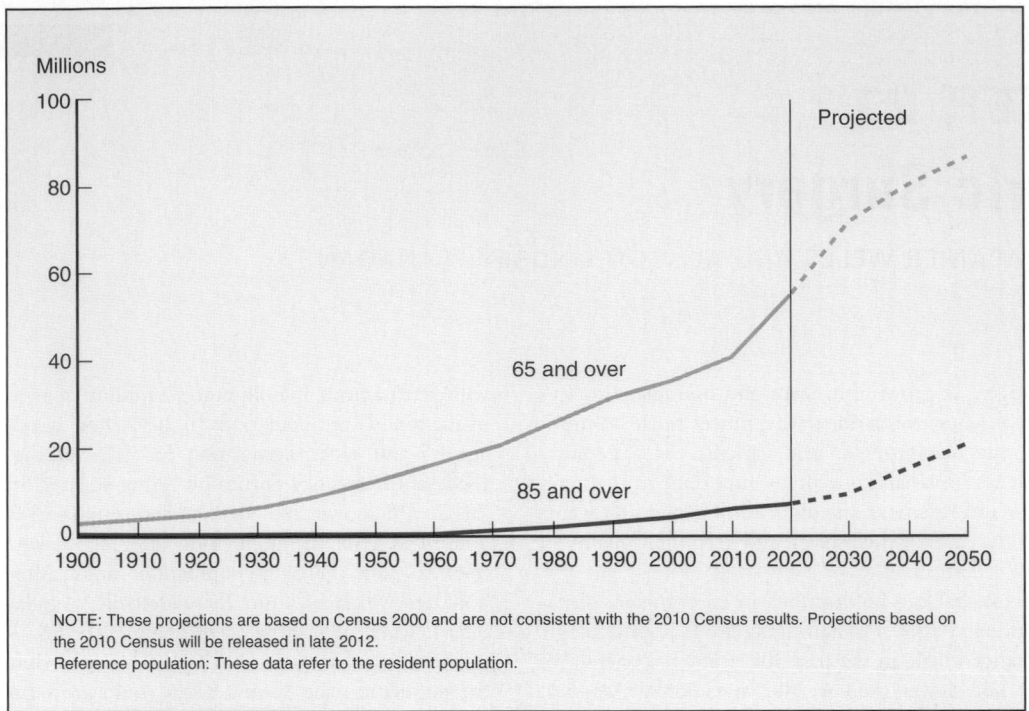

NOTE: These projections are based on Census 2000 and are not consistent with the 2010 Census results. Projections based on the 2010 Census will be released in late 2012.
Reference population: These data refer to the resident population.

FIGURE 27-1 Actual and projected population data for people age 65 years and older and 85 years and older. Selected years are 1900-2010; projected years are 2020-2050.

than ever. By 2050 programs and services for older people will require greater flexibility to meet the needs of a more diverse population. In 2010 non-Hispanic whites accounted for 80% of the U.S. older population; African Americans accounted for 9%; Asians 3%; and Hispanics (of any race), 7%. Projections are that by 2050 the composition of the older population will change to 58% non-Hispanic white, 20% Hispanic, 12% African American, and 9% Asian. The older Hispanic population is projected to grow the fastest, from just under 3 million in 2010 to 17.5 million in 2050, and to be larger than the older African American population. In 2010 over 1 million older Asians lived in the United States; by 2050 this population is projected to be 7.5 million (FIFARS, 2012). Figure 27-2 illustrates resident population by racial and ethnic composition.

Those older than 85 are the fastest-growing age group among the U.S. population. According to the U.S. Census Bureau, in 2010, 3.1% of the U.S. population was at least 100 years old, compared with 0.1% in 1901. The total number is expected to increase by 400% by 2030. Translating these demographics into healthcare trends produces even more startling implications for perioperative patient care. As a result of the "graying of America," healthcare will never be the same. Most older adults have at least one chronic condition, and many have multiple conditions. Chronic diseases that are rarely cured, such as heart disease, stroke, cancer, and diabetes, are among the most common and costly health conditions. These long-term health conditions negatively affect quality of life, contributing to declines in functioning and the inability to remain in the community. Although chronic conditions can be prevented or modified with behavioral interventions, six of the seven leading causes of death among older Americans are chronic diseases (FIFARS, 2012) (Figure 27-3 lists the percentages of chronic diseases by gender). Between 1992 and 1999, the hospitalization rate

in the older population increased from 306 hospital stays per 1000 Medicare enrollees to 365 per 1000. In 2009 the rate decreased to 320 per 1000 enrollees, and the average length of stay decreased from 8.4 days in 1992 to 5.4 days in 2009. The number of Medicare enrollees staying in skilled nursing facilities increased from 28 per 1000 in 1992 to 80 per 1000 in 2009. The utilization rates for many services change based on changes in medical technology and physician practice patterns (FIFARS, 2012). The dramatic growth in elderly surgical patients punctuates the necessity for perioperative nurses to recognize the special needs of these patients. Understanding how normal aging changes and chronic disease affect the successful outcome of any surgical procedure is critical and is therefore the emphasis of this chapter.

Perioperative Nursing Considerations

Preliminary Evaluation

Before an elderly patient actually arrives in surgery, the physician considers many factors to determine whether the benefits of surgery outweigh the potential risks. In the past, elders were not considered good candidates for surgery merely because of age. Uncertainty about the value of surgery in elders and about the operative risks prevailed. Because surgical morbidity and mortality increase with age and complexity of disease conditions, a thorough understanding of the physiology of aging is necessary when considering surgery on older patients (Evidence for Practice). Although improvements in technology, monitoring techniques, and anesthesia have made surgery safer for older adults, age remains a significant risk factor. Nevertheless, adequate assessments of the functional age and the physiologic reserve of the elderly surgical patient are of paramount importance (Wold, 2012).

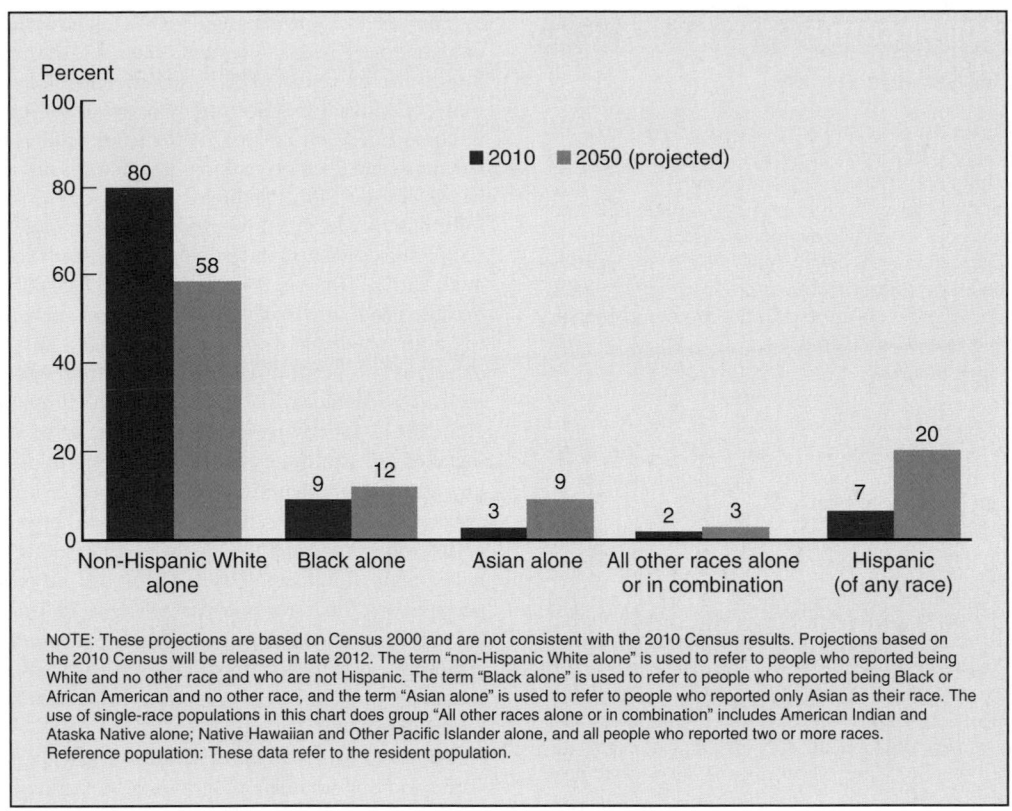

FIGURE 27-2 Ethnic population data for people age 65 years and older for 2010 and projected for 2050.

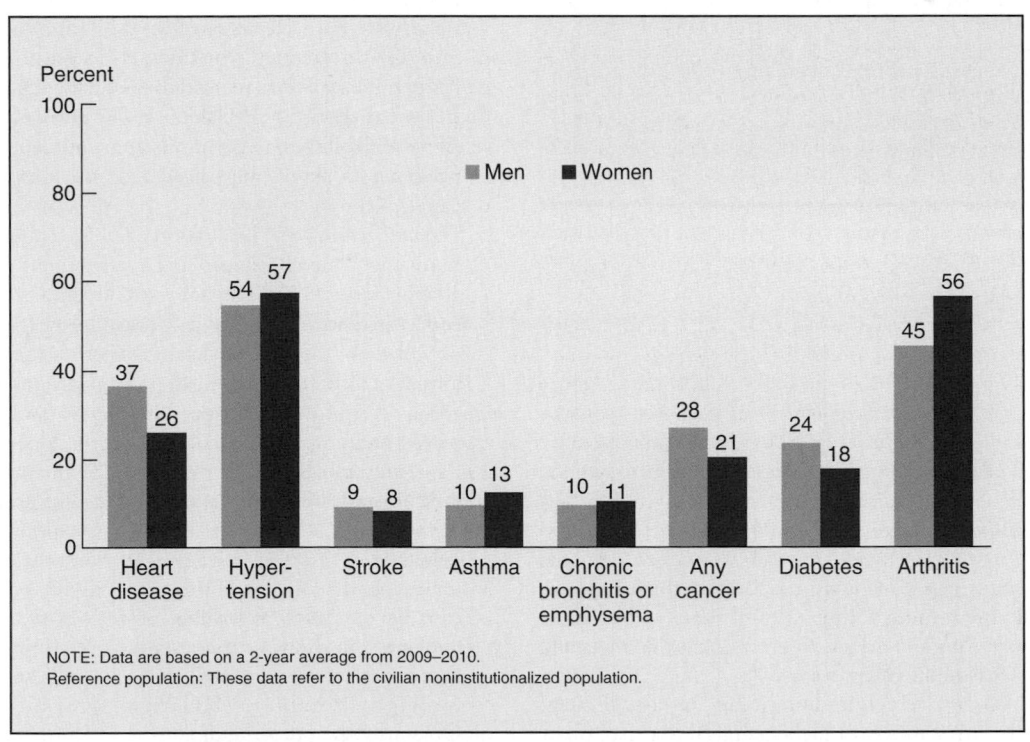

FIGURE 27-3 Chronic disease by gender in people ages 65 years and older.

Considerations for Geriatric Surgery

The following principles can be used when evaluating the geriatric patient prior to surgery. After a complete history and physical, the following assessments are strongly recommended:

- Assess cognitive ability and capacity to understand the anticipated surgery. Cognitive dysfunction is common in the geriatric patient postoperatively but difficult to quantify without a baseline status documented. The nurse should asses for the patient's ability to provide informed consent.
- Screen for depression. Depression is associated with higher pain perception and increased postoperative analgesic use.
- Screen for alcohol and substance abuse. Alcohol and substance abuse in the older adult is associated with increased rates of mortality and complications. These patients should be on a perioperative multivitamin.
- Ensure the patient has had a preoperative cardiac evaluation. Older patients are more vulnerable to postoperative cardiac events.
- Identify risks for pulmonary complications. Pulmonary complications are common in the geriatric patient and contribute to mortality and morbidity.
- Determine functional status and history of falls. The nurse needs a baseline functional status on the geriatric surgical patient. Immobility puts patients at an increased risk for delirium postoperatively and complications such as surgical site infections.
- Determine baseline frailty score. Geriatric patients have a decreased physiologic reserve and resistance to stressors. This leaves patients more vulnerable to bad postoperative outcomes including falls and decreased mobility.
- Record an accurate medication history. A detailed history of the medications the geriatric patient is currently taking will help minimize the risk for adverse reactions by identifying medications that should be discontinued prior to surgery.
- Determine treatment goals and expectations of outcomes. The nurse should ensure the surgeon has discussed advanced directives with the patient and a health care proxy has been established if necessary.
- Determine the patient's support system. Make sure the patient has someone at home to help care for him or her after surgery.

From Chow WB et al: Optimal preoperative assessment of the geriatric surgical patient: a best practices guideline from the American College of Surgeons National Surgical Quality Improvement Program and the American Geriatrics Society, *J Am Coll Surg* 215(4):453–466, 2012.

According to Kim and Zenilman (2007), the occurrence of perioperative mortality in geriatric surgical patients is influenced by three factors—presence of coexisting disease, emergency surgery, and site of surgery:

1. *Presence of coexisting disease as quantified by the American Society of Anesthesiologists (ASA) Physical Status Classification.* Patients with an ASA status of IV or V are consistently found to have greater mortality than those with a physical status of I or II.
2. *Emergency surgery.* Surgical risk in elders increases dramatically when the surgery is of an emergent nature.
3. *Site of surgery.* Major vascular, intrathoracic, and intra-abdominal procedures are reported to have a higher surgical risk than other surgical procedures in elders.

Surgical decision-making regarding elders can be difficult. As the baby-boomers become seniors, they will be very different from healthcare consumers of the past. They will tolerate less and expect more. In clinical practice today, patients are increasingly involved in clinical decision making. Patients are willing to actively participate in shared decision making. Emphasis is on patient involvement in medical decision making as a result of the growing amount of information available through the Internet, patient education materials, advertisements, and public quality reporting databases (Slover et al, 2012). The age structure in the United States is changing because people are living longer. The aging baby-boomers are creating a greater demand for surgical services, and this presents challenges to the healthcare system. Surgeons will have to meet the increased demands while guaranteeing high-quality care (Zenilman et al, 2011). Elderly patients have an increased tendency for slower metabolism, multiple chronic diseases, and a decreased reserve capacity of their organs to respond to stress, as compared to younger patients (Dardik et al, 2012). What should be considered is the risk of not operating and the quality of life expected. Although the recommendation for surgery is within the purview of the physician, perioperative nurses should be aware of its implications. Surgical intervention and management should be tailored to the patient's symptoms, overall functional and health status, and the predicted advantage of palliative intervention. Important factors that need to be evaluated are:

- *Disease course versus life expectancy:* Surgical intervention may not be appropriate if the prognosis of the disease is poor. However, if the patient has several years of life expectancy left and is likely to outlive the condition with minimal morbidity, surgical treatment may be the treatment of choice.
- *State of independence:* The patient's right to self-determination and making healthcare decisions should always be considered. The need for independence is of utmost importance to elderly adults, and most of them are far more interested in maintaining health and independence than longevity. Complications of surgery are not well tolerated by elders and can quickly develop into life-threatening situations. If surgical intervention will further incapacitate an already debilitated person, alternative treatment should be considered. However, if surgery will help alleviate debilitating conditions and improve or maintain independence, it should be considered an appropriate modality of care.
- *Personal motivation:* Evaluation of the elderly patient's level of motivation must be considered when surgery is planned. Many elderly patients are reluctant to undergo surgery because of concerns that the surgery will not improve their quality of life or will make them more dependent or destine them to a life in a care facility. In addition, they do not want to withstand the pain, discomfort, and rigors of surgery and the recuperative period necessary to treat a condition that does not really bother them very much or that they have "learned to live with." This lack of motivation can have a negative influence on the results of the surgery. Conversely, some elders expect and in some cases demand the best of care. They believe that the money they spend on taxes and healthcare entitles them to the very best that healthcare has to offer, regardless of its practicality. Nonetheless, patients who show a strong sense of determination in doing all that is necessary to get well and stay well are better candidates for surgery than those who believe illness is a prelude to death. Obviously the outcome of surgery is enhanced if the patient is motivated to have a positive result.

- *Surgical risk versus medical management:* Deciding between the risks of medical or nonoperative management and surgical intervention can be difficult for elderly patients. Surgical and anesthetic risks increase in proportion to the emergent nature of the patient's condition. When an acute emergency condition taxes an already overburdened physiologic state, survival is less likely. Patients may die even if the surgery was considered successful because of complications resulting from the complexity of the patient's comorbid condition. Nonetheless, healthcare providers need to be sensitive to this possibility when communicating with family members. To increase the chances of survival from a surgical procedure, the elderly person must be in optimum condition and adequate preoperative assessment and preparation must precede an elective procedure.

The following considerations should be included when deciding to proceed with surgery in elders (Dardik et al, 2012):

- Is there a clear indication for surgery, including a likelihood of disease progression?
- What practical limitations will be imposed on the patient with the progression of the disease?
- How much improvement can be expected after the surgical procedure?
- What is the expectation for quality of life with or without the surgery?
- How aware is the patient and the patient's family about the problem and proposed solutions?
- What risks are there for negative outcomes related to the procedure and the presence of comorbid conditions?
- Has an adequate preoperative assessment and preparation preceded an elective procedure?

There are many important considerations related to the extent of surgical treatment. Therefore, the decision for surgery relies heavily on the patient's physical status at the time of surgery and on the extent of disease progression. When treating patients who are nearing the end of life, attention should shift from solely maximizing survival to maximizing the quality of life and dignity while minimizing suffering. Early identification of problems with aggressive, preventive surgical treatment is considered more appropriate than waiting for problems to develop.

Perioperative nurses have a unique opportunity to assess and screen for signs of emotional and physical abuse in elderly patients during their preoperative assessment and while assisting with surgical positioning. Box 27-2 lists signs that may indicate abuse. If such signs are present, the perioperative nurse should report the suspected abuse to the appropriate authority. Reporting laws and regulations vary by state and facility.

Assessment

In elderly people a preoperative medical assessment is conducted to determine present physiologic functioning. When compared with younger people, the geriatric population may be more vulnerable to certain adverse events that may significantly affect their outcomes (Zenilman et al, 2011). Predicting surgical risk in the elderly can be challenging. According to Zenilman and colleagues (2011), frailty describes the global phenotype of a patient with decreased physiologic reserve and ability to withstand stress. Frailty is becoming an increasingly recognized tool to measure a patient's physiologic reserve. Frailty status is categorized in a standardized way as "frail," "intermediately frail," and "non-frail." Frailty is determined using a five-domain assessment tool including shrinking, weakness, exhaustion, lower physical activity, and slowness. Shrinking is

---

BOX 27-2

Signs That May Indicate Elder Abuse

- The older person demonstrates *excessive* agreement or compliance with the caregiver.
- The older person shows signs of poor hygiene, such as body odor, uncleanliness, or soiled clothing or underpants.
- The older person has malnutrition or dehydration.
- The older person has burns or pressure sores.
- The older person has bruises in various stages of healing that may indicate repeated injury.
- The older person lacks adequate clothing or footwear.
- The older person has not received adequate medical attention.
- The older person verbalizes lack of food, medication, or care.
- The older person verbalizes being left alone or isolated in some way.
- The older person verbalizes fear of the caregiver.
- The older person verbalizes his or her lack of control in personal activities or finances.

From Wold GH: *Basic geriatric nursing,* ed 5, St Louis, 2012, Mosby.

---

considered an unintentional weight loss of 10 pounds or more in the past year. Weakness is determined by assessing grip strength. Exhaustion and lower physical activity are assessed by giving the elderly patient a questionnaire. Slowness is assessed using a series of walking trials (Zenilman et al, 2011). Not all elderly people are frail and not all frail people have active disease, but measuring frailty provides surgeons with a tool to predict postoperative outcomes. Solely using chronologic age as a predictor of a patient's response to surgery is not a reliable measurement. It gives little indication of the physiologic or biologic age and condition of a person. For example, a 75-year-old person can be in better physical and mental condition for surgery than a 65-year-old. Biologic age as a measurement criterion is much more reliable. Establishing biologic age, however, becomes the greatest challenge. One tool, the Comprehensive Geriatric Assessment (CGA), is a multidimensional evaluation that scrutinizes medications, functional ability, comorbid conditions, cognitive ability, mental function, nutritional status, and socioenvironmental factors. The CGA may be used both to identify at-risk individuals and to guide interventions. When evaluated as a screening tool in the geriatric community, it has been shown to detect new and unsuspected problems in 76% of elderly persons living at home. In geriatric medical studies the CGA has been found to be potentially beneficial in reducing the incidence of hospitalization, falls, delirium, and readmission. It is predictive of both morbidity and mortality in older patients (Kim and Zenilman, 2007).

Evaluation of functional status typically includes assessment of the patient's ability to perform activities of daily living (ADLs) (personal care tasks) and instrumental activities of daily living (IADLs) (everyday tasks). The scoring system that is employed for assessing comorbidity in surgical patients is the American Society of Anesthesiologists Physical Status Classification (see Chapter 5). Additional measures of comorbidity include the Cumulative Illness Rating Scale for geriatrics and the Charlson Comorbidity Index (Kim and Zenilman, 2007) and the American Geriatrics Society (AGS) clinical management guidelines (2012). The AGS guidelines promote a patient-centered approach (Patient-Centered Care).

PATIENT-CENTERED CARE

As noted throughout this chapter, older adults are a vulnerable population due to many factors.

The nurse's role as health advocate is the heart of patient-centered care, which fosters a shared decision-making model to involve the patient in all aspects of care. The presence of multiple morbidities in the elderly can hinder the provision of care. The American Geriatrics Society (AGS) proposes the concepts listed below as a basis for involving the elderly patient in the decision-making process when multimorbidity is present:

- Inquire about the patient's primary concern (and that of the family and/or friends) and any other objectives.
- Conduct a complete review of the plan of care of older adults with multiple morbidities, or focus on a specific aspect of care, asking about current medical conditions and interventions. Is there adherence/comfort with the treatment plan?
- Consider the patient's preference. Is relevant evidence available regarding important outcomes?
- Consider the prognosis.
- Consider interactions within and among treatments and conditions.
- Weigh benefits and harms of components of the treatment plan.
- Communicate and decide for or against implementation or continuation of intervention/treatment.
- Reassess at selected intervals for benefit, feasibility, adherence, and alignment with the patient's preferences.

Modified from American Geriatrics Society (AGS) Expert Panel on the Care of Older Adults with Multimorbidity: *Patient-centered care for older adults with multiple chronic conditions: a stepwise approach from the American Geriatrics Society*, 2012, available at www.americangeriatrics.org/files/documents/MCC.stepwise.approach.pdf. Accessed February 3, 2013.

BOX 27-3

Preanesthesia Evaluation Data

Preanesthesia evaluation data include but are not limited to the following:

- Complete medical history with systems' review and anesthetic history, including self or family difficulty with anesthesia
- Complete surgical history
- Proposed surgical procedure
- Allergies—drug, food, environmental, latex
- Routine medications—prescription, over-the-counter (OTC), herbal, diet, recreational
- Current physical information—height, weight, baseline vital signs
- Social history—cultural and religious beliefs, alcohol and tobacco use
- Mental status—emotional clues; learning barriers; sensory, sight, or speech impairments
- Prosthetics—dentures, glasses or contacts, hearing aids, assistive devices (walker, wheelchair), implanted devices, prosthetics, body piercings
- Socioeconomic issues—transportation, home support
- Advance directives—living will, do not resuscitate (DNR) directive

Modified from Woogler JM: Preoperative testing and medication management, *Clin Geriatr Med* 24:573–583, 2008.

Impaired nutritional status is highly prevalent among the elderly; as many as 12% of men and 8% of women in the healthy geriatric population are considered undernourished. Higher rates of surgical complications and increased postoperative mortality have been observed in patients with poor nutritional status, as determined by a low body mass index, weight loss, a low preoperative serum albumin level, or a low Mini Nutritional Assessment score. Preoperative cognitive dysfunction has been associated with increased postoperative complications and worse survival in elderly surgical patients. Cognitive ability can be assessed with the Mini-Mental State Examination (MMSE) (Kim and Zenilman, 2007).

Depression and the lack of social support are also linked to adverse outcomes in older surgical patients. A tool that is commonly used in screening for depression in the elderly is the Geriatric Depression Scale. Several tools are available for quantifying social support resources in elderly patients. One such tool is the Medical Outcome Study Social Support Survey, which yields a score on a scale of 0 to 100 and includes "emotional" and "tangible" subscales. Another commonly used measure of social support is the Seeman and Berkman Social Ties Score, which measures social ties in four different areas.

An interdisciplinary approach is necessary to consider the complex health needs of the elderly patient in an effort to provide quality care. Application of these findings identifies operative risk, minimizes postoperative complications, and establishes the presence and status of any concomitant disease process that could negatively affect the outcome of the surgery. The preoperative nursing assessment is conducted to plan patient care throughout the perioperative period. In particular, assessment data are used to establish presurgical baseline data so that health status changes, primarily during the intraoperative and postoperative periods, are more readily recognized. The nurse's data collection includes the standard assessment information with considerations of coexisting conditions and a review of the patient's medication list (Box 27-3). Polypharmacy is an issue for many elderly patients and is a concern because of the physiologic changes associated with aging that lead to susceptibility to alterations in pharmacokinetics and vulnerability to adverse drug reactions.

Chronic conditions may interfere with the elderly person's ability to distinguish between recent and long-standing ailments. Therefore, the preoperative interview should be conducted in a quiet, relaxed environment with as few distractions as possible. The elderly person should be allowed to respond to each question independently without prompting from a spouse or other family members unless absolutely necessary. This helps maintain the patient's dignity, independence, and control, which are extremely important to the older adult.

Normal Age-Related Changes. Aging is a biologic process characterized by the inevitable, progressive, predictable evolution and maturation until death. Aging is not the accumulation of disease, although the two are related in subtle, complex ways. A fundamental principle is that biologic age and chronologic age are not the same. Different individuals age at different rates. Physical aging occurs in different organ systems at different rates, influenced by lifestyle choices and socioeconomic status. In general, the aging process imposes a decline in organ functions, atypical responses to pain and temperature, alterations in pharmacokinetics (Surgical

SURGICAL PHARMACOLOGY

Medication and the Elderly

Perioperative nurses caring for older adults must consider factors that affect the choice of medications and the effects of those medications on this population. Older adults may not tolerate the standard dosages used for younger adults and are at higher risk for side effects and toxicity. Dosages of drugs may initially be smaller than those used for the general adult population and then titrated based on the patient's response and therapeutic effect. Older adults have less reserve, and chronic disease may contribute to drug reactions. Physiologic changes may affect the absorption, distribution, metabolism, and excretion of medications. Older adults also have a higher prevalence of nonprescription drug use (e.g., analgesics, antacids, laxatives, supplements). A complete medication history should be obtained including prescription and over-the-counter medications including vitamins and herbal products. The nurse should partner with the surgeon and anesthesia provider to ensure that drug therapy is individualized based on the patient's baseline condition, actual physiologic impairments, and severity of preexisting illness. Identify medications that should be discontinued prior to surgery. Consider medications that should be started prior to surgery to reduce the risk of an adverse cardiac event. A medication history will help identify any renal function medications that need to be adjusted prior to surgery. The nurse should monitor for polypharmacy and potential adverse interactions. The addition of new medications postoperatively should be kept to a minimum.

Common adverse drug reactions in older adults include the following:
- Edema
- Dizziness
- Nausea and vomiting
- Urinary retention
- Anorexia
- Diarrhea
- Dry mouth
- Constipation
- Fatigue
- Confusion
- Weakness

Age-related changes that may affect medication administration in the perioperative period are as follows:
- *Changes in Absorption*
  - Increased gastric pH
  - Decreased gastric blood flow
  - Decreased gastrointestinal motility
- *Changes in Drug Distribution*
  - Decreased amounts of total body water
  - Increased ratio of adipose tissue to lean body mass, causing storage of lipid-soluble drugs and decreased plasma drug levels
  - Decreased albumin levels
  - Decreased cardiac output
- *Changes in Metabolism and Excretion*
  - Decreased liver size
  - Decreased hepatic blood flow
  - Decreased liver enzyme activity
  - Decreased renal blood flow
  - Reduced glomerular filtration rate, leading to slower excretion times for medications and allowing serum drug levels to rise

For patients at increased risk for delirium:
- Avoid starting new prescriptions for benzodiazapines and reduce current prescriptions when possible.
- Avoid using meperidine (Demerol) for pain control. Make sure pain is well controlled to avoid postoperative delirium.
- Caution when prescribing antihistamine H antagonists such as Benadryl and other medications with strong anticholinergic effects.

Modified from Hodgson BB, Kizior RJ: *Saunders nursing drug handbook 2013,* St Louis, 2013, Saunders; Ignatavicius DD: Common health problems of older adults. In Ignatavicius DD, Workman ML, editors. *Medical-surgical nursing: patient-centered collaborative care,* ed 7, St Louis, 2013, Saunders; Chow WB et al: Optimal preoperative assessment of the geriatric surgical patient: a best practices guideline from the American College of Surgeons National Surgical Quality Improvement Program and the American Geriatrics Society, *J Am Coll Surg* 215(4):453–466, 2012.

Pharmacology), and atypical signs and symptoms of disease, all of which may vary from one elderly person to the next. Having a clear understanding of normal age changes helps establish appropriate nursing diagnoses and develop a plan of care (Box 27-4). The following review of systems focuses on age-specific changes of particular importance to the perioperative plan of care.

Physiologic Changes

Integumentary System. The nails become thick and tough related to a decrease of circulation in the hands and feet (Table 27-1). A nick or cut can lead to a serious infection. Color and texture of hair change, and the loss of pigmentation results in graying of hair. Decrease in oil content makes the hair dull and lifeless, and the amount of hair decreases. The skin loses elasticity and subcutaneous fat and becomes more prone to shear force and pressure injury. Because of the thinness of the skin and small-vessel fragility, bruising and hemorrhaging are common. Dry skin develops because of decreased oil and sweat production from sebaceous and sweat glands, respectively (Research Highlight). As a result, skin breakdown and pressure ulcers, as well as wound infections, develop more easily. The vascular system of the skin has nutritional and protective roles. It is necessary for body heat regulation, provides defenses against microbial and physical damage, provides nutrient

BOX 27-4

Age-Related Physiologic Changes

Hematopoietic and Lymphatic System
- Increased plasma viscosity
- Decreased red blood cell production
- Increased immature T cells

Respiratory System
- Decreased tissue elasticity, resulting in pooling of secretions in lower lung bases
- Increased calcification of cartilage, leading to increased rigidity of the rib cage, decreased lung capacity, and reduced cough efficiency
- Less ciliary activity by bronchial lining
- Reduction in number of capillaries, resulting in decreased gas exchange and drying of mucous membranes

Cardiovascular System
- Changes in cardiac muscle tone and blood vessel elasticity, leading to decreased tissue oxygenation and decreased venous return
- Dysrhythmias; rapid or slow heartbeat
- High blood pressure related to atherosclerosis
- Chest pain or shortness of breath on exertion
- Decreased cardiac output, causing decreased circulation to extremities

Digestive System
- Dental issues (e.g., tooth loss, periodontal disease), leading to chewing issues
- Decreased saliva production
- Relaxation of esophageal muscle tone, increasing the prevalence of esophageal reflux
- Decreased gastric secretions
- Bowel dysfunction from decreased peristalsis

Urinary System
- Loss of nephron units
- Decline in renal tissue growth
- Reduced kidney size
- Reduced bladder capacity
- Increased prostate size in men
- Weakened bladder muscles with consequent postvoid residual

Musculoskeletal System
- Progressive loss of muscle strength from decreased muscle mass
- Decreased fluid in intervertebral disks
- Postural changes, such as curvature of the spine from decreased bone calcium
- Joint and back pain/stiffness
- Bone breakdown overcomes bone building, with resultant osteoporosis
- Decreased tissue elasticity, resulting in decreased mobility and flexibility

Nervous System
- Loss of neurons, leading to decreased reflexes
- Slower reaction time from loss of nerve fibers
- Changes in sleep patterns; less rapid eye movement (REM) and deep sleep
- Decreased amounts of neuroreceptors, resulting in decreased perception of stimuli

Sensory System
- Decreased tear production
- Increased lens discoloration, which decreases color perception
- Decreased muscle tone in eye, leading to decreased pupil diameter, decreased night vision, increased refractive errors, increased sensitivity to glare
- Loss of hair cells in inner ear, leading to balance problems
- Decreased joint mobility in bones of inner ear
- Decreased number of papillae on tongue

Endocrine System
- Decreased pituitary secretions (growth hormone), leading to decreases in muscle mass
- Reduction in the production of thyroid-stimulating hormone
- Decreased production of parathyroid hormone
- Increased prevalence of diabetes mellitus

Reproductive System
Female
- Decreased estrogen levels
- Decreased tissue elasticity
- Increased vaginal alkalinity

Male
- Decreased testosterone levels
- Circulatory changes

Modified from Wold GH: *Basic geriatric nursing*, ed 5, St Louis, 2012, Mosby.

TABLE 27-1

Age-Related Skin Changes

Physiologic Change	Results
Decreased vascularity of dermis	Increased pallor in white skin
Decreased amount of melanin	Decreased hair color (graying)
Decreased sebaceous and sweat gland function	Increased dry skin; decreased sweating
Decreased subcutaneous fat	Increased wrinkling
Decreased thickness of epidermis	Increased susceptibility to trauma
Increased localized pigmentation	Increased prevalence of brown spots (senile lentigo)
Increased capillary fragility	Increased purple patches (senile purpura)
Decreased density of hair growth	Decreased amount and thickness of hair on head and body
Decreased rate of nail growth	Increased brittleness of nails
Decreased peripheral circulation	Increased longitudinal ridges on nails, increased thickening and yellowing of nails
Increased androgen/estrogen ratio	Increased facial hair in women

From Wold GH: *Basic geriatric nursing*, ed 5, St Louis, 2012, Mosby.

RESEARCH HIGHLIGHT ||

Using the Braden Scale to Predict Risk for Postoperative Complications in Older Surgical Patients

Individuals 65 years and older comprise an increased proportion of surgical patients. Older surgical patients generally have a higher mortality and morbidity rate than do younger patients. These adverse reactions can often be attributed to postoperative complications. To prevent these serious complications early detection and quick response is key. Patients who are at an increased risk must be identified early, and awareness must be heightened for these individuals.

The Braden Scale is a tool used to assess the risk of developing pressure ulcers. Six domains are assessed including sensory perceptions and communication, moisture, activity, mobility, nutrition, and skin friction and shear. The sum of each domain score correlates to a low or high risk for developing a pressure ulcer. According to Cohen and colleagues (2012), a lower Braden Scale score postop was associated with postoperative complications. The study identified the Braden Scale as an independent predictor of the incidence of complications within the first 30 days after surgery for patients ages 65 and older. The Braden Scale may be used to identify surgical patients who are at a higher risk for postoperative complications. More research is needed to determine the Braden Scale's efficacy at determining postoperative complications.

Modified from Cohen RR et al: Exploring predictors of complications in older surgical patients: a deficit accumulation index and the Braden Scale, *J Am Geriatr Soc* 60(9):1609–1615, 2012.

supply to the avascular epidermis, and promotes wound healing. Having an intact vascular system to maintain these skin role characteristics is extremely important for a patient undergoing surgical intervention. However, papillary capillaries, responsible for epidermal nourishment and heat dissipation, degenerate with aging. What is left is only the horizontal arteriovenous plexus lying beneath the skin surface. This progressive impairment of vascular circulation and tissue nutrition and the loss of subcutaneous tissue predispose to a feeling of cold, especially in cool environments such as the operating room (OR). Therefore, the ability to maintain thermoregulation is compromised in elders and must be controlled through external measures.

Respiratory System. Pulmonary complications in the elderly account for nearly 50% of postoperative complications in the total population of surgical patients (Wold, 2012). Lungs lose elasticity, which contributes to a decrease in functional residual capacity, residual volume, and dead space. Lungs increase in size and are lighter in weight with aging. A rigid chest wall is the result of calcification of costal cartilages, osteoporosis, and dorsal kyphosis. Muscles responsible for inhalation and exhalation may be weakened, resulting in a diminished ability to increase and decrease the size of the thoracic cavity. All these changes contribute to a minimal tidal exchange, which makes the elderly patient more susceptible to pulmonary complications, such as acute respiratory distress syndrome (ARDS), pneumonia, and aspiration. Lung changes are not usually obvious at rest. However, when the person becomes active, breathing may be more difficult. The ability to cough and clear the upper airway is lessened, and such reduction may increase the chance of respiratory tract infections and diseases, some of which can be severe enough to be life-threatening.

Cardiovascular System. A decrease in coronary artery blood flow is more likely in older adults. Because of a shift in blood flow, there is a greater decrease in circulation to the kidneys and liver than to the brain and heart. Blood pressure rises as a result of increased arterial resistance. When the elderly person is at rest, the heart rate remains approximately the same as that of a younger person. However, the older heart requires a longer recovery time after each beat, which means that it reacts poorly to stress and anxiety-produced tachycardia. In general, the capacity of the cardiovascular system to tolerate and buffer insults is limited. Activity, exercise, excitement, and illness increase the body's need for oxygen and nutrients. The older heart may be unable to meet these needs. Arteries lose their elasticity and become narrow, causing a weakened heart to work harder. As a result, less blood flows through the arteries, causing poor circulation in many parts of the body. Elders have an increased risk for aortic arch disruption, myocardial contusion, and aneurysm development. A complete, comprehensive cardiac workup should be performed before the elderly patient is scheduled for any surgical procedure (Workman, 2013).

Digestive System. As a person ages digestive glands decrease the amount of secretions; mucus becomes thicker, causing dysphagia; and saliva becomes more alkaline. Loss of teeth or poorly fitted dentures make chewing difficult, resulting in digestion problems. Foods that are difficult to eat are avoided, and such avoidance can affect overall nutrition. Decrease in peristalsis and a reduction of gastric motility—the results of muscle tone loss—cause a delay in stomach emptying. Potential traumatic injuries to the bowel and mesenteric infarction are more likely to occur (Wold, 2012). The absorption of drugs is affected because of a reduction of blood flow to abdominal viscera, a reduction in the amount of hydrochloric acid secreted, and delayed gastric emptying. Decreases in the levels of total body water and plasma volume result in a smaller volume of distribution for water-soluble drugs. Because the percentage of body fat increases and the lean body mass decreases, the storage of lipophilic drugs, such as diazepam and lidocaine, is enhanced. These factors are of particular importance for assessing the patient's response to preoperative, anesthetic, and postoperative medications.

Urinary System. Nephrons decrease in function with age, so by 75 years of age a person has probably lost one third to one half of original nephron function. Elasticity and tone are lost in the ureters, bladder, and urethra, which lead to incomplete emptying of the bladder. Benign prostatic hyperplasia is the most common condition in men, with a significant increase in prevalence with age—from 20% in men ages 41 to 60 to 90% in men older than age 80 (Ebersole et al, 2012). Difficulty in voiding and retention of urine are common with this condition. Total bladder capacity also declines, so elderly persons experience a more frequent and urgent need to urinate. Because blood flow to the kidneys is decreased, patients are at greater risk for fluid overload, fluid and electrolyte imbalance, and alterations in the elimination of medications. During the perioperative phase of the patient's hospital stay, the greatest number and variety of drugs are given; the cumulative effect increases the chances for adverse and consequential results.

Musculoskeletal System. Changes to the elderly person's skeleton, such as the loss of bone mass, contribute to skeletal instability and make fractures of the hip, rib, distal radius, and vertebrae common. Curvature of the spine and arthritis of the joints are also common. Pain as a fifth vital sign is routinely evaluated for all patients. In elders, long-standing conditions such as arthritis, neuralgia, and ischemic disorders produce chronic pain. Back pain is related to dehydration and decreased flexibility of the vertebral disks. These changes result in a gradual loss of height, loss of strength, and decreased mobility. Poor posture tends to be proportional to the degree of back pain experienced and may greatly compromise internal organ function. Joint range of motion is impaired to varying degrees and may affect surgical positioning. The nurse takes extra care in positioning elderly patients in the OR, ensuring appropriate padding and joint protection (Wold, 2012).

Nervous System. Although not functionally significant, a steady loss in the number of neurons begins at about 25 years of age. An inappropriate or slow response to stimuli is primarily a result of a decrease in some organ systems' ability to send reliable messages to the brain and spinal cord. Nerve cells are particularly sensitive to lack of oxygen. Because older adults may have, in varying degrees, cerebral arteriosclerosis and atherosclerosis, decreased blood flow and nervous system deficits, such as insomnia, irritability, visual motor deficits, and memory loss, may occur. These patients are more likely to experience subdural hematomas or closed head injuries from falls. Other neurologic changes significant to perioperative care include a loss of position sense in the toes, decreased tactile sense, and atypical response to pain. In addition, aging is associated with disruption of thermoregulation (Wold, 2012); inadvertent hypothermia (temperature less than 96.8°F [36°C]) is a common problem in elders. (See Chapter 5 for a full discussion of preventing unplanned hypothermia in adult surgical patients.) In the OR, maintaining balance between heat gain (e.g., metabolic production, muscular contraction, hot ambient temperature) and heat loss (e.g., radiation, convection, evaporation, ventilation, cold fluid infusion, blood loss, antithermoregulatory drugs, impaired heat production) can be difficult in older surgical patients.

Sensory Changes. Changes in vision, hearing, taste, smell, and touch may influence the patient's response to care. If preadmission communication is done, the perioperative nurse may ask about vision and hearing and remind patients to bring their glasses and hearing aids to the facility (Clayton, 2008). Farsightedness, or presbyopia, in the aging person is a result of the lens becoming more rigid and less pliable. Consequently, visual acuity and accommodation are decreased. Color perception changes as a result of a yellowing of the lens, which makes distinguishing blue, green, and purple more difficult. Of particular importance in the OR is an awareness of the older person's difficulty in adapting to changes in light. Moving patients from a dimly lit holding area to the bright lights of the OR can cause momentary "blindness."

Presbycusis, or loss of hearing sensitivity, is irreversible, bilateral, and primarily sensorineural, although metabolic and mechanical causes are also possible. It is the most frequent cause of hearing loss in the geriatric patient. Hearing loss, which appears to be greater in men than in women, is mostly within the higher frequencies (above 1000 Hz). In addition, cerumen thickens and the eardrum becomes less pliable, and such changes also contribute to diminished hearing. Often geriatric patients are labeled "confused" or "senile" because they respond inappropriately to questions they did not hear or they describe what they see inaccurately because of poor vision.

Changes in taste and smell begin to occur at approximately 60 years of age and become more pronounced with advanced age. Older adults have two to three times more difficulty in detecting flavors than do young adults. Oral hygiene, dental disease, and decreased salivary function may also alter tasting ability. There is a close association between the sense of smell and human behavior. Smell can affect emotions when a person recalls a particular odor.

Other functions include protection of the individual by warning of danger in the air, such as smoke or gas fumes; assistance in digestion; and helping a person to remember or recollect. In elders, the sense of smell can be reduced, as well as the ability to identify odors (Wold, 2012).

Changes in sensitivity to touch often accompany the aging process, but the degree of change varies among individuals. In some cases, losses can be related to neuropathy caused by disease, injury, or circulatory problems. Decreased sense of touch can affect the elderly person's ability to localize stimuli and can reduce the speed of reaction to tactile stimulation. For example, an older person may have difficulty differentiating among coins, fastening buttons, or grasping small items.

Psychologic Changes. Physiologic and psychologic stress may result in an acute state of confusion or delirium in the geriatric patient that is analogous to convulsions as a stress reaction in the pediatric patient. In elders, mental change can be a warning of some underlying problem. It is of pivotal importance to determine the patient's interpretation of pain in the assessment phase. Confusion or delirium should therefore not be dismissed as an expected behavior of the geriatric patient. Delirium occurs in more than 80% of intensive care patients and patients at the end of life and in as many as 50% of hospitalized elders (Research Highlight). It is associated with increased length of stay, increased morbidity, poorer functional outcomes, increased risk of nursing home placement, and increased patient care costs. Several studies suggest that delirium is lessened when pain is appropriately managed, as determined in the study by Robinson and colleagues (2008) of hip fracture patients. The most important assessment factor is determining whether the confusion is chronic or acute. Chronic conditions, such as depression and Alzheimer disease, can make communication with the patient difficult. Depending on the stage of disease, patients may not be able to understand explanations. Family members are the best resource to determine the patient's ability to comprehend and respond to questions and instructions. Behavioral changes such as aggressiveness, agitation, and paranoia are not uncommon. Soft restraints

---

RESEARCH HIGHLIGHT

Delirium in Elderly Hip Fracture Patients

Hip fractures are associated with high incidences of complications. Delirium is a common complication of a hip fracture, and has been associated with a greater mortality and morbidity rate, longer hospital stay, and greater risk of institutionalization. Delirium incidence rates are up to 53.3%. Premorbid cognitive impairment is the most common risk factor for delirium after a hip fracture. Few studies have made a distinction between patients who had dementia preoperatively. Dementia patients are often frail and knowledge of risk factors is necessary to develop strategies to prevent delirium and further the decline of cognitive and physical health in elderly hip fracture patients.

According to the author, the incidence of delirium postoperatively on hip fracture patients in their study was 36.4%. Patients who had a body max index (BMI) of less than 20 were found to be at an increased risk, indicating that malnutrition is associated with postoperative delirium. Delay in surgical intervention was also associated with postoperative delirium in this study. Delay in surgery could be caused by patients who are underweight and might constitute targets for further intervention studies.

Modified from Juliebo V et al: Risk factors for preoperative and postoperative delirium in elderly patients with hip fracture, *J Am Geriatr Soc* 57(8):1354–1361, 2009.

BOX 27-5

Strategies for Communicating with Impaired Elderly Adults

When communicating with elderly adults who have cognitive impairments, perioperative nurses and surgical technologists should consider the following strategies:

- Try not to startle the person when starting a communication.
- Approach from the front, knock, or announce your presence by calling the person's name.
- Approach patients who have a left-sided hemiparesis from the right side and vice versa.
- Identify yourself.
- Communicate when the person is most alert.
- Eliminate or reduce noise and distractions.
- Make sure you have the person's attention before speaking.
- Try to use a variety of words or descriptions until meanings are clear.
- Ask clear, specific questions.
- Ask only one question at a time.
- Pay attention to the emotional context of conversation.
- Use pictures and gestures in addition to words.
- Have the person sit up for conversation whenever possible.
- Keep messages simple and repeat as needed.
- Be patient and do not interrupt. Slow down the pace of communication.
- Treat the person as normally as possible.

Modified from Wold GH: *Basic geriatric nursing*, ed 5, St Louis, 2012, Mosby.

BOX 27-6

Mnemonic for Assessing Pain in Demented and Nonverbal Elders

B   What **Behaviors** did you see?
O   How **Often** did the behaviors occur?
D   What was the **Duration** of behaviors?
I   How **Intense** were the behaviors?
E   How **Effective** was the treatment, if given?
S   What made the behaviors **Start or Stop**?

Modified from Ferris M: Pain in the cognitively impaired elderly: guidance for clinicians, *Adv Pract Nurse* eJournal posted May 15, 2008, available at http://geroresourcenurse.org/grn/download/GRN%20Council/pain%20in%20cognitively%20impaired%20older%20adult%20print.pdf. Accessed November 15, 2012.

---

may be necessary during local procedures in the OR to ensure patient safety. Taking the time to talk slowly, being deliberate in movements, getting to know the patient, and developing a trusting relationship before surgery can help to lessen the patient's anxiety and control the combative outbursts that occur in some Alzheimer patients (Box 27-5). A mnemonic for pain assessment in demented and nonverbal elders is described in Box 27-6. The American Society of Pain Management Nursing (ASPMN) has created guidelines for assessing pain:

- Ask the patient about pain.
- Search for potential causes of pain.
- Observe behaviors.
- Seek surrogate reports of pain.
- Do an empiric analgesic trial (Ferris, 2008).

Acute confused states or delirium in elders can be precipitated by a number of conditions and may be the sole manifestation of a

---

BOX 27-7

Preoperative Risk Factors for Postoperative Delirium in Elders

- Age 80 years or older
- Decreased education level
- Decreased functional status
- Alcohol or sedative-hypnotic withdrawal
- Depression
- Drug interaction or polypharmacy; duration of anesthesia
- Endocrine and metabolic problems
- History of dementia-like symptoms
- Low mobility
- Presence of multiple diseases
- Sensory impairments
- Surgical procedures considered major in nature
- Emergent or urgent surgical procedures
- Dehydration
- Low serum albumin level
- Abnormal preoperative serum sodium, glucose, or potassium level
- American Society of Anesthesiologists (ASA) class III or IV
- Uncontrolled pain
- Urinary elimination problems

Modified from Duthie EH et al, editors: *Practice of geriatrics*, ed 4, Philadelphia, 2007, Saunders; Bargi AS et al: Evaluation and management of elderly patients at risk for postoperative delirium, *Clin Geriatr Med* 24:667–686, 2008.

---

life-threatening complication. Delirium in elders may be evidenced by alteration in level of consciousness, inattention, disorganized thinking, or an acute onset of mental status change.

Some of the most common predisposing factors for confusion or delirium are noted in Box 27-7. Among the most predictive risk factors for delirium are immobility, functional deficits, use of restraints or catheters, medications, acute illness, infections, alcohol or drug abuse, sensory impairments, malnutrition, dehydration, respiratory insufficiency, surgery, and cognitive impairment (Touhy, 2012). Even the disruption of relocation into the hospital, which brings the patient into an unfamiliar environment, can cause acute confusion, particularly during the postoperative period. Validation of the patient's previous mental state with a relative or significant other can help determine if the onset occurred since hospitalization.

Routine Laboratory and Diagnostic Tests. The physiologic changes of aging do not significantly alter the diagnostic values of complete blood count (CBC), differential cell count, platelets, urinalysis, and blood chemistry results; therefore, abnormalities should be evaluated. A slight increase may be noted in the levels of potassium, fasting blood glucose, postprandial blood glucose, oral glucose tolerance, total cholesterol, and thyroid-stimulating hormone. A decrease in the amounts of vitamin B_{12}, folic acid, magnesium, vitamin D, and albumin as well as decreased creatinine clearance also may be noted. A chest x-ray film may reveal increased anteroposterior diameter, osteopenia, and degenerative joint disease. The heart size should appear normal, even in elders. Cardiomegaly can contribute to postoperative complications and should be evaluated. The electrocardiogram (ECG) may show P-wave notching, ST-segment depression or left ventricular hypertrophy, and T-wave flattening or inversion that are associated with an increased risk of myocardial ischemia (Dardik et al, 2012). An increase in bundle branch block, hemiblock, and first-degree block also may be noted, largely as a result of degenerative disease of the conduction system. Opinion about the number of preoperative laboratory tests to be ordered varies. Use of a focused history and physical examination yields important information regarding which preoperative tests are indicated. Preoperative testing should be based solely on the history, physical examination, and planned surgical procedure.

Medications. Because many elderly patients take several medications, assessing their drug history is important. The patient's physician will determine which medication should be withheld during the preoperative period and which should be administered with a sip of water the morning of surgery. A patient undergoing minor surgery who has been taking 10 mg or more per day of prednisone will need 25 to 100 mg of hydrocortisone at induction and can resume the normal regimen the next day. A patient undergoing major surgery will need 100 mg of hydrocortisone every 8 hours for 24 hours, and then the dose should be decreased rapidly. Oral therapy can be resumed when gastrointestinal (GI) function resumes. Patients undergoing ambulatory procedures will need 100 mg intravenously at discharge and a prescription of a rapid taper of prednisone or resumption of previous dose (Kuwajerwala, 2008).

Control of diabetes is often difficult during the perioperative period. For patients taking oral hypoglycemic agents, the medication is generally withheld, and serum glucose and urinary glucose levels are closely monitored. Diabetic patients treated with long-acting parenteral insulin typically discontinue it on the day of surgery, and regular insulin is given during the preoperative period. Diabetic patients who are fasting the morning of surgery should take their insulin as directed by the anesthesia provider and have an intravenous (IV) line inserted for infusion of 5% dextrose and water on admission to the OR.

Additional Assessment Data. Additional data regarding the patient can be gained from observing appearance, behavior, dress, and language. For instance, does the patient's apparent age (how old the patient looks) match the chronologic age? Facial expressions and contradictory behaviors can help the nurse assess the patient's mental status. Perioperative nurses in the preoperative area can gather additional data by noting the patient's clothing. For example, does the clothing size indicate signs of weight loss? Is clothing stained or burned? What is the condition of the patient's shoes? The patient's use of language and communication skills should also be assessed when formulating a teaching plan.

Another important but often overlooked area of assessment is dental and oral health evaluation. Disorders of the oral cavity can affect the patient's nutritional condition. Many elderly people simply do not attempt to eat because of ill-fitting dentures or poor oral health. In addition, the condition of the patient's temporomandibular joint and the presence of an oral disorder, including loose teeth and dentures, can make the difference between a smooth and safe anesthesia induction and a disastrous anesthesia experience.

The risk for impaired nutritional intake is exacerbated by other factors, such as reduced salivary gland activity, receding gums, and thinner tooth enamel, with concomitant brittleness in the teeth. Esophageal mobility is reduced, and a more relaxed cardiac sphincter slows emptying in the esophagus. Moreover, weakened intestinal musculature and slower peristalsis in the lower GI tract may lead to constipation. The confluence of these factors often results in poor nutrition. For the elderly surgical patient this can have deleterious effects, especially for wound healing.

Life changes can also affect nutritional status. Of particular importance are the losses endured with aging, such as the loss of one's spouse, family, or friends through death or relocation; loss of a prior standard of living through retirement; and loss of physical or mental well-being. These changes can affect older people to the point that they either cannot afford to buy nutritious foods or lose the ability or interest to prepare food. The ultimate effect, among other things, is a nutritionally debilitated patient. Any nutritional deficits should be corrected before surgery because the success of the operative procedure, the rate of wound healing, and the length of hospital stay are directly related to the nutritional state.

Determination of Operative Risk. After assessment of the patient is completed, conditions that can add to the patient's operative risk may be identified (Box 27-8). Medical disorders (including cardiac, abdominal, and thoracic) as well as multiple operations performed on an emergency basis significantly increase operative risk. Whenever possible, medical conditions are treated before surgery. Sometimes correction is not possible, and the risk of forestalling surgery outweighs any other medical problem. The determination of operative risk for the patient is generally based on the ASA Physical Status Classification (Sieber and Pauldine, 2009). Although the anesthesia provider performs the actual classification of the patient, it is important for the perioperative nurse to understand the significance of the classifications. Refer to Chapter 5 for more information on ASA classifications.

The most common surgical procedures in the elderly population that pose a greater risk of death are as follows:
- Acute intestinal vascular insufficiency
- Fracture of neck of femur
- Malignant neoplasm of colon
- Perforated diverticulum of colon
- Peripheral arterial occlusive disease
- Ruptured abdominal aortic or thoracic aneurysm

Other factors that are considered in determining operative risk are the patient's cognitive and functional states. Surgeons and anesthesia providers can assess the patient's cognitive state through the use of tools such as the MMSE, which evaluates four areas: orientation, registration, attention/calculation, and language. Points are assigned to each area; a perfect score is 30. A score below 24 indicates cognitive impairment, which may increase operative risk and increase the likelihood for postoperative complications. Functional status can be assessed through scoring the patient's ability to perform physical tasks. Each task is assigned a metabolic equivalent (MET). Tasks range from the ability to feed and dress oneself (1 MET) to the ability to participate in strenuous activity, such as football or skiing (10 METs). The inability to function above 4 METs is associated with increased perioperative cardiac events and long-term risk (Dardik et al, 2012).

Nursing Diagnosis

In evaluating, synthesizing, and prioritizing the data collected during the preoperative assessment, the perioperative nurse can formulate nursing diagnoses that will form the basis of the plan of care.

Nursing diagnoses related to the care of geriatric surgical patients might include the following:
- Risk for Deficient Fluid Volume
- Ineffective Thermoregulation
- Risk for Impaired Skin Integrity
- Risk for Perioperative Positioning Injury

BOX 27-8

Risk Factors for Surgery in Elders

Surgical Risks
- Emergency surgery
- Site of surgery
  - Vascular
  - Aortic
  - Intrathoracic
  - Intraperitoneal
- Duration of procedure (more than 3.5 hours)

Anesthetic Risks
- American Society of Anesthesiologists (ASA) classifications III to V
- Age older than 75 years
- Preexisting medical disease (hypertension; diabetes mellitus; cardiac, renal, liver, or respiratory disease)

Disease-Related Risks
- Cardiovascular
  - Angina
  - Previous myocardial infarction
  - Congestive heart failure
- Pulmonary
  - Bronchitis
  - Pneumonia
- Cigarette smoking
- Digestive
  - Poor nutritional status or malnutrition
  - Protein deficiency
  - Cirrhosis
  - Active peptic ulcer
- Endocrine
  - Adrenal insufficiency
  - Hypothyroidism

Cognitive Impairment
- Dementia
- Acute confusional state (delirium)
- Alzheimer disease

Other Factors
- Dehydration
- Anemia
- Recent stroke
- Malignancy
- Low albumin level
- Impaired mobility
- Patient living in institutional care

Modified from Kim SS, Zenilman ME: The elderly surgical patient. In Souba W et al, editors: *ACS surgery principles and practices*, ed 6, Ontario, Canada, 2007, BC Decker.

- Risk for Injury related to medication safety
- Risk for Infection

Outcome Identification

Outcomes identified for the selected nursing diagnoses could be stated as follows:
- The patient will maintain age-appropriate fluid volume levels intraoperatively and postoperatively.
- The patient will maintain normothermia ±1°F throughout the perioperative period.
- The patient's skin integrity will remain intact intraoperatively.
- The patient will be free from perioperative positioning injury.
- The patient receives appropriate medication or medications, safely administered during the perioperative period.
- The patient is free from signs and symptoms of infection.

Planning

As a result of anatomic and physiologic effects of aging, geriatric patients have, in varying degrees, a general decline in organ function and an altered ability to recover from stressful events. In addition to normal age changes, many older adults experience one or more chronic conditions that influence the risk of surgery. Successful surgical outcomes in the geriatric patient depend on elective versus emergency surgical procedures, optimum physical condition of the patient, thorough preoperative assessment, close intraoperative and postoperative monitoring, and preventive measures to decrease the likelihood of complications. Collaboration with the entire surgical team can create an environment that is safe, efficient, and caring and provides for a positive patient outcome.

A Sample Plan of Care for a geriatric surgical patient is shown on page 1094.

Implementation

Perioperative geriatric patient care is very similar to the care provided to younger adults. However, modifications that involve consideration of age-specific differences between the two groups are made. The perioperative nurse who recognizes the special needs of the elderly patient during what may be the most critical period of hospitalization helps to enhance the course of surgical intervention and postoperative recovery (Patient Safety). All members of the surgical team must work together in all phases of the perioperative continuum to provide an environment that focuses on the needs of the patient.

Preoperative Evaluation Guidelines

The American College of Surgeons and the AGS have issued a best practice guidelines for preoperative evaluation of patients at least 65 years of age who are undergoing surgery. The major objective of these guidelines is to help surgeons and the entire perioperative care team improve the quality of surgical care for elderly patients. The evidence-based guidelines will enhance surgical practice by setting higher standards and performance measures for surgeons and the entire perioperative care team. Another impetus behind these recommendations is the number and severity of underlying medical conditions that often require multidisciplinary management. The guidelines highlight 13 important areas in geriatric patients: cognitive impairment and dementia, decision-making ability, postoperative delirium, alcohol and substance abuse, cardiac assessment, pulmonary assessment, functional status, mobility and fall risk, frailty and nutritional status, medication regimen, counseling, preoperative testing, and patient family and social support system. Caring for the elderly is a team approach. Everyone should be of same accord in providing good quality care.

The guidelines strongly recommend the following preoperative assessments for every geriatric patient:
- Performing complete history and physical examination
- Conducting cognitive assessment, including the patient's ability to understand the purpose and likely outcomes of the planned surgical procedure
- Screening for depression
- Determining risk factors for postoperative delirium
- Screening for substance abuse/dependence, including alcohol

SAMPLE PLAN OF CARE

Nursing Diagnosis
Risk for Deficient Fluid Volume related to nothing-by-mouth (NPO) status and intraoperative blood and body fluid losses secondary to age-associated decrease in total body water and plasma volume

Outcome
The patient will maintain age-appropriate fluid volume levels intra-operatively and postoperatively.

Interventions
- Review medical history for presence and number of chronic diseases.
- Review, document, and communicate significant abnormal labo-ratory findings.
- Monitor and record intraoperative intake and output.
- Monitor and calculate estimated blood loss on sponges and in suction canisters.
- Distinguish between blood and irrigation fluid amounts in suction canister or canisters.
- Ensure visibility of the urine drainage bag.
- Ensure availability of blood and fluid replacement products as needed.
- Monitor and report intake and output to the anesthesia provider, surgeon, and postanesthesia care unit (PACU) nurse.

Nursing Diagnosis
Ineffective Thermoregulation related to poikilothermy secondary to age-associated physiologic decompensation

Outcome
The patient will maintain normothermia (±1°F) throughout the peri-operative period.

Interventions
- Identify risk factors for unplanned hypothermia.
- Use warm blankets during transport to the OR, and replenish as needed throughout the perioperative period (include the patient's feet within blanket covering).
- Adjust and maintain ambient room temperature at comfortable levels.
- Place a warmed sheet on the OR bed before patient transfer.
- Use active warming intraoperatively by applying forced-air warming system.
- Monitor the patient's temperature.
- Provide additional head covering (cloth, plastic, or reflective) during surgical procedures.
- Minimize exposure of the patient.
- Use warmed irrigation and preparation solutions (as recom-mended by manufacturer).
- Administer warmed blood and blood products and intravenous fluids at room temperature.
- Remove wet linens before transport to the PACU.

Nursing Diagnosis
Risk for Impaired Skin Integrity related to preoperative and intra-operative procedures secondary to alterations in skin turgor, sensa-tion, peripheral tissue perfusion, and skeletal prominence

Outcome
The patient's skin integrity will remain intact intraoperatively.

Interventions
- Review risk factors for intraoperative pressure ulcer development.
- Assess potential pressure areas before anesthesia induction and positioning, noting bruises, sores, skin tears, rashes, lesions, and pressure ulcers.
- Avoid friction and shearing forces by using a four-person lift, a lift sheet, or lifting device when transferring patient to or from

the OR bed and turning the patient to the desired surgical position.
- Prevent wrinkling of linen under the patient or positioning devices.
- Place electrosurgical dispersive pad in the most appropriate area while avoiding bony prominences.
- Avoid pooling of solutions under the patient.
- Apply tape sparingly to prevent skin injury during removal. If tape must be used, consider paper tape or a nonadherent dressing on fragile skin. Gauze wrap, stockinette, or tape alternatives may also be considered.
- Position the patient.
- Evaluate for signs and symptoms of physical injury to skin and tissue.

Nursing Diagnosis
Risk for Perioperative Positioning Injury related to positioning procedures secondary to musculoskeletal changes and associated chronic pain

Outcome
The patient will be free from perioperative positioning injury.

Interventions
- Assess pain and skeletal/range-of-motion limitations before anesthesia induction and positioning.
- Assess potential pressure areas before anesthesia induction and positioning.
- Place safety strap above the knees; prevent undue pressure on the popliteal space and heels.
- Ensure that armboards are maintained at less than a 90-degree angle.
- Provide adequate padding to protect potential pressure areas.
- Maintain body alignment within restrictions imposed by chronic pain and musculoskeletal age-related changes.
- Use gentleness during positioning and turning.
- Keep head and neck in a comfortable position that limits hyperextension.

Nursing Diagnosis
Risk for Injury related to medication safety

Outcome
The patient receives appropriate medications, safely administered during the perioperative period.

Interventions
- Administer prescribed antibiotic therapy and immunizing agents as ordered.
- Administer prescribed medications and solutions.
- Administer prescribed prophylactic treatments.
- Label all medications on the sterile field.
- Validate medication orders with perioperative team.

Nursing Diagnosis
Risk for Infection

Outcome
The patient is free from signs and symptoms of infection.

Interventions
- Implement aseptic technique.
- Monitor for signs and symptoms of infection.
- Initiate traffic control.
- Administer care to invasive device sites.
- Assess susceptibility for infection.
- Protect from cross-contamination.

PATIENT SAFETY

Preventing Deep Vein Thrombosis in the Elderly

Providing safe care for older adults in the perioperative setting requires the nurse and scrub person to have a thorough knowledge of the changes associated with aging and the risk factors for surgical complications. One change associated with aging is the increased risk for the development of deep vein thrombosis (DVT). The chances for developing DVT increase with age and double each decade of life over the age of 40 years. For example, a person who is 80 years old is twice as likely to develop DVT as someone who is 70 years old and 16 times more likely as someone who is 40 years old. The incidence of DVT is more than 150-fold higher among hospitalized patients than those in the community.

DVT is triggered by the Virchow triad: venostasis, hypercoagulability, and vessel wall inflammation, which leads to intravascular coagulation and the formation of a structureless mass of red blood cells, fibrin, and other cellular components. Several risk factors may increase the likelihood of DVT in an older person and include the following:

- Immobility; physical limitations that influence ambulation and movement
- Congestive heart failure
- Hypertension
- Use of diuretics, which contribute to dehydration and hypercoagulability
- Obesity
- Smoking
- Varicose veins
- Atherosclerosis

Prevention of DVT in the older person begins in the preoperative phase of care. Whenever possible, the nurse should contact the patient well in advance of the planned procedure to begin education on DVT precautions. Before surgery, patients should avoid long airline travel or immobility. Walking and increasing the activity level before surgery can improve the patient's venous return as well as

overall health state. Unless contraindicated by the patient's condition or physician's order, the nurse should advise patients to drink adequate fluids up until the time of their nothing-per-mouth (NPO) status to help maintain hydration. Whenever possible, the patient should be instructed about leg exercises (e.g., ankle rolls, leg lifts) to be performed before and after the surgery.

When the patient arrives in the preoperative area, the nurse should consult with the surgeon to ensure that antiembolic stockings or sequential compression sleeves are ordered for the patient. Antiembolic stockings improve venous return by squeezing and closing venous valves, preventing pooling and stagnation of blood in the lower extremities. Intermittent pneumatic compression devices, which alternately inflate and deflate, serve to push the blood in the extremities back toward the heart. The nurse should demonstrate the leg exercises to be performed in the postoperative period and assess the patient's understanding and mastery through return demonstration and also discuss the benefits of early ambulation.

Before anesthesia induction, the nurse ensures the patient's antiembolic stockings are placed correctly with no wrinkles or rolling that might impede venous return and verifies that the intermittent pneumatic compression device is functioning normally. If the patient's feet are accessible during long procedures, the nurse should perform periodic passive range-of-motion exercises to maximize venous blood return (if possible without compromising the sterile field).

The nurse encourages the patient to move his or her legs and perform the recommended exercises as soon as possible in the postanesthesia care unit (PACU). The PACU staff should reinforce the preoperative teaching about DVT prevention and ensure that the patient's caregiver also understands the instructions.

Pharmaceutical prophylaxis for DVT may be considered in some patients.

Modified from Jaffer AK et al: Prevention of venous thromboembolism after surgery, *Clin Geriatr Med* 24(4):635–639, 2008; *Understanding deep vein thrombosis,* available at www.clotcare.com/dvt.aspx. Accessed November 16, 2012.

- Performing cardiac evaluation following the American College of Cardiology/American Heart Association algorithm for patients undergoing noncardiac surgery
- Assessing risk factors for postoperative pulmonary complications and implementing suitable preventive strategies
- Documenting functional status and fall history
- Calculating frailty score at baseline
- Assessing nutritional status and considering implementation of preoperative interventions for high-risk patients
- Taking a complete medication history, making needed perioperative adjustments, and monitoring for polypharmacy
- Identifying the patient's treatment goals and expectations in light of anticipated and unexpected treatment outcomes
- Assessing the family and social support system
- Performing suitable diagnostic tests as needed for elderly patients (Chow et al, 2012)

Preoperative Preparation. The preoperative period is an opportune time to evaluate the patient's psychosocial status and educational needs. As mentioned, the motivation of the patient can affect operative risk and successful surgical outcomes. Awareness of psychologic and emotional status is as important as awareness of physiologic status. Often the patient's concerns are focused on the spouse

or other family members rather than on the impending surgery. An unexpected hospitalization can be very disruptive to an elderly patient who perhaps was the sole caretaker of an ill spouse, parent, or even a pet. In addition, the concern for quality of life and the fear of institutionalization after surgery can be extremely upsetting. This population has the highest morbidity and mortality in the adult population. Using the assistance of a discharge planner or case manager to arrange for resources may help allay the patient's concerns.

Sensory deficits, occurring either as a result of age-related changes or merely because eyeglasses and hearing aids are removed, can make communication with geriatric patients more difficult. Unresponsive or uncooperative behavior may be inappropriately diagnosed as dementia, expected as part of aging, and ignored. As discussed, acute confusion or delirium in elders is the most important indicator of possible underlying conditions that could seriously and adversely affect surgical intervention and outcomes. Knowing whether the patient's cognitive impairment is recent or chronic will provide direction for planning postoperative care.

The perioperative nurse should take advantage of the time spent in the preadmission interview, presurgical care unit, preoperative holding area, or the surgical corridor to introduce herself or himself and explain events to follow. Because a surgical mask is generally not required in these areas, this is the most opportune time for talking with the older adult. Once the patient is taken into the OR, a reassuring touch and remaining close to the patient, particularly during anesthesia induction, can help decrease anxiety.

Anesthesia Induction. The perioperative nurse shares with the anesthesia provider any pertinent assessment data that may affect anesthesia. A medical history of asthma, previous patient or family anesthesia problems, abnormal laboratory data, and physical limitations affecting induction or airway management are important findings. The following anesthetic issues contribute to the morbidity and mortality of the older population:

- Active or unstable concurrent diseases
- Decreased mobility
- Intubation difficulties
- Gravity of the surgical procedure
- Myocardial depression from anesthetic agents
- Potentially altered respiratory and cardiac reserves

Elderly patients frequently have changes in airway anatomy that make appropriate ventilation difficult. Changes in facial contour from sunken cheeks or lack of dentition can result in an inadequately fitting anesthesia mask. Keeping dentures in place often offsets this problem; however, if intubation is planned, the anesthesia provider usually removes the dentures. The joints of the head and neck may exhibit limited range of motion, making intubation and airway management more difficult in elders. Identification of these potential problems before anesthetic administration facilitates a smooth induction period.

The choice of anesthesia in the elderly patient depends on physiologic status, length of the operative procedure, and preference of the anesthesia provider. IV sedation with local anesthesia may be selected for herniorrhaphy or other procedures that do not entail complicated manipulation of organs. Regional anesthesia (e.g., spinal, femoral, brachial, axillary, or peribulbar blocks) may be chosen over general anesthesia for specific surgical procedures (e.g., cataract extraction, transurethral resection of the prostate [TURP]) because blood loss, deep vein thrombosis, and pulmonary embolism are less likely to occur (Sieber and Pauldine, 2009). The use of spinal anesthesia may be effective for orthopedic surgical procedures, such as hip fractures or knee replacements. Flexibility of the elderly patient or the presence of arthritic problems must be considered before attempting administration of a spinal anesthetic. In patients undergoing vascular or abdominal procedures, an epidural catheter may be considered for postoperative pain management.

Accurate predictions of how the elderly patient will respond to drugs or anesthetics are difficult to make because of a decrease in systems' function. Older patients have both an altered pharmacodynamic (relation between plasma concentration and drug effect) and an altered pharmacokinetic (distribution and elimination of drugs) response to drugs. These physiologic changes can affect medication administration because of a longer or shorter duration of action and less predictable effects. The increasing age of the patient decreases the dose requirement of anesthetic. This includes agents that induce anesthesia (e.g., thiopental sodium, etomidate, propofol) and narcotics. The induction dose of a barbiturate required for a 70-year-old patient will be less than that for patients 20 to 30 years old. Minimal blood levels of a drug may produce undesired side effects before therapeutic levels are reached. Likewise, reduced liver and kidney function, altered body composition, decreased albumin level, and decreased cardiac output all modify the aged person's ability to eliminate drugs from the body.

Age-related changes in homeostatic mechanisms affect the older adult's ability to deal with physiologic stresses of surgery, such as fluid depletion, volume overload, or hypoxemia. Mild hypothermia of only 1° to 3° F below normal can increase postoperative myocardial ischemia and ventricular tachycardia. The incidence of hypothermia is greatest with combined epidural-general anesthesia (Sieber and Pauldine, 2009). The perioperative nurse should be prepared to respond quickly in assisting the anesthesia provider to stabilize the patient when adverse reactions occur.

Positioning. Protection of skin integrity is of utmost importance. Loss of subcutaneous fat, poor skin turgor, and tissue fragility can worsen a postoperative skin problem. Elderly patients should be lifted into position, rather than slid or dragged, to prevent shearing injuries. Aging changes in the musculoskeletal system accentuate bony prominences and decrease the range of motion. These skeletal changes coupled with limitations imposed by chronic pain make positioning one of the most important considerations of care. The provision of appropriate positioning devices is pivotal to the protection from injury for this population of surgical patients. Arms are placed on padded armboards with the palms up and fingers extended. Armboards are maintained at less than a 90-degree angle to prevent brachial plexus stretch. If there are surgical reasons to tuck the arms at the side, the elbows are padded to protect the ulnar nerve, the palms face inward, and the wrist is maintained in a neutral position (Denholm, 2009). A drape secures the arms. It should be tucked snuggly under the patient, not under the mattress. This prevents the arm from shifting downward intraoperatively and resting against the OR bed rail.

Often, because of musculoskeletal deformity and chronic pain, elderly patients cannot fully extend the spine, neck, or upper and lower extremities. Using padding devices to compensate for these limitations not only makes the patient more comfortable during the procedure but also prevents residual pain or injury postoperatively. Depending on the situation, positioning the patient before anesthesia induction may be best so that the patient can direct positioning efforts in regard to comfort.

Skin Preparation and Thermoregulation. Aging skin is more susceptible to rashes, infection, and inflammation. A common complaint of the elderly is dry skin that may be part of the natural aging process or can be related to diseases such as anemia, malignancy, kidney disease, or diabetes. Medications, such as corticosteroids, may cause skin to become more fragile. Changes in the dermal receptor cells can alter the ability of the elderly to perceive sensations of pressure and touch, as well as changes in temperature.

Decreased muscle tissue and activity, reduced subcutaneous fat, and diminished peripheral circulation are some of the changes in aging that can have a negative effect on thermoregulation (Wold, 2012). The perioperative environment can expose the elderly patient to cool temperatures and hazardous chemicals, thus requiring the perioperative registered nurse to assume extra caution in this environment.

Aseptic Techniques and Safety Measures. Age-related changes in functioning of the immune system and some age-associated diseases have a detrimental effect on the aging body's ability to appropriately respond to infection. One out of every 10 to 20 patients hospitalized in the United States develops a hospital-acquired infection. Central line–associated bloodstream infections, ventilator-associated pneumonia, catheter-associated urinary tract infections, and surgical site infections are targeted by hospitals' prevention efforts. Two specific organisms, methicillin-resistant *Staphylococcus aureus* (MRSA) and *Clostridium difficile* (C-diff), are also targeted because of their increasing incidence and morbidity rates (Yokoe et al, 2008).

Immobility and drug therapy alter flora in the intestines. Infection and delayed wound healing are poorly tolerated and sometimes fatal in debilitated elderly patients. In addition to adherence to aseptic technique, there are other measures used in the OR to protect aging patients from the risk of infection. Because length of surgical procedure is related to incidence of infection, the nurse should ensure that needed supplies and equipment are readily available to avoid delays or prolonging the procedure. The scrub person, who may be a registered nurse or surgical technologist, should be familiar with the procedure being performed to maximize efficiency to prevent unnecessary delays, decrease exposure of the surgical site, and reduce the length of time the elderly patient is anesthetized.

Fluctuations in fluid volume are common in aging patients. Volume deficits occur as a natural course of aging, whereas volume excess can occur from intraoperative fluid replacement. The age-related failure of homeostasis to adjust for stressful disturbances has been demonstrated by changes in fluid balance. Large variability in the way different organs are affected by dehydration results in atypical symptoms in older adults. Table 27-2 provides important clues for assessing dehydration. Careful measurement of intake and output is essential. Communication among team members regarding blood loss during the procedure can prevent complications. The nurse and scrub person must collaborate to ensure accuracy in irrigation distributed to the sterile field and used during the procedure. The team closely monitors discarded sponges, suction canister contents, and urinary output as part of volume assessment. During the hand-off report, the nurse reports intraoperative IV fluid volumes, estimated blood loss, and other parameters to the postanesthesia care unit (PACU) staff for their continued assessment and evaluation.

Evaluation

Because of the relatively fine line between stability and development of postoperative complications, the elderly patient's response to surgery must be closely evaluated. Before transporting the patient to the PACU, the perioperative nurse should assess the care provided intraoperatively by evaluating expected versus actual outcomes. Specific outcome criteria established for each nursing diagnosis provide the basis for evaluation of care. Many of the nurse's actions at the end of the intraoperative phase provide data for evaluation of care.

The nurse collaborates with the anesthesia provider to complete and record the patient's intake and output measurements. Because of the consequences of postoperative dehydration or fluid volume overload in the elderly patient, fluids are increased or decreased accordingly. Blood loss is carefully evaluated, recorded, and reported.

The wound is closely observed for bleeding before dressing application and postoperatively because the elderly person's ability to recover from hemorrhage and shock is extremely poor. Anticipated frequency of dressing change, as in a draining wound, should govern the method used to secure the dressing. A minimal amount of tape should be used because its removal can cause additional skin trauma. Depending on the wound site and character, rolled gauze, stockinette, or similar bandaging over the primary dressing may be the best choice so that tape is not applied directly to the skin. Another alternative is the use of Montgomery straps. For smaller

wounds, the least possible amount of hypoallergenic tape should be used. Because infection is poorly tolerated, the choice of dressing should maximize wound protection while being the least irritating to the skin.

The nurse examines the patient for signs of injury, particularly over bony prominences and under the electrosurgical dispersive pad. To prevent skin injury postoperatively the patient should be carefully lifted from the OR bed to the stretcher. Pain is assessed and compared with preoperative levels. Evaluation of musculoskeletal pain will determine intraoperative positioning effectiveness.

Evaluation of body temperature is particularly important in elders because postoperative hypothermia is quite common and can precipitate agitation and confusion or delirium. To prevent any adverse response, the nurse covers the patient with warmed blankets and uses a forced-air warming unit until the patient is transported to the PACU.

Depending on the patient's level of consciousness, the nurse should explain the impending transfer to the PACU as a form of reality orientation for the patient. As appropriate, the nurse

---

TABLE 27-2

Important Clues in the Initial Assessment of Dehydration in Older Adult Patients

Clinical Indicator	Water Deficiency	Water + Electrolyte Deficiency
Medical history	Recent >3% weight loss Impaired water intake Increased perspiration (fever, tachypnea, heat)	Recent >3% weight loss Vomiting, diarrhea, diuretic, drug use, diabetes, bleeding
Physical Examination		
Tongue dryness	Present	Present
Longitudinal tongue furrows	Present	Present
Dry mucous membranes, mouth	Present	Present
Upper body muscle weakness	Present	Present
Confusion	Present	Present
Speech difficulty	Present	Present
Sunken eyes	Present	Present
Blood pressure	Unchanged or decreased	Highly decreased
Pulse rate	Unchanged or decreased	Highly decreased
Laboratory Tests		
Serum creatinine	Increased	Increased
Serum urea	Increased	Highly decreased
Tonicity	Highly decreased	Unchanged or decreased
Urinary output	Decreased	Decreased, unchanged, or highly decreased
Urinary sodium concentration	Decreased	Decreased, unchanged, or highly decreased

Modified from Faes MC et al: Dehydration in geriatrics, *Geriatr Aging* 10(9):590–596, 2007.

should introduce the patient to the PACU nurse and explain what to expect in the unit. Explanations should always precede any procedure. Often the elderly person is reluctant to cooperate simply because no one has taken the time to explain what is going to happen.

Verbal communication between the perioperative and PACU nurses should include any pertinent preoperative and intraoperative information that could affect postoperative care outcomes. This information includes pain levels; physical and sensory limitations; intake and output measurements; allergies; type and location of catheters, drains, packing, and implantable devices; anesthetics and medications received; and any unusual occurrences that could affect the patient's recovery. Perioperative nurses should be aware of the risk for the phenomenon known as postoperative delirium, a condition that can occur in elderly patients. Box 27-8 (p. 1093) lists the most frequently identified preoperative risk factors for postoperative delirium.

Documentation of outcome evaluation can be phrased as follows:

- Fluid balance was maintained; urinary output was within normal limits; the patient's forehead skin was checked and had good turgor; and vital signs were stable.
- Temperature was ±1° F of normal range; skin was warm to touch; and patient verbalized comfort.
- Skin integrity was maintained free from redness, bruises, and abrasions; patient reported no pain or impairment of the skin; and there were no apparent signs or symptoms of infection.
- The patient accurately perceived and interpreted environmental stimuli, expressed and demonstrated understanding of procedures, and responded appropriately to auditory and verbal stimuli.
- Perioperative positioning injury was effectively prevented and patient had no compromise in musculoskeletal ability or range of motion from preoperative levels. Patient had no complaints of increased pain.
- Medications used during the intraoperative procedure caused no apparent adverse reaction.
- Patient shows no signs or symptoms of infection.

The type and extent of surgery may affect postoperative pain. Elderly persons may not complain of pain, but this does not mean that pain does not exist. Those patients with cognitive impairment may experience pain but may be unable to verbalize it. Box 27-9 lists key elements of pain assessment and management in older adults.

Contemporary pain control delivery systems and techniques offer a variety of treatment routes and modalities. Various routes may be used to deliver medication for pain control: oral, intramuscular, IV, regional (i.e., spinal or epidural), or patient-controlled analgesia (PCA). Cognitive modalities that may be used are distraction, relaxation (i.e., biofeedback), or hypnosis. Physical modalities that may be used are cold, exercise, heat, immobilization/rest, massage, positioning, or transcutaneous electrical nerve stimulation (TENS).

Clinical management of pain should be multimodal and individualized for the patient, procedure, and circumstance. Evaluation of the balance between pain control and side effects should be documented, timely, routine, and specific.

Patient and Family Education and Discharge Planning

Education should be conducted at a time when the patient is at rest rather than during preoperative or postoperative procedures. Too

---

BOX 27-9

Pain and Older Adults

Prevalence of Pain
Recognize that older adults are at great risk for undertreated pain.

Beliefs About Pain
In addition to receiving less analgesia than younger adults, older adults tend to report pain less often. These findings may be related to beliefs and concerns about pain and the reporting of pain. Many older people hold the following beliefs and concerns about pain:
- Pain is something that must be endured; it is part of life.
- Expressing pain is unacceptable or is a sign of weakness.
- Complaining of pain will result in being labeled as a "bad" patient.
- Nurses are too busy to listen to complaints of pain.
- Pain signifies a serious illness or impending death.

Nurses should be aware of the beliefs of older patients regarding pain management. Nurses and other caregivers often undermedicate these patients and are sometimes reluctant to administer the prescribed analgesics.

Assessment
- Ask about present pain only.
- Use a standard scale, such as the numeric faces or Iowa thermometer rating scale.
- Explain the scale each time it is used.
- Use verbal descriptions other than pain, such as "ache," "sore," and "hurt."
- Use visual representations of pain measures rather than mental images of pain rating scales. Be sure that the patient is wearing glasses and hearing aids if needed and available.
- Alter a written pain scale to include large lettering, adequate space between the lines, nonglossy paper, and appropriate color for increased visualization.
- Provide adequate lighting and privacy to avoid distracting background noise.

Consideration for Cognitively Impaired Patients
- Assess for nonverbal indications of pain (facial expressions, grimacing, vocalizations, body movements, behavioral changes).
- Remember to "assume pain is present" in cognitively impaired patients in the perioperative setting.
- Consider an analgesic trial.

Management of Pain
- Be aware of adverse effects of acetaminophen (hepatotoxicity and nephrotoxicity) and nonsteroidal antiinflammatory drugs (NSAIDs) (gastrointestinal [GI] bleeding and nephrotoxicity).
- Start low and go slow with opioid dosing.
- Avoid the use of meperidine and codeine.
- Use methadone and tramadol with caution.
- Older adults and those with renal disease should not take meperidine because of the prolonged half-life of its drug metabolite, normeperidine.
- Use nondrug pain-relief measures.

Modified from Ignatavicius DD: Pain: the fifth vital sign. In Ignatavicius DD, Workman ML, editors: *Medical-surgical nursing: patient-centered collaborative care*, ed 7, St Louis, 2013, Saunders.

---

many stimuli from outside sources can interfere with the patient's ability to concentrate and motivation to learn. The nurse ensures the patient's physical comfort and privacy. Education will be ineffective in the patient who is uncomfortable or in pain. Age-related changes can affect the elderly patient's ability to learn new material;

therefore modification of traditional teaching approaches should be used to enhance effectiveness. Patient education should consider health literacy and be individualized based on how the patient will best understand the information.

A comprehensive discharge plan should identify and address communication barriers, incorporate the patient's current mental and physical condition, address environmental issues that can be improved to support recovery, and diminish the social support challenges. Sensory changes in vision and hearing, cognitive impairment, and literacy level can be communication barriers that interfere with the patient's ability to understand and retain information. Giving the patient postoperative instructions in written form helps with retention, and modifications using large, easy-to-read typeface on matte-finish paper of warm tones (yellow, tan) make the instructions easier to read. It may be helpful to have a magnifying glass available and supplemental light on the object or surface involved in the teaching/learning activity. Family members or significant others who are present should be included in the educational session so that they can provide reinforcement at home.

The discharge plan should consider the patient's ability to perform ADLs, ambulate, and manage his or her preexisting medical condition after surgery. The older person's basic medical condition does not change because of surgery. Content should focus only on relevant information about surgical procedures or postoperative recoveries; relating it to previous life experiences helps the patient grasp the concepts more readily. The nurse should provide the most important information first. If motor skills (i.e., crutch walking, dressing change) are involved, all steps should be taught one at a time, and mastery should be demonstrated before moving to the next step. Increased time is often necessary when teaching motor skills.

Discharge planning begins during the preoperative assessment. Sufficient time is needed to make appropriate decisions about postdischarge care to prevent complications, reduce the risk of rehospitalization, and minimize stress to the patient and the caregivers. Consideration should be given to the environment to which the patient will be transferred following the surgery. The patient considers relocation as a disruption after discharge. Although the plan should consider that older adults prefer to keep their autonomy, the postoperative care may require special facilities, such as a rehabilitation center or long-term care facility, at least for a time.

Transitions between care settings are periods of vulnerability for the elderly. The reasons include the involvement of multiple caregivers and errors in communication and information transfer. Some type of communication tool and electronic health care record across all phases of patient care is recommended to support effective communication for all patients (Nelson and Carrington, 2011).

The type of surgery and expected postoperative recovery period determine the extent of resources and social systems needed, such as durable medical equipment, home health and homemaker services, extended care, social and community services, and physical rehabilitation. The success of postdischarge outcomes in elders is influenced by the patient's self-assessment of health as good or excellent, the complexity of the patient's medical condition, the patient's history of being able to maintain responsibility for his or her own health, and the patient's family or social networks. Many elders undergo procedures on an ambulatory basis (Ambulatory Surgery Considerations). Discharge needs of the patient should be evaluated as early as possible so that appropriate education, referrals, and home preparation can be completed before the patient leaves the hospital or ambulatory facility.

AMBULATORY SURGERY CONSIDERATIONS

Procedures of the Eye

Cataract surgery is among the most common ophthalmic surgical procedures performed in older adults. Some degree of cataract formation is expected in all people older than 70 years of age. The majority of these procedures are performed in an ambulatory setting, with patients returning home the day of surgery. Cataracts are associated with factors including trauma, inflammation, genetic predisposition, metabolic disease, and cigarette smoking, but aging is by far the most common factor. Most eye surgery patients make the decision to have the procedure done after months of deliberation and slow, progressive loss of vision. The overall risk of death is low and does not significantly change whether local or general anesthetic is used. Intraocular lenses can be safely implanted in the majority of patients. Microsurgical wound closure ensures a secure incision that allows immediate ambulation. The surgical stress is considered so low and visual rehabilitation so rapid that severe visual impairment is considered a reasonable indication to perform surgery even if the patient is debilitated. (See Chapter 18 for an in-depth description of cataract surgery.)

Surgical Interventions

The elderly account for the majority of cancer patients. Cancer disproportionately affects those 65 years and older and that number will increase substantially in the coming decades as a result of the increasing life expectancy, thus creating a challenge for cancer specialists. The optimum treatment must be determined while paying special attention to comorbidity, physical reserves, disabilities, and geriatric conditions (Hamaker et al, 2012). Colorectal cancer is one of the most common malignancies and the second cause of cancer death in the United States, with a great number of these patients being elderly (Beretta et al, 2012). Women 65 years and older have a rate of breast cancer of 404 per 100,000. Women 70 years and older comprise 30% to 40% of all breast cancer patients (Jones et al, 2012).

Surgical procedures that are common among the geriatric population are governed more by pathologic condition than by anatomy and are directly related to the common diseases affecting older adults. Healing is an important consideration in the decision to perform surgery on this population. The level of tissue oxygen is the main factor in determining wound healing and is influenced by factors such as cardiovascular status and anemia. Other factors are included in Box 27-10. In the text that follows, some surgical procedures that are commonly seen in elderly patients are briefly discussed. Reference is made to other sections of the text for a more in-depth description of the technical aspects of the procedures. Surgical interventions take place in various types of venues. Operative and invasive procedures can be performed in ORs, cardiac catheterization laboratories, ambulatory surgery centers (ASCs), doctors' offices, and any other facility deemed appropriate for a surgical intervention.

Common Surgical Procedures in Geriatric Patients

It is becoming common for patients well past 85 years of age to have surgery with relatively good outcomes. Decisions are no longer based solely on surgical risk but rather on optimal disease management and the preservation of quality of life. This shift in thinking has taken us beyond just getting the patient through the surgery and has produced a genuine concern about what the surgery will do for patients in the remaining years of life.

The advent of advanced technology has led to a decreased length of time for surgical procedures for the elderly patient. Namely, an open abdominal aortic aneurysm (AAA) surgery has been replaced with an endoscopic AAA, an open coronary artery bypass graft (CABG) has been replaced with a minimally invasive CABG, and an open total knee replacement has been replaced with minimally invasive robotic knee replacement, to name a few. These procedures also decrease infection rates and length of stay.

Thyroid Surgery

In the elderly population, thyroid gland dysfunction is common and associated with significant morbidity because the symptoms are often subtle, absent, or confused with coexisting diseases. Thyroid disorders are highly prevalent, with the highest incidence being in aging women (Bensenor et al, 2012).

Typical symptoms of thyroid disorders may be absent or erroneously attributed to comorbid conditions or normal aging. The polypharmacy used in the treatment of elderly patients can interfere with normal thyroid function. Drugs such as lithium or amiodarone may cause primary hyperthyroidism. For example, an elderly man taking medication for hypertension, congestive heart failure, and atrial fibrillation with complaints of fatigue, weakness, constipation, and weight gain may be considered to have these symptoms because of medication or medical conditions, whereas the symptoms also could be caused by hypothyroidism.

A rare complication of hypothyroidism, myxedema coma, affects patients older than 75 years. Confusion, disorientation, lethargy, thinning eyebrows and hair, hoarse voice, bradycardia, cardiomegaly, pericardial effusion, hypothermia, hyponatremia, and pseudomyotonic reflexes characterize this condition.

The great masquerader in the elderly population is hyperthyroidism and can easily be missed in patients older than 60 years. It can be severe and even life-threatening. Elderly patients may not have a goiter, exophthalmos, or other ophthalmopathy. Hyperthyroidism may also cause osteoporosis. Almost any condition that can make a person ill can cause euthyroid sick syndrome; so elders are more susceptible because of their comorbid conditions. Medication to suppress hormone secretion by the gland, surgery to remove the hyperfunctioning tissue, and radioactive iodine (RAI) to destroy the gland are the three treatment options. Although surgery is a less attractive option, it must be used when RAI is ineffective in the presence of a single nodule or multinodular toxic goiter or when the patient has dysphagia, tracheal compression, or suspected malignancy. Following surgery, the perioperative nurse must be aware of the possibility of a hyperthyroid storm that can be precipitated by the stress of the procedure, systemic infections, and anesthesia induction. (See Chapter 16 for an in-depth description of operations of the thyroid.)

Abdominal Surgery

Accurate diagnosis of abdominal disease is important in elders to plan timely and appropriate surgical interventions. However, clinical signs of abdominal disease, such as tenderness, pain, muscle rigidity, and fever, are frequently less obvious in elderly patients. The common use of nonsteroidal antiinflammatory drugs (NSAIDs) may mask symptoms or even predispose elderly patients to acute abdominal disease.

The most common causes of acute abdominal complaints in older patients are biliary tract disease, intestinal obstruction, GI hemorrhage, hernia, diverticulitis, and appendicitis. Common abdominal procedures in people older than 65 years include cholecystectomy, lysis of adhesions, appendectomy, and partial excision of the small bowel (Wold, 2012).

Most often, surgery is performed for complications of calculus disease and less often for malignant obstruction of the bile ducts. The prevalence of gallstones increases with age. Because laparotomy is a stressor in older ill patients, laparoscopic cholecystectomy is considered the preferred surgical approach in elderly patients with both symptomatic and asymptomatic gallstone disease. (See Chapter 12 for an in-depth description of operations of the biliary tract.)

The age group older than 65 years has seen an increase of ulcer disease. Many believe that the higher incidence of *Helicobacter pylori* infection, prevalent use of NSAIDs, and prevalence of cigarette smoking in elders account for the age-related differences. Up to 80% of peptic ulcer–related deaths occur in patients older than 65 years (Dardik et al, 2012).

GI bleeding is a frequent indication for hospitalization affecting a substantial number of elderly people. A coordinated approach to diagnose and manage these patients can optimize favorable outcomes. Per Yachimski and Friedman (2008), key points to remember include the following:

- Immediate attention should be focused on hemodynamic stabilization followed by diagnostic assessment to identify the source of bleeding.
- Outcomes are influenced by the use of anticoagulant therapy, the presence of medical comorbidities, and the nature of the lesion.
- Peptic ulcer disease is usually the most frequent source of upper GI bleeding. Rebleeding and morbidity can be reduced with gastric acid suppression and endoscopic hemostatic therapy.
- Diverticular disease is the most frequent source of lower GI bleeding. Urgent colonoscopy to identify the bleeding site and perform hemostasis is indicated. Persistent, recurrent diverticular bleeding may necessitate emergency colectomy that is associated with higher morbidity and mortality.
- Tolerance of procedural sedation must be critically considered in providing safe, effective endoscopy for elderly patients.

In selecting the procedure to correct the source of GI bleeding, the surgeon considers the patient's overall condition, history of chronic versus acute symptoms, and bleeding location. Elderly patients tolerate a surgical procedure better than they tolerate prolonged or recurrent bleeding. (See Chapter 11 for an in-depth description of ulcer surgery.)

Hernia Surgery

The estimated incidence of abdominal wall hernia in persons older than 65 years is 13 per 1000, with a fourfold to eightfold increase in the incidence in men. Fifty percent of all hernias are indirect inguinal, 20% are direct inguinal, 10% are ventral, 6% are femoral, 3% are umbilical, and 1% are esophageal-hiatal (Dardik et al, 2012). The elective repair of inguinal and femoral hernias is strongly advised because of the risk of incarceration with subsequent emergency surgery. Many hernia repairs in elderly patients are emergency procedures because of incarcerations and small bowel obstruction. When elective, the operation may be performed as an ambulatory procedure; IV sedation and local anesthesia provide a very satisfactory alternative to general or spinal anesthesia.

Laparoscopic techniques for hernia repair have gained popularity because of associated shorter hospital stay, minimal pain postoperatively, and early recovery. However, the necessity for general anesthesia makes this approach one that may not be advisable in elders. Decisions for local versus spinal or general anesthesia are made based on the patient's overall physiologic status and surgical risk.

In elderly men the coexistence of inguinal hernia and prostatism is fairly common. Depending on the size of the prostate, the hernia repair should be postponed until after the prostate surgery.

Large, neglected scrotal hernias are not an unusual finding in elderly men. The repair of these hernias is not routine, in that the abdominal wall defect may be so large that primary repair cannot take place without tension. Synthetic abdominal wall replacements are helpful in the management of such large hernias. The repair of huge scrotal hernias can have a tremendous benefit on the personality of the geriatric patient, who is much relieved after removal of what can be considered an accessory appendage that is offensive, difficult to clean, and often an impedance to daily activities. (See Chapter 13 for an in-depth description of herniorrhaphy.)

Genitourinary Surgery

The predominant reason for urologic surgery in elderly men is benign prostatic hypertrophy (BPH). BPH may be silent or have minimal symptoms in the presence of severe bladder decompensation. As part of history taking, the nurse should determine if symptoms such as dysuria, straining at micturition, and hematuria exist. Prostate surgery, especially TURP, is relatively safe and generally well tolerated. Other surgical procedures for prostate include high-intensity–focused ultrasound, prostatic stents, and transurethral electrovaporization. The majority of BPH operations are performed to relieve symptoms, such as nocturia, slow stream, intermittency, and double voiding. TURP is indicated if the surgeon believes that total resection can be accomplished in 1 hour and that no bladder disease or impairment to urethral access is present. Alternatives to TURP surgery are discussed in Chapter 15.

Genitourinary (GU) procedures may also be performed to correct incontinence. Incontinence in elderly men can result from nerve-damaging events such as radical prostatectomy and spinal cord injury. Surgical treatments can include artificial sphincter creation, formation of a bulbourethral sling, and a urinary diversion procedure (Men's Guide to Urinary Incontinence, 2008).

Older women experience urinary incontinence more frequently than younger women. Sneezing, coughing, and laughing may cause urine to leak from the bladder. The decision to have surgery should always be based on appropriate diagnosis, evaluation of all treatment modalities, and realistic expectations from surgical intervention. Surgical choices can include urethral sling, retropubic suspension, and tension-free vaginal tape surgery. Factors that can impair a positive outcome include, but may not be limited to, obesity, radiation therapy, aging, chronic cough, poor nutrition, low estrogen level, postmenopausal, and strenuous physical activity (Women's Guide to Urinary Incontinence in Females, 2008). (See Chapter 15 for an in-depth description of GU procedures.)

Ophthalmic Surgery

Because of elders' long life span, undergoing eye surgery (most commonly for cataracts) is more likely than other surgical procedures. Most ophthalmic procedures are minimally invasive and have a high success rate. Because elderly patients may have concurrent systemic disease, even a low-stress procedure should not be treated lightly. Age-related changes, such as hearing loss and musculoskeletal disease, may pose a challenge during ophthalmic surgery because the patient must lie still for long periods and be able to follow verbal instructions. Patients with chronic lung disease lying in the supine position may experience coughing, which can increase intraocular pressure and jeopardize the outcome of the surgery.

Orthopedic Surgery

Osteoporosis is the most obvious skeletal change that occurs with advancing age. It leads to susceptibility to fracture, which doubles every 5 years after 50 years of age. An approximate loss of 25% to 40% of the mineral content of the bone must be present before detectable change is evident on x-ray films. To some degree, osteoporosis is related to a lessening of physical activity, but other risk factors are female gender, Northern European ancestry, multiparity, lean body build, and excessive alcohol intake (Ignatavicius, 2013). Osteoporosis is also related to decreased hormonal secretion; thus postmenopausal women are more prone to develop the condition and therefore more likely to sustain a hip fracture.

Age-related changes in bone increase the prevalence of displaced femoral and intertrochanteric fractures of the upper femur. The prevalence of hip fracture increases with advancing age, is more common in women, and is higher in institutionalized patients. Because the usual cause of death in patients with upper femur fracture is pulmonary embolus, surgery is designed to relieve the severe pain, allow movement in and out of bed, and return the patient to his or her former environment as quickly as possible with minimal debilitation. Only 50% to 60% of patients with hip fractures will recover their prefracture ambulation abilities in the first year post fracture. Older adults who fracture a hip have a five to eight times' increased risk of mortality during the first 3 months after the fracture (Ebersole et al, 2012). A displaced femoral neck fracture must be surgically repaired or healing will not occur. In patients 70 years and older, prosthetic replacement is usually done because it allows for early ambulation and will last throughout the remaining years of the patient's life. Intertrochanteric and subtrochanteric fractures are best treated with internal fixation. These methods also allow for early mobility.

Degenerative joint disease (osteoarthritis) and inflammatory polyarticular disease (rheumatoid arthritis) are the primary indications for total joint replacement in the hip and knee. In these patients, pain that disrupts normal daily activities and interrupts sleep is the major reason for surgery regardless of the patient's age. Octogenarians and nonagenarians achieve successful pain relief and report satisfaction after the procedure. Methyl methacrylate bone cement is often used in orthopedic procedures in spite of its cardiotoxic effect. Cardiac arrest from cement insertion is a possible risk for frail patients. Supplemental inspired oxygen at the time of insertion, irrigation of the bone to remove excessive marrow elements, and retrograde insertion of the cement are methods to prevent the risk of adverse effects (Burlingame and Blanchard, 2009). Usually knee replacement procedures are elective, and patients have better functional status and a higher bone mass than those with hip fracture. (See Chapter 20 for an in-depth description of hip and knee surgery.)

Vascular and Cardiovascular Surgery

The most frequent vascular conditions treated surgically in the older population are abdominal aortic aneurysms, carotid artery disease, and peripheral vascular disease. In patients 65 and older, the mortality from elective aneurysm repair is less than 5% in spite of existing comorbidities. Emergency repair for ruptured aneurysm carries an operative mortality of more than 50% (Dardik et al, 2012). Peripheral vascular surgery for limb salvage can be safely performed in patients older than 80 years and may be indicated for ischemic rest pain and nonhealing ulcers.

Cardiovascular disease is a significant cause of death in older patients. More than 55% of CABG procedures are performed on patients older than 65 years. Several risk factors associated with increased mortality include emergency procedure, severe left ventricular dysfunction, mitral insufficiency requiring combined procedure, elevated preoperative creatinine level, chronic obstructive pulmonary disease (COPD), anemia, and prior vascular surgery. Factors associated with morbidity in the elderly population include obesity, diabetes mellitus, aortic stenosis, and cerebrovascular disease (Dardik et al, 2012). (See Chapters 24 and 25 for a more in-depth description of vascular and cardiac surgery, respectively.)

Additional Considerations

Regardless of the age of the patient every surgical procedure possesses a certain amount of risk. With increasing life expectancy, the number of surgical procedures performed on older adults will increase. Nonetheless, just as comorbidity and emergent surgery increase surgical risk, so do the physiologic deficits of aging. Procedures that are performed in the thorax or the peritoneal cavity are considered high risk. Procedures of moderate risk include vascular and hip procedures, and low-risk procedures include prostatectomy and mastectomy. However, any procedure, even those considered low risk, can have poor outcomes, depending on the patient's overall condition. Caution is advised even with the ever-increasing numbers of minimally invasive surgeries (e.g., laparoscopy). It seems logical that elders would benefit from smaller incisions that produce less postoperative pain, atelectasis, and ileus. However, the extent of hemodynamic and pulmonary consequences of CO_2 pneumoperitoneum is still unclear. In patients with severe cardiac or pulmonary disease, recommendations include invasive monitoring to maintain adequate volume loading and use of alternate gas sources or gasless techniques.

An ethical consideration with elderly surgical patients centers on the dilemma of do not resuscitate (DNR) orders. The organization's policy must give the patient a voice in the intraoperative area. Even though the patient may have made end-of-life decisions, the fact that the patient has signed the surgical informed consent implies that he or she seeks to improve quality of life, which is incompatible with withholding cardiopulmonary resuscitation (CPR). It is difficult to differentiate between a cardiac arrest precipitated by anesthesia and one that is spontaneous. The anesthetic agent itself promotes cardiovascular instability. Consideration should be given to the medical indications for the procedure with the goal of treatment to alleviate pain and morbidity and provide for the patient's comfort. The guiding principle in the decision to maintain or suspend DNR orders should be respect for the patient's autonomy. Elderly patients have the right to participate in the process for making end-of-life decisions.

As more procedures are performed, there are ways to assist perioperative nurses to prepare for the care of the elderly population:
- Educate staff members by reviewing the special needs of this age group.
- Develop a separate process for preoperative assessment, and use multiple screens for evaluation of older patients.
- Improve communication and collaboration among healthcare providers.

Understanding the age-specific needs of the older surgical patient is critical to successful outcomes for these patients. High rates of medical errors have become serious challenges in the healthcare industry. As a result of their role in providing the majority of direct patient care, nurses' performance is closely tied to the quality of healthcare services. Fatigue has been associated with stress, safety, and nurses' performance. Nurses who work more than 12.5 hours per day are three times more likely to commit an error (Barker and Nussbaum, 2011). Challenges in the healthcare system such as nursing shortages, increased patient loads, and decreased resources place a high demand on nurses. Understanding the relationship between the work environment, fatigue, and the environment is essential.

An organizational culture of safety must include a blame-free response to medical mistakes. Potential for errors must be recognized as opportunities to review process and policy to prevent future mistakes. Perioperative nurses have the responsibility to contribute to the creation of a culture of safety in the workplace to improve safety in the workplace for patients and nurses.

To ensure that older Americans receive high-quality appropriate care, the Institute of Medicine recommends the following steps:
1. Enhance the competence of all healthcare personnel involved in the delivery of geriatric care instead of depending on specialists.
2. Provide stronger incentives to recruit and maintain geriatric practitioners.
3. Apply more flexible models of care to enable self-care for patients and informal caregivers (Institute of Medicine, 2008).

Technical advances in surgery and anesthesia will continue to provide for beneficial surgery performed on older and older patients. The perioperative nurse who approaches the care of elders with this in mind not only will enhance the surgical outcome but also significantly affect the patient's overall quality of life.

KEY POINTS

- Although the age of 65 is often used for reporting demographics of older patients, being 65 or older does not make a person necessarily "old."
- The majority of patients 65 or older have one or more chronic health conditions that may be a risk factor for perioperative mortality.
- Perioperative nursing assessment should take into consideration normal age-related changes.
- Age alone should not be a barrier to surgery in elders.

- Elderly persons with conditions treatable by surgery have as much right as younger patients to benefit from modern surgery, anesthesia, and medical and intensive care techniques.
- Medical and surgical techniques that can enhance the older person's life should be equally available to patients regardless of age.
- Elderly patients have special needs because of their atypical presentation of disease, multiple medical disorders or comorbidity, impaired homeostasis, and altered drug response.
- Most elderly patients are mentally competent and should therefore always be involved in making decisions about their plan of care.

CRITICAL THINKING QUESTION

When reviewing the surgery schedule, you note you are caring for a 91-year-old female who is scheduled for removal of a skin lesion with a possible local flap. When you interview her in the preoperative area, you discover she is alert, oriented, a good health historian, and generally experiencing only normal age-associated changes. What factors would you incorporate in your perioperative plan of care? Note the critical assessment factors you would include and perioperative nursing interventions to address them.

ⓔvolve *The answers to the Critical Thinking Question can be found at http://evolve.elsevier.com/Rothrock/Alexander.*

REFERENCES

American Geriatrics Society (AGS) Expert Panel on the Care of Older Adults with Multimorbidity: *Patient-centered care for older adults with multiple chronic conditions: a stepwise approach from the American Geriatrics Society*, 2012, available at www.americangeriatrics.org/files/documents/MCC .stepwise.approach.pdf. Accessed February 3, 2013.

Barker L, Nussbaum M: Fatigue, performance and the work environment; a survey of registered nurses, *J Adv Nurs* 67(6):1370–1382, 2011.

Bensenor I et al: Hypothyroidism in the elderly: diagnosis and management, *Clin Interv Aging* 7:97–111, 2012.

Beretta M et al: Oxaliplatin-based chemotherapy in the treatment of elderly patients with metastatic colorectal cancer (CRC), *Arch Gerontol Geriatr* 55(2):271–275, 2012.

Burlingame B, Blanchard J: Bone cement implantation syndrome, *AORN J* 89(2):399–400, 2009.

Chow W et al: Optimal preoperative assessment of the geriatric patient: a best practice guideline from the American College of Surgeons National Surgical Quality Improvement Program and the American Geriatrics Society, *J Am Coll Surg* 215(4):453–466, 2012.

Clayton JL: Special needs of older adults undergoing surgery, *AORN J* 87(3):557–570, 2008.

Dardik A et al: Surgery in the geriatric patient. In Townsend CM et al, editors: *Sabiston textbook of surgery*, ed 19, Philadelphia, 2012, Saunders.

Denholm B: Tucking patients' arms and general positioning, *AORN J* 89(4):755–757, 2009.

Ebersole P et al: *Toward healthy aging: human needs and nursing response*, ed 8, St Louis, 2012, Mosby.

Federal Interagency Forum on Aging-Related Statistics: *Older Americans 2012: key indicators of well-being*, Federal Interagency Forum on Aging-Related Statistics, Washington, DC, June 2012, U.S. Government Printing Office.

Ferris M: Pain in the cognitively impaired elderly: guidance for clinicians, *Adv Pract Nurse* eJournal posted May 15, 2008, available at http://geroresourcenurse.org/grn/download/GRN%20Council/pain%20in%20 cognitively%20impaired%20older%20adult%20print.pdf. Accessed November 15, 2012.

Jones E et al: Adjuvant therapy of breast cancer in women 70-years of age and older: tough decisions, high stakes, *Oncology* 26(9):793, 2012.

Hamaker M et al: Frailty screening methods for predicting outcome of a comprehensive geriatric assessment in elderly patients with cancer: a systematic review, *Lancet Oncol* 13(10):437–444, 2012.

Ignatavicius DD: Care of patients with musculoskeletal problems. In Ignatavicius DD, Workman ML, editors: *Medical-surgical nursing: patient-centered collaborative care*, ed 7, St Louis, 2013, Saunders.

Institute of Medicine: *Retooling for an aging America: building the health care workforce*, Washington, DC, 2008, The National Academies Press, available at www.iom.edu/CMS/3809/40113/53452.aspx. Accessed November 5, 2012.

Kim SS, Zenilman ME: The elderly surgical patient. In Souba W et al, editors: *ACS surgery principles and practices*, ed 6, Ontario, Canada, 2007, BC Decker.

Kuwajerwala NK: *Perioperative medication management*, available at www .emedicine.medscape.com/article/28480. Updated 2008. Accessed December 30, 2012.

Men's guide to urinary incontinence, available at www.webmd.com/urinary -incontinence-oab/mens-guide/urinary-incontinence-in-men-surgery. Updated July 21, 2008. Accessed November 5, 2012.

Nelson JM, Carrington JM: Transitioning the older adult in the ambulatory care setting, *AORN J* 94:348–358, 2011.

Robinson S et al: Aging and delirium: too much or too little pain medication, *Pain Manag Nurs* 9(2):66–72, 2008.

Sieber FE, Pauldine R: Geriatric anesthesia. In Miller RD, editor: *Miller's anesthesia*, ed 7, vol 2, Philadelphia, 2009, Churchill Livingstone.

Slover J et al: Shared decision making in orthopaedic surgery, *Clin Orthop Relat Res* 470(4):1046–1053, 2012.

Touhy TA: Cognition and caring for persons with cognitive impairment. In Ebersole P et al, editors: *Toward healthy aging: human needs and nursing response*, ed 8, St Louis, 2012, Mosby.

Wold GH: *Basic geriatric nursing*, ed 5, St Louis, 2012, Mosby.

Women's Guide to Urinary Incontinence, available at www.webmd.com/urinary-incontinence-oab/womens-guide/urinary-incontinence-in-women-surgery. Updated September 17, 2008. Accessed November 3, 2012.

Workman ML: Assessment of the eye and vision. In Ignatavicius DD, Workman ML, editors: *Medical-surgical nursing: patient-centered collaborative care*, ed 7, St Louis, 2013, Saunders.

Yachimski PS, Friedman LS: Gastrointestinal bleeding in the elderly, *Nat Clin Pract Gastroenterol Hepatol* 5(2):80–93, 2008.

Yokoe DS et al: A compendium of strategies of prevent healthcare associated infections in acute care hospitals, *Infect Control Hosp Epidemiol* 29(1):12–21, 2008.

Zenilman M et al: New developments in geriatric surgery, *Curr Probl Surg* 48(10):670–754, 2011.

Trauma Surgery

DAVID P. GAWRONSKI

Trauma is ranked as one of the foremost public health issues in the United States. Unintentional injury related to trauma is the fifth leading cause of death and the leading cause of death for people ages 1 to 44 years (Barclay, 2009). Whether the injury is a result of a motor vehicle collision, violence, crime, or is a work-related injury, trauma occurs unplanned and without warning. The unpredictable nature of trauma poses a major challenge to the perioperative nurse and the patient care team.

The potential for injury has existed since the beginning of humanity. Many of the major advances in care of critically injured patients have been accomplished through experience in the military. Clearly the shorter the response time, the greater the survival rate for casualties. This was demonstrated by the success of the mobile army surgical hospital (MASH) units during the Korean conflict and again during the Vietnam conflict; MASH brought the necessary supplies, equipment, and personnel closer to the battlefields and consequently improved patient outcomes.

Eventually this concept was applied to the civilian population and is commonly referred to as the "golden hour" of trauma care. More specifically, the golden hour refers to the time immediately after the injury when rapid and definitive interventions can be most effective in the reduction of morbidity and mortality. The golden hour starts at the scene, where prehospital personnel determine the severity of injury, initiate medical treatment, and identify the most appropriate facility to which to transport the patient. Traumatic deaths may occur in three phases, or timeframes. The first occurs immediately after the injury. In this phase, death is usually a result of lacerations to the heart or aorta or brainstem injury. These patients rarely survive transport to the hospital, and die at the scene. The second phase occurs within the first 1 to 2 hours after the injury. These patients have injuries to the spleen, liver, lung, or other organs that result in significant blood loss. This is the group in which definitive trauma care (i.e., appropriate and aggressive resuscitation with adequate volume replacement) may have the most significant effect (the golden hour). The third phase occurs days to weeks after the injury, often during the intensive care phase, and is usually caused by complications or a failure of multiple organ systems.

The wars in Iraq and Afghanistan have resulted in some changes in the way traumatic injuries are managed; the military has not set up convalescence centers as in Vietnam and Desert Storm. Rather, the doctrine of "essential care in theater" is followed. Physicians and nurses have been trained to provide immediate care, keeping in mind the treatment resources that will be available at the next level of care. Soldiers with upper body injuries are surviving because of body armor. However, there is no protection for upper extremities; therefore, many amputations are performed, including above-elbow and shoulder disarticulations. The new philosophy is to stress continuity of care with the goal of returning the soldier to the highest possible level of function.

Time is of the essence in providing definitive care to the critically injured person. A significant number of patient deaths can be prevented if rapid transport is provided from the scene to a facility equipped to provide resuscitation and treatment in an efficient and timely manner. This concept is reflected in the national development of the emergency medical services (EMS) system. Facilities and resources are allocated and coordinated to provide specific interventions for a group of patients. For example, facilities that meet certain criteria to accommodate the specialized needs of the critically injured patient are designated as *trauma centers*. Communities establish transfer and triage protocols that allow for a trauma patient to reach the appropriate facility with the least out-of-hospital time possible. This may be accomplished by a helicopter with a specially trained flight crew or by the use of ground transport with an advanced life support (ALS) ambulance team (Figure 28-1).

Trauma centers (TCs) are classified based on the scope of available services and resources. A level I TC is capable of providing total care for every type of injury. Accepting this designation commits the TC to providing qualified personnel and equipment necessary for rapid diagnosis and treatment on a 24-hour basis. A level II TC provides comprehensive care for all injuries but lacks some of the specialized clinicians and resources required for the level I designation. A level II facility may provide surgical intervention if the critical nature of the injury dictates immediate intervention before transfer to a level I facility. A level III facility provides prompt evaluation, resuscitation, emergency surgery, and stabilization, as needed, before transfer to a higher-level facility. The American College of Surgeons (ACS) recommends that in level II and III centers, an operating room (OR) team be readily available at all times. Depending on the population served and the volume of urgent cases, this requirement may be met with on-call staff. A level IV trauma center has the ability to provide advanced trauma life support before patient transfer. These facilities may be located in rural areas with limited access and may be a clinic or a hospital.

Although the risk for death is 25% lower for a severe injury treated in a level I TC (Barclay, 2009), not all patients require the services of a level I TC and thus may be transported to the closest emergency department (ED) for care. New guidelines and recommendations for triage, first developed as a position statement by the ACS in 1986, have been published (Barclay, 2009). Known as the Decision Scheme, this algorithm guides EMS personnel through the following four decision points: physiologic parameters, anatomic parameters, mechanism of injury (MOI), and other special considerations. Personnel review physiologic parameters. Patients with a Glasgow Coma Scale (see Table 21-2) score less than 14, systolic blood pressure less than 90 mm Hg, or respiratory rate less

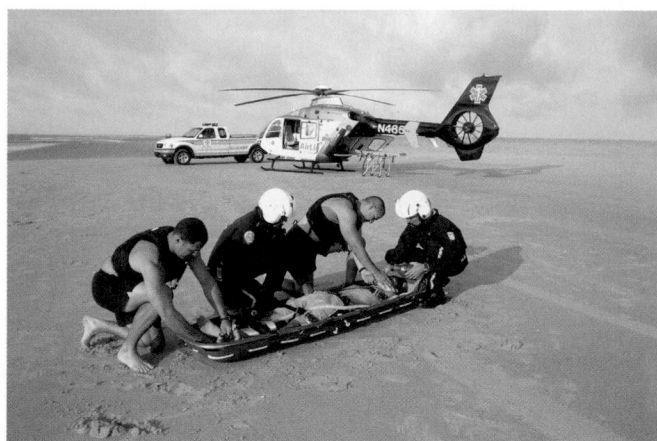

FIGURE 28-1 New Hanover Health Network EMS Air Link rescue at the beach.

TABLE 28-1	
Biomechanics in Trauma	
Mechanisms of Injury	**Phases of Injury**
Vehicle of transfer of energy from environment to human host	**Examples** Falls Motor vehicle collisions Bullets Stabbing instruments Blasts/bombs
Deceleration Forces Decrease in speed of a moving object or person	**External Forces** Victim strikes steering column Victim impacts ground
Acceleration Forces Increase in speed of a moving object or person	Pedestrian thrown when struck by moving vehicle
Blast Forces Heat, light, pressure Low- and high-velocity missiles Human body's response to kinetic energy load	Bomb explosion Bullets Stabbing instruments **Internal Forces** Stress Cells separate, stretch, compress, or shear Strain Tissue damage or deformation from stress
Describing for clinical and diagnostic purpose	**Types of Injuries** Blunt vs. penetrating Closed vs. open Primary vs. secondary Direct vs. indirect

Modified from Emergency Nurses Association (ENA): *Trauma nursing core course,* ed 6, Des Plaines, IL, 2007, Author.

than 10 breaths per minute or greater than 29 breaths per minute should be transported to the highest level facility available. The anatomic parameters include specific types of injuries, such as penetrating injuries of the neck or torso, flail chest, or proximal long bone fracture; these patients are also transported to the highest level facility available. The MOI and other special considerations, such as age or prior medical history, are also reviewed to determine to what level facility the patient is transported.

Trauma patients require immediate access to the OR 24 hours per day, 365 days per year. A sudden influx of a large number of trauma patients to a trauma center may necessitate triage or classification of those less seriously injured as less urgent, allowing immediate access for the critically injured patients. The elective surgery schedule may need to be interrupted to expedite care for the trauma patient or patients. Scheduling policies and procedures are established collaboratively by the departments of surgery, trauma, anesthesia, and perioperative nursing services. Consequently, the perioperative nurse and scrub person (who may be a registered nurse or surgical technologist) need to be familiar with supplies and equipment located in the OR designated for trauma or in the ORs that are used most frequently for these patients.

Perioperative Nursing Considerations

Preliminary Evaluation: Mechanism of Injury

Because of the unpredictable timing of trauma, it is often the on-call perioperative nursing team who cares for injured patients requiring surgical intervention. In contrast to an elective surgical procedure, little information may be known about trauma patients and preparation time is often abbreviated. A working knowledge of the MOI is essential to assist the perioperative nurse in rapid patient assessment.

MOI, or kinematics, involves the action of forces on the human body and their effects. Knowing the forces applied provides valuable information in evaluation of the patient and injuries that may be present. The first EMS team to respond to the scene of an injury must carefully evaluate the patient in relation to the MOI. For example, the position of the victim in a car, whether the person was the driver or a passenger seated in the back seat or front seat, estimated velocity of the vehicle, location of impact, and use of a seat

belt or air bag are all pieces of information used to determine the index of suspicion about the probable causes of injuries to the patient. After immediate threats to life are addressed, the MOI can provide valuable clues as to probable cause of injuries. This systematic approach can reduce morbidity and mortality (Table 28-1).

The MOI is a product of the type of injuring force and the resulting tissue response. The velocity of the collision, the shape of the object, and the tissue's flexibility influence the magnitude of the injury sustained. For example, long bone tissue has little or no flexibility. A strong collision involving a long bone most often results in a fracture of some type. In contrast, soft tissue injury from a colliding force may result in a contusion because this tissue has greater flexibility.

Blunt trauma is injury resulting from a combination of forces, such as acceleration, deceleration, shearing, and compression that do not result in a break of the skin. Morbidity and mortality may be greater than with penetrating trauma because identification of injuries is more difficult when injuries are less obvious. Causes of blunt trauma include motor vehicle collisions (MVCs), contact sports injuries, aggravated assault, and falls. Even low-energy trauma, such as that associated with low-level falls, can produce significant injuries.

RESEARCH HIGHLIGHT ‖

BMI and Risk for Upper Body Injury Following an MVC

Individuals with a high BMI have an increased amount of adipose tissue; the adipose distribution differs between men and women. Obese women tend to have excess fat around the hips, thighs, and buttocks, whereas obese males typically have more adiposity in the upper body. A recent study explored the differences in body shape among obese men and women in relation to the severity of injuries sustained following an MVC.

The study obtained data from the Crashworthiness Data System of the National Automotive Sampling System and computer crash simulation data to examine the injury patterns. The researchers found obese males to be at a higher risk for injuries to the head, face, thorax, abdomen, and spine. Obese females have a decreased risk for injuries to the face and an increased risk of injury to the thorax, abdomen, and lower extremities. Obese males are more vulnerable to serious upper body injuries due to the fat distribution, body shape, and a higher center of gravity.

Studies found obese males to be at a higher risk for injury related to a combination of factors including momentum effects, comorbidities associated with obesity, and the body's response to the crash. Furthermore, the vehicle's cabin is designed for a male with a BMI of 24.3, which is not optimal for an obese male.

BMI, Body mass index; *MVC*, motor vehicle collision.
Modified from Zhu S et al: BMI and risk of serious upper body injury following motor vehicle crashes: concordance of real-world and computer-simulated observation, 2010, *PLoS Med*, available at www.plosmedicine.org/article/info%3Adoi%2F10.1371%2Fjournal .pmed.1000250. Accessed October 21, 2012.

FIGURE 28-2 The three collisions of a head-on motor vehicle crash: the car hits an object; the occupant's body impacts on some surface within the motor vehicle; and the result is a collision between internal tissues and the rigid body surface structures.

Acceleration and deceleration injuries occur most frequently in blunt trauma. A ruptured thoracic aorta is an example of an injury that occurs as a result of these types of forces. In an MVC the large vessels are stopped or decelerated rapidly, resulting in vessel damage caused by stretching that exceeds the vessel's elastic ability. This affects the aorta at the ligamentum arteriosum, the anatomic point where it is affixed tightly to the chest wall, just below the origin of the subclavian artery. This shearing below the attachment site causes a rupture as the aorta continues to move in a forward motion after the chest wall motion has stopped.

MVCs account for a high degree of blunt trauma (Research Highlight). During an MVC, actually three collisions occur (Figure 28-2). The first collision is that of a car into another object. The second collision is the impact of the occupant's body on the vehicle's interior. The third collision occurs when an internal body structure hits a rigid bony surface. A coup-contrecoup injury of the brain, for example, is the result of an acceleration force to one area of the brain and a deceleration force to an opposite area. Front and side air bag deployment along with the use of seat belts can decrease the severity of traumatic injury.

Falls also cause a significant number of traumatic deaths in the United States. Injuries are most commonly associated with children experiencing falls more than twice their height. In adults, falls more than 10 to 15 feet are usually accompanied by significant injury. Deceleration forces in falls produce forces of stretching, shearing, and compression. Consequently, aortic injuries are also suspect in this group of patients. Skeletal injuries occur as well, because of the compressive forces present.

Penetrating trauma is a result of the passage of a foreign object through tissue. The degree or extent of tissue injury is a function of the energy that is dissipated to the tissue and the surrounding areas. The anatomic structures most often injured include the liver, intestines, and vascular system. The extent of the injury relates to the nature of the foreign object (e.g., bullet caliber, knife size), distance from the weapon, structures penetrated, and amount of energy dissipated to the structures.

The velocity of a bullet is responsible for the degree of injury or cavitation to the tissue. A low-velocity bullet is one that travels at a lower speed (1000 feet per second or less) and disrupts only the bullet tract and its immediate surrounding area. A high-velocity weapon, such as used by the military, fires a bullet traveling at a greater speed (3000 feet or more per second) and causes significantly more damage and tissue destruction because the bullet tract involves more extensive surrounding tissue (Figure 28-3). The distance from the weapon also influences the degree of injury because the velocity is greatest when the bullet leaves the weapon and decreases as it travels. In addition, the type of bullet (e.g., shotgun shells with multiple pellets and hollow-point bullets, which mushroom on impact) influences the degree of injury. Commonly the entrance wound is smaller than the exit wound because of the dissipation of energy, but an exit wound may not always be present. If the bullet completely fragments or is lodged in an internal structure, there will not be an exit wound. Depending on the position of the bullet and any injury that could be caused by attempting to remove it, bullets are not always removed.

Stab and impalement wounds are considered to be low-velocity wounds. The associated injuries usually correspond to the path of the penetrating object. Factors such as the object's width and length assist in identifying the possible occurrence of injuries. A single injury site may penetrate several different organs or cavities.

High-velocity wound profile

Low-velocity wound profile

FIGURE 28-3 Potential injury path of high- and low-velocity bullets.

TABLE 28-2

Mechanisms of Blast Injuries

Category	Areas Affected	Types of Injuries
Primary: Caused by blast itself	Gas-filled organs most susceptible:	
	• Eye	Rupture of globe
	• Middle ear/ tympanic membrane	Rupture and permanent deafness possible
	• Lungs	Pneumothorax, alveolar rupture, air embolus
	• GI tract	Abdominal hemorrhage, contusions, rupture
	• Central nervous system	Diffuse cerebral hemorrhage, cerebral air embolism, concussion syndrome (injury without physical signs)
Secondary: Caused by debris and projectiles	Any body part	Varies depending on size of projectiles: penetrating or blunt injury
Tertiary: Caused by victim being thrown against stationary objects	Any body part	Similar to those seen in motor vehicle collisions: fractures, traumatic amputations, closed/ open brain injury
Quaternary: Exacerbation or complications of existing conditions	Any body part	Burns, crush injuries, inhalation of dust or toxic gases causing exacerbation of asthma or COPD, angina

COPD, Chronic obstructive pulmonary disease; *GI,* gastrointestinal.
Modified from Emergency Nurses Association (ENA): *Trauma nursing core course,* ed 6, Des Plaines, IL, 2007, Author.

Penetrating injuries located at or below the nipple line may cause both chest and abdominal injuries. This is attributable to the diaphragmatic excursion that occurs with inspiration and expiration. Impaled objects should not be removed at the scene or in the ED. The impaled object provides a tamponade effect to injured blood vessels and is removed only when the ability to control potential bleeding from those vessels is present. Wound debridement may also be necessary. Therefore, these objects are removed in the OR, where the needed supplies and instrumentation are located.

Injuries that result from explosions are related to the effects of the blast. With the threat of domestic terrorism on the rise, the treatment of blast victims may become more frequent in trauma settings. Blast injuries are capable of inflicting a variety of injuries. Primary blast injury is the result of a direct pressure wave on the body, most likely to affect the lungs, gastrointestinal (GI) tract, tympanic membrane, or blood vessels. Secondary blast injuries are often present as penetrating organ injury and result from airborne shrapnel and debris. Tertiary injuries result from the blast wind moving bodies and debris (Kumar, 2010). The type of injury sustained and its intensity are directly related to factors such as the size of the blast and the proximity of the victim or victims. Patients from a blast explosion may present with penetrating injury, contusions, lacerations, amputations, abrasions, avulsions, evisceration, and various degrees of burns (Table 28-2).

Thermal and electrical tissue damage and inhalation injuries may occur from an explosion or as a sole mechanism of injury. These patients are usually resuscitated and require operative intervention for debridement on a nonemergent basis, unless the injury is limb- or life-threatening.

Injuries can be scored objectively according to their severity. This scoring system assists medical personnel in more effective triage and provides a universal method of communication among facilities, departments, and nursing personnel. The ACS guidelines, as published by the National Expert Panel on Field Triage, now recommend the use of the Decision Scheme (Table 28-3).

Assessment

The resuscitative process begins with arrival of emergency personnel on the scene and ends when the patient has been stabilized, received definitive care, and undergone a complete and thorough physical examination to determine all injuries sustained. When the patient arrives in the ED, the trauma team initiates a primary assessment and secondary assessment. This is a logical, orderly process of patient assessment for potential life threats. These assessment activities are based on established protocols for advanced trauma life support (ATLS). The mnemonic used for the primary assessment is "ABCDE," representing assessment of the following:

- *A*irway (with cervical spine precautions)
- *B*reathing
- *C*irculation
- *D*isability (brief neurologic examination)
- *E*xposure (to reveal all life-threatening injuries) and *e*nvironmental control (thermoregulation)

Airway interventions may include manual maneuvers (chin-lift, jaw-thrust), insertion of oral or nasopharyngeal airways, or

TABLE 28-3

Decision Scheme Recommendations*

Steps	Transition	Recommendations
Step 1		Transport to TC for any of the following: GCS <14, systolic BP <90 mm Hg, respiratory rate <10 or >29 breaths/min
	1 to 2	These patients have potentially serious injuries and should be transported to highest level TC available
Step 2		Transport to TC for any of the following: penetrating injuries of head, neck, torso, and extremities proximal to elbow and knee; flail chest; 2 or more proximal long bone fractures; crushed, degloved, or mangled extremity; amputation proximal to wrist and ankle; pelvic fracture; open or depressed skull fracture; paralysis
	2 to 3	If yes to any criteria, transport to highest level TC available; if patient does not meet step 2 criteria, proceed to step 3
Step 3		Transport to TC for any of the following: falls >20 feet for adults, >10 feet or 2-3 times child's height; motor vehicle collision with partial or complete ejection of occupant; auto vs. pedestrian/bicyclist thrown; motorcycle crash at speeds >20 mph
	3 to 4	If yes to any criteria, transport to closest TC
Step 4		Consider transport to TC for the following: age >55 or <15, anticoagulation and bleeding disorders, burns, time-sensitive extremity injury, end-stage renal disease requiring dialysis, pregnancy, or provider judgment

*The Decision Scheme is an essential component of the trauma system, guiding EMS providers in transporting injured patients to the most appropriate facility, ensuring proper treatment, and thus reducing death and disability.

BP, Blood pressure; *GCS,* Glasgow Coma Scale; *TC,* trauma center.

Modified from Barclay L: *Guidelines issued for field triage of injured patients,* Medscape Medical News, 2009, available at www.medscape.org/viewarticle/587385. Accessed October 20, 2012.

intubation. The trauma team may also perform emergent procedures, such as tracheotomy or needle cricothyrotomy, to secure the patient's airway. Pulse oximetry and capnography monitoring are used. If cervical spine precautions were not implemented before arrival at the hospital, the team initiates them before performing any other procedures on the patient. A trauma team member can stabilize the head and neck, if necessary, until a cervical collar is placed. Once placed, the team does not remove it until an examination and cervical radiograph confirms there is no neck injury.

During this time, the surgeon or ED physician and trauma team identify and correct life threats that are present before progressing to the next part of the examination. A patient requiring immediate surgery is transported to the OR, undergoes surgical intervention, and then is transferred to the postanesthesia care unit (PACU) or intensive care unit (ICU), depending on his or her condition. On the other hand, a patient may have a penetrating wound with evisceration of abdominal contents. However, correcting the obvious defect, which is currently not life-threatening, is postponed until the trauma team is assured that the patient has a patent airway and an effective breathing pattern and cervical spine precautions have been implemented. An evisceration needs to be corrected, but an inadequate airway is an immediate life threat and assumes priority.

Depending on the patient's injury, the surgeon may order an arterial blood gas (ABG) measurement. This test provides an accurate assessment of the ventilatory status of the patient and evaluates resuscitative airway and breathing interventions. Metabolic acidosis or a large base deficit (pH <7.35 or >7.45), with all other causes ruled out, may indicate internal bleeding. The surgeon may check for coagulopathy using thromboelastography (TEG). Rapid TEG testing can provide valuable information about the depleted component within the clotting cascade, allowing for direct therapy to correct the coagulopathy (Jeger et al, 2009).

After the trauma team completes the primary assessment and corrects any immediate life threats, they perform a secondary assessment. The purpose of the secondary assessment is to identify all injuries present. Sometimes the secondary assessment may be completed by the perioperative nurse, the PACU nurse, or the critical care nurse. The mnemonic used for the secondary assessment is "FGHI," representing assessment of the following:

- *F*ull set of vitals/focused adjuncts/facilitate family presence
- *G*ive comfort measures
- *H*istory/head-to-toe assessment
- *I*nspect posterior surfaces

This assessment begins with a full set of vital signs, including a rectal or tympanic temperature, unless contraindicated, and placement of noninvasive monitoring devices. Often during resuscitation the nurse will insert a Foley catheter to monitor urine output and fluid resuscitation efforts. The nurse should inspect the urinary meatus for the presence of blood before inserting the catheter. If blood is noted, the nurse notifies the surgeon and does not insert the catheter. The patient may have a ruptured bladder or a urethral injury, either of which is commonly associated with a fracture of the pelvis. The surgeon may wish to perform a retrograde urethrogram to examine the bladder and urethra for the presence of tears or disruption. After catheter insertion, urine is obtained for a urinalysis and urine drug screen. The identification of specific drugs in the urine may assist in further diagnosis and treatment. The urine will also be tested to determine the presence of red blood cells (RBCs). Depending on the amount of hematuria present, a renal contusion or other renal injury may be present. In addition, a nasogastric tube may be inserted at this time. The nurse prepares to provide comfort measures by assessing the patient's pain by using a pain scale (if indicated, orders for pain medication should be obtained).

The history and past medical history begin with information generated from the patient; if the patient is unable to provide the history, the team obtains the information from the family or significant others when possible (Emergency Nurses Association [ENA], 2007). This history is referred to as the "AMPLE" history and may be obtained even after the patient is transferred to the OR by the ED personnel. The history includes the following:

- *A*llergies
- *M*edications
- *P*ast medical history

- *L*ast meal, *L*ast menstrual period (if appropriate)
- *E*vents or *E*nvironment leading to the accident or injury

If the history is obtained after the initiation of surgery, it is important to communicate it to the surgeon and the anesthesia providers.

The head-to-toe evaluation of the patient—inspection, palpation, percussion, and auscultation—is used in the complete head-to-toe assessment to reveal any deformities, open injuries, tenderness, or swelling. The assessment begins at the head and face and then moves to the neck (including the spine), the chest, the abdomen, and the pelvis. The four extremities are next; distal pulses, motor function, and sensation are assessed. The final check is the back; the patient is carefully log-rolled to the side for a full visual and tactile assessment (Evidence for Practice).

Routine Laboratory Tests. Laboratory values aid the trauma team in evaluating the patient's status (see Appendix A). Appropriate laboratory tests include a minimum of a complete blood count (CBC), hemoglobin and hematocrit (H&H) value, blood alcohol level (BAL), and a blood type and screen; other tests may be requested during evaluation. The results of the laboratory studies should be reviewed and communicated as appropriate. An abnormal level of RBCs may signify dehydration, hypovolemia, or fluid overload (dilutional). An elevated white blood cell (WBC) count, indicating the presence of infection, may be related to inflammation, tissue necrosis, or immunocompromise. H&H values also are important to note. Caution is recommended when evaluating an H&H drawn in the ED. The time delay between bleeding and a drop in the H&H value can be significant. It is only after hemodilution occurs (from shock compensation or crystalloid replacement) that hematocrit level drops. Frequently, abnormal values in the patient with blunt trauma alert the team to the possibility of internal bleeding.

BAL also assists the trauma team in their evaluation. If the patient's level is significantly high, the physical examination and response may be unreliable. In addition, the neurologic status of patients with high BALs is very difficult to assess. Abnormal clotting studies are of obvious significance in trauma patients. These results may be attributable to anticoagulant medication the patient is taking or the effects of profound hypothermia. Clotting times may also be prolonged in the presence of excessive alcohol ingestion or the use of anabolic steroids. Clotting times may decrease with the use of antihistamines and diuretics.

A blood type and screen shortens the time needed by the blood bank to obtain a crossmatch, if needed later. Most trauma centers have several units of type O-negative blood (universal donor) available in the event that a blood transfusion is required before a type and crossmatch (T&C) can be performed. Because of regional shortages of O-negative blood, O-positive blood can be used in male patients and adult female patients of non-childbearing age. Initially, trauma patients are fluid-resuscitated with warmed crystalloid solutions, such as lactated Ringer's solution or normal saline solution. If the patient's blood pressure responds, the diagnostic examination continues. However, if the hypotension returns, blood transfusions may be initiated and the patient may be transported immediately to the OR for exploratory surgery.

Many trauma centers are implementing massive transfusion policies for the clinical management of patients experiencing massive hemorrhage and to coordinate interdisciplinary and interdepartmental resources. Massive transfusion is defined as the replacement of one or more blood volumes within a 24-hour period,

EVIDENCE FOR PRACTICE

Assessing Neurovascular Status in Patients with Musculoskeletal Trauma

Trauma patients frequently present to the OR with fractures or other musculoskeletal injuries. A thorough assessment of the patient's neurovascular status is imperative to establish a baseline for nursing and surgical interventions.

Assessment Technique	Normal Findings
Skin Color	
Inspect the skin distal to the injury.	There is no change in pigmentation compared with other parts of the body.
Skin Temperature	
Palpate the area distal to the injury (the dorsum of the hands is the most sensitive to temperature).	The skin is warm.
Movement	
Ask the patient to move the affected area or the area distal to the injury (active motion).	The patient can move without discomfort.
Move the area distal to the injury (passive motion).	There is no difference in comfort compared with active movement.
Sensation	
Ask the patient if numbness or tingling is present (paresthesia).	There is no numbness or tingling.
Palpate with a paper clip (especially in the web space between the first and second toes or the web space between the thumb and forefinger).	There is no difference in sensation in the affected and unaffected extremities. (Loss of sensation in these areas indicates perineal nerve or median nerve damage.)
Pulses	
Palpate the pulses distal to the injury.	Pulses are strong and easily palpated; there is no difference between the affected and unaffected extremities.
Capillary Refill (Least Reliable)	
Press the nailbeds distal to the injury until blanching occurs (or the skin near the nail if nails are thick and brittle).	Blood return (to usual color) is within 3 seconds (5 seconds for older people).
Pain	
Ask the patient about the location, nature, and frequency of the pain.	Pain is usually localized and is often described as stabbing or throbbing. (Pain out of proportion to the injury and unrelieved by analgesics may indicate compartment syndrome.)

Modified from Ignatavicius DD: Care of patients with musculoskeletal trauma. In Ignatavicius DD, Workman ML, editors: *Medical-surgical nursing: patient-centered collaborative care*, ed 7, St Louis, 2013, Saunders.

or 50% of estimated blood volume in 3 hours or less (Nessen et al, 2008). This volume is approximately equal to the transfusion of 10 units of RBCs. Transfusion guidelines recommend a balanced administration of blood products. Replacing a patient's circulating volume with packed RBC/plasma/platelet ratios of 1 : 1 : 1 improves outcomes by preventing and treating coagulopathy due to massive hemorrhage (Johansson et al, 2012). This simple ratio not only is easy to use but also has the benefit of administration of higher plasma and platelet volumes.

Diagnostic Procedures

Radiology. Depending on the trauma center protocol, a blunt trauma radiographic series may be ordered during the resuscitative phase. The series minimally includes a lateral view of the cervical spine and an anteroposterior (AP) view of the chest. In addition, the patient also undergoes lateral thoracic and lumbar spine films and an AP view of the pelvis. Any area with deformity, swelling, or pain may also be examined by x-ray. Trauma patients are always treated as if they have a cervical spine injury until proven otherwise. When reviewing the cervical spine films for cervical spine injury clearance, the clinician should consider any existing factors that place the patient at high risk for spine injury. These include age older than 65 years, a dangerous MOI, and paresthesias in the extremities. Patients with penetrating trauma injuries usually are transferred immediately to the OR for exploratory laparotomy.

If the resources are available, the trauma center protocol may also include a computed tomography (CT) scan as a diagnostic or screening tool. Depending on the MOI, such as a fall, CT scans of the head and abdomen may be performed. Because injuries in blunt trauma are very difficult to diagnose, the CT scan is frequently done before patient transfer to the OR. A high index of suspicion is maintained for other injuries until proven otherwise. Bowel injuries may be missed during initial scanning. A CT scan of the brain revealing an injury incompatible with life may alter the course of definitive treatment for a patient.

A CT-angiogram may be indicated in diagnosis of vascular injuries. If the patient is hemodynamically stable, this test is of great value in determining the extent of the injury. It is particularly beneficial in the diagnosis of a ruptured thoracic aorta, in which extravasation of the dye at the area of aortic fixation to the chest wall is noted. Other uses include evaluation of penetrating wounds, especially in the extremity. Vessel injury can be noted and the need for surgical intervention determined.

Other Diagnostic Tests. Cardiac monitoring is another component of the initial phase of trauma care and is particularly important in blunt trauma. Early detection of ventricular dysrhythmias may indicate a myocardial contusion, or bruising of the heart. An electrocardiogram (ECG) is obtained when indicated by the mechanism of injury or the patient's symptoms. Undiagnosed heart disease, as evidenced by an abnormal ECG, is noteworthy in a patient requiring operative intervention.

Focused assessment with sonography in trauma (FAST) may assist with diagnosis in difficult situations. FAST is a portable, noninvasive scan that can determine the presence of free fluid in the chest or abdomen. The typical FAST scan consists of chest, pelvic, and four abdominal scans. The chest scan examines right and left chest views and can determine the presence of pericardial fluid. The upper right abdominal scan evaluates the hepatorenal area, the first area that shows the presence of air. The left upper scan examines the splenorenal area. The left and right paracolic gutters are also scanned. The pelvic scan assesses for free fluid near the bladder.

TABLE 28-4

Comparison of DPL, FAST, and CT Scans

Diagnostic Peritoneal Lavage (DPL) Documents Bleeding	Focused Assessment with Sonography in Trauma (FAST) Documents Fluid	Computed Tomography (CT) Scan Documents Organ Injury
Advantages		
Early diagnosis	Early diagnosis	Most specific to
Performed rapidly	Noninvasive	injury
98% sensitive	Performed rapidly	92% sensitive
Detects bowel injury	86%-97% accurate	98% accurate
	Repeatable	
Disadvantages		
Invasive	Operator dependent	Increased cost
Low specificity	Bowel gas and	and time
Misses diaphragmatic	subcutaneous air	Misses diaphragm,
and retroperitoneal	distortion	bowel, and
injuries	Misses diaphragm,	some pancreatic
	bowel, and	injuries
	pancreatic injuries	

Modified from Emergency Nurses Association (ENA): *Trauma nursing core course*, ed 6, Des Plaines, IL, 2007, Author.

FAST is also used in pregnant patients with blunt abdominal trauma; it is both faster and safer than a CT scan, which is contraindicated in the pregnant patient because of the use of iodinated contrast medium and ionizing radiation (Cunningham, 2008).

Although FAST is useful in diagnosing free fluid, it cannot determine damage to solid organs; therefore, it complements rather than replaces other imaging scans. Diagnostic peritoneal lavage (DPL) may be performed to determine the presence of abdominal injury. This tool is of particular benefit when evaluation of the abdomen is difficult, such as when the patient is intoxicated, unconscious, or hemodynamically unstable. DPL can be performed in the ED, OR, PACU, or ICU. Nonetheless, retroperitoneal blood may be missed with a DPL, whereas the FAST approach may be quicker and visualize more structures, even pericardium; it is also less expensive and noninvasive. Thus FAST may be used with patients who are unstable and need a quick approach without the risk of a false-positive tap (Table 28-4).

Internal compartment pressures may be measured with an injury to the extremity as well as to the abdomen. Swelling of the muscles below the fascia covering may compromise circulation and result in the eventual loss of the extremity because of tissue necrosis. This is known as *compartment syndrome*. There are multiple compartments in the lower extremity that may be affected (Figure 28-4). Surgeons may measure compartment pressures with a manometer/stopcock/syringe or a commercial compartment pressure–measuring device. Normal compartmental pressures are less than 20 mm Hg. Pressures more than 30 mm Hg require a fasciotomy. Symptoms include severe pain, paresthesia, and a decrease in motor movement in the involved extremity, especially on passive movement (Table 28-5).

Massive intestinal edema may occur with trauma patients, causing compromise to internal organs and development of a different type of compartment syndrome. Abdominal compartment syndrome, also called abdominal hypertension, is characterized by increased intra-abdominal pressure (IAP). An increase in IAP can have a negative effect on the respiratory, splanchnic, and cerebral functions. It contributes to sepsis or multiple organ failure seen in many trauma patients. Normal IAP is approximately 5 to 7 mm Hg; elevation to 25 mm Hg is often seen in patients with septic shock and correlates with high mortality (Vegar-Brozovic et al, 2008). IAP is graded from I to IV based on a 12 to more than 25 mm Hg scale. Adverse effects on organ function may manifest as decreased cardiac output, oliguria, and hypoxia. Elevated intrathoracic pressure reduces left ventricular compliance, causing limitations in effective ventilation, often requiring ventilator support. Elevated IAP may cause an increase in intracranial pressure related to obstruction of cerebral venous blood outflow and increased intrathoracic and central venous pressure. Delay in treatment of IAP may lead to brain deterioration and damage.

Management involves a decompressive laparotomy. After a decompression the greatest nursing priority is wound management. The swelling may render the abdomen difficult or impossible to close. If the abdomen is closed, IAP may rise to a level greater than 25 cm of H_2O, at which point it may lead to significant organ dysfunction (Kulaylat and Dayton, 2012). IAP monitoring is accomplished with the use of a nasogastric tube in the stomach or a Foley catheter in the bladder. Simple water-column manometry is done at 2- to 4-hour intervals, although it is possible to connect a pressure transducer to a Foley catheter by way of the sampling port (Figure 28-5). By establishing a water column of urine in the Foley catheter with a clamp distal to the port, a pressure gradient is established. After zero-balancing the transducer, an 18-gauge needle is placed on the end of the pressure tubing and inserted into the sampling port. Using the pressure tubing and a 60-mL syringe, 50 to 60 mL of normal saline is then instilled into the Foley. On

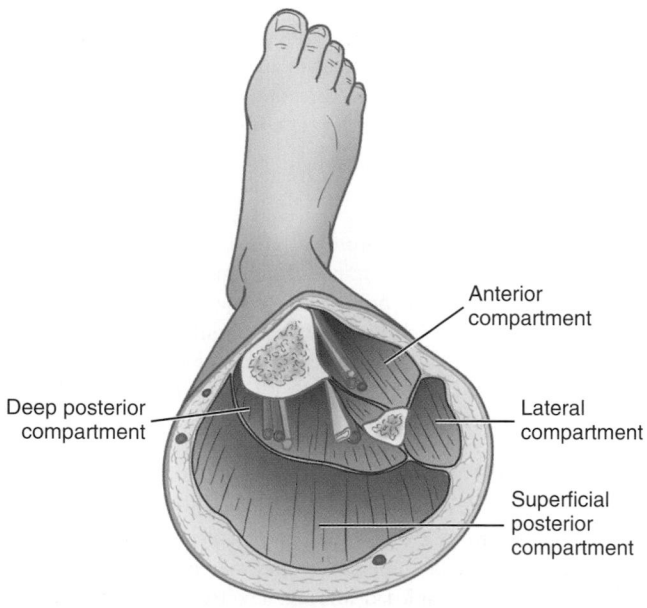

FIGURE 28-4 Compartments of the lower leg.

FIGURE 28-5 Setup for measuring abdominal compartment syndrome using a two-way Foley catheter and a pressure monitoring system.

TABLE 28-5

Signs and Symptoms Associated with Compartmental Syndromes

Compartment	Location of Sensory Changes	Movement Weakened	Painful Passive Movement	Location of Pain or Tenseness
Lower Leg				
Anterior	First web space	Toe extension	Toe flexion	Along lateral side of anterior tibia
Lateral	Dorsum (top) of foot	Foot eversion	Foot inversion	Lateral lower leg
Superficial posterior	None	Foot plantar flexion	Foot dorsiflexion	Calf
Deep posterior	Sole of foot	Toe flexion	Toe extension	Deep calf—palpable between Achilles tendon and medial malleoli
Forearm				
Volar	Volar (palmar) aspect of fingers	Wrist and finger flexion	Wrist and finger extension	Volar forearm
Dorsal	None	Wrist and finger extension	Wrist and finger flexion	Dorsal forearm
Hand				
Intraosseous	None	Finger adduction and abduction	Finger adduction and abduction	Between metacarpals on dorsum of hand

Modified from Warme WW, Matsen FA: *Compartmental syndromes*, 2011, available at www.orthop.washington.edu/?q=patient-care/articles/shoulder/compartmental-syndromes.html. Accessed November 3, 2012.

instillation of the saline, the waveform on the monitor is correlated to the existing bladder pressure. Normal IAP is zero, or subatmospheric. A pressure of more than 25 cm of H_2O is considered diagnostic of abdominal compartment syndrome (Kulaylat and Dayton, 2012). Postoperatively these patients are susceptible to fluid and heat loss. Continuous hemodynamic monitoring is essential in the critical care phase of treatment.

Admission Assessment. The perioperative nurse may not obtain information concerning the trauma patient until the patient arrives in the OR for surgical intervention. If the patient's condition permits, the perioperative nurse should obtain a brief, precise report from the ED nurse that contains the following information: MOI, an AMPLE history (if available), condition on arrival (e.g., level of consciousness), availability of and prior administration of blood or blood products, spine clearance, injuries present, and any other pertinent information (e.g., family present, completion of secondary assessment). If the injury is life- or limb-threatening, implied surgical consent is assumed (i.e., if the patient were able, consent would be given).

Additional data are collected as the perioperative nurse accompanies the patient to the OR. The status of the airway, as well as breathing patterns and circulatory condition, can be observed. The ED record also provides information concerning amount and type of intravenous (IV) fluid received, vital signs, core temperature, and laboratory and other diagnostic examinations performed. A quick visual and physical survey of the patient when the perioperative nurse is preparing the patient for the procedure enables identification of other sites of injury that might require attention.

The patient's psychologic status also can be assessed. If the patient is conscious, the perioperative nurse is challenged to allay fear and anxiety. The trauma patient has endured a very frightening experience and is in need of support. The perioperative nurse is often the best member of the surgical team to communicate with the patient and explain the interventions occurring before anesthesia induction. A touch or handhold is an important aspect of this communication process, demonstrating the nurse's caring behaviors and offering comfort.

Nursing Diagnosis

Nursing diagnoses related to the care of trauma patients undergoing operative intervention might include the following:

- Anxiety and Fear (patient and family) related to unpredictable nature of condition
- Deficient Fluid Volume related to hemorrhage, fluid shifts, alteration in capillary permeability, alteration in vascular tone, or myocardial compromise
- Hypothermia related to rapid infusion of IV fluids, decreased tissue perfusion, and exposure
- Acute Pain related to effects of trauma/injury agents, experience during invasive procedures or diagnostic tests
- Risk for Aspiration related to reduced level of consciousness secondary to injury or concomitant substance abuse; impaired cough and gag reflex; trauma to head, face, or neck; and secretions and debris in airway

Outcome Identification

Outcomes identified for the selected nursing diagnoses could be stated as follows:

- The patient and family will experience decreasing anxiety and fear, as evidenced by orientation to surroundings, ability to verbalize concerns and ask questions of the healthcare team, decreased fear-related behaviors (e.g., crying, agitation), and use of effective coping skills.
- The patient will have an effective circulating volume as evidenced by strong, palpable peripheral pulses; warm, dry skin of normal color; stable vital signs appropriate for age; maintenance of hematocrit level of 30 mL/dL or hemoglobin level of 12 to 14 g/dL or greater; and control of external hemorrhage.
- The patient will maintain a normal core body temperature, as evidenced by a core temperature measurement of 98° to 99.5° F (36.6° to 37.5° C) and warm, dry skin of normal color.
- The patient will experience relief of pain, as evidenced by diminishing or absent level of pain through his or her self-report, absence of physiologic indicators of pain (e.g., tachypnea, pallor, diaphoretic skin, increasing blood pressure), and ability to cooperate with care as appropriate.
- The patient will not experience aspiration, as evidenced by a patent airway; clear and equal bilateral breath sounds; regular rate, depth, and pattern of breathing; clear chest radiograph without evidence of infiltrates; and ability to handle secretions independently.

Planning

Because of the unexpected nature of trauma, planning perioperative care is of the utmost importance. Equipment, instruments, and supplies that have a high probability of use must be immediately available. Autologous blood salvage units should also be considered during patient care preparation, because blood salvage will be done if not contraindicated by the nature of the injury. (A Sample Plan of Care for a trauma patient is shown on page 1113.)

Implementation

Multiple Operative Procedures. Depending on the severity of the injuries, the multiple trauma patient may require many surgical interventions. Some of these procedures may be performed simultaneously. This is determined through a collaborative effort among the surgeons, anesthesia provider, and perioperative nurse. If a patient has sustained severe head and abdominal trauma, a surgeon will need to place an intracranial pressure (ICP) monitoring device (Surgical Pharmacology). However, the abdominal exploration is also emergently indicated. Consequently, the severe condition of the patient may require performance of both of these procedures at the same time.

Multiple procedures, either simultaneously or in succession, require a great deal of preparation by the perioperative nurse, scrub person, and the trauma team. The order of procedures is determined by the presence or absence of life threats. The usual order of priority is chest, abdomen, head, and extremities. However, this priority is determined for each patient's situation and adjusted accordingly. Performance of simultaneous procedures is preferable when physically possible. Anesthesia time is decreased for the critically ill patient, and definitive surgical interventions are accomplished more rapidly.

Increased Risk for Infection. Many trauma patients have wounds that are contaminated with roadside debris, dirt, grass, or automobile parts. Others have a perforated full stomach, and food particles are released into the peritoneum, increasing the risk of peritonitis. Consequently many patients are at high risk for infection. Sterile technique may be compromised secondary only to immediate life threat. Pouring an antimicrobial solution across the surgical site

SAMPLE PLAN OF CARE

Nursing Diagnosis

Anxiety and **Fear** (patient and family) related to unpredictable nature of condition

Outcome

The patient and family will experience decreasing anxiety and fear, as evidenced by orientation to surroundings; ability to verbalize concerns and ask questions to healthcare team; decreased fear-related behaviors (e.g., crying, agitation); and use of effective coping skills.

Interventions

- Monitor the patient's level of anxiety by assessing the state of alertness, ability to comprehend, and ability to comply with requests.
- Facilitate the family's presence.
- Assist the family in identifying coping mechanisms; facilitate and support their use.
- Reassure the patient and family during interactions by touch (when welcomed) and empathic verbal and nonverbal communication.
- Explain the perioperative environment to patient and what to expect to assist in reduction of anxiety.
- Discuss the patient's postoperative appearance (i.e., drains, tubes, equipment) with the patient and family.

Nursing Diagnosis

Deficient Fluid Volume related to hemorrhage, fluid shifts, alteration in capillary permeability, alteration in vascular tone, or myocardial compromise.

Outcome

The patient will have an effective circulating volume as evidenced by strong, palpable peripheral pulses; warm, dry skin of normal color; stable vital signs appropriate for age; maintenance of hematocrit level of 30 mL/dL or hemoglobin level of 12 to 14 g/dL or higher; and control of external hemorrhage.

Interventions

- Manage any uncontrolled bleeding by doing the following:
  - Applying direct pressure over bleeding site
  - Elevating extremities
  - Applying pressure over arterial pressure sites
- Ensure trauma profile laboratory work is complete.
- Verify that requested blood and blood replacement components are available in the OR.
- Prepare laboratory request slips as required; document time and type of analysis requested.
- Collaborate with anesthesia provider in monitoring cardiovascular changes suggestive of hypovolemia.
- Assist in accurate monitoring of intake and output during the surgical procedure.
- Administer blood and blood components as indicated.

Nursing Diagnosis

Hypothermia related to rapid infusion of intravenous (IV) fluids, decreased tissue perfusion, exposure

Outcome

The patient will maintain a normal core body temperature, as evidenced by a core temperature measurement of 96.8° to 99.5° F (36° to 37.5°C) and warm, dry skin of normal color.

Interventions

- Warm IV solutions and blood products using approved warming devices.
- Minimize body exposure during all phases of perioperative care.
- Use forced-air warming units and warm blankets to facilitate normothermia.
- Ensure irrigant solutions are warm.
- Monitor body temperature for signs of hypothermia, and report to anesthesia provider.

Nursing Diagnosis

Acute Pain related to effects of trauma/injury agents, experience during invasive procedures or diagnostic tests

Outcome

The patient will experience relief of pain, as evidenced by diminishing or absent level of pain through self-report, absence of physiologic indicators of pain (e.g., tachypnea, pallor, diaphoretic skin, increasing blood pressure), and ability to cooperate with care as appropriate.

Interventions

- Collaborate with anesthesia provider and surgeon regarding pain management therapy to increase the patient's level of comfort if condition permits.
- Assess nonverbal cues regarding level of pain and discomfort.
- Assume that pain is present or that procedures will cause pain if the patient is unable to provide verbal or nonverbal cues.
- Use a visual or numeric pain scale to assess pain levels and change in comfort if the patient is conscious and able to respond.

Nursing Diagnosis

Risk for Aspiration related to reduced level of consciousness secondary to injury or concomitant substance abuse; impaired cough and gag reflex; trauma to head, face, or neck; and secretions and debris in airway

Outcome

The patient will not experience aspiration, as evidenced by a patent airway; clear and equal bilateral breath sounds; regular rate, depth, and pattern of breathing; clear chest radiograph without evidence of infiltrates; and ability to handle secretions independently.

Interventions

- Ensure operation of suction apparatus preoperatively, and maintain one open suction line solely for use by the anesthesia provider.
- Provide assistance with cricoid pressure under the direction of the anesthesia provider.
- Assist with placement of nasogastric or orogastric tube to evacuate stomach contents.

---

may be the only surgical skin prep undertaken when an immediate life threat exists. The use of antimicrobial prophylaxis shortly before skin incision has become the standard of care for surgical procedures. Perioperative nurses are in a position to ensure the timely administration of antibiotics.

Wounds may need to be grossly decontaminated before the surgical skin prep. Sterile scrub brushes or a mechanical

irrigation-under-pressure device may be used preoperatively and intraoperatively. Care must be exercised to remove as much contamination as possible, without creating further damage to the wound or body part. Perioperative personnel must wear personal protective equipment (PPE) during irrigation under pressure to prevent splashes and contamination from the lavage system. Traffic in the OR should be limited to essential personnel. Increased traffic

SURGICAL PHARMACOLOGY

Commonly Used Medications by the Anesthesia Provider to Decrease ICP

Medication/Category	Dosage/Route	Purpose/Action	Adverse Reactions	Nursing Implications
Thiopental (Pentothal) *Pharmacotherapeutic:* Barbiturate	*Adults:* 1.5-3.5 mg/kg IV bolus	Reduce intraoperative elevations of intracranial pressure	Respiratory depression, hypotension, bronchospasm, and cardiac arrhythmias	Monitor for hypotension, ECG.
Propofol (Diprivan) *Pharmacotherapeutic:* General anesthetics	*Adults:* Induction 20-40 mg every 10 sec until induction onset *Children 3-16 yr:* Induction 2.5-3.5 mg/kg over 20-30 sec	For general anesthesia induction, reduce cerebral blood flow and the cerebral metabolic rate for oxygen	Respiratory depression, apnea, hypotension, and sinus bradycardia	Monitor respiratory rate, BP, heart rate, O₂ saturation, ABGs.
Esmolol (Brevibloc) *Pharmacotherapeutic:* Beta-blocker	*Adults:* Initially give a loading dose of 250-500 mcg/kg IV over 1 min, then begin a maintenance infusion of 50-100 mcg/kg/min IV for 4 min	Blunt systemic hypertension caused by laryngoscopy	Hypotension, bradycardia, dizziness, syncope, drowsiness, breathing difficulty, bluish fingernails or palms of hands, seizures	Monitor hypotension, ECG, heart rate; assess pulse for quality, irregular rate, bradycardia.
Mannitol (Osmitrol) *Pharmacotherapeutic:* Osmotic diuretic	*Adults:* Initial dose 0.5-1 g/kg IV, then maintenance dose 0.25-0.5 g/kg IV q4-6 hr *Children:* Initial dose 0.25-1 g/kg IV, then maintenance dose 0.25-0.5 g/kg IV q4-6 hr	Elevates osmotic pressure of glomerular filtrate, inhibiting tubular reabsorption of water and electrolytes, resulting in increased flow of water into interstitial fluid/plasma	Pulmonary edema, CHF, excessive diuresis may produce hypokalemia, hyponatremia	Monitor urinary output to determine therapeutic response. Monitor serum electrolytes, BUN, renal/hepatic function tests, assess vital signs.
Furosemide (Lasix) *Pharmacotherapeutic:* Diuretic	*Adults:* 20-40 mg IV; may increase by 20 mg/dose q1-2 hr; maximum single dose 160-200 mg *Children:* 1-2 mg/kg IV q6-12 hr; maximum single dose 6 mg/kg	Excretion of sodium, chloride, potassium by direct action at ascending limb of loop of Henle; produces diuresis; lowers BP, ICP	Hypokalemia, hyponatremia, dehydration, sudden volume depletion may result in increased risk of thrombosis, circulatory collapse, sudden death	Check vital signs, BP, pulse; assess baseline serum electrolytes, especially for hypokalemia.

ABGs, Arterial blood gases; *BP,* blood pressure; *BUN,* blood urea nitrogen; *CHF,* congestive heart failure; *ECG,* electrocardiogram; *ICP,* intracranial pressure; *IV,* intravenous.
Modified from Drugs: *Thiopental,* available at www.nursingconsult.com/nursing/drugs/monograph?tab=generic&drug_id=604&firstpage=1&secondpage=1&firstsort_by=title&firstsort_order=asc&secondsort_by=&secondsort_order=&firsttitle=Thiopental&secondtitle=&firstdrugsRequestUri=quick-find&monotype=full. Accessed October 28, 2012; Hall M: Increased intracranial pressure and traumatic brain injury. In Duke J, editor: *Anesthesia secrets,* ed 4, Denver, 2011, Mosby; Hodgson BB, Kizior RJ: *Saunders nursing drug handbook 2013,* St Louis, 2013, Saunders.

in the room increases chances for contamination in an already compromised patient, as well as potentially interferes with the delivery of expedient care.

Procedure Preparation. Most level I trauma centers have a designated trauma OR that contains all equipment and supplies potentially needed for trauma patients. Many hospitals maintain an emergency abdominal procedure set, craniotomy procedure set, and chest procedure set either obtainable in the OR's sterile supply area or immediately available in the central supply department. This streamlines preparation for the surgical procedure and allows for rapid preparation in those instances in which the patient bypasses the ED on arrival and is transported directly to the OR.

After the perioperative nurse is notified of the surgical procedure, OR determination is made in consultation with the anesthesia provider and surgeon. Considerations include the following:

- Equipment required by the surgeon or surgeons to perform the surgical procedure
- Room availability

- Room size (to accommodate equipment, staff, and multiple procedures)
- Need for additional staff
- Capability for autologous blood salvage
- Availability of emergency procedure supplies (including power equipment)
- Selection of OR bed

Additional diagnostic procedures are often required during multiple trauma procedures. A fluoroscopic electric OR bed provides increased flexibility in patient management. The bed can be rotated on its base to facilitate two teams operating at once. The fluoroscopic capabilities allow for additional radiographs and arteriograms as needed. The bed should easily accommodate different positions, such as lithotomy or lateral rotation. If a fluoroscopic bed is not available, arrangements must be made in advance to perform diagnostic radiologic procedures intraoperatively.

Before transfer of the patient to the OR bed, the perioperative nurse must ascertain if the spinal column has been cleared by the surgeon or attending physician as free from injury. If the spine has not been cleared, the surgeon must be consulted before removal of the patient from the backboard. Safe transfer of the patient from the transport vehicle to the OR bed can be accomplished using the log-rolling technique.

Positioning the patient is based on the surgical approach. Ascertaining the type and location of the wound (anterior or posterior) and type of operative procedure dictates the patient's position. For example, an aortic injury may be approached through a thoracotomy or a median sternotomy incision. The thoracotomy requires lateral positioning devices, and the sternotomy necessitates a supine position.

If several procedures are being performed, positioning may change intraoperatively. Changing the anesthetized patient's position is accomplished under the supervision of the anesthesia provider, with particular attention to maintain the airway. The patient is moved slowly, allowing for assessment of vital sign changes in response to the position movement. All precautions regarding positioning are re-executed, with special attention given to the electrosurgical grounding pad. This pad may loosen during patient repositioning and require replacement to ensure adequate pad contact.

When the trauma patient is transferred to the OR, the extent of injury is not always known. The perioperative nurse should prep the patient from the suprasternal notch to the midthigh. This allows for rapid access to the chest to clamp the aorta should massive hemorrhage control be indicated; it also allows for exposure of the femoral arteries for potential cannulation and access to the thigh for harvesting a saphenous vein.

Established policies for counting soft goods, instruments, and sharps should address surgical procedures of an emergent nature within the institution. Every attempt is made to verify appropriate numbers of counted items without compromising the timeliness of intervention in a life-threatening situation. If a preprocedural count is not performed, the perioperative nurse must document the occurrence and rationale used in accordance with established hospital policies and procedures. Some institutions require an x-ray examination postoperatively to examine the patient for the presence of a retained object. If counted soft goods are intentionally left in the patient (e.g., in a damage control procedure at a level II, III, or IV center before transfer to a level I facility), the number and type of soft goods left in the wound should be documented on the perioperative nursing record and communicated when there is a transfer in patient care (Association of periOperative Registered Nurses [AORN], 2013). The operative dictation by the surgeon should also verify the presence of retained soft goods, their type, and their number. This allows for accurate counts in subsequent procedures and prevents the potential for inadvertently retained soft goods.

In the presence of clotting difficulties or specific types of organ injuries with continuous oozing of blood, the surgeon may elect to pack the surgical site with soft goods and close the site as a temporary measure. After a period of 24 to 48 hours, the patient returns to the OR for removal of the soft goods and primary closure if possible. In such instances the perioperative nurse must document and record accurately the number of soft goods used for packing, as noted. When the soft goods are removed, the exact number is verified and they are isolated and contained in accordance with established hospital policy and procedure.

Autotransfusion. Considering the high blood loss associated with traumatic injuries, autotransfusion has become a vital asset in trauma care. Preoperative blood loss that is associated with an isolated hemothorax is collected in a designated chest-drainage device for reinfusion within 4 hours to avoid bacterial contamination. Intraoperative blood loss is collected, filtered, and reinfused to the patient. This provides immediate volume replacement, decreases the amount of bank blood used, and reduces the possibility of transfusion reactions or risk of transfusion with bloodborne pathogens.

The autologous blood salvage unit requires specialized training for operation. Institutional policies vary regarding appropriate personnel designated for operation of the equipment. Capabilities for autotransfusion should be considered during procedure preparation because additional qualified personnel may be required.

During autologous blood salvage the scrub person squeezes out additional blood and fluid from saturated soft goods before discarding them from the surgical field. The blood salvage suction is used whenever possible to maximize the amount of blood salvaged. However, care must be taken to ensure that the blood collected in the salvage unit is free from contamination. For instance, if the abdomen is contaminated with free food particles or colonic perforation is present, the blood cannot be used. Similarly, once antibiotic irrigation is initiated, the blood salvage unit is not used.

Evidence Preservation. If the injury to the patient is a result of a violent crime, the team must give special attention to preservation of evidence during the course of patient care. Physical evidence (e.g., bullets, bags of powder, weapons, pills, and other foreign objects), trace evidence (e.g., hair and fibers), biologic evidence (e.g., body fluids and blood), and clothing are types of evidence to be preserved. Specific procedures on handling of evidence may differ by institution and law enforcement agencies.

Clothing must be handled properly. When clothing is removed from the patient, the person removing it should cut along the seams or around the bullet or stab wound holes. The shape of the hole may help identify the weapon used. Clothing is placed in paper bags, labeled appropriately, and given to law enforcement personnel. Plastic bags trap moisture and may facilitate growth of mold, which could destroy evidence. The transport vehicle sheet should also be handled in a similar manner because evidence may be present. The nurse must ensure that descriptions of wound appearances, body markings consistent with gang or cult activity, and statements from the patient are accurately recorded.

The chain of custody for all evidence, including clothing, is followed. This process allows for identification of all people handling the evidence. Documentation must verify that the evidence has been in secure possession at all times. Records should be kept of all evidence discovered, including its site of origin and when and to whom the evidence was given. A system of documentation using receipts or a specific form should be established to ensure appropriate compliance.

Gunpowder residues, tissue, hair, or other valuable information may be present on the hands of a trauma patient. This evidence can be preserved by placing the patient's hands in a paper bag and securing it with tape. Washing the hands should be avoided until evidence is collected, or until directed to do so by the police.

Bullets and retained implements offer valuable evidence and may assist in identifying the assailant. The weapon firing the bullet and the bullet itself can be matched by the specific grooves and markings placed on the bullet when the gun was fired. Most bullets are composed of soft lead, and handling with metal instruments can interfere with the markings. Therefore, the surgeon should avoid using metal instruments to handle bullets. Some of the newer exploding types of bullets can present a risk to perioperative team members during wound exploration. Care should be exercised to avoid sterile glove tears because these types of bullets are extremely sharp. Once a bullet is removed, the scrub person should place it in dry, clean gauze in a plastic specimen container and pass it off the sterile field to the perioperative nurse. Using the chain-of-custody procedures, the perioperative nurse should label the container appropriately and dispose of the bullet according to established institutional policies.

Deep Vein Thrombosis Prophylaxis. Because of the prolonged immobilization anticipated for the trauma patient, along with the frequency of orthopedic or lower extremity surgery, trauma patients are at high risk for developing venous thromboembolic events (VTE). Placement of a intermittent pneumatic compression device preoperatively is ideal. These pneumatic compression devices assist in decreasing the possibility of deep vein thrombosis (DVT), and their effect is optimized when applied before surgical intervention. Preoperative placement is subject to the physician's preference; clinical research regarding similar devices and demonstrated product effectiveness is ongoing. The incidence of DVT and pulmonary embolism (PE) in trauma patients varies widely. In the approximately 235,000 cases of traumatic brain injury (TBI) that occur every year, up to 54% who do not receive any intervention will develop DVT or PE (Phelan, 2012).

Currently, in patients with traumatic brain injury, the only recommended prophylaxis is the use of an intermittent pneumatic compression device because of concerns with the use of heparin leading to bleeding complications. Subsequently, an inferior vena cava filter (VCF) may be inserted in high-risk patients to prevent pulmonary embolus. Risk factors for PE include prolonged immobility, multiple pelvic and lower extremity fractures, previous history of PE, severe head trauma, and incomplete spinal cord injury with paralysis. However, the placement of a VCF is associated with inferior vena cava obstruction and recurrent DVT. Contraindication to pharmacologic prophylaxis is generally limited to a short period after the initial trauma, and long-term vena cava filtration is rarely necessary.

Anesthesia Implications. Depending on institutional protocol, the anesthesia team may be directly involved in resuscitation of the trauma patient immediately after arrival at the ED. The anesthesia provider maintains the airway and intubates the patient if necessary. A critically injured patient may be transferred directly to the OR, whereas some interventions may be performed in the ED of a trauma center. These interventions vary from insertion of an ICP monitor to an emergent exploratory thoracotomy.

However, if diagnostic evaluation can be accomplished without intubation and sedation, the patient may be conscious on arrival in the OR. A trauma patient is assumed to have a full stomach; thus these patients are at high risk for aspiration and resultant pneumonia. Under the direction of the anesthesia provider, the perioperative nurse applies cricoid pressure (Sellick maneuver) (see Figure 5-4). This pressure is maintained over the cricoid area until the cuff on the endotracheal (ET) tube is inflated and tube placement verified by the anesthesia provider. This type of intubation is often referred to as a "crash induction."

In addition, the patient may require intubation for protection of the airway before radiologic examination of the cervical spine. If the cervical spine is not cleared or if the radiographic screening examination is not performed before intubation, ET intubation is done while cervical spine precautions (i.e., in-line intubation) are

---

BOX 28-1

Rapid-Sequence Intubation Steps

Preparation	Assist anesthesia care provider as needed. Ensure all equipment is available.
Preoxygenation	Administer 100% oxygen.
Pretreatment	Assist anesthesia provider in medication administration, as indicated (atropine, lidocaine, etomidate).
Paralysis with induction	Stand by while anesthesia is induced (midazolam, fentanyl), provide support while patient loses consciousness and neuromuscular agent is administered (succinylcholine).
Protection and positioning	Use Sellick maneuver to provide cricoid pressure. Prepare to apply pressure continuously and until anesthesia provider asks to have pressure released to avoid aspiration.
Placement with proof	Inflate cuff; check placement with exhaled carbon dioxide detector and by listening to lungs with stethoscope.
Postintubation management	Secure tube, verify ventilator settings, and monitor per routine.

Modified from Emergency Nurses Association (ENA): *Trauma nursing core course,* ed 6, Des Plaines, IL, 2007, Author.

---

maintained. The anesthesia provider may decide to use rapid-sequence intubation (RSI), which involves administering 100% oxygen, an analgesic, and a neuromuscular relaxant; applying cricoid pressure; and inserting a cuffed ET tube. Etomidate (Amidate) is the most commonly used induction agent (ENA, 2007). It acts in about 1 minute and lasts about 5 minutes and is often used in trauma patients because it does not cause an increase in ICP or worsening of hypotension. Succinylcholine (Anectine) is the most frequently used neuromuscular relaxant. The perioperative nurse can facilitate RSI by ensuring availability of all intubation and resuscitation equipment, assisting with monitoring devices, and confirming correct ET-tube placement (Box 28-1).

In injuries of the face where midface fractures are present, nasal intubation and nasogastric tube placement are avoided. Tube placement in the brain through a fracture of the cribriform plate is a well-known complication. To avoid this, oral ET intubation is the technique of choice. The anesthesia provider places an oral gastric tube to achieve stomach decompression. An oral intubation on a conscious patient is often necessary because anesthetics and muscle relaxants can result in the loss of any remaining airway in the presence of facial trauma.

Large-bore IV access used with rapid-infusion fluid warmers may be used in the ED. These fluid warmers can deliver high volumes of crystalloid solution at body temperature. Use of the fluid warmer may continue during the intraoperative phase to facilitate volume replacement and help maintain normothermia. A number of factors may influence a trauma patient's response to fluid loss. These factors include age, severity of injury, type and location of injury, time lapse from injury to treatment, prehospital fluid therapy, prehospital use of a pneumatic antishock garment (PASG), and medications taken for chronic conditions. Fluid resuscitation should be initiated when early signs of blood loss are suspected. A classification system can be useful in determining the needs of the patient (Table 28-6).

TABLE 28-6

Estimated Fluid and Blood Losses Based on Patient's Initial Presentation*

	Class I	Class II	Class III	Class IV
Blood loss (mL)	Up to 750	750-1500	1500-2000	>2000
Blood loss (% blood volume)	Up to 15%	15%-30%	30%-40%	>40%
Pulse rate (beats/min)	<100	>100	>120	>140
Blood pressure	Normal	Normal	Decreased	Decreased
Pulse pressure	Normal or increased	Decreased	Decreased	Decreased
Respiratory rate (breaths/min)	14-20	20-30	30-40	>35
Urine output (mL/hr)	>30	20-30	5-15	Negligible
Central nervous system (CNS)/mental status	Slightly anxious	Mildly anxious	Anxious, confused	Confused, lethargic
Fluid replacement (3:1 rule)	Crystalloid	Crystalloid	Crystalloid and blood	Crystalloid and blood

*The guidelines are for a 70-kg man. They are based on the 3:1 rule. This rule derives from the empiric observation that most patients in hemorrhagic shock require as much as 300 mL of electrolyte solution for each 100 mL of blood loss. Applied blindly, these guidelines can result in excessive or inadequate fluid administration. For example, a patient with a crush injury to the extremity may have hypotension out of proportion to his or her blood loss and require fluids in excess of the 3:1 guidelines. In contrast, a patient whose ongoing blood loss is being replaced by blood transfusion requires less than 3:1. The use of bolus therapy with careful monitoring of the patient's response can moderate these extremes.
Modified from American College of Surgeons: *ATLS program for doctors,* ed 8, Chicago, 2008, Author; Boswell SA, Scalea TM: Initial management of traumatic shock. In McQuillan KA et al, editors: *Trauma nursing: from resuscitation through rehabilitation,* ed 4, St Louis, 2009, Saunders.

TABLE 28-7

Maternal Adaptation During Pregnancy and Relation to Trauma

System	Alteration	Clinical Responses
Respiratory	↑ Oxygen consumption ↑ Tidal volume ↓ Functional residual capacity Chronic compensated alkalosis ↓ $PaCO_2$ ↓ Serum bicarbonate	↑ Risk of acidosis ↑ Risk of respiratory mismanagement ↓ Blood-buffering capacity
Cardiovascular	↑ Circulating volume, 1600 mL ↑ Cardiac output ↑ Heart rate ↓ Systemic vascular resistance (SVR) ↓ Arterial blood pressure	Can lose 1000 mL of blood No signs of shock until blood loss >30% of total volume ↓ Placental perfusion in supine position Point of maximal impulse, fourth intercostal space Heart displaced upward to left
Renal	↑ Renal plasma flow Dilation of ureters and urethra Bladder displaced forward	↑ Risk of stasis, infection ↑ Risk of bladder rupture
Gastrointestinal	↓ Gastric motility ↑ Hydrochloric acid production ↓ Competency of gastroesophageal sphincter	↑ Risk of aspiration Passive regurgitation of stomach acids if head lower than stomach
Reproductive	↑ Blood flow to organs Uterine enlargement	Source of ↑ blood loss Vena caval compression in supine position
Musculoskeletal	Displacement of abdominal viscera Pelvic venous congestion Cartilage softened Fetal head in pelvis	↑ Risk of injury, altered rebound response; altered pain referral ↑ Risk of pelvic fracture Center of gravity changed ↑ Risk of fetal injury
Hematologic	↑ Clotting factors ↓ Fibrinolytic activity	↑ Risk of thrombus formation

Modified from Dorman KF: Obstetric critical care. In Lowdermilk DL et al, editors: *Maternity & women's health care,* ed 10, St Louis, 2012, Mosby.

Pregnancy. Trauma in pregnancy is a leading cause of nonpregnancy-related maternal deaths and fetal demise. An estimated 6% to 7% of pregnancies are complicated by MVCs, falls, violent assaults, and burn injuries (Reddy et al, 2012). It is most important to remember that two patients are being treated.

The normal physiologic changes that occur during pregnancy increase the challenge of evaluation and treatment when these individuals are victims of trauma. The pelvis protects the uterus and fetus during the first trimester; after 12 weeks, the uterus expands into the peritoneal cavity, increasing the risk for injury. Furthermore, intra-abdominal organs change position as pregnancy progresses, increasing the risk for GI injury when the MOI is a stabbing or gunshot wound (Reddy et al, 2012).

It is also important to note that the pregnant trauma patient has a much larger circulatory volume (Table 28-7). The cardiac output may be increased by as much as 40%. Oxygen requirements are increased. Heart rate increases over the prepregnant state. The usual clinical indicators of hypovolemic shock are unreliable in the

TABLE 28-8

Signs of Hypovolemic Shock in Pregnancy

	Circulating Blood Volume Deficit	
	Early (20%)	**Late (25%)**
Pulse rate	<100 beats/min	>100 beats/min
Respiratory rate	12-20 breaths/min	>20 breaths/min
Blood pressure	Normal	Hypotensive
Skin perfusion	Warm, dry skin	Cool, ashen skin
Capillary refill time	<2 seconds	>2 seconds
Level of consciousness	Alert	Agitated, lethargic
Urine output	>30-50 mL/hr	<30-50 mL/hr
Fetal heart rate (normally 120-160 beats/min)	High, low, late decelerations	High, low, absent, late decelerations

pregnant trauma patient (Table 28-8). The team must assume that the pregnant trauma victim is in shock until proven otherwise. Early aggressive treatment is essential. The uterus is enlarged and no longer a pelvic organ, and it elevates the bladder out of the pelvis as well. Supine position for the pregnant patient can result in a decrease in cardiac output as a result of compression of the inferior vena cava. If the patient is close to term, cardiac output can be reduced by as much as 30% as a result of compression on the inferior vena cava. Consequently, patients who are 20 weeks or more into their pregnancy should be placed in the left lateral decubitus position to avoid a hypotensive episode and maintain blood flow to the uterus and placenta. If this is not possible, manual displacement of the uterus by lateral abdominal pressure should be attempted. As a result of the physiologic changes just described, the pregnant patient is at risk for aspiration. Rapid-sequence induction, along with the Sellick maneuver, is the preferred method for intubation.

Ultrasound studies are conducted to determine viability of the fetus when possible. In the event of a ruptured uterus, a cesarean delivery and hysterectomy may be required if the fetus is viable. Neonatal resuscitation is of the utmost importance immediately on delivery of the fetus.

Pregnant patients requiring surgery also need fetal assessment performed intraoperatively. Any fetal movement should be noted. In addition, fetal monitoring is continuous. This includes fetal heart rate and uterine contractions. Fetal monitoring provides information on the condition of the fetus and the response to uterine contractions, if present. Fetal heart rate can usually be obtained after 10 weeks of gestation. Abnormalities in fetal heart rate can be an early sign of maternal compromise because the pregnant uterus is viewed as a nonessential peripheral organ in states of hypovolemic shock. Personnel qualified in the interpretation of fetal heart rate patterns must be present. This expertise may be provided by the obstetric nursing staff.

Perimortem (postmortem) cesarean delivery may be performed in the event of the sudden death of the mother and the presence of a viable fetus.

Pediatric Trauma Patients. Special considerations related to the care of infants and children who have sustained a trauma are described in Chapter 26. Table 26-7 details a modified Glasgow Coma Scale for children.

Elderly Trauma Patients. As the number of adults older than 65 years continues to grow, so does the number of elderly patients requiring surgical intervention related to trauma. The physiologic effects of aging combined with the preinjury health status of many elderly patients significantly affect their ability to respond to initial treatment for traumatic injuries and subsequent surgical intervention. Consequently the mortality for elderly trauma patients is significantly higher than that in younger patients with the same level of injury. Preexisting medical conditions, medication use, decreased physiologic reserves, and the physical and psychologic stress experienced during surgical interventions place elderly trauma victims at increased risk for perioperative complications (Plummer, 2009). (See Chapter 27 for the physical and psychologic changes that occur in elderly patients.)

Bariatric Trauma Patients. There has been a notable increase in admissions of bariatric patients in all healthcare facilities. Bariatric medicine is defined as the care of the extremely obese patient, as measured by body mass index (BMI). The World Health Organization (WHO) defines obese as a BMI greater than 30 and severely obese as a BMI greater than 40 (Muir and Archer-Heese, 2009). The obese patient often has several comorbid conditions, including cardiac disease, hypertension, respiratory disease, diabetes, osteoarthritis, and stress incontinence. Because of their size and their decreased self-esteem, the needs of bariatric patients are different from those of other patients. Societal prejudice against obesity is well established. Studies show that nurses are often less attentive to the needs of the obese patient and are often worried about the possibility of personal injury related to positioning the patient (Patient Safety). Furthermore, the patient's BMI may prohibit CT and MRI scans due to the limitations of the equipment (Sherwood et al, 2009).

Invasive Emergency Department Interventions. If a patient has shown a very recent deterioration of vital signs, either en route to the hospital or on arrival at the ED, the surgeon may elect to perform an emergency thoracotomy in the ED. A left-sided approach is usually performed because this allows rapid access to the heart for external cardiac massage and exposure of the great vessels for clamping in the event of severe blood loss (Figure 28-6). The incision can be extended to the right side by cutting across the sternum; this approach is commonly referred to as the clam shell thoracotomy. This procedure can be used to gain control in hemorrhage of the great vessels, to access the heart, or, in a grave situation, as a final effort to save a life. The procedure is used more often in penetrating injuries in which a laceration to a ventricle or other potentially treatable, life-threatening injury may be present.

Because of the perioperative nurse's knowledge of surgical instrumentation and procedures, his or her assistance in this procedure in the ED is often required. Rapid access to the heart and great vessels is the goal. The patient is then transported to the OR for additional interventions once hemorrhage is controlled.

In a similar fashion, an exploratory laparotomy can be initiated in the ED to control abdominal hemorrhage, especially when a splenic rupture is suspected and the patient is severely compromised.

If all other techniques of airway access are unsuccessful, the surgeon performs a cricothyrotomy. The surgeon makes a vertical incision through the skin, and incises the cricothyroid membrane. An ET or tracheostomy tube can be inserted through the membrane to create an airway. In the event a tube is not immediately available, a large-bore needle can be inserted into the membrane and the catheter left in place. This provides a temporary airway access

PATIENT SAFETY

The Bariatric Trauma Patient

Patient safety in the trauma OR is important for all patient populations. The perioperative team must be familiar with equipment weight limits, proper positioning, and safe patient handling techniques for the bariatric patient population. An obese trauma patient is also at an increased risk for respiratory complications and deep vein thrombosis (DVT). The perioperative nurse and scrub person must ensure the appropriate equipment and supplies are ready for the bariatric trauma patient to prevent delays in patient care.

Most OR beds have a weight limit of 500 pounds; newer OR beds are capable of supporting patients up to 1000 pounds. The newer OR beds may come with side extensions to accommodate the excess girth of the patient. If these are unavailable the OR team may use armboards attached to the lower end of the table to support the lower extremities. In addition, a footboard may be used to decrease the risk of peroneal and tibial nerve damage. To secure the patient to the OR bed, place one safety strap across the thighs and another across the lower legs.

Recommended methods for transferring the patient to the OR bed include using an air-assisted lateral transfer device, friction-reducing sliding aids, motorized lateral transfer aids, or a slide-and-roll board. The nurse must be familiar with the devices used in their OR and assess the patient to determine what transfer device is safest for the patient and staff members. The OR team must ensure adequate staff members are present to assist with the patient transfer to avoid injury.

Chronic obstructive pulmonary disease (COPD), sleep apnea, hypoxemia, and hypercapnia are common respiratory conditions associated with obesity and can rapidly cause decompensation because oxygen desaturation occurs three times faster in patients who are obese as a result of reduced functional residual capacity. Furthermore, patients with sleep apnea have an increased risk for failed endotracheal intubation. The perioperative nurse must be ready to assist the anesthesia provider with intubation and have the difficult airway cart immediately available.

In addition to these recommendations the bariatric trauma patient should have subcutaneous heparin and intermittent pneumatic compression devices for DVT prophylaxis. Intermittent pneumatic compression devices are usually indicated for this patient population and should be applied to the lower extremities.

Modified from Al-Benna S: Perioperative management of morbid obesity, *J Perioper Pract* 21(7):225–233, 2011; Evans DC et al: Obesity in trauma patients: correlations of body mass index with outcomes, injury patterns, and complications, *Am Surg* 77(8):1003–1008, 2011; Graham D et al: Preventing perioperative complications in the patient with a high body mass index, *AORN J* 94(4):334–344, 2011; Rowen L et al: Managing obese patients in the OR, *OR Nurse* 6(2):26–35, 2012, available at http://journals.lww.com/ornursejournal/Fulltext/2012/03000/Managing_obese_patients_in_the_OR.7.aspx. Accessed October 20, 2012.

measure but is inadequate to effectively ventilate the patient without a jet oscillating ventilator.

Successive Surgical Interventions. Often the multiple trauma patient requires a multitude of surgical procedures—either specialty-related or as a stepwise progression in the primary treatment of the initial injury. Initially the trauma patient is critically ill and requires intensive care facilities. When surgery is scheduled, the perioperative nurse may need additional assistance in transporting the patient as transport monitoring of the ECG, arterial line, and blood pressure is performed. Oxygen administration and mechanical ventilation with an Ambu bag are necessary for the intubated patient.

FIGURE 28-6 Emergency clam shell thoracotomy performed in the emergency department.

Acalculous cholecystitis is often a secondary complication of the trauma patient's postoperative course that requires cholecystectomy. Fixation of initially undiscovered fractures, debridements, secondary wound closures, flap constructions, and other reconstructive procedures make up the majority of follow-up procedures. Depending on the patient's condition, some procedures may be performed after discharge on an outpatient basis (Ambulatory Surgery Considerations).

Evaluation

The evaluation of the patient should reflect the effectiveness of the interventions. Did the patient remain free from untoward complications? Was there progress toward the expected outcomes as described in the perioperative plan of care? The following are examples of evaluation statements in relation to the sample plan of care:

- The patient demonstrated a decreased level of anxiety; he or she verbalized less apprehension, maintained eye contact, and was able to comply with requests even though anxiety persisted.
- The patient remained hemodynamically stable; fluid resuscitation was undertaken, blood pressure and pulse rate measurements were adequate considering the patient's status, and the H&H values were within acceptable ranges.
- The patient achieved and maintained normothermia in the OR.
- The patient reported reasonable relief from pain during preparatory maneuvers in the OR.
- The airway was maintained, and induction of anesthesia proceeded without complication.

On completion of the procedure or procedures, the perioperative nurse is afforded an opportunity to further assess the trauma patient as well as evaluate the plan of care implemented. If the patient sustained numerous injuries and remains critically injured, the PACU may be bypassed and the patient may be transferred directly to the ICU. The perioperative nurse should accompany the patient, along with the anesthesia provider, to the ICU. Once the anesthesia report is given, the perioperative nurse can provide a wealth of information to the critical care nurse. At this point, family members may have been contacted or are present, allowing more specific medical history information to be obtained. However, the mechanism of injury and events surrounding the trauma are still significant. A high index of suspicion remains during postoperative care

AMBULATORY SURGERY CONSIDERATIONS

Outpatient Follow-up Procedures

Because of the extensive nature of some traumatic injuries, many trauma patients need further surgeries. Often follow-up procedures are performed on an outpatient basis. The perioperative nurse's care and planning for these patients must include an awareness of the physiologic and psychologic effects of the previous trauma. Preoperative teaching should include an assessment of the knowledge acquired by the patient and caregiver(s) from previous admission as well as the coping strategies they have been using. Maintaining the same routine as much as possible will help with the psychologic adjustment to yet another procedure. Pain assessment by the perioperative nurse is critical and must consider the patient's current medication use, including the duration of use as well as the medication's effectiveness. It is imperative to consider that this procedure will likely change the focus and severity of the pain and that additional or different medications may be necessary postoperatively.

Modified from Association of periOperative Registered Nurses (AORN): Preoperative patient care in the ambulatory setting guideline. In *Perioperative standards and recommended practices*, Denver, 2012, The Association.

of the patient sustaining multiple injuries. Attention can be diverted from a less significant injury in the presence of a highly visible or obvious trauma. Once the obvious trauma undergoes intervention, pain or discomfort from other injuries becomes more apparent. In the care of a patient with neurologic deficit, physical assessment and continued evaluation are essential because patient self-report is nonexistent.

The nurse should also report the status of progress in the secondary assessment. Any additional laboratory work or interventions that have yet to be completed should be discussed. It is imperative in a thorough examination to view the back of the patient in an effort to locate all injuries.

Additional diagnostic procedures may be required after completion of the surgical procedure if the patient's condition is stable. The perioperative nurse may be requested to accompany the patient to the diagnostic department with the anesthesia provider. In addition, respiratory care personnel may assist in patient transport and maintenance of the airway.

Patient and Family Education and Discharge Planning

Traumatic injury to a family member or significant other occurs without warning. Patients may be traveling or visiting out of town or state at the time of injury. Families or friends involved in a MVC may be triaged to several different facilities based on severity of injury or age. A family member or significant other may not be contacted until several hours or even days after the injury. Sometimes the patient's identity either is unknown or must be kept confidential to prevent further harm. Both the patient and the family member are truly victims of traumatic injury. Consequently, patients and family members are in a time of crisis.

Some families may handle the crisis with ease, whereas others become dysfunctional. Coping strategies may be inappropriate at times as the patient and family attempt to reestablish patterns of function. A family system already taxed before the event may be overwhelmed with the additional stress of a sudden traumatic event. On the other hand, family members may wish to be present during resuscitation efforts. Family presence requires a facilitator to explain

procedures and the accompanying sights, sounds, and smells that may occur. Nurses base their decisions on medical concerns, which may be very different than patient and/or family concerns. In trauma situations, nurses do not know their patient's preferences and may even be unaware that differences in opinion exist. Care may be improved when understandable terms are used to explain the situation, to provide realistic expectations, and to relay when clinicians will be available to answer questions (Murray, 2008).

The perioperative nurse must be prepared for a variety of responses, both from the patient and from the family or significant others. Interaction with the patient before surgical intervention may be impossible because of the severity of the injury, prior intubation, or hemodynamic instability. The perioperative nurse will need to offer brief, simple instructions and explanations if the patient is conscious. These may include the following:

- Background noise as caregivers prepare for emergent intervention
- Perception of cold within the OR room
- Placement of safety and restraining straps, armboards, warming devices, and pneumatic compression stockings, for example
- Invasive interventions, such as additional IV access or arterial line monitoring

A reassuring touch or holding the patient's hand may be the only communication possible. Touch, placement of warm blankets, a gentle squeeze of the hand, and softly spoken words of reassurance are important comfort measures.

In accordance with hospital policies and procedures, the perioperative nurse may call the surgical waiting room with periodic updates on the patient's condition. The information shared is subject to the surgeon's discretion and is usually concise in nature, such as, "At this time the extent of injury is unknown; his/her condition is critical." When implemented, these contacts with family members are appreciated because frequently they were unable to see or speak with the patient before surgery.

All of the patient's injuries and possible subsequent complications may not be known at the time of operative intervention. The multiply injured patient frequently requires rehabilitation or an extended stay in a skilled nursing facility before discharge to home. In addition to coping with physical changes, some patients may experience post-traumatic stress disorder. Continued therapy, such as neuropsychology (for cognitive impairment) or occupational and physical therapy, may be provided on an outpatient basis. Consequently, information regarding recovery and rehabilitation is limited on admission to the hospital. Many facilities have access to or provide support groups for patients and families related to the type of injury and its subsequent lifelong effects.

End-of-Life Care

Unfortunately some accidental injuries result in death. Many facilities have a chaplain or social worker available to assist family members during this time of crisis. These caregivers assist in the initial family contact and provide immediate support. Providing end-of-life care for patients and family is relevant, even in trauma situations. Trauma is different in that the patient and family do not have a prior relationship with the healthcare team. This makes it difficult for the team to know and/or understand the wishes and values of the patient and family.

The Trauma End-of-Life Optimum Support (TELOS) best practice model was developed to provide a framework for optimum support to dying patients and their families. It was designed to be carried out in the prehospital setting, ED, and the ICU; however, it can be implemented in any healthcare setting. The foundations of the best practices are engagement, ethics, education, economics, and evaluation. They direct healthcare workers to act in the best interest of the patient and to engage in authentic relationships that are patient-centered. Furthermore, TELOS requires healthcare professionals to comply with the continuing education requirements in order to remain current with evidence-based research to maximize patient outcomes (Burns et al, 2011).

Critical Incident–Stress Debriefing

When the end result of a traumatic injury is death, it can be particularly difficult for the perioperative team because most surgical interventions are of a curative or restorative nature. In many emergency medical systems is a critical incident–stress debriefing team. It is composed of mental health professionals and specially trained volunteers who are also professionals and peers in the healthcare field. Police officers, firefighters, paramedics, ED nurses, and ICU nurses also may be on the team. In the event of a particularly tragic death of a patient, the team can be contacted, and a meeting with that patient's care providers is arranged. The benefit of this team is enhanced when intervention is timely for the care providers. Opportunity for them to discuss their feelings and emotions is provided and encouraged as each provider discusses feelings related to personal participation in the care of the patient. There are many benefits of critical incident–stress debriefing for the individual staff member and the organization. The debriefing provides the individual with information and resources to assist in coping with the traumatic situation. At the organizational level the debriefing fosters a therapeutic environment to discuss the emotional and cognitive responses to the incident (Blacklock, 2012).

Surgical Interventions

Damage Control Surgery

Damage control surgery is a well-recognized surgical strategy that sacrifices complete, immediate repair to adequately address the physiologic impact of trauma and surgery. Damage control surgery is a series of operations performed to accomplish definitive repair of abdominal injuries with consideration of the patient's physiologic tolerance. The focus is on control of hemorrhage and contamination to stop bleeding and control any intestinal, biliary, or urinary leak into the abdominal cavity. Indications for the potential need for damage control surgery include hemodynamic instability, hemorrhagic shock, coagulopathy, hypotension, tachycardia, tachypnea, inaccessible major anatomic injury, concomitant major injury, and altered mental status.

Abdominal packing is the foundation principle of damage control surgery, first reported in the early twentieth century. Later reports detailed survival of patients with severe liver injuries that were packed. In 1981 a report described operative management that included initial abandonment of laparotomy, use of intra-abdominal packing, correction of coagulopathy and metabolic acidosis, and later reoperation for definitive repair (Germanos et al, 2008). The term *damage control* was first used in 1993 along with a detailed approach. The components are stop bleeding, close perforations; continue resuscitation, emphasizing correction of coagulopathy, acidosis, and hypothermia; plan reoperation for definitive repair.

There are five decision-making stages for damage control.
- *Stage 1:* Patient selection and decision to perform damage control: The emphasis is on early recognition for potential

damage control surgery, including rapid transport to the hospital and early decisions related to control of hemorrhage.
- *Stage 2:* Operation and intraoperative reassessment of laparotomy: This consists of control of hemorrhage and contamination with rapid packing and temporary abdominal closure.
- *Stage 3:* Physiologic restoration in the ICU: The focus here is restoration of physiologic status, which may include rewarming and fluid replacement.
- *Stage 4:* Return to OR for definitive procedures: The focus is on removal of packing, repair of injuries, and closure. Indications for emergency reoperation include massive ongoing bleeding, evidence of bowel leak or ischemic organ, and presence of abdominal compartment syndrome.
- *Stage 5:* Abdominal wall closure/reconstruction: It is not always possible to close the abdominal wall in stage 4, necessitating further repair.

Injuries of the Head and Spinal Column

Trauma to the head is responsible for half of all trauma deaths. Brain injury occurs either as a direct result of the trauma to the tissue or as a complication. Often forces of energy from the impact are tolerated by the rigid skull, but the soft tissue of the brain is traumatized, resulting in the formation of subdural (Figure 28-7), epidural, or intracerebral hematomas. Blood clots are classified by their location in the brain and range from mild to life-threatening. A clot under the skull but on top of the dura is an epidural hematoma, which often results from a tear in an artery under the skull. A clot under the skull and dura but outside the brain is a subdural hematoma, often resulting from a tear in a vein or from a cut on the brain itself

FIGURE 28-7 Subdural hematoma causing increased intracranial pressure with shifting of tissue.

Temporal bone fracture

Temporoparietal epidural hematoma

Uncal herniation with accompanying lateral brainstem compression

Midline shift

Ipsilateral dilation of pupil caused by compression and stretching of third cranial nerve

Displacement of midbrain causing compression of pyramidal tract resulting in contralateral hemiparesis (or hemiplegia) and plantar extensor responses (Babinski)

FIGURE 28-8 Cross section showing herniation of lower portion of temporal lobe (uncus) through tentorium caused by temporoparietal epidural hematoma. Herniation may occur also in cerebellum. Note mass effect and midline shift.

PATIENT-CENTERED CARE

You are the nurse caring for a trauma patient in the OR, who is having a craniotomy for evacuation of a subdural hematoma. The patient's family just arrived; they are in the waiting room and are asking for information. It's important to remember this is a stressful time for family members and that communication needs to be very basic to meet their needs; their capacity for understanding may be compromised by the critical surroundings, concern for their loved one, and prior healthcare experiences.

Keeping the patient first, the nurse should first let the surgeon and anesthesia provider know that the family members are in the waiting area and requesting information. The nurse should ask what information is appropriate to report to the family at this time. It may be beneficial to find out what the family has been told about the situation by the social worker or case manager. When providing the family with the update from the surgeon, the nurse explains the procedure in layman's terms. Rather than saying the patient has a subdural hematoma, the nurse might explain to the family that the patient had a head injury that resulted in a collection of blood over the surface of the brain and that the blood needs to be drained to relieve the pressure on the brain. The nurse assesses the family's understanding by asking them to repeat the information back and inviting further questioning.

(Patient-Centered Care). An injury to the brain itself, a contusion, is an intracerebral hematoma, a result of a skull fracture or other blood clot causing swelling inside the brain. In addition, cerebral swelling can result in herniation of the brain despite treatment (Figure 28-8).

A baseline neurologic examination is extremely important. The pupils are examined, and the presence or absence of posturing is noted. The Glasgow Coma Scale (see Table 21-2) provides a universally accepted mechanism to assess the baseline data for the trauma team. However, in the presence of alcohol or drug intoxication or chemical paralysis, the scale cannot be used. For patients with a score of 8 or less, intubation with controlled ventilation is the immediate treatment of choice. In the highly combative patient, intubation may also be performed to allow adequate assessment of the extent of injury.

Previously, hyperventilation was routinely used to decrease ICP in the initial management of patients with neurologic deterioration. No studies have shown improved outcomes for these patients, and other methods of assessment have shown that hyperventilation can cause significant constriction of cerebral vessels and may reduce cerebral blood flow to an ischemic level. Occasionally, hyperventilation may be necessary with persistently high ICP unresponsive to other treatment modalities.

An osmotic diuretic, such as mannitol, can be used to treat increased ICP. Osmotic effects take place in 15 to 30 minutes (Hodgson and Kizior, 2013) and instigate an osmotic gradient to extract water from neurons. Osmotic diuretics such as mannitol have proven benefits in lowering ICP without reducing cerebral blood flow. They are given by bolus administration to create an acute reduction phase in ICP. These agents are excreted in the urine and cause a rise in serum and urine osmolality. Patients with serum osmolalities higher than 320 mOsm/kg (Kulaylat and Dayton, 2012) are at risk of acute tubular necrosis. Hypovolemia should be avoided with the infusion of isotonic fluids as necessary. Because such agents act quickly, fluid intake and output and the potential for fluid and electrolyte imbalances mandate close hemodynamic monitoring. Elevating the head of the bed 30 degrees and keeping the patient's head midline (to promote venous drainage) also can be beneficial.

Skull fractures usually do not require operative intervention when there is no displacement and the fracture is linear. Depressed fractures or the presence of bone in the brain frequently requires elevation and debridement (Figure 28-9). Hematoma evacuation is based on the location as well as the size and number of hematomas

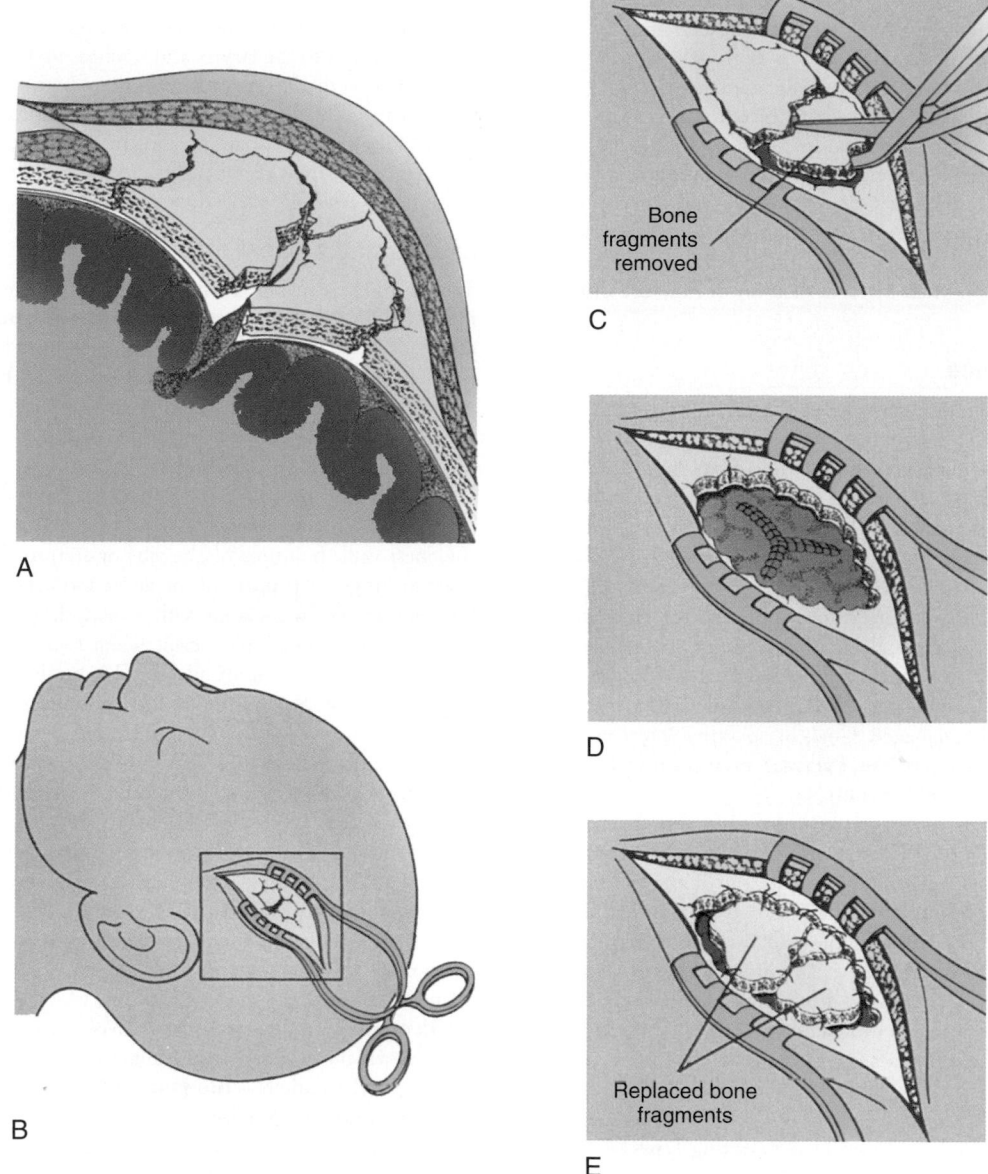

A

B

C

Bone fragments removed

D

E

Replaced bone fragments

FIGURE 28-9 Treatment of compound depressed fracture of skull. **A,** Depressed skull fracture and scalp injury. **B,** Incision to expose fracture and remove the portion of the scalp that is devitalized. **C,** Removal of impacted bone by burr hole to locate and identify normal dura, followed by resection of bone fragments. **D,** Watertight closure of dura after brain debridement. **E,** Replacement and fixation of bone fragments.

present. Before performing a craniotomy or drilling a burr hole, the CT scan, the neurologic status of the patient, the morbidity or mortality associated with the procedure, and the presence of other injuries or underlying medical problems, if known, are evaluated. An ICP monitor may be placed in the patient who is at risk for increased ICP. (Chapter 21 discusses neurosurgical procedures.)

The patient with a cervical spine injury at or near C3 to C5 is at great risk for respiratory difficulties because this is the area of diaphragmatic innervation. There is also the possibility of swelling above the area of injury, and the perioperative nurse should be alert for the potential of respiratory distress even if it is not initially present. A 24- to 48-hour dose of methylprednisolone (Solu-Medrol), calculated by body weight, is considered to decrease initial cord swelling.

The standard indicators of possible cord injury are absence of rectal tone and bradycardia in the presence of hypotension. The body's normal response is to increase heart rate in the presence of decreased blood flow or hypotension. These responses are not present in injury of the spinal cord, and vagal control results in bradycardia.

Injuries involving the spinal cord can range from a contusion of the cord to complete transection, without hope of recovery. Fractures or dislocation of a vertebra can result in the protrusion of small pieces into the spinal canal. This is known as a *burst fracture*. Several vertebrae may be fractured or have fractured components. The decision to surgically treat vertebral fractures is based on many factors. In patients with minimal compression and no neurologic signs or symptoms, spinal bracing may be an option. Cerebral arteriography may be used to screen patients with cervical vertebral fractures for blunt vertebral artery injuries (BVIs). According to deSouza and colleagues current literature recommends CT angiography as the preferred method for screening patients with BVIs. Patients are treated with anticoagulant therapy if not contraindicated; contraindications include patients with active bleeding or patients with multiple trauma including the head (deSouza et al, 2011).

Treating spinal column fractures can involve surgery. Stabilizing the fracture may be necessary, depending on the severity of the injury. For cervical spine fractures, traction may be used initially to reduce the fracture, followed by surgical intervention as soon as the patient's condition permits. Internal fixation devices are discussed in Chapter 20.

Injuries of the Face

MVCs account for about 60% of maxillofacial injuries. Mandibular fractures alone are highly associated with assault as the MOI. In the patient who presents with facial injury, the airway must be secured. This requires ensuring patency and removing any items that pose the threat of aspiration. If a midface fracture is present, the anesthesia provider avoids nasogastric tube placement and nasotracheal intubation. A tracheostomy may need to be performed before initiation of the operative procedure. Control of scalp or facial hemorrhage can be achieved through a pressure dressing until surgical intervention is possible because exsanguinations can occur. Treatment of the fracture may be delayed until the immediate life threats have been successfully managed. Goals of operative intervention are to reduce and immobilize the fracture, prevent infection, and restore facial cosmesis and function.

Facial fractures can be categorized into Le Fort I, II, or III (see Figure 22-24). A Le Fort I fracture is the most common maxillary fracture. It involves a horizontal interruption of the anterior and lateral wall of the maxillary sinus. Le Fort II is a pyramidal fracture along the maxilla and lacrimal bones and through the infraorbital rim. Le Fort III is otherwise known as *craniofacial disjunction.* The midface is completely disengaged from the cranial base, resulting from a fracture across the frontomaxillary sutures. (Specific information regarding these injuries is in Chapter 22.)

Injuries of the Eye

Eye injuries can result from blunt or penetrating types of trauma. Penetrating objects in the globe are stabilized and not removed until the patient is in the OR. These injuries threaten loss of vision because of the injury itself, inflammation, or infection. Blunt injury to the eye can result in hematomas and accompanying fractures. A blow-out fracture is the result of a blunt force to the eye that pushes soft tissue through the thin bony orbital floor. The eye recedes into the orbit and the patient loses the ability to gaze upward. Surgical repair is often indicated. (Chapter 18 discusses ophthalmic procedures.)

Injuries of the Neck

Injury to the neck and soft tissue structures is most commonly a result of penetrating trauma. The neck can be divided into three zones with respect to injury and consequence. Zone I is the base of the neck below the clavicles. Anatomic structures located in this region are the great vessels and aortic arch, innominate veins, trachea, esophagus, and lungs. Zone II is the area in the middle of the neck between the clavicles and the mandible. Structures located in this area include the carotid artery, internal jugular vein, trachea, and esophagus. Zone III is located between the angle of the mandible and the base of the skull. The primary target of evaluation in these injuries is vascular structures.

Zone II injuries may necessitate an otorhinolaryngologist. Penetrating injuries to the larynx and trachea can be primarily repaired. Blunt force to the larynx can result in a fracture and impose immediate airway obstruction. These patients require immediate tracheotomy followed by repair of the fracture when it is unstable or displaced. Chapter 19 provides specific information concerning otorhinolaryngologic procedures.

Injuries of the Chest and Heart

Trauma to the chest area is the primary cause of death in approximately 20% to 25% of trauma victims (Mancini, 2012). Blunt trauma is most often associated with high-speed MVCs. Penetrating traumas may be associated with violent crimes. Penetrating injuries at or immediately below the nipple line or level of the scapular tips are evaluated for both chest and abdominal involvement. Diaphragmatic injury is also a possibility.

Deceleration injury, such as that occurring from a fall or from striking the steering wheel in a MVC, may cause contusions of the chest wall, fractures of the ribs or sternum, contusions of the heart or lungs, or rupture of the aorta and other major vessels. Rib fractures are also associated with a hemothorax or pneumothorax. A flail-chest segment may result when two or more adjacent ribs are broken in two or more places. This results in paradoxical chest wall movement as a result of loss of bony support; that is, the affected segment of the chest wall moves in the opposite direction. If respiratory distress and diminished breath sounds are present, a chest tube is indicated immediately; an autotransfusion chest drainage device is also considered. Chest tube output must be closely monitored intraoperatively because accumulation of 1000 to 1500 mL of blood is an indication for chest exploration. Penetrating wounds, as a result of either gunshot or stab injuries, may cause hemothorax and pneumothorax as well. Lacerations or perforation of the lung, heart, great vessels, trachea, esophagus, and bronchus is possible.

Myocardial contusion usually involves the right ventricle and can be evidenced by dysrhythmias on patient arrival or shortly thereafter. The patient is monitored on a telemetry unit, and surgical intervention is not required. Rupture of a heart valve can occur, depending on the timing of the contusion in relation to the phase of the cardiac cycle. If valve rupture has occurred, surgical repair is necessary. Heart sounds should be evaluated during the secondary assessment to document the presence or absence of murmurs. Heart valve rupture can occur as a late complication of myocardial contusion. Pericardiocentesis is performed for signs and symptoms of pericardial tamponade (Figure 28-10), which include jugular venous distention, muffled heart sounds, and a narrowing pulse pressure. Patients may present to the OR for a pericardial window either emergently or during the recovery phase.

An emergency thoracotomy may be indicated in the patient with penetrating trauma to the chest in full arrest or pulseless electrical activity on ECG. If a laceration to the heart is suspected and the patient is rapidly deteriorating, the surgeon may perform a thoracotomy in the ED. The laceration may be primarily repaired and the patient transferred to the OR for irrigation, wound debridement, and closure. Otherwise, surgical intervention is initiated in the OR. Wounds located across the mediastinum accompanied by hemodynamic instability, massive penetrating lung injuries, and disruption of the trachea, bronchus, or esophagus also require surgical intervention. Rupture of the thoracic aorta is another injury

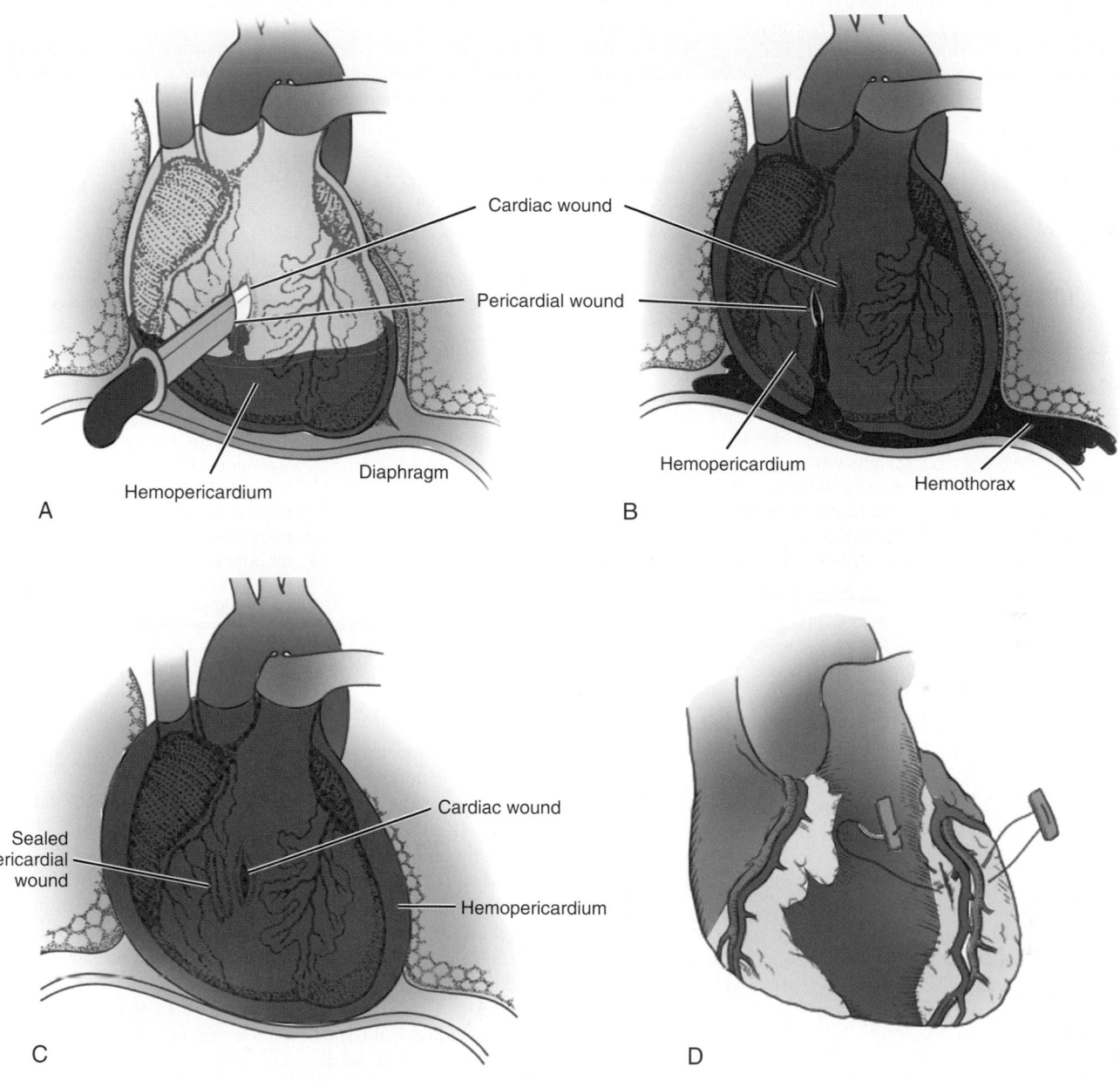

FIGURE 28-10 **A,** Cardiac injury with pericardial disruption. **B,** Bleeding from heart through pericardial tear into pleural space. **C,** Self-sealing of pericardial wound resulting in pericardial tamponade. **D,** Sutured cardiac wound.

requiring surgical intervention and includes the use of extracorporeal bypass. This injury is an obvious life threat but may be difficult to diagnose. An arch aortogram is indicated in trauma patients who may have sustained such an injury. Rupture of the thoracic arch is associated with first rib or sternal fractures. (Chapters 23 and 25 provide additional information about associated surgical procedures in thoracic and cardiac surgery, respectively.)

Injuries of the Abdomen

The spleen is the most common organ injured in blunt trauma, and the liver, because of its large size, is the most common organ injured in penetrating trauma. Historically, initial efforts were aimed at performing splenectomy in response to splenic injury. However, because of the role of the spleen in the body's defense against infection, the surgeon makes every effort to control hemorrhage in the spleen and avoid its removal. Treatment is determined by the condition of the spleen and of the patient. Injury to the spleen occurs with deceleration injuries, resulting in fracture of the organ because of its multiple fixation points. Splenic injury may be associated with fractures of the left tenth through twelfth ribs. The patient may exhibit left shoulder pain (Kehr sign), upper left quadrant tenderness, abdominal wall muscle rigidity, spasm or involuntary guarding, or signs and symptoms of hemorrhage and hypovolemic shock. Splenic injuries (Table 28-9) range from laceration of the capsule to ruptured subcapsular hematomas or parenchymal laceration. The most serious injury is a severely fractured spleen or vascular tear, producing massive blood loss and splenic ischemia. Rupture of the spleen can be immediate or delayed. Splenic

TABLE 28-9

Splenic Injury Scale

Grade	Type of Injury	Description of Injury
I	Hematoma	Subcapsular: <10% of surface area
	Laceration	Capsular tear: <1 cm parenchymal depth
II	Hematoma	Subcapsular: 10%-50% of surface area; intraparenchymal: <5 cm in diameter
	Laceration	Capsular tear: 1-3 cm; parenchymal depth that does not involve a trabecular vessel
III	Hematoma	Subcapsular: >50% of surface area or expanding; ruptured subcapsular or parenchymal hematoma; intraparenchymal hematoma: >5 cm or expanding
	Laceration	>3 cm parenchymal depth or involving parenchymal vessels
IV	Laceration	Laceration involving segmental or hilar vessels, producing major devascularization (>25% of spleen)
V	Laceration	Completely shattered spleen
	Vascular	Hilar vascular injury that devascularizes spleen

Modified from Martin RS, Meredith JW: Management of acute trauma. In Townsend CM et al, editors: *Sabiston textbook of surgery*, ed 19, Philadelphia, 2012, Saunders.

TABLE 28-10

Liver Injury Scale

Grade	Type of Injury	Description of Injury
I	Hematoma	Subcapsular: <10% of surface area
	Laceration	Capsular tear: <1 cm parenchymal depth
II	Hematoma	Subcapsular: 10%-50% of surface area; intraparenchymal: <10 cm in diameter
	Laceration	Capsular tear: 1-3 cm parenchymal depth; <10 cm in length
III	Hematoma	Subcapsular: >50% surface area of ruptured subcapsular or parenchymal hematoma; intraparenchymal hematoma: <10 cm or expanding
	Laceration	>3 cm parenchymal depth
IV	Laceration	Parenchymal disruption involving 25%-75% of hepatic lobe or 1-3 of 8 Couinaud segments
V	Laceration	Parenchymal disruption involving >75% of hepatic lobe or >3 of 8 Couinaud segments within a single lobe
	Vascular	Juxtahepatic venous injuries (i.e., retrohepatic vena cava/central major hepatic veins)
VI	Vascular	Hepatic avulsion

Modified from Martin RS, Meredith JW: Management of acute trauma. In Townsend CM et al, editors: *Sabiston textbook of surgery*, ed 19, Philadelphia, 2012, Saunders.

lacerations may be treated nonoperatively by close monitoring and bed rest or operatively for lacerations of a more severe nature. The surgeon creates a midline incision, which allows for exposure of all abdominal contents. Topical hemostatic agents are also used with success, as well as suturing and the argon laser in some instances. In some cases, angiographic embolization may be attempted. A laceration involving the splenic hilum or complete shattering of the organ usually necessitates splenectomy.

The severity of hepatic injury ranges from controlled hematoma to severe vascular injury of the hepatic veins or hepatic avulsion (Table 28-10). Because liver tissue is so friable and has an extensive blood supply as well as blood storage capacity, hepatic injuries often result in profuse hemorrhage and require surgical control of bleeding. The patient usually exhibits upper quadrant pain, abdominal wall muscle rigidity, involuntary guarding, rebound tenderness, hypoactive or absent bowel sounds, and signs of hemorrhage or hypovolemic shock. Nonoperative treatment is indicated in minor capsular and subcapsular injuries. This can be accomplished with bed rest and close monitoring. Topical hemostatic agents and suturing are used in management of minor injuries. Fibrin glue is also used in some institutions as a topical hemostatic agent. Some surgeons may request to use a kaolin-based gauze. This type of gauze speeds up the clotting cascade process and hemostasis is usually achieved within 3 to 5 minutes (Z-Medica, 2012). More severe injuries with active expanding hematomas or lobe disruption require surgical exploration and may necessitate hepatic resection or ligation of associated vasculature. With massive hemorrhage, control of bleeding is the primary concern. Packing with soft goods may be indicated, along with manual compression of the organ if intraoperative hypotension becomes severe. The surgeon may apply a pressure dressing and temporary wound closure until associated coagulopathies, hypothermia, and hemodynamic instability can be corrected. The patient usually returns to the OR within 24 to

72 hours postoperatively or when his or her condition permits further exploration and removal of the soft goods.

Injuries to the GI system are also associated with abdominal trauma. Bowel injuries may be missed on abdominal CT scan during the initial diagnostic period. The small bowel is frequently injured because deceleration may lead to shearing, which causes avulsion or tearing. The most commonly affected areas of the small bowel are areas relatively fixed or looped. Associated with any perforation of the GI tract is a chance for peritonitis and sepsis or compartment syndrome from increased pressure. Crystalloid resuscitation and capillary leakage contribute to tissue swelling. The resulting abdominal edema creates a pressurized compartment that must be explored to render relief to the compromised organs.

If the abdomen is difficult to close, alternative wound closure techniques may be used to prevent the occurrence of abdominal compartment syndrome. One such method is to use a silo-bag closure, in which heavy plastic is trimmed to fit and sutured to skin edges (Figure 28-11). A sterile absorbent drape may also be placed inside the abdomen to absorb fluid.

In the event of a penetrating injury, the trajectory of the missile or the implement is examined, and organs within the area are considered potentially injured. Exploration is indicated, and the surgeon thoroughly examines all components of the GI system for any perforations, contusion, hemorrhage, or compromise of vasculature, such as a mesenteric hematoma. When an injury is identified, suturing, stapling, or segmental excision may be indicated. (Chapter 11 discusses GI surgery, and Chapter 12 addresses surgery of the liver, biliary tract, pancreas, and spleen.)

Diagnostic laparoscopy is frequently used for direct visualization of abdominal organs to decrease the need for open abdominal exploration. This procedure allows the surgeon to effectively evaluate the presence of any injury and develop an appropriate plan of

FIGURE 28-11 Alternative technique using plastic for temporary closure of the abdomen.

TABLE 28-11

Renal Injury Scale

Grade	Type of Injury	Description of Injury
I	Contusion	Normal urinalysis except possible microscopic or gross hematuria
	Hematoma	Subcapsular, no parenchymal laceration
II	Hematoma	Perirenal, confined to renal retroperitoneum
	Laceration	>1 cm depth of renal cortex
III	Laceration	>1 cm parenchymal depth of renal cortex
IV	Laceration	Extends through cortex, medulla, and collecting system
	Vascular	Involves main renal artery or vein
V	Vascular	Completely shattered kidney
		Includes avulsion of renal hilum, which devascularizes kidney

Modified from Emergency Nurses Association (ENA): *Trauma nursing core course,* ed 6, Des Plaines, IL, 2007, Author.

treatment in the stable patient. However, there is some concern that bowel injuries may not always be identified. Some therapeutic interventions may also be performed through the laparoscope so that the more invasive open approach is avoided. Increased IAP required in laparoscopic insufflation may create an adverse ventilatory effect. In the presence of abdominal vein injury with low pressures, CO_2 could leak into the vasculature and result in CO_2 emboli to the heart or lungs. Tension pneumothorax may be created in patients with a diaphragmatic injury. Consequently, indications for these procedures in the trauma setting continue to be evaluated.

Injuries of the Genitourinary System

Laceration of the kidney is closely associated with fracture of the ribs and transverse vertebral processes (Table 28-11). Because the kidney is retroperitoneal, the presence of bleeding may not be observed on diagnostic peritoneal lavage. Renal contusions often produce hematuria. Gross clots may also be seen in more serious injury, but it should be noted that hematuria is not present in a complete avulsion injury. Management of renal contusions can be nonoperative with monitoring of hematuria. Lacerations involving the collecting system, severe crush injuries, or pedicle injuries necessitate surgical intervention (Figure 28-12). Nephrectomy may be indicated with severe injury of the pedicle or massive hemorrhage.

Rupture of the bladder and urethral injury are most often associated with pelvic fractures. Both blunt trauma and penetrating trauma are causative factors. The type of bladder injury is a direct result of the amount of urine present in the bladder at the time of injury. Blunt forces applied to a full bladder result in an intraperitoneal rupture. This type of rupture is closely associated with alcohol consumption because of alcohol's diuretic effect. Pelvic fracture is associated with an extraperitoneal bladder rupture. Most often these patients present with gross hematuria. A small extraperitoneal rupture may be managed by urinary catheter drainage. A large extraperitoneal rupture and intraperitoneal rupture require surgical intervention. The surgeon may place a suprapubic cystostomy tube, and repair the bladder. Pelvic fracture reduction and fixation are also performed.

Urethral injuries require exploration and primary repair. These types of injuries are more common in the male because the male

A

B

FIGURE 28-12 Renal injuries. Acceleration-deceleration injury may produce disruption of the **(A)** renal artery and **(B)** the ureteropelvic junction.

FIGURE 28-13 Complete urethral injury as demonstrated on urethrogram.

urethra is longer and less protected than the female urethra (Figure 28-13). A fall or straddle type of injury is usually responsible. This injury is detected by the presence of blood at the urinary meatus. In these instances an indwelling urethral catheter should not be inserted. Blood at the urinary meatus may indicate a tear in the anterior urethra. A retrograde urethrogram may be performed to evaluate for extravasation of urine and potential injury. Suspicion of a pelvic fracture raises the index of suspicion of a concomitant urethral injury. (Chapter 15 provides additional information on urologic procedures.)

Skeletal Injuries

Trauma to the skeletal system usually results in contusion or fracture. After stabilization of the patient, radiographs are taken of any body part that is distorted, edematous, painful, or highly suspicious for fracture or dislocation. Treatment of fractures is aimed at restoring function with a minimum of complications. Immobilization of fractures can be accomplished by casting, bracing, splinting, application of traction, or hardware fixation. Femur fractures in particular can be associated with a high risk of hemorrhage and require traction before surgical repair. Closed and open reductions, application of internal and external fixators, and some types of traction may be performed in the OR (Patient and Family Education). The perioperative nurse involved in care of the trauma patient must have a working knowledge of orthopedics. Fractures must be repaired in a timely manner to avoid untoward complications; however, immediate life threats are corrected first. Open fractures are at an increased risk of infection. (Chapter 20 contains information on the surgical procedures used in fracture management.)

Pelvic fractures may pose an additional challenge to the perioperative team. Fractures within the pelvic ring are associated with significant internal blood loss and shock. Systemic peripheral vascular resistance is increased. A method to quickly minimize or tamponade blood loss in severe pelvic fractures is the application of a PASG or PASG trousers to provide stabilization of the fracture and reduce associated hemorrhage. The use of PASG trousers may be effective in patients who are 20 to 40 minutes away from the hospital and have pelvic fracture, hypotension, and decompensated shock (Adler, 2011). If a PASG is applied, the patient may be transported to the OR with the trousers still inflated. The perioperative nurse must be familiar with deflation procedures. The attending anesthesia provider directs deflation in collaboration with the surgeon. Blood pressure and other vital signs are closely monitored. The abdominal compartment is deflated first. Deflation continues slowly while IV fluids are infused to maintain blood pressure. A 5 mm Hg drop in blood pressure requires fluid resuscitation of approximately 200 mL before deflation of the next compartment. If the patient remains stable after 5 minutes of rest, each leg compartment is deflated slowly. The legs must be deflated one at a time, with a resting period of 5 minutes between deflations; if one leg is injured, begin deflating the uninjured leg first (Adler, 2011).

Some trauma centers apply external fixator devices in the ED during initial resuscitation. A pelvic C-clamp, sheet wrap, or a commercially available support binder may be used for initial stabilization of pelvic fractures. Severe hemorrhage associated with the fracture may be controlled by arterial embolization performed in the radiology department if surgical intervention for fracture fixation must be delayed.

Soft tissue injuries of an extremity are subject to compartment syndrome. This is a result of swelling of the soft tissues and muscles encased in the fascia. With a significant amount of swelling, pain is increased and the surrounding circulation may be compromised. The patient may experience a decrease in motor and sensory function. This injury must be treated surgically by a fasciotomy. Incising the fascia allows space for tissue swelling. Several days later the patient returns to the OR for closure, which may require skin grafting for complete coverage.

Hypothermia

When trauma is involved, hypothermia often begins at the time of injury, related to heat loss through conduction and convection. A core body temperature of 89.6° F (32° C) is associated with a nearly 100% mortality rate (Moore, 2008). Moore (2008) reviewed a study designed to determine if trauma nurses check the patient's temperature during the secondary assessment. Only 40% of the patients had their temperature checked and of these 33% were hypothermic. Starting hypothermia prevention at the trauma scene and continuing measures to prevent hypothermia throughout surgery (Research Highlight) and into the ICU continue to be the recommended best practice.

For purposes of definition, generalized hypothermia is considered to be present when the core temperature is below 96.8° F (36° C). (See Chapter 10 for a discussion of the prevention of inadvertent hypothermia in adult surgical patients.) Hypothermia can be classified into three types. *Mild hypothermia* is a core temperature between 89.6° and 96.8° F (32° and 36° C). These patients may appear gray and are cool to the touch. Some alterations in level of consciousness can be present. If the patient's clothing is wet, the nurse should remove it and cover the patient with warm blankets.

RESEARCH HIGHLIGHT ||

Intraoperative Hypothermia and Surgical Site Infection

The Centers for Disease Control and Prevention (CDC) reports, approximately 30 million surgical procedures take place in the United States annually. Furthermore, surgical site infections (SSIs) comprise 38% of all healthcare-associated infections (HAIs). Research has shown that patients requiring emergency trauma procedures are at a greater risk for developing an SSI than patients who have elective surgery.

Patients undergoing emergent laparotomy procedures are hypothermic, coagulopathic, and are at an increased risk for developing an SSI. Research suggests that one intraoperative temperature of 95° F (35° C) during an emergent laparotomy can double a patient's risk for acquiring a postoperative SSI. When a patient is hypothermic the sympathetic nervous system increases serum norepinephrine levels, leading to peripheral vasoconstriction of the skin and subcutaneous tissues. The decrease in oxygen caused by vasoconstriction leads to decreased wound oxygen tensions and wound hypoxia, thus altering the host immune defense system.

Researchers suggest using an aggressive approach to intraoperative warming to prevent SSI and improve patient outcomes. Common methods to prevent hypothermia during a trauma laparotomy are to increase operating room temperature to 78.8° F (26° C), warm water blankets underneath the patient, forced-air warming unit, intravenous fluid, and blood warmer devices using high-flow tubing.

Modified from Seamon MJ et al: The effects of intraoperative hypothermia on surgical site infection: an analysis of 524 trauma laparotomies, *Ann Surg* 255(4):789–795, 2012.

Treatment is aimed at passive rewarming of the patient by means of warm ambient room temperature, warm fluids, and infrared radiant energy lights. *Moderate hypothermia* is characterized as core temperatures between 86° and 89.6° F (30° and 32° C). Warmed fluids are given by IV line and also by gastric or peritoneal lavage. In addition, a warming blanket, such as a forced-air warming device, may be used. Immersion in a Hubbard tank filled with warm water has also been successful. An irritable myocardium may cause dysrhythmias to be present. Shivering may or may not be present. If the patient is intubated, warmed, humidified gases can be administered. *Severe hypothermia* is diagnosed in the patient with a temperature below 86° F (30° C). The heart rate and the respiratory rate are greatly decreased. This patient is comatose, often appears deceased, and requires active rewarming processes. It is advisable to warm the core first to avoid complications associated with rewarming. This can best be accomplished by using cardiopulmonary bypass (CPB), which directly warms internal vital organs, including the heart. The patient should be handled gently during transfers to avoid further tissue injury and stimulation of an irritable myocardium.

In the trauma patient, hypothermia may be potentiated by hypovolemia, hypotension, and shock. Cold hemoglobin cannot release oxygen to tissue as readily as normothermic hemoglobin, and decreased circulating volume related to hemorrhage reduces oxygen delivery to the tissues. The combination of hypothermia, acidosis, and coagulopathy is known as the trauma triad of death (Mitra, 2012). The three parts of the triad have a complex relationship; each may be influenced by the other and often results in high mortality if not interrupted. In hypoperfusion, cells burn glucose for energy (lactic acidosis), which increases total blood acidity (metabolic acidosis). Hypoperfusion may also halt the coagulation cascade (coagulopathy), thus triggering the triad. Hypothermia also affects other body systems already compromised by the trauma. At a core temperature of less than 86° F (30° C), atrial fibrillation is common; when the core temperature is less than 77° F (25° C), the heart automatically converts to ventricular fibrillation (Moore, 2008). Cerebral blood flow is highly sensitive to hypothermia, and the patient may appear to be dead. Resuscitation measures are ceased if the patient is rewarmed to at least 97° F (35° C) and cardiac functions remain nonexistent.

Thermal Injuries

Heat and cold exposure injuries require prompt initial management in the ED setting. Some institutions transfer pediatric burn patients and severely burned adult patients to a burn center for treatment once the patients' conditions are stabilized. In addition to treatment of the site of injury to decrease further tissue damage, fluid management is of the utmost importance in these patients. After hemodynamic stabilization of the patient, burn and frostbite wounds usually require a series of procedures. These patients may have multiple surgical debridement procedures before skin grafting and cosmetic interventions. Restoration of function is important. Circumferential burns may restrict the neurovascular structures during eschar formation. Chest burns with eschar may restrict movement of the chest wall and ventilatory function. An escharotomy (incision of the eschar) may be performed to alleviate the constriction. If necessary, this procedure may be performed at the bedside and the perioperative team may be asked to assist.

Organ and Tissue Procurement

As noted, trauma primarily affects young people. In the event that resuscitation efforts or surgical interventions are not successful, the patient may be declared dead. Depending on the cause of death and preexisting medical conditions, the patient may be an organ-donor candidate. Both federal and state laws mandate that local organ-procurement facilities are notified of potential donors and that families are informed that organ donation exists as an option. Organ-donation agencies can be contacted early and will assist in assessing the potential donor, as well as providing a protocol for donor management once the patient is declared dead. The organ donation agency will also confirm the patient's enrollment in the organ donation registry. The organ donation agency will assist the family members in understanding the organ donation process and convey the patient's consent for organ donation if wishes were unknown to the family.

Brain death criteria for organ donation began around 1968, attributed to the Harvard Ad Hoc Committee on Brain Death. Most organ donations in this country are from patients who experience brain death. In 1980 the Uniform Declaration of Death Act offered an additional option: cardiopulmonary death, defined as irreversible cessation of circulatory and respiratory function. This may present an ethical dilemma to some perioperative nurses. With brain death, withdrawal of support can occur in the ICU or the OR depending on hospital policy. The patient has 60 and 90 minutes to expire. If the patient continues into cardiopulmonary arrest, the team must wait an additional 2 to 5 minutes to ensure autoresuscitation does not occur and then the physician can declare the patient's death (Everidge, 2012). During this timeframe, the organ procurement team and OR staff are present in the surgical suite waiting for the patient to arrive to begin the procurement. Definitions of brain and cardiopulmonary death are not uniform throughout the United States. The perioperative nurse should be familiar with the state's definitions of brain and cardiopulmonary death and the institution's criteria for the declaration.

After a patient is declared dead and becomes a potential organ donor, the patient's family does not incur any financial costs acquired from that point. The patient is not disfigured in any way that will interfere with bereavement rituals.

A transplantation coordinator assists in managing the organ-donor patient in the ICU setting until the procurement teams arrive. The perioperative nurse must prepare for the organ-procurement procedure. The procurement of organs and tissue may take several hours. Different organ-procurement agencies will provide a surgical team, but additional scrub and circulating personnel are needed. The transplantation coordinators actively seek tissue and organ recipients during the procurement procedure. Most organ-transplantation agencies contact the institution and provide follow-up information regarding the ultimate success of the transplantation procedures and information about the recipients.

The heart is removed first, followed by the lungs, pancreas, liver, and kidneys. Tissue dissection is performed in such a manner as to allow for optimal organ transplantation. Sterile technique remains important. In addition, traffic control is of concern during these procedures. Traffic should be limited to essential personnel. Bone, skin, and corneas can also be removed. Some procurement agencies remove bone and corneas in the morgue rather than in the OR.

KEY POINTS

- Understanding the mechanism of injury will assist the perioperative nurse with patient assessment.
- A pregnant trauma patient who is 20 weeks or more into pregnancy should be placed in the left lateral decubitus position to avoid a hypotensive episode and maintain blood flow to the uterus and placenta. If this is not possible, manual displacement of the uterus by lateral abdominal pressure should be attempted.
- Osmotic diuretic such as mannitol have proven benefits in lowering intracranial pressure (ICP) without reducing cerebral blood flow.
- The perioperative nurse must become familiar with the primary and secondary assessments performed with trauma patients. There may be times when the perioperative nurse has to complete the secondary assessment following the interventions to correct the immediate life threats.

CRITICAL THINKING QUESTION

You are the on-call nurse working in the OR when the trauma surgeon calls over to tell you a patient is arriving for an exploratory laparotomy, now. The ED charge nurse calls to give report and explains the patient was an unrestrained driver involved in a high-speed, frontal impact MVC. The vehicle's airbag did not deploy and the patient has bruises on the chest and abdomen. The OR room was just opened and you hear the trauma team entered the holding area. What information would you expect to be reported off during the transfer of patient care? How would you assess this patient? Note the critical assessment factors you would include and perioperative nursing interventions to address them.

ⓔvolve *The answers to the Critical Thinking Question can be found at http://evolve.elsevier.com/Rothrock/Alexander.*

REFERENCES

Adler AP: *Pneumatic anti-shock garment: deflation and removal*, 2011, CINAHL Nursing Guide, available at http://search.ebscohost.com/login.aspx?direct=true&db=nrc&AN=5000013383&site=nrc-live. Accessed October 7, 2012.

Association of periOperative Registered Nurses (AORN): Recommended practices for prevention of retained surgical items. In *Perioperative standards and recommended practices*, Denver, 2013, The Association.

Barclay L: *Guidelines issued for field triage of injured patients*, 2009, Medscape Medical News, available at www.medscape.com/viewarticle/587447. Accessed October 20, 2012.

Blacklock E: Interventions following a critical incident: developing a critical incident stress management team, *Arch Psychiatr Nurs* 1(26):2–8, 2012.

Burns KJ et al: A time for trauma end-of-life optimum support, *J Trauma Nurs* 18(2):97–101, 2011.

Cunningham AR: FAST scan: ultrasound's role in trauma, *Radiol Technol* 79(5):455–457, 2008.

deSouza RM et al: Blunt traumatic vertebral artery injury: a clinical review, *Eur Spine J* 20:1405–1416, 2011.

Emergency Nurses Association (ENA): *Trauma nursing core course*, ed 6, Des Plaines, IL, 2007, Author.

Everidge CS: Donation after cardiac death: ethical dilemmas and implications for advanced practice nurses, *Dimens Crit Care Nurs* 31(4):228–234, 2012.

Germanos S et al: Damage control surgery in the abdomen: an approach for the management of severely injured patients, *Int J Surg* 6:246–252, 2008.

Hodgson BB, Kizior RJ: *Saunder's nursing drug handbook*, St Louis, 2013, Saunders.

Jeger V et al: Can rapid TEG accelerate the search for coagulopathies in the patient with multiple injuries? *J Trauma* 66(4):1253–1257, 2009.

Kumar M: Blast injuries, *Med J Armed Forces India* 66(4):309–311, 2010.

Kulaylat MN, Dayton MT: Surgical complications. In Townsend CM et al, editors: *Sabiston textbook of surgery*, ed 19, Philadelphia, 2012, Saunders.

Johansson PI et al: Current management of massive hemorrhage in trauma, *Scand J Trauma Resusc Emerg Med* 20(1):47, 2012.

Mancini M: *Blunt chest trauma*, 2012, available at: http://emedicine.medscape.com/article/428723-overview. Accessed November 3, 2012.

Mitra B et al: Trauma patients with the "triad of death," *Emerg Med J* 29(8):622–625, 2012.

Moore K: Hypothermia in trauma, *J Trauma Nurs* 15(2):62–64, 2008.

Muir M, Archer-Heese G: Essentials of a bariatric patient handling program, *Online J Issues Nurs* 14(1), 2009.

Murray MA: A question of evidence: decision-making in palliative care nursing, *Int J Palliat Nur* 14(1):45–46, 2008.

Nessen S et al: Acute resuscitation and critical care: massive blood transfusion in patient with hemoperitoneum. In Nessen S et al, editors: *War surgery in Afghanistan and Iraq: a series of cases, 2003–2007*, USA, 2008, Department of the Army.

Phelan HA: Pharmacologic venous thromboembolism prophylaxis after traumatic brain injury: a critical literature review, *J Neurotrauma* 10(29):1821–1828, 2012.

Plummer E: Trauma in the elderly. In McQuillan KA et al, editors: *Trauma nursing: from resuscitation through rehabilitation*, ed 4, St Louis, 2009, Saunders.

Reddy SV et al: Trauma during pregnancy, *J Obstet Anaesth Crit Care* 2(1):3–5, 2012.

Sherwood SF et al: Emergency management of obese patients with blunt trauma, *Bariatric Nurs Surg Patient Care* 4(4):287–293, 2009.

Vegar-Brozovic V et al: Intra-abdominal hypertension: pulmonary and cerebral complications, *Transplant Proc* 40:1190–1192, 2008.

Z-Medica: *How QuikClot works, FAQs*, 2012, available at www.z-medica .com/healthcare/How-QuikClot-Works/FAQs.aspx. Accessed October 17, 2012.

CHAPTER 29

Interventional and Image-Guided Procedures

JENNIFER SCHAADT

Interventional Radiology

Image-guided procedures use medical imaging to plan, perform, and evaluate surgical procedures and therapeutic interventions. Interventional techniques began in 1953 when Dr. Sven-Ivar Seldinger performed percutaneous vascular access using a hollow-core needle guidewire and catheter (Mauro, 2009). This development led to the specialties of interventional radiology (IR) and interventional cardiology and is the catalyst for today's minimally invasive procedures. IR is the medical subspecialty of radiology using minimally invasive, imaging-guided procedures to diagnose and treat disease. The IR procedure scope includes 10 major service areas (Box 29-1), is therapeutic, and is considered a clinical discipline (Mauro, 2009). Interventional radiologists have expertise in diagnostic imaging, radiation safety, image-guided minimally invasive techniques, and patient evaluation and management associated with these procedures (Society of Interventional Radiology [SIR], 2010). This less invasive combination results in lower risks, less pain, and shorter recovery time compared with open surgery (SIR, 2010). Interventional radiologists complete a residency in diagnostic radiology, then a fellowship in vascular and interventional radiology. Further specialization includes interventional neuroradiology and pediatrics. Additionally, IR categorizes procedures into vascular or nonvascular categories. Although this chapter focuses on IR, vascular procedures are not exclusive to IR and vice versa. Depending on the institution, interventional radiologists, vascular surgeons, and interventional cardiologists also perform peripheral vascular work, endovascular aortic stenting, inferior vena cava (IVC) filter placement, arteriovenous (AV) fistulas, and other similar procedures.

IR team members include nurses, physician extenders (e.g., nurse practitioners, physician assistants), radiology technologists (RTs), radiology assistants, and when required, anesthesia providers (American College of Radiology [ACR]. 2009). IR uses radiography, computed tomography (CT), ultrasound, magnetic resonance imaging (MRI), fluoroscopy, and nuclear medicine (NM). NM typically is a distinct hospital department and not discussed in this chapter.

Imaging and the Operating Room

The most common imaging in the operating room (OR) is ultrasound and portable C-arm fluoroscopy. Ultrasound does not emit ionizing radiation, and is used for pelvis, prostate, testicle, abdomen, obstetrics, and pediatric studies. Other applications of ultrasound include transcranial Doppler, intravascular ultrasound (IVUS), and transesophageal echo (TEE). The traditional angiography system in the OR is a portable C-arm, used primarily as an adjunct to surgical procedures, producing limited imaging and quality views (Katzen et al, 2010). Relative to intraoperative CT and MRI, a few large academic centers have these in an OR. Potential applications are for

trauma, neurosurgery (Research Highlight), and stroke treatment, but the cost and facility constraints limit its overall adoption. The traditional care path for imaging and surgery is diagnostic imaging, surgery, repeat imaging with discharge, or additional surgery. Advances in imaging and percutaneous techniques have changed this sequenced care path to an integrated single episode, theoretically meaning a shorter length of stay, less-invasive procedures, customized care at the point of diagnosis, quicker recovery time, and a single anesthesia encounter. This integrated care requires effective collaboration of multiple staff members and physicians on all levels and interdisciplinary cooperation surrounding the new technology. As the adaption matures and becomes conventional in more specialties, some procedure overlap occurs. Vascular medicine exemplifies this trend performing diagnostic, percutaneous interventions and open surgeries overlapping the traditional medical, cardiologic, radiologic, and surgical disciplines (Bashore et al, 2012). This paradigm continues relative to the new physician fellowships and specialties such as interventional nephrology, interventional pain, minimally invasive surgery-gastroenterology, image-guided therapy, advanced or interventional endoscopy, and endovascular neurosurgery.

Radiology Terminology

The specialty of radiology has its own vernacular, detailed here and in the text (Box 29-2). Terminology differences include the use of *physician* rather than surgeon or interventionalist because various specialists perform these procedures. IR uses the term *procedure* when referring to a case, rather than surgery. Many faculties use the term *special procedures* or *specials lab* versus IR. This terminology carries through in patient communication as well. Staff in the holding room area prepare and recover patients. *Modality* is a general term meaning imaging technology. Radiology does not use the term *table;* modalities have tables and table tops. The term *scanner* means either a CT scanner or an MRI scanner; likewise *scanning* refers to the process of image acquisition for a CT or MRI. *Magnet* is another term for MRI scanner. Fluoroscopy is an imaging technique displaying continuous X-ray imaging blood flow in vessels (angiography). A fluoroscope is the modality inherent to the IR suite or specials lab, as well as the cardiac catheterization lab, electrophysiology (EP) lab, neurointerventional labs, and hybrid ORs.

Hybrid OR

A hybrid OR has a fixed angiography system (versus mobile C-arm) performing open surgical and catheter-based interventions (Figure 29-1). Hybrid ORs vary in equipment configuration; however, the universal element inherent to a hybrid OR is its advanced imaging and reconstruction capabilities. These applications enable physicians to optimize their approach percutaneously, distinguish organ

BOX 29-1

Interventional Radiology Procedures

Ablations
- Endovenous
- Sclerotherapy
- Radiofrequency
- Tumor (renal and hepatic)

Angiography angioplasty (see stent)

Biopsies
- Abdominal
- Breast
- Chest, lung, and mediastinum
- Musculoskeletal

(Central) venous access procedures, PICC

Coiling-aneurysms

Dialysis
- Grafts, studies, and repairs

Drainage
- Abscess
- Cysts
- Intrathoracic
- Lymphocele

Embolizations
- Chemoembolization
- Uterine fibroid
- Solid organ
- Radioembolozation
- Vessel (pulmonary, uterine, varicocele, portal vein)

Ischemic stroke-clot retrieval

Pain

Percutaneous
- Biliary interventions
- Gastrostomy, jejunostomy, cecostomy
- Nephrostomy

Thrombectomy and thrombolysis
- Acute limb ischemia
- Dialysis grafts
- Deep vein thrombosis
- Shunts
- Transjugular intrahepatic portosystemic shunts (TIPs)

Stents (angioplasty)
- Hepatic
- Mesenteric
- Renal
- Pelvic
- Lower limb

Vena cava filter insertions

PICC, Peripherally inserted central catheter.

RESEARCH HIGHLIGHT

Intraoperative MRI Guidance in Neurosurgery

The development of image-guided neurosurgery represents a substantial improvement in the microsurgical treatment of tumors, vascular malformations, and other intracranial lesions. One of the most important contributions is the availability of intraoperative magnetic resonance imaging (iMRI). iMRI permits the neurosurgeon to increase the extent of resection while providing physiologic and biologic data of the brain and tissue as well as the intraoperative detection of complications, particularly in glioma surgery. The use of iMRI is relevantly influencing the operative strategy in 30% to 50% of glioma surgeries, resulting in more radical resections and improved neurologic function compared with traditional or standard navigation methods. Outcomes include prolonged overall survival, increased progression-free survival, and preserved neurologic function. Examining age-adjusted death rates at 1, 2, and 5 years for patients undergoing surgical resection using iMRI were 1.9%, 3.6%, and 17.6%, respectively, which is significantly lower than rates reported in former publications without the use of iMRI. Caveats of the technology are its cost and installation within an OR. Currently the question whether the implementation of a costly highly technical navigational tool remains restricted to a very small number of neurosurgical centers or whether it will be a major breakthrough in current neurosurgery cannot be answered, with the exception of surgery on cerebral glioma.

Modified from Schulz C et al: Intraoperative image guidance in neurosurgery: development, current indications and future trends, *Radiol Res Pract* Epub 197364, 2012.

FIGURE 29-1 Hybrid OR containing a fixed angiography system.

pathology, navigate instrument placement, ensure accurate device implantation and function, and convert to an open procedure if warranted. The image processing is done by a skilled RT or physician. Some of the advanced imaging techniques used in a hybrid OR include digital subtraction angiography (DSA), roadmapping, and rotational angiography. DSA is a computer-assisted fluoroscopy technique subtracting out the images of bone and soft tissue to view the vessels. DSA is useful in the diagnosis and treatment of peripheral arterial and venous occlusions, carotid artery stenosis, pulmonary embolisms, acute limb ischemia, renal arterial stenosis, and cerebral aneurysms and arteriovenous malformations (AVMs).

Roadmapping is the superimposition of a live fluoroscopic image on a previously stored digitally subtracted angiogram. Roadmapping facilitates catheter and wire placement in complex and small neuroendovascular procedures such as aneurysm coiling, advanced stroke interventions, AVMs, and carotid stenting. Rotational angiography uses the rotation of the C-arm around the patient to reconstruct three-dimensional, cross-sectional CT-like images from standard two-dimensional angiography. Uses for rotational angiography include visualization of endovascular stent placement, complex surgeries of the aortic arch, transcatheter aortic valve replacement (TAVR), atrial fibrillation ablations, embolization

BOX 29-2

Glossary Terms

Absorbed dose: Energy imparted per unit mass by ionizing radiation; unit is the gray (Gy)

CIN: Contrast-induced nephropathy: most commonly defined as acute renal failure occurring within 48 hours of exposure to intravascular radiographic contrast material not attributable to other causes

Control room: A separate, nonsterile room for data processing

Contrast media: Substances used to enhance the visibility of blood vessels, fluid, and other structures

CT: Computed tomography: imaging method that uses x-rays to create cross-sectional pictures of the body

CTA: Computed tomographic angiography: a test combining a CT scan with angiography to create detailed images of the blood vessels in the body

CTDI and CTDI vol: CT dose index: metric to quantify the radiation output from a CT examination

Deterministic effect: Radiation effect characterized by a threshold dose; the effect is not observed unless the threshold dose is exceeded

DAP: Dose area product; a surrogate measure for the entire amount of energy delivered to the patient by the beam. The dose multiplied by the area of the tissue irradiated; expressed as $Gy*cm^2$

Dosimeter: A small portable device recording the total accumulated dose of ionizing radiation received

DSA: Digital subtraction angiography: a computer-assisted fluoroscopy technique that subtracts images of bone and soft tissue to view the vessels only

Effective dose: The sum of weighted equivalent doses, over specified tissues, of the products of the equivalent dose in a tissue and its tissue weighting factor. Measured in sieverts (Sv)

Equivalent dose: Measures the biologic damage to living tissue as a result of radiation exposure. Also known as the "biologic dose." Unit is the sievert (Sv).

Fluoroscopy: A type of medical imaging showing a continuous x-ray image on a monitor, much like a movie

Gray (Gy): The international system unit (SI) of radiation dose, expressed as absorbed energy per unit mass of tissue. Gray describes any type of radiation (e.g., alpha, beta, neutron, gamma), but it does not describe the biologic effects of different radiations

Gauss: Historic unit for magnetic field strength, the unit tesla (T) is used. (1 tesla = 10,000 gauss)

High-osmolarity contrast media (HOCM): Media composed of salts dissociating into cations and anions

Kerma: Acronym for kinetic energy released in matter; the amount of energy transferred from the x-ray beam to charged particles per unit mass in the medium of interest (air, tissue, bone). Measure is in gray (Gy).

Low-osmolarity contrast media (LOCM): Contrast media not composed of salts; does not dissociate

MRA (magnetic resonance angiogram): A type of magnetic resonance imaging (MRI) scan to image blood vessels

MRI (magnetic resonance imaging): A test using a magnetic field, pulses of radiowave energy, and a computer to image organs and structures inside the body

PACs (picture archiving and communications systems): Hardware and software to store, retrieve, manage, distribute, and view images. PACs replace film with digital images

Peak skin dose: Highest radiation dose at any portion of the patient's skin; includes scatter radiation

Reference dose: An approximation of the total radiation (gray) dose to the skin

Roadmapping: The overlaying of a stored image superimposed on a current fluoroscopic image

Rotational angiography: An imaging technique in which a fixed C-arm rotates around the patient and acquires a series of x-ray images manipulated by software algorithms

RIS (radiology information system): Software for managing radiology, imaging, and scheduling

Scatter radiation: Radiation occurring when the x ray beam intercepts an object, causing the scatter of x-rays

Sievert (Sv): Measures the biologic effects of radiation (former term, "rem"). Sievert is calculated as follows: gray multiplied by the radiation weighting factor (also known as the quality factor) associated with a specific type of radiation.

Stochastic effect: Radiation effect in which probability of occurrence increases with increasing dose; severity of effect is independent of total delivered dose; example is radiogenic cancers

Tesla: SI unit for magnetic field strength approximately 20,000 times as strong as the earth's magnetic field (1 tesla = 10,000 gauss)

Threshold dose: The minimum radiation dose at which a specific deterministic effect can occur

Transient erythema: Mild observable skin reaction to radiation resembling sunburn

---

techniques for tumor treatment, punctures, and drainages. Additional procedures performed in a hybrid OR requiring basic fluoroscopy include arteriograms or venograms, angioplasty and stenting, thrombectomies, arrhythmia device implantation, high-risk percutaneous coronary intervention (PCI) for unprotected left main coronary artery disease, and other complex and high-risk morphology. Combination interventional and surgical procedures performed in a hybrid OR include hybrid revascularization cardiac bypass graft (CABG), and PCI in the same setting, and congenital, structural and heart valve interventions.

Location. The location of a hybrid OR depends on the facility design, physicians, and procedures. New construction tends to locate a hybrid OR near the cardiac catheterization lab, IR, OR, or vascular lab. Such adjacencies bring economies of scale because

these services use the same support space, imaging equipment, anesthesia, recovery, and supplies, as well as shared expertise (Schaadt and Landau, 2013). Facilities retrofitting typically convert an existing OR or interventional or catheterization lab into a hybrid room. Planning considerations regarding hybrid OR placement in a facility include procedure diversity, physicians, building constraints, and technology. In addition to imaging are numerous adjunctive technologies requiring advanced and expert planning prior to installing a hybrid OR (Landau, 2011).

Personnel and Staffing Requirements for a Hybrid OR. Hybrid ORs are complex work environments. There are no specific regulations or practices regarding skill sets and staffing patterns for a hybrid OR. Team representatives typically have a blended skill set of IR, surgery, and radiology. Although team members vary, an underlying key success factor is the interdisciplinary collaboration required to work in the room and optimize patient care. The personnel profile should include an open-minded attitude toward innovation, excellent communication skills, and a willingness to change traditional processes. Process change is perhaps the biggest obstacle to overcome because the standard workflow and processes inherent to each specialty must merge. There may be significant changes regarding the procedure approach, equipment, and environment depending on the core skill sets of staff. Moreover, in some cases the procedures are evolving, and best practice or standard workflow has not yet been established. When the processes, roles, and responsibilities become defined and standardized the benefits of a hybrid OR can be realized.

Radiology Nursing

The role of the nurse in radiology varies according to the site, modality, and department organization and the level of expertise. The practice analysis of radiology nursing (Center for Nursing Education and Testing [CNET], 2010) defined nine broad areas of nursing practice within both diagnostic IR roles.

1. Access patient and plan care.
2. Administer, monitor and evaluate therapeutic interventions.
3. Teach patient and family.
4. Provide a supportive environment.
5. Provide a safe environment.
6. Manage emergency situations.
7. Participate in quality assurance improvement activities.
8. Participate in facility interdisciplinary activities including clinical, legal, and ethical issues.
9. Participate in professional practice activities.

While the nurses' focus has always been on patient safety and advocacy, today's radiology nurse expands this focus across the entire continuum of radiology services, beginning with scheduling through follow-up postdischarge. The nursing process is intertwined with carefully designed, interdisciplinary protocols ensuring patient safety in a regulatory compliant and cost-effective environment (Kandarpa and Machan, 2011).

There is no specific academic educational preparation for radiology nursing. Typical qualifications are prior experience in critical care nursing, emergency nursing, the cardiac catheterization lab, conscious sedation, advanced cardiac life support (ACLS), and pediatric advanced life support (PALS) (ACR and Society of Interventional Radiology [SIR], 2010.) Nursing practice should be in accordance with the American Nurses Association (ANA) and the Association for Radiologic and Imaging Nursing (ARIN) standards, and other established nursing guidelines. The ANA recognizes ARIN as a specialty with its own certifying exam, using the credentials certified radiology nurse (CRN). As always, nurses must practice within their scope of professional practice as per state licensing, national associations, regulatory agencies, and institutional policies and procedures.

Interventional Radiology Nursing

There is a clear delineation between the physician practice of diagnostic radiology and IR, but not necessarily for nursing. Depending on the institution, physician expertise, and case load, nurses may rotate or float from diagnostic radiology to IR. In other institutions, diagnostic and IR registered nurses (RNs) are separate departments, with different reporting structure, physician oversight, and dedicated staff. Nurses working within radiology may also work in the holding area. Because IR is procedure based, it requires a higher

standard of patient care than general radiology. The scope of IR nursing practice is diverse and includes patient education, preprocedure planning, circulating, scrubbing, administering conscious sedation, patient recovery, and postprocedure discharge planning. The procedures performed encompass many different organ systems, various pathologies, and disease processes and are performed in different environments using a variety of imaging technology. As with traditional surgery, patient safety, procedural setup, instrumentation, medications, conscious sedation-monitoring, patient assessment, and complication management are IR nursing responsibilities. In IR the concomitant use of various imaging modalities creates a different environment and new dimension of patient care.

Imaging Overview

The field of IR incorporates the same imaging technology (modalities) inherent to diagnostic radiology (e.g., radiography, CT, ultrasound, MRI, and fluoroscopy). IR is therapeutic, requiring a higher standard of care than diagnostic radiology. In many instances the modality establishes nursing practice. Hence, a high level understanding of each imaging technology, contrast agents, and radiation physics is important for the perioperative nurse.

Radiography. Radiography is the most common study ordered in hospitals. The correct terminology for radiologic images is radiography, films or images, not x-ray. Historically radiography studies required film. Today most radiography systems are filmless, known as computed radiography (CR) or digital radiography (DR). Instead of film, a photosensitive layer on a flat detector absorbs the energy, and converts it into photons captured for interpretation as a pixel. A computer converts the digital data into an image. X-rays can alter cellular activity resulting in damage to deoxyribonucleic acid (DNA). For this reason it is imperative to consider the benefit-versus-risk ratio when ordering medical imaging studies using ionizing radiation (Erkonen and Smith, 2009).

CT Scan. A CT scan enables the clinician to review anatomic cross sections (slices) and three-dimensional images of the body using a combination of x-rays, x-ray detectors, and a computer. X-ray beams pass through sections of the patient as the patient traverses through the scanner. The detectors rotate, collecting a large amount of data reconstructed via computer to generate an image. CT studies are fast and rule out or determine the extent of any type of acute trauma, bleed, or injury as well as ongoing progression or resolution of a disease or condition. CT imaging assists with the planning and administering of radiation cancer treatments, surgical planning, guiding biopsies, and other minimally invasive procedures. CT contrast agents are either barium, for GI studies, or an iodine-based contrast injection given intravenously.

Fluoroscopy. Fluoroscopy is real-time continuous x-ray. Ionizing radiation passes through the patient collected by an intensifier or flat detector and digitally recorded and transmitted into moving images on a screen. Cardiac catheterization labs, electrophysiology (EP) labs, IR, and vascular and hybrid ORs use fluoroscopy for diagnostic and therapeutic procedures to determine catheter and device placement using iodine-based contrast agents.

MRI. MRI is a radiology technique using magnets, radio waves, and a computer to produce images of body structures. The MRI scanner is a tube surrounded by a giant circular magnet with the patient placed on a movable table inserted into the magnet. The magnet

RESEARCH HIGHLIGHT

Whole-Body MRI for Evaluation of Atherosclerosis in Asymptomatic Individuals

Various diagnostic methods are available to evaluate the presence of atherosclerosis; however, only some are suitable for asymptomatic patients. This study examined the use of whole-body magnetic resonance imaging (MRI) and magnetic resonance angiography (MRA) in the screening of 138 asymptomatic individuals, 118 males and 20 females, with a mean age of 54. There was no report or documentation of any cardiovascular (CV) and malignant disease by patients and their healthcare practitioners. Relevant findings were those leading to a physician referral and further diagnostic workup or therapy. Approximately 25% of the patients had vascular abnormalities. Significant luminal narrowing was apparent in 12.3% of the study population. Mild to severe narrowing was apparent in 0.7% of subjects in the renal arteries, 5% in the carotids, 2.2 % in the pelvic and upper leg, and 12.3% of arteries in the lower leg. Cardiac function and perfusion imaging revealed 4.3% of patients with ventricular wall motion disorders. The first evidence of CV disease may be a fatal event such as myocardial infarction or stroke. Thus early detection and diagnosis of CV disease permit the initiation of secondary preventive measures. MRI and MRA represent a compelling noninvasive modality, lacking ionizing radiation and a lower risk of nephrotoxicity compared with iodinated contrast agents used in other imaging modalities.

Modified from Laible M et al: Whole body MRI and MRA for evaluation of the prevalence of atherosclerosis in a cohort of subjectively healthy individuals, *Insights Imag* 3(5):485–493, 2012.

creates a strong magnetic field aligning the protons of hydrogen atoms, which are then subject to radio waves. This spins the various protons of the specific body part being imaged producing a faint signal detected and amplified by coils. A computer receives and processes these signals generating an image. A magnetic resonance angiogram (MRA) is a type of MRI scan using a magnetic field and pulses of radio wave energy to image blood vessels. MRI scan times range anywhere from 30 minutes to several hours depending on the number of studies, requirement for contrast, and area of the body imaged. It is excellent for soft tissue anomalies and musculoskeletal studies as well as the abdomen, pelvis, brain, and spine and in other diagnostic applications (Research Highlight). The generation of a magnetic field requires a closed space, resulting in noise. Claustrophobic patients may require sedation. Contraindications for MRI include patients with implanted metal devices (e.g., pacemakers, defibrillators, plates, screws, and aneurysm clips or any foreign body [shrapnel]). Although MRI does not use ionizing radiation, it is crucial for those working in the environment to adhere to the ferrous metal guidelines protecting the patient and staff from injury (Patient Safety).

Ultrasound. Ultrasound produces sectional images or slices in multiple planes much like CT and MRI. Ultrasound uses the interaction of high-frequency sound waves to form the image. As these sound waves strike different tissue densities, a transducer measures the sound waves and an image results by converting the echoes into electrical impulses. Ultrasound does not use ionizing radiation. Applications include obstetrics, vascular studies, and abdominal studies (kidney, liver, gallbladder, pancrease) and for visualization during fluid drainage or biopsy procedures. Color flow Doppler

uses ultrasound technology to quantify the direction and velocity of blood flow in vascular and cardiac diagnostic and surgical applications.

Radiation Physics

Ionizing Radiation. Radiation is present naturally in the environment and is manmade. The use of medical imaging began with the discovery of x-ray in 1895. An x-ray is a form of ionizing radiation present within the portion of the electromagnetic spectrum (Figure 29-2). The ions liberated may produce cell injury by damaging the DNA molecules through the ionizing effects on DNA or indirectly through the formation of free radicals. The categories of radiation effects are deterministic and stochastic effects (Holmes, 2011). A deterministic effect occurs when individuals receive greater than a threshold radiation dose, with the severity of the effect depending on the amount of radiation and tissue exposed (Table 29-1). Stochastic effects refer to the probability of suffering a disease due to the cumulative exposure of radiation over years, for example, radiation-induced cancers, such as leukemia.

The U.S. population's total exposure to ionizing radiation has nearly doubled over the past two decades (National Council on Radiation Protection and Measurements [NCRP], 2009) as a result of increased exposure from CT, nuclear medicine, and interventional fluoroscopy. The NCRP (2009) estimates the increased incidence of radiation-induced skin injury cases will grow resulting in regulatory concerns regarding radiation exposure (Evidence for Practice).

Units of Measurement. It is important for the perioperative nurse to understand the basics of radiation physics and radiation dose metrics to effectively communicate with colleagues and patients, as well as for documentation, monitoring, and quality assurance. Different units of measure describe radiation dose. The Health Physics Society Position Statement (2012) advocates the exclusive use of the international system of units (SI) for radiologic quantities, which are the gray (Gy), sievert (Sv) and millisievert (mSv). For conversion purposes:

$$1\,Gy = 1\,Sv \text{ and } 1\,mSv = 0.001\,Sv$$

Dose refers to radiation to the tissues. A dosimeter measures the amount of x-rays or radiation absorbed in a given period. The terms used to describe dose are *absorbed dose, equivalent dose*, and *effective dose* (Holmes, 2011). The unit for absorbed dose is Gy and is a simplistic definition referring to the amount of energy deposited in a kilogram of matter. The Gy does not take into account the type of radiation or tissue damage. The equivalent dose unit is the Sv, and refers to the damage caused by the type of radiation on a specific tissue using a weighting factor. The effective dose (Sv) measures both the type of radiation and the biologic effect of radiation on all the exposed organs (Holmes, 2011).

Radiation dose varies by modality, with CT and fluoroscopy higher than radiography. For example, the adult effective dose from a CT exam of the head is equivalent to the adult effective dose from roughly 100 chest x-rays. The adult effective dose from a CT exam of the abdomen is roughly equivalent to the adult effective dose from roughly 400 chest x-rays (Table 29-2). The portion of the x-ray passed through the patient is the primary source. However, x-rays scatter on contact when interacting with various materials, producing scatter radiation, known as secondary radiation.

Fluoroscopic Dose Measurement. Four metrics exist for radiation dose estimation in fluoroscopic procedures: peak skin dose,

PATIENT SAFETY

Magnetic Resonance Imaging Safety

There is no ionizing radiation exposure with magnetic resonance imaging (MRI); however, the MRI suite is potentially dangerous subsequent to the strong magnetic field. Hazards include metal projectiles, implantable devices, systemic and localized heating of the body, and high-level acoustic noise. MRI generates an image via computer by exposing a specific body part to a magnetic field. The unit of measure for a magnetic field is tesla (T). U.S. Food and Drug Administration (FDA)–approved magnet strengths are 1T, 1.5T, and 3T, with higher magnet strengths yielding better image resolution. For comparison, the earth's natural magnetic field is 0.5 gauss (G). There are 10,000 G in 1 tesla; therefore, a 1.5T magnet is 30,000 times stronger than the earth's magnetic field. The magnetic strength to pick up cars in junkyards is about that of a 1.5T to 2T MRI (Jerrolds and Keene, 2009). An MRI can pull heavy-duty floor buffers, stretchers, carts, and oxygen cylinders across the room to the magnet exceeding speeds of 40 mph, resulting in serious injury or traumatic death. Prohibiting ferrous objects and devices in the proximity of the MRI scanner reduces these risks (Jerrolds and Keene, 2009).

Safety is a universal goal for anyone working within the MRI suite. The magnetic field extends in all directions outside the confines of the magnet. The field strength intensifies the closer to the magnet and is weakest on the outside edge known as the fringe field. Restricted access is characterized by zones. Zone 1 is usually the reception or waiting area. Zone 2 is the patient changing area, restricting public access. Zone 3 is the control room. Zone 4 is the MRI suite, containing the magnet. The standard safety reference point is the 5 gauss line within zone 4. Access within this line is limited to MRI-trained clinical staff. The magnet is always on; therefore, prohibited items in the MRI area include cards with a magnetic strip such as ID badges, credit cards, hotel keys, analog and digital watches, cell phones, pagers, hearing aids, keys, hair clips, pens, and paper clips. Medical equipment, including intravenous pumps, poles, patient monitors, ventilators, and oxygen tanks, must be MRI compatible. The patient must be transferred from a wheelchair, stretcher, or gurney prior to entering the room, unless the transport equipment is MRI compatible. If a patient has a cardiac arrest during a scan, resuscitation occurs outside the MRI suite (ASA, 2009.)

MRI schedulers query patients for metal implants prior to scheduling, with a thorough screening done by MRI staff on patient arrival. Some implantable devices are MRI compatible. If compatibility is unknown, the MRI staff must obtain the patient's operative report, which includes make and model of the implant, and determine if the implant is MRI compatible. It should not be assumed that devices compatible on a 1.5T MRI are compatible on a 3T MRI. If access to the medical record is not possible, or the patient or family is unsure of implant compatibility, the scan is at the discretion of the MRI physician department head.

Fluctuations in radiofrequency energy during the MRI generate heat. The most common sources of thermal exposure are looped or unlooped medical equipment, electrocardiogram (ECG) leads, MRI accessories, and sensors. These include conductive loops touching the patient or crossing the extremities, clothing, and metalized drug delivery patches (over the counter or prescription). Care must be taken when positioning the patient because these items can transmit heat, resulting in burns. MRIs also generate considerable acoustic noise up to 140 decibels (dB) depending on the MR sequence and the magnet strength (Schmidt et al, 2011). Patients undergoing MRI studies must wear disposable foam earplugs and/or headphones. Earplugs can reduce noise by 30 dB. Other individuals in the room while scanning must also wear earplugs.

The four zones of an MRI suite. Zone one is the patient registration area, zone two is the changing area, zone three is the control room, zone four is in the MRI suite, and the 5 gauss line is around the magnet.

Modified from Jerrolds J, Keene S: MRI safety at 3T versus 1.5T, *Internet J World Health Societ Pol*, 2009, available at www.koppdevelopment.com/articles/MRI%20Safety%20at%20 3T%20VS%201-5T.pdf. Accessed June 13, 2012; American Society of Anesthesiologists (ASA) Task Force on Anesthetic Care for Magnetic Resonance Imaging: Practice advisory on anesthetic care for magnetic resonance imaging, *Anesthesiology* 110:459–479, 2009; Schmidt T et al: Lows and highs: 15 years of development in intraoperative magnetic resonance imaging, *Acta Neurochir* 09:s17–s20, 2011.

reference dose, dose area product [DAP]), and fluoroscopy time (Miller et al, 2012). Peak skin dose, measured in Gy, is the highest radiation dose at any portion of the patient's skin during the procedure. This measurement includes radiation from the primary x-ray beam and scatter. The skin dose varies by procedure as well as other factors (Table 29-3). Reference dose measured in Gy is the approximation of the total radiation dose to the skin and does not incorporate scatter. All fluoroscopes sold in the United States must display the reference dose at the operator's working position. The DAP is a measure for the entire amount of x-ray energy delivered to the patient by the beam and is expressed as Gy*cm2. The DAP

uses a device in front of the x-ray tube to measure radiation entering the body (Figure 29-3). Fluoroscopy time is a surrogate measure for documenting approximate radiation dose. Fluoroscopy time measures the time the x-ray beam is on and does not incorporate information about dose rate or entrance ports.

CT Dose Measurement. For CT the best radiation dose descriptors are CT dose index volume (CTDIvol) and dose length product (DLP) (Halliburton et al, 2011). Current CT scan technology uses multiple slices and spiral rotations of the x-ray tube to acquire an image. CT dose index (CTDI) measures ionizing radiation exposure per slice of data acquisition. The CTDIvol represents the total

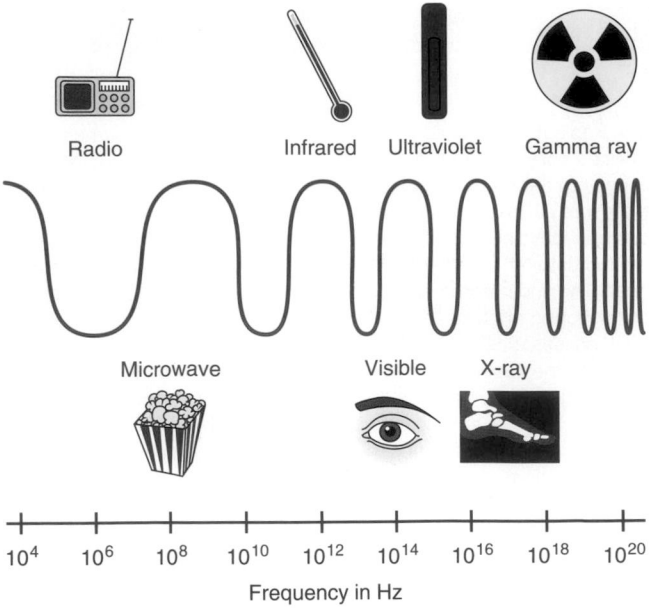

FIGURE 29-2 The electromagnetic spectrum.

TABLE 29-1

Dose Threshold for Deterministic Effects

Tissue	Total Acute Dose Threshold (Gy)	Time to Develop Effect
Detectable opacities	0.5-2	>1 year
Cataract formation	5.0	>1 year
Skin reddening	3-6	1-4 weeks
Temporary hair loss	4	2-3 weeks
Skin death and scarring	5-10	1-4 weeks
Temporary sterility	0.15	3-9 weeks
Permanent sterility	3.5-6	3 weeks
Mucosa lining loss	6	6-9 days
Reduced RBC production	0.5	1-2 months

RBC, Red blood cell.
Modified from International Commission on Radiation Protection: Recommendations of the International Commission on Radiological Protection (users edition), *ICRP publication 103 (users edition)*, Ann. ICRP 37, 2007.

TABLE 29-2

Dose Comparison

	Average Adult Effective Dose (mSv)	Estimated Dose Equivalent (Number of Chest X-Rays)
Dental x-ray	0.005-0.01	0.25-0.5
Chest x-ray	0.02	1
CT scan	2-16	100-800
Nuclear medicine	0.2-41	10-2050
Fluoroscopy	5-70	250-3500

CT, Computed tomography.
Modified from U.S. Food and Drug Administration: *Initiative to reduce unnecessary radiation exposure from medical imaging,* available at www.fda.gov/Radiation-emittingProducts/RadiationSafety/RadiationDoseReduction/default.htm. Accessed March 5, 2012.

EVIDENCE FOR PRACTICE

Strategies to Manage Radiation Dose to Patients and Operators

Immediate

Optimize Dose to Patient
- Radiologists should ensure the proper dosing protocol is in place for the patients being treated.
- Keep extremities out of the beam.
- Maximize the distance between the x-ray tube and patient.
- Minimize the distance between the patient and image receptor.
- Minimize fluoroscopy time.
- Vary the beam angle to minimize exposure to any single skin area.
- Use last-image-hold and stored fluoroscopic image settings to review findings.
- Use collimation to the fullest extent possible.
- Consider the use of other diagnostic technologies such as MRI and ultrasound.

Minimize Dose to Operators and Staff
- Keep body parts out of the field of view at all times.
- Use movable shields; wear adequate protection: lead apron, leaded eyeglasses, thyroid shield.
- Maximize the distance from the x-ray source, when possible using remote hand switch for acquisitions.
- Institute a process for annual education review and competency testing for physicians and technologists.

Long Term
- Incorporate dose-reduction technologies and dose-measurement devices in equipment.
- Establish a facility quality improvement program that includes an appropriate x-ray equipment quality assurance program, overseen by a medical physicist.
- Ensure that the recommended quality control testing (daily functional tests) and preventive maintenance functions are performed in accordance with the manufacturer's guidelines.
- Review dosing protocols annually or every 2 years.
- Establish appropriate dose ranges for high-volume and high-dose diagnostic imaging studies.

Documentation and Follow-Up
Measure and record patient radiation dose as part of the study summaries report findings:
- Inform patients who have received high doses to examine the x-ray beam entrance site for skin erythema.
- Develop methods to quantify late effects.
- Design medical records to clearly document the number and types of interventional procedures received by the patient.
- Maintain a database of all patients with procedure and dose information.
- Investigate patterns outside the range of appropriate doses.
- Participation in a national registry to track radiation doses as the start of a process to identify optimal and reference doses.

MRI, Magnetic resonance imaging.
Modified from The Joint Commission: *Sentinel event alert, issue 47: radiation risks of diagnostic imaging,* 2011, available at www.jointcommission.org/sea_issue_47. Accessed May 23, 2012.

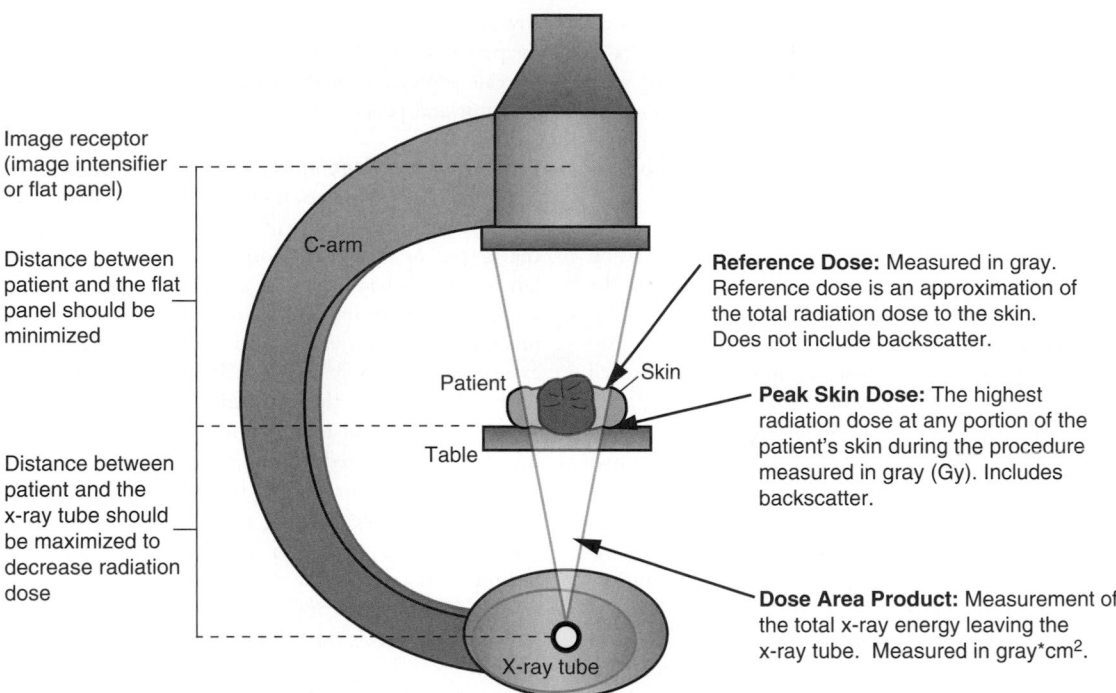

Image receptor (image intensifier or flat panel)

Distance between patient and the flat panel should be minimized

C-arm

Distance between patient and the x-ray tube should be maximized to decrease radiation dose

Patient

Skin

Table

X-ray tube

Reference Dose: Measured in gray. Reference dose is an approximation of the total radiation dose to the skin. Does not include backscatter.

Peak Skin Dose: The highest radiation dose at any portion of the patient's skin during the procedure measured in gray (Gy). Includes backscatter.

Dose Area Product: Measurement of the total x-ray energy leaving the x-ray tube. Measured in gray*cm².

FIGURE 29-3 Components of a C-arm fluoroscopy system and key terms relating to radiation dose and fluoroscopy.

TABLE 29-3	
Skin Dose Approximation	
Procedure	**Approximate Skin Dose**
TIPS	2168 mGy
Nephrostomy	258 mGy
Neuroembolization—head	1977 mGy
Neuroembolization—spine	3739 mGy
IVC filter placement	193 mGy
Biliary drainage	781 mGy
Hepatic embolization	1959 mGy
PCI	2 Gy
PTCA and CA	1407 mGy

CA, Coronary artery; *IVC*, intravenous catheter; *PCI*, percutaneous coronary intervention; *PTCA*, percutaneous transluminal coronary angioplasty; *TIPS*, transjugular intrahepatic portosystemic shunt.
Modified from Conference of Radiation Control Program Directors, Inc: *Monitoring and tracking fluoroscopic dose*, 2010, available at www.crcpd.org/Pubs/Handout-Monitoring AndTrackingFluoroDosePubE-10-8.pdf. Accessed July 3, 2012.

absorbed dose in and outside the slices with a unit of milligray (mGy). The DLP factors in dose along the actual length of the body part being scanned; units are mGy*cm. As an example, the DLP for a CT scan of the head will be smaller than the DLP for a CT scan of the chest and abdomen because the surface area is smaller.

Radiation Dose Factors. Patient size is a key factor governing the dose of radiation. Obese patients, as well as those with larger chests, require higher radiation doses to adequately penetrate tissues to yield a quality image. Radiation exposure to staff occurs as a result of scatter (Figure 29-4). The amount of scatter radiation varies

FIGURE 29-4 Effect of scatter radiation on the operator and other personnel in the room.

directly with patient size (i.e., the scatter produced from pediatric procedures is lower than adult procedures). Other determinates of scatter are the duration of radiation exposure, the field of view (FOV), the intensity of the x-ray beam, and the angulation of the x-ray beam. It is important to recognize that measures to control the patient radiation dose also control the dose received by the operator and staff (Klein et al, 2009).

ALARA. The "as low as reasonably achievable" (ALARA) radiation safety principle focuses on minimizing ionizing radiation doses. The three major principles inherent to ALARA are:

1. *Time*—minimizing the time of exposure (also known as "on beam" time) directly reduces radiation dose to the patient as well as the staff exposure to scatter radiation
2. *Distance*—doubling the distance between the staff member's body and the radiation source will divide the radiation exposure by a factor of 4, also known as the inverse square law
3. *Shielding*—using absorber materials such as Plexiglas for beta particles and lead for x-rays and gamma rays

These principles apply to ionizing radiation in general, but are more relevant to fluoroscopy than CT. Regarding time and distance, CT scans take seconds, with the distance between the CT's x-ray source and the patient remaining relatively constant. The technologist is in a control room outside the CT scanner, shielded from radiation by lead-lined walls and doors. Exposure to fluoroscopy is longer (minutes) and varies by procedure. Distance is a primary method providing protection because radiation exposure follows the inverse square law. With fluoroscopy the distance between the patient and the x-ray tube varies. The team ensures the patient is positioned as far from the x-ray tube and as close to the image intensifier as possible for optimal image quality and minimal radiation dose (Mauro, 2009). Prolonged procedures using fluoroscopy should change the beam's entry point to reduce repeated exposure to the same area. Staff members in the control room do not wear lead. Staff members in the procedure room during fluoroscopy wear lead in addition to radiation protection provided by table-side lead apron drapes, ceiling-suspended lead acrylic shields, and movable lead acrylic shields (Figure 29-5). Wrap-around lead aprons and

thyroid shields with a minimum of 0.5 mm of lead must be worn by personnel in the room during fluoroscopy. Leaded eyeglasses provide protection against cataract development for the equipment operator and personnel adjacent to the operator.

Protection and Regulation. Personnel radiation monitoring is an important part of radiation safety. Personal radiation dosimeters are worn on the trunk (under the apron) and at the collar level (outside the apron) to measure exposure. These dosimeters should not be left on aprons because this would cause inaccurate readings when an apron is worn by another user. The Nuclear Regulatory Commission (NRC) states that no occupationally exposed personnel exceed 50 mSv per year (NRC, 2012). Dosimeter frequency monitoring depends on the institution's policies and procedures and governing laws. Outside the hospital, regulatory and manufacturer initiatives exist to reduce radiation exposure. The U.S. Food and Drug Administration (FDA) requires that fluoroscopy equipment produce an audible warning sound after 5 minutes of fluoroscopy. Other radiation reduction techniques and applications include beam collimation (Figure 29-6), pulsed versus continuous fluoroscopy, digital fluoroscopy imaging techniques, and specific dose-reduction protocols for CT and fluoroscopy.

Pregnancy and Radiation. The preferred modality for the pregnant patient does not use ionizing radiation (e.g., ultrasound and MRI). All efforts should be made to minimize the exposure, with consideration of risk versus benefit for each clinical scenario. There is potential for the embryo or fetal radiation exposure during diagnostic or therapeutic procedures for pregnant women undergoing x-ray, fluoroscopy, or CT scans. Risk depends on the gestational age at the time of exposure, fetal cellular repair mechanisms, and the absorbed radiation dose level (Brent, 2011). With CT, the fetal radiation dose varies with the proximity of the uterus to the scanning plane, patient thickness, depth of the fetus, and imaging techniques. Lead shielding is at the discretion of the practitioner if it will not interfere with the scan field, although the dose from

FIGURE 29-5 Ceiling mounted lead shield at the nurse's station in a hybrid OR.

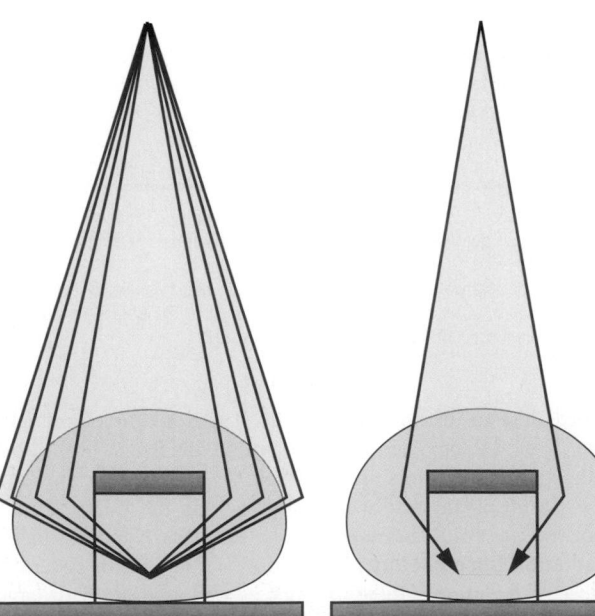

FIGURE 29-6 One strategy to reduce radiation dose is by collimating the x-ray beam to decrease the exposure area.

external scattered radiation is minimal (Radiological Society of North America [RSNA], 2007).

Nursing Care of the Interventional Radiology Patient

Preliminary Evaluation

Depending on the institution, the perioperative nurse initiates patient contact to schedule the procedure and perform an assessment, either by telephone or at the hospital. The nurse provides clear verbal instructions regarding preprocedure lab work or special studies: the time, date, and place to arrive on the day of the procedure; advance directives; insurance information; and nothing per mouth (NPO) status. Most patients are NPO after midnight, although angiography patients receiving contrast may continue water as prophylaxis against the dehydrating effects of contrast. Patients undergoing MRI have additional metal screenings. Same-day procedure patients must adhere to the prerequisites for same-day discharge. The determination of special needs (e.g., interpreters, claustrophobia, transportation) and the corrective or preventive actions are also components of the preprocedure phone call or visit. Most institutions use a checklist for the initial screening.

Assessment

The assessment and preparation for IR patients includes a complete medical history and physical, nursing assessment with care plan, informed consent, patient teaching, and the development of procedural sedation or analgesia planning. Due to the broad scope of IR, it is important to establish interdisciplinary patient preparation protocols. These include the requirement and completion of specific consultations (e.g., nephrology, oncology, anesthesia, orthopedics, gynecology, urology, etc.) as well as specific laboratory testing, urinalysis, and other required screenings and tests. Previous radiologic studies should be available for evaluating and planning procedure specifics. The physician performing the procedure determines protocol specifics including the access site, side and approach, imaging modality, contrast use, and device selection. Other considerations include specific medications, anesthesia plan, premedication for history of contrast reactions, antibiotic requirements, blood products, and use of closure devices.

Assessment includes obtaining the patient's height and weight, a brief history of the present illness, and past history, including renal dysfunction, coagulopathies, and allergies (including contrast medium allergy). The nurse verifies the patient's current weight for medication dose calculation and to ensure compliance with the manufacturer's modality table weight tolerance. For bariatric patients, the ARIN position statement on bariatric patient safety (2011) states preadmission planning for the bariatric patient includes careful screening for comorbidities and determining special equipment needs and history of past procedure sedation. Preadmission information includes height, weight, and body mass index (BMI) calculation. Depending on the patient's body habitus, he or she may be within weight tolerance but the girth prohibits the scan. The average CT and MRI gantry size (bore opening) is 70 cm but does not factor in the table or instruments for a procedure. The nurse or technologist can use an appropriate diameter hula hoop to determine if a patient will fit in the scanner. The nurse performs and marks the initial distal pulse assessments' presence or absence and quality for patients undergoing angiography before and after the procedure. An 18- or 20-gauge angiocath is standard for administering medications, contrast, and hydration. Intravenous (IV) placement is usually antecubital but varies depending on the

procedure, patient positioning, and vascular access. For neuroangiography procedures, the nursing neurologic assessment should include notation of difficulty with speech, visual disturbances, facial weakness, and any motor or sensory loss in the extremities, prior to the procedure start. This assessment provides a comparison during the procedure and recovery. Timing and selection of preprocedure antibiotics should be in accordance with regulatory agencies and facility and professional association guidelines.

Labs. Please refer to Appendix A for standard labs. The referring physician and interventionalist collaborate to determine when and if to stop anticoagulants. Physician collaboration is essential regarding the use of aspirin-containing medication; nonsteroidal antiinflammatory drugs (NSAIDs) and antiplatelet medications. Some patients require bridging protocols (e.g., short-acting injected low-molecular-weight heparin) to wean oral anticoagulants while maintaining necessary anticoagulation until the procedure. The nurse provides clear instructions to the patients on continuing and discontinuing medications prior to the procedure. On admission the nurse measures the appropriate coagulation profiles prior to the start of the procedure according to hospital policy.

Cardiopulmonary. All patients undergoing cardiac or pulmonary procedures and patients with a history of cardiopulmonary disease should have electrocardiograms (ECGs). The nurse gives specific dosing instruction to patients taking any hypertensive, antiarrhythmic, and cardiac medications prior to surgery. Patients with asthma should take their medications the day of the procedure and bring their inhalers. When appropriate, the anesthesia department should be consulted regarding airway management. The nurse should note any history or suspected problems with sleep apnea. Patients using continuous positive airway pressure (CPAP) or bilevel positive airway pressure (BiPAP) at home should bring their own machines due to the possibility of inducing sleep during sedation. Patients receiving sedation should undergo evaluation for obstructive sleep apnea (OSA) as per the American Society of Anesthesiologists' guidelines to identify adverse sedation reaction risk (Minokadeh et al, 2011).

Diabetes. Diabetic patients who take oral hypoglycemic medications should take their routine dose on the morning of the procedure. The nurse obtains blood glucose on arrival to the procedure room via a fingerstick and consults the appropriate physician for insulin adjustment if the blood sugar is greater than 250 mg/dL. Additional screening of diabetic patients for metformin and medications containing metformin is critical (Box 29-3). These medications

---

BOX 29-3

Medications Containing Metformin

- Actoplus Met (metformin and pioglitazone)
- Avandamet (metformin and rosiglitazone)
- Glucovance (metformin and glyburide)
- Janumet (metformin and sitagliptin)
- Kombiglyze XR (metformin and saxagliptin)
- Metaglip (metformin and glipizide)
- PrandiMet (metformin and repaglinide)

Modified from Hodgson BB, Kizior RJ: *Saunders nursing drug handbook 2013*, St Louis, 2013, Saunders.

should be discontinued for 48 hours after the procedure in patients receiving contrast due to the risk of lactic acidosis. The ARIN clinical practice guideline (2006) recommends evaluating renal function before resuming metformin or metformin-containing medications. It is not necessary to discontinue metformin or drugs containing metformin prior to gadolinium-enhanced MRI studies using normal dosage regimens (0.1 to 0.3 mmol/kg of body weight). The ACR (2009) does recommend withholding metformin and drugs containing metformin with large doses of gadolinium, due to potential nephrotoxicity.

Renal Disease. Preexisting renal disease and hydration status increase the risk of nephrotoxicity. The nurse obtains serum creatinine and glomerular filtration rates prior to contrast administration in patients with history of kidney disease or surgery, family history of kidney failure, diabetes, paraproteinemia syndromes or diseases (e.g., multiple myeloma), collagen vascular disease (e.g., scleroderma, systemic lupus erythematosus), metformin-containing medications, chronic or high doses of NSAIDs, or regular use of nephrotoxic medications, such as aminoglycosides. Preprocedural considerations for renal disease patients include adequate hydration, coordination of contrast media volume, and type to preprocedure kidney function tests (Naidu et al, 2012). If risk exceeds benefit, the physician may substitute another imaging modality.

Contrast Allergies and Other Considerations. The nurse determines and documents any prior exposure to, or history of, contrast media allergic reactions. Predisposing allergic risk factors include asthma, renal insufficiency, significant cardiac disease, anxiety, paraproteinemia, particularly multiple myeloma. Common pretreatment protocols for contrast allergies are steroids—32 mg methylprednisolone 12 hours before and 2 hours prior to the procedure or 50 mg prednisone orally 13 hours, 7 hours, and 1 hour prior to procedure; and IV diphenhydramine 25 to 50 mg as per the physician's order. Beta-blockers may increase the risk of reaction to contrast media or increase the severity of a reaction. Thyroid disease may increase the risk of delayed hyperthyroidism, and contrast media may be a contraindication in patients with thyroid cancer. The physiologic and emotional status of the patient contributes to the incidence and severity of adverse reactions. Often the procedure diagnosis is the source of anxiety more so than the procedure. Patients may experience claustrophobia when undergoing CT or MRI, or any IR procedure in which sterile draping around the head, face, and neck occurs. Reassurance that sedation and analgesia will be available may help to allay fears. Other alternatives include complementary or alternative therapies, such as verbal relaxation techniques, music distraction, and therapeutic presence.

Consent. The ACR and SIR (2011) *Practice Guideline on Informed Consent for Image-Guided Procedures* advocates obtaining consent for invasive diagnostic and therapeutic procedures requiring moderate sedation. The physician or other qualified personnel assisting the physician should explain the procedure, answer all questions, and arrange for appropriate documentation of informed consent. In the consent discussion, the physician should explain the likelihood and characteristics of radiation injury, particularly for procedures associated with higher levels of radiation (e.g., transjugular intrahepatic portosystemic shunt [TIPS], embolization, stroke therapy, biliary draining, visceral angioplasty, stent placement, vertebroplasty, and radiofrequency ablation [RFA]). The ACR guideline (2011) notes the omission of IV contrast consent is in accordance

to state law, institutional and departmental policy, and surrounding community practice.

Nursing Diagnosis

Nursing diagnoses related to the care of patients undergoing IR procedures might include the following:
- Risk for Impaired Comfort
- Anxiety related to the procedure
- Deficient Knowledge related to procedure and postprocedure period
- Ineffective Breathing Pattern related to pain or conscious sedation
- Ineffective Peripheral Tissue Perfusion related to sedation, procedural fluid imbalance, or postprocedure bleeding
- Risk for Injury related to radiation exposure

Outcome Identification

Outcomes for the selected nursing diagnoses could be stated as follows:
- The patient will experience relief of pain, verbalize relief of pain, and demonstrate less autonomic responses to pain.
- The patient will verbalize decreased anxiety.
- The patient will verbalize understanding of the procedure and postprocedure expectations.
- The patient's airway will be maintained and oxygen saturation will be within normal limits.
- The patient will maintain vital signs within acceptable limits, maintain peripheral pulses as expected, and demonstrate no evidence of excessive bleeding.
- The patient's skin remains intact, is not reddened, and is free from blistering.

Planning

Planning for an interventional procedure consists of the standard elements of perioperative care, as well as considerations relevant to the imaging modality. Some procedures, such as vascular access, drainage procedures, and biopsies, are done bedside with ultrasound. Sterile techniques for bedside procedures vary by facility. Because ultrasound incorporates the imaging unit and probes near or within the sterile field, additional sterile drapes are used when required as different configurations, probe sizes, length and position of the probes may drape over the field. The nurse ensures the imaging screen is within the operator's line of sight. Procedures performed in the CT or MRI suites must consider the space required for the sterile field. Planning should include appropriate clearance of needles and catheters during scanning and movement of the imaging table. When planning for interventional procedures the nurse must consider the table and the modality (CT, MRI, fluoroscopy) as "integrated." The table is a specific component of the imaging system. Tables have a dedicated motor, are fixed to the floor, and are not interchangeable. Imaging tables are significantly longer and narrower than standard OR tables, with minimal or no padding (Figure 29-7). CT tables and angiography tables are made of radiolucent carbon fiber containing no metal joints to reduce imaging artifacts. MRI tables contain no metal. In a standard IR suite that performs only interventions, the table is a nonissue. However, the table becomes an important planning consideration for hybrid ORs if the intent is to do interventional and open surgeries (Schaadt and Landau, 2013). Surgeries requiring elaborate patient positioning are not compatible with an imaging table. Alternatives include bringing in an articulated surgical bed while

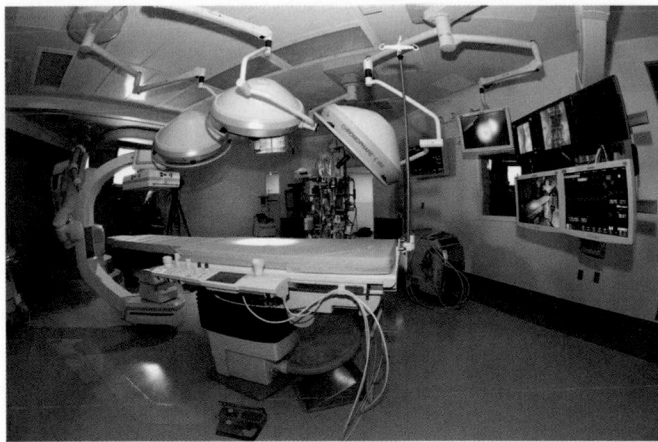

FIGURE 29-7 Radiolucent nonbreakable imaging table fixed to the floor, with table controls mounted tableside.

pivoting the radiolucent table out of the way, or purchasing a core table base with changeable table tops to accommodate various surgery and interventions. As with traditional OR beds, imaging tables, and table tops have weight tolerances. The mobility and range of movement of imaging tables for fluoroscopy is extensive, including vertical, float, stepping, tilt, and cradle rotation to accommodate visualization of the vasculature. Table controls are modular consisting of table side panels, touch screens, and joysticks to position the table, as well as the C-arm and detectors. Physicians may operate the table via table side controls, or the RT may use a remote trolley or foot-mounted controls (outside the sterile field). Because of the table's power and extensive range of motion, the nurse ensures nothing is underneath the fluoroscopy table that could cause significant damage to the table, carts, or supplies. For rotational angiography cases, the C-arm rotates around the patient for image acquisition. Prior to the rotation, all IV poles, tables, patient lines, monitoring equipment, and ventilator tubing must be out of the path of the C-arm. The scrub person should use a plastic sterile drape to cover the image intensifier or flat detector if it will be in the sterile field during the procedure. The nurse places imaging acquisition foot pedals in waterproof plastic bags to prevent damage from inadvertent fluid leakage from the field. A best practice is to use a wireless foot switch to reduce tripping hazards and charge foot switches when not in use. Grounding pads must be as close to the operative site but not in the field of view because they impair image quality. Adequate planning for these issues at case setup is optimal because the physician may request to dim the lights during image acquisition. A Sample Plan of Care is shown on page 1144.

Implementation

The perioperative nurse verifies that all personal equipment, instrumentation, supplies, and radiation safety precautions are in place prior to the procedure.

Positioning. Patient positioning for interventional and image procedures depends on the procedure and modality. Positioning is key because the quality of imaging depends on proper patient positioning and minimal patient movement. Complications from positioning include nerve injury, dyspnea, eye or ear injury, hemodynamic compromise, and soft tissue injury. Patients are positioned supine for the abdomen, pelvis, chest, cervical and thoracic spine, skull,

and peripheral procedures. The nurse pads all bony prominences and uses pillows to relieve pressure points and support the lower back. The arms are tucked at the sides in a neutral position to prevent brachial plexus stretch and ulnar nerve injuries. Patients are placed prone for nephrostomy tube placement or spinal procedures, either with the head turned to one side or facing down. When patients are prone, their arms should be placed in a neutral position at their side or next to their head, extended less than 90 degrees. The nurse pads and flexes the legs slightly at the knee and hips (Dean and Scoggins, 2012). Pressure points include the ear or eye on the dependent side of the head, or on the forehead or eyes if the patient is face down. This position may be difficult for elderly or acutely ill patients to tolerate and may cause hemodynamic changes in patients with preexisting cardiac or pulmonary disease. The lateral recumbent position is used for procedures involving the skull, femoral head and neck, hips, shoulder, pelvis, and sacrum as well as biopsies and drainages (affected side up). The patient lies on his or her side balanced with anterior and posterior support with a pillow or padding to protect bony prominences (e.g., the knees and ankles). Additional pressure points include the shoulder, pelvis, and trochanter (Dean and Scoggins, 2012.) When positioning patients the nurse checks to make sure no tension exists on drainage tubes, IV lines, or catheters to accommodate anticipated table movement. All sponges, wedge pillows, or other positioning or monitoring devices and grounding pads must be out of the field of view for imaging. Any equipment used in MRI must be MRI compatible or kept a certain distance from the magnet (see Patient Safety, p. 1137).

Prepping. For femoral access the nurse preps the skin with a solution of chlorhexidine gluconate 2% and isopropyl alcohol 70%. The physician drapes the patient in the standard fashion using a disposable interventional drape. For nonvascular IR procedures (e.g., biopsies, ablations, embolizations) the patient is positioned, prepped, and draped per the specific site and procedure.

Equipment

Control Room. A separate lead-lined room for data processing of the images outside the scanner (CT or MRI) or fluoroscope (Figure 29-8), the control room is a nonsterile area containing various computers accessing the picture archiving and communication system (PACs), radiology information systems (RISs), and imaging processing software. Control rooms are standard in CT, MRI, cardiac catheterization labs, and IR suites. Many institutions position two IR suites with a shared control room between them. Hybrid ORs or EP labs may or may not have a separate control room.

Angiography Equipment Configuration. In the angiography suite the C-arm(s) and the table move for image acquisition; however, the base of the system does not. The "system configuration" refers to the base location, either the floor or ceiling. Physician preference, procedure, facility structural limitations, and other regulations determine system configuration. Cardiac catheterization labs and IR typically use ceiling-mounted systems resulting in more floor space and easier foot traffic. For hybrid ORs, however, ceiling-mounted systems compete with "air space" subsequent to monitors, lights, and booms. Effects on positive air pressure and air exchange may also prohibit ceiling-mounted systems. Other concerns specific to a ceiling-mounted system in a hybrid OR are the location and cleaning of the support rails that extend over the open operative field. Floor-mounted systems eliminate ceiling congestion and potential airflow issues. Placement of floor-mounted systems is at

SAMPLE PLAN OF CARE

Nursing Diagnosis
Risk for Impaired Comfort

Outcome
The patient will experience relief of pain, verbalize relief of pain, and demonstrate less autonomic responses to pain.

Interventions
- Assess characteristics of pain: location, severity on a scale of 1 to 10, type, frequency, precipitating factors, relief factors.
- Eliminate factors that precipitate pain.
- Offer analgesics per physician's orders.
- Teach the patient to request analgesics before pain becomes severe.
- Explore nonpharmacologic methods for reducing pain and promoting comfort.

Nursing Diagnosis
Anxiety related to the procedure

Outcome
The patient will verbalize decreased anxiety.

Interventions
- Monitor the patient's level of anxiety by assessing the state of alertness, ability to comprehend, and ability to comply with requests.
- Facilitate the family's presence.
- Assist the family in identifying coping mechanisms; facilitate and support their use.
- Reassure the patient and family during interactions by touch (when welcomed) and empathic verbal and nonverbal communication.
- Explain interventional radiology (IR) environment to patient and what to expect to assist in reduction of anxiety.
- Discuss the patient's postoperative appearance (e.g., drains, tubes, equipment) with the patient and family.
- Have the interventional team include the physicians and technologists, meet the patient and family prior to the procedure, and give ample time for questions.

Nursing Diagnosis
Deficient Knowledge related to the procedure and postprocedure pain

Outcome
The patient will verbalize understanding of the procedure and postprocedure expectations.

Interventions
- Assess the patient's desire to learn.
- Assess the preferred learning mode (e.g., auditory, visual) and literacy level.

- Provide orientation to the preprocedure unit, procedural area, and postprocedure unit.
- Provide health teaching and written or video/DVD instructions.
- Plan and share necessity of learning outcomes with the patient.

Nursing Diagnosis
Ineffective Breathing Pattern related to pain or conscious sedation

Outcome
The patient's airway will be maintained and oxygen saturation will be within normal limits.

Interventions
- Note risk factors for respiratory compromise.
- Assess for signs and symptoms of respiratory distress.
- Administer oxygen as ordered.
- Monitor respiratory rate, pulse oximetry, and capnography (when available) parameters.

Nursing Diagnosis
Ineffective Peripheral Tissue Perfusion related to sedation, procedural fluid imbalance, or postprocedure bleeding

Outcome
The patient will maintain vital signs within acceptable limits, maintain peripheral pulses as expected, and demonstrate no evidence of excessive bleeding.

Interventions
- Monitor the patient's vital signs and assess cardiac rhythm.
- Assess peripheral pulses and compare to preprocedure pulse assessment.
- Observe for signs of bleeding.
- Assess the patient for the underlying cause and contributing factors.
- Correct the underlying cause.
- Maintain patency of all intravenous (IV) and other invasive lines.
- Provide psychosocial support for the patient and family members.

Nursing Diagnosis
Risk for Injury related to radiation exposure

Outcome
The patient's skin remains intact, is not red, and is free from blistering.

Interventions
- Implement protective measures to prevent injury caused by radiation sources.
- Minimize the time of exposure to radiation.
- Maximize the distance from the radiation source if possible.
- Evaluate patient for signs and symptoms of radiation injury.

---

the head of the bed, and generally offset at an angle to permit anesthesia workflow. A biplane configuration has two C-arms—one on the ceiling and one on the floor (Figure 29-9). Biplane, as the name suggests, acquires images from two reference points at the same time. Clinical settings for biplane imaging include neuroangiography, congenital and/or structural cardiac abnormalities, and complex EP mapping procedures.

Contrast Injectors. Radiographic contrast is administered by a handheld syringe or a power injector. A power injector allows the operator to bolus contrast media at a rapid preset flow rate, triggered

by a hand or foot switch. The physician selects the quantity, type of contrast media, dilution, and injection rate. Location of the power injectors is either free standing or table mounted.

Imaging Monitors. Image displays for CT and MR are on computers in the procedure and control room. In IR suites, typically two monitors provide live fluoroscopy and reference imaging. Another monitor displays C-arm positioning and angulation, or this information is integrated into an existing monitor. Monitor placement in IR and the catheterization lab is usually across from the operating physician. This is not necessarily the case with the

FIGURE 29-8 The control room is a nonsterile room adjacent to the procedure area that is used for image processing and data achieving.

FIGURE 29-9 Hybrid OR containing a biplane (two C-arms) angiography system.

FIGURE 29-10 Mobile cart for a hybrid OR to store sheaths, catheters, and guidewires.

hybrid OR. In the hybrid OR there are additional physicians and monitors displaying ultrasound, reconstructed images, vital signs, and hemodynamics in addition to the standard monitors. The number and arrangement of monitors varies by procedure, physician(s), and approach. Monitors must be easily movable, particularly in hybrid ORs. Staff members must be cognizant when working in the room to avoid collisions involving monitors, operating lights, booms, and other ceiling-mounted equipment.

General Supply with Disposables. IR suites and hybrid ORs need additional supply space for catheter-based interventions (Figure 29-10). A reasonable number of various sized sheaths, catheters, guidewires, and implants must be available in the room, control room, or in an adjacent clean core. In dedicated IR suites or newly constructed hybrid ORs, custom cabinetry accommodates a large variety of catheter, introducer, and sheath lengths. In smaller rooms or hybrid ORs, mobile carts transport interventional supplies into the room, reducing storage space requirements. Because some interventional suites and hybrid ORs are the end destination for stroke patients, emergency supplies and medications are specifically set aside or available in the room for timely setup.

Supplies and Instrumentation. Needles, guidewires, sheaths, catheters, and vascular closure devices are inherent to most interventions. A Seldinger needle (18 gauge, 2¾ inches) is standard for groin access (see the Seldinger technique, page 1153). Smaller-gauge needles or micropuncture sets are used for axillary or brachial artery punctures, or pediatric cases. Guidewires range from 0.010 to 0.038 inch in diameter and 5- to 300 cm in length. Guidewire selection depends on its purpose and physician preference. Guidewires have tapered tips easing insertion. There are steerable and nonsteerable guidewires, as well as introducing and exchange guidewires. Coated guidewires decrease friction when wet, facilitating advancement. Flexible-tipped guidewires navigate past tortuous vessels. After each introduction into the body, the scrub person wipes the guidewire with saline solution-soaked gauze. The buildup of blood, clot, fibrin or dried contrast impedes the guidewire's ability to advance or results in sticking inside the catheter and possible emboli. Because guidewires can dislodge during catheter exchanges, frequent fluoroscopy verifies proper guidewire position.

Placement of sheath and dilator assemblies at the arterial or venous puncture sites is over the guidewire as described in the Seldinger technique. Sheaths protect the puncture site and vessel from damage and increase patient comfort during multiple sheath and dilator exchanges. Sheaths have a valved end to prevent backflow of arterial blood and a side arm to infuse heparinized saline solution. Selection of dilators depends on the procedure, vessel, and anatomy. After the appropriate dilation and sheath insertion the physician removes the dilator and guidewire together while retaining the sheath hub in place. If a sheath is to be left in place for another procedure or thrombolysis, the physician sutures it to the skin and covers with a sterile dressing.

Catheters are made from a variety of materials in ranges of lengths and shapes sized by the French system. In general the French size is the size in mm divided by 3. Flow rates vary according to catheter types, configuration, and lumen size. A pigtail catheter delivers a larger amount of contrast medium because of additional side holes, compared to a catheter with one end hole. Microcatheters (coaxial catheters) provide access to very small vessels. Balloon catheters have angioplasty balloons. Careful technique during the procedure prevents the introduction of inadvertent air or coagulation of blood in the catheter, resulting in thrombus. Thrombus formation depends on the size of the catheter's outer diameter, with respect to the vessel's inner diameter and indwelling time (Kandarpa and Machan, 2011). The physician flushes the catheters frequently; usually after removing the wire and every few minutes when in the vessel and again on removal to reduce the incidence of thrombus. Interventional procedures require pressure bags with heparinized normal saline, high-pressure tubing, connectors, and three-way stopcocks and manifolds within the flush line for the drawing up and discard of flush, contrast medium, or blood.

Medications and Contrast Agents. A variety of medications are used in IR (Surgical Pharmacology). In addition to becoming familiar with standardized medications, the perioperative nurse working in IR must also have a broad knowledge of contrast agents.

SURGICAL PHARMACOLOGY

Medications Used in Interventional Radiology Settings

Medication	Dosage/Route	Purpose	Adverse Reactions	Nursing Considerations
Lidocaine hydrochloride (Xylocaine)	For local subQ infiltration: 1%-4% solution, maximum 7 mg/kg with epinephrine, 4.5 mg/kg without, up to 300 mg (30 mL of a 1% solution)	Local anesthetic	Drowsiness is an early sign of high blood level of lidocaine	Plasma half-life is approximately 2 hr.
Heparin	IV: Mix 50,000 units of heparin in 500 mL NS or D$_5$W (= 100 international units/mL) Bolus: 5000 units IV (2500-5000 units IV if <70 kg) Infuse: 800-1500 units/hr (reduce rates for older patients, especially females). Maintain PTT at 1.5-2.5 times normal. Check PTT at 4 hr, then 2-4 hr until therapeutic, then four times a day	Anticoagulant preventing the conversion of fibrinogen to fibrin	Hemorrhage, acute thrombocytopenia, hypersensitivity	Reverse using protamine sulfate 10 mg/1000 units of heparin. Drip slowly using caution in diabetic patient taking neutral protamine Hagedorn NPH insulin; very high incidence of allergic reaction with possible anaphylaxis.
Warfarin sodium (Coumadin)	Dose is titrated to INR based on procedure or disease process	Long-term oral anticoagulant	Patients at risk for hemorrhage from serious trauma, pregnancy	If intravascular procedure is contemplated, it is best to discontinue 3-5 days prior to invasive procedure. If necessary, IV heparin may be given instead of warfarin until 3-6 hr prior to procedure.
Low-molecular-weight (LMW) heparins, (enoxaparin, fondaparinux)	Parentally every 12 hr (enoxaparin) or every 24 hr (fondaparinux)	Anticoagulation, DVT, PE prophylaxis	Generally the same with heparin	Tests are less commonly available for measuring the effect of LMW heparin; administered on a weight-based dosing schedule.
Direct thrombin inhibitors (bivalirudin, dabigatran, desrudin, hirudin, lipirudin)	IV continuous infusion: 1.75 mg/kg/hr	Short-term anticoagulation for patients with contraindications to heparin	Bleeding	These medications have a short half-life (<30 min) so they must be administered by infusion. No specific test for measuring efficacy is available; dosage is weight based.

SURGICAL PHARMACOLOGY

Medications Used in Interventional Radiology Settings—cont'd

Medication	Dosage/Route	Purpose	Adverse Reactions	Nursing Considerations
Ketorolac tromethamine (Toradol)	IM: 30-60 mg loading dose followed by half loading dose every 6 hr as needed	Short-term pain management	Reversible platelet dysfunction	May prolong bleeding time, should not be given >72 hr.
Glucocorticoids (dexamethasone, prednisone, methylprednisolone)	Methylprednisolone: PO 32 mg the evening prior to procedure and 1-2 hr before contrast infusion	Prophylaxis against contrast agents and drug hypersensitivity	Hyperglycemia, hypertension	Recommended to be administered before the procedure; however, appropriate timing has not been established. Contrast prophylaxis may include diphenhydramine 25-50 mg.
Aspirin (ASA)	Low dose: PO 75-100 mg once daily as long-term therapy	Platelet inhibition during and after percutaneous transluminal angioplasty (PTA)	Bleeding, GI distress	ASA is cleared from the body within a few hours but its effect on platelets is irreversible and lasts for the lifetime of the platelet (several days).
Clopidogrel bisulfate (Plavix)	PO: 75 mg once daily. May be given as a loading dose of 300 mg	Reduction of atherosclerotic events (MI, stroke, and vascular death) in patients with atherosclerosis	Bleeding, neutropenia, agranulocytosis	The drug is nonreversible; platelet transfusion is necessary to reverse the effect.
Reteplase (Retavase)	Bolus into thrombus 50,000 international units. Infuse 5000 international units/hr for 12 hr, then 2500 international units/hr for duration of therapy	Treatment of peripheral arterial thrombolysis	Bleeding, allergic reactions	Systemically heparinize patient to prevent clot formation around catheter.
Urokinase	Inject into thrombus 30,000-60,000 international units. Infuse 4000 international units/min for 2 hr, then 2000 international units/min for 2 hr, then 1000 international units for 8 hr	Thrombolysis for peripheral arterial thrombolysis, IA infusion	Bleeding, mild bronchospasm or skin rash, fever	Systemically heparinize patient to prevent clot formation around catheter.
Epinephrine (1:1000)	Renal arteriography: 3-6 mcg/ 10 mL, NS IA (followed by 5-10 mL saline flush). Renal venography, celiac and mesenteric arteriography: 10-12 mcg IA followed by NS flush	To differential normally vasoconstricting vessels from abnormal ones whose response is variable; for renal arteriography and venography	Palpitations, dizziness, headache, anxiety, respiratory difficulty	Contraindications are individuals with organic brain damage, narrow-angle glaucoma.
Vasopressin (Pitressin)	Infuse at a rate of 60 mL/hr or 0.2 unit/min	IA infusion for GI bleeding control	Hypertension, angina, and CNS symptoms	Contraindicated in chronic nephritis and angina pectoris.
Nifedipine (Procardia)	For peripheral angioplasty: PO 10 mg	A vasodilator used during angioplasty to prevent or treat vasospasm caused by catheter or wire manipulation	Hypotension	Relaxes and prevents arterial spasm.
Nitroglycerin (Nitro-Bid IV)	During angioplasty: 100-200 mcg bolus into artery	A vasodilator used during angioplasty to prevent or treat vasospasm caused by catheter or wire manipulation	Headache, tachycardia	Plasma half-life is approximately 1-4 min.

Continued

SURGICAL PHARMACOLOGY

Medications Used in Interventional Radiology Settings—cont'd

Medication	Dosage/Route	Purpose	Adverse Reactions	Nursing Considerations
Tolazoline hydrochloride (Priscoline)	Give 25 mg IA (diluted) prior to contrast injection. Give over 2 min	Used during peripheral arteriography to elicit hyperemic pressure gradients and better visualize the portal venous systems during visceral arteriography or peripheral vessels in extremity arteriography	Systemic hypotension, tachycardia	Direct peripheral vasodilator; decreases peripheral resistance and increases venous capacitance.
Diphenhydramine (Benadryl)	Give 25-50 mg PO, IV or IM. Maximum dose during a 2-hr study should be limited to 100 mg	Sedation, treatment of contrast-induced urticaria, precontrast prophylaxis in high-risk patients	Sedation, epigastric distress, urinary retention	Should not be used to treat lower respiratory tract symptoms, including asthma, in conjunction with MAOIs.
Glucagon	IV 0.5-1.0 mg a few minutes prior to study	Used to decrease bowel peristaltic activity during digital subtraction angiography (DSA), or gastrostomy tube placement	Nausea, vomiting	Relaxes smooth muscles of stomach, duodenum, small bowel and colon.

ASA, Acetylsalicylic acid; *CNS*, central nervous system; *DVT*, deep vein thrombosis; *GI*, gastrointestinal; *IA*, intraarterial; *IM*, intramuscular; *INR*, international normalized ratio (prothrombin); *IV*, intravenous; *MAOIs*, monoamine oxidase inhibitors; *MI*, myocardial infarction; *NS*, normal saline; *PE*, pulmonary embolism; *PO*, per mouth (orally); *PTT*, partial thromboplastin time; subQ, subcutaneous.
Modified from Kandarpa K, Machan L: *Handbook of interventional radiology procedures*, ed 4, Philadelphia, 2011, Lippincott Williams & Williams.

Contrast. Contrast visualizes blood flow and structures such as a blood vessel, part of the urinary tract, or body cavities (Box 29-4). The healthcare professional (e.g., certified and or licensed RT, nurse, physician assistant, physician, or other appropriate credentialed professional) under the supervision of the radiologist or physician designee may give contrast if the practice is in compliance with institution or state regulations (ACR, 2012). State regulations, institutional policy, and licensure status govern who administers contrast. The total rate, volume, and type of contrast depend on the study, physician preference, and injection site. Contrast agent classification is by effect, either positive or negative. A negative contrast agent is a substance with a lower density than the body tissues being investigated (e.g., carbon dioxide, air). A positive contrast agent has a higher density than the body tissue being investigated (e.g. iodine-based contrast media, barium sulfate, and gadolinium).

Carbon Dioxide. CO_2 is a contrast agent for arterial and venous studies and assists in a variety of endovascular interventions including central venography of the upper extremity, wedged hepatic venography to visualize the portal venous system before TIPS and for fine-needle TIPS procedures (Cho and Lin, 2011). There are no nephrotoxicity or allergic reactions with CO_2; after it is injected into the blood, CO_2 metabolizes into bicarbonate and bicarbonate reverts to CO_2, which the lung exhales. Contraindications include arterial studies above the diaphragm due to the risk of gas embolization of the spinal, coronary, and cerebral arteries. Likewise CO_2 may enter the arterial system in the presence of cardiac defects, resulting in embolism. CO_2 is used with caution in patients with pulmonary insufficiency or pulmonary hypertension because it may increase pulmonary artery pressure. The nurse avoids excess sedation and monitors ECG, pulse oximetry, blood pressure, respiratory rate, and heart rate. End-tidal CO_2 ($ETCO_2$) is monitored in intubated patients.

Iodinated Contrast. Fluoroscopy and CT use iodine-based media. Iodine absorbs x-rays, resulting in a lighter appearance in areas containing contrast. Classification of iodine contrast is by chemical structure, iodine content, osmolarity, and ionization in solution (Siddiqi and Lin, 2012. Types of iodinated contrast media are ionic high osmolarity contrast media (HOCM) and both ionic and nonionic low osmolarity contrast media (LOCM). HOCM dissociates in solution, yielding an anion and cation and produces undesirable side effects (e.g., vascular pain, nausea and vomiting, bradycardia, and disturbances in the blood-brain barrier). These adverse effects lead to the development of LOCM. There are three types of LOCM: high osmolar (>1200 mOsm/kg H_2O), low osmolar (600 to 1000 mOsm/kg H_2O), and iso-osmolar (280 mOsm/kg H_2O), the approximate osmolarity of blood. Although LOCM reduces side effects, serious contrast reactions and complications still occur. Patients likely to benefit from LOCM are those with a previous adverse effect from contrast media; patients with asthma; patients with renal insufficiency, particularly those with diabetes; patients with known cardiac dysfunction; and severely debilitated patients as determined by a physician. Other circumstances warranting consideration for LOCM are patients with sickle cell disease, pheochromocytoma, or myasthenia gravis; patients very anxious about receiving contrast; and patients at risk for aspiration (ACR, 2012).

BOX 29-4

Indications for Use of Iodinated Contrast Media—ACR Manual on Contrast Media

Intravenous
- Computed tomography
- Digital subtraction angiography
- Epidural venography
- Intravenous urography
  - Extremities
  - Venography (phlebography)
- Other venous sites

Intra-Arterial
- Angiocardiography
- Aortography
- Visceral and peripheral arteriography
- Pulmonary angiography
- Coronary angiography
- Digital subtraction angiography

Body Cavity Use
- Herniorrhaphy
- Peritoneography
- Vaginography
- Hysterosalpingography
- Arthrography
- Endoscopic retrograde cholangiopancreatography
- Cholangiography
- Nephrostography
- Pyelography—antegrade, retrograde
- Urethrography—voiding, retrograde
- Cystography
- Sialography
- Ductography (breast)

Central Nervous System
- Cerebral, vertebral, and spinal angiography

Other Indications
- Computed tomography
- Miscellaneous
- Sinus tract injection

Modified from American College of Radiology (ACR): *ACR manual on contrast media,* 2012, available at www.nxtbook.com/nxtbooks/acr/contrastmediamanual2012. Accessed October 10, 2012.

Gadolinium-MRI Contrast. Gadolinium is a magnetically active compound and the contrast medium for MRI. Although the type of contrast agents between CT, fluoroscopy, and MRI differ (x-ray absorbing versus magnetic), the outcome is similar. Both agents cause lesion enhancement or brightening of the area versus the surrounding tissues.

Contrast Complications

Contrast-Induced Nephrotoxicity. Contrast-induced nephrotoxicity (CIN) results from administering iodine contrast agents. The exact mechanism is not well understood. The ACR (2012) states there is no standard definition for CIN; commonly accepted definitions include a percent change in the baseline serum creatinine (a 20% to 50% rise) and absolute elevation from baseline (an increase of 0.5 to 2 mg/dL). Levels begin rising within 24 hours, and peak within 2 to 4 days. The glomerular filtration rate (GFR) is the rate glomeruli filter impurities in the blood per unit time, and estimates renal function. Creatinine levels remain normal until

BOX 29-5

Estimated Glomerular Filtration Rate

The modification of diet in renal disease (MDRD) study equations are serum creatinine–based equations used to estimate glomerular filtration rate (GFR). In adults the recommended equation for the estimated glomerular filtration rate (eGFR) from serum creatinine is the MDRD study equation and is reported in mg/dL.

$$\text{GFR (mL/min/1.73 m}^2) = 175 \times (S_{cr})^{-1.154} \times (\text{Age})^{-0.203}$$
$$\times (0.742 \text{ if female}) \times (1.212 \text{ if African American})(\text{conventional units})$$

Population Mean eGFRs

Age (Years)	Mean eGFR*
20-29	116 mL/min/1.73 m^2
30-39	107 mL/min/1.73 m^2
40-49	99 mL/min/1.73 m^2
50-59	93 mL/min/1.73 m^2
60-69	85 mL/min/1.73 m^2
70+	75 mL/min/1.73 m^2

*For diagnostic purposes the National Kidney Disease Education Program (NKDEP) recommends laboratories report eGFR values greater than or equal to 60 as "≥60 mL/min/1.73 m^2," not as an exact number.
Modified from National Kidney Foundation: *Laboratory evaluation,* available at http://nkdep.nih.gov/lab-evaluation/gfr-calculators.shtml. Accessed June 3, 2012.

the GFR, as least as reflected in the creatinine clearance, decreases by nearly 50%. Direct GFR measurement is not possible. The GFR is estimated (eGFR) using the modification of diet in renal disease (MDRD) formula (Box 29-5). The incidence of CIN is negligible with normal renal function but increases 4% to 11% with mild to moderate insufficiency alone, defined as a plasma creatinine 1.5 to 4 mg/dL. The incidence rises to 9% to 38% with diabetes, and more than 40% in patients with advanced renal dysfunction, marked volume depletion, advanced heart failure, or multiple contrast studies within a 72-hour period; and more than 50% if baseline plasma creatinine exceeds 4 mg/dL, particularly in patients with diabetic neuropathy (Michael and Breall, 2012.) Management of CIN involves maintaining fluid and electrolyte balance. Because no specific treatment for CIN exists, the best treatment is prevention and the use of an unenhanced (no contrast) examination or alternative imaging. Preventive action against CIN is hydration. If the patient cannot tolerate oral hydration it is appropriate to infuse 0.9% sodium chloride at 100 to 200 mL/hr as early as 24 hours prior to contrast and continue the infusion 24 hours after administering contrast. The severity of CIN depends on the baseline renal function, dehydration status, and other risks. Patients may develop permanent renal failure, particularly in the setting of multiple risk factors.

Iodine-Based Contrast Reactions. Determining the incidence of adverse effects after the administration of iodine-based contrast media is difficult because signs and symptoms are synonymous with local anesthetic administration, needle, sheath and catheter insertions, and anxiety. There are three categories of contrast reactions: mild, moderate, and severe (Box 29-6). Fortunately serious contrast reactions are rare, occurring in 1 or 2 per 1000 intravascular injections of HOCM and in 1 or 2 per 10,000 IV injections of LOCM (ACR, 2012). Severe reactions are life-threatening if not recognized and treated promptly. Although most serious reactions occur in the immediate postinjection period, delayed reactions can occur (ACR,

Classification of Severity and Manifestations of Adverse Reactions to Contrast

Mild

Signs and symptoms appear self-limited without evidence of progression (e.g., limited urticaria with mild pruritus, transient nausea, one episode of emesis) and include:

- Altered taste
- Anxiety
- Chills
- Cough
- Diaphoresis
- Dizziness
- Flushing
- Headache
- Nasal stuffiness
- Pallor
- Shaking
- Swelling (eyes, face)
- Warmth

Treatment: Requires observation to confirm resolution or lack of progression but usually no treatment. Patient reassurance is usually helpful. The patient should be monitored for 20 to 30 minutes to ensure that the symptoms do not worsen.

Moderate

Signs and symptoms are more pronounced. Moderate degree of clinically evident focal or systemic signs or symptoms, including:

- Bronchospasm, wheezing
- Dyspnea
- Generalized or diffuse erythema
- Hypertension
- Laryngeal edema
- Mild hypotension
- Tachycardia or bradycardia

Treatment: Clinical findings in moderate reactions frequently require prompt treatment. These situations require close, careful observation for possible progression to a life-threatening event. Moderate reactions require close monitoring (vital signs every 5 minutes, pulse oximeter in place and continuous observation by staff). Treatment may include diphenhydramine for symptomatic hives, leg elevation for hypotension, use of a beta-agonist inhaler for bronchospasm, or epinephrine for laryngeal edema.

Severe

Signs and symptoms are often life-threatening, including:

- Cardiopulmonary arrest
- Clinically manifest arrhythmias
- Convulsions
- Laryngeal edema (severe or rapidly progressing)
- Profound hypotension
- Unresponsiveness

Treatment: Requires *prompt* recognition and aggressive treatment; manifestations and treatment frequently require hospitalization.

NOTE: These classifications (mild, moderate, severe) do not attempt to distinguish between allergic-like and nonallergic-like reactions. Rather, they encompass the spectrum of adverse events that can be seen following the intravascular injection of contrast media.

Modified from ACR: *ACR manual on contrast media,* 2010, available at www.acr.org/media/ACR/Documents/PDF/QualitySafety/Resources/ContrastManual/2013_Contrast_Media.pdf. Accessed May 11, 2012.

2012). Thorough documentation of all contrast reactions, as well as notification of the patient's primary care provider and referring physicians of contrast media reactions is advisable. The nurse informs the patient of the reaction, and emphasizes the importance in communicating his or her history of reaction and verbalizing contrast when asked about allergies. Pretreatment with steroids and diphenhydramine (Benadryl) is recommended for patients with known or suspected past reactions to contrast media; however, premedication does not guarantee against a reaction. All patients are observed for the possibility of a contrast reaction after injection, and the nurse should maintain IV access until there is reasonable certainty that there is none. If the nurse suspects a reaction, the contrast injection should be stopped and no additional fluids or medications administered in tubing containing residual contrast media. All personnel in the area should be knowledgeable about, and know their role in, treating reactions.

Gadolinium-Based Contrast Reactions. The majority of contrast reactions are mild and include coldness at the injection site, nausea with or without vomiting, headache, warmth or pain at the injection site, paresthesias, dizziness, and itching. Reactions resembling an "allergic" response are atypical with a frequency from 0.004% to 0.7% (ACR, 2012). Reactions of this type manifest as a rash or urticaria, and very rarely bronchospasm. Acute adverse gadolinium reactions are less frequent than reactions with iodinated contrast media. Severe, life-threatening anaphylactoid or nonallergic anaphylactic reactions are rare (0.001% to 0.01%). The frequency of acute adverse reactions is about eight times higher in patients with a previous reaction, with the severity of the reaction increasing with each exposure (ACR, 2012). Gadolinium is radiodense, and can be used at much higher doses instead of iodinated contrast media in CT and angiography but should still be used with caution when extrapolating the lack of nephrotoxicity. Treatment of moderate to severe acute gadolinium reaction is similar to reactions with iodinated contrast.

Nephrogenic systematic fibrosis (NSF) is one risk associated with the administration of gadolinium-based contrast media. It is a fibrosing disease primarily of the skin and subcutaneous tissues but also involves the lung, esophagus, heart, and skeletal muscles. Initial symptoms develop rapidly and include skin thickening and or pruritus. The relative risk of NSF development after the use of gadolinium-based contrast media is unknown. Empiric data suggest not all gadolinium-based contrasts have identical risk factors for developing NSF. The incidence of NSF occurs in patients receiving high contrast doses, as well as in patients receiving higher cumulative lifetime doses, and patients with chronic kidney disease, severe renal failure, and transient acute renal failure. The highest-risk patients are those between the ages of 30 and 70, with chronic kidney disease level IV or V, or recently on dialysis (ACR, 2012). The only way to reverse NSF is to improve renal function, or obtain a kidney transplant. In many cases the disease is progressive, leading to thickened, painful skin, paresthesias, contractures, and loss of function. Patients with a history of renal disease, those who are older than age 60, and patients with hypertension and diabetes should have a GFR test 6 weeks prior to the scan as well as consideration of the risk-to-benefit ratio (ACR, 2012).

Contrast Media Extravasation of Iodinated Contrast. Extravasation is contrast medium injection or leakage into soft tissue. Tissue damage is a result of the toxicity of the agent or through pressure (e.g., compartment syndrome). The use of power injectors increases the risk for extravasation as do certain medical conditions such as circulatory problems of an extremity, history of radiation, or surgery. Infiltration risk increases with IV lines in place longer than 24 hours. To prevent extravasation, the nurse establishes a reliable peripheral injection site and assesses the site before injection. Commercial extravasation detector devices are available but are not a substitute for patient site assessment, observation, and communication. The nurse should instruct the patient to report any burning, stinging, swelling, or tight feeling occurring with the injection of the contrast agent. The ACR (2012) recommends close follow-up for any extravasation because the initial evaluation may not reveal the extent of the problem. Treatment includes limb elevation and warm or cold compresses as per the physician. It may take up to 2 weeks for tissue damage, discoloration, blistering, and sloughing to occur following extravasation. Compartment syndrome is often identifiable within 24 hours. Symptoms include coolness in the extremity and continuing swelling after the initial extravasation. Loss of pulses is a medical emergency, requiring a fasciotomy.

Contrast Media Extravasation of Gadolinium-Based Contrast. According to laboratory animal studies, gadolinium-based agents are much less toxic to the skin and subcutaneous tissues than iodinated contrast (ACR, 2012). Furthermore, the smaller volumes injected limit the chances for compartment syndrome. The likelihood of a significant injury from extravasated MR contrast media is extremely low.

Moderate Sedation and Analgesia. The amount and type of analgesia and sedation depend on patient and procedure factors. Moderate sedation and analgesia (conscious sedation) facilitates imaging acquisition during the procedure by decreasing patient movement, and preventing motion artifact, distorted images, and repeat scans. In many cases the level of sedation must be appropriate to enable the patient to comprehend and perform specific breathing instructions and repositioning or tolerate a painful maneuver (e.g., dilation or catheter advancement). ACR-SIR practice guidelines for analgesia and sedation (2010) state that emergency and monitoring equipment must be available to accommodate all ages and sizes of patients. Additional equipment includes oxygen delivery equipment with a backup oxygen supply, airway maintenance, intubation, emergency medications, defibrillators, and physiologic monitoring. Selection of only MRI-compatible monitoring and emergency equipment is mandatory in the MRI environment.

Site Marking. The nurse is often responsible for ensuring the Universal Protocol for preventing wrong site, wrong procedure, wrong person surgery. The time-out must involve the whole team including the patient when possible and is performed before the procedure starts. All procedures involving an incision, percutaneous puncture, or insertion of an instrument require site marking. Exemptions from site marking include those procedures having no predetermined site of insertion, where imaging guidance is an inherent part of the procedure (e.g., angiography, central line insertion). Other exemptions include procedures using a midline approach intended to treat a single midline organ or lesion and endoscopy without intended laterality (Kandarpa and Machan, 2011). Universal Precautions, infection control measures, and the use of personal protective equipment are in accordance with the institution.

Documentation. The nurse documents patient identification, allergy assessment, surgical procedure verification, and any other intervention performed. A brief mental status and neurologic assessment is important for patients with neurologic conditions or those at high risk for stroke. Documentation should include the integrity of the patient's skin, presence or absence of peripheral pulses, positioning, use of positioning devices, fluid intake, output measurements, contrast usage and the achievement of patient goals. If administering moderate sedation and analgesia the nurse documents the patient's level of consciousness, anxiety and pain levels, and incremental doses of sedative medication.

The nurse ensures all medications, medication containers, and other solutions on and off the sterile field in perioperative and other procedural settings are labeled (TJC, 2012). The labels should be verified by two qualified individuals if the person preparing the medication is not administering it. The nurse is responsible to document the type size, serial number, and lot number of implantable devices according to institutional policy. The nursing report should include information about the procedure, all procedure-specific instructions, and information about possible equipment, device, and catheter care.

Radiation Dose Documentation. The ACR-SIR practice guideline (2009) recommends, if technically possible, all radiation dose data provided by the fluoroscopy unit or CT scanner be transferred and archived with the images from the procedure. This is usually an automatic electric data transfer from the fluoroscopy unit or CT scanner to the PACs done by the technologist or physician on study completion. Archiving of radiation dose data is of particular importance if repeat procedures are probable or the patient received a clinically significant radiation dose. The use of PACs systems to record dose has several drawbacks. PACs systems are typically radiology department specific and do not interface with the facility's electronic medical record (EMR). In some institutions the cardiac catheterization lab, EP lab, hybrid OR, special procedures, and IR each have their own PAC system, with no interdepartmental access. System configurations such as this do not offer insight into a patient's total exposure across hospital departments. Other forms of documentation include the radiology technician manually recording radiation doses into log books or the nurse documenting in the patient's medical record the dose information provided by the physician or radiology technologist.

With the increasing rates of radiation exposure, the ACR launched an initiative for the collection of dose-related indices and registries for CT and fluoroscopy (FDA, 2012). As of yet, no national standards exist for the recording-reporting of radiation dose information. For hospitals, TJC published a sentinel event alert on the radiation risks of diagnostic imaging containing suggested actions to mitigate risk (TJC, 2011). Some states have legislation regarding the documentation, reporting, and verification of dose as well as error reporting (CA Dept of Public Health, 2011). Radiation dose monitoring, auditing, and reporting should be a component of the facility's quality assurance and quality improvement processes along with periodic reviews of protocols for radiation dose optimization. A process should also be in place to notify patients receiving significant radiation doses and a mechanism for patient follow-up of potential adverse effects.

Evaluation

During the evaluation phase of care the nurse determines if the outcomes established for the patient were met and revises outcomes and interventions accordingly. The evaluation period provides opportunities to improve nursing interventions through careful reflection and analysis of outcomes. The following are possible evaluation statements relating to the Sample Plan of Care (see page 1144):

• The patient verbalized an acceptable level of pain as defined with a 1 to 10 pain scale.

- The patient demonstrated a decreased level of anxiety, verbalized less apprehension, maintained eye contact, and was able to comply with requests even though anxiety persisted.
- The patient verbalized understanding of the procedure and described the actions to take after discharge.
- The patient's airway was maintained and oxygen saturation was within preprocedure baseline limits.
- The patient's vital signs were within acceptable limits, peripheral pulses returned to baseline, and there was no evidence of excessive bleeding.
- The patient's skin was intact with no reddened areas or lesions.

Postprocedural Care. Postprocedural nursing care involves ensuring hemostasis of the puncture site through patient discharge. After the procedure the nurse monitors vital signs, and assesses the puncture site and distal pulses with the patient remaining flat as per institutional protocol. The catheter or sheath removal time, closure method, and catheter size are documented. Time to ambulation and elevation of the head of bed (HOB) depends on the procedure, diagnostic or interventional, vascular access, arterial or venous, and puncture site. During this time the nurse checks the groin site frequently for evidence of bleeding or hematoma. Hemostasis methods include manual pressure, compression devices, vascular suturing, or collagen plug devices according to procedure and physician preference. Compression should be firm but should not obliterate the distal pulses. The nurse monitors the appropriate distal pulse based on the access vessel (e.g., radial or femoral artery). If brachial access was used for the procedure, blood pressure measurement is not undertaken in the affected arm. The nurse observes the affected limb for changes in color, temperature, pain, and pre- and post-pulse quality to detect acute arterial occlusion. Pseudoaneurysm formation, nerve damage, and infection are complications from arterial punctures. The nurse monitors neurologic function in patients undergoing head and neck arteriography. Observation is increased to 6 hours in patients with hypertension, or those with a hematoma postprocedure. The nurse encourages patients receiving contrast to drink large amounts of clear liquids and/or increase the administration rate of IV fluids. Contrast agents act as an osmotic diuretic, thus additional fluid counteracts dehydration as well as prevents contrast-induced nephropathy. Patients receiving contrast or experiencing contrast-related complications must receive appropriate discharge instructions and follow-up directions. Patient recovery and monitoring are in accordance with the amount of sedation and analgesia received, pain level, and vital signs. The type of interventional procedure performed determines additional monitoring criteria, including distal pulses for angiography; neurologic, motor, and sensory signs of the lower extremities after vertebroplasty; urine output following nephrostomy; and bleeding post biopsy.

Patient and Family Education and Discharge Planning

Patient and family education includes providing basic information about the procedure, table, room, and staff members and the identification and procedure verification process when appropriate. The nurse discusses the use of sedation to address the patient's expected level of procedure sedation versus realistic level of sedation and informs the patient of the need to remain still to avoid motion artifact resulting in repeating the study. Included in the discussion is information about the procedure process, requirement for cooperation (e.g., breath holds, positioning, contrast administration, and staff activities). The nurse reviews that during CT and MRI procedures that staff members will exit the room during scanning, and

voice communication with the patient will be maintained via intercom. Additional information that is reviewed includes anticipated recovery time, discharge criteria, postprocedure care, and follow-up instructions (Patient and Family Education).

Discharge assessments should be in accordance with facility policy. For inpatients, appropriate discharge criteria includes stable cardiovascular and airway status, stable vital signs, and no evidence of bleeding, drainage, or hematoma at puncture site. On stabilization, inpatients are transferred to the designated location per

---

PATIENT AND FAMILY EDUCATION
Discharge Instructions for Contrast Media Injection

Always provide the patient and the caregiver with verbal and written instructions. Provide them with the name and telephone number of the physician or nurse to call if questions arise. Review the physician's explanation of postdischarge care and evaluate the patient's response to the instructions provided.

General Instructions after Injection of Contrast Media
- Drink two to four glasses of water within 4 hours of your scan to help your kidneys pass the contrast media (x-ray dye).
- Call your physician if any of the following occur:
  - You have any worsening of the pain or symptoms you were having before the procedure.
  - The place where the contrast media was injected, or the catheter was put into your skin, begins to bleed or swell, or it becomes more painful.
  - Your arm, leg, or foot becomes cool or cold.
  - You have slurred speech, balance problems, or trouble using your arm or leg.
  - You develop a rash, itching, sweating, or trouble breathing.

Instructions for Contrast Media Reactions
- Call the radiology nursing station if your symptoms do not resolve, or you develop new symptoms such as hives or a rash, itching, prolonged or frequent vomiting, chest tightness, shortness of breath, dizziness, or swelling. Take the medications prescribed to treat your reaction. Oral antihistamines, such as diphenhydramine (Benadryl), may make you too drowsy to drive or operate machinery safely. They can affect concentration and interfere with children's learning in school. These medications should be taken only as long as directed.
- If you do not respond to the treatment prescribed for your reaction, it is important that you see a medical professional for reevaluation.
- Do not attempt to treat or "wait out" severe reactions at home. Go immediately to a hospital emergency department. *Seek immediate medical care if you develop breathing problems, swelling in the throat, or wheezing.* If no one is available to drive you right away, call an ambulance for emergency medical transport.
- Obtain and wear a MedicAlert bracelet and carry an identification card describing your allergy.
- Inform healthcare providers about your allergy before any procedures are performed.
- Follow up with your healthcare provider to let him or her know about your reaction. At this follow-up appointment, he or she can evaluate your recovery from the reaction and adjust any medications.

Modified from Mosby's Nursing Consult: *Patient education instructions; drug rash, use of contrast media, CT scanning, angiography,* available at www.nursingconsult.com. Accessed August 6, 2012; Siddiqi NH, Lin EC: Contrast media reactions, available at http://emedicine.medscape.com/article/422855-overview. Accessed June 30, 2012.

AMBULATORY SURGERY CONSIDERATIONS

Discharge Criteria

The following criteria should be met before patients are discharged after outpatient interventional radiologic procedures:

- Patient has stable vital signs (resembling baseline vital signs), including SpO$_2$ level.
- Patient shows no evidence of respiratory depression.
- Patient is oriented per baseline to person, place, and time.
- Patient can take fluids, if appropriate, without nausea.
- Patient can void, if a procedure-specific criterion.
- Patient can ambulate with/without assistance as appropriate, and has no dizziness.
- Pain has been addressed/managed.
- Bleeding is not present; drainage is per procedure expectation.
- Written discharge instructions including medication reconciliation with phone number to call have been given to patient (patients are informed how to obtain necessary supplies, if applicable).
- A responsible person is available to escort patient to home or stay with patient.

FIGURE 29-11 Seldinger technique using a hollow needle and guidewire to obtain vessel access for percutaneous procedures. **A.** Insertion of needle. **B.** Placement of needle in lumen of vessel (inner cannula removed). **C.** Insertion of guidewire. **D.** Removal of needle (guidewire remains in place). **E.** Threading of catheter over guidewire. **F.** Removal of guidewire.

institutional policy. Neurointerventional procedure patients may go to intensive care. The IR nurse provides written documentation and verbal report to the receiving unit as well as notifies them of special patient needs, equipment, supplies, level of care, and expected time of transfer.

The nurse reviews postprocedure instructions with the patient and family if teaching is appropriate. Discharge criteria for outpatients is according to assessment criteria as per the facility's policy and procedure (Ambulatory Surgery Considerations). The physician or nurse reviews discharge instructions with the patient (or responsible adult) and provides supplies and written prescriptions if needed. The patient is provided with the physician's name and emergency contact numbers for problems or questions for 24 hours postprocedure.

Discharge instruction forms should be procedure specific and include activity restrictions, possible complications and when and whom to call for help, diet, medications, specific care related to procedure, driving restrictions, signs of infection, and follow-up care plan and appointment. Patients with arterial punctures receive precise instructions in case of hemorrhage or other puncture site complication. Patient and family teaching with return demonstrations for procedures such as tube care, drainage bags, tube-catheter flushing, and sterile technique is essential.

The decision to admit a patient after an outpatient procedure is at the discretion of the physician. Indications include the following:

- Complication resulting from the procedure including any significant change in pulse in the affected extremity, neurologic changes, persistent bleeding, or persistent nausea and vomiting postprocedure
- Significant findings on the diagnostic examination warranting further therapy requiring an inpatient admission

Procedures

Interventional Access with the Seldinger Technique

The Seldinger technique changed IR because it provided a less invasive and safer means of access to vessels. Most IR procedures

are initiated with the Seldinger technique (Figure 29-11). After sterile preparation and draping, the physician administers a local anesthetic over the intended entry site, usually the groin, for an angiogram that uses the retrograde femoral artery approach. A needle (Seldinger 18-gauge, 2¾-inch or other) with stylet is used to gain vascular access, and then the stylet is removed. A pulsatile backflow of blood will be noted with arterial access. The physician passes a guidewire several centimeters into the needle, then removes the needle while compressing the puncture site and leaving the guidewire in place. A small incision is made, and the surgeon places an introducer with a dilator over the guidewire. The guidewire and dilator are removed and an introducer sheath is used to advance the catheter. Puncture location is crucial. High arterial punctures above the inguinal ligament may result in bleeding, whereas low arterial punctures may yield pseudoaneurysm. Fluoroscopy over the femoral head helps confirm access. Ultrasound facilitates vessel access in patients with altered anatomy, obesity, or scarring caused by previous vascular surgeries, multiple catheterizations, and previous insertion of intra-aortic balloon pumps. Femoral access alternatives include brachial or axillary artery punctures. Translumbar punctures are rare. The nurse documents the presence and quality of distal extremity pulse before the procedure. Potential complications of arterial puncture and catheterization include hemorrhage, distal embolization, and pseudoaneurysm development. Complications of femoral venous puncture-catheterization include puncture-site infection, phlebitis, and hematoma.

Diagnostic Procedures

Angiography. Angiography uses fluoroscopy and contrast to image anatomic and pathologic changes in vascular anatomy. Angiography determines occlusive disease, aneurysms, AVM, and AV fistulae, as well as localizes small vascular tumors. Angiography may be performed as a single procedure or may precede an intervention. Classification of angiography is either coronary or noncoronary. Only interventional cardiologists perform PCI. Noncoronary angiography procedures include peripherally inserted central catheters (PICCs), vascular access procedures, organ-based therapies using fluoroscopic guidance for biopsies, tumor ablations, and various embolizations. Angiography and interventions on the cerebral vessels remain exclusive to the neurointerventionalist and usually use a biplane system.

Universal screening for angiography patients includes coagulation status, contrast allergies, metformin use, existing renal dysfunction or failure, anemia, and diabetes. Generally all patients are NPO except for extra fluids for hydration and renal dysfunction prevention subsequent to contrast. To avoid accidental contamination during the procedure, the nurse secures the patient's arms at the sides using wristbands or armboards. Good image quality requires a motionless field, thus a variety of soft restraints and bands ensure minimal patient movement. The nurse performs baseline assessment of the appropriate pulse site including axillary, brachial, radial, femoral, popliteal, and dorsalis pedis before needle entry. Arterial access sites include the femoral artery, as well as brachial, radial or axillary artery, translumbar, and subclavian. Venous access routes include brachial, femoral, internal jugular, and subclavian. Contrast injection occurs after the catheter is in the target vessel for catheter navigation. With an arterial puncture the injector system, tubings, and catheters must be free of air bubbles. Patients may feel a transient warmth or hot sensation in the injection area, or the sensation of incontinence with catheters positioned in vessels near or in the lower abdomen or pelvis.

Biopsy. Imaging used for biopsies include fluoroscopy, ultrasound, CT, and MRI. Modality selection is per the physician, site, and results of prior imaging studies. Specimens undergo preparation and handling according to established policy and procedures. After administering a local anesthetic the physician makes a small puncture with a scalpel to aid the passage of the needle followed by imaging to check for placement. Biopsy needle selection depends on the lesion location, size and depth, the suspected diagnosis, access route, and the amount of tissue required for study. Biopsies involving a specific area or small lesion are more labor intensive than random tissue sampling. Complications vary depending on the biopsy site.

Chest Biopsy. Thorax needle biopsies rule out suspicion of malignancy; evaluate nodules, lesions, and masses; obtain tissue staging samples; and determine localized infections. Patient positioning depends on the location of the lesion and the path the physician uses to reach it. Modality selection is CT, fluoroscopy, or ultrasound based on the biopsy site and lesion size. Access is via the Seldinger technique. Adequate anesthesia levels are essential to minimize discomfort and chest wall motion. Common complications include pneumothorax confirmed by CT or x-ray and minor bleeding resulting in hemoptysis. Patients must abstain from strenuous exercise for several days and go to the emergency department if dyspnea develops.

Liver Biopsy. Transcutaneous liver biopsies diagnose tumors and determine etiology. Some physicians perform liver biopsies at the bedside, but an increasing number use ultrasound or CT for image guidance. Indications for liver biopsy are patients with massive ascites and coagulopathies. Access is by the jugular vein using angiography. Bleeding is a common complication subsequent to the impaired clotting mechanisms in liver disease. Serious bleeding or bile leaks are complications causing acute abdomen, hypovolemia, and sepsis.

Kidney Biopsy. Kidney biopsies determine disease and rejection status in transplant patients as well as adrenal gland tumors. The physician isolates the tumor by CT scan or ultrasound guidance and obtains a sample for analysis. Caution is advised with adrenal biopsies because of the possibility of a pheochromocytoma. This tumor secretes adrenaline and other catecholamines resulting in paroxysms of hypertension, tachycardia, headache, nausea, and diaphoresis. Bleeding is the most common complication subsequent to the long sampling needles.

Therapeutic Interventions

Percutaneous Transluminal Angioplasty (PTA). Angioplasty is a nonsurgical means to open atherosclerotic vessels using fluoroscopy guidance to inflate a balloon-tipped catheter compressing atherosclerotic plaque. Peripheral angioplasty refers to vessels outside the coronary and cerebral vasculature, most notably the aortoiliac, infrapopliteal, superior femoral artery (SFA), and other lower-extremity vessels. Indications for peripheral angioplasty include lifestyle-limiting claudication, chronic leg ischemia, restenosis of a previous graft anastomoses, treatment pre- or post-bypass surgery, tissue ulceration, and necrosis. After establishing vessel access, the patient receives heparin to achieve the desired anticoagulation status. The surgeon advances the appropriate guidewire across the stenosis or occlusion and positions the balloon catheter in the affected area using radiopaque markers and fluoroscopy. The balloon is inflated with a mixture of sterile saline and contrast medium to a specific atmosphere of pressure. Dilation may require several inflations. A postprocedure angiogram is performed to assess the technical success of the procedure and vessel patency. Complications are rare and include vessel trauma, hematoma, thrombosis, and vessel reocclusion.

Peripheral Vascular Stents. Stents are common adjuncts to angioplasty, acting as a mechanical scaffold to maintain vessel patency. Vascular stents come in various sizes, lengths, and materials and include a variety of coatings as well as drug-eluting capabilities. After angioplasty the physician directs the stent to the desired location using an introducer catheter with radiopaque markers under fluoroscopy and then deploys the stent. Contraindications include patients with bleeding disorders, patients not able to take anticoagulants, circumstances in which stent placement would exacerbate arterial leakage, and when stenoses prohibits the passage of the delivery catheter. Complications include hematoma formation, thrombosis, pseudoaneurysm formation, and stent migration.

Dialysis and Fistula Graft Repair. Long-term dialysis requires a surgical AV shunt, composed of native vessels or synthetic grafts or a combination of both bridging an artery and vein. Problems inherent to maintaining vascular access include poor flow, increased resistance during dialysis, prolonged bleeding, arm swelling and collateral vein development. Restoring patency by PTA is possible through the graft itself or via arm or femoral venous access. Strictures at venous anastomoses may be particularly severe, warranting prolonged inflation with high-pressure balloons and higher doses of IV analgesics and sedatives. Other options to restore patency include mechanical thrombectomy devices to aspirate blood clots, or injection of thrombolytic agents, recombinant tissue plasminogen activator (rt-PA) to lyse, or dissolve, the clot. Complications include vein rupture, bleeding subsequent to thrombolysis, pulmonary artery, or arterial embolization.

Peripherally Inserted Central Catheters. A PICC is a long, thin venous access device inserted into the brachial or cephalic vein, terminating in the superior vena cava or right atrium. PICC lines provide long-term therapies such as antibiotic and narcotic administration and total parenteral nutrition (TPN). Physicians, physician assistants, radiology assistants, nurse practitioners, or specially trained RNs and RTs may insert PICC lines. PICC placement is a sterile procedure but can be done at bedside. After placement, the position of the catheter tip is confirmed using fluoroscopy or chest x-ray. Outpatients receive instruction on how to care for the PICC line, including flushing the line, when to change the dressing, and when to shower. Patients must inspect the site daily for any irregularities such as swelling, redness, leakage, or pain and report them to a healthcare professional immediately.

Drainage Procedures. The development of cross-sectional imaging enables drainage of deep body cavities without open surgery. Image guidance for abdominal, pelvic, or other soft tissue fluid collections and abscesses use CT, ultrasound, or fluoroscopy. Indications include diagnostic fluid evaluation, treatment of abscess or sepsis, and palliation of symptoms for patients with tense ascites resulting in dyspnea, pain, or compromised renal function. Visceral collections include treatment for abscess and cysts of the liver, spleen, and pancreas. Depending on the drainage site, the approach can be subphrenic, transgluteal, transrectal, or transvaginal. A preliminary CT determines the optimal path for catheter placement. Therapeutic drainages use two techniques depending on the size of the collection, location, physician preference, and imaging modality. Large superficial drainages use a trocar technique in conjunction with CT or ultrasound imaging. Small collections remotely situated or with limited assess use the Seldinger technique. Catheter size and configuration selection depends on the site and fluid drained. Imaging is performed immediately before catheter removal to document emptying of the cavity, then the catheter is withdrawn and the site covered with a dry, sterile dressing. Drainage catheters left in place must be safely secured and dressed by the nurse or IR technologist. Physician orders specify catheter care and measurement and emptying of the drainage chambers. Patients discharged with the catheter in place receive instructions on catheter care and an appointment for catheter removal.

Endoscopic Retrograde Cholangiopancreatography (ERCP). ERCP is an interventional procedure combining endoscopy and fluoroscopy to treat or diagnose biliary or pancreatic disease. A multidisciplinary team of interventionalists, surgeons, gastroenterologists, and medical oncologists performs ERCP under fluoroscopy with surgical assistance from the OR staff. The patient receives moderate sedation, and the physician passes an endoscope through the mouth, the upper GI tract to the opening of the hepatopancreatic ampulla. Contrast material and fluoroscopy visualize the ducts, anatomy, and presence of stones, blockages, or other lesions. Endoscopic treatment includes stone removal, cytology, sphincter dilation, tumor removal, and stenting. Contraindications for ERCP are acute pancreatitis and coagulation and bleeding disorders. Complications include hemorrhage and pancreatitis.

Percutaneous Transhepatic Cholangiogram (PTC). PTC visualizes drainage of the biliary system and accesses the biliary tree in cases in which ERCP was unsuccessful. PTC is characteristically palliative for patients with nonresectable malignant disease, although percutaneous treatment of biliary stone disease with or without choledochoscopy occurs in selected cases. Other applications include cholangioplasty for biliary strictures, biopsy of the biliary duct, and management of complications from laparoscopic cholecystectomy and liver transplantation. Contraindications include diffuse hepatic metastasis, liver failure, or a shortened life expectancy. After the initial workup, ultrasonography, MRI, or CT are done to determine the etiology of the obstruction. Patients receive prophylactic antibiotics 24 hours prior to a PTC. The patient is positioned supine, prepped, draped, and administered a local anesthetic. The physician selects the level to insert the needle between adjacent ribs, avoiding the lung. A 21- or 22-gauge needle is guided along into the liver under fluoroscopy, with the exact position determined by contrast injection. PTC is more invasive and painful than ERCP, warranting additional doses of sedatives and opioids before the liver capsule is punctured. The physician exchanges various wires and introducers under fluoroscopy until the proper drainage catheter is in place. Bile may be sent to the laboratory for culture and sensitivity. Drainage may be external or internal. The bile drains into the duodenum and an external bag, or internal via stent placement in the small intestine. Initial drainage can be external until the bile is clear and debris free, then capped for internal drainage only. Catheters are changed every 4 to 6 weeks in an ambulatory setting and oral antibiotics are given prior to catheter changes. Complications include sepsis, peritonitis, hemorrhage, and pneumothorax when using a right-sided approach.

Uterine Fibroid Embolization (UFE). UFE treats uterine leiomyomata or fibroids by blocking perfusion to the benign tumors, resulting in degeneration, scar tissue formation, and fibroid shrinkage. This procedure appeals to many women because of its minimally invasive nature and outpatient setting. A complete blood count, electrolytes, and pregnancy test are obtained before the procedure. Moderate sedation and local anesthesia or epidural anesthesia may be used. The physician performs arteriography of the pelvic vasculature under fluoroscopy to determine uterine artery blood flow and then embolizes the uterine arteries by injecting the agent through the catheter until proximal arterial flow or reflux of contrast material no longer occurs. Particles (either PVA or microspheres) are the embolic agents most often used in patients with uterine fibroids. Particle sizes of 355-500 μm and 500-710 μm are used most commonly (Konez and Cho, 2011). Collateral circulation maintains the blood supply to the myometrium. Pain is moderate to severe depending on the degree of occlusion. Some institutions add pretreatment with steroids as well as the use of an epidural and intraoperative ketorolac or ketorolac tromethamine administration. Patient-controlled anesthesia with IV narcotics is standard in the immediate postoperative phase, transitioning to oral medications prior to discharge. Procedure success is according to patient symptomatology before and after the procedure, 6 weeks and 6 months at gynecologic follow-up (Patient-Centered Care). Overall, 85% to 95% experience a reduction in symptoms, with reintervention needed in approximately 5% to 10% due to lack of symptom improvement (Kandarpa and Machan, 2011). The main complication is postembolization syndrome, which is most likely the result of an inflammatory response to necrotic tissue postembolization. Signs and symptoms include pain, fever, malaise, nausea,

PATIENT-CENTERED CARE

Patient-centered care has been identified by the Institute of Medicine (IOM) as a critical element within the six domains that characterize quality care (e.g., effectiveness, patient-centeredness, timeliness, safety, efficiency, equity) and further defines it as "health care that establishes a partnership among practitioners, patients, and their families (when appropriate) to ensure that decisions respect patients' wants, needs, and preferences and that patients have the education and support they need to make decisions and participate in their own care" (Iowa Department of Health, 2010). Clancy (2008) notes, the essence of patient-centered care is captured in the maxim, "Nothing about me without me."

Effective communication between patients and healthcare providers essential to establishing partnership and as the patient-centered care movement has gained momentum, a variety of campaigns have been launched to foster communication and partnership, such as the National Patient Safety Foundation's (NPSF) Ask Me 3 patient education program. The campaign seeks to simplify the communication process by encouraging patients to focus on understanding the answers to three questions when facing healthcare decisions (NPSF, 2013). The questions can be asked by the patient and can be used by the healthcare provider to check understanding. The questions are:

1. What is my main problem?
2. What do I need to do?
3. Why is it important for me to do this?

The NPSF has brochures that can be downloaded as well as a printable form for patients to take to record their answers. Nurses can facilitate the Ask Me 3 approach by making patients aware of the campaign and providing the brochure or website address. An example of how a nurse might use the Ask Me 3 approach in the interventional radiologic setting follows:

Mrs. G. is a 46-year-old who is scheduled for a uterine fibroid embolization. When she went to the facility for her preoperative labwork she saw an Ask Me 3 brochure in the waiting room and took it home with her. She used the questions during a phone call with the physician as a way to get more information about her procedure. When Mrs. G. was admitted to the facility the nurse assessed Mrs. G.'s understanding of the procedure, asking her questions in the context of the Ask Me 3 framework. When asked, "Can you tell me what problem you're being treated for with this procedure?" Mrs. G. responded that she had fibroid tumors on her uterus that were causing her pain, discomfort, and heavy bleeding. Mrs. G. went on to say that she understood the physician would put a catheter in her groin and would inject particles through it to block blood flow to the fibroid, causing it to shrink. When asked, "What do you expect to happen after your procedure?" Mrs. G. accurately describes the expected postprocedure course including the side effects she might experience from the procedure, and the possibility that she could require overnight admission. Without prompting, Mrs. G. also shares with the nurse that she realizes she will need to lie flat for 6 hours after the procedure to prevent bleeding from the puncture site (thereby demonstrating understanding of the answer to question 3 without the nurse's asking it). She also notes that she is looking forward to resolution of her symptoms within the next 6 months.

Modified from Iowa Department of Health: *Patient-centered: what does it look like?* April 2010, available at www.idph.state.ia.us/hcr_committees/common/pdf/clinicians/1005_mhsac.pdf. Accessed April 1, 2013; Clancy C: How patient-centered healthcare can improve quality, *Patient Saf Qual Healthc*, March/April, 2008, available at www.psqh.com/marapr08/ahrq.html. Accessed April 1, 2013; National Patient Safety Foundation (NPSF): *Ask Me 3*, 2013, available at www.npsf.org/for-healthcare-professionals/programs/ask-me-3. Accessed March 31, 2013.

and vomiting lasting approximately 2 to 7 days (Sisken and Sekhar, 2011).

Embolization for Obstetric Hemorrhage. Potential life-threatening hemorrhagic conditions amenable to embolization include abdominal and cervical pregnancy, placenta previa, and placenta accreta. Placenta accreta is a potential life-threatening condition when the placenta invades and is inseparable from the uterine wall. Incidence is about 1 in 2150 pregnancies (American College of Obstetricians and Gynecologists [ACOG], 2012). Optimal treatment is delivery by elective cesarean section under controlled planning involving anesthesiology, obstetrics, a pelvic surgeon, an intensivist, maternal fetal medicine specialists, neonatologists, a urologist, a hematologist, and IR (Garmi and Salim, 2012). In cases incorporating IR, the procedure occurs either in the IR suite or in an OR capable of advanced imaging. Prior to delivery of the infant, the physician prophylactically places balloon catheters in the anterior division of the both internal iliac arteries. After the delivery the physician inflates the balloon catheters achieving temporary hemostasis and allowing for complete selective embolization of the uterine arteries. Uncontrolled bleeding warrants a hysterectomy. When hemostasis is achieved, the catheters are removed and the patient is transferred to the postprocedure area or postanesthesia care unit (PACU). Although current evidence is insufficient to make a firm recommendation on the use of balloon catheter occlusion or embolization to reduce blood loss and improve surgical outcome, individual situations may warrant their use (ACOG, 2012).

Transjugular Intrahepatic Portosystemic Shunt. TIPS is a nonoperative therapeutic option for management of variceal bleeding from portal hypertension. Mostly commonly seen in patients with cirrhosis, these vessels enlarge, become tortuous, and bleed due to pressure buildup. A percutaneous stent is placed to dilate a tract between the hepatic and portal vein. The stent creates a shunt, lowering the portal vein pressure. All patients undergoing TIPS receive prophylactic broad-spectrum antibiotics. The physician confirms portal vein patency preoperatively by ultrasound and assesses coagulation profiles. Vascular access is through the internal jugular vein using ultrasound guidance. A guidewire is placed into the right atrium followed by a sheath for pressure recording. The physician then places a catheter into the hepatic vein under fluoroscopy. A balloon forming a shunt from the portal vein to the hepatic vein creates a dilated tract. Stent deployment occurs using angiographic verification to assess stent position. Repeated serial dilation of the stent occurs until pressures are satisfactory, followed by catheter removal. Major complications include hemorrhage and bile duct trauma. Other complications include hepatic encephalopathy, recurrent portal hypertension, and shunt thrombosis or stenosis.

Balloon-Occluded Retrograde Transvenous Obliteration (BRTO). BRTO is an adjunctive or alternative treatment to TIPS, in the management of gastric varices. BRTO occludes the outflow veins of the portosystemic shunt using an occlusion balloon following by the injection of a sclerosing agent. Successful BRTO relies on integral knowledge of gastric variceal anatomy. Patients undergoing BRTO are usually cirrhotic for either bleeding gastric varices or hepatic encephalopathy. Management of the BRTO patient is complex and requires a team approach including a hepatologist, an endoscopist, and IR (Sauer et al, 2011). The anatomy of the varix dictates the treatment approach and correlates with the degree of difficulty (Sabri et al, 2010). The most common approach is the right femoral vein; however, if there is a history of TIPS, the internal jugular vein is used. The physician positions an access sheath in the IVC or renal vein, enabling balloon occlusion venography of the left renal vein to determine anatomy and varix type. With the occlusion balloon inflated, a microcatheter is advanced in the varix and a sclerosing agent is instilled under fluoroscopic guidance filling the varix and the draining shunt. The occlusion balloon remains in place and the patient waits 4 hours in recovery or as indicated by the physician. The patient is returned to the procedure area to assess embolization. If obliteration is not complete, the patient may undergo further BRTO. Balloon deflation or rupture may require an additional intervention. When the obliteration is complete, the physician deflates the balloon, removes the sheath, and establishes hemostasis. Postprocedure monitoring consists of assessing vital signs, checking the puncture site for bleeding or hematoma, and observing for signs for GI bleeding and pulmonary emboli. Obliteration of the varices is confirmed using computerized tomographic angiography (CTA), MRI, or endoscopy ultrasound before discharge. Complications include fever, chest or epigastric pain, hemoglobinuria, transient hypertension, nausea or vomiting, and pulmonary embolus in the case of balloon rupture (Sauer et al, 2011).

Image-Guided Tumor Ablation. Image-guided tumor ablation is the direct application of chemical or thermal therapies in an attempt to eradicate or substantiate tumor destruction. The imaging modalities used for ablations include ultrasound, CT, MRI, and fluoroscopy. Chemical ablations use ethanol and acetic acid, resulting in coagulation necrosis and tissue destruction. Thermal ablations, categorized by energy, use RF, cryotherapy, laser, microwave, and ultrasound (Webb et al, 2011). Although "needle" is the nonspecific term for the application devices, correct terminology is electrodes to deliver RF energy, antennas to deliver microwave applicators, fibers for laser application, cryoprobes for cryoablation, and probes to deliver high-intensity ultrasound (Webb et al, 2011). Energy source selection depends on multiple variables, with certain pathologies more responsive to specific energy sources. Pulmonary and hepatic RFA proves feasible and efficacious in treating lung and hepatocellular carcinomas. Laser ablations are standard for the ablation of incompetent saphenous veins and other venous pathology. Cryoablation or RF energies ablate renal tumors. Microwave, RF, or cryoablations provide palliative treatment for pain associated with bone cancer (Kandarpa and Machan, 2011). Uterine fibroids and the treatment of cancers of the brain, breast, liver, and bone are amenable to high-frequency ultrasound. For most ablations moderate sedation is sufficient, although general anesthesia is best for bone ablations for pain management. Specific positioning, procedure considerations, lab data, modality selection, and complications depend on the organ being ablated, energy source, and pathology. In general, postprocedure nausea, vomiting, fever, and pain are common after ablations due to the body's reaction to the damaged tissue.

Intraoperative MRI. There have been numerous advances in neurosurgery; however, one of the most important developments is intraoperative MRI (iMRI). The iMRI suite permits real-time MRI imaging that allows the surgeon to distinguish tumors from normal tissue, ensuring complete tumor excision. Complete versus subtotal versus partial resection is of ongoing debate regarding the balance between oncologic and functional status of patients. iMRI is a very important development in the field of neurosurgery (Schmidt et al, 2011).

The iMRI configuration is a ceiling-mounted MRI scanner housed in a diagnostic room adjacent to a standard OR separated by a locked sliding door. In these procedures a standard craniotomy and tumor resection occurs in the OR. After the resection, preparation of the room and patient for the MRI scan begins. On completed preparation, the MRI technologist opens the door and the MRI moves into the OR via ceiling rails. The MRI scan lasts about 30 minutes and is done with or without contrast. If the resection is complete, the MRI returns to the diagnostic room, the door closes, and surgery proceeds. If additional pathology remains, sub- or partial resections may warrant further tissue removal and reimaging.

The MRI and the OR remain separately functioning areas when not being used for iMRI. As with traditional MRI, safety considerations with iMRI require extensive training, preparation, and team work throughout all aspects of the case. All clinical staff must be current in iMRI safety training (indicated by stickered badges) to access this room. During case setup, the nurse ensures that all non–MRI-compatible equipment is tagged and placed underneath the scanning table with string for visibility and easy removal prior to bringing in the magnet and performs an additional instrument count prior to prepping and draping the patient for the scan. The anesthesia provider performs a separate instrument-needle count accounting for all needles, angiocaths, syringes, stylets, blades, and other related equipment, and stores used needles and syringes in needle mats. Scanning does not occur if any counts are incorrect. The perioperative nurse and the MRI technologist position, pad, and prep the patient. Grounding pads, hypothermia, and compression devices are removed. MRI coil cables must be off the floor and attached to bed rails. All IV lines, leads, Foley catheters, and wires must not be looped or in contact with the skin (Figure 29-12). The nurse tapes the patient's earplugs into place. The urinary catheter system is positioned as far away from the magnet as possible and tucked under the mattress (many contain metal). With the patient prepped, the technologist and nurse check the diameter of the patient using a 70-cm hula hoop to confirm that the patient will fit into the 70-cm bore (opening) of the magnet before unlocking the doors. Prior to opening the door, the team moves all booms, lights, tables, microscopes, kick buckets, foot pedals, and other metal

FIGURE 29-12 Patient specifically prepped for intraoperative magnetic resonance imaging (iMRI) scan. MRI is mounted on ceiling rails and travels into the OR after careful room and patient preparation.

equipment that is not MRI safe behind the 5 gauss line. All anesthesia carts, supply carts, and IV infusion pumps are locked and secured. With additional staff, this preparation takes between 20 and 45 minutes to complete. The nurse documents and verbalizes the completion of all checklists and counts. The MRI travels into the OR on ceiling rails. All other doors providing OR access are locked during scanning. The anesthesia provider, an additional MRI tech, and the perioperative nurse remain in the room during the scan for patient safety, monitoring purposes, and contrast injection.

Percutaneous Nephrostomy (PCN). PCN is a procedure to drain the renal collecting system in cases of obstruction and is often performed in partnership between a urologist and IR physician. PCN refers to an external drainage catheter and collection system placed via a flank approach positioned in the renal pelvis. Nephroureteral or nephreuterostomy catheters drain externally and internally via a catheter in the bladder. Ureteral stents are internal and extend from the renal pelvis to the bladder. Indications for PCN include obstructive uropathy (kidney and bladder stones, tumor obstructions) or tract creation for device insertion (e.g., antegrade ureteral stenting), extracorporeal shock wave lithotripsy, tumor biopsies, and stricture dilation. For concurrent procedures the interventionalist establishes drainage, and the urologist proceeds with stone removal via the PCN tract. Nephrostomies performed for future stone removal may plug the drainage until stone removal. Preprocedural imaging includes ultrasound of the kidney along with nuclear medicine and CT scans. Local anesthesia with moderate sedation is typical; however, excessive dilation may warrant general anesthesia. Prophylactic antibiotic treatment varies with clinical practice and bacterial culture status. The nurse positions the patient prone with both arms above the head or one arm up and the other at the noninvolved side. Catheter insertion site is via the right, left, or bilateral flank, pubis, or right or left lower quadrant of the abdomen of renal transplant patients. The site is prepped and draped and local anesthetic is infiltrated. The physician makes a small puncture, then using ultrasound or fluoroscopic guidance directs the needle toward a lower calyx of the kidney. When the tip of the needle is in a dilated portion of the collecting system, urine flows back from the needle on stylet removal. If urine does not flow, the needle is retracted in small increments while aspirating with a 20-mL plastic syringe until urine emerges. The needle is exchanged over a guidewire, followed by upsizing of various dilator and introducer systems. The final trocar and catheter assembly, typically an 8 French, terminates in the renal pelvis. The trocar and the guidewire are removed when the catheter is positioned correctly. Internal or external drainage determines catheter selection. Additional criteria, such as catheter material, configuration, coating, and locking mechanism are per physician. If PCN was performed for obstruction, the nurse should be aware that a profuse diuresis may result warranting IV volume replacement and monitoring of input and output. Antibiotic therapy is administered after the procedure to prevent infection. Hematuria may be present up to 48 hours postprocedure. Complications include hemorrhage, but the risk decreases with smaller needle sizes, as well as catheter dislodgement, blockage, or infection. Tube changes are scheduled for every 6 to 12 weeks. If the PCN is for decompression, the external drainage continues until achievement of the desired outcome occurs and urine flows naturally down the ureter.

Antegrade Ureteral Stent Placement. Ureteral stents maintain patency in a stenosed portion of the ureter. Obstruction can be iatrogenic, neoplastic, or inflammatory as a result of pressure necrosis from a ureteral stone, trauma, radiation therapy, surgical manipulation of the ureter, inflammatory disease, and chronic transplant rejection. Urologic stent placement typically occurs during cystoscopy via a retrograde approach. The antegrade approach, however, requires a PCN. Recommendations are to wait at least 1 week following the placement of a nephrostomy tube stent to decrease the likelihood of stent occlusion due to clot or debris (Kandarpa and Machan, 2011). Preparation is similar to a PCN. The physician obtains guidewire access and places a sheath through the skin into the renal pelvis to reduce friction when passing guidewires, dilators, and stents. A guidewire is placed distal to the obstruction and advanced into the bladder. This may require various guidewires due to the configuration of the ureter and obstruction type. The physician sizes the stent and positions it using contrast injection and fluoroscopy. Additional sedation may be required for supplemental dilations or balloon angioplasties if the stent cannot pass a stricture. When the stent is in the proper location, the physician deploys it, removes the sheath and guidewire, and replaces the nephrostomy tube. The draining nephrostomy catheter remains for 1 to 2 days after internal stent placement, allowing draining urine to flush normal operative debris from the stent. Postprocedure follow-up consists of an antegrade contrast injection through the nephrostomy tube to assess patency of the ureter and implanted stent. Contrast seen traversing the stent and collecting in the bladder justifies nephrostomy tube removal. Complications include perforation of the renal collecting system or ureter. After the site heals, the urologist removes the stent in the cystoscopy room with urologic instruments. When the stent must remain in place, the urologist may be able to exchange it through a retrograde cystoscopy procedure.

KEY POINTS

- Due to the broad scope of IR, it is important to establish interdisciplinary patient preparation protocols, according to procedure and modality selection. Imaging selection is according to physician; however, distinct nursing considerations exist for each modality.
- Radiography exposes the patient to ionizing radiation and is the most common imaging diagnostic.
- Fluoroscopy is moving x-ray, used to determine catheter placement in various procedures and clinical settings by different physician specialties. It requires iodinated contrast agents, which may result in an allergic reaction. The nurse needs to understand precipitating factors as well as management and prophylaxis regarding these reactions.
- CT scans also use ionizing radiation, and some scans require iodinated contrast agents. Diagnostic CT scans are very short in duration. Those using CT for procedures require preoperative planning to accommodate patient positioning and equipment positioning as well as potential contrast allergies.
- MRI scans are much longer in duration. This modality does not require ionizing radiation; however, MRI-guided procedures warrant meticulous monitoring because ferrous objects are attracted to the magnet and represent a safety issue. Some MRI studies and procedures use contrast. MRI contrast issues, however, are much less frequent than CT.
- Ultrasound is a portable technology, using sound waves. Ultrasound does not emit ionizing radiation. The use of ultrasound is common in urogynecologic and obstetric procedures. Considerations when using ultrasound are the use of probes and cables and their location to the sterile field.

- Positioning. The field of IR is diverse. Depending on the procedure, the approach, and modality selection, patient positioning is highly variable. Because the quality of imaging is contingent on the patient being still, adequate procedure knowledge and preparation by the nurse to ensure patient comfort and positioning tolerance is important.
- Radiation safety is an important aspect in IR nursing. A basic understanding of the principles of radiation is needed to safely work in this environment as well as provide patient care.

CRITICAL THINKING QUESTION

When reviewing the special procedures schedule you learn you are scheduled to care for a 65-year-old female transferred to your institution to have an AV node ablation with pacemaker insertion. The electrophysiologist ordered an upper extremity venogram prior to the ablation procedure because the patient had an upper-extremity thrombus approximately 6 months ago after a PICC placement. Her medical history includes atrial fibrillation-flutter with uncontrolled ventricular response, moderate chronic obstructive pulmonary disease, type 1 diabetes, and renal insufficiency. Her creatinine was 1.2 with a GFR of 45 mL/min/1.73 m^2 on her preadmission testing performed yesterday. Routine medications include aspirin, insulin, warfarin, prednisone, metoprolol, and a metered-dose inhaler. She is allergic to sulfa and lorazepam. You need to set up her prescreening call. What factors would you incorporate in your perioperative plan of care?

ⓔvolve *The answers to the Critical Thinking Question can be found at http://evolve.elsevier.com/Rothrock/Alexander.*

REFERENCES

The American College of Obstetricians and Gynecologists (ACOG): Placenta accreta, *Committee Opin Number* 529:1–5, 2012.

American College of Radiology (ACR): *ACR manual on contrast media*, 2012, available at www.nxtbook.com/nxtbooks/acr/contrastmediamanual2012. Accessed October10, 2012.

American College of Radiology (ACR) Society of Neurointerventional Surgery (SNIS), Society of Interventional Radiology (SIR): *ACR-SIR-SNIS practice guideline for interventional clinical practice*, 2009, available at www.sirweb.org/clinical/cpg/41A31d01.pdf. Accessed March 2, 2012.

ACR-SIR: *ACR-SIR practice guideline on informed consent for imaging guided procedures*, 2011, available at www.acr.org/-/media/ACR/Documents/PGTS/guidelines/Informed_Consent_Image_Guide.pdf. Accessed April 2, 2012.

ACR-SIR: *ACR-SIR Practice Guideline for the Reporting and Archiving of Interventional Radiology Procedures*, 2009 available at http://www.acr.org/-/media/B6AD9A7E4D5E411DA9C3E19E86F9311F.pdf. Accessed August 13, 2013.

ACR-SIR: *ACR-SIR practice guideline for sedation/analgesia*, 2010, available at www.acr.org/-/media/ACR/Documents/PGTS/guidelines/Adult_Sedation.pdf. Accessed April 14, 2012.

Association for Radiologic and Imaging Nursing (ARIN): *Clinical practice guideline: metformin therapy and lactic acidosis risk*, 2006, available at www.arinnursing.org/dmdocuments/ARIN_ClinicalGuideline_Metformin%20Therapy%20and%20Lactic%20Acidosis%20Risk.pdf. Accessed May 5, 2012.

ARIN: *Position statement on bariatric patient safety in the imaging environment*, 2011, available at https://www.arinnursing.org/dmdocuments/10123_Bariatric PatientSafety_PositionStatement_final.pdf. Accessed April 13, 2012.

Bashore TM et al: Angiography and interventions expert consensus document on cardiac catheterization laboratory standards update, *JACC* 59:2221–2305, 2012.

Brent R: *Pregnancy and radiation exposure*, 2011, available at http://hps.org/hpspublications/articles/pregnancyandradiationexposureinfosheet.html. Accessed September 11, 2012.

California Department of Public Health: *Information notice regarding Senate bill (SB) 1237, California Health and Safety (H&S) Code Section 115113*, 2011, available at www.cdph.ca.gov/certlic/radquip/Documents/RHB-SB1237-FAQ.PDF. Accessed June 25, 2012.

Center for Nursing Education and Testing (CNET) Inc., Radiological Nursing Certification Board Inc.: Practice analysis of radiology nursing, *J Radiol Nurse* 29:109–128, 2010.

Cho KJ, Lin EC: *Carbon dioxide angiography*, 2011, available at http://emedicine.medscape.com/article/423121-overview. Accessed August 27, 2012.

Dean ER, Scoggins ML: Essential elements of patient positioning: a review for the radiology nurse, *J Radiol Nurse* 31:42–52, 2012.

Erkonen WE, Smith WL: *Radiology 101: the basics and fundamentals of imaging*, Philadelphia, 2009, Lippincott Williams & Williams.

Garmi G, Salim R: *Epidemiology, etiology, diagnosis and management of placenta accreta, Obstet Gynecol Int*, 2012, available at www.hindawi.com/journals/ogi/2012/873929. Accessed September 2, 2012.

Halliburton SS et al: SCCT guidelines on radiation dose, *J Cardiovasc Comput Tomogr* 5:198–224, 2011.

Health Physics Society: *Exclusive use of SI units to express radiological quantities. Position statement of the Health Physics Society*, 2012, available at http://hps.org/documents/SIunits_ps025-0.pdf. Accessed March 31, 2013.

Holmes EB: *Ionizing radiation exposure with medical imaging*, 2011, available at http://emedicine.medscape.com/article/1464228-overview#showall. Accessed April 22, 2012.

Kandarpa K, Machan L: *Handbook of interventional radiology procedures*, ed 4, Philadelphia, 2011, Lippincott Williams & Williams.

Katzen BT et al: Hybrid interventional radiology, *Periop Nurs Clin* 5:215–227, 2010.

Klein LW et al: Joint inter-society task force on occupational hazards in the interventional laboratory, *J Vasc Interv Radiol* 20:147–153, 2009.

Konez O, Cho K: *Vascular lesion embolization imaging*, 2011, available at http://emedicine.medscape.com/article/419614-overview. Accessed September 12, 2012.

Landau B: Hybrid operating rooms and R.T.s, *Radiol Technol* 82:1–2, 2011.

Mauro MA: Interventional radiology: an ever changing landscape, *Am J Radiol* 104:920–921, 2009.

Michael M, Breall JA: *Understanding contrast induced nephropathy*, 2012, available at www.dicardiology.com/article/understanding-contrast-induced-nephropathy. Accessed July 1, 2012.

Miller DL et al: Quality Improvement guidelines for recording patient radiation doses in the medical record for fluoroscopically guided procedures, *J Vasc Interv Radiol* 23:11–v18, 2012.

Minokadeh A et al: Obstructive sleep apnea, anesthesia, and ambulatory surgery, *Anesthesiol News Guide Airway Manage*, 2011, available at www.anesthesiologynews.com/download/OSA_ANGAM11.pdf.

Naidu SS et al: *Clinical expert statement on best practices in the cardiac catheterization laboratory: Society for Cardiovascular Angiography and Interventions*, 2012, available at www.scai.org/Publications/Guidelines.aspx. Accessed April 20, 2012.

National Council on Radiation Protection and Measurements (NCRP): NCRP report No.160:242–243, 2009.

Nuclear Regulatory Commission: *Fact sheet on biological effects of radiation*, 2012, available at www.nrc.gov/reading-rm/doc-collections/fact-sheets/bio-effects-radiation.html. Accessed June 21, 2012.

Radiological Society of North America (RSNA). *Radiation exposure and pregnancy: when should we be concerned?* 2007, available at http://radiographics.rsna.org/content/27/4/909.full. Accessed September 11, 2012.

Sabri SS et al: Balloon occluded retrograde transvenous obliteration of gastric varices, *Endovasc Today*, 2010, Available at http://bmctoday.net/evtoday/2010/04/article.asp?f=balloon-occluded-retrograde-transvenous-obliteration-of-gastric-varices. Accessed September 2, 2012.

Sauer BG et al: Balloon-occluded retrograde transvenous obliteration (BRTO): follow up and postprocedural imaging, *Semin Intervent Radiol* 28:325–332, 2011.

Schaadt J, Landau B: Hybrid OR: a primer for the nurse, *AORN J* 97:81–100, 2013.

Schmidt T et al: Lows and highs: 5 years of development in intraoperative magnetic resonance imaging, *Acta Neurochir* 09:s17–s20, 2011.

Siddiqi NH, Lin EC: *Contrast medial reactions*, 2012, available at http://emedicine.medscape.com/article/422855-overview. Accessed June 30, 2012.

Siskin GP, Sekhar KP: *Uterine fibroid embolization and imaging*, 2011, available at http://emedicine.medscape.com/article/421734-overview#aw2aab6b2. Accessed September 3, 2012.

Society of Interventional Radiology (SIR): SIR/multisociety consensus statement global statement defining interventional radiology, *J Vasc Interv Radiol* 21:1147–1148, 2010.

The Joint Commission (TJC): *National patient safety goals effective Jan 1*, 2012, available at http://www.jointcommission.org/assets/1/18/2011-2012_npsg_presentation_final_8-4-11.pdf. Accessed August 13, 2013.

TJC: *Sentinel Event Alert Issue 47*, 2011, available at http://www.jointcommission.org/assets/1/18/sea_471.pdf. Accessed August 13, 2013.

U.S. Food and Drug Administration: *Initiative to reduce unnecessary radiation exposure from medical imaging*, available at http://www.fda.gov/Radiation-EmittingProducts/RadiationSafety/RadiationDoseReduction/default.htm. Accessed March 5, 2012.

Webb H et al: Thermal ablation, *Semin Roentgenol* 46(2):133–141, 2011.

CHAPTER 30

Integrative Health Practices: Complementary and Alternative Therapies

RACHAEL LARNER

Energy Therapies History and Background

An accurate presentation of the history of medicine in the United States needs to include influences from the botanic cultural traditions of Asia, India, Europe, and the First Nations. Our current medical system, referred to as *biomedicine,* began to dominate sometime in the mid-1800s with the discovery that microorganisms were responsible for disease and pathologic damage and that antitoxins and vaccines could improve the body's ability to oppose the effects of pathogens. Armed with this knowledge, scientists and clinicians were able to refine surgical procedures and treat previously serious and fatal infections.

As biomedicine dominated the healthcare system, it became the mainstream or "conventional" approach, establishing the standards for diagnosis and treatment of illness. By the 1990s, however, consumer faith and trust in this system began to falter, and many Americans sought complementary or alternative treatments for their healthcare. Complementary and alternative medicine (CAM), known currently as "integrative health practices," has grown to constitute a significant percentage of American healthcare dollars and visits. This growth is sustained by patients who desire to be more empowered healthcare consumers and the availability of media information about the many alternatives to mainstream, conventional Western biomedical approaches to healthcare.

Myths and misconceptions initially prevented investigation and development of promising therapies outside the biomedical regimen. In response to growing consumer pressure, anecdotal evidence, and a small body of published scientific results, the U.S. Congress established the Office of Alternative Medicine (OAM) within the office of the director, National Institutes of Health (NIH), in 1992. This office was given responsibility for: (1) facilitating fair, scientific evaluation of alternative therapies that showed promise in health promotion, and (2) reducing barriers to the acceptance and utilization of those alternative therapies that showed promise.

In 1998 the OAM became the National Center for Complementary and Alternative Medicine (NCCAM, 2012a). This expansion into a center allowed more substantial funding for and initiation of research projects, providing more sound information about integrative health practices. The annual budget for NCCAM has grown significantly, as has the sophistication of research designs of studies being funded by the center. The NCCAM adheres to guidelines set forth in public policy.

Many integrative health practices and therapies stem from a philosophy of wholeness, with intent to treat the entire person (body-mind-spirit) (Evidence for Practice). This is in contrast to the current gold standard of randomized, controlled clinical trials, which may not be the best, or indeed appropriate, way to measure the effectiveness of many integrative health practices and therapies. Conventional scientists and physicians and the proponents of integrative health practices and CAM often debate the appropriate forms of research to determine efficacy and safety of alternative therapies. A reason for this disparity stems from divergent theoretic models. The *comprehensive approach* takes into account multidimensional factors that may not easily or appropriately be studied independently. The comprehensive approach is more congruent with the philosophic underpinnings of most integrative health practices and CAM. The *biomedical approach,* on the other hand, is concerned with a disease orientation, suggesting that a specific agent or variable is responsible for a specific disorder or illness.

The NCCAM has categorized the many integrative health practice modalities into five major domains: alternative medical systems, mind-body medicine, biologically based therapies, manipulative and body-based methods, and energy therapies (Figure 30-1). Numerous treatments and systems are within each category. The remainder of this chapter discusses the major domains and provides examples of each.

Major Categories of Integrative Health Practices and Complementary and Alternative Medicine

Alternative Medical Systems

An estimated 10% to 30% of human healthcare is delivered by practitioners such as surgeons and nurses who have been trained in the mainstream, conventional Western biomedical model. The remaining 70% to 90% involves care given in a healthcare system that is based on alternative traditions—self-care based in folk practice or practices that range somewhere between alternative and traditional healthcare. Many of these integrative health therapies are culturally, ethnically, spiritually, or religiously derived. Among the diverse values, beliefs, and practices found in the many cultural groups in the United States are those relating to health, illness, professional healthcare, and folk healthcare (Box 30-1). They include well-known and respected Asian systems of medicine. Many Asian medicine techniques or systems are widely known in the United States. The most well-known and popular of these include herbal medicines, massage, energy therapy, acupressure, acupuncture, and qi gong (Figure 30-2). This integrative, alternative medicine system has a wide range of applications from health promotion to the treatment of illness. A significant aspect of Asian medicine is an emphasis on diagnosing and treating disturbances of *qi* (pronounced "chee"), or vital energy, and restoring its proper balance (Micozzi, 2010).

EVIDENCE FOR PRACTICE

Evaluating Complementary and Alternative Medicine Therapies

According to the National Center for Complementary and Alternative Medicine (NCCAM), millions of Americans use some form of complementary and alternative medicine (CAM). In discussing the use of CAM with perioperative patients, nurses have a unique opportunity to advise patients on best practices to adopt when considering using CAM therapies and should include the following advice:

- Take charge of your health by being an informed consumer. Investigate the therapy to determine what studies have been done on its safety and effectiveness. Check to see if the federal government has useful information on the therapy. Visit the U.S. Food and Drug Administration (FDA) website (www.fda.gov) to see if information has been provided on this therapy.
- The Internet is a good source to find information about CAM. In evaluating information on the Internet you should always ask the following questions:
  - Who runs the website? Is it a government, university, or reputable medical or health-related association? Is it sponsored by a manufacturer of products, drugs, and so on? It should be easy to clearly identify the sponsor.
  - What is the purpose of the site? Is it to educate the public or sell a product? The purpose should be clearly stated.
  - What is the basis of the information? Is it based on scientific evidence with clear references?
  - Check with the Federal Trade Commission at www.ftc.gov to see if there are any enforcement actions for deceptive advertising for this therapy.
  - How current is the information? Is it reviewed and updated frequently?
- Visit the NCCAM website (NCCAM.nih.gov) for information on specific CAM therapies with links to other online services and information. You can also find information from NCCAM on Facebook, Twitter, and YouTube.
- If you do not have access to the Internet, contact the NCCAM clearinghouse at 1-888-644-6226 for assistance.
- Visit your local library or medical library to search for scientific information about CAM.
- Discuss CAM with your healthcare provider before making any decision about care. Ask questions about any possible interactions with medications you currently take or therapy you are undergoing. If your physician cannot answer your questions, he or she may be able to refer you to someone who can.
- Before taking herbal supplements:
  - First, talk to your physician.
  - Talk to a licensed pharmacist if you have questions about the supplement, and discuss any potential reactions with any prescription or nonprescription medications (over-the-counter [OTC] medications) you currently take.
  - Read labels carefully. Buy only supplements that are approved by the American Botanical Council's Commission E.
  - Buy products from a reputable herbal company. Be cautious about products for sale through magazines, TV, radio, or the Internet.

Modified from *Are you considering using complementary and alternative medicine (CAM)?*, available at http://nccam.nih.gov/health/decisions/consideringcam.htm. Accessed September 11, 2012.

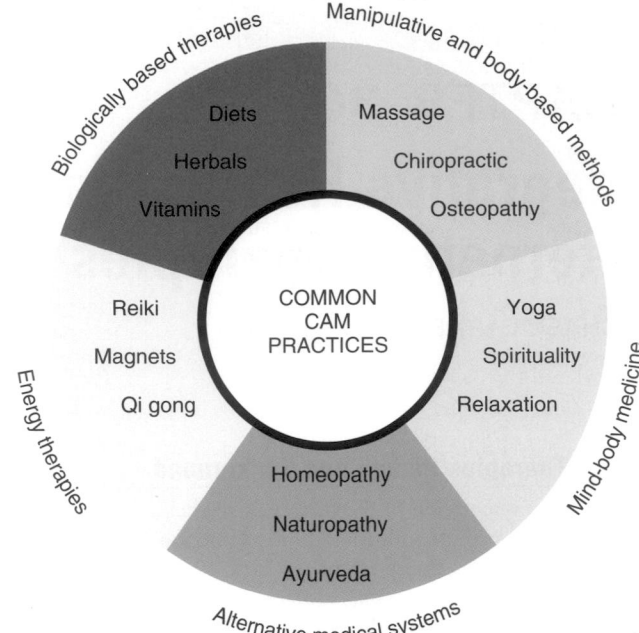

FIGURE 30-1 The National Center for Complementary and Alternative Medicine (NCCAM) groups complementary and alternative medicine (CAM) practices into five domains, recognizing that there can be some overlap among them. Often these systems have evolved apart from and earlier than the conventional medical approach used in the United States.

Ayurveda is a traditional system from India that strives to restore the innate harmony of the individual while placing equal emphasis on body, mind, and spirit. Ayurvedic practitioners use many products and techniques to cleanse the body and restore balance. Key foundations are universal connectedness (e.g., that all living and nonliving things are joined together, health will be good if one's mind and body are in harmony, disease arises when a person is out of harmony with the universe), the body's constitution or *prakriti* (e.g., the person's unique physical and psychologic characteristics and how the person functions to maintain health), and life forces, or *doshas*. Each person has a combination of three doshas; each dosha has a particular relationship with a bodily function and can be upset for a variety of reasons. Treatment is tailored to each person's constitution and predominant dosha. Practitioners expect patients to be active participants because many ayurvedic treatments require changes in diet, lifestyle, and habits (NCCAM, 2012b).

Native American, Middle Eastern, Tibetan, Central and South American, and African cultures have developed other traditional medical systems (Micozzi, 2010). Additional examples of complete integrative health practice and alternative medicine systems are naturopathic and homeopathic medicine systems. Homeopathic medicine is based on the principle that "like cures like" (i.e., a substance that in large doses produces the symptoms of a disease will, in a very diluted dose, cure the patient). Small doses of plant extracts and minerals specially prepared are given to stimulate the body's defense mechanisms and encourage healing processes. Careful evaluation of symptoms enables the practitioner to determine a patient's specific sensitivity and to select the appropriate remedy.

Naturopathic medicine is one of the most recent alternative approaches to have developed as a health system across North

BOX 30-1

Cultural Characteristics Related to the Balance of "Hot" and "Cold"

A naturalistic or holistic approach often assumes that there are external factors (some good, some bad) that must be kept in balance if we are to remain well. The balance of "hot" and "cold" is a part of the belief system in many cultural groups, such as the Arab, Chinese, Filipino, and Hispanic cultures. To restore a disturbed balance (i.e., to treat) requires the use of opposites (e.g., a hot remedy for a cold problem). Different cultures may define hot and cold differently. It is not a matter of temperature, and the words used might vary; for example, the Chinese have named the forces yin (cold) and yang (hot). Western medicine cannot ignore the naturalistic view if many of its patients are to have appropriate treatment for illness as well as disease.

HOT CONDITIONS AND THEIR CORRESPONDING TREATMENTS

Hot Conditions	Cold Foods	Cold Medicines and Herbs
Fever	Fresh vegetables	Orange flower water
Infection	Tropical fruits	Linden
Diarrhea	Dairy products	Sage
Kidney problem	Meats such as goat,	Milk of magnesia
Rash	fish, chicken	Bicarbonate of soda
Skin ailment	Honey	
Sore throat	Cod	
Liver problem	Raisins	
Ulcer	Bottle milk	
Constipation	Barley water	

COLD CONDITIONS AND THEIR CORRESPONDING TREATMENTS

Cold Conditions	Hot Foods	Hot Medicines and Herbs
Cancer	Chocolate	Penicillin
Pneumonia	Cheese	Tobacco
Malaria	Temperate-zone fruits	Ginger root
Joint pain	Eggs	Garlic
Menstrual period	Peas	Cinnamon
Teething	Onions	Anise
Earache	Aromatic beverages	Vitamins
Rheumatism	Hard liquor	Iron preparations
Tuberculosis	Oils	Cod liver oil
Cold	Meats such as beef,	Castor oil
Headache	waterfowl, mutton	Aspirin
Paralysis	Goat's milk	
Stomach cramps	Cereal grains	
	Chili peppers	

Modified from Seidel HM et al: *Mosby's guide to physical examination*, ed 7, St Louis, 2010, Mosby.

FIGURE 30-2 Acupuncture is one tool a traditional Chinese medical doctor uses to shift a person's vital energy. It involves the insertion of thin, solid, stainless steel needles into specific points on the body. Acupuncture points can also be stimulated manually without the use of needles; this approach may be better suited for children or the elderly.

currents; therapeutic counseling; and pharmacology (Pizzorno and Snider, 2010).

Mind-Body Interventions

A growing scientific movement has explored the mind's ability to affect the body. The clinical application of this relationship is categorized as *mind-body medicine.* Some mind-body interventions (e.g., cognitive-behavioral therapy), formerly categorized as CAM therapies, have been assimilated into conventional mainstream medicine. Progressive relaxation techniques, biofeedback, meditation, and cognitive-behavioral approaches have a well-documented theoretic basis with supporting scientific evidence. Other mind-body interventions still considered "alternative" by some include hypnosis, music, dance, art therapy, prayer, and mental healing.

Biologically Based Therapies

The integrative health practices category of biologically based therapies includes biologically based and natural-based practices, products, and interventions, some of which overlap with mainstream medicine's use of dietary supplements. Herbal, orthomolecular, individual biologic therapies and special dietary treatments are encompassed in biologically based therapies.

Herbs are plants or parts of plants that contain and produce chemical substances that act on the body. Some diet therapies are believed to promote health and prevent or control health. Proponents of diet therapies include religious factions such as Seventh-Day Adventist, or Jewish Kosher. Veganism, vegetarianism, raw food diets, and diets promoted by Drs. Atkins, Pritikin, and Weil are other examples of therapeutic nutrition. Orthomolecular therapies use differing concentrations of chemicals or megadoses of vitamins aimed at treating disease. Many biologic therapies are available but not currently accepted by mainstream medicine, such as the use of cartilage products from cattle, sheep, or sharks for treatment of cancer and arthritis or the use of bee pollen to treat autoimmune and inflammatory diseases.

Manipulative and Body-Based Methods

Methods that are based on the movement or manipulation of the body include chiropractic, osteopathy, and massage. Touch and

America. In practice, modern naturopathic is eclectic, drawing on different systems and models (e.g., Chinese medicine, homeopathy, and manual therapies) to fit the patient profile and clinical problem with the appropriate techniques (Micozzi, 2010). Naturopathic medicine emphasizes health restoration as well as disease treatment based on the belief that disease is a manifestation of alterations in the body's natural healing processes. Naturopathic physicians use multiple modalities, including clinical nutrition and diet; acupuncture; herbal medicine; homeopathy; spinal and soft tissue manipulation; physical therapies involving ultrasound, light, and electric

The Use of Palpation in Physical Examination

Palpation involves the use of your hands and fingers to gather information through the sense of touch. Certain parts of your hands and fingers are better than others for specific types of palpation. The palmar surface of the fingers and finger pads is more sensitive than the fingertips and is used whenever discriminatory touch is needed for determining position, texture, size, consistency, masses, fluid, and crepitus. The ulnar surface of the hand and fingers is the most sensitive area for distinguishing vibration. The dorsal surface of the hands is best for estimating temperature; of course, this estimate provides only a crude measure and is best used to detect temperature differences in comparing parts of the body.

Touch is in many ways therapeutic, and palpation is the actuality of the "laying on of hands." It is the moment at which health practitioners begin their physical invasion of the patient's body. The oft-repeated advice that the approach to palpation be gentle and the practitioner's hands be warm is not only practical but also symbolic of respect for the patient and for the privilege the patient gives.

Modified from Seidel HM et al: *Mosby's guide to physical examination*, ed 7, St Louis, 2010, Mosby.

manipulations with the hands have been used in healing and medical practice since the beginning of the history of medicine. At one time, the physician's hands were considered the most important diagnostic and therapeutic tool. This remains true today, despite sophisticated diagnostic equipment and modalities (Box 30-2). Manual healing methods are based on the principle that dysfunction of a part of the body often affects secondarily the function of other discrete, possibly indirectly connected body parts. Theories have developed for correction of these secondary dysfunctions by realigning body parts or manipulating soft tissues. Chiropractic science is concerned primarily with the relationship between structure (spine primarily) and function (nervous system primarily) of the human body to preserve and restore health. Osteopathic medicine incorporates an extensive body of work that supports the use of osteopathic techniques for both musculoskeletal and nonmusculoskeletal problems. Massage therapy is one of the oldest methods known in the practice of healthcare. One experimental pilot showed that using massage with music therapy during the perioperative period reduced postoperative prolactin levels and anxiety (Selimen and Andsoy, 2011). Many different massage techniques are aimed at helping the body heal itself through the use of manipulation of the soft body tissues.

Energy Therapies

Energy therapies have been categorized into two groups: biofield therapies (those that focus on fields believed to originate within the body) and electromagnetic fields (those that originate from other sources). The existence of energy fields that originate within and around the body has not yet been definitively proven. However, many studies have examined the experiences of recipient or practitioner and the outcomes of this type of energy therapy. Examples of therapies with a biofield basis include acupuncture, reiki, qi gong, therapeutic touch (TT), and healing touch. Therapies that involve electromagnetic fields use unconventional pulsed fields, magnetic fields, alternating current fields, or direct current fields. These therapies have been clinically applied with patients who have arthritis, cancer, and pain (Kolthan, 2009).

Integrative Health Practices Use and Surgery

Energy Therapies

Patients have choices in how to manage their healthcare. However, surgery is the most invasive of all options. As healthcare consumers become more knowledgeable about their health they often seek complementary modalities to augment traditional Western medical therapies. Using the term *alternative* is actually misleading, which is why the field formerly known as CAM is more appropriately termed integrative health practices. Many progressive medical facilities embrace a holistic patient focus, exploring and integrating nontraditional healing modalities to support an individualized surgical experience. Biofield therapies represent a nonpharmacologic anxiolytic for surgical patients that may be integrated with an allopathic treatment plan.

Many ancient cultures refer to a human biofield or "life force." Sometimes referred to as "energy work," biofield therapeutics are a range of interventions sharing common beliefs. First is the existence of a "universal force" or "healing energy" arising from God (as the person understands this being), the cosmos, the earth, or another supernatural source. Second, the human biofield, as part of the "universal field," is dynamic, open, complex, and pandimensional. Human biofields are constantly changing and interacting with each other, the environment, and the universal force field. Third, the ability to use one's biofield for healing is considered to be universal, although few people are aware of it without specific training. Last, practitioners intend to positively affect the patient's biofield, either by direct contact or by using the hands in proximity, similar to the ancient practice of laying on of hands (Jackson and Keegan, 2008) (Table 30-1).

Therapeutic Touch. Therapeutic touch (TT) is the contemporary interpretation of several ancient healing modalities. Dolores Krieger and Dora Kunz developed TT in the early 1970s. The practice, like others that form part of the body of CAM, consists of learned skills for the conscious manipulation of human energies. In practice it is not necessary for the practitioner (healer) to actually touch the recipient (healee), because the energy field can be "felt" several inches away from the physical body. TT helps to aid in relaxation, reduces pain, promotes deeper and easier breathing, improves circulation of blood and movement of lymph fluids, reduces blood pressure, and strengthens the immune system.

To work within biofields, the practitioner uses a model or map to focus the healing energy. Chakras, or energy centers, described by the Upanishads in the Vedas, the oldest literature of the East Indian people, are often used as a reference point. Although the most detailed descriptions are in the Upanishads, the attributes are found in the teachings of other cultures as widely geographic as the Sufis of the Middle East to the First Nations, particularly from the North American Southwest (Figure 30-3).

TT practice lends itself well to the fast-paced surgical environment. The skills learned through study of TT provide a trained practitioner with the ability to center quickly and use intention to calm both himself or herself and others nearby in stressful situations. Research design, methods, techniques, and sample sizes are considerations for future studies into how biofield therapeutics may benefit surgical patients. Replicating past studies, as well as new research based on physiologic data and quantitative studies, is necessary (Research Highlight). It has become evident that the concepts involved in energy therapies need consistent definitions. If the concepts do not have preestablished definitions, they cannot be

TABLE 30-1

Comparisons of Selected Biofield Therapies

Therapy	Practice Initiated	Developers	Hand Placement	Theoretic Basis and Intent
Healing Touch	1981	American Holistic Nurses Association	Both on and off the body	Uses elements of healing science and therapeutic touch in conjunction with crystal and dowsing to treat whole person and specific disorders
Qi gong	Traditional	Chinese	At meridian points or short distance from the body	Qi follows meridians and body patterns to heal biologic disorders.
Reiki	Traditional 1800s 1936	Buddhist Japan—Hawayo Takata United States—Mikao Usui	A few standardized hand placements on the physical body	Spiritual energy from universe is channeled by "masters" to heal the spiritual body, which in turn heals the physical body
Therapeutic touch	1972	Dolores Krieger and Dora Kunz	Primarily off the body 2-4 inches	Aligning Kunz's Human Energy Field model with Martha Rogers's Science of Unitary Human Beings, the centered practitioner assesses, directs, and modulates biofield energy to achieve relaxation response for healing of whole person
Reflexology	Traditional	Ancient method of treatment for ailments dating back to Egyptians and beyond	Application of pressure to sites on foot, hands, ears, and so on that correspond with organs and nerves to cause a reflex arc of stimulation to area in need	Promotes balance and wellness through nerve stimulation

Modified from Engebretson J, Wardell D: Energy-based modalities, *Nurs Clin North Am* 42:243–259, 2007; National Center for Complementary and Alternative Medicine: *Energy medicine: an overview,* available at http://nccam.nih.gov/health/whatiscam. Accessed October 7, 2012.

	English Name	Situation
1	Root or basic chakra	At the base of the spine
2	Spleen or splenic chakra	Over the spleen
3	Navel or umbilical chakra	At the navel, over the solar plexus
4	Heart or cardiac chakra	Over the heart
5	Throat or laryngeal chakra	At the front of the throat
6	Brow or frontal chakra	In the space between the eyebrows
7	Crown or coronal chakra	On the top of the head

FIGURE 30-3 Chakras.

RESEARCH HIGHLIGHT

Time, Touch, and Compassion: Effects on Autonomic Nervous System and Well-Being

This study tested the feasibility of delivering two strategies (tactile and nontactile) and two lengths of time (10 and 20 minutes) for a practitioner to nonverbally communicate compassion to subjects.

Twenty healthy volunteers (all younger than age 40) were informed that the study would test the effects of time and touch on the autonomic nervous system. During tactile interventions the practitioner placed hands on the subjects' arms, legs, and hands. During nontactile interventions the practitioner pretended to read. The practitioner also meditated healing thoughts to the subjects during all interventions. Along with having the subjects' heart rates monitored, they completed visual analogue scales before, immediately postintervention, and after postintervention rest.

Overall, the subjects were shown to have a lower heart rate with the tactile interventions, along with the longer time periods, than compared with nontactile interventions. The autonomic nervous system was affected by nonverbal communication. Although this study was limited in scope, it does open the doors to further study in this area.

Modified from Shaltout H et al: Time, touch, and compassion: effects on autonomic nervous system and well-being, *Explore* 8(3), 2012.

quantified or measured in meaningful ways. However, interest is high and research continues in an effort to better understand a phenomenon that seems to provide meaningful relief to the patient.

Perioperative Medical Hypnotherapy

Use of medical hypnotherapy in hospitals and clinics for perioperative care is not uncommon. Patients are seeking an active role in their treatment and are better informed regarding surgical options. Participating in perioperative medical hypnotherapy allows patients to take shared responsibility for their healing process, giving them a measure of control, because all hypnosis is self-hypnosis. Meaningful and active participation empowers a patient to enter into anesthesia and surgery with confidence.

Surgery is a life-changing event, and each perioperative medical hypnotherapy patient is unique. The initial assessment serves to determine goals and explore questions relative to emotional as well as physical concerns. The hypnotherapist, working within the patient's belief system, helps acknowledge areas of the patient's concern as a multidisciplinary partnership of healing is forged in a patient-centered manner.

As the hypnotherapist guides the patient into relaxation and induces hypnosis, both therapist and patient journey into the body, together addressing predetermined issues. Fear of the unknown, preprocedure anxiety, changes in body image, anticipated pain or nausea, loss of organs, and transplantation of new organs are some examples of issues that may be addressed in the perioperative setting (Gurgevich, 2012).

Hypnosis compassionately allows a patient to explore emotions without judgment or expectation of those feelings. The practice of emotional awareness, of being present with feelings, and of holding those feelings sacred can bring a sense of peace and healing insights during a time of profound stress, such as that experienced by many surgical patients. Predetermined suggestions or affirmations may increase confidence in the healthcare team, increase compliance with the treatment plan, decrease blood loss, maintain intraoperative homeostasis, reduce the need for sedation or pain medication, decrease postoperative nausea or vomiting, and increase patient satisfaction. In a study done on patients undergoing upper abdominal surgery, it was found that preoperative relaxation techniques helped with postoperative pain and increased healing time (Topcu and Findik, 2012).

Postoperative hypnotherapy sessions reinforce continued participation of patients in their healing process. This may take the form of establishing metabolic gauges in the "control room" or show a symbolic shield of protection, holding or sending color, light, or a certain feeling of safety to a specific part of the body. It may be expressing gratitude to and confidence in the medical and nursing community. Follow-up sessions allow both patient and hypnotherapist to evaluate attainment of preoperative goals, consider postoperative outcomes, and explore issues relevant to the ongoing healing process.

Guided Imagery

Another therapy closely related to hypnosis is guided imagery. Imagery, or thinking in pictures, is the natural language of the unconscious mind and is used by the autonomic nervous system as a primary mode of communication. The autonomic nervous system controls unconscious body functions such as heart rate, immune function, digestion, blood flow, smooth muscle tension, and pain perception (Figure 30-4). Guided imagery for surgical patients may be in the form of pre-scripted tapes that lead the patient through relaxation exercises and provide healing suggestions. In other instances the perioperative nurse may assist the patient with guided imagery through the use of a calming, monotone voice; a smooth speaking delivery; and the use of relaxing images, such as a place in nature. The perioperative nurse coaches the patient to see, feel, smell, sense, and hear the imagined scene. Imagery may help patients build a "tool" to help in the postoperative period and lead

to quicker recovery. According to Selimen and Andsoy (2011), benefits of guided imagery for surgery patients may include:

- Decreased anxiety
- Decreased pain perception
- Improved focus and concentration
- Relieved apprehension

Aromatherapy in Perioperative Services

Aromatherapy involves the therapeutic use of fragrance (e.g., aromatic plant extracts and essential oils) applied to the patient's body through inhalation or topical methods, or rarely ingestion. Long before Western medicine, use of aromatherapy and herbs was part of physicians' practice and prescriptive use and was taught in all of the original Nightingale schools (Radzyminski, 2007). Clinical aromatherapy is gaining acceptance with consent and participation of patients. It is practiced by certified clinical aromatherapy practitioners (CCAPs), knowledgeable about the specific properties of essential oils and how they interact with patients and the therapeutic environment. CCAPs use clinical-grade essential oils in a controlled way for specific, measurable outcomes. These may affect the patient on a psychologic, physiologic, or cellular level. The choice of essential oil is based on the chemistry of that essential oil and its proven effects (Table 30-2).

As pharmacology combines medications to potentiate effect, aromatherapy may act synergistically with traditional treatment, or it may be offered in concert with other complementary modalities to relieve discomfort, thereby reducing dosages of analgesics or sedatives. Using specific scents postoperatively, such as peppermint, has decreased nausea and vomiting (Lane et al, 2012).

The nursing process of aromatherapy begins with obtaining consent for use of aromatics and collecting pertinent information. Assessment of the patient, the physical environment, and the team of caregivers defines the healing environment. Along with review of the medical and nursing histories, allergies, vital signs, and laboratory values, subjective data are relevant, such as how to offer treatment. The plan of therapy may include direct inhalation (on a cotton ball or through a diffuser), compresses, topical application, or massage. As with all nursing interventions, postprocedure follow-up with the patient is imperative to assess efficacy of this intervention (Research Highlight).

Additional well-designed research is required to provide data substantiating the value of clinical aromatherapy as another component of holistic perioperative nursing practice.

Music and Surgery

The therapeutic and healing properties of music have been recognized throughout history. Music has been shown to reduce stress and can block out unwanted noises around the patient during all perioperative phases, which makes the environment more enjoyable for the patient. Music can be used to stimulate the left and right side of the brain simultaneously and therefore can stimulate and organize muscle response, which can be a large benefit to patients with neuromuscular disorders. Patients who listen to music 30 minutes before a surgery or within 1 hour following surgery have lower pain and anxiety levels, which provides a more therapeutic environment for the patient (Selimen and Andsoy, 2011).

Music has been shown to increase metabolism; increase or decrease muscular energy, breathing rate, blood volume, pulse rate, and blood pressure; and lower sensory stimuli thresholds. Music can touch patients deeply and thus transform their anxiety and discomfort into relaxation and healing.

FIGURE 30-4 Locations of neurotransmitters and receptors in the autonomic nervous system. In all pathways, preganglionic fibers are cholinergic, secreting acetylcholine *(Ach)*, which stimulates nicotinic receptors in the postganglionic neuron. Most sympathetic fibers are adrenergic **(A)**, secreting norepinephrine *(NE)*, thus stimulating alpha- or beta-adrenergic receptors. A few sympathetic postganglionic fibers are cholinergic, stimulating muscarinic receptors in effector cells **(B)**. All parasympathetic postganglionic fibers are cholinergic **(C)**, stimulating muscarinic receptors in effector cells.

TABLE 30-2

Essential Oils and Their Properties

Property	Essential Oils
Antiemetic	Chamomile, lavender, lemon, peppermint, ginger
Antiseptic	Bergamot, clove, eucalyptus, lavender, juniper, thyme, tea tree
Anxiolytic	Benzoin, bergamot, chamomile, jasmine, lavender, neroli, rose, sandalwood, verbena, ylang-ylang
Analgesic	Lavender, West Indian lemongrass, peppermint, Turkish oregano, Brazilian mint
Sedating	Bergamot, chamomile, jasmine, lavender, neroli, rose, ylang-ylang
Stimulating	Basil, black pepper, eucalyptus, peppermint, rosemary
Antiinflammatory	German chamomile, rosemary, black pepper, helichrysum

Modified from Mantle F, Tiran D: *A-Z of complementary and alternative medicine*, London, 2009, Churchill Livingstone; Steflitsch W, Steflitsch M: Clinical aromatherapy, *J Men Health* 5(1):74–85, 2008.

Anxiety and pain are common perioperative nursing diagnoses identified in the sample plans of care in Unit 2 in this book. Because anxiety and pain lead to increased stress and stress may cause detrimental physiologic reactions, many nursing interventions are undertaken to reduce patients' anxiety. Music is a nursing intervention that is easy to administer, relatively inexpensive, and noninvasive.

Music is therapeutic if used in a manner that enables its elements and their influences to aid in integration of the body, mind, and spirit of the patient during the treatment of an illness or disability. When selecting music to invoke physiologic and psychologic changes, it is important to note the attributes of music. Factors that need to be considered are the various elements of music (e.g., tempo, mode, pitch, rhythm, harmony, melody); listener characteristics (e.g., age, language, culture, education, musical preferences); and the mode of delivery (e.g., headphones, speakers). Slow, quiet music without lyrics tends to lower the physiologic responses associated with stress and anxiety. Fast tempos tend to increase tension, and slow tempos can cause suspense. A tempo of 60 to 72 beats per minute appears to promote relaxation and decrease anxiety, as theorized by matching the normal heart rate of humans. Research also demonstrates the importance of patient-selected music that is familiar, desirable, and meaningful, which often leads to positive responses from patients. The use of headphones blocks unpleasant

Evaluation of Controlled Breathing With or Without Peppermint Aromatherapy for Postoperative Nausea and Vomiting Relief

This study worked with postoperative participants who suffered from nausea and vomiting in the recovery period after general anesthesia and elective surgery. Subjects were randomly assigned to receive aromatherapy while experiencing postoperative nausea and vomiting (PONV). The subjects would rate their level of nausea 0 to 10 and then be instructed to breathe through their nose and hold the breath, then release for 3 seconds. Subjects would be given the peppermint aromatherapy concurrently. If after 5 minutes, the PONV was not relieved, another round of peppermint aromatherapy was given. If after a following 5 minutes subjects were still experiencing PONV, they would be given medications. Intervention effectiveness equaled absence of symptoms, whereas efficacy was defined as resolution of symptoms, that is, no rescue with antiemetics, at endpoint.

Subjects were enrolled over 18 months (N = 331); analysis was performed on subjects completing the study (N = 220). Controlled breathing alone proved 46.2% effective and 61.5% efficacious, whereas aromatherapy with controlled breathing was 38.5% effective and 55.6% efficacious.

The treatment of PONV with either controlled breathing alone or combined with peppermint aromatherapy was efficacious for more than 50% of PONV episodes. An inexpensive, readily available alternative to prescribed medications with no known side effects can successfully relieve PONV. Further studies could evaluate the cost-effectiveness and other delivery routes of aromatherapy.

Modified from Johnson N et al: Evaluation of controlled breathing with or without peppermint aromatherapy for postoperative nausea and/or vomiting relief, *J Perianesth Nurs* 27(3), 2012.

environmental sounds, a common occurrence in busy preoperative holding areas and operating room (OR) suites. Compact disks or MP3 players provide consistent, uninterrupted music, which is critical to the success of the ongoing therapeutic reactions that music affords. Best of all, music therapy can be used preoperatively, intraoperatively, and postoperatively.

Anticipation of surgery commonly produces anxiety. The preoperative waiting period may be more stressful and anxiety-provoking for some patients than the anticipated surgical intervention. High levels of anxiety cause negative physiologic manifestations, such as elevated blood pressure, that can lead to postoperative complications, such as increased cardiac workload. High levels of preoperative anxiety may result in postoperative complications such as depression, fear, and anger, and the use of music during the preoperative phase can decrease anxiety and significantly lessen complications in the postoperative phase of recovery. Emotions are altered, apprehension and tension are reduced, and sympathetic stimulation and adrenocortical activation are more controlled. Therefore, changes in vital signs, such as elevated blood pressure and increased heart rate, are minimal. Studies have shown that patients listening to music have a decrease in anxiety and pain during the perioperative stay (Wakim et al, 2010).

Patients undergoing surgery in which local or regional anesthetics are administered have an acute awareness of the environment found within the OR. The OR may appear threatening, with unfamiliar machines, equipment, noises, and smells. Physical positioning and exposure of body parts intensify anxiety. Unfamiliar sounds, bright lights, and technical language add to the stressors of the surgical experience. During surgery, patient-selected music reduces anxiety by providing the patient some autonomy through self-selected musical choices, while distracting the patient from what is happening within the environment. The music not only blocks the various sounds in the room but also provides an escape through imaginative thought. Researchers support the idea that musical vibrations have an effect on the subconscious mind. Older patients have reported comfort and strength by listening to hymns and other music of spiritual or psychologic support. Daydreaming, imagery, escape, and fantasizing are common to listeners. This creates a release of tension and is a way of focusing attention away from threats. Intraoperative music may decrease the patient's anxiety and consequently minimize the need for patient-controlled conscious sedation and analgesia. Music can have a positive effect during general anesthesia when delivered through headphones or earpieces, as long as care is exerted to prevent pressure points and volume increases.

Pain is a common problem in the postanesthesia care unit (PACU). Pain results in negative respiratory, cardiovascular, gastrointestinal, renal, neuroendocrine, and autonomic nervous system consequences for patients. The traditional means to providing pain relief in the PACU has been through medication administration. Because the effects of medication differs from person to person, using nonpharmacologic interventions along with traditional medications may serve to lower a patient's anxiety and pain throughout all perioperative phases (Schultz et al, 2012).

Noise levels contribute to the patients' discomfort (Nightingale, 1859). The level of noise typically encountered during the surgical experience is potentially harmful to patients because of the undesirable effects of a release of stress hormones on the cardiovascular system, including increased vasoconstriction, heart rate, and blood pressure. Noise also increases psychologic stress and discomfort, and patients' ability to cope is reduced. Soothing music delivered through a headset can block out external noises and can serve as a distraction from the noise of the PACU.

When using music as a nursing intervention to promote physiologic and psychologic well-being, the nurse prepares both the patient and the environment. The nurse should inform the patient of the purpose of the music experience and interview the patient about musical preferences, allowing the patient to listen to portions of selected music to ensure the music will afford the therapeutic purpose. The use of music therapy is documented in the medical record. A library of different types of music selections should be available. When compiling these collections, it is important that attention is given to the tempo, rhythm, melody, and harmony of the music (as noted earlier). In addition to implementing the music intervention, nurses monitor patients' responses to ensure that intended outcomes are achieved, making adjustments as necessary.

Psychoneuroimmunology

Psychoneuroimmunology studies the relationship between the brain and immune function. Thus perioperative nursing interventions that seek to reduce stress influences have the potential to improve immune system function. This involves how perioperative nurses communicate with patients as well as their behaviors, the attitudes they convey, the language they use, and their being "present" and totally engaged with their patients (Table 30-3) (Patient-Centered Care).

Early animal conditioning studies showed links on a molecular level (immune regulators: neurotransmitters and hormones) that act to stimulate nerves or trigger physiologic changes. Further, the perception of stress is known to lead to a reduced ability to fight infection. Because measurement of immune function is a complicated process, much remains to be learned about the precise mechanism of how psychosocial or emotional factors affect susceptibility to disease.

Herbs and Surgery

The use of herbal and botanic products is common. Patient surveys have shown 12% of Americans use herbal medications (Wong and Townley, 2011). However, many patients do not communicate this information to their conventional medical physicians or nurse caregivers, because they are unsure of the reaction of conventional caregivers to their use of alternative substances.

Botanicals are marketed as food supplements in the United States. Manufacturers are not allowed to make claims about health benefits for these products because they are not FDA-approved. Since 1994, when the Dietary Supplement Health and Education Act (DSHEA) was passed, the definition of dietary supplements has broadened. A product that contains a vitamin, mineral, herb, amino acid, or other botanic or dietary substance used to supplement the diet is considered a dietary supplement; this includes concentrates, metabolites, constituents, extracts, and combinations of listed ingredients. These supplements are no longer subject to premarket safety evaluations by the FDA. Once a supplement is marketed, under the DSHEA, the FDA can restrict its use only if it can be shown that the product is unsafe.

There are no regulations establishing criteria for purity, manufacturing procedures, or identification of ingredients for these supplements. Therefore, the potential exists for high variability in the potency of different batches of the same botanic product. In addition, impurities and unknown substances may also be present in these products. Because herbal products are so readily available and have such widespread media attention, many people think that they can safely self-medicate (Patient and Family Education). Another mistaken assumption is that dietary supplements are safer than prescribed or over-the-counter drugs.

Botanicals may initiate a pharmacologic response within the body and therefore should be considered as medications from a medical or nursing perspective. Many herbal products have actions that could be dangerous during surgery. Some herbal supplements may accentuate the toxicity of anesthetics or interfere with drug metabolism or clearance (Surgical Pharmacology). Herbal supplements may also have a role in the perioperative setting and are an important consideration for nurses.

Coagulation Interactions. Anesthesia providers are concerned about the potential increased risk of instability intraoperatively resulting from inhibition of coagulation with the use of ginger, ginseng, feverfew, ginkgo, and garlic (Skidmore-Roth, 2010). One difficulty with analyzing case reports is the lack of laboratory analysis of the purported botanicals. In some reported cases in which prolonged or excessive bleeding occurred, the patient had been taking multiple herb supplements and drugs. Many plants contain anticoagulant components, including ginger, ginseng, feverfew, and others (Box 30-3); however, it is unknown if the danger posed is clinically significant.

TABLE 30-3

Languaging for Nurses: Enhancing Patient-Centered Communication

Positive, Therapeutic Language	Negative, Toxic Language
We're giving you the medication that will let you gently go to sleep.	We're going to put you to sleep now.
We are well trained in how to take care of you.	Don't be afraid.
I'll be with you the entire time to make sure you stay asleep and comfortable.	Don't worry; you won't wake up during surgery.
Focus your energy on healing.	Don't give up.
You might feel pressure; some people don't feel anything.	This isn't going to hurt.
	Just a little bee sting.

Modified from Eslinger MR: The power of suggestion, languaging for nurses, AHNA beginnings, *Am Holist Nurs Assoc* 29(2):22–23, 2009.

PATIENT-CENTERED CARE

Surgical patients are considered communication-vulnerable, and therefore perioperative nurses should ensure they use plain language when providing information and engaging the patient in teaching. An example of using plain language in the context of eliciting information about the use of integrative therapies might be, "I have reviewed the list of medicines you take from the pharmacy on a regular basis. I'm also interested in hearing about any medication you take that you don't need a prescription to buy," or "I see that you've been taking pain medicine because the knee you're having surgery on is constantly hurting. Is there anything else you do to help you cope with your knee pain? What makes it better? What makes it worse?" Asking patients to answer open-ended questions in their own words provides a basis for the nurse to gauge understanding of the patients' knowledge of their condition.

BOX 30-3

Herbs That Affect Bleeding

Certain herbal preparations are known to affect bleeding. Careful preoperative screening for these substances is essential:

- Ajoene
- Birch bark
- Cayenne
- Chinese black tree fungus
- Cumin
- Evening primrose oil
- Feverfew
- Garlic
- Ginger
- Ginkgo biloba
- Ginseng
- Grapeseed extract
- Milk thistle
- Omega-3 fatty acids
- Onion extract
- St. John's wort
- Turmeric
- Vitamins C and E

Modified from University of Wisconsin Hospitals and Clinic Authority: Medications and herbs which affect bleeding, available at www.uwhealth.org/healthfacts/B_EXTRANET _HEALTH_INFORMATION-FlexMember-Show_Public_HFFY_1126651115765.html. Accessed October 24, 2012.

PATIENT AND FAMILY EDUCATION

Advising Patients About Integrative Therapies

Nurses traditionally act as guides for patients as they navigate through the healthcare system, providing support, counseling, and advice. When providing education to patients about integrative therapies, the nurse should consider the overwhelming amount of information available via the Internet and popular media. The Internet is a popular source of information regarding the use of herbal and dietary supplements and other integrative therapies, but caution must be used in evaluating the validity of the information that is accessed. Nurses can use the following tips from the National Institutes of Health (NIH) to educate their patients on accessing reliable information from the Internet. These tips are also useful for nurses to use when evaluating consumer information from the Internet.

Consider the Source—Use Recognized Authorities

- Determine if the website has the Health on the Net (HON) certificate, which verifies that the website, at the date of certification, complied with and pledged to honor the eight principles of the HON Code of Conduct as drawn up by the HON Foundation
- Know who is responsible for the content.
- Look for an "about us" page. Check to see who runs the site: Is it a branch of the federal government, a nonprofit institution, a professional organization, a health system, a commercial organization, or an individual?
- Scrutinize the source of the content. There is a big difference between a site that says, "I developed this site after my heart attack" and one that says, "This page on heart attack was developed by health professionals at the American Heart Association."
- Look for a way to contact the organization or webmaster for the site. If the site provides no contact information, or if you cannot easily determine who runs the site, use caution.

Focus on Quality—All Websites are Not Created Equal

- Question whether the site has an editorial board. Is the information reviewed before it is posted? This information is often on the "about us" page, or it may be under the organization's mission statement or be part of the annual report.
- Determine if the board members are experts in the subject of the site. For example, a site on osteoporosis whose medical advisory board is composed of attorneys and accountants is not medically authoritative.
- Look for a description of the process of selecting or approving information on the site. It is usually in the "about us" section and may be called "editorial policy," "selection policy," or "review policy." Sometimes the site will have information "about our writers" or "about our authors" instead of an editorial

policy. Review this section to find out who has written the information.

Be a Cyberskeptic—Quackery Abounds on the Web

- Be skeptical if the site makes health claims that seem too good to be true. Does the information use deliberately obscure, "scientific"-sounding language? Does it promise quick, dramatic, miraculous results? Is this the only site making these claims?
- Beware of claims that one remedy will cure a variety of illnesses, that it is a "breakthrough," or that it relies on a "secret ingredient."
- Use caution if the site uses a sensational writing style (lots of exclamation points, for example). A health website for consumers should use simple language, not technical jargon.
- Get a second opinion! Check more than one site.

Look for the Evidence—Rely on Medical Research, Not Opinion

- Check to see if the site identifies the author for the content. Does it rely on testimonials?
- Look for the author of the information, either an individual or an organization. Good examples are "Written by Jane Smith, RN," or "Copyright 2012, American Cancer Society."
- Use caution when reading case histories or testimonials on the website. Look for contact information such as an email address or telephone number. If the testimonials are anonymous or hard to locate (e.g., "Jane from California"), be watchful.

Check for Currency—Look for the Latest Information

- Determine if the information is current.
- Look for dates on documents. A document on coping with the loss of a loved one does not need to be current, but a document about the latest treatment of AIDS needs to be current.
- Click a few links on the site. If there are many broken links, the site may not be kept up-to-date.
- Beware of bias: What is the purpose? Who is providing the funding?

Ask WHO Pays for the Site

- Check to see if the site is supported by public funds, by donations, or by commercial advertising.
- Review any advertisements carefully. Advertisements should be labeled and should say "Advertisement" or "From Our Sponsor."
- Look at a page on the site, and see if it is clear when content is derived from a noncommercial source and when an advertiser provides it. For example, if a page about treatment of depression recommends one drug by name, see if you can tell if the company that manufactures the drug provides that information. If it does, you should consult other sources to see what they say about the same drug.

AIDS, Acquired immunodeficiency syndrome.
Modified from *MedlinePlus guide to healthy web surfing,* available at www.nlm.nih.gov/medlineplus/healthywebsurfing.html. Accessed October 7, 2012.

Sedative Interactions. Some botanicals have significant sedative actions. Anesthesia providers are concerned about the potential for valerian and St. John's wort to prolong or potentiate the sedative effect of anesthetic agents. Valerian has been associated with central nervous system (CNS) depression and muscle relaxant effects in animals; large doses of valerian may contribute to delirium and high-output cardiac failure on emergence from general anesthesia. Although St. John's wort has been found to inhibit the binding of naloxone, to date no cases have been reported of excessive sedation

when combined with narcotics. In addition, there is concern about the monoamine oxidase inhibitor (MAOI) activity of St. John's wort, although no cases of MAOI effects in humans have been reported (Skidmore-Roth, 2010).

Cardiovascular Interactions. Hypertension and cardiac dysrhythmias are potential adverse events that may result from the sympathetic stimulation that occurs during intubation and surgery. Ephedra has been associated with cardiovascular effects, including

SURGICAL PHARMACOLOGY

Herbs: Effects and Precautions/Recommendations

The use of herbal and dietary supplements (HDS) has become increasingly popular as people become more educated consumers and take a more active interest in their health. Because herbal supplements and other nutriceuticals are available without prescription, patients may not reveal their use of these therapies unless specifically questioned. The perioperative nurse must always consider the possibility that the patient is taking supplements, and assess for their use. As with other medications the patient may be taking, the nurse is responsible to know the potential for interaction with medications used in the perioperative period. The information that follows offers a source for broadening the perioperative nurse's knowledge of commonly used herbal supplements.

Herb (Scientific Name) and Other Names	Purpose/Action	Adverse Reactions	Nursing Implications
Black cohosh (*Cimicifuga racemosa*) Rattle root Squaw root	Antihypertensive; lowers cholesterol; reduces mucus production; induces labor to aid in childbirth; relieves menopausal symptoms (hot flashes)	May lead to premature labor if used in pregnancy	Avoid use in pregnancy.
Cayenne (*Capsicum annuum*) Hot chili pepper Paprika	*External use:* Muscle spasm or soreness *Internal use:* GI disorders	*External:* Skin irritation, especially if used longer than 2 days *Internal:* Lower GI discomfort; overdose may cause hypothermia	
Dong quai (*Angelica polymorpha*)	Relieves menstrual disorders; increases effects of ovarian and testicular hormones	Dizziness, headache, nausea, miscarriage, dermatitis, GI upset, photosensitivity	Avoid use in pregnancy.
Echinacea (*Echinacea purpurea, E. pallida, E. angustifolia*) Purple coneflower	Antiinfective; antiinflammatory; enhances immune function; may prevent or minimize symptoms and duration of common cold, upper respiratory infection (URI); enhances wound- and burn-healing process	May activate T cells Cross-allergic reaction Immune suppression if taken long term	Discontinue as far in advance preoperatively as possible. Should not be used by patients with autoimmune diseases. Should not be used by patients with allergy to sunflower. Avoid use for transplant patients or those with liver dysfunction.
Ephedra (*Ephedra sinica*) Ma huang Mexican or Mormon tea Desert tea Natural ecstasy Natural fen-phen Ephedrine Chinese joint fir	Stimulant; bacteriostatic; antitussive; decongestant; bronchodilator; used for weight loss	Hypertension (HTN), tachycardia, dysrhythmias, cardiac arrest, myocardial infarction, nausea, vomiting, decreased GI motility, mydriasis, diuresis, anxiety, constipation, dizziness, headache, insomnia, psychosis, urine retention, seizure, stroke, uterine contractions	Do not use with cardiac glycosides, guanethidine, MAOI medications. Do not use for patients with anxiety, HTN, glaucoma, enlarged prostate, or heart disease. Discontinue use at least 24 hr preoperatively. Limit use to 7 days.
Feverfew (*Tanacetum parthenium*) Featherfew Midsummer daisy	Antipyretic; relieves arthritis, fever, headache, and migraine pain; increases fluidity of respiratory mucus; promotes menses and uterine contractions	Oral lesions, GI tract irritation Rebound headache with sudden cessation Hypersensitive reaction in those allergic to ragweed, asters, chrysanthemums, or daisies May increase clotting time	Causes increased bleeding risk. Avoid use preoperatively.
Garlic (*Allium sativum*) Clove garlic Ajo Poor man's penicillin	Antioxidant; antibiotic; lowers low-density lipoproteins (LDLs) to prevent atherosclerosis; has antihypertensive, antiplatelet, and antithrombolytic properties	May prolong bleeding or clotting time, potentiate effects of antihypertensive or anticoagulant drugs	Large doses (>5 cloves) may cause gastrointestinal (GI) upset, garlic breath/flatus. Discontinue use at least 7 days preoperatively.
Ginger (*Zingiber officinale*) African ginger Black ginger	Prevents nausea caused by motion sickness, pregnancy, chemotherapy, and anesthesia; antispasmodic	Heartburn Inhibition of platelet aggregation	Causes increased bleeding risk. Avoid use preoperatively.
Ginkgo (*Ginkgo biloba*) Duck foot Kew tree Maidenhair tree Silver apricot Fossil tree	Antioxidant; anticlotting; enhances blood flow (especially to brain); reduces cellular lesions, retinal edema; treats symptoms of peripheral vascular disease and dementia; inhibits platelet-activating factors; used to enhance brain function and memory; treats headaches, depression, vertigo, and tinnitus	Headache, GI upset, palpitations, dizziness, or skin reactions	Causes increased bleeding risk by inhibiting platelet activity, lowering fibrinogen levels, and decreasing plasma viscosity. May potentiate anticoagulant therapy. Discontinue use at least 36 hr preoperatively.

Continued

Herbs: Effects and Precautions/Recommendations—cont'd

Herb (Scientific Name) and Other Names	Purpose/Action	Adverse Reactions	Nursing Implications
Ginseng American ginseng (*Panax quinquefolius*) Chinese ginseng or Korean ginseng (*Panax ginseng*) Siberian ginseng (*Eleutherococcus senticosus*)	Antioxidant; enhances memory and immune function; increases stamina; decreases fatigue; reduces stress response; lowers blood glucose level; inhibits clotting	Usually mild and dose-related: nervousness, dizziness, mastalgia "Ginseng abuse syndrome" (>15 g/day) = insomnia, hypotonia, and edema Siberian ginseng may falsely elevate digoxin levels; potentiate monoamine oxidase inhibitors (MAOIs)	Contraindicated for patients with hypoglycemia, hypertension, and cardiac disorders. Avoid with other stimulants; may lead to tachycardia or hypertension. May decrease effectiveness of warfarin (decreased international normalized ratio [INR]). May cause postmenopausal bleeding. Discontinue use at least 7 days preoperatively.
Goldenseal (*Hydrastis canadensis*) Orange or yellow root Ground raspberry Turmeric root Eye root	Antibacterial, antiinflammatory properties; diuretic (no sodium excreted); laxative; improves immune function; aids digestion; regulates menses	Hypotension, nausea, vomiting, abdominal cramping May exacerbate edema or hypertension May potentiate effects of insulin	May cause electrolyte imbalance, seizures, respiratory paralysis. Avoid use preoperatively.
Hawthorn (*Crataegus oxyacantha*) May bush May blossom Whitethorn	Antihypertensive; dilates coronary blood vessels; improves cardiovascular function (inotropic and beta-blocking effect); lowers cholesterol	Nausea, fatigue, sweating, headache, hypotension, mild central nervous system (CNS) depression	Use caution with cardiac glycosides, CNS depressants, antihypertensives, and nitrates.
Huang qi (*Astragalus membranaceus*)	Antibacterial; increases production of white blood cells (WBCs); immunostimulant; cardiotonic; energy tonic (strengthens *wei qi*); regulates water metabolism	Inhibits platelet aggregation and fibrinolysis	Causes increased bleeding risk.
Kava kava (*Piper methysticum*) Awa, kawa Intoxicating pepper Tonga	Anxiolytic; mild sedative; muscle relaxant; sleep aid	Adverse effect on motor reflexes and judgment	Potentiates sedative/hypnotics. Discontinue use at least 24 hr preoperatively.
Licorice (*Glycyrrhiza glabra*) Sweet root	Antipyretic; antiviral; demulcent; expectorant; beneficial for chronic fatigue, allergies, asthma, bronchitis, depression, emphysema, herpes, and hypoglycemia; treats gastritis and gastric and duodenal ulcers	May cause headache, muscle flaccidity, lethargy, edema, HTN, hypokalemia, or other electrolyte imbalance, and electrocardiogram (ECG) changes (prolonged QT interval) Pseudoprimary aldosteronism a possible complication	Contraindicated for chronic liver conditions, renal insufficiency, hypertonia, or existing hypokalemia. Avoid use for more than 7 consecutive days.
Saw palmetto (*Serenoa repens*) Sabal cabbage palm	Relieves benign prostatic hypertrophy; has antiandrogenic and antiexudative properties	Headache, increased appetite	Causes additive effects with other hormone therapies.
Senna (*Cassia senna*)	Stimulating laxative	Abdominal cramping; affects absorption in GI system	Causes potential electrolyte imbalance.
St. John's wort (*Hypericum perforatum*) Amber touch-and-heal Goatweed Klamath weed	Anxiolytic; antidepressant (mild to moderate symptoms), may take 4-6 wk for effect; relieves dyspepsia and insomnia; mechanism: inhibits uptake of neurotransmitters	Photosensitization, skin irritation, restlessness, fatigue May prolong effects of anesthesia and potentiate meperidine or other narcotics Possible peripheral neuropathy, serotonergic crisis	
Valerian (*Valerian officinalis*) All heal Setwell Vandal root	Mild anxiolytic, muscle relaxant, hypnotic and sedative; may ease symptoms of benzodiazepine withdrawal	Headache, excitability, nausea, visual disturbance Potentiates sedative/hypnotics Long-term use may increase anesthesia tolerance Sudden cessation may cause withdrawal symptoms	Potentially prolongs anesthesia recovery time. Treat withdrawal symptoms with benzodiazepines. If possible, taper dose over 1-2 wk preoperatively; if not, continue use until surgery.
Vitamin E (D-α-tocopherol)	Antioxidant used for cardiovascular disease	Reduced platelet adhesion and aggregation	Causes increased bleeding risk.
Yohimbe (*Pausinystalia yohimbe*)	Increases blood flow (particularly to genitalia) and libido	Anxiety, hallucinations, HTN, elevated heart rate, headache, dizziness, flushing	Avoid use by patients with psychologic or renal disorders.

Modified from Skidmore-Roth L: *Mosby's handbook of herbs & natural supplements*, ed 4, St Louis, 2010, Mosby; Tsai HH et al: Evaluation of documented drug interactions and contraindications associated with herbs and dietary supplements—a systematic literature review, *Int J Clin Pract* 66(11):1056–1078, 2012.

hypertension, palpitations, tachycardia, stroke, and seizures. The long-term use of licorice may cause hypertension, dysrhythmias, or hypokalemia, which can potentiate muscle relaxants and cause adverse cardiovascular effects (Skidmore-Roth, 2010).

Because the use of botanic supplements may increase the risk of adverse herb-drug interactions, patients should be counseled to discontinue herbs preoperatively. Generally anesthesiologists recommend that patients stop taking any herbal supplement at least 2 weeks preoperatively (Wong and Townley, 2011). Most patients, however, do not see an anesthesia provider until the day of surgery or a few days before surgery, so the implementation of this recommendation is challenging. Clinical research is insufficient to quantify the actual dangers of these herbal supplements. Nonetheless, because individuals vary in their absorption, distribution, and clearance of the drugs administered during anesthesia, adding unknown chemicals into an already complex and fast-acting mix of drugs is likely an unnecessary risk.

Integrative Health Practices and Perioperative Patient Care

A variety of factors influence the perioperative patient's experience. Well-informed healthcare consumers increasingly choose a blend of traditional and nontraditional healing modalities with sensitivity to cultural, spiritual, and health education needs. Public involvement and legislative policy decisions are just beginning to equalize emphasis between the traditional biomedical model of care and a holistic comprehensive focus. Integrating health and wholeness incorporates elements of self-responsibility for wellness and self-awareness to inner changes on the part of the patient.

A collaborative partnership of professionals involved in an individual's care optimizes resources that promote comprehensive, effective, less-invasive, and nonpharmacologic adjuncts to allopathic medical treatment (Patient Safety). Perioperative nurses using available resources on interactions among prescriptions, dietary supplements, and herbals ensure preoperative medication safety. Seeking out and participating in appropriate research methodologies are essential for grounding the diverse components of our practice in evidence-based knowledge.

Documenting integrative health practices may involve noting herbals or the dietary supplement regimen the patient followed preoperatively. The nurse should also note whether these were discontinued and, if so, when. Nurse energy work practitioners who comply with a patient's request for energy treatment may refer to the North American Nursing Diagnosis Association (NANDA International) diagnosis Disturbed Energy Field when comfort measures such as TT, healing touch, or reiki are provided by the perioperative nurse.

Integrative health practices and therapies have a place in each perioperative nurse's practice (Ambulatory Surgery Considerations).

AMBULATORY SURGERY CONSIDERATIONS

Supporting Integrative Health Practices in the Ambulatory Surgical Setting

As advocates using the holistic approach, perioperative nurses play an important role in supporting patients who desire to use integrative health practices in ambulatory perioperative settings. It is important to balance the use of conventional and nonconventional interventions in respecting the patient's wishes and providing safe care. Many integrative interventions are well suited to the ambulatory setting, including music therapy, relaxation exercises, aromatherapy, and energy interventions. The perioperative nurse ensures that any healthcare personnel using integrative practices do so under the institution's policies and procedures. The nurse also documents use of these interventions in the perioperative nursing record along with the patient's response.

In the educator role, the nurse may be able to partner with patients to empower them to research the safety and efficacy of the techniques they are using. The preoperative assessment offers a prime opportunity for the nurse to identify possible safety risks for the perioperative patient. Whenever possible, the preoperative assessment should be conducted a few days before the planned surgical procedure to allow ample time to gather data and begin patient teaching in a controlled, unhurried setting versus the typical fast pace that occurs on the patient's day of admission to the ambulatory surgery setting. The nurse can use this time to educate patients about the effect of integrative health practices in the perioperative period and beyond. By obtaining information in advance about the patient's use of medications, herbs, vitamins, dietary supplements, and the like, the nurse can effect safe care by advising the patient to consult with the surgeon and modify the treatment regimen to avoid anesthetic complications.

Preoperative assessments also allow a forum to educate patients about the need to obtain reliable information about integrative health practices. The nurse reminds the patient that results should be supported by clinical trials and that information on the Internet may be commercial in nature rather than scientific (see Patient and Family Education box on p. 1170). Patients who use integrative practices need to notify their physician if any side effects occur.

PATIENT SAFETY

Encouraging the Patient/Physician Relationship

Perioperative nurses can encourage safety in patients who use integrative health practices by promoting the National Center for Complementary and Alternative Medicine (NCCAM) *Time to Talk* education campaign. The goal of the campaign is to ensure safe and coordinated care for patients while helping minimize the risks of interaction with any conventional therapy in which the patient may be engaged. The campaign also seeks to inform and educate patients so they are empowered to make better healthcare decisions and more effectively manage their health. Nurses can provide the following advice from NCCAM to patients as a starting point:

- Include all therapies and treatments you use when completing patient history forms. Make a list in advance. Also note all medical specialists or integrative practitioners you see. Take the list with you whenever you visit a healthcare provider.
- Tell your healthcare providers about all therapies or treatments, including over-the-counter and prescription medicines as well as herbal and dietary supplements.
- Take control. Do not wait for your providers to ask about your use of integrative therapies.
- Ask questions any time you are considering a new therapy; ask your healthcare providers about its safety, effectiveness, and possible interactions with medications (both prescription and over-the-counter).

Modified from National Center for Complementary and Alternative Medicine: *Time to talk,* available at http://nccam.nih.gov/timetotalk/backgrounder.htm. Accessed October 7, 2012.

Modified from Caspi O: Evidence-based medicine and clinical decision making. In Rakel RE, Rakel DP, editors: *Integrative medicine,* ed 3, Philadelphia, 2012, Saunders; Dossey BM, Guzzetta CE: Holistic nursing practice. In Dossey BM et al, editors: *Holistic nursing, a handbook for practice,* ed 6, Boston, 2012, Jones & Bartlett.

Nursing history demonstrates a philosophic attitude of altruism and compassion, founded in creating an environment of healing. Awareness of how vital self-care practices are to sustaining a caregiver role may ultimately benefit our practice. Self-care learning and meditative experiences may come full circle by enhancing the caregiver's therapeutic use of self through presence, compassion, and holistic assessment skills.

KEY POINTS

- The *comprehensive approach* takes into account multidimensional factors that may not easily or appropriately be studied independently. The comprehensive approach is more congruent with the philosophic underpinnings of most integrative health practices.
- The *biomedical approach* is concerned with a disease orientation, suggesting that a specific agent or variable is responsible for a specific disorder or illness.
- The NCCAM has categorized the many integrative (CAM) modalities into five major domains: alternative medical systems, mind-body interventions, biologically based therapies, manipulative and body-based methods, and energy therapies.
- Naturopathic medicine emphasizes health restoration as well as disease treatment based on the belief that disease is a manifestation of alterations in the body's natural healing processes.
- Touch and manipulations with the hands have been used in healing and medical practice since the beginning of the history of medicine.
- To use the term *alternative* is actually misleading. Many progressive medical facilities embrace a holistic patient focus, exploring and integrating nontraditional healing modalities to support an individualized surgical experience.
- As pharmacology combines medications to potentiate effect, aromatherapy may act synergistically with traditional treatment; or it may be offered in concert with other complementary modalities to relieve discomfort, thereby reducing dosages of analgesics or sedatives.
- Because the use of botanic supplements may increase the risk of adverse herb-drug interactions, patients should be counseled to discontinue herbs preoperatively. Generally anesthesia providers recommend that patients stop taking any herbal supplement at least 2 weeks preoperatively.
- Well-informed healthcare consumers increasingly choose a blend of traditional and nontraditional healing modalities with sensitivity to cultural, spiritual, and health education needs.
- Documenting integrated care may involve noting herbals or the dietary supplement regimen the patient followed preoperatively. The nurse should also note whether these were discontinued and, if so, when.

CRITICAL THINKING QUESTION

While assessing your preoperative patient undergoing thyroid surgery, you notice she is visibly upset and worried about the operation. She is particularly upset about waking up during surgery, postoperative pain, and postoperative nausea and vomiting. Otherwise she is oriented, alert, and educated on what her surgery entails. What holistic nursing interventions would you consider in your plan of care? How would you communicate with this patient to help to decrease her anxiety prior to surgery?

℮volve *The answers to the Critical Thinking Question can be found at http://evolve.elsevier.com/Rothrock/Alexander.*

REFERENCES

Gurgevich S: Self-hypnosis techniques. In Rakel D, editor: *Integrative medicine*, ed 3, Philadelphia, 2012, Saunders.

Jackson C, Keegan L: Touch. In Dossey BM et al, editors: *Holistic nursing: a handbook for practice*, ed 5, Boston, 2008, Jones & Bartlett.

Kolthan D: Introducing complementary and alternative therapies, *J Nurs Pract* 5(1):18–20, 2009.

Lane B et al: Examination of the effectiveness of peppermint aromatherapy on nausea in women post C-section, *J Holist Nurs* 30(2):90–104, 2012.

Micozzi MS: Translation from conventional medicine. In Micozzi MS, editor: *Fundamentals of complementary and integrative medicine*, ed 4, St Louis, 2010, Saunders.

National Center for Complementary and Alternative Medicine (NCCAM): *Important events in NCCAM history*, 2012a, available at www.nih.gov/about/almanac/organization/NCCAM.htm. Accessed September 11, 2012.

National Center for Complementary and Alternative Medicine (NCCAM): *Ayurvedic medicine: an introduction*, 2012b, available at http://nccam.nih.gov/health/ayurveda/introduction.htm. Accessed September 11, 2012.

Nightingale F: *Notes on nursing*, London, 1859, JB Lippincott.

Pizzorno JE, Snider P: Naturopathic medicine. In Micozzi MS, editor: *Fundamentals of complementary and integrative medicine*, ed 3, St Louis, 2010, Saunders.

Radzyminski S: Legal parameters of alternative-complementary modalities in nursing practice, *Nurs Clin North Am* 42:189–212, 2007.

Selimen D, Andsoy I: The importance of a holistic approach during the perioperative period, *AORN J* 93(4):482–487, 2011.

Skidmore-Roth L: *Mosby's handbook of herbs & natural supplements*, ed 4, St Louis, 2010, Mosby.

Topcu SY, Findik UY: Effect of relaxation techniques on postoperative pain, *Pain Manag Nurs* 13(1):11–17, 2012.

Schultz N et al: Surgery with music: our evidence based practice rocks! *J Perianesth Nurs* 27(3):e35, 2012.

Wakim JH et al: The efficacy of music therapy, *J Perianesth Nurs* 25(4):226–232, 2010.

Wong A, Townley SA: Herbal medicines and anaesthesia, *Contin Educ Anaesth Crit Care Pain* 11(1):14–17, 2011.

APPENDIX A
Laboratory Values

Analyte	Conventional Units	SI Units
Acetoacetate plus acetone		
Qualitative	Negative	Negative
Quantitative	0.3-2 mg/dL	30-200 µmol/L
Acid phosphatase, serum (thymolphthalein monophosphate substrate)	0.1-0.6 units/L	0.1-0.6 units/L
ACTH (see Corticotropin)		
Alanine aminotransferase (ALT), serum (SGPT)	1-45 units/L	1-45 units/L
Albumin, serum	33-52 g/L	33-52 g/L
Aldolase, serum	0-7 units/L	0-7 units/L
Aldosterone, plasma		
Standing	5-30 ng/dL	140-830 pmol/L
Recumbent	3-10 ng/dL	80-275 pmol/L
Alkaline phosphatase (ALP), serum		
Adult	35-150 units/L	35-150 units/L
Adolescent	100-500 units/L	100-500 units/L
Child	100-350 units/L	100-350 units/L
Ammonia nitrogen, plasma	10-50 µmol/L	10-50 µmol/L
Amylase, serum	25-125 units/L	25-125 units/L
Anion gap, serum calculated	8-16 mEq/L	8-16 mmol/L
Ascorbic acid, blood	0.4-1.5 mg/dL	23-85 µmol/L
Aspartate aminotransferase (AST), serum (SGOT)	1-36 units/L	1-36 units/L
Base excess, arterial blood, calculated	0 ± 2 mEq/L	0 ± 2 mmol/L
Bicarbonate		
Venous plasma	23-29 mEq/L	23-29 mmol/L
Arterial blood	21-27 mEq/L	21-27 mmol/L
Bile acids, serum	0.3-3 mg/dL	0.8-7.6 mmol/L
Bilirubin, serum		
Conjugated	0.1-0.4 mg/dL	1.7-6.8 µmol/L
Total	0.3-1.1 mg/dL	5.1-19 µmol/L
Calcium, serum	8.4-10.6 mg/dL	2.10-2.65 mmol/L
Calcium, ionized, serum	4.25-5.25 mg/dL	1.05-1.30 mmol/L
Carbon dioxide, total, serum or plasma	24-31 mEq/L	24-31 mmol/L
Carbon dioxide tension (Pco_2), blood	35-45 mm Hg	35-45 mm Hg
β-Carotene, serum	60-260 mcg/dL	1.1-8.6 µmol/L
Ceruloplasmin, serum	23-44 mg/dL	230-440 mg/L
Chloride	96-106 mEq/L	96-106 mmol/L
Cholesterol, serum or EDTA plasma		
Desirable range	<200 mg/dL	<5.20 mmol/L
Low-density lipoprotein (LDL) cholesterol	60-180 mg/dL	1.55-4.65 mmol/L
High-density lipoprotein (HDL) cholesterol	30-80 mg/dL	0.80-2.05 mmol/L
Copper	70-140 mcg/dL	11-22 µmol/L
Corticotropin (ACTH), plasma, 8 AM	10-80 pg/mL	2-18 pmol/L
Cortisol, plasma		
8:00 AM	6-23 mcg/dL	170-630 µmol/L
4:00 PM	3-15 mcg/dL	80-410 µmol/L
10:00 PM	<50% of 8:00 AM value	<50% of 8:00 AM value

Continued

REFERENCE INTERVALS* FOR CLINICAL CHEMISTRY (BLOOD, SERUM, AND PLASMA)—cont'd

Analyte	Conventional Units	SI Units
Creatine, serum		
Males	0.2-0.5 mg/dL	15-40 µmol/L
Females	0.3-0.9 mg/dL	25-70 µmol/L
Creatine kinase (CK), serum		
Males	55-170 units/L	55-170 units/L
Females	30-135 units/L	30-135 units/L
Creatine kinase MB isoenzyme, serum	<5% of total CK activity	<5% of total CK activity
	<5 ng/mL by immunoassay	<5 ng/mL by immunoassay
Creatinine, serum	0.6-1.2 mg/dL	50-110 µmol./L
Erythrocytes	145-540 ng/mL	330-120 nmol/L
Estradiol-17 β, adult		
Males	10-65 pg/mL	35-240 pmol/L
Females		
Follicular	30-100 pg/mL	110-370 pmol/L
Ovulatory	200-400 pg/mL	730-1470 pmol/L
Luteal	50-140 pg/mL	180-510 pmol/L
Ferritin, serum	20-200 ng/mL	20-200 mcg/L
Fibrinogen, plasma	200-400 mg/dL	2-4 g/L
Folate, serum	3-18 ng/mL	6.8-41 nmol/L
Follicle-stimulating hormone (FSH), plasma		
Males	4-25 mU/mL	4-25 units/L
Females, premenopausal	4-30 mU/mL	4-30 units/L
Females, postmenopausal	40-250 mU/mL	40-250 units/L
Gastrin, fasting, serum	0-100 pg/mL	0-100 mg/L
Glucose, fasting, plasma or serum	70-115 mg/dL	3.9-6.4 nmol/L
γ-Glutamyltransferase (GGT), serum	5-40 unitsL	5-40 units/L
Growth hormone (hGH), plasma, adult, fasting	0-6 ng/mL	0-6 mcg/L
Haptoglobin, serum	20-165 mg/dL	0.20-1.65 g/L
Immunoglobulins, serum (see table, Reference Intervals for Tests of Immunologic Function)		
Iron, serum	75-175 mcg/dL	13-31 µmol/L
Iron-binding capacity, serum		
Total	250-410 mcg/dL	45-73 µmol/L
Saturation	20%-55%	0.20-0.55
Lactate		
Venous whole blood	5-20 mg/dL	0.6-2.2 mmol/L
Arterial whole blood	5-15 mg/dL	0.6-1.7 mmol/L
Lactate dehydrogenase (LD), serum	110-220 units/L	110-220 units/L
Lipase, serum	10-140 units/L	10-140 units/L
Lutropin (LH), serum		
Males	1-9 units/L	1-9 units/L
Females		
Follicular phase	2-10 units/L	2-10 units/L
Midcycle peak	15-65 units/L	15-65 units/L
Luteal phase	1-12 units/L	1-12 units/L
Postmenopausal	12-65 units/L	12-65 units/L
Magnesium, serum	1.3-2.1 mg/dL	0.65-1.05 mmol/L
Osmolality	275-295 mOsm/kg water	275-295 mOsm/kg water
Oxygen, blood, arterial, room air		
Partial pressure (PaO$_2$)	80-100 mm Hg	80-100 mm Hg
Saturation (SaO$_2$)	95%-98%	95%-98%
pH, arterial blood	7.35-7.45	7.35-7.45
Phosphate, inorganic, serum		
Adult	3-4.5 mg/dL	1-1.5 mmol/L
Child	4-7 mg/dL	1.3-2.3 mmol/L
Potassium		
Serum	3.5-5 mEq/L	3.5-5 mmol/L
Plasma	3.5-4.5 mEq/L	3.5-4.5 mmol/L
Progesterone, serum, adult		
Males	0-0.4 ng/mL	0-1.3 mmol/L
Females		
Follicular phase	0.1-1.5 ng/mL	0.3-4.8 mmol/L
Luteal phase	2.5-28 ng/mL	8-89 mmol/L

REFERENCE INTERVALS* FOR CLINICAL CHEMISTRY (BLOOD, SERUM, AND PLASMA)—cont'd

Analyte	Conventional Units	SI Units
Prolactin, serum		
Males	1-15 ng/mL	1-15 mcg/L
Females	1-20 ng/mL	1-20 mcg/L
Protein, serum, electrophoresis		
Total	6-8 g/dL	60-80 g/L
Albumin	3.5-5.5 g/dL	35-55 g/L
Globulins		
α_1	0.2-0.4 g/dL	2-4 g/L
α_2	0.5-0.9 g/dL	5-9 g/L
β	0.6-1.1 g/dL	6-11 g/L
γ	0.7-1.7 g/dL	7-17 g/L
Pyruvate, blood	0.3-0.9 mg/dL	0.03-0.10 mmol/L
Rheumatoid factor	0-30 IU/mL	0-30 kIU/L
Sodium, serum or plasma	135-145 mEq/L	135-145 mmol/L
Testosterone, plasma		
Men	300-1200 ng/dL	10.4-41.6 nmol/L
Women	20-75 ng/dL	0.7-2.6 nmol/L
Pregnant	40-200 ng/dL	1.4-6.9 nmol/L
Thyroglobulin	3-42 ng/mL	3-42 mcg/L
Thyrotropin (hTSH), serum	0.4-4.8 µIU/mL	0.4-4.8 mIU/L
Thyrotropin-releasing hormone (TRH)	5-60 pg/mL	5-60 ng/L
Thyroxine free (FT_4), serum	0.9-2.1 ng/dL	12-27 pmol/L
Thyroxine (T_4), serum	4.5-12 mg/dL	58-154 nmol/L
Thyroxine-binding globulin (TBG)	15-34 mcg/mL	15-34 mg/L
Transferrin	250-430 mg/dL	2.5-4.3 g/L
Triglycerides, serum, 12-hr fast	40-150 mg/dL	0.4-1.5 g/L
Triiodothyronine (T_3), serum	70-190 ng/dL	1.1-2.9 nmol/L
Triiodothyronine uptake, resin (T_3RU)	25%-38%	0.25%-0.38%
Troponin I	0.05-0.50 ng/mL	0.05-0.50 ng/mL
Urate		
(FT_4) Males	2.5-8 mg/dL	150-480 µmol/L
(FT_4) Females	2.2-7 mg/dL	130-420 µmol/L
Urea, serum or plasma	24-49 mg/dL	4-8.2 nmol/L
Urea nitrogen, serum or plasma	11-23 mg/dL	8-16.4 nmol/L
Viscosity, serum	1.4-1.8 ∞ water	1.4-1.8 ∞ water
Vitamin A, serum	20-80 mcg/dL	0.70-2.80 µmol/L
Vitamin B_{12}, serum	180-900 pg/mL	133-664 pmol/L

*Reference values may vary depending on the method and sample source used.
EDTA, Ethylenediaminetetraacetic acid; *SI,* International System of Units.

REFERENCE INTERVALS* FOR CLINICAL CHEMISTRY (URINE)

Analyte	Conventional Units	SI Units
Acetone and acetoacetate, qualitative	Negative	Negative
Albumin		
Qualitative	Negative	Negative
Quantitative	10-100 mg/24 hr	0.15-1.5 µmol/day
Aldosterone	3-20 mcg/24 hr	8.3-55 nmol/day
δ-Aminolevulinic acid (δ-ALA)	1.3-7 mg/24 hr	10-53 µmol/day
Amylase	<17 units/hr	<17 units/hr
Amylase-to-creatinine clearance ratio	0.01-0.04	0.01-0.04
Bilirubin, qualitative	Negative	Negative
Calcium (regular diet)	<250 mg/24 hr	<6.3 nmol/day
Catecholamines		
Epinephrine	<10 mcg/24 hr	<55 nmol/day
Norepinephrine	<100 mcg/24 hr	<590 nmol/day
Total free catecholamines	4-126 mcg/24 hr	24-745 nmol/day
Total metanephrines	0.1-1.6 mg/24 hr	0.5-8.1 µmol/day
Chloride (varies with intake)	110-250 mEq/24 hr	110-250 mmol/day
Copper	0-50 mcg/24 hr	0-0.80 µmol/day

Continued

REFERENCE INTERVALS* FOR CLINICAL CHEMISTRY (URINE)—cont'd

Analyte	Conventional Units	SI Units
Cortisol, free	10-100 mcg/24 hr	27.6-276 nmol/day
Creatine		
Males	0-40 mg/24 hr	0-0.30 mmol/day
Females	0-80 mg/24 hr	0-0.60 mmol/day
Creatinine	15-25 mg/kg/24 hr	0.13-0.22 mmol/kg/day
Creatinine clearance (endogenous)		
Males	110-150 mL/min/1.73 m^2	110-150 mL/min/1.73 m^2
Females	105-132 mL/min/1.73 m^2	105-132 mL/min/1.73 m^2
Cystine or cysteine	Negative	Negative
Dehydroepiandrosterone		
Males	0.2-2 mg/24 hr	0.7-6.9 µmol/day
Females	0.2-1.8 mg/24 hr	0.7-6.2 µmol/day
Estrogens, total		
Males	4-25 mcg/24 hr	14-90 nmol/day
Females	5-100 mcg/24 hr	18-360 nmol/day
Glucose (as reducing substance)	<250 mg/24 hr	<250 mg/day
Hemoglobin and myoglobin, qualitative	Negative	Negative
Homogentisic acid, qualitative	Negative	Negative
17-Hydroxycorticosteroids		
Males	3-9 mg/24 hr	8.3-25 µmol/day
Females	2-8 mg/24 hr	5.5-22 µmol/day
5-Hydroxyindoleacetic acid		
Qualitative	Negative	Negative
Quantitative	2-6 mg/24 hr	10-31 µmol/day
17-Ketogenic steroids		
Males	5-23 mg/24 hr	17-80 µmol/day
Females	3-15 mg/24 hr	10-52 µmol/day
17-Ketosteroids		
Males	8-22 mg/24 hr	28-76 µmol/day
Females	6-15 mg/24 hr	21-52 µmol/day
Magnesium	6-10 mEq/24 hr	3-5 mmol/day
Metanephrines	0.05-1.2 ng/mg creatinine	0.03-0.70 mmol/mmol creatinine
Osmolality	38-1400 mOsm/kg water	38-1400 mOsm/kg water
pH	4.6-8	4.6-8
Phenylpyruvic acid, qualitative	Negative	Negative
Phosphate	0.4-1.3 g/24 hr	13-42 mmol/day
Porphobilinogen		
Qualitative	Negative	Negative
Quantitative	<2 mg/24 hr	<9 µmol/day
Porphyrins		
Coproporphyrin	50-250 mcg/24 hr	77-380 nmol/day
Uroporphyrin	10-30 mcg/24 hr	12-36 nmol/day
Potassium	25-125 mEq/24 hr	25-125 mmol/day
Pregnanediol		
Males	0-1.9 mg/24 hr	0-6 µmol/day
Females		
Proliferative phase	0-2.6 mg/24 hr	0-8 µmol/day
Luteal phase	2.6-10.6 mg/24 hr	8-33 µmol/day
Postmenopausal	0.2-1 mg/24 hr	0.6-3.1 µmol/day
Pregnanetriol	0-2.5 mg/24 hr	0-7.4 µmol/day
Protein, total		
Qualitative	Negative	Negative
Quantitative	10-150 mg/24 hr	10-150 mg/day
Protein-to-creatinine ratio	<0.2	<0.2
Sodium (regular diet)	60-260 mEq/24 hr	60-260 mmol/day
Specific gravity		
Random specimen	1.003-1.030	1.003-1.030
24-hr collection	1.015-1.025	1.015-1.025
Urate (regular diet)	250-750 mg/24 hr	1.5-4.4 mmol/day
Urobilinogen	0.5-4 mg/24 hr	0.6-6.8 µmol/day
Vanillylmandelic acid (VMA)	1-8 mg/24 hr	5-40 µmol/day

*Values can vary depending on the method used.
SI, International System of Units.

REFERENCE INTERVALS FOR TESTS PERFORMED ON CEREBROSPINAL FLUID (CSF)

Test	Conventional Units	SI Units
Cells	<5/mm^3; all mononuclear	<5 × 10^6/L; all mononuclear
Protein electrophoresis	Albumin predominant	Albumin predominant
Glucose	50-75 mg/dL	2.8-4.2 mmol/L
	(20 mg/dL less than in serum)	(1.1 mmol less than in serum)
IgG		
Children less than 14 yr	<8% of total protein	<0.08 of total protein
Adults	<14% of total protein	<0.14 of total protein
IgG index	0.3-0.6	0.3-0.6
Oligoclonal banding on electrophoresis	Absent	Absent
Pressure, opening	70-180 mm H$_2$O	70-180 mm H$_2$O
Protein, total	15-45 mg/dL	150-450 mg/L

Ig, Immunoglobulin; *SI,* International System of Units.
From *Mosby's dictionary of medicine, nursing, and health professions,* ed 9, St Louis, 2013, Mosby.

Illustration Credits

Chapter 1

1-1, Courtesy University of Pennsylvania School of Medicine, Philadelphia; **1-4,** From Titler MG et al: The Iowa model of evidence-based practice to promote quality care, *Crit Care Nurs Clin North Am* 13(4):497-509, 2001; **1-5,** From Baker JD: Nursing informatics, *Periop Nurs Clin* 7(2):151-160, 2012.

Chapter 2

2-1, 2-2, 2-3, 2-5, Courtesy Christiana Care Health Services, Newark, DE; **2-4,** From Beare PG, Myers JL: *Principles and practices of adult health nursing*, ed 3, St Louis, 1998, Mosby.

Chapter 3

3-1, From Waters T et al: AORN ergonomic tool 1: lateral transfer of a patient from a stretcher to an OR bed, *AORN J* 93(3):334-339, 2011; **3-2,** From Nancy Hughes, 2009, American Nurses Association; **3-3, 3-4,** From International Healthcare Worker Safety Center, 2005, University of Virginia.

Chapter 4

4-1, From Huether SE, McCance KL: *Understanding pathophysiology*, ed 4, St Louis, 2008, Mosby; **4-2,** Courtesy Charleston Area Medical Center, Charleston, WV; **4-4,** From Fuller JR: *Surgical technology*, ed 6, St Louis, 2013, Saunders; **4-5,** From Fuller JR: *Surgical technology*, ed 4, St Louis, 2005, Saunders; **4-6, 4-8,** Courtesy STERIS Corp, Mentor, OH; **4-9A and B,** Reprinted with permission from Advanced Sterilization Products. STERRAD is a registered trademark of Advanced Sterilization Products, Division of Ethicon, Inc.

Chapter 5

5-4, Redrawn from Whitten C: *Anyone can intubate,* ed 4, San Diego, 1997, K-W Publications.

Chapter 6

6-1, From Loeper JM et al: *Therapeutic positioning and skin care*, Minneapolis, 1986, Sister Kenny Institute; **6-2, 6-3, 6-4,** Courtesy Molnlycke Health Care US, LLC; **6-5, 6-6, 6-12, 6-13,** Courtesy Kendall-LTP; **6-9, 6-16, 6-27, 6-32, 6-38,** From Miller RD et al: *Miller's anesthesia*, ed 7, Philadelphia, 2009, Churchill Livingstone; **6-10,** Modified from Martin JT: *Positioning in anesthesia and surgery*, ed 2, Philadelphia, 1987, Saunders; **6-17,** From Munro D: The perioperative nurse's role in table-enhanced anterior total hip arthroplasty, *AORN J* 90(1):57, 2009; **6-18,** Courtesy Mizuho OSI, Unionville, CA; **6-21,** Courtesy HoverTech International, Fountain Hill, PA; **6-23,** From Chitlik A: Safe positioning for robotic-assisted laparoscopic prostatectomy, *AORN J* 94(1):39, 2011; **6-24,** From Shveiky D et al: Brachial plexus injury after laparoscopic and robotic surgery, *J Minim Invasive Gynecol* 17(4):419, 2010; **6-29,** From Bennicoff G: Perioperative care of the morbidly obese patient

in the lithotomy position, *AORN J* 92(3):297-312, 2010; **6-30,** Courtesy Allen Medical Systems, Acton, MA; **6-31, 6-35, 6-36,** From St-Arnaud D: Safe positioning for neurosurgical patients, *AORN J* 87(6):1167, 2008; **6-37,** Courtesy SchureMed, Abington, MA.

Chapter 7

7-2, 7-14, From Ethicon Endo-Surgery, Cincinnati, OH; **7-3, 7-7, 7-17, 7-24,** From Phillips N: *Berry & Kohn's operating room technique*, ed 12, St Louis, 2013, Mosby; **7-4, 7-5, 7-6, 7-9, 7-10, 7-12,** From Davis and Geck: *Surgical atlas and suture guide*, ed 2, Wayne, NJ, 1992, American Cyanamid Co; **7-11,** Courtesy Intuitive Surgical Inc, Sunnyvale, CA; **7-13,** Courtesy 3M, St. Paul, MN; **7-15, 7-26,** From Beth Israel Deaconess Medical Center, Boston; **7-16, 7-19, 7-20, 7-22, 7-23,** Courtesy Codman & Shurtleff, Inc, Randolph, MA; **7-18,** Courtesy Miltex Instrument Co; **7-21,** Courtesy Shirley M. Tighe, Lake Havasu City, AZ.

Chapter 8

8-2, 8-5, 8-6, 8-9, 8-10, 8-13, 8-17, 8-18, 8-20, 8-35, 8-37, 8-43, 8-65, 8-68, 8-69, 8-76, From Ball KA: *Endoscopic surgery*, St Louis, 1997, Mosby; **8-3, 8-42, 8-46, 8-47,** Courtesy Gyrus-ACMI, Southborough, MA; **8-4,** Courtesy HGM Medical Laser Systems, Santa Clara, CA; **8-7, 8-33, 8-38, 8-41,** Courtesy Olympus Surgical America, Orangeburg, NY; **8-8,** Courtesy Endoscopy Support Services, Inc, Brewster, NY; **8-11,** From Brooks-Tighe SM: *Instrumentation for the operating room*, ed 6, St Louis, 2003, Mosby; **8-12,** From Tighe SM: *Instrumentation for the operating room*, ed 8, St Louis, 2012, Mosby; **8-14, 8-19, 8-21, 8-24, 8-27,** Copyright © 2010 Covidien. All rights reserved. Used with the permission of Covidien; **8-16,** From Applied Medical Inc., Rancho Santa Margarita, CA; **8-22, 8-23, 8-55, 8-74, 8-75,** Courtesy Ethicon Endo-Surgery, Cincinnati; **8-29,** Courtesy Medivators, a Minntech Corporation Business Group, Minneapolis, www.medivators.com; **8-31,** Courtesy Circon ACMI, Santa Barbara, CA; **8-39,** From New Wave Surgical Corp, Coral Springs, FL; **8-45, 8-70,** Courtesy I.C. Medical Inc, Phoenix; **8-48, 8-49, 8-51,** Courtesy Valleylab, Inc; **8-50,** From Spruce L, Braswell ML: Implementing AORN recommended practices for electrosurgery, *AORN J* 95:373-384, 2012; **8-52,** From Megadyne Medical Products Inc, Draper, UT; **8-53, 8-54,** Courtesy Megadyne Medical Products Inc, Draper, UT; **8-57, 8-58,** Courtesy Encision, Boulder, CO; **8-71,** From ConMed Electrosurgery, Centennial, CO.

Chapter 9

9-1, From Herlihy B: *The human body in health and illness*, ed 5, St Louis, 2014, Saunders; **9-2, 9-6,** From Ignatavicius DD, Workman ML: *Medical-surgical nursing: patient-centered collaborative care*, ed 7, St Louis, 2013, Saunders; **9-3,** From Townsend CM et al: *Sabiston textbook of surgery*, ed 19, Philadelphia, 2012, Saunders; **9-4,** From Harkreader H et al: *Fundamentals of nursing: caring* *and clinical judgment,* ed 3, St Louis, 2007, Saunders; **9-5,** Courtesy KCI, San Antonio, TX; **9-7C and D,** Courtesy CR Bard, Inc, Murray Hill, NJ.

Chapter 10

10-1, 10-2, From Litwack K: *Post anesthesia care nursing,* ed 2, St Louis, 1995, Mosby; **10-3, 10-4,** From Monahan FD et al: *Phipps' medical-surgical nursing: health and illness perspectives,* ed 8, St Louis, 2007, Mosby; **10-5,** Reproduced with permission. Copyright © 2010 Arizant Healthcare, Inc. All rights reserved; **10-6,** From Nagelhout JJ, Plaus K: *Nurse anesthesia,* ed 5, St Louis, 2014, Saunders; **10-7, 10-8, 10-9,** From American Society of PeriAnesthesia Nurses PONV/PDNV Strategic Work Team: ASPAN's evidence-based clinical practice guideline for the prevention and/or management of PONV/PDNV, *J Perianesth Nurs* 21(4):243-245, 2006; **10-10,** From Acute Pain Management Guideline Panel: *Acute pain management in adults: operative procedures: quick reference guide for clinicians,* AHCPR Pub No. 92-0019, Rockville, MD, 1992, Agency for Health Care Policy and Research; **10-11A-C,** From Acute Pain Management Guideline Panel: *Acute pain management in adults: operative procedures: quick reference guide for clinicians,* AHCPR Pub No. 92-0019, Rockville, MD, 1992, Agency for Health Care Policy and Research; **10-11D,** From Hockenberry MJ, Wilson, D: *Wong's essentials of pediatric nursing,* ed 9, St Louis, 2013, Mosby. Used with permission. Copyright Mosby; **10-12,** From Prospect Working Group: PROSPECT: Procedure Specific Postoperative Pain Management at www.postoppain.org; **10-13,** From Long BC et al: *Medical-surgical nursing: a nursing process approach,* ed 3, St Louis, 1993, Mosby.

Chapter 11

11-3, 11-4, 11-14, 11-17, 11-18, From Thompson JC: *Atlas of surgery of the stomach, duodenum, and small bowel,* St Louis, 1992, Mosby; **11-6, 11-10, 11-25, 11-26, 11-27, 11-28, 11-29, 11-30, 11-31, 11-32,** From Bauer JJ: *Colorectal surgery illustrated,* St Louis, 1993, Mosby; **11-8,** Modified from Thibodeau GA, Patton KT: *Anthony's textbook of anatomy and physiology,* ed 20, St Louis, 2013, Mosby; **11-19,** Courtesy of Inamed Health, Inc, Santa Barbara, CA. In Townsend CM et al: *Sabiston textbook of surgery: the biological basis of modern surgical practice,* ed 17, Philadelphia, 2004, Saunders; **11-20, 11-21, 11-22,** From Townsend CM et al: *Sabiston textbook of surgery: the biological basis of modern surgical practice,* ed 18, Philadelphia, 2007, Saunders; **11-23, 11-24,** From Marceau P et al: Malabsorptive obesity surgery, *Surg Clin North Am* 81:1113-1127, 2001. In Townsend CM et al: *Sabiston textbook of surgery: the biological basis of modern surgical practice,* ed 17, Philadelphia, 2004, Saunders.

Chapter 12

12-6, From Townsend CM et al: *Sabiston textbook of surgery,* ed 16, Philadelphia, 2001, Saunders; **12-7,** From Daly JM, Cady B: *Atlas of surgical oncology,* St Louis, 1993, Mosby; **12-13,** From Zuidema G, editor: *Shackelford's surgery of the alimentary tract,* ed 3, Philadelphia, 1996, Saunders; **12-17,** Modified from Moody FG, editor: *Surgical treatment of digestive disease,* ed 2, St Louis, 1990, Mosby; **12-18,** Modified from Larson-Wadd K, Belani KG: *Anesthesiol Clin North Am* 22:663, 2004; **12-19, 12-20, 12-21,** Copyright © 1990 Lahey Clinic, Burlington, MA; **12-22,** From Simmons RL et al, editors: *Manual of vascular access, organ donation, and transplantation,* New York, 1984, Springer-Verlag.

Chapter 13

13-1, From Ignatavicius DD, Workman ML: *Medical-surgical nursing: patient-centered collaborative care,* ed 7, St Louis, 2013, Saunders; **13-2,** From Harkreader H et al: *Fundamentals of nursing: caring and clinical judgment,* ed 3, St Louis, 2007, Mosby; **13-12,** From Seidel HM et al: *Mosby's guide to physical examination,* ed 7, St Louis, 2011, Mosby; **13-14,** From Schumpelick V: *Atlas of hernia surgery,* Toronto, 1990, BC Decker; **13-16,** From Liechty RD, Soper RT: *Synopsis of surgery,* St Louis, 1985, Mosby.

Chapter 14

14-1, 14-13B, 14-14B, From Seidel HM et al: *Mosby's guide to physical examination,* ed 7, St Louis, 2011, Mosby; **14-2, 14-8,** From Lowdermilk DL, Perry SE: *Maternity and women's health care,* ed 10, St Louis, 2012, Mosby; **14-4,** From Dalrymple NC et al: *Problem solving in abdominal and pelvic imaging,* Philadelphia, 2009, Mosby; **14-5,** From Standring S: *Gray's anatomy,* ed 40, London, 2008, Churchill Livingstone; **14-6,** From Gabbe SG et al: *Obstetrics: normal and problem pregnancies,* ed 6, Philadelphia, 2012, Saunders; **14-7,** From DiSaia PJ, Creasman WT: *Clinical gynecologic oncology,* ed 8, Philadelphia, 2012, Saunders; **14-9,** From Bristow R, Armstrong DMD: *Early diagnosis and treatment of cancer series: ovarian cancer,* Philadelphia, 2010, Saunders; **14-10, 14-30, 14-41,** From Bieber EJ et al: *Clinical gynecology,* Philadelphia, 2006, Churchill Livingstone; **14-11,** From Townsend CM et al: *Sabiston textbook of surgery: the biological basis of modern surgical practice,* ed 18, Philadelphia, 2008, Saunders; **14-12,** From Ignatavicius DD, Workman ML: *Medical-surgical nursing: patient-centered collaborative care,* ed 6, St Louis, 2010, Saunders; **14-15,** Redrawn from Symmonds RE: Relaxation of pelvic supports. In Katz VL et al: *Comprehensive gynecology,* ed 5, Philadelphia, 2007, Mosby; **14-16, 14-17,** From Lentz GM et al: *Comprehensive gynecology,* ed 6, St Louis, 2012, Mosby; **14-23, 14-27, 14-35, 14-43,** From Ball TL: *Gynecologic surgery and urology,* ed 2, St Louis, 1963, Mosby. Daisy Stillwell, medical illustrator; **14-24,** From Nucci MR, Oliva E: *Gynecologic pathology,* London, 2009, Churchill Livingstone; **14-26,** Courtesy Dr. Henry J. Norris, Orlando, FL. From Robboy SJ et al: *Robboy's pathology of the female reproductive tract,* ed 2, London, 2009, Churchill Livingstone; **14-28,** From Emond RT: *Colour atlas of infectious diseases,* ed 4, St Louis, 2003, Mosby; **14-31,** From Hacker NF et al: *Essentials of obstetrics and gynecology,* ed 4, Philadelphia, 2004, Saunders; **14-32, 14-33, 14-34,** From Edwards SK et al: Surgery in the pregnant patient, *Curr Prob Surg* 38(4):213-292, 2001; **14-36,** From Ignatavicius DD, Workman ML: *Medical-surgical nursing: patient-centered collaborative care,* ed 7, St Louis, 2013, Saunders; **14-37, 14-44, 14-45,** From Nichols DH: *Gynecologic and obstetric surgery,* St Louis, 1993, Mosby; **14-39,** From Hacker NF et al: *Hacker & Moore's essentials of obstetrics and gynecology,* ed 5, Philadelphia, 2010, Saunders; **14-42,** From Voet RL: *Color atlas of obstetric and gynecologic pathology,* St Louis, 1997, Mosby; **14-48, 14-49,** Courtesy Marjorie Pyle, RNC, Lifecircle, Costa Mesa, CA. In Lowdermilk DL, Perry SE: *Maternity and women's health care,* ed 10, St Louis, 2012, Mosby.

Chapter 15

15-1, 15-6, 15-7, Modified from Seidel HM et al: *Mosby's guide to physical examination,* ed 7, St Louis, 2011, Mosby; **15-3, 15-11, 15-20, 15-24, 15-31, 15-36, 15-37, 15-51, 15-64,** From Nagle GM: *Genitourinary surgery,* St Louis, 1997, Mosby; **15-8, 15-49,** Courtesy Bard Urological, Covington, GA; **15-10,** Courtesy CR

Bard, Urological Division, Covington, GA. In Nagle GM: *Genitourinary surgery*, St Louis, 1997, Mosby; **15-12, 15-46,** Courtesy Gyrus-ACMI, Southborough, MA; **15-13, 15-25, 15-47,** From Williamson MR, Smith AY: *Fundamentals of uroradiology*, Philadelphia, 2000, Saunders; **15-14,** Courtesy Circon Corp, Santa Barbara, CA. In Nagle GM: *Genitourinary surgery*, St Louis, 1997, Mosby; **15-16B, 15-62,** From Tighe SM: *Instrumentation for the operating room*, ed 4, St Louis, 1994, Mosby; **15-19, 15-21, 15-22, 15-57A,** Courtesy American Medical Systems, Minnetonka, MN; **15-29,** Courtesy Ethicon, Inc, Somerville, NJ; **15-32,** Courtesy Omni-Tract Surgical, St. Paul, MN; **15-33, 15-34, 15-38, 15-39, 15-55, 15-56, 15-57B, 15-63, 15-65,** From Droller MJ: *Surgical management of urologic disease*, St Louis, 1992, Mosby; **15-41, 15-42,** From Wein AJ et al: *Campbell-Walsh urology*, ed 9, Philadelphia, 2007, Saunders; **15-44,** Courtesy Circon Corp, Santa Barbara, CA; **15-48, 15-50,** From Raz S: *Atlas of transvaginal surgery*, ed 2, Philadelphia, 2002, Saunders; **15-58, 15-59,** From Gillenwater JY et al: *Adult and pediatric urology*, ed 3, St Louis, 1996, Mosby; **15-60,** From Gray M: *Genitourinary disorders,* St Louis, 1992, Mosby; **15-61,** Copyright © Karl Storz Endoscopy America, Inc.

Chapter 16

16-2, From Drake RL et al: *Gray's anatomy for students*, ed 2, Philadelphia, 2010, Churchill Livingstone; **16-3,** From Wein RO, Weber RS: Parathyroid surgery, *Neuroimaging Clin N Am* 18(3):554-555, 2008; **16-4,** From Netter Anatomy Illustration Collection, © Elsevier, Inc. All rights reserved, www.netterimages.com; **16-5,** From Goldman L, Schafer AI: *Goldman's Cecil medicine*, ed 24, Philadelphia, 2012, Saunders; **16-6,** From Fakhran S et al: Parathyroid imaging, *Neuroimaging Clin N Am* 18(3):538, 2008; **16-7,** From Kukora JS et al: Thyroid nodule. In Cameron JL, editor: *Current surgical therapy*, ed 7, St Louis, 2001, Mosby; **16-8, 16-9, 16-10, 16-11,** From Dhingra JK, Raval T: Minimally invasive surgery of the thyroid, eMedicine.com, June 13, 2008, WebMD; **16-12,** From Healy J, Hodge J: *Surgical anatomy*, ed 2, Philadelphia, 1990, BC Decker.

Chapter 17

17-1, 17-10, 17-12, From Townsend CM et al: *Sabiston textbook of surgery*, ed 19, Philadelphia, 2012, Saunders; **17-2, 17-3,** From Isaacs JH: *Textbook of breast disease*, St Louis, 1992, Mosby; **17-4,** From Standring S et al, editors: *Gray's anatomy*, ed 40, London, 2008, Churchill Livingstone; **17-5,** From Townsend CM: *Sabiston textbook of surgery*, ed 16, Philadelphia, 2001, Saunders; **17-6,** Courtesy Wende W. Logan, MD, Rochester, NY and the Breast Clinic of Rochester; **17-7A,** From Don Bliss, artist, National Cancer Institute (NCI), www.cancer.gov; **17-7B,** From Ignatavicius DD, Workman ML: *Medical-surgical nursing: critical thinking for collaborative care*, ed 5, St Louis, 2006, Saunders; **17-8,** From Townsend CM et al: *Sabiston textbook of surgery: the biological basis of modern surgical practice*, ed 18, Philadelphia, 2008, Saunders; **17-9,** From Hueske RD: *Mosby's PDQ for surgical technology*, St Louis, 2008, Mosby; **17-11,** From Ignatavicius DD, Workman ML: *Medical-surgical nursing: patient-centered collaborative care,* ed 7, St Louis, 2013, Saunders; **17-13,** Redrawn from Zollinger RM: *Atlas of surgical operations*, ed 6, NY, 1988, MacMillan.

Chapter 18

18-1, 18-2, 18-4, Courtesy Eyemaginations, Towson, MD; **18-5,** From Seidel HM et al: *Mosby's guide to physical examination*, ed 7, St Louis, 2011, Mosby; **18-6,** From Thompson JM et al: *Mosby's clinical nursing*, ed 5, St Louis, 2002, Mosby; **18-7A and B, 18-8, 18-11, 18-12, 18-15,** Courtesy Todd Bauders; **18-7C, 18-13, 18-14, 18-18,** Courtesy National Eye Institute, National Institutes of Health; **18-16,** Courtesy Alcon Laboratories, Inc, Fort Worth, TX; **18-17, 18-25, 18-26,** From Lindquist TD, Lindstrom RL: *Ophthalmic surgery: looseleaf and update service*, St Louis, 1990, Mosby; **18-19, 18-21,** From Federman JL et al: *Retina and vitreous*, London, 1994, Mosby; **18-22,** From Ryan SJ et al: *Retina*, ed 4, St Louis, 2006, Mosby; **18-30,** From Swartz MH: *Textbook of physical diagnosis*, ed 6, Philadelphia, 2010, Saunders; **18-33, 18-34, 18-36, 18-37,** From Tenzel RR: *Textbook of ophthalmology*, vol 4, *Orbit and oculoplastics*, London, 1993, Gower; **18-35,** From Massry GG: Ptosis repair for the cosmetic surgeon, *Facial Plast Surg Clin North Am* 13(4):533-539, 2005; **18-38,** Courtesy June Nichols, Board Certified Ocularist, Diplomate, American Society of Ocularists.

Chapter 19

19-1, 19-2, From Ignatavicius DD, Workman ML: *Medical-surgical nursing: patient-centered collaborative care*, ed 7, St Louis, 2013, Saunders; **19-3,** From DeWeese DD et al: *Otolaryngology: head and neck surgery*, ed 7, St Louis, 1988, Mosby; **19-5, 19-17A and C,** From Saunders WH et al: *Nursing care in eye, ear, nose, and throat disorders*, ed 4, St Louis, 1979, Mosby; **19-7,** From Seidel HM et al: *Mosby's guide to physical examination*, ed 7, St Louis, 2011, Mosby; **19-8,** Redrawn from Thompson JM et al: *Mosby's clinical nursing*, ed 5, St Louis, 2002, Mosby; **19-9,** From Marino LB: *Cancer nursing*, St Louis, 1981, Mosby; **19-10, 19-16, 19-17B,** From Myers EN: *Operative otolaryngology: head and neck surgery*, ed 2, St Louis, 2008, Saunders; **19-11, 19-26, 19-35, 19-36, 19-37, 19-49,** From Cummings CW et al: *Otolaryngology: head and neck surgery*, ed 3, St Louis, 1993, Mosby; **19-13,** Courtesy Medtronic Xomed; **19-19, 19-20,** Courtesy Cochlear, Ltd; **19-21, 19-22, 19-23,** Courtesy Entific Medical Systems; **19-25, 19-31,** From DeWeese DD, Saunders WH: *Textbook of otolaryngology*, ed 6, St Louis, 1982, Mosby; **19-28,** From Schuller DE, Schleuning AJ: *Otolaryngology: head and neck surgery*, ed 8, St Louis, 1994, Mosby; **19-29, 19-30,** Courtesy Entellus Medical, Plymouth, MN; **19-39,** Modified from LaFleur Brooks M: *Exploring medical language: a student-directed approach*, ed 8, St Louis, 2012, Mosby; **19-40,** From Luckmann J: *Medical-surgical nursing*, ed 3, Philadelphia, 1987, Saunders; **19-42, 19-43,** From Ignatavicius DD, Workman ML: *Medical-surgical nursing: critical thinking for collaborative care*, ed 5, St Louis, 2006, Saunders.

Chapter 20

20-1, 20-4, 20-5, 20-6, 20-8, 20-9, From Patton KT, Thibodeau GA: *Anatomy and physiology*, ed 8, St Louis, 2013, Mosby **20-2,** From Patton KT, Thibodeau GA: *Anatomy and physiology*, ed 7, St Louis, 2010, Mosby; **20-3,** Redrawn from Lewis RC: *Primary care orthopedics*, NY, 1988, Churchill Livingstone; **20-7A, 20-12, 20-13, 20-88,** From Thibodeau GA, Patton KT: *Anatomy and physiology*, ed 3, St Louis, 1996, Mosby; **20-11, 20-37, 20-65, 20-69,** Courtesy Zimmer, Inc, Warsaw, IN; **20-14,** Courtesy Tenet Medical, Dallas; **20-15,** Courtesy Innomed, Savannah, GA; **20-16, 20-57,** Courtesy Acufex Microsurgical, Inc, Mansfield, MA; **20-17,** Courtesy OSI, Union City, CA; **20-18, 20-25, 20-34, 20-35, 20-44, 20-55, 20-71, 20-73,** From Gregory B: *Orthopaedic surgery*, St Louis, 1994, Mosby; **20-19, 20-48,** Courtesy Zimmer Traction Handbook, 1989, Zimmer, Inc, Warsaw, IN; **20-21,** From Mourad LA: *Orthopedic disorders*, St Louis, 1991, Mosby; **20-23,** From Monahan FD et al: *Phipps' medical-surgical nursing*, ed 8, St Louis,

2007, Mosby; **20-24,** Courtesy EBI, Parsippany, NJ; **20-26,** Courtesy Synthes USA, Paoli, PA; **20-27,** Courtesy Prototech AS, Bergen, Norway; **20-28, 20-46, 20-47,** From Gustilo RB et al: *Fractures and dislocations,* vol 2, St Louis, 1993, Mosby; **20-29,** Courtesy LTI Medica and the Upjohn Co. Illustration by Beverly Kessler, 1982, Learning Technology, Inc; **20-30, 20-39, 20-50,** From Canale ST, Beaty JH: *Campbell's operative orthopaedics,* ed 11, St Louis, 2008, Mosby; **20-31,** Courtesy Biomet, Inc, Warsaw, IN; **20-33,** Redrawn from Rockwood CA et al: *Fractures in adults,* ed 2, Philadelphia, 1984, Lippincott; **20-36,** Redrawn Neerii CS: Displaced proximal humeral fractures: part I: classification and evaluation, *J Bone Joint Surg Am* 52(6):1077-1089, 1970; **20-40, 20-42,** From Crenshaw AH: *Campbell's operative orthopaedics,* ed 8, St Louis, 1992, Mosby; **20-41,** From Knight RA: *AAOS Instructional Course Lecture* 14:123, 1957; **20-43, 20-59,** From Muller ME et al: *Manual of internal fixation: techniques recommended by AO-ASIF group,* ed 3, Berlin, 1990, Springer-Verlag; **20-45,** Redrawn from Sprague HH, Howard FM: *Contemp Orthop* 16:18, 1988; **20-49,** Courtesy OsteoMed, Addison, TX; **20-51,** Courtesy Exactech, Inc, Gainesville, FL; **20-52,** From Gustilo RB: *The fracture classification manual,* St Louis, 1991, Mosby; **20-53,** Redrawn from Muller ME et al: *The comprehensive classification of fractures of long bones,* Berlin, 1990, Springer-Verlag; **20-54,** Redrawn from Schatzker J et al: *Clin Orthop* 138:94, 1979; **20-56,** From DePuy ACE Medical Co, El Segundo, CA; **20-58,** From Canale ST: *Campbell's operative orthopaedics,* ed 9, St Louis, 1998, Mosby; **20-60,** From Richards V: *Surgery for general practice,* St Louis, 1956, Mosby; **20-62, 20-64, 20-70,** Courtesy Howmedica, Inc, Rutherford, NJ; **20-66,** Courtesy Stryker, Kalamazoo, MI; **20-67,** Redrawn from Gristina AG, Webb LX: *Proximal humeral and monospherical glenoid replacement: surgical technique,* Rutherford, NJ, 1983, Howmedica, Inc; **20-68,** Courtesy Smith & Nephew, Memphis; **20-72,** Courtesy College of Southern Idaho, Twin Falls; **20-74, 20-75, 20-76, 20-77, 20-80,** Courtesy ConMed Linvatec, Utica, NY; **20-78,** From Browner BD et al: *Skeletal trauma,* ed 4, Philadelphia, 2009, Saunders; **20-79,** From Canale ST, Beaty JH: *Campbell's operative orthopaedics,* ed 12, Philadelphia, 2013, Mosby; **20-81,** Courtesy Johnson & Johnson; **20-85,** Courtesy Smith & Nephew Dyonics, Andover, MA; **20-86,** From Kim DH et al: *Surgical anatomy and techniques to the spine,* St Louis, 2006, Saunders; **20-87,** Courtesy NuVasive, Inc, San Diego; **20-89,** From Bradford DS et al: *Moe's textbook of scoliosis and other spinal deformities,* ed 2, Philadelphia, 1987, Saunders; **20-90,** Courtesy Medtronic Sofamor Danek, Memphis; **20-91, 20-92, 20-93, 20-94,** Reprinted with permission from Synthes Spine LP; **20-95,** From Ortiz A: Vertebral body reconstruction: review and update on vertebroplasty and kyphoplasty, *Appl Radiol* 37(12):10-24, 2008.

Chapter 21

21-1, 21-24, From Thibodeau GA, Patton KT: *Structure and function of the body,* ed 13, St Louis, 2008, Mosby; **21-2, 21-3, 21-4, 21-6,** From Thibodeau GA, Patton KT: *Anatomy and physiology,* ed 3, St Louis, 1996, Mosby; **21-5,** Photograph by Sarah-Jane Smith. Artwork modified from Lumley JSP: *Surface anatomy,* ed 3, Edinburgh, 2002, Churchill Livingstone. In Standring S: *Gray's anatomy,* ed 40, Edinburgh, 2008, Churchill Livingstone; **21-7, 21-9, 21-10, 21-12, 21-26,** From Conway-Rutkowski BL: *Carini and Owens' neurological and neurosurgical nursing,* ed 8, St Louis, 1982, Mosby; **21-8, 21-19,** From Anthony CP, Thibodeau GA: *Textbook of anatomy and physiology,* ed 11, St Louis, 1983, Mosby; **21-11,** Photograph by Kevin Fitzpatrick on behalf of GKT School of

Medicine, London. In Standring S: *Gray's anatomy,* ed 40, Edinburgh, 2008, Churchill Livingstone; **21-13,** Modified from Thibodeau GA, Patton KT: *Anatomy and physiology,* ed 5, St Louis, 2003, Mosby; **21-14, 21-28, 21-29, 21-31, 21-43, 21-44, 21-45, 21-46, 21-47, 21-48, 21-50,** From Rengachary SS, Ellenbogen RG: *Principles of neurosurgery,* ed 2, Edinburgh, 2005, Mosby Ltd; **21-15, 21-16, 21-17,** From Rengachary SS, Wilkins RH: *Principles of neurosurgery,* London, 1994, Wolfe/Mosby Europe Ltd; **21-18,** From Patton KT, Thibodeau GA: *Anatomy and physiology,* ed 8, St Louis, 2013, Mosby; **21-20,** From Standring S: *Gray's anatomy,* ed 40, Edinburgh, 2008, Churchill Livingstone; **21-21, 21-22,** From Mettler FA: *Neuroanatomy,* ed 2, St Louis, 1948, Mosby; **21-30,** Provided by Shaun Gallagher, GKT School of Medicine, London; photograph by Sarah-Jane Smith. In Standring S: *Gray's anatomy,* ed 40, Edinburgh, 2008, Churchill Livingstone; **21-32,** Courtesy Dr. Justin Lee, Chelsea and Westminster Hospital, London. In Standring S: *Gray's anatomy,* ed 40, Edinburgh, 2008, Churchill Livingstone; **21-33,** Courtesy Integra LifeSciences Corp, Plainsboro, NJ; **21-35,** From Barker E: *Neuroscience nursing,* St Louis, 1994, Mosby; **21-40, 21-41, 21-42,** Courtesy Codman, a Johnson & Johnson Co, Raynham, MA; **21-49,** From Sachs E: *Diagnosis and treatment of brain tumors and the care of the neurosurgical patient,* ed 2, St Louis, 1949, Mosby; **21-51,** From Carini E, Owens G: *Neurological and neurosurgical nursing,* ed 6, St Louis, 1974, Mosby.

Chapter 22

22-1, From Townsend CM et al, editors: *Sabiston textbook of surgery,* ed 18, Philadelphia, 2008, Saunders; **22-2, 22-3, 22-10, 22-19, 22-20, 22-26, 22-30, 22-34,** From Fortunato N, McCullough SM: *Plastic and reconstructive surgery,* St Louis, 1998, Mosby; **22-4,** Courtesy Carl Zeiss, Oberkochen, Germany; **22-5,** Used with permission from LifeCell Corporation; **22-6, 22-16, 22-17, 22-21,** Courtesy Ramasamy Kalimuthu MD, FACS, Oak Lawn, IL; **22-7, 22-9,** From Thibodeau GA, Patton KT: *The human body in health and disease,* ed 5, St Louis, 2010, Mosby; **22-8, 22-12,** From Ignatavicius DD, Workman ML: *Medical-surgical nursing: patient-centered collaborative care,* ed 7, St Louis, 2013, Saunders; **22-15,** Courtesy Inamed Aesthetics, Santa Barbara, CA; **22-18, 22-39, 22-40,** Courtesy Marc A. Drimmer, MD; **22-22,** From Weinzweig N, Weinzweig J: *The mutilated hand,* St Louis, 2005, Mosby; **22-24,** From Flint PW et al: *Cummings otolaryngology head and neck surgery,* ed 5, St Louis, 2010, Mosby; **22-25,** From Fonseca RJ et al: *Oral and maxillofacial trauma,* ed 3, Philadelphia, 2005, Saunders; **22-27, 22-33,** From Kaminer MS et al: *Atlas of cosmetic surgery,* ed 2, St Louis, 2009, Saunders; **22-35,** From Capella JF: Body lift, *Clin Plast Surg* 35(1):28, 2008; **22-36,** From Aly A et al: Brachioplasty in the massive weight loss patient, *Clin Plast Surg* 35(1):146, 2008; **22-37,** From Cram A, Aly A: Thigh reduction in the massive weight loss patient, *Clin Plast Surg* 35(1):170, 2008; **22-41,** From Wilkinson TS: *Atlas of liposuction,* Philadelphia, 2005, Saunders.

Chapter 23

23-4, From Schottelius BA, Schottelius DD: *Textbook of physiology,* ed 18, St Louis, 1978, Mosby; **23-5,** From Townsend CM et al: *Sabiston textbook of surgery,* ed 16, Philadelphia, 2001, Saunders; **23-7,** From Johnson J, Kirby CK: *Surgery of the chest,* ed 4, Chicago, 1970, Year Book; **23-8,** Courtesy Teleflex Medical, Research Triangle Park, NC; **23-9,** From Baumgartner FJ: Surgical approaches and techniques in the management of severe hyperhidrosis, *Thorac Surg Clin* 18(2):167-181, 2009; **23-10,** From Kernstine KH et al: Robotic lobectomy, *Op Tech Thorac Cardiovasc Surg* 13(3):204.

e1-204.e23, 2009; **23-11,** From Damjanov I, Linder J, editors: *Anderson's pathology,* ed 10, St Louis, 1996, Mosby; **23-12, 23-18,** From McCance KL, Huether SE: *Pathophysiology—the biologic basis for disease in adults and children,* ed 6, St Louis, 2010, Mosby; **23-21,** From Sellke F et al: *Sabiston & Spencer's surgery of the chest,* ed 8, Philadelphia, 2010, Saunders.

Chapter 24

24-1, 24-4, From Patton KT, Thibodeau GA: *Anatomy and physiology,* ed 8, St Louis, 2013, Mosby; **24-2,** From Thibodeau GA, Patton KT: *Anatomy and physiology,* ed 5, St Louis, 2003, Mosby; **24-3,** From Kumar et al: *Robbins and Cotran pathologic basis of disease,* ed 8, St Louis, 2010, Saunders; **24-5,** From Dettenmeier PA: *Radiographic assessment for nurses,* St Louis, 1995, Mosby; **24-10,** From Townsend CM et al: *Sabiston textbook of surgery,* ed 17, Philadelphia, 2004, Saunders; **24-11,** From Haimovici H: *Vascular surgery: principles and technique,* ed 4, Oxford, 1995, Blackwell Science; **24-13, 24-16,** From Hershey FB, Calman CH: *Atlas of vascular surgery,* ed 3, St Louis, 1973, Mosby; **24-14, 24-15,** From MacVittie BA: *Vascular surgery,* St Louis, 1998, Mosby; **24-20, 24-22, 24-23,** From Wilson SE: *Vascular access: principles and practice,* ed 3, St Louis, 1996, Mosby; **24-21,** From Calne R, Pollard SG: *Operative surgery,* London, 1992, Gower; **24-24,** From Ballinger PW: *Merrill's atlas of radiographic positions and radiologic procedures,* ed 8, vol 2, St Louis, 1995, Mosby; **24-25, 24-26,** From Townsend CM et al: *Sabiston textbook of surgery,* ed 18, Philadelphia, 2010, Saunders.

Chapter 25

25-1A, 25-6A, From Thibodeau GA, Patton KT: *Anatomy and physiology,* ed 5, St Louis, 2003, Mosby; **25-2, 25-6B and C,** From Seifert PC: *Cardiac surgery,* St Louis, 1994, Mosby. Drawings by Peter Stone; **25-4,** From Pappano AJ, Wier GW: *Cardiovascular physiology,* ed 10, St Louis, 2013, Mosby; **25-5,** From Thompson JM et al: *Mosby's clinical nursing,* ed 5, St Louis, 2002, Mosby; **25-8, 25-11,** From Canobbio M: *Cardiovascular disorders,* St Louis, 1990, Mosby; **25-9A, 25-33,** From Braunwald E et al, editors: *Heart disease,* ed 6, Philadelphia, 2001, Saunders; **25-9B, 25-32B and C, 25-40A,** From Seifert PC: *Cardiac surgery,* St Louis, 1994, Mosby; **25-10,** Courtesy Edward A Lefrak, MD, Annandale, VA; **25-12,** From Kinney M, Packa D: *Andreoli's comprehensive cardiac care,* ed 7, St Louis, 1995, Mosby; **25-13,** From Brooks-Tighe SM: *Instrumentation for the operating room,* ed 4, St Louis, 1994, Mosby; **25-14,** Courtesy Scanlan International, St. Paul, MN; **25-15,** Courtesy Rultract, Inc, Cleveland; **25-16,** Courtesy Pilling Co, Fort Washington, PA; **25-17,** Courtesy Hewlett-Packard Co, Medical Products Group, Andover, MA; **25-18, 25-34, 25-36, 25-37, 25-41, 25-44, 25-45, 25-52, 25-56, 25-58, 25-59, 25-61, 25-62, 25-63, 25-65, 25-66, 25-70, 25-71, 25-72, 25-73, 25-74, 25-77, 25-78,** From Waldhausen JA et al: *Surgery of the chest,* ed 6, St Louis, 1996, Mosby; **25-19, 25-20,** Courtesy Meadox Medicals, a division of Boston Scientific Co; **25-21,** Courtesy WL Gore & Associates, Inc, Flagstaff, AZ; **25-22,** Courtesy of St. Jude Medical, Inc, St. Paul, MN; **25-23,** Courtesy Sulzer Carbomedics, Inc, Austin, TX; **25-24, 25-25, 25-31, 25-46, 25-76,** Copyright Medtronic, Inc, Minneapolis; **25-26, 25-32A,** Courtesy Baxter Healthcare Corp, Edwards CVS division, Santa Ana, CA; **25-27, 25-79,** Courtesy ATS Medical, Minneapolis, MN; **25-28, 25-67,** From Medtronic Cardiovascular, Mounds View, MN; **25-29, 25-30,** Courtesy CryoLife, Inc, Marietta, GA; **25-35, 25-39,** Courtesy Terumo Cardiovascular Systems Corporation. All rights reserved;

25-38, 25-43, 25-48, 25-54, 25-55, 25-57, 25-75, From Townsend CM et al: *Sabiston textbook of surgery,* ed 19, Philadelphia, 2012, Saunders; **25-47,** Courtesy Heartport, Inc, Redwood City, CA; **25-49,** From Doty DB: *Cardiac surgery: operative technique,* St Louis, 1997, Mosby; **25-50,** From Lytle BW et al: Coronary artery bypass grafting with the right gastroepiploic artery, *J Thorac Cardiovasc Surg* 976:826, 1989; **25-51, 25-69,** From Zipes DP et al: *Braunwald's heart disease: a textbook of cardiovascular medicine,* ed 7, Philadelphia, 2005, Saunders; **25-61,** From David TE et al: Long-term results of mitral valve repair, *J Thorac Cardiovasc Surg* 115(6):1279-1286, 1998; **25-68,** From Cleveland Clinic Center for Medical Art & Photography © 2006-2013. Reprinted with permission. All rights reserved; **25-80,** From Seifert PC et al: Surgery for atrial fibrillation, *AORN J* 86(1):23-40, 2007.

Chapter 26

26-3, 26-4, 26-5, 26-7, 26-8, 26-9, From Children's Hospital of Philadelphia; **26-6,** From Schalamon J et al: Minimally invasive correction of pectus excavatum in adult patients, *J Thorac Cardiovasc Surg* 132(3):524-529, 2006; **26-10, 26-11, 26-12, 26-19, 26-24,** From Coran AG et al: *Surgery of the neonate,* Boston, 1978, Little, Brown; **26-13, 26-16, 26-28, 26-30, 26-37, 26-38, 26-72,** From Holcomb GW, Murphy JP: *Pediatric surgery,* ed 5, Philadelphia, 2010, Saunders; **26-14,** Modified from Gross RE: *An atlas of children's surgery,* Philadelphia, 1970, Saunders; **26-15, 26-21, 26-22, 26-25, 26-40,** From Spitz L et al: *A colour atlas of paediatric surgical diagnosis,* London, 1990, Mosby Ltd; **26-17,** Modified from Boley SJ: An endorectal pull-through operation with primary anastomosis for Hirschsprung's disease, *Surg Gynecol Obstet* 127(2):253, 1986; **26-18,** From Chessell G et al: *Diagnostic picture tests in clinical medicine,* vol 2, St Louis, 1984, Mosby; **26-20,** From DeVries PA: Posterior sagittal anorectoplasty. In Holmann von Kap S, editor: *Anorektale fehlbildungen,* Stuttgart, 1984, Gustav Fischer-Verlag; **26-23,** Courtesy Dr David Clark, NeoPIX, Albany, NY; **26-26,** From Davenport KP et al: Pediatric malignancies: neuroblastoma, Wilms tumor, hepatoblastoma, rhabdomyosarcoma and sacrococcygeal teratoma, *Surg Clin* 92(3):745-767, 2012; **26-27,** From Townsend CM et al: *Sabiston textbook of surgery,* ed 18, Philadelphia, 2008, Saunders; **26-29,** Courtesy H. Gil Rushton, MD, Children's National Medical Center, Washington, DC. In Hockenberry MJ, Wilson D: *Wong's nursing care of infants and children,* ed 8, St Louis, 2007, Mosby; **26-31, 26-32, 26-36,** Modified from Droller MJ: *Surgical management of urologic disease,* St Louis, 1992, Mosby; **26-33,** From Devine CJ, Jr: Chordee and hypospadias. In Glenn JF, Boyce WH, editors: *Urologic surgery,* ed 3, Philadelphia, 1983, Lippincott; **26-39,** From Fuhrman BP, Zimmerman J: *Pediatric critical care,* ed 4, Philadelphia, 2011, Mosby; **26-41,** Courtesy Albert Biglan, MD, Children's Hospital of Pittsburgh. In Zitelli BJ et al: *Zitelli and Davis' atlas of pediatric physical diagnosis,* ed 6, Philadelphia, 2012, Saunders; **26-42,** From Neurosurgery wound closure, Ethicon, Inc; **26-48, 26-49,** From Zitelli BJ et al: *Zitelli and Davis' atlas of pediatric physical diagnosis,* ed 6, Philadelphia, 2012, Saunders; **26-50,** From Zitelli BJ, Davis HW: *Atlas of pediatric physical diagnosis,* ed 5, Philadelphia, 2007, Saunders; **26-51,** Courtesy Emory University School of Medicine, Atlanta; **26-52, 26-53, 26-54, 26-55,** Katowitz JA, editor: *Pediatric oculoplastic surgery,* Philadelphia, 2002, Springer; **26-56A,** Redrawn from Chameides L: *Pediatric advanced life support,* Dallas, 1988, American Heart Association; **26-56B,** From Barkin RM, Rosen P: *Emergency pediatrics: a guide to ambulatory care,* ed 3, St Louis, 1990, Mosby; **26-57, 26-59, 26-61, 26-63, 26-67,** From Nichols DG, Cameron

DE: *Critical heart disease in infants and children*, ed 2, St Louis, 2006, Mosby; **26-58, 26-62, 26-64, 26-66, 26-68,** From Hockenberry MJ, Wilson D: *Wong's nursing care of infants and children*, ed 9, St Louis, 2013, Mosby; **26-60,** From Cooley DA, Norman JC: *Techniques in cardiac surgery*, Houston, 1975, Texas Medical Press; **26-65, 26-69, 26-70, 26-71,** From Nichols DG et al: *Critical heart disease in infants and children*, St Louis, 1994, Mosby.

Chapter 27

27-1, 27-2, 27-3, From Federal Interagency Forum on Aging-Related Statistics, *Older Americans 2012: key indicators of well-being*, Federal Interagency Forum on Aging-Related Statistics, Washington, DC: U.S. Government Printing Office, June 2012, available at www.agingstats.gov/Main_Site/Data/2012_Documents/docs/EntireChartbook.pdf. Accessed March 7, 2013.

Chapter 28

28-1, Courtesy New Hanover Health Network EMS Air Link, EMS, Emergency Medical Services, Wilmington, NC; **28-2, 28-12,** From McQuillan KA et al: *Trauma nursing*, ed 4, St Louis, 2009, Saunders; **28-3, 28-10,** From Neff JA, Kidd PS: *Trauma nursing: the art and science*, St Louis, 1993, Mosby; **28-6,** From Cothren CC, Moore EE: Emergency department thoracotomy for the critically injured patient: objectives, indications, and outcomes, *World*

J Emerg Surg 1(4):1-13, 2006; **28-7,** From Cosgriff H, Jr, Anderson DL: *The practice of emergency care*, ed 2, Philadelphia, 1984, Lippincott; **28-8,** Redrawn from Kintzel KC: *Advanced concepts in clinical nursing*, ed 2, Philadelphia, 1997, Lippincott; **28-9,** Redrawn from Becker DP et al: Diagnosis and treatment of head injury. In Youman JR, editor: *Neurological surgery*, ed 3, Philadelphia, 1990, Saunders; **28-11,** Courtesy Haim Paran, MD; **28-13,** From Townsend CM et al: *Sabiston textbook of surgery*, ed 18, Philadelphia, 2008, Saunders.

Chapter 29

29-1, 29-7, 29-10, From St. Peter's Hospital, Albany, NY; **29-5, 29-8, 29-9,** From Massachusetts General Hospital, Boston; **29-11,** From Bontrager KL, Lampignano JP: *Textbook of radiographic positioning and related anatomy*, ed 8, St Louis, 2014, Mosby; **29-12,** From University of Utah Medical Center, Salt Lake City.

Chapter 30

30-1, From Rakel RE, Rakel DP: *Textbook of family medicine*, ed 8, Philadelphia, 2011, Saunders; **30-2,** From Hochberg MC et al: *Rheumatology*, ed 5, Philadelphia, 2011, Mosby; **30-3,** From Jonas WB: *Mosby's dictionary of complementary and alternative medicine*, St Louis, 2005, Mosby; **30-4,** Modified from Patton KT, Thibodeau GA: *Anatomy & physiology*, ed 7, St Louis, 2010, Mosby.

Index

Page numbers followed by "f" indicate figures, "t" indicate tables, and "b" indicate boxes.

Special Features